Modern Synopsis of
Comprehensive Textbook of
PSYCHIATRY/II
Second Edition

Modern Synopsis of
Comprehensive Textbook of
PSYCHIATRY/II
Second Edition

ALFRED M. FREEDMAN, M.D.

Professor of Psychiatry and Chairman of the
Department of Psychiatry, New York Medical College;
Director of Psychiatric Services, Metropolitan Hospital and
Flower and Fifth Avenue Hospitals, New York, New York;
Chairman, Department of Psychiatry
Grasslands Hospital, Valhalla, New York.

HAROLD I. KAPLAN, M.D.

Professor of Psychiatry and Director of Psychiatric
Education and Training, New York Medical College;
Attending Psychiatrist, Flower and Fifth Avenue Hospitals;
Visiting Psychiatrist, Metropolitan Hospital, and Bird S. Coler
Memorial Hospital and Home, New York, New York.

BENJAMIN J. SADOCK, M.D.

Professor of Psychiatry, Director, Division of Group Process,
and Director, Continuing Education in Psychiatry, New York Medical College;
Attending Psychiatrist, Flower and Fifth Avenue Hospitals;
Visiting Psychiatrist, Metropolitan Hospital, New York, New York.

The Williams & Wilkins Co. / BALTIMORE

Library of Congress Cataloging in Publication Data

Freedman, Alfred M
  Modern synopsis of Comprehensive textbook of psychiatry, II.

  Includes bibliographies and index.
  1. Psychiatry. I. Kaplan, Harold I., joint author. II. Sadock, Benjamin J., 1933–   joint author. III. Freed-
man, Alfred M. Comprehensive textbook of psychiatry, II. IV. Title. [DNLM: 1. Mental disorders. WM100
F855m]
RC454.F742 1976   616.8′9   76-22737
ISBN 0-683-03370-0
ISBN 0-683-03371-9 pbk.

Composed and Printed at the
Waverly Press, Inc.
Mt. Royal and Guilford Aves.
Baltimore, Md. 21202, U. S. A.

Dedication

TO OUR FAMILIES

Preface

The *Comprehensive Textbook of Psychiatry/ II*, which is 2,707 pages long and composed of 226 contributions by the outstanding behavioral scientists in the United States, is admirably serving the uses of psychiatrists, psychologists, psychiatric social workers, and other mental health professionals. However, the book is too voluminous, especially for the medical student who requires a text that can be integrated into the medical school curriculum. For this reason the authors of the *Modern Synopsis*/II decided to abbreviate, condense, and modify the contents of the *Comprehensive Textbook of Psychiatry*/II. In order to accomplish this, we have deleted sections deemed less necessary for medical student education in particular, introduced new subjects, and brought up to date certain key sections. As the authors of the Synopsis, we wish to acknowledge our great and obvious debt to the contributors to the original text. At the same time, we must accept responsibility for the modifications and possible shortcomings of the new work. Since the first edition of *Modern Synopsis* appeared in 1972, the expansion in psychiatric knowledge has been so great—even explosive—that the second edition has had to be approximately two times the size of the first edition. A great variety and a tremendous number of new subject areas have been added. Because of the many content changes, which have exceeded 75 per cent, the second edition can truly be considered a new textbook based on the tradition and built on the matrix of the first edition.

Philosophy

The second edition of *Modern Synopsis* of the *Comprehensive Textbook of Psychiatry*/II has evolved from our experience in establishing undergraduate, graduate, and postgraduate continuing-education programs in psychiatry. The responsibility for preparing a teaching program for students of psychiatry at every level has made us acutely conscious of the expansion of the field and of the many important additions to the traditional body of the discipline.

The superstructure of clinical psychiatry has expanded and strengthened: thus, the practitioner now has at his disposal a great deal of new information in various major areas of behavioral science, information that he must incorporate into the existing theoretical and therapeutic knowledge in psychiatry. Among these areas are the basic science, such as neurophysiology and neuropharmacology; the social sciences that pertain to individual persons; and those that concern the behavior of groups and of systems. Knowledge in these areas is important not merely as an intellectual exercise but because it is a vital part of the practice of psychiatry. It is, in fact, a prerequisite for clinical competence. The perplexing array of therapeutic drugs, for example, demands that the practitioner have a full understanding of their properties—in particular, their effects on the central nervous system—so that he may dispense them in the most sophisticated manner possible. Similarly, increasing awareness of the contribution of social factors to the development and the continuance of mental illness requires that the student be systematically trained in pertinent aspects of the social sciences. The interplay between the individual person and the social structure is especially important in such disorders as drug addiction, alcoholism, deliquency, and educational disabilities—problem areas that psychiatry can no longer avoid.

Modern psychiatric practice should evolve in a manner complex enough to allow for new inputs and sufficiently flexible to adapt to a rapidly changing social scene. Such a structure permits taking into account certain features of American life that distinguish it from life in other highly developed countries.

Pluralism. This textbook is organized according to principles derived from certain distinctive characteristics of American life that are rooted in our history and that form the guidelines for the development of our social institutions. The first of these characteristics is pluralism. American communities are composed of a multitude of governmental structures and private groups, each with a measure of power and strength. Sometimes these structures and groups cooperate, but often they act in competition with one another. Each has its own responsibilities, and the fulfillment of these responsibilities gives rise to diffuse goals. The operation of such groups is seldom conducive to the formation of unified conceptual systems, and the history of American psychiatric schools is no exception to this rule. This diversity is caused not only by the steady growth of knowledge within the United States but also by the constant enrichment of American intellectual life through immigration. New ideas brought here by our colleagues from abroad have taken root and flourished. Much of this new knowledge is now incorporated into the body of American psychiatry and has enhanced it immeasurably. To present this diversity in all its richness and contradiction, one must be truly eclectic. It has been our aim in this textbook to include all the major contributions and trends that are now influencing the direction of the discipline.

Pragmatism. If pluralism is a feature of American life that demands recognition, then pragmatism is one that requires compensation. Although truth needs testing by the practical consequences of belief, commonplace American pragmatism often goes beyond empiricism to a disregard for theory. Thus, American psychiatry has shown strength in the development and application of treatment methods while neglecting nosology and clinical description. Nosology is of relatively minor interest when psychiatric therapies are nonspecific; indeed, classification is not of practical use for those who are wedded to single general-purpose therapies. To compensate for these weaknesses, we have stressed the development of theoretical models, the presentation of adequate clinical description, and the importance of classification schemes. To the same end, we have emphasized the behavioral science materials, the full comprehension of which is required not only for practice but for the expansion of theoretical understanding.

Traditional societies have revered what is old, but Americans are typically engaged mainly by what is new. A veneration for change gives rise to a galloping faddism in intellectual life. We have attempted to deal with this problem conservatively by preserving significant knowledge developed over a period of time while presenting new approaches. We have applied this principle not only to treatment methods but also to theoretical issues that are not immediately translated into therapeutic technique.

As a result of the fascination with change, new ideas become superimposed on older ones that are still viable. Thus, one sees change by accretion. New hypotheses and treatment methods are promulgated before older ones have been either validated or discarded. Because both old and new exist at the same time, they must both be presented in a comprehensive psychiatric text, even at the risk of overinforming the reader. American psychiatry cannot be presented adequately in a simple fashion. To oversimplify what is complex would be a disservice to the student and a backward step in the field. It is hoped that this textbook will be an organizing statement for the multitude of relevant variables and an initial approach to a complex model. More parsimonious statements must await further research and developments in the field. In the meantime, it is important not to exclude any aspect of psychiatry and to encourage constant evaluation methods.

Implementation

The organization and orientation of this book were determined in large measure by our assessment of the distinctive characteristics of modern American psychiatry and philosophy, as expressed above. In addition, our efforts were guided by certain practical considerations. As a manual of instruction, this textbook's prescribed aim is to foster professional competence. Accordingly, the content follows the psychiatric curriculum recommendations of the National Board of Medical Examiners and the American Board of Psychiatry and Neurology. On the other hand, the presentation of the material we consider essential to competence in this field was subject to certain restrictions, imposed by limitations of time and space.

To translate our ideals into the reality of a textbook we had to resolve many practical problems, which required some basic decisions. Specifically, we decided that the approach would be comprehensive in scope—that is, it would include contributions on topics fundamental to psychiatry in addition to the traditional clinical material, and be eclectic.

Eclectic orientations. Since psychiatry is currently in a state of rapid development and change, commitment to any one approach would be unwise at this time and in our opinion would constitute a disservice to the discipline and to the young student, who bears the responsibility for its progress. To avoid premature closure, we have included different theoretical models or schools of thought and contributions from various related disciplines, such as neurophysiology, psychology, and sociology.

We have tried to pursue this eclectic orientation throughout the textbook, although our approach has varied, depending on the material under consideration. For example, in the part of the book that deals with the fundamental topics, the various theoretical models and disciplines stand side by side, and their very juxtaposition transmits the message of eclecticism. In the sections covering clinical material, the dynamics and treatment of a given disorder may be presented with emphasis on the particular theoretical orientation that is most widely accepted at the present time. However, in each instance alternate approaches and assumptions are also delineated.

Comprehensive scope. We feel that psychiatry can no longer be taught as a technical trade. Obviously, clinical competence is an essential goal of training, but it is not the only goal. As stated earlier, knowledge of the behavioral sciences and of underlying theoretical models is fundamental to theoretical understanding and clinical skills in psychiatry. Moreover, psychiatry is currently faced with the challenge of distributing its services to previously unreached populations. Therefore, in addition to clinical material on the description and treatment of the various disorders that constitute the content of the traditional psychiatric text, this book includes germane biological, psychological, and sociological information; presentations of current concepts and theoretical models; and discussions of various aspects of community psychiatry and of the delivery of mental health services.

Although the basic organization of the second edition of *Modern Synopsis*/II may appear similar to that of the first edition, so many new subjects have been added to each conceptual area that they have, in effect, created a new book. For example, in the behavioral sciences, major new contributions have been added in the area of circadian rhythm, general systems theory, aggression, biofeedback, and psychiatric statistics. In personality theory, new in-depth studies have been written on Rado, Maslow, and Berne, among others. Major changes have also been made in the clinical areas. For example, in the area of schizophrenia, recent treatment trends and a complete evaluation of treatment methods and outcome studies have been added. In all clinical areas, much new case material, including the problems of patient management, has been added to provide a more dynamic and descriptive presentation.

Recognizing the major importance of psychiatry in the political, philosophical, and humanistic trends of today's society, we have added new sections on current topical subjects, such as prison psychiatry, poverty, psychohistory, creativity, psychopolitics, interracial relations, the women's movement, psychiatry and urban problems, sexuality, the economic and health insurance apsects of psychiatry, religion, and ethics.

A detailed and expanded glossary of psychiatric and psychological terminology has been included at the end of the book. Finally, we have carefully illustrated the text to add yet another dimension to the learning experience.

Acknowledgments. Accomplishing a task of this magnitude required 4 years of work and an accomplished, dedicated, and devoted staff. Norman Sussman, M.D., Robert Gelfand, and Nancy Barrett provided important literature research and assistance. Susan Goldhush served as picture editor. In charge of the secretarial staff was Lois Baken, assisted by Eva Washington. Proofreading was directed by Batya Bauman. Special thanks are extended to Joan Welsh, head of editorial supervision, for her excellent talents and the key role she played in the difficult synopsizing task. Virginia A.

Sadock, M.D., served admirably as assistant to the editors and deserves particular mention and thanks not only for her excellent and original contributions but also for her active help in the many editorial decisions in which she participated. At Williams & Wilkins, Charles Reville, James Gallagher, Dick Hoover, Andrea Albrecht, Norman Och, and their production staff were, as usual, of great help.

New York, May 15, 1976   A. M. F.
                                            H. I. K.
                                            B. J. S.

Acknowledgments

The authors wish to acknowledge the following individuals, most of whom contributed to the *Comprehensive Textbook of Psychiatry*, second edition, and whose material was synopsized, providing much of the basis for this book.

Harry S. Abram, M.D.
Richard Abrams, M.D.
Gerald Adler, M.D.
Anne Anastasi, Ph.D.
E. James Anthony, M.D.
Theus N. Armistead, M.D.
Haroutun M. Babigian, M.D.
Hrair M. Babikian, M.D.
Arthur J. Bachrach, Ph.D.
Stewart L. Baker, Jr., M.D.
Anita K. Bahn, M.D., Sc.D.
Samuel H. Barondes, M.D.
Arthur L. Benton, Ph.D.
Irving N. Berlin, M.D.
Victor Bernal y del Rio, M.D.
Grady L. Blackwood, Jr., B.A.
Eugene L. Bliss, M.D.
Jeannette D. Branch, M.A.
Bertram S. Brown, M.D.
Robert N. Butler, M.D.
Arthur C. Carr, Ph.D.
Raymond B. Cattell, Ph.D., D.Sc.
Morris E. Chafetz, M.D.
John A. Clausen, Ph.D.
Robert A. Cohen, M.D., Ph.D.
Jonathan O. Cole, M.D.
C. Keith Conners, Ph.D.
Constance Hellyer Corning, B.A.
Peter A. Corning, Ph.D.
Joseph B. Cramer, M.D.
Raymond R. Crowe, M.D.
Leon Cytryn, M.D.
Allan J. D. Dale, M.D.
Michael Joe Daly, M.D.
Robert S. Daniels, M.D.
John M. Davis, M.D.
Thomas P. Detre, M.D.

John M. Dusay, M.D.
Lloyd O. Eckhardt, M.D.
Leon Eisenberg, M.D.
Rudolf Ekstein, Ph.D.
David Elkind, Ph.D.
Jean Endicott, Ph.D.
George L. Engel, M.D.
W. Dennis Engels, M.D.
Margaret E. Ensminger, M.A.
Frank R. Ervin, M.D.
Dana L. Farnsworth, M.D.
Sherman C. Feinstein, M.D.
Ronald R. Fieve, M.D.
Stuart M. Finch, M.D.
Stephen Fleck, M.D.
Vincent J. Fontana, M.D.
Hamilton Ford, M.D.
Jerome D. Frank, M.D., Ph.D.
Abraham N. Franzblau, M.D., Ph.D.
Alfred M. Freedman, M.D.
Arnold P. Friedman, M.D.
George E. Gardner, M.D., Ph.D.
Mark A. Geyer, Ph.D.
Eli Ginzberg, Ph.D.
Bernard C. Glueck, M.D.
Milton Greenblatt, M.D.
Robert B. Greenblatt, M.D.
Roy R. Grinker, Sr., M.D.
Lester Grinspoon, M.D.
Ernest M. Gruenberg, M.D.
Jay Haley, M.A.
David A. Hamburg, M.D.
Harry F. Harlow, Ph.D.
Robert J. Harmon, M.D.
Saul I. Harrison, M.D.
D. James Henderson, M.D.
Marvin I. Herz, M.D.

Marc H. Hollender, M.D.
Herbert Holt, M.D.
Frederick J. Humphrey II, D.O.
Paul E, Huston, M.D., Ph.D.
Elizabeth Janeway, B.A.
David Jenness, Ph.D.
Edward D. Joseph, M.D.
Anthony Kales, M.D.
Joyce D. Kales, M.D.
Lothar B. Kalinowsky, M.D.
Francis J. Kane, Jr., M.D.
Harold I. Kaplan, M.D.
Frederic T. Kapp, M.D.
Sheppard G. Kellam, M.D.
Harold Kelman, M.D., D.Md.Sc.
Otto F. Kernberg, M.D.
Seymour S. Kety, M.D.
Mitchell L. Kietzman, Ph.D.
Herbert E. Klarman, Ph.D.
Susan T. Kleeman, M.D.
Gerald L. Klerman, M.D.
Peter H. Knapp, M.D.
Lorrin M. Koran, M.D.
Irvin A. Kraft, M.D.
David J. Kupfer, M.D.
Maurice W. Laufer, M.D.
Heinz F. Lehmann, M.D.
Molly Apple Levin, B.A.
Melvin Lewis, M.B., B.S. (Lond.)
Harold I. Lief, M.D.
Robert Jay Lifton, M.D.
Louis Linn, M.D.
Zbigniew J. Lipowski, M.D.
Samuel Livingston, M.D.
Reginald S. Lourie, M.D.
John E. Mack, M.D.
Paul D. MacLean, M.D.
Robert B. Malmo, Ph.D., LL.D. (Hon.)
Arnold J. Mandell, M.D.
Edward C. Mann, M.D.
Judd Marmor, M.D.
Maurice J. Martin, M.D.
Jules H. Masserman, M.D.
Philip R. A. May, M.D.
Alan A. McLean, M.D.
Virginia P. McNamara, M.D.
John F. Meeks, M.D.
William Walter Meissner, S.J., M.D.
James G. Miller, M.D., Ph.D.
Neal E. Miller, Ph.D.
Herbert C. Modlin, M.D.
George Mora, M.D.

Jacob L. Moreno, M.D. (deceased)
Loren R. Mosher, M.D.
Donald W. Mulder, M.D.
Patrick Mullahy, M.A.
Evelyn S. Meyers, B.A.
John C. Nemiah, M.D.
Peter B. Neubauer, M.D.
William G. Niederland, M.D.
Daniel Offer, M.D.
Mortimer Ostow, M.D., Med. Sc.D.
Anita Werner O'Toole, R.N., Ph.D.
Helene Papanek, M.D.
Lydia L. Pauli, M.D.
Anne C. Petersen, Ph.D.
Gerald C. Peterson, M.D.
Chester M. Pierce, M.D.
Phillip Polatin, M.D.
Alvin F. Poussaint, M.D.
Dane G. Prugh, M.D.
John D. Rainer, M.D.
Louis S. Reed, Ph.D.
Herbert S. Ripley, M.D.
Carl R. Rogers, Ph.D.
Jurgen Ruesch, M.D.
Melvin Sabshin, M.D.
Benjamin J. Sadock, M.D.
Virginia A. Sadock, M.D.
Robert L. Sadoff, M.D.
Eugene C. Sandberg, M.D.
Burton A. Sandok, M.D.
Raul C. Schiavi, M.D.
Abraham Schmitt, D.S.W.
Helen Schucman, Ph.D.
Arthur H. Schwartz, M.D.
Elvin V. Semrad, M.D.
Robert A. Senescu, M.D.
Charles Shogass, M.D.
David Shainberg, M.D.
David Shakow, Ph.D.
Taranath Shetty, M.D.
Edwin S. Shneidman, Ph.D.
Albert J. Silverman, M.D.
William Simon, Ph.D.
Iver F. Small, M.D.
Joyce G. Small, M.D.
Solomon H. Snyder, M.D.
Raymond Sobel, M.D.
Albert J. Solnit, M.D.
Philip Solomon, M.D.
Herbert Spiegel, M.D.
John P. Spiegel, M.D.
Robert L. Spitzer, M.D.

Marvin Stein, M.D.

Robert L. Stewart, M.D.

Robert J. Stoller, M.D.

Charles F. Stroebel, M.D., Ph.D.

Hans H. Strupp, Ph.D.

Robert L. Stubblefield, M.D.

Albert J. Stunkard, M.D.

Norman Sussman, M.D.

Joseph D. Teicher, M.D.

William N. Thetford, Ph.D.

Danielle Turns, M.D.

Edward A. Tyler, M.D.

Montague Ullman, M.D.

Anthony F. C. Wallace, Ph.D.

Andrew S. Watson, M.D.

Jack Weinberg, M.D.

Herbert Weiner, M.D.

Avery D. Weisman, M.D.

Charles E. Wells, M.D.

Louis J. West, M.D.

W. Donald Weston, M.D.

Otto Allen Will, Jr., M.D.

Paul T. Wilson, M.D.

George Winokur, M.D.

E. D. Wittkower, M.D.

Jack A. Wolford, M.D.

Lyman C. Wynne, M.D., Ph.D.

Leon J. Yarrow, Ph.D.

Hans H. Zinsser, M.D. (deceased)

Joseph Zubin, Ph.D.

Jack Zusman, M.D.

Contents

xvi   Contents

xviii   Contents

1

Historical and Theoretical Trends in Psychiatry

1.1. HISTORICAL AND THEORETICAL TRENDS IN PSYCHIATRY

Introduction

Psychiatry was the last specialty to be incorporated into the over-all field of medicine, about a century and a half ago. Before that time, mental diseases were considered the province of philosophy; further back, from early times to the Middle Ages, the mentally ill, when not ignored, were usually taken care of—that is, sheltered, punished, or exorcised—by medicine men and clergymen.

Preliterate Cultures

Common to many cultures of the eastern Mediterranean, pre-Columbian America, and African areas was the belief that mental diseases, like other diseases, were sent by a god or by gods, thus justifying all sorts of propitiatory and expiatory rituals. In addition, all kinds of misfortunes were attributed to the actions of devils; to control them, practices of so-called white magic—that is, permissible magic—and of black magic—that is, forbidden magic, such as the evil eye and spells—were used. Prognosis was based on the study of numbers, of astrology, of the configuration of the interiors of animals (especially hepatoscopy), of divination by some persons endowed with extrasensory powers, and of the interpretation of dreams.

A few basic postulates appear to be common to the beliefs of preliterate cultures (a term preferable to primitive cultures): the liberation of immaterial forces by divine power or magical arts; the principle of solidarity or contagion,

implying a continuity between the human being and his surroundings; the belief in sympathetic, imitative forms of magic occurring by telepathy and in the synergic or antagonistic interactions between similar elements, such as homeopathic medicine's method of treatment by similars; the symbolism of certain elements, such as the purifying role of water; and, especially, the power attributed to the utterance of certain words. Other therapeutic practices consist of the prescription of drugs, obtained either from vegetables or from animals, quite often combined in a complex and secret way, and prepared according to certain rituals.

Some procedures are based on substitute methods—that is, on transferring a disease to a scapegoat, usually an animal, as in cases of expiatory sacrifice. The prevention of diseases is assured by the use of magic objects, mainly amulets that protect the person, talismans that symbolize power, and fetishes that represent the protecting deity. Mental diseases or, rather, diseases considered to be mental by Western observers are mainly attributed to the violation of taboos, the neglect of ritual obligations, the loss of a vital substance from the body (mainly the soul), the introduction of a foreign and harmful substance into the body (possession by spirits), and witchcraft.

Trepanation of the Skull

Trepanation of skulls was performed during the Neolithic period. It is believed that this practice was carried on in Eastern Mediterranean and North African countries as early as 4,000 to 5,000 years ago, that it was widespread—not, however, in China, Japan, or

Egypt—and that it reached its highest development in Stone-Age Peru of 1,000 to 2,000 years ago, especially in connection with surgical traumas during wars. The relevance of this procedure for psychiatry lies in the opinion that the operation was done to liberate the evil spirits supposedly causing the symptoms. This opinion was subsequently enlarged to include, as other reasons for the procedure, combat of sorcery, a way of permitting something to enter the body of the person, and interest in obtaining a piece of bone (rondelle) for magic-religious purposes.

Shamanism

In contrast to the trepanation of skulls, shamanism is still widely practiced in many cultures of the world. The most commonly held picture of the shaman is that of an inspiration-type medicine man who is quite vulnerable to possession by spirits and through whom the spirits communicate with human beings (see Figure 1). Typically, the shamanistic séance takes place in the presence of a selected group of participants. It involves a progressively increasing state of excitement on the part of the shaman; this state of excitement is induced by heavy smoking, drinking, and the use of drugs, accompanied by rhythmic music, especially drums, to the point of paroxysm, characterized by partial loss of consciousness and unusual movements. The shaman reveals the presence of the spirits through utterances and violent actions. Mentally disturbed patients, in the course of active participation in the ceremony, may confess their sins or ask for the removal of certain disturbances specifically attributed to an evil spirit. The excursion of the shaman into the realm of the spirits is symbolic of the restoration of the patient's peace of mind through sacrifices and other symbolic means. Frequently, the patient's liberation from the evil spirit is expressed concretely through the actual expulsion of an object—such as a stone, insect, or hair—from the mouth of the shaman.

The opinion most commonly held is that the shaman is not psychotic or epileptic, as originally believed, but is essentially neurotic. As such, he may find an outlet for his own emotional instability through the séance. Eligibility for the role of shaman requires a particular state of receptivity to dreams and other psychological phenomena, elicited with the help of drugs and medicinal plants; a novitiate period is passed in

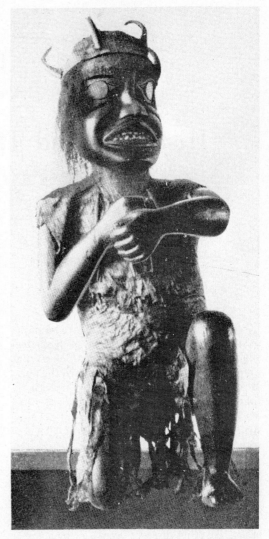

FIGURE 1. Wooden statue of shaman. North Pacific coast.

isolation from the community. With regard to the patients who ask for the shaman's help, their symptoms, although difficult to translate into current psychiatric terminology, appear to range widely from depression to withdrawal; for the most part, their symptoms appear to be acute.

The Dawn of Civilization

Egyptian Culture

In the Egyptian culture, life was viewed as a balance between man's static experience and his relationship to the universe—that is, as an interaction between internal and external forces. This balance gave rise to rhythmic and cyclic happenings from birth to death. Emphasis on the supernatural, especially communication with the dead, such as the spirits of the Pharaohs, was possible through a healing sleep induced by incubation techniques. It is likely that the treatment of mental disorders involved the integration of physical, psychic, and spiritual factors, accomplished through identification with positive, constructive forces.

Indian Culture

In the Indian culture, the earliest source of psychiatric interest is found in the magic formulas against demons and their human representatives contained in the Atharva-Veda (700 B.C.), the most important document of Vedic medicine. The theory of the transmigration of the soul at death was the dominant feature of the Vedantic concept of psychic function; the theory was based on the belief that the soul never dies. Also, the brain was differentiated from the mind, and, as in Aristotle, the heart was considered the center of sensations and consciousness.

Dreams were believed to carry important prognostic indications. Insanity was attributed to the prevalence of passion and darkness, which cause an imbalance in the constitution of the person. Mental diseases were divided into endogenous and exogenous, grossly corresponding to today's schizophrenia and manic-depressive psychosis.

Treatment included four methods: (1) psychotherapy based on the chanting of songs; the performance of auspicious rites, sacrifices, and expiatory ceremonies; fasting and purification rituals performed in the temples; and divine messages conveyed through dreams; (2) drugs obtained from plants or animals, particularly sarpagandha (rauwolfia serpentina) as a sedative and tranquilizer; (3) divine agents, such as the sun, air, and water; and (4) drugs made by man. Physical and mental shocks were also considered therapeutic in some cases.

Chinese Culture

In the Chinese culture, old philosophical thoughts expressed in Confucian writings center on three main tenets: (1) The world was not created by a divine or supernatural being but by tao, an abstract principle, which turned into an active moral guide after creation was accomplished. (2) Man is composed of the same elements as the universe and reflects in himself the principles of the macrocosm. (3) Mental functions are not conceived distinct from physical functions and are not localized in any part of the organism, although the heart is given particular importance as a guide for the mind.

Both deviation from filial piety and loss of face were believed to be important contributing factors in acute psychosis, leading even to suicide. Evidence of knowledge of other mental diseases is substantiated by the number of ideographs describing them. Also, in the medical textbook *The Yellow Emperor's Classic of Internal Medicine* (about 1000 B.C.), reference is made to insanity, dementia, violent behavior, and convulsions. It is likely that mentally ill persons, when not violent, were left wandering in the country.

Folk beliefs and practices centered on superstitious causation of disease as related to the invasion of the mind by noxious spirits, a notion that presupposes a consideration of body and soul as separate entities. Special priests acted as exorcists and performed ceremonies especially geared to propitiating the ancestors.

Judaic Culture

In one of the oldest books of the Bible, Deuteronomy, it is said that God will punish those who violate His commands with "madness, and blindness, and astonishment of heart"—that is to say, with mania, dementia, and stupor.

Perhaps the most famous episode of insanity in the Bible refers to the case of Saul, who, after some disturbed behavior early in life, developed abnormal irritability, great suspiciousness (especially toward David), and uncontrollable impulses that ended in suicide; apparently, he was affected by manic-depressive psychosis. In his case, in line with a long tradition that can be followed in many cultures, music was used to alleviate his emotional condition.

Also, Nebuchadnezzar, king of Babylon, became very depressed, irritable, and uncontrollable and finally fell into a condition called lycanthropy—a form of mental disorder in which the patient imagines himself to be a wolf or other wild beast—which is probably a form of melancholia.

Prophecy was a form of ecstasy that belonged

to borderline psychological states. In line with the over-all biblical tradition, prophecy was an expression of the power of words, as illustrated by blessings and curses.

Aside from evil spirits, the causes of mental illness included inheritance, physiological processes, lewdness and improper sexual relations, dirt, and idleness. Essentially, these various causes can be divided into two main groups—unprovoked occurrences of madness by divine decree and punishment for something done by the person.

It is likely that the margin of tolerance for mental abnormalities was rather wide. Well-to-do patients were probably kept confined at home; others were left wandering on their own. Mentally ill persons could not take part in religious ceremonies and, when judged incompetent, were assigned a guardian. The attitude of the Judaic culture toward mental illness vacillated between an enlightened approach and an intolerant attitude, but, in any case, it was influenced by the strong belief that man remains in the image of God, even when he becomes mentally ill.

Greek and Roman Cultures

Greek Concepts of Madness

Essentially, the description of madness in Greek culture derives from three main sources: popular opinion, medical knowledge, and literary-philosophical works.

Popular Concept. Characteristic of the popular view was the belief in the supernatural causation of mental disorders. Persons so afflicted were believed to be possessed by evil spirits, personified by the dread goddesses Mania and Lyssa, that had been sent by angry gods. The habit of wandering around and proneness to violence were especially considered signs of mental disorder. However, persons who manifested behavioral aberrations and who were, therefore, believed to be possessed by evil spirits may also have been regarded as sacred, as was the case in primitive cultures. Presumably, this belief was based on an unconscious fear of death, for the spirits represented the cult of the dead and their persisting influence on the living.

This popular view provided no facilities for the treatment of the mentally ill. Mild cases were simply left to fare for themselves as objects of contempt, ridicule, and abuse. Those who

were considered violent were kept at home, often in chains, on the assumption that the same gods who made people mad could cure them of it; this was in line with the homeopathic trend of Greek medical thinking. Therapeutic techniques—in addition to the various cures by purification and participation in the mysteries—included a number of animal and vegetable substances which were considered specific for the treatment of madness and epilepsy. No clear legal status was outlined for the mentally ill person. Since his antisocial behavior was viewed as punishment by the gods, the mentally ill criminal was relieved of any legal responsibility for his actions and was exiled from his city voluntarily or was forced to flee and to undergo purification rites. There was no psychiatric examination, except in cases involving slaves; in controversial cases—such as those involving marriage, divorce, and adoption—appeal on psychiatric grounds was made to the guardians of the law, rather than to physicians.

Medical Concepts. The medical concept of madness, as elaborated in the Hippocratic writings (4th century B.C.), centered on the interactions of the four bodily humors—blood, black bile, yellow bile, and phlegm—which resulted from the combination of the four basic qualities in nature—heat, cold, moisture, and dryness. Persons were classified according to four corresponding temperaments—sanguine, choleric, melancholic, and phlegmatic—which classification was considered to indicate their prevailing emotional orientation. Personality functioning reached an optimal level when crasis—that is, the appropriate interaction of internal and external forces—had been achieved. Conflict between these forces, termed dyscrasia, indicated the presence of excessive bodily humor, which had to be removed by purging.

A radical change in the concept of madness began to emerge at this time. This change was first expressed by Hippocrates (460–355 B.C.) in the introduction to his treatise on epilepsy:

I do not believe that the "sacred disease" is any more divine or sacred than any other disease but, on the contrary, has specific characteristics and a definite cause.

And, from a more general perspective, he states:

Men ought to know that from nothing else but thence [from the brain] come joys, delights, laughter, and sports; and sorrows, griefs, despondency, and lamentations. And by this in an especial manner, we acquire vision and knowledge, and we see and hear. And by the same organ we become mad and delirious, and fears and terrors assail us, some by night and some by day. . . . All these things we endure from the brain, when it is not healthy.

Literary-Philosophical Concepts. In the time of Homer (10th and 9th centuries B.C.), no definition of personality was advanced that might be equated with current concepts of personality. Thinking had not yet been separated from its physical substratum, the brain. Psyche was conceptualized as the breath of life, the force that kept the human being alive. Moreover, it persisted after life as the spirit of the dead.

In the *Iliad*, human beings lacked personal motivation; instead, they were possessed by sudden feelings of power, almost comparable to states of temporary insanity. Typically, infatuation sent by a god was used to explain the aberrant behavior and thoughts of the heroes. In general, mental activity was regarded not as something intrinsically private and inaccessible to others but rather as something resulting from the interchange among several characters, either human or divine; and gods were often portrayed as initiating human action by putting into a man a drive or an idea, so that the Homeric man experienced himself as a plurality, rather than a unity, with uncertain boundaries.

In the *Odyssey*, however, there were implications of moral criticism; and in time the concept of *hybris* (arrogance) became prominent in terms of its link with success, complacency, sin, and guilt. In other words, the literary and philosophical works of the period began to evidence an awareness of the fact that moral principles—that is, conscience—were internalized. They further stressed the relationship between the violation of these principles and consequent punishment by the gods as an inevitable part of man's destiny.

Development of Greek Psychiatry

The concept of the soul divorced from the qualities of the body and its physical organs was expressed for the first time by Heraclitus (540–475 B.C.). In time, a distinction between *soma* (body) and *psyche* came to the fore. Dreams came to be considered as liberating the person from adverse external forces and, later

on, from the impediment of his own body—the orphic tradition—and, thus, to have a therapeutic function. Furthermore, the highly emotional group rites in praise of Dionysius—the Greek god of fruitfulness and vegetation, especially wine—came to be replaced by mystic individualistic expressions, as typified by the puritanic community established by Pythagoras (6th century B.C.), which emphasized vegetarianism and purification by ritual means. Typically, such rituals included recollection, to the degree that, in time, catharsis was considered the only means of salvation.

Even more important for cathartic liberation from disturbing emotions was the function of the theatre, which in the Greek culture was attended by the entire community at intervals. The actions performed in the theatre portrayed the conflict between various contrasting and instinctual tendencies, and the chorus represented the instances of a collective superego.

In some of the most important dramatic productions, the key figures were afflicted with madness vividly pictured on the stage. In Sophocles (ca. 496–406 B.C.), the madman lived in an unreal, rather than a supernatural, world. But in Euripides (ca. 484–407 B.C.), behavioral expressions of madness, such as hallucinations, were purposely exaggerated for dramatic effect.

Plato's Concepts. Plato's (428–348 B.C.), tripartite subdivision of the soul in *The Republic* into appetite, reason, and temper has been compared by many to the psychoanalytic subdivision of the psyche into id, ego, and superego, the main differences being that the appetite, in contrast to the id, is largely conscious and that the superego, although largely irrational and punitive, is not limited to the emotions.

Also well known is the concept of health as harmony between body and mind, which has led to the conception that mental health was Plato's invention. Conversely, it is said in *Timaeus* that disharmony between body and mind causes mental aberrations based on either mania or gross ignorance. In *Phaedrus* Plato described four kinds of madness: prophetic, telestic or ritual, poetic, and erotic. Prophetic madness was defined as a unique form of temporary insanity that was reserved for the few persons who were able to reach the paroxysm of enthusiasm characteristic of the shamanistic trance, as typified by the ecstatic prophecy of Apollo's oracle at Delphi and as immortalized in Aeschylus' (525–456 B.C.) *Cassandra*. Telestic or ritual madness typically signified freedom from instinctual needs, and it was achieved collectively during the Corybantic religious rites. These rites were characterized by orgiastic dances performed to music, especially flute and drum in the Phrygian mode, accelerated to the point of paroxysm, and they served a cathartic function. According to Plato's *Laws*, the Corybantic rites and the practice of rocking babies were based on the same therapeutic principle. Poetic madness, due to possession by the muses, was described as a state of particular inspiration that was bestowed by the gods on the artist in order to facilitate the process of creation. Erotic madness was associated with human love, which in the Greek culture included homosexual as well as heterosexual relationships.

In the *Laws* psychiatric issues are openly discussed. Mentally ill persons presenting psychopathic behavior were to be sentenced by the judge to a house of correction for a term of not less than 5 years, during which time their contact with the community was to be kept to a minimum. After the term of confinement expired, the prisoner was to be freed if he had improved, or, if not, he was to be put to death. Lunatics were to be kept in safe custody at home, and stiff penalties were to be given to relatives who did not take care of them. Definite rules were also to be followed in matters of competency in relation to marrying, leaving a will, and other legal issues.

Aristotle's Empirical Psychology. Plato made an impressive effort to explain irrational events and behavior as an inevitable part of human life, rather than as the result of noxious influences. Concurrently, he attempted to subject them to the rational control of the mind. In contrast, Aristotle (384–322 B.C.) approached the various expressions of human behavior from an empirical viewpoint, which is more in keeping with today's psychology.

Like others, Aristotle supported the view that the black bile caused disturbed sensory perception and hallucinations. In Aristotle, the mediating aspect of the bile between the body and the mind offered one more argument in support of his organicistic philosophy of body-mind unity.

He conceived of the mysteries as ritual happenings in the course of which mental disorder could be healed. In accordance with the basic orphic theme, which Plato subscribed to as well, Aristotle believed that the disordered movement of the mysteries was ultimately conducive to order. Nor did he deviate substantially from general belief in his identification of the three irrational elements presented in these rituals——enthusiasm, a state of temporary madness, related to sexuality; divination through dreams; and divination through chance. However, whereas according to the classical Pythagorical tradition the music that accompanied such rituals was considered to evoke harmony, Aristotle postulated that its therapeutic function was to arouse passions. This was the first clear statement that the release of repressed emotions or passions—that is, abreaction—was an essential prerequisite for the effective treatment of mental illness, a viewpoint that was to serve as the basis for the moral treatment of the early 19th century.

Aristotle further advocated the use of catharsis, wine, aphrodisiacs, and music, since, in the final analysis, they were all found to produce similar effects, especially in people with melancholic constitutions. In summary, Aristotle discussed catharsis from a naturalistic viewpoint. In contrast to Plato, he did not emphasize the occult and supernatural character of catharsis; rather, he conceived of it as a natural outlet for disturbing passions. In fact, passions must be purged consistently to avoid violence. The use of the theater as a civic and collective cathartic device in Greek culture may be attributed largely to the wide acceptance of this belief.

Aristotle's empirical psychology did not undergo further development by his disciples. Instead, *ataraxia*, a mental state of imperturbability, became the ideal of the Epicureans and Stoics during the 3rd century B.C., and the foundation of psychology became much more rationalistic.

Roman Concepts of Madness

In the succeeding two centuries, Rome acquired increasing political importance, but Greek culture continued to dominate those aspects of Roman life that related to philosophy and art. The popular and medical concepts of madness, as well as literary and philosophical writings, repeated the Greek themes for the most part, with minor variations.

Superstitious practices continued to determine the popular attitude toward the mentally ill, who were neglected, banned, or persecuted.

They were deprived of freedom of action and were judged incompetent to control their own personal and business affairs.

Roman physicians continued to believe in the premonitory value of dreams and, in general, continued to be influenced by Greek concepts. In the 1st century B.C., Asclepiades rejected the doctrine of vital fluids and built his theories on the atomic hypotheses of Democritus. He described phrenitis as a fever accompanied by mental excitement and mania as continuous excitement without fever. Anticipating Esquirol, Asclepiades further differentiated illusions from hallucinations and prescribed treatment in light rooms for patients afflicted with hallucinations because of their characteristic fear of the dark. Treatment also emphasized the proper use of food and wine, physiotherapy, and other activities that imposed minimal physical restrictions, and it included such psychotherapeutic techniques as music and intellectual stimulation; patients were encouraged to form emotional relationships with others.

In the 1st century A.D., Celsus, the author of the classic eight-volume *De Re Medica*, dealt at length with mental diseases. The originality of Celsus' approach lay in the emphasis he placed on the value of the individual doctor-patient relationship. Celsus proposed that such a relationship might evolve from the use of specific techniques to cheer depressed patients and to quiet those who are manic; furthermore, he advocated the proper use of language and music and, possibly, some group activities, such as reading groups. Once again, Aristotelian passions were recognized as constituting the essential ingredient for the treatment of the mental patient.

Cicero (106–43 B.C.) must be credited with the first detailed description of passions. He used the word "libido" (violent desire) in a psychological sense for the first time. Cicero further stated that excessive perturbation might give rise to *morbi*, actual diseases of the soul, and that, basically, they were caused by a contempt or abuse of *ratio*—that is, by errors in judgment. In essence, the concepts elaborated by Cicero were based on the philosophical doctrine of Stoicism.

Seneca (4–65 A.D.) considered reason as basic for proper human behavior and passions as perturbations of the soul, to be differentiated from mental diseases. He advocated, as medicine of the soul, the rationalization of morbid processes—that is, philosophical examination of the realities of death, pain, and infirmity—and the cultivation of wisdom and of friendship.

Galen (ca. 130–200 A.D.) was undoubtedly the greatest physician of Roman times. He pointed out that the retention of male sperm or the delay of uterine discharges contributed to psychic imbalance and to manifestations of anxiety. He was aware of the correlation between hysterical symptoms and the absence of sexual relations, and he noted the curative effect of sexual relations and the release of tension provided by masturbation.

Galen attempted to disprove the Stoic dogma that psychological deviations were due to defects of reason. He maintained that the health of the soul depended on the proper harmony of the rational, irrational, and lustful parts of the soul. When errors in judgment were made unconsciously, they might be corrected by proper education.

Roman Contribution to Forensic Psychiatry

It is in relation to the legal aspects of mental illness that the Romans made their most important contributions to psychiatry. Previously, the various terms that defined the mentally ill had been used interchangeably. In contrast, the classic legal text of the late Roman times, *Corpus Juris Civilis*, detailed the various conditions—insanity, drunkenness, and so on—that, if present at the time the criminal act was committed, might decrease the criminal's responsibility for his actions. Apparently, however, the state of mind of the defendant was determined by a judge; physicians were not consulted in such matters. And, for the most part, those persons who were considered to be mentally ill, including those who might be diagnosed as criminal psychopaths today, were placed under the custody of relatives or guardians appointed by legal authorities. In addition, laws were passed that defined the ability of the mentally ill to contract marriage, to be divorced by a spouse, to dispose of their possessions, to leave a will, and to testify. During the rule of the emperor Justinian (483–565 A.D.), a number of mentally ill patients, for whom facilities had not been provided earlier, were admitted to institutions for the poor and infirm, perhaps as a result of the influence of Christianity.

Roman Treatment of Mental Illness

Aretaeus of Cappadocia (1st century A.D.), who belonged to the pneumatic school of thought, described forms of melancholia that terminated in mania, thus anticipating the manic-depressive syndrome. Of particular interest is the psychological insight Aretaeus demonstrated in defining the influence of the emotions on mental functioning—for example, the influence of love on melancholia.

Soranus (1st to 2nd centuries A.D.) described the ideational content of mental disturbances and of various forms of stupor. However, Soranus is known in particular for the truly humanitarian principles he applied in the treatment and management of the mentally ill. Rooms were to be kept free from disturbing stimuli; visiting by relatives was restricted; the personnel responsible for the care of the patients were instructed to be sympathetic; during lucid intervals mental patients were encouraged to read and then to discuss what they had read, to participate in dramatic performances—tragedy was prescribed to counteract mania, comedy to counteract depression—and to speak at group meetings.

Ancient Therapeutic Methods

Among the various psychotherapeutic interventions for emotional disorders in antiquity, three stand out because of their widespread use for many centuries in various cultures in the Near East and the Mediterranean areas—the interpretation of dreams, incubation techniques, and therapy with words.

Three types of dreams can be differentiated: dreams that served as a vehicle for the revelation of a deity and that might or might not require interpretation, dreams that foretold future events, and dreams reflecting the state of mind of the dreamer, which was implied but never recorded. Initially, dreams were thought of as real events. Subsequently, the dream was thought to be the creation of the gods, who used it as a mode of communicating with the dreamer. Still later, the dream was recognized as the product of the dreamer, and it was further recognized that the events portrayed therein might be interpreted in the light of their symbolic meaning.

The phenomenon of incubation consisted of several stages: Postulants, who were afflicted with a variety of physical and psychic diseases, were first subjected to ritual purification, special diet, and fumigations with various sleep-inducing drugs. They then went to sleep in the temple in underground corridors constructed to form a maze in which music was played. While the patient slept, the god Asclepias appeared in his dreams as a man or a child or as a snake or a dog; he then touched the sick part of each patient's body, after which he disappeared. The patient awoke healed and had his dream decoded by an interpreter. The patient's dream and his subsequent recovery were regarded as a reward for his devotion to the god Asclepias, to whom he would then make further votive offerings.

In *Poetics* Aristotle called catharsis the purgation that certain words, especially those of the tragic poems, can produce in the whole reality of the human being. He described three distinct types of logos: dialectical or convincing; rhetorical or persuasive, related to verbal psychotherapy; and purgative or cathartic, related to medicine.

The Middle Ages

A philosopher and a theologian, St. Augustine (354–430) was not interested in psychology proper and even less in mental disorders. Yet his observations in many areas—on educational methods, on the nature of children, on the joy of being with friends, on the sense of power one derives from doing what is forbidden—reveal great psychological insight.

In regard to the causes of mental disorders, increasing attention was given to the notion of localizing imagination in the forebrain, understanding in the midventricles of the brain, and memory in the back part of the brain (see Figure 2). Considerable difficulty surrounded the traditional pathogenic view of the black bile. Throughout the early Middle Ages many attempts were made to view the humoral doctrine from a Christian perspective. Another concept relevant to psychopathology that came to the fore during the Middle Ages was the doctrine of temperaments.

Clinical Concepts and Practices

Throughout the Middle Ages, melancholia continued to be the term most frequently used in describing all kinds of mental disorders,

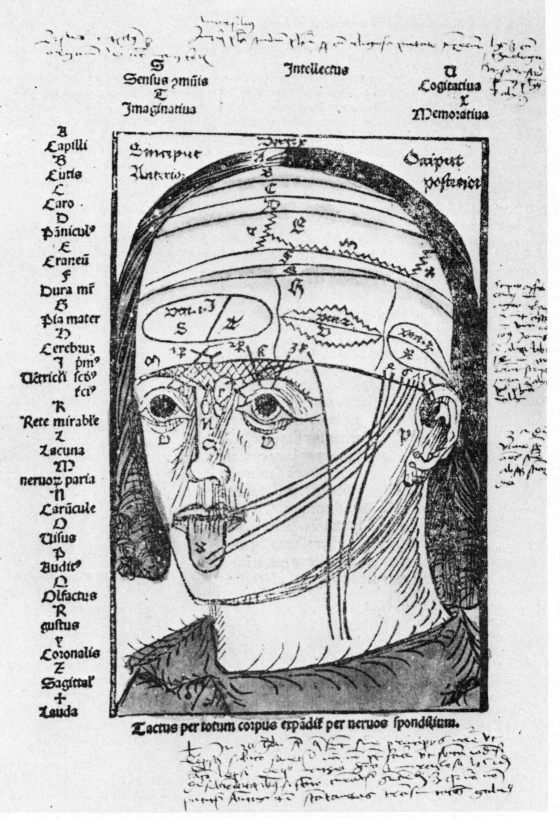

FIGURE 2. The functions of the brain. From *Anthropologium de hominis dignitate natura et proprietatibus . . .* (1501) by Magnus Hundt the Elder.

many of which would today be labeled as schizophrenic symptoms. Some people were impressed by the cyclic occurrence of mental disorders. The Byzantine physician Alexander of Tralles (525–605) described a condition that is not simply melancholia but turns into mania in a cycle—apparently the first description of circular insanity. Epilepsy, identified by a variety of names, was frequently mentioned by medieval writers, probably because of its dramatic manifestations.

Incubus (from the Latin *in cubitum*, on the couch), corresponding to the English "nightmare," was attributed to various causes but most often to a male demon attacking chaste girls, as opposed to the succubus—that is, a female demon molesting men. Also related to sexuality was the picture of effeminacy or pathic disorder in a man, attributed by Avicenna to a degraded mind, a vicious nature, and bad habits. Lycanthropy, a species of melancholy in which the patient wanders about at night—in sepulchers, woods, and elsewhere —imitating wolves and wild animals, was also mentioned.

In regard to treatment, bloodletting and purgatives continued to prevail throughout the Middle Ages. Skull trepanation was apparently practiced in cases of epilepsy and dementia (see Figure 3).

The Byzantine physician Paulus of Aegina (7th century) advised that the mentally ill be swung in a wicker basket bed suspended from the ceiling. Bartholomeus Salernitanus (12th century) prescribed silence and solitary confinement for the mentally ill; quite to the contrary Bernard of Gordon (13th century) recommended a bright and light facility filled with fragrant odors and located in pleasant and cheerful surroundings. The Arabian Rhazes was in favor of frequent sexual intercourse and the moderate use of alcohol.

Arab Contributions to Psychiatry. A humanistic attitude toward the mentally ill prevailed in Arab countries. Their approach to mental diseases was largely influenced by Greek medical science, by the tenets of Christianity, and by the enlightened Byzantine administration. Arabs translated into Arabic many Greek classic texts and established flourishing medical schools and a number of asylums. Travelers returning to Europe reported on the enlightened treatment mental patients received in these institutions. The atmosphere was relaxed and the therapeutic regimen included special diets, baths, drugs, perfumes, and concerts at which the instruments were tuned in a special way so they would not jar the patients' nerves. An outpatient clinic and a medical school, where teaching was conducted in the Greek tradition, were attached to each hospital. The same treatment facilities were available to rich and poor patients alike, the majority of whom appear to have been manic-depressive psychotics.

At the root of this humanitarian attitude was the Moslem belief that the insane person is loved by God and is particularly chosen by Him to tell the truth. The difference between insanity and possession was thought to be minimal, and the mentally ill were frequently worshipped as saints. From a modern viewpoint, it appears that this attitude might facilitate the patient's recovery, since it permitted the free expression of his sexual and aggressive instincts.

School of Salerno. Constantinus Africanus (ca. 1020–1087) is recognized as the founder of the medical school of Salerno, near Naples, which enjoyed great renown in the late Middle Ages. His *De melancholia* was based on the amalgamation of classic and Arab influences. Typically, an excess of bile, which was attributed to an imbalance of the systems of the body, could cause melancholia. The recommended treatment included proper diet, kind and sensible words, music, baths, cathartics, rest, physical exercise, and sexual gratification. He described for the first time the symptoms that characterized this syndrome—sadness (due to loss of the loved object), fear (of the unknown), withdrawal (staring into space), delusions surrounding siblings and parents (which today would be attributed to ambivalence), and intense fear and guilt in religious people. Africanus also advanced certain hypotheses regarding prognosis that are generally accepted today—for example, the prognosis was more favorable in acute reactive conditions and when the patient had not reached an extreme state of withdrawal.

The 13th Century

Outstanding among the thinkers of the 13th century were Albert the Great (1193–1280) and Thomas Aquinas (1225–1274). Aside from Aristotle's teaching, both were influenced by the

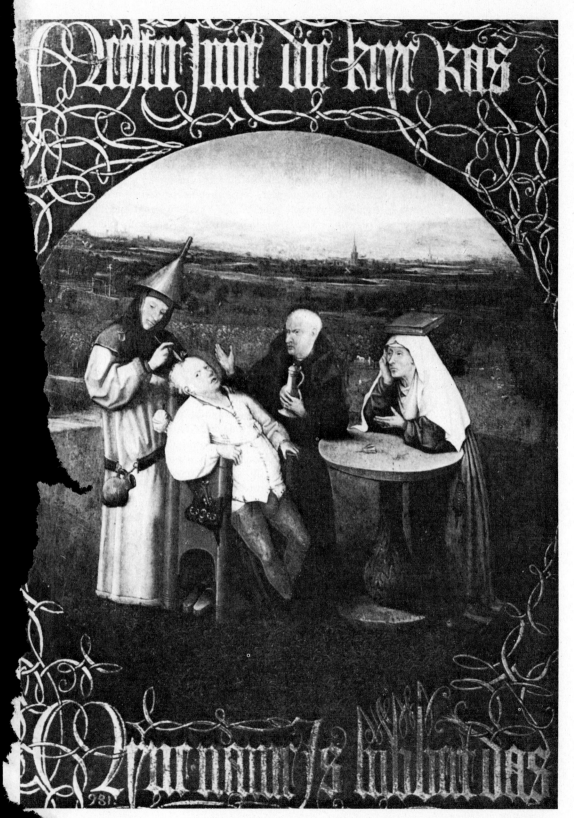

Figure 3. Cutting for stone in head. By Hieronymus (Jerome) Bosch (1450–1516). Prado Museum, Madrid.

views of Hippocrates, Galen, and the Arabs, according to whom the body, conceived of in terms of the four classic elements, influenced all psychic phenomena, and the soul was the form of the body.

The structure of the psyche was conceived of as comprising three levels—anima vegetativa, anima sensitiva, and anima intellectiva. The anima vegetativa referred to physiological functions. The anima sensitiva was concerned with the external and the internal senses. The anima intellectiva alluded to those qualities in the senses that made possible the cognitive functions.

Central to the theory of psychopathology postulated by Albert the Great and Thomas Aquinas was the notion that the soul could not become sick. Therefore, insanity was primarily a somatic disturbance. Mental disturbance was attributed to the deficient use of reason, which was due to one of two factors: either passions were so intense that they interfered with proper reasoning, or reason could not prevail because of the peculiar functioning of the physical apparatus—in dream states or states of intoxication, for example. Even the pathological character traits described by Albert—such traits as timidity, arrogance, resentment, and impulsiveness—were attributed to somatic factors.

Both Albert and Thomas Aquinas described various psychotic symptoms, such as hallucinations, and different types of mental patients; these descriptions, although highly intuitive, show a lack of clinical experience. In addition to melancholia, which he attributed to altered body humors, Thomas Aquinas described mania (pathological anger), organic psychosis (loss of memory), and epilepsy, which he attributed to an increased formation of vapors in the brain.

Although mental patients might have lucid intervals, they were, from a legal viewpoint, incapable of distinguishing right from wrong; therefore, they could not be held responsible for any crimes they committed. Sleep and baths were recommended treatment procedures. However, even Albert the Great and Thomas Aquinas believed that the cause and the treatment mental illness depended largely on astrologi influences on the psyche and on the evil po of demons.

Popular Attitudes toward Mental Disorder

The ignorant population, which repres the great majority, were influenced by all of mystic and occult beliefs, mainly of E origin. There are written records by Bed other historians of charms and of cerer involving idolatry, the worship of demor cult of the dead, the worship of   and and fire, augury, and divination. "L vil' meant pagan deity, rather than spirit of

Possession of the mind of the menta person by an evil spirit, with or without of the subject, resulting in all manifestations and abnormal be' be accepted as a common c disorders. The exorcising of persons alleg possessed by harmful intruders became a quent practice in the Middle Ages.

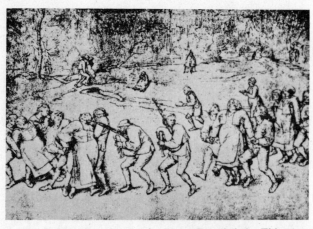

FIGURE 4. Dance epidemics of 1564. Pen drawing by Pieter Breughel the Elder (ca. 1525–1569). Albertina Collection of Vienna.

nsanity was alienation. But alienation had two opposite meanings—on the one side, failure to love God and refusal to adhere to the order e had given; on the other side, lack of involvement in this world for the purpose of being warded in the other world. Madmen, left wandering on their own, were a testimony to the eatness of God and the frailty of man. Probably they were not mistreated or neglected but imply viewed as a necessary, although at times noying, part of the community. Many may ve found relief from their overwhelming aggive and sexual impulses through participation in religious wars and crusades and in long images; others preferred to embrace emolly charged heretic movements. Typical estations of disorder available to large s of the population were religious dances, the famous dance epidemics of the 14th (see Figure 4).

The Renaissance

aft Mo a

ccus based on suspicion or rumor be brought to the Inquisition authorities; ular power would apprehend the alleged articular marks supposedly made by the h birthmarks and patches of anesound; under tortures of various would confess the pact with devil. Quite often she would be found guilty entenced to a cruel death. Conservative estes put the figure of executed men, women, children a ore than 100,000 in Germany a similar number in France. In England, ere the pagan Anglo-Saxon law persisted, ording to which a person was innocent unless oved guilty, very few people were killed; in in, too, the attack on witchcraft was reicted because of the nationalistic and indeent attitude of the Spanish Inquisition.

everal treatises on witchcraft began to appear in the early 15th century, and they contributed to the spread of this belief, with the help of the newly discovered system of printing. The most influential treatise was *Formicarius* (*Ant Heap*), published in 1437 by the Dominican Johann Nider. In that treatise the supposed sexual activities between women and the devil are discussed in detail. The highest peak in herence to the tenets of witchcraft was d in 1484, when Pope Innocent VIII

MALLEVS
MALEFICARVM,
MALEFICAS ET EARVM
haeresim framea conterens,

EX VARIIS AVCTORIBVS COMPILATVS,
& in quatuor Tomos iustè diftributus,

*QVORVM DVO PRIORES VANAS DÆMONVM
verſutias, praſtigioſas eorum deluſiones, ſuperſtitioſas Strigimagarum
cæremonias, horrendos etiam cum illis congreſſus; exactam demque
tam peſtiferæ ſectæ diſquiſitionem, & punitionem complectuntur.
Tertius praxim Exorciſtarum ad Dæmonum, & Strigimagarum male-
ficia de Chriſti fidelibus pellenda; Quartus verò Artem Doctrinalem,
Benedictionalem, & Exorciſmalem continent.*

TOMVS PRIMVS.
Indices Auctorum, capitum, rerumque non deſunt.

Editio nouiſſima, infinitis penè mendis expurgata; cuique acceſſit Fuga
Dæmonum & Complementum artis exorciſticæ.

*Vir ſiue mulier, in quibus Pythonicus, vel diuinationis fuerit ſpiritus, morte moriatur
Leuitici cap. 10.*

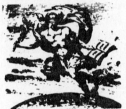

LVGDVNI,
Sumptibus CLAVDII BOVRGEAT, ſub ſigno Mercurij Galli.

M. DC. LXIX.
CVM PRIVILEGIO REGIS.

FIGURE 5. Title page of the *Malleus Maleficarum*, 1486, by the two Dominicans Jacob Sprenger and Heinrich Kramer.

issued the bull *Summis Desiderantes Affectibus*, which aimed to remove any possible hesitation in persecuting those accused. It was followed shortly thereafter by the unfortunately famous *Malleus Maleficarum* (*The Witches' Hammer*) by the two Dominicans Jacob Sprenger and Heinrich Kramer, published in Cologne in 1486 (see Figure 5). Zilboorg (1933) had pointed out that this book was so replete with sexual details that at times it may well be considered a handbook of sexual psychopathies.

The belief of Western civilization in witchcraft, based on elements of religion and magic common to all cultures, underwent a transformation from a probable fertility cult, the so-called society of Diana of women in the early Middle Ages, to a definite ritual sanctioned by ecclesiastic authorities. This transition occurred at a particular period of great social upheavals. In such circumstances, men subjected to all kinds of frustrations tend to discharge their pent-up aggression on a scapegoat. The crystallization of the belief in witchcraft made possible the establishment of a system of counterwitchcraft—that is, of an attempt to apply a system of putative knowledge to maintain order in the world—a fact that explains why all the rulers of that period, feeling their status threatened, actively contributed to the belief in witchcraft.

In the compact and socially rigid society of the time, witchcraft acquired the characteristic of alienation—that is, of repudiation of the existing order. Because of the theocentric view of the world, such a repudiation was expressed essentially through religious means.

Even more important is the fact that, in most instances, women were involved in the witchcraft rituals. At the base of this phenomenon is the overwhelmingly antifeminine trend of the Judeo-Christian traditions. From the very beginning, sin entered the world through Eve, and the demons originally fell because they lusted after the daughters of men; later on, from St. Augustine and St. Jerome to all the other Christian fathers, sexuality was viewed as degrading for men, even in the context of marriage. In the Middle Ages, the traditional image of the woman as a passive being bearing children and tending to the house split into contrasting images—on the one side, the courtly lady of the troubadours and of the heroes, almost a mundane version of the Virgin Mary; on the other side, a dangerous creature ready to use and misuse sex to control men or to lead them into perdition. The fact that many more women than men were involved in heretical movements and in witchcraft rituals may then be viewed as a form of rebellion against the male establishment.

Emergence of Humanism

The confluence of witchcraft and the position of women in the Middle Ages and the Renaissance is also reflected in the work of some great humanists of the time—notably Vives, Agrippa, and Weyer. It is significant that, in direct opposition to the belief in witchcraft, these three men held enlightened views about the role of women and about the mentally ill.

In 1524 Juan Luis Vives (1492-1540) wrote a treatise on the education of women, a pioneering concept at that time, and dedicated it to the daughter of Catherine of Aragon, wife of Henry VIII. The next year he published *On Poor Relief*, in which he advanced modern views on welfare, stating that particular attention should be given to those who are sick in the mind, for whom the authorities should build special hospitals.

In 1538 Vives published *De Ánima et Vita*. Among the many interesting points in the book are his awareness of psychological associations and recognition of their emotional origin, the emphasis given to the role of instinct in human behavior, and belief in the ambivalent aspect of certain emotions. Called the father of modern empirical psychology, Vives should also be recognized as the forerunner of dynamic psychology.

The wandering scholar Cornelius Agrippa (ca. 1486-1535) was even more outspoken in his opposition to misogyny. *On the Nobility and Pre-eminence of the Feminine Sex* was written in 1509 as a general defense of women. Furthermore, in 1519 he underscored his beliefs by risking his life in Metz to liberate a woman who had been accused of witchcraft.

Johann Weyer. Johann Weyer (1515-1588) turned his interest from general medicine to the study of individual human behavior—in particular, to the study of women who had been accused of witchcraft. The conclusions he reached in the course of his investigations were ultimately incorporated into *De Praestigiis Daemonum*, which was published in Basel in 1563.

Weyer began with an adamant rejection of the belief in witchcraft and a strong condemnation of the clergy who supported it. He proceeded to explain a variety of the so-called supernatural signs by which witches were usually identified. When medical knowledge proved inadequate, as in the case of hallucinations, he attributed such phenomena to a combination of natural and supernatural factors. Weyer had extensive clinical experience, which enabled him to describe a wide range of diagnostic entities and associated symptoms, including toxic psychoses, epilepsy, senile psychoses, nightmares, hysteria, delusions, paranoia, *folie à deux*, and depression.

However, it is in the realm of psychotherapy that Weyer's contribution to psychiatry is truly outstanding and unique. For example, he recommended that nuns in convents who manifested psychological symptoms, frequently of an erotic nature, be isolated first and then permitted to return to their own families. Above all, he insisted that the needs of the individual, rather than the rules of the institution, must be given primary consideration.

Weyer recognized the importance of the therapeutic relationship and of the kindness and understanding the therapist must extend toward his patient. However, he further postulated that, to be truly effective, this benevolent attitude must be based on scientific principles—that is, careful psychiatric examination and observation.

Weyer's radical approach was completely alien to the thinking of his times. As a result, his work evoked hostility at first and then was simply ignored by theologians, philosophers, physicians, and lawyers alike—the very audience to whom his book had been directed. Weyer's contributions are of such importance that he has been called "the first psychiatrist."

Humanism of Paracelsus and Cardan

The Swiss-born physician Paracelsus (ca. 1493–1541) advocated a more humane approach to all patients, including those who were afflicted with mental illness. He presented a dynamic view of the personality and emphasized its total involvement in each mental illness; he attempted to clarify definite clinical pictures of mental diseases—especially manic-depressive psychoses, psychopathic personality, and mass psychic contagion—he posited that mental illness is a deviation from normality, with a consequent search for causative factors and for therapeutic methods to reintegrate the patient to his original state of health; and he held the basic tenet that the mental patient is neither a criminal nor a sinner but a sick person in need of medical help. From the perspective of psychodynamics, Paracelsus anticipated the concepts of projection, ambivalence, unconscious self-destructive trends, and the economy of the libido.

Paracelsus adhered strictly to the notion that psychic conditions should be treated with psychic methods. Consequently, he practiced a method of psychotherapy based on counseling, suggestion, reasoning, and encouraging the patient.

Jerome Cardan (1501–1576)—a mathematician, philosopher, and physician—was among the first to use his personal experiences as the basis for his efforts to understand psychological phenomena. In his *Autobiography*, which he completed in 1570, Cardan described in detail the emotional disorders he underwent during his childhood (nightmares and stuttering, which he ascribed to his father's pathological influence) and as an adolescent (sexual impotence, hallucinations, and grandiose ideas). He opposed persecution of people for so-called witchcraft, detailed the prerequisites for mental health, and described various character types and their somatic correlations.

Physiognomy and Morphology

An attempt to correlate character type with somatic variables properly includes physiognomy, a field of study that became popular during the Renaissance at the time of the "discovery" of anatomy by Vesalius (1514–1564) and the concomitant emphasis on man as a microcosm that reflected the macrocosm. Many volumes on physiognomy were published in the late 15th century, but none acquired such wide popularity as *De Humana Physiognomia* by Giambattista della Porta (1538–1615), a Neapolitan writer on scientific or pseudoscientific subjects. The main thesis of his book was that the physical resemblance of man to animals may be extended to apply to behavioral characteristics as well—for instance, sharpness of sight, cautiousness, and aggressiveness.

Juan Huarte (ca. 1530–1592), in his book *The Examination of Men's Wits*, published in 1574, advanced the thesis that variations in the intellectual capacity of men may be attributed to differences in temperament. Thus, Huarte came even closer to modern character analysis and the concepts of vocational orientation.

Pioneer Hospital Treatment

Despite advances in psychology and psychiatry, the attitude of the general public toward mental illness remained essentially the same as the attitude that had prevailed in ancient and medieval times. This phenomenon was due to the lag between persisting medieval social institutions, on the one hand, and advancing individual creativity, on the other. This basic discrepancy accounted for the lack of community responsibility and humanitarian attitudes that characterized this period. The general belief was that mental patients were cured by supernatural forces—that is, the intercession of saints. In fact, there was a similarity with the ancient practice of incubation, for such intercession was held to occur for the most part while the patient was asleep. When the saints failed to intervene, physical treatment methods—such as cathartics, emetics, and bloodletting—were used.

By the 14th century, several institutions had been established for the care or, more accurately, the custody of mental patients in Metz (1100), Uppsala (1305), Bergamo (1325), and Florence (1385). Furthermore, the town of Gheel in Belgium had become a center for the care of mental patients during the Middle Ages. Traditionally, however, the founding of the first mental hospital, in Valencia in 1409, is attributed to Father Gilabert Jofré (1350–1417), a Spanish priest. Between 1412 and 1489 five similar institutions were established in various cities in Spain, and in 1567, under Spanish influence, the first mental hospital was established in Mexico City.

The Arabs exerted a major influence in shaping the new attitude of the Spaniards toward mental patients. This fact is borne out by the many similarities between these early mental hospitals and some of the Arab institutions that were apparently devoted to mental patients.

When mentally ill patients were kept at home, their families frequently resorted to the use of chains. And, with few exceptions, the conditions to which the hospitalized mental patient was exposed were equally deplorable.

Apparently, hospital administrators shared the popular view of mental illness, for, until the 19th century, mental patients were regularly placed on exhibition at Bethlehem Hospital in London, (see Figure 6), where they could be viewed by the public for a few pennies.

Laymen's View of Mental Illness

Contrasting and at times opposing etiological factors in mental diseases based on the humoral theory, on a mysterious correspondence between human behavior and the planets, and on other unproved notions are typical of the so-called Elizabethan malady, described with unwarranted frequency in the English literature from the late 16th century to the middle 17th century.

However, recognition of the importance of passion as an internal force that, when it was not regulated by reason, could produce melancholia through the mediating action of the body, suggests that the foundation had been laid for a more modern view of human psychological functioning as representing a continuum that ranged from normality to disease. The Renaissance picture of the fool slowly faded, and in its place modern conscience slowly advanced.

The 17th and Early 18th Centuries

The 17th century represents a period of transition from uncritical dependence on the ancients' belief in the gods, which in the Renaissance had found expression in the witchcraft mania, to the specification and application of methodological criteria in science. In psychol-

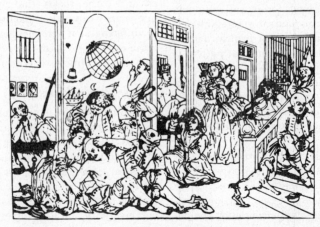

Figure 6. Sketch of Bedlam (Bethlehem Hospital) by William Hogarth (1697–1764). (From *A Rake's Progress*, Plate VIII.)

ogy, a word coined in 1590 by the German philosopher Göckel (1547-1628), the emphasis was placed on the organs that mediated between passions and body humors—namely, on the body-mind relationship.

In line with the contemporary taxonomic trend in many fields of science, a preoccupation with the classification of mental disorders emerged. The first medical textbook published in the 17th century to deal with psychiatry, *Praxis Medica*, written in 1602 by the Swiss physician Felix Platter (1536-1614), begins with a 75-quarto-page introduction on the classification of mental diseases. Like his contemporaries, Platter subscribed to a theory of organic humoral causation; however, this view did not necessarily rule out the devil as a causative factor, at least in some cases of possessed female patients.

Legal Psychiatry

Paolo Zacchia (1584-1659), who is generally regarded as the father of legal medicine, wrote that only a physician was competent to judge the mental condition of a person. He suggested that such an examination should be based on observation of the person's behavior, language, actions, ability to exercise sound judgment, and emotional state. Zacchia stressed that the person, rather than the law, was to be given primary consideration. Thus, manic patients who had lucid intervals could be held only partly responsible for their criminal acts; marriage might be beneficial for some melancholics, who could also hold positions with limited responsibilities. Persons who committed crimes of passion should be acquitted; alcoholics should be studied carefully; epileptics should be made to undergo a period of intensive study and observation before they were accepted into religious orders. In cases of malingering, one should keep in mind that not all symptoms are known to the patients and can be reproduced by them. And melancholia led possessed persons to believe they were persecuted by the devil.

Advances in Clinical Observation

Thomas Sydenham (1624-1689) is generally thought to have initiated the clinical approach in modern medicine. Although Sydenham was not specifically interested in diseases of the mind, he had, in the course of his clinical experience, become aware of the importance of neurotic and hysteric symptoms and the frequency with which they occurred among his patients. He described these symptoms in detail. He pointed out that, contrary to popular belief, hysteric manifestations were not restricted to women but might be observed in men and children as well. Moreover, hysterical illness might include a wide range of symptoms, such as vomiting, convulsive coughing, spasm of the colon, pain in the bladder and back, and retention of urine. Sydenham's importance derives from the fact that, whereas psychiatry had focused exclusively on psychotic phenomena, now, for the first time, attention was drawn to the symptoms of neurosis.

Throughout the 17th and 18th centuries, other workers adopted the clinical approach initiated by Sydenham for the observation and description of emotional disturbances. But the advances in psychiatric knowledge achieved during these two centuries consisted of isolated descriptions of symptoms and clinical pictures.

Laymen's Concepts of Mental Disorders

In *Anatomy of Melancholy* (1621) Robert Burton (1577-1640), a divine at St. Thomas near Oxford, elucidated the psychological and social causes of insanity—for example, jealousy, solitude, fear, poverty, unrequited love, excessive religiosity. This emphasis on emotional factors in the causation of mental illness, combined with rejection of supernatural factors and occult practices, marked a new stage in the development of a more humane and understanding concept of man.

This trend was similarly reflected in the spiritual and moral Christian guidance movement that developed during the 17th century as an expression of Protestant piety and of the Catholic counterreformation and the religious orders that evolved from it. In brief, concern for the moral and spiritual welfare of the soul could not be divorced from consideration of psychological factors, as typified by the casuistry of the Jesuits, which was based on counseling and on establishing a relationship with the person. On the philosophical level, the Jewish philosopher Baruch Spinoza (1632-1677) provided the foundation for an integrated approach to physical and psychological phenomena by considering them as two aspects of the same living organism; in so doing, he anticipated some concepts of the dynamic unconscious.

Contradictions in Attitudes toward the Mentally Ill

With the rise of liberalism in economy and Puritanism in religion, labor became equated with morality and idleness with sin. The king of each European nation was idealized as a benign father figure who was responsible not only for the safety of his subjects but also for their health, mental as well as physical. Accordingly, general hospitals for the care of elderly people, people with venereal diseases, epileptics, and the mentally ill were built in several cities in France and in Germany. These installations, each one containing several thousand inmates, combined the characteristics of a penal institution, an insane asylum, a sheltered workshop, and a hospital.

Madness was confined to the realm of the absurd and irrational, as portrayed in Molière's comedies. The glorification of reason and the concomitant lack of tolerance for the irrational culminated in a complete rejection of the mentally ill from a philosophical viewpoint. Although passions were discussed to an increasing extent in the literary salons and in the lucid prose of the French moralists, they were also considered a great potential evil when they were not controlled by reason. Reason took the place of the medieval God; but in the eyes of God, madness had had to be exposed; in the eyes of reason, madness had to be hidden.

The fear of madness grew out of proportion, and there was a basic contradiction in the attitude toward mental illness. On the one hand, the mentally ill were rejected by medical and other professional societies. On the other hand, the impressive scientific and social accomplishments during this period led to the establishment of modern science. Even as cultivated men all over Europe were engaged in philosophical discussion of the human mind and its functions and of social and economic theories, mental patients continued to be objects of ridicule and neglect.

Yet some progress was made in the understanding and treatment of mental disorders. The Elizabethan Poor Law Act of 1601, which placed the responsibility for the care of the poor—and frequently the insane—on local authorities, had led to their exile from one community after another. The obvious inequities of this situation finally gave rise to some concern for the mentally ill and, concurrently, efforts to devise improved methods for their treatment. In 1744, Britain established rules for the commitment of mental patients. In 1750 St. Luke's Hospital was opened at Moorsfield, England.

The religious order of St. Vincent de Paul founded Saint Lazare in 1632, and the Brothers of Charity founded the Charité de Senlis in 1668 for the care of the insane and of patients who today would be called juvenile delinquents or psychopaths, primarily in need of supervision and rehabilitation. Both open and closed wards were provided for the patients, depending on their condition. They received both physical and psychological treatment, consisting of isolation, reading, personal interviews with the religious staff, spiritual exercises, and controlled contact with their families.

The Late 18th and Early 19th Centuries

Vincenzo Chiarugi

The rulers of Florence during the 17th and 18th centuries continued to encourage scientific research, especially in biology and medicine. Italian enlightenment, in contrast to that of the French and the English, acquired a practical character, which crystallized under the rule of the Grand Duke Peter Leopold (1747–1792) in a number of economic, financial, judiciary, educational, and religious reforms. The law on the insane—which established the specific rules, including a mental examination, to be followed in cases of proposed commitment—was passed in 1774. In 1785 the Grand Duke began the construction of the Hospital Bonifacio, which was opened 3 years later under the medical direction of a young physician, Vincenzo Chiarugi (1759–1820). The 1789 regulations of the hospital, which were obviously prepared under Chiarugi's supervision, specifically stated:

It is a supreme moral duty and medical obligation to respect the insane individual as a person.

Accordingly, neither physical force nor cruel methods of restraint were to be applied to patients, except for the occasional use of a straitjacket, designed so that it would not cause the patient undue discomfort. Hygienic and safety measures were also described in the regulations, and, despite their unpretentious character, these represented a radical change in the treatment of the mentally ill.

William Tuke

While these developments were taking place in Florence, the Society of Friends held a series of meetings in York, England, that were motivated by a desire to find ways of

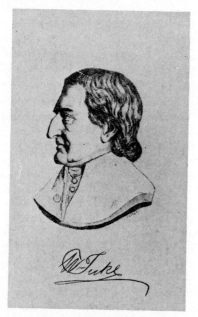

FIGURE 7. William Tuke (1732–1819), Founder of the Retreat at York, England.

mitigating the misery and restoration of those who are lost to civil and religious society.

Under the leadership of the elderly but still vigorous William Tuke (1732–1819) (see Figure 7), the Retreat was opened at York in 1796 for about 30 patients, who were treated as guests, with kindness and understanding, in a friendly atmosphere free from any mechanical restraint—and also from any direct medical influence. Rather, manual work was considered beneficial and was greatly encouraged. This treatment philosophy was continued by William's son, Samuel Tuke, and the Retreat served as a model for several institutions that were opened in the United States in the early 19th century.

Philippe Pinel

In 1793, Philippe Pinel (1745–1826) became superintendent of the Bicêtre (for male patients) and later of the Salpêtrière (for females), where criminals and mentally retarded patients, as well as the mentally ill, were housed. One of Pinel's first accomplishments at the Bicêtre was to free the mentally ill from their chains (see Figure 8).

Pinel is remembered for two other major contributions to psychiatry: his attempt to analyze and categorize symptoms and his appli-

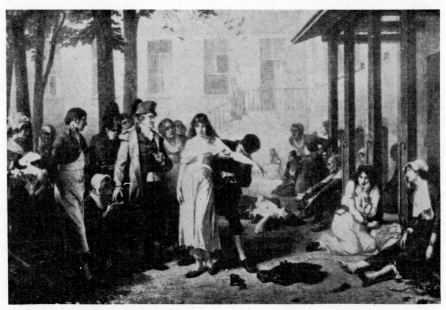

FIGURE 8. Philippe Pinel (1745–1826), the founder of modern psychiatry, liberating mental patients at the Salpêtrière in 1795. (From the painting by Robert Fleury.)

cation of moral treatment. Pinel described clinical symptoms in a very simple manner but with great clarity. He described four types of insanity: (1) melancholia (disturbance in intellectual functioning), (2) mania (excessive nervous excitement with or without delirium), (3) dementia (disturbance in thought processes), and (4) idiocy (obliteration of intellectual faculties and affects). Detailed data were accumulated for each patient.

More important than environmental factors were those factors that were thought to indicate a predisposition to the later development of insanity; among these, passions were considered of particular importance. Accordingly, moral treatment was based on Aristotle's concept of mental health as dependent on the balance of passions, a word that in 18th century literature corresponded to the present use of the word "emotions." Moreover, in anticipation of later theories of psychosomatic functioning, passions (emotions) were considered the link between mind and body. With regard to specific therapeutic techniques, the doctor initially had to exert the greatest firmness in his approach to the patient and hold his attention and control his will with his eyes. Once the patient was subdued and had been completely dominated by the doctor, treatment consisted of a combination of kindness, firmness, and coercion. The patient's participation in various activities within a structured environment greatly contributed to the success of Pinel's moral treatment.

Phrenology

Franz Josef Gall (1758–1828), the founder of phrenology, was a distinguished physician from Vienna who taught brain physiology there for several years. On the basis of physiognomic concepts, especially those developed by the Swiss pastor Johann Kasper Lavater (1741–1801), Gall postulated that mental faculties were innate and that they depended on the topical structures of the brain, to which corresponded particular protuberances of the external cranial surface. Eventually, he identified 27 organs in the human brain—19 of which were found in animals as well. These organs corresponded to an equal number of faculties that, being fixed from birth, could not be modified by education. Gall was accused of materialism and was ultimately forced to leave Vienna for Paris.

His phrenological teaching was carried on by his pupil Johann Casper Spurzheim (1776–1832), who lectured extensively on phrenology in the United States. Eventually, phrenological societies and journals were founded in several American cities, and the movement became increasingly popular. It did not decline in popularity until the latter half of the century.

Mesmerism

Mesmerism was initiated by Franz Anton Mesmer (1734–1815), who in 1766, in his doctoral dissertation at the University of Vienna Medical School, subscribed to the concept that planets influence physiological and psychological phenomena. In a later publication, entitled *Memory on the Discovery of Animal Magnetism* (1779), Mesmer hypothesized that man was endowed with a special magnetic fluid, a kind of sixth sense, that, when liberated, could produce amazing healing effects. Mesmer himself claimed to have magnetized and cured many patients, but controversy forced him to leave Vienna and to move to Paris in 1778. There he achieved great success (see Figure 9), and elicited the support of many distinguished and wealthy people—and an equal amount of opposition from the medical profession. Mesmer retired to Switzerland, where he died in poverty and oblivion. However, his pupils continued to practice mesmerism, and eventually the Marquis du Puységur (1751–1825) came to the conclusion that mesmerized patients were actually in a trance state. This observation was subsequently confirmed by James Braid (1795–1860), who coined the word "hypnosis." Even as the teaching of mesmerism flourished in Germany, the physicians James Esdaile (1808–1859) and

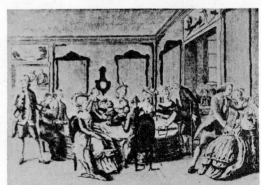

FIGURE 9. A mesmeric séance held around the baquet in Mesmer's clinic in Paris around 1780.

John Ellioston (1791–1868) made good use of mesmerism as a method of anesthetizing surgical patients in India and in England, respectively. The importance of mesmerism for psychiatry lies in the fact that it represented the most notable attempt to focus on neurotic phenomena, as opposed to psychoses.

Treatment in the United States

During the Colonial period, insanity was linked to superstitious beliefs of all kinds, including belief in witchcraft. In 1647, in Connecticut, the first alleged witch was hanged. Under the influence of narrow Puritanism and obviously misogynic views, the community of Salem, Massachusetts, was filled with terror of the invisible world—that is, unexplainable phenomena. The accusations of some suggestible young girls resulted in the Salem witchcraft trials in 1692, when 250 persons were arrested and tried: 50 were condemned, 19 were executed, 2 died in prison, and 1 died of torture. The next year Governor Phips released from custody all persons accused of witchcraft, but superstitious beliefs persisted.

A few mentally ill persons were left at home or boarded for a lump sum in private homes, where they were likely exploited. Violent and dangerously sick persons were put in jails. Other mentally ill persons were either sold on the auction block or simply taken to the town line and left to wander on their own. The basic attitude of the general population toward the mentally ill was uncharitable and punitive.

In the late 18th century, however, under the influence of the Enlightenment, a more optimistic view of man as innately good and as possessing perfectibility slowly came to prevail. The Quakers played a paramount role in fostering a humanitarian approach to the mentally ill. In 1756 the first group of mentally ill patients were admitted in the cellar of the new Pennsylvania Hospital. Great faith was placed in work as a way to restore health. Patients were cared for by cell-keepers—that is, attendants. When violent, the patients were restrained by handcuffs, ankle-irons, or the madd-shirt, a strait waistcoat. As in England, the patients could be exhibited on Sunday to curious sightseers for a set admission fee. Eventually, in 1796, a new wing was erected especially for the mental patients. Meanwhile, in 1773 the first American asylum exclusively for the mentally ill was opened under government auspices and with the support of the state in Williamsburg, then the flourishing capital of Virginia. The therapeutic approach used there was benign and humanitarian, and considerable use was made of agricultural work and recreational programs, mainly music and reading.

Benjamin Rush. The early treatment of the mentally ill at Pennsylvania Hospital is closely connected with the work of Benjamin Rush (1745–1813), who is called the father of American psychiatry and whose picture is reproduced in the seal of the American Psychiatric Association. In 1783 he became a regular member of the staff of the Pennsylvania Hospital, and for many years he was in charge of the mental patients housed there. Slowly, through his own observation and under the influence of Pinel and others, he developed his psychiatric concepts and finally presented them in 1812 in *Medical Inquiries and Observations upon the Diseases of the Mind*, which remained for 70 years the only American textbook on psychiatry (see Figure 10). Rush regarded insanity as a disease of the brain. He classified the remote and exciting causes of mental disorders in two groups, those acting directly on the body or the brain—congenital malformations, cerebral diseases, systemic diseases affecting the central nervous system—and those acting on the body or the brain through the medium of the mind—intensive study, strong emotional impressions, or moral preoccupations, such as guilt feelings. Rush listed as predisposing factors to mental diseases: heredity, young age, female sex, single status, intellectual occupations, excesses of climate, certain forms of government, revolutions, and particular religious tenets.

Rush's importance lies not in his elaborate classification but in the role he attributed to the derangement of passions—love, grief, fear, anger, joy, envy, malice, and hatred—and of the sexual appetite, in his lengthy discussion about dreams and sleep, and in his description of certain clinical pictures, such as hysteria. Regardless of his conviction of the organic nature of insanity, in actuality he believed in the psychogenic origin of many forms of mental disorders.

Rush advocated two types of treatment, one intended to act directly on the body and another intended to act indirectly on the body through the medium of the mind. To the first type

MEDICAL INQUIRIES

AND

OBSERVATIONS,

UPON

THE DISEASES OF THE MIND.

BY BENJAMIN RUSH, M. D.
Professor of the Institutes and Practice of Medicine, and of Clinical
Practice, in the University of Pennsylvania.

PHILADELPHIA:

PUBLISHED BY KIMBER & RICHARDSON,

NO. 237, MARKET STREET.

Merritt, Printer, No. 9, Watkin's Alley.

1812.

FIGURE 10. Title page of the textbook on mental diseases by Benjamin Rush (1745–1813).

belonged bloodletting (of which he made great use), purges, emetics, reduced diet, drugs, and, in particular cases, the use of two curious mechanical devices: the tranquilizer, a chair to which the patient was strapped hand and foot, and the gyrator, a modification of a circulating swing, a rotating board to which the patient was strapped with the head farthest from the center in an attempt to cause the blood to rush to the head. To the second and more enlightened type of treatment belonged the attempt to eliminate all old associations and ideas through removal of the patient from his family and from all remote and exciting causes, the writing of a personal account of the symptoms, a complete change of activities, encouragement to memorize passages of verse and prose, and the use of work, amusements of various types, and travel.

In the hospital the physician was urged to listen sympathetically to patients and thus give them the opportunity to relieve their minds and their consciences while he exercised control over them through his eye, his voice, and his countenance, so as to secure their obedience; very noisy and disturbing patients were to be housed in separate buildings; patients were to be divided by sexes; intelligent men and women were to be hired as attendants; and visitors were to be rigidly excluded.

Mental Hospitals. Strongly influenced by optimistic and humanitarian trends in beliefs about human nature, some community leaders took the initiative in opening a few mental hospitals early in the 19th century. Under private auspices, the Friends Asylum at Frankford, Pennsylvania, was opened in 1817 by some Quakers; the Bloomingdale Asylum in New York was opened in 1821 (under the auspices of the New York Hospital, founded in 1771) by the layman Thomas Eddy, a Quaker merchant; the McLean Asylum in Massachusetts was opened in 1818 under the leadership of Rufus Wyman, the first physician appointed to this post in America; the Hartford Retreat in Connecticut was opened in 1824; the Brattleboro Retreat in Brattleboro, Vermont, was opened in 1836; and the Butler Hospital in Providence, Rhode Island, was opened in 1847. Among the earliest state-supported institutions were the Eastern State Hospital at Lexington, Kentucky, opened in 1824; the Manhattan State Hospital in New York City, opened in 1825; the Western State Hospital in Staunton, Virginia, opened in 1828; and the South Carolina State Hospital in Columbia, South Carolina, opened in 1828. In contrast with the private or corporate hospitals, in which moral treatment was applied, these state institutions remained largely custodial.

Within 30 years, 18 hospitals were built; from 1825 to 1865 the number of asylums grew from nine to sixty-two. The first state institution that relied on moral treatment and one that carried a brilliant tradition in American psychiatry was the Worcester State Hospital in Worcester, Massachusetts, founded largely through the efforts of Horace Mann. Ten years later, in 1843, the New York State Lunatic Asylum was opened in Utica, New York.

Moral Treatment. The foundations of the Protestant ethic were at the base of the pioneers' philosophy of moral treatment: a humanistic background, an enlightened and humanitarian approach toward other men, middle-class values, and a community-oriented way of operating. There was a widespread conviction that mental aberrations did not affect the immortal soul, a theory in line with the Christian tradition. Necessarily, mental diseases had to be diseases of the brain, which could be caused by physical factors or by psychological factors.

The main causes leading to mental disorders were considered to be psychological and environmental and were divided into predisposing and precipitating, then called "exciting." Among the causes were heredity, passions, unhappy childhood, faulty education based on too much strictness or leniency, excessive masturbation, sudden shocks, frightening and lustful novels, lack of sleep, rapid changes of habits (related to wars, revolutions, or economic recessions), religious overemphasis, and, in general, the many dangers of civilization, ranging from political freedom to the appearance of industry, the growth of cities, and economic uncertainties.

Moral treatment attempted to prevent, treat, and correct these various causes of mental disorders. Among the preventive measures were compliance with phrenological and eugenic principles. The therapeutic and corrective measures consisted of a therapeutic milieu in which the emphasis was on building up the self-esteem and self-control of the patient through the rational use of rewards and punishments in the context of a strong emotional relationship with a doctor. This doctor, viewed by the patients as a father figure, was expected to be intelligent, courageous, firm but kind, understanding, hopeful and cheerful, and able to achieve dominance over the patient tactfully. In summary, moral treatment was a method of re-educating the patient in a proper environment.

Moral treatment was a movement well supported by the community; it was applied to relatively small numbers of patients in each hospital, then housing a maximum of 200 patients; almost all patients were from homogeneous New England middle-class or upper-class backgrounds; and there were some differences in the treatment of the patients, depending on their symptoms (violent patients were confined in separate wards and were not expected to do manual work).

National Trends

In France, where the most important developments occurred, psychiatrists stressed the clinical study of the patient—that is, the clarification of symptoms and their detailed description, the close relationship between psychiatry and neurology, and the medicolegal aspects of psychiatry. A continuous effort was made to improve institutions and hospitals for the mentally ill. The contributions of Jean Etienne Esquirol (1772–1840), who was Pinel's favored pupil, were particularly significant. Esquirol's textbook *Des Maladies Mentales*, which was published in 1837, soon became a classic because of its clarity and the inclusion of statistics in the presentation of clinical matters.

Esquirol clearly defined hallucinations and monomania, a symptom that is currently termed paranoid ideation; emphasized the role of the emotions in the etiology of mental illness; fostered a therapeutic philosophy based on the combined action of the milieu of the institution and the use of proper passions to replace the disturbed ones; developed programs involving group activities in various mental hospitals; taught the first course on psychiatry in 1817; and was largely responsible for the lunacy bill of 1838, which delineated commitment procedures for prospective mental patients and influenced similar legislation in other countries.

German psychiatry was strongly influenced by the romantic movement, especially by the philosopher Schelling, and by theological principles. German psychiatrists during this period had little actual clinical experience. Their writings lack scientific objectivity; although there is occasional evidence of good insight, such insights were, for the most part, blunted by sentimental pathos and by religious and metaphysical expressions.

Nevertheless, there were exceptions. Johann Christian Heinroth (1773–1843), the first psychiatrist to use the word "psychosomatic," stressed the unity of mental phenomena—that is, total personality. He attached particular importance to psychological conflict, which he identified as the cause of guilt and, ultimately, of mental illness.

British psychiatry was characterized by a practical orientation, as evidenced by the well-built hospitals provided for mental patients. This orientation was in accordance with the respect for the individual that was emphasized in the English philosophical works of the period.

The Italian layman Pietro Pisani (1760–1837), who was superintendent of the mental hospital in Palermo, applied advanced methods of treatment that anticipated current concepts of milieu therapy. The Belgian Joseph Guislain (1797–1860) became well known for his textbooks and for his many activities on behalf of mental patients in his own country.

The Late 19th Century

Wilhelm Griesinger's (1817–1868) *Pathology and Therapy of Mental Diseases*, which was published in Germany in 1845, was soon considered the most authoritative textbook in psychiatry. Griesinger maintained that mental diseases could be explained only on the basis of physical changes in the nervous system. However, he also advanced views that anticipated recent developments in ego psychology. Griesinger's organic approach was adopted by other leading German psychiatrists, such as Leidesdorf, Westphal, and Meynert, who earned a place in history primarily because he was one of Freud's teachers.

In its extreme form, this organic viewpoint found expression in France in the work of Benedict Morel (1809–1873) and Valentin Magnan (1835–1916), who postulated that mental disease was evidence of a degenerative hereditary strain that would become progressively severe in successive generations, causing their extinction. In Italy, Cesare Lombroso (1836–1909), considered the founder of criminal anthropology, was particularly impressed by the degenerative stigmata and atavistic types of delinquents and, in general, of all sorts of people who demonstrated a wide range of physical and psychological abnormalities. However, the main psychiatric literature of the time, particularly the works of Krafft-Ebing (1840–1902) and Forel (1848–1931), reflected the concerns that occupied the Victorian mind—that is, the influence of noxious factors (sex, alcohol, infections, industrialization, and social progress) on personality.

American Psychiatry

In private hospitals and in a few state hospitals, the philosophy of moral treatment continued to prevail for some time. But most of the state hospitals rapidly became overcrowded with paupers, criminals, alcoholics, and vagrants. All these persons constituted a burden on the taxpayers, leading to a negative reaction against the use of moral treatment and to a justification for excluding them from the mental hospitals.

The movement toward institutionalizing the mentally ill was enhanced by several lay crusaders motivated by humanitarian reasons, notably Dorothea L. Dix (1802–1887). By 1861 there were 48 asylums in the United States—1 federally run in the District of Columbia, 27 state-supported, 5 maintained by cities and counties, 10 corporate institutions, and 5 privately owned. The total number of hospitalized patients was about 8,500 in a United States population of more than 27 million. On October 16, 1844, in Philadelphia, 13 superintendents of mental hospitals (The Original Thirteen) founded the Association of Medical Superintendents of American Institutions for the Insane, later called the American Medico-Psychological Association and now the American Psychiatric Association, the oldest national medical association in this country (see Figure 11). The same year the *American Journal of Insanity*, now entitled the *American Journal of Psychiatry*, was founded by Brigham and published for many years at the New York State Lunatic Asylum in Utica.

Almost all American psychiatrists came to believe in the physiopathological cause of mental disorders. Postmortem examinations became more important than individual contacts with patients, physicians progressively lost contact with the families of their patients and with the community, and the psychiatric guild found itself more and more isolated from the stream of medicine and the public. An aura of pessimism seemed to pervade psychiatry.

One effect of the large number of medical casualties during the Civil War was to focus attention on the importance of neurology. Apart from their contributions to this discipline, William Hammond, E. C. Spitzka, and S. Weir Mitchell (1829–1914) were the neurologists whose names are most frequently associated with progress in psychiatry during this period: Hammond and Spitzka for their textbooks on psychiatry; Mitchell for his outspoken criticism of the isolation of psychiatry from medicine and of the lack of interest in research and training, and for his rest cure method, which he considered particularly beneficial in the treatment of neurotic women and which was a logical outgrowth of the concept of neurasthenia, developed by George Beard in 1880.

Toward the end of the century, refreshing signs of a more positive and individualized

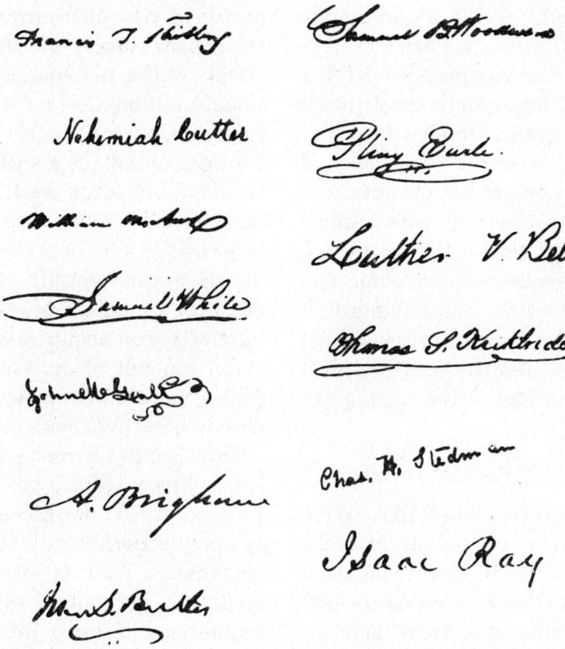

FIGURE 11. Signatures of the original 13 founders of the American Psychiatric Association, 1844.

approach to the mentally ill were becoming evident. Functional insanity was linked to faulty habits of life; separate facilities for acute cases were advocated; new forms of physical therapy—diet, massage, hydrotherapy, electrotherapy—were introduced; family care and the cottage system were initiated; and training courses for nurses and attendants were established.

As a reaction to Mitchell's criticism, a few psychiatrists became interested in research, and this interest led to the founding in 1895 of the Pathological Institute of New York Hospital, which later became the New York State Psychiatric Institute. A few years later, in 1902, the young Swiss psychiatrist Adolf Meyer (1866–1950) was appointed to the staff of the Institute, where he remained until 1913, when he became director of the newly built Henry Phipps Psychiatric Clinic at The Johns Hopkins University.

One other event during this period was of particular importance for the development of psychiatry: Clifford Beers, a distinguished businessman, published *A Mind That Found Itself* in 1908, after his recovery from a mental breakdown. In so doing, he launched the mental hygiene movement.

Kraepelin

Although he was Freund's contemporary, Emil Kraepelin (1855–1926) can be considered the last representative of the predynamic school of psychiatry. Kraepelin attempted to identify definite clinical syndromes by following and statistically recording their signs, their course, and their outcome. This method was objective and limited to the patient—that is, it took no consideration of his family and environment. On the basis of the voluminous data gathered, Kraepelin clearly differentiated manic-depressive psychosis from dementia precox, which was characterized by a weakening of emotional activities and a loss of inner unity. Unfortunately, this differentiation was carried one step further than necessary, and dementia precox patients came to be considered incurable. Kraepelin's classification was accepted all over the world; consequently, schizophrenia acquired a fatalistic connotation.

Constitution and Personality

From earliest times, man has attempted to correlate constitution—that is, the intrinsic physical endowment—with personality type, temperament, and emotional disorder. Kretschmer correlated the short, stocky, round pyknic habitus with extroversion, cyclothymic (cycloid) tendencies, and manic-depressive psychosis; the thin, asthenic, leptosomic constitution with introversion, schizoid tendencies, and schizophrenia; and the abnormally proportioned dysplastic habitus with endocrine and pituitary disorders. According to Sheldon, who applied the methodology of anthropometrics, the endomorph is temperamentally viscerotonic (sociable, relaxed; enjoys eating), the ectomorph is temperamentally cerebrotonic (antisocial, hypersensitive, secretive), and the mesomorph is somatonic (energetic, competitive, action-oriented) (see Table I).

Psychoanalysis and Recent Trends

The psychiatric events described above refer, for the most part, to psychotic or, at least, grossly disturbed patients. In fact, even those workers, such as Mesmer and his followers, who did attempt to describe and treat neurotic symptoms were largely unaware of the true origins of these symptoms in the unconscious. But interest in the unconscious, which may be attributed primarily to the romantic movement, was evident throughout the 19th century. The concept of the dynamic unconscious was developed as a concomitant of hypnosis by a number of physicians of the French school.

Jean Martin Charcot (1825–1893), a neurologist and literary man, was attracted by the puzzling symptoms of hysteria and investigated it thoroughly from the psychological perspec-

tive. He described hysterical stigmata, hysterogenous zones, the attacks, and the labile affect of the patients, characterized by emotional indifference (*la belle indifférence*). Eventually, Charcot came to recognize that a trauma, mainly of a sexual nature, quite often touched off ideas and feelings that become unconscious. Symptoms similar to hysteria, such as the idea of a paralysis, could be reproduced experimentally through hypnosis. Because of Charcot's prestige at the Salpêtrière, hypnosis soon acquired wide popularity and an equal amount of opposition from the medical profession. Charcot believed that hysteria could be cured by hypnosis.

Opposed to Charcot's thesis that only hysterical subjects could be hypnotized were two physicians, A. A. Liébeault (1823–1904) and Hippolyte Bernheim (1837–1919), of the school of Nancy. They stressed that anybody who could be influenced by suggestion could be hypnotized. After a bitter controversy and in spite of the prestige carried by Charcot, the school of Nancy eventually proved to be right.

Pierre Janet (1859–1947) developed the notion of psychological automatism—that is, the appearance of lower psychological functions when the higher functions are impaired. He excelled in clinical descriptions of hysteria, amnesia, fugues, anorexia, tics, and other syndromes. Common to most of these syndromes was the emergence of subconscious contents related to forgotten dimensions of the psyche, with which contact could be established in

TABLE I

Schools of Constitutional Typology*

Nationality of School	Name of Main Investigator	Name of Constitutional Types			
		Type I	Type II	Type III	Type IV
Greek	Hippocrates	Apoplecticus	Phthisicus		
Roman	Galen	Sanguine	Melancholic	Phlegmatic	Choleric
French	Rostan	Digestive	Respiratory cerebral	Muscular	
Italian	De Giovanni	Megalosplanchnic	Microsplanchnic	Normosplanchnic	
	Viola	Brachymorphic	Dolichomorphic	Eumorphic	
German	Gall-Beneke	Hyperplastic	Hypoplastic		
	Kretschmer	Pyknic	Asthenic	Athletic	Dysplastic
Anglo-American	Stockard	Lateral	Linear		
	Rees-Eysenck	Eurymorphic	Leptomorphic	Mesomorphic	
	Sheldon	Endomorphic (viscerotonic)	Ectomorphic (cerebrotonic)	Mesomorphic (somatotonic)	Dysplastic

* Adapted from F. J. Kallmann. *Heredity in Health and Mental Disorder*, p. 56. W. W. Norton, New York, 1953.

particular situations of suggestibility. Central to his theory of psychopathology was the concept of psychasthenia, which he described as loss of "the function of the real," partial dissociation, and inability to keep ideas in full consciousness owing to weakness of the highest integrative activities. The fact that Janet was influenced by the concepts related to hysteria and hypnosis developed by Charcot undoubtedly explains the many similarities between his own publications in clinical psychiatry and those of Freud at the end of the 19th century.

In addition to the great influence exercised on the development of modern psychiatry by the French clinicians at the turn of the century, brief mention should be made of the Swiss school, notably represented by the mental hospital Burghölzli in Zurich. The Burghölzli Hospital, founded in the mid-19th century, achieved great renown under the leadership of August Forel (1848–1931), who studied hypnosis extensively, vigorously fought against alcoholism, and presented enlightened views on sex in *The Sexual Problem* (1905). He was succeeded as director of Burghölzli by Eugen Bleuler (1857–1939) who, during his tenure there (1898–1927), coined the word "schizophrenia" (from the Greek words for split mind—that is, dissociation between thoughts and affects); classified the disorder into hebephrenic, catatonic, and paranoid; differentiated the primary disturbances, essentially loose associations, from the secondary disturbances, such as autism and hallucinations; under the influence of psychoanalysis focused on the content of the syndrome, such as displacement and condensation; and presented a much more optimistic view of its outcome than the one held by Kraepelin.

The physician Hermann Rorschach (1884–1922) also worked at Burghölzli. Under the influence of Jung's studies on associations and the complex, Rorschach published *Psychodiagnostik* in 1921, a fusion of clinical psychiatry, psychoanalysis, and applied psychology.

Burghölzli was the first mental hospital to accept psychoanalysis as a modality of treatment because of Eugen Bleuler, Carl Jung, and Ludwig Binswanger. As a number of physicians from many countries, including the United States, trained at Burghölzli early in the 20th century, the therapeutic methods used there were soon practiced elsewhere. Among these methods were emphasis on work therapy and the placement of patients in colonies and halfway houses.

Psychoanalytic Movement

Freud. Significantly, the 20th century opened with the publication of Sigmund Freud's (1856–1939) *The Interpretation of Dreams* (1900), a milestone in the history of psychology. Although the book at that time passed almost unnoticed, it represented a major breakthrough in the understanding of the human mind on three different grounds: (1) It introduced a strict methodological technique in the study of dreams. (2) It relied on the introspective study of the self. (3) It posed the basis for a foundation of psychology in which normality and pathology were conceived of as an uninterrupted continuum.

As a medical student, Freud held an apprenticeship in the scientific investigation of physiology under Ernest Brücke. After having obtained a medical degree in 1881, Freud, beset by financial difficulties, turned to neurology, did research in Meynert's psychiatric institute, and became *Privatdozent* in 1885. In the next two years he published two books, one on infantile cerebral paralysis and one on aphasia. In 1886 he studied in Paris under Charcot and, on his return to Vienna, became a vigorous defender of the value of hypnosis. He was influenced by the Viennese internist Joseph Breuer (1842–1925), who in 1880 had successfully treated a young woman affected by hysterical symptoms with a new talking cure, catharsis. After a second period of study in Nancy, France, in 1889, under Hippolyte-Marie Bernheim, Freud became convinced that suggestion was the psychological foundation of hypnosis. In *Studies on Hysteria* (1895) Breuer and Freud related the cure of hysteric symptoms to the release of blocked emotions. The same year Freud discovered the method of free association and gave up hypnosis completely. He called his method "psychoanalysis" for the first time in 1896.

Around that time Freud shared his most intimate thoughts related to his work with the German otorhinolaryngologist, Wilhelm Fliess. In retrospect, it is clear that through this relationship Freud underwent a sort of personal analysis, which eventually resulted in *The Interpretation of Dreams*.

For the next two decades Freud dedicated himself entirely to clinical matters, which he presented with great care in a number of books and articles. In *Psychopathology of Everyday Life* (1901), he described, in succession, primary process, condensation, displacement, and such other phenomena as slips of the tongue and parapraxias. Impressed by the importance of sexual disturbances in neuroses and by a hint at the Oedipus complex through his own analysis, Freud posed the foundations of the libido theory in *Three Essays on the Theory of Sexuality* (1905). In line with evolutionary concepts, he described an oral, an anal, and a phallic phase, all preceding the genital phase of maturity. He also described the fixation and regression that are typical of neurotic and psychotic symptoms.

Some young physicians were attracted by Freud's ideas, and in 1907 the first formal psychoanalytic society was formed in Vienna. Its original members were Alfred Adler, Wilhelm Stekel, Sandor Ferenczi, Otto Rank, Carl Jung, Karl Abraham, and Max Eitington. These last three were on the staff of the Burghölzli Psychiatric Hospital of Zurich, whose director, Bleuler, was originally well disposed toward psychoanalysis.

In 1910 Freud published *A General Introduction to Psychoanalysis* (English translation 1920), in which he dealt extensively with defense mechanisms, such as overcompensation, reaction formation, rationalization, projection, and displacement. Neurotic symptoms were considered unsuccessful attempts to achieve self-healing—unsuccessful because of the handicaps posed by the defense mechanisms themselves.

The second decade of the 20th century marked the publication of Freud's metapsychological—that is, theoretical—writings. In *Beyond the Pleasure Principle* (1920), he differentiated between ego drives and sexual libido, proposing a new theory of two primary instincts, the life instinct (eros) and the death instinct (thanatos); the life instinct deals with the preservation of the individual, and the death instinct deals with the preservation of the race. Three years later, in *The Ego and the Id*, Freud continued to elaborate on a general theory of personality: the id is the common matrix of the unconscious from which each person, from birth on, gradually develops his own ego, progressively substituting the reality principle for the pleasure principle. This substitution takes place under the influence of the superego, which consists of largely unconscious parental and social mores and rules; ultimately, the function

of the ego is to harmonize the needs of the instincts with external expections. In *Inhibitions, Symptoms, and Anxiety* (1925), Freud replaced the earlier notion of anxiety as a product of frustrated sexual libido with a new concept of anxiety as a signal of approaching internal danger; in contrast to anxiety, fear is a signal of approaching external danger. Anxiety, rather than sexuality, became paramount in the pathogenesis of neurosis, and the importance of the ego slowly began to overshadow the earlier emphasis on the unconscious.

The last group of Freud's writings deals with cultural phenomena and represents the beginning of the trend of applying psychoanalysis to the social sciences. In *Totem and Taboo* (1913), under the influence of James Frazer's emphasis on the universality of taboos against incest and against the killing of the totem animal, Freud explained the origin of society as related to the ancestral killing of the father by the jealous sons, with the consequent rise of fraternal guilt and of worship of the totem, which represents the killed father.

In *Group Psychology and the Analysis of the Ego* (1920), Freud, under the influence of the studies of the French sociologist Gustave Le Bon, attributed the cohesion and dynamics of any group to the libidinous relationship of each individual member to the leader, who can exercise a positive or a negative influence. Under stress, the group tends to regress to an extreme level of disorganization in conditions of panic.

Progressively, Freud's interest in social factors broadened to include the whole of society. A few years later, Freud published *The Future of an Illusion* (1927), in which he related the universal need for a religion to dependency needs. In *Civilization and Its Discontents* (1929), Freud attributed the dynamics of society to a balance between aggressive impulses and the need of its individual members for security. Necessarily, freedom has to be limited in order to obtain security, and this limitation arouses guilt feelings that are unavoidable in any society.

The theme of Moses fascinated Freud for years and culminated in the publication of his final book, *Moses and Monotheism* (1939), which combined his two interests, the study of the individual personality and the study of society. Freud's theory was that Moses was originally an Egyptian who embraced monotheism while in Egypt and then converted the Jews to this belief. Later on, however, Moses was murdered by his followers, and this murder is the origin of the unconscious feeling of guilt that is a pervasive characteristic of the Jews and that is cyclically re-enacted—typically, in the death of Christ.

From a historical perspective, undoubtedly Freud's work has the characteristics and originality of genius. Nevertheless, some of his basic concepts can be followed throughout the development of medical and cultural history. The value of catharsis was recognized in ancient Greek culture. Symptoms were believed to represent a compromise between opposing forces —unconscious, sexual, life, and death—during the romantic movement and in early 19th century medicine. The unconscious was thought to play an essential role as conducive to self-knowledge by the French moralists of the 18th century and the philosophers and biologists of the 19th century. The interpretation of dreams was part of ancient tradition and was essential to the technique of incubation. Descriptions of the gradual unfolding of the sexual instinct and the developmental nature of neuroses may be found in the evolutionary concepts of Goethe, Darwin, and others. The teleological, sexual, and self-preservation aims of the instincts were fundamental to Plato's basic concept of the immutability of things and their mythical return to an earlier state. Freud's concept of regression was stated earlier by Hughlings Jackson as part of his neurological concept of dissolution. The scientific character of psychoanalytic technique and its concept of behavior as predetermined are evident in the deterministic and experimental frame of reference of 19th century medicine. And Freud's belief that the cure depended on the insight gained by the patient was in the Platonic and orphic tradition.

Adler. Alfred Adler (1870–1937) belonged to Freud's small psychoanalytic circle from 1902 to 1911. In *Studies of Organ Inferiority* (1907) he submitted that, as a reaction to an organ inferiority due to organic or functional causes, the patient develops a compensation that often takes neurotic form—typically, masculine protest in women.

Because of his many conflicts with Freud, which were related mainly to Adler's denial of the sexual element in neuroses, he departed from Freud in 1911. The next year he published *The Nervous Character*, rich in ideas and clinical data, in which he stated that neurosis stems from feelings of inferiority brought forth by social factors and that the emphasis should be on the individuality of the person viewed in the temporal dimension.

He further elaborated on his concepts in *Understanding Human Nature* (1927), which was based on concrete psychology. In it he stressed various principles: the indivisibility of the human being, the dynamism of the psyche, and the style of life of each person. He paid special attention to the dynamics of interpersonal relations—typically, the position of a person vis-à-vis his siblings—out of which inferiority feelings, educational errors, and, eventually, social disorders may develop.

By 1932 the tenets of his psychotherapeutic methods had reached full expression. The emphasis was on the patient's gradually becoming aware of his fictitious life goals and lifestyle and being motivated to change them in the context of a cooperative patient-doctor relationship.

Adler's work represents a pioneering effort in some fields, notably in psychosomatic medicine (organ inferiority), in group therapy and community psychiatry (social factors in psychopathology), and in existential psychiatry (lifestyle). Moreover, the primacy he attributed to the aggressive drive over the libido has been considered favorably by many.

Jung. Carl Gustav Jung (1875–1961) was assistant to Bleuler at the Burghölzli Hospital in Zurich from 1900 to 1909. At the suggestion of Bleuler, Jung did extensive research on word association and published a book on it in 1906, *Studies in Word Association*. In the next year *The Psychology of Dementia Praecox* appeared, the first monograph in which the new dynamic psychology was applied to a psychotic patient.

During that period Jung was greatly influenced by Freud's principles, which, with Bleuler's encouragement, were then applied at Burghölzli. Soon, however, the discrepancies between Freud and Jung, characterized by mutual ambivalence, came to the fore. Freud expected that Jung would remain his faithful disciple; instead, Jung revealed independence of thinking in rejecting the Oedipus complex and the exclusively sexual origin of the libido. In Jung's *Metamorphosis and Symbols of the*

Libido (1911-1912), translated into English as *The Psychology of the Unconscious*, which was based on comprehensive study of myths from early times up to the present, he considered the libido as psychic energy, manifesting itself in three stages in the development of the child up to sexual maturity. Psychotherapy was to be based largely on the analysis of dreams, and the psychoanalyst was to undergo analysis himself —apparently, the first statement to this effect.

In the period from 1913 to 1919, Jung apparently went through a personal crisis, during which he forced unconscious material to the fore of his personality through dreams, fantasies, and other psychological forms. At the end of this period, Jung emerged as head of the new school of analytic psychology and a famous therapist. In 1921 he published *Psychological Types*, in which, on the basis of a contrast between the psychological syndromes of hysteria and of schizophrenia, he presented an entirely new system of dynamic psychiatry, centered on the two opposite concepts of extroversion and introversion, for which he found confirmation in philosophy, theology, and literature.

From then on, Jung developed the various original concepts with which analytical psychology has been especially identified: psychic energy stemming from the instincts; the collective unconscious from which universal archetypes emerge, regardless of cultures and historical periods; the structure of the human psyche as a composite of persona (social mask), shadow (hidden personal characteristics), anima (feminine identification in man), animus (masculine identification in woman), and self (the innermost center of the personality); the individuation, the slow process of achieving wisdom in the second half of life through the emergence of an archetypal image of the self; and, at variance with Freud's analytic-reductive therapy, Jung's synthetic-hermeneutic therapy of helping the patient achieve individuation.

Rank. Otto Rank (1884-1939) wrote in his first book, *The Artist* (1907), that creativity was a constructive outlet for neurotic conflicts.

In his early twenties, he developed a filial sort of relationship toward Freud. In *The Myth of the Birth of the Hero* (1909) he submitted that the son's rebellion against the father is provoked by the hostile behavior of the father. In 1912 he published *The Incest Motive in Poetry and Saga*, a thorough study of the Oedipus conflict

in literature, pointing to the unconscious gratification derived by the artist through his creation. Also in that year, he and Sachs started to edit the journal *Imago*, devoted to the application of psychoanalysis to literature and art. Shortly thereafter, Rank began to act as private secretary to Freud on many occasions.

In 1913 Rank co-authored with Sachs *The Significance of Psychoanalysis for the Mental Sciences*; the next year, he published *Doppelgänger (The Double)*, in which he discussed the mirror reflection of the person described by many authors and considered by him a narcissistic protection against the destruction of the ego. It was followed by *Don Juan* (1922), in which the theme of the gallant man is related to his search for an ideal woman. Shortly thereafter, in spite of the antagonism that developed between him and Abraham and Jones, Rank published with Ferenczi *The Development of Psychoanalysis* (1923), in which the notion of acting out is mentioned for the first time in psychiatric literature.

The same year, 1924, marked the publication of *The Trauma of the Birth* and the beginning of Rank's separation from the psychoanalytic movement. In this book Rank minimized the importance of the Oedipus conflict and considered the separation anxiety connected with birth (primary anxiety) as the most important element in the future development of the person and also as the source of neurosis. Freud was initially inclined to absorb this new notion into the psychoanalytic doctrine, but, in the face of strong rejection by all his colleagues, eventually repudiated it in 1926.

In 1935 Rank moved to New York, where he worked on his later books—*Art and Artist* (1932), *Modern Education* (1932), *Will Therapy* (1936), *Truth and Reality* (1936), and his posthumously published *Beyond Psychology* (1941). In them, therapy was viewed as an emotional rather than an intellectual change, taking place only in the present situation.

Other Exponents of Psychoanalysis. Hanns Sachs (1881-1947), a lawyer by training, joined Freud's group in 1909. In 1913 he co-authored with Rank *The Significance of Psychoanalysis for the Mental Sciences*. From his long-standing interest in literary works came his volume *Creative Unconscious* (1942). In 1944 he published *Freud, Master and Friend*, a biography for which he is mostly remembered today.

Ernest Jones (1879-1958), a Welshman, is

considered the most faithful of the pupils of Freud. He is best remembered for his three-volume biography of Freud, which is based on much unpublished material and praised for its thoroughness but is criticized for the uncritical idealization of his hero.

Edward Hitschmann (1871–1957) wrote *Freud's Theories of the Neuroses*, a well-organized presentation of psychoanalytic concepts, in 1909. His name is connected especially with the psychoanalytic studies that he wrote on literary figures of the past.

Paul Federn (1871–1950) became Freud's personal deputy in 1924, after a decade of didactic analyses. His most original contribution lies in his emphasis on ego psychology and in his belief that the psychoses are due to a deficient ego.

Sandor Ferenczi (1873–1933) became closely associated with Freud. Soon recognized as an outstanding therapist, Ferenczi was among the first to link homosexuality to the pathogenesis of paranoia. In his classic essay "Stages in the Development of the Sense of Reality" (1913), he anticipated the later emphasis on ego psychology and attempted to define the succession of stages progressively leading from magic-hallucinatory omnipotence to magic thoughts and words and finally to acceptance of reality. His active therapy is described in the book he co-authored with Rank, *The Development of Psychoanalysis* (1923). In active therapy the patient was encouraged to act and behave in a way to mobilize unconscious material.

Karl Abraham (1877–1925) became acquainted with Freud while studying under Bleuler at Burghölzli in Zurich. His main contribution lies in the study of character formation. On the basis that the character is formed in the pregenital stage of the development of the personality, he opposed the expansive oral character to the constricted anal character and assumed an anal, sadistic fixation for the obsessional neuroses and an oral fixation for melancholia.

Oscar Pfister (1873–1956), a clergyman, was the first educator to apply psychoanalytic concepts to education. By the time Pfister published *The Psychoanalytic Method* in 1917, he had developed a deep friendship with Freud. His work greatly contributed to the dissemination of psychoanalytic ideas among educators and clergymen. After his retirement, he published *Christianity and Fear* (1944).

Victor Tausk (1877–1919) has stirred recent controversies about Freud's supposed envy of him and the vicissitudes of his personal analysis, which allegedly drove him to suicide at the age of 42. But Tausk is remembered most for his paper "On the Origin of the 'Influencing Machine' in Schizophrenia." By linking the symbol of the machine to the patient's unconscious sexual fantasies, he opened the way to the psychoanalytic study of psychosis.

Geza Róheim (1891–1953) was early influenced by psychoanalysis through Ferenczi while studying anthropology in Leipzig and Berlin. He pioneered the introduction of psychoanalysis into anthropological thinking.

Georg Groddeck (1866–1934) conceived of illness as a physical reaction of the body to trauma and also as a symbolic creation, expressing the inner needs of the "it"—that is, the unknown forces influencing human beings. The term "it" was eventually accepted by Freud in the modified form of "id." Groddeck appears to have anticipated the theory and practice of natural childbirth and some contemporary methods of psychotherapy of the psychoses.

Abraham Brill (1874–1948), while working at Burghölzli in Zurich under Bleuler, came in contact with Freud, toward whom he developed strong feelings of veneration. Between 1908 and 1910 Brill was the only analyst in New York City. In 1938 he published *The Basic Writings of Sigmund Freud*. His most original contribution consists of the book *Lectures on Psychoanalytic Psychiatry* (1946).

Sandor Rado's (1890–1971) most original contribution concerns adaptational psychodynamics, which has many similarities to psychoanalytic ego psychology. Adaptational psychodynamics is an attempt, based on evolutionary biological concepts, to stress the integrative act of instinctual urge and reality testing leading to purposeful adaptive behavior.

Theodor Reik's (1888–1969) most important publications are his psychoanalytic studies of the couvade, an old practice in which the husband of a woman in labor takes to his bed, as if he were bearing the child; of the puberty rites of savages, such as circumcision and death rites; and of criminals—in particular, the criminal's unconscious need to confess.

Helene Deutsch, born in 1884, became an ardent follower of Freud and, in 1918, a full member of the Vienna Psychoanalytic Society. Her original contributions to clinical psychoanalysis were gathered in her book *Psychoanal-*

ysis of the Neuroses (1930). Her name, however, is mainly associated with her two-volume *The Psychology of Women* (1944-1945). Challenging Freud's statement that the enigma of the woman could be fully understood neither by men nor by women—a chauvinistic statement in line with the over-all masculine orientation of the psychoanalytic movement—her work represented the culmination of two decades of intensive research on the subject. The entire life cycle of woman, from prepuberty to climacterium, is thoroughly presented from a comprehensive physiological, psychological, and socio-historical perspective: the essential passive-masochistic disposition of woman, the early identification of the girl with the mother and then the libidinal relationship to the father, the slow transition at puberty from a clitoral to a vaginal orientation, the meaning of the sexual act, the orientation of libidinal forces during pregnancy and after delivery, and the maternal role.

Felix Deutsch (1884-1964) established in 1919 the first clinic on organ neurosis and presented the first seminar on this subject at the Vienna Psychoanalytic Institute. He continuously stressed the principle of the homeostatic balance and reciprocal interaction between organic functions and psychic processes. Specific methods advocated by him in *Applied Psychoanalysis* (1949) include the activation of the autonomic nervous system to release emotional conflict and the use of associative anamnesis, to which he later added sector psychotherapy—that is, the aim of keeping the material brought forth by the patient centered on certain symptoms or certain conscious and unconscious conflicts to avoid an unnecessary spread of energy.

Ernst Simmel (1882-1947), in his book *On the Psychoanalysis of War Neuroses* (1918), discussed the military ego—that is, the substitution of the parental superego by the military unit—the value of group identity for the support of the ego, and other phenomena and advocated a therapeutic method based on cathartic abreactions under the influence of hypnosis, which was later used again during World War II. He emphasized the removal of the patient from his neurotic constellation and the infantile gratification provided by the analyst in the hospital setting. In his late years Simmel became interested in the problems of addiction, which he attributed to a protection against the depression resulting from the introjection of a disappointing love object, and of anti-Semitism, a prejudice that he related to a defense against latent homosexuality.

Siegfried Bernfeld (1892-1953), in *Sisyphus or the Boundaries of Education* (1925), emphasized the sociological and psychological dimensions of education. *The Psychology of the Infant* (1925) was presented exclusively from the viewpoint of the unconscious, with no regard for ego psychology, and thus it is outdated today.

Wilhelm Reich (1897-1957) was director of the prestigious Seminar for Psychoanalytic Therapy from 1924 to 1930. In some studies published during that period he advanced views at variance with those of his more orthodox colleagues; for instance, he did not hesitate to encourage genital masturbation as a step toward genital maturity. His most important contribution to psychiatry during that period is *Character Analysis* (1928), essentially a phenomenological description of character formation as an outgrowth and development of oral, anal, and genital ego types. In this book Reich convincingly proved that the characterological substructure of the personality, based on the repression of instinctual demands, serves as a compact defense mechanism and as a resistance against therapeutic efforts; this fact justifies the therapist's eliciting of a negative transference in the patient as a way to overcome such a resistance.

In line with his official adherence to Marxism, Reich expressed his dissatisfaction with Freud's neglect of social factors in the etiology of neuroses. It was Reich's contention that Marx's concept of alienation should be broadened to include the sexual realm, as reflected in the inability of people to come to grips with their life situations because of sexual repression. He linked sexual blockage to the performance of boring, mechanical work by most people in a capitalist society in the interest of the society's maintaining its existing class structure by perpetuating sexual repression with the help of education, the family, and, in general, the prevailing ideology. Reich's philosophy is not, as many erroneously believed, to advocate free sexual intercourse but to make possible a satisfactory love life.

Karen Horney (1885-1952) advocated a greater role for cultural factors in the development of neuroses. For instance, she reversed Freud's view that penis envy is of basic importance in the psychological development of the girl; she favored a view that the widespread male dread of women comes from a basic dread of the vagina. Later on, she challenged the universality of the Oedipus complex, again on cultural grounds. In her later books, written especially for the general public, she elaborated on the concepts of the neurotic process as moving toward, moving away, and moving against; of the major solutions of self-efface-ment, expansiveness, and resignation; and of the clinical pictures of masochistic, perfection-istic, and narcissistic characters. Moreover, she anticipated today's notion of alienation.

Paul Ferdinand Schilder (1886–1940), under the influence of the philosopher Edmund Hus-serl, the founder of phenomenology—that is, of the philosophical movement based on the study of phenomena as they are experienced or pres-ent themselves in consciousness—carried on many studies of the body image in man's relation to himself, to his fellow human beings, and to the world around him, culminating in his classic *The Image and Appearance of the Human Body* (1935). At variance with Freud's tendency to think in terms of opposites and dichotomies, as well as with the static approach of Gestalt theory, Schilder constantly pointed to the simultaneous and integrated aspects of the psychological and the somatic viewpoints and to the constructive and world-oriented fundamental attitude of human beings, above the narrow interest of self-preservation. Typi-cally, perception, rather than being passive, had to be viewed as a continuous process of construction and reconstruction, and the body image had to be viewed as a dynamic process of interrelationship between a person's libidinous drives and his social experiences.

Franz Alexander (1891–1964), in his first book, *Psychoanalysis of the Total Personality* (1929), proposed that conversion hysteria, obsessive-compulsive neurosis, and manic-depressive disease are different forms of dis-turbances in the interplay between the repres-sive functions of the ego and the repressed tendencies. In 1929 he published *The Criminal, the Judge, and the Public* with Hugo Staub; there he presented a psychoanalytic study of criminology, emphasizing the unconscious mo-tivations prevailing in the criminal's sense of justice, in the judge's attitude, and in the public's expectations.

Alexander stressed the role of countertrans-ference and advocated a flexible technique, including short-term therapy, leading to a re-experiencing of past reactions in the new and different setting of the patient-physician rela-tionship, a process he called "corrective emo-tional experience." He developed an extensive program of research in psychosomatic medicine, introduced the concept of vector analysis—that is, the wish of the organs of the body to receive, to retain, or to eliminate in the context of loving or, conversely, aggressive and hateful connotations—and introduced the notion of specificity—that is, of a specific correlation between a particular conflict and a psy-chosomatic disorder—for instance, chronic, in-hibited rage in cases of patients with essential hypertension. Also important is his concept of surplus energy discharged through sexuality, generativity, and creativity after physical growth has reached its peak in late adolescence.

Anna Freud, the daughter of Sigmund Freud, was born in 1895. Originally a teacher, she devoted herself to the psychoanalytic study of children. Her major contribution is *The Ego and the Mechanisms of Defense* (1937), a contin-uation and refinement of Sigmund Freud's 1926 work "Inhibitions, Symptoms, and Anx-iety," in which the concept of the signal func-tion of anxiety implied the concept of the adap-tation of reality. Her book was essentially an attempt to investigate the ego processes as re-vealed by the defense mechanisms that the ego uses against drive impulses. She discussed sev-eral mechanisms—such as regression, repres-sion, projection, introjection, and reaction for-mation—but, essentially, repression continued to be the chief factor at work in the genesis of neuroses. She stressed the educational compo-nent of child analysis and the substantial differ-ences between adult analysis and child analysis, especially the inability of children to develop a full-fledged transference neurosis.

Melanie Klein (1882–1960) is known for her ideas about the fantasies and anxieties ex-pressed by children in play and about the feasibility of analyzing children outside of the educational context. She postulated that pro-jective and introjective mechanisms, based on the internalization by the child of parts of the mother (breast, face, hands) and of the splitting of impulses and objects into good and bad aspects, are essential for the building of the child's internal world and of an embryonic superego; a depressive position, related to the infant's awareness of his mother as a separate person, is normal; a paranoid-schizoid position can inhibit the capacity to form and use symbols and can lead to a fixation in psychotic illness. These concepts, by stressing the preoedipal cause of psychopathology, were in direct contrast with Freudian psychoanalysis. Also unorthodox were her beliefs that children can be helped by being given direct interpretations of unconscious motivations and that a transference neurosis can develop between the therapist and the child.

Psychiatry in the Past Three Decades

The great number of psychiatric casualties during World War II had the effect of bringing the attention of many—including legislators—to the problem of mental illness and emotional disorders in general. In the United States the need for a treatment and rehabilitation program for many servicemen and veterans led to the establishment of vast psychiatric services by the Veteran's Administration, out of which eventually emerged a pioneering effort toward the systematic training of psychiatrists. This training was facilitated by the high standards of the examining body, the American Board of Psychiatry and Neurology, that was established in 1934 by the American Psychiatric Association, the American Medical Association, and the American Neurological Association. The National Mental Health Act was passed in 1946, resulting in the opening of the National Institute of Mental Health in Bethesda, Maryland, in 1949 for the purposes of research, training, and assistance to the states in providing preventive, therapeutic, and rehabilitative services.

From the Mid-1940's to the Mid-1950's. During this period the development of psychiatry, especially in this country, was characterized by a rather strong dichotomy between the biological orientation and the dynamic orientation.

The biological school had a brilliant tradition, especially in European countries. Histopathological, biochemical, and genetic studies had opened the path for the scientific understanding and treatment of a number of psychiatric conditions. Constitutional theories linking the leptosome or asthenic type to schizophrenia and the rotund, pyknic type to manic-depres-

sive psychosis had acquired ample renown in the 1920's, mainly through the work of the German Ernst Kretschmer (1888–1964), the author of *Physique and Character*, which was translated into English in 1925. These theories were followed in this country by the studies of William Sheldon, who described the mesomorph, the ectomorph, and the endomorph types. Important research on the heredity of mental disease was carried on for many years at the New York Psychiatric Institute by Franz Kallmann (*Heredity in Health and Mental Disorders*, 1953), who studied schizophrenic identical twins. The introduction of shock treatment and psychosurgery in the late 1930's and the 1940's had had the effect of offering a more optimistic outlook for the treatment of severe mental disorders; however, after the initial period of unrealistic expectations, the indications for shock treatment and psychosurgery were limited to specific clinical conditions.

Historically, this biological orientation represented a return to the emphasis on the study and treatment of psychoses, which had been replaced by the emphasis on neuroses with the advent of the psychodynamic schools. Still under the over-all influence of Watson's behaviorism and of Cannon's main ideas—the concept of homeostasis and the study of the autonomous reactions (fight or flight) of the organism under stress—new concepts were brought forward: James Papez's theory of emotions, Paul MacLean's visceral brain, Giuseppe Moruzzi's and Horace Magoun's reticular system, Donald Hebb's sensory deprivation, Wilder Penfield's stimulation of the cerebral cortex, John Fulton's effects of the ablation of the frontal lobes, and, from a comprehensive perspective, Hans Selye's stress syndrome and general adaptational syndrome. Other studies dealt with the biological dimensions of anxiety—for example, Stewart Wolf's and Harold Wolff's studies of the effects of anxiety on gastric secretion and Daniel Funkenstein's distinction between fear and anger through the assessment of the levels of epinephrine and norepinephrine.

Research in psychosomatic medicine received great impetus in the 1940's and 1950's. At the Chicago Psychoanalytic Institute, under the influence of Alexander's vector theory, a specificity was found in the psychodynamic constellation of six chronic diseases: ulcerative colitis, asthma, hypertension, rheumatoid arthritis, neurodermatitis, and hyperthyroidism. Other researchers established a correlation between phases of the ovarian cycle and emotional attitudes, particularly the content of dreams, in a group of women (Therese Benedek); still others identified the somatic factor in duodenal ulcer as a constitutional tendency to gastric hypersecretion (I. Arthur Mirsky).

In the psychoanalytic field proper, Jules Masserman's studies on experimentally induced neuroses in the 1930's were followed by research in the area of the mother-child relationship. Early in the 1940's Leo Kanner attributed the syndrome of autism in children to a lack of maternal emotional involvement; David Levy studied the detrimental consequences of maternal overprotection for personality development; Réné Spitz described hospitalism in children raised in an environment void of proper maternal stimulation and anaclitic depression in children who, as infants, were denied proper maternal care. Along similar lines in England, John Bowlby identified three phases—protest, despair, and detachment—in children separated from their mothers, and he related these phases to mourning and to later psychopathology. New theoretical notions in the field of psychoanalysis were advanced by Thomas French, who considered psychoanalysis as a process of progressive adaptation on the part of the personality moved by a chain of motivation to achieve a complex process of integration, and by Sandor Rado, who described his adaptational psychodynamics as a study of behavior focused on the motivational context and on the interplay of emotions and leading to flexible therapeutic techniques.

However, it was in the area of ego psychology that a significant development took place in the 1940's and 1950's. The shift of emphasis from the unconscious to the ego in psychoanalysis can be traced back to the basic study *Ego Psychology and the Problem of Adaptation* (1939) by Heinz Hartmann (1894–1972). In his monograph he distinguished two groups of ego functions, those specifically involved in conflict and those that develop outside of conflict and that constitute the conflict-free ego sphere. These functions of the ego, independent of instinctual drives and outside reality, are of fundamental importance in a person's adaptation to his environment and have a survival value and a biological purposefulness in terms of the average expectable environment. In the early 1950's these concepts were further defined by Hartmann in association with Ernst Kris (1900–1957) and Rudolf M. Loewenstein, born in 1898. These men further developed the concepts of primary autonomous ego functions, secondary autonomous ego functions, and neutralized energy as desexualized and aggression-free energy.

Further contributions to the study of ego psychology came from the research carried on by David Rapaport (1911–1960). He postulated for the optimal functioning of the organism a constant balance of mutually controlling factors, ego autonomy from the id and ego autonomy from the environment.

Historically, ego psychology signifies a trend toward rapprochement with genetic psychology, as represented by the work of Heinz Werner (1890–1964) and of Jean Piaget (born in 1896), the author of many books on child development and a pioneer in the field of genetic epistemology.

Thus, the trend of ego psychology emerged as a further elaboration of psychoanalytic tenets related to the development of the individual personality and of neuroses on the part of some European-born researchers. It was only natural that in this country, where behaviorism had flourished in the 1920's and the social sciences in the 1930's, trends more consonant to the social dimensions in life should emerge. Several psychiatric schools of thought, apparently unrelated, have in common this emphasis on the social component. Karen Horney's concern with environmental influences in the causation of neuroses is an example.

Even more original and fruitful are the concepts developed by Harry Stack Sullivan (1892–1949), the only American-born psychiatrist founder of an independent school during this period. Trained in Meyer's psychobiology and in classical psychoanalysis, he was influenced by such social scientists as Ruth Benedict, Margaret Mead, Edward Sapir, L. Cattrell, and Harold Lasswell. Central to his thinking is the emphasis on a behavioristic approach in psychopathology, based on the interpersonal theory, which was at variance with the strictly individual emphasis in psychoanalysis. Still appealing are his concepts of anxiety as related to feelings of disapproval by others, of stages of personality development as an outgrowth of interpersonal experiences, and of psychopathological phenomena as substitutive (neurotic) or disintegrative (psychotic) processes in the distressing effects of anxiety. His main contribution, however, consists of his pioneering method of psychotherapy of the psychoses. He aimed at the understanding and correction of the patient's distorted communication process in the context of a patient-therapist relationship based on a reciprocal learning situation.

Eventually, the psychotherapy of the psychoses received great impetus from Frieda Fromm-Reichmann (1899–1957), author of *The Principles of Intensive Psychotherapy* (1950). This work was followed shortly thereafter by John Rosen's method of direct analysis for schizophrenic patients (*Direct Analysis*, 1953), a method that has remained controversial.

Even more influenced by social and anthropological ideas are the concepts expressed by the exponents of the culturalistic and neo-Freudian schools. Ruth Benedict (1887–1948), who wrote *Patterns of Culture* (1934), studied the influence of the culture, defined as a consistent cohesive ideological pattern, on child rearing and mental development; and Margaret Mead, who was born in 1901, showed in many of her publications, such as *The Balinese Character* (1942) and *Male and Female* (1949), how individual and family traits are culturally determined.

Also typically American and again related to the social dimension has been the field of group psychotherapy. Anticipated in Vienna in the 1920's by Jacob Moreno's use of dramatic classes with disturbed children and in this country by the lecture classes for mental patients organized by Edward Lazell in Washington in 1919 and, later on, by L. Cody Marsh in New York, group psychotherapy acquired momentum in the 1940's and 1950's. Moreno, born in 1892, developed a method he called "psychodrama," which allows the patient to act out his conflicts on the stage through the use of particular techniques (auxiliary ego, mirror, double, and role reversal). Samuel R. Slavson (*An Introduction to Group Therapy*, 1943, and other volumes) used play therapy in his group work with children.

Dissatisfied with the empirical and intuitive approach to psychotherapy, a few researchers attempted to introduce a more objective method in the therapeutic process. Carl Rogers

is mainly associated with client-centered therapy, which is characterized by genuineness, unconditioned positive regard for the patient, and accurate empathic understanding.

Even old forms of therapy were revitalized and made the subject of fresh investigation. Hypnosis, for instance, after the pioneering study by Clark Hull (*Hypnosis and Suggestibility: An Experimental Approach*, 1933), was critically presented by Lewis Wolberg and later by Milton Erickson, Jerome Schneck, and others. Under the influence of the learning theories in psychology—that is, stimulus-response theories and cognitive theories—others attempted to subject the psychoanalytic tenets to an experimental approach. Notably, John Dollard and Neal E. Miller at Yale, after their original study *Frustration and Aggression* (1939), showing that hostility in animals results from frustration, attempted to correlate learning theories and psychoanalysis (*Personality and Psychotherapy*, 1950). Still others tried to introduce a mathematical terminology in human behavior by making use of the field-theory system developed by Kurt Lewin (1890–1947). Lewin developed a topological system, according to which the life-space of a person is the result of the interplay of positive (reward-giving) and negative (punishment-giving) values. The aforementioned reawakened interest in the schools of academic psychology (see Table II).

Quite apart from these attempts to objectify psychiatry, some new concepts slowly started to emerge in the early 1950's. Mainly influenced by the works of two exponents of existentialism—the German Martin Heidegger, born in 1889, and the Swiss Ludwig Binswanger (1881–1966)—the American psychologist Rollo May, born in 1909, published *The Meaning of Anxiety* in 1950. In it he considered anxiety as a threat to the very foundation of existence. Shortly thereafter appeared *The Courage to Be* (1953) by the German-born Paul Tillich (1886–1965). The courage to be is authenticity as a search for the ultimate individual potentialities, despite the threat it presents of not being. By that time some works of Erich Fromm—a social philosopher born in Germany in 1900—had become known. Fromm presented with dramatic pathos the situation of malaise of the person aspiring to freedom but having to comply with the overwhelming collective sys-

TABLE II

Schools of Academic Psychology (1870–1930)

School of Psychological Thought	Workers	Specific Emphasis
Structuralism	Wundt, Titchener	The study of conscious experience through introspective experimentation. Elementary psychological states—such as sensations, images, and feelings—that make up consciousness are observed and analyzed.
Functionalism	Titchener, Dewey, Angell	Like structuralism, functionalism emphasizes the study of consciousness but in relation to environmental adaptation through application to education (educational psychology) and people (clinical psychology).
Associationism	During the 17th century, philosophers like Hobbes, Berkeley, Locke, Brown, Hartley, Mills and Bain. In the early 19th century, Herbart. From 1885 on, psychologists like Ebbinghaus, Pavlov, Thorndike, Skinner.	The study of learning and memory, as exemplified by Thorndike's law of effect, Pavlov's law of reinforcement, and Skinner's study of learning in animals and human beings, through application of the "Skinner box."
Behaviorism	Watson, Meyer, Weiss, Hunter, Lashley, Tolman, Hull, Skinner	The objective study of human and animal behavior. "Mental" concepts, such as sensation and emotion, are replaced by concepts of stimulus, response, learning, habit, and receptor and effector function. Even the study of consciousness is avoided.
Gestalt psychology	Wertheimer, Koffka, Köhler, Lewin	The total perceptual configuration and the interrelation of its parts are studied. Total experience or behavior is considered to represent more than the sum of its parts. Perception and memory are studied through introspection and observation.
Purposive or hormic psychology	McDougall	The study of goal-seeking behavior. Emphasizes striving and foresight. Human propensities (instincts) constitute the ultimate, primary motivation for behavior. Observations on social behavior stimulated the field of social psychology.
Organismic psychology	Coghill, Kurt Goldstein, Kantor	The holistic, biological study of the individual.
Personalistic psychology	Calkins, Stern	The holistic, social study of the individual.

tems. Taking issue with some of the basic Freudian postulants, he delineated several personality types: the receptive, exploitive, hoarding, maketing, and productive.

These various authors, however, have remained somewhat peripheral to the central core of psychiatry. Much more relevant for psychiatry has been the work of the German-born Erik H. Erikson, born in 1902. As a result of his thorough studies on the psychological development of the person in the 1930's and 1940's, he published *Childhood and Society* in 1950. In this book he presented a psychosocial theory of development based on the interplay of the biological epigenesis with societal dimensions and encompassing a total life cycle from birth to senescence through the progressive unfolding of eight polarities. As is usual in the case of pioneers, it was some time before Erikson's innovating formulations had a significant impact on psychiatry. During the 1940's and 1950's the prevailing theoretical frame remained the psychoanalytic one, progressively influenced by the trend of ego psychology.

Teaching in psychiatry—first enhanced by the Veteran's Administration and supported by such private foundations as the Rockefeller Foundation, the Commonwealth Fund, and the Menninger Foundation—progressively became more formal and homogeneously organized because of the requirements of the American Board of Psychiatry, established in 1934. After some conferences on psychiatric education held at Cornell University in the early 1950's and proposals advanced by the Committee on Medical Education of the Group for the Advancement of Psychiatry, an active group of research-oriented and teaching-oriented psychiatrists established in 1946, psychiatry came to play an increasing role in medical schools, both at the undergraduate level and at the graduate level. The National Institute of Mental Health, founded in 1949, has since its inception given priority to training, as well as research, in psychiatry by establishing a program of fellowships that in time extended to many centers in the country. The philosophy of teaching was based mainly on the understanding of psychodynamics and the acquisition of psychotherapeutic skills with the help of individual supervision. A personal analysis was strongly recommended in many training centers as a way of achieving better insight and self-knowledge.

From the Mid-1950's to the Mid-1960's. By the mid-1950's some early signs indicated that psychiatry was entering a new stage, although the psychoanalytic ideology, increasingly tinged with ego psychology, remained prevalent. Particularly significant was the interest in the psychodynamics and psychotherapy of schizophrenia. In 1955 Silvano Arieti's *Interpretation of Schizophrenia*, a comprehensive presentation of this condition, appeared. In this study, the emphasis was put for the first time on the formal mechanisms—that is, on how rather than on what the patients think—in line with previous studies by Jacob S. Kasanin (*Language and Thought in Schizophrenia*, 1946) and Ellhard von Domarus. Shortly thereafter, in 1956, Erikson introduced the concepts of ego identity, ego diffusion, and identity crisis to explain the complex development of the personality in passing from childhood to adulthood.

Some early signs of dissatisfaction with prevailing theories and methods came to the fore from psychoanalytic quarters themselves. The issue of incorporating psychoanalytic didactic training into the over-all psychiatric training was discussed by many, especially by Franz Alexander in *Psychoanalysis and Psychotherapy* (1956). Research on the various dimensions of psychoanalytic therapy was initiated in some quarters. Considerable interest, mixed with accusations of secession by some orthodox analysts, accompanied the introduction of brief psychotherapy by Alexander and a few others.

Much more important, however, were the introduction of psychopharmacology and the revolution that took place in mental hospitals. Tranquilizers and psychic energizers were introduced in the early 1950's. After the discovery of the beneficial effect of chlorpromazine in psychotic and agitated mental patients by the Frenchmen Pierre Deniker, Henri Leborit, and Jean Delay in 1953, meprobamates, synthesized by Frank Berger and B. Ludwig in 1950, were introduced in clinical practice in 1954; lysergic acid, first accidentally discovered by Albert Hoffman, was made the subject of clinical investigation by Joel Elkes and others; reserpine, empirically used in India for centuries, was synthesized by Hugo Bein and R. Kuhn in 1956; chlordiazepoxide was first used by I. Cohen in 1960; and lithium was successfully used by J. Cade in the 1960's.

These developments in psychopharmacology meant that, beginning in the early 1950's, many mental patients were able to function in a more integrated and acceptable way in institutional settings, and, even more important, many of them could avoid hospitalization or could be returned earlier to their families and communities. Around that same time a new atmosphere of innovation and hopefulness became noticeable in some mental institutions. Social psychiatry, a term coined by Thomas Rennie in 1956, acquired quick prominence in its various environmental, socio-cultural, ecological, interdisciplinary, and cross-cultural dimensions. To be sure, social factors in relation to psychopathology and treatment had been anticipated by some pioneering educational and sociological influences—such as settlement houses, visiting nurses, and juvenile courts—early in the century under the influence of the progressive movement and with the support of private organizations. Even the initial child guidance movement in the 1920's had been affected by those trends. The main field of psychiatry, however, still consisted of institutionalized patients in mental hospitals that had remained largely isolated from their communities and from the mainstream of medicine. The mental hygiene movement, launched by Clifford Beers, had acquired a more scientific aspect through the leadership of Thomas Salmon, and the First International Congress on Mental Hygiene was held in Washington in 1930, but the movement was still largely limited to layman participation. The application of the social sciences to psychology in the 1930's, mainly at the University of Chicago, had not gone beyond theoretical studies. The wide acceptance of long-term individual treatment, based on psychoanalytic ideas and administered mainly to neurotic middle-class and upper-class patients from urban areas, had further contributed to the isolation of psychiatry from mental hospitals.

In the mid-1950's, some innovating concepts and procedures, introduced in England a few years before, became known in this country: the open-door policy; the tenets of the therapeutic community, based on a better staff-patient relationship and increased patient participation in the therapeutic program; and the beginning attempts to try new methods, such as halfway houses, family care, aftercare services, and the involvement of volunteers in mental institutions. All these developments generated considerable hope and helped to open new vistas in this country, too. In 1954 appeared the monograph by Alfred Stanton and Morris Schwartz, *The Mental Hospital*, a study of the social structure of the Chestnut Lodge Hospital in Rockville, Maryland. This monograph was followed shortly thereafter by the collaborative books edited by Milton Greenblatt and others, *From Custodial to Therapeutic Patient Care in Mental Hospitals* (1955) and *The Patient and The Mental Hospital* (1957). In 1958 August Hollingshead and Frederick Redlich published *Social Class and Mental Illness*, a report of a sociological investigation carried on in New Haven that unequivocally showed that middle-class and upper-class people tended to make use of outpatient clinics and of private practitioners and that lower-class patients tended to use hospitals.

By this time, with typical American enthusiasm and urge for action, the issue of mental illness was becoming national. With the strong support of the National Institute of Mental Health, of the Governors Conference on Mental Health, and of many private organizations and professional associations, the Mental Health Study Act was passed in 1955. It established the Joint Commission on Mental Illness and Health for the purposes of establishing priorities and viable methods of services for the mentally ill throughout the country. After 5 years of intensive work, the commission came to the conclusion that the present psychiatric manpower and the network of mental hospitals were totally inadequate to serve the country. The final report of the commission, *Action for Mental Health* (1961), was essentially a proposal for a concerted attack on mental illness through a better distribution and a community-oriented philosophical reorientation of psychiatrists; increasing participation of many lay people at various levels in a massive program of prevention, treatment, and rehabilitation of the mentally ill; a progressive shift of emphasis from institutional to community services; and plans for shared federal, state, and local funding of community mental health centers.

In the next 2 years, with the help of many professionals and laymen, including some prominent legislators, the community mental health movement was launched. On February 5, 1963, President John F. Kennedy, in a message to the 88th Congress, clearly identified the national aspect of the problem of mental illness and the need for returning mental illness to the mainstream of American medicine and for upgrading mental health services. On October 31, 1963, the Community Mental Health Act was passed, mandating the National Institute of Mental Health to establish and fund community mental health centers, each one located in a homogeneous catchment area of about 75,000 to 200,000 people.

Research has centered on biological dimensions (chemotherapy, sensory deprivation, electroencephalography, biochemistry of schizophrenia and depression, neurophysiology of dreams, genetic aspects of the deoxyribonucleic acid molecule and of ribonucleic acid, and identification of inborn errors of metabolism, enzymatic defects, and chromosexual abnormalities), on epidemiological dimensions (large epidemiological surveys with the help of up-to-date statistical techniques, the definition of the concept of normality, the application of computing techniques to psychiatry), on psychosomatic aspects, and on child development, such as Harry Harlow's studies on the mother-child relationship in monkeys.

Family therapy came to be viewed as a treatment of choice in many cases. In the broad context of communication theory, transactional analysis—essentially an abridged combination of psychoanalysis, Adler's life-style, and Reich's character analysis—was developed and popularized by Eric Berne in *Games People Play* (1964). Group psychotherapies of various kinds, including psychodrama, became increasingly popular, partly because of their relatively low cost. Milieu therapy, which focused on the strengthening of the ego in a suitable therapeutic setting, became the center, rather than the context, of the psychotherapeutic process. And brief psychotherapy, in the past considered as a modality of psychoanalysis, became an independent technique that was especially useful for many reactive and acute conditions and for crisis intervention.

The general system theory initiated by Ludwig von Bertalanffy postulated a reciprocally influencing system of homeostasis, transaction, and communication among all aspects of life, leading to optimal function or, conversely, dysfunction in particular circumstances. On the practical side, rapid growth marked the introduction of behavior therapy, essentially a combination of Pavlov's Russian reflexology and Thorndike's and Hull's American instrumentalism, popularized mainly by the psychiatrist Joseph Wolpe.

From the Mid-1960's to the Present and into the Future. By the mid-1960's it appeared that psychiatry was going to enjoy an increasingly favorable condition in this country, with the massive support of the federal government and growing acceptance by the general population. However, a number of stressful and interrelated events challenged this optimistic view—the Vietnam War, the outbreak of violence in urban and academic settings, the racial confrontations that were characterized by the broad issues of school integration and black militancy, the women's movement, the endemic spread of all sorts of drugs of the mind, the less inhibited attitudes toward sex and marriage, the concern with environmental problems of ecology and survival, and the rise of the third world among Afro-Asian nations.

Initially, the reaction of most psychiatrists was rather defensive, on the assumption that these trends were outside the realm of psychiatry proper. Increasingly, however, many psychiatrists have become involved in a number of social issues in different ways. The success of the historical overtures to psychoanalysis offered by Erikson in *Young Man Luther* (1958) and *Gandhi's Truth* (1969) was an expression of this new attitude by many. Since then, there has been a noticeable change in the self-image of psychiatrists and in the perception of psychiatry by the general population—more involvement in community affairs, less emphasis on didactic analysis and psychoanalysis, more inclination toward an eclectic approach to theory and practice, and a closer relationship with other professionals and lay people concerned with mental health.

The field of psychiatry is now in a state of uncertainty and restlessness, unable to abandon the traditional theoretical models and unprepared to face the challenge of the great social issues at stake. Yet, some progress is being made, at least in psychiatrists' increased flexibility of approach toward new ideas. B. F. Skinner's operant conditioning; Herbert Marcuse's one-dimensional man; Kenneth Keniston's uncommitted youth; Thomas Szasz's myth of mental illness; Abraham Maslow's third force psychology; Claude Levi-Strauss' structuralism and new integration of Piaget's work in psychology; Konrad Lorenz's ethology; R. D. Laing's bold views on schizophrenia; William Masters' and Virginia Johnson's new approach to the treatment of sexual disorders; more enlightening views on parapsychology, on legal matters, and even on clinical matters (typically, homosexuality); an entire new range of psychotherapeutic techniques, from sensitivity training to encounter and marathon groups; and self-hypnotic ascetic practices, derived mainly from Yoga and Zen Buddhism—these are some of the most remarkable developments that have taken place in psychiatry in the past few years. Other matters that are relevant to psychiatry are the "right to treatment" laws, the psychology of assassination attempts, the Watergate scandal, and the use of psychiatry by government such as the Central Intelligence Agency.

All these developments point to a growing sense of social responsibility on the part of the psychiatrist, perhaps as a result of the apparent decline of traditional institutions, the change of mores, and the search for new values. This sense of responsibility is being enhanced by the decrease of governmental financial support in the past few years. On a broader scale, the rapidly spreading concern that many issues—wars, poverty, famine, endemic diseases, environmental contamination, and now depletion of sources of energy—can be coped with only through international effort points to the need for an entire reevaluation of the ideology of psychiatry. Far from being molded by the prevailing social forces of a few affluent nations, such an ideology may be increasingly influenced by many other cultures and nations of the world. History, however—by pointing to the similarities between now and the past, to the apparent cyclic occurrence of attitudes and customs, and to the basic constancy of human needs and ways of solving problems—may offer much needed guidelines for the future.

REFERENCES

Ackerknecht, E. H. *Short History of Psychiatry*, ed. 2, Hafner Press, New York, 1968.

Alexander, F., and Selesnick, S. T. *The History of Psychiatry*. Harper and Row, New York, 1966.

Back, K. W. *Beyond Words: The Story of Sensitivity Training and the Encounter Movement*. Russell Sage Foundation, New York, 1973.

Deutsch, A. *The Mentally Ill in America*, ed. 2. Columbia University Press, New York, 1948.

Deutsch, H. *Confrontations with Myself: An Epilogue*. W. W. Norton, New York, 1973.

Ellenberger, R. *The Discovery of the Unconscious: The History and Evolution of Dynamic Psychiatry*. Basic Books, New York, 1970.

Frank, J. D. *Persuasion and Healing: A Comparative Study of Psychotherapy*, ed. 2. Johns Hopkins University Press, Baltimore, 1973.

Havens, L. H. *Approaches to the Mind: Movement of the Psychiatric Schools from Sects toward Science*. Little, Brown, Boston, 1973.

Jones, E. *The Life and Work of Sigmund Freud*. 3 vols. Basic Books, New York, 1953–1957.

Jung, C. G. *C. G. Jung's Letters*, vol. 1. Princeton University Press, Princeton, 1973.

Misiak, H., and Saxton, V. S. *Phenomenology, Existentialism, and Humanistic Psychologies. A Historical Survey*. Grune & Stratton, New York, 1973.

Nunberg, H., and Federn, E., editors. *Minutes of the Vienna Psychoanalytic Society*, 3 vols. International Universities Press, New York, 1962–1974.

Siegel, R. E. *Galen on Psychology, Psychopathology, and Function and Diseases of the Nervous Systems*. S. Karger, New York, 1973.

Simon, B., and Weiner, H. Models of mind and mental illness in ancient Greece. J. Hist. Behav. Sci., 2: 303, 1966; 8: 389, 1972; 9: 3, 1973.

Szasz, T. S. *The Age of Madness: The History of Involuntary Mental Hospitalization Presented in Selected Texts*. Doubleday, Garden City, N. Y., 1973.

Wyckhoff, J. *Wilhelm Reich: Life Force Explorer*. Fawcett, Greenwich, Conn., 1973.

Zilboorg, G. *A History of Medical Psychology*. W. W. Norton, New York, 1941.

1.2. GENERAL SYSTEMS THEORY

Introduction

General systems theory asserts that the universe is composed of a hierarchy of concrete systems, defined as accumulations of matter and energy organized into co-acting, interrelated subsystems or components and existing in a common space-time continuum. General systems behavior theory is concerned with a subset of all such systems, the living systems. It provides a conceptual framework within which the content of biological and social sciences can be logically integrated with that of the physical sciences. It is not a new discipline but, rather, seeks to eliminate the firm discipline boundaries that obscure the orderly relationships among pacts of the real world and lead many to overlook their shared characteristics. In psychiatry it provides a new resolution of the mind-matter dilemma, a new integration of biological and social approaches to the nature of man, and a new approach to psychopathology, diagnosis, and therapy.

Applications to Psychiatry

Conceptual Issues

Mind-Matter Dilemma. Psychiatry has long been segregated from the other medical specialties because the classical distinction between mind and matter has separated mental disease from physical disease. This conceptual dichotomy is also manifested in the gap that exists between the usually objective, biological study of humans and the frequently subjective, psychosocial study of humans.

General systems theory provides a resolution for this unhealthy situation. The proper dichotomy is not between mind and matter but between information processing and matter-energy processing.

There is no mind-matter dichtomy in computer science. Often the the behavior of a computer is pathological—its output is incorrect. Then computer operators diagnose the reasons for the maladaptive performance and try to cure or correct it, just as psychiatrists do.

Decoding and Encoding. Like perception of the environment, the comprehension of language is a complex information-processing function in which certain patterns of input signals are decoded to other patterns that represent them in the ensemble of an internal code of the nervous system. Studies of patients suffering from aphasia indicate that damage to the temporoparietal lobe of the dominant side of the brain can render the patient unable to comprehend symbolic inputs (damage to the decoder) or to produce normal linguistic outputs (damage to the encoder or, perhaps, to the output transducer) or both. Understanding which of the multiple information-processing subsystems are involved clarifies the findings in aphasia.

Humans beings and higher animals can receive and decode information that comes to them, often simultaneously, over different bands. Each band has its characteristic variables. Since multiple bands may be used simultaneously, supplementary and even contradictory messages can be received from the same source. When a watchdog growls and wags its tail at the same time, the interpretation is difficult.

The auditory band carries verbally coded messages as well as expressive tones and sounds, such as cries and whimpers and the sound communications of animals. Human speech also carries messages encoded in other ways than in words. When a contentless flow of recorded low frequency (100 to 550 cycles per second) vowel tones is played, produced by filtering out the high frequency sounds of consonants which carry most of the semantic information in speech, there is reasonably good agreement among judges on the speaker's emotional state. Singing, with or without words, also carries emotional content.

A General Systems Theory of Personality. A personality theory proposed by Karl Menninger describes normal personality function and psychopathology in systems theory terms. He relates classical psychoanalytic concepts to present-day systems theory. A central feature of his approach is a detailed analysis of internal information-adjustment processes that he calls coping devices, which are much like Freudian defense mechanisms or the adjustment processes of general systems theory. His theory deals with four major issues: adjustment or individual-environment interaction; the organization of living systems; psychological regulation and control, known as ego theory in psychoanalysis; and motivation, which in psychoanalysis is often called instinct theory. Like other systems

theorists, Menninger makes a salient point of the principle of homeostasis. He considers the maintenance of steady states to be basic to both psychological and physical processes. Also, he contends that certain forces cause living systems to search for new and unsettled states. He agrees with Ali Ibn Hazm, who lived from 994 to 1064, that all men are constantly attempting to escape anxiety. Also, Menninger believes that negative feedbacks maintain the steady states in living systems, which he calls their vital balance. He interprets Freudian personality theory in terms of this systems approach. The ego, he says, is the central executive. The instincts of the id are dual drives that alter adjustments in either of two opposite directions. The one drive, sex, tends toward positive relationships with other organisms, human and nonhuman. The other drive, aggression, tends toward disruption of such relationships. The introjected superego is concerned with the governance of the organism's suprasystem.

Noting that stresses on organisms and strains within them are different orders of magnitude, Menninger asserts the validity for the human organism of the general systems principle that the greater a threat or stress on a system is, the more of the system's components are involved in adjusting to it. When no further components with new adjustment processes are available, the function of the system collapses.

Diagnosis

A number of aspects of general systems theory can contribute to improved psychiatric diagnosis. One principle is that every process should, when possible, be identified with the structure that carries it out. If, as is currently true, not all neural structures that mediate behavior can be identified, then a reasonable hypothesis can be proposed until research identifies the structure.

A second principle is to include, as part of diagnosis, a tracing of the routes of all separate sorts for matter-energy and information transmissions, including feedbacks, from inputs to outputs, of systems and subsystems. This principle requires greater precision than is possible when one uses the common terms "stimulus" and "response." Each sort of transmission can be traced through the system to determine whether the relevant variables are within normal ranges or to locate the places where they are not—the loci of pathology. Also, research can reveal the quantitative relationships of the variables.

A third principle, the existence of 19 critical subsystems in all living systems, gives a basis for agreement among diagnosticians as to what are the basic parts and processes of the system. The variables of each subsystem can be tested to determine whether they are within normal steady state ranges. If they are not, the controlling feedbacks can be tested to determine why the relevant adjustment processes are not working properly.

Therapy

Identification of the type and location of the pathology can indicate to the clinician the proper sorts of therapy to use. If the basic fault is in matter-energy processing, perhaps that can be corrected by diet, by drugs that affect metabolism, or by surgery that alters matter-energy flows. If the basic fault is in information processing, the clinician can use psychotherapy that alters neurotic habits or drugs that block pathological signals.

Pathology

Just as the previous levels of living systems have comparable adjustment processes, so they have comparable pathologies. Since people most commonly live in families or other groups and participate in numerous organizations that are part of total societies, it is important that the pathology be identified according to the level on which it occurs. This is recognized by many psychiatrists, who find that they cannot treat one member of a family in isolation from the others because the pathology is in the family interrelationships.

Cell Level. Addictive drugs like heroin apparently create abnormalities in internal cellular information processes by altering enzymatic controls. At least some behavioral changes follow from these cellular alterations. Also, inputs to vertebrate cells of hormonal molecules, such as thyroxine, bearing chemically coded information, at ordinary rates convey signals that promote the normal functions of those cells by regulating the rates of certain enzymatic processes. Abnormally high rates of hormonal inputs can produce thyrotoxicosis; when they affect neural cells, such excess inputs can produce toxic psychoses. Furthermore, various neuropsychiatric disease syndromes result from inputs of maladaptive genetic information, as in the DNA of the human chromosomes. One of these maladaptive inputs is mongolism or Down's syndrome.

Genes act on cells by controlling the synthesis of enzymes that perform the production of substances required by the cells. An aberration in the genetic signal, therefore, can affect the synthesis of some specific substance or substances required by the system for normal growth, repair, or function. This is an inborn error of metabolism. Phenylketonuria is an example of such an error.

Certain psychoses may be determined by aberrations in the genetic signal. Some studies of schizophrenic patients and their relatives have been interpreted as showing such inheritance, but the exact nature of the genetic defect, the gene or genes involved, and the probability that the disease will appear in a relative of a schizophrenic patient are not clear.

Organ Level. A blood clot or tumor can produce a lack of matter inputs, such as oxygen from the blood stream, into a component of the brain and cause a stroke. Shrapnel (excess matter inputs) in the temporoparietal area of the cortex can cause aphasia. In addition, endocrine and neural information-processing components are subject to the effects of trauma, infection, tumors, and other types of abnormalities in internal matter-energy processes. These abnormalities may or may not cause illnesses.

Organism Level. *Pathological Adjustment Processes.* According to Menninger, normal adjustments to ordinary matter-energy and information lack and excess stresses and the resultant strains include such information processes as general irritability, feelings of tension, overtalkativeness, repeated laughter, frequent losses of temper, restlessness, sleepless worrying at night, and fantasies about solutions to real problems. Beyond these normal adjustments, in response to stresses and strains of greater magnitude, more costly and more pathological adjustments are resorted to. They are pathological if more expensive adjustment processes are used when less costly ones would suffice.

A great variety of symptoms—including pain, paralyses, and anesthesias of parts of the body—are seen in patients with neurotic conflicts. They often have only a superficial resemblance to symptoms resulting from damage to neural or muscular components.

Some kinds of hypertension, rheumatic diseases, arthritis, kidney diseases, vascular diseases (including, possibly, atherosclerosis), and a number of other illnesses have been classified by Selye as diseases of adaptation, brought about by the excess of anterior pituitary and adrenocortical hormones that characterizes bodily responses to stresses. Overdosages with such hormones can cause the formation and eventual perforation of a peptic ulcer. These hormones are assumed to accelerate the flow of the gastric juices as a result of more rapid secretion of acethylcholine and consequent increased vagal activity.

Anxiety. This unpleasant emotional experience, like pain, may be viewed as information, a signal that a steady state has been or threatens to be seriously disturbed. In the absence of an excessive stress or threat, the intensity of the anxiety probably signals the relative strengths of the stress or threat, on the one hand, and the adjustment processes available to counter it, on the other hand. Either an increase in the stress or threat or a decrease in the adjustment processes as perceived by the organism can produce this signal. Anxiety can be pathological in some patients, but it is often like pain—a useful signal in normal people that a steady state does not exist because available adjustment processes appear inadequate to cope with a potential or actual stress.

When a person experiences anxiety, physiological measures often indicate that he is under stress. The anxiety signal is transmitted up to and through the frontal lobes of the brain. It can be blocked by tranquilizers, sedatives, and other psychoactive drugs. It can also be blocked by operative techniques that separate the prefrontal areas from their related thalamic nuclei. Although this destructive procedure is followed by profound personality changes, it has sometimes been carried out in the hope of ending the anxiety signal of patients suffering intractable pain from terminal cancer.

Adjustment Processes to Lacks of Information Inputs. Information input underload is a lack stress. Under normal conditions most people are able to adjust information flows to confortable levels by seeking or avoiding other people, shifting attention, increasing physical activity, or making adjustments in the environment, such as lowering window shades or turning on lights. A minimum rate of information inputs to a system must be maintained for it to function normally, and organisms strive to get such inputs.

The effects of social isolation and lack of variability in information inputs on people—like truck drivers who must spend long hours driving alone, prisoners in solitary confinement, patients in respirators, and explorers alone on the sea or in the wilderness—have been described as an isolation syndrome. Rather extreme subjective experiences, such as hallucinations, have been reported with even relatively mild sensory deprivation, such as is experienced in a long drive alone at night. Experimental subjects have experienced similar symptoms.

The isolation syndrome has a number of stages, commonly including the following: At first, the person is able to pass time thinking, but he finally becomes sleepy and may fall asleep. As time goes on, he is unable to direct his thoughts or to think clearly. He becomes irritable, restless, and hostile. Then he may make an explicit attempt to use fantasy material as an adjustment process to substitute for needed information inputs. Later, he becomes childlike in his emotional variability and behavior. A stage of vivid visual, auditory, or kinesthetic hallucinations follows, succeeded by a final stage in which there is a sensation of otherness. He may "see" his subjective experience as a bright area in darkness. Termination of the information input lack stress does not immediately return the person to normal. He slowly readjusts to society. Hallucinations and blank periods may continue to bother him. He often finds it difficult to concentrate attention, and he must take care to keep his fantasies out of his speech.

An organism experiencing information input lack stresses can increase its activity in the environment to speed the rate of information inputs to it. Most of the adjustments that subjects in such experiments can use, however, concern internal information processing. A person or animal can move his joints and so send signals from his internal transducer through his nervous system. One can also sleep. In sleep, time passes quickly while the sleeper dreams and is unaware of the lack of information inputs. Organized thought, possible during early deprivation, also maintains a flow of information that is fairly comfortable for the subject. When such organized thought breaks down, fantasies and hallucinations take over.

The bulk of the research evidence is that drastic curtailment of information inputs has an important influence on behavior. There are individual differences in the optimal rate of information input for a person to maintain arousal, think well, act effectively, and feel good.

Adjustment Processes to Excesses of Information Inputs. Information input overload can produce major pathology in organisms. Various sorts of pathology in rats in crowded pens, as Spitz concluded from Calhoun's work, arose from the fact that each animal was subjected to an excessive rate of information inputs. These rapid inputs elicited various abnormal internal cognitive and affective processes and overt behaviors, particularly frenetic activity and pathological withdrawal. According to Spitz, repeated interruptions before completion of normal input-output sequences by new inputs produce this pathology. In his view, infants are particularly susceptible to such pathogenic processes.

Such states of information input overload are like those that Toffler calls "future shock." In severe or irreversible form, this condition has been explicitly identified by Lipowski as a form of pathology. He explains its origins as follows: Today's affluent, technical society is characterized by an excess of attractive information inputs. Social influences pressure the individual person to choose among these attractive inputs, creating in him conflicts as to which of several desirable behaviors he should carry out. Anxiety is associated with these conflicts. The person attempts to cope with them by such adjustment processes as filtering, escape, repeated approaches to many different goals or sources of information inputs, aggressive or violent behavior, and passive surrender. The young appear to be more vulnerable to excesses of information inputs because they have not learned how to choose among attractive alternatives and to strive in a sustained manner for selected goals.

There is also suggestive clinical and experimental evidence that overloads of information may have some relation to schizophrenic behavior. In schizophrenia a genetically determined metabolic fault or some other source of increased neural noise may lower the capacities of certain as yet unidentified channels involved in cognitive information processing. Various studies suggest that input channels are particularly affected.

On the basis of work on information overload, Luby et al have suggested that schizophrenic withdrawal, manifested in its most extreme form as schizophrenia, may be an attempt by the patient to use escape as an adjustment process to reduce the rate at which information impinges on him, in order to prevent overload and keep the rate within a range he can handle. This may be why a psychotic beachcomber or vagrant or hippie shuns much human contact. Also, a catatonic schizophrenic may be unable to respond to information inputs because they overload him and create confusion.

Various case histories of schizophrenic patients, together with a large mass of other observations and experiments on schizophrenics, make it apparent that they have difficulty in ordering and organizing the large fluxes of information inputs that impinge on their input channels. Chapman and McGhie showed that schizophrenics did as well as normal subjects on tasks involving distraction but were worse when selective attention was involved, particularly when information was put in simultaneously on competing sensory channels. Schizophrenics, they contend, are unable to use the adjustment process called "filtering" to shut out irrelevant information inputs. Consequently, their short-term memory is overloaded. One indication of this overload is that schizophrenics are as good as normal subjects in repeating sentences of low redundancy, but they do not improve as much as normal subjects when repeating sentences of higher redundancy. In normal speech, actually, redundant words are distractors for a schizophrenic. His channel capacity is lowered, according to Pishkin et al. He takes longer than a normal person to perceive single and multiple units of inputs, according to Harwood and Naylor. And his use of the filtering adjustment process is abnormal, according to Payne et al.

Research findings, as well as other data, suggest that the differences in speech between schizophrenics and normal subjects arise from overloading some information-processing component or components that in schizophrenia have abnormally low channel capacity. Consequently, schizophrenics cannot process signals as quickly or as correctly as normal persons can.

At usual rates of information input, schizophrenics make omissions and errors and otherwise behave as normal people do under forced-paced inputs. Evidence suggests that schizophrenia, by some as yet unknown process that increases neural noise or distortion, lowers channel capacity. Infections, trauma, or other events that, as Menninger has indicated, can precipitate schizophrenia may perhaps further lower channel capacity biochemically, exacerbating abnormal states that were themselves caused by some prior lowering of channel capacity of uncertain origin.

Group Level. Conflict may arise in a group like a family if there is a lack of matter-energy inputs, such as a shortage of food, water, or clothing. Excess or unwanted matter-energy inputs, like the destruction of a house or the arrival of a chronic invalid in a home, can also subject a family to severe strains. Lacks of information inputs, like sensory deprivation to a team of astronauts during a long space journey or inadequate income to feed a family, can produce pathological behavior. Also, when certain arrangements of the channel and net subsystems of groups centralize communications in one or a few members and they consequently tend to suffer from excesses of information inputs, frequently one member of a group—like the chairman of a committee, the quarterback of a football team, or the ranking officer of a command post—takes on an undue proportion of the total information processing being carried out by his group. Under such circumstances, pathological group processes can easily arise. Undue physical aggressiveness and unfair acquisitiveness, resulting in inputs of inappropriate forms of matter-energy and abnormalities in internal information processes, can also produce group pathology.

Organization Level. Inadequate food in a community or insufficient food, drugs, and other supplies in a hospital are lacks of matter-energy inputs that can result in pathological functioning of the system. Excesses of matter-energy inputs, like overpopulation in a city and overcrowding of hospitals and prisons, cause organizational pathology, such as delays in providing essential services. Pollution and accumulated wastes in cities are inputs of inappropriate forms of matter-energy that cause them to function unsatisfactorily.

Lacks of information inputs about the suprasystem in which it exists can result in the inadequate performance of an organization. A psychiatric hospital can serve the needs of the community best only if it carefully and continuously assesses those needs by direct study of the community. Persons in the primary communication nodes of large organizations, particularly the executives, are often overloaded by excesses of information inputs. Such overloads fatigue those who suffer from them. They also delay communications and decisions, make them erratic or wrong, and may result in their not being made or being made by persons not properly equipped to do so. All these causes can produce pathological effects in cities, hospitals, corporations, armies, and other types of organizations.

Abnormalities in internal matter-energy processes include requiring laborers to work in unattractive surroundings, prisoners to live under inhumane conditions, and outpatients to wait idly for hours to be treated. Abnormalities in internal information processes include management styles of administrators that neglect worker needs and produce poor organizational morale. Breakdowns in communications between component units are common causes of inadequate performance in all types of organizations. Similar breakdowns in information flows among ethnic groups destroy the relationships among citizens in a city. Such forms of pathology must be dealt with by psychiatrists who care for patients who live or work in organizations.

REFERENCES

Cramer, E. H., and Flinn, D. E. *Psychiatric Aspects of the SAM Two-Man Space Cabin Simulator.* USAF School of Aerospace Medicine, Brooks Air Force Base, San Antonio, Texas, 1963.

Freud, S. Inhibitions, symptoms, and anxiety. In *Standard Edition of the Complete Psychological Works of Sigmund Freud,* vol. 20, pp. 87-175. Hogarth Press, London, 1959.

McClearn, G. E., and Meredith, W. Behavioral genetics. Ann. Rev. Psychol., *17:* 515, 1966.

Menninger, K. A. *The Vital Balance.* Viking, New York, 1963.

Miller, J. G. Psychological aspects of communication overloads. In *International Psychiatry Clinics: Communication in Clinical Practice.* R. W. Waggoner and D. J. Carek, editors, pp. 201-224, Little, Brown, Boston, 1964.

Miller, J. G. Living systems: The organism. Q. Rev. Biol., *48:* 92, 1973.

Spitz, R. A. The derailment of dialogue: Stimulus overload, action cycles, and the completion gradient. J. Am. Psychoanal. Assoc., *12:* 752, 1964.

Toffler, A. *Future Shock.* Random House, New York, 1970.

2

Science of Human Behavior:
Contributions of the Biological Sciences

2.1. GENETICS AND PSYCHIATRY

Classical Genetics

In classical genetics, it is assumed that single genetic traits are determined by paired genes, one of which is derived from the male germ cell and the other from the female germ cell. One may speak of the total genetic constitution of a person as his genotype and of his appearance at any given time as his phenotype. A person receiving a given gene from both parents is called a homozygote for that particular gene, and, under proper environmental conditions, he is certain to show its characteristics. If a person receives the given gene from one parent and a different gene at the corresponding locus from the other parent, he is known as a heterozygote. In some cases, the heterozygote displays traits intermediate between those represented by homozygotes; in other cases he displays the trait as a homozygote does. In the latter instance, the trait is known as dominant. In still other cases, he does not display the trait; in this instance, the trait is known as recessive—that is, it is expressed only if both genes are present.

Simple dominant traits are transmitted in the direct line of descent by inheritance from one parent. They appear in about 50 per cent of the offspring (see Figure 1).

In simple recessive traits, inheritance from both parents is necessary. The parents themselves are frequently unaffected, since they are usually heterozygotes. If two heterozygotes mate, each child has a 25 per cent chance of being a homozygote and, therefore, affected (see Figure 2).

Certain traits are determined by the interaction of several or many genes. This type of inheritance is called polygenic, with contributions made in a cumulative manner by a number of genes that by themselves produce only minor effects.

Biochemistry of Genetic Substance

By 1952 chemists had determined that the genetic material transferred from generation to generation and carrying genetic information is not protein but deoxyribonucleic acid (DNA). Chromosomes are composed of DNA and protein, but DNA appeared to be the primary genetic material.

In 1953, the structure of this molecule was proposed by Watson and Crick. It was known that DNA contains deoxyribose (a 5-carbon sugar), phosphate, and four nitrogenous bases—two purines (adenine and guanine) and two pyrimidines (cytosine and thymine)—and that the number of adenine molecules equals that of thymine, the number of guanine molecules equals that of cytosine. Watson and Crick suggested that DNA consists of two sugar-phosphate chains and that the chains are twisted around each other in the form of a double helix. From each sugar on one chain to a corresponding sugar on the other there is a hydrogen bond linkage through either adenine on one chain and thymine on the other or guanine on one and cytosine on the other. A DNA molecule may consist of thousands of such nucleotide linkages.

In the framework of the modern theory of gene action, a mutation may be considered as a

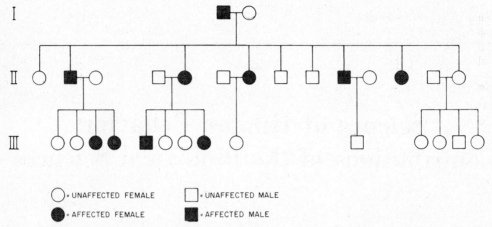

FIG. 1. A pedigree of Huntington's chorea, illustrating dominant inheritance. (From the Department of Medical Genetics, New York State Psychiatric Institute.)

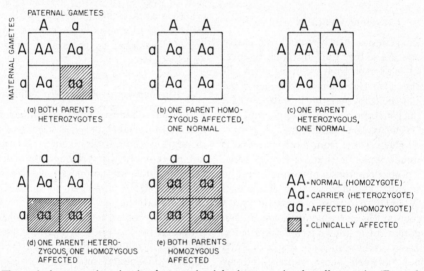

FIG. 2. Theoretical expectations in simple recessive inheritance as in phenylketonuria. (From the Department of Medical Genetics, New York State Psychiatric Institute.)

change in the sequence of nucleotides in the DNA. Such changes may take place through a mistake in the replication process at the time the cell divides, possibly through the action of certain chemicals or as a result of high energy radiation. The changes may consist of the addition of an extra nucleotide pair, the subtraction of a nucleotide, the substitution of one nucleotide for another, or various rearrangements of the nucleotide sequence.

Human Cytogenetics

Until recently, most textbooks stated that the total number of chromosomes in each normal human cell was 48. The number is now estab-

lished as being 46. And, although it was known that females had two X chromosomes and males one X and one Y, it was erroneously thought that the Y chromosome was inactive, sex being determined by the number of X chromosomes.

In 1949 Barr and Bertram found a dark-staining mass of chromatin in the nuclei of many cells in females. From 30 to 60 per cent of the cells of the normal woman show this dark-staining mass, which is now referred to as sex chromatin or, after its discoverer, a Barr body (see Figure 3).

In 1954 a second difference between male and female cells was discovered. A drumstick like appendage attached to one of the lobes of the nucleus of polymorphonuclear leukocytes was consistently noted in about 5 per cent of cells in females and in an insignificantly small number of cells in males.

Normal Human Karyotype

In 1956 Tjio and Levan found, by tissue culture methods, that the number of chromo- somes in man is 46. It was possible, by enlarging the photograph of the microscopic field and cutting each chromosome out, to arrange the chromosomes in descending order of size, thus producing a visual representation of the chromosome complement or karyotype. Since the chromosomes are photographed after replica- tion, they appear as two chromatids attached at

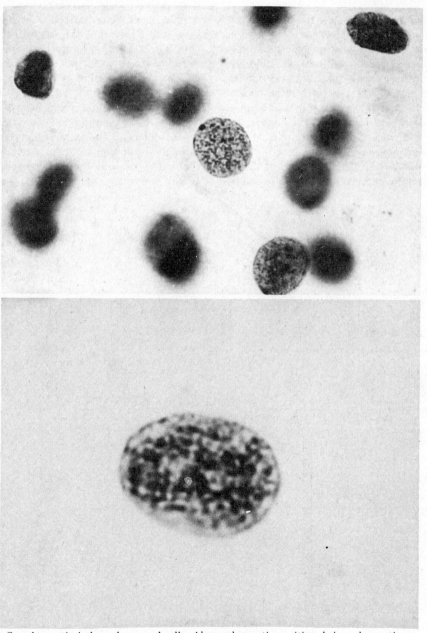

Fig. 3. Sex chromatin in buccal mucosal cells. *Above*, chromatin-positive; *below*, chromatin-negative.

one point called the centromere. The chromosomes are distinguishable within size groups by the position of this centromere.

In 1960 the numbering system was standardized, the first 22 pairs of autosomes being divided into seven groups (see Figure 4) labeled A to G and numbered 1 to 22. The 23rd pair represents the sex chromosomes—XX in women, XY in men.

Chromosomal Aberrations

Nondisjunction Leading to Trisomy. One group of aberrations is marked by the presence of an extra chromosome, so that there are 47 rather than 46 chromosomes in the karyotype. The extra chromosome represents the presence of three, rather than two, of a given chromosome. Such an anomaly arises through a process of nondisjunction, usually in the formation of the sperm or the egg cell. In the splitting of the cell, one chromosome of each pair ordinarily goes to each of the daughter cells. If the two chromosomes of a given pair remain joined and enter one of the daughter cells together, that cell has an extra chromosome. When that daughter cell combines in fertilization with a normal gamete, a zygote is formed with the extra chromosome, a condition known as trisomy.

Three viable types of nondisjunction causing trisomic conditions have been described in which the autosomes, as distinguished from the sex chromosomes, are involved. The first of these is the trisomy of a chromosome in group G in mongolism, better termed Down's syndrome. It is very likely that this condition arises by nondisjunction in the formation of the maternal ovum, related somehow to the age of the mother. A second autosomal trisomy is the trisomy 17-18 (Edward's) syndrome. The third trisomy found in living infants involves one of the chromosomes in group D.

Mosaicism. If the extra chromosome is lost through disjunction in the early cell divisions of the zygote, two cell lines may persist, one with 46 and one with 47 chromosomes.

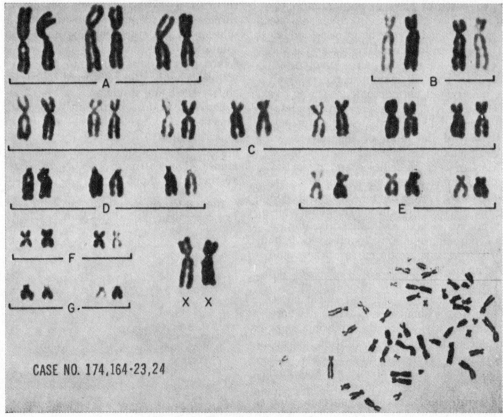

FIG. 4. Karyotype of a normal man.

Translocation. In a mongoloid child born to a young mother Poloni found a normal chromosome count of 46, but one of the chromosomes in group D turned out to be longer than normal. This oversized chromosome consisted of the long arm of a D chromosome plus that of an extra G chromosome; in such cases, there are effectively, three G chromosomes. In about half of such cases, the mother or the father also has such a long D chromosome, but the added unit is balanced by the absence of one of the unattached G chromosomes, leaving the parent with a total number of 45 chromosomes. Such a parent is a carrier; his children theoretically have one chance in three of being affected, although empirically the risk is acutally about 10 per cent if the mother is a carrier and 2 to 3 per cent if the father has the aberration. In Down's syndrome translocation may also occur between two chromosomes in the G group.

The difference between trisomy and translocation is important. Especially for older mothers, having a child with Down's syndrome produces a small risk of a second affected child; the risk is 1 in 600; for mothers under 35 it may be 1 in 1,000, but it is about 1 in 50 for mothers over 45. If a parent is a translocation carrier, however, the risk may be considerably higher.

Deletion. In deletion, part of a chromosome breaks off during cell replication and is lost, so that future cells have a smaller-sized chromosome than usual. The *cri-du-chat* syndrome is associated with a deletion of part of the short arm of a B-group chromosome.

Abnormalities Involving Sex Chromosomes. Chromatin-positive male patients with Klinefelter's syndrome generally have 47 chromosomes. They have two X chromosomes and a Y chromosome. The two X chromosomes are sufficient to cause the appearance of the Barr body, but the Y chromosome causes them to have male gonads and essentially male genitals. Such an anomaly may be brought about by the union of an abnormal XY sperm with a normal ovum or by the union of an abnormal XX ovum with a normal Y-bearing sperm. In each case the abnormal gamete is the result of nondisjunction.

Most girls with Turner's syndrome and no Barr body are found to have a karyotype containing only 45 chromosomes; they have only one X chromosome. Nondisjunction in a sperm cell or, less frequently, in an ovum results in a gamete containing neither an X nor a Y chromosome; the union of such deficient cell and an X-bearing gamete results in the anomaly.

Other abnormalities involving the sex chromosomes are seen in females having 47 chromosomes, with three X chromosomes and two Barr bodies, and in males with an extra Y chromosome (XYY) (see Figure 5).

Methods of Genetic Investigation

Pedigree Method

Genetic data obtained from individual pedigrees or individual pairs of siblings or twins are useful in the study of rare pathological conditions that are fairly constant in their penetrance and clinical expression. Such data are not calculated to furnish conclusive proof about the operation of heredity or about the mode of inheritance involved. Since family histories are often published only if there is a concentration of affected persons, the data are not statistically representative of the population.

Census Method

Total population surveys by the census method are valuable but difficult to conduct. The populations must be sufficiently cooperative and not too large, and the traits under investigation must be relatively uncomplicated ones.

Family-Risk Studies

The contingency method of statistical prediction aims to compare the expenctancy of a given medical condition developing among relatives of affected persons with the expectancy in the general population. The condition in question must be well-defined, so that a number of independent observers may accurately diagnose persons coming into the study. And the original group of patients whose relatives are to be investigated must be either a consecutively reported series representing a complete ascertainment or a random sample thereof.

Twin-Family Method

The use of twins in genetic research is based on the occurrence of two genetically different types of twins: those derived from one fertilized ovum and those derived from two fertilized ova. Comparisons are made between one-egg

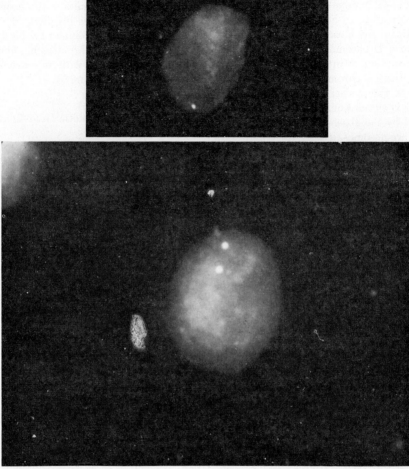

FIG. 5. Fluorescent Y chromosome in buccal mucosal cells. *Above*, normal male; *below*, male with XYY karyotype.

twins, two-egg twins of the same sex, two-egg twins of opposite sexes, full siblings, half siblings, and step siblings. Comparisons can be made between one-egg twins brought up and living together and two-egg twins under the same conditions. It is more difficult to find one-egg twins who have been raised apart and who present a particular syndrome.

Adoption Studies

A useful method of separating biological from rearing influences is the study of children cared for since early infancy by nonrelated foster or adoptive parents. It is possible to compare psychopathology in adopted children whose biological parents were ill with children with unaffected biological parents; to compare psychopathology in the biological parents and the adoptive parents of affected children; to compare parents, biological and adoptive, of affected adopted children with parents of control adoptees without psychopathology.

Longitudinal Studies

Longitudinal studies are, perhaps, the most valuable approach to the understanding of genetic interaction in psychiatry. Although these studies can be retrospective, there is much chance for bias in sampling and in the data remembered or recorded; prospective observation of high-risk groups, particularly the children of one or two affected parents, can best provide data on early signs—behavioral, neurological, psychophysiological, biochemical—and provide leads for prevention.

Pharmacogenetics

There may be inherited differences in response to drugs. In the first place, the therapeutic value of certain drugs may vary with the genetic form of a given syndrome; for example, response to lithium may be correlated with genetically distinct forms of cyclic mood disorder. Secondly, side-effects of drugs may depend quantitatively or qualitatively on genetic differences. Persons with atypical forms of the enzyme pseudocholinesterase may show a prolonged reaction to the administration of succinylcholine. Used before electroconvulsive treatment, this muscle relaxant may cause prolonged apnea in a patient with this rare (1 in 3,000), gene-controlled metabolic disorder. Hereditary predisposition to phenothiazine-induced parkinsonism has been described, and the acute paralytic effect of barbiturates in persons with porphyria is of clinical importance.

At the level of the gene and the chromosome, the mutagenic effects of ionizing radiation and various chemicals in the natural or the man-created environment may lead to somatic changes or hereditary damage. In addition, certain substances have been implicated in causing chromosome damage *in vivo* and *in vitro*. Lysergic acid diethylamide (LSD) has been found to increase the number of chromosome breaks when added to lymphocyte cultures in low concentration. Other more commonly used agents—such as aspirin, caffeine, and ergonovine maleate—have also been shown to cause chromosome breaks when added to cultures.

Psychiatric Genetics

Schizophrenia

Early studies of schizophrenia in relatives of schizophrenic patients, as compared with the general population, give strong evidence that genetic factors are necessary, although not sufficient, in the pathogenesis of schizophrenia. In his large family study conducted in Berlin, Kallmann (1938) investigated the families of 1,087 patients; the over-all expectancy rate for sibs was 11 per cent, but it was higher for the sibs of nuclear (catatonic, hebephrenic) cases than of peripheral (paranoid, simple) ones. In a combined series of 25 investigations, Zerbin-Rüdin presented 8.7 per cent as the minimal expectancy in sibs. For children of index cases, where one parent was schizophrenic, the expectancy rate in the combined series was 12 per cent, in Kallman's 16.4 per cent, with about 20 per cent for the nuclear group and 10 per cent for the peripheral. With both parents schizophrenic, the range of expectancy in children was between 35 and 68 per cent in the various studies. Regarding the mode of inheritance, Kallmann assumed that a single unit factor was responsible for schizophrenia and that this factor was autosomal recessive in nature and subject to modification by other genes conferring a greater or lesser degree of resistance. Other hypotheses that have been advanced include a dominant mode of inheritance with incomplete penetrance of heterozygotes, a polygenic form of inheritance with a threshold, and a heterogenetic model specifying a variety of separate genes, dominant or recessive, any one of which might be involved in the etiology of schizophrenia. Environmental stress as an interacting factor is presumed in all these hypotheses.

Twin Studies. The concordance for monozygotic twins of schizophrenic patients in studies between 1928 and 1961 is 65 per cent and for dizygotic twins about 12 per cent, close to the figure for all sibs. Kallmann's figures (1946), based on the largest series of index cases, were 69 per cent and 10 per cent, respectively; with age correction these yielded the well known expectancies of 86 and 14 per cent. While twin studies cannot establish the mode of inheritance, one aim of these studies was to explore the nature of the protective factors at work in discordant pairs. Foreshadowing later findings were the differences in concordance rates even in Kallmann's series, where the over-all expectancies given above masked the wide range depending on the severity of illness in the index case. With little or no deterioration in the index case, the monozygotic twin expectancy rate was as low as 26 per cent and the dizygotic 2 per cent, whereas for those with extreme deterioration, the rates were as high as 100 and 17 per cent, respectively. In a 1967 study based on all the 25,000 pairs of twins born in Norway between 1901 and 1930, concordance rates for pairs with schizophrenia in one twin ranged from 25 to 38 per cent for monozygotic pairs and

4 to 10 per cent for dizygotic. Gottesman and Shields, studying all twins treated as outpatients or short-stay inpatients at the Maudsley Hospital in London between 1948 and 1964, found over-all concordance expectancy rates of 50 per cent for monozygotic twins and 10 per cent for dizygotic. Pollin and Stabenau studied discordant pairs and found that it was the smaller and physiologically less competent twin at birth who later developed schizophrenia.

Many formulations have been made in the attempt to assess the meaning of the various twin studies in conceptualizing the role of heredity in schizophrenia. The same results have been interpreted as evidence for and against a strong genetic component.

Adoption Studies. In studying the parents—biological and adoptive—of matched groups of schizophrenic patients, Wender and his group found a considerable increase in severity of psychopathology among the biological parents. In a similar study conducted in Denmark by Kety and his group, a significantly higher prevalence of schizophrenia and related disorders was found in the biological relatives of adopted schizophrenic patients than in the biological relatives of nonschizophrenic adoptee controls. In the adoptive families, the prevalence of these disorders was lower and was randomly distributed between the relatives of patients and controls. Two studies by Heston and Denney and by Rosenthal and his group suggest higher rates for schizophrenia and related pathology in the children of schizophrenic parents than in the children of nonschizophrenic parents, even when both groups were raised not by their biological parents but in comparable adoptive homes.

Depressive Illness

Manic-Depressive Illness. The general population rate for manic-depressive psychosis in most European and American populations has been not more than 0.4 per cent. In the case of parents, siblings, and children of manic-depressive index cases, the rates are much higher. Stenstedt in Sweden conducted a population study from 1949 to 1952 and found morbidity risks of 12.3 per cent for siblings, 7.4 per cent for parents, and 9.4 per cent for children. Kallmann in New York found that the expectancy of manic-depressive psychosis varied from 16.7 per cent for half siblings to 22.7 and 25.5 per cent for

siblings and two-egg co-twins, respectively, and 100 per cent for one-egg co-twins. Parents of index cases showed a rate of 23.4 per cent. Stenstedt and Kallmann concluded that manic-depressive psychosis followed a dominant type of inheritance with incomplete penetrance and variable expressivity of a single autosomal gene.

There has recently been a tendency to subdivide affective disorders into two clinical groups —one with alternating periods of mania and depression (bipolar) and the other with recurrent depression alone (unipolar). Higher morbidity risks have been found in relatives of bipolar cases than in families of unipolar cases, with both unipolar and bipolar disease found in the first-degree relatives of the former and unipolar illness alone among relatives of the latter.

In Kallmann's study of manic-depressive illness in families, no twins were found with a schizophrenic psychosis in one partner and a cyclic psychosis in the other, and the morbidity risk for schizophrenia among families of manic-depressive index cases was not statistically different from that in the general population.

Involutional Melancholia. Kallmann found no increase in involutional melancholia among the families of manic-depressives. In the families of 96 involutional twin index cases, the risk of involutional melancholia was increased (6.4 per cent for parents, 6 per cent for full siblings, 6 per cent for dizygotic co-twins, and 60.9 per cent for monozygotic co-twins). The risk for schizophrenia was somewhat elevated (5.5 per cent in parents and 4.2 per cent in siblings), but the risk for manic-depressive psychosis was hardly raised at all. Finally, the expectancy of involutional melancholia among the parents and siblings of schizophrenic twin index cases was increased to 6.6 per cent.

Neurosis

Slater found an increase in neurotic illnesses and neurotic personality traits of a like kind among relatives of obsessional neurotics, anxiety neurotics, and persons diagnosed as hysterics, with the evidence much stronger in the first of these than in the last. The evidence supported a multifactor type of inheritance with continuous and probably multidimensional variation in traits.

In a twin sample tested with the Minnesota Multiphasic personality Inventory, Gottesman found either a low genetic component or none in neuroses with hypochondriacal and hysterical elements, but he found a substantial genetic component in those with elements of anxiety, depression, obsession, and schizoid withdrawal.

Male Homosexuality

Some of the highest monozygotic twin concordance rates have been those for homosexual behavior in men. In Kallmann's series of 40 male homosexuals with identical twins, almost perfect concordance was found, whereas in 45 dizygotic male homosexual twins, the degree of concordance in the co-twin was no higher than what might be anticipated on the basis of Kinsey's statistics for the general population. These findings were interpreted as suggesting a gene-controlled disarrangement between male and female psychosexual maturation patterns. In this formulation, homosexuality would appear to be a part of the personality structure, rather than directly determined by the gonadal apparatus.

A few one-egg twin pairs discordant for homosexual behavior also showed important similarities, principally in psychological test findings that indicated sexual confusion and body-image distortion. Divergent patterns of experience may be influenced by such factors as differences in the twins' relationships with their parents, frustration in heterosexual contacts, and poor masculine identification in the case of the homosexual twin.

Criminal Behavior

Studies of twins showing criminal behavior have tended to show high concordance rates for both monozygotic and same-sex dizygotic twins, leading to the conclusion that there is a large environmental role in the pathogenesis of criminal behavior.

Intelligence

Although intelligence scores, largely consisting of I.Q.s, show remarkable correlation with genetic closeness, it is not yet clear what factors are measured by the various tests or how their results are affected by environmental factors. Specific genetic factors and obvious infectious or birth-traumatic incidents account for barely half of all persons with I.Q.s below 70. Polygenic inheritance is probably responsible for most of the others, with social deprivation usually playing a secondary or modifying role.

Chromosomes and Behavior

Aside from Down's syndrome (marked by mental deficiency but no specific behavior disturbance), most major chromosomal aberrations in persons surviving past infancy involve the sex chromosomes.

Klinefelter's syndrome includes weak libido, mental subnormality, and nonspecific personality disorders ranging from inadequate personality and delinquency to schizophrenia like behavior.

In Turner's syndrome, the typical patient is a short and sexually undeveloped female. These girls and women have been described as resilient to adversity, stable in personality, and maternal in temperament.

The 47-chromosome XYY genotype seems to occur to excess among aggressive, impulsive, and criminally inclined persons, who also tend to be tall and of low intelligence. Those who have been studied appear to show episodic violence and are often the only delinquent members of their families.

Disorders of Aging

There is evidence of genetic transmission in presenile psychoses, with the dominant mode suggested in the case of Pick's disease. In senile disease, a higher frequency of chromosome loss has been noted in peripheral leukocyte cultures taken from women with organic brain syndrome without evidence of cerebral arteriosclerosis than in women without organic brain syndrome. The same findings were not evident in men.

SOCIAL PROBLEMS

Reproductivity of Schizophrenics

With the decrease in length of hospital stay and more flexible social attitudes toward former patients, an increase in marital and reproductive rates of schizophrenic patients between the mid-1930's and the mid-1950's was found in a large-scale study in New York. This gain represents a real decline in the selective disadvantage previously associated with schizophrenia. The developmental hazards of children born into homes in which one or both parents are schizophrenic include overwhelming proportions of broken homes, displacements, and chaotic lives during many rehospitalizations of the parents, in which both the child and the parent are harmed.

Genetic Counseling

Genetic counseling may represent a short-term course of psychotherapy based on psychological understanding and conducted according to established techniques of psychiatric interviewing. The counselor must be well-versed in the medical, legal, and psychological implications of such procedures as amniocentesis, contraception, sterilization, abortion, artificial insemination, and adoption.

REFERENCES

Bartalos, M., and Baramki, T. A. *Medical Cytogenetics.* Williams and Wilkins. Baltimore, 1967.

Gottesman, I. I., and Shields, J. *Schizophrenia and Genetics: A Twin Study Vantage Point.* Academic Press, New York, 1972.

Kallmann, F. J. *Heredity in Health and Mental Disorder.* W. W. Norton, New York, 1953.

Rainer, J. D. Genetic counseling, social planning and mental health. In *Social Psychiatry*, F. Redlick, editor. Williams & Wilkins, Baltimore, 1969.

Rosenthal, D., and Kety, S., editors. *The Transmission of Schizophrenia.* Pergamon Press, Oxford, 1968.

Slater, E., and Cowie, V. *The Genetics of Mental Disorder.* Oxford University Press, London, 1971.

Watson, J. D. *Molecular Biology of the Gene.* ed. 2. W. A. Benjamin, New York, 1970.

2.2.   PSYCHOPHARMACOLOGY

Neurotransmitters

Acetylcholine has the longest history of investigation as a neurotransmitter, followed in close historical sequence by norepinephrine (see Figure 1). Interactions of psychotropic drugs with the catecholamines norepinephrine and dihydroxyphenylethylamine (dopamine) have been discovered by numerous investigators and appear to account for the actions of numerous drugs. Accordingly, some people have gained the impression that the catecholamines and acetylcholine, along with the indoleamine serotonin, account for the bulk of synaptic transmission in the brain. Quantitatively, these compounds are all only minor transmitters in the brain, although they may have particular importance in the areas of the brain concerned with emotional behavior.

It is likely that a variety of amino acids are transmitters at the major excitatory and inhibitory synapses. In various brain regions γ-aminobutyric acid (GABA) probably accounts for transmission at between 25 and 40 per cent of synapses. GABA inhibits the firing of neurons and is, therefore, a major inhibitory transmitter. In the spinal cord and brain stem the amino acid glycine, in addition to its other metabolic functions, appears to be a prominent inhibitory transmitter at about the same percentage of synapses as GABA. A given neuron presumably uses only a single neurotransmitter. Thus, GABA and glycine are transmitters at distinct synapses. The identity of the major excitatory neurotransmitters is somewhat less certain. However, glutamic and aspartic acids, which uniformly excite neurons, satisfy many characteristics demanded of the prominent excitatory transmitters.

Amine Tracts

In the histochemical fluorescence method, serotonin can be distinguished from the catecholamines by the wave length of fluorescence, which varies in such a way that serotonin appears bright yellow and the catecholamines appear bright green. Although both dopamine and norepinephrine fluoresce green, they can be differentiated by their response to drugs. What are the pathways of the monoamine neuronal systems? The cell bodies of all of them are within the brain stem. Axons ascend or descend throughout the brain and into the spinal cord. For each of the amines, there are several separate and distinct tracts (see Figure 2).

Norepinephrine. There are two major norepinephrine tracts. The ventral pathway has cell bodies in several locations in the brain stem and axons that ascend in the medial forebrain bundle to give off terminals predominantly in the hypothalamus and limbic system. The cell bodies of the dorsal norepinephrine pathway are discretely localized in a single nucleus of the brain stem, the locus ceruleus. Its axons also ascend in the medial forebrain bundle but more dorsally than those of the ventral pathway. Terminals of the dorsal pathway are located predominantly in the cerebral cortex and hippocampus. Some axons from the locus ceruleus descend to give off nerve terminals synapsing upon the Purkinje cells of the cerebellum. Certain cells from the locus ceruleus give off axons that bifurcate, sending one branch to the cerebral cortex and another to the cerebellum. In this way a single neuron can influence widely separated parts of the brain.

Other norepinephrine pathways have cell

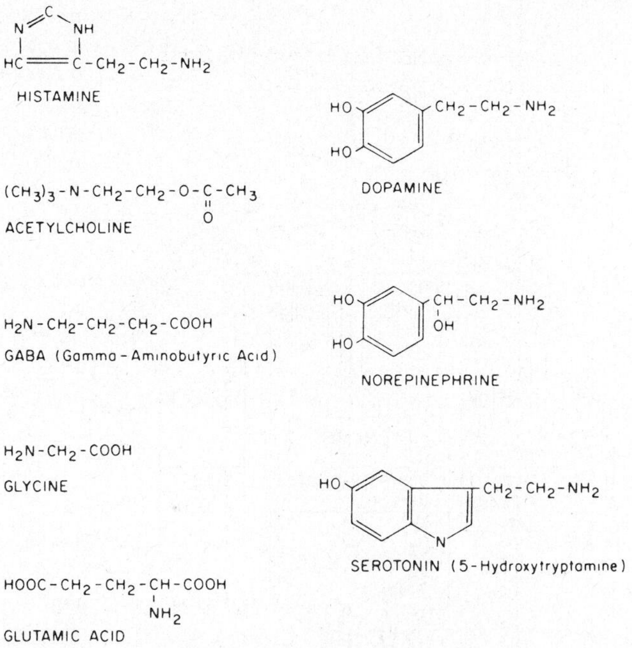

FIGURE 1. Structures of neurotransmitter candidates in the brain.

bodies in the brain stem and axons that descend in the lateral sympathetic columns of the spinal cord, terminating at various levels. These neurons influence a variety of spinal cord reflexes.

Dopamine. There are several discrete dopamine pathways. The most prominent pathway has cell bodies in the substantia nigra and gives rise to axons that terminate in the caudate nucleus and putamen of the corpus striatum. Other dopamine pathways in the brain have cell bodies close to the substantia nigra, just dorsal to the interpeduncular nucleus, with terminals in the nucleus accumbens and olfactory tubercle, both parts of the limbic emotional areas of the brain. There are also dopamine neurons in the cerebral cortex. A dopamine pathway with cell bodies in the arcuate nucleus of the hypothalamus and terminals in the median eminence probably regulates release of hypothalamic trophic hormones, which then act on the pituitary gland. There are also dopamine neurons in the retina.

Serotonin. All cell bodies of the serotonin-containing neurons are localized in a series of nuclei in the lower midbrain and upper pons that are called the raphe nuclei. Axons of these cells ascend primarily in the medial forebrain bundle and give off terminals in all brain regions, but with the majority in the hypothalamus and the fewest in the cerebral cortex and cerebellum.

Amine Metabolism

The amino acid tyrosine is the dietary precursor of the catecholamines (see Figure 3). The first enzyme in the biosynthetic pathway of the catecholamines is tyrosine hydroxylase, which converts tyrosine into dihydroxyphenylalanine. Tyrosine hydroxylase is considered to be the major rate-limiting enzyme in catecholamine biosynthesis, because increasing or decreasing its activity produces corresponding changes in the levels of the catecholamines. Dopa is then decarboxylated by the enzyme dopa-decarboxylase to dopamine. Dopa-decarboxylase is often referred to as aromatic amino acid decarboxylase because it is relatively nonspecific and can decarboxylate any aromatic amino acid, with important consequences when certain amino acids are used as drugs.

In norepinephrine neurons, dopamine is converted to norepinephrine by the addition of a hydroxyl group by the enzyme dopamine-β-hydroxylase.

Under normal conditions, when a neuron fires and releases a molecule of a catecholamine, the

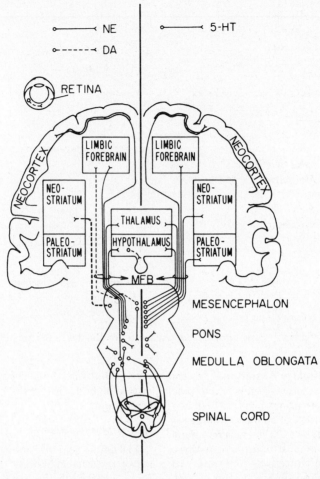

FIGURE 2. Pathways of serotonin (5-HT), norepinephrine (NE), and dopamine (DA) neuronal systems in the central nervous system. (Adapted from Anden et al., 1966.)

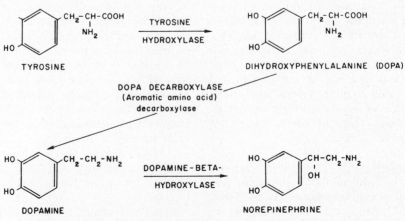

FIGURE 3. Pathways of catecholamine synthesis. (From Snyder, 1967.)

neuron must synthesize a new catecholamine molecule to replace the one just released. Accordingly, when the firing rate of catecholamine neurons is accelerated, there is a parallel increase in the conversion of tyrosine to new catecholamines.

Catecholamines can be metabolically degraded primarily by two enzymes, monoamine oxidase and catechol-O-methyltransferase (COMT). Monoamine oxidase oxidatively deaminates dopamine or norepinephrine to the corresponding aldehydes. These, in turn, can be converted by aldehyde dehydrogenase to corresponding acids. The aldehydes may also be reduced to form alcohols. Dietary factors, such as the ingestion of ethanol, can determine the relative amounts of catechol acids or alcohols formed from the catecholamines because ethanol also competes for aldehyde dehydrogenase.

Catecholamines can be methylated by COMT, which transfers the methyl group of S-adenosylmethionine to the meta (3 position) hydroxyl of the catecholamines. COMT acts on any catechol compound, including the aldehydes and acids formed from the action of monoamine oxidase on the catecholamines. When norepinephrine is methylated by this enzyme, the product is called normetanephrine.

Like COMT, monoamine oxidase is relatively nonspecific and acts on any monoamine—including serotonin, normetanephrine, and 3-O-methyldopamine—converting these first into their respective aldehydes and then into acids or alcohols. Thus, an O-methylated alcohol or acid results from the combined actions of monoamine oxidase and COMT. In the peripheral sympathetic nervous system, the O-methylated acid product of norepinephrine degradation is called vanillylmandelic acid. Its levels are measured in clinical laboratories as an index of

sympathetic nervous function and to diagnose tumors that produce norepinephrine or epinephrine, such as pheochromocytomas and neuroblastomas. Dopamine O-methylation and deamination gives rise to homovanillic acid.

In the brain, reduction of the aldehyde formed from the action of monoamine oxidase on norepinephrine or normetanephrine predominates, so that the major metabolite in the brain is an alcohol derivative called 3-methoxy-4-hydroxylphenylglycol (MHPG). The MHPG formed in the brain is conjugated to sulfate.

Serotonin. Tryptophan, the dietary amino acid precursor of serotonin, is hydroxylated by the enzyme tryptophan hydroxylase to form 5-hydroxytryptophan (see Figure 4). 5-Hydroxytryptophan is decarboxylated to serotonin by 5-hydroxytryptophan decarboxylase, which is also referred to as aromatic amino acid decarboxylase, since its range of substrate preference is the same as that of dopa-decarboxylase. Serotonin is destroyed by monoamine oxidase, which oxidatively deaminates it to the aldehyde, just as this enzyme does with the catecholamines. The aldehyde formed from serotonin is predominantly oxidized to 5-hydroxyindoleactic acid, although a limited amount is reduced to the alcohol, 5-hydroxytryptophol.

Reuptake Inactivation. After discharge at synapses, acetylcholine is inactivated through hydrolysis by the enzyme acetylcholinesterase. None of the enzymes that degrade serotonin or the catecholamines appear to be responsible for their synaptic inactivation. Instead, these amines are predominantly inactivated by reuptake into the nerve terminals that released them (see Figure 5). It appears likely that reuptake inactivation is the universal mechanism for neurotransmitter inactivation and that enzymatic degradation in the case of acetylcholine

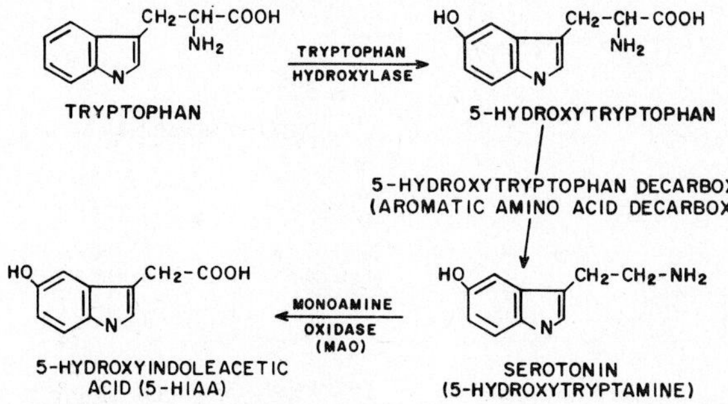

FIGURE 4. Pathways of serotonin synthesis and degradation. (From Snyder, 1972.)

is an exception to the rule. Interference with reuptake inactivation is a major mechanism of action of several psychotropic drugs.

Psychotropic Drug Action

Stimulants

Amphetamines and related stimulants bear striking structural resemblances to the catecholamines (see Figure 6). Amphetamine causes a direct release of catecholamines into the synaptic cleft and, hence, onto postsynaptic receptor sites. Amphetamine can also efficiently block the reuptake inactivation mechanism of the catecholamines, thus prolonging the effects of synaptically released norepinephrine and dopamine.

Amphetamine can be metabolized by a variety of routes. The most prominent ones involve the introduction of a hydroxyl group on the ring opposite (para) to the side chain and the deamination of the side chain nitrogen by a

SYNAPTIC
CLEFT

CATECHOLAMINE
REUPTAKE
INACTIVATION
blocked by
amphetamine

PHENOTHIAZINES
BLOCK CATECHOLAMINE
RECEPTORS

NERVE
ENDING

POST SYNAPTIC
RECEPTOR

CATECHOLAMINES RELEASED
INTO SYNAPSE BY NERVE
IMPULSE OR AMPHETAMINE

FIGURE 5. Diagram of catecholamine synapse.

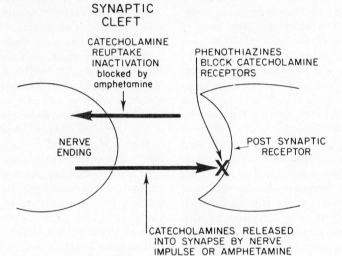

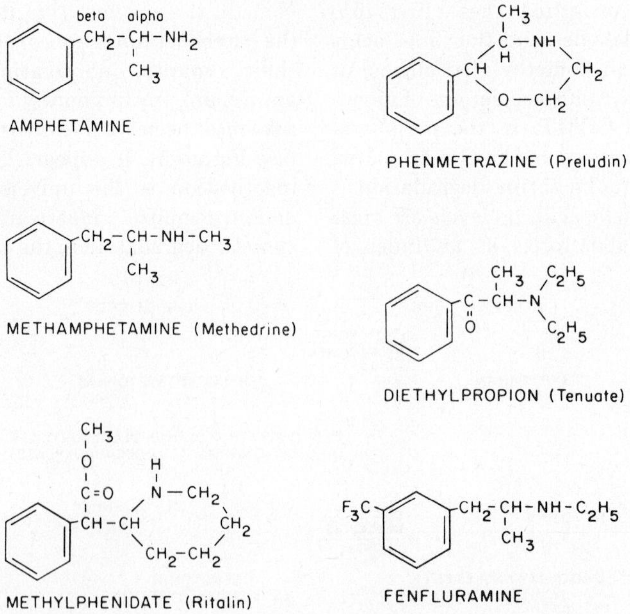

AMPHETAMINE

PHENMETRAZINE (Preludin)

METHAMPHETAMINE (Methedrine)

DIETHYLPROPION (Tenuate)

METHYLPHENIDATE (Ritalin)

FENFLURAMINE

FIGURE 6. Structures of amphetamine and related drugs.

drug-metabolizing system in the liver that is different from monoamine oxidase. However, metabolic pathways are not especially prominent in man, and a major amount of amphetamine is excreted in the urine unchanged. Because amphetamine is an amine, it is un-ionized at alkaline pH values and, accordingly, predominantly reabsorbed into the circulation from the kidney tubules and poorly excreted. To facilitate amphetamine excretion, one would want to increase the positive charge on the amine nitrogen by acidifying the urine—for example, by treating the patient with ammonium chloride.

Antidepressant Drugs

There are two major classes of antidepressant drugs, the monoamine oxidase inhibitors and the tricyclic antidepressants. Monoamine oxidase inhibitors comprise a group of agents that have widely varying chemical structures but that have in common the ability to inhibit monoamine oxidase. Inhibition of this enzyme results in an accumulation of the monoamines norepinephrine, dopamine, and serotonin within nerve terminals. At a certain point the amines start leaking out into the synaptic cleft so that the drugs facilitate the actions of all monoamines.

The tricyclic antidepressants are potent inhibitors of the reuptake inactivation mechanism of catecholamine and serotonin neurons. The chemical structures of the tricyclic antidepressants closely resemble those of the phenothiazines. These antidepressants were initially developed as antischizophrenic drugs, although they were relatively ineffective in treating schizophrenic patients. Like certain phenothiazines, the tricyclic antidepressants, such as imipramine (Tofranil) and amitriptyline (Elavil), tend to sedate normal people and yet, paradoxically, relieve depression. In the treatment of depression, these drugs, as well as the monoamine oxidase inhibitors, require a latency period of 1 to 3 weeks before they are fully effective.

Both the tricyclic antidepressants and the monoamine oxidase inhibitors presumably owe their clinical actions to the facilitation of the synaptic actions of norepinephrine or serotonin in the brain. These drugs also facilitate the effects of norepinephrine released at sympathetic synapses in the peripheral nervous system. This action can give rise to major side effects associated with enhanced sympathetic function. In some patients these drugs produce marked hypertension. Since the two classes of drugs facilitate norepinephrine effects in different ways, they enhance the activities of each other in a synergistic fashion. Extremely severe, even fatal, hypertensive crises have occurred in certain patients treated simultaneously with monoamine oxidase inhibitors and tricyclic antidepressant drugs.

Tricyclic antidepressants block the metabolism of amphetamine and slow its disappearance from the brain. Accordingly, these drugs potentiate the central stimulant effects of amphetamine. There is some limited evidence that amphetamines retard metabolism of the tricyclic antidepressants and in this way facilitate their therapeutic actions.

Antischizophrenic Drugs

Phenothiazines have been used as tools to discern abnormal brain mechanisms in schizophrenia. The phenothiazines are complex 3-ringed structures with side chains, quite similar in structure to the tricyclic antidepressants (see Figures 7 and 8). The butyrophenones, such as haloperidol (Haldol), differ markedly from the phenothiazines in chemical structure but have extremely similar pharmacological activities.

In 1962 the Swedish pharmacologist Arvid Carlsson observed that phenothiazines that are effective antischizophrenic agents tend to elevate brain levels of methoxydopamine, but clinically ineffective phenothiazines do not. This observation suggested that effective antischizophrenic drugs cause an increased release of dopamine and, to a lesser extent, of norepinephrine. Subsequently it was found that phenothiazines and butyrophenones accelerate the formation of dopamine from tyrosine in proportion to their clinical efficacy. Haloperidol, which is about 100 times as potent as chlorpromazine, is also about 100 times as potent in accelerating dopamine formation, but promethazine, which is ineffective in the treatment of schizophrenia, does not accelerate dopamine formation. An acceleration of norepinephrine synthesis occurs with these drugs but correlates much less with their antischizophrenic activity.

The phenothiazines and butyrophenones all share an antischizophrenic action. In addition, they possess several other clinically useful actions, which vary among the drugs. Phenothia-

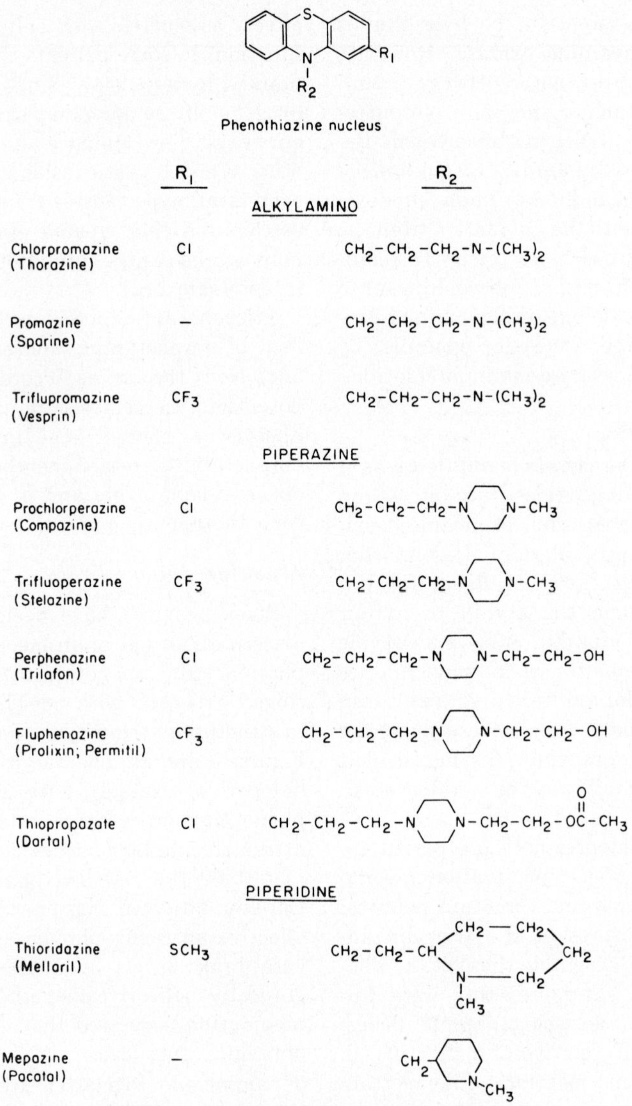

Phenothiazine nucleus

	R₁	R₂

ALKYLAMINO

Chlorpromazine (Thorazine)	Cl	$CH_2-CH_2-CH_2-N-(CH_3)_2$
Promazine (Sparine)	—	$CH_2-CH_2-CH_2-N-(CH_3)_2$
Triflupromazine (Vesprin)	CF₃	$CH_2-CH_2-CH_2-N-(CH_3)_2$

PIPERAZINE

Prochlorperazine (Compazine)	Cl	$CH_2-CH_2-CH_2-N\diagup\diagdown N-CH_3$
Trifluoperazine (Stelazine)	CF₃	$CH_2-CH_2-CH_2-N\diagup\diagdown N-CH_3$
Perphenazine (Trilafon)	Cl	$CH_2-CH_2-CH_2-N\diagup\diagdown N-CH_2-CH_2-OH$
Fluphenazine (Prolixin; Permitil)	CF₃	$CH_2-CH_2-CH_2-N\diagup\diagdown N-CH_2-CH_2-OH$
Thiopropazate (Dartal)	Cl	$CH_2-CH_2-CH_2-N\diagup\diagdown N-CH_2-CH_2-O\overset{O}{\overset{\|}{C}}-CH_3$

PIPERIDINE

| Thioridazine (Mellaril) | SCH₃ | $CH_2-CH_2-CH\diagup\diagdown$ piperidine ring with N—CH₃ |
| Mepazine (Pacatal) | — | $CH_2\diagup\diagdown$ piperidine ring with N—CH₃ |

FIGURE 7. Structures of phenothiazine drugs.

zines elicit postural hypotension, and some of these drugs are quite sedating. Most phenothiazines exert an antiemetic effect by acting directly on the chemoreceptor trigger zone in the brain stem. Some phenothiazine derivatives are marketed primarily for their antiemetic actions. The alkylamino and piperidine side chain phenothiazines produce more hypotensive and sedating effects than the piperazine side chain phenothiazines. By contrast, the piperazine phenothiazines are more potent antiemetics and provoke more extrapyramidal side effects than the alkylamino and piperidine phenothia-

zines. The butyrophenones tend most to resemble the piperazine phenothiazines in their side effects.

The extrapyramidal side effects of the phenothiazines frequently resemble the symptoms of Parkinson's disease, with akinesia, rigidity, and tremor. In addition, there are other extrapyramidal effects, such as akathisia, which refers to a peculiar sort of restlessness, almost a muscular itchiness, in which patients cannot sit still and so pace up and down the floors of the hospital. Other extrapyramidal symptoms include abnormal muscular movements, such as torticollis. The symptoms of idiopathic Parkinson's disease are presumed to result from a deficiency of dopamine because of the degeneration of the dopamine neurons in the corpus striatum. The extrapyramidal side effects of phenothiazine drugs appear to result from dopamine receptor blockade. By blocking dopamine receptors in the corpus striatum, phenothiazines can produce a pharmacological model of Parkinson's disease.

Patients treated for a long period of time with phenothiazines develop a side effect that seems to be the opposite of parkinsonianlike side effects of the drugs, namely tardive dyskinesia. This side effect consists of a hypermotility of facial muscles and the extremities. Even though tardive dyskinesia follows prolonged phenothiazine treatment, phenothiazines and butyrophe-

nones relieve the symptoms of tardive dyskinesia.

Phenothiazines can be metabolized by a large number of pathways. More than 100 metabolites of chlorpromazine have been reported in the urine. There are wide individual variations in blood levels of chlorpromazine after fixed doses, suggesting that there are wide variations in phenothiazine metabolism.

Psychedelic Drugs

The psychedelic drugs comprise a wide range of chemical structures that, despite their marked chemical differences, produce a strikingly similar set of profound subjective effects. Humphrey Osmond coined the word psychedelic, which is derived from the Greek meaning "mind-manifesting," to emphasize the extraor-

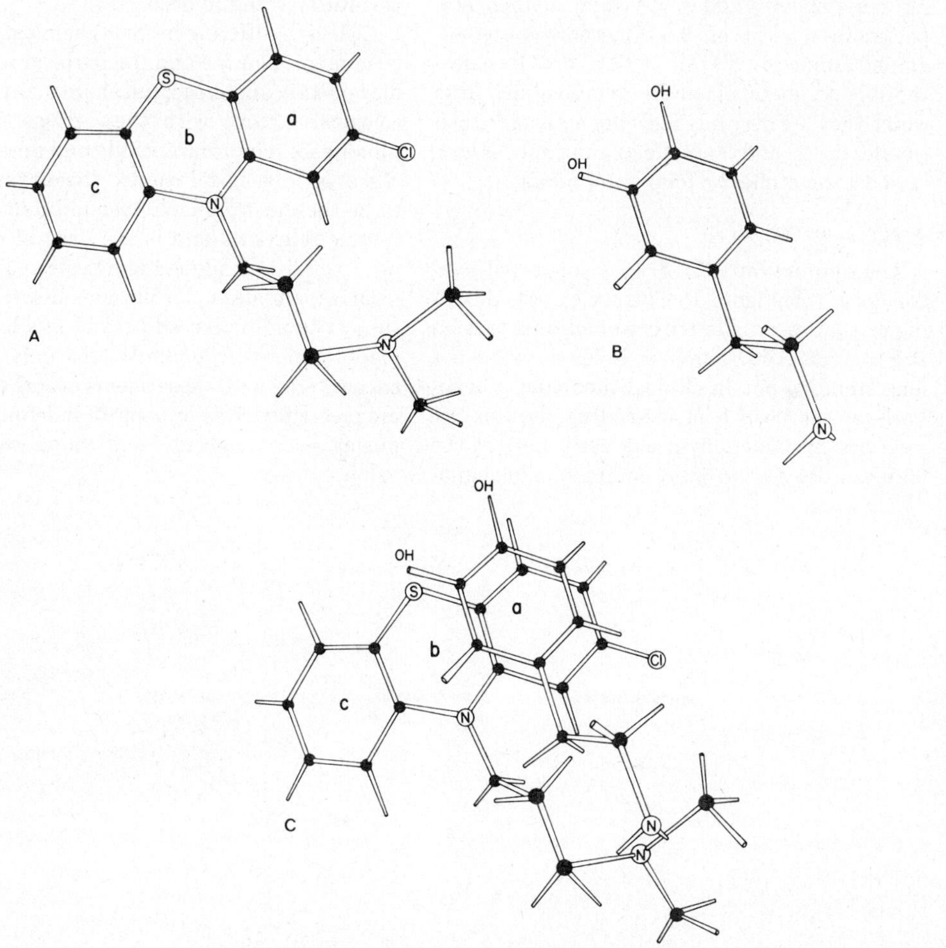

FIGURE 8. Diagrams of chlorpromazine (*A*) and dopamine (*B*) in their optimal conformations, as determined by X-ray crystal analysis, and their super-imposition (*C*). (From Horn and Snyder, 1971.)

dinary changes in state of consciousness brought about by these agents. By mind-manifesting, he really meant mind-expanding.

The chemical structure of LSD (lysergic acid diethylamide) possesses certain similarities to that of serotonin. One dramatic effect of LSD closely parallels its clinical actions: reduced firing of serotonin neurons.

The various psychedelic drugs differ from each other in certain nuances of their subjective effects and in their duration of action. However, their effects are far more similar than they are dissimilar. Most work by mouth, although dimethyltryptamine (DMT) is not active by mouth and is usually injected or inhaled. LSD effects persist about 8 hours; mescaline is a little longer-lasting. DMT is the shortest acting psychedelic drug; its effects persist for only about 1 hour. Certain methoxyamphetamines, such as 2,5-dimethyl-4-methylamphetamine or DOM (STP), are less susceptible to metabolism than mescaline, from which they are derived. They are active in much smaller doses, and their effects continue for long periods, sometimes as long as 24 hours.

Antianxiety Agents

The term antianxiety drug is somewhat controversial (see Figure 9). The notion of prescribing a sedative drug to reduce emotional tension and produce mild skeletal muscle relaxation is a long standing one in clinical medicine. Phenobarbital has been a favorite drug for this use since its introduction in the early part of the 20th century. Of the many commercially availa-

ble barbiturates, phenobarbital appears to be the most valuable drug, primarily because of its slow onset and long duration of action. Barbiturates with steep dose-response curves, such as secobarbital, are better sleeping medications but less satisfactory as tranquilizers. Drugs such as phenobarbital, with relatively shallow dose-response curves, produce calming without drowsiness, sleep, ataxia, or slurred speech over a wide range of doses. Phenobarbital has a more shallow dose-response curve than other barbiturates because it is more slowly metabolized, excreted, and absorbed into the brain.

Meprobamate can be addicting, although it may not be as addictive as barbiturates, and there have been numerous suicides with meprobamate. However, it is true that the lethal dose of the drug is proportionately greater than barbiturates' lethal dose.

Although differing in their chemical structure from meprobamate and the barbiturates, chlordiazepoxide and diazepam share many pharmacological actions with these drugs. Like meprobamate, chlordiazepoxide and diazepam are effective muscle relaxants. Diazepam appears to be the most clinically useful of all available muscle relaxants and is the drug of choice for most conditions involving muscle spasm.

Diazepam and chlordiazepoxide are both less subject to addictive abuse and less lethal than meprobamate. Apparently, the only difficulty encountered with these agents occurs when they are prescribed for a prolonged, indefinite period, during which considerable tolerance can develop.

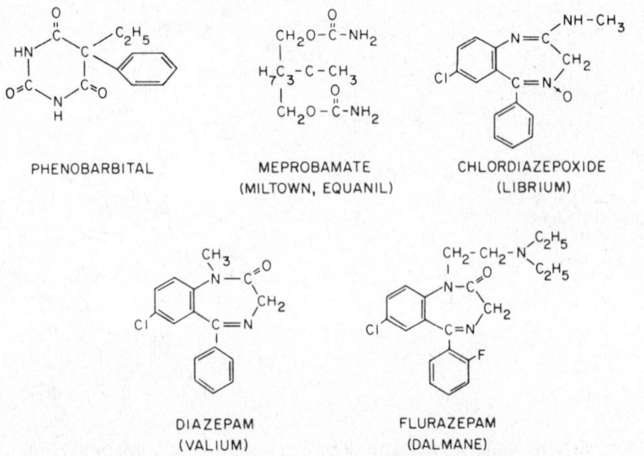

PHENOBARBITAL   MEPROBAMATE   CHLORDIAZEPOXIDE
                     (MILTOWN, EQUANIL) (LIBRIUM)

DIAZEPAM   FLURAZEPAM
(VALIUM)   (DALMANE)

FIGURE 9. Structures of antianxiety drugs.

The mechanism of action of these agents is not clear. Pharmacologically, there is considerable overlap between alcohol, barbiturates, meprobamate, chlordiazepoxide, and diazepam. The symptoms of withdrawal from all these drugs are almost the same, with insomnia, tremulousness, great anxiety, convulsions, and a confusional psychosis resembling delirium tremens. For this reason, one can relieve withdrawal symptoms from one drug by administration of any of the others. Diazepam is highly effective in treating the symptoms of delirium tremens or of barbiturate withdrawal and may well be the drug of choice in this regard because of its general over-all safety.

Within the brain, these drugs produce a number of effects, particularly a general slowing of oxidative metabolism and depression of synaptic transmission. These effects are not confined to any single neuronal system. As yet, there is no evidence of a selective action for barbiturates. Conceivably, their therapeutic action may be related to an over-all depression of neuronal function. Diazepam, chlordiazepoxide, and related benzodiazepine drugs appear to exert their muscle relaxant and antianxiety effects by mimicking glycine at its receptor sites in the spinal cord and brain stem.

The barbiturates stimulate liver drug-metabolizing enzyme systems, including those that metabolize barbiturates. This effect explains, in part, tolerance to barbiturates. There must, in addition, be a tolerance at receptor sites in the brain because, even at identical brain levels of barbiturates, an animal that has received the drugs chronically displays less of a pharmacological response than does a naive animal. Since meprobamate and barbiturates induce a wide variety of drug-metabolizing enzymes, metabolic tolerance to them is associatzd with metabolic tolerance to other drugs.

REFERENCES

Aghajanian, G. K., and Bunney, B. S. Central dopamine neurons: Neurophysiological identification and responses to drugs. In *Frontiers in Catecholamine Research*. E. Usdin and S. H. Snyder, editors. Pergamon Press. Oxford, 1973.

Aghajanian, G. K., Foote, W. E., and Sheard, M. H. Action of psychotogenic drugs on single midbrain raphe neurons. J. Pharmacol. Exp. Ther., *171:* 178, 1970.

Anden, N. E., Dahlström, A., Fuxe, K., Larsson, K., Olson, K., and Ungerstedt, U. Ascending monoamine neurons to the telencephalon and diencephalon. Acta Physiol. Scand., *67:* 3131, 1966.

Davis, J. M., and Janowsky, D. Amphetamine psychosis. In *Frontiers in Catecholamine Research*. E. Usdin and S. H. Snyder, editors. Pergamon Press, Oxford, 1973.

Klein, D. F., and Davis, J. M. *Diagnosis and Drug Treatment of Psychiatric Disorders*. Williams & Wilkins. Baltimore, 1969.

Maas, J., Dekirmajian, H., and Jones, F. The identification of depressed patients who have a disorder of norepinephrine metabolism and/or disposition. In *Frontiers in Catecholamine Research*, E. Usdin and S. H. Snyder, editors. Pergamon Press, Oxford, 1973.

Snyder, S. H. Catecholamines and serotonin. In *Basic Neurochemistry*, R. W. Albers, G. I. Siegal, R. Katzman, and B. W. Agranoff, editors, p. 89. Little, Brown, Boston, 1972.

Young, A. B., Zukin, S. R., and Snyder, H. Interaction of benzodiazepines with central nervous glycine receptors: Possible mechanism of action. Proc. Natl. Acad. Sci. U. S. A., **71:** 2246–2250, 1974.

2.3. SLEEP AND DREAMS

Introduction

The current picture of sleep as a composite of repeated cycles representing different phases of brain and body activity has been determined largely by researchers working in more than two dozen sleep laboratories in the United States. Methods for study are based on electroencephalographic (EEG), electro-oculographic, and electromyographic (EMG) tracings on subjects studied nightly for 8- to 10-hour periods. Standard electrode placements are made on the scalp to detect brain activity, at the outer canthus of each eye to record eye movements, and beneath the chin to determine muscle tonus. Other electrodes monitor heart and respiratory rate. These electrical potentials are then transmitted to recorders; later, the massive accumulation of data is subjected to rigid statistical analysis and evaluation.

Normal Sleep

Sleep Stages

In the 1950's, Aserinsky, Dement, and Kleitman discovered that sleep consisted of a series of qualitatively different events recurring periodically throughout the night. One of these sleep stages was characterized by a series of rapid eye movements (REM) readily observable beneath the closed lids of the sleeper. Temperature was found to be elevated, metabolic rates increased, and electrical patterns of the brain strikingly akin to those seen during the height of arousal. Such findings prompted many to call REM sleep active or activated sleep, as compared with the quiet sleep of the remaining sleep stages. Sleep was divided into two major categories: REM sleep and nonrapid eye movement (NREM) sleep. Later, NREM sleep was further divided into stages 1, 2, 3, and 4.

Sleep Cycle

In a young adult, a typical night of sleep (see Figure 1) begins with stage 1 and is followed by stages 2, 3, and 4. Then there is a return from stage 4 to stages 3 and 2. About 70 to 100 minutes after sleep onset, the person enters the first period of REM sleep. From this REM stage, the sleeper re-enters stages 2, 3, and 4, swings back through stages 3 and 2, and returns to the REM stage. This cycling from the onset of one REM stage through to the onset of the next REM stage is repeated throughout the night. Each cycle is similar to the others, except that during the last part of the night REM periods lengthen, and the descent of sleep only reaches stage 3, from which there is the inevitable return to REM sleep.

The number of cycles and the number of REM periods varies between four and six nightly, depending on the length of sleep. The total time spent in the REM stage constitutes about 20 to 25 per cent of the total sleep time; stage 2 constitutes 50 per cent; stages 3 and 4 constitute 20 per cent; and stage 1 constitutes 5 to 10 per cent (see Figure 1).

Kleitman has indicated that the 90-minute REM-NREM sleep cycle is a part of the 24-hour, basic rest-activity cycle. The basic rest-activity cycle represents a basic biological rhythmicity of about 90-minute periods, within which there are regularly occurring periods of waxing and waning activity of the central nervous system.

Age and Sleep Patterns

Sleep is correlated with age in three areas—length, distribution in a 24-hour day, and sleep stage patterns. Average sleep length decreases

from 16 hours at birth to 9 hours at 12 to 17 years. Total sleep time continues to decrease with age, with young adults averaging 8 hours and the elderly averaging significantly less because of frequent and prolonged awakenings.

In terms of sleep distribution, the sleep of the neonate is polyphasic; by the third week, only 60 per cent of sleep occurs between 9 P.M. and 8 A.M., and by the twenty-sixth week 75 per cent of sleep occurs during this period. By the first year, naps tend to consolidate into a single afternoon nap and are usually eliminated by age 5. Frequently, napping reoccurs to varying degrees in the elderly, often making an assessment of their total sleep time difficult.

In general, premature and newborn infants show the highest levels of active or REM sleep, ranging from 84 per cent at 29 weeks conceptional age to 38 per cent at 43 weeks. REM sleep decreases to 20 or 25 per cent of total sleep time by the end of the first year of life. This level remains almost constant throughout life, although there is a progressive lengthening of the first three REM periods. In children, the combined stages 3 and 4 range from 20 to 30 per cent and in young adults from 10 to 15 per cent. In middle-aged and elderly subjects, the percentage of REM sleep remains in the range of 18 to 25 per cent. REM periods are fairly uniform in length, and there is a decrease in stage 4 sleep to as much as 4 per cent or as little as none (see Figure 2).

BIOCHEMISTRY

A number of theories have been advanced as to the neurophysiological and biochemical regulation of sleep. Presently, the role of the monoamines is receiving the greatest amount of attention, and controversy exists as to which amines are of paramount importance.

Physiology

Measurements of pulse, respiration, and blood pressure show wide variations during REM sleep, in contrast with slight changes during NREM sleep. There is also a high correlation between the occurrence of penile erections and REM sleep. Erections begin and end in close temporal relation to the onset and termination of REM periods.

Neuroendocrinology

Several hypothalamic-pituitary hormones have been found to be closely related to the

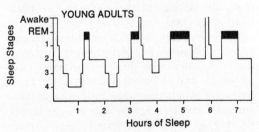

FIGURE 1. Sleep cycle of a normal young adult.

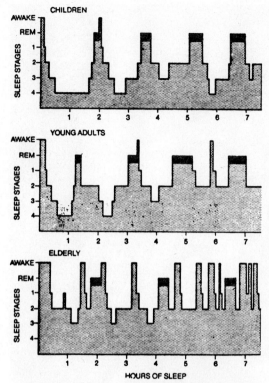

FIGURE 2. Sleep cycles and the effect of age. This illustration compares the sleep cycles of normal subjects in different age groups (children, young adults, and the elderly). The amount of REM sleep shows little variation among the three groups, but stage 4 sleep decreases with age. In addition, the elderly have frequent awakenings and a marked increase in the total wake time.

24-hour sleep-waking cycle. Studies of urinary and plasma corticosteroids demonstrated that there is a peak in these levels in the last part of the night, when REM sleep predominates. Growth hormone is secreted during the first 2 hours of sleep, suggesting a relation with stages 3 and 4. Blood levels of prolactin show a clear increase 60 to 90 minutes after sleep onset and are increased during the entire night's sleep. Luteinizing hormone secretion is affected by such factors as maturation, sex differences, and the menstrual cycle. Plasma testosterone levels increase during sleep, with peak levels occurring in relation to REM sleep.

Dreaming

Aserinsky and Kleitman found that vivid dreams were recalled 74 per cent of the time when subjects were awakened from REM-sleep periods but only 7 per cent of the time from NREM awakenings. Dreaming can also occur during NREM sleep, but REM-sleep dream recall most often closely resembles what persons ordinarily regard as a dream, whereas recall from NREM awakenings is more thoughtlike.

Detailed, vivid, and visual dream recall is more likely to occur from REM periods late in the night, when these periods are longer and sleep is lighter, than early in the night. Dream recall is further facilitated if the awakening from REM sleep is abrupt, rather than gradual. An inability of some persons to recall dreams may be the result of an over-all greater depth of sleep and a lack of awakenings from REM periods, which are necessary for memory consolidation of dream recall. Thus, the inability to recall dream may have physiological bases, as well as a psychological base—that is, anxiety and repression—whereas the forgetting of dreams is related more to psychological factors (see Fig. 3).

Deprivation

Persons who go without sleep for extended periods frequently exhibit disorders of thought and perception that are sometimes indistinguishable from those observed in schizophrenia.

Dement used selective deprivation of REM sleep by arousing experimental subjects just after the onset of each REM period. He observed that the frequency of the REM periods increased at a rate greater than normal throughout each night and that they became more marked during each successive night of REM-sleep deprivation. The subjects exhibited significant elevations in the percentage of time spent in REM sleep, as compared with their previous base line levels, when they were allowed to sleep undisturbed on subsequent recovery nights. Some psychological changes were reported in all subjects during the REM-sleep deprivation period in the form of increased appetite, anxiety, irritability, and difficulties in concentrating. Dement concluded that there was a specific need for REM sleep that must be made up at a later time, when it was allowed to occur naturally.

Behavioral changes during total sleep deprivation are often dramatic as well as incapacitating. Most often reported or observed are increasing fatigue, instability, feelings of persecution, misperception, and disorientation. Illusions and hallucinations, when present, are usually visual and tactile, in contrast to the

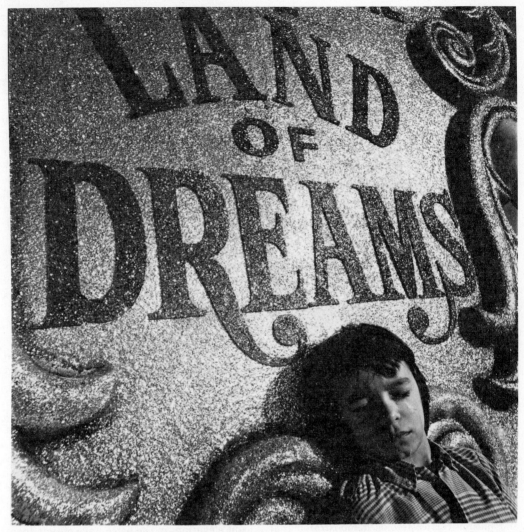

FIGURE 3. Dreams are the royal road to the unconscious. They are also the guardians of sleep. (Courtesy of Arthur Tress for Magnum Photos, Inc.)

auditory hallucinations of schizophrenic patients. These changes become more evident after about 100 hours of total sleep deprivation, become more intense as sleep loss progresses, and are usually more pronounced in the early morning hours, the period when the subject is usually asleep. In spite of these often dramatic changes, once the subjects are allowed to recover sleep they quickly reconstitute, and no permanent psychopathological effects extend beyond the period of sleep deprivation.

Psychological and Physiological Processes in Dreaming

The state in which dreaming can occur, REM sleep, is a universal and regularly occurring process. The cyclical patterns of REM sleep represent a basic biological process on which the psychological process of dreaming may be superimposed.

The association between penile erections and REM sleep illustrates the relation between the psychological and the physiological processes of dreaming. Penile erections begin several minutes before the onset of REM sleep, suggesting that a neurophysiological mechanism initiates the penile erection before the development of a dream.

Throughout REM sleep, muscle tonus is markedly decreased, although there are periodic, brief bursts of body motility, especially at the beginning and the termination of REM sleep. Thus, in REM sleep, motor expression of the dream content is definitely inhibited but not completely absent, thus supporting Freud's conclusion that during dreaming there is a motor paralysis that permits the safe expression of generally unacceptable, unconscious impulses. In addition, the visual system is activated during REM sleep. This activation lends neurophysiological support to Freud's theory that during dreaming there is a regression from motor discharge to hallucinatory perception.

Sleep Disturbances

Psychiatric Disorders

Raybin and Detre reported a 20 per cent incidence of some form of sleep disturbance in a presumably normal population. The incidence of sleep disturbances in the general population appears to increase with age and with the presence of significant levels of anxiety or depression. Sleep disturbance is an extremely common complaint of patients with psychiatric disorders. A rough correlation has been observed between the severity of sleep disturbance and the severity of psychopathology.

Schizophrenia. Schizophrenic patients have markedly varying degrees of sleep disturbances, depending on whether the process is acute or chronic. The chronic schizophrenic patient or the patient in remission often does not present with any sleep difficulty. In acute schizophrenic episodes, severe sleep disturbances are frequent, often to the point of total insomnia.

In the sleep disturbances that accompany schizophrenia, phenothiazines with sedative effects, such as chlorpromazine (Thorazine) and thioridazine (Mellaril), are most helpful.

Depression. Sleep disturbance is one of the most consistent symptoms of depressive illness. In neurotically depressed patients, sleep disturbances are frequently found but are highly variable in type. Frequently, there is difficulty in falling asleep; difficulty in staying asleep, early morning awakening, and even hypersomnia may occur.

There have been many sleep laboratory studies of neurotic and psychotic depressed patients. These patients have less total sleep time and varying decreases in REM and stage 4 sleep. The decrease in stage 4 sleep is the most consistent finding.

In sleep disturbances associated with re-

tarded depressions, a tricyclic antidepressant with an energizing effect is used in divided doses during the day, together with 15 or 30 mg. of flurazepam (Dalmane) at bedtime. In agitated depressions, tricyclic antidepressants with sedating effects or thioridazine (Mellaril) may be used for treating both the depressive process and the accompanying symptoms of insomnia.

Insomnia. Insomnia may consist of difficulty in falling asleep, difficulty in staying asleep, too-early final awakening, or a combination of these. Transitional or situational insomnia is a universal phenomenon that is highly individualized and may occur in response to a variety of emotional or physical stresses, such as the loss of a loved one, job pressures, anxiety over examinations, anticipation of major life changes, and extended travel across time zones.

Insomnia is often a symptom associated with medical disorders, including any condition in which pain and physical discomfort are significant symptoms. When insomnia is associated with medical conditions, both physical and emotional factors must be considered, since it can be assumed that there is always an emotional response to a disease process.

The experience of Kales *et al.* has been that the majority of insomnia cases are secondary to psychological disturbances. More than 85 per cent of Kales' patients who were tested with the Minnesota Multiphasic Personality Inventory had one or more major scales in the pathologic range. The most frequently elevated scales were those for depression sociopathy, obsessive-compulsive features, and schizophrenic trends.

When patients who had been taking sleep medication chronically (months to years) were evaluated in the sleep laboratory while they continued to take their bedtime medication in the accustomed manner and dose, the patients experienced considerable difficulty in both falling asleep and staying asleep. These data, as well as clinical observations, suggest that these drugs are quite ineffective when used chronically.

The chronic use of multiple doses of hypnotic drugs was also found to result in a marked decrease in REM sleep and a marked decrease to complete absence of stages 3 and 4. During gradual withdrawal of the drugs, there was an immediate and marked increase in REM sleep, associated with an increase in the frequency and intensity of dreaming. With gradual withdrawal, the insomnia of the patients did not worsen, and in some cases sleep improved (see Figure 4).

The majority of patients with chronic or severe insomnia fall within the diagnostic category of the neuroses or personality disorders and have a history of chronic anxiety or anxiety mixed with depression. For these patients, best results are obtained with a combination of psychotherapy and pharmacological treatment. The authors recommend flurazepam as the pharmacological treatment for difficulty falling asleep, difficulty staying asleep, or both. For most patients, treatment is initiated with a dosage of 15 mg. at bedtime. Studies have shown that the drug is more effective on the second, third, or fourth night of consecutive use.

Insomniac patients often have difficulty in expressing or controlling their aggressive feelings. To many of these patients, going to sleep represents a loss of control, whereas the insomnia is a defense against this fear. Often, this need for control results in the insomniac patient's attempting to control or manipulate his sleep medication contrary to the physician's recommendations.

In cases of transient insomnia resulting from situational disturbances, pharmacological treatment with flurazepam may be used if the insomnia is severe or if the situational stress is likely to persist for a protracted period. In medical conditions, pharmacological treatment of the insomnia is often indicated in addition to treatment of the primary disease process.

Insomniac patients are encouraged to increase gradually their activity and exercise levels during the day but are also instructed not to exercise near their bedtime. Exercise several hours before sleep increases stage 4 sleep, but exercise just before bedtime may have an excitatory effect. Patients are encouraged to establish a regular bedtime hour, but they are advised not to remain in bed if they cannot sleep. Patients are also instructed to maintain relaxing mental activities before bedtime, since engaging in complex mental activity before bedtime can aggravate an insomniac condition. In cases of mild insomnia, these measures may be sufficient in themselves. In moderate to severe insomnia, these measures are not adequate in themselves but are useful adjuncts to the psychotherapy and pharmacological treatment.

Sleep Disorders

Most sleep disorders occur with the greatest frequency in childhood. During the period from birth through latency, isolated incidents of sleep disorders are universal.

During the first year of life, tensions in the child from any cause may be reflected in either a sleeping or an eating disturbance. Disturbances in sleep patterns between 1 and 3 years often relate to separation anxiety, with the child resisting sleep unless his mother remains in the room until he is asleep.

Between 12 and 18 months of age, there may be periods of refusal to go to sleep. These periods are felt to be related to the child's reluctance to give up the pleasures of the day during this period of growing motor mastery and progressive discovery of the world about him. During toilet training, the child resists sleep,

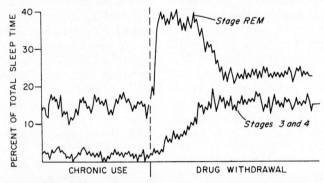

FIGURE 4. Sleep patterns during chronic drug use and after drug withdrawal. With many hypnotic drugs, chronic use, especially in multiple doses, produces a suppression of both REM and stages 3 and 4 sleep. When the drugs are withdrawn abruptly, there is often marked insomnia. When the subjects do fall asleep, there is a marked increase in REM sleep, associated with an increase in the frequency and intensity of dreaming. Nightmares may occur. These disturbances of sleep may result in even further insomina.

since conscious control of his bladder and activity is lessened with sleep and he fears that loss of control may result in a loss of parental approval, which is equated with a loss of love.

From 3 to 6 years, there is an increased frequency of nightmares, associated with the stresses and fears of the phallic-oedipal period, complicated by the young child's cognitive inability to distinguish among reality, fantasies, and dream content.

At latency, sleep patterns generally stabilize, although nightmares and insomnia still occasionally occur. The older the child the greater the relation between these sleep disturbances and significant psychopathology.

Somnambulism. Sleepwalking is not a rare nocturnal disturbance; its incidence in the general population is estimated to be from 1 to 6 per cent. It occurs predominantly in males and more commonly in children than in adults, and often there is a positive family history. Sleepwalkers have a significantly higher incidence of enuresis than does the general population.

Sleepwalking incidents occur exclusively during NREM sleep, especially stages 3 and 4 sleep, when dreaming is least likely to occur. During the incidents, experimental subjects have exhibited low levels of awareness, reactivity, and motor skill. The sleepwalkers in the sleep laboratory were totally amnesic for the events on awakening.

Follow-up studies demonstrated that most of the somnambulists had outgrown the disorder after several years, suggesting a delayed central nervous system maturation in these children and adolescents. Superimposed on this basic maturational process underlying somnambulism is the influence of environmental and psychological factors. Parents of child somnambulists report that often there is an increased incidence of sleepwalking events under conditions of stress, excitement, and environmental change.

Psychological disturbances are not primary factors in child and adolescent somnambulism. In adult somnambulists, psychological disturbances are frequent.

Somnambulistic incidents of one degree or another are universal. It is only when sleepwalking episodes are persistent and frequent that management is considered. The most important consideration in managing the child and adult sleepwalker is to protect him from injury. Pro-phylactic measures—such as locking doors and windows, removing potentially dangerous objects, and having him sleep on the first floor, if possible—are essential to the safety of the sleepwalker.

Night Terrors and Nightmares. The night terror—pavor nocturnus in children and incubus in adults—is characterized by intense anxiety, extreme levels of autonomic discharge, motility, vocalization, and little recall. Night terrors occur more frequently in children than in adults, and it is common for somnambulism and night terrors to occur in the same person, often simultaneously.

The nightmare that represents the ordinary, frightening dream is much more frequent than is the night terror. Nightmares occur at all ages. In a nightmare, as compared with the night terror, there is much less anxiety; autonomic changes, if present, are light; the person is more easily aroused; and the content recalled is more lengthy and developed.

Night terrors occur during stage 4 sleep, early in the sleep period, often as early as 15 to 30 minutes after sleep onset. The entire episode lasts for only a minute or two. Follow-up studies have shown that most children with night terrors eventually outgrow this disorder, suggesting a delayed central nervous system maturation. Psychological disturbances are not frequent in children with night terrors, but are common in adults with this disorder.

The nightmare characterized by detailed, unpleasant, and frightening recall usually occurs during normal REM sleep patterns. Nightmares in children are usually transient and situational. When nightmares persist in children or adults, they are frequently accompanied by other symptoms of psychopathology.

Conservative management and treatment are indicated in children with night terrors. Psychological evaluation and treatment are often indicated for adult patients with night terrors and for children and adults with persistent nightmares.

Enuresis. About 10 to 15 per cent of all children between 4 and 5 years of age continue to wet the bed. Even within the age range of 17 to 28 years, the incidence of enuresis may be as high as 1 to 3 per cent.

In the case of primary enuresis (since infancy, the patient has not been consistently dry for at least one period of several months), there is often a family history of the disorder. Organic disease, such as urological obstruction or epispadias, is occasionally the cause.

Secondary enuresis (patient has been consistently dry for at least one period of several months and then relapses) is often secondary to psychological factors. Occasionally, relapses are the result of organic factors, such as polyuria with diabetes, infection, or a degenerative neurological disorder.

Enuresis occurs predominantly during NREM sleep. Although the bed-wetting incidents occur throughout the night, there is some preponderance in the first third of the night.

In treating this disorder, the physician must first establish whether the enuresis is primary or secondary. In the case of primary enuresis, the probability of a maturational lag should be considered. In the case of secondary enuresis, psychological evaluation is often indicated. In both primary and secondary enuresis, young children should not be considered for urological procedures unless there is a specific indication of possible uropathology, since the psychological effects of these procedures may be quite detrimental.

Parents of enuretic children are invariably deeply concerned, but they should be educated to recognize the consequences of overreacting. They should be informed that, with patience and understanding, children generally outgrow this disorder. This counseling is extremely important in preventing the superimposition of severe guilt and anxiety on the enuresis problem through parental mishandling of the bed-wetting incidents. A number of investigators have reported that imipramine is effective in reducing enuretic frequency, especially if the dosage is properly adjusted. However, patients show a tendency to relapse when the drug is withdrawn. Whether the drug is effective with prolonged use and, if so, whether such potent pharmacological treatment should be used chronically in young children are matters that need to be evaluated. A promising physiological treatment consists of bladder training exercises in which the child drinks large amounts of fluid and delays micturition as long as possible. The child practices bladder control by stopping in midstream and then resuming.

Narcolepsy. Narcolepsy is characterized by irresistible sleep attacks of relatively short du-

ration, usually less than 15 minutes. In addition to the sleep attacks, there may be three auxiliary symptoms: cataplexy, sleep paralysis, and hypnagogic hallucinations. The sleep attacks are more frequent after meals, in monotonous situations, and as the day progresses. After a sleep attack, the patient usually awakens refreshed, and there is a refractory period of 1 to 5 hours until the next sleep attack occurs. Cataplexy, the most frequent auxiliary symptom, is a partial or complete loss of muscle tone that occurs largely in response to emotional or sudden stimulation; laughter is the most common instigator. The cataplectic attack may result in serious falls and injuries. Sleep paralysis occurs during the transition between wakefulness and sleep. It is more frequent when the patient is falling asleep, but may occur when the patient is waking. Hypnagogic hallucinations are false visual or auditory perceptions that occur just before falling asleep. They often occur simultaneously with sleep paralysis.

Establishing the diagnosis in this disorder is critical. Otherwise, the narcoleptic patients and their relatives, friends, and employers frequently misconstrue the symptoms as indicative of laziness, irresponsibility, or emotional instability. All-night EEG studies can assist in distinguishing narcolepsy with cataplexy from narcolepsy alone. Other laboratory tests, such as those for thyroid function and glucose tolerance, can be useful in differentiating narcolepsy from other disorders.

Narcoleptics whose attacks cannot be controlled by medication should not be allowed to perform certain potentially dangerous activities—for example, driving an automobile and operating certain industrial machinery.

Stimulant drugs, such as dextroamphetamine sulfate and methylphenidate HCl (Ritalin), are effective in the treatment of the sleep attacks of narcolepsy. Imipramine (Tofranil) is an effective treatment for the auxiliary symptoms but a relatively ineffective one for the sleep attacks. The combination of imipramine and the amphetamines to treat both cataplexy and sleep attacks may be dangerous.

Hypersomnia. Excessive sleep is characteristic of hypersomnia. In contrast to narcolepsy, the sleep is not irresistible but is usually much longer, lasting from many hours to several days. There are no auxiliary symptoms, as in narcolepsy. Postawakening or postdormital confusion is the most characteristic symptom of hypersominia.

Two periodic forms of hypersomnia are the Klein-Levin syndrome, associated with bulimia, and the Pickwickian syndrome, associated with obesity and respiratory insufficiency. Chronic hypersomnia may be a symptom of a central nervous system abnormality, such as occurs in head injuries, brain tumor, and cerebrovascular disorders. Chronic hypersomnia may also be a symptom of a psychological disorder, such as depression; as such, it represents an escape from the stresses of everyday life.

Hypersomniac patients should be evaluated

TABLE I
Sleep Disorders

Disorder	Sleep Laboratory Findings	Psychological Evaluation	Management and Treatment
Somnam-bulism	Incidents occur out of stage 4 sleep. Critical skills and reactivity are impaired during the incident.	In children, psychiatric disturbances are infrequent, but in adults they are frequent.	Prophylactic measures. Children frequently outgrow disorders. Psychiatric evaluation for adults.
Enuresis	Occurs out of all sleep stages. Misconception of dreaming as a frequent causal factor is explained.	Psychiatric disturbances are infrequent with primary enuresis. Psychological evaluation is often indicated for secondary enuresis.	Parental counseling and reassurance is critical so parental mishandling does not create psychiatric problems. Pharmacological treatment (Tofranil) may be indicated in older children.
Night Terrors	Occur out of stage 4 sleep. Characterized by extreme vocalizations, motility and autonomic response. Recall is minimal or absent.	Psychiatric disturbances are infrequent in children and frequent in adults.	Reassure parents that children frequently outgrow the disorder. For adults, psychological evaluation is often indicated. Use of stage 4 suppressants is under investigation.
Night-mares	Occur out of REM sleep. Characterized by less motility and autonomic response. Recall is frequent and elaborate.	Frequent nightmares in children or adults may indicate psychopathology.	Reassure parents that nightmares in children are often transient. If frequent in children or adults, psychological evaluation is indicated.
Narco-lepsy	Sleep attacks of narcolepsy may be accompanied by 3 auxiliary symptoms: cataplexy, sleep paralysis, and hypnogogic reverie. Cataplexy is accompanied by sleep onset REM periods.	Sleep attacks may be misinterpreted for laziness, irresponsibility, or emotional instability.	Establishing the diagnosis is critical. Stimulants are effective for sleep attacks. Imipramine is effective for auxiliary symptoms. There is danger in using both drugs simultaneously.
Hyper-somnia	Sleep stage patterns are normal but sleep is extended. Associated with postdormital confusion and difficulty in awakening. Autonomic parameters are increased.	Often is a symptom of psychological disorder, e.g., depression.	Stimulant drugs are effective. Neurological and psychological evaluation is important in establishing a diagnosis.
Insomnia	Complaints of insomniac patients have been verified in the sleep lab. Sleep of insomniacs is more aroused, i.e., heart rate and respiration are increased. Most hypnotic drugs lose their effectiveness within 2 weeks.	Insomnia is most often a symptom of psychological disturbance, and not a primary disorder. Depression is a common feature.	When insomnia is secondary to medical conditions, pharmacological treatment may be useful. If psychological factors are primary, pharmacological therapy should be combined with psychotherapy.

to determine whether a significant neurological or psychological disturbance exists; if a disorder is found, it should be treated appropriately. The stimulant drugs used in narcolepsy are also effective in the treatment of hypersomnia.

Sleep Apnea. Sleep apnea has been reported to be a universal occurrence in normal infants between 1 and 3 months of age. The incidence of the disorder in sudden infant death syndrome siblings is reported to be 5 times greater than in the normal population.

Sleep apnea in infants occurs most frequently during REM sleep. Sleep apnea has also been noted in hypersomnia, narcolepsy, and insomnia and has been shown to occur during both REM and NREM sleep. Guilleminault and associates (1973) suggest that as many as 10 per cent of all insomniacs may have associated sleep apnea. However, Kales and Kales (1974) report that in 50 insomniac patients studied in their laboratory none was found to have sleep apnea. This suggests that the incidence of sleep apnea in insomnia is much lower and may be restricted to patients with specific central or cardiopulmonary defects.

Table I summarizes the sleep laboratory findings, the results of psychological evaluation, and recommendations for management and treatment of the most prevalent sleep disorders.

Neurological Conditions

Mental Retardation. Feinberg et al. evaluated sleep variables of mongolian and phenylpyruvic oligophrenia (PKU) patients. The amount of REM sleep in the retardates, compared with control subjects, showed only an equivocal reduction. However, the retardates had markedly lower amounts of eye movement activity. In a further study, Feinberg demonstrated a significant positive correlation between the amount of REM sleep and estimates of intellectual level in a group of both retarded and normal subjects—that is, the lower the intelligence quotient, the lower the amount of REM sleep.

Other investigators evaluated the sleep of mentally retarded patients ranging in age from 3 months to 62 years and found that the patients between 3 and 35 years, as compared with the controls, showed a definite decrease in total sleep time.

Chronic Brain Syndrome. In comparing young and aged normal subjects and patients with chronic brain syndrome (CBS), Feinberg and associates noted that normal aging is associated with decreased total sleep, decreased stage 4 sleep, and a tendency toward decreased REM sleep. Pathological aging, as manifested by the CBS group, resulted in an accentuation of these changes. Within the CBS group, total sleep time was highly and significantly correlated with scores of intellectual function— that is, with lowered intellectual functioning, there was less total sleep time. In addition, several CBS subjects awakened regularly from REM sleep in states of agitation and delirium lasting 5 to 10 minutes, and they had to be physically restrained.

Epilepsy. Seizures are frequent during sleep; some patients have seizures only during sleep. Ross, Johnson, and Walter obtained all-night recordings from 13 patients with petit mal attacks or grand mal seizures or both. No differences were noted in the over-all sleep patterns of these patients, as compared with nonepileptic subjects, indicating that the discharges had little effect on general sleep measurements.

Parkinson's Disease. Patients with parkinsonism were studied in the sleep laboratory before the administration of L-dopa and during initial, short-term, long-term, and chronic usage. The results with these parkinsonian patients clearly indicate that before drug administration they sleep very poorly and have difficulty in falling asleep and in staying asleep. As their condition improves after the administration of L-dopa, these patients may become much more aware of their pre-existing sleep difficulties.

REFERENCES

Broughton, R. J. Sleep disorders: Disorders of arousal? Science, *159:* 1070, 1968.

Fisher, C. Psychoanalytic implications of recent research on sleep and dreaming. J. Am. Psychoanal. Assoc, *13:* 197, 1965.

Fisher, C., Kahn, E., Edwards, A., and Davis, D. M. A psychophysiological study of nightmares and night terrors. The suppression of stage 4 night terrors with diazepam. Arch. Gen. Psychiatry, *28:* 252, 1973.

Guilleminault, C., Eldridge, F. L., and Dement, W. C. Insomnia with sleep apnea: A new syndrome. Science, *181:* 856, 1973.

Hartmann, E. Sleep requirements: Long sleepers, short sleepers, variable sleepers, and insomniacs. Psychosomatics, *14:* 95, 1973.

Kales, A., Bixler, E. O., Tan, T. L., Scharf, M. B., and Kales, J. D. Chronic hypnotic use: Ineffectiveness, drug withdrawal insomnia and hypnotic drug dependence. J. A. M. A., *227:* 513, 1974.

Kales, A., and Kales, J. D. Sleep disorders: Recent findings in the diagnosis and treatment of disturbed sleep. N. Engl. J. Med., *29:* 487, 1974.

Rechtschaffen, A., and Dement, W. C. Narcolepsy and hypersomnia. In *Sleep: Physiology and Pathology*, A. Kales, editor, p. 119. J. B. Lippincott, Philadelphia, 1969.

Zarcone, V. Narcolepsy. N. Engl. J. Med., *288:* 1156, 1973.

2.4. NEUROCHEMISTRY AND BEHAVIOR: AN OVERVIEW

Introduction

Neurochemistry is concerned with describing the chemical contents of the brain—their synthesis and degradation and how some regulate the metabolism of others. Its units are molecules and chemical reactions. The challenge to neurochemistry is to explain how the molecules and chemical reactions in the brain give rise to behavior.

Chemical Components of the Brain

The first step in developing a chemistry of the nervous system is to identify its chemical constituents. The nervous system is extremely rich in lipids. This richness is due to the high concentration of lipids in the extensive membrane surface of neurons and glia. The gangliosides appear to be associated primarily with neurons. An abnormality in the degradation of gangliosides is responsible for Tay-Sachs disease, a genetic disorder of infancy associated with severe mental retardation.

Acetylcholine was found in the vagus nerve. The catecholamines were first identified in the adrenal gland. Studies of the brain have yielded important compounds like the amino acid gamma-aminobutyric acid and the tripeptide thyrotropin-releasing factor, obtained respectively by extraction of the whole and specific regions of the brain. Prostaglandins, unusual lipids that influence neuronal function, were first found in the male reproductive tract.

There are thousands of brain proteins, many of which are shared with other organs. Some control specific brain functions. Acetylcholine and norepinephrine are synthesized neurotransmitter compounds. S-100 is found only in tissues of the nervous system and has been shown to be associated with astroglia. Another protein, tubulin, is present in all organs but is most highly concentrated in the nervous system, where it is the subunit of the tubules found in neurites.

Metabolism of Brain Constituents

All metabolic processes are catalyzed by specific proteins, the enzymes. One metabolic process that is particularly active in the brain oxidizes glucose, the brain's major source of energy. Hypoglycemia, like brain anoxia due to cerebral vascular disease, illustrates how general metabolic abnormalities in the brain may cause mental disturbances. General depression of over-all brain function leads not only to a general reduction in brain function but also to specific symptoms.

In recent years, the metabolism of many other brain constituents—neurotransmitters, lipids, proteins, and nucleic acids—has been studied. The relationship between behavior and the metabolism of some of these compounds, particularly catecholamines and indoleamines, is under extensive investigation. But the fact that drugs that affect amines may have behavioral effects is far more specific and provocative than the finding that hypoglycemia or anoxia may have behavioral effects.

Regulation of Metabolism

Two major classes of regulatory mechanisms have been discovered. One involves an alteration in the rate of synthesis of the enzyme involved in a specific metabolic reaction. The other is based on a structural change of an existing enzyme that changes its activity.

The synthesis of specific enzymes in mammalian cells is controlled not only by specific substrates but also by regulatory compounds, such as hormones. The hormones associate with specific receptor proteins present on the surface of those cells that are targets for the hormone.

Structural changes in proteins can be produced in a variety of ways. For example, regulatory molecules may bind reversibly to an enzyme and thereby change its state of activity. An example in the nervous system is the interaction of norepinephrine with the enzyme tyrosine hydroxylase. Feedback inhibition plays a role in regulating the rate of synthesis of norepinephrine.

Other examples of structural changes in proteins that alter function involve the covalent addition of residues to the proteins. For example, the addition of phosphate groups to proteins by enzymes called protein kinases may activate these proteins.

Evidence suggests that neurotransmitters in

nervous system tissue may catalyze the phosphorylation of specific proteins, which may play an important role in regulating the resultant activity of the cells in question.

Regulation of Intercellular Relationships

Neurons are specialized to communicate only with a restricted group of cells that they physically contact at synapses. By releasing a neurotransmitter, the presynaptic cell alters the state of activity of the postsynaptic cell. The process of neural transmission may set in motion alterations in the synthesis or state of activity of specific proteins in the postsynaptic cell.

If the neurons that innervate a cell are destroyed, it may undergo profound metabolic changes and may even die. Some evidence indicates that neurotransmitter release and the resultant activity of the postsynaptic cell are necessary and sufficient for maintaining the availability and specific enzymatic composition of the postsynaptic cell. In addition, factors other than neurotransmitters may be released by the presynaptic cell and influence the postsynaptic cell.

Cells may influence each other not only by secreting regulatory molecules but also by specifically sticking to each other without exchange of materials. It seems likely that when neurons form synapses with each other such reactions occur. Through interaction between surface molecules, the metabolism of both cells may be regulated.

Still another problem in the regulation of intercellular relationships involves the question of how cells specifically choose to associate with specific others. For example, it is important to determine how motor neurons from the spinal cord come to innvervate certain muscles. Schizophrenia may not be an enzymatic abnormality but, rather, one of a faulty wiring diagram.

Regulating the Function of Neuronal Circuits

Since the nervous system is organized in terms of specific intercellular interactions, behavioral changes are expected if the efficacy of these interactions are changed. This concept is the basis of psychopharmacology. Many of the drugs used to modify human behavior are known to change the state of activity of enzymes involved in the metabolism of neurotransmitter compounds or of the postsynaptic receptors for these neurotransmitters. The altered balance in the state of activity of the neuronal pathways leads to behavioral changes.

Another behavioral problem, memory storage, has also been examined, using a neurochemical strategy. Since many of these processes depend on the synthesis of proteins, attempts were made to block memory by injecting drugs that block brain protein synthesis. For example, mice have been trained after injections of cycloheximide that block about 95 per cent of brain protein-synthesizing capacity. The drug persists for several hours, and training was done while it was exerting its maximal effect. The mice were then tested at various times thereafter to determine whether they remembered what they had learned. If brain protein synthesis is required for memory storage, memory should be impaired.

The results of these experiments clearly indicated that protein synthesis is not required for the *learning* of simple tasks in the mouse. Thus, mice whose brain protein synthesis was markedly inhibited learned as well as controls did. Furthermore, in many situations, memory was normal when the animals were tested one or several hours after training. This finding suggests that memory for this period of time is also independent of brain protein synthesis. However, in many experiments it has been shown that memory beyond this time was strikingly impaired if brain protein synthesis was inhibited at the time of training. Therefore brain protein synthesis appears necessary for long term memory but not for memory for several hours after training. Presumably, the mechanism of memory storage during learning, and for hours after training was based on a structural change in a pre-existent protein. Such structural changes in proteins are not affected by the inhibition of protein synthesis.

The relevance of these experiments to this discussion is in emphasizing that application of the increasing general understanding of biological regulatory processes is, indeed, pointing the way to an analysis of behavioral problems through biochemical experiments. The ultimate problem, understanding how regulation of chemical processes controls behavior, seems approachable.

REFERENCES

Albers, R. W., Siegel G., Katzman, R., and Agranoff, B. W., editors. *Basic Neurochemistry*. Little, Brown, Boston, 1972.

Barondes, S. H., editor *Cellular Dynamics of the Neuron.* Academic Press, New York, 1969.

Lajtha, A., editor. *Handbook of Neurochemistry*, 7 volumes. Plenum Press, New York, 1969.

Quarton, G. C., Melnechuck, T., and Schmitt, F. O., editors. *The Neurosciences: A Study Program*, Rockefeller University Press, New York, 1967.

Schmitt, F. O., editor. *The Neurosciences: A Second Study Program*, Rockefeller University Press, New York, 1970.

Schneider, D., editor. *Proteins of the Nervous System*, Raven Press, New York, 1973.

2.5. NEUROCHEMISTRY OF BEHAVIOR: RECENT ADVANCES

Metabolism

Brain metabolism is characterized by an exceedingly high consumption of oxygen and an almost exclusive use of glucose as a source of energy.

Normal Respiration

As blood traverses brain tissue, compounds used for metabolic purposes are extracted from the arterial blood, and the end products of metabolism are discharged into the venous circulation. The measurement of arteriovenous differences in the composition of cerebral blood reveals the characteristic aspects of brain respiration (see Table I). The fall in oxygen concentration is significantly greater in the brain than in other organs.

The respiratory demands of the brain are underscored by the disproportionate share of blood provided to the brain. Although this organ constitutes only 2.5 per cent of the adult body weight, it receives 15 per cent of cardiac output, extracting 25 per cent of the blood oxygen in the process.

Altered Brain Metabolism

Brain death. Matakas and his associates (1973) make reference to the increasingly common issue of brain death. The introduction of artificial life-support systems and intensive care units creates a condition in which the organism survives after cerebral circulation is completely and permanently disrupted, a situation defined as brain death. Matakas et al. suggest that angiography is the most reliable method of determining the arrest of cerebral circulation. Ouaknine et al. (1973) describe a combination of procedures that can be relied upon to confirm brain death.

Brain tissue can tolerate a 10 to 20 per cent decrease in the oxygen content of ambient air without cerebral respiratory change. This tolerance is due in part to compensatory increase in cranial blood flow. Different parts of the brain vary in their sensitivity in oxygen deprivation. Neurons of the globus pallidus, cerebellum, and

TABLE I
Changes in Blood on Its Passing through the Brain*

Constituent	Blood Levels		Venous-Arterial Levels ±Standard Deviation
	Arterial	Venous	
Oxygen			
Content (ml./100 ml.)	19.6	12.9	−6.7 ± 0.8
Capacity (ml./100 ml.)	20.9	20.8	−0.1
Saturation (%)	93.9	61.8	−31.7 ± 3.9
Carbon dioxide			
Content (ml./100 ml.)	48.2	54.8	+6.6 ± 0.8
Tension (mm. Hg)	39.9	49.9	+10.0 ± 1.2
Glucose (mg./100 ml.)	92.0	82.0	−9.8 ± 1.7
Lactic acid (mg./100 ml.)	9.9	11.5	+1.6 ± 0.9
Free amino acids (mg. α-amino-N/100 ml. plasma)	6.16	6.02	−0.14
pH at 38°C	7.42	7.37	−0.05
Inorganic phosphate (mg./100 ml.)	3.4	3.4	0
Total base (meq./liter serum)	152.9	154.1	+1.2 ± 1.2

* The blood content of the brain is relatively low at about 3 to 3.5 per cent of the total volume, compared with the cerebrospinal fluid content of some 9 per cent, and is renewed rapidly. In the adult human, with a total body blood volume of 5,500 ml., the blood flows through the brain at a rate of 750 ml. per min. (From H. McIllwain and H. S. Bachelard, *Biochemistry and the Central Nervous System*. Williams & Wilkins, Baltimore, 1971.)

cerebral white matter are the most readily affected by anoxia.

Normal blood glucose concentrations are 80 to 100 mg. per 100 ml. When there is a drop to 50 to 70 mg. per 100 ml., human beings experience changes in sensation, impaired behavior, and coma. There are concomitant alterations in the electrical activity of the brain. The compensatory increase in blood flow seen during anoxia does not take place during episodes of hypoglycemia. The provision of mannose and maltose to hypoglycemic individuals restores normal behavior, a consequence of the conversion of these compounds to glucose. Prolonged periods of low blood sugar, seen in periods of starvation, result in the adaptation of the brain to the use of other oxidizable substrates.

Occlusion of the blood supply to the brain for more than 5 minutes at 37° C. produces tissue damage. If the temperature is lowered to 25° C., tissue can survive for periods of 15 to 20 minutes. During neurosurgery, the blood supply to the brain has been cut off for nearly 45 minutes at 15° C. without observable damage. Oxygen consumption is markedly below normal in these episodes. General anesthetics also decrease brain respiration.

The cerebral respiration rate is increased after sympathetic discharge and anxiety reactions. The infusion of sufficient epinephrine to cause a 20 per cent rise in mean arterial blood pressure induces active neural metabolic activity.

The diseases of aging—such as organic dementia, cerebral atherosclerosis, and senile psychoses—are associated with decreased rates of cerebral blood flow and respiration. The presence of nitrogenous metabolites in the blood of patients with renal failure appears to produce intoxication. Brain respiration is decreased by 35 per cent in the confusional state, but the general metabolic rate is normal. Coincident with the confusional state and coma seen in uncontrolled diabetes is a decrease of as much as 50 per cent in cerebral oxygen uptake.

Severe damage to the liver, with subsequent accumulation of numerous toxic substances in the cerebrospinal fluid, may lead to hepatic coma. In this condition cerebral respiration may decrease to 65 per cent of the normal value.

Arteriovenous oxygen differences and cerebral respiratory rates remain within normal limits of schizophrenic patients. However, this lack of observed change does not exclude the possibility of focal changes in metabolism.

Composition

Amino Acids and Proteins

Amino acids are nitrogen-containing compounds that serve as the building blocks of protein. Cerebral amino acids and proteins participate in all aspects of neural function. More than two-thirds of the free amino nitrogen in the brain is represented by glutamic acid, glutamine, N-acetylaspartic acid, and γ-aminobutyric acid (GABA). Amino acids, free or as proteins, account for nearly half the dry weight of the brain. GABA and N-acetylaspar-

TABLE II

Free Amino Acids and Related Compounds of the Brain*

Compound	Content (μmoles/100 g.)	Ratio Brain/ Blood Plasma
N-Acetylaspartate	470–974	
Alanine	14–94	2.5
β-Alanine	7	
γ-Aminobutyrate	83–227	300
Ammonia	16–26	5
Arginine	7–16	*c*. 1
Asparagine	11	
Aspartate	153–272	300
Citrulline	2.5	
Cystathionine	4–18	
Cystine	4	
Glutamate	781–1250	*c*. 150
Glutamine	215–560	10
Glutathione	90–340	
Glycine	55–146	
Histidine	6–9	*c*. 1
Isoleucine	6–9	
Leucine	7–14	0.7
Lysine	11–22	0.7
Methionine	8–10	
Ornithine	4–5	
Proline	6–12	
Phenylalanine	5–9	1.4
Serine	39–177	6
Taurine	125–535	40
Threonine	9–29	2
Tryptophan	2·5	
Tyrosine	3–11	1.4
Urea	340–417	0.7
Vahne	12–18	*c*. 1

* From H. McIllwain and H. S. Bachelard, *Biochemistry and the Central Nervous System*. Williams & Wilkins, Baltimore, 1971.

tic acid are derivatives of dietary amino acids, formed by enzymatic action within the central nervous system. Because of their high concentration within the brain, they are considered characteristic of the organ. Other amino acids and related compounds are present only in trace amounts (see Table II).

In the human brain, S-100, a protein specific to the nervous system, is found primarily in white matter and is highly concentrated within glial cells. It appears to be related to learning.

A low molecular weight polypeptide termed scotophobin has been isolated in the brains of animals that had been trained to avoid the dark. The intracerebral injection of scotophobin into control animals resulted in a similar avoidance of the dark.

More than 30 inherited disorders of amino acid metabolism have been found to produce abnormal formation or functioning of the nervous system (see Table III). Mental retardation is a common feature. Convulsions, ataxia, and disorders of speech are also frequently observed. The primary abnormality in these disorders may involve systemic changes in enzyme activity, the complete absence of an enzyme, changes in enzymatic kinetic properties, or disturbances in the absorption of dietary amino acids. Abnormalities of absorption reflect the involvement of membranes in the inherited amino acid disorders. In contrast with other metabolic genetic diseases, the severe disabilities in mental and neurological function caused by these diseases are often prevented by dietary restrictions.

Lipids

Cholesterol is the only sterol of quantitative importance in the brain, and it is the single most abundant constituent in the organ, after water. Most cerebral cholesterol is synthesized locally and is most concentrated in the myelin nerve sheaths.

The brain is rich in lipids but low in its concentration of fatty acids and simple glycerides. The presence of these compounds in higher concentrations in other tissues, where they may be used to provide metabolic energy, reflects the inability of cerebral tissue to replace carbohydrates with fat in order to support its function.

The phosphorus-containing lipids of the brain represent about 50 per cent of total brain lipids, and the plasmalogens constitute between 18 and 30 per cent of the cerebral phospholipids. Myelin is high in plasmalogen content.

The major sphingolipids in the brain are sphingomyelin, cerebroside, sulfatide, and ganglioside. Also recognized are compounds known as ceramide oligohexosides.

The term "lipidoses" or "lipodystrophies" describes a group of inherited neurometabolic disturbances that result in the accumulation of normal and abnormal sphingolipids in the brain

TABLE III

*Mental Defect or Disorder Associated with Abnormal Metabolism of Amino Acids**

Disease	Amino Acid Involved	Enzymatic or Equivalent Defect	Chemicals Augmented in Urine
Argininosuccinic aciduria	Arginine	Argininosuccinase	Argininosuccinic acid
Citrullinemia	Citrulline	Argininosuccinic acid synthetase	Citrulline
Cystathioninuria	Methionine	Cystathionase	Cystathionine
Hartnup disease	Tryptophan	(Intestinal absorption)	Many amino acids and indoles
Histidinemia	Histidine	Histidase	Histidine
Homocystinuria	Methionine	Cystathionine synthetase	Homocystine
Hyperammonemia	Ornithine	Ornithine transcarbamylase	Ammonia
Maple syrup urine disease	Leucine Isoleucine Valine	Oxidative decarboxylation of corresponding branched chain α-oxo-acids	Branched chain α-oxo-acids and α-hydroxy acids
Phenylketonuria	Phenylalanine	Phenylalanine hydroxylase	Phenylpyruvic acid; other metabolites

* From H. McIllwain and H. S. Bachelard, *Biochemistry and the Central Nervous System.* Williams & Wilkins, Baltimore, 1971.

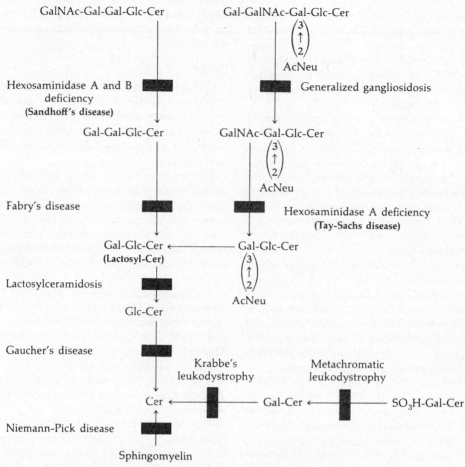

FIGURE 1. Catabolism of major glycosphingolipids and of sphingomyelin in man. The absence of a hydrolase in a specific known disorder is indicated by a *solid bar*. The following abbreviations are used: Cer, ceramide; Gal, galactosyl; Glc, glucosyl; GalNAc, *N*-acetylgalactosaminidyl; AcNeu, *N*-acetylneuraminidyl. (From White, A., Handler, P., and Smith, E. S., *Principles of Biochemisty*. Copyright © 1973 by McGraw-Hill, Inc. Used with permission of the McGraw-Hill Book Co.)

and in various other organs of the body. The deficiency of a hydrolase enzyme results in a disorder (see Figure 1). Different clinical syndromes arise, depending on the enzyme involved and the lipid accumulated. The outstanding feature of these disorders is neural degeneration as an early presenting sign, followed by death before the age of 5 years (see Table IV).

Prostaglandins have been identified in the human brain in association with microsomes and nerve-ending particles. Because of their presence in the brain, these acidic lipids are being investigated as possible neurotransmitters.

Electrolytes

Electrolytes play an important role in forming the internal environment by which the human nervous system responds to external events. Ionic compounds participate in the synapse and in the changes associated with neuronal conduction of impulses. The metabolism of the neurotransmitters depends on electrolytes.

The familial disorder Wilson's disease, hepatolenticular degeneration, is the most widely discussed disturbance of copper metabolism. Monoamine oxidase (MAO) and dopamine-β-hydroxylase are copper-dependent. The white

TABLE IV

The Sphingolipodystrophies

Disease	Enzyme Defect	Accumulated Sphingolipid
Tay-Sachs	Hexosaminidase A	Monosialoceramidetrihexoside (ganglioside GM_2)
Gaucher's	β-Glucosidase (glucocerebrosidase)	Ceramide glucoside (glucocerebroside)
Fabry's	α-Galactosidase	Ceramide trihexoside
Niemann-Pick	Sphingomyelinase	Sphingomyelin
Globoid leukodystrophy (Krabbe's disease)	β-Galactosidase (galactocerebrosidase)	Ceramide galactoside (galactocerebroside) (galactosylceramide)
Metachromatic leukodystrophy	Sulfatidase	Sulfatide (ceramide-galactose-sulfate)
Generalized gangliosidosis	β-Galactosidase	Monosialoceramidetetrahexoside (ganglioside GM_1)
Sandhoff's (variant of Tay-Sachs)	Hexosaminidase A and B	Globiside plus ganglioside GM_2
Lactosylceramidosis	β-Galactosidase (β-galactosyl hydrolase)	Ceramide lactoside (lactosylceramide)

matter of the central nervous system undergoes severe degeneration in states of copper deficiency.

A deficiency of manganese elicits bizarre behavior, primarily because of faulty mucopolysaccharide production. Hyperirritability is a prominent feature.

Behavioral changes develop in iron-deficient persons, but these changes appear to be the result of impaired hemoglobin function with secondary hypoxia or anoxia in the brain.

Anorexia, apathy, decreased sexual activity, and lethargy are associated with low body zinc levels. Task performance and emotionality are also decreased.

There is an increase in sodium retention during depression, and nonpsychiatric patients have been reported to experience psychotic episodes because of low sodium levels of body fluids.

The release of acetylcholine and norepinephrine depends on the presence of calcium. Nerve membrane changes that permit sodium to enter the cell and potassium to leave the cell during the propagation of impulses appear to be sensitive to calcium concentration.

Enzymes

Enzymes are proteins whose function is the catalysis of chemical reactions. Disorders of amino acid, carbohydrate, and lipid metabolism may be ascribed to enzyme disturbances.

Most but not all metabolic steps require a highly specific enzyme. Many of the enzymes specific to the brain are involved in the synthesis and degradation of neurotransmitters.

Enzymes associated with acetylcholine activity are the best understood neurotransmitter catalysts. Through the action of these enzymes, acetylcholine effects are limited in their duration, and fresh supplies are readily available for release.

Attention is also focused on the enzymes of catecholamine synthesis and degradation. Deficiencies in the amount and function of these enzymes, as well as the presence of abnormal enzymes, have been associated with mental illness. Platelet MAO activity in schizophrenic patients is markedly lower than in normal persons.

The enzyme adenyl cyclase catalyzes the conversion of ATP to cyclic AMP. Because it has the highest tissue concentration of adenyl cyclase, the brain has the greatest capacity to synthesize cyclic AMP. The involvement of this compound in neural activity is reflected by increased cellular levels of cyclic AMP after neural and electrical excitation, alterations in membrane potentials, administration of psychotomimetic agents, and release of neurotransmitter compounds, especially norepinephrine, histamine, and serotonin.

Urinary concentrations of cyclic AMP increase during manic episodes and decrease during periods of depression. Norepinephrine has been reported to increase brain levels of cyclic AMP, a phenomenon that is inhibited by some psychoactive drugs. Electroconvulsive therapy raises the levels of cyclic AMP.

Vitamins

The vitamins are required for metabolic processes. Numerous enzyme systems depend on vitamins as cofactors. Vitamin deficiencies produce defects in neurological and mental functions. Thiamine deficiency, for example, results in the Wernicke-Korsakoff syndrome and beriberi. A lack of vitamin B_{12} can cause subacute degeneration of the spinal cord.

Neurotransmitters and Neurosecretion

The currently accepted candidates for designation as neurotransmitters include acetylcholine, dopamine, histamine, GABA, norepinephrine, glycine, glutamic acid, and serotonin (5-hydroxytryptamine). These substances are synthesized and released by nerve cells. Neurosecretions are released by glandlike neurons that are anatomically and functionally related to endocrine functions. Such neuroendocrine relations are best seen in the hypothalamohypophyseal system.

Two neurosecretory centers, the supraoptic and paraventricular hypothalamic nuclei, have been identified as the sites of synthesis of vasopressin (antidiuretic hormone) and oxytocin. These hormones are stored at the axon terminals. Neurophysin is a carrier protein that binds vasopressin and oxytocin and, thus, mediates the storage and release of these hormones.

Myelin

Myelin is the material that covers axons of some cells and gives them their white appearance. The lack of observed ionic movement through the myelin sheath reflects its role as an electrical insulator. Some movement of ions does take place at interruptions in the covering—termed nodes or clefts—permitting rapid conduction of impulses.

A disorder such as metachromatic leukodystrophy, which produces degeneration of myelin secondary to the accumulation of granules in the myelin-forming Schwann cells, is not considered a demyelinating disease. Multiple sclerosis (disseminated sclerosis) is such a disorder and is the most common nervous system disease in the Northern hemisphere.

Blood-Brain Barrier

A series of barriers serve to create and maintain the internal milieu of the central nervous system. The blood-brain barrier refers to the interface between the capillary wall and the brain substance, and the blood-cerebrospinal fluid (CSF) barrier is represented by the choroid

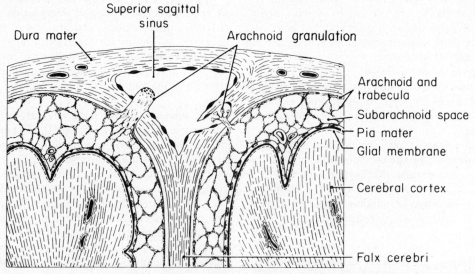

FIGURE 2. Diagram of meningeal-cortical relation. Arachnoid granulations may penetrate dural sinus or terminate in lateral lacuna of sinus. The pia is firmly anchored to the cortex by the glial membrane. (From Truex, R. C., and Carpenter, M. B., *Human Neuroanatomy*. Williams & Wilkins, Baltimore, 1969.)

plexus. A third barrier, between the CSF and the brain, mediates the transfer of this fluid into the brain through the ventricular lining or pia-glial membrane. The CSF-blood barrier is concerned with the exchange of the fluid directly into the blood vessels of the subarachnoid space (see Figure 2). When the blood-brain barrier is destroyed, as occurs in excised tissue, materials penetrate the brain indiscriminately at the cut surface.

Cerebrospinal Fluid

The intracellular compartment of the central nervous system is represented by the neurons and glia. The extracellular compartment is composed of spaces filled with blood, cerebrospinal fluid, or extracellular fluid. The extracellular fluid, also called the interstitial fluid, immediately surrounds the cells of the brain and constitutes 25 per cent of the cerebral volume. The CSF serves as a protective cushion against trauma and acts as a pathway by which substances are transported to and removed from the central neural tissue.

REFERENCES

Banik, N. L., and Davison, A. N. Isolation of purified basic protein from human brain. J. Neurochem., *21:* 489, 1973.

Barbeau, A. G.A.B.A. and Huntington's chorea. Lancet, *2:* 1499, 1973.

Bickerstaff, E. R. *Neurological Examination in Clinical Practice*. Blackwell, Oxford, 1973.

Bogoch, S. *The Biochemistry of Memory*. Oxford University Press, London, 1968.

Dekaban, A. S., and Herman, M. M. Childhood, juvenile, and adult cerebral lipidoses. Arch. Pathol., *97:* 65, 1974.

Glen, A. I. M., and Reading, H. W. Regulatory action of lithium in manic-depressive illness. Lancet, *2:* 1239, 1973.

Greep, R. O., and Weiss, L. *Histology*. McGraw-Hill, New York, 1973.

Haglid, K. G., and Starrou, D. Water-soluble and pentanol-extractable proteins in human brain normal tissue and human brain tumours, with special reference to S-100 protein. J. Neurochem., *20:* 1523, 1973.

Hawkins, D., and Pauling, L., editors. *Orthomolecular Psychiatry*. W. H. Freeman, San Francisco, 1973.

Lipton, M. A. Schizophrenia: A dubious approach. Med. World News, 41, 1973.

Marx, J. L. Biomedical science: Immunology and neurobiology to the fore. Science, *182:* 1329, 1973.

Matakas, F., Cervos-Navarro, J., and Schneider, H. Experimental brain death: Morphology and structure of the brain. J. Neurol. Neurosurg. Psychiatry, *36:* 497, 1973.

McIlwain, H., and Bachelard, H. S. *Biochemistry of the Central Nervous System*. Williams & Wilkins, Baltimore, 1971.

Meckler, J., editor. *Introduction to Neuroscience*. C. V. Mosby, St. Louis, 1972.

Ouaknine, G., Kosary, I. Z., Braham, J., Czerniak, P., and Nathan, H. Laboratory criteria of brain death. J. Neurosurg., *39:* 429, 1973.

Pampiglione, G., and Harden, A. Neurophysiological identification of a late infantile form of "neuronal lipidosis." J. Neurol. Neurosurg. Psychiatry, *36:* 68, 1973.

Prockop, L. D. Disorders of cerebrospinal fluid and brain extracellular fluid. In *Biology of Brain Dysfunction*, G. E. Gaull, editor, vol. 1, p. 229. Plenum Press, New York, 1973.

Schultz, J., and Daly, J. W. Adenosine 3′,5′-monophosphate in guinea pig cerebral cortical slices: Effects of α- and β-adrenergic agents, histamine, serotorin, and adenosine. Science, *21:* 573, 1973.

Seiler, N. Enzymes, In *Handbook of Neurochemistry*, A. Latjha, editor, vol. 1, p. 325. Plenum Press, New York, 1969.

Singer, I., and Rotenberg, D. Mechanisms of lithium action. N. Engl. J. Med., *289:* 254, 1973.

Smythies, J. R. Nicotinamide treatment of schizophrenia. Lancet, *2:* 1450, 1973.

Vergara, F., Plum, F., and Duffy, T. E. Ketoglutaramate: Increased concentrations in the cerebrospinal fluid of patients in hepatic coma. Science, *183:* 81, 1974.

White, A., Handler, P., and Smith, E. S. *Principles of Biochemistry*. McGraw-Hill, New York, 1973.

Zimmerman, E. A., Carmel, P. W., Husain, M. K., Ferin, M., Tannenbaum, M., Frantz, A. G., and Robinson, A. G. Vasopressin and neurophysin: High concentrations in monkey hypophyseal portal blood. Science, *182:* 925, 1973.

2.6. THE BRAIN AND PSYCHIATRY

Introduction

The brain consists of the mass of nervous tissue contained within the cranium; it includes the cerebrum, cerebellum, midbrain, pons, and medulla oblongata. The field of psychiatry—seeking to understand feelings, perception, intellect, memory, and affect—has often avoided such anatomical designations, making reference, instead, to that faculty of the brain by which these functions are mediated—the mind or psyche. In recent years, however, there has been a revival of interest in theories that propose neurobiological disorders as the basis of emotional and behavioral dysfunction. Increasingly sophisticated and precise research techniques are enabling investigators to probe the deepest aspects of the brain and to observe events that correlate with observed behavior. The rapidly expanding body of information provided by such efforts is obscuring the boundaries of interest between psychiatry and other disciplines.

Neuroanatomy

Forebrain

The external surface of an intact brain is represented by the cerebral hemispheres. Numerous furrows—sulci or fissures—are present on the cerebral surface, along with elevated regions called gyri. On the basis of these landmarks, the cerebral hemispheres are divided into five areas: frontal, parietal, occipital, temporal, and insular lobes. With the exception of the insular lobe, which is buried beneath the lateral fissure, each lobe is visible on the surface of the brain (see Figure 1). The two cerebral hemispheres are almost completely separated by the longitudinal fissure; they communicate with each other primarily through the corpus callosum, which forms the floor of this fissure. The outer covering of the hemispheres is formed by the cerebral cortex, which consists of some 14×10^9 nerve cells. Beneath the cortex are several areas of white matter and nuclear masses. Prominent are the basal ganglia, made up of the caudate, lenticular, and amygdaloid nuclei and the claustrum (see Figure 2). Because of their striated appearance, the caudate and lenticular nuclei are called the corpus striatum. Below the basal ganglia, structures derived from the diencephalon are seen. These are the thalamic and hypothalamic nuclei. They are closely associated with the ventricular system, representing the floor and lateral walls of the third ventricle.

Midbrain

Internally, the midbrain can be divided into three parts: the tectum, the tegmentum, and the crura cerebri. The crura cerebri contain numerous descending fibers. The tegmentum, which runs into the midbrain from the spinal cord, contains a diffuse aggregate of cells and fibers called the reticular formation. The tectum forms the roof of the midbrain.

Externally, the mesencephalon is characterized by the superior and inferior colliculi, nuclei involved with the relay of visual and auditory impulses, respectively.

Hindbrain

The medulla, pons, and cerebellum constitute the hindbrain. The medulla and the pons are rich in discrete ascending and descending tracts and in cranial nerve nuclei. In addition, the pons provides connections to the cerebellum and other parts of the nervous system.

Neurophysiology

Neuron

The neuron is the anatomical and functional unit of the nervous system. Individual neurons,

arranged in simple or complex circuits, exist in a wide variety of sizes and shapes throughout the peripheral and central nervous systems. However, 90 per cent of all neurons are found in the brain. Despite their diverse morphology, all nerve cells have three common parts: cell body, dendrite, and axon (see Figure 3).

The cell body (soma, cyton, perikaryon) contains the machinery essential to cell life. Dendrites are branchlike neuron processes that receive and conduct impulses toward the cell body. Most neurons have multiple dendrites, although some cells may have none at all. Axons transmit impulses away from the cell body. Usually only one axon is found in each neuron.

Nuclei and Tracts

Masses of nerve cell bodies are gray in appearance and are called gray matter. When they occur outside the central nervous system, such concentrations of cell bodies are called ganglia; within the brain and the spinal cord, they are called nuclei. The term nucleus in this instance and the term nucleus used in discussing the architecture of an individual cell have different meanings. Bundles of fibers within the central nervous system, usually subserving special sensory or motor functions and existing in discrete regions, are commonly termed tracts or fasciculi. Since fibers in these tracts are covered by myelin, they take on a white color, giving these areas the designation white matter.

Conduction of Impulses

The prime function of the nervous system is to transmit excitatory messages from one point in the body to another. Initial stimulation may be electrical, thermal, chemical, or mechanical. If the stimulus reaches a threshold value, it creates an excitatory state, initiating a propagated impulse within the neuron. This process is called conduction and is accomplished by the movement of ions into and out of the nerve cell. This movement creates alterations in the electrical charge on the axon membrane. In the normal intact nerve cell, impulses are transmitted in one direction—away from the cell body and toward the synaptic knobs at the end of the axon.

Synaptic Transmission

Once the propagated nerve impulse reaches the terminal end of the axon, it initiates a series

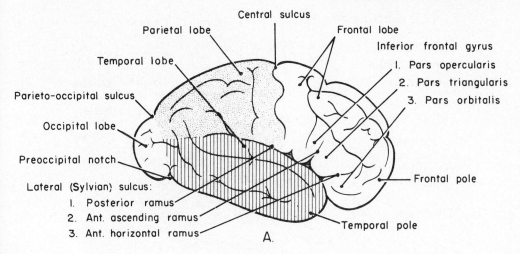

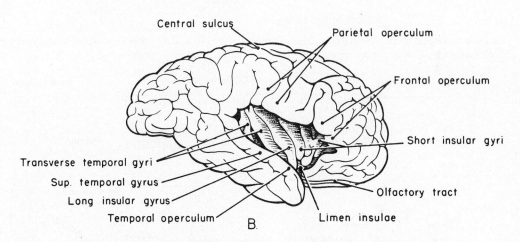

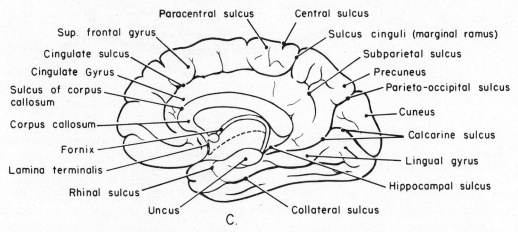

FIGURE 1. Right cerebral hemisphere. *A*, Lateral surface showing lobes of the brain. *B*, Lateral surface with the lips (*opercula*) of the lateral sulcus drawn apart to expose the insula. *C*, Medial surface showing principal gyri and sulci. (From R. C. Truex and M. B. Carpenter, *Human Neuroanatomy*. Williams & Wilkins, Baltimore, 1969.)

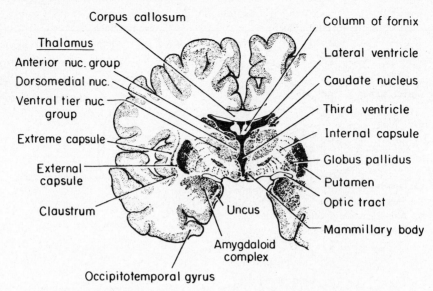

FIGURE 2. Frontal brain section passing through the basal ganglia and diencephalon. (From R. C. Truex and M. B. Carpenter, *Human Neuroanatomy*. Williams & Wilkins, Baltimore, 1969.)

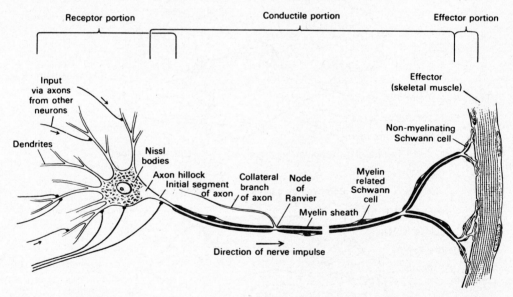

FIGURE 3. The receptor, conductile, and effector portions of a typical large neuron. The effector endings on skeletal muscle identify this as a somatic motor neuron; in many neurons the effector endings are applied to the receptor portions of other neurons. The presence of the myelin sheath on the conductile portion of the neuron (the axon) increases conduction velocity. The axon is shown as interrupted, for it is much longer than can be illustrated here. Note the numerous axons communicating with the dendritic zone. *Arrows* indicate the unidirectional nature of the impulse. (From W. M. Copenhaver, R. P. Bunge, and M. B. Bunge, *Bailey's Textbook of Histology*. Williams & Wilkins, Baltimore, 1971.)

of events that transfer that impulse to a second neuron. This event takes place at a structure called the synapse. The synapse is composed of the presynaptic axon terminus and a postsynaptic membrane. There is a discontinuity, termed the synaptic cleft, between communicating neurons (see Figure 4).

Electrical depolarization of the presynaptic

membrane permits release of chemical transmitters stored in presynaptic vesicles. These substances cross the synaptic cleft and combine with a postsynaptic receptor system. The action of the mediators may cause either a depolarization of the postsynaptic membrane, resulting in excitation of the second neuron, or a hyperpolarization, resulting in an inhibitory situation.

Chemical Mediators

Acetylcholine is present in the synaptic vesicles of certain peripheral nervous system axons, as well as in the brain. Neurons that release acetylcholine are termed cholinergic. In the peripheral nervous system, acetylcholine and norepinephrine are by far the most important neurotransmitters. Within the brain, however, these agents are of quantitatively minor importance. Acetylcholine has an uneven distribution, having its lowest concentration in the cerebellum and its highest concentration in the brain stem. The injection of this compound into either the ventricles or the gray matter produces excitatory effects and profound behavioral alterations.

Norepinephrine and dopamine are collectively called the catecholamines and are derived from a common precursor–phenylalanine. Norepinephrine is essentially a peripheral compound, but in the central nervous system it is found abundantly in the hypothalamus and brain stem reticular formation. Dopamine is found in high concentrations in the corpus striatum and substantia nigra. Most catecholamines are recycled by an amine pump, but a small percentage that is not taken up is broken down through the action of two enzymes, catechol–O-methyltransferase and monoamine oxidase (MAO).

Serotonin (5-hydroxytryptamine) has long been recognized as being present in cells of the intestine and in blood platelets. Only recently has this biogenic amine been described as a central neurotransmitter. The pineal gland, the

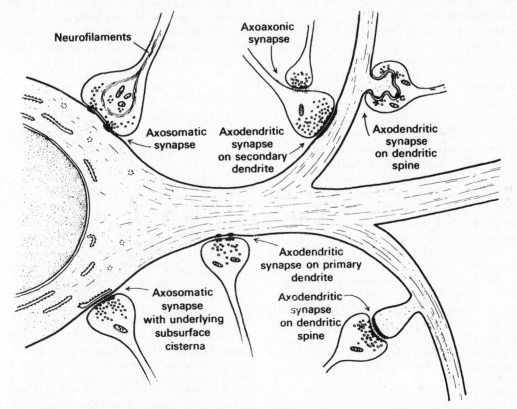

FIGURE 4. Schematic representation of the types of synapses occurring on various parts of a single neuron. (From W. M. Copenhaver, R. P. Bunge, and M. B. Bunge, *Bailey's Textbook of Histology*. Williams & Wilkins, Baltimore, 1971.)

hypothalamus, and a group of mesencephalic and pontine nuclei, the raphe nuclei, are especially high in serotonin content. This substance is synthesized from tryptophan, then degraded by MAO. Inhibitors of MAO block the breakdown of serotonin and have been shown to cause a twofold increase of serotonin in the brain less than an hour after administration. Currently, many theories link serotonin to mental illness, sleep, autonomic disorders, and migraines.

The removal of the carboxyl group from the amino acid glutamate results in γ-aminobutyric acid (GABA). Brain tissue has been shown to perform this function. In certain regions GABA may represent 40 per cent of all synapses. GABA is an inhibitory transmitter, and several forms of induced convulsions have been shown to result from its decreased concentration in the brain.

Aspartic acid (aspartate) and glutamic acid (glutamate) are two amino acids currently believed to serve as neurotransmitters. Glutamic acid has been shown to be as excitatory as acetylcholine when injected into neurons. Another amino acid, glycine, is also present in the brain and has been reported as inhibiting neuronal transmission in the spinal cord.

Other chemicals that seem to act as neurotransmitters are epinephrine, octopamine, and histamine.

Reticular Activating System

On the basis of changes in electroencephalogram (EEG) activity, those areas of the brain stem and diencephalon that produce arousal or altered consciousness on stimulation are called the reticular activating system (RAS). The most extensive portion of this system is the reticular formation.

The reticular formation is that region of the brain stem, extending from the caudal medulla to the diencephalon, occupying a central location and characterized structurally by numerous diffusely arranged neurons. If the RAS were to be divided into both anatomical and physiological portions, the reticular formation would represent its caudal segment, and the diencephalon centers would be at the cephalic pole.

Structure-Function Relationships

All aspects of RAS function derive from the structure of the system's neurons and their connections. Individual cells are able to send impulses rostrally into the brain, caudally into the spinal cord, and collaterally to other RAS neurons and are able to do so with marked variations in speed.

The RAS differs from classical sensory pathways in two respects. The first difference relates to the routes taken by sensory impulses to the cerebral cortex. For example, there is a direct pathway system, such as the spinothalamic tract, that converges on the thalamus before going to other areas of the brain (see Figure 5). The RAS represents an indirect route, with many of its fibers bypassing the thalamus as they diffusely project to the cortex. The second difference involves specificity of sensory input. Because of the complex neuron network, any specificity of sensory input is quickly abolished, so that different sensory stimuli produce equal activation.

Stimulation of the RAS can have both facilitory and inhibitory effects. All forms of movement can be affected, muscle tone altered, and respiration increased or decreased, and the circulatory system can experience pressor or depressor effects. Besides playing a central role in sleep and arousal, the RAS appears to be involved with attention, memory, and habituation.

Clinical Syndromes

The hyperkinetic syndrome in children is characterized by attention weakness, distracti-

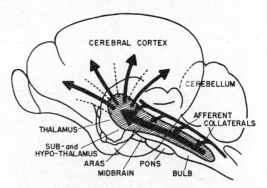

FIGURE 5. Outline of the brain of the cat, showing general location of the activating mechanism in the tegmentum of the brain stem and its relation to principal afferent systems and projections via thalamus to cerebral cortex. Starzl et al., cited from Magoun, 1952. (From J. R. Brobeck, Neural control systems. In *Best and Taylor's Physiological Basis of Medicine*, J. R. Brobeck, editor. Williams & Wilkins, Baltimore, 1973.)

bility, overactivity, irritability, impulsiveness, low frustration tolerance, and poor school performance. Although no single cause of this syndrome has been shown, some disorder in the function of the reticular formation is suggested. It is also presumed that some disorder of the reticular system produces the characteristic behavior seen in narcolepsy. And numerous researchers have suggested mechanisms of schizophrenia based on failure of the RAS integrating activities.

Limbic System

In his classic paper, Papez attempted to point out that emotion is not a magic product but "a physiologic process which depends on an anatomic mechanism." A group of structures associated with an arcuate convolution on the medial surface of the cerebral hemisphere known as the limbic lobe, Papez suggested, "deal with the various phases of emotional dynamics, consciousness, and related functions." This seat of emotion includes a portion of the cerebral cortex—the septal region, amygdaloid complex, and hippocampus—which connects with the anterior thalamic nuclei, mammillary bodies, and the hypothalamus. These form part of a circuit by which impulses are transferred from the hypothalamus to the cortex and returned by the cortex to the hypothalamus.

This interconnecting network of nuclei and tracts, involving separate structural areas, can be viewed as a closed circuit that permits the projection of impulses to and from higher cortical centers. It provides pathways through which regions in the neocortex influence events in the limbic structures and, conversely, permit processing by these structures before relaying emotionally colored impulses into the cortex.

The Papez hypothesis is remarkable in the context of what little functional neuroanatomy relating to behavior and emotion was known at the time. In the years since 1937, evidence in support of the proposal has grown, and another element of the Papez theory—that emotional experience and emotional expression are separate phenomena—has gained general acceptance. Many workers have built on the initial suggestion of Papez and have clarified the role of structures regulating emotional behavior. In the forefront of these researchers has been MacLean, who suggested (1952) that an ex-

panded group of structures related to emotional functions be termed the limbic system. The MacLean system, also known as the visceral brain because of its intimate relationships to visceral function through the hypothalumus, is composed of several structures—the subcallousal, eingulate, and parahippocampal gyri and the hippocampus proper. Collectively, these are designated the limbic lobe (see Figure 6). Included as well are associated subcortical nuclei, such as the amygdaloid complex, septal nuclei, hypothalamus, epithalamus, anterior thalamic nuclei, and parts of the basal ganglia (see Figure 7).

Structure-Function Relationships

No component of the limbic system appears to exert a single effect. As a unit, the system exerts a restraining force on the cortex. This force is demonstrated in experiments in which the neocortex is totally removed, resulting in extreme rage reactions. If the cortex is partially resected, with the limbic cortical areas left intact, behavior is markedly placid.

The amygdala consists of a group of nuclei occupying a dorsomedial position in the temporal lobe (see Figure 8). Removal of the amygdalae in dominant male monkeys transforms them into submissive animals. Stereotactic lesions in the amygdaloid nuclei of man have produced marked reduction in emotional excitability, normalization of social behavior, and adaptation in patients with severe behavior disturbances.

The dentate gyrus, the hippocampus proper, and the parahippocampal gyrus are commonly termed the hippocampal formation. The rostromedial portion of the parahippocampal gyrus is called the uncus. Lesions and stimulation of the hippocampus in cats have induced behavioral changes similar to those observed in psychomotor epilepsy. This area has an extremely low seizure activity threshold.

The hippocampus plays a major role in memory functions. Bilateral hippocampal damage results in permanent arrest of recent memory and is related to several amnestic syndromes. The manifest disorder is in the registration of memories.

Stimulation of the cingulate gyrus produces an arrest reaction, an immediate cessation of other activities. Localized stimulation of the posterior cingulate areas produces sexual and

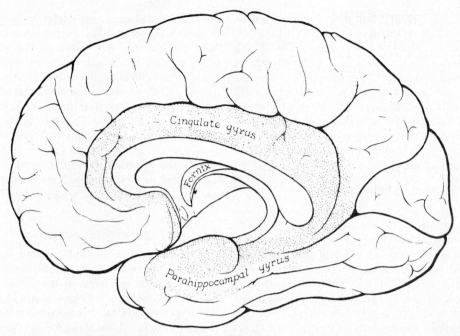

FIGURE 6. The medial surface of the hemisphere. *Shading* indicates the limbic lobe, which encircles the upper brain stem. Although the cortical areas designated as the limbic lobe have some common structural characteristics, the extent to which they form a functional unit is not clear. (From R. C. Truex and M. B. Carpenter, *Human Neuroanatomy.* Williams & Wilkins, Baltimore, 1969.)

pleasurable reactions. Spontaneous changes in behavior result from lesions in the anterior cingulate region of monkeys. Previously aggressive animals become placid, and anxious animals become calm.

The septal region acts as a pleasure center. Animals with electrodes implanted in this area deliver as many as 5,000 self-stimulatory shocks within an hour. Septal stimulation in cats produces penile erection.

Septal lesions have been shown to increase emotional reaction. Electrical stimulation has halted epileptic seizures, dulled intractable pain, and brought relief from anger and frustration. It is suggested that the septum exerts an inhibitory influence on emotion, thus opposing the effects of the amygdala.

Clinical Syndromes

Bilateral temporal lobe destruction—involving total destruction of the amygdaloid complex and destruction of major sections of the parahippocampal gyrus, the hippocampus proper, and the temporal neocortex—produces the Klüver-Bucy syndrome, characterized by psychic blindness or visual agnosia, compulsive licking and biting, the examination of all ob-

jects by mouth, an inability to ignore any stimulus, docility, hypersexuality, and hyperphagia.

Destruction of the mammillary bodies produces Korsakoff's psychosis. Patients with this syndrome suffer from profound amnesia, which the patient denies and is, in fact, unaware of. This condition is disguised by confabulation and pseudoremembrance. Apathy, indifference, poor initiative, and inertia are also present. The syndrome is caused by thiamine deficiency and represents late changes of Wernicke's encephalopathy seen in alcoholics. If untreated, this process may progress to irreversible dementia. Response to thiamine therapy is dramatic.

In a patient with damage exclusively to the limbic system, Gascon and Gilles report behavioral alterations identical to those seen in classic demented states. They suggest that this syndrome be termed "limbic dementia."

A constellation of changes seen in temporal lobe epilepsy arise from involvement of the uncus and are collectively grouped as uncinate fits. The characteristic olfactory aura, involuntary movements, and sensations of *déjà vu* and *jamais vu* are accompanied by the changes of behavior seen in schizophrenia. Rage, fear, and depression may be present. Penfield and Japer report such changes during electrical stimulation of limbic structures in patients undergoing neurosurgery.

A possible anatomical unit responsible for the signs and symptoms of schizophrenia has been offered by Stevens. On the basis of the link between antipsychotic and antiparkinsonism drugs, as well as certain histochemical findings, she suggests

that the principle terminus of the brain stem DA (dopamine) system, the corpus striatum, and in particular its most anterior extremity, the limbic striatum, are concerned fundamentally in the schizophrenic process.

On the basis of reciprocal relationships between the frontal cortex and limbic system, a team of English physicians have performed stereotactic surgery in patients with intractable psychiatric illness. These operations interrupted connections between the frontal cortex and the limbic system and destroyed a portion of the system itself by placing a lesion in one of the main circuits in the anterior cingulate gyrus. Of 40 patients involved, over-all improvement was reported in 67 per cent.

Hypothalamus

The hypothalamus (see Figure 9) is directly or indirectly involved in the physical manifesta-

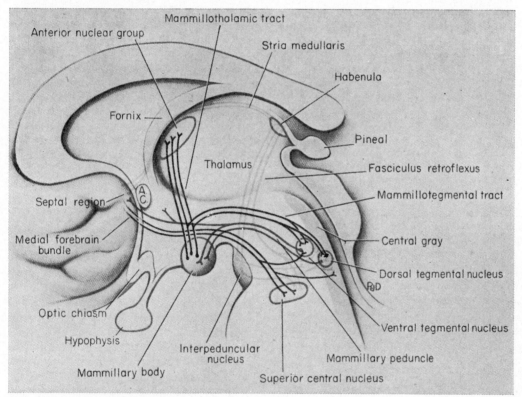

FIGURE 7. Limbic pathways interrelating the telencephalon and diencephalon with medial midbrain structures. The medial forebrain bundle originates from the septal and lateral preoptic region, traverses the lateral hypothalamic area, and projects into the midbrain tegmentum. The mammillary princeps divides into two bundles, the mammillothalamic tract and the mammillotegmental tract. Ascending fibers of the mammillary peduncle arise from the dorsal and ventral tegmental nuclei. Most of these fibers pass to the mammillary body, but some continue rostrally to the lateral hypothalamus, the preoptic regions, and the medial septal nucleus. Fibers arising from the septal nuclei project caudally in the medial part of the stria medullaris to terminate in the medial habenular nucleus. Impulses conveyed by this bundle are distributed to midbrain tegmental nuclei via the fasciculus retroflexus. (Based on Nauta. From R. C. Truex and M. B. Carpenter, *Human Neuroanatomy*. Williams & Wilkins, Baltimore, 1969.)

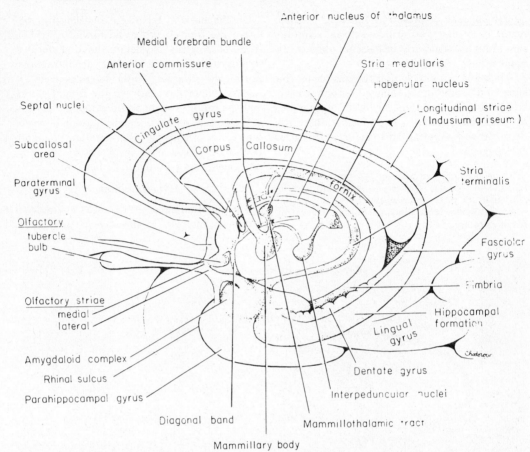

Anterior nucleus of thalamus

Medial forebrain bundle

Anterior commissure

Stria medullaris

Habenular nucleus

Septal nuclei

Longitudinal striae
(Indusium griseum)

Subcallosal
area

Cingulate gyrus

Corpus Callosum

Paraterminal
gyrus

fornix

Stria
terminalis

Olfactory
tubercle
bulb

Fasciolar
gyrus

Olfactory striae
medial
lateral

Fimbria

Hippocampal
formation

Lingual
gyrus

Amygdaloid complex

Rhinal sulcus

Dentate gyrus

Parahippocampal gyrus

Interpeduncular nuclei

Diagonal band

Mammillothalamic tract

Mammillary body

FIGURE 8. Rhinencephalic structural relationships as seen in medial view of the right hemisphere. Both deep and superficial structures are indicated. (Modified from a drawing by Krieg. From R. C. Truex, and M. B. Carpenter. *Human Neuroanatomy*. Williams & Wilkins, Baltimore, 1969.)

tions of emotion. By virtue of its control over the sympathetic and parasympathetic portions of the autonomic nervous system, as well as its influence on the endocrine system, the hypothalamus is able to mediate the physiological changes associated with fear, anger, hunger, thirst, sex, and pleasure. At the same time, the hypothalamus is an integral part of both the RAS and the limbic system. Controversy revolves about which comes first, the emotional experience or the visceral reaction.

Connections

The richness of fiber connections between hypothalamic nuclei and other brain structures reflects its pivotal role in emotional expression. Several afferent pathways connect the hypothalamus with parts of the limbic system.

Efferent hypothalamic fibers from the mammillary bodies travel cephalically and caudally as the mammillothalamic and mammillotegmental tracts. The former is important since it connects with the anterior thalamic nuclei, which then form part of a hypothalamic-thalamic-cingulate circuit.

Behavioral Changes

The most dramatic behavioral changes associated with hypothalamic function are the related expressions of fear and rage. Both responses are closely tied to the visceral and somatic processes evident during periods of danger or stress and represent the organism's instinctive efforts at self-preservation. The familiar concept of flight-or-fight reactions refers to these fear-induced or defensive changes.

The hypothalamus also appears to influence passive behavior. The loss of affective response is especially marked by lesions restricted to the posterior regions.

Both the frontal lobe and the amygdala connect with the hypothalamus and share with it a regulatory function over hunger. Lesions of the ventromedial nucleus of the hypothalamus result in voracious eating, causing hypothalamic obesity. Stimulation of the same nucleus abolishes the desire to eat.

Stimulation of the medial forebrain bundle and associated hypothalamic areas results in penile erection and mating behavior in monkeys. Conversely, lesions in the anterior hypothalamus completely abolish sexual interest.

The hypothalamus is but one of many parts in the sleep-waking mechanism of human beings. It is presently felt that some pathological sleep behavior is a consequence of widespread neural activity involving parts of the thalamus and the RAS.

Biochemistry

The causes and the chemical alterations underlying behavioral and emotional disturbances remain an enigma. At best, it has been demonstrated that certain changes are associated with behavioral disorders. Many findings support theories but do not confirm them.

Schizophrenia

Indolamine Hypothesis. A defect in the metabolism of indolamines, most notably serotonin, is currently being investigated as a possible cause of schizophrenia. The hallucinogens bufotenine and dimethyltryptamine are the

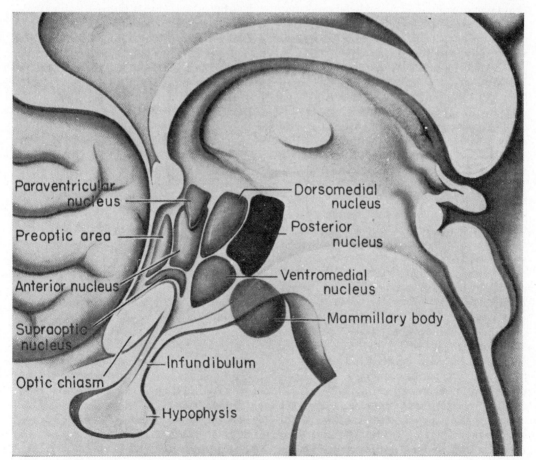

FIGURE 9. The medial hypothalamic nuclei. (From R. C. Truex and M. B. Carpenter, *Human Neuroanatomy*. Williams & Wilkins, Baltimore, 1969.)

N-methylated derivatives of serotonin and tryptamine, respectively. The human brain has recently been found to contain an enzyme that mediates this reaction, further enhancing the feasibility of this hypothesis. Moreover, clinical studies support this theory. Normal persons given large doses of the two amino acids tryptophan and methionine or a combination of the two experience an excited state. The same regimen in schizophrenics produces recurrence and exacerbation of psychosis, with the disorder being more severe if there is concurrent administration of a monoamine oxidase (MAO) inhibitor.

One group of investigators have found bufotenine in the urine of schizophrenics but not in control subjects, with or without the addition of MAO inhibitors. Levels of bufotenine were also observed to rise with the severity of psychotic episodes. Of particular interest are findings that chlorpromazine inhibits N-methylation of several amino acids, suggesting a possible connection between the indolamine hypothesis and the action of antipsychotic drugs.

Transmethylation Hypothesis. Harley-Mason proposed that schizophrenia may result from abnormal transmethylation of catecholamines, yielding dimethoxyphenylethylamine (DMPEA), a compound closely related to mescaline. Ten years later, Friedhoff and Van Winkle reported finding DMPEA in the urine of schizophrenics and not in normal control subjects, and they were also able to demonstrate the conversion, in vitro and in vivo, of dopamine in schizophrenic patients to the urinary excretion product of DMPEA. But subsequent research by other workers has failed to confirm these early findings. Kuehl et al. found no relationship between urine DMPEA and schizophrenia. The most serious challenge is the finding that DMPEA in the urine is closely related to diet.

Amine Hydroxylation Theory. Stein and Wise provide evidence that 6-hydroxydopamine (6-HD), an aberrant dopamine metabolite, produces schizophrenic symptoms by causing "a prolonged or permanent depletion of brain catecholamines" through the specific degeneration of epinephrine-containing nerve terminals. The behavioral result of 6-HD injected intraventricularly into rat brains was a suppression of self-stimulation in animals with electrodes implanted in the medial forebrain bundle. This finding is the basis of the postulated link with schizophrenia, where there is a selective destruction of the reward system. That 6-HD is formed at all, Stein and Wise suggest, is the result of a genetic defect. The possibility is also explored that chlorpromazine may exert its antipsychotic effect by preventing 6-HD destruction of the nerve terminal (see Figure 10). Szara has presented other evidence that 6-HD may produce schizophrenia by interfering with the action of serotonin.

Taraxein Hypothesis. Heath and his coworkers reported evidence of a protein that they called taraxein in the blood of schizophrenics. This agent reportedly blocks the action of acetylcholine in the limbic system, especially in the septal region, resulting in a lack of ability to experience pleasure or pain. The injection of taraxein into volunteers produced characteristic schizophrenic symptoms.

It is hypothesized that taraxein is the consequence of a genetic disorder most manifest in periods of stress, when it is liberated. The validity of the taraxein hypothesis remains clouded. Most attempts by independent researchers to duplicate the findings of Heath have proved unsuccessful.

Dopamine Hypothesis. Horn and Snyder note that central dopaminergic receptors are blocked by all effective antipsychotic drugs, such as chlorpromazine, and X-ray crystallography indicates that these drugs have a molecular configuration similar to that of dopamine. Janowsky and his associates have provided data consistent with this theory.

Affective Disorders

Biogenic Amine Hypothesis. Some, if not all, depressions are associated with an absolute or relative deficiency of catecholamines, particularly norepinephrine, at functionally important receptor sites in the brain. Elation, conversely, may be associated with an excess of such amines. Drugs such as the MAO inhibitors and tricyclic antidepressants, which potentiate or increase brain catecholamines, cause behavior stimulation and excitement and have an antidepressant effect. Conversely, drugs that deplete or inactivate central amines produce sedation or depression.

Evidence linking the central action of serotonin to depression has come from studies that

NORMAL

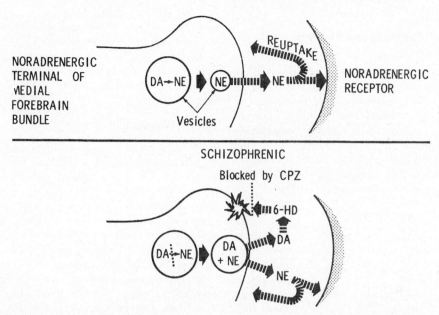

FIGURE 10. Hypothetical diagram of noradrenergic transmission in normal and schizophrenic brain. *Normal:* Virtually all dopamine (DA) is converted to norepinephrine (NE) by dopamine-β-hydroxylase. *Schizophrenic:* Pathological gene causes reduced synthesis or abberant formation of dopamine-β-hydroxylase, resulting in only incomplete conversion of DA to NE. Hence, nerve impulses release both DA and NE into synaptic cleft. Autoxidation or enzymatic conversion of dopamine produces 6-hydroxydopamine, which, when taken up by noradrenergic terminal, destroys it. (From L. Stein and D. Wise. Possible etiology of schizophrenia: progressive damage to the noradrenergic reward system by endogenous 6-hydroxydopamine. In *Neurotransmitters*, I. K. Kopin, editor. Williams & Wilkins, Baltimore, 1972.)

demonstrate below normal concentrations of the principal serotonin metabolite, 5-hydroxyindoleacetic acid, in the lumbar spinal fluid of depressed patients.

Other studies suggest a role for dopamine. The administration of L-dopa has been shown to increase brain dopamine and norepinephrine. It appears likely that dopamine is responsible for the production of symptoms in certain patients.

However, the complex relationship of the catecholamines to other elements of the body chemistry leads to the conclusion that the biogenic amine hypothesis may represent an oversimplification of the mood mechanism.

Endocrine Factors. Sachar et al. have been pursuing evidence suggesting that norepinephrine is the neurotransmitter that regulates the release of growth hormone from the pituitary gland and that a similar role is played by dopamine with regard to prolactin release. Several reports have shown that there is inade-

quate growth hormone response in depressed patients.

Sachar demonstrated that a relationship does exist between such a central neurochemical imbalance and unipolar depression as measured by endocrine function. Other correlations among physiological levels of female steroid hormone levels, altered tryptophan metabolism, and depression have been suggested.

Neurochemical Antagonism. Antagonistic adrenergic and cholinergic systems in the central nervous system may influence behavior. Janowsky and his co-workers report that opposite effects were observed when methylphenidate (an adrenergic stimulating agent) and physostigmine (a cholinomimetic agent) were administered to a group of patients. Adrenergic stimulation intensified manic symptoms in manic patients, worsened psychoses in schizophrenic patients, and produced a marked increase in activation in all patients. Conversely, physostigmine produced an inhibitory syndrome that was similar to the psychomotor retardation seen in endogenous depression.

Learning and Memory

Disorders of remote and short-term memory result from bilateral temporal lobe destruction, and the hippocampus is involved in the registration of recent memories. But numerous attempts to locate neural regions that act primarily as learning centers or memory centers have·been unsuccessful. It is currently held that learning and memory functions are performed in a diffuse fashion in many areas of the cortex, with many areas of overlapping activity.

Ribonucleic Acid (RNA)

Early biochemical experiments of memory involved worms. Planarians were trained, then killed and fed to untrained planarians. The untrained worms, when trained identically as the worms they had eaten, learned more readily. Moreover, when RNA was extracted from trained worms and injected into untrained worms, the untrained worms were observed to possess the conditioned behavior of the trained worms. Subsequent findings have also suggested RNA involvement in long-term memory.

Cholinergic Agents

Deutsch and his associates have used diisopropylphosphorofluoridate, an anticholinesterase, to study the role of cholinergic drugs in memory. Rats injected with diisopropylphosphorofluoridate suffer from memory losses. These losses involve recently learned tasks and appear to be concerned with the process of memory retrieval. Eserine, another anticholinesterase, has similarly been found to inhibit the learning of passive avoidance reactions in rats. O,O-Diethyl-S-ethylmercaptothiophosphate, an insecticidal anticholinesterase, increases problem-solving errors in rats.

Proteins

It is difficult to separate concepts of protein synthesis from RNA activity. This is especially true of ribosomal RNA, a nucleic acid that is primarily involved in the formation of proteins. Rats that are being trained to perform new tasks, for example, are found to have increased amounts of nervous system ribosomal RNA,

indicating that protein synthesis is occurring. Direct evidence of protein involvement in learning and memory comes from two recently isolated compounds, S-100 and scotophobin. Inhibitors of protein synthesis, such as acetoxycycloheximide and puromycin, provide indirect evidence of a role for proteins. Under certain conditions, these compounds have decreased memory functions.

Electrophysiology

Spontaneous or evoked brain electrical activity has been explored as a reflection of previous experience. By using evoked potential techniques, workers have found that released patterns of electrical activity may reflect the activation of specific memories. It has also been observed that cerebral potentials normally elicited by a specific event are recorded even when the specific event fails to occur.

Evoked response waveshapes are identical for identical stimuli. When a novel stimulus is presented, a waveshape similar to the initial evoked response is recorded. As both stimuli are repeatedly presented, the similarity between waveshapes decreases.

REFERENCES

Axelrod, J. Neurotransmitters. Sci. Am., *230:* 58, 1974.

Brobeck, J. R. Neural control systems. In *Best & Taylor's Physiological Basis of Medical Practice,* J. R. Brobeck, editor, sect. 9, p. 1. Williams & Wilkins, Baltimore, 1973.

Brodie, K. H., and Sabshin, M. An overview of trends in psychiatric research: 1963–1972. Am. J. Psychiatry, *130:* 1309, 1973.

Carpenter, M. B. *Core Text of Neuroanatomy.* Williams & Wilkins, Baltimore, 1972.

Frazer, A., Ghanshyam, P. N., and Mendels, J. Metabolism of tryptophan in depressive disease. Arch. Gen. Psychiatry, *29:* 528, 1973.

Gascon, G. G., and Gilles, F. Limbic dementia. J. Neurol. Neurosurg, Psychiatry, *36:* 421, 1973.

Goodwin, F. K., and Bunney, W. E. A psychobiological approach to affective illness. Psychiatr. Ann. *3:* 19, 1973.

Janowsky, D. S., El-Yousef, M. K., Davis, J. M., and Sekerke, H. J. Antagonistic effects of physostigmine and methylphenidate in man. Am. J. Psychiatry. *130:* 1370, 1973.

John, E. R., Bartlett, F., Shimokochi, M., and Kleinman, D. Neural readout from memory. J. Neurophysiol. *36:* 893, 1973.

Kelly, D., Richardson, A., and Mitchell-Heggs, N. Stereotactic limbic leucotomy: Neurophysiological aspects and operative technique. Br. J. Psychiatry, *123:* 133, 1973.

Kelly, D. Richardson, A., Mitchell-Heggs, N., Greenup, J., Chen, C., and Hafner, R. J. Stereotaxic limbic leuctomy: A preliminary report on forty patients. Br. J. Psychiatry, *123:* 141, 1973.

Langman, J. *Medical Embryology.* Williams & Wilkins, Baltimore, 1969.

MacLean, P. D. The hypothalamus and emotional behavior. In *The Hypothalamus,* W. Haymaker, E. Anderson, and W.

J. Nauta, editors, p. 659. Charles C Thomas, Springfield, Ill., 1969.

Mandell, A. J., and Segal, D. S. The psychobiology of dopamine and the methylated indolamines with particular reference to psychiatry. In *Biological Psychiatry*, J. Mendels, editor, p. 89. John Wiley, New York, 1973.

Romano, J. Psychiatry and medicine, 1973. Ann. Intern. Med., *79:* 582, 1973.

Schwartz, I. L. General physiological processes. In *Best & Taylor's Physiological Basis of Medical Practice*, J. R. Brobeck, editor, p. 1-1. Williams & Wilkins, Baltimore, 1973.

Stevens, J. R. An anatomy of schizophrenia? Arch. Gen. Psychiatry, *29:* 177, 1973.

Truex, R. C., and Carpenter, M. B. *Human Neuroanatomy.* Williams & Wilkins, Baltimore, 1969.

2.7. CHRONOPSYCHOPHYSIOLOGY

Chronopsychophysiology

Implicit in much of the current research in chronopsychophysiology is the hypothesis that disturbances in periodic processes contributing to psychopathology may not be apparent at the surface level of clinical description and observation, and that measurement and elucidation of such latent periodic processes may be crucial in advancing psychobiological understanding of psychiatric illness, just as insight into latent unconscious mental processes was crucial for the development of psychodynamics. The rationale for this hypothesis is the observation that virtually every physiological process has demonstrated a 24-hour periodicity. The orderly sequence of crest and trough of these component rhythms, not all in phase, creates a unique succession of internal physiological states that is repeated once every 24-hours. This orderly sequence can be viewed as the body's own timing mechanism or biological clock.

Rhythms underlie much of what is assumed to be in the range of constant homeostasis in people and the world. In health, a human being has an appearance of stability that cloaks an inner symphony of biological rhythms—a spectrum ranging from microseconds for biochemical reactions, milliseconds for unit nerve activity, about a second for the heart rhythm, the 90-minute rapid eye movement cycle of dreaming, the major 24-hour rest-activity cycle, and the 27-day menstrual cycle to, finally, the single life-span cycle. A schematic spectrum of bioperiodicities is shown in Figure 1. The normally unconscious regularity of these inner rhythms becomes apparent only when there is discord caused by trauma, disease, chronic stress, or erratic external synchronization.

An example of erratic external synchronization that has dramatically drawn attention to chronopsychophysiology is the 4-to 5-day period of fatigue and adjustment needed after a transcontinental flight to resynchronize the inner clock system with the activity cycle of the new time zone.

External cues—light cycle, social regimen—serve to synchronize circadian rhythms through the hypothalamic-pituitary axis and adrenal steroid hormone system. Night people differ from day people simply in using a different set of cues to synchronize their rhythms with their environment. Without such cues, the rhythms approximate a 24-hour period, keeping neither a precise solar-day cycle (24 hours) nor a precise lunar cycle (24.8 hours). In the complete absence of external synchronizers a rhythm drifts, gaining or losing a few minutes each day, a condition known as free running. This free-running condition has been advanced as one possible explanation for certain forms of insomnia.

Rhythms shorter than 24 hours have been designated as ultradian, those longer than 24 hours as infradian. Repeated measurements are needed to observe periodicities.

Although documentation of human circadian rhythms is tedious for both subjects and experimenters, the list of body functions identified as circadian is steadily growing, making possible circadian rhythm maps or norms under conditions of health and disease (see Figure 2).

In view of documented circadian fluctuations in levels of consciousness and liver and kidney function, it is not unreasonable to think that the body also varies cyclically in its ability to tolerate stress or to detoxify and excrete toxins, poisons, and drugs. Numerous studies, usually in animals, have identified circadian susceptibility rhythms to such agents. Chronobiologists are investigating a wide variety of chemotherapeutic agents, particularly anticancer drugs, to determine whether an optimal time exists for administering the drug each day to maximize its therapeutic principle and to minimize its undesirable side-effects. The circadian peaks for a number of human susceptibility variables have been analyzed by Halberg and his colleagues, as shown in Figure 3.

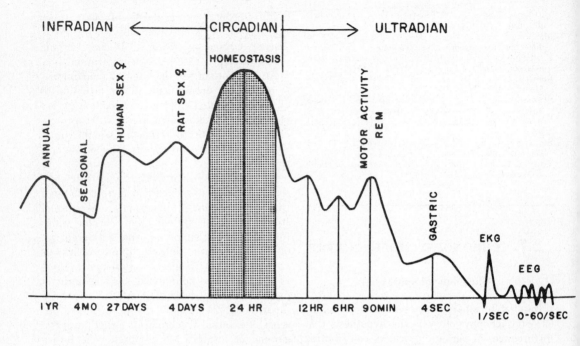

FIGURE 1. Schematic spectrum of biological periodicities along a continuum, with more reactive rhythms on the right. (Reprinted from C. F. Stroebel. Behavioral aspects of circadian rhythms, in *Comparative Psychopathology*, J. Zubin and H. F. Hunt, editors, 1967, by permission of Grune & Stratton.)

Susceptibility to ECT and Conditioned Fear

Two applications of the circadian susceptibility design are of particular interest for psychiatry. McGaugh and Stephens measured the degree of retrograde amnesia produced by electroconvulsive therapy (ECT) treatments in rats at different times over a 24-hour period. Amnesia was significantly greater when the ECT was administered during the active period, as opposed to the quiescent period (see Figure 3).

Stroebel evaluated a variety of animal-learning paradigms commonly used in psychopharmacological research for a possible circadian susceptibility effect. He administered training trials to each of four identical groups of rats at one of four times each day. The results for acquisition of a conditioned emotional response revealed a significant circadian susceptibility effect with faster acquisition of unavoidable fear—a median of six learning trials at the onset of the activity period, as opposed to a median of

11 for the group receiving training at the onset of the rest period.

Experiments strongly suggest that cognitive cerebral behaviors are minimally influenced by circadian variations but that emotional behaviors dominated by conflict are strongly influenced and, further, are highly correlated with the level of steroid hormones in the blood, possibly by influencing the cyclic adenosine monophosphate-norepinephrine sensitivity of neuroendocrine receptors on effector organs. Personal experience seems to verify these findings; most persons can bring themselves to a level of attention fairly quickly at any point in the 24-hour span, even awakening from sleep; they can intelligently converse, abstract, and reason. Emotionally, however, most of us sense that our moods, irritability, and empathy vary consistently and significantly over each 24-hour period.

These findings are directly applicable to animal psychopharmacology. Experimental procedures must include rhythm synchronization

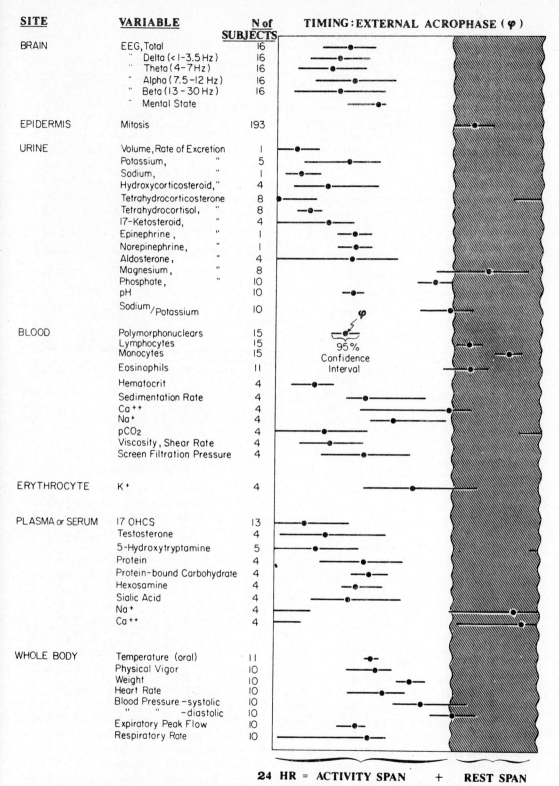

SITE	VARIABLE	N of SUBJECTS	TIMING: EXTERNAL ACROPHASE (φ)
BRAIN	EEG, Total	16	
	" Delta (<1-3.5 Hz)	16	
	" Theta (4-7 Hz)	16	
	" Alpha (7.5-12 Hz)	16	
	" Beta (13-30 Hz)	16	
	" Mental State		
EPIDERMIS	Mitosis	193	
URINE	Volume, Rate of Excretion	1	
	Potassium, "	5	
	Sodium, "	1	
	Hydroxycorticosteroid, "	4	
	Tetrahydrocorticosterone	8	
	Tetrahydrocortisol, "	8	
	17-Ketosteroid, "	4	
	Epinephrine, "	1	
	Norepinephrine, "	1	
	Aldosterone, "	4	
	Magnesium, "	8	
	Phosphate, "	10	
	pH	10	
	Sodium/Potassium	10	
BLOOD	Polymorphonuclears	15	
	Lymphocytes	15	
	Monocytes	15	
	Eosinophils	11	
	Hematocrit	4	
	Sedimentation Rate	4	
	Ca++	4	
	Na+	4	
	pCO2	4	
	Viscosity, Shear Rate	4	
	Screen Filtration Pressure	4	
ERYTHROCYTE	K+	4	
PLASMA or SERUM	17 OHCS	13	
	Testosterone	4	
	5-Hydroxytryptamine	5	
	Protein	4	
	Protein-bound Carbohydrate	4	
	Hexosamine	4	
	Sialic Acid	4	
	Na+	4	
	Ca++	4	
WHOLE BODY	Temperature (oral)	11	
	Physical Vigor	10	
	Weight	10	
	Heart Rate	10	
	Blood Pressure —systolic	10	
	" " —diastolic	10	
	Expiratory Peak Flow	10	
	Respiratory Rate	10	

95% Confidence Interval

24 HR = ACTIVITY SPAN + REST SPAN

FIGURE 2. Map of human circadian rhythms, as analyzed by the chronobiology laboratory at the University of Minnesota. The rhythm peak (acrophase) is indicated by a dot surrounded by lines indicating the 95 per cent confidence interval. (Reprinted from G. Luce, *Biological Rhythms in Medicine and Psychiatry*, 1970, by permission of Gay Luce and the U. S. Public Health Service.)

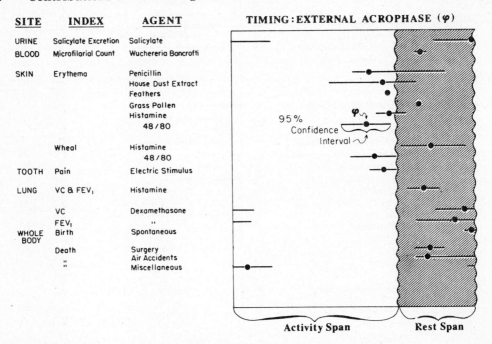

SITE	INDEX	AGENT
URINE	Salicylate Excretion	Salicylate
BLOOD	Microfilarial Count	Wuchereria Bancrofti
SKIN	Erythema	Penicillin
		House Dust Extract
		Feathers
		Grass Pollen
		Histamine
		48/80
	Wheal	Histamine
		48/80
TOOTH	Pain	Electric Stimulus
LUNG	VC & FEV₁	Histamine
	VC	Dexamethasone
	FEV₁	"
WHOLE BODY	Birth	Spontaneous
	Death	Surgery
	"	Air Accidents
	"	Miscellaneous

TIMING: EXTERNAL ACROPHASE (φ)

95% Confidence Interval

Activity Span   Rest Span

FIGURE 3. Map of circadian rhythms in the human for birth, death, morbidity, susceptibility, and reactivity, as analyzed by the chronobiology laboratory at the University of Minnesota. (Reprinted from G. Luce, *Biological Rhythms in Medicine and Psychiatry*, 1970, by permission of Gay Luce and the U. S. Public Health Service.)

with a light-dark cycle, control for time of training trials, and designs sensitive to drug-susceptibility rhythms.

Memory of Acquired Fear

A succession of internal physiological states is created by the 24-hour sequence of component rhythms. It is almost as if the body rhythm system assigns a sequence of priorities, a metabolic timetable, directing resources to important functions in a preset order. Current data suggest that specific organ systems are given priority to replicate once each day—for example, liver mitoses at the onset of activity or corneal epithelial mitoses at the onset of rest. It is possible that the escape of a cell or organ from the endocrine-circadian priority system may be one of the mechanisms involved in cancer, since the cells could presumably replicate repeatedly, out of control as outlaws. Although highly speculative, abnormal rhythm functioning may provide a link to explain the frequent reports of a personality change in a family member months before a malignancy manifested itself clinically.

Emotional Memory Substrate

Emotional memory, previously demonstrated to be circadian-dependent, may be directly linked to specific body clock times, much like the vault of a bank that opens only at preset hours.

Emotional responses acquired at the same time each day—for example, the indigestion and frustration felt by a secretary when her tyrannical boss storms into the office each day at 8:30 A.M.—may be optimally accessible to conscious memory and to deconditioning only at that time. Emotional behaviors randomly acquired at many points in the biological rhythm cycle may be particularly resistant to behavior therapy procedures unless the therapy sessions are conducted at many points in a 24-hour span. And daily repetition of the internal states associated with the memory of an emotional behavior may serve as unconscious practice of that behavior, even in the absence of the usual external cues—that is, even on Saturday and Sunday, when the secretary is not confronted by her boss, her biological rhythms are cycling through the same circadian-determined internal stimulus conditions normally occurring at 8:30 A.M. each day.

Replication Problem

Except for the catecholamine hypothesis for affective disorders, the replication status of virtually every physiological correlate or explanation of mental disorder is uncertain at present. Findings in the original laboratory are only rarely confirmed in a second setting.

Some major source of previously unidentified variance must be present in these studies to account for the discrepant findings. The ubiquitous nature of rest-activity disturbances in human emotional illness, coupled with their appearance as a common denominator in most models of psychopathology, clearly make biological rhythm variation a possible candidate for the missing variance.

Psychophysiological Chronotography

Halberg advocates the daily measurement of a number of biological rhythm variables as a focal tool for preventive medicine. Significant changes in body timing are sensitive early warning signs of pathology and could be used to alert the patient and the clinician that a careful medical examination is warranted. Halberg has developed a concept, called autorhythmometry, in which persons are trained to make computer-scorable measurements—such as blood pressure, pulse, temperature, mood scale, grip strength, and time estimation—on themselves with relatively inexpensive instruments.

Autorhythmometry will provide an enormous prospective data base on the population who cooperate, willingly carrying their instruments and scoring sheets with them wherever they go. It may also produce a new population suffering from heightened hypochondriasis. Another problem with current autorhythmometry procedures is their relative insensitivity to the richness of psychic life—that is, unreported feelings of love on a beautiful spring day may account for variations in the measured variables.

In a practical attempt to make rhythm measurement palatable to as large a segment of the population as possible, Stroebel and colleagues have developed a computer-scored daily record of moods, body changes, and life events called the psychophysiological diary. Previous successes in automating behavioral observations

have already demonstrated the potential power of repeated behavioral observations as a means for detecting underlying periodic functioning. One example is the automated psychiatric nursing note.

The procedure for routine charting of psychiatric nursing notes was computerized at the Institute of Living in 1967. Nursing reports are made on each patient twice daily by routine nursing personnel on a special IBM 1232 mark-sense form that is designed for computer scoring. Eleven areas of noninferential patient behavior are rated on the front side of the form. Temperature, pulse, blood pressure, the nature of the patient's daily activities, and his physical complaints are reported in a similar fashion on the reverse side of the form. The computer produces two types of output from each report: The first is a narrative summary to be filed in the patient record as a legal document; the second is a set of 20 daily factor scores, describing the patient's behavior numerically, as compared with his hospital residence unit.

Psychophysiological chronotography represents an apparently practical means for extending the knowledge of rhythmic processes clinically as they relate to emotional functioning. A psychophysiological chronotogram will help identify those specific components of behavior and physiology that progressively evolve over time in health, in psychic development, and in disease. It will provide a new kind of laboratory precision to prospective analysis in psychiatry and preventive medicine, perhaps complementing and improving on the traditional retrospective approaches.

REFERENCES

Halberg, F., Halberg, J., Halberg, F., and Halberg, E. Reading, 'riting, 'rithmetic . . . and rhythm: A new "relevant" "R" in the educative process. Perspect. Biol. Med., *17:* 128–141, 1973.

Halberg, F., Haus, E., et al. Toward a chronotherapy of neoplasia: Tolerance of treatment depends on host rhythms. Experientia, *29:* 909, 1973.

Halberg, F., Johnson, E. A., Nelson, W., and Sothern, R. Autorhythmometry: Procedures for physiologic self-assessment and their analysis. Physiol. Teach., *1:* 1, 1972.

Luce, G. *Biological Rhythms in Medicine and Psychiatry.* U. S. Department of Health, Education, and Welfare, Chevy Chase, Md., 1970.

Reinberg, A., and Halberg, F. Circadian chronopharmacology. Am. Rev. Pharmacol., *11:* 455, 1971.

Stroebel, C. F. Behavioral aspects of circadian rhythms. In *Comparative Psychopathology,* J. Zubin and H. F. Hunt, editors, pp. 158–172. Grune & Stratton, New York, 1967.

Stroebel, C. F. Biologic rhythm correlates of disturbed behavior in the rhesus monkey. In *Circadian Rhythms in*

Nonhuman Primates, F. H. Rohles, editor, p. 20. Karger, New York, 1969.

Stroebel, C. F. Autorhythmometry methods for longitudinal evaluation of daily life events and mood: Psychophysiologic chronotography. In *Chronobiology*. Igaku Shoin, Tokyo, 1974.

Stroebel, C. F., and Glueck, B. C. Biofeedback treatment in medicine and psychiatry: An ultimate placebo? In *Seminars in Psychiatry*. Grune & Stratton, New York, 1973.

2.8. BIOCHEMISTRY OF THE MAJOR PSYCHOSES

Introduction

In both schizophrenia and manic-depressive psychosis, new evidence indicates the importance of genetic factors in their transmission. New drugs have been discovered with considerable specificity against the cardinal features of schizophrenia and the affective disorders, and the accumulation of fundamental knowledge has made possible the productive exploration of their mechanisms of actions.

Affective Disorders

Recent Genetic Information

In family studies extending over several years, Winokur and his associates were unable to support the traditional separation of these disorders into endogenous and reactive types on the basis of either clinical symptoms or family history. On the other hand, manic-depressive illness, recently designated bipolar, seems to form a distinct subtype both genetically and clinically. In patients with this disorder, a curious absence of transmission of the affective illness from father to son suggested the existence of an X-linked dominant gene. Families were found in which another X-linked trait, such as color-blindness or Xg blood type, was significantly associated with an affective disorder in individual members, providing strong evidence for the hypothesis.

Electrolyte Changes

Several studies have noted significant changes in body weight, body water, and exchangeable sodium ion during recovery from depression, and studies with Na^{22} and total body counting confirm the retention of sodium during depression and its release during recovery. There is some evidence that in mania an even greater retention of sodium ion occurs than during depression. Under controlled electrolyte and fluid intake in humans, the administration of lithium in therapeutic doses produces an early sodium, potassium, and water diuresis, followed by retention of sodium and water. The therapeutic effectiveness of lithium in mania may be related to these changes.

Endocrine Changes

The severe alterations in mood, libido, emotionality, activity, sleep, and autonomic function that are found in affective disorders strongly suggest an involvement of the limbic system, hypothalamus, and pituitary and resultant influences on the peripheral endocrines. Severe alterations in cortisol excretion paralleling the mental changes have often been reported in the affective disorders. The diurnal curve of corticosteroid production in depression shows more peaks during the 24-hour cycle and a lower amplitude than normal. During the few days before a suicide or attempted suicide, there is often a marked increase in cortisol excretion. Cortisone and other corticosteroids are important regulators of electrolyte metabolism and undoubtedly play some role in the electrolyte changes that accompany affective disorders. Thyroxine is capable of potentiating the antidepressant action of imipramine in women, and the injection of the thyrotropin-releasing factor of the hypothalamus has been reported to produce a prompt, brief, and perceptible improvement in mood.

Biogenic Amines

Shore and his collaborators found that the administration of reserpine to animals was followed by a marked increase in 5-hydroxyindoleacetic acid excretion and a depletion of serotonin in the brain. This tranquilizing drug, which produced symptoms of severe depression in some patients who received it, interfered with the capacity of axonal endings to store a variety of putative neurotransmitters, including norepinephrine and dopamine, as well as serotonin. The excitant properties of iproniazid and its effectiveness as an antidepressant were found to be related to its inhibition of monoamine oxidase, an observation that was readily confirmed by the development of a large number of monoamine oxidase inhibitors that had antidepressant properties.

Attention shifted from serotonin to the catecholamines when it was demonstrated that the administration of L-dopa was capable of reversing the depressant effects of reserpine in animals, whereas 5-hydroxytryptophan was relatively ineffective. This finding was followed by evidence that amphetamine and the tricyclic antidepressant drugs may increase the concentration of norepinephrine at central synapses by favoring its release or blocking its reuptake by the presynaptic terminal. At the present time, a large number of observations are compatible with the involvement of epinephrine or of serotonin in mood and affective disorders in human beings.

Norepinephrine. Some depressions may be associated with an absolute or relative deficiency of catecholamines, particularly norepinephrine, at functionally important receptor sites in the brain, whereas manias may be associated with an excess of such monoamines. Drugs that elevate mood or relieve depression in human beings appear to increase the concentration of norepinephrine at central synapses, but drugs that cause severe depression in human beings deplete norepinephrine in those regions.

The pharmacological evidence of an increase or a decrease in norepinephrine at central synapses is necessarily indirect. Increased synthesis, release from presynaptic endings, and decreased inactivation of the amine are factors that would be expected to increase its synaptic concentration. An increased synthesis has been inferred from a more rapid turnover of the amine in the brain and by demonstrating an increased activity of the rate-limiting enzyme, tyrosine hydroxylase. An increased release, which has not been demonstrated directly at central synapses, has been inferred from an increased concentration of the O-methylated derivative, normetanephrine, which appears to be formed by catechol-O-methyltransferase acting postsynaptically. Release has been more directly but less physiologically measured in stimulated brain slices in vitro. The major mechanism for synaptic inactivation of norephinephrine is by its reuptake into the presynaptic ending, which may be indicated by the rate of uptake of labeled norepinephrine injected into the cerebrospinal space.

A decreased synaptic concentration is inferred from a decrease in synthesis or an increase in the inactivation of the amine in the presynaptic terminal, making less of it available for release. Presynaptic inactivation is accomplished largely by monoamine oxidase and has been estimated by the concentration of deaminated metabolites.

Evidence has been accumulated that amphetamine—a well known euphoriant agent that increases arousal, exploratory activity, and appetitive behavior in animals—inhibits monoamine oxidase, favors the release of norepinephrine, and inhibits its reuptake at the presynaptic ending. The monoamine oxidase inhibitors that are effective antidepressants diminish the presynaptic inactivation of norepinephrine and produce a substantial increase in noremetanephrine in the brain, thus indicating the likelihood of an increased concentration of norepinephrine at the synapse. The tricyclic antidepressants appear to block the reuptake of norepinephrine by the presynaptic ending.

The quite specific effect of lithium ion in mania may be related to its ability to diminish the release of norepinephrine by brain slices and to increase the uptake of the amine by nerve endings. Its administration is accompanied by some increase in deaminated metabolites of norepinephrine in the brain.

An electroconvulsive shock appears to cause the release of norepinephrine in the brain. A series of such shocks over a period of a week results in an increased turnover of norepinephrine and a slight increase in the activity of tyrosine hydroxylase in the brain; the increase in activity persists for 24 hours after the last shock.

These findings associated with shock and with the drugs that affect mood are all compatible with an involvement of norepinephrine in their action. However, this does not constitute proof that the action on norepinephrine is the major or the only mechanism involved in the clinical antidepressant effects. Conclusive evidence has not been obtained of an inadequacy of norepinephrine in the brain of depressed patients or of an excess in those with mania. A number of studies of the urine show a decrease in the excretion of norepinephrine and normetanephrine in patients with retarded depression and an increase of these metabolites in patients with mania and hypomania. However, a small fraction of these urinary amines represent the release or metabolism of norepinephrine in the brain, and these findings must be regarded as measures of peripheral autonomic and adrenal medullary activity that may parellel changes in mood. On the other hand, there is reason to believe that 3-methoxy-4-hydroxyphenylglycol (MHPG) is a major metabolite of norepinephrine in the brain and that much of what appears in the urine is derived from that source. In subhuman primates, it has been shown that about 50 per cent of the urinary MHPG originates in the brain. In man, urinary levels of this metabolite parallel the mood changes induced by terminating prolonged amphetamine usage, whereas other metabolites of norepinephrine do not. Measurement of urinary MHPG in affective disorders indicates a tendency for levels to be low in depression and elevated in hypomania, although this finding is not always the case. In some patients with agitated depression, MHPG has been depressed in the urine, even though other norepinephrine metabolites have been elevated, suggesting a closer approximation of MHPG excretion to the central state.

In blood, a reduction in catecholamine-O-methyltransferase in erythrocytes of women with unipolar depression has been observed; this reduction was independent of the phase of illness or recovery. In two studies, monoamine oxidase in platelets was found to be increased in depression. This enzyme appears to increase in platelets and in the brain with advancing age above 35 years and also seems to be higher in women, suggesting a possible relation with the higher incidence of depression in middle age and in women.

In an attempt to get closer to the metabolism of norepinephrine in the brain, some investigators have examined cerebrospinal fluid for catecholamine metabolites in patients with affective disorders. In one study, MHPG was low in depression and unchanged in mania; in another study, that metabolite was unchanged in depression but markedly elevated in mania. An interesting control group was included in the latter study—that of simulated mania. In such subjects, there was no change in MHPG, but there was an increase in homovanillic acid and in 5-hydroxyindoleacetic acid. Homovanillic acid, the major metabolite of dopamine, has been found in several studies to be decreased in depressed patients but to be unchanged or decreased in those with hypomania and mania.

A greater sensitivity may be obtained in cerebrospinal fluid studies by the use of probenecid, which blocks the transport of acid aminemetabolites, permitting them to accumulate in the cerebrospinal fluid at a rate that may serve to reflect the rate of the release or metabolism of the parent amine. In two studies with this agent, a decreased accumulation of homovanillic acid has been found in depressed patients.

Neuroendocrine studies have been used by Sachar and associates in an ingenious approach to the study of norepinephrine synapses in the hypothalamic functions of depressed patients. The hypothalamic regulation of growth hormone release from the anterior pituitary appears to depend on central norepinephrine activity. The infusion of that amine into the ventricle causes growth hormone release in animals, and the blockade of catecholamine synthesis inhibits the normal growth hormone response to insulin, as does the administration of an α-adrenergic antagonist. On the other hand, a single oral dose of L-dopa stimulates growth hormone release in human beings. The release can also be blocked by an α-adrenergic antagonist. Whereas only 7 per cent of young normal subjects showed an inadequate growth hormone release after a standard dose of L-dopa, 36 per cent of normal subjects between 48 and 68 years of age and 77 per cent of depressed patients gave an abnormally low response. Insulin, which normally stimulates growth hormone release, failed to induce an adequate release in 5 of 13 depressed patients, whereas all 23 age-matched, nondepressed patients gave a normal response. These findings are compatible with diminished function of norepinephrine-mediated activity in the hypothalamus of some patients with depressive illness.

Serotonin. The monoamine oxidase inhibitors affect levels of serotonin in the brain and presumably its synaptic activity to a greater extent than that which can be shown for norepinephrine. The tricyclic antidepressants also block the reuptake of serotonin by presynaptic endings, and one of them, amitriptyline, may even have a greater effect on serotonin than on norepinephrine. Repeated electroconvulsive shocks increase serotonin levels in the brain.

Elevating serotonin activity by the administration of its immediate precursor, 5-hydroxytryptophan, produces drowsiness, sedation, and lethargy in animals; blockade of serotonin synthesis by para-chlorophenylalanine, which inhibits tryptophan hydroxylase, produces an increase in aggressive behavior, locomotion, and sexual excitation. An agent that appears to destroy serotonergic endings, 5,6-dihydroxytryptamine, produces similar effects. Lesions of the serotonin-containing raphe nuclei of the brain stem deplete serotonin, increase motor activity and arousal, and inhibit sleep. These effects can be counteracted by 5-hydroxytryptophan. Clinical use of para-chlorophenylalanine in human beings has been reported to produce anxiety, arousal, and psychotic manifestations reminiscent of effects sometimes reported with L-dopa. In fact, these effects of L-dopa may result from an interference with serotonin action on the basis of competition with the serotonin precursor for transport into the brain or for decarboxylation, and serotonin has been found to be decreased by as much as 60 to 80 per cent in the brain after large doses of L-dopa. Elevation of serotonin in the brain increases the threshold of pain; depletion of serotonin lowers that threshold.

In general, these studies do not support a hypothesis that increased or decreased serotonin activity elevates or depresses mood, respectively. Instead, there is the suggestion of another type of involvement for serotonin at central synapses and in affective states.

Several studies of the urinary excretion of 5-hydroxyindoleacetic acid (5-HIAA), the major metabolite of serotonin, reveal no consistent pattern in the affective disorders, which is not unexpected. Practically all the serotonin in the body is present in the gut, and the metabolite found in the urine undoubtedly originates there, rather than in the brain.

In the cerebrospinal fluid, most observers have found a decrease in 5-HIAA in depressed patients, although a few studies do not confirm this finding. There appear to be some differences between diagnostic subgroups; for example, unipolar depressives show lower levels than do bipolar depressives, and psychotic depressives have lower levels than do those who are nonpsychotic. In mania and hypomania, four studies showed a decrease in this metabolite, and three studies showed no change or an increase. The decrease may be more impressive, in view of the results obtained in sham mania, in which levels of this metabolite in the cerebrospinal fluid were increased.

An interesting finding reported by Coppen is that the low levels of this metabolite found in depression appear to persist after recovery. He studied 18 patients with mania and 31 with depression, of whom eight were restudied after recovery, and compared his findings with values obtained from 20 hospitalized control subjects with no psychiatric disturbances. In both the manic and the depressive groups, including the patients in remission, there was 50 per cent less 5-HIAA in the cerebrospinal fluid in comparison with the control group. This persistence in both types of affective disturbance and after recovery diminishes the likelihood that irrelevant artifacts are operating and if it were confirmed would suggest the presence of some constitutional factor common to both depression and mania.

The accumulation of 5-HIAA in cerebrospinal fluid after probenecid, was found to be decreased in four studies of depression and two studies of mania.

The effects of precursor administration in the case of serotonin appear to be more consistent than those reported with L-dopa. The first investigators who administered 5-hydroxytryptophan to depressed patients reported no effects or conflicting results. After a report that schizophrenics treated with monoamine oxidase inhibitors and substantial doses of tryptophan showed an elevation of mood and loosening of association, two groups evaluated the same combination in patients with depression, and both reported significant improvement. There have been five additional studies in which improvement has been reported after large doses of tryptophan with or without monoamine oxidase inhibitors, but four studies report no beneficial effects.

The evidence for the involvement of serotonin in affective disorders is no less provocative than that for norepinephrine and, in the case of the clinical studies, seems somewhat more consistent. Although the findings are quite controversial, a tentative hypothesis seems permissible: Serotonin activity may be decreased in the brain in both depression and mania, and the effect appears to be more characteristic of the patient than of his particular stage of affective disorder of recovery. The rate-limiting hydroxylation of tryptophan may be impaired in depressed patients.

Synthesis

Recent genetic evidence strongly suggests that one or more biochemical disturbances play important roles in a major segment of the serious affective disorders. Research over the past two decades has shown some reasonably reproducible biochemical changes that are associated with affective disorders. Significant alterations undoubtedly occur in electrolyte balance and in cortiscosteroid secretion. Although their role need not be secondary, no parsimonious concept has as yet emerged relating these changes to the pathogenesis of the affective disorders. On the other hand, fundamental knowledge of the biochemistry and pharmacology of the biogenic amines, their localization and distribution in the brain, and their interrelationships with behavior and clinical states strongly suggests that further study of these areas should elucidate some of the underlying biological processes in depression and mania.

The two major hypotheses that have been advanced—implicating norepinephrine and serotonin—are not mutually exclusive. By combining them, one may account for some of the discrepancies. Behavioral studies in animals as well as clinical findings are compatible with the thesis that norepinephrine pathways are involved in mood, with deficiency producing depression and overactivity resulting in euphoria, hypomania, or mania. Similar types of observations with serotonin suggest that its rôle may be to exert a reciprocal or, more likely, a stabilizing or damping effect on synapses, including those that may be associated with mood. There is some clinical evidence that serotonin or its activity is reduced in the brain of many patients suffering from affective disorders, whether they be depressed or manic or in remission. It is possible that a deficiency of serotonin at central synapses is an important genetic or constitutional requirement for affective disorder, permitting what might otherwise be normal and adaptive changes in norepinephrine activity and the resultant mood states to exceed the homeostatic bounds and progress in

an undamped fashion to depression or excessive elation. The symptomatic extremes of depression or mania would thus be attributable to high or low norepinephrine synaptic activity, and the predisposition to them or the extent to which those changes overrun their adaptive bounds would depend on a constitutional deficit in serotonin activity.

Schizophrenia

Recent Genetic Information

Several studies that have used adopted persons and their biological and adoptive families as a means of disentangling genetic from environmental contributions have adduced compelling evidence that genetic factors operate significantly in the transmission of schizophrenia. These studies have found, with great consistency, a significant incidence of schizophrenia in persons genetically related to schizophrenics but reared in different environments.

In one of these studies (Kety et al., 1974), the finding of a high incidence of schizophrenia in the biological paternal half-siblings of schizophrenics who had been adopted and who did not share with them the same environment, including even the in utero environment and early mothering experience, may represent the most conclusive evidence for genetic factors that has been obtained (see Table I). Whether schizophrenia is a homogeneous entity or a phenomenologically similar group of illness with different causes remains to be determined, although there is some evidence that latent or borderline schizophrenia is genetically related to more severe forms of the illness. Two hypotheses related to the biological substrates of schizophrenia are the foci of considerable current research activity.

Transmethylation

In 1952 Harley-Mason speculated that the newly delineated process of biological transmethylation may somehow be involved in schizophrenia. He singled out one substance, 3,4-dimethoxyphenylethylamine, as being of special interest, since it had been reported to produce catatonic behavior in animals.

In 1961 the hypothesis was tested by the administration of methionine to schizophrenic patients in conjunction with a monoamine oxidase inhibitor. In about a third of the patients,

TABLE I
*Prevalence of Schizophrenia in Biological and Adoptive Relatives**

	Biological Relatives of		Adoptive Relatives of	
	Schizophrenic Adoptees	Control Adoptees	Schizophrenic Adoptees	Control Adoptees
Relatives				
Total identified	173	174	74	91
Diagnosed as				
Definite schizophrenia	14	4†	1	2
Definite or uncertain schizophrenia	29	8‡	3	5
Paternal half-siblings				
Total identified	63	64	2	0
Diagnosed as				
Definite schizophrenia	8	1†	0	0
Definite or uncertain schizophrenia	14	2‡	0	0

* Table is based on psychiatric interviews and hospital records. The relatives are parents, siblings, and half-siblings of 33 adoptees who became schizophrenic and of their matched control subjects (Kety et al., 1974).
† $P < 0.02$.
‡ $P < 0.001$.

there was a brief exacerbation of psychosis, and this phenomenon has been reported in several subsequent studies. In one of these studies, it was found that methionine alone, without monoamine oxidase inhibition, can produce the same effect in schizophrenic patients. Normal subjects who receive the same dose of methionine experience no such effect. The ability of large doses of methionine to elevate S-adenosylmethionine levels in the brain and reports that methionine administration in schizophrenics caused an increase in the excretion of dimethyltryptamine, a well-known hallucinogen, were compatible with the hypothesis.

In 1962 the presence of a substance that produced a pink spot on paper chromatography and that was identified as 3, 4-dimethoxyphenylethylamine was reported in the urine of schizophrenic patients. This finding was followed by a large number of attempts to replicate it, most of which were successful in demonstrating the pink spot in the urine of schizophrenics and, to a considerably smaller extent, in the urine of normal persons. However, the fact that phenothiazines produce metabolites that also yield a pink spot in a similar position confused the issue. More recently, 3, 4-dimethoxyphenylethylamine has been demonstrated by mass fragmentography in the urine of normal subjects and schizophrenics, and evidence adduced that it is of exogenous origin. The issue has not yet been resolved.

Evidence for an enzyme, indoleamine-N-methyltransferase, in the brain has been obtained. That enzyme is capable of methylating tryptamine to dimethyltryptamine, although it does not methylate serotonin.

In 1972 it was shown that 5-methyltetrahydrofolic acid (MTHF) could serve as a methyl donor in the N-methylation of dopamine to epinine. Banerjee and Snyder have since reported that MTHF can serve as the methyl donor in the methylation of both indoleamines and phenethylamines. They showed that serotonin and dimethylserotonin were actively methylated on the 5-hydroxyl group, with MTHF serving as the methyl donor to form the corresponding 5-methoxy compound. One of these, 5-methoxy-N,N-dimethyltryptamine, is a potent hallucinogen, considerably more active than the parent substance, bufotenin.

Dopamine

Since the discovery in 1951 that chlorpromazine is beneficial in the treatment of schizophrenic patients, a number of phenothiazine derivatives have been prepared, many of which have antipsychotic properties. Haloperidol, a butyrophenone not chemically related to the phenothiazines, was also found to be effective in the treatment of schizophrenic patients. As both groups of drugs became widely used, it soon became evident that an important side-effect of both was the development of symptoms like those of Parkinson's disease. With the discovery that dopamine is deficient in the caudate nucleus of patients suffering from Parkinson's disease, an action on that amine became a possibility for explaining the extrapyramidal effects of the antipsychotic drugs.

Carlsson and Lindqvist, in 1963, first suggested that these drugs act by a blockade of dopamine receptors. They speculated that there is an increased release of dopamine in the case of the active antipsychotic drugs, brought about by some feedback mechanism in response to a blockade of dopamine receptors.

Several pharmacological studies have confirmed the increased synthesis and turnover of dopamine in the brain in response to psychoactive congeners, and a blockade of dopamine receptors has been demonstrated physiologically by microelectrode recording and biochemically on dopamine-sensitive adenylate cyclase of brain.

The phenothiazines have rather specific effects on the cardinal features of schizophrenia. Whereas sedative agents, like the barbiturates, and antianxiety drugs, like diazepam, were no more effective than a placebo in the treatment of schizophrenics, chlorpromazine in large-scale controlled studies produced significant improvements in thought disorder blunted affect, withdrawal, and autistic behavior.

Although LSD commanded considerable interest because of its ability to produce a toxic psychosis thought to resemble schizophrenia, it has been known for some time that the psychosis induced by an overdosage of amphetamine is much closer to schizophrenia and is often confused with that disorder, even by experienced clinicians. Chronic amphetamine toxicity is characterized by a paranoid psychosis with auditory hallucinations and stereotyped behavior with little delirium or confusion. Schizophrenic patients have been reported readily able to recognize an LSD psychosis as different from their usual symptoms but unable to differentiate an amphetamine psychosis. Furthermore, amphetamine, methylphenidate, and L-dopa can precipitate active schizophrenia in schizophrenic patients during remission.

There is evidence to suggest that the psychosis of amphetamine is mediated through its release and potentiation of dopamine at its receptors in the brain. The stereotyped behavior induced in animals by amphetamine can be prevented by lesions of the dopamine pathways. Dopamine itself or apomorphine, which is known to stimulate dopamine receptors, produces stereotypy when injected into the brain. Behavioral and biochemical observations suggest that d-amphetamine is considerably more potent in potentiating norepinephrine than is l-amphetamine; both isomers of amphetamine have equivalent actions on dopamine synapses. In human beings the d-form is about 5 times as potent as the l-form of amphetamine in its arousal and euphoriant effects, suggesting that these effects are mediated by noradrenergic pathways, but the two forms of amphetamine are almost equipotent in producing psychosis. Further suggesting that the amphetamine psychosis is the result of an activation of dopamine synapses is the observation that chlorpromazine and haloperidol are very effective in preventing or aborting the psychosis.

There is a remarkable convergence on dopamine synapses in the brain on the part of several types of agents. The drug that produces a psychosis most closely resembling schizophrenia appears to act by potentiating dopamine at its synapses in the brain, whereas a large number of drugs in two distinct chemical classes that have in common their ability to block dopamine receptors also have quite specific effects on the cardinal features of schizophrenia, leading to the hypothesis that an overactivity of dopamine synapses may play a crucial role in the pathogenesis of schizophrenia.

Dopamine-Norepinephrine Imbalance

Although a hyperactivity of dopamine could explain certain features of schizophrenia—such as stereotyped behavior, paranoid delusions, and auditory hallucinations—it would hardly in itself account for other features of schizophrenia, such as anhedonia, withdrawal, autism, and flatness of affect. These manifestations appear to involve behavioral components that in animals have been related to the activity of norepinephrine. Thus, there is indirect evidence that norepinephrine pathways are involved in appetitive or reward behavior, in exploratory activity, and in elevated mood. It is possible that the corresponding manifestations of anhedonia, withdrawal, and flatness of affect represent a lessened activity of norepinephrine at its synapses. A parsimonious mechanism exists that could produce both the increase in dopamine activity and the decrease in norepinephrine activity which the more complete explanation of the symptoms requires. That mechanism may be the enzyme dopamine-β-hydroxylase, which converts dopamine to norepinephrine at the noradrenergic endings in the brain. A throttling of that enzyme could conceivably result in the release of dopamine at the expense of norepinephrine. Some evidence is compatible with such a hypothesis.

REFERENCES

Banerjee, S. R., and Snyder, S. H. Methyltetrahydrofolic acid mediates N- and O-methylation of biogenic amines. Science, *182:* 74, 1973.

Carlsson, A., and Lindqvist, M. Effect of chlorpromazine or haloperidol on formation of 3-methoxytyramine and normetanephrine in mouse brain. Acta Pharmacol. Toxicol., *20:* 140, 1973.

Carroll, B. J. Monoamine precursors in the treatment of depression. Clin. Pharmacol. Ther., *12:* 743, 1971.

Coppen, A. Indoleamines and affective disorders. J. Psychiatr. Res., *9:* 163, 1972.

Davison, K., and Bagley, C. R. Schizophrenia-like psychoses associated with organic disorders of the central nervous system: A review of the literature. In *Current Problems in Neuropsychiatry*, R. N. Harrington, editor, p. 113. Royal Medico-Psychological Association, London, 1969.

Fink, M., Kety, S. S., and McGaugh, J., editors. *The Psychobiology of Electroconvulsive Therapy*, V. H. Winston & Sons. Washington, 1974.

Kety, S. S. Biochemical theories of schizophrenia. A two-part critical review of current theories and of the evidence used to support them. Science, *129:* 1528, 1959.

Kety, S. S., Rosenthal, D., Wender, P. H., Schulsinger, F., and Jacobsen, B. Mental illness in the biological and adoptive families of adopted individuals who have become schizophrenic: A preliminary report based upon psychiatric interviews. In *Genetics and Psychopathology*, R. Fieve, H. Brill, and D. Rosenthal, editors. Johns Hopkins Press, Baltimore, 1974.

Lipton, M. A., Ban, T. A., Kane, F. J., Levine, J., Mosher, L. R., and Wittenborn, R. *Megavitamin and Orthomolecular Therapy in Psychiatry*. American Psychiatric Association, Washington, 1973.

Matthysse, S. Antipsychotic drug actions: A clue to the neuropathology of schizophrenia. Fed. Proc., *32:* 200, 1973.

Matthysse, S., and Kety, S. S., editors. Catecholamines and their enzymes in the neuropathology of schizophrenia. J. Psychiatr. Res., *11:* 107–113, 1974.

Matthysse, S., and Pope, A. The approach to schizophrenia through molecular pathology. In *Molecular Pathology*, R. Goode and S. Day, editors. Charles C Thomas Publisher, New York, 1974.

Nicol, S., Seal, V. S., and Gottesman, I. I. Serum from schizophrenic patients: Effect on cellular lactate stimulation and tryptophan uptake. Arch. Gen. Psychiatry, *29:* 744, 1974.

Prange, A. J., Wilson, I. C., Lynn, C. W., Alltop, L. B., and Stikeleather, R. A. L-Tryptophan in mania. Arch. Gen. Psychiatry, *30:* 56, 1974.

Schildkraut, J. J. *Neuropsychopharmacology and the Affective Disorders*. Little, Brown, Boston, 1970.

Wise, C. D., and Stein, L. Dopamine beta-hydroxylase deficits in the brains of schizophrenic patients. Science, *181:* 344, 1973.

Wyatt, R. J., Murphy, D. L., Belmaker, R., Cohen, S., Donnelly, C. H., and Pollin, W. Reduced monoamine oxidase activity in platelets: A possible genetic marker for vulnerability to schizophrenia. Science, *179:* 916, 1973.

3

Science of Human Behavior: Contributions of the Psychological Sciences

3.1. COGNITION AND PERCEPTION

Cognition

Classification, Concepts, and Concept Learning

The basis of classification is the notion that each individual object or event is, at the same time, a kind of object or event. Concepts are sets of objects, events, beings, acts, conditions, representations, and the like that belong together behaviorally, reflecting the ways human beings categorize their experience and classify the stuff of their perceptual-cognitive worlds.

Generally speaking, concepts are expansible, admitting of additional members to the set; modifiable through experience and by taking context into account; and constructed or learned, reflecting cultural and personal experience, rather than being *a priori*. Some logical categories or mathematical relationships may not meet all these specifications, but only certain concepts are logical. Concepts are also interrelated, either hierarchically—for example, species, genera, and higher taxa—or in their range of reference. Concepts can ordinarily be defined in terms of not only what they include but what they omit or the alternatives they imply, and these omissions or alternatives are themselves conceptualized.

To experimental psychologists, concept learning occurs when a number of distinct stimuli come to be treated the same way—that is, elicit the same response—either on the basis of commonalities inherent in them or on the basis of functional equivalence. To cultural anthropologists and some sociologists, a reper-tory of concepts, particularly the pattern of their interrelations, expresses the cognitive structure of a culture or group. To developmental psychologists, the attainment of particular concepts demonstrates a stage of mental growth in the child. To contemporary cognitive psychologists, achieved conceptual categories are part of the mental structure that represents the patterns and stages by which information is processed in humans and behavior organized. And to some philosophers and linguists, certain concepts are epistemological necessities or givens, without which thought and thinking about thought could not proceed.

A concept is formed when relevant attributes are identified and the appropriate rule for treating them is understood. When the definition and formation of concepts involves verbal-symbolic mediation and superordinate and subordinate categorical relations, concepts become more and more abstract—although any concept, by definition, involves generalization and thus abstraction to some degree. Highly abstract concepts are typically formed not on the basis of sorting experiments with objects but from the highly symbolic operations of language and other representational modes. Such concepts, which may even be imaginary—for example, atoms and electrons, unicorns and griffins—tend to be unstable and inexact because of the complexity or the contingent nature of the rules of formation or because of the intangibility of criterial attributes. For example, of what hardness and hue is a unicorn's horn? Concepts involving essentially abstract attributes are difficult because of the absence of appropriate symbolic mediators, such as images

110

and words. Most instances of concept formation are highly abstract, without recourse to concrete or pictorial aids. Even so, many of the same operations obtain.

In principle, the creation of any category implies the existence of at least one other (a, not a); but in practice, concepts are often better learned, defined, and integrated with other concepts when positive instances are used. This tendency may be partly cultural and partly logical. The total set of positive instances may be intuitively smaller than that of negative instances. In many circumstances, positive examples are more informative.

Problem Solving and Other Higher Behavior

Generally, in problem-solving situations all the elements are present at once; the behavior demanded is a more goal-oriented, transactional behavior than is the typical concept-formation situation; and what is required is not the forming of concepts but the discovery of implicit relations among them by means of the novel manipulation or recombination, in a step-by-step fashion, of concepts and rule systems (strategies) already attained. Most problem solving is cumulative, a matter of dealing with experience already organized conceptually. Moreover, most real-life problems have a certain goal-defined character. The cardinal question in conceptual behavior is: What goes with what? In problem solving the cardinal question is: What leads to what?

Problem solving and other somewhat similar kinds of behavior, like creative or productive thinking and decision making, are of classical status in psychology but have never been as systematically studied as has concept formation. Part of the reason seems to be that problem-solving behavior has a certain unique or arbitrary character. Such behavior is identified by its end result, subject to consensual judgments in specific contexts. A certain example of verbal artifact—a witty turn of phrase, say—may show that creative thinking has taken place, but an equally unlikely verbal specimen is regarded as a slip of the tongue or a schizophrenic flight of ideas. A particular manual behavior is regarded as solving a problem, but another manual behavior is taken as random movement, even though it may have exactly the same physical consequences, largely because the context has not been identified by others as problematical. Then, too, it is difficult to deal experimentally with behaviors regarded as infrequent or verging on the unique. When someone supplies multiple examples of a formal algebraic solution, he ceases to be regarded as solving a problem but, rather, is regarded as running off a routine or applying an algorithm.

Concepts versus Conceptions

Since concepts refer to classes of stimuli, they always represent a certain level of abstraction. Concepts vary in their degree of abstractness; for example, one says that "rock" and "hardness" are concrete and abstract, respectively, but it is evident that "rock" represents a concept that is already considerably abstracted.

Is classification in this sense the predominant way in which one brings order to his experience? Philosophers and psychologists have been sporadically interested in other possible kinds of conceptions, defined here as single instances of abstract mental representation. These conceptions are of various kinds but share the quality of seeming to be to some extent *sui generis*, forming categories of one or varying in their degree of category membership. For most people, "home" or "mother" has a special personal meaning; to decompose that meaning would violate one's sense of reality. Other conceptions, especially those based on images, are highly embedded in an associative network, from which it is difficult to disentangle them. If one's image of architectural beauty is the Parthenon, it is probably the Parthenon from a particular angle of vision or bathed in moonlight, as one first saw it. Other conceptions simply seem to be best examples. A turkey is somehow less of a bird than a robin. Some conceptions seem *sui generis* because they have a hypothetical or nonanalyzable referent: unicorn, God. The natural color categories that all human beings possess are difficult to explain in terms of the usual characteristics of concept formation. Category boundaries shift markedly with context, and there seem to be focal colors, common across many or perhaps all cultures, that are better exemplars of particular color categories than are other values.

Whether these conceptions are thought of as prototypes, prime exemplars, canonical forms, critical features, or best figures, they all share the quality of having a central value surrounded by a range of variation or a core meaning surrounded by examples of lesser degrees of membership. This quality makes them essentially analog categories, as opposed to the digital categories of concept formation (atribute: relevent/irrelevent; value: present/absent).

Developmental Approaches

Piaget. The major unified body of work on cognitive ontogenesis is that of Jean Piaget; this work has been developed over a period of nearly 50 years. Piaget's investigations focus on the achivement of mental structures, which are systems of operations and transformations that reveal the logical principles of a particular range of actions—at the highest level, internalized actions. The operations and transformations themselves have logicomathematical qualities—for example, reversibility, commutability, and substitutability—within a situation of invariance of identity. Whatever the form of a particutar structure, it is a sufficient code for an interaction between the person and the objective environment.

Structures, taken together, are comprehensive; at any given stage, they represent the mental organization. However, in the course of development, imperfect structures are continually modified and replaced, following fixed sequences, until the highest epistemological level is reached. In general, the ontogenetic process involves the parallel movement from the concrete and particular to the general and abstract, from the static to the dynamic, and from the egocentric to the decentered, when objective reality is fully comprehended as independent of the person's particular or momentary situation.

The many stages through which these processes extend are sometimes grouped into the sensorimotor period (up to about the age of 18 months), the representational period (through middle or late childhood), and the mature operational period. The sensorimotor period is one of elementary action and exploration of the surround, with little mentation. The representational period is primarily one of increasingly stable organized perceptions, the result of the accumulation of the child's experience; but these perceptions are largely untested in the effective environment in terms of actions. Such perceptions are prelogical, egocentric, and solipsistic. The operational period is one of relat-ing specific perceptions to the transactional demands of the outside world, of testing strategies and constructing logical principles, and of the increasing ability to handle abstract relationships, conjecture, and hypothetical thinking.

Structures, also called schemes, are continually modified, at least until fully mature equilibration is achieved. Each structural level is dynamically built on the preceding one, but the transitions tend to appear discontinuous. A given structural level is fairly stable as long as the contemporary processes of assimilation and accommodation are successful. In confronting a new experience in whatever stage or mode—concrete versus abstract, manipulative versus observational—the person attempts to interpret or act toward the environment in accord with existing structures, to assimilate new information into the present organization. If this attempt is unsuccessful, the scheme itself is modified so as to accommodate external reality. The new scheme is then of a higher or more general logical order than was the earlier scheme.

Piaget's system is based on action, with the result that it is sometimes regarded as a motor theory of thought. Structures are not emergent but are constructed, and behavior comes before structure. A scheme is a summary of possible actions—environmental transactions—and is formed on the basis of such actions, which, when internalized in the course of assimilation and accommodation, amount to the experience that the structure encodes. Action may range from primitive, episodic manipulation of objects to highly sustained symbolic processes.

The description of Piagetian stages—sensorimotor, representational, and operational—inevitably reminds one of developmental stages of psychodynamic theory and the tripartite basis of personality structure. Yet Piaget regards cognitive ontogenesis as conflict-free and has little interest in motivational and affective factors, partly because his theory is essentially unilinear, cumulative, and comprehensive, leaving no room for divisions of function or unintegrated—neurotic—patterns of behavior.

Bruner. Another influential body of developmental research of importance to cognition is that of Bruner and his associates. Bruner's system is rather like Piaget's in that it involves orderly stages and necessary sequences in cognitive growth. Bruner, for example, cites cognitive stages called the enactive, the ikonic, and the symbolic. However, Bruner's work has a wider experimental basis than does Piaget's and is more solidly empirical. Probably because of this fact, Bruner—who is keenly interested in general formal abilities, such as the rule-governed behavior—has by no means ignored specific contents and context in investigating children's actual attainments. Furthermore, for Bruner, cognitive stages succeed each other—that is, appear in an orderly sequence in development—but do not replace each other. Adults have access to all three modes, and the full richness and productivity of adult thinking are due to the interplay and simultaneous processing among these modes. And Bruner attaches far more importance to language than does Piaget. For Bruner, the basic structure of thought is linguistic, involving fundamental experiential relations, such as agent/object, transitive/intransitive, active/passive, discrete/continuous. In his view, language develops in advance of other forms of cognitive behavior and acts as a catalyst for their development; in adulthood, language is the primary form in which thought is conducted, so that it guides and amplifies thought. Bruner probably would not find the question, "How do I know what I think until I hear what I say?" a trivial or unrealistic one. Although Bruner does not claim that all thought is conducted linguistically, he points out that much information is imparted and acted on entirely by linguistic means, especially but not exclusively in adulthood. Consider story telling and its part in the cognitive development of the child, as well as the prevalent character of instruction in higher education. He holds that the conflict between description of reality and perceived reality causes cognition to alter or to advance—to be restructured or for subsuming principles to be found—and that often it is only by verbalizing the problem that many problems are conceptualized, let alone solved. With the former claim, at least, Piaget would, no doubt, diametrically disagree.

Language and Cognition

In the past two decades, the development of psycholinguistics has resulted in a sophisticated approach to describing the underlying intuitive linguistic knowledge that enables the speakers of a language to communicate with each other. Linguists refer to this knowledge as the grammar of a language.

First-language acquisition involves a standard developmental sequence, in which the order of mastery of various phonological, syntactical, and lexical elements but not necessarily the age of mastery is nearly invariant in children in normal social environments. This is true both within a given language and, given suitable comparisons, across at least a wide variety of languages from a number of different language families. During language learning, children repeatedly produce sentences or other utterances that they have demonstrably never before heard and, for the most part, do so appropriately—that is, recognizably moving toward closer and closer approximation of grammatical regularity. Children, in other words, actively construct (discover, infer) the rules that govern language, and they do so in an orderly and to some extent autonomous fashion. This is shown not only by the fact that they produce, on their own initiative and without specific instruction, more and more elaborate grammatical utterences but also by their commission of certain kinds of plausible errors—for example, "hisself" and "I seed the sheeps"—that show the child working out for himself certain basic grammatical rules without knowledge of obligatory exceptions. Up to ages 3 to 5, at any rate, children ignore much grammatically inconsequential variation, such as hesitations in the speech they actually hear, in inferring the rules of language, and they are remarkably resistant to explicit shaping or correction by parents and other linguistic caretakers—at least, shaping of syntactical elements.

Chomsky's Theory. Chomsky's linguistic theory, called transformational-generative (TG) grammar, goes beyond earlier theories, which attempted to account only for the grammatical relations manifest in sentences as they are produced by speakers (the surface structure). Chomsky's theory goes to a deeper level of explanation, involving deep or base structure in an attempt to make explicit the implicit grammatical relations among semantically related synonymous sentences. Deep structures are limited in number, and they express basic and ultimately cognitive relations; surface structures are more various and more determined by context, style of discourse, and the like—that is, by nongrammatical factors.

TG theory is transformational in that particular surface structures reflect a given underlying deep structure, sometimes directly but generally by a series of transformations that yield the appropriate surface form. The obvious examples here are active and passive sentence forms. "The truck hit the boy" and "The boy was hit by the truck" are held to express the same proposition and, therefore, to share the same base-grammatical form, but they differ somewhat in emphasis and in the way they fit into an ongoing pattern of discourse. Other normal transformations of the basic sentence account for the tense of the verb, noun number, the presence of modifiers, the replacement of nouns with pronouns, negation, forming the interrogative, and so on.

TG theory is generative in two senses. First, from possessing the mastery of a relatively few basic syntactical principles and at least a finite number of syntactical rules or transformations, the competent user of a language can both produce and understand the infinite set of grammatical sentences of which any language is composed. Second and more subtle, syntax is an aspect of the basic structure of the human mind; it is inconceivable that a child, by empirical processes alone, could effectively analyze the surface structures of the sentences he hears into the necessary body of syntactical rules—owing, among other things. to ambiguity. Hence, to achieve the miraculous accomplishment of an infinite capacity from a finite experience in a few years, the child must be presumed to apply actively a native endowment, to possess structural models to account for and go beyond the speech he hears. In fact, so runs the argument in its extreme form, in order to cope with language, he must have perfect knowledge of a universal grammar, since the native-endowment premise implies that all human languages are basically alike in their underlying syntactical organization.

Generative Semantics. A current linguistic movement toward generative semantics involves a fundamentally different set of assumptions but retains the idea of deep versus surface interpretations and the idea of transformations.

In brief, those identified with the semantic movement, either in current linguistics or in cognitive psychology, give priority in grammar to the meaning of the utterance, holding that syntactical, lexical, and phonological rules are developed primarily to express meaning. To the syntacticist, uncovering the deep structure of the sentence, "They are eating apples," ac-

counts for the ambiguity without specifying the semantic interpretation. To the semanticist, the most obvious way to determine the syntactic structure is to take account of the meaning; in fact, if the meaning cannot be accounted for, the syntactic structure cannot be determined. As for actives and passives, the semanticist points precisely to the subtle shades of meaning revealed in each form. "The boy was hit by the truck" is held to emphasize the kind of thing that hit the boy, in a way that the active form, "The truck hit the boy," does not impart. The passive sentence form is usually processed psychologically in a more laborious or inexact way than is the active form, supporting the idea that it is less basic, that it is transformed. But under appropriate contextual circumstances this is not the case, suggesting that actual cognitive processing of these passives by reduction to and then retransformation from the base structure is not necessary.

TG theorists hold that semantic interpretation is a relatively late or subsidiary stage of the generation or comprehension of sentences. Furthermore, specific semantic evaluations, as required by syntactical form, are relatively trivial and are handled by a separate means. Lexical entities, in the course of experience, become marked with the appropriate semantic properties. Thus, "boy" carries with it the necessary implications of male, human, young.

Research by Clark and Card suggests that lexical marking is an important phenomenon but that syntactic theoy does not necessarily handle it. For example, in many paired terms (man, woman; large, small), one term is more general (man, large) in its range of reference, and the other is narrower in its range or more distinctive (woman, small)—hence, marked in a second sense. The comprehension of sentences and probably their construction in spontaneous language reflect these subtle referential differences. Then, too, the TG position that semantic interpretation is a separate and relatively superficial domain and that it consists of the user's learning necessary properties or features implies that sentences like "My son is a young boy" are, formally, tautologies and hence meaningless. This implication is questionable. The semantic domain is limitless, and no lexical item can ever be finally and definitively marked. Much of what is involved in constructing sentences—length, complexity, word order, and syntax—may be an accommodation to semantic imperatives—associations, implications, presuppositions—of the meaning that is to be conveyed.

The semantic position presently seems more open to explanations involving gradual, situationally relative, or environmentally directed processes than does TG grammar.

To generative semanticists, meaning units combine and condition each other, and the role of syntactic transformations is primarily to coordinate meanings in well-formed sentences. The sequential, hierarchical, and implicatory coordination of meaning that language provides, if this model is at all correct, may remind one of the familiar notion that thinking is a matter of coordinating concepts (reordering, collapsing, combining) or that having an idea involves fitting a particular example to a pre-existing structure, thereby slightly altering the structure. In the notion of semantic features or markedness, there may be suggestive parallels to the kind of distinctive conceptions, as opposed to logical classes.

Semantic Memory

It has long been suggested that there must be more than one kind of long-term memory—for example, background versus foreground memory, master versus focal memory, semantic versus episodic memory. In all these formulations, the second term refers to memory that deals with specific experiences of a particular spatial-temporal character. Whether in the encoding or the retrieval phase, such memory is tied to exact occasions, particular media, temporal order, and so on. The first term refers to memory that is, in some sense, the cumulative mental thesaurus, an encyclopedia rather than a word list. This is a noncompartmentalized, infinitely searchable, recombinatory, lattice structure of associations, tacit knowledge, implications, inferences, and relations.

Psychopathology

Disorders of thinking have been described for centuries in relation to a number of forms of psychopathology; indeed, thought disorder still serves as the hallmark of the most recalcitrant of the functional psychoses, schizophrenia. However, very little persuasive experimental work has been done on abnormal cognitive functioning, particularly in psychosis, because of the inaccessible nature of cognition, the difficulties of working with the mentally ill, and the enormous and unstable range of signs and symptoms evinced in the various conditions and syndromes. It has often proved to be impossible to separate cognitive malfunctioning from impaired motivation, the effects of treatment or maintenance of patients, and the understandable inability of the patient to understand or engage fully in the experimental task.

Cognitive behavior is characteristically refractory to explanation, unless the entire past history of the patient is taken into account. At the same time, the tremendously variegated manifestations of illness, even within one diagnostic category, reflect to a large degree inevitably different courses of illness. These two considerations suggest that progress in the study of cognitive functioning in relation to psychopathology may depend largely on the provision of longitudinal and prospective studies.

Categorizing and Conceptual Behavior. According to Whitehead, abstraction has two general meanings. In one sense it refers to the analysis of actual objects, events, and relations into attributes, like redness or sphericity. This he calls "abstraction from actuality." He has suggested the expression "abstraction from possibility" for the process by which an abstractive hierarchy is erected from attributes by a consideration of possible relations among attributes. Abstraction from possibility is the recognized method for extracting implications from assumptions, as in logic, law, philosophy, and mathematics.

Many schizophrenics can evolve rather elaborate logical constructs (abstraction from possibility) but fail on conceptual tests because they are unpredictable in abstraction from actuality, often defining category boundaries in an unusual fashion or selecting an incidental attribute as a basis for classification, rather than a commonly recognized property. In this respect, their behavior shows high eccentricity but not necessarily low abstract ability.

Word Association. Idiosyncratic word associations are among the most striking and most noted aspects of schizophrenic behavior. Systematic studies over many years have demonstrated that, compared with responses in normal persons, schizophrenics' responses in word association tasks are unusual (but not meaningless) and variable—from test to test in the same subject and in schizophrenics taken as groups compared with normal groups. Their clinical value aside, these phenomena by themselves are of little more than descriptive interest until they are related to theoretical models, such as those dealing with categorizing or concept usage, or until they are related to a broader behavioral context. Such a context is provided by the connected speech of schizophrenics, in which it has long been noted that seemingly unnatural verbal associations and intrusions break into the progress of directed discourse.

Schizophrenic Speech. The disordered speech of schizophrenics is unmistakable yet elusive. Transcribed samples of such speech can be reliably identified as seriously abnormal by university students. Yet schizophrenic speech is not frequent; many patients rarely or never show disordered speech, and those who do by no means do so in all their utterances but only in connection with certain situations or topics, often those that are emotionally toned. The most dramatic and oft-recorded forms of schizophrenic speech—such as echolalia and word salad and, for that matter, muteness—are very rare in modern times; given the ease with which particular speech patterns can be operantly conditioned in psychotics and normals, one can reasonably suspect that these forms owe much to special circumstances, including the interest and attention historically paid to such speech by others.

Brown suggests that there is nothing wrong with schizophrenic speech, only with schizophrenic thinking. He says that schizophrenic speech is recognizable as such because the speakers say things that others in the language community know cannot be true, even metaphorically or hypothetically, and that in such speech others recognize a profound failure of reality testing and knowledge of the world.

The overriding difficulty seems to lie in the semantic realm, dealing with meaning and content, but one must not ignore stable structural aspects of the speech itself. For example, schizophrenic speech is tangential. Sentences emitted by schizophrenics are less referentially well-knit than are those of normal people. Schizophrenics begin dealing with one subject matter but never do quite deal with it, and they end dealing with another one entirely.

Perception

Perception, according to a generally acceptable definition, is the process of organizing and interpreting sensory data by combining them with the results of previous experience. This definition indicates that perception is a complex process involving the past as well as the present and involving an external stimulus as well as an internal response.

Perception stretches from the biological sciences on one side to the social sciences on the other, and it includes data and ideas from physics and philosophy. The study of perception involves the physical properties of stimuli, the individual's nervous system, and his background and experiences. The physical properties of stimuli—wave lengths of light, frequencies of sound, and the like—are fundamental in determining the nature of the sensory data. The individual's nervous system is the locus of the sensation and the perception, and its functional strengths and deficiencies relate to what is sensed and what is perceived. The individual's family background and general social milieu and experiences contribute to his interpretation of the sensory data that he receives.

There are various sense modalities through which organisms are stimulated, and the sense organ that is stimulated yields only a particular type of sensation. This last point was enunciated first as the doctrine of the specific energy of nerves by Johannes Müller in the 19th century.

Organization

A great deal of the work on the influence of the stimulus field in perception has been done in the visual area. This is probably because what is perceived visually is strongly determined by the ordering of the stimulus components in space, and this ordering is rather easy to manipulate. For example:

****

is a row of 16 asterisks. By manipulating the spatial relationships, one can enhance the probability that they will be seen as eight pairs of asterisks:

** ** ** ** ** ** ** **

Such situations led to the enunciation of a principle to the effect that the whole is different from the sum of its parts. One explanation of this principle defines stimulus organization, or

Gestalt, as an additional property of the stimulus field (Figure 1).

Selectivity

Far more stimuli than the individual can be aware of or respond to are impinging on him at any given instant. These stimuli impinge simultaneously through many different channels, but the perceptual process is a central one, and only a limited amount of this information can be processed at one time. Therefore, a process of selectivity becomes operative. Some stimuli are perceived, and some are not; some that are perceived are responded to, and some are not.

Some objective and many subjective factors govern the operation of this selectivity; both the stimulus field and the attributes of the perceiver determine what will be perceived. One important objective factor is the strength of the stimulus. A strong stimulus is more likely to be perceived than a weak one. Another objective factor that governs what is perceived is timing. A stimulus that begins an instant before another may be perceived at the expense of the second.

Neurophysiology of Perception

The intactness of the sense organs and tracts is a necessary precondition for accurate perception. For example, color blindness interferes with the perception of color. However, the perception of physical stimuli involves more than simply the sensory pathways specific to a particular modality of stimulation. Recent work has placed considerable emphasis on the role of the reticular formation in the perception of stimuli.

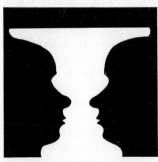

FIGURE 1. Figure and ground. The drawing demonstrates that the individual organizes visual sensations into perceptions. The simple pattern can be organized in two ways, and the viewer does both, alternately perceiving a white goblet against a ground of two silhouettes of faces.

This activating system is apparently essential to arousal, which must precede the reception of a stimulus from any modality.

Individual Development and Experience

One tends to perceive the more important stimuli rather than the less important. Since the attribute of importance is based on individual experience and interests, two people in the same situation may perceive very different things, and yet both may be accurate. What each perceives is a function of his own learning and experience. For example, the letter A would be simply a collection of lines to someone who does not know how to read.

An experience that predisposes an individual to certain types of perceptions is called a set. The more ambiguous the stimulus, the more its perception is determined by the set or proclivities of the subject. And the stronger the set of the individual, the more it determines his perception. The meaning attributed to a particular stimulus by an individual is a function of the ambiguity of the stimulus and the strength of his set.

The major application of these principles in psychiatry has been in projective testing, in which ambiguous stimuli are presented to individuals and their responses are analyzed in terms of their emphasis and patterning. Extrapolated from this analysis is a description of the individual's personality in terms of his perceptual proclivities. Perhaps the best known projective test is the Rorschach test, a collection of 10 inkblots.

The needs of the individual influence the content of what is perceived. Overall psychological needs as well as immediate physical needs influence perception. The Thematic Apperception Test (TAT) is based on this proposition. The stimuli for this test consist of pictures of people in various situations. The situations are ambiguous enough to allow for a variety of interpretations. The subject is asked to tell a story about each picture, and his story is interpreted in terms of his particular needs and drives.

Many experiments have indicated that people can be influenced in their own perceptual judgments by the judgments of others. The degree of influence depends on the consistency of others' judgments, the status of the other judges, and the expertise attributed to them.

Much of perception is learned behavior.

Senden reports a series of studies of people who were blind from birth and who, at varying ages, underwent successful surgery for the removal of cataracts. Studies of their visual perception indicated that they had great difficulty in perceiving objects and even greater difficulty in distinguishing one object from another. Most of the young subjects were able to acquire adequate visual perception with time and practice, but many of the older subjects sustained an apparently permanent visual handicap.

Some psychiatric patients display unique or malfunctioning sensory and perceptual behavior. The more obvious differences between patients and nonpatients in such sensory phenomena as hallucinations illustrate this fact. The literature, both scientific and autobiographical, contains numerous examples of patients' reports of profound changes during psychiatric illness, particularly during the early stages. In the course of psychiatric illness, from its onset to periods of remission or recovery, sensory changes of a variety of types may be displayed by patients. However, numerous complex difficulties arise when scientific attempts are made to measure these differences precisely and to interpret their significance.

Difficulties and Limitations

Perceptual responses, by their very nature, are subjective; the interest is in what the subject experiences. Therefore, to obtain measures that are truly sensory or perceptual, one must use indirect techniques; an objective response measure does not always represent the best or even the most appropriate way to measure sensation or perception. It has been suggested that the most valid way to measure what is intrinsically subjective is to design experiments that use converging operations to measure the sensory and perceptual responses of interest.

To evaluate sensory-perceptual research in psychopathology, one must ask the fundamental question: Is there any evidence that unequivocally demonstrates sensory and perceptual differences between psychopathological patients and normal subjects? Or instead: Is it not usually the case that apparent sensory differences are simply due to differences in such factors as motivation and cooperation or to various response biases of the subjects?

In the area of experimental psychopathology,

there has been an increasing recognition that many of the previously reported sensory differences between patients and normal subjects may not, in fact, have been true sensory differences at all but, instead, nonsensory differences related to a variety of subject variables, including response criterion. There has also been a recognition of a need in this area of research for a refined methodology that eliminates, controls, or even measures contaminating nonsensory variables. Recently, certain investigations using more refined methodological procedures have indicated that genuine sensory differences in psychiatric patients can still be demonstrated experimentally.

Another problem in sensory-perceptual research with patients stems from the fact that there is increasing evidence that, if sensory differences do exist between psychiatric patients and normal subjects, they may be small but significant effects. Small effects require the use of optimum procedures, the best and most precise equipment, the cooperation of the subject, and the best experimental designs to eliminate possible sources of confounding. A further complication is that the human subject is an incredibly sensitive observer and that small stimulus fluctuations or changes can lead to marked performance differences. The implication is that adequate sensory and perceptual studies require sophisticated physical apparatus with precise ancillary calibrating and monitoring equipment.

If sensory research with motivated, cooperative normal subjects is difficult, then similar research with unmotivated, uncooperative, and emotionally disturbed psychiatric subjects is virtually impossible. In traditional psychophysical experiments a single observer makes hundreds and sometimes thousands of observations extending over days and weeks. This procedure enables the investigator to obtain the most precise measures of the sensory factor that he is exploring and to determine whether there are systematic changes over time. Unfortunately, many patients cannot be expected to cooperate to this extent. For this reason the investigator must devise techniques that do not involve such a high degree of cooperation.

In this regard two fairly recent developments in the field of perception are worth noting, since they enable precise sensory measurement for a wide variety of observers, including infants and subhuman subjects. The first technique involves eye movement measurement in relation to complex perceptual phenomena. The second is the use of operant conditioning procedures for purposes of training subjects to make discriminations.

Advantages

Despite the difficulties involved in sensory-perceptual research with psychiatric patients, there are several advantages in using sensory psychology as a point of departure for psychiatric research. One advantage is that the large amount of scientific information available about sensation and perception can be used as a base line. In the practical realm, this advantage means that an investigator has a number of established sensory and perceptual methods and techniques available.

Besides the practical considerations of having base line data to refer to and techniques to use, a more basic question is involved. Much psychiatric research entails the manipulation of subject variables. In such research, instead of using independent variables involving manipulation of physical factors, like those of experimental psychology, one indirectly manipulates some characteristic of the groups being compared. For example, a psychotic group may be compared with a normal group on some dependent variable, such as a test score. In this case the psychiatric status of the persons tested is the subject variable that is being manipulated. The difficulty with this procedure is that, if a response difference is obtained between the groups of subjects tested, it is unclear whether the difference is caused by the subject variable that was manipulated or by some other subject variable that was related to the subject variable being manipulated.

Another potential advantage of sensory-perceptual research is the possibility that demonstrated behavior differences between patients and normal subjects may actually reflect differences that are in some way fundamentally related to the psychiatric illness. An alternative but perhaps related exploration of the relation between sensory differences and psychopathology suggests that a fundamental impairment in behavior pathology is in the person's information processing. In this case, sensory and perceptual responses would provide excellent techniques for investigating such an impairment, and differences in sensory and perceptual responses may help to clarify the nature of the information-processing disorder.

Approaches

Perceptual-Personality Approach. This approach to psychopathology has emphasized research using certain perceptual responses to measure aspects of personality. Generally, this personality-through-perception approach has stressed the investigation of normal subjects, although an implicit assumption is that there is a relation between the personality of the subject and his behavior, be it normal or abnormal. More directly held is the assumption that personality factors may be important in explaining abnormal behavior.

One way to evaluate the perceptual-personality approach is to consider the tenability of the assumptions made by the researchers in this field. How reasonable are these assumptions in the light of the available empirical evidence? The first and foremost assumption made by workers in this field is that perception is determined more by a person's internal or inward state than by the external stimuli.

The next closely related major assumption of the perceptual-personality approach is that the differences in perception or in the errors of perception reflect stable individual differences that can be related either to personality characteristics or to psychiatric illness. The important fact, so the argument goes, is that people perceive the same things differently. It seems well-established that individual differences in perception do exist. Less clear is the evidence that these differences are caused only by personality differences. It is likely that the major individual differences have multiple causes.

The final assumption is that differences in perception are responsible for the performance differences displayed by the subjects. This assumption entails the problem of how to determine whether differences in performance are correctly interpreted as indicating true perceptual differences and not simply as reflecting other nonperceptual differences. Admittedly, the study of perception necessarily involves the study of behavior. It is possible, at least abstractly, to conceive of a situation in which the perceptions of a group of subjects are essentially the same and yet the resulting behavior differs.

In recent years, the perceptual-personality approach has lost some of its initial promise; consequently, relatively few investigators are engaged today in research on these problems. In part, the disenchantment may be related to the major conclusion of the numerous studies of perceptual defense and subliminal perception, topics that come from the tradition represented by the perceptual-personality approach. What the investigations of perceptual defense and subliminal perception found was that these phenomena were largely attributable to methodological artifacts, rather than to real perceptual differences.

Sensory-Physiological Approach. A second sensory-perceptual approach to psychopathology, by far the oldest approach, is based on the underlying assumption that psychiatric illnesses have physiological bases and that it is possible to tap such physiological differences by using a sensory or perceptual measure. In its boldest form, this approach uses sensory behavior as an indicator of central nervous system malfunctioning associated with or responsible for psychopathology. A milder version of this approach is held by the investigator who hypothesizes that, although psychiatric illness is not necessarily caused by physiological differences between patients and normal subjects, the illness has definite physiological correlates, and sensory measures can be used as indicators of what these physiological correlates are. In this approach the main objective is to determine genuine sensory and, therefore, physiological, differences; there is little concern about the significance of these differences, if they exist.

Sensory-Perceptual Processing Approach. Presently, it is fashionable in all areas of experimental psychology to use what is loosely called an information-processing approach. The prevalent general notion of this approach is that the human organism has information-processing capacities and that different persons display differences with respect to these processing capacities. In this approach to psychopathology, the working assumption is that there is some deviation or breakdown in the information-processing capacities of the patient population and that this deficit may help to explain the psychopathology. The deficit is not necessarily interpreted as causing the illness.

Experiments exemplifying this approach stress the notion that sensory and perceptual research provides a means for investigating the processing capacities of the observer. Since the nature of the processes after stimulus presentation are both complex and little understood, a major problem is how behavioral techniques can be used to obtain reliable and unequivocal measures of such events. The assumption is that, by using proper experimental techniques, the investigator can obtain measurements of these events. To date, research in the field, both empirical and theoretical, is still primarily speculative and illustrative, rather than definitive.

REFERENCES

Bourne, L. E., Jr. *Human Conceptual Behavior*. Allyn & Bacon, Boston, 1966.
Broen, W. E., Jr. *Schizophrenia: Research and Theory*. Academic Press, New York, 1968.
Brown, R. *A First Language: The Early Stages*. Harvard University Press, Cambridge, 1973.
Brown, R. Schizophrenia, language, and reality. Am. Psychol. *28:* 395, 1973.
Bruner, J. S., Goodnow, J. J., and Austin, G. A. *A Study of Thinking*. Wiley, New York, 1956.
Clark, W. C. Pain sensitivity and the report of pain: An introduction to sensory decision theory. Anesthesis., *40:* 272, 1974.
Emmerich, D. S., and Levine, F. M. Phenothiazine dosage levels and auditory signal detection in schizophrenia. Science, *179:* 405, 1973.
Eriksen, B. A., and Eriksen, C. W. *Perception and Personality*. General Learning, Morristown, N. J., 1972.
Frith, C. D. Abnormalities of perception. In *Handbook of Abnormal Psychology*, H. J. Eysenck, editor, ed. 2, p. 284. R. R. Knapp, San Diego, 1973.
Goldiamond, I. Perception. In *Experimental Foundation of Clinical Psychology*, A. J. Bachrach, editor, p. 280. Basic Books, New York, 1962.
Kimura, D. The asymmetry of the human brain. Sci. Am., *228:* 70, 1973.
Milner, B. Introduction: Hemispheric specialization and interaction. In *The Neurosciences, Third Study Program*, F. O. Schmitt and F. G. Warden, editors, p. 375. M.I.T. Press, Cambridge, 1974.
Neisser, U. *Cognitive Psychology*. Appleton-Century-Crofts, New York, 1966.
Payne, R. W. Cognitive abnormalities. In *Handbook of Abnormal Psychology*, H. J. Eysenck, editor, p. 193. R. R. Knapp, San Diego, 1973.
Piaget, J. *The Construction of Reality in the Child*. Basic Books, New York, 1954.
Salzinger, K. *Schizophrenia: Behavioral Aspects*. Wiley, New York, 1973.
Sutton, S. Fact and artifact in the psychology of schizophrenia. In *Psychopathology*, M. Hammer, K. Salzinger, and S. Sutton, editors, p. 197. Wiley, New York, 1973.

3.2.   LEARNING THEORY

Definition

Learning is defined as a change in behavior potential resulting from reinforced practice.

Thorndike indicated that rewarded responses are always strengthened but that punished responses do not always diminish in strength, thus leading to an emphasis on reward as a primary determinant of behavior.

Conditioning

It is fairly traditional to view conditioning as a case of learning. Most theorists accept a rough dichotomy between two types of conditioning: classical (Pavlovian) and instrumental.

Classical Conditioning

Ivan Pavlov, a Russian physiologist, observed in his work with gastric secretions in dogs that stimuli that were often present at the time the dogs were offered food came to evoke salivation in the animals, even in the absence of food. In a typical Pavlovian experiment, a stimulus that, before training, had no capacity to evoke a particular type of response becomes able to do so. For example, under normal circumstances, a bell sounded near an animal will probably do no more than evoke exploration, such as a turning of the head toward the sound or, at most, a startle response. Also, under normal circumstances, a hungry animal may be expected to salivate in the presence of food. In Pavlov's conditioned reflex experiment, the previously neutral stimulus of a bell was paired with the food to evoke the response of salivation. To diagram this:

Preconditioning: $S \leftrightarrow R$
      (bell)   (exploration)

      $S \leftrightarrow R$
      (food)   (salivation)
Conditioning: S (bell)$\leftrightarrow S$ (food)$\leftrightarrow R$ (salivation)

Bell sounds are followed by the presentation of food. The animal salivates at the sight of the food and ultimately pairs S (bell) and S (food).

Postconditioning: S (bell) $\rightarrow R$ (exploration)

      $\lfloor$ conditioned
           $\downarrow$

      S (food) $\rightarrow R$ (salivation)
      (unconditioned stimulus)
           (unconditioned response)

Because the food naturally produces salivation, it is referred to as an unconditioned stimulus. Because the bell was originally unable to evoke salivation but came to do so when paired with food, it is referred to as a conditioned stimulus.

In the process of conditioning, Pavlov noted that animals would respond to stimuli similar to the stimulus to which they were conditioned. This event was called by Thorndike "response by analogy" and by Pavlov "generalization."

Generalization is at the basis of higher learning, inasmuch as it is possible through stimulus generalization to learn similarities. For a balance in learning, stimulus discrimination must also occur. For example, a child may refer to any quadruped as "doggie," but he learns to discriminate among quadrupeds so that he can differentiate a dog from a cow from a cat and, ultimately, as finer discrimination occurs, a boxer from a beagle from a basset.

A good deal of disordered behavior illustrates problems of this balance between generalization and discrimination. A patient may have affective reactions to a person with a moustache, presumably based on a traumatic earlier experience. A faulty generalization to *all* men with moustaches shows that discrimination training has not been successful.

Instrumental Conditioning

In contrast to classical conditioning, in which the organism is usually restrained (in a Pavlovian harness, for example) and in which the response is elicited by the experimenter, instrumental conditioning is an experimental technique in which a freely moving organism emits behavior that is instrumental in producing a reward. For instance, a cat in a Thorndike puzzle box must learn to lift a latch to escape from the box.

Generally, it is assumed that most learning occurs as a result of instrumental responding, rather than as an elicited consequence of classical conditioning.

Hull's Learning Theory

Hull's approach to learning theory is strongly mathematical and neurophysiological. For Hull, the process of learning consists in the strengthening of certain receptor-effector connections or in the setting up of new connections. These connections occur internally and are mediated by nervous system stimulation. The establishment of a connection occurs as:

$$S \rightarrow s \rightarrow r \rightarrow R$$

An external stimulus, S, has as its function the stimulation of an efferent system, s, which effects a motor impulse, r, within the nervous system. The final response, external R, does not have to occur for learning to take place: The critical connection is the s-r connection, leading to a habit.

Habit Family Hierarchy

The habit, for Hull, is an established connection within the nervous system, but these connections are not limited. The concept of the habit family hierarchy allows for transfer of learning or generalization to occur. Thus, a given stimulus, S, may evoke a number of different responses in varying levels of strength, but this stimulus evokes a response or set of responses within the nervous system that anticipate a goal response. For Hull, the goal response is antedated by fractional responses in the establishment of a habit. Thus, r may become a fractional response, an element of R, called a "fractional anticipatory goal response," or r_G, which in itself is stimulating. The fractional response then becomes a mediating element between S and R. An example of this is salivation occurring before the consummatory goal response to eating.

Because there is variability in response sequences leading to a goal as a result of varying environmental conditions, Hull postulated that "since all the alternative behavior sequences have led to the same goal, all of the component acts of all the sequences will alike be conditioned to the same fractional anticipatory goal-reaction stimulus (s_G), and in this sense will constitute a family."

Drive

Thorndike's law of effect used the concept of satisfaction to account for reinforcing effects of certain responses. Hull attempted to make the satisfying element less subjective. The reinforcing state of affairs, Hull believed, represented the "diminution in a need (and the associated diminution in the drive)." This principle of primary reinforcement is clearly a drive reduction approach. Attaining the goal response reduces the drive associated with the aroused need, strengthening the behaviors that led to the reduction in tension. This strengthened sequence becomes the habit.

Inhibition

Hull postulated that neural impulses (afferent receptor discharges) "occurring at about the same time interact and so modify each other." He called this afferent interaction and viewed it as a basis for the reduction or elimination of a response through the presence of an "extra or alien stimulus in a conditioned stimulus compound which can reduce the excitatory potential." Hull saw it as equivalent to Pavlov's external inhibition. Pavlov's concept of internal inhibition is similar to Hull's conditioned inhibition, which is an interfering set of events.

Wolpe's Conditioning Theory

Wolpe defined neurotic behavior as behavior that "consists of persistent habits of learned (conditioned) unadaptive behavior acquired in anxiety-generating situations." He reflects a neural approach to learning when he notes that "learning is subserved by the development of conductivity between neurons in anatomical apposition."

Wolpe also reflects a Hullian orientation in his principle of reciprocal inhibition, which may account for anxiety drive reduction: "If a response inhibitory to anxiety can be made to occur in the presence of anxiety-evoking stimuli, it will weaken the connection between these stimuli and the anxiety responses." Relaxation, for example, is considered to be incompatible with and therefore inhibitory to anxiety.

Wolpe used Hull's concept of habit family hierarchy when he established anxiety hierarchy relationships among anxiety-evoking stimuli. Assuming that various stimuli may evoke the response of anxiety, Wolpe asks his patient to imagine (usually under hypnosis) the least disturbing item of a list of potential anxiety-evoking stimuli, then to proceed up the list to the most disturbing stimuli. For example, a patient with a fear of death might rank the sight of a coffin lower in the hierarchy than a corpse.

Wolpe's technique of desensitization is a counterconditioning technique in which responses designed to inhibit the anxiety response are evoked at each level along the hierarchy. Reciprocal inhibition of the fear response is thus conditioned.

Skinner's Learning Theory: Operant Conditioning

Instead of dealing with the repression of unacceptable thoughts, as psychoanalysts do, Skinner suggests that it is more important to avoid the inner causes and to emphasize the questions that ask why the response was emitted in the first place, why it was punished, and what current variables are active.

The term "operant" refers to a class of responses emitted by the organism rather than elicited by some known stimulus. Operant responses are also referred to as voluntary, as opposed to involuntary or reflex behavior. Reflex responses are elicited, as in classical conditioning, and are called "respondents." Thus, respondents, such as pupillary reflexes, are differentiated from operants. An example of an operant response is reaching for a telephone. An operant has some effect on the environment.

A key concept in operant conditioning is reinforcement. The term "positive reinforcement" is used to describe an event consequent upon a response that increases the probability that the response will recur. A negative reinforcement is an event likely to decrease the probability of that response's recurrence. A negative reinforcement is an event that strengthens the response that removes it.

The frequency with which a response is emitted is a clear, observable measure of behavior. Aggressive behavior is emitted by most people; to say that a person is hostile suggests that this class of response occurs with a higher level of frequency than is usually expected.

By shaping, the experimenter, having specified the response he desires from the organism, brings the organism closer to the chosen terminal behavior. For example, if an experimenter wishes a pigeon to peck at a translucent plastic key on a wall of an experimental box, he most likely starts by reinforcing the pigeon for facing the wall on which the key lies. Then he reinforces the pigeon when he moves toward the wall, when he ultimately pecks at the wall, and, finally, when the pigeon pecks at the plastic key. The terminal response of key pecking was shaped from a large number of possible responses. The reinforcement must occur immediately after the response, since a delay in reinforcement may be accompanied by other responses that are not desired, and these may be reinforced adventitiously.

In chaining, each response becomes the reinforcing event for the previous response and the stimulus for the succeeding response. In this manner all complex behavior, particularly in skills that appear to be fluid responses, may be shaped and perceived as a chain of individual stimulus and response units.

There is reason to assume that, although behavior is established through reinforcement in a stimulus situation, the maintenance of once-established behavior is more a function of stimulus control than of continuing reinforcement. Assume that you have been sitting in room A and need an object located in room B. You go to room B and, when you enter the room, forget what it was you went to get, whereupon you return to room A, where the object is not but where the stimuli that evoked the searching behavior are.

There are times when responses are reinforced adventitiously (or accidentally) by coincidental pairing of response and reinforcement. Adventitious reinforcement can be linked to responses of the organism accidentally paired with reinforcing contingencies, as well as incidental stimuli. The latter may play a role in the development of phobic responses. Adventitious association of sensory stimuli with punishing or rewarding events appears to be closely related to superstitious responding. The adventitious association of certain consequences to responses may be at the basis of much of what is referred to as neurotic behavior, which persists as though it were contingent on certain responses and events.

Mowrer's Two-Factor Learning Theory

Mowrer theorized that much learning could be explained on the basis of acquired fear (anxiety) and that responses that reduce this anxiety are learned and maintained.

Mowrer suggested that anxiety responses are learned by contiguity. A stimulus that in itself is not fear-evoking is accidentally presented at the same time as a painful stimulus; by simple conditioning, the neutral stimulus becomes a conditioned aversive stimulus. Any response that results in the avoidance or elimination of such a conditioned aversive stimulus (as an anxiety-producing event) is reinforced, even in the absence of other reinforcement, because the response reduces anxiety (drive). Once learned, these avoidance responses persist.

Mowrer felt that conditioned anxiety responses did not need the reinforcement of repetition of the original trauma. Although the responses were conditioned by contiguity, they were maintained by the reinforcing effects of drive reduction. Classical conditioning of fear by contiguity was maintained by the subsequent conditioning (instrumental) of avoidance behavior by drive reduction.

Mowrer assumed that fear responses are entirely autonomic. Emotional responses are involuntary and largely autonomic; instrumental responding is voluntary and largely under the control of the central nervous system. The classically conditioned fear response learned under contiguity was physiologically differentiated from the instrumentally conditioned avoidance responses maintained by anxiety reduction.

Mowrer has also invoked a model in which the stimuli conditioned to the onset of painful events acquire certain drive (anxiety) characteristics, but those stimuli associated with the avoidance of or escape from pain become positively reinforcing. Mowrer described these two events as responses of fear and hope. In recent years, Mowrer's theorizing has centered largely on the development of neurosis and, in particular, the centrality of guilt and anxiety in emotional disorders.

Autonomic Conditioning and Biofeedback

Research has indicated that the distinction between the voluntary and the involuntary nervous systems is not as clear as was once believed and that responses of the autonomic nervous system may be brought under control in a fashion similar to those of motor and skeletal behaviors. In addition, certain behaviors under the autonomic nervous system can be modified through operant conditioning techniques. Experiments have shown that heart rate, blood pressure, hand temperature, and alpha activity can be brought under control in a laboratory situation.

REFERENCES

Hilgard, E. R. *Theories of Learning.* Appleton-Century-Crofts, New York, 1956.

Hull, C. L. *Principles of Behavior: An Introduction to Behavior Theory.* Appleton-Century-Crofts, New York, 1943.

Keller, F. S. *Learning: Reinforcement Theory.* Random House, New York, 1969.

Kimble, G. A. *Hilgard and Marquis' Conditioning and Learning,* ed. 2. Appleton-Century-Crofts, New York, 1961.

Skinner, B. F. *The Behavior of Organisms.* Appleton-Century-Crofts, New York, 1938.

Skinner, B. F. *Science and Human Behavior.* Macmillan, New York, 1953.

Wolpe, J. *Psychotherapy by Reciprocal Inhibition.* Stanford University Press, Palo Alto, Calif., 1958.

3.3.   MOTIVATION AND AFFECTIVE AROUSAL

Motivation

Animal Motivation

In the mediation of learning and perception in mammals, the cerebral cortex plays a major role, but the limbic system—the hypothalamus, in particular—and midbrain mechanisms appear to hold the main keys to understanding basic biological mechanisms responsible for motivating behavior.

Homeostatic Mechanism for Water Regulation. The problem of water regulation requires analysis at two levels: physiological reflexive and behavioral.

At the physiological reflexive level, water deprivation causes a release of the antidiuretic hormone, vasopressin, which, in its action on the kidneys, reduces urine flow to a minimum, thus conserving water. Crucial for understanding this mechanism and other fluid-regulating homeostatic mechanisms is the *milieu intérieur* concept of Claude Bernard. In the case of water regulation, *milieu intérieur* refers to critical physicochemical relations between internal conditions of certain cells, called receptor cells or sensors, and the extracellular fluids surrounding them.

The critical physicochemical changes are increment in effective osmotic pressure in extracellular fluids and intracellular volume changes. Cells specialized for sensing and signaling such intracellular volume changes are called osmoreceptors. Apparently, the osmoreceptors are not stimulated by a rise in total fluid osmolarity per se but, rather, by a change in the extracellular fluid, involving such substances as sodium salts, the molecules of which have low mobility through the semipermeable cell membranes.

Verney suggested that there were nerve cells in or near the supraoptic nucleus of the hypothalamus that monitored blood osmolarity and effected appropriate release of antidiuretic hormone. Actually, there appear to be two types of receptors: (1) osmoreceptors, which are responsive to changes in the effective osmolarity of the extracellular fluids, and (2) receptors that respond chiefly to reduction in intravascular fluid volume (hypovolemia). Both kinds of receptors may be viewed as points of origin in a cycle that leads back to the optimal *milieu intérieur*. However, the firing of single osmoreceptors has been recorded electrophysiologically and, consequently, their precise role in the cycle is clearer at the present time than is that of the other receptors.

Osmoreceptors, mainly in the supraoptic nucleus of the hypothalamus, are involved in the production and release of vasopressin from the posterior lobe of the pituitary. The end result of the reflexive chain, beginning with discharge of the osmoreceptors, is conservation of water by the kidneys, effecting return to more nearly optimal physiological conditions.

Neurophysiological Approach to Thirst-related Behavior. The behavior chain is enormously more complicated than the reflex chain. In the behavior chain, the osmoreceptor is the first-order neuron. One can call them thirst osmoreceptors to distinguish them from the reflex osmoreceptors.

The close proximity of the reflex osmoreceptors in the supraoptic nucleus to the pituitary gland is an obvious advantage. There is good evidence that thirst osmoreceptors are located elsewhere.

From behavioral observations of water-deprived animals, one can make some predictions about how the thirst osmoreceptors must interact with higher order neurons. Contrary to some older notions about drive, the thirsty animal does not necessarily become more active. If the animal is confined in a cage where there is no water or any cue that had previously been associated with water, it will not increase its activity as a rule and, in fact, may decrease it. Thus, deprivation of a basic need and the accompanying increased firing of sensor neurons in the brain can occur without necessarily increasing the level of behavioral activity. The potential push from an internal need must interact with the pull from relevant environmental stimulation for motor activity to be generated. "Incentive" is the term for this external pull.

The second-order neurons activated by concomitant bombardment by (1) osmoreceptors reacting to increased concentration of sodium in extracellular fluids and (2) sensory input from tongue or other receptors signaling the availability of water. The second-order neurons bring into activation a neural sequence that gains

facilitation of the motor mechanisms of drinking.

Homeostatic Mechanism for Drug Addiction. Drug dependence appears to involve some kind of acquired homeostatic mechanism. The only requirement for establishing dependency on morphine is that the administration be kept up regularly, day after day, until some objective criterion of dependency has been reached, usually the appearance of withdrawal symptoms. It is conceivable that certain brain cells, not already specialized for detecting dehydration or other such primary need states, may somehow undergo modification during the course of continuous morphine administration, thereby acquiring a sensitivity to the physicochemical conditions that underlie withdrawal symptoms.

Two theories about dependency may be distinguished. Both models postulate a form of cellular adaptation, and they are not mutually exclusive. According to one theory, the mechanism of adaptation requires that the drug be present on the neuron itself. According to the other theory, it is simply necessary that neurohumoral input be reduced; in other words, the reduction of nervous activity and not the exposure of neurons to the drug itself is directly responsible for the development of withdrawal hyperexcitability.

Interaction between internal and external instigations is an important key to the problem of relapse. There appears to be an internal push that remains after withdrawal, and, although weaker than before withdrawal, in interaction with external sources of pull it is strong enough to cause relapse. Physiological consequences of previous physical dependence have been observed to persist long after thorough withdrawal treatment.

The importance of the external pull factor in relapse has been experimentally demonstrated. It is easier to readdict rats in the same environment in which they were originally addicted than in a different environment. Stimuli in the familiar environment most likely exert pull on the rat.

This fundamental concept of interaction between central activation and external stimulation is useful in overcoming the mind-body dichotomy inherent in the distinction between physical and psychological dependence.

Alcoholism. The classic syndrome that is generally meant when the term "alcoholism" is used depends on the repeated ingestion of large quantities of ethanol over a considerable period of time. One hypothesis suggests that the continuous ingestion of large quantities of ethanol cause deviations in the normal metabolism of alcohol, resulting in the formation of compounds capable of producing physical dependence. According to another hypothesis, sudden abstinence after heavy and continuous ethanol intake produces a state of disuse supersensitivity. The two hypotheses are not mutually exclusive.

General Drive, Activation, Arousal

Current terminology applied to general aspects of motivation is not rigidly fixed. Terms such as "general drive," "activation," and "arousal" are used interchangeably in the current literature.

Research in the Area of Activation. The term activation is useful chiefly in referring to research in which level of physiological activation is studied in relation to interacting factors, such as internal and external factors. Researchers have found that food deprivation and cues associated with food had to be operative *together* for heart rate to show a rise. Even though the animal was deprived of food or water, heart rate did not increase in the absence of appropriate external cues.

There is a level of activation that is optimal for performance. On either side of this optimum, there is a performance decrement: The greater the departure from the optimum, the greater the decrement in performance. It is probable that the freezing reaction in frightened animals represents impairment of normal motor sequences by overactivation. Although inactive, an animal paralyzed with fear is, nevertheless, highly activated.

According to the activation or arousal concept, the kind of neural activity considered here feeds impulses into organized neural cell assemblies, supporting the firing of their units in delicately timed sequences. The optimal level of activation is that level of background firing that provides the optimal facilitations of the organized neural activities. Too little or too much background firing of cells in the arousal system is deleterious with regard to organized neural firing (mediating performance).

Nonhomeostatic Mechanisms of Motivation. When an animal is hungry or thirsty, its behavior is largely dominated by cues associated through learning with these organic needs. However, when the animal's basic needs are satisfied, its behavior is often directed by cues that have nothing whatever to do with seeking food or water or escaping from painful stimulation. Thorough experimental documentation of this point comes from extensive work on the curiosity drive in monkeys. Harlow and his associates demonstrated that monkeys will work for hours on mechanical puzzles with no reward other than solving them. Far from seeking reduction in level of activation or arousal, animals will look for excitement. Even lower mammals, like the rat, manifest exploratory behavior that seems to have little or nothing to do with food-seeking.

Another strongly motivated activity that does not depend on the animal being in a deprived state is the Olds-Milner phenomenon of intracranial self-stimulation. Electrical stimulation of certain areas of the brain is clearly rewarding. Rather complicated, well directed patterns of behavior can be elicited by means of stimulation through chronically implanted electrodes in the brains of awake animals.

In the higher mammals, especially in the chimpanzee but to some extent even in the dog, copulatory behavior is more complicated than the stimulus-bound subcortically mediated behavior in lower mammals. The relative importance of the cerebral cortex in mating behavior increases in the mammalian series from rat to man.

Human Motivation

Extremes of Motivation and Overarousal

The previous discussion of impairment produced by overactivation was concerned mainly with the impairment of response manifested in slow performance or failure to respond at all. Apparently this is the most prevalent kind of impairment in disaster situations. This kind of impairment is generally manifested in errors of omission.

As Spences noted, increasing the level of drive increases the advantage of a strong response over a weaker response in the competition for control of overt expression. If the strongest response happens to be wrong, then an error of commission will be made.

The concept of overarousal is currently in the

focus of various studies of chronic schizophrenia. According to Shagass, one of the most prevalent interpretive ideas about certain schizophrenic disorders is that they involve a chronic state of cerebral overstimulation or hyperarousal.

Physiological Gradients

Results from a substantial number of studies have revealed electromyographic (EMG) gradients from certain muscles depending on the task commencing with the onset of the behavior sequence and terminating at its conclusion.

Evidence from a significant number of studies indicates that the steepness of the rise in muscle tension is an indication of degree of motivation, interest, and the like. The gradients do not appear to reflect increasing motivation mounting steadily *during* the task or other sequence. The gradients appear to reflect some supportive central mechanism that is required to ensure the steady running off of a behavioral sequence. It seems that, in order for the behavioral sequence to proceed without breaking down, its central mechanism must receive an ever-increasing facilitation from the supportive central mechanism, whose peripheral facilitation is reflected in the EMG and other physiological gradients.

Whatever the mechanisms are that furnish the support for continuous productive mental activity, they seem to depend partly on normal exteroceptive sensory stimulation, since, under prolonged conditions of sensory isolation, mental activity suffers markedly. To this extent, at least, the peripheral components, sensory and motor, are critically important for operation of central activities.

Other Motivational Phenomena

The hypothesis that the strength of achievement motivation can be gauged in a meaningful and useful way by analyzing the content of stories told from pictures, such as those in the Thematic Apperception Test (TAT), underlies the extensive investigative work of McClelland and his associates. The research began with a demonstration that college students, given instructions designed to heighten their intensity of motivation to perform well on certain tests, produced in the stories they wrote from the TAT pictures more responses having to do with future achievement than students who were in a relaxed state at the time of writing TAT stories. The next stage in the experimental program was guided by the general hypothesis that persons who obtain high TAT need (n) achievement scores under controlled conditions are normally more intensely motivated to achieve than are persons who obtain low (n) achievement scores under the same condition.

Intensity of motivation to achieve at any task in any particular situation is determined by at least two factors: (1) the achievement motive—that is, desire to achieve—and (2) expectancy of probable success or failure.

There are marked individual differences with respect to values placed on certain objects or goals. Some students strive for A's; others depreciate the importance of grades, placing high values mainly on intellectual satisfactions or on extracurricular activities. The expectancy factor refers to the subjective probability that, with the expenditure of sufficient effort, the object may be acquired or the goal reached.

Milner has found that frontal-lobe patients break test rules more often than other patients do. It seemed they just could not control their impulsiveness. When progress toward the goal came into conflict with rules, the value system normally respecting rules was shown to be abnormally weak in the frontal-lobe patients.

Level of aspiration involves a procedure in which the subject is asked to say how he will do on the next trial of a task.

Cognitive dissonance means incongruity or disharmony with respect to such matters as expectation and actuality. In general, dissonance occurs when there is a palpable disparity between two experimental or behavioral elements. It is postulated that cognitive dissonance produces a tension state (like hunger) that is motivating.

The chief distinguishing feature of a cognitive approach to motivation is that the cognitive motivation theorists focus on perceptual and informational aspects of the total stimulating situation. They tend to deal with physiological arousal in terms of stimuli generated by the physiological processes.

Attribution theory is also a cognitive approach, and in essence it is concerned with how people perceive the motivations of others. According to Kelley, the basic assumption here is that man is motivated "to attain a cognitive mastery of the causal structure of his environment."

Freud's writings were probably the most powerful single influence initiating scientific investigations of human motivation. From Freud's observations, it was plain that a full understanding of the causes of human behavior could not be gained from conscious introspections. Clearly, much of behavior is determined by unconscious mental activities, activities that the person is unaware of and consequently cannot report on.

Physiological Concomitants of Affective Arousal

Careful physiological recordings made with sensitive instruments invariably show measurable changes concomitant not only with reaction to an emotion-producing situation but with reaction to any significant change in the environmental situation. When subjects in one experiment were injected with adrenalin, which produced a state of physiological arousal, but were given an inappropriate explanation of the effects by a physician, their reactions were determined by the environmental situation, whereas, with an appropriate explanation, there was no such dependence on the environmental events.

It seems unlikely that subjective differences between emotions could be based mainly on differentiation between autonomic nervous system patterns of reaction, as some early writers thought. This is not to say, however, that sensory feedback from the autonomic nervous system does not ever enter significantly into the picture. Indeed, in the case of some psychiatric patients with somatic symptoms, when stress evokes a symptom reaction, such as tachycardia and palpitations, the sensations associated with this physiological reaction can be frightening, even terrifying if there is fear of impending death.

There are distressing sensations from muscles tensing under stress in patients prone to muscular discomfort in specific muscular groups. A 42-year-old female psychiatric patient complained of muscular discomfort localized in the left thigh. While the patient was engaged in a tracking task, EMGs were recorded from various muscles over the body. When a loud distracting noise was presented during tracking,

tension in the left thigh rose to a very much higher level than that recorded from the right thigh. As a matter of fact, tension in the thigh muscles on the right (nonsymptom) side of the body actually fell slightly under the activating conditions. When tracking was performed under distraction-free conditions, no tensional difference between right and left thighs was observed.

A depressed single woman of 28 complained of a painful tightness on the right side of her neck. At the time the EMG recordings were made, the patient had been suffering from this tension for some weeks. This young woman feared contact with men, a fear that may have been caused in part by severe punishment that she received as a child from her mother, who believed that the patient and her brother had been engaging in sex play. During EMG recording, she was resting quietly when a male research assistant began to remove cloth electrode holders from her arm. In so doing, he happened to take her hand in his, whereupon the EMGs from her right neck muscles suddenly increased in level while the EMGs from the opposite side of her neck showed little or no change. It was established that the rise in right neck muscle tension was not an artifact of head turning or of any other kind of head movement. By taking her hand in his, the male assistant evidently embarrassed her by an unintended act of intimacy, at the same time triggering her specific tensional reaction.

Physiological recordings that have been successfully taken from patients under test conditions or during psychiatric interview include cardiovascular, respiratory, skin conductance, gastrointestinal, electromyographic, and electroencephalographic. Changes are generally polyphasic in character; a change in one direction is followed by a compensatory change in the opposite direction. In some cases, the compensatory reaction may predominate over the initial reaction.

Individual Differences

Some people tend to show what has been called sympathetic dominance; others tend to show parasympathetic dominance. The majority of persons show a fairly equal balance, and only a few persons show extremely high sympathetic or extremely high parasympathetic dominance.

Another kind of individual difference is determined by particular physiological measures that show the greatest relative changes under standard conditions of stimulation. Specificity of physiological reaction to stress is observed with remarkable clarity in patients with complaints of bodily discomfort, such as tachycardia, palpitations, precordial pain referred to the cardiovascular system, and tensional discomfort (including muscular pains and tension headache) referred to the skeletal-motor system.

Pathological Anxiety

Pathological anxiety—the emotional responses of pathologically increased intensity and duration that may be observed in certain neurotic patients—has been objectively defined for research purposes as a tensional state of such severity that work efficiency is interfered with and medical advice is sought. It is characterized by one or more of the following complaints: persistent feelings of tension or strain, irritability, unremitting worry, restlessness, inability to concentrate, and feelings of panic in everyday life situations. Patients with these symptoms have been found to be physiologically hyperactive. Proneness to overreaction appears to involve a physiological alteration that renders the patient overly sensitive to a wide range of relatively innocuous and insignificant stimuli and situations.

Startle induced by a strong auditory stimulus was found to be an effective form of stimulation for physiological differentiation of anxiety patients and normal persons. EMG recording under these circumstances revealed no difference between patients and controls in the immediate reflex reaction to the startling sound; the differences in the EMG reactions of patients and controls came after the primary period of reflex startle. In view of results from neurophysiological experiments, a likely explanation of the abnormally high afterreaction observed in anxiety patients is that the sustained tension is due to the failure of some central homeostatic mechanism, possibly located in the reticular systems. Experiments with animals have demonstrated that, by stimulating certain parts of the thalamic reticular system, one can inhibit motor afterdischarge.

Other kinds of physiological dysfunction observed in anxiety patients compared with controls under experimental conditions include irregularities in motor action, such as finger tremor and respiratory irregularity, and autonomic nervous system overreactivity, such as reactions of blood pressure and heart rate.

Any phasic reaction must be judged in relation to the tonic level prevailing at the time. A physiological function that is already highly activated generally reacts less to further stimulation than does a function that is less activated at the outset. Chronic, excessive physiological activity, phasic *or* tonic, is evidence for defective physiological regulation in anxiety patients. Which action predominates depends on the precise conditions, before, during, and after testing.

The chronic character of pathological anxiety, its persistence for months or longer after stress has been removed, must be due to a breakdown, for a time, in certain parts of complexly interacting mechanisms. Such a pathological state may develop in a number of different ways: for instance, by chiefly constitutional metabolic and neural deficiencies or an extraordinarily stressful life situation that starts the pathological chain of physiological events by, perhaps, causing a greatly increased flow of adrenalin over a long period of time.

REFERENCES

Ellis, F. W., and Pick, J. R. Experimentally induced ethanol dependence in rhesus monkeys. J. Pharmacol. Exp. Ther., *175:* 88, 1970.

Engel, B. T. Response specificity. In *Handbook of Psychophysiology*, N. S. Greenfield and R. S. Sternbach, editors, p. 571. Holt, Rinehart and Winston, New York, 1972.

Greenfield, N. S., and Sternbach, R. A., editors. *Handbook of Psychophysiology*. Holt, Rinehart and Winston, New York, 1972.

Hahn, W. W. Attention and heart rate: A critical appraisal of the hypothesis of Lacey and Lacey. Psychol. Bull., *79:* 59, 1973.

Lader, M. H. Psychophysiological aspects of anxiety. In *Studies of Anxiety*, M. H. Lader, editor, p. 53 (Br. J. Psychiatry, Spec. Publ. No. 3). Headley Brothers, Ashford, Kent, 1969.

Malmo, R. B. Studies of anxiety: Some clinical origins of the activation concept. In *Anxiety and Behavior*, C. D. Spielberger, editor, p. 157. Academic Press, New York, 1966.

Malmo, R. B. Overview. In *Handbook of Psychophysiology*, N. S. Greenfield and R. A. Sternbach, editors, p. 967. Holt, Rinehart and Winston, New York, 1972.

Malmo, R. B., and Belanger, D. Related physiological and behavioral changes: What are their determinants? Res. Publ. Assoc. Res. Nerv. Ment. Dis., *45:* 288, 1967.

Pert, C. B., and Snyder, S. H. Opiate receptor: Demonstration in nervous tissue. Science, *179:* 1011, 1973.

3.4. BIOLOGICAL ASPECTS OF AGGRESSIVE BEHAVIOR

The biological contribution to aggressive behavior is significant. In some cases of antisocial violence, biological abnormalities may even be the most important single variable. Biological factors may be involved in human aggressive behavior at several levels: genetic programing, learning, intraspecies variation, and through indirect sociological linkages. In theory, these levels are distinct, but, in practice, they permeate and interact with each other.

In some animal species, aggressive behavior is at least in part genetically preprogramed (instinctual). This behavior may consist of stereotyped and apparently innate behavior patterns that occur in response to certain sign stimuli or releasers. If there is a degree of human preprograming, at least in the young child, cross-cultural contrasts indicate that it can be overridden by training. More likely, the genetic contribution will be found to be not so much in the form of innate, preprogramed responses as in predispositions and preparedness to learn, with considerable openness as to the particular program learned.

Each species has a unique complex of learning aptitudes that are genetically based. Each species is more or less prepared to acquire certain skills and information and to learn them by certain mechanisms—such as conditioning, modeling, insight, and imprinting—at certain periods in its life and to forget or extinguish them more or less easily. Human beings, it appears, readily learn certain aggressive behaviors that have survival value for primates living beyond the fringes of the sheltering forest. On the other hand, human beings also have a demonstrated capability to learn nonviolent ways of responding. A significant positive correlation has been found between the use of violence in punishment and aggressive behavior, at least in adolescent boys. Presumably, the child is more influenced by the violent behavior of the parent (model) than by punishment (negative reinforcement).

Biological factors are also significant on an intraspecies level and are implicated in sex differences, age differences, and individual differences. Biological differences may affect ease of learning or thresholds of aggressivity. Hormonal patterns and brain anomalies appear to be significantly involved.

Juvenile delinquents include a disproportionate share of poor readers, and a high proportion of disfiguring scars and deformities has been noted among prison populations. It is likely that persons so handicapped are victims of social rejection or educational humiliation; the resulting personal frustration and unhappiness increase the likelihood of deviant behavior, including antisocial aggression.

Kinds of Aggression

Moyer has tentatively proposed eight distinct classes of aggression: predatory, fear-induced, irritable, territorial, maternal, sex-related, intermale, and instrumental. These classes are most readily distinguished on the basis of the stimulus configurations that evoke them. Aggressive behavior in most species is stimulus-bound; it is elicited only by highly specific stimulus situations. It also appears that the basic physiological mechanisms involved in at least some of the proposed categories can be similarly differentiated.

Fear reactions have been reduced by lesions in the temporal lobe and the amygdala and by amygdalectomies and anterior cingulectomies. Conversely, septal lesions may facilitate fear-induced aggression. There also appears to be some involvement of the hypothalamus, and Romaniuk suggests the possibility of escape-aggression reactions being organized in the hypothalamus on a dorsal ventral basis.

Although irritable aggression can be increased in many but not all species by increases in other drive states, other precursor events may also contribute—fatigue, lack of sleep, population density or crowding, pain, and other forms of aversive stimuli. There is some evidence that the ventro-medial hypothalamus and medial nucleus of the amygdala are involved. Androgenic hormones also appear to play a role in the interindividual variations observed in response to irritating or aversive stimuli. Likewise, the effects of population density and the pituitary-adrenal axis have been explored, and there appear to be linkages between adrenal function and irritable aggression.

A critical element in intermale aggression,

unlike some other forms of aggression, is the male androgens.

Learning may never be entirely absent from aggressive behavior. The apparently innate territoriality of some species, for instance, depends for its expression on the acquired attachment to a particular territory. However, the category of instrumental aggression is thought by Moyer to include those aggressive behaviors that are called into play primarily as a result of learning. The biological correlates of this category of aggression are, in theory, the same that contribute to preparedness for learning and the physiological changes that take place in the learning process.

The usefulness of a given category of aggression varies according to the particular survival strategy used by any given species, and each species has its own particular aggressive repertoire. Even within the lifetime of a single animal, the potential for a given category of aggressive behavior may fluctuate, according to seasonal or other considerations. Most experiments indicate that aggressive behavior is not appetitive but is evoked mainly in situations in which it is likely to have survival advantages.

Sex Differences in Aggressivity

Although human females are known to engage in violence, the frequency of violent acts by males is far higher. Cultural conditioning and expectations are, of course, significantly different for the two sexes (see Figure 1). However, the predominance of males as perpetrators of violence is so consistent across cultures that biological influences must be suspected. Marked sexual differences in agonistic behavior are also common in other species, often appearing at an early age.

The presence or absence of male sex hormones (androgens) appears to be a critical variable in these sexual differences in apparent aggressiveness. The removal of the hormone-producing gonads renders young males relatively mild and tractable. However, experiments with castrated mice show that normal

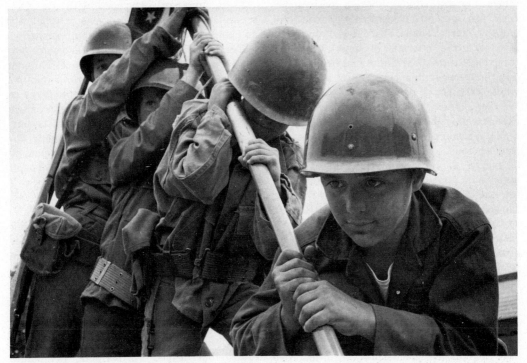

FIGURE 1. In most societies young boys are conditioned to assume an attitude toward life by means of role-playing. In this picture the raising of the flag at the battle of Iwo Jima during World War II is portrayed. (Courtesy of Roger Malloch for Magnum Photos, Inc.)

aggressive (and sexual) behavior can be restored by the injection of the missing testosterone or other androgens. Conversely, some researchers have been able to suppress at least some forms of fighting behavior in intact (uncastrated) males through the administration of estrogens.

The earlier in life that castration occurs, the more feminized is the behavior of a genetically male animal and the less likely he is to exhibit normal behavior, even when male hormones are administered. The prenatal and immediately postnatal period is particularly critical to the normal physical development and sexual behavior of male animals.

Androgenized female mouse pups engage in the rough-and-tumble play typical of male pups, and they display male mounting (sexual) behavior. The same is true of monkeys.

In some cases, such an abnormal hormonal situation has existed for a female human fetus, with androgens present to an unusual degree in the prenatal period. Studies of girls with such a history indicate that their behavior and interests, as described by both themselves and others, are distinctly tomboyish, with preferences for vigorous outdoor sports, rough play, and toys, such as guns, that are usually associated with the interests of boys. The adult behavior of these girls cannot now be predicted, but the strong influence of social and family values must not be discounted.

Other studies examined the effects of intrauterine estrogen and progesterone on psychosexual development in boys. Although the subjects were not, at the age of 6, significantly less aggressive than the controls, marked differences had appeared by the time they were retested at the age of 16. At that time the boys showed themselves to be less assertive and aggressive than the controls.

Only a small minority of violent acts are attributed to women, but these few outbreaks tend to cluster during the premenstrual week, when levels of progesterone and the estrogens are at their lowest.

The general conclusion to be drawn is that the male hormones increase the likelihood of aggressive behavior and that the female hormones have the opposite effect. However, in maternal and predatory aggression the hormones do not necessarily have this effect or may even have an opposite effect. Hormonal changes associated with lactation may heighten the aggressive potential of females.

Interindividual Variation

Genetics and Aggression

By far the greatest source of data on inherited differences in aggressivity has been the laboratory rodents—mice and rats. And in these species, the heritability of aggression is rather high, although not unalterable by training.

The evidence for the heritability of aggressivity in man is still fragmentary. A gross chromosomal abnormality, the XYY syndrome, has received a great deal of publicity in connection with crimes of violence. When the frequency of this chromosomal abnormality in institutionalized populations was compared with the frequency among newborns in the population at large, Hook noted that there was "a definite association between the XYY genotype and presence in the mental-penal settings." However, neither the nature nor the extent of this association has yet been determined. Hook's impression is that "increased impulsiveness, rather than greater aggressivity per se" may be the more relevant behavioral factor.

As is apparently the case with the XYY syndrome, the link between genetic variability and behavioral manifestations in human beings will probably prove to be indirect and subject to considerable environmental influence. Through differences in preparedness to learn, irritability and tolerance of frustration, receptiveness to arousal, or even such physical attributes as size and strength—all of which influence the outcome of learning experiences—the genetic differences may be found to express themselves by increasing or decreasing the probability of overt aggressive behavior.

Testosterone Levels

A series of hormonal assays of normal children showed both sex differences and wide individual differences in prepubertal children in blood plasma levels of testosterone. Moreover, between the ages of 10 and 15, testosterone levels in boys increase dramatically, as much as 10-fold.

Monkeys with strikingly aggressive behavior have been found to have higher than average testosterone levels. Furthermore, dominance rank was positively correlated with testosterone concentrations, although the most aggressive animals in the group were not always the most dominant, nor were the least aggressive necessarily lowest in dominance. The correlation between testosterone and aggression and dominance was significant but other factors were also involved, including other morphological characteristics of the animal and, frequently, its previous experience in the environment.

Whether correlations between hormone levels and human dominance or aggresivity exist has been little investigated.

Brain Anomalies

Researchers have been able to switch violence on and off through the stimulation of selected brain sites. And psychosurgeons have sought, by the removal or destruction of any of several brain areas, to pacify individual human beings exhibiting pathological, uncontrolled violence. It is not always clear, however, whether the parts of the brain so excised were themselves abnormal or whether the consequent lessening of hostility was achieved by a general sedating effect or by removal of parts of the brain that merely mediate or facilitate aggressiveness motivated and organized elsewhere in the brain.

It is likely, however, that brain abnormalities of some sort are directly involved in at least a portion of the cases of pathological violence. Certain known brain diseases—such as brain tumors, temporal lobe epilepsy, and such viral infections as encephalitis—are associated with violent behavior. And there appears to be a higher incidence of abnormal encephalographic readings among persons who exhibit motiveless violence and those who are labeled as severe psychopaths.

REFERENCES

Bandura, A. *Aggression: A Social Learning Analysis.* Prentice-Hall, Englewood Cliffs, N. J., 1973.

Berkowitz, L., editor. *Roots of Aggression: A Re-Examination of the Frustration-Aggression Hypothesis.* Altherton, New York, 1969.

Clemente, C. D., and Lindsley, D. B., editors. *Aggression and Defense: Neural Mechanisms and Social Patterns.* University of California Press, Los Angeles, 1967.

Daniels, D. N., Gilula, M. F., and Ochberg, F. M., editors. *Violence and the Struggle for Existence.* Little, Brown, Boston, 1970.

Garattini, S., and Sigg, E. B., editors. *Aggressive Behavior.* Wiley, New York, 1969.

Hook, E. B. Behavioral implications of the human XYY genotype. Science, *179:* 139, 1973.

Mark, V. H., and Ervin, F. R. *Violence and the Brain.* Harper & Row, New York, 1970.

Moyer, K. E. *The Physiology of Hostility.* Markham, Chicago, 1971.

St. John, R. D., and Corning, P. A. Maternal aggression in mice. Behav. Biol., *9:* 635, 1973.

3.5.   COLLECTIVE AGGRESSION

Causes

A number of attempts have been made to extrapolate from various presumed causes of individual aggression to collective aggression. For instance, in 1932 Freud suggested that group violence derives from a simple extension of the individual death or destructive instinct. Social learning, likewise, has been advanced by several behavioral scientists as the main cause of warfare. Frustrations, both individual and collective, have also been linked to collective violence. Individual frustrations may lead to collective violence through a process of displacement or projection.

Collective aggression also involves variables associated with the dynamics of organized group behavior. The research of Tajfel, for instance, suggests that polarizations and antagonisms may arise, in part, as an outcome of the very process of forming within-group bonds, independently of any external grounds for conflict. Likewise, the work of Milgram on obedience to authority indicates that leader-follower relations and the commands of an authority figure may play an important role in collective aggression.

Another factor is the role of cognitive and problem-solving processes, more or less conscious and rigorous cost-benefit analyses by leaders and followers of the relative utilities of collective aggression as an instrumentality for attaining group goals as defined by the leadership.

There is some evidence that, in civil violence and revolutions, relative socio-economic deprivations or systemic frustrations may play a role, but the influence of such factors is complex and apparently mediated by a number of other considerations, including the role of leadership and perceptions as to the legitimacy of the existing institutions and of their capacity to maintain order.

The causes of warfare have been studied for a longer period of time, and data are more extensive. No single factor stands out as being of overriding importance, although leadership—the personalities, perceptions, and pressures operating on political leaders—is assuming an important place in the thinking of social scientists.

Conclusion

Warfare represents a form of collective coping behavior closely associated with basic, survival-related pressures. In this view war is not in the genes in the sense of being a spontaneous and appetitive behavior but is a product of the relationships between man and the environment. Thus, the most effective means for reducing the probability of war appears to be intervention in the man-environment relationship in such a way as to mitigate those preconditions that make war more likely to occur.

REFERENCES

Carneiro, R. L. A theory of the origin of the state. Science, *169:* 733, 1970.
Choucri, N., and North, R. C. Dynamics of international conflict: Some implications of population, resources, and technology. World Polit. *24 (Suppl.):* 80, 1972.
Milgram, S. Some conditions of obedience and disobedience to authority. Hum. Relations, *18:* 57, 1965.
Scott, J. P. *Aggression.* University of Chicago Press, Chicago, 1958.

3.6. ETHOLOGY

Introduction

The dictionary defines ethology as the systematic study of animal behavior. Originally, ethologists were primarily interested in the detailed analysis of the behavior of intact animals in their natural environment or closely related environments, using direct observation as the basic technique for behavioral measurement. With the passage of time, ethologists added experimental modifications to the natural environment and initiated experimental laboratory investigations.

Contributions to Psychiatry

Ethological data and theory have allegedly been used to support basic constructs of psychoanalysis. Freud postulated psychic energy as the basic motivating force underlying human behavior. It has been suggested that an objective explanation or description of psychic energy may be provided in terms of Lorenz's action-specific energy hypothesis, which implies that external inhibition of instinctive behavior patterns acts as a powerful intrinsic motivational factor insofar as the behavior is concerned.

Once an animal's specific reservoir of energy is completely drained or depleted as a result of continuous activation of a particular response, a time interval is required for the energy supply to be replenished.

Accordingly to Hess, the action-specific energy hypothesis is illustrated by the phenomenon of displacement, in which a conflict between two instinctive behavior patterns results in the release of a third instinctive behavior pattern. In the stickleback, conflict between attack and flight is often resolved by nest-building behavior. According to Kaufman, the transition from the purely physical behavior patterns of animals to the physical and psychic relationships characterizes the developmental motivational changes from the animal to the human level. Furthermore, at the human level, the psychic energy that may be invested in the sexual and aggressive drive may be cathected to the mental representations of these objects, as determined by individual experience.

A complex interpretation of displacement activity has been presented by Ostow. He hypothesizes that the gratification of sexual instincts takes different forms during different periods of development and that the mechanism that leads from one form to another functions in the same way that displacement activities function in lower animals. As one form of gratification is inhibited, the instinct accepts another form of gratification.

Hess has strongly indicated that Freudian theory is closely related to ethology by way of the concept of imprinting, which places an enormous emphasis on the importance of early learning. Imprinting refers to the early, rapid, specific, and persisting learning, seen particularly in birds (Figure 1), by which the neonatal animal becomes attached to the mother and, by generalization, to members of the animal's own species. The term "imprinting" was given to this phenomenon by Lorenz, although the phenomenon or a similar phenomenon had previously been described. Unlike most learning, imprinting is facilitated by punishment or painful experience.

Body contact or some similar mechanism is now generally accepted as *a* primary, if not *the* primary, mechanism binding the baby to the mother. However, analysts are unwilling to accept any further ethological-psychological affectional theory, since it contradicts or does not

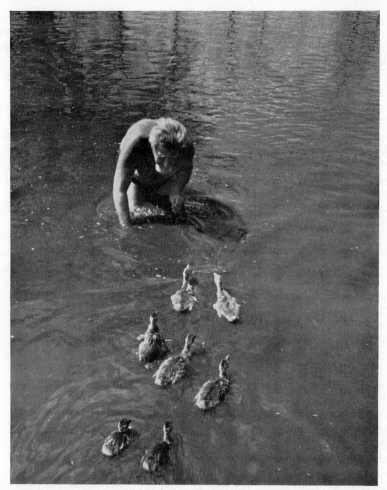

FIGURE 1. In a famous experiment, Lorenz demonstrated that goslings would respond to him as if he were the natural mother. (Reprinted by permission from Hess, E. H. Imprinting: An effect of early experience. Science *130:* 133, 1959.)

relate to Freud's four developmental stages: oral, anal, phallic, and genital. Another matter of concern to analysts is that biological theories assume generalization, whereas analytical treatment is an individual matter of more concern to the analysts than are generalized scientific laws.

On the basis of observation and study of normal and autistic children, the Tinbergens explicated basic rules, long employed in ethological practice, that they felt should be observed in socially contacting and treating the autistic human infant. Social approach and contact with the child should be achieved by aversion of the face, since this is a biologically threatening gesture. Also, any successful ges-

tural approach should be followed and extended by cautious step-by-step procedures. The Tinbergens believed that every attempt should be made to avoid overintimidation of the autistic child, that intense observation and attention should be given to nonverbal interactions, and that intense social bonding should be achieved without extreme or sudden intrusion.

Induced Subhuman Psychopathology

The first scientist to study induced psychopathology in a laboratory animal was the neurophysiologist Pavlov in Russia. Pavlov inadvertently produced the abnormal phenomenon, which he labeled "experimental neurosis," by use of a conditioning technique. He taught dogs to discriminate between a circle and an ellipse and then progressively diminished the ratio between the diameter of the circle and the length of the ellipse. When the difference was reduced to approximately 10 per cent, the neurotic symptoms of extreme and persistent agitation, with continual struggling and howling, appeared and apparently remained for a long time in most animals. Pavlov attributed the neurosis to a collision in time or space of the processes of excitation, or reinforcement, and inhibition, or nonreinforcement.

Other investigators, using a wide variety of animals, have succeeded in attaining more precise liminal discriminations in a wide variety of visual problems without severe psychopathology. It is true that driving an animal to achieve liminal discriminations may produce some emotional stress, but the Pavlovian technique has never become the method of choice for achieving nonhuman psychopathology or experimental neuroses.

Gantt and Liddell in America used similar techniques to produce behavior disorders in subhuman animals forced into conflictual learning situations. Gantt used the term "behavior disorders" to describe his dogs' complex and variegated autonomic responses. Liddell described the stress responses he obtained in sheep, goats, and dogs as "experimental neurasthenia," and this condition was obtained in some cases by merely doubling the number of daily test trials in an unscheduled manner. It was also achieved by conflict between food and pain. Liddell believed that the experimental neurasthenia represented a primitive, relatively undifferentiated state, rather than mimicking any human psychopathological condition.

Massermann studied abnormal behavior produced by motivational conflict situations in cats and monkeys. The subjects were trained to obtain food pellets from boxes and were then subjected to blasts of air on an irregular schedule when they approached food. Masserman also studied methods designed to extinguish the abnormal behaviors through disuse, stimulus satiation, reconditioning, and alcoholic therapy.

Nurturance of Normality

The only way to demonstrate induced psychopathic behavior in laboratory animals is to compare the abnormal animals with others that are normal or, at least, as normal as can be achieved. The Harlows have defined the social, as contrasted to the physical, essentials that create a normal environment—laboratory or feral. These essentials are provided by particular people as gifts of affection.

An obvious criterion for the social adequacy of any particular environment is the degree to which it prohibits or limits social interactions, particularly affectional interactions, between or among its inhabitants during or throughout any or all stages of social development. Doubtless there are many other variables of secondary importance, particularly those relating to the physical environment.

Throughout most of the primate order, there exist five basic affectional systems. One is the system of mother love. A second, closely synchronized system is that of infant love for the mother. The third system is peer love or agemate love or playmate love. The fourth system develops from and is a normal sequence of peer love and is heterosexual love. In primates heterosexual love in normal form depends on the establishment of the antecedent affectional systems. The fifth love or affectional system is that of paternal love.

Most feral environments provide opportunities for the development of all these forms of love or affection to the members of the primate order. No monkey laboratory environment made all these forms of love available to all monkey participants until the creation of the nuclear family apparatus by the late Margaret K. Harlow. This apparatus produced nuclear families of rhesus monkeys with a single father and mother and their infants. The family members lived in such a manner that both parents were accessible to each other and to all the parental groups.

The structure of the nuclear family apparatus is illustrated in Figure 2. Four nuclear families (Figure 3) were housed in each apparatus. The nuclear family apparatus provides all family members full opportunity for social and sexual expression, and the primary missing feral variable is the predator.

The Harlows have studied the effects of various forms of social environment on the social development of young monkeys. These studies have convinced them that development must be a combined function of emotional learning, social learning, and maturation.

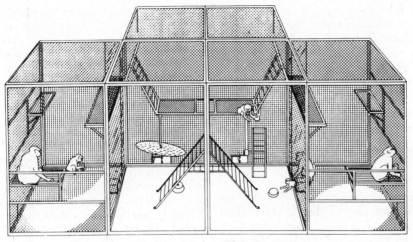

FIGURE 2. Nuclear family apparatus.

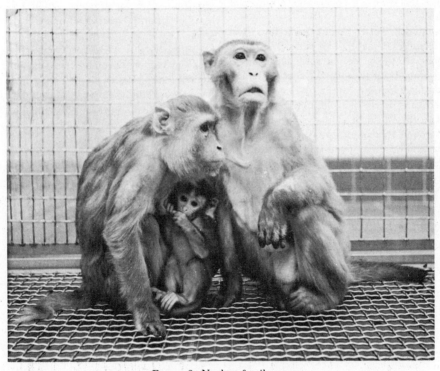

FIGURE 3. Nuclear family group.

By and large, monkeys mature 4 or 5 times as fast as humans in many aspects, and at birth a monkey is comparable to a 1-year-old human being in terms of body and bone structure. Female monkeys are sexually mature at about 3 years of age, even though most females must wait another year for the advent of their offspring. Male monkeys are spermatically competent at an equal age, even though the anatomical adornments of maturity, the large canine teeth and temporal muscles, do not achieve pubertal perfection for 6 or 7 years.

Like people, monkeys attain full intellectual age at approximately full sexual age. Curiosity in the monkey matures by 30 days of age, even though its full potentialities have not yet been realized, and early curiosity is regulated and restrained by maternal ministrations. The all-important primate behavior pattern of play matures at approximately 90 days of age, as shown in Figure 4. Social fears appear at approximately 80 to 100 days of age, similar to Spitz's 9-month anxiety in human beings, an anxiety that really matures between 6 and 13 months of age.

Advent of Abnormalities

Total Social Isolation

Probably the most dramatic and destructive abnormal environment is that of total social isolation. Monkeys may be raised from birth onward under such conditions. Here, for some predetermined period of time, an animal has no social partners and can consummate no social interactions.

Three-month Total Social Isolation. Two studies conducted at the Wisconsin Primate Laboratory on the effect of total isolation in monkeys from birth through the first 3 months of life yielded similar results. When removed from their early world of social nothingness and exposed to the world of monkeys and manipulanda, some of the infants went into a state of deep shock. Two died of self-imposed anorexia, and another was on the verge of starvation until saved by forced feeding.

The infants that survived, and most did,

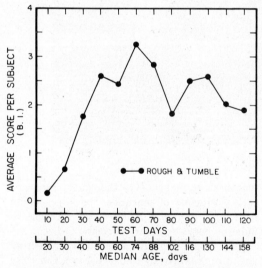

FIGURE 4. Development of social play behavior in monkeys.

made a remarkable social adjustment by the development of play. When allowed to interact with equal-age, normally reared rhesus monkeys, the isolates were playing effectively within the first week or so. By the end of the first month and throughout the second month, the behavior of the 90-day isolates was normal, as indicated by the frequency of play and threat gestures.

Six-month Total Social Isolation. Raising monkeys in total social isolation from birth throughout the first 6 months of life produced dramatic developmental differences in the isolated monkeys. The early infantile responses of self-clasp and huddle remain consistently low in socially raised monkeys. But these infantile behaviors increased progressively in the isolated monkeys and attained a level that was clearly abnormal and significantly greater than the level of infantile responses made by the controls.

Similar results were obtained for the level of rocking responses and stereotype responses. Rocking responses remained at a near-normal level throughout the first 4 isolation months and then exploded upward with increasing frequency. Stereotypy progressively increased from the second month onward. Neither rocking nor stereotypy is a normal infant response; both apparently depend on prolonged deprivation.

When removed from the isolation chambers, these 6-month isolates were terrified by relatively normal social age-mates. Representatives from the normal and abnormal groups were then tested 5 days a week for 2 months in social groups of two isolates and two controls in a standardized playroom situation.

The isolate monkeys exhibited a very low level of threat responses, whereas the controls showed a high incidence of threat. Situational and social fears had matured in all the animals, but the isolates had had no social opportunities to develop natural and normal defense mechanisms. One cannot learn in a social vacuum. Threat responses were essentially nonexistent in the isolate monkeys. Levels of threat behavior by the isolate and control subjects remained essentially unchanged during the first and second months.

Play in the isolates was essentially nonexistent. The failure of the isolate monkeys to develop any play probably stems from the isolates' fear of their normal age-mates. The lack of play was not the result of aggressive physical assault on the part of the normal monkeys, since this was not observed. Aggression, even relatively weak aggression, does not mature in monkeys until or slightly after the end of the first year of life. However, social fears had matured long before these isolate monkeys were allowed any social interaction with peers. Play requires freedom of movement and freedom of social interaction, and play and fright give rise to antithetical responses. Play can be inhibited almost as effectively by the threat of aggression as by aggression itself.

Representative members of the 6-month totally isolated monkeys were maintained in the laboratory under conditions of partial social isolation for 3 or more years, and, when they were socially tested under these inadequate social conditions, their social responses to each other became more impaired. When these long-term isolates were paired with equal-aged macaques or even monkeys half their age, they assumed violent and grotesque postures of terror such as the monkey lying on its back supine and frozen with terror (see Figure 5). This is a posture never assumed by a normal monkey. Similarly, a group of isolates is shown in Figure 6 with two of them holding their heads in their hands. A third totally abnormal posture of terror is illustrated in Figure 7.

The long-term effects of 6 months of total social isolation produced the paradoxical position of creating adolescent monkeys that were both abnormally aggressive and abnormally fearful. The 6-month isolates aggressed or attempted to aggress against all other monkeys. They aggressed or threatened infants, an activity beneath the dignity of any normal rhesus monkey. Furthermore, during these acts of threat or assault, the isolates indicated, by their gestures, feelings of fear and apprehension. The isolates aggressed against age-mates who were far more physically adept. These aggressions were fraught with fear, and the physical encounters were massacres. Even worse, the 6-month isolates often made one suicidal aggressive assault against a member of a group of large, mature, aggressive males, illustrating the ultimate combination of paradoxical fear and hate. Such aggressions seldom occurred twice since even the isolate monkeys could learn in this situation to compensate for their emotional deficiencies or hypersufficiencies.

Twelve-month Total Social Isolation. Rowland isolated a group of macaque monkeys for the first 12 months of life, a period roughly equivalent to 5 or 6 human years. These monkeys were totally unresponsive to the new physical and social world with which they were presented when the screens of their isolation world were raised (Figure 8). The researchers measured play of the most nonsocial type—that of individual or activity play. The control monkeys showed a high level of activity throughout the entire 10-week test period, whereas the 12-month isolates started with a very low level, which progressively languished with the passage of time. Since the isolates were devoid of play,

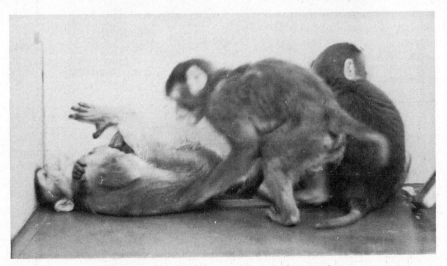

FIGURE 5. Abnormal fear posture in isolate monkey.

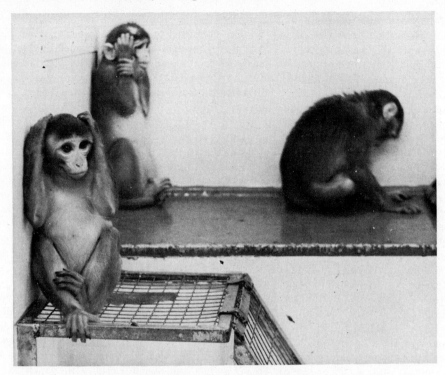

FIGURE 6. Frozen fear postures in isolate monkeys.

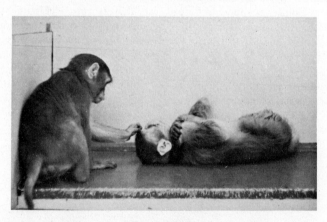

FIGURE 7. Terrified isolate monkey posture.

the researchers did not expect them to be full of passion, and they were correct. Nevertheless, the researchers tested these isolates for both threats and social play and obtained the expected—nothing.

Partial Social Isolation

Under partial social isolation, each animal lives in a wire cage that is usually one in a rack of several cages, as shown in Figure 9. Actually,

monkeys, and doubtless other animals, have been housed in this manner for many decades without thought being given to the fact that these animals were being socially deprived. Indeed, before the researchers at Wisconsin became aware of the social predicament of monkeys raised in partial social isolation, the monkeys were described as control subjects or even normal subjects for various experimental groups.

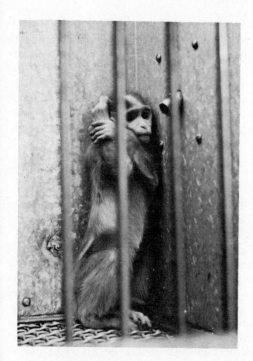

FIGURE 8. Twelve-month total social isolate upon removal of isolation screen.

Monkeys raised in partial social isolation can see, hear, and doubtless smell other monkeys. But partially isolated monkeys can never make any physical contact with other monkeys, and without physical contact monkeys can experience none of the normal affectional or love sequences.

During the first and second years of life by partially isolated monkeys, totally infantile responses of rock and huddle and self-mouth wane with age, whereas self-bite and stereotypy wax. In other words, the extremely infantile responses drop out and are superseded by more complex responses.

Totally isolated monkeys tend to exhibit a depressive-type posture, including such patterns as self-clutch, rocking, and depressive huddling. Partially isolated monkeys assume, with increasing frequency, postures that are more schizoid. These postures may include extreme stereotypy and sitting at the front of the cage and staring vacantly into space, as illustrated in Figure 10. Occasionally, the arm of a monkey starts to rise, and, as it extends, the wrist and fingers flex. While this takes place,

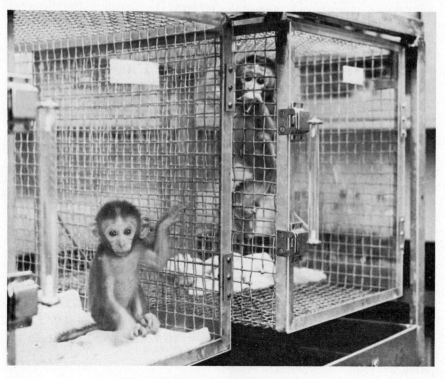

FIGURE 9. Partial social-isolate monkeys.

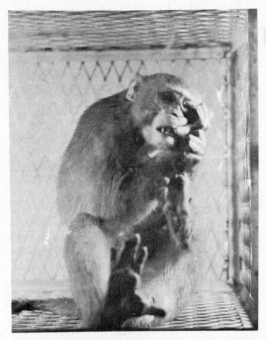

FIGURE 10. Partial social-isolate monkey attacking offending appendage.

the monkey ignores the arm, but, when it is extended, the monkey may suddenly respond to the arm, jump as if frightened, and even attack the offending appendage.

Maturation of aggression progresses systematically in monkeys raised in bare wire cages over a period of years—both externally directed aggression and self-directed aggression. All monkeys were tested in two conditions, a passive condition, when the observers sat 8 feet from the subjects and only observed and scored, and an active condition, when an experimenter ran a large black rubber glove over the cage top.

Externally directed aggression was apparent in the male at 2 years and not apparent in the female until year 4. The frequency of aggressive responses matured progressively in the male and the female, but aggression was stronger in the male before the fifth year of life. Self-aggression matured later than did externally directed aggression in both the male and the female, and it was never as frequent as was externally directed aggression.

Privation and Deprivation

In privation, the animal experiences no social companionship from birth until some predeter-

mined period. Deprivation results when animals are isolated after social relationships have been established. Invariably, deprived or late-isolate groups have shown far less behavioral deficit than the early-isolate or privation animals. Furthermore, when the late-isolate deprivation monkeys returned to social living, they often appeared to be meaninglessly hyperaggressive.

Induction of Depression

Anaclitic Depression

The first formal Wisconsin study of induced nonhuman anaclitic depression was conducted by Seay et al. The test situation, illustrated in Figure 11, was designed so that each of two mother-infant pairs lived in home cages, with an infant play area in between. The infants were free to wander at will from the home cages to the mutual play area, but the mothers were restrained in the home cages by the size of the apertures into the play area. Play by these infants, like all rhesus infants, matured at about 90 days of age and was near maximal at 180 days, which was the age chosen to begin maternal separation. This separation was achieved by dropping transparent Plexiglas screens in front of both home cages while the two infants were romping in the play area.

All monkeys tested in this situation exhibited a complete or nearly complete picture of human anaclitic depression. At initial separation the rhesus infants exhibited a protest stage, as illustrated by violent attempts to regain maternal contact, plaintive vocalization, and a persistent high level of random behavior. The protest stage changed to despair during the subsequent 48 hours. Despair was characterized by a drastic reduction in vocalization and movement and by the frequent assumption of prone postures, with the head and body

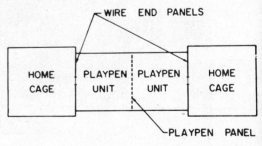

FIGURE 11. Mother-infant separation apparatus.

wrapped in the arms and legs. The most dramatic measure of the despair stage was that of the near-total suppression of play. Play was almost abolished during the 3-week period of maternal separation and then rose rapidly after maternal reunion.

When many human children are reunited with their mothers, their responses toward the maternal figure are those of rejection; Bowlby called this reunion stage "detachment." This phenomenon of detachment is far less common and far less intense in monkey infants than in the human infants reported by Bowlby. One of the first infant monkeys tested showed some maternal detachment upon reunion, and one mother showed some transient reluctance to accept her infant. Temporary detachment by the infant to the mother was exhibited by one of four infants in a replication study. However, the separated monkey infants typically reattached to the monkey mother vigorously and rapidly when the separation phase ended. Bowlby has more recently expressed doubts about the universality of the detachment stage in human infants.

The effect of maternal separation in macaque monkeys was replicated by a second study, differing only in that the partitions separating mother and infant were opaque instead of transparent and each stage was measured for only 2 instead of 3 weeks. The infant's distress was slightly less when the view of the mother was totally obscured—perhaps a case of out of sight, out of mind. Play was again dramatically and significantly reduced during the depression stage.

In later experiments, infants living with mothers and peers were first separated from the mothers at about 180 days of age and then separated from their peers at 205 days. This procedure produced a double despair syndrome, first elicited by maternal separation and then by playmate or peer separation. It is clear that anaclitic depression may be induced by the loss of any social object to which the animal is deeply attached, and not only by loss of the mother.

Species Differences. In a series of studies, Kaufman and Rosenblum compared the separation reactions of infant pigtail monkeys with infant bonnet macaques. In their studies they removed the mother from the infant and from a relatively large housing group consisting of several adult females, an adult male, and infants of assorted ages. Most of the pigtail infants went through a conventional protest and despair stage that began to lift after a week and fluctuated during the next month. But the comparably treated bonnet infants showed little indication of anaclitic depression. Instead, the separated bonnets found surcease from sorrow by attaching to the remaining adults, particularly the females who reciprocated their affectional advances. They solved their sorrow by attachment to substitute mothers.

The behaviors of the infant and mother pigtail and bonnet monkeys were totally in keeping with the normal behaviors for their species before any separation procedures had been instituted. Bonnet macaque monkeys are born to be receptive to group maternal administrations. From the first month of life onward, bonnet mothers allow their infants to wander forth and accept female social advances from other female members of the bonnet group. Thus, removal of the biological mother produced only extenuated maternal loss. But pigtail mothers are physically demanding and restrict the social adventures of their infants for at least several months. Lacking experience with other mothers, the maternally separated pigtail infants suffered intense pigtail-type anaclitic depression. Anaclitic depression is not produced by mere physical manipulations; it is produced by social loss.

Repeated Separation of Infant Monkey Peers. Suomi et al., measured the effects of repeated separation of infant pairs that had been separated from their mothers and raised in a spacious cage as part of a group of eight infants. At 90 days of age, the first of a series of 20 separations was begun, with monkeys being separated for 4 days and reunited for 3 days in each of the 20 separations completed over a 6-month period.

During the course of every separation, the separated age-mate pairs displayed the three conventional stages of anaclitic depression— protest, despair, and reattachment (detachment). However, infantile behaviors of self-mouth and self-clasp, which normally drop out by the fourth month, persisted in undiminished frequency and remained throughout the 9-month test period. Furthermore, complex social behaviors of environmental exploration and particularly play, which should become progressively more frequent and precise from 3 months to 9 months, remained unchanged in their formlessness and remained at a near-nonexistent frequency throughout the entire 9-month period. Thus, multiple peer separations did more than cause distress and depression. The separations eradicated the entire normal behavioral maturaltional process.

Depression in Adolescent Monkeys

McKinney, measured the effects of age-mate separation in one group of socially sophisticated monkeys more than 3 years of age and also measured the effect of vertical chamber confinement in a similar group.

Age-mate separation produced no depression in the socially sophisticated adolescents. Positive but slightly puzzling results were obtained from the vertically chambered animals. After release, these monkeys tended to show depressed locomotions, and the members of a pair frequently sat close to each other without attempting effective social interactions and without showing the conventional infantalized responses of self-clasp, huddle, rock, and stereotypy.

Behavioral Rehabilitation

Time

An approach to psychopathology that may be considered either a method or a control is the manipulation of no variable other than time. It is doubtful whether time is ever the therapeutic method of primary choice. Time's efficacy may be an illusory factor, since in many cases it is the natural and normal social forces acting on the animal during the temporal interval that facilitate the cure, rather than time itself.

After 6 months of social isolation, monkeys placed with normal peers were socially inadequate. Subsequently, the isolates lived alone for 3 or more years. Time alone worked wonders for these animals, but in a negative direction: the original behavioral deficits not only remained but were exaggerated. Actually, there is no objective record of a monkey psychopathology being cured by time.

Treatment of Specific Symptoms

All basic affectional patterns of mother love, infant love, peer love, heterosexual love, and even paternal love are based on responses involving bodily contact. Social isolation denies the monkey any contact comfort during both its personal and its social development. When social contact became accessible to isolated rhesus monkeys after isolation had ended, they did not make systematic attempts to achieve or maintain bodily contact with their simian associates. In fact, they went out of their way to avoid contact with fellow-species members.

To test contact comfort rehabilitation, Suomi first placed a group of rhesus monkeys in total isolation for 6 months. The isolates were then put in individual cages with a heated, simplified surrogate. Subsequently, six pairs of isolates and their surrogates were placed in a large group living cage for 8 weeks. The data showed that the monkeys given surcease from social sorrow by surrogate satisfaction subsequently showed a marked decrease in self-directed disturbance activities, including self-clasp, self-mouth, rock, and stereotypy. Contingent on the reduced frequency of display of these behaviors, there was an increase in frequency of environmental exploration and peer contact.

Obviously, increased frequency of environmental exploration and peer contact is not total rehabilitation, which should involve multiple peer interactions, various forms of peer play, and real or or at least attempted heterosexual behavior. It appears that experience with the warm surrogate imparted considerable social security to the isolated monkey, as it can impart security during the social development of the normal infant. Contact with surrogates changed the isolated monkeys from animals devoid of security when with their confreres into animals capable of maintaining some social contacts. Social contact training, nevertheless, failed as a total rehabilitation process. The isolated monkeys never achieved the full gamut of monkey realization, involving active, sex-typed play and appropriate sexual responsiveness.

Social Behavior Therapy

Four males were reared for the first 6 months of life in total social isolation, then removed and allowed to interact with four normal female "therapist" monkeys that were housed in quad cages, shown in Figure 12. Each of the normal monkeys had previously had 2 daily hours of early social experience with another infant, and the pairings of social partners were systematically rotated.

When first socially tested in the home cage,

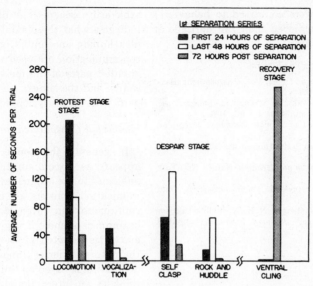

FIGURE 12. Quad cages—combined living-experimental cages.

the isolates were 180 days of age and the "therapists" were 90 days of age. This age differential was deliberately chosen so that the isolated monkeys would not be terrified by their new companions. Also, increasingly complex play develops in normal monkeys from 90 days onward, and these behaviors were judged best to gradually indoctrinate isolate monkeys into increasingly complex social interactions.

At this time two "therapist" females and two isolate monkeys were housed in diagonal corners of the home cage, and a "therapist" and an isolate were allowed 2 daily hours of social interaction, the various members of each group being systematically rotated. The quad cages were home cages when rehabilitation was instituted, and home cages are minimally disturbing environmental situations. Pairs of normal and isolate monkeys were subsequently tested in strange playrooms for 2 hours a day with increasing frequency throughout the rehabilitation process.

Successful therapy in the home cage was indicated by the progressive reduction of abnormal behaviors by the isolate monkeys of self-clasp, huddle, rock, and sterotypy. All these infantile or abnormal behaviors were progressively reduced under behavior therapy, and the frequency of these deviant derelictions fell to a normal level in the relatively strange playroom situation.

Although the decrease in frequency of abnor-

mal behaviors is an indicator of rehabilitation, the most important measure of successful behavior therapy is that of the development of adequate, positive social behaviors, such as social contact, particularly play. Social contact by the isolated monkeys in both the home cage and playroom environments reached normal levels by the end of the preplanned period of rehabilitation.

Although frequency of play progressively increased throughout the 6-month preplanned rehabilitation period, it did not quite attain normal levels in the playroom. Since there had been no rationale for the period of therapy, an additional 6-month period of behavior therapy was instituted. At the end of the 12-month period of therapy, no differences existed between isolated and control monkeys in the observed frequency of any behavioral forms, including social behaviors of social contact and play.

Through accidents of time of birth, the four "therapists" were females and the four isolates were males. Normative monkey studies have shown that males and females play differently. Male play is rough, tough, and contactual; female monkey play is gentle, chasing, and basically noncontactual. The only play the female "therapists" could have taught the isolates was gentle, noncontact play; but, when the male monkeys were rehabilitated, their play was masculine, contactual monkey play. Thus, when the males were converted to behavioral normality, they achieved their full heritage of monkey masculinity.

REFERENCES

Bowlby, J. *Attachment and Loss. Vol. I. Attachment.* Basic Books, New York, 1969.

Harlow, H. F., and Novak, M. A. Psychopathological perspectives. Perspect. Biol. Med., *16:* 461, 1973.

Jolly, A. *The Evolution of Primate Behavior.* Macmillan, New York, 1972.

Lorenz, K. Der Kumpan in der Umwelt des Vogels. J. Ornithol., *83:* 137, 289, 1935.

Masserman, J. B. *Behavior and Neurosis.* Hafner, New York, 1964.

Spitz, R. A. Anaclitic depression. *Psychoanal. Study Child,* 2: 313, 1946.

Tinbergen, E. A., and Tinbergen, N. Early childhood autism: An ethological approach. *J. Comp. Ethol., 10* (*Suppl.*)*:* 9, 1972.

3.7.   COMMUNICATION

Introduction

Communication can be defined as the process that links discontinuous parts of the living world to one other. It is made possible by three basic properties of living organisms: perception, decision making, and expression. In machines and large organizations these properties are sometimes referred to as input, central functions, and output.

Characteristics of Human Communication

A human being's communicative operations are based on two fundamentally different symbolization systems: nonverbal communication rests on the analogue principle, and verbal codification rests on the digital principle. The inner experience of what is going on at any moment involves nonverbal images that in some way reflect the total situation. Bodily movements and spontaneous, immediate reactions require an analogical appreciation of events. A person thus develops within himself a small-scale model of the world based on the recognition of similarities or differences. This method is used for gaining a bird's-eye view of events and for implementing quick reactions necessary for survival. But when a person has time to analyze a situation he uses words or numbers, which are capable of denoting detailed aspects of events without recourse to analogies. In the digital-verbal system, numbers or letters are arbitrarily assigned to events and a legend indicates what these symbols refer to. In complex human encounters, verbal and nonverbal communication are used together. The object-oriented parts of the message are expressed in words, and the subject- or participant-oriented parts are expressed nonverbally.

Nonverbal Communication

In general, the nonverbal denotation unit appears as a configuration that bears some analogies to the original event. Nonverbal communication consists of movements that are continuous and often do not have discrete beginnings or ends; it is governed by principles and rules dictated by biological necessities or the natural order of things. Because nonverbal denotation is based on self-evident analogies, it provides an international, intercultural, interracial, and interspecies language (see Figure 1). As far as temporal characteristics are concerned, nonverbal denotation is extremely flexible. A movement can be carried out slowly or quickly, or successive events can be indicated simultaneously. Nonverbal denotation is excellent for indicating timing and coordination in the present mode, but it is inadequate for describing elapsed time or the past. Inasmuch as movements and material objects used for communication require a predetermined amount of space, nonverbal denotation is spatially rather demanding; however, it is the method of choice for the representation of three-dimensional configurations by means of sketches, photographs, or small-scale models.

Nonverbal expressions are controlled by the phylogenetically older structures of the nervous system. These movements are learned early in life. They usually involve a large number of muscles.

The development of nonverbal communication in the child depends on the reactions of the parents and other adults. In the first year of life, all expression must occur through nonverbal means, but specialized movements of which the infant is capable are limited. As long as sucking, biting, and clutching are the only available expressions, communication, by necessity, is interpersonal and is carried on at close range. Later, when locomotion develops, the child's statements are expressed through creeping, walking, and running.

Although speech gradually takes on more and

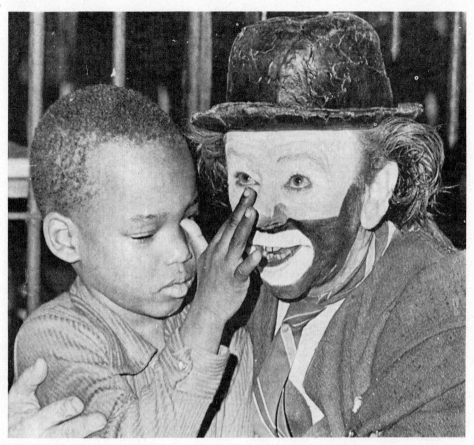

FIGURE 1. Clowns are a universal symbol of nonverbal communication. They convey a wide range of emotions and attitudes through a series of precise body movements and facial expressions (UPI photo).

more importance, communication mediated through action continues to be of significance until the child reaches the age of 8 or 10. By this time, the assistance given by the adult involves more and more information and less and less direct action. By adolescence, action codifications have been largely relinquished, and the verbal, gestural, and symbolic means of communication predominate. In adult life, nonverbal communication is retained to denote events for which words are inadequate—the speaker's emotions, state of health, attitudes. For details, the reader is referred to the sources listed in Table I.

Verbal Communication

The biological foundations of verbal denotation are mostly associated with the phylogenetically younger structures of the brain, particularly the cortex. Verbal denotation is learned only after nonverbal denotation has been mastered, and the two systems, to a large extent, use separate neural pathways. Verbal language facilitates information storage and retrieval, influences thinking, and is essential for planning. Logic is inconceivable without digital and verbal denotation. Mastery of verbal communication requires decades of training, particularly because the referential property of words is based on prior agreements that differ from culture to and from group to group.

Verbal communication depends on the development of speech, which depends on the maturation of the central nervous system. Most normal children have begun to speak by the time they are 3 ½ years old; all speech sounds have developed by the time the child is 7. At the age of 8 or 9, he beings to use language for purposes of strategy.

The unit of denotation, be it number or letter,

TABLE I

Source Material on Nonverbal Communication

Topic	Description	Source
Review	Paralinguistics, kinesics, and cultural anthropology	LaBarre
Anthology	A reader in interpersonal, intercultural, and political communication	Bosmajian
Evolution of language	The origins and prehistory of language	Revesz
History	From cave painting to comic strip (with illustrations)	Hogben
Culture	Space, time, value orientation, and assumptions made by various cultures	Hall
Theory	Gesture, posture, situational context, and traces of action (illustrated with review of older literature)	Ruesch and Kees
Human development	Genesis of nonverbal communication	Spitz
Kinesics	Body motion communication (review of recent literature)	Birdwhistell
	The regulation and control of interpersonal behavior (with illustrations)	Scheflen
Indicators of nonverbal behavior	Emblems, illustrations, affect displays, regulators, adaptors, and other categories of analysis	Ekman and Friesen
Gesture	Varieties of gestures (review of older literature)	Critchley
Facial expression	The origins of facial expression	Andrew
Human sounds	The acoustic communication of emotions	Ostwald

cannot be broken down further. Verbal and digital codifications are arbitrary and discontinuous, and the marks have a discrete beginning and end. Inasmuch as verbal denotation consists of a serial alignment of signs and signals, simultaneous events must be listed successively. In addition, words have to be spoken at a given speed; when produced too slowly or too quickly, they become unintelligible. Verbal denotation is clumsy when used to indicate spatial arrangements, except for the description of boundaries. It is also unsuitable for indicating timing and coordination, but it is excellent for indicating elapsed time.

Words exert an intellectual appeal and are suitable for reaching agreements. Most words refer to things that can be heard and seen or about which man can think. But those events that are perceived by means of the mechanical and chemical proximity receivers—that is, touch, smell, taste, pain, and temperature— have hardly any verbal representation at all. Because verbal codification is most suited for distance communication, it has a vocabulary that refers primarily to events in the world around us. The vocabulary for events occurring inside the organism and for bodily experiences is rudimentary. For these reasons, artists often resort to nonverbal expression to represent inner experience (see Figure 2). For details concerning verbal communication, the reader is referred to Table II, which lists the principal sources.

Communication Network

A communication network is made up of at least two communicating entities, which may comprise persons, machines, or groups. Each of these entities is characterized by input (perception); by central functions consisting of data scanning (recognition), data processing (thinking), and data storage (memory); and by output (expression and action). Input, central functions, and output enter into decision making, which steers subsequent action.

Two or more communicating entities are related to each other by a variety of connecting processes. The network is defined by the pathways that the messages take as they travel from one communicating entity to the other. The code, which in the human situation is language, must be shared by the participants. The metacommunicative processes, which are those devices that instruct the participants as to how to phrase or interpret a given message, must also be shared by the participants. Feedback corrects information, links information to action, and facilitates planning and organization. Feedback, which joins the physical with the symbolic universe, steers behavior in man, animal, and machine. When feedback no longer operates effectively, the survival of the communicating entity is in doubt.

Words have multiple meanings; therefore, it is essential to determine which meaning is applicable in a given message. To understand meaning, the participants must share the knowledge of sets, and to do this takes decades of careful learning.

Communication between participants is influenced by the presence of an observer or reporter. Unable to gaze into the communicating entities and rarely knowing their intentions, the scientific observer must usually confine himself to the assessment of effects. In such an analysis, the exchange of messages is related to the effect that a given communication has produced. In enterprises in which action is of the essence, the scientific observer is replaced by a manager, who manipulates the message exchange. By assigning positions to the participants, and by instructing them to report to supervisors and to receive reports from peers

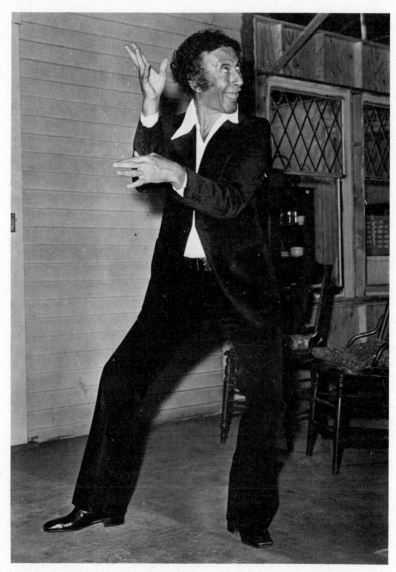

FIGURE 2. Mime is the essence of communication elevated to an art form. Here, Marcel Marceau, the world's foremost mime, displays his amazing talents of nonverbal expression (UPI photo).

TABLE II
Source Material on Verbal Communication

Topic	Description	Source
Scientific aspects of human communication	A reader on the mathematical, social, linguistic, semantic, and technical aspects of communication	Smith
Humanistic aspects of communication	A reader on dialogue, rhetoric, and interaction	Matson and Montagu
Decision making	A reader on theory, probability, risk, and scientific models	Edwards and Tversky
Review of theories	Contributions of various disciplines to the field of communication	Dance
Psycholinguistics	A reader on the various approaches to speech and language problems	Saporta
History	The story of language	Pei
Human development	Infant speech	Lewis
Speech	The biological foundations of language	Lenneberg
Semiosis	The processes involving signals, signs, and symbols	Morris
Cognition	Experimental data, perception, decision making, memory, and stress	Broadbent
Operant conditioning	The conditioning of verbal behavior	Skinner
General semantics	The meaning of language in thought and action	Hayakawa
Neuropsychology	Languages of the brain	Pribram
Neurophysiology	The relationship of behavior and the nervous system (collected papers)	McCulloch
	Information processing in the central nervous system (transactions of meetings)	Gerard and Duyff: Leibovic
Mass media	The understanding of radio, television, and other mass media	McLuhan
Social network	Attitudes, opinions, and beliefs	Lin

and subordinates, he controls the flow of messages. This process is called organization. Whereas the term "management" indicates interventions with the connecting processes, the word "treatment" refers to intervention with the communicating entities.

The communication process that connects person with person or the social conflict that disrupts relationships can best be studied through observation of the ways and means of a message exchange. After establishing the general context of a set of circumstances and after having selected a situational label, the observer may use certain questions as guidelines in assessing a network: *Who* (status, role, identity) said *what* (content) to *whom* (status, role-identity), *when* (chronological, biological, elapsed time), *where* (situation) *how*, (language), with what *effect* (feedback).

Disturbed Communication

Western thought, including scientific logic, has been largely based on the Aristotelian approach, which is rooted in Greek grammar and its subject-predicate language structure. Within such a structure, the subject of discourse must be stated and the level of abstraction defined. In the evolution of language, the separation of the pronoun (actor) or noun (subject) from the verb (action) was a necessary step toward development of the notion of process; the separation of adjectives from nouns and adverbs from verbs made scientific measurement possible.

The separation of various aspects of an event that occur together in nature is responsible for some serious distortions. If a word exists, some people are inclined to attribute body and substance to its referent. Through this process of reification, people forget that some words used in the sciences and professions reflect abstractions or intervening constructs that do not refer to real events but have been created for convenience.

Distortion in the Use of Words

Distortions can occur before and during the process of verbalization. In a person's perception or awareness, there may exist distortions of natural events. In the assignment of vocal sounds to a percept, the words selected may not be sufficiently discriminating to separate it from other percepts, or perhaps the usage of the term is not sufficiently uniform. Several people have to agree as to the meaning of a word, and the definition has to be incorporated in some sort of a dictionary to remain relatively stable over time. The term itself must belong to a language that is suitable for the purpose at hand.

Disturbances of the Communicating Entity

In the older textbooks, disturbances of the communicating entity were listed under the heading of psychopathology in terms of disturbances of thinking, association, feeling, judgment, expression, and action. At present, these empirical observations are more succinctly integrated under the heading of disturbed communication. In the case of a person, we call the cause of the malfunction trauma or disease; in the case of a machine, we refer to it as technical malfunction; and in the case of a group, we label it disorganization. Organic conditions usually produce massive, quantitative deviations in perception, judgment, and expression, but other conditions result in subtle qualitative deviations. If a person has led a restricted life and experienced one-sided exposure to people and situations, he may lack communicative skills. Or he may have been the victim of overly rigid or inadequate reinforcement of desirable behavior. In either case, his learning of certain communicative behavior patterns is faulty.

Disturbances of the Connecting Processes

In disturbances of the connecting processes, the individual entity functions, but the connection with other communicating entities is the disturbing factor. The participants may not share the same language; or, if they do, they may engage in idosyncratic, nonshared interpretations of content. Perhaps the verbal aspects of communication function adequately, but the non-verbal, metacommunicative devices are underdeveloped. Communication within a system may be disturbed if feedback processes are not functioning properly, as evidenced by lack of acknowledgment, delayed response, or replies that are not relevant to the original statement. But, perhaps more than anything else, overload

exerts a disorganizing effect. Underload, although frustrating, is less damaging, provided it does not last too long. In addition, messages that imply a real or imagined threat are highly disturbing, as is the failure to reach some agreement with opponents who, under certain circumstances, may force an agreement by resorting to coercion or violence.

Messages that are too intense or too weak, that arrive too early or too late, that are repeated too often or not often enough, or that are inappropriate to the situation become sources of stress, giving rise in the person to all the bodily manifestations of alarm.

Disturbances Introduced by Observer or Therapist

An observer, physician, or therapist may disturb the existing network. The psychiatrist uses communication to explore the patient's experiences, to gather his personal history, to explain procedures, and to give instructions. The disturbance that follows the diagnostic exploration may be used for therapeutic purposes, forcing the patient to change his habitual methods of communication. If the treatment is organic, it is aimed at restoring perception, decision making, and expression that have been distorted by trauma or disease. If the treatment is psychological, the process of communication is used to exert a communicative influence on the patient.

Stabilization of Pathology

The human being is a herd animal, linked to other human beings by means of communication. If the message exchange is gratifying, anything that threatens this linkage upsets the person and the people with whom he is connected. If a communicative exchange is frustrating, the feedback and steering devices that control the exchange tend toward a weakening or dissolution of the connection. Disturbed communication is characterized by the fact that these regulatory mechanisms do not operate. In spite of frustration, the communicators continue to participate in the same network, sometimes because separation is too painful, sometimes because they are unable to find new connections.

Disturbed or pathological communication is stabilized by mutually inflicted frustration. In the process, the participants become interdependent on other family members or friends, and they find it hard to communicate in networks that do not observe the paradoxical rules. It is the task of the psychiatrist to explore the highly complex principles that govern such abnormal exchanges in an attempt to introduce normal, self-steering qualities.

Disturbed Communication and Overt Behavior

Erroneous information leads to ineffective or deviant action. If the intrapersonal and interpersonal feedback devices function and a person is capable of correcting his body of information, he is; in spite of mistakes, eventually able to engage in action that is both gratifying to him and tolerated by the group. But if the feedback devices for correcting information do not operate effectively, the person acquires a distorted body of information, leading to unsuccessful and unrewarding action that may not be tolerated by the group. The repetitive sequence of communicative exchanges that originally led to an erroneous body of information is eventually responsible for failure in action. Such an experience may induce the person to withdraw from social contact, to doubt his ability to engage in realistic thinking, and to give up the testing of assumptions in action. Instead, he may rely on fabricated or imagined responses of others, a body of information that has not been tested, and action behavior that is unintelligible to others. As a result, the link between the body of information, the perception of the response of others, and subsequent action becomes looser and, eventually, these aspects may become disunited. The person is then said to be psychotic.

Functional Psychoses

The functional psychoses are characterized by disturbances of perception, decision making, and expression. Cognition is distorted, judgment is clouded, and, in some cases, the ability to make decisions is altogether absent. Expression is idiosyncratic and inappropriate to the circumstances. Recall from memory may be chaotic in that events that just happened are not recorded, but past events, which may have no connection with the present, are recalled in great detail. Above all, the perspective of placing present events in the light of past experiences gets lost. In the functional psychoses,

then, feedback and correction are disturbed across the board.

Neuroses and Personality Disorders

The neuroses and personality disorders are characterized by perception and cognition that are functioning satisfactorily except for systematic biases that induce the person to pay more attention to one set of phenomena than to another. Judgment, therefore, may not be the best, and the person may not always select the option that insures his survival or solves the problem at hand. Usually, expression is not affected, except for occasional inefficient implementation of expressive movements, gestures, and speech. Feedback and correction operate except in the area of the neurotic conflict.

Psychosomatic Conditions

Involvement of the whole body in communication is usually abandoned between the second and third years of life; when speech and the striated muscles take over the communicative task. On the whole, people who suffer from psychosomatic conditions have remained infantile. This tendency is reflected in the evaluation of events in which information received from the chemical and mechanical sensory end organs is unduly weighted. The maturational shift in emphasis from the proximity receivers (touch, taste, smell, pain, temperature, vibration) to the more complex distance receivers (vision and hearing) is delayed. Signals that impinge on the proximity receivers, therefore, remain more significant that those relating to the distance receivers, and contraction of the smooth muscles plays a greater role than speech. Because of their limitations in communicative skills, these patients often engage in symbiotic relationships, whereby some aspects of perception, decision making, or expression are delegated to the other person. Both people then operate together, as if they were one person or one communicative entity.

A brief survey of the principal sources bearing upon disturbed communication is given in Table III.

Therapeutic Communication

The psychiatrist influences his patients by intervening with the human instruments of communication, as in psychosurgery, electro-

TABLE III
Communication and Psychiatric Disorders

Topic	Description	Source
Review	Contributions of psychiatry to the study of human communication	Meerloo
Theories	Value theory, information theory, codification, and metacommunication in the field of psychiatry	Ruesch and Bateson
	Axioms, premises, paradoxical communication, and general systems approaches	Watzlawick et al.
	The double blind theory of schizophrenia	Bateson
	Outline of a general theory of communication	Shands
Speech and hearing	Development of language and thought of the child	Piaget
	Mannerisms of speech and gesture in everyday life	Feldman
	Psychological and psychiatric aspects of speech and hearing disorders	Barbara
	Voice disorders, auditory perceptual disorders, stuttering, stammering	Weston
	Aphasia, apraxia, agnosia	Brain
	Reading disability and word-blindness	Hermann
Communication with patients	Interviewing	Bird
	Relating to various kinds of patients	Waggoner and Carek
Disorders of communications	Selected problems of disordered communication (transactions of scientific meetings)	Assoc. Res. Nerv. Ment. Dis; Hoch and Zubin
	Disturbed communication, a systematic treatise	Ruesch (1972a)
	Review of communication disorders in psychiatric conditions	Spiegel
	Thought disorders and family relations of schizophrenics	Wayne and Singer
Psychotherapy	Therapeutic communication, a systematic treatise	Ruesch (1973)
	Social environment, culture and mental disease (collected papers on social communication)	Ruesch (1972b)
	Various aspects of psychotherapy	Shands

shock, and drug therapy. He may attempt to change the patient's body of information by deliberately imparting new information, or he may try to mobilize, inside the patient, information of which the patient was not aware. He may attempt to alter the patient's ways of responding, as in the social therapies, through changes brought about either in the impersonal environment or in the relationship with other persons.

In a one-to-one setting, the communication system is symmetrical, reply is instantaneous, and the time between stimulus and response is minimal. Therefore, communication may be used to increase the person's awareness of himself to verbalize silent assumptions, to abandon unnecessary assumptions, to modify attitudes, to increase the tolerance for the behavior of others, to formulate goals of action, and to clarify the personal style of life.

In the group setting, the communication system is asymmetrical, and reply is often delayed, but the impact of a person's communications and actions on other people receives more attention. Therefore, communication here may be used for clarifying rules, specifying roles, and discussing organization.

In both two-person and group settings, communication may be either verbal or nonverbal. In verbal communication, words slice human experience into segments; they rearrange simultaneous events and bring them into successive order; and, through the process of abstraction, they condense multivaried behavior. Nonverbal communication, in contrast, is essentially subject-oriented rather than object-oriented. Nonverbal expressions tell how a person feels. Nonverbally, a therapist can convey his own feelings to a patient without explicit commitment. He can indicate whether he has hope and is optimistic, whether the situation is grave, and whether he likes or dislikes what is happening. If verbal communication is used to explore a subject matter, nonverbal communication is used to steer the encounter.

Neither individual nor group therapy can be limited to the achievement of understanding and insight unless the communicative exchange has an influence on action. In preparation for action, the therapist resorts to a communicative task called programing, which in essence, organizes future action.

In both interpersonal and group contexts, the psychiatrist gains leverage and exerts influence through acknowledgment, understanding, and agreement. Acknowledgment refers to the therapist's reply to the patient's presence and intention to communicate. Understanding refers to the establishment of an accurate model of the patient's behavior in the mind of the therapist. Agreement implies the isolation of a certain topic within the universe of discourse and the establishment of correspondence of information between the participants. To be acknowledged is pleasant; to be understood is even more gratifying; and to reach an agreement makes cooperation possible.

In all therapeutic situations, the therapist relies on the fact that, on the whole, every person strives to belong to a number of diverse groups at the same time and that he attempts to remain a distinctly separate entity within each group. The individual achieves balance by controlling the type and magnitude of social differences that exist between himself and others. Excessive differences that may produce tensions can be decreased. Insufficient differences that may produce tension can be increased.

If a balance cannot be achieved between personal uniqueness and shared group characteristics, the ensuing tension usually exerts a disruptive influence on both the individual and the group. This tension can be reduced to a tolerable level if one or more persons adapt pathologically. If a person neglects his own needs and overadapts, his behavior is diagnosed as a neurosis or a personality disorder. If he resists or rebels and the group uses coercive measures to bring him into line, his behavior is called psychopathic or sociopathic.

Regardless of diagnosis, the communication therapies aim at restoring the link between the patient and other people. In this sense, the communication therapies are not aimed at removing the cause of the disturbance. Instead, they are intended to restore those maintenance processes that enable a person to acquire and correct information, to establish a workable model of himself and others, to respond to the messages and actions of others, and to participate with others in tasks he cannot carry out alone.

Selected references bearing on electronic aids for the psychiatrist are given in Table IV.

Conclusion

Constructive and destructive processes inside a person are reflected in his human relations

TABLE IV

Source Material on Electronic Aids

Topic	Description	Source
Operations research	Analysis of systems and problems	Ackoff and Sasieni
Content of communication	Theories and computer techniques	Gerbner et al.
Biomedical research	Computers and mathematics in the life sciences	Stacy and Waxman
Computer programs	Description and tabulation of data, and various types of statistical analysis in clinical medicine and psychiatry	Dixon
Psychiatric research	Computers and electronic devices in psychiatry	Kline
Psychiatric records	Automated recording of data	Spitzer and Endicott
MEDLARS	Medical literature analysis and retrieval systems (computerized abstracts)	Austin
Computers in psychiatry	Various practical applications of computer sciences in psychiatry	Amer. Psychiatr. Assoc.

and vice versa. In extreme cases—for example, in solitary confinement and the exposure of children to disorganized communication of adults—the relationship between communication and subsequent behavior is clear. However, where the contact is discontinuous, evaluation is more difficult because memory traces can prolong an initially short impact.

On the whole, it is best to view communication as a buffer system. The better it works, the better the person is protected; the worse it works, the more vulnerable the person becomes. Communication serves as a corrective, attenuating, or aggravating force that connects the person with his surroundings and enables him to influence others and to be influenced by them. Personality is, in effect, the long-term product of a large number of communicative experiences. Normal and abnormal action behavior is steered by information stored by the person and acquired through the process of communication.

REFERENCES

Association for Research in Nervous and Mental Disease. *Disorders of Communication* (Proceedings of the Association, December 1962). Williams & Wilkins, Baltimore, 1964.

Brain, W. R. *Speech Disorders (1961)*, Ed. 2. Butterworths, Washington, 1965.

Lin, N. *The Study of Human Communication.* Bobbs-Merrill, New York, 1973.

Ruesch, J. *Therapeutic Communication (1961)*, Ed. 2. W. W. Norton, New York, 1973.

Scheflen, A. E. *Body Language and the Social Order.* Prentice-Hall (Spectrum), Englewood Cliffs, N. J., 1972.

Shands, H. C. *Semiotic Approaches to Psychiatry.* Mouton, The Hague, 1970.

Smith, A. G., editor. *Communication and Culture.* Holt, Rinehart and Winston, New York, 1966.

3.8.   APPLICATIONS OF LEARNING AND BIOFEEDBACK

Introduction

Certain applications of the principles of learning and behavior theory are believed to be particularly relevant to psychiatry and to other branches of medicine—fear, how symptoms may be learned or unlearned, conflict behavior, ways in which learning may influence emotions, the bodily effects that these emotions can produce, visceral learning, and biofeedback.

To the extent that neuroses and psychoses are functional—in other words, instrumental in serving a need—they must be learned. Putting the emphasis on learning does not denigrate genetic and other organic factors; all behavior is a result of an interaction among genetic, organic, and learned factors. Conversely, emphasizing the organic factors does not eliminate the learned ones. For example, pareis caused by brain damage in the late stages of syphilis produces delusions, but the specific content of these delusions varies with the history of the times and of the person and hence must be learned.

Fear and Learning

The fact that fear can be learned quickly, can be a strong drive, and can motivate the learning of new habits allows it to be responsible for behavior in one experimental rat that is different from that of other rats. Clinical evidence also indicates that fear—or anxiety, as it is called when its source is vague or unknown—can play an important role in a considerable range of abnormal behavior. Removal of the drive of fear is analogous to the goal of various types of psychotherapy, be they Freudian or behavioral.

In combat neurosis the source of fear is usually quite clear, and the fear-reducing value of the symptom that allows escape from combat provides a clear explanation for the reinforcement of that symptom. The impaired depth perception of a pilot or the hysterical paralysis of the trigger finger or the legs of an infantryman are examples.

Studies of combat show that the average person's response to extreme fear runs the entire gamut of virtually all neurotic and many psychotic symptoms. These reactions are a pounding heart and rapid pulse, a strong feeling of muscular tension, trembling, exaggerated startle response, dryness of the throat and mouth, a sinking feeling in the stomach, perspiration, a frequent need to urinate, irritability, aggression, an over-powering urge to cry or run and hide, confusion, feelings of unreality, feeling faint, nausea, fatigue, depression, slowing down of movements and thoughts, restlessness, loss of appetite, insomnia, nightmares, interference with speech, the use of meaningless gestures, the maintenance of peculiar postures, and sometimes stuttering, mutism, and amnesia. Presumably, most of these reactions are innate responses to fear.

Once strong fear is learned, any of the foregoing symptoms can appear as a direct consequence of it. But, if one of these symptoms is followed by a decrease in fear, one may expect it to be rewarded and hence to become relatively more dominant. Indeed, the first stages of combat neurosis are likely to be characterized by a kaleidoscopic array of diverse symptoms that come and go. With the passage of time, one type of symptom usually becomes predominant. It is exactly what one would expect if the patient were showing trial-and-error learning.

A great deal is known about how fear can be learned as a strong drive that motivates further learning. But any other strong drive could be the basis for similarly reinforcing the learning of a symptom. Indeed, there is evidence that the reward for a given symptom often comes from a number of drives. An incomplete list of such drives includes guilt (which seems to be closely related to fear and is perhaps a special kind of fear), anger, sex, and the needs for self-esteem, love, and social approval.

Conflict and Displacement

Conflict plays a key role in many forms of mental disorder. A common form of conflict is that in which a subject is motivated both to approach and to avoid a given desired but feared goal.

The analysis of such conflicts is based on a number of assumptions: (1) The tendency to approach a goal is stronger the nearer the subject is to it. (2) The tendency to avoid a feared stimulus is stronger the nearer the subject is to it. (3) The strength of avoidance increases more rapidly with nearness than does the strength of approach. (4) The strength of the tendency to approach or avoid varies directly with the strength of the drive on which it is based. Therapy can come about readily by natural increases in the drive to approach or be facilitated by associates who use various means to enhance the attractiveness of the goal and to encourage the subject.

Many strong fears are realistic. In these cases a person either suffers severe punishment if he achieves a dangerous goal or strong fear and conflict if the punishment just barely keeps him away from it. In such a situation, attempting to decrease fear and avoidance produces a nega-tive therapeutic effect; conversely, a positive therapeutic effect may be produced by increasing the strength of fear and avoidance to the point where the subject remains far enough away from the dangerous goal so that he is not tempted and hence not in any conflict.

In the analysis of conflict, one is dealing with distance from the dangerous goal object. A similar analysis applies to displacement, in which the relevant dimension is similarity to the original dangerous goal object. In many cases, changes in the stimulus situation or in the goal object reduce the generalized fear more than the generalized approach, so that the subject may be able to achieve the same goal under altered conditions or a somewhat similar goal under the same conditions. In behavior therapy the construction of hierarchies is often based on the principle of a stimulus-generalization decrement in fear as the stimulus conditions are altered.

Functional Amnesia and Repression

The most easily understood type of repression is the combat amnesia produced by extremely terrifying circumstances without any head injury. Learning theory predicts that the intense fear aroused by the terrifying memories should motivate the victim to stop thinking about them, and the consequent relief should reinforce the inhibition of such thoughts. If someone who has a mild fear of heights had to jump across a 4-foot gap from the roof of a skyscraper to a ledge 2 feet wide, he might well run up to the edge and suddenly find himself physically unable to jump. The hypothesis of Dollard and Miller is that a train of thought is a sequence of responses, just like running, and that stopping a specific train of thought is a response, just like stopping running. To carry the analogy further: If a person were given a drug that reduced his fear enough, it is conceivable that he would be able to jump to the precarious ledge but that, once there, the stimuli confronting him would elicit far more fear than he was experiencing when he was unable to jump before taking the drug.

Grinker and Spiegel found that giving victims of combat amnesia an intravenous injection of sodium amobarbital, a drug that reduces fear, frequently enabled them to recover their memories, which acted as stimuli to elicit intense fear. The terrifying memories that occur when the fear-motivating combat amnesia is reduced by a drug may be related to the terrifying thoughts that sometimes occur to certain patients whose fears are reduced by deep relaxation.

According to the hypothesis of Dollard and Miller, other forms of repression are motivated and reinforced in much the same way as combat amnesia is. When the subject loses his ability to remember and to think about certain topics, he loses his ability in the area of repression to make fine discriminations, including those between realistic and unrealistic dangers. He also loses the ability to use his higher mental processes in achieving creative thought, foresight, and sophisticated problem solving. Similarly, the social and voluntary controls involving language and thought are lost. In short, the patient's behavior in the area affected by repression becomes more childlike.

Methods of Reducing Fear

One way of reducing fear is by drugs, but a number of difficulties should be borne in mind. One expects the reduction in fear to reinforce the taking of the drug, and there is good experimental evidence that this can occur. Furthermore, one does not expect a drug to differentiate between realistic and unrealistic fears. Thus, a person who uses alcohol to reduce his unrealistic fear of normal self-assertiveness at a party may not be cautious enough in driving home. And there is the problem of transfer from the drugged to the nondrugged state, so that it may be desirable to reduce the dose gradually and take special steps to help the patient cope after withdrawal.

In contrast to the effects of a drug, learning can be made very specific. A patient can be taught the discrimination of not being afraid of appropriate self-assertiveness but of being cautious about inappropriate aggression. Learning this discrimination may reduce chronic fear.

One way of getting rid of an unrealistic fear is to expose the subject to the fear-inducing cues without having the fear be reinforced by any aversive event. Students of learning call this procedure experimental extinction. But the extinction is often slow.

There is some evidence that the process of extinction can be hastened by the procedure of counterconditioning—namely, by pairing a fear-inducing stimulus with some stimulus that has a stronger tendency to elicit a response

incompatible with fear. Giving food to a hungry child and giving specific training in relaxation to an adult have been used as counterconditioning measures. Expressions of love and support from an important person or group can produce a strong counterconditioning effect.

Effects of Learning on Fear

Observations of people in dangerous situations, such as combat, suggest that two of the factors reducing fear are learning exactly what to expect and learning exactly what to do about it. These observations have been confirmed by experiments showing that, when the physical strength of painful electric shock is held constant, these purely psychological factors of learning when to expect the shock and how to cope with it can produce a great difference in chronic fear as measured by a variety of indices, including gastric lesions.

Compared with nonshocked controls, animals that had an opportunity to perform a successful response had an elevated level of norepinephrine in their brains, but their helpless yoked controls had a depressed level. This result is particularly suggestive because the drugs that are useful in treating many clinical cases of depression are those that increase the effectiveness of norepinephrine and possibly other monoamines at the synapse where these amines serve as neurotransmitters. Conversely, the drugs that have the opposite effect of reducing the effectiveness of norepinephrine and possibly other monoamines at the synapse also have the opposite effect of causing or intensifying depressions if they are given to the wrong patient. Schildkraut has advanced the hypothesis that situationally produced depressions may involve a similar reduction of the effectiveness of norepinephrine at the synapse.

Implications for Medicine

If animals are given exactly the same physical strength of painful electric shock, purely psychological factors can make a great difference in the amount of fear elicited and in the consequent gastric lesions. These animal experiments confirm the clinical observation that psychological factors can play a role in the production of stomach lesions.

Additional clinical evidence suggests that the effects of such psychological factors may not be limited to the types of disease frequently considered to be psychosomatic. For example, the death rates from a variety of diseases of people between the ages of 25 and 34 who have suffered the loss of a spouse by death are markedly higher than those of a group who have not suffered such a loss. Such stresses as fear-inducing electric shocks increase the mortality of animals exposed to standardized doses of specific viruses or given transplants of malignant tumors. Also, avoidance learning and other psychosocial variables, such as the housing arrangements of the animals, affect the antibody level after a challenge by a specific foreign protein. Other aspects of the immune response, such as asthmatic attacks, can also be affected.

Another clinical observation is that fear or other strong emotions can contribute to the sudden death of patients who are subject to premature ventricular contractions.

Implications for Psychotherapy

Turning away from danger and suppressing or repressing thoughts about it are natural types of response, which are rewarded by a temporary reduction in fear. This type of habit may be useful when there is nothing at all that can be done about the danger. But it often interferes with a more adaptive response when something can be done about the danger. Short-sighted maladaptive behaviors are maintained because immediate rewards or punishments are more effective than delayed ones.

Also, a person who is frustrated in his work may let his anger motivate him to perform sly types of maladaptive sabotage. The therapist's task may be to teach him to remove the frustration by standing up for his reasonable rights.

Although a theoretical prescription of teaching a more adaptive response is simple, one needs to discover more powerful practical techniques for achieving it. Some techniques are: classical conditioning, imitation (recently renamed "modeling"), verbal instruction (once the relevant units have been learned), reasoning, and trial and error. Students of Skinner have powerfully improved on trial and error by emphasizing the process they call "shaping," which consists of producing successively better approximations of the desired behavior by closely observing and immediately rewarding small spontaneous variations in the desired direction. Another contribution of this group

has been the study of schedules of reinforcement, which enables behavior to be maintained when rewarded only occasionally. Such schedules of reinforcement can account for the maintenance of either maladaptive or adaptive behaviors.

Placebo Effects

Evidence of the potent effects of psychological factors comes from clinical observations on the effects of a placebo—in other words, a pill containing a therapeutically inert substance, such as sugar, or a type of treatment that has no specific effects on the particular illness involved. Some but not necessarily all the effects of a placebo may be related, perhaps by stimulus generalization, to the fear-reducing effects of coping responses and of safety signals. Other reassuring effects of the doctor-patient relationship may come from innately programed fear-reducing mechanisms, analogous to those that cause primate and human infants to be less fearful when clinging to their mothers. Indeed, anxiety is one of the conditions believed to predispose patients to placebo effects. Whatever their mechanisms, placebo effects are not limited to verbal testimonials; they can produce clinically significant changes in physiological functions. The effectiveness of drugs—including those that subsequently are discovered to be, in fact, placebos—depends on the enthusiasm of the physician administering them.

Placebo effects can be quite specific. For example, Luparello et al. showed that the effects on airway resistance of a drug that produced bronchial dilation were about twice as great when asthmatic subjects were told that it was going to produce this effect than when they were told it would have the opposite one. Similar effects of expectation occurred with a drug that produced bronchial constriction. Furthermore, isotonic saline produced the appropriate effects when it was described as a drug that produces bronchial dilation on some administrations and as a drug that produces constriction on other administrations. In another study, Sternbach found that, when subjects were given a pill containing nothing but a little magnet used to measure their stomach motility, this activity increased, decreased, or remained constant according to the effects they were led to expect the pill would produce.

The results of these studies indicate that

Alexander underestimated the autonomic nervous system when he claimed that, since psychosomatic symptoms are under its control, they necessarily cannot be subject to the higher type of symbolic control involved in other symptoms.

Biofeedback

The development of improved instrumentation and programing equipment has made the moment-to-moment measurement of an increasing number of physiological processes much more readily accessible to the experimenter and the clinician. These developments, plus the emergence of the idea that processes hitherto thought of as being completely outside the domain of instrumental learning might be subject to such learning, has encouraged investigators to try various unconventional types of training. The common element in these new studies is the use of instrumentation to provide the subject with information about his performance, information that would otherwise be either completely unavailable to him or available only in an inaccurate and less perspicuous form. In the terminology of servo systems, such information is currently called "feedback." Recent studies frequently supply analogue information on the amount of change toward or away from the goal. For the subject who is interested in improving, the information that he is changing in the right direction serves as a reward, with larger improvements serving as greater rewards.

A decade ago the instrumental learning of visceral responses was so firmly believed to be impossible that it was difficult to get anyone to work on that problem, but now the interest in this and related extensions of the domain of learning is so strong that is possible to summarize only a sample of key studies. The swing from disbelief to enthusiasm has been extreme in popular news media descriptions of possible therapeutic applications of this work. Having learned that it is wasteful to design time-consuming controls for effects that are not there, the investigators trying to make therapeutic applications have first concentrated on seeing whether they can get any effects at all. But now that some effects have been obtained, it is essential to put in controls for placebo effects. Unless specifically mentioned in studies of therapy, such controls, which unfortunately are absent in many areas of psychotherapy, should be assumed to be missing.

Relaxation

Jacobson has devised techniques of verbal instruction to teach patients suffering from anxiety and stress-related disorders to relax their skeletal musculature progressively. Luthe has extended this procedure with a series of exercises emphasizing the imagery of heaviness and warmth. This is called autogenic training. He presents examples of physiological changes, presumably produced by autogenic training, in such variables as temperature, heart rate, and blood pressure. Wolpe and other behavior therapists have used somewhat similar techniques to produce deep relaxation, which they believe is incompatible with anxiety and hence helps to countercondition it. In experiments with a total of 30 tension headache patients, roughly 75 per cent showed significant declines in headache activity.

Brudny et al. and Korein et al. have used electromyograph feedback to train nine patients to control their spasmodic torticollis. Nine out of nine patients showed improvement, three of them to the point of remaining symptom-free for several months to more than a year. Since these three patients had had the symptoms for 3, 10, and 15 years, respectively, and had not responded to previous treatments, a placebo effect seems unlikely. At the present time, three other patients can maintain control without feedback for several hours, and the remaining three can maintain control for 5 to 10 minutes.

Certain characteristics of the electroencephalogram can be modified by using instrumentation that measures the occurrence of the desired characteristic and immediately rewards the subject for either increasing or decreasing its occurrence. A series of studies has shown that, if people are given feedback indicating the amplitude or incidence of the α component (8 to 11 cps) in their EEG, they can learn in one way or another to control the amount of α recorded.

Visceral Learning

Work on classical conditioning in the Soviet Union showed that a large number of visceral responses can be classically conditioned—for example, salivation, contractions of the intestine, contractions of the uterus, ejection of red blood cells from the spleen, formation of urine by the kidney, secretion of bile, changes in temperature, and vasomotor responses (see Figure 1).

The strong traditional belief has been that the autonomic nervous system responsible for visceral responses is fundamentally less perceptive than the somatic one, so that visceral responses can be learned only by classical conditioning. However, new evidence indicates that this view is not valid, that visceral responses can be instrumentally learned and reinforced by rewards or secondary gains. This newer view is consonant with neurophysiological evidence showing that the visceral organs are represented at the highest level of the brain, the cortex.

Applications. A specific instrumental learning situation can produce a relatively specific

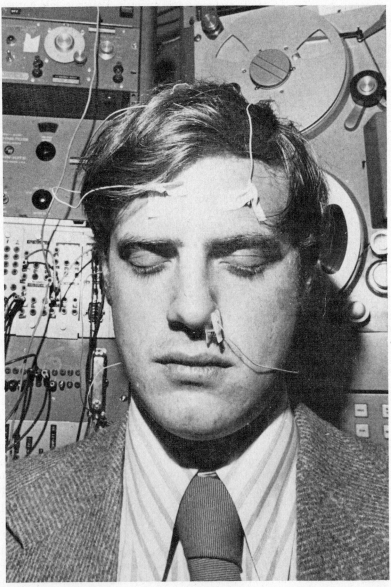

FIGURE 1. This experimenter is able to monitor his own physiological changes during altered states of consciousness. Similar biofeedback experiments may eventually enable patients to control certain body functions such as respiration and heartbeat, which have always been thought of as involuntary (UPI photo).

visceral response. This fact removes the main basis for assuming that psychosomatic symptoms involving the autonomic nervous system are fundamentally different from those functional symptoms, such as hysterical symptoms, that involve the somatic nervous system; it means that psychosomatic symptoms can be reinforced by the full range of rewards, including escape from aversive stimulation, known as secondary gains. In stressful situations in which any symptom of illness is likely to be rewarded, the symptom to which a person is innately predisposed is the one most likely to occur, be rewarded, and thus be strengthened additionally by learning.

At present, the practical application of visceral learning to the reduction of hypertension awaits development of either superior methods for selecting the rare patients who can benefit from current techniques or the development of considerably improved techniques of training. In either event, the results must be validated by controls for placebo effects and by tests for transfer to life situations.

One of the most convincing therapeutic applications of visceral training to date has been in the treatment of cardiac arrhythmias. In a typical training situation, the patient is confronted by three lights: a green one that is a signal for him to try to speed his heart, a red one that is a signal to slow his heart, and a yellow one that tells him he is performing correctly. In addition, there is a percentage-time meter, which runs whenever the subject has met the criterion and thus provides an additional incentive believed to be important during the early stages of training.

The patients are first trained to alternately speed and slow their heart rates a few beats a minute. (The alternations between training in two directions convince the patients that they are able to control their hearts.) Next, the patients are given training in holding their heart rates within a narrow range. The feedback is gradually phased out by omitting it on a progressively greater proportion of trials, a procedure believed to be important in helping the subjects feel without aid whether their hearts are beating correctly or incorrectly and, thus, transfer their training from the laboratory to daily life.

Six of the nine patients studied to date have learned to control their premature ventricular contractions (PVCs) in the laboratory; the three failures had the most seriously damaged hearts. Five patients showed persistence of lowered PVC activity on clinical tests outside the laboratory for the considerable number of months they were followed up. One patient was found to have good control 1 year after, and another patient had good control 5 years afterward.

Training in Visceral Perception. One's perception of the external world is sharpened by checking one modality against another and by training in social communication. Most people receive no training in the perception of visceral events, and such perceptions are notoriously inaccurate. Modern instrumentation provides new opportunities for the feedback necessary to train such perceptions, and work from Eastern Europe shows that both animals and people can be trained to make much better discriminations of visceral sensations. Training in better visceral perception should enable a patient to substitute his own direct perceptions for feedback from elaborate instrumentation and thus help in the transfer from the laboratory to the life situation.

Some of the avenues to be tried in improving visceral learning are training in visceral perception, use of imagery, use of classical conditioning to initiate a response that is later instrumentally rewarded, use of mediating skeletal responses that can be phased out later, use of hypnosis, and the investigation of various means of supplying feedback and of various types of motivation, reward, and other parameters known to be relevant to learning and motor skill. And there is an urgent need for the studies that appear to have produced therapeutic effects to be repeated with better controls for placebo effects, with controlled comparisons with other techniques, and with longer term follow-ups.

REFERENCES

Brener, J. A general model of voluntary control applied to the phenomena of learned cardiovascular change. In *Cardiovascular Psychophysiology*, P. A. Obrist, editor, p. 321. Aldine, Chicago, 1974.

Brener, J., Eissenberg, E., and Middaugh, S. Respiratory and somatomotor factors associated with operant conditioning of cardiovascular responses in curarized rats. In *Cardiovascular Psychophysiology*, P. A. Obrist, editor, p. 117. Aldine, Chicago, 1974.

Budzynski, T. H., Stoyva, J. M., Adler, C. S., and Mullaney, D. J. EMG biofeedback and tension headache: A controlled outcome study. Psychosom. Med., *35:* 484, 1973.

Carmona, A., Miller, N. E., and Demierre, T. Instrumental learning of gastric tonicity responses. Psychosom. Med., *36:* 156, 1974.

Dollard, J., and Miller, N. E. *Personality and Psychotherapy.* McGraw-Hill, New York, 1950.

Engel, B. T., and Bleecker, E. R. Application of operant conditioning techniques to the control of the cardiac arrhythmias. In *Cardiovascular Psychophysiology*, P. A. Obrist, editor, p. 430. Aldine, Chicago, 1974.

Harris, A. H., Gilliam, W. J., Findley, J. D., and Brady, J. B. Instrumental conditioning of large-magnitude, daily, 12-hour blood pressure elevations in the baboon. Science, *182:* 175, 1973.

Korein, J., Levidow, L., and Brudny, J. Self-regulation of EEG and EMG activity using biofeedback as a therapeutic tool. EEG Clin. Neurophysiol., *36:* 222, 1974.

Lown, B., Verrier, R., and Corbalan, R. Psychologic stress and threshold for repetitive ventricular response. Science, *182:* 834, 1973.

Miller, N. E. Liberalization of basic S-R concepts: Extensions to conflict behavior, motivation, and social learning. In *Psychology: A Study of a Science*, S. Koch, editor, study 1, vol. 2, p. 196. McGraw-Hill, New York, 1959.

Miller, N. E. Learning of visceral and glandular responses. Science, *163:* 434, 1969.

Miller, N. E., and Dworkin, B. R. Visceral learning: Recent difficulties with curarized rats and significant problems for human research. In *Cardiovascular Psychophysiology*, P. A. Obrist, editor, p. 218. Aldine, Chicago, 1974.

Obrist, P. A., editor. *Cardiovascular Psychophysiology.* Aldine, Chicago, 1974.

Raskin, M., Johnson, G., and Rondestvedt, J. W. Chronic anxiety treated by feedback-induced muscle relaxation. Arch. Gen. Psychiatry, *28:* 263, 1973.

Roberts, A., Kewman, D. G., and Macdonald, H. Voluntary control of skin temperature: Unilateral changes using hypnosis and feedback. J. Abnorm. Psycho., *82:* 163, 1973.

Shapiro, D. Operant-feedback control of human blood pressure: Some clinical issues. In *Cardiovascular Psychophysiology*, P. A. Obrist, editor, p. 232. Aldine, Chicago, 1974.

Shapiro, D., Barber, T. X., DiCara, L. V., Kamiya, J., Miller, N. E., and Stoyva, J., editors. *Biofeedback and Self-Control 1972.* Aldine, Chicago, 1973.

Sterman, M. B. Neurophysiological and clinical studies of sensorimotor EEG biofeedback training: Some effects on epilepsy. In *Seminars in Psychiatry*, L. Birk, editor, p. 507. Grune & Stratton, New York, 1973.

Stoyva, J., and Budzynski, T. Cultivated low arousal: An anti-stress response? In *Recent Advances in Limbic and Autonomic Nervous System Research*, L. V. DiCara, editor, p. 43. Plenum, New York, 1973.

4

Science of Human Behavior: Contributions of the Sociocultural Sciences

4.1. ANTHROPOLOGY

Introduction

What is recognized as pathological in behavior is usually a matter of common consensus within a society. But the standards of consensus vary from one society to another. The anthropologist, who studies human societies in an evolutionary and cross-cultural perspective, explains such differences as the results of differences in culture.

Culture, in the anthropologist's sense, is the sum of what the individual members of a community have learned from generations of accumulated social experience. It includes manners, customs, tastes, skills, language, beliefs, and all the other patterns of behavior that are part of organized social life. Just as cultures differ in technology, kinship practices, and religious belief, so they differ in the behaviors classified as normal and abnormal.

Cultural Similarities and Differences

Change in any one sector of culture—for instance, in technology or the economic system—is apt to produce a series of changes in other sectors, such as family structure, religious belief, and values. Studies also show that certain assortments of culture elements are more congenial than others and are most likely to be found together in a society; for instance, strong belief in witchcraft tends to occur in societies with poorly developed governmental systems of social control. The implication for psychiatry is that the folk definition of behavior disorder, the precise symptoms of that disorder, the stresses contributory to its development, onset, and course, and the methods of social response to the disorder are likely to be more or less direct functions of many cultural factors, such as economic system, family structure, political organization, and religious belief and practice.

Several generalizations can be made about deviant behavior in the simpler cultures: (1) There are always folk criteria for distinguishing behavior that is normal from that which is abnormal. (2) Abnormal—as distinct from merely wrong or criminal or even pathological—behavior is always explained as a result of interference by disease or by supernatural agencies with the normal functioning of the organism. (3) Conventional therapeutic or extrusive procedures are always available and believed to be effective to end any unwanted interference and thereby to restore the victim's behavior to normal or at least to minimize its disrupting effect on the community. (4) There are no human societies in which mental disorders of one sort or another never occur. (5) In most human societies, the same major symptom clusters can be recognized.

Societies seem to differ markedly in preferred style of symptoms, in the incidence and prevalence of major types of disorder, and, slightly, in total psychiatric census. Furthermore, societies exotic to Western eyes may display dramatically different ethnic psychoses, whose symptoms may, at first glance, appear strange to Western eyes: *amok* in Southeast Asia (a homicidal rampage), *latah* in Malaya (echopraxia), and *piblokto* among the polar Eskimos (an endemic convulsive disorder).

For example, the *windigo* psychosis repeatedly described among the Algonkian hunters of northeastern North America, is superficially unique. The victim of the *windigo* psychosis gradually becomes convinced that he is possessed by a supernatural monster, the *windigo*, whose taste for human flesh is notorious in mythology. However, his unique decisions and occasional accompanying hallucinations appear to follow the same sort of mental process that in Western society may accompany fears of homosexuality. The basic structure of a paranoid process involving fear, defense against the fear, and powerful but disallowed impulses in a progressively delusional set of defense mechanisms is apparent.

Causes of psychiatric disturbances appear to be more diverse than the basic symptomatic structures. Social structures and even political structures provide different opportunities for stress and for particular kinds of symptomatic relief. Religious beliefs, too, are notoriously variable from culture to culture; they condone, reward, or taboo human impulses in a remarkably irregular way.

Many anthropologists and psychiatrists have suggested that each culture is associated with a common or at least widely shared national character or basic or modal personality structure. This character is particularly adapted to the prevailing social structure and belief system and is, at the same time, particularly vulnerable to certain stresses. From this point of view, the type of neuroticism that Freud was able to define as common among his patients—focusing on an oedipal conflict involving a nuclear family in which the father holds the position of supreme authority and the mother is the nurturant figure—is by no means universal. Large modern nations like the United States are polycultural. They display a diversity of socio-economic classes, geographic regions, and ethnic origins.

Institutionalizing Symptoms

Most societies have traditional means for accommodating themselves to episodes of disturbed behavior. In a sense, the task of the culture is to institutionalize and channel the symptoms of an endemic disease in such a way that the symptoms do not disrupt orderly community life.

Denial of Illness

Although ignoring or denying even gross symptoms may be deplored where more effective means of treatment are available, such a procedure has the probable advantage of not adding to the sick person's difficulties the burden of being publicly branded as incompetent. Where the condition is widespread, where there is no reliable and inexpensive treatment, and when the symptoms are episodic and not severely threatening to community welfare, such a policy has even more merit.

In our own culture, the ignoring of emotional disorders associated with menstrual periods seems to be dictated by such considerations. Among the polar Eskimos, *piblokto* (fits of convulsive hysteria whose cause is not fully understood) is apparently treated with a similar indifference. On the other hand, in some other cultures, menstruating women are taboo and physically isolated because of beliefs concerning the dangerous nature of menstrual contamination. And, in our culture, episodic convulsive disorders are often regarded as serious, requiring heroic measures of treatment.

Special Roles for the Ill

In many societies, including sectors of our own, a person suffering from a chronic condition such as schizophrenia is allowed to take on or is even encouraged to take on the role of shaman. He is regarded as a person who has a special skill in communicating with or manipulating supernatural powers and beings and who, for a fee, performs such services as divining the location of missing objects, foretelling the future, curing illness, and persuading a divinity to bestow benefits on a client.

Rituals for Episodic Illness

Religious rituals in almost all societies may give symptomatic relief in episodes of acting out to persons suffering from chronic but not necessarily grossly disabling emotional conflicts. In many cultures, rituals are cathartic; impulses that cannot be readily satisfied in the workaday world may find expression in ritual. Rituals may also be repressive, intended to strengthen the capacity of the person to reduce the anxiety of conflict by supporting defense mechanisms. For instance, rituals in which a scapegoat is condemned and destroyed have the effect of enabling the conflict-ridden person to say, "It is not I, but he, who is guilty of such and such wishes."

Specific treatment of mental disturbance in primitive societies commonly involves one of four principles: exorcising a possessing spirit (see Figure 1), recalling the victim's wandering soul, making reparations for the violation of taboo, or countering the spell cast by witch-craft.

The ritual procedures may be based on a faulty conception of the nature and causes of mental illness, but such procedures are not necessarily inefficacious. Sharing a belief system with the shaman that defines his ritual as effective, the victim is apt to be relieved of the fear that his case is hopeless and must end in death or the destruction of his identity. Further-

more, some shamans interview the patient to discover the nature of the taboo violation or the possible occasion for witchcraft. In the inter-view, the shaman may directly encounter the patient's unconscious conflicts, help him to verbalize them, and thus, in the manner of any good psychotherapist, bring them into a state of consciousness, where the ego can begin to deal with them.

Prophylactic Rituals

In what may be called preventive psychother-apy, most primitive societies tend to rely on what are called rites of passage. These are the rituals, often supported by more or less elabo-rate religious beliefs, in which a person is separated from an earlier social role and intro-duced to a new one. They are performed on occasions of life crisis: birth, puberty, marriage, military undertakings, bereavement, and so on. The particular pattern of occasions selected for

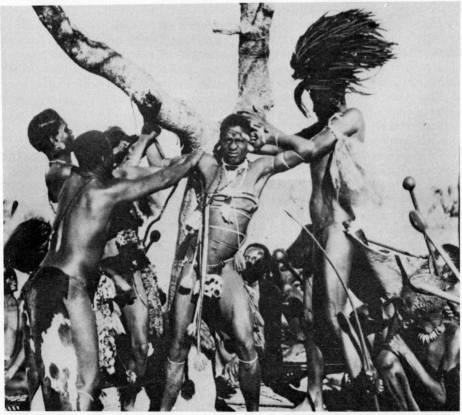

FIGURE 1. Primitive societies often resort to elaborate exorcism rituals in order to cope with physical and mental illness. The patient above endures a cure at the hands of tribal witchdoctors and excited tribesmen (UPI photo).

ritual treatment and the content of the rituals vary with the culture.

A major function of such rituals is to minimize the duration and depth of internal psychic conflict accompanying major changes in social role. The agonizing conflicts concerning roles, values, motives, and responses commonly observed in many members of Western societies at times of life crisis seem to be, in part, a consequence of the unavailability of *effective* rites of passage.

Puberty Ceremonies

The rites of passage most relevant to the interests of modern psychiatry are the puberty ceremonies performed on boys and girls, usually in the early stages of puberty, to mark the transition from childhood to adolescence or even adulthood. What is involved is usually more than a mere celebration of the change in social role. In the classic instances, such as the initiation rituals of the Australian aborigines and the bush schools of West Africa, a class of initiates, particularly males, is physically removed from the community and imprisoned in a special compound. There they are instructed in the secrets of manhood and are subjected for days or weeks to prolonged and various forms of hazing at the hands of elder males. The climax of the ritual is the public occasion on which genital mutilation—generally circumcision, but among some Australian aborigines subincision also—is performed on the youth. This marks the completion of the process of transformation. The child is considered to have died, to have been reconceived and held in embryonic isolation, and finally, to have been reborn a man. Comparable ceremonies are, more rarely, also conducted for girls.

The unconscious meanings of the acts performed in such rituals are subject to multiple interpretations. The Australian circumcision and subincision ritual has been interpreted as a symbolic castration by jealous elders of young males who potentially compete for their women. It has also been interpreted as the satisfaction of an unconscious womb envy on the part of males, who by the operation of subincision acquire the simulacrum of a vagina.

Among the more interesting programs of research with initiation ceremonies have been those in the cross-cultural tradition. Whiting and his associates, in a series of papers, advanced the argument that initiation rituals for males function to revise an early cross-sex identification. Initially they argued that the boy's original identification with his mother was a consequence of libidinal ties intensified by mother-son sleeping arrangements that excluded the father. Later they argued that it was the envy of the mother, as the highest status object available to a boy when his father slept away from them, that was responsible for the cross-sex identification. In any case, the statistics demonstrate convincingly that initiation ceremonies with genital mutilation tend to occur in societies where the father sleeps apart and the mother and infant son sleep together (see Table I). Along the same lines, of the 12 societies in the above sample where the *couvade* was practiced (i.e., the husband mimics childbirth and postnatal care during his confinement), 10 had the exclusive mother-son sleeping arrangement, suggesting that those societies did indeed provide the male with status envy of the female and a consequent optative female identification. As one might expect, societies with mother-son exclusive sleeping arrangement tend also to be societies where polygyny is common or at least regarded favorably, where females contribute importantly to the subsistence economy, where there is a long postpartum sex

TABLE I

Initiation with Genital Multilation	Mother-Son Exclusive Sleeping	
	Present	Absent
Present	13	0
Absent	8	35

taboo, and, paradoxically, where there are *female* initiation ceremonies also.

A competing argument, however, has been presented by Young and Cohen, who suggest that the formation of such ceremonies is to dramatize masculine status in societies that have exclusive male organizations (such as men's clubs) or unilinear male descent groups. Young's data are just as convincing as Whiting's, as shown in Table II. These approaches seem to dispense with personality as a variable, but in fact they agree substantially with Whiting's in arguing that the adult male groups see the entering youths as inadequately gender-socialized males who require the additional benefit of ritual before they can be considered nondisruptive recruits.

TABLE II

Male Initiation Ceremony	Exclusive Male Organization	
	Present	Absent
Present	16	4
Absent	2	32

Hospitals as Cultural Systems

In recent years, many social scientists, including anthropologists, have studied the social and cultural milieu of the mental hospital, its customs and procedures, and their possible unintended effects on patients.

Characteristic types of social conflict are built into the social system of the hospital staff: the castelike division of the staff into hierarchically ranked categories, the militarylike pattern of authority, characterized particularly by the phenomenon of multiple subordination, and the tendency for the patient to be effectively stripped of his outside identity and to display the syndrome of hospitalism.

However indispensable rational conversation may be to the therapeutic process at some points, much of the emotionally significant interchange between therapist and patient involves the mutual communication of affects by autonomic signs, culturally patterned gestures and postures, and para-language—intonation, voice, quality, and so forth. The availability of multiple modes of communication also facilitates those ambiguous and contradictory exchanges described by such terms as the double bind and the identity struggle, which some investigators have regarded as possibly pathogenic.

Marked differences in social class, education, and ethnic background between staff and patient may directly interfere with communication because the staff simply does not know what the patient is talking about and may more subtly block agreement on the goals and nature of treatment because the patient's tacit expectations are at variance with the physician's. Segregated ethnic minorities may entertain a world view very different from the middle-class psychiatrist's.

Psychiatric Disorders

Misconceptions

Happy-Primitive Misconception. One popular delusion about human nature is probably inherited from romantic Rousseauistic notions of the happy primitive. Mental disorder is regarded as a disease of civilization that regularly increases in frequency as civilization progresses. But mental difficulties are not recent afflictions of mankind. They could probably be traced, if records were available, far back in human phylogeny to a time when technological and social simplicity, comparable to that of modern primitives, was the general condition.

Sick-Society Misconception. A related popular misconception is that whole societies can be diagnosed as suffering from paranoid or other psychoses. This pseudoscientific attitude is apt to flourish most exuberantly when scientists feel the need to condemn their own or their nation's enemies without seeming to exhibit prejudice.

Inherited-Neuroses Misconception. There is little to support the argument that neurotic guilt and the consequent Oedipus neurosis began with some primal parricide, as suggested by Freud, and that the nucleus of the Oedipus conflict is a genetically inherited constant in human nature. There are some startling uniformities in symbolism and mythology across otherwise widely differing cultures, but these can readily be interpreted as the consequences of common features of the human condition, such as prolonged infancy. Or they may be the results of the historical diffusion of culture content. Nor can one support the idea that in neurosis and psychosis the human mind recapitulates the stages of barbarism and savagery through which our ancestors passed tens of thousands of years ago.

Social Reactions to the Mentally Ill

Hunting and gathering cultures have a work rhythm characterized by periods of intense, exacting effort alternating with periods of rest and relaxation. A person's contribution to the welfare of such groups is better measured by what he can do when he is at his best than by how constantly he remains at a standard level of performance. Thus, simple societies can and do tolerate episodic disorders more readily than the more complex societies do.

Agricultural and, particularly, industrial societies depend far more heavily on continuous, reliable, day-after-day performance of routine tasks, frequently involving intricate machinery and complexly arranged social relationships. Here, reliability of performance over long periods of time, even at a mediocre level, may be more important than the high peaks of efficiency during occasions of intense effort. The interruption of the routine by episodes of behavioral disorder in such societies may present serious problems and attract therapeutic efforts or sanctions far more intense than in the hunting and gathering societies.

REFERENCES

Chance, M. R. A., and Jolly, C. J. *Social Groups of Monkeys, Apes, and Men*. E. P. Dutton, New York, 1970.

Hsu, F. L. K., editor. *Psychological Anthropology*. Dorsey Press, Homewood, Ill., 1972.

Kiev, A. *Transcultural Psychiatry*. The Free Press (Macmillan), New York, 1972.

Opler, M., editor. *Culture and Mental Health*. Macmillan, New York, 1959.

Spiro, M. Ghosts, Ifaluk, and teleological functionalism. Am. Anthropol., *54*: 497, 1952.

* Textor, R. *A Cross Cultural Summary*, HRAF Press, New Haven, Conn., 1967.

4.2.   SOCIOLOGY

Introduction

Man is at the same time an organism, a member of society, the bearer of a culture, and a person or personality. Human potentialities become manifest only in society, and the bent they take in any particular society can be fully understood only in the context of the culture and the social organization of that society. The self arises in the process of social interaction, and the structuring of goals and motives in the person is likewise a product of interaction within a framework of norms and values basic to a culture.

Basic Formulations

The relationship of the indivudual to society and group life is the core problem of social psychology. Sociological interest in this field has centered on such issues as the rise of the self in social interaction, the process of socialization (whereby a person takes on the way of life of his society and becomes a competent par-

ticipant in it), and the operation of processes of social control on the one hand and the genesis and stabilization of deviance on the other. The dominant perspective of sociologists presently working on these issues is that of symbolic interactionism.

Central to symbolic interactionism is the concept of the self, which comes into being through interaction between the small child and his caretakers. By virtue of language and antecedent gesture and role taking in play and games, the child is able to get outside himself and to take the perspective of significant others toward himself. Once a symbol system has been mastered, the great bulk of human action is built up by people noting and interpreting the actions of others in social situations. Behavior is not a release but a construction. Collective action always entails an aligning of individual actions, and, conversely, individual actions are a consequence of definitions and interpretations of social situations and the actions of others.

Symbolic interactionism focuses on the person's interpretation of his own behavior, as well as the behavior of others. It tends, therefore, to give primary consideration to the rational, consciously purposive aspects of behavior. Nevertheless, it provides a framework for examining the subjective representation of interaction.

Role

The concept of role has long been used to characterize coherent patternings in behavior, but its current use in the behavioral sciences focuses on behaviors expected of people because of their positions in groups or networks of social ties. The terms father, mother, son, and daughter designate not merely biological relationships but culturally defined sets of obligations, duties, and privileges between specified social positions. Similarly, the doctor-patient role relationship is defined in terms of general expectations that have been built up historically and that serve as guidelines for interaction. Each participant expects the other to know the guidelines and to follow them. However, role enactment tends to show considerable variation around the normative definitions of roles, largely because each enduring role relationship involves the construction of a new social reality through the give and take of interaction. Equally important, a person's identity tends to be linked with his role and with the set of definitions by which it is sustained.

Social Structure, Socialization, and Personality

At every stage of life, a person is enmeshed in a structure of relationships and expectations that influences how he defines his goals and his self-image. The infant is born into a matrix of social relationships, as well as into an ongoing cultural order. They provide him with his initial orientations and train him for expected performances. Within this matrix, the child develops characteristic ways of interpreting and responding to others. Position in society also carries an implicit social stereotype of attributed characteristics. Other people define the child partly in terms of his family's reputation, his social class, his ethnic group, and his religion.

As he moves from the family into relationships in the larger community, the child brings to each new situation or social role behavioral tendencies that are typical for him, most of which were built up in previous social roles with parents, siblings, and other important caretakers. The child must somehow incorporate and integrate experience from one situation or setting to another, discerning what is expected by various co-participants and coping with conflicting demands. Sometimes it is possible to compartmentalize conflicting demands by varying roles across settings. At other times the child may be forced to choose between parties exerting claims on him—often before he knows what his choice entails or has the cognitive maturity to act on rational grounds.

The concept of social class has been variously formulated in terms of economic power, social prestige, political identification, and patterns of association. In American society, class position is most frequently characterized by occupation and education. White-collar occupations, especially when coupled with education beyond high school, tend to place one in the middle class; blue-collar occupations tend to place one in the working class. Income differences between the classes may be minimal, but life-styles, aspirations, and, even, to a degree, cognition and modes of personality coping and defense tend to differ by class.

Working-class parents tend to stress conformity to external standards; middle-class parents place greater stress on self-direction and responsibility. Working-class parents appear to punish their children on the basis of the direct consequences of the children's actions; middle-class parents seem to act more often on the basis of the child's intent. Praise and encouragement of the child also seem to be more prevalent in the middle class, and this is especially true with respect to the father-son relationship.

Studies have found a sharper differentiation of sex roles in the working class, less involvement of the father in child rearing, and a greater tendency toward authoritarian parental behaviors. Education goals and cognitive skills are more emphasized in the middle class, and feelings of personal efficacy (of being in control of one's destiny as against being subject to external controls) are more characteristic in the middle class than in the working class. Denial is more frequent as a working-class defense mechanism, and intellectualization and projection appear to be more common in the middle class.

Family size and authority structure, the homogeneity or heterogeneity of one's childhood neighborhood, the consonance of values and goals presented to the child in home and school—these and many other aspects of socialization are influenced not only by class but by religion, ethnic background, community of residence, and parental personalities.

At each developmental stage, the socialization process entails changing goals, agents, and techniques. The tasks of early childhood socialization are basic to all later stages, but both socialization and personality change continue through the life course. By adolescence, most people are to a large extent selecting or at least modifying their own socialization opportunities, but they are being selected or recruited for later roles as well. In Western societies, where occupation is the most potent single predictor of attitudes, values, and life styles generally, educational selection in adolescence is the most potent single predictor of occupational success. Those who fail to achieve occupational success have lower self-esteem, show more physiological symptoms, and, in general, exhibit many more forms of deviant behavior than do those who are highly successful in their occupations.

Social Control and Deviance

Behavior that contravenes the norms of the society gives rise to negative sanctions in all societies. Social control is maintained in part by the person's internalizing the norms and values of his society and in part by the institutionalization of mechanisms for punishing deviation. In complex societies, however, norms and values are themselves subject to variation among class strata, subcultural groups, and other bases of differentiation. Such differentiation is often associated with a good deal of mobility, both geographical and social. Some people or groups may be marginal to the major social groupings of the society and not incorporated into enduring social structures. Recent migrants, devalued ethnic groups, and persons alienated from the dominant way of life of the society are especially subject to stress, lacking in resources for dealing with such stress, and peculiarly vulnerable to being publicly labeled as deviants.

Both the forms that deviance takes and the responses of others to the deviant are strongly influenced by social status and ethnic membership. For example, there are marked class and ethnic differences in the likelihood of being sent to prison for theft, of being hospitalized if one manifests psychotic behavior, or of being retained for a long period in a mental hospital.

To be labeled delinquent, homosexual, or mentally ill is to be stigmatized. Mental patients are not, in general, regarded as sick but as crazy, unreliable, or morally degraded. Indeed, recent studies suggest that, among the general population in present-day urban America, to consult a psychiatrist is to threaten one's public identity as a responsible person. Regardless of what led to a person's being defined as mentally ill, the labeling itself calls into question his ability to control himself and his relationships. The patient tends to be accorded a stereotyped role. Often, the patient's problem is then made more acute, and a secondary deviation occurs as a result of labeling and of stigmatization.

Social Competence

Mental health is often equated in popular thinking with personal adjustment. Implicit in the concept of adjustment is the assumption that existing social arrangements are either optimal or inevitable and that people should accept them as such. But an examination of such phenomena as delinquency and drug abuse in urban areas or of the educational opportunities available to many minority group children clearly reveals that these problems are group phenomena. Most juvenile delinquency in the city is learned behavior for which there is substantial social support in the pre-existing peer culture. Indeed, the delinquent may be better adjusted to his milieu than the nondelinquent, if one takes the perspective of members of that milieu. He may, however, lack the kind of competence that is needed for successful functioning in conventional society.

Competence is the ability to attain and perform in social roles, both those to which one is assigned and those to which one aspires. The development of competence rests on perception of the self as causally important and on at least moderately favorable levels of self-esteem. Its acquisition also appears to be favored by early stimulation, enhancing cognitive development, and by continuity of experience and consistency in the presentation of valued goals. Where gross discontinuities occur or the child is not given adequate orientation and preparation for expected roles, early difficulties with role performance can be anticipated.

Social Processes and Mental Disorder

The preponderance of evidence suggests that both treated mental disorder and the symptoms of psychological discomfort are found more frequently in the lower class than in the upper and middle classes, among persons who are not incorporated in meaningful social ties, among those who do not have useful social roles, and among those who have suffered traumatic loss of significant social ties.

Assessment

Efforts to establish rate differentials in mental disorder among population segments most often either rely on records of treated mental disorder or attempt to make a direct assessment of mental health status in a carefully selected sample of the population. Studies of various forms of deviance have demonstrated, however, that the frequency with which deviants come to official attention is seldom an adequate index of the incidence of deviance. The representation of population segments in a treatment facility is as likely to reflect knowledge about the facility and attitudes toward it as to reflect differences in the incidence of the problems presented for treatment.

Lower-class and minority members come to treatment through the police, the courts, and welfare agencies, whereas upper-middle-class persons come more often as a result of self-referrals or referrals by the family and the family physician.

Before ataractic drugs, how long a patient remained in most public mental hospitals was strongly influenced by his social status. The lower the status, the longer the stay. An unskilled worker diagnosed as schizophrenic was likely to remain in the hospital two or three times as long as a middle-class college graduate with the same diagnosis. The unskilled worker was thereby more likely to become a chronic schizophrenic, whatever his level of disorder. This can hardly be taken as evidence that working-class life produces schizophrenia.

Attempts to assess untreated mental disorder confront a different but somewhat similar set of sociocultural contingencies. First of all, there is the problem of gaining access to a cross-section of the population. Since the prevalence of severe mental disorder at any given time is relatively low and since persons who are suspicious or upset are less likely to make themselves available for interviews, it is likely that seriously distressed persons are underrepresented in population surveys.

Moreover, the data elicited in a survey interview are unlikely to be adequate for diagnostic assessment. Furthermore, efforts to induce people to present themselves for psychiatric assessment cannot, in general, hope to succeed with more than one-half to two-thirds of the population. When a structured interview is used, the meaning of any given question and of the response to it depends on the person's personal experiences, his willingness to disclose his own feelings, and the subcultural norms that govern the reporting of particular kinds of feelings or experiences.

Distribution

The first systematic study of the distribution of severe mental disorder within a community was the investigation undertaken in Chicago by Faris and Dunham in the mid-1930's. The highest rates of mental disorder clustered toward the center of the city and in areas of low socio-economic status, high population turnover, and a high incidence of other social problems. Mental disorder was associated with poverty, with recent migration to the city, with social disorganization, and with other forms of social pathology.

Urban Life and Social Change

It is widely believed that life in urban industrial societies affords less sense of belonging and less social integration than did life in earlier, simpler societies, But there is evidence that urban life is no more productive of mental disorder than is rural life.

Social change is often disruptive of relationships and life patterns, but it appears that long-term social change is not a major cause of mental disorder. On the other hand, changes that deprive a person of employment or other meaningful roles appear frequently as precursors of mental disorder.

Social Class

Hollingshead and Redlich found the highest prevalence of mental hospital inpatients in the lowest class (largely unskilled and semiskilled workers) and, in general, decreasing prevalence as one moves up the status ladder. In large part, the prevalence differences derived from the greater duration of hospitalization of lower-status patients, who received the least treatment and were accorded the poorest prognoses. But even rates of initial hospitalization, which should come closer to reflecting the actual incidence of disorder, showed significant class differences. Entry into care for schizophrenia was 3 times as frequent in the lowest class as in the upper classes.

Half of the upper-middle-class neurotics entered treatment after referral by a private physician, and more than a third were either self-referrals or came at the urging of family and friends. Lower-working-class patients, on the other hand, were most often referred by social agencies or clinics; only 5 per cent were self-referred or family-referred. The class differences in source of referral were equally great for psychotics.

The Midtown Manhattan research of Srole and his associates was designed to assess the prevalence of symptoms of mental disorder, using a structured interview of a cross-section of the population. Symptoms were much more widespread among persons of lowest social status, of whom nearly half were rated impaired, as against only about an eighth of persons in the highest stratum. Srole and his associates found that middle-class persons who were rated impaired were either currently receiving outpatient therapy or had been under psychiatric treatment in the past, whereas only a fifth of the impaired members of the working class were or had been psychiatric patients, and most of these had been hospitalized. This study and other similar surveys show that the frequency of emotional upset and other symptoms of mental distress is greater among the poor and deprived segments of the population. It is less clear, however, that diagnosable psychoses, such as schizophrenia, are as closely linked with social status.

The Midtown Manhattan study also documented that upward and downward social mobility are highly related to the prevalence of symptoms. Persons who move up the ladder tend to show a lower prevalence of symptoms of emotional distress than do those who remain at the same initial status. But persons who drop in status—that is, who move into less prestigous occupations—show more than the level of symptoms expected for persons of their origins.

Thus, the meaning of social status is ambiguous, since it reflects attainment as well as origins. Nevertheless, there are real differences in symptoms associated with childhood social class. Attempts to explain such differences most frequently focus on the more stressful conditions of working-class life or on differences in childhood socialization.

Life Crises

Studies of life crises suggest that specific life changes in the weeks immediately before breakdown frequently serve as precipitants of the onset of schizophrenia. It is not clear whether the effect of such life changes rests primarily on a general demand for adaptation or on their meaning in terms of ego involvement. Nor has there been adequate examination of the social networks of persons who are overwhelmed by life change as compared with those who seem able to adapt.

Mental Hospitals

Studies of large state hospitals revealed as the central feature the sharp dichotomy between the inmate world and the world of the attendants who made up the great bulk of the staff and who are often fearful of patients and authoritarian in outlook. In such hospitals, the attendants maintained a repressive control over the ward and even over access of patients to physicians.

Sociological research on mental hospitals has dealt with the splitting of supervision of professional and maintenance operations, with the consequences of limited access to advancement for attendants and aides, and with the different ideologies about mental illness and its treat-

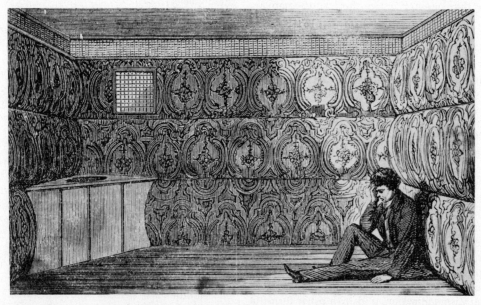

FIGURE 1. Before the twentieth century mental illness was viewed with great horror and embarrassment. Patients were frequently locked away for life in attics and padded rooms with no thought to their rehabilitation (Culver Pictures).

ment prevailing in different segments of the staff.

Mental Patients

The stigma of mental illness seems inevitable in a society that puts heavy emphasis on instrumental achievement and devalues excesses of emotional expression. In such a society, immobilization through neurotic anxiety or psychotic episodes is likely to lead to occupational difficulties and to the disruption of other role relationships. Hospitalization exacerbates the situation by symoblizing role failure (see Figure 1).

Relatively few patients come into treatment with the directness that is found for most physical illness. Before the patient's initial treatment, there is typically a high level of conflict in the family. Treatment comes only when other ways of coping—including consultation with clergymen, physicians, and lay confidants have failed to produce a change in the patient's situation.

Most patients represented at commitment proceedings by counsel are released, whereas most of those equally symptomatic but not represented by counsel are committed. Changed social circumstances are perhaps more important precipitants of hospitalization in the mental disorders of old age than are changes in the symptoms of the disorder.

Release from hospitalization depends at times on the willingness of the family to have the patient back. As the duration of hospitalization decreases and hospital facilities become more attractive, there are evidences that patients' decisions to enter or leave the hospital may rest on considerations other than psychopathology.

In general, instrumental performance and symptoms are highly related, and it is the direct effect of level of symptoms, rather than tolerance of deviance, that appears to account for the retention of patients in the community. For chronic schizophrenic patients, community tenure is enhanced when there is less emotional involvement between the patient and those with whom he lives.

Social Policy

The community mental health movement was given great impetus by the demonstration that long-term stays in large mental hospitals led to incapacity and by the development of drugs that provided alternatives to hospitaliza-

tion. In the early rush of enthusiasm over the availability of Federal support for the development of community mental health services, however, there was far too little consideration of social science knowledge and, in the view of many social scientists, a rather blithe tendency to assume that psychiatry had the answers to everyone's needs. The diversity of problems that lead persons to feel despairing or anxious or unable to control their thoughts and impulses is such that many different psychological and social processes are implicated. Various forms of skill training may be more important than psychotherapy and drug therapy for dealing with the problem of some patients from deprived backgrounds.

REFERENCES

Braginsky, B. M., Braginsky, D. D., and Ring, K. L. *Methods of Madness: The Mental Hospital as a Last Resort.* Holt, Rinehart and Winston, New York, 1969.

Clausen, J. A. Faulty socialization and social disorganization as etiological factors in mental disorder. In *Social Psychiatry.* J. Zubin and F. A. Freyhan, editors, p. 42, Grune & Stratton, New York, 1968.

Elder, G. H. *Children of the Depression.* University of Chicago Press, Chicago, 1974.

Faris, R. E., and Dunham, H. W. *Mental Disorders in Urban Areas.* University of Chicago Press, Chicago, 1939.

Hollingshead, A., and Redlich, R. C. *Social Class and Mental Illness.* John Wiley, New York, 1958.

Langner, T. S., and Michael, S. T. *Life Stress and Mental Health: The Midtown Manhattan Study.* The Free Press (Macmillan), New York, 1963.

Roman, P. R., and Trice, H. M. *Schizophrenia and the Poor.* Cayuga Press, Ithaca, N. Y., 1967.

Srole, L., Langner, T. S., Michael, S. T., Opler, M. K., and Rennie, T. A. C. *Mental Health in the Metropolis: The Midtown Manhattan Study.* McGraw-Hill, New York, 1962.

4.3.   THE FAMILY

Introduction

The family is the universal primary social unit. Every human group has devised traditional prescriptions and proscriptions to make sure that the family fulfills its biological and enculturating tasks. The family is both a link between generations that ensures the stability of the culture and a crucial element in culture change.

Marriage

Purposes of Marriage

A universal biopsychosocial need for completion and fulfillment of oneself through intimate life with another exists among humans and some other species, and two people may undertake marriage solely for their mutual satisfaction, without intent or capacity to establish a family. On the other hand, marriage may be undertaken solely for the purpose of procreation, and in some religions it is so prescribed, even if not always practiced.

Depending on the partners' culture, they unite in marriage because they want to, because it has been arranged for them by their parental families, or because of a combination of these prescriptions. Among the less conscious motivations and unrealistic factors that lead to marriage are many neurotic tendencies and needs. Most common among these is probably the use of marriage to achieve independence from the family of procreation. This brings to the marriage some dependency needs that are likely to result in expecting parental care from the spouse. Another factor is social pressure, especially on girls, from families or peers, who see marriage at a certain age as an essential earmark of success. Not all unconscious or external determinants need be unsound; the choice of a marital partner is a complex process, and a certain intuitive sense of personality fit between two people seems to operate effectively at times, even if neither spouse can account for it explicitly. One of the chief criteria for a successful marriage is that it furthers individual growth and growth as a unit, especially as a parental team (see figure 1).

The personalities and the sociocultural values that two people bring to a marriage determine the nature of their relationship more than do their hopes, dreams, and intentions during courtship. This is particularly so now in industrialized societies, where marriage has shifted during this century from being an economic advantage and even a necessity to being an economic liability. The basis for marriage and/or marital continuity has changed to companionship, encompassing physical, intellectual, affectional, and social facets. Although the partners may share the economic burdens, they rarely can do so side by side, as they would have in working on complementary tasks on the farm. Maintaining a house and household can be reduced to a minimum of labor, leaving as the major shared goal family life itself, together with the care of the offspring. Sharing family responsibilities, however, has been made more difficult by the absence of the husband during working hours, and, if he is ambitious, working hours may approach the entire waking hours of the family on many days.

Marital Coalition

The marital coalition may be defined as those interactional patterns that the spouses evolve to provide at first for their mutual satisfaction.

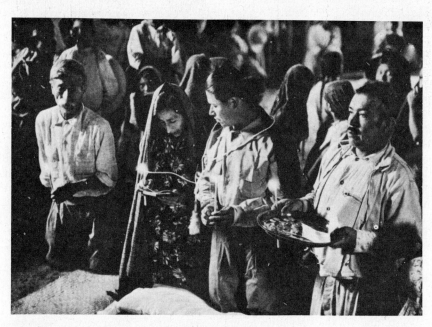

FIGURE 1. A beginning.

Later, this coalition must serve the age-appropriate needs of the children and still maintain an area of exclusive relationship and mutuality between the parents. One of these parental sectors is sexual activity, interdicted to children in our society.

An important function of this coalition is the mutual reinforcement of the spouses' complementary sex-linked roles. As parents, they represent culture-determined masculinity and feminity. Another facet of the coalition is the conjugal role divisions and reciprocities the spouses establish for themselves. These role allocations and the decision-making methods vary with socio-economic class.

Currently, sex-linked roles and role paradigms are changing rapidly in response to two significant forces. One is the women's liberation movement, and the other is the tendency toward small families.

Industrialization and social and geographic mobility have isolated the nuclear family, adding to the critical importance of the marital coalition in the life of the family. Because the marital partners usually become the sole or at least the major sources of identification for their young, the spouses' personalities and the marital coalition are much more critical today for the personality development of the children than in the past. Living isolated from close relatives deprives the spouses of the advantage of sharing parental functions with an extended family group and leaves each child with little alternative but to view his parents and their relationship as exemplary. Problems in the isolated nuclear family, therefore, tend to become circular: marital difficulties affect children adversely, and a difficult or ill child strains the marital coalition.

In a free society, spouses depend on their inner resources because, compared with other cultures, there are relatively few social rules or rituals concerning marriage. In the West, society and religion concern themselves primarily with the beginning of marriage and with death and divorce. Aside from registration of the newborn, society intervenes with a family only if gross undercare or mistreatment of the young is made evident.

Marital Problems

Marriage in the United States now depends primarily on the personalities the spouses bring to it. Their personalities are shaped largely by their parents and by the marital modes to which they have been exposed, modes that often do not serve or suit a younger generation of newlyweds. Because marital and familial maladjustment tends to be encapsulated, the spouses in need of help must seek it actively outside the family.

Although a marriage between two distrubed partners can be satisfactory to them, it does not ensure a good prognosis for a healthy family. Furthermore, a marital coalition adequate for the nurturance of a few children may deteriorate if the family enlarges every year.

Premarital and extramarital sexual intercourse must not be confused with normality or morality. Societies that permit complete freedom of sexual activity after puberty are no less stable or less successful than we are in living up to their cultural norms and preserving their continuity. The same is true of societies that condone extramarital sexual activity, implicitly or explicitly. The changes in premarital sexual activities in our society may be less marked in practice than are the attitudes toward such practice.

Clinically, there is no evidence that premarital sexual relationships either promote or detract from successful marital adjustment. However, one reason for early marriage seems to be the desire for legitimate sexual union, even though emotional and socio-economic independence may not have been achieved by the couple. They may become parents while still dependent on others; also they may not be as mature and certain in their identities as they might be a few years later, when they might seek different partners. In general, the younger the marital partners are at the start, the less good is the prognosis for marital success and stability.

Sexual adjustment in marriage is not static or a single given or symptom but varies with the evolution of a marriage. Partners must learn how to communicate with each other about their sexual experiences, which is also an important preparation for the sex education of children. When sexual dissatisfaction becomes a complaint, it is rarely an isolated problem in the marriage and, if so, is readily remediable by appropriate discussion with both spouses and by specific instruction.

Divorce

Divorce is popularly considered as a barometer of familial and societal stability. But divorce as a social phenomenon is susceptible to customs, to legalistic vogues and changes in the law, and to religious codes.

It is fashionable to point out that the divorce rate in this country has risen 5-fold in this century from 0.7 to 3.7 per 1,000 population and that the number of divorces has risen more than seven times. But these figures must be considered in the light of the changed basis for marriage, the modern risks to marital stability, and the freer attitudes toward the dissolution of marriages so beset by problems and suffering that present-day counseling or therapeutic agencies find them beyond salvage.

From the over-all statistical standpoint, the divorce-risk time has doubled because, with an increased life expectancy in this century of from 47 to 70 years, the duration of marriage (over 90 per cent of which take place before the age of 30) has more than doubled. Also the proportion of the population ever married has increased 20 per cent. The lowering of the average marriage age requires a further correction. Therefore, the corrected rate increase may be only a third of the gross 5-fold rate increment. And since 10 per cent of the population will require temporary psychiatric hospital care and most but not all divorces involve one or two emotionally unstable partners, the present divorce rate is not even commensurate with the estimated prevalence of emotionally disturbed persons.

Family Structure and Dynamics

Here the term "family" refers to the Western nuclear family, the isolated family of industrial society, unless otherwise specified.

From the sociodynamic standpoint, the family is a small group to which most small group dynamics apply, but the parents form the generation that leads and are implicitly obligated to relate sexually to each other. Sexual relations are interdicted to all other members by the archetype of all taboos, the taboo against incest. The offspring follow and learn from the parents as gender-typical models.

As a group, the family moves from the parental dyad to a triad and larger group, and later contracts again. Because the family is divided into two generations, each child's relationship to the parents is, to some degree, exclusive and unique and can be represented by an inverted triangle. The family consists of a series of overlapping triangles, and these triangular relationships are not identical (see figure 2).

One important task of the marital coalition consist in mastering the family's evolutionary transitions or crises. Besides the arrival of children, such critical phases include each child's oedipal phase, school beginnings, puberty, adolescence, and eventual emancipation as he leaves his family of origin physically and emotionally. Adversities such as illnesses or economic or political misfortunes may produce other crises and even temporary or permanent separations.

These evolutionary crises can also be viewed as a succession of separations that all family members must learn to master. Some separations are intangible, as when a child in early adolescence withdraws from closeness to parents. Family life requires the capacity to

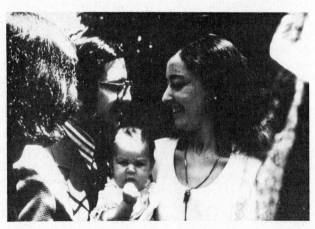

FIGURE 2. Becoming a triad.

forgo individual gratifications for the sake of the group, whose cohesion depends on the example being set by the parents' forgoing some degree of their individuality and certain gratifications for the benefit of the marital condition and of the family.

Role divisions

Compared with the Victorian prototype of the autocratic patriarch, the role of the father in present-day America has weakened, but more in appearance than in substance. Typically, the father's role is still that of the leader; his activities, his productivity, and his education usually determine the position of the family in the community and larger society. He provides the instrumental model of how things are done in society in matters of acquisition and survival. The fact that the father's activities today occur mostly away from home, unshared and unobserved by the family, is a disadvantage.

The mother's primary role concerns the affective life of the family, and she also tends to its biological needs in health and sickness. She identifies affective needs and helps the children to learn about and understand feelings and, therefore, is more responsible for their self-expressive communication. She also guides the child toward self-awareness.

Parental role divisions should be flexible and complementary rather than fixed, because, in crises, role complementarity may be essential, and even temporary role reversal may be necessary. Permanent role reversal of the spouses may be mutually satisfactory to the parents, but it provides offspring with unsuitable models for their future life in society. Parents must provide gender-typical role models that are in some harmony with the larger society in which they live.

Personality Development

Dynamically, the triangular structure of the family is epitomized by the oedipal phase of each child. Its adequate and appropriate resolution depends more on the family structure and

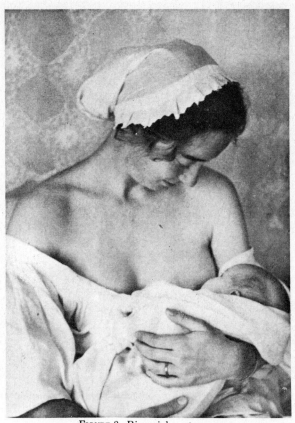

FIGURE 3. Biosocial nurturance.

behavior than on biological determinants. This appears to be true of all phases of psychosocial development, although parental attitudes and behavior are both reactive and interactive with the child, so that a child's equipment at birth, his temperament, and the parents' capacity to cope with infantile needs all coincide to establish the family's interactional patterns. Personality development depends as much on the parents' individual characteristics as on their correlated marital and familial interactive behavior. The child observes and absorbs the defensive modes of those around him.

After a child has learned body awareness and body management, including communicative facility, his relational learning begins. The task for the family is to help each child establish his place in the family and to make him feel so secure in it that he can begin to move beyond the family circle without undue anxiety (see Figure 3). To attain this place of nearly equal emo-

tional distance from both parents, he must not only master body competence but also desexualize his close primary object relations to his parents. Only then can he turn to his peers as an increasingly important source of relationships. This step, in one sense the internalization of the incest taboo, the family must accomplish with him. The parents' personalities, especially the degree of security in sexual identity that they bring to their union, and their coalition are more crucial to this task than in any other phase of family life, most of which can be more explicit and verbally directed.

Further personality development of the child is less directly dependent on family structure and dynamics. But in subtle and not so subtle ways, the oedipal issues are relived in adolescence in terms of dependence-independence issues. To achieve a workable ego integration and identity, the offspring must be able to overcome his negativistic stances, which serve

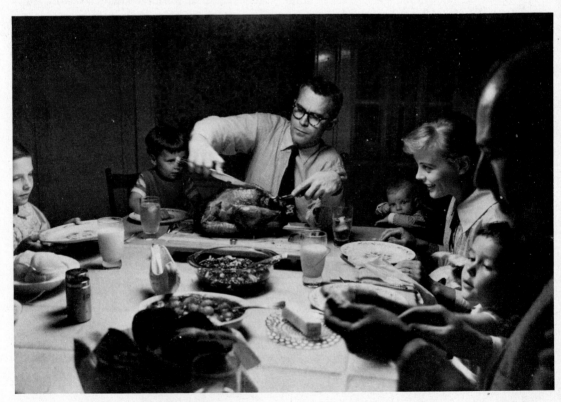

FIGURE 4. Mealtimes serve the important function of maintaining cohesion among family members. A feeling of security and well-being is essential to normal child development. (Courtesy of Elliott Erwitt for Magnum Photos, Inc.)

the separation from his elders but do not serve in themselves the reintegration of an independent and inner-directed personality.

Family Functions

Marital Functions

Marriage must serve the respective needs and satisfactions of the spouses and enable them to effect an appropriate family constellation to fulfill their tasks. Beyond the familial obligations, the marital partners must jointly prepare to renounce their close ties to their children when they are ready to emancipate themselves physically and emotionally from the family.

Nurturant Functions

The nurturant functions of the family encompass more than nursing and food supply, although these are basic at first. Beyond nursing, the helpless infant needs other forms of physical care. Their performance requires the mother's motivation and some degree of security on her part in performing these tasks.

The less specific nurturant activities of the mother continue throughout the life of the family. Eating together as a family at least once a day is not only a caloric ritual but a significant landmark in family life for communication, learning, interacting as a group, and relaxing together (see Figure 4).

Relational Functions

Weaning is part of nurturing but implies more than withdrawing bottle or breast. The intimate physical closeness with the mother must be decreased and an increasingly non-physical intimacy established with all family members. Both the process of weaning and its accomplishment are foundation stones in the acquisition of ego boundaries. In all these functions the mother plays the dominant role, but

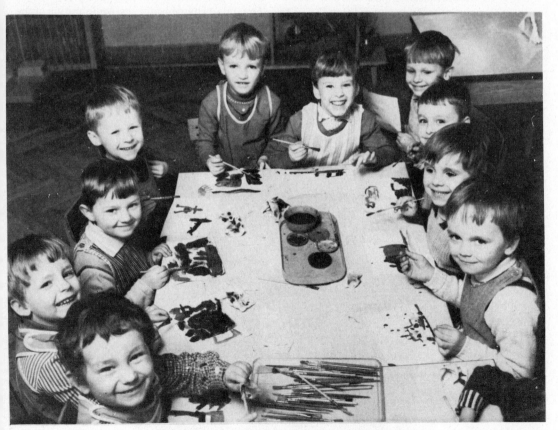

FIGURE 5. The nursery school offers a child an introduction into peer group relationships and is the beginning of the socialization process (UPI photo).

the entire family atmosphere and interaction are also crucial.

After the child has been helped to find his place in the family, permitting him to feel comfortable and safe in intrafamilial relationships, his relational learning turns to peer groups (see Figure 5). Here familial guidance becomes more distant and indirect, but familial facilitation and support of peer relationships are as essential as restraint against undue familial intrusion into peer activiteis. After 6 or 7, the child's relational learning depends increasingly on extrafamilial examples and on the family's social activities with relatives and friends.

Communicative Functions

The central element in the family's educative mission concerns communicative competence. This includes nonverbal and verbal interchange, and there must be culture-typical congruence between the two. Talking with the child about his earliest internal and external experiences is essential to his beginning to talk and to communicate meaningfully. Only through language and the symbols basic to it does body awareness become body knowledge, and only through language can the basic trust of the mother-infant relationship be reinforced and broadened to include other family members and people outside the family. Without language or equivalent symbols, prediction and a grasp of the future are almost impossible.

Familial communication must be related to the communication styles and symbol usages of the family's community. Language reflects the culture's conceptual heritage and determines thought and concept organization across the generations—that is, the cultural system of logic and institutionalized beliefs.

Emancipative Functions

The ultimate goal for each child is to grow up and take his place as a full-fledged member in the society in which his family has placed him. The process of emancipation of each child demands a compensatory re-equilibration of the

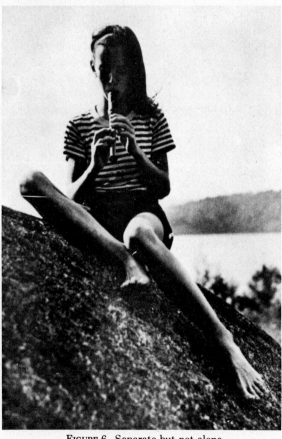

FIGURE 6. Separate but not alone.

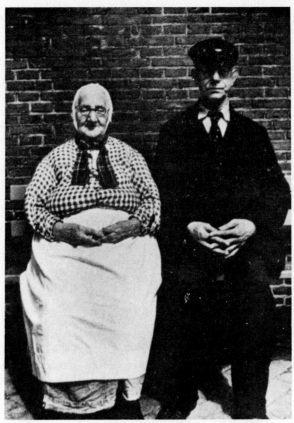

FIGURE 7. Grandparents.

family after each departure until the spouses return to a dyadic existence, free to enjoy parental prerogatives as grandparents without the continuing responsibilities of a nuclear family. Each step toward emancipation poses the recurrent issue of separation, until it is final and definitive, ideally without rupture of emotional ties (see Figure 6). The degree of mastery of the earlier and more limited separations—beginning with weaning and later the beginning of school, separate vacations, and possible hospitalizations of members—indicates and to some extent determines the ease or difficulty experienced by the family when a child leaves for college, to get married, or for military service.

Geographic separation is only a part of the issues to be mastered; more important are the emotional components, the sense of loss experienced by all involved, and the inner capacity of each member and the capacity of the family as a group to do the work of mourning appropriately without becoming pathologically depressed.

The modern family is handicapped with regard to total separation experiences, as the death of a parent or child within the life span of the nuclear family is now rare, whereas it was rather common only 50 years ago. And grandparents often live at a distance, so that the impact of their deaths on the nuclear family does not carry the immediacy and intensity of the permanent loss of a regular participant in family life. The time when the first child leaves may be the first occasion for all family members to mourn together (see Figure 7).

Recuperative Functions

The family must provide for the relaxation of its members—relaxation of manners and behavior and even of defenses essential to interaction in the community. In the family circle, parents shed formal attire, actually and symbolically. If a man's home is his castle, his family is the one group in which he can be king or at least president, but in which he can also exhibit dependency needs. The same is true for the wife, especially if she works outside the home.

To some degree the family also permits its members to engage in creative or other activities that afford relief by contrast from the monotony of many jobs. By setting limits on relaxing activities, the family as a group also demands and teaches impulse control—in games, for instance—and all members may have to defer individual hobbies to family group activities at times.

Family Impoverishment

If familial resources are limited primarily by external social and economic circumstances, such families should be considered impoverished, as opposed to pathological. Both types of families may benefit from family group treatment, but the impoverished family needs many communal supportive and remedial measures, and treatment for tissue abnormalities and defects may be as urgently needed as restoration of family function competence.

One-Parent Families

Widowed parents must cope with the loss of spouses and also with the children's grief and sorrow. If not adequately resolved, the ensuing depression, whether masked or overt, may become pathological for that family member and a pathological focus for the family as a whole. The problem varies depending on the age of the children, the circumstances of the death, and other factors, such as support resources from outside the family, including possible remarriage. The crucial issue, however, is the surviving parent's mode of dealing with the loss and mourning and his or her representation of the decreased parent to the children.

Divorce or desertion presents a different problem, although the sense of loss may be equally intense. The remaining spouse may have great difficulty in representing the absent parent realistically, and opportunities abound for the children to be confused about what each parent is really like.

Parenthood outside marriage is an increasing occurrence and is class-related in that its prevalence is highest in the lowest socio-economic class, although its incidence is increasing in the middle and higher classes. The impoverishment is often not only that of single parenthood but is compounded by the characteristics of family life in the poverty sector of the population.

Poverty

Economically and educationally underendowed parents are handicapped in their enculturating missions. Nurturance in such families is often distorted by a literalness, in that all discomfort in infants and children is sought to be alleviated by feeding. Relational issues are met tangibly and often orally or by verbal or physical punishments, thus interfering with emotional growth, communicative development, and the capacity to postpone need-satisfaction, which is basic to the attainment of long-range goals.

Cultural Deprivations

Further enculturating deficiencies in poor families are the lack of toys and of play space and the common disinterest or inability of adults to interact meaningfully with children beyond infancy. In a one-parent family, that parent often is working, and the child is left to the care of a grandmother or aunt or older sibling, none of whom is as motivated to stimulate and interact with the child as a mother could be if supported by a spouse who shares parental tasks. Racial or other group discrimination may further impair the slim opportunities for developing self-esteem and hope for mastery over one's fate.

Children ill-prepared to begin shcool are not only hampered or discouraged by their own backwardness but are likely to be stamped as poor students from the beginning, which leads to educational neglect in many school systems. The feedback from school to family then further depreciates an already underendowed family, enhancing their pessimism and likely apathy toward education and social betterment.

The salient family dynamics are those of predominantly reactive interaction and defective development of thought and language because of disbelief and even mistrust in the utility of abstract and symbolic mentation and communication. Moreover, there is impaired capacity for pleasures that are not immediate; generally, such family members know and exploit how to make one another feel bad, but not how to make each other feel good except by granting immediate satisfaction, regardless of long-range consequences (see Figure 8).

Family Pathology

Psychiatric Disturbances

If a psychiatric condition requires institutionalization, the family deserves therapeutic attention because it may be involved in the genesis of the illness. If this is so, the patient should not return to his family unless the other members are helped to change. Also, the hospitalization of a family member is a crisis that affects all members and that demands therapeutic consideration.

Mental subnormality tends to run in families apart from genetic factors. Below certain intelligence levels, parental functioning, especially the communicative performance, does not suffice to accomplish the enculturation of offspring. Educational inadequacies and inferior social position in a given subculture can also result in ineffectual family structure and dynamics, especially if the family belongs to a group against which the surrounding community discriminates actively.

Parental overinvestment in the achievement of children, especially parents' social prestige aspirations, is commonly found in the backgrounds of depressive and manic-depressive patients. Such parental attitudes are introjected and predispose the child to intense ambivalence and a sense of being loved and worthy only on the basis of superior performance and achievement. Resentment and punitive attitudes toward the self supervene when failure in terms of internalized overstringent expectations occurs.

Asocial behavior is often associated with family pathology; children have been found to carry out covert or overt needs or wishes of parents. Emphasis on proper appearance and denial of any problem in the face of evident malfeasance by a family member is often encountered in the families of psychopaths.

Addictive behavior, especially alchoholism, is also related to certain family problems. In general, parental examples of unrestrained indulgence in smoking or drinking or drug intake to alleviate habitually acute or chronic discomfort and stress are likely to be followed by offspring, although not necessarily in the identical form of overindulgence.

Families with schizophrenic offspring evidence faulty structure and functioning in almost every parameter of essential family tasks.

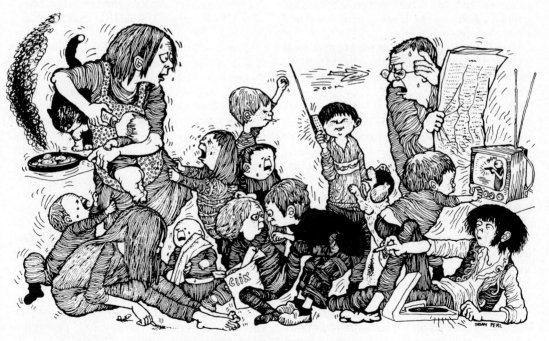

FIGURE 8. A family beyond its resources.

In some cases the parental model paradigms are so irreconcilable that the offspring must fail in integrating an identity.

Defects in Organization and Dynamics

A disturbed or immature parent may or may not satisfy the spouse but is apt to blur the generation boundaries, besides being a poor model for the same-sexed child. Parental communication inadequacies pervade the family and handicap children or encourage them to continue a life in fantasy, uncorrected by reality presentation from the older generation.

Severe immaturity may lead one spouse to seek a dependent position in the family akin to that of an offspring. Such a spouse expects parental care from the partner or even from a child. Almost any form of neurosis or psychosis in one parent is apt to produce defective parental coalitions, which handicap the nurturant and enculturating tasks on which the children depend.

Inability or failure of a parent to serve adequately as a gender model appropriate to the larger society leads to increased developmental vicissitudes for a child of the same sex. The insecure gender identity of a parent predisposes the same-sex child to gender uncertainty and confusion and to social ineptness, important elements in the development of perversions and schizophrenia.

Parents with severe hysterical or obsessional or other neurotic characteristics are apt to produce offspring with like defensive structures if not symptoms.

The surreptitious need for an extended family system occurs overtly or covertly when one parent or both remain primarily attached to and dependent on their parents or a parental substitute. The center of gravity for authority, decision-making, and emotional investment rests outside the nuclear family group. This distorts family structure and functions.

Family boundaries can be impaired in the form of undue rigidity or excessive porosity or undue elasticity. A departing member may be engulfed by an extension of the family, which allows no one to leave it. Overly rigid boundaries are established by some pathological families, leading to isolation from and fear of the larger community. Porous and inadequate boundaries are found in ghetto and broken families. Often

such defective external boundaries coincide with or reflect chaotic internal organizations of the family.

Broken families are the grossest but not necessarily the psychiatrically most devastating form of family pathology. Broken families are disproportionately frequent in the backgrounds of sociopaths, unmarried mothers, and schizophrenics, regardless of whether the fracture is through death, desertion, or divorce.

Probably more pathogenic than actual parental separation is family schism. Here, the family is divided overtly or covertly into warring camps, usually because of chronic conflict and strife between the parents. The children are forced to take sides, to the detriment of their personality development and integration. This type of family pathology is found in the background of schizophrenic patients.

In a skewed marital relationship one spouse expects the other to be a parent to him or her, or one disturbed parent dominates the other and family life absolutely and rigidly. Such a marital coalition often pre-empts parental functions and emotional resources, and the children's affective and psychological needs, are neglected. However, a family may be skewed when a dyad other than the parental one dominates the group emotionally and often tangibly. Most often this is a symbiotic mother-child relationship.

In both schismatic and skewed families violations of the generation boundary abound, and in both, the intense relationship between one parent and one child may have seductive and incestuous components.

Overt incest is evidence of gross parental psychopathology and of defective family structure. Father-daughter incest is commonest, but both parents are psychologically involved, since incest often bespeaks a tenuous equilibrium in a family that seeks to avoid overt disintegration. The involved daughter has assumed many parental functions, and the parents maintain a facade of role competence. The family often breaks up after incest is brought out into the open, usually by the involved child.

Deficits in Family Tasks

Nurturant deficiency occurs because of parental neglect and disinterest. The worst manifestation is the battered-child syndrome, although such victims are not necessarily malnourished. More discrete nurturant disturbances occur because of maternal illness or anxiety and empathy failure. Such mothers tend to overfeed the baby or try to do so, thus coupling pain and discomfort with oral input. It is likely that the marital coalition is also deficient in such families.

Failure in separation mastery may begin with a mother's inability to wean a child effectively. The offspring is prone to develop one of the classical neuroses. If coupled with other family function deficits, the defective separation competence may be important in the development of schizophrenia and is a handicap at all stages of personality development.

Aberrant communication is a common finding in families with psychiatric problems. Young children learn the defective communication modes, which distort their linguistic development, perception, and concept formation. If communication is confusing within the family and ineffectual as expressive or instrumental tools, children are deprived of a critical socializing instrument outside the family.

Severely amorphous or fragmented modes of communicating have been found in families of schizophrenic patients and may be pathognomonic for schizophrenia. Parental examples of paralogical thinking and of fear and mistrust of their social environment affect offspring by creating confusion and anxiety, and children may internalize the faulty ideation and mistrust of the world and externalize their problems by habitual projection.

Scapegoating is discernible only if the family as a unit is considered and studied. The scapegoat—regardless of whether he is schizophrenic, psychopathic, an underachiever, or neurotic—serves to bind family anxiety and to mask family deficiences. The scapegoat diverts parents from their own conflicts or provides an alibi for deficient parenting of all offspring in terms of warmth and nurturant care. The scapegoated child suffers because his needs are neglected and he is made to feel that it is all his fault. His siblings suffer insufficient care and attention and either learn a distorted view of the scapegoat or must covertly oppose the parents' view, leading to conflict and a sense of guilt. In addition, the scapegoat may cause the family tangible harm and suffering.

Clinical Evaluation

Symptoms aside, the clinician seeks information about the basic elements of family structure, notably the maintenance of the generation boundary and the gender-linked role divisions and complementarities, and about the manner in which the family copes with its major tasks and functions. He pays special attention to their communication modes.

Ideally, the individual histories and statements of all family members are combined and examined for confluent and contradictory data. These individual records are complemented by participant observation of the family as a group.

The referential framework begins with an examination of the marital relationships, the pertinent data concerning the spouses' respective backgrounds, their personal developments, educational levels, socio-economic class positions, and the cultural and ideological value patterns of their respective families of origin. Significant discrepancies in these parameters should alert the examiner to potential conflict areas.

Data about family structure can be obtained through inquiries about living and sleeping arrangements, activities of the family as a group and as part-groups, role divisions incident to various family tasks and crises, and the decision-making processes. As far as possible, these items should also be examined directly through group observations, as should the possible existence and nature of dominant dyads other than that of the parents. In observing the family as a group, the diagnostician gains impressions about the effectiveness of the parental coalition and the integrity of generational division. Gender appropriateness in manners and conversational content can be established impressionistically in family interviews.

The normal crises of family evolution are important sources for understanding the family's coping patterns, coping reserves, and coping deficiencies. Among such crises are possible resistance or reservations of the spouses' families to the marriage, the first pregnancy, the original triad formation, subsequent pregnancies and births, evolutionary separations, economic misfortunes, and deaths of relatives or friends.

The nature of the family's social network

should be examined to establish social isolation or the nature of family relatedness within the community. The network must fit to some degree the class position and the patterns of the community and subculture of which the family is a part. The involvement with the spouses' families of origin and collaterals must also fit to some degree their cultural pattern, or conflict should be presumed and the resolution of it examined.

Related to the issue of the family's social interactions is the issue of how family boundaries are managed. Properly permeable boundaries permit age-appropriate exit from and entry into the family circle without undue conflict.

Evaluation of the children depends on their respective ages. Pediatric histories including well-child care data, may be the only source of information available from outside the family. For older children, kindergarten and school adjustments, records from recreational agencies, and information from neighbors and friends as to the socialization of a child can be utilized.

REFERENCES

Ackerman, N. W. *The Psychodynamics of Family Life.* Basic Books, New York, 1958.

Anthony, E. O., and Benedek, T., editors. *Parenthood: Its Psychology and Psychopathology.* Little, Brown, Boston, 1970.

Howells, J. G. *Theory and Practice of Family Psychiatry.* Brunner-Mazel, New York, 1971.

Lidz, T. *The Person.* Basic Books, New York, 1968.

Parsons, T. *Social Structure and Personality.* The Free Press (Macmillan), New York, 1964.

Rainwater, L., *Family Design.* Aldine Publishing Company, Chicago, 1965.

5

Science of Human Behavior: Quantitative Experimental and Research Methods

5.1.   EPIDEMIOLOGY

Introduction

Epidemiology relates the distribution, incidence, and duration of disorders to the physical, biological, and social environment in which people live. It is the basic science of preventive medicine and, therefore, of preventive psychiatry.

The proportion of a population that has a condition at one moment in time is called the prevalence rate. The proportion of a population that begins an episode of a disorder during a year's time (new cases) is called the annual incidence rate. In a stable situation the prevalence rate is approximately equal to the annual incidence rate times the average duration, measured in years, of the condition. The risk of acquiring a condition at some indefinite time in the future represents the accumulation of age-specific annual incidence rates over a period of time.

Historical Trends

Epidemiologists need to know whether an illness is on the wane or is a growing health problem. A growing problem gets more attention than a waning problem in planning preventive measures, services, clinical specialist training, and research funding.

Disappearing Conditions

The consensus of psychiatrists surveyed in the 1960's was that general paresis, pellagra psychosis, and conversion hysteria were on the wane.

New cases with a diagnosis of general paresis coming to hospital care each year can be taken as an index of the number of new cases arising in the population. First admissions with general paresis to New York State hospitals between 1911 and 1951 dropped from 8.2 to 2.1 cases per 100,000 population. This decline may be attributed to technical advances—the treatment of syphilis with arsphenamine and later with penicillin and other drugs. It was not due to a decline in the annual incidence of syphilis, which had been rising.

Some declines are due neither to medical advances nor to public health efforts. Pellagra and its associated psychoses declined in frequency after the 1920's presumably because of changes in eating habits, nutritional value of foods, and, after 1939, the rising standard of living.

The conclusion that conversion hysteria has become less common is based entirely on the consensus of expert opinion and the drop in journal articles on the condition. The decline may be due to decreasing public credulity toward pseudolosses of function.

The absence of statistical data in this last example carries several lessons. First, it is possible to draw epidemiological inferences in the absence of statistical data. Second, historical trends are particularly hard to measure. Incidence, prevalence, severity, duration, and outcome of an illness are difficult enough to evaluate now. One must compare these measures with old data, often gathered for another purpose and filled with unknown errors and bias. Changes in labels or categories may have occurred, necessitating a translation. The presenting symptoms of clinical entities vary over time. One must beware of the effects of fashions in medical diagnosis and treatment. The general population may have changed not only in size and socio-economic level but also in attitudes toward deviant behavior. The availability of treatment centers and diagnostic, preventive, and therapeutic technology have also changed.

Conditions on the Increase

Paradoxically, medical advances can lead to a rise in the frequency of disorders. Since the widespread use of antibiotics, the life expectancy of mongoloid (Down's syndrome) newborns has been extended dramatically. Hence, the number of living mongoloid persons is rising. The prevalence rate of mongolism has risen, although the annual incidence rate may not have changed.

The same thing has presumably also happened with senile brain disease and arteriosclerotic psychoses. Most of these disorders were in the past terminated by lobar pneumonia, which has been treated successfully since the discovery of sulfanilamid in 1936 (see Figure 1).

Advances in industrial chemistry and psychopharmacology have created new conditions, such as the toxic psychoses due to pesticide sprays, cortisone, and amphetamines. Psyche-

delics contribute their share of drug-induced psychoses, and heroin, methadone, barbiturates, and some minor tranquilizers have created new subvarieties of drug addition.

Community Diagnosis

Community diagnosis seeks to ascertain the nature and relative size of a health problem. The simplest way to get a comprehensive picture of the cases of mental disorder in a community is to summarize all the cases in treatment by public agencies and private practitioners (see Figure 2). However, the cases in clinical care represent something like the tip of an iceberg; below the clinical horizon are several times as many cases.

To determine whether psychoses treated and untreated, occur at higher rates among the least affluent part of a community, epidemiologists need a technique that distinguishes the neuroses from the psychoses in household surveys. Communities examined directly by psychiatrists are relatively small, homogeneous communities, where the clinician could obtain rapport with the population. In these communities, socioeconomic status does not vary as widely as it does in large metropolitan centers, so the surveys provide little information on rates by socioeconomic status. Studies in large cities with great contrasts in socioeconomic status

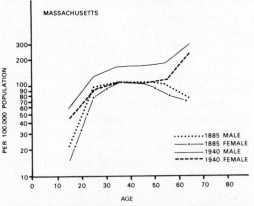

FIGURE 1. First mental hospital admission rates. Logarithmic curve reproduced from Gruenberg, E. M. Epidemiology of mental disorders and aging. (From Goldhamer and Marshall's data.) in *The Neurological and Psychiatric Aspects of Disorders of Aging.* Williams & Wilkins, Baltimore, 1956.

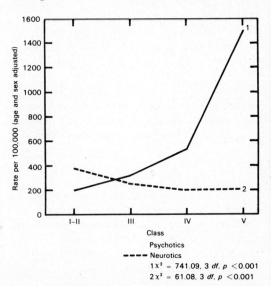

FIGURE 2. Prevalence of neurotic and psychotic disorders per 100,000, adjusted for age and sex by class. (Reproduced from Hollingshead, A. B., and Redlich, F. C. *Social Class and Mental Illness.* Wiley, N. Y., 1958.)

tend to use indirect methods, which make diagnostic distinctions uncertain.

Serious mental disorders rise in prevalence with age. Mental disorders as a whole are found more commonly in women, but organic syndromes are commoner in men. Unmarried people are at higher risk of many mental disorders. Poverty is associated with a higher proportion of people in treatment and with a higher prevalence of organic syndromes and major psychoses. These are loose generalizations not applicable to certain specific conditions. For example, suicide in the age group 20 to 64 is commoner among the most affluent than among the poor (see Table I).

Community morbidity surveys for mental disorders have produced only broad outlines for a community diagnosis. They have tried to do too much when seeking to identify every type of mental disorder and have tended to do too little in stating testable hypotheses.

Health Services

The selection of patients who come to treatment is influenced by factors other than the presence and nature of mental disorders. The admission rate to a mental hospital is high if the population it serves lives close by and low if the population lives far away. Administrative criteria for admission also influence admission rates. Within a city, admission rates may be a function of housing conditions. Single-family home areas have low rates in all economic groups, and multiple-family dwelling areas have high rates, regardless of economic level. However, the poorest people tend to have higher first-admission rates to treatment. General hospital psychiatric units tend to concentrate on white and relatively well-to-do patients; state and county hospitals do the opposite. The nonwhite and the poor tend to be assigned the more serious diagnoses.

There has been a long-term trend toward rising admission rates for the elderly. This trend began to change in the mid-1960's; since then, the numbers of over-65 patients admitted to and resident in mental hospitals have been declining (see Figure 3). Presumably, this trend was due to the rapid expansion of nursing homes.

Social Policy and Health Services

Since the 1950's national governments and many states have adopted a policy of reducing mental hospital censuses in the middle years of life. The drop in census of younger patients (ages 16 to 65) was achieved by rapidly lossening criteria for admission and release simultaneously in such a way that the drop in average length of stay outstripped the rapid rise in admission rates.

Registers

Psychiatric registers, which record all persons receiving psychiatric treatment in a community, can be useful tools in studying admission patterns, ratios for different population segments, changes over time, and diagnostic distributions. They can also be used as a case-finding source for other studies (see Figure 4). One of the drawbacks of registers is that, in providing a complete list of mentally ill people, they are a source of confidential information of potential harm to patients. The registers are also costly in relation to their research products.

Individual Risks

Calculating a person's risk of contracting a specific disease in his lifetime is a useful epidemiological tool. For example, the likelihood of a child's being a mongoloid rises with his mother's age. The risk in the 40-and-over age group is one in 50, compared with one in 1,000 in the youngest maternal age groups. Identifying a population at risk is helpful in terms of organizing screening services, counseling services, and primary prevention.

Hagnell calculated that 5.5 per cent of men and 13.7 per cent of women would have a mental disorder lasting more than 3 years by the time they were 60. Psychoses account for only a small proportion of the risk, but men do have a higher risk of becoming psychotic and of organic syndromes, even though women have a higher over-all risk of mental morbidity. The risk of admittance to a mental hospital for the first time was estimated at 4.1 per cent for men and 5.5 per cent for women up to age 60.

Currently, about half of the under-65 admissions to public facilities are readmissions. The rate of readmission within a year varies with age, length of hospitalization, and diagnosis. Chances of readmission increase dramatically with the number of previous admissions.

The individual risk of developing a mental illness or of being hospitalized for the first time increases along with life expectancy.

TABLE I
Mental Disorder Prevalence Rates per 1,000

Author	Site and Date	Total Mental Disorders	Psychoses	Schizophrenia	Affective Psychoses	Neuroses	Personality Disorders	Mental Retardation	Impaired	Comments
Treated Cases Only										
Kramer et al.	U.S., 1959–61	2.97	1.79 (functional)	1.51	0.23	0.04	0.06	0.26		Annual average resident patient rate (age adjusted) in public hospitals
Hollingshead, Redlich	New Haven, 1950	8.3*	6.3*			2.0*				Inpatient and outpatient care. Crude rate.
Rennie, Srole	Midtown Manhattan Treatment Census, 1953–54	12.90								5.02 for inpatients and 7.88 for outpatients.
Unpublished Treated Cases plus Identified through Nonmedical Records or Key Informants										
	Dutchess County, 1972	4.98		0.73	0.13	1.00	1.00	0.40		Point prevalence, outpatients only.
Cohen, Fairbank	Eastern Health District, 1933	44.5	8.18 (age over 15)			2.0				After Plunkett and Gordon table.
Lemkau et al.	Eastern Health District, 1936	60.5	6.6			3.10	4.61*			Age-adjusted rates. Population age over 10.
Same plus Intensive Survey of Subsample Population										
Rosanoff	Nassau County, 1916	13.74	2.39* (functional)					5.46		Intensively surveyed area's total mental disorder rate: 36.4.
Roth, Luton	Tennessee, 1938	69.4	6.32*	1.73*	1.65*	4.0*	37.8*	8.20*		Intensively surveyed area's total mental disorder rate: 123.7.
Lin	Formosa, 1946–48	10.8	3.8	2.1	0.7	1.2	0.5	3.4		Persons with more than one symptom pattern were counted for each, and diagnoses' specific rates exceed total rate.
Leighton	Bristol, 1952	690	10			570	290	110	420	
Surveys of Total Populations										
Bremer	Norway fishing village, 1939–1944	232.4	35.9			58.0	93.5	55.6	193.6 (chronic)	
Essen-Möller	Lundby, Sweden, 1947	Evident and probable 179.0 Conceivably ill	19.5*	7	10.2*	58.8*	Major 64* Minor 210*	9.8		Lifetime prevalence rates calculated on total population.
Hagnell	Lundby, Sweden, 1957	180	17			131		12		Lifetime prevalence rates.
Eaton, Weil	Hutterites, 1950	46.5*	12.4*	2.1	9.3	16*		12*		Base population 15 and over. Lifetime prevalence.
Surveys of Probability Sample Populations										
Leighton	Stirling County, 1948–50	570							240	Population over 18.
Rennie, Srole	Midtown Manhattan, 1953–54	815							234	Interviewed population's age: 20–59.

* Gruenberg and Turns calculation.

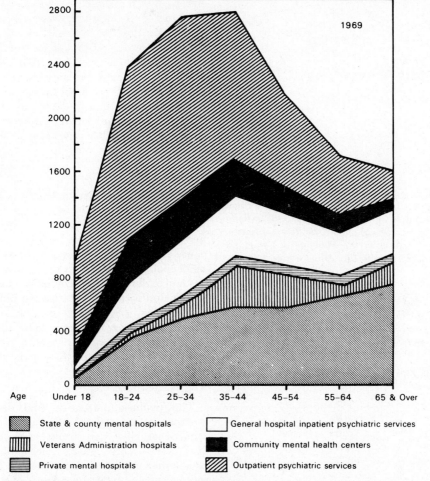

1969

Age	Under 18	18–24	25–34	35–44	45–54	55–64	65 & Over

State & county mental hospitals

Veterans Administration hospitals

Private mental hospitals

General hospital inpatient psychiatric services

Community mental health centers

Outpatient psychiatric services

FIGURE 3. Number of patient care episodes per 100,000 population in psychiatric facilities by type of facility, by age, United States 1969. (Reproduced from Kramer, M., et al., *The Role of a National Statistics Program in the Planning of Community Psychiatric Services in the United States.* 1972.)

The Clinical Picture and Syndrome Identification

The clinical picture of a condition may be significantly altered when the perspective is broadened by searching out cases not in active treatment. Patients may be followed after they have stopped treatment, or cases that have not come to clinical attention may be located (see Table II).

The word "schizophrenia" implies for many clinicians an ineluctable dismal outcome. Yet M. Blueler, who followed for 22 years 208 schizophrenics admitted to his clinic in 1920, showed that the most catastrophic outcomes of schizophrenia became rarer than in a previous cohort (see Figure 5).

Without systematic data gathering, clinicians sometimes think of manic-depressive illness as relatively benign. Yet some 9 per cent of a cohort followed by Lundquist developed a chronic course. And in the early 1930's, Derby found a death rate of 22 per cent in hospitalized acute manic cases. Lundquist found the risk for multiple attacks to be higher for manics, particularly those who had an onset before age 20.

Institutional neurosis develops after years of institutional life have robbed the patient of dignity and initiative. It is characterized by indifference, apathy, passive compliance, self-neglect, and occasionally aggressive behavior.

The social breakdown syndrome includes a variety of decompensations in personal and

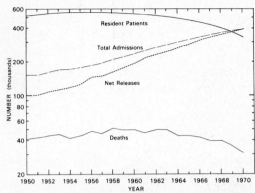

FIGURE 4. Number of resident patients, total admissions, net releases, and deaths, state and county mental hospitals United States, 1950 to 1970. (Reproduced from Kramer, M., et al. *The Role of a National Statistics Program in the Planning of Community Psychiatric Services in the United States.* 1972.)

TABLE II

Re-entry Rates (Percentage of Releases* Returned within 6 Months) by Length of Hospital Stay before Release, New York State Hospitals and Children's Hospitals, Year Ended March 31, 1971.

Length of Stay before Release	Number	Per cent	Re-entry Rate, within 6 Mos.
Total	42,308	100.0	27.7
Less than 3 Mos	27,925	66.0	27.9
3 to 5 Mos	5,522	13.1	27.6
6 to 11 Mos	3,257	7.7	29.1
1 to 2 Yrs	1,805	4.3	29.8
2 to 5 Yrs	1.476	3.5	26.2
5 Yrs. and over	2,323	5.5	21.9

* Direct discharges plus placements on convalescent care.

Reproduced from Weinstein, A. S., DiPasquale, D., and Winsor, F., Relationships between length of stay in and out of the New York mental hospitals. Am. J. Psychiatr., *130:* 904, 1973.)

social functioning. Most episodes of social breakdown syndrome are short-lived, start in the community, and end shortly after a hospital admission. But some cases last for years, representing extreme social disability and wasted lives. This kind of picture is characteristic of chronically deteriorated psychotic patients.

Psychiatric patients have more physical disorders than do most people. Babigian and Odoroff found the relative risk of death in the mentally ill to be 2½ to 3 times that of the gen-

eral population. When the chronically ill, the aged, and the alcoholics, who are high-risk groups, are removed, the relative risk remains 1½ to 2 times that of the general population.

Some features of the deteriorated functioning previously thought to be an ineluctable consequence of psychosis have been shown to be largely preventable sociogenic complications. On the other hand, mental disorders may be only one facet in the spectrum of ill health suffered by some patients.

Causes

Clinical observations, laboratory research, and epidemiology feed one another with new knowledge, new investigative techniques, and new insights into disease pathogenesis. Sometimes the breakthrough comes through purely epidemiological data. This was true with pellagra and fetal rubella's causation of fetal anomalies, including mental retardation. More often, epidemiology comes in when clinical observations or laboratory findings need field testing to implement programs designed to reduce the impact of a condition on the population.

Preventive trials

The planned preventive trial determines whether a planned modification of circumstances actually lowers the incidence of disease. It provides more definite information about causes than any other kind of method. It generally comes as the last in a series of investigations that have clarified a causal hypothesis, but preventive trials can also come very early in the course of investigations.

Another form of preventive trial occurs when a major reform is introduced with the intent of preventing a specific form of disorder. It cannot be designed to include a control group because the reform involves the reorganization of all the mental health services of a community.

Stress

Stress is an ill-defined concept used in different ways by researchers of various scientific backgrounds who do not always explain their specific meaning. This lack of definition produces methodological difficulties.

In recent years, attention has been focused on life events. Whether they are good or bad, life events demand adaptive changes. Persons with many significant life events are more likely to become ill than are those who experience few and minor events.

Early Physical Environment

Knobloch and Pasamanick demonstrated the relationship between prenatal factors and mental retardation and between organic and functional disorders in children. They also correlated season of birth and incidence of mental deficiency. Significantly more children born in the winter months were admitted to the Columbus State School in Ohio. This finding was particularly true for those children born in years when the average temperature in the third month after their conception had been the highest of the summer. This finding suggests that pregnant women may then have decreased their protein intakes to levels low enough to impair the developing brains of their unborn children. Malnourished populations have been

shown to have handicaps of central nervous system development.

Sociopsychological Hypotheses

Faris and Dunham found a concentric distribution of schizophrenia rates, with the highest rates at the center of Chicago and the lowest at the periphery of the city. Manic-depressive psychoses had a random pattern throughout the city, and there was a tendency for such cases to come from a higher socio-economic level than did schizophrenics. Organic psychoses, alcoholic psychoses, and drug addiction had different patterns. The authors advanced the hypothesis that social isolation produced the abnormal traits of behavior and mentality characteristic of schizophrenia.

The drift hypothesis, which holds that impaired persons slide down the social scale because of their illness, was not supported by their data. Young patients who had little time to drift

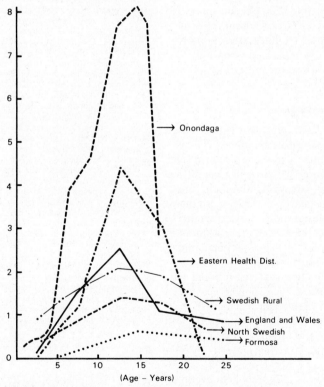

FIGURE 5. Long courses of the schizophrenias according to catamneses of 316 schizophrenics completed in 1941. (Reproduced from Bleuler, M. A 23-year longitudinal study of 208 schizophrenics and impressions in regard to the nature of schizophrenia, in *The Transmission of Schizophrenia*, D. Rosenthal and S. S. Kety, Editors, pp. 3–12. Pergamon Press, N. Y., 1968.)

were concentrated in the same manner as older patients. More recently, Wender et al. in their study of the socio-economic status of schizophrenic adoptees and their biological and adoptive parents found that only part of their data supported the drift hypothesis.

The hypothesis of differential tolerance explains higher schizophrenic admission rates in some communities on the basis of familial and cultural attitudes. The segregation hypothesis holds that, instead of helplessly drifting downward, the schizophrenic actively seeks city areas where anonymity and isolation protect him against the demands that more organized societies make. Another sociogenic hypothesis is that belonging to a lower social class with the problems that it entails fails to inhibit and possibly triggers or exacerbates existing psychopathology.

In 1897 Durkheim related increasing industrialization and urbanization to a rise in secularism and individualism and a decreased sense of community affiliation. He coined the term "anomie" to describe this phenomenon. He believed that suicide rates were an index of a population's anomie. He and later Halbwachs showed that suicide rates across nations and over time increased with Protestantism and secularization.

Familial Aggregations

Clinicians have been impressed with the high frequency of mental disorders among the relatives of their patients. It was long assumed that, when family histories of particular conditions were being studied, one was studying the transmission of genetic material through the germ plasm. The earliest morbidity surveys tended to show the existence of a very definite familial aggregation of cases of schizophrenia and of manic-depressive psychosis.

When it became clear that the familial patterns of schizophrenia could not be accounted for by any simple Mendelian mechanism, psychogenetic theories became more popular and persuasive. By the end of World War II, a spate of articles of familial rearing patterns in relationship to the later development of schizophrenic syndromes in children had begun to appear. These investigators tended to ignore the fact that parents and children come from the same genetic pool and have more in common than their emotional relationships to one another.

Böök postulated that familial clusters of schizophrenia could be accounted for by a recessive gene with very low penetrance. A low penetrance implies that environmental factors play important roles in determining which persons carrying the gene become affected. The data produced by Kety and his associates on adopted children of schizophrenics supported the genetic hypothesis.

It is known that genetic factors play a crucial role in the etiological complex responsible for schizophrenia and manic-depressive illness. It is also known that somatic insults—such as stress, prematurity, and malnutrition—and such unfavorable environmental circumstances as poverty and emotional deprivation are associated with psychopathology.

REFERENCES

Faris, R. E. L., and Dunham, H. W. *Mental Disorders in Urban Areas: An Ecological Study of Schizophrenia and Other Psychoses.* University of Chicago Press, Chicago, 1939.

Hagnell, O. *A Prospective Study of the Incidence of Mental Disorder.* Svenska Bokförlaget, Norstedts, Lund, 1966.

Hollingshead, A. B., and Redlich, F. C. *Social Class and Mental Illness: A Community Study.* John Wiley, New York, 1958.

Kramer, M., Rosen, B. M., and Willis, E. M. Definitions and distribution of mental disorders in a racist society. In *Racism and Mental Health*, C. V. Willie, B. M. Kramer, and B. S. Brown, editors. University of Pittsburgh Press, Pittsburgh, 1973.

Leighton, D. C., Harding, J. S., Macklin, D., Macmillan, A. M., and Leighton, A. H. *The Character of Danger, Vol. III, The Sterling County Study of Psychiatric Disorder and Socio-cultural Environment.* Basic Books, New York, 1963.

Morris, J. N. *Uses of Epidemiology*, ed. 2. E. & S. Livingston, London, 1970.

Schimel, J. L., Salzman, L., Chodoff, P., Grinker, R. R., and Will, O. A. Changing styles in psychiatric syndromes: A symposium. Am. J. Psychiatry, *130:* 146, 1973.

Srole, L., Langner, T. S., Michael, S. T., Opler, M. K., and Rennie, T. A. C. *Mental Health in the Metropolis, Vol. I, The Midtown Manhattan Study.* McGraw-Hill, New York, 1962.

Stein, Z., Susser, M., and Guterman, A. V. Screening programme for prevention of Down's syndrome. Lancet, *1:* 305, 1973.

Weinstein, A. S., DiPasquale, D., and Winsor, F. Relationships between length of stay in and out of New York State mental hospitals. Am. J. Psychiatr., *130:* 904, 1973.

Wender, P. H., Rosenthal, D., Kety, S. S., Schulsinger, F., and Welner, J. Social class and psychopathology in adoptees. Arch. Gen. Psychiatry, *28:* 318, 1973.

5.2.   COMPUTERS

Introduction

Some of the most extensive and sophisticated attempts at computerizing patient records have been undertaken by psychiatric hospitals. The multivariate nature of psychiatric illness, with its lack of specific causative agents and wide range of treatment techniques, provides ample motivation for improved methods for dealing with the enormous mass of information represented by the record of even a single patient.

Computer Compared with Clinician

Information is stored and used in computers as bits (a contraction of "binary digit"). A bit is defined as the standard unit of information, and it corresponds to a single binary alternative, such as on-off, zero-one, or true-false. The rapid-access memory of the average medium-size computer available today is approximately 1.3×10^5 bits. Now available are large random-access, mass memory systems that provide storage capacity as high as 10^{12} bits, with a retrieval time of less than 50 milli-seconds. By contrast, the human brain has been estimated to possess a rapid, random-access memory capacity of approximately 10^{20} bits (see Table I).

The computer has a small number of exceedingly reliable and fast circuits and is designed to perform many simple tasks—one or perhaps a few at a time. The computer is immensely faster than the human brain. By contrast, the brain has a huge number of relatively slow circuits, operating in parallel, and is, therefore, better equipped to cope with large amounts of information presented for simultaneous processing. The human brain is superior in pattern recognition.

The brain, more or less on its own, can organize the information it receives into an elaborate multidimensional model of the outer world, using this model to arrive at intelligent decisions. The fact that computing systems lack such a global model for the environments to which they are interfaced has imposed a ceiling on their intellectual abilities.

The clinician does poorly with serial presentation. The computer does poorly with the recognition of complex patterns, which implies parallel presentation of data.. Attempts to program computers to interpret patterns such as X-rays, electrocardiograms, and chromosomal patterns are at various stages of development.

In recent years, two important developments have made it especially practicable to use the computer to assist the physician with a variety of medical decisions. One is the advent of programing languages that can manipulate strings of text according to the rules of syntax, just as the more widely used computer languages manipulate numbers according to the rules of arithmetic. The other is the development of interactive or conversational computer programs that communicate with the user not through a batch of punched cards but through a suitable terminal, such as a teletypewriter/video-tube display that exchanges messages with the computer over ordinary telephone lines. Light pens can be used at video terminals to entirely eliminate the need for typing skills.

Diagnostic Applications

Clinical applications of computers in psychiatry are being reported with increasing frequency. Most such applications can be classified into one of five general areas: (1) data collection about the patient, including numerous rating scales, automated history, and mental status procedures, (2) attempts to identify objectively symptom clusters that may be designated as syndromes or diagnoses, (3) formal assignment of diagnosis, treatment form, and prognosis by computer, (4) computer evaluation of patient progress and treatment outcome, (5) treatment per se.

Within the traditional medical model, each of the first four areas may be viewed as a part of a diagnostic process undergoing continuous refinement. Adequately programed, computers can perform the diagnostic process as well as or better than skilled clinicians.

Before the computer can be employed to significant advantage in diagnosis, precise procedures must be formulated to deduce the clinical state of the patient from observed signs and symptoms. One can try to use the processes the physician employs in a sufficiently precise manner to allow for their simulation by a

TABLE I
Comparison of a Medium-Size Computer with the Human Brain

	PDP-15 Computer	Human Brain
Number circuits	10^4	10^{10}
Weight (pounds)	2,300	3
Size (cubic feet)	225	$\frac{1}{20}$
Memory (bits)	1.3×10^5	10^{20}
Speed (conduction rate)	10^7	10^3
Serial 7's (seconds)	3.0×10^5	30
Pattern recognition	Minutes	Seconds

computer program. Unfortunately, there are several drawbacks to this approach. The most obvious is the current lack of understanding of the processes used by physicians. It seems highly unlikely that the diagnostic processes of doctors would be those most applicable for computers (see Figure 1).

characteristic of a given patient. Semiobjective rating instruments are organized to ensure completeness and also to augment reliability by requiring observation of behavior in noninferential, phenomenologically small units; scored as numerical indices, they allow quantitative assessment of reliability and validity.

Step 1: Measurement-Assessment

Diagnosis starts with the identification of the historical and presenting signs and symptoms

Step 2: Diagnostic Schemata—Models

Clinicians gain knowledge of which signs, symptoms, and therapeutic modalities cluster

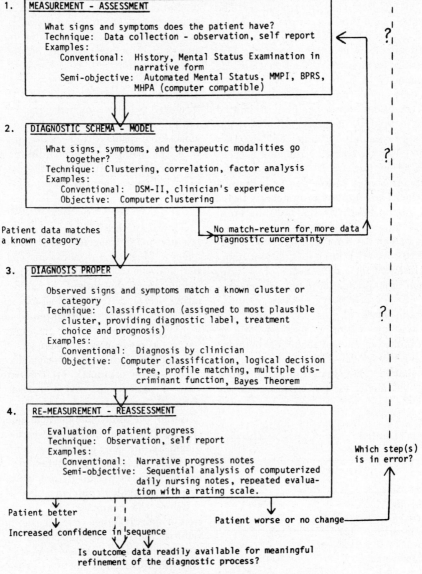

FIGURE 1. Four steps in the diagnostic process.

together by way of training and experience. *Diagnostic and Statistical Manual of Mental Disorders*, second edition (DSM-II), the official American Psychiatric Association diagnostic system, is a formal basis for continuing empirical refinement of the diagnostic process. Investigators are using computerized clustering processes to pursue new synthetic diagnostic schemata for ultimate comparison with the present DSM-II. Essentially, this is an endeavor to start with no *a priori* knowledge of current symptom-clustering to build a diagnostic schema. A large set of generally appropriate measurements and tests is made on a sizable number of patients, furnishing a multiple-variable data set of signs and symptoms, which is analyzed by a computer algorithm in an attempt to identify a latent organization by grouping patients into a diagnostic schema. In effect, the computer attempts to determine which patients seem to cluster together on the basis of available signs and symptoms, to which subsequent diagnostic labels may be applied. A prevailing objection to nearly all computer-clustering or classification programs is that they seldom include any patient history data.

Step 3: Diagnosis Proper

Objective computer techniques of diagnosis (assignment of classification) have been developed that are in accord with empiric clinical diagnosis, at least as well as clinicians agree among themselves. A prime effort has been given over to the development of parallel methods that modify a set of test results. measurements, or symptom ratings into a diagnosis in one stage. However, consider the cost in terms of patient time and money for a thorough medical diagnostic system if all possible measurements and all possible laboratory tests had to be made before computer assessment of a diagnosis. Recognition of this dilemma has led to the development of a sequential approach that takes into account the relative cost of sign, symptom, and laboratory information and the cost of misdiagnoses, as does a clinician in his work-up of a patient. Sequential methods can be compared with the game of 20 questions, in which the answer to a question is the determinant of the next question to be asked. In contrast, parallel methods pose all 20 questions at once and evaluate the answers simultaneously to reach a decision. Sequential methods,

such as the diagnostic tree, are gainfully employed when each of the component questions is answered consistently for all members of a given category. However, when there is a scattering of answers, which is common when dealing with psychiatric data, sequential methods may take too many wrong turns.

Regardless of the approach taken—whether an empirical model of diagnosis, as is provided by DSM-II and an expert clinician or an objective clustering model of diagnosis—classification-assignment techniques are now at hand for diagnostic labeling of psychiatric patients with an accuracy (validity) that matches that of expert clinicians and with a reliability nearing 100 per cent. However, a disturbing fact is the inability of any general classification method (expert clinician or computer program) to accomplish more than 70 to 75 per cent interrater reliability in the prediction of psychopathological criteria.

Step 4: Reassessment—Re-evaluation

New rating instruments expedite routine quantitative measurement of treatment outcome. What is needed now are reassessment-remeasurement techniques that are routine, quantitative, and semiobjective. Toward this end, Stroebel and Glueck have constructed a system in which factor scores secured on a regular daily basis for each patient from computer-scored nursing notes are subjected to a graphic statistical process called sequential analysis to produce computer global decisions of "significantly better," "worse," or "unchanged" without special research techniques. The advantages of this approach are that it is automated and has built-in statistical guides for assessing patient progress over time on a daily basis (see Figure 2). When a significantly better decision is made, there is an increase in confidence in the whole diagnostic sequence, Steps 1 to 4. When the patient remains unchanged or gets worse, there is uncertainty as to which of the preceding steps may be wrong.

Other Clinical Uses

Fink and Itil have provided impressive evidence that classes of clinically used psychoactive drugs may be differentiated by using computer-based period analysis, suggesting that new drugs can now be evaluated by EEG criteria.

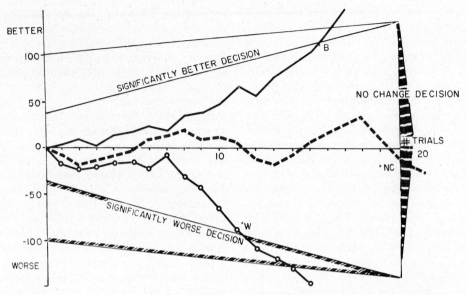

FIGURE 2. Computer global judgments.

Bickford and co-workers have developed a computer-based pictorial display technique that compresses EEG frequency-spectrum information from a 30- to 40-minute clinical recording into one page. Recent innovations in Bickford's procedure permit detection of spike-and-wave activity.

Psychophysiology has gained significant relevance as a basic medical science of psychiatry through the use of computer techniques that permit analysis of multiple and complex variables, such as averaged evoked responses. Notable has been the widespread adoption of variations of the Massachusetts Institute of Technology-developed computer, LINC (Laboratory Instrument Computer). The widespread availability of these small but powerful computers has facilitated the sharing of software and programs among laboratories and has improved the clinical relevance of laboratory investigations. For example, longitudinal studies where changes over time are important variables, although of paramount importance in psychiatry, have often been neglected because of the overwhelming amount of data and analysis involved. Halberg and co-workers have developed computer-based techniques, termed autorythmometry, that make such longitudinal analyses practicable in resolving subtle variations, even within a 24-hour period.

The psychophysiologists' use of computers in psychiatric settings very likely provides a new kind of data base for psychiatry. Longitudinal psychophysiological multiphasic screening is available as psychiatric clinical laboratory data for enhancing diagnostic, treatment, and preventive decision processes.

User Acceptance

A number of attempts have been made to provide viable hospital information systems. The fact that most have failed is partially due to problems of user acceptance. A major factor in these difficulties has been the failure of the various parties involved to develop adequate lines of communication in the early stages of the project. Most attempts to develop hospital information systems have originated with the electronic engineers and systems technicians. In addition, most hospitals that have started computer operations have done so through the medium of the business office. As a result, business applications—such as payroll, patient billing, and inventory control—have been given priority in the development of hospital computer systems, and the system design has centered on these familiar applications rather than considering, at the outset, changes that may have to be made for appropriate clinical use.

When clinicians have been approached about automation, the approach has usually been made by electronics experts, with the clinicians being told. "This is the way the system runs; now how will you modify your procedures to fit the system?" The usual answer has been, "I won't" or "I can't and therefore i'm not interested in the wonders of your computer system."

The hospital information systems that have survived have done so in large part because the clinical users of the system were consulted from the outset. The way they performed their tasks was carefully evaluated, and attempts, not always successful, were made to try to modify the computer system to fit the clinical needs and usual mode of operation.

Another critical factor in determining acceptance of an automated system is the usefulness of the system to the clinical users. If the system requires large amounts of more or less precise information from the users but gives little in return, it is quickly abandoned. However, if the computer applications are designed so that automation makes the user's job easier or more accurate and provides immediate return of more sophisticated information than the user has fed into the system, then acceptance is rapid and usually enthusiastic.

Medical-Legal Considerations

One of the important constraints in the development of computer-based hospital information systems is the effect of the system on a wide range of medical-legal issues that necessarily concern the hospital board, the medical staff, and the hospital administrators. Of immediate concern is the question of danger of the confidentiality of the doctor-patient relationship. A second consideration is the concern that accreditation from the various agencies that now monitor hospital operations will be jeopardized because of the introduction of electronic medical record storage.

A number of intricate coding schemes have already been devised to insure a high degree of confidentiality and security for automated information systems. Given time, however, any of these systems could be unscrambled by a determined expert. Ultimately, confidentiality in both automated and nonautomated procedures depends on trustworthy personnel.

The early concerns about accreditation have diminished as the development of medical computer systems have progressed. Of particular importance is the recent impact of the changes in the Social Security laws, which require the development of Professional Standards Review Organizations (PSROs). Persons working on these problems are convinced that adequate automation of patient information is the only way in which the PSROs can possibly function effectively. As a greater and greater portion of medical care costs are covered by various third-party payers, the need for adequate data to document the necessity for medical care is bound to increase. As a result, the various accrediting agencies have updated their standards to include electronic patient data storage along with other forms of data storage, provided adequate safeguards are taken to ensure accuracy and completeness of the information.

The most significant stumbling block at present is the lack of provision of some electronic alternative for the signature of medical and nursing staff members. Several approaches to the problem of positive personal identification are being investigated. These include devices to measure the geometry of the hand, thumb or fingerprint comparisons and voice print comparisons. However, current devices for converting the prints into computer-readable form are still much too expensive to be considered for use at every computer terminal. One of the devices for reading the hand measurements is considerably less expensive but does not have the unique identifying ability of the fingerprints and voice prints. It is, in addition, still much too expensive for availability at every terminal in a multiterminal hospital system.

REFERENCES

Feinstein, A. R. *Clinical Judgement.* Williams & Wilkins, Baltimore, 1967.
Laska, E., Weinstein, A., Logemann, G., Bank, R., and Breuer, R. The use of computers at a state psychiatric hospital. Compr. Psychiatry, *8:* 476, 1967.
Sines, J. O. Acturial versus clinical prediction in psychopathology. Br. J. Psychiatry, *116:* 129, 1970.
Sletten, I., Ulett, G., Altman, H., and Sundland, D. The Missouri Standard System for Psychiatry (SSOP). Arch. Gen. Psychiatry, *23:* 73, 1970.
Spitzer, R. L., and Endicott, J. DIAGNO II: Further developments in a computer program for psychiatric diagnosis, Am. J. Psychiatry, *125:* 12, 1969.
Stroebel, C. F., and Glueck, B. C. Computers in medicine. In *Practice of Medicine,* vol. 2, chap. 61. Harper & Row, Hagerstown, Md., 1972.

5.3. EXPERIMENTAL NEUROSIS

Introduction

Experimental psychopathology attempts to investigate abnormal behavior systematically under conditions that are more or less known or controlled. Controlling conditions may be manipulations of physical and psychological aspects of the environment, administration of drugs and chemicals, and ablation of tissues by surgery.

The central assumption in experimental psychopathology is that laboratory models of clinical disorder can be created and that investigation of such models will yield information relevant to the nature of the disorders. The animal model must be confirmed by showing that laws governing the animal behavior are applicable to man. The validity of human experimental models depends on those predictions derived from their study that can be generalized to the clinical situation.

Experimental Neuroses in Animals

Hebb defines human neurosis in behavioral terms, without use of verbal report of the subjective state, so that the definition can be used at the animal level. His definition is: "Neurosis is in practice an undesirable emotional condition which is generalized and persistent; it occurs in a minority of the population and has no origin in a gross neural lesion."

Pavlov

Pavlov formulated three possible causes for experimental neurosis. (1) excessive stimulation of inhibitory processes, (2) overstrain of the excitatory process by extraordinarily strong or unusual stimuli, and (3) conflict between cortical inhibitory and excitatory processes.

Gantt

The Pavlovian laboratory at the Johns Hopkins Medical School, directed by W. Horsley Gantt, has been a principal American contributor to the study of experimental neurosis. An outstanding feature of the work is the provision of detailed case histories.

Gantt introduced two fundamental theoretical concepts: schizokinesis and autokinesis. Schizokinesis implies a cleavage in response between the emotional and visual systems and the skeletal musculature. The concept originated in observations suggesting that cardiac conditioned responses are formed more quickly than motor responses, are of comparatively greater intensity, and are more resistant to extinction. Gantt considers schizokinesis to be a built-in unacquired mechanism, the function of the normal organism.

Autokinesis refers to the internal development of responses on the basis of old excitations. This is seen in the spontaneous restoration of extinguished conditioned responses and the appearance of signs of experimental neurosis long after the causal conflict has been removed. Gantt also distinguishes between negative and positive autokinesis. The development of new symptoms in a neurotic animal is negative, whereas improvement occurring some time after a specific therapeutic procedure, such as a drug, has been administered may be considered positive.

Liddell

The Cornell University group, led by H. S. Liddell, succeeded in producing chronic abnormal states in several animal species using conditioned reflex techniques (see Figure 1). Single animals were observed for as long as 12 years. Anderson and Parmenter described three types of procedure: (1) difficult differentiations, (2) experimental distinctions, and (3) rigid time schedules.

The many manifestations of experimental neurosis included hyperirritability, tenseness, and restlessness during the experiment; inhibitory motor reactions; change in diurnal activity cycle; respiratory and cardiac changes; changes in micturition and defecation patterns; and social and emotional changes.

Liddell did not agree with Pavlov's hypothesis that the cause of abnormal behavior is a clash between intense cortical excitations and inhibitions. He assigned considerable importance to the factor of restraint, introduced by negative conditioned stimuli, and showed that animals allowed to run at will in a maze while attempting to solve difficult problems never developed disturbances. He thought the experimental neurosis was caused by the equivalent of a human conflict situation. The animal must decide whether or not to respond, and, if the decision is too difficult, there is a drastic change in nervous system functioning, resulting in signs of neurosis.

Liddell also emphasized the importance of vigilance in experimental neurosis. Trained sheep and goats had initially struggled to escape from their restraining harnesses but had learned to restrict their movements. Their autonomic

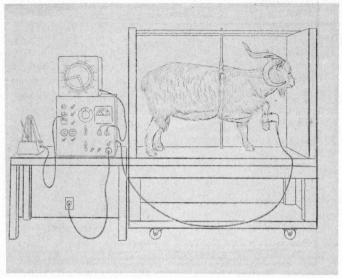

FIGURE 1. Conditioned reflexes were produced by means of this apparatus in the Cornell University Behavior Farm Laboratory. Attached to the right foreleg of the goat are two electrodes through which a mild electric shock can be administered after the click of the metronome at the *left*. After the animal has come to associate the two stimuli, it raises its leg in anticipation of the shock. (From Liddell, H. S. Conditioning and emotion. Sci. Am., *190:* 49, 1954.)

functioning, however, suggested a strong emotional undertow.

Liddell concluded that the conditioned reflex described by Pavlov was not an example of ordinary learning. He saw it as an emotionally charged episode of behavior bracketed between two primitive stereotyped reactions, the vigilance reaction and the unconditioned reaction the reinforcement of the conditioned stimulus by food or electric shock. He equated the conditioned reflex with the emergency reaction as a persisting apprehensive watchfulness in the animal.

Masserman

Masserman's biodynamic approach is associated with a long series of experiments in which experimental behavior disturbances were produced in conditioning situations. The basic experiment requires learning to open a food box in response to a sensory signal. The usual technique of inducing neurotic behavior was to present a traumatically deterrent stimulus during the execution of the well-learned response. Stimuli were electric shock, a startling air blast across the food box, or, even more effective in the case of monkeys, the sudden appearance of the head of a toy snake when the food reward

was about to be taken. If the traumatic stimulus was repeated several times, behavioral aberrations appeared.

Masserman has described severe but transitory emotional disturbances that were produced in monkeys by delayed auditory feedback of their own vocal productions or by varying the sequence and timing of the switches operated in a learned task. He also drew attention to species differences in symptomatic manifestations of experimental neurosis.

Stroebel

In Stroebel's experiments, animals were subjected to a long period of noxious stimuli but they did not become disturbed until the lever that signified their control over such stimuli was made unavailable to them, even though the unpleasant stimuli were no longer given. The symptoms were similar to those produced by Masserman, but they were generated by removing a way of dealing with traumatic stimuli, rather than by imposing such stimuli.

Conditioned Emotional Response Versus Specific State

It has been suggested that experiments of the Masserman type, which involve inhibition of feeding responses by the introduction of fear-arousing stimuli, should be regarded as eliciting conditioned emotional responses. Such responses carry no implication of a specific abnormal state. Masserman has argued against this interpretation, contending that the generalization of anxiety reactions to many other situations only remotely or symbolically associated with the original one is characteristic of human neurosis and not of a simple conditioned response.

The view that experimental neurosis is learned behavior is favored by Wolpe and is supported by the results of his experiments. These were carried out on cats in a situation like that used by Masserman but were distinguished by use of a control group, which received no initial training to feed on hearing a signal. Nevertheless, electric shock produced behavioral disturbances in all animals.

One striking difference between the results of Pavlov, Gantt, and Liddell on one hand and Masserman and Wolpe on the other is that disturbances were produced in all animals by the latter workers and only in some by the former. The clearly traumatic stimuli used in the Masserman procedure present an obvious difference. It appears that the need for inhibition or restraint brings out much greater individual differences in susceptibility of animals to experimental neurosis than does exposure to traumatic stimuli.

If susceptibility to experimental neurosis could be shown to depend on constitutional factors, this would reinforce the hypothesis that they reflect a specific central state. Pavlov noted the appearance of neurotic behavior only in dogs of the melancholic type—timid and docile with predominance of inhibitory processes—or of the choleric type—aggressive and excitable with excitatory predominance. Initially well-balanced animals did not develop chronic disturbances in behavior.

Pavlov found that temporary administration of bromides resulted in apparently permanent improvement of dogs with neuroses of the excitatory type. Treatment of the inhibitory type of neuroses was unsuccessful until he used a very small dose, only a fraction of that beneficial to the excitatory type. These observations indicate that the manifestations of a disorder are related to drug reactivity, and they favor Pavlov's theory of types, since it is easy to consider drug

reactivity as an aspect of constitutional make-up.

Learned Helplessness

The experiments of Seligman and his associates have provided an animal model that appears relevant to depressive reactions in humans. The model psychopathology is created by exposing a dog to unavoidable and uncontrollable electric shocks while it is restrained in a Pavlovian hammock. Later the animal is placed in a shuttle box divided in half by a shoulder-high partition. If the animal jumps over the partition, the shock stops. Experimentally naïve dogs, when first exposed to the shuttle box situation, run frantically about, defecating, urinating, and howling, until they accidentally scramble over the barrier and so escape the shock. They quickly learn to escape shock altogether.

Although the initial reaction of dogs previously exposed to inescapable shock is quite similar to that of the naïve animal, they soon stop running and howling and sit whining quietly until shock terminates. They do not cross the barrier and escape from shock but seem to give up and passively accept it.

Seligman calls the phenomenon learned helplessness. The essential condition leading to the learned helplessness is the experience of being unable to control the trauma by responding. If even a minimal degree of such control is provided, subsequent helplessness is avoided.

Seligman believes that learned helplessness may parallel human depression, particularly reactive depression, in several ways. Depression is characterized by reduced response initiation and a hopeless attitude about the potential effectiveness of one's own responses.

Psychosomatic Disorders in Animals

Various physiological disturbances frequently accompanied the behavioral manifestations of experimental neuroses. Often they were the most convincing signs of disturbance. One could argue that the experimental neurosis is a psychophysiological reaction.

Gastrointestinal Disorders

Mahl carried out a series of studies on the effects of chronic fear. He concluded that sustained fear is accompanied by increased HCl secretion in dogs, monkeys, and humans and that conditioned fear stimuli evoked increased HCl secretion in the absence of pain stimulation. By contrast, HCl secretion is inhibited during episodic fear stimulation.

Mahl found no evidence of stomach lesions in his animals, but other investigators have been able to produce lesions and to study the relevant conditions (see Figure 2). Brady's results place emphasis on the role of gastric acidity after stress and on the particular timing of this local factor, but there is evidence that sustained central nervous system excitation can also produce lesions. French and associates showed that prolonged electrical stimulation to the hypothalamic region produced duodenal ulceration in monkeys.

Stress does not lead to gastric ulceration in all animals. Sines and McDonald indicate that more than half of the variability in stress ulcer responsiveness of the rat may be genetically determined. Whether or not a given stress results in a gastric lesion seems to depend on interactions among the stress, constitutional factors (heredity, sex, intrauterine history), predisposing life circumstances (early handling, housing), and current organismic state (nutrition, bodily activity cycle).

Asthma

It is possible to induce asthma experimentally in the guinea pig by sensitizing the animal to egg white; asthmatic attacks then occur in response to a spray of homologous antigen. Ottenberg and co-workers found that consistently reactive guinea pigs displayed attacks when placed in the experimental chamber in the absence of the egg white spray. The asthmatic attacks of these animals appeared to be a conditioned response to the chamber.

The respiratory pattern associated with pain-fear response to electric shock resembles that found in experimental allergic asthma but involves different mechanisms. Schiavi and associates found bronchiolar obstruction in experimental allergic asthma, whereas no increased airway resistance was found in the animals exposed to electric shock.

Arterial Hypertension

Systolic blood pressure increases with age in many but not all human populations. Henry and associates concluded that, in a constant external environment, systemic arterial pres-

sure reflects the symbolic stimuli received during social interaction and that early experience plays a role in determining the arousal value of the stimuli perceived. They demonstrated that mice exposed to a high level of social stimulation showed increases in adrenal weight and adrenal noradrenaline and adrenaline, as well as elevated blood pressure.

In long-term experiments lasting 7 to 14 months, Forsyth found that elevations of both systolic and diastolic blood pressures occurred in all but one of six monkeys after 4 to 6 months of normal pressure or even hypotension. However, autopsy revealed no consistent pathological findings.

Changes in arterial blood pressure were produced in the squirrel monkey by Morse and co-workers. They point to the similarities between behavioral hypertension in the squirrel monkey and essential hypertension in humans. In both cases, transient episodes of elevated pressure over a period of months are followed by sustained hypertension.

Developmental Intervention in Animals

The proposition that the adult is significantly shaped by experience during infancy and childhood is generally accepted. There is also widespread acceptance of the related idea that experiential deprivation during development results in abnormal behavior. Since planned interference with normal development of human infants is not ethically permissible, animal experimentation provides a major source of scientific information. The general technique is to intervene in the normal course of development by removing some important factors from the environment.

Sensory Restriction

Animals reared under conditions of sensory deprivation generally show deficits in perceptual and learning performance. Hymovitch showed that problem-solving behavior in rats at maturity was superior when they were reared in a free environment box than when their development took place in individual enclosures that severely restricted sensory input. He also found that the effects of environmental restriction were greater when it occurred during early life, rather than later on. He concluded that problem-solving activities at maturity depend on early opportunity for perceptual learning and

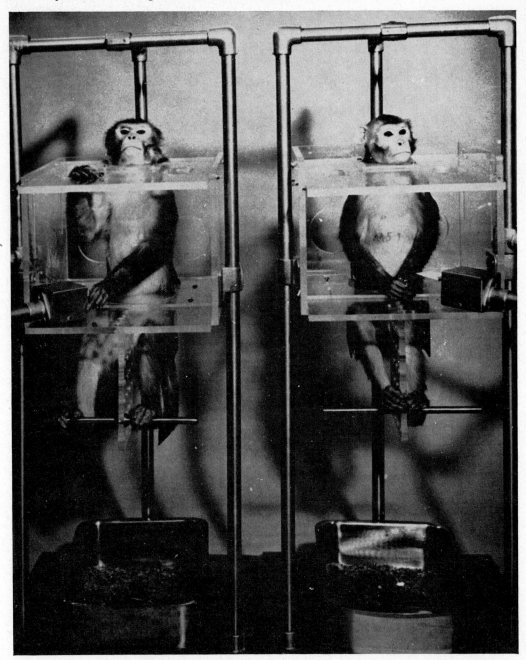

FIGURE 2. The monkey on the left, known as the executive monkey, controls whether or not both will receive an electric shock. The decision-making task produces a state of chronic tension. Note the more relaxed attitude of the monkey on the right. (United States Army Photographs.)

that the impairments of restricted animals appear to be relatively permanent and possibly irreversible.

Fuller outlined three major theoretical interpretations of changes in perception, learning, and emotional reactivity consequent on sensory restriction. (1) They reflect a need for perceptual learning. (2) Isolation has destructive or interfering effects on previously organized processes; this is supported by observations that, after isolation, dogs often perform more poorly than they did before. (3) The changes result more from competing emotional responses than from inferior behavioral organization during isolation or from loss of established patterns.

There are probably large individual differences in the persistence of postisolation deficits. Persistent psychopathological effects related to early experiential deprivation in humans may occur mainly in those who are rendered vulnerable for other reasons, such as genetic defect or nutritional deficit.

Social Deprivation

The best-known studies of social deprivation in animals are those conducted under the direction of Harry F. Harlow (see Figure 3). In later life, monkeys reared in social isolation exhibited behavioral abnormalities rarely seen in wild-born animals brought to the laboratory as adolescents. Perhaps the most striking difference between socially isolated and normal monkeys was in sexual behavior. At 2 years of age, the laboratory-born animals were not lacking in

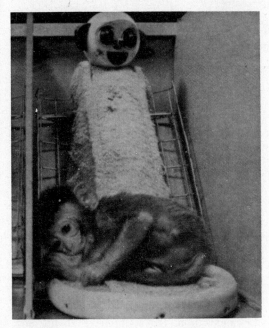

FIGURE 3. Infant rhesus with cloth surrogate "mother." (From Harlow, H. F., and Harlow, M. K. Psychopathology in monkeys. In *Experimental Psychopathology: Recent Research and Theory*, H. D. Kimmel, editor, p. 204. Academic Press, New York, 1971.)

sex drive, but they did not orient themselves correctly and did not succeed in mating.

In monkeys, the damaging effects of early social isolation do not seem to result specifically from absence of the mother, since her absence may be overcome by the presence of peers. Total social isolation for several months, which eliminates both mothering and peer interaction, results in irreversible abnormalities of social behavior.

Social isolation leads to marked and lasting physiological abnormalities in addition to severe behavioral incapacity. I. A. Mirsky has studied some of Harlow's monkeys that had been raised in total isolation for 12 months. These monkeys were found to manifest polydypsia and polyuria; they drank and excreted nearly three times as much as wild-born controls. It appeared that the mechanism involved a derangement in regulation of the water satiety mechanism of the hypothalamus.

Other studies revealed that the isolates excreted larger quantities of various substances than did the controls. Mirsky considers the biochemical aberrations exhibited by these socially isolated monkeys to bear some similarity to chemical deviations observed in humans suffering from schizophrenia.

The effects on infant monkeys of being separated from their mothers for intervals ranging from a few minutes to several weeks have been studied by a number of workers. The reaction to separation appears to have two stages: violent protest and despair. The latter stage is characterized by less activity, little or no play, and occasional crying. Kaufman and Rosenblum related the separation reaction to the anaclitic depression of human infants after separation (see Figure 4).

Studies of Neuroses in Humans

A number of experimental strategies have been used to obtain observations relevant to the problems of neurosis and psychophysiological dysfunction in humans. One approach is to compare persons who clearly suffer from the condition now under examination with controls not so afflicted. However, although functional differences between sickness and health may be ascertained by this approach, the findings leave uncertain the antecedents of illness. Another approach is to reproduce the manifestations of

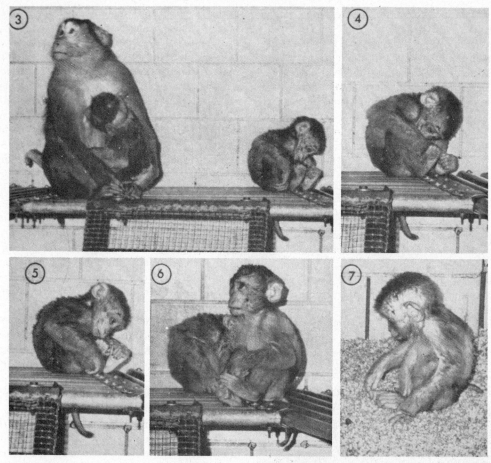

FIGURE 4. *3,* Depressed pigtail infant showing characteristic hunched over posture with flexion throughout. He is completely disengaged from mother and infant nearby in ventral-ventral contact. *4,* Depressed pigtail infant showing characteristic posture including head between legs. Note slightly opened eyes as he sucks his penis. *5,* Depressed pigtail infant showing characteristic posture and dejected facies. *6,* Two depressed pigtail infants. The one in the rear shows characteristic hunched over posture. The one in the front has lifted his head to look across the pen. Despite their passive contact they are quite disengaged from each other. *7,* Depressed infant showing aimless, tentative exploration of bedding during early stages of recovery. (From Kaufman, I. C., and Rosenblum, L. A. The reaction to separation in infant monkeys: Anaclitic depression and conservation-withdrawal. Psychosom, Med., *29:* 655, 1967.)

illness in healthy subjects in a temporary and fully reversible fashion.

Hypnotically Induced Conflicts and Emotions

The Russian psychologist Luria used hypnotic induction, together with a special method of recording motor effects, for the study of human conflicts. In a typical experiment, a hypnotized subject was told a story; according to the story he had committed a reproachable act, one that was contrary to his usual personality trend. A number of critical words were taken from this story and placed in a list of control words not specifically related to the story. The list was then presented as an association experiment. With each verbal response, the subject was required to press on a tambour with his preferred hand. Voluntary pressure curves, verbal reaction time to the words, involuntary movements from the nonpreferred hand, and respiration were recorded. The signs of conflict consisted of irregular hand pressures, lengthened reaction times, and irregular respiration.

Wittkower produced X-ray evidence of fluctuations in the size of the heart. Salivary secretions were altered both in quantity and in chemical constitution. Gastric motility and acidity were either increased or decreased. Wittkower demonstrated changes in the amount of bile and the chemical constitution of bile, alterations of leukocyte counts, and changes in the serum calcium, potassium, and chloride content. He also observed changes in the urine, in the blood iodine content, and in the galvanic skin response. He drew attention to the need for integrating observations of multiple reaction systems if one is to understand the total emotional reaction.

One study of respiratory responses showed that increased ventilation and oxygen consumption followed meaningful hypnotic suggestions of situations eliciting anxiety, anger, exercise, and head pain. Anger, anxiety, and exercise —all of which involve an orientation toward action—were contrasted with depression, the suggestion of which resulted in no respiratory changes. Depression does not involve an action orientation.

Hypnotic techniques have also been used to provide evidence for the specificity of attitude hypothesis in psychosomatic disease. The hypothesis states that each attitude toward a disturbing situation is associated with its own specific disease or set of physiological changes.

Luparello and his co-workers used techniques based on suggestion to elucidate mechanisms influencing airway reactivity in asthmatic subjects. All subjects were lead to believe that they were inhaling irritants or allergens that cause bronchoconstriction, although the inhaled substance was a nebulized solution of physiological saline. Of 40 asthmatics, 19 reacted with significant increase in airway resistance, and 12 developed attacks of bronchospasm. The attacks were reversed with saline placebo. Subjects in control groups did not react. Also, bronchodilator and bronchoconstrictor drugs exerted a greater effect when the pharmacological action was in accord with the expectations suggested to the subject than when the drug action and subject's expectations were discordant.

Conditioning

Much recent research in the Soviet Union has provided experimental demonstrations that a large number of bodily functions obey Pavlovian laws of conditioning. These experiments provide a basis for relating visceral dysfunctions to symbolic cues that have acquired meaning on the basis of previous experience. Furthermore, Razran's experiments on semantic conditioning indicate that bodily reactions may be elicited in response to verbal cues that are different in form from the initial stimuli but that have a similar meaning or a strong, previously formed, associational bond.

Experimental Stress

The idea that disturbed behavior and bodily reactions occur in response to severely taxing environmental conditions is in accord with general human experience and is widely accepted. Since environmental demands or stimuli that place strain on reserve capacities of the organism are relatively easy to produce in the laboratory, much experimental work has used this method.

Among the most biologically meaningful procedures for studying stress are those that involve complete or partial frustration of basic organismic needs for food, sleep, or environmental stimulation. Partial starvation over a prolonged period of time may result in various neurotic manifestations. Bizarre behavior in connection with food was almost universal and often took the form of compulsive rituals. The disturbances were reversible with restoration of an adequate diet.

A dangerous sport provides a natural situation for studying the effects of stress and mechanisms used in coping with stress. The autonomic responses (galvanic skin response, respiration, and heart rates) of sport parachutists have been studied before and after the jump. Novice parachutists showed gradual increase in reactivity until the last point immediately before the jump; experienced jumpers showed their increase early in the jump sequence, and their arousal had decreased nearly to normal at the time of the jump. The good performers had patterns like those of the more experienced jumpers.

In general, it appears that persons with already-established illness or proneness to anxiety tend to react to moderate pain stimulation with greater physiological disturbance in various organ systems than do persons who are free of illness. Similar differentiations may be obtained by nonpainful stresses, such as those requiring the execution of difficult tasks. Furthermore, the physiological system that is particularly responsive to experimental stress is more likely to be one habitually involved in the patient's illness.

A laboratory stress technique that has been gaining increasing favor involves the use of motion picture films likely to induce particular kinds of emotional reactions. Investigators have been able to relate the nature of the reactions to some personality variables and to the kind of psychological mechanisms used to deal with emotionally disturbing stimuli.

Another technique has been the deliberate manipulation of events in a laboratory situation to arouse emotions the investigator wanted to study. For example, Funkenstein et al. deliberately created a situation in which the subject was required to carry out computational problems at a very rapid rate while the experimenter became critical and demanding. The subject's behavioral reaction was classified as reflecting anger in, anger out, or anxiety. Significant differences in various cardiovascular measures were found between the anger in and the anger out groups.

Interviews that deliberately focus on emotionally charged material so that related bodily reactions may be studied represent another variant of experimental stress. Although this procedure involves numerous methodological difficulties, it has yielded data concerning the participation of physiological response systems in symptom mechanisms.

REFERENCES

Broadhurst, P. L. Abnormal animal behavior. In *Handbook of Abnormal Psychology*, H. J. Eysenck, editor, p. 726. Basic Books, New York, 1961.

Gantt, W. H. *Physiological Bases of Psychiatry*. Charles C Thomas, Springfield, Ill., 1958.

Harlow, H. F., and Harlow, M. K. Psychopathology in monkeys. In *Experimental Psychopathology: Recent Research and Theory*, H. D. Kimmel, editor, p. 204. Academic Press, New York, 1971.

Luria, A. R. *The Nature of Human Conflict*. Liverwright, New York, 1932.

Masserman, J. H. *Behavior and Neurosis: An Experimental Psychoanalytic Approach to Psychobiologic Principles*. University of Chicago Press, Chicago, 1943.

Seligman, M. E. P. Learned helplessness. Ann. Rev. Med., *23:* 407, 1972.

Young, L. D., Suomi, S. S., Harlow, H. F., and McKinney, W. T. Early stress and later response to separation in rhesus monkeys. Am. J. Psychiatr., *130:* 400, 1973.

5.4.   EUPHOROHALLUCINOGENS

Introduction

Much myth and prejudice concerning the euphorohallucinogens grows from the definition of the drug category. If one conceptualizes the definitive drug effects only on the basis of phenomena (hallucinatory psychoses) associated with high doses, it it reasonable to define such drugs as psychotomimetic or psychotogenic compounds, and it makes sense to use phrases that have been associated with functional psychoses to describe their effects. However, in low doses these compounds produce euphorigenic activation of a very complicated sort; in intermediate doses, they activate a wide range of physical functions.

A number of drug categories go through the euphorigenic mode of action at some dose level. Only with the drugs in the euphorohallucinogenic category is a wide range of experimentation and transcendent experience possible without the threat of death from overdose. Bad trips and potential psychical dangers from euphorohallucinogenic drugs can be associated with toxicity or idiosyncratic responses, rather than with inherent parameters of drug action. These drugs are particularly sensitive to individual differences in personality and environmental set.

Human Pharmacology

Phenylethylamines

The simplest family of drugs in the euphorohallucinogenic category is made up of substituted phenylethylamines. The prototype compound, mescaline (3,4,5-trimethoxyphenylethylamine) (see Figure 1), comes from a cactus of the species *Lophophora williamsii* found in the southwestern United States and northern Mexico. Although mescaline is one of the least active drugs in the category (the active dose range is about 200 to 500 mg.), it has become the compound of reference. Mescaline bears a remarkable structural resemblance to the catecholamines norepinephrine and dopamine and to one candidate for the role of endogenous hallucinogen, 3,4-dimethoxyphenylethylamine.

mescaline

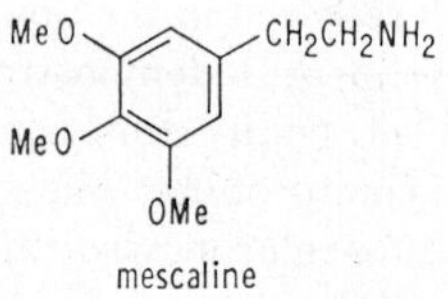

FIGURE 1. The major phenylethylamine hallucinogen.

Indolealkylamines

A more complex family of euphorohallucinogens is made up of indolealkylamines (see Figure 2). The simplest one is *N,N*-dimethyltryptamine (DMT), which is found in a number of snuffs in South America. An enzyme has been reported in human brain that synthesizes the *N,N*-dimethyl derivatives of tryptamine and serotonin. Such an enzyme may play a role in some phenomena of natural behavior. 5-Methoxy-*N,N*-dimethyltryptamine is also a component of some snuffs and is relatively potent in humans in the milligram dose range. Most of these compounds are active when given parenterally. Other derivatives of this family include a 4-hydroxy compound, psilocybin, and the *N,N*-dimethyl derivative of serotonin, bufotenin.

Ergot Alkaloids

LSD, which is active in doses of 25 to 200 $\mu g.$, is the most potent of the ergot alkaloids. There is considerably less potential for productive structural alterations to LSD than to the mescaline or amphetamine derivatives; most changes in the structure appear to weaken the euphorigenic activity of the compound. The indolealkaloids with a larger ring structure include ibogaine, which produces confusion, drunkenness, and hallucinations if taken in large doses.

Cannabinols

The active components of the plant *Cannabis sativa* are characterized either by a three-ring system or by a system that is easily convertible to three rings (see Figure 3). Although the dose-response characteristics of the active principle, Δ-3-tetrahydrocannabinol (THC), resemble those of LSD, they differ in one significant

FIGURE 3. Cannabinol.

way. With increasing doses and over longer periods of time, the drug user, instead of being activated, gets sleepy and experiences frequent bursts of dreaming during several hours of drug-induced sleep. Another way that THC differs on a dose-response basis from other euphorohallucinogens has to do with the giggling and uncontrollable laughter associated with the euphoria. The structure of the cannabinols differs significantly from the aromatic amine constellation of the other families of euphorohallucinogens.

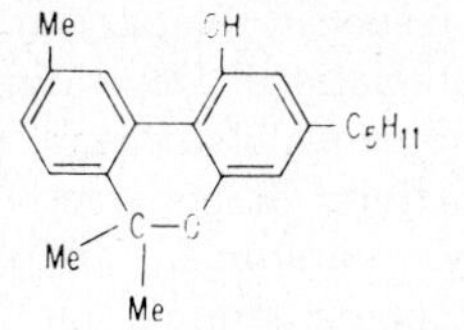

Glycolate Esters

A number of compounds have been synthesized and tested in which the substituted glycolic acid side chains are meta instead of para to the nitrogen of the piperidine ring. These changes have resulted in a large series of euphorohallucinogens, including 1-methyl-3-piperidylcyclopentylphenylglycolate, the most powerful, and Ditran, the best known. These compounds can cause delusional thinking, disorientation, and hallucinations.

Another piperidine derivative is phencyclidine (PCP). It has effects at low doses that mimic the primary signs of schizophrenia—including flattened affect, thought disorder, and emotional withdrawal—without the secondary signs, such as delusions or hallucinations.

Anticholinergics

Atropine does not produce a significant phase of euphoria at low doses, and at high doses the hallucinatory and delusional states are associated with amnesia. Human reactions to the anticholinergics include confusion, delirium, and hallucinations.

Behavioral Effects

Because of the limitations of research with euphorohallucinogens in human beings, the development of animal models for the assessment of behavioral effects has been prerequisite to investigations of structure-function relation-

N, N-dimethyltryptamine

bufotenin

psilocin

α-methyltryptamine

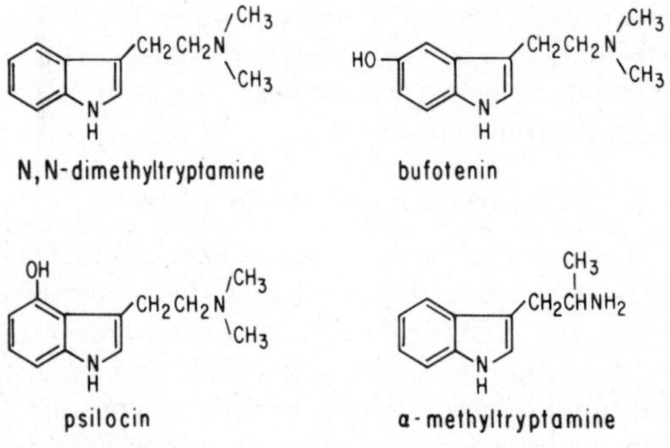

FIGURE 2. Some hallucinogenic indoleamines.

ships, dose-response comparisons, and pharmacological interactions. Depending on dose and species, euphorohallucinogens variously produce hypoactivity or hyperactivity, aggression or docility, catatonia, peculiar postures, marked autonomic stimulation, incoordination, and hypersensitivity to sensory stimuli. Large, toxic doses are generally necessary to produce such marked effects in animals, in contrast to the exquisite potency of these agents in humans. Except in the realm of perceptual alterations, the multitude of animal behavior studies have failed to provide any coherent picture of the psychological variables affected by euphorohallucinogens.

In sufficient doses, LSD produces some impairment in most psychomotor tasks involving sustained, goal-directed responses. Distractability, physiological arousal, and the generally reported increase in reaction time may contribute to the effect. Operant response rate maintained by positive reinforcement is reduced by LSD. Generally, operant behavior maintained by aversive contingencies has been resistant to the actions of euphorohallucinogens, with results varying both quantitatively and qualitatively with different species or paradigms.

Because of the variety of perceptual changes reported by human beings after LSD, many tests of auditory and, especially, visual functions have been made in animals. In monkeys, spatial disorientation and impaired visual size-discrimination have been reported. Other tests have indicated that either increases or decreases in the accuracy of visual discrimination can be demonstrated, depending on the animal and the dose range. One of the most pervasive effects of low doses of euphorohallucinogens in animals is a decreased ability to habituate to sensory stimuli. This effect has been demonstrated for most sense modalities. Similar findings have been obtained with a variety of psychophysical tests in human beings.

Neurophysiology

Excluding the anticholinergics, euphorohallucinogens have a number of physiological and neurophysiological effects in common, usually including mydriasis, elevated heart rate, elevated blood pressure, hyperreflexia, tachypnea, increased muscle tension, occasional ataxia, nausea and vomiting, salivation, lacrimation, leukocytosis, and increased reaction to internal and external stimuli. Most of these phenomena are concomitants of general physiological arousal.

Both in animals and in humans, these compounds alter the electroencephalogram, although not dramatically. Except at high doses, the EEG is typically characterized by low-amplitude, high-frequency activity after a dose of LSD, mescaline, or a similar compound. LSD has been reported to increase the duration of rapid eye movement (REM) sleep periods in man.

A number of workers have shown abnormal activity in the limbic system to be a result of euphorohallucinogenic drug action. Studies in man have also shown the temporal lobe limbic rhythms to be altered by LSD.

Working with microelectrodes, several investigators have found that euphorohallucinogens, particularly LSD, at very low doses suppress the firing rates of neurons in the dorsal and median raphe. These raphe nuclei contain many of the serotonergic cells in mammalian brain and may include other indoleamine transmitters as well. Generally, LSD suppresses the spontaneous firing activity of some neurons in most areas of the brain, including the lateral geniculate. One exception has been reported: the spontaneous activity of the retinal ganglion cells increases after administration of LSD or certain other euphorohallucinogenic drugs.

Much neurophysiological explanation of euphorohallucinogens has sprung from the similarity of one or another of these compounds to natural neurotransmitters in the brain. The indolealkylamines and the indole moiety of LSD seem to work by blocking receptor sites or interfering with normal transmission in the serotonergic pathways. Methoxyamphetamines or phenylethylamines apparently alter dopaminergic transmission. The anticholinergic compounds resemble acetylcholine. However, attempts to relate specific transmission in these systems to neurophysiological responses have been far from satisfactory.

Neurochemical Mechanisms

The system of serotonergic neurons in the brain consists of cell bodies in the midbrain, pons, and medulla (the raphe nuclei) and projections into the forebrain (striatum and limbic forebrain structures) and the lumbosacral cord. This neurotransmitter system has been the one most studied in relation to the euphorohal-lucinogens, initially because of the indole nucleus common to serotonin and LSD. LSD can block the agonistic actions of serotonin. Relatively small doses of LSD dramatically inhibit the spontaneous firing of the cells of the dorsal and median raphe nuclei. Major perturbations and adaptive changes occur in the serotonergic system after the administration of narcotic euphorigens, and the responses of this system to psychoactive drugs are dampened by lithium.

Impairment of a biogenic amine neurotransmitter system often results in behavioral responses that may reflect denervation or decentralization supersensitivity. For example, pretreatment with reserpine or tetrabenazine, which release much of the vesicular store of serotonin and lead to depletion of the transmitter, enhances the effects of a threshold dose of LSD in rats.

Hemispheric Brain Function and Drug Effects

The left side of the brain is characterized as verbal, analytical, symbolical, and propositional. The right hemisphere appears to be more perceptual, analogical, synthetical, and appositional. The most characteristic effects of right-hemispheric damage in humans are visuospatial and temporal disorganization. Neurological observations and subtle tests of information processing in commissurotomized patients indicate that the left hemisphere processes input in a sequential analytical manner, and the right side integrates material more nearly simultaneously.

After systematic observations of the effects of LSD and mescaline, Masters and Houston listed the following: "Changes in visual, auditory, tactile, olfactory, gustatory, and kinesthetic perception; changes in experiencing time and space; changes in the rate and content of thought; body image changes; hallucinations; vivid images—eidetic images—seen with the eyes closed; greatly heightened awareness of color; abrupt and frequent mood and affect changes; heightened suggestibility; enhanced recall or memory; depersonalization and ego dissolution; dual, multiple, and fragmentized consciousness; seeming awareness of internal organs and processes of the body; upsurge of unconscious materials; enhanced awareness of linguistic nuances; increased sensitivity to non-verbal cues; sense of capacity to communicate much better by non-verbal means; . . . and, in general, apprehension of a world that has slipped the chains of normal categorical ordering."

The common effects of these drugs may be comprehensible in terms of a shift in the relative activities of the cerebral hemispheres in man. By virtue of the left brain's explicit verbal capacities, its rational, analytical processing is strongly emphasized and consistently reinforced in Western culture. Similarly, euphorohallucinogens may effect the emergence of right-hemispheric modes of consciousness.

The most typical effects of both euphorohallucinogens and right-hemispheric disturbances are heteromodal changes in perception. Visual functions and spatial orientations are foremost on both lists. Difficulty in describing verbally the effects of euphorohallucinogens is a common lament. The increased reliance on nonverbal communication may result from a combination of diminished linguistic capacity and augmented perception of the facial expressions of others. The simultaneous influx of multimodal perceptions produced by increased attentiveness and decreased habituation to sensory stimuli may overwhelm the systematic sequential processing of the language hemisphere. The more analogical integrative processing of the right hemisphere seems better suited to the task of consolidating this perceptual flood.

The appreciation of music and art, another dimension of right hemispheric functioning, is dramatically emphasized in most subjective descriptions of the euphorohallucinogenic experience. The increases in artistic creativity and understanding claimed by some to be common with LSD may result from distortions of visual perception and reduced habituation to visual stimuli.

Drug Effects and Psychopathology

The euphorohallucinogenic drugs often produce important new feelings from apparently chance connections between freely floating emotional cathexes and cognitive associations. The patient or experimental subject often reports new insights about old matters. These random relationships between feelings and thoughts resemble the phenomena that characterize schizophrenia, yet they differ. They appear more under control and far more productive and available for adaptive use than do the split affect and thoughts of the schizophrenic. The drug experience manifests many of the features of creativity. The moment of insight or creation against a background of high, unstable emotional tone is a feature of temporary post-turmoil stabilization in acute schizophrenia, but, again, it appears less malignant and destructive in drug subjects. The drug subject often reaches for new thoughts, new relationships with people, or a new metaphysic to deal with the ambiguity of his altered perceptions. This slide through a number of psychological mechanisms is also consistent with the early picture of functional psychosis but lacks its desperation.

Compared with functional psychotics, patients who were ill from drugs were more disorganized, less retarded in motor movement, less blunted in affect, and more excited; they had better prior histories of socialization, were more intelligent, had better premorbid work records, and had considerably lower incidences of Schneider's signs. In short, as a psychiatric population, they had a good prognosis for a high rate of remission of their psychoses and later social cure. The average length of their hospitalizations was considerably shorter than that of functionally ill patients. Outside of impulsive self-destructive behavior, the prolonged psychotic reactions induced by euphorohallucinogens seem to be more benign than naturally occurring psychoses in course and in prognosis.

An issue of complexity and theoretical import concerns people who use large amounts of euphorohallucinogens frequently during the developmental periods of adolescence and young adulthood. Although there is a paucity of hard data on this subject, most clinicians agree that a syndrome emerges that includes passivity, lack of competitiveness, and a tendency to escape rather than cope actively with normal impediments to successful functioning in interpersonal relationships and the marketplace. These and other changes are rationalized as changes in value systems.

REFERENCES

Bogen, J. E. The other side of the brain II: An appositional mind. Bulletin Los Angeles Neurol. Soc., *34:* 135, 1969.

Cole, J. O., Freedman, A. M., and Friedhoff, A. J., editors. *Psychopathology and Psychopharmacology.* The Johns Hopkins University Press, Baltimore. 1973.

Efron, D. H., editor. *Psychotomimetic Drugs.* Raven Press, New York, 1970.

Klüver, H. *Mescal and Mechanisms of Hallucinations.* University of Chicago Press, Chicago, 1966.

Mandell, A. J. Neurobiological barriers to euphoria. Am. Sci., **61:** 565–573, 1973.

Mandell, A. J., editor. *New Concepts in Neurotransmitter Regulation.* Plenum, New York, 1973.

Smythies, J. R., editor. *The Mode of Action of Psychotomimetic Drugs,* NRP Bulletin, Volume 8. MIT Press, Boston, 1970.

Sugerman, A. A., Goldstein, L., Marjerrison, G., and Stolzfuss, N. Recent research in EEG amplitude analysis. Dis. Ner. Syst., *34:* 162, 1973.

5.5   SENSORY DEPRIVATION

Introduction

Instances of aberrant mental behavior in explorers, shipwrecked sailors, and prisoners in solitary confinement have been known for centuries. Toward the end of World War II, startling confessions induced by brainwashing in prisoners of war caused a rise of interest in the psychological phenomena brought about by deliberate diminution of sensory input.

In controlled experiments, volunteer subjects—under conditions of visual, auditory, and tactile deprivation (see Figures 1 through 4) for periods of up to 7 days—reacted with increased suggestibility and showed symptoms that have since become recognized as characteristic of the sensory deprivation state: anxiety, tension, inability to concentrate or organize one's thoughts, vivid sensory imagery—usually visual, sometimes reaching the proportions of hallucinations with delusionary quality—body illusions, somatic complaints, and intense subjective emotional accompaniment.

Theoretical Explanations

Suppression of the secondary process (perceptual contact with reality) brings about emergence of the primary process—regression, confusion, disorientation, fantasy formation, primitive emotional responses, hallucinatory activity, and pseudopathological mental reactions.

Presumably the maintenance of optimal conscious awareness and accurate reality testing depends on a necessary state of alertness, which depends on a constant stream of changing stimuli from the external world, mediated through the ascending reticular activating system. In the absence or impairment of such a

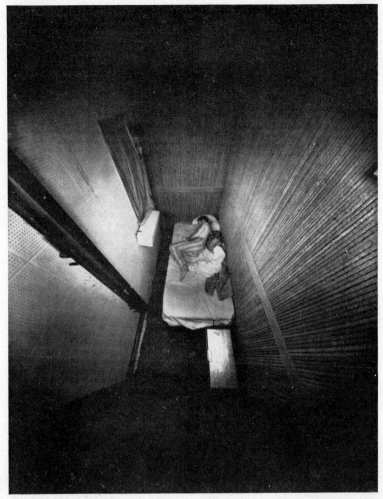

FIGURE 1. A volunteer subject in a sensory deprivation experiment. The special room is soundproofed and pitch-black (the photograph was taken with the use of infrared light). The subject wears gloves to blunt the sense of touch. (Yale Joel, Life Magazine, ©Time, Inc.)

stream, as occurs in sensory deprivation and in sensory monotony, alertness falls away, direct contact with the outside world diminishes, and the balance of integrated activity tilts in the direction of increased relative prominence of impulses from the inner body and the central nervous system itself. Material previously repressed and relatively unconscious is given an impetus to appear in consciousness.

Personality theories attempt to explain the variation in phenomena from subject to subject. Instinctual drive or need theories are based on hypothecated specific needs or drives built into the organism, allied to inquisitiveness, curiosity, investigative or search behavior, and information-seeking. Expectation hypotheses involve social influences, including the important role played by the experimenter.

Cognitive theories lay stress on the organism as an information-processing machine whose purpose is optimal adaptation to the perceived environment. With insufficient information, the machine cannot form the cognitive map against which to match current experience, and there is resultant disorganization and maladaptation.

Applications

The phenomena of sensory deprivation are evoked increasingly to explain puzzling industrial and military accidents. They have been implicated in plane crashes and truck crashes on long hauls over monotonous superhighways.

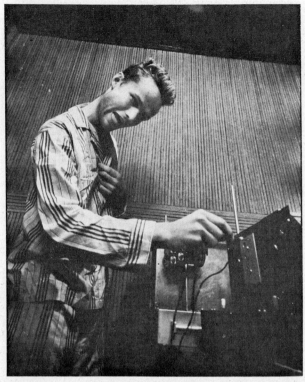

FIGURE 2. Just after his release the subject tries in vain to hold a small rod in a hole without touching the sides. (Yale Joel, Life Magazine, ©Time, Inc.)

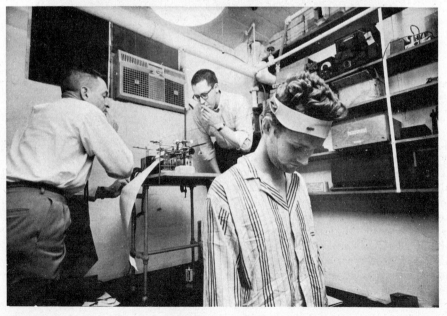

FIGURE 3. Immediately after his release, the volunteer subject was subjected to a battery of tests. Although most volunteers could perform simple memorization in confinement, tests showed their comprehension ability to be impaired just after release. It took most volunteers about a day to return to normal. (Yale Joel, Life Magazine, ©Time, Inc.)

HYDROHYPODYNAMIC ENVIRONMENT

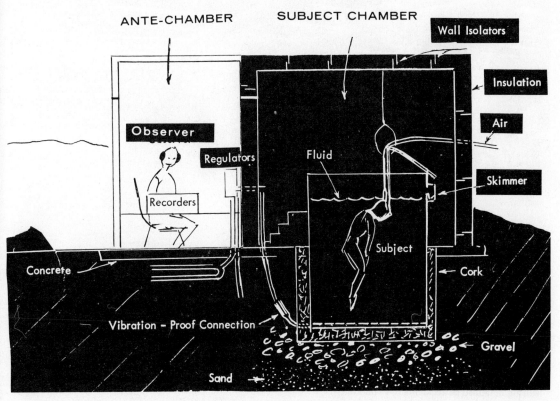

FIGURE 4. Diagram of laboratory used by Jay T. Shurley for sensory deprivation experiments. Volunteer subjects are immersed in tepid water, breathe through blacked-out masks, and are observed and monitored. (Courtesy of J. T. Shurley, M.D.)

Modern industrial and business plants sometimes produce an environment devoid of sensory stimulation for workers. Assembly-line production, with its boredom, may bring about similar results and increased accident rates (see Figure 5).

Patients with respiratory paralysis treated in a tank-type respirator experience hallucinatory states that disappear promptly on the patient's removal from the respirator. The states are produced by sensory deprivation. Patients with so-called cardiac psychosis may be suffering from the effects of sensory deprivation. Too much rest, silence, solitude, and darkness loosen the patients' hold on reality and make them prey to fantasy. Arthritics and chronic invalids too carefully protected from environmental stimulation may be afflicted similarly.

Black-patch psychosis, which occurs postoperatively in patients after cataract and other eye operations, is often characterized by a frenzied confusion and disorientation. Bandaging only one eye or allowing a central peephole is often corrective or preventive. Patients in total body casts or immobilized by head tongs or other severely restricting apparatus may develop disturbing psychotic behavior (see Figure 6). The provision of private nursing, frequent visitors, radio, and television may be effective in relief. Postoperative isolation in exaggerated form, especially in open-heart cases, can bring about postoperative psychosis.

Sensory deprivation is surely important in delirium tremens and is probably a vital factor in the deterioration of the chronic back-ward inmate. When sensory deprivation is neutralized by the many attentions that accompany a new drug study, some previously neglected patients seem to get well. When wards for chronic patients are emptied, the resultant flood of unaccustomed stimulation may have a nonspecific beneficial effect.

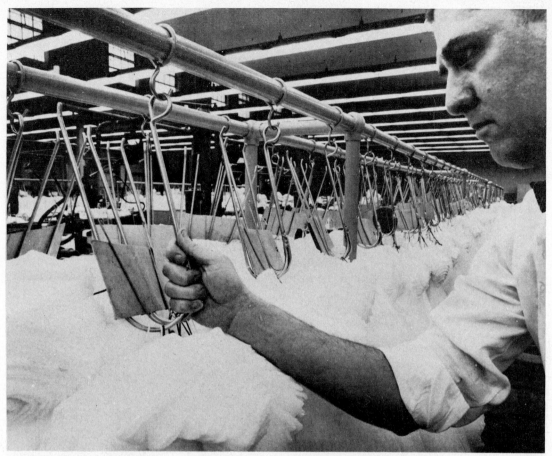

FIGURE 5. A lack of varied stimuli on an assembly line job can cause boredom and mental fatigue, often resulting in industrial accidents (UPI photo).

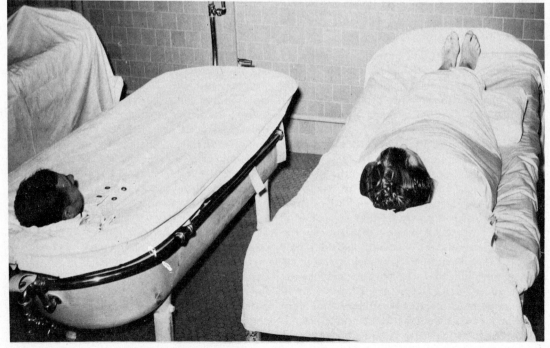

FIGURE 6. A patient who is restrained for prolonged periods of time is likely to suffer sensory deprivation. The use of bindings and isolation is potentially counterproductive to therapy (Culver Pictures).

A variegated sensory environment is necessary for the normal development of the infant. Mental retardation may be the result of sensory deprivation as well as of biochemical or physiological factors. Animal studies have also shown that early sensory deprivation leads to lowered resistance to stress in later life.

Psychological functions in the elderly may deteriorate as the result of pitiable social isolation and sensory deprivation. Sensory deprivation may make some psychotic and depressed patients more susceptible to certain treatment methods. The associated regression, for example, favors the anaclitic approach.

REFERENCES

Bexton, W. H., Heron, W., and Scott, T. H. Effects of decreased variation in the sensory environment. Can. J. Psychol., 8: 70, 1954.

Kubzansky, P. E. The effects of reduced environmental stimulation on human behavior: A review. In *The Manipulation of Human Behavior: The Case for Interrogation,* A. D. Biderman and H. Zimmer, editors, p. 51. Wiley, New York, 1961.

Rossi, A. M., Fuhrman, A., and Solomon, P. Arousal levels and thought processes during sensory deprivation. Abnorm. Psychol., 72: 166, 1967.

Solomon, P., et al., editors. *Sensory Deprivation.* Harvard University Press, Cambridge, Mass., 1961.

Thomson, L. R. Sensory deprivation: A personal experience. Am. J. Nurs., 73: 266, 1973.

Wilson, L. M. Intensive care delirium: The effect of outside deprivation in a windowless unit, Arch. Int. Med., 130: 225, 1972.

Zubek, J. P., editor. *Sensory Deprivation: Fifteen Years of Research.* Appleton-Century-Crofts, New York, 1969.

5.6.   NORMALITY

Introduction

Normality serves as a base line for all behavior, whether pathological or not. However, the concept of normality is ambiguous, has a multiplicity of meanings and usages, and is burdened by being value-laden.

Four Perspectives of Normality

Normality as Health

Most physicians equate normality with health and view health as an almost universal phenomenon. As a result, behavior is assumed to be within normal limits when no manifest psychopathology is present. If one were to put all behavior on a continuum, normality would encompass the major portion of the continuum, and abnormality would be the small remainder.

Health in this context refers to a reasonable rather than an optimal state of functioning.

Normality as Utopia

The second perspective conceives of normality as that harmonious and optimal blending of the diverse elements of the mental apparatus that culminates in optimal functioning. Such a definition emerges clearly when psychiatrists or psychoanalysts talk about the ideal person.

Normality as Average

The third perspective is commonly used in normative studies of behavior and is based on the mathematical principle of the bell-shaped curve. This approach conceives of the middle range as normal and of both extremes as deviant. Variability is described only within the context of groups and not within the context of one person.

Normality as Transactional Systems

The fourth perspective stresses that normal behavior is the end result of interacting systems. It stresses changes or processes, rather than a cross-sectional definition of normality, and encompasses variables from the biological, psychological, and social fields—all contributing to the functioning of a viable system over time.

Research on Normal Populations

One can conceptualize four different levels of investigations into the psychological functioning and development of healthy or normal people—cross-sectional, follow-up, longitudinal, and predictive. In general, the first two levels correspond to either normality as health or normality as average. The last two levels are more likely to correspond to either normality as utopia or normality as transactional systems. All the studies were of middle-class if not upper-middle-class populations. There are no studies of minority-group populations. Also, the majority of the subjects studied were males.

Cross-sectional studies involve the assessment of individual psychological functioning at one point in time. The methods vary from survey techniques, questionnaires, and psychological tests to in-depth psychiatric interviews. Relatively more studies use the cross-sectional approach than any other method.

These studies clearly demonstrate that non-patient populations function psychologically on a different behavioral and affective level than do patients. The structure of the ego in the nonpatient group is different from that in the patient group. The nonpatients have fewer identity problems, and they move slowly and cautiously in the direction of independence and maturity.

One major limitation of cross-sectional studies is the difficulty in obtaining reliable and valid data regarding background factors leading to these findings, and one wonders whether these nonpatients will stay healthy in the future.

Follow-up studies cover two different points in time. The methods vary, as in the cross-sectional studies. Follow-up studies usually have a specific aim in mind.

Follow-up studies provide significant support for the hypothesis that continuity does exist in the realm of psychological functioning. In many ways, follow-up studies confirm the validity of cross-sectional studies. They leave unanswered the question: How does this process take place? More specific micropsychological analysis of behavior and feeling states of persons across time is necessary before one can begin to answer this question.

In longitudinal studies, the subjects are studied over time by appropriate methods. The purpose of these studies is usually to determine the factors that influence the functioning and adjustment of persons over time. The subjects are studied on at least three occasions. The advantage of multiple observations is that they tend to eliminate errors or biases.

Longitudinal studies can be undertaken at any stage of the life cycle.

The major findings suggest that stability rather than change involves successive adaptation throughout the life cycle. The coping styles and psychological reactions in the different stages of development are similar.

Predictive studies are conceptually difficult to organize because one does not know what the right questions or variables are. They are empirically difficult to undertake because of the expense, commitment, and time involved. Such studies are particularly difficult to start because it is almost impossible to know which intervening variables will have the most influence on the functioning of persons in the future. At times, one can use retrospective studies by deciphering crucial from noncrucial variables and identifying those variables with potential predictive power.

Normality and Emergent Social Movements

Recently, the women's movement in the United States has criticized psychiatry for its portrayal of the normal psychology of women. Indeed, the statement is often made that psychiatry's characterizations of feminine behavior have been derived from a male perspective and are decidedly sexist in nature. There is much recent evidence that calls into question prior hypotheses and concepts. In reality, women appear to be less vulnerable, less fragile psychologically, and more able to cope with developmental and situational vicissitudes than many concepts seem to acknowledge.

In a similar manner, there has been frequent criticism of psychiatry's tendency to emphasize psychopathology in minority groups. The portrayal of psychological issues related to blacks has appeared especially tinged with an overemphasis on pathology.

Much of the criticism raised against psychiatry by blacks and by women illustrates a strong reaction against stereotyping. Psychiatrists have also been accused of stereotyping by age, by social class, and by geography.

Conclusion

Is a profile emerging that reliably describes the normal man or woman? Definitely not. The more one studies normal populations, the more one becomes aware that healthy functioning is as complex and coping behavior as varied as the psychopathological entities. Normality and health cannot be understood in the abstract. Rather, they depend on the cultural norms, society's expectations and values, professional biases, individual differences, and the political climate of the time, which sets the tolerance for deviance.

REFERENCES

Futterman, E., and Hoffman, I. Crisis and adaptation in the families of fatally ill children. In *The Child and His Family*, E. J. Anthony and C. Koupernick, editors, vol. 2, p. 127. Wiley, New York, 1973.

Grinker, R. R., Sr., Grinker, R. R., Jr., and Timberlake, J. A study of "mentally healthy" young males (homoclites). Arch. Gen. Psychiatry 6: 405, 1962.

Kagen, J., and Moss, M. A. *Birth to Maturity: A Study in Psychological Development.* Wiley, New York, 1962.

Offer, D. *The Psychological World of the Teen-ager: A Study of Normal Adolescent Boys.* Basic Books, New York, 1973.

Offer, D., and Offer, J. L. *Youth: A Study of Normal Young Men.* Basic Books, New York, 1974.

Offer, D., and Sabshin, M. *Normality: Theoretical and Clinical Concepts of Mental Health.* Basic Books, New York, 1966.

Smith, M. B. Normality: For an abnormal age. In *Modern Psychiatry and Clinical Research*, D. Offer and D. X. Freedman, editors, p. 102. Basic Books, New York, 1972.
White, R. W. *Lives in Progress*. Dryden, New York, 1952.

5.7 STATISTICS

Data Collection

Statistical aspects of a study must be considered in the early planning stages in order to (1) sharpen the question that the study is designed to answer, (2) appraise whether the question can be answered practically by valid and reliable data, (3) clarify the unit of population to be studied, (4) select the relevant aspects about the groups on which data should be sought, (5) help delineate the data essential for the objectives of the study, and (6) prepare an outline of the proposed tabulations of the data and of the methods of analysis to ensure that the end result will be satisfactory.

The questionnaire and interviewing techniques must be standardized. For example, open-ended questions should be replaced by categorical, objective choices to ensure precise, valid data.

Precision (reliability) is concerned with the repeatability or consistency of data. Validity, on the other hand, is directed to the question: Are the data measuring what is intended to be measured? Validity is also concerned with whether the instruments are measuring accurately and without bias.

Bias may be defined as systematic error—that is, the difference between the true value and the value obtained through data collection attributable to all causes other than sampling error or variability. Bias may enter the data through the manner in which the question is asked, how the response is judged, problems of recall, and nonresponse.

Another aspect of validity is the sensitivity and specificity of screening tests and procedures for detecting a disease or condition in the general population. A highly sensitive test is one that, when applied to a group, identifies as positive a large proportion of those with the disease; relatively few with the disease are labeled as not having the disease (false negatives). A highly specific test is one that identi-

fies as negative a large proportion of those without the disease; relatively few without the disease are labeled as having the disease (false positives). Setting the cutoff point between normal and abnormal so as to increase the sensitivity of a test automatically decreases its specificity and vice versa.

A critical decision is the choice of the universe (population) appropriate for study. The selective factors that influence the admission of patients to a hospital reflect both societal forces (such as admission policies, geographic and referral patterns) and patient-determined forces (such as acceptance of care). Therefore, the patients in any one hospital are rarely representative of all such patients in the community. Conclusions based on autopsy series are also suspect.

After the universe or sampling frame of subjects is determined, a random sample may be selected from it. A foolproof system (simple random sampling) is to number each case folder in sequence and then select a sample by use of a table of random numbers.

Alternately, the terminal digit of the previously assigned case numbers may be used for selection, such as every case number ending in 3. This method is called systematic sampling. It is unbiased if the case numbers had been assigned sequentially to patients in turn, if the terminal digit bears no special significance, and if there is no periodicity to the way patients turned up. Sampling on the basis of surname (alphabetical sampling) must be avoided, since surnames are highly correlated with ethnicity.

When the population is very heterogeneous—that is, when persons differ markedly from each other with respect to the characteristics being studied—the investigator may wish to stratify them into subgroups, such as short-term and long-term clinic cases, and sample from each stratum or subgroup separately. Stratified sampling assures that each subgroup is represented in the sample, thus tending to reduce sampling error. Other types of sampling, such as multistage sampling and area sampling, can be employed to reduce travel costs or to increase efficiency.

Before embarking on a survey, the investigator should estimate the minimum size of the sample needed to answer the question with a specified degree of precision or sampling error. He may find that a survey to detect a rare psychiatric disease or to estimate a population value requires an impractically large number of interviews.

Descriptive Statistics

After the data are collected, they must be summarized or reduced to a manageable and easily comprehended form. Tabulating devices varying in complexity from simple index cards to key-sort cards, electrical sorters and tabulators, and electronic machines (computers) are used, depending on the amount and complexity of the data and the analyses.

Qualitative versus Quantitative Data

Qualitative data deal with enumerative or categorical data, data that are readily divided into discrete groups or categories, such as those with or without a certain characteristic. Data of this type include "yes" or "no" responses, categories of "improved" or "not improved," and classification by sex. The data may be binomially distributed, consisting of only two categories, as in the above examples, or multinomially distributed, consisting of more than two categories, such as data collected in the form "improved," or "no change," or "condition worse."

In quantitative data, also referred to as measurement data, the data are usually continuous. That is, there are an infinite number of points in the measurement of blood pressure, height, weight, hormone output, and so on. Occasionally, the data are discrete. The number of teeth is an example of a discrete quantitative variable. Measurement data, however, can be condensed into qualitative (categorical) form.

It is simpler to describe distributions of qualitative data than of quantitative data. For example, a binomial population can be completely described by only one parameter. That parameter would be the proportion (p) with a certain attribute. The proportion (q) without that attribute is always $(1 - p)$ (see Figure 1).

Populations of quantitative data, on the other hand, may assume any shape. Figure 2 illustrates: (A) a normal or Gaussian population, (B) a symmetrical non-normal population (in this case a bimodal distribution), (E) and (F) a log-normal population (that is, the logarithms of the data are normally distributed), and other skewed populations (C and D).

Most quantitative populations require a minimum of two parameters for adequate description: (1) a measure of central tendency (or average) and (2) a measure of variation or dispersion of individuals around that average.

Measures of Central Tendency

The three most common measures of central tendency are the mean, the mode, and the median (see Figure 2).

The mean is the arithmetic average. For example, the mean of 6, 6, 8, 10, and 15 = 45/5 = 9.

The mode is the most frequent value (point of maximum concentration). In the above example, the mode is 6.

The median is the middle value of data ordered from the lowest to highest. In the above example, the median is 8.

In normally distributed populations the mean, the mode, and the median coincide, as shown in Figure 2A.

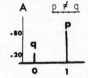

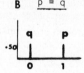

O   Attribute absent

1   Attribute present

FIGURE 1. Binomial populations showing the proportions with an attribute present (p) or not present (q). *A*, The proportion with the attribute is greater than the proportion without the attribute. *B*, The proportion with the attribute and the proportion without the attribute are equal. (From A. K. Bahm, *Basic Medical Statistics*. Grune & Stratton, New York, 1972.)

A. Symmetrical Normal

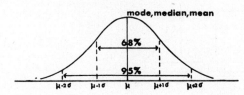

B. Symmetrical Non-Normal [1]
(in this case a bimodal curve)

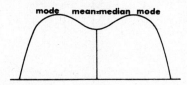

C. Non-Symmetrical with right tail skewness [2]

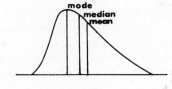

D. Non-Symmetrical with left tail skewness [3]

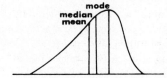

E. Non-Symmetrical Log Normal

F. Transformation of Log Normal

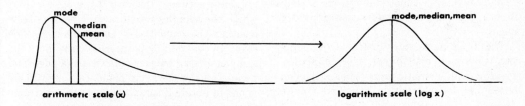

arithmetic scale (x)

logarithmic scale (log x)

[1] The bimodality of this population suggests that it is not homogeneous and should be divided into subgroups for analysis.

[2] Same as positive skewness.

[3] Same as negative skewness.

FIGURE 2. Hypothetical examples of continuous distributions. (From A. K. Bahn, *Basic Medical Statistics*. Grune & Stratton, New York, 1972.)

The mean is generally the most useful measure of central tendency. For skewed populations, however, the mean is misleading, since it is greatly affected by extreme values. In such cases as data on income, size of family, and many biological data, the median is more appropriate.

Measures of Variation

Three common measures of variation are the range, the variance, and the standard deviation.

The range is the difference between the highest and the lowest values. In the above example, the range is 15 minus 6 = 9.

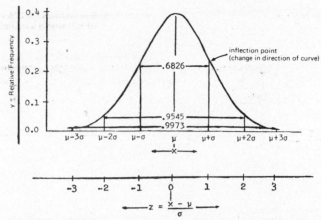

FIGURE 3. The normal frequency distribution and proportionate areas included within various multiples of σ. (From A. K. Bahn, *Basic Medical Statistics*. Grune & Stratton, New York, 1972.)

The variance is the average squared deviation of individual values around the mean value. In the above example, the mean is 9, so the variance is $(6-9)^2 + (6-9)^2 + (8-9)^2 + (10-9)^2 + (15-9)^2 = 56/5 = 11.2$.

The standard deviation (SD) is the square root of the variance. In the above example, the SD is $\sqrt{11.2} = 3.3$.

A principal disadvantage of the range is that it is affected by sample size; it tends to be larger when the sample is larger, since then more extreme observations are likely to be selected. This disadvantage is not found in the SD, since it is a type of average deviation around the mean.

The SD is particularly useful if the population is normally distributed. Then, as shown in Figure 3, characteristic proportions of the population are located within specified standard deviations around the mean. The mean $\pm$ 1 SD includes 68 per cent of the population. The mean $\pm$ 2 SD includes 95 per cent of the population. The mean $\pm$ 3 SD includes 99.7 per cent of the population.

Inferential Statistics

Most knowledge is based on sample observations only. Generalization beyond the sample to the population from which it was drawn is possible only if the sample was selected by appropriate random methods.

With random methods, inference to the population from a sample is possible, since the sample mean is then an unbiased estimate of the population mean, and the sample variance is an unbiased estimate of the population vari-ance. "Unbiased" refers to the fact that the average of all such sample estimates equals the true (population) value. However, any single sample outcome may differ from the true population value just by chance (sampling error).

Null Hypothesis

In the general procedure for significance testing, one sets up a straw man—the null hypothesis—and then determines whether it can be knocked down. One asserts that there is no true difference—that is, the difference is null or zero—between the two populations from which the samples were drawn. One then tests whether this hypothesis holds. That is, one asks: If the null hypothesis is true and the samples were, in fact, drawn from identical populations or the same population, how likely is one to obtain a sample difference as extreme as the one observed or more extreme?

The probability of finding a sample outcome as extreme or more extreme is determined in two steps: (1) Generation of a sampling distribution under the null hypothesis—that is, a distribution of differences between two random samples drawn repeatedly from the same population. This can be done mathematically or experimentally. (2) Location of the observed sample difference on this chance distribution to determine the probability of such an outcome or of one more extreme.

Type I and Type II Errors

One may make an arbitrary a priori decision that, if the probability of a difference as extreme as that observed or more extreme under the null hypothesis is less than 0.05 (P < 0.05), one will reject the null hypothesis, and the difference will be called significant. The arbitrary level of significance chosen a priori (in this case 0.05) is called alpha (α). If the probability (P) is greater than 0.05, one accepts the null hypothesis, and the difference is labeled not significant. In either case, one is at risk of making an error in the decision, depending on the actual situation. A false claim of a true difference is called type I or α error. And falsely accepting the null hypothesis when, in fact, there is a true difference is called type II or β error.

These two error risks are inversely related. The risk of the type I error is established by the a priori level of significance (for example, α = 0.05 or 0.01). The risk of the type II error is more difficult to measure but can be minimized by sufficiently large sample sizes.

Standard Error

Just as the standard deviation of a population indicates how variable individuals are, the standard deviation of a sampling distribution, called a standard error, indicates how variable (reliable) the sample statistic is. Thus, the standard error of the mean (SE$\bar{x}$) is a measure of the variability or error of the sample mean as an estimate of the true mean. Similarly, the standard error of the difference between two sample means is a measure of the variation or error of sample (chance) differences around a true difference of zero. In practical application, the SE is important because it is the denominator of the critical ratio used for significance testing. Therefore, the larger the SE, the smaller is the critical ratio and the less significant the result.

The standard error of the mean (SEM or (SE$\bar{x}$) is obtained by dividing the standard deviation of the population by the square root of the number of individuals in the sample:

$$\text{SEM} = \frac{\text{SD}_{pop}}{\sqrt{n}} \left(\text{or SE}_x = \frac{\sigma_{pop}}{\sqrt{n}} \right)$$

The corresponding formula for the standard error of the proportion is SE$p = \sqrt{\frac{pq}{n}}$.

The size of the standard error of the difference between two sample means (SE$p_1 - x_2$) or two sample proportions (SE$p_1 - p_2$) is directly related to the standard deviation of the population and inversely related to sample sizes.

In any test of significance, one uses a sampling distribution—such as a distribution of the means of many samples drawn from the same universe—under the null hypothesis. One then locates the sample observation on this curve by use of a critical ratio and notes the area in the tails of the distribution. This area indicates the probability (P) of a chance observation as extreme as that observed or of one more extreme if the null hypothesis is true. If the chance observation could occur relatively frequently, such as more than 5 per cent of the time when sample(s) are selected from the same universe, one then says that chance alone could likely explain the outcome, and the difference is declared not significant. On the other hand, if such a chance outcome occurs relatively rarely, one calls the outcome significant.

Tests of significance against a normal distribution of sample outcomes under the null hypothesis are called z tests. The use of the normal distribution requires that the variance of the population be known. This is rarely the situation. Instead, one must estimate the population variance from the sample variance. One then must test against the t distribution. The t distribution is similar to the normal distribution but for small samples has more area in the tails. The t distribution approaches the normal distribution as the size of sample increases. The shape of the t distribution depends on the number of degrees of freedom.

The χ^2 test is an alternative test for evaluating the significance of sample proportions. Most χ^2 tests can be called tests of association because they answer the question: Is there an association between a factor (or attribute) and an outcome? The formula for the χ^2 test is:

$$\chi = \Sigma \, \frac{(\text{observed number} - \text{expected number})^2}{\text{expected number}}$$

The expected number of frequency is usually derived from the sample data under the assumption of the null hypothesis of no true difference between groups.

The χ^2 test can be used for multinomial data —that is, for data classified into more than two categories or for comparing more than two samples. The χ^2 distribution can also be used to test whether a sampling distribution follows some theoretical distribution, such as the normal distribution or the binomial distribution, or a particular population distribution. Such tests are called χ^2 goodness of fit tests.

In the two-sample tests discussed so far, the assumption is made that the samples are independent of each other. This is the situation, for example, when samples of patients from each of two psychiatric wards are compared with each other or when a sample of schizophrenic patients and a sample of manic-depressive patients are compared. The following types of samples, however, are not independent of each other but are most likely correlated: patients and control subjects matched individually on the basis of a large number of variables, such as age, sex, position in the family, and socio-economic status; a sample of patients and a control sample composed of the patients' siblings; before and after measurements on the same persons; and littermates. In these situations, the significance test must take into account the nonindependence of the samples, or pairing.

The advantage of such pairing is that the heterogeneity (or variance) between the two groups is reduced. Because the groups are homogeneous (alike), they tend to differ only in the factor being tested, such as treatment effect. If successful pairing has been carried out, the reduced variance may make it possible to use a smaller sample size to demonstrate a significant difference, if one does exist.

The test for paired data requires a modification of the t test or of the χ^2 test.

Interval Estimation

After one finds that a significant difference exists, one should like to know within what bounds the true difference may lie—that is, the problem is to estimate a confidence interval for the true population value. However, it is also possible to estimate a confidence interval for a population parameter without first conducting a test of significance. In this case, the interval itself is used to perform a significance test.

The sample provides a point estimate that is the most likely value. The interval estimate includes all possible values for the parameter that are consistent with the data at a specified probability or confidence level.

In general, the confidence interval for any true (population) parameter can be constructed from:

Sample value or statistic $\pm$ [(factor)
    $\times$ (standard error of the statistic)]

The factor (such as 1.96 or 2.58) is determined by (1) the level of confidence (95 per cent or 99 per cent) that one wishes to achieve in including the true parameter within the interval estimate and (2) the appropriate sampling statistic (such as z or t).

Two-Variable Analysis

Until now the discussion has been of the analysis of one variable. Regression and correlation are concerned with association among measurements of two variables.

In regression, one variable is considered as the independent (x) (for example, caloric intake) and the other (for example, fasting blood sugar) as the dependent variable (y). If the relationship is that of a straight line, linear regression methods are used to obtain the best estimate of the dependent variable when the independent variable is fixed or is otherwise known. That is, a regression line is fitted to the data by inspection or mathematically.

In correlation neither variable is necessarily assumed to be the independent one. Correlation is used to measure the degree of linear relationship between two variables. Even if a correlation coefficient is large and significant, this does not prove a cause-and-effect relationship. Before a causal relationship is asserted, various alternative interpretations of a high correlation must be ruled out; for example, there may be a spurious correlation, or each variable may be independently related to a common third factor (indirect association). Five criteria may be used for judging the evidence for a causal association: strength of the association, consistency of the association in different places and study groups, temporally correct association, specificity of the association, and coherence with existing knowledge.

Analysis of Variance (ANOVA)

The t test is applicable for the comparison of only two sample means. When more than two sample means are to be compared, it is necessary to use analysis of variance and the F test. The F test for two sample means is equivalent to the t test, since $F = t^2$ and gives identical P values.

In the simplest analysis of variance (ANOVA) model, the over-all variance of an experiment can be partitioned into the variance between treatment groups and the variance within the treatment groups—that is, the variance between means and within means. Each of these variance terms is considered as an independent estimate of the population variance.

If the estimate between treatment groups is significantly greater than that within groups, this suggests that not all the population means (treatment group means) are equal. One can then employ a multicomparison technique to determine which means are significantly different.

Design of Experiments

In evaluating a single-factor intervention, such as treatment with only one drug and a placebo, one may randomly assign half of the subjects to each of two regimens. Alternatively, one arranges the subjects into clinically homogeneous groups, blocks, or pairs of individuals that are considered likely to respond in a similar manner to the intervention. Within such pairs, patients are allocated at random to the treatment or to the placebo. (Or the patient may serve as his own control in a cross-over study).

In the first design, called completely randomized, the unpaired t test may be used. In the second, the randomized block design, the paired t test would be appropriate. Any extension of these models, however, including the cross-over design, or a comparison of the effects of two or more separate treatments and a placebo would require analysis of variance.

If several factors are to be investigated simultaneously, the experiment is multifactorial, and the design and analysis become more complex.

The interaction among the factors also must be examined.

Even though random methods are used for the allocation of patients to groups, by chance these groups may turn out to be significantly different with respect to one or more important variables at the onset. Therefore, to ensure alikeness at the start of the study, the experimenter should always compare the characteristics of the groups before the experiment is begun.

It is often desirable for ethical reasons to test for significance periodically during the course of an experiment. In this way any untoward added hazard experienced by a particular experimental group may be detected. Certain kinds of experiments are particularly suited for sequential tests. Sequential tests also permit termination of an experiment with the minimum number of patients after a significant result has been achieved.

Measures of Disease Frequency and Prognosis

Rate Analysis

Measures of disease frequency are qualitative data in which the number of cases enumerated is related to the denominator or population base in the form of a ratio or rate. There are two major types of morbidity rates: prevalence and incidence.

Prevalence. Suppose that it were possible to conduct a survey in two communities, A and B, and identify all persons who meet the diagnostic

Point prevalence as of January 1, 1970

$$A: \frac{30 \text{ cases}}{6{,}000 \text{ persons in population}} = 5.0 \text{ cases per } 1{,}000 \text{ population} \qquad B: \frac{40 \text{ cases}}{10{,}000 \text{ persons in population}} = 4.0 \text{ cases per } 1{,}000 \text{ population}$$

$$\text{Point prevalence} = \frac{\text{number of existing cases of schizophrenia}}{\text{population}} \text{ at a point in time}$$

FIGURE 4. Prevalence rate of schizophrenia in two communities at a given point in time.

Incidence rate during 1970

$$A: \frac{10 \text{ cases}}{5{,}970 \text{ persons}} = 1.7 \text{ cases per } 1{,}000 \text{ persons} \qquad B: \frac{25 \text{ cases}}{9{,}960 \text{ persons}} = 2.5 \text{ cases per } 1{,}000$$

$$\text{Incidence rate} = \frac{\text{number of new cases of schizophrenia}}{\text{population at risk}} \text{ over a period of time.}$$

FIGURE 5. Incidence rate of schizophrenia in two communities over a period of time.

criteria for schizophrenia. Suppose, further, that 30 persons in A and 40 persons in B meet these criteria. Although the number of schizophrenics is of interest, comparison of the two communities requires that one relate the number of cases to the number of persons in the population (denominator) in the form of a prevalence rate. Thus, in Figure 4, although B has numerically more cases, A has the higher (point) prevalence rate.

Other prevalence measures may be used, such as (1) period prevalence—cases existing during a period of time, such as a year, instead of on one day—and (2) lifetime prevalence—patients who have ever been ill at any time in their lives.

Incidence. The prevalence rate does not answer the question: What is the risk of developing schizophrenia? That answer requires an incidence rate, the number of new cases per 1,000 persons.

The incidence rate includes in the numerator only cases that have occurred for the first time during some defined period, such as one year, and includes in the denominator only those persons who do not already have the disease and, therefore, are at risk of developing it.

In Figures 4 and 5, one sees that, although A has the higher point prevalence rate, B has the higher incidence rate—that is, persons in B appear to be at greater risk of developing the disease than do persons in A.

Incidence indicates the rate at which new illnesses occur, whereas prevalence measures the residual of such illness, the amount existing at a point in time.

Adjusted Rates. Suppose the age composition of the two communities were markedly different, with B having relatively more persons in the ages 15 to 44, when the risk of developing schizophrenia is greatest. One needs an age-adjusted total rate, in which the difference in age composition between the two populations has been removed. Similar adjustments could be made for differences in sex distribution and in other characteristics, but differences in age are usually the most important. Two methods of age adjustments are used.

Direct Age Adjustment. A common age-structured population is used as the standard to which are applied the observed age-specific rates in A and B. One thus derives expected cases at each age. The resulting adjusted total rates reflect solely the difference in observed age-specific rates.

Indirect Age Adjustment. The expected cases are obtained by applying the more stable age-specific rates of the larger (standard) population to the age structure of the smaller population. The result yields a ratio of observed to expected cases known as the standard morbidity ratio (SMR):

Standard morbidity ratio
$$= \frac{\text{observed cases in a population}}{\text{expected cases in a population}}$$

A comparable adjustment for death rates is called the standard mortality ratio.

Cohort Analysis

In the study of the prognosis of chronic diseases, such as schizophrenia, the long time that patients must be kept under observation may result in the attrition of cases from loss to follow-up or migration. Outcome rates are, therefore, difficult to derive, and special analytical techniques, such as the cohort life table, are necessary. This technique makes maximal use, without bias, of all available information on persons followed for unequal periods of observation.

REFERENCES

Bahn, A. K. Some methodologic issues in psychiatric epidemiology and some suggested approaches. In, *Psychiatric Epidemiology and Mental Health Planning*, R. Monroe, G. D. Klee, and E. Brody, editors, p. 69, Psychiatric Research Report 22. American Psychiatric Association, Washington, 1967.

Bahn, A. K. *Basic Medical Statistics.* Grune & Stratton, New York, 1972.

Kramer, M., Pollack, E. S., Redick, R., and Locke, B. Z. *Mental Disorders: Suicide.* Vital and Health Statistics Monographs, American Public Health Association, Harvard University Press, Cambridge, Mass., 1972.

Mausner, J. A., and Bahn, A. K. *Epidemiology: An Introductory Text.* W. B. Saunders, Philadelphia, 1974.

Snedecor, G. W., and Cochran, W. G. *Statistical Methods*, ed. 6. Iowa State University Press, Ames, 1971.

World Health Organization. *Statistical Principles in Public Health Field Studies*, Technical Report Series No. 510. Fifteenth Report of the WHO Expert Committee on Health Statistics. World Health Organization, Geneva, 1972.

6

Theories of Personality and Psychopathology: Freudian Schools

6.1. SIGMUND FREUD AND CLASSICAL PSYCHOANALYSIS

Introduction

Psychoanalytic concepts have so widely permeated the training and practice of modern psychiatry that they have come to be regarded as a fundamental part of the understanding and approach to mental and emotional disorders. One cannot, therefore, understate the importance of a clear understanding of psychoanalytic theory in an approach to mental illness and, particularly, an understanding of the basic contributions of the founder of psychoanalysis, Sigmund Freud (see Figure 1).

Psychoanalysis had undergone a continual remodeling and reorganizing of its basic concepts at almost every step of its progress. The ferment of rethinking and recasting was a dynamic manifestation of Freud's own struggles in bringing understanding to his ever-growing clinical experience. Since his passing from the scene, the struggle has continued.

The basic investigative tool of classical psychoanalysis is free association. The psychoanalyst does not deliberately undertake to elicit specific information from his patient on any sort of organized plan. Rather, the psychoanalyst seeks to enable his patient to present verbal expressions of his own inner experiences and mental processes as spontaneously and in as completely uncensored a way as is possible.

Freud's Early Years

Freud was a convinced empirical scientist of his era. His early training was in the best scientific centers of his time. Consequently, he brought to his study of psychological processes a

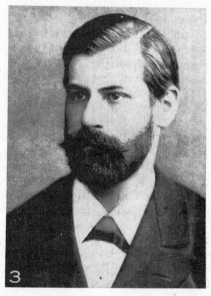

FIGURE 1. Sigmund Freud as a young man. (Austrian Information Service, New York, N. Y.)

strong belief that scientific law and order would ultimately permit an understanding of the apparent chaos of mental processes. He believed that brain physiology was the definitive scientific approach to this objective. Even though, in

227

the course of his experience, Freud had to modify and mitigate that basic scientific credo, he nonetheless maintained it throughout his long career.

Formative Influences

One of the most significant influences on Freud's theories came from the Helmholtz school of physiology. It stated that all processes were determined by causal laws and sequences. Scientific laws, it held, could ultimately be reduced to the laws of physics.

Freud's neurological training and his experience in neurological research were also important influences. His neurological background allowed him to understand psychological functioning in terms of a series of organizations, which were hierarchically and topographically superimposed on each other. It also influenced his conception of the nervous system as composed of associative networks that were organized in terms of contiguity on one level but also more fundamentally by drive influences. Also from this source came his basic approach to the understanding of neurodynamics in terms of the dynamics of the nervous system. Even when forced to abandon this point of view, he maintained the assumption in the form of a belief that psychodynamics could ultimately be placed on a more solid footing by an understanding of neurochemical or biochemical processes.

Another important influence in his thinking was the Darwinian heritage. Darwin's influence was reflected in the genetic aspects of Freud's own thinking particularly in his concern for the relationship between phylogenesis and ontogenesis. Other important scientific influences came from the work of the psychologist Herbart and also, to a lesser extent, from Hering.

Another considerable influence was Freud's immersion in and intense fascination with literature, particularly with the works of Shakespeare and Goethe. It was Freud's readiness and capacity for discerning the meaning behind meaning and for unraveling the symbolic dimension of human cognitive functioning that laid the cornerstone for that aspect of psychoanalysis that is perhaps most characteristic of it, the mephasis on symbolic interpretation. Related to this influence is Freud's rooting in the Jewish tradition. And one must also remember that Freud lived for most of his life in Victorian Vienna, where an emphasis on sexual conflicts and vicissitudes was a pervasive element.

Freud's Career

Sigmund Freud was born on May 6, 1856, in the small Moravian town of Freiburg. The territory has since been incorporated as part of Czechoslovakia. His father was a Jewish wool merchant who enjoyed moderate financial success. When Sigmund was 4 years old, the family moved to Vienna, where his life and career were centered. He was forced to flee to England in the face of the impending Nazi persecution in 1938. He died in 1939 (see Figures 2–6).

Medical Training. Freud's education followed a somewhat erratic course, with the result that it took him nearly 3 years longer than the average medical student of his day to earn his medical degree. It was during this period that the work of Darwin and his associates in biology and the physiological and physical investigations on the part of Helmholtz and his school were producing a new and vigorous scientific climate. Freud became a dedicated and convinced adherent of the new empiricism.

During these years of medical study, Freud worked in the physiological laboratory of Ernst Brücke, who was one of the founders of the Helmholtz school of medicine. Helmholtz postulated that the only forces active in biological organisms were reducible to the physical chemical forces inherent in matter and were reducible to the forces of attraction and repulsion. Freud was strongly influenced by these basic principles, and even more particularly by the man Brücke himself, who seemed to embody the qualities Freud most admired—a capacity for scientific discipline and complete intellectual integrity.

The other figure who dominated Freud's early scientific world was Theodor Meynert. Freud was also strongly influenced by, even though somewhat competitive with, Sigmund Exner, who also worked in Brücke's laboratory.

Medical Career. Freud continued to work in Brücke's laboratory for a year after he graduated from medical school. His experience in Brücke's laboratory allowed him to develop the physiological framework that played a prominent role in the casting of his psychological theories.

During the year Freud spent in Brücke's institution, his attention was primarily directed

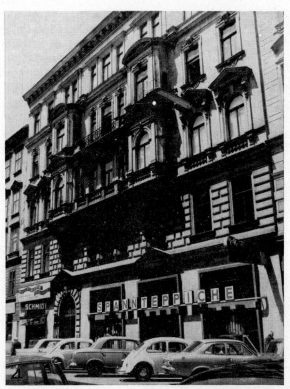

FIGURE 2. Berggasse 19, the building in which Freud had his offices and which now houses the Freud Museum. (Austrian Information Service, New York, N. Y.)

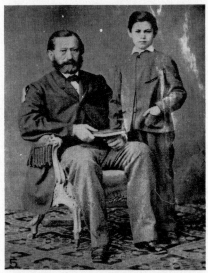

FIGURE 3. Sigmund Freud and his father. (Austrian Information Service, New York, N. Y.)

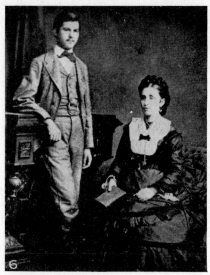

FIGURE 4. Sigmund Freud and his mother in 1872. (Austrian Information Service, New York, N. Y.)

to neurological and neuroanatomical research. Freud found painstaking research work much to his liking and was ambitious to continue it, but financial considerations made this course in- creasingly difficult. In the meanwhile, he be- came enamored of Martha Bernays, and the prospects of marriage and family pressed them- selves on him. He left Brücke's laboratory in

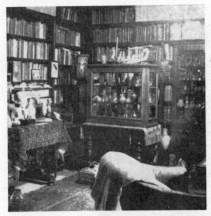

FIGURE 5. Sigmund Freud's office in Vienna. (Austrian Information Service, New York, N. Y.)

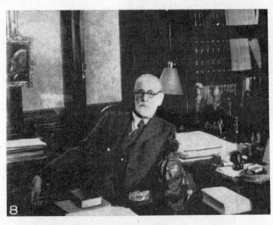

FIGURE 6. Sigmund Freud at his desk in his Vienna office. (Austrian Information Service, New York, N. Y.)

1882 to begin work as a general physician in the Vienna General Hospital.

He served first on the surgical service and later in Theodor Meynert's psychiatric clinic. Meynert had the reputation of being the most prominent brain anatomist of his time. Freud's study of Meynert's amentia (acute hallucinatory psychosis) undoubtedly made a vivid impression on him and contributed to his own views on wish fulfillment, which later became a basic part of Freud's own theory of the unconscious.

On Meynert's service, Freud's neurological knowledge of brain disorders grew by leaps and bounds. He obtained permission from Meynert to use his laboratory for an extensive study of neonatal brain disorders. In 1885 he received a traveling grant that allowed him to visit Paris, where he studied for about 19 weeks in the neurological clinic of the French neurologist Jean-Martin Charcot in the Salpêtrière, the famous French hospital (see Figure 7). During his experience in Charcot's clinic, Freud was exposed to a fascinating variety of neurological syndromes and to the charismatic personality of Charcot himself. Under Charcot's influence, Freud became deeply interested in the problem of hysteria and became firmly convinced that hysterical phenomena were a genuine form of pathology worthy of careful study and understanding.

Charcot himself had not undertaken any psychological explanation of hysterical phenomena. However, the possibility that hysterical phenomena were psychological in origin was suggested to Freud by the fact that Charcot was able to precipitate and reproduce hysterical paralyses, seizures, and other characteristic hysterical manifestations through the use of hypnotic suggestion.

Charcot firmly believed that the ultimate basis of hysteria was neurological, and he attributed it specifically to a congenital degeneration of the brain. But he also held that the form of the symptoms manifested in hysterical seizures was psychogenic in origin—that is, symptoms were produced by specific ideas in the patient's mind. By the same token, he believed that hysterical symptoms could be cured by ideas. It was probably under the influence of Charcot that Freud began to suspect the connection between hysterical pathology and sexuality. The use of hypnosis in the study of hysteria was to provide one the most significant points of origin for psychoanalysis.

Liébault, a French country doctor in Nancy, used hypnotic induction to relieve the neurotic symptoms of large masses of peasants. The technique was basically one of hypnotic suggestion. Freud became particularly interested in the work of Hippolyte Bernheim, who was associated with Liébault in the use of hypnosis as a therapeutic technique. Bernheim concluded that suggestibility could be identified in patients with a wide variety of neurotic disorders, as well as in normal persons.

Freud spent several weeks during the summer of 1889 studying in Liébault's clinic in Nancy. He was profoundly impressed by the relationship that Liébault was able to establish with his patients and by the effects Bernheim was able

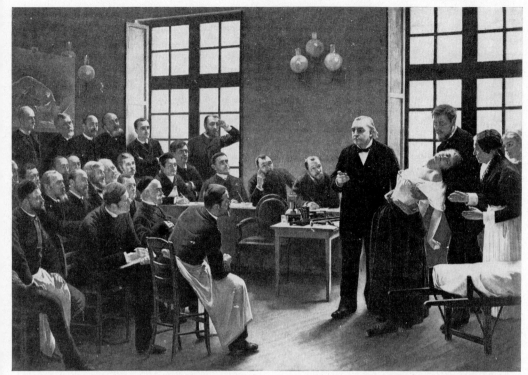

FIGURE 7. A clinical lecture by Jean Charcot at the Salpêtrière. (Culver Pictures, New York, N. Y.)

to produce in hospitalized patients through the use of hypnotic suggestion. Freud, became profoundly impressed by the possibility that mental events may take place outside of the range of consciousness and may have powerful effects on human behavior and psychopathology.

Beginnings of Psychoanalysis

From 1887 to 1897, the period in which Freud began to study seriously the disturbances of his hysterical patients, psychoanalysis can be said to have taken root. These slender beginnings had a three-fold aspect: the emergence of psychoanalysis as a method of investigation, as a therapeutic technique, and as a body of scientific knowledge based on an increasing fund of information and basic theoretical propositions. These early researches flowed out of Freud's initial collaboration with Joesph Breuer and then increasingly out of his own independent investigations and theoretical developments.

The Case of Anna O.

Perhaps the decisive influence that drew Freud toward the study of psychopathology came from Joesph Breuer, a distinguished and

established practitioner in the Viennese community. Knowing of Freud's interests in hysterical pathology, Breuer told him about an unusual case of a woman he had treated from December 1880 to June 1882.

Anna O.—in reality, Bertha Pappenheim—was an intelligent and strong-minded woman of about 21 years of age who had developed a number of hysterical symptoms in connection with the illness and death of her father. These symptoms included paralysis of the limbs, contractures, anesthesias, visual disturbances, disturbances of speech, anorexia, and a distressing nervous cough. Her illness was also characterized by two distinct phases of consciousness: one was relatively normal, but in the other she seemed to assume a second and more pathological personality. The transition between these two states seemed to be brought about by a form of autohypnosis. Breuer became able to manipulate the transition between these two states by placing her in a hypnotic state.

Anna had been very close to and very fond of her father. She and her mother had shared the duties of nursing him on his death bed. During her altered states of consciousness, she was able to recall the vivid fantasies and intense emotions she had experienced while nursing her father. When she was able to recall, with the associated expression of affect, the scenes or circumstances under which her symptoms had arisen, the symptoms could be made to disappear. Anna described this process as the "talking cure," also calling it "chimney sweeping." Once the connection between talking through the circumstances of the symptoms and the disappearance of the symptoms themselves had been established, Anna proceeded to deal with each of her many symptoms, one after another.

In the course of the somewhat lengthy treatment of Anna O., Breuer had become increasingly preoccupied with his fascinating and unusual patient, and his wife had grown increasingly jealous and resentful. As soon as Breuer began to realize this, the sexual connotations of it frightened him, and he abruptly terminated the treatment. Only a few hours later, however, he was recalled urgently to Anna's bedside. He had felt that she was greatly improved as a result of the treatment, but he found her in a stage of acute excitement. She had never alluded to the forbidden topic of sex during the course of her treatment, but she was now experiencing hysterical childbirth. The phantom pregnancy was the logical termination of the sexual feelings she had developed toward Breuer in response to his therapeutic efforts. He had been quite unaware of this development, and the experience was quite unnerving to him. He was able to calm Anna down by hypnotizing her, but then he left the house in a cold sweat and immediately set out with his wife for Venice on a second honeymoon.

Studies on Hysteria

The collaboration with Breuer finally brought about the publication of the "Preliminary Communication" in 1893. Essentially, Freud and Breuer extended Charcot's concept of traumatic hysteria to a general doctrine of hysteria. Hysterical symptoms were related to determined psychic traumata, sometimes clearly and directly and sometimes symbolically.

The authors observed that individual hysterical symptoms seemed to immediately disappear when the event that provoked them was clearly brought to life and the patient was able to describe the event in great detail and put the accompanying affect into words. The basis of hysteria was described as a state of dissociated consciousness.

The "Preliminary Communication" was followed in 1895 by the *Studies on Hysteria*, in which Breuer and Freud reported on their clinical experience in the treatment of hysteria and proposed a theory of hysterical phenomena. The volume included the "Preliminary Communication," a report by Breuer of his work with Anna O., a series of cases reported by Freud, a lengthy theoretical section written by Breuer, and, finally, a section on the psychotherapy of hysteria, which was contributed by Freud.

Out of his cases, Freud constructed the following sequence of steps in the development of hysteria:

1. The patient has undergone a traumatic experience, one that stirred up intense emotion and excitation and that was intensely painful or disagreeable to the patient.

2. The traumatic experience represented to the patient some idea or ideas that were incompatible with the dominant mass of ideas constituting the ego.

3. This incompatible idea was intentionally dissociated or repressed from consciousness.

4. The excitation associated with the incompatible idea was converted into somatic pathways and resulted in the hysterical manifestations and symptoms.

5. What is left in consciousness is merely a mnemonic symbol that is connected with the traumatic event only by associative links, which are frequently disguised links.

6. If the memory of the traumatic experience can be brought into consciousness and if the patient is able to release the strangulated affect associated with it, the affect is discharged, and the symptoms disappear.

Technical Evolution

Freud began to use hypnosis intensively in treating his patients when he opened his own practice in 1887. In the beginning, his use of hypnosis was primarily as a means of getting the patient to rid himself of his symptoms by means of hypnotic suggestion. It was soon obvious, however, that, even though the patient responsed to hypnotic suggestion and acted, under hypnosis, as if the symptoms did not exist, the symptoms asserted themselves during the patient's waking experience.

By 1889, Freud was sufficiently intrigued by Breuer's cathartic method to attempt to use it in conjunction with hypnotic techniques as a means of retracing the histories of neurotic symptoms, as Breuer had done with Anna O. The first time he used Breuer's method was in his treatment of Emmy von N. The goal of treatment was restricted to a removal of symptoms through the recovery and verbalization of suppressed feelings with which the symptoms were associated. This procedure has since been described as abreaction.

Once again, however, the beneficial effects of the hypnotic treatment seemed to be effective only as long as the patient remained in contact with the physician. Freud suspected that the alleviation of symptoms was, in fact, dependent in some manner on the personal relationship between the patient and the physician. In his account of Emmy von N., Freud had begun to feel that inhibited sexuality may have played a role in the production of the patient's symptoms. Freud's suspicion of a sexual aspect in the treatment of such patients was amply confirmed one day when a patient awoke from a hypnotic sleep and suddenly threw her arms around his neck. Freud suddenly found himself in the same position that Breuer had found himself in during his earlier treatment of Anna O. Perhaps bolstered by Breuer's experience and apparently able to learn from it, Freud did not panic or retreat in the face of this sexual advance. Rather, he was able to treat this phenomenon as a scientific observation.

Freud began to understand that the therapeutic effectiveness of the patient-physician relationship, which had seemed so mystifying and problematical, could be attributed to its erotic basis. These observations were to become the basis of the theory of transference, which he later developed into an explicit theory of treatment. In any event, these experiences served to reinforce his dissatisfaction with hypnotic techniques. Freud felt that a cure that did not involve some understanding on the part of the patient of the origins and significance of symptoms and that did not base itself on some more scientific approach to the problem could not be expected to be a reliable cure but was, at best, only a temporary expedient.

In addition, Freud had discovered that many patients were refractory to hypnosis. Only gradually did he recognize that what seemed to be his inability to hypnotize a patient might be due to a patient's reluctance to remember traumatic events. He was later able to identify this reluctance as resistance.

Concentrations. Bernheim had observed that, although certain experiences appeared to be forgotten, they could be recalled under hypnosis and then recalled consciously·if the physician asked the patient leading questions and urged him to produce these critical memories. In Freud's method of concentration, the patient was asked to lie down on a couch and to close his eyes. He was then instructed to concentrate on a particular symptom and to recall the memories associated with it. Freud would press his hand on the patient's forehead and urge him to recall the unavailable memories.

Free Association. Elizabeth von R., one of Freud's patients, remarked that she had not expressed her thoughts because she was not sure what he was expecting to hear. This observation made him realize the extent to which his interventions had been a form of suggestion akin to the basic suggestion involved in the hypnotic technique. Freud decided that he would not try to direct the patient's thinking but would, instead, encourage her to express every idea that occurred to her mind, no matter how insignificant, irrelevant, shameful, or embarrassing it might seem to her, ignoring all censorship and suspending all judgment.

Moreover, she complained that Freud's continual attempts to question her and to push her to respond only served to interrupt her train of thought. She even found his somewhat magical and suggestive technique of pressing his hand against her forehead a distraction.

By the end of the century, Freud had more or less established his free association technique. In *The Interpretation of Dreams*, he describes it in the following terms.

This involves some psychological preparation of the patient. We must aim at bringing about two changes in him: an increase in the attention he pays to his own psychial perceptions, and the elimination of the criticism by which he normally shifts the thoughts that occur to him. In order that he may be able to concentrate his attention on his self-observation, it is an advantage for him to lie in a restful attitude and to shut his eyes. It is necessary to insist explicitly on his renouncing all criticism of the thoughts that he perceives. We therefore tell him that the success of the psychoanalysis depends on his noticing and reporting whatever comes into his head and not being misled, for instance, in suppressing an idea because it strikes him as unimportant or irrelevant or because it seems to him meaningless. He must adopt a completely impartial attitude to what occurs to him, since it is precisely his critical attitude which is responsible for his being unable in the ordinary course of things to achieve the desired unraveling of his dream or obsessional idea, or whatever it may be.

Theoretical Innovations

Causes of Hysteria. Freud felt that the basic causes of neurosis had to be located in sexual factors. Usually, the neurotic picture was mixed, and the purer forms of either hysterical or obsessional neurosis were relatively rare. Freud did not regard all hysterical symptoms as psychogenic in origin, and he felt they could not all be effectively treated by a psychotherapeutic procedure. He found that a significant number of patients could not be hyponized, even when the diagnosis of hysteria seemed to be clearly established. In these cases, Freud felt that he had to overcome a certain psychic force in the patient that was set in opposition to any attempt to bring the pathogenic idea into consciousness.

The pathogenic idea, despite the force of resistance, could be reached by relatively easily accessible associations. The patient seemed to be able to get rid of such an idea by verbally describing it. Freud discovered that the patient's train of memories extended well beyond the traumatic events that were responsible for precipitating the onset of illness. Indeed, he found that his patients were able to produce the memories of childhood experiences, events, and scenes that had long been lost to memory. This finding led Freud to the conclusion that such memories had frequently been inhibited because they involved sexual experiences or other incidents in the patient's life that seemed painful.

The recollection of such experiences could evoke intense affects of agitation, moral conflict, self-reproach, remorse, fear of punishment, and guilt. Freud concluded that, since these childhood experiences retained such a vivid quality, they must exert a predisposing influence on the development of neurotic manifestations.

Freud did not abandon the congenital point of view—namely, that heredity must be accorded a major role as a predisposing factor to neurosis. However, he postulated that hysteria can also be acquired. Even further, he postulated that emotionally disturbing experiences can play a major causative role in acquired hysteria, in which the hereditary factors seem to be of minor importance.

Resistance. Freud discovered that his patients were often quite unwilling or unable to recall traumatic memories. He defined this reluctance as resistance. As his clinical experience expanded, he found that, in the majority of patients he treated, resistance was not a matter of reluctance to cooperate. Frequently, the patients who were most distressed by their symptoms seemed most hampered in treatment by the presence of resistance. Freud's conclusion was that resistance was a matter of the operation of active forces in the mind, of which the patients themselves were often quite unaware and which resulted in the exclusion from consciousness of painful or distressing material. Freud described the active force that worked to exclude particular mental contents from conscious awareness as repression.

Repression. Freud described the mechanism of repression in the following terms: A traumatic experience or a series of experiences, usually of a sexual nature and often occurring in childhood, had been forgotten or repressed because of their painful or disagreeable nature. But the excitation involved in the sexual stimulation was not extinguished, and traces of it persisted in the unconscious in the form of repressed memories. These memories could remain without pathogenic effect until some contemporary event—for example, a disturbing love affair—revived them. At this juncture, the strength of the repressive counterforce was diminished, and the patient experienced what Freud termed "the return of the repressed." The original sexual excitement is revived and finds its way by a new path, which allows it to manifest itself in the form of a neurotic symptom. Repression and the return of the repressed are conceived of in terms of conflicting forces—the force of the repressed idea struggling to express itself against the counterforce of the ego seeking to keep the repressed idea out of consciousness.

Infantile Sexuality. Invariably, in digging into the past histories of his hysterical patients, Freud found that the repressed traumatic memories that seemed to lie at the root of the pathology had to do with sexual experiences. His attention became increasingly focused on the importance of these early sexual experiences, usually recalled in the form of a sexual seduction occurring before puberty and often rather early in the child's experience.

Freud took literally the accounts his patients gave him in the form of forgotten but revived memories of sexual involvements. The patients provided him with tales of outrage committed by fathers, nursemaids, and uncles. But little by little he began to have second thoughts about these so-called memories. He had gained additional insight into the nature of pathological processes as a result of his clinical experience and his increasing awareness of the role of fantasy in childhood. And he found it hard to believe that there could be so many wicked and seductive adults in Viennese society.

While he was attempting to come to terms with the subjective experience of his patients, Freud found himself drawn to look inward and to find within himself the reflections of what he had been able to identify in his patients. He began, therefore, the laborious process of his own self-analysis. He was able to survey his own history, to revive repressed memories from quite early levels of his childhood experience, and, particularly, to focus his attention on the content of dreams. As this self analysis progressed, Freud began to have more and more reason to call the seduction hypothesis into question.

The abandonment of the seduction hypothesis, with its reliance on actual physical seduction, forced Freud to turn with new realization to the inner fantasy life of the child. What emerged from this shift in direction was a dynamic theory of infantile sexuality, in which the child's own psychosexual life played the significant and dominant role.

The Interpretation of Dreams

Freud became aware of the significance of dreams when he realized that, in the process of free association, his patients frequently reported their dreams. He discovered that dreams had a definite meaning, though that meaning was often hidden and disguised. Moreover, Freud found that, when he encouraged his patients to associate freely to the dream fragments, what they reported was frequently more productive of pertinent, repressed material than the associations to events of their waking experience.

The data derived from Freud's clinical exploration of his patients' dreams and the profound insights derived from his investigation of his own personal dreams was distilled into the landmark publication in 1900 of *The Interpretation of Dreams*. Freud presented a theory of the dream that paralleled his analysis of neurotic symptoms. The dream was viewed as a conscious expression of an unconscious fantasy or wish that is not readily accessible to conscious waking experience. Thus, dream activity was considered a normal manifestation of unconscious processes.

Freud felt that the dreaming experience of any normal person in sleep bore a significant resemblance to the pathological conscious organization of the thought processes in psychotic patients. The dream images represented the unconscious wishes or thoughts disguised through a process of symbolization and other distorting mechanisms.

Analysis of Dream Content

Freud's view of the dream material was that the content had been repressed or excluded from consciousness by the defensive activities of the ego. The dream material, as it is consciously recalled by the dreamer, is simply the end result of the unconscious mental activity that takes place during sleep. Freud felt that the upsurge of unconscious material was so intense that it threatened to interrupt sleep itself. Instead of being awakened by these ideas, the sleeper dreams. Freud regarded the conscious experience of such thoughts during sleep as dreaming.

The manifest dream, which embodies the experienced content of the dream and which the sleeper may or may not be able to recall after waking, is the product of the dream activity. The unconscious thoughts and wishes that, in Freud's view, threaten to awaken the sleeper are described as the latent dream content. Freud referred to the unconscious mental operations by which the latent dream content is transformed into the manifest dream as the dream work. In the process of dream interpretation, Freud was able to move from the manifest content of the dream by way of associative exploration to arrive at the latent dream content, which lies behind the manifest dream and which provides it with its core meaning.

In Freud's view, a variety of stimuli initiated dreaming activity—nocturnal sensory stimuli, day residues, and repressed infantile drives. Contemporary understanding of the dream process, however, suggests that dreaming activity takes place more or less in conjunction with the psychic patterns of central nervous system activation that characterize certain phases of the sleep cycle. What Freud thought to be initiating stimuli may, in fact, be incorporated into the dream content.

Significance of Dreams

The study of dreams and the process of their formation became the primary route by which Freud gained access to the understanding of unconscious processes and their operation. He maintained that every dream somehow represents a wish fulfillment, a form of gratification of an unconscious instinctual impulse in fantasy form. In the state of suspended motility and regressive relaxation induced by the sleep state, the dream permits a partial and less dangerous gratification of the instinctual impulse.

Dream Work

The theory of dream work became the fundamental description of the operation of unconscious processes. Unconscious instinctual impulses that were continually pushing for discharge had been repressed because of their unacceptable or painful nature. These impulses had to be attached to neutral or innocent images to be allowed into conscious expression. This was made possible by selecting apparently trivial or insignificant images from the residues of the dreamer's current psychological experience and linking these trivial images dynamically with the latent unconscious images, presumably on the basis of some resemblance that allowed the associative links to be established. The dream work used a variety of mechanisms, including symbolism, displacement, condensation, projection, and secondary revision (see Figure 8).

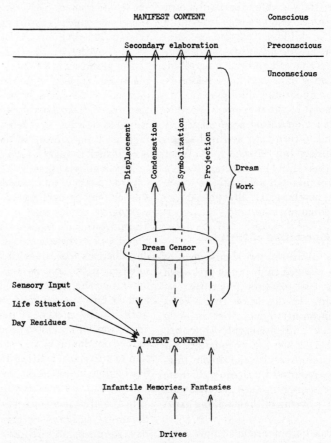

FIGURE 8. The dream process, as explained by Freud. (Modified from H. Ellenberger, *The Discovery of the Unconscious*, p. 491, Basic Books, New York, 1970.)

Symbolism is a complex process of indirect representation. The symbol is a manifest expression of an idea that is more or less hidden or secret. Freud discovered that the ideas or objects represented in this way were highly charged with inappropriate feelings and burdened with conflict. The forbidden meanings of these symbols remained unconscious. Although the symbol disguises what is unacceptable, it can also offer partial gratification of underlying wishes or can signify, and thus partially retain, lost objects.

Displacement refers to the transfer of energy from an original object to a substitute or symbolic representation of the object. Because the substitute object is relatively neutral, it can pass the borders of repression more easily. Whereas symbolism can be taken to refer to the substitution of one object for another, displacement facilitates the distortion of unconscious wishes through the transfer of affective energy from one object to another. For example, the mother may be represented visually by an unknown female figure or, at least, by one who has less emotional significance for the dreamer, but the naked content of the dream continues to derive from the dreamer's unconscious instinctual impulses toward the mother.

Condensation is the mechanism by which several unconscious wishes, impulses, or attitudes can be combined and attached to a single image in the manifest dream content. In a child's nightmare, an attacking monster may come to represent not only the dreamer's father but also some aspects of the mother and even some of his own primitive hostile impulses.

Projection allows the dreamer to perceive his own unacceptable wishes or impulses as emanating in the dream from another person or independent source. The figure to whom these unacceptable impulses are ascribed in the dream often turns out to be the figure toward whom the dreamer's own unconscious impulses are directed. For example, the man who has a strong repressed wish to be unfaithful to his wife may dream that his wife has been unfaithful to him.

Secondary revision uses intellectual processes that closely resemble organized thought processes governing states of consciousness. Through the process of secondary revision, logical mental operations are introduced into and modify dream work.

Repressed emotions may not appear in the manifest dream content at all or may be experienced in a considerably altered form. For example, repressed hostility or hatred toward another person may be modified into a feeling of annoyance or mild irritation in the manifest dream expression, or it may even be represented by an awareness of not being annoyed, a conversion of the affect into its absence. Or the latent affect may be directly transformed into an opposite in the manifest content, as when a repressed longing is represented by a manifest repugnance.

Symbol formation, displacement, condensation, projection, and secondary revision serve a dual purpose. They facilitate the discharge of unconscious drive impulses, and they are primitive defense mechanisms that prevent the direct discharge of instinctual drives. They thereby protect the dreamer from an excessive discharge of unconscious impulses and from the excessive anxiety and pain that accompany it. However, if an element of the latent dream content has succeeded in forcing its way into the manifest dream content in a form that is too direct, too little disguised, and too readily recognized for the ego to tolerate it, the ego reacts to this direct expression of repressed impulses with anxiety.

In the punishment dream, the ego anticipates a condemnation on the part of the superego (conscience) if repressed impulses find direct expression in the manifest dream content. The demands of the superego for punishment are satisfied in the dream content by giving expression to punishment fantasies.

Topographic Theory

Freud's thinking about the mental apparatus in 1900 was based on the classification of mental operations and contents according to regions or systems in the mind. These systems were specified in terms of their relationship to consciousness. Any mental event that occurred outside of conscious awareness and that could not be made conscious by the effort of focusing attention was said to belong to the deepest regions of the mind, the unconscious region or system. Mental events that could be brought to conscious awareness through an act of attention were said to be preconscious. The mental events that occurred in conscious awareness were regarded as belonging to the perceptual consciousness system and were conceived of as located on the surface of the mind.

The topographic model has essentially fallen into disuse in terms of its utility as a working model of psychoanalytic processes, largely because it has been surpassed and supplanted by the structural theory. However, the topographic viewpoint is still useful in terms of descriptively classifying mental events in terms of the quality and degree of awareness.

Freud conceived of the psychic apparatus in the context of the topographic model as a kind of reflex arc, in which the various segments have a spatial relationship. The arc consisted of a perceptual or sensory end, through which impressions were received; an intermediate region, consisting of a storehouse of unconscious memories; and a motor end, closely associated with the preconscious, through which instinctual discharge could occur. In early childhood, perceptions were modified and stored in the form of memories.

According to this theory, the mental energy associated with unconscious ideas seeks discharge through thought or motor activity in ordinary walking life, moving from the perceptual end to the motor end. However, under certain conditions, such as external frustration or sleep, the direction in which the energy travels along the arc is reversed, and it moves from the motor end to the perceptual end. It thereby reanimates childhood impressions in their earlier perceptual forms and results in dreams during sleep or hallucinations in mental disorders. Although Freud subsequently abandoned this model of the mind as a reflex arc, the central concept of regression was retained and applied later in a somewhat modified form in the theory of neurosis.

Instinct Theory

Freud regarded the sexual instinct as a psychophysiological process that has both mental and physiological manifestations. He used the term "libido" to refer to "that force by which the sexual instinct is represented in the mind."

Freud recognized early that the sexual instinct does not originate in a finished form, as represented by the stage of genital primacy. Rather, it undergoes a complete process of development, at each phase of which the libido has specific aims and objects that diverge in varying degrees from the simple aim of genital union. The libido theory came to include the investigation of all these manifestations and the complicated paths they follow in the course of psychosexual development.

Infantile Sexuality

Freud had become convinced of the relationship between sexual trauma and disturbances of sexual functioning. He originally viewed these conditions as related to the misuse of sexual function.

As his clinical experience increased, Freud was able to reconstruct the early sexual experiences and fantasies of his patients. These data provided the framework for a developmental theory of childhood sexuality. Perhaps an even more important source of information was his own self-analysis, which he had begun in 1897. The realization of the operation of infantile sexual longings in his own experience suggested to Freud that these phenomena might not be restricted to the pathological development of neurosis but that essentially normal persons may undergo similar developmental experiences.

Freud used the term "sexuality" in a more or less familiar sense to refer to the erotic life of the person, but he also extended the general concept to include those sensations and activities that could be described as sensual, in the sense that they are a source of pleasure and gratification but are not generally considered as sexual. Freud was able to show, in terms of levels of development, the connection between such sensual behaviors and activities and libidnal gratification.

The earliest manifestations of infantile sexuality, as Freud described them in *Three Essays on the Theory of Sexuality*, arise in relation to bodily functions that are basically nonsexual, such as feeding and the development of bowel and bladder control. Freud divided these stages of psychosexual development into a succession of developmental phases, each of which was thought to build on and subsume the accomplishments of the preceding phases. The oral phase occupied the first 1 to 1½ years of the infant's life, the anal phase the period up until about the age of 3, and the phallic phase from the third until about the fifth year (see Table I). For each of the stages of psychosexual development, Freud delineated specific eroto-

TABLE I
Stages of Psychosexual Development

Oral Stage

Definition	This is the earliest stage of development. The infant's needs, perceptions, and modes of expression are primarily centered in the mouth, lips, tongue, and other organs related to the oral zone.	Objectives	To establish a trusting dependence on nursing and sustaining objects, to establish comfortable expression and gratification of oral libidinal needs without excessive conflict or ambivalence from oral-sadistic wishes.
Description	The oral zone maintains its dominant role in the organization of the psyche through approximately the first 18 months of life. Oral sensations include thirst, hunger, pleasurable tactile stimulations evoked by the nipple or its substitute, sensations related to swallowing and satiation. Oral drives consist of two separate components: libidinal and aggressive. States of oral tension lead to a seeking for oral gratification, typified by quiescence at the end of nursing. The *oral triad* consists of the wish to eat, to sleep, and to reach that relaxation which occurs at the end of sucking, just before the onset of sleep. Libidinal needs (*oral erotism*) are thought to predominate in the early parts of the oral phase; they are mixed with more aggressive components later (*oral sadism*). Oral aggression may express itself in biting, chewing, spitting, or crying. Oral aggression is connected with primitive wishes and fantasies of biting, devouring, and destroying.	Pathological traits	Excessive oral gratification or deprivation can result in libidinal fixations that contribute to pathological traits. Such traits can include excessive optimism, narcissism, pessimism (often seen in depressive states), and demandingness. Oral characters are often excessively dependent and require others to give to them and to look after them. Such persons want to be fed but may be exceptionally giving in order to elicit a return of being given to. Oral characters are often extremely dependent on objects for the maintenance of their self-esteem. Envy and jealousy are often associated with oral traits.
		Character traits	Successful resolution of the oral phase provides a basis in character structure for capacities to give to and to receive from others without excessive dependence or envy, a capacity to rely on others with a sense of trust and with a sense of self-reliance and self-trust.

Anal Stage

Definition	This stage of psychosexual development is prompted by maturation of neuromuscular control over sphincters, particularly the anal sphincters, thus permitting more voluntary control over retention or expulsion of feces.		parent over retaining or expelling feces in toilet training give rise to increased *ambivalence*, together with a struggle over separation, individuation, and independence. *Anal erotism* refers to the sexual pleasure in anal functioning, both in retaining the feces and in presenting them as a gift to the parent. *Anal sadism* refers to the expression of aggressive wishes connected with discharging feces as powerful and destructive weapons. These wishes are often displayed in children's fantasies of bombing and explosions.
Description	This period, which extends roughly from 1 to 3 years of age, is marked by a recognizable intensification of aggressive drives mixed with libidinal components in sadistic impulses. Acquisition of voluntary sphincter control is associated with an increasing shift from passivity to activity. The conflicts over anal control and the struggle with the	Objectives	The anal period is essentially a period

TABLE I (*continued*)

Anal Stage (continued)

	of striving for independence and separation from dependence on and control by the parent. The objective of sphincter control without overcontrol (fecal retention) or loss of control (messing) is matched by the child's attempts to achieve autonomy and independence without excessive shame or self-doubt from loss of control.		are less effective, the anal character reveals traits of heightened ambivalence, messiness, defiance, rage, and sadomasochistic tendencies. Anal characteristics and defenses are most typically seen in obsessive-compulsive neuroses.
		Character traits	Successful resolution of the anal phase provides the basis for the development of personal autonomy, a capacity for independence and personal initiative without guilt, a capacity for self-determining behavior without a sense of shame or self-doubt, a lack of ambivalence, and a capacity for willing cooperation without either excessive willfulness or sense of self-diminution or defeat.
Pathological traits	Maladaptive character traits, often apparently inconsistent, are derived from anal erotism and the defenses against it. Orderliness, obstinacy, stubborness, willfulness, frugality, and parsimony are features of the anal character derived from a fixation on anal functions. When defenses against anal traits		

Urethral Stage

Definition	This stage was not explicitly treated by Freud but is envisioned as a transitional stage between the anal and the phallic stages of development.		quently have regressive significance that reactivates anal conflicts.
		Objectives	It is not clear whether or to what extent the objectives of urethral functioning differ from those of the anal period.
Description	The characteristics of the urethral phase are often subsumed under those of the phallic phase. Urethral erotism, however, refers to the pleasure in urination and to the pleasure in urethral retention analogous to anal retention. Similar issues of performance and control are related to urethral functioning.	Pathological traits	The predominant urethral trait is that of competitiveness and ambition, probably related to the compensation for shame due to loss of urethral control.
	Urethral functioning may also be invested with a sadistic quality, often reflecting the persistence of anal-sadistic urges. Loss of urethral control, as in enuresis, may fre-	Character traits	Urethral competence provides a sense of pride and self-competence derived from performance. The resolution of urethral conflicts sets the stage for budding gender identity and subsequent identifications.

Phallic Stage

Definition	The phallic stage of sexual development begins sometime during the third year of life and continues until about the end of the fifth year.		considered as evidence of castration. The phallic phase is associated with an increase in genital masturbation, accompanied by predominantly unconscious fantasies of sexual involvement with the same-sex parent. The threat of castration and its related castration anxiety arises in connection with guilt over masturbation and oedipal wishes. During this phase, the oedipal involvement and conflict
Description	The phallic phase is characterized by a primary focus of sexual interest, stimulation, and excitement in the genital area. The penis becomes the organ of principal interest to children of both sexes, with the lack of a penis in the female being		

TABLE I (*continued*)

Phallic Stage (continued)

Objectives	are established and consolidated. The objective of this phase is to focus erotic interest in the genital area and genital functions. This focusing lays the foundations for gender identity and serves to integrate the residues of previous stages of psychosexual development into a predominantly genital sexual orientation. The establishing of the oedipal situation is essential for the furtherance of subsequent identifications that serve as the basis for important and enduring dimensions of character organization.		against both of these, and the patterns of identification that emerge from the phallic phase are the primary determinants of the development of human character. They also subsume and integrate the residues of previous psychosexual stages, so that fixations or conflicts that derive from any of the preceding stages can contaminate and modify the oedipal resolution.
Pathological traits	The derivation of pathological traits from the phallic-oedipal involvement is so complex and subject to such a variety of modifications that it encompasses nearly the whole of neurotic development. The issues, however, focus on castration in males and on penis envy in females. The other important focus of developmental distortions in this period derives from the patterns of identification developed out of the resolution of the oedipal complex. The influence of castration anxiety and penis envy, the defenses	Character traits	The phallic stage provides the foundations for an emerging sense of sexual identity, of a sense of curiosity without embarrassment, of initiative without guilt, of a sense of mastery not only over objects and persons in the environment but also over internal processes and impulses. The resolution of the oedipal conflict at the end of the phallic period gives rise to powerful internal resources for regulation of drive impulses and their direction toward constructive ends. This internal source of regulation is the superego, and it is based on identifications derived primarily from parental figures.

Latency Stage

Definition	This is the stage of relative quiescence or inactivity of the sexual drive during the period from the resolution of the Oedipus complex until pubescence (from about 5 or 6 years until about 11 to 13 years).		things and persons around them. It is a period for development of important skills. The relative strength of regulatory elements often gives rise to patterns of behavior that are somewhat obsessive and hypercontrolling.
Description	The institution of the superego at the close of the oedipal period and the further maturation of ego functions allow for a considerably greater degree of control over instinctual impulses. Sexual interests during this period are generally thought to be quiescent. This is a period of primarily homosexual affiliations for both boys and girls and a sublimation of libidinal and aggressive energies into energetic learning and play activities, exploring the environment, and becoming more proficient in dealing with the world of	Objectives	The primary objective in this period is the further integration of oedipal identifications and a consolidation of sex-role identity and sex roles. The relative quiescence and control of instinctual impulses allows for development of ego apparatuses and mastery skills. Further identificatory components may be added to the oedipal ones on the basis of broadening contacts with other significant figures outside the family—teachers, coaches, and other adult figures.

TABLE I (*continued*)

Latency Stage (continued)

Pathological traits | The danger in the latency period can arise from either a lack of development of inner controls or an excess of them. The lack of control can lead to a failure of the child to sublimate his energies in the interests of learning and development of skills. An excess of inner control, however, can lead to premature closure of personality development and the precocious elaboration of obsessive character traits.

Character traits | Important consolidations and additions are made to the basic postoedipal identification. It is a period of integrating and consolidating previous attainments in psychosexual development and of establishing decisive patterns of adaptive functioning. The child can develop a sense of industry and a capacity for mastery of objects and concepts that allow him to function autonomously and with a sense of initiative without running the risk of failure or defeat or a sense of inferiority. These important attainments need to be further integrated as the basis for a mature adult life of satisfaction in work and love.

Genital Stage

Definition | The genital or adolescent phase of psychosexual development extends from the onset of puberty in about the eleventh to thirteenth years until the adolescent reaches young adulthood.

Description | The physiological maturation of systems of genital (sexual) functioning and attendant hormonal systems leads to an intensification of drives, particularly libidinal drives. This intensification produces a regression in personality organization, which reopens conflicts of previous stages of psychosexual development and provides the opportunity for a reresolution of these conflicts in the context of achieving a mature sexual and adult identity.

Objectives | The primary objectives of this period are the ultimate separation from dependence on and attachment to the parents and the establishment of mature, nonincestuous, heterosexual object relationships. Related to these objectives are the achievement of a mature sense of personal identity and acceptance and integration of a set of adult roles and functions that permit new adaptive integrations with social expectations and cultural values.

Pathological traits | The pathological deviations due to a failure to achieve successful resolution of this stage of development are multiple and complex. Defects can arise from the whole spectrum of psychosexual residues, since the developmental task of the adolescent period is in a sense a partial reopening, a reworking, and reintegrating of all these aspects of development. Previous unsuccessful resolutions and fixations in various phases or aspects of psychosexual development produce pathological defects in the emerging adult personality. A more specific defect from a failure to resolve adolescent issues has been described by Erikson as identity diffusion.

Character traits | The successful resolution and reintegration of prior psychosexual stages in the adolescent, fully genital phase sets the stage normally for a fully mature personality with a capacity for full and satisfying genital potency and a self-integrated and consistent sense of identity. Such a person has reached a satisfying capacity for self-realization and meaningful participation in areas of work and love and in the creative and productive application to satisfying and meaningful goals and values.

genic zones that, when stimulated, give rise to erotic gratification.

During infancy and early childhood, erotic sensations emanate, for the most part, from the mucosal surfaces of a particular body part or organ. During the earliest years of life, the mucous membranes of the mouth, anus, or external genitalia are the appropriate primary focus of the child's erotic life. The focus varies, depending on the phase of psychosexual development. Sexual activity in normal adults is dominated by the genital zone. Nonetheless, the pregenital or prephallic erotogenic functioning of the oral and anal zones retains a place in sexual activity, specifically in preliminary mating activities of foreplay. Stimulation of such zones elicits preliminary gratification (forepleasure), which precedes coitus. In normal adults who have achieved a level of mature genital potency, the sexual act culminates in the pleasure of orgasm.

Freud described the erotic impulses arising from the pregenital zones as component or part instincts. Kissing, stimulation of the area surrounding the anus, and biting the love object in the course of lovemaking are examples of activities associated with these part instincts. Ordinarily, these component instincts undergo repression or persist in a restricted fashion in sexual foreplay. The young child is characterized by a polymorphous-perverse sexual disposition; his total sexuality is relatively undifferentiated and encompasses all the part instincts. However, in the normal course of development to adult genital maturity, these part instincts presumably become subordinate to the primacy of the genital region. The failure to achieve genital primacy may result in various forms of pathology. If, for example, the libido becomes too firmly attached to one of the pregenital erotogenic zones or a single part instinct becomes predominant, a perversion such as fellatio or voyeurism, which under ordinary circumstances is limited to the preliminary stages of lovemaking (foreplay), replaces the normal act of sexual intercourse, and orgastic satisfaction is derived from it. The persistent attachment of the sexual instinct to a particular stage of pregenital development is called a fixation.

Freud discovered that in the psychoneuroses only a limited number of sexual impulses that had been repressed and were responsible for neurotic symptoms were of a normal kind. Usually, the repressed and pathogenic impulses were the same impulses that were given overt expression in the perversions. He regarded the neurosis as the negative of a perversion. However, Freud's theory was unable to explain the outcome of fixation in a particular case. The resolution of this problem had to await the development of later parts of the theory, particularly those concerning defense mechanisms, the functions of the ego and the superego, and the nature and role of anxiety in mental functioning.

Development of Object Relations

Throughout his descriptions of the libidinal phases of development, Freud made constant references to the significance of the child's relationships with crucial figures in his environment. He postulated that the choice of a love object in adult life, the love relationship itself, and object relationships in other spheres of interest and activity depend largely on the nature and quality of the child's object relationships during the earliest years of life.

At birth, the infant's responses to external stimulation are relatively diffuse and disorganized. Even so, the infant is quite responsive to external stimulation, and the patterns of response are quite complex and relatively organized, even shortly after birth. At the beginning of life, however, the infant is not responding specifically to objects. More development of perceptual and cognitive apparatuses and more differentiation of sensory impressions and integration of cognitive patterns are required before the child is able to differentiate between the impressions belonging to himself and those derived from external objects.

Oral Phase. In the first months of life, the human infant is considerably more helpless than any other mammal, and his helplessness continues for a longer period of time. He cannot survive unless he is cared for, and he cannot achieve relief from the painful disequilibrium of inner physiological states without the help of external caretaking objects. Object relationships of the most primitive kind begin to be established only when the infant first begins to grasp this fact of his experience. In the beginning, the infant cannot distinguish between his own lips and the mother's breast, nor does he initially associate the satiation of painful hunger pangs with the presentation of the extrinsic breast. Because he is aware only of his own inner tension and relaxation and is unaware of the external object, the longing for the object exists only in the degree that the disturbing stimuli persist and the longing for satiation remains unsatisfied in the absence of the object. When the satisfying object finally appears and the infant's needs are gratified, the longing also disappears.

This experience of unsatisfied need, together with the experience of frustration in the absence of the breast and need-satisfying release of tension in the presence of the breast, forms the basis of the infant's first awareness of external objects. The first awareness of an object in the psychological sense comes from the longing for something that is already familiar, for something that actually gratified his needs in the past but is not immediately available in the present. It is basically the infant's hunger that initially compels him to recognize the outside world. His first primitive reaction to objects becomes understandable insofar as he wants to put them all in his mouth. He judges reality in terms of oral gratification—that is, whether something provides relaxation of inner tension and satisfaction and should, therefore, be incorporated and swallowed, or whether it creates inner tension and dissatisfaction and, consequently, should be spit out.

The mother-infant interaction not only keeps the child alive but sets a rudimentary pattern of his experience, within which he can build a basic trust that allows him to rely on the benevolence and availability of caretaking objects. The mother's administrations and responsiveness to the child help to lay the foundations for the most rudimentary and essential basis for the subsequent development of object relations and the capacity for entering the community of human beings.

As the differentiation between the limits of self and object is gradually established in the child's experience, the mother is acknowledged and recognized as the source of gratifying nourishment as well as the erotogenic pleasure the infant derives from sucking on the breast. In this sense, she becomes the first love object. The quality of the child's attachment to this primary object is of the utmost importance. From the oral phase onward, the whole progression in psychosexual development reflects the quality of the child's attachment to the crucial figures

in his environment and his feelings of love or hate or both toward these important persons. If a fundamentally warm, trusting, and affectionate relationship has been established between mother and child during the earliest stages of the child's life, then, at least theoretically, the stage is set for the development of trusting and affectionate relationships with other human objects during the course of his life. The mother's nursing and caretaking interaction with the child can become the focus for a variety of conflicts and pathological influences deriving from disturbances in the mother-child relationship or from the mother's own personal inadequacies or psychopathology.

The stage of oral eroticism is succeeded by an increase of oral sadistic impulses in the biting phase. Inevitably, the frustration associated with the latter part of the oral period—particularly with the weaning process, which to the child signifies the imminent loss of gratification and rejection—can evoke biting and cannibalistic impulses toward the object. When such impulses are excessive, as they may be under conditions of maternal rejection or unresponsiveness, they can serve as a prelude for later, more serious impairments of object relations.

Anal Phase. During the oral stage of development, the infant's role is not altogether passive, since he is caught up in a process of mutual interaction, in which he contributes by eliciting certain responses from the mother. However, his control over the mother's feeding responses is relatively limited. The primary onus remains on the mother to gratify or frustrate his demands.

In the transition to the anal period, the child acquires a greater degree of control over his behavior, particularly over his sphincter function. Moreover, during this period the demand is placed on him to relinquish some aspect of his freedom for the first time. He is expected to accede to the parental demand that he use the toilet for evacuation of feces and urine. However, the primary aim of anal eroticism is the enjoyment of the pleasurable sensation of excretion. Somewhat later, the stimulation of the anal mucosa through retention of the fecal mass may become a source of even more intense pleasure. One of the important aspects of the anal period, therefore, is that it sets the stage for a contest of wills over when, how, and on what terms the child achieves his gratification.

The connection between anal and sadistic

drives may be attributed to two factors. First, the feces themselves become the object of the first anal-sadistic activity. The expulsion of the fecal mass is perceived as a sadistic act. Subsequent to this experience, the child can begin to treat objects as he had previously treated the feces. The sense of social power that evolves from sphincter control provides the second sadistic element. The child exerts his power over the mother by means of his control over evacuatory functions. He can exert power over her by yielding and giving up the fecal mass or by refusing to yield and withholding the fecal mass. If his attempts to withold are excessively punished or his loss of control is excessively shamed, the child may regress to more primitive oral patterns of relating to the mother.

The first anal strivings are autoerotic. Pleasurable elimination and, later, pleasurable retention do not require any outside help from an object. At this stage of development, defecation is accompanied by a sense of omnipotence, and the feces, which are the agency of this pleasure, become a libidinal object. Although they become external in the act of defecation, they have a high degree of narcissistic cathexis, since they represent an object that was once part of one's own body. The child wishes to retain or regain the lost feces in order to restore the narcissistic equilibrium. In this way, the feces become an ambivalently loved object: they are loved and retained or desired on one hand, or they are hated, pinched off, and expelled on the other.

During this period, the ministrations of the mother, such as diaper changes, are also associated with pleasurable anal sensations. The quality of maternal care, in combination with conflicts surrounding toilet training, can alter the direction of object strivings. There is a tendency for the attitudes toward feces to be displaced toward objects. For example, in an obsessive-compulsive neurotic, the compulsive neatness characteristic of this syndrome reflects the patient's regression to the anal phase of development and serves to express his wish to dominate. The ambivalence characteristic of the obsessive neurotic is derived from the anal eroticism, which reflects itself in the child's developmental tendency to treat his feces in a contradictory manner. He alternately expels it from his body and retains it as a loved object.

Phallic Phase. The fundamental task of the phallic phase is the finding of a love object. The establishment of genital love relationships in this period lays down the pattern for subsequent and more mature object choices. The phallic period is also a critical phase of development for the budding formation of the child's sense of his own gender identity as decisively male or female, based on the child's discovery and realization of the significance of anatomical sexual differences. The events associated with the phallic phase also set the stage for the developmental predisposition to later psychoneuroses. Freud used the terms "Oedipus complex" to refer to the intense love relationships that are formed during this period between the child and his parents, together with their associated rivalries, hostilities, and emerging identifications (see Figure 9).

In boys the development of object relations is relatively less complex than in girls, since the boy remains attached to his first love object, the mother. In addition to the child's attachment to and interest in the mother as a source of

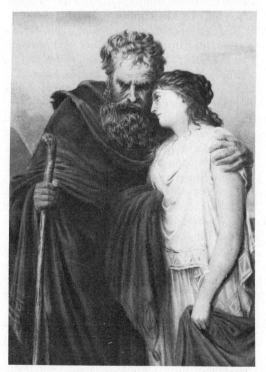

FIGURE 9. Antigone comforts her father Oedipus. He unwittingly killed his father Laius, married his mother Jocasta and sired Antigone. The oedipal complex is based on this myth (Culver Pictures).

nourishment, the boy develops a strong erotic interest in her and a concomitant desire to possess her exclusively and sexually. These feelings usually become manifest about the age of 3 and reach a climax in the fourth or fifth year of life.

With the appearance of the oedipal involvement, the boy begins to show his loving attachment to his mother almost as a lover might—wanting to touch her, trying to get in bed with her, proposing marriage, expressing wishes to replace his father, and devising opportunities to see her naked or undressed. Competition from siblings for his mother's affection and attention is intolerable. Above all, he wants to eliminate his arch rival—the mother's husband, his father. The child anticipates retaliation for his aggressive wishes toward his father, and these expectations give rise to a severe anxiety. The boy begins to feel that his sexual interest in his mother will be punished by removal of his penis. Freud identified this idea of mutilation of the male organ in retaliation for incestuous wishes as the castration complex. Confronted with this threat of castration and the anxiety related to it, the boy renounces his oedipal love for his mother, identifies with the father, and internalizes the father's prohibitions and restraints.

Under certain circumstances, the reversal of the typical oedipal triangle may have serious implications for the child's future development. Homosexual development, for example, is often characterized by an unsatisfied longing for closeness with the father and a strong identification with the mother, derived from an unresolved, negative oedipal involvement.

Like the little boy, the little girl forms an initial attachment to the mother as a primary love object and source of fulfillment of vital needs. For the little boy, the mother remains the love object throughout his development, but the little girl is faced with the task of shifting this primary attachment from the mother to the father in order to prepare herself for her future sexual role.

When the girl discovers that her clitoris is inferior to the male counterpart, the penis, the typical reaction is an intense sense of loss, narcissistic injury, and envy of the male penis. At this point, the little girl's attitude toward the mother changes. The mother is held responsible for bringing the little girl into the world with inferior genital equipment. With the further discovery that the mother also lacks the vital penis, the child's hatred and devaluation of the mother become even more profound. In a desperate attempt to compensate for her inadequacy, the little girl turns to her father in the vain hope that he will give her a penis—or a baby in place of the missing penis.

The little girl's sexual love for her father and her hope for a penis-child from him undergo a gradual diminution as a result of her continuing disappointment and frustration. The wish to be loved by her father may foster an identification with her mother, whom father loves and to whom he gives children. Ultimately, the little girl must renounce her father in order to reattach her libido to a suitable, nonincestuous love object.

Narcissism

The notions of self-love, autoeroticism, and narcissism were not newly coined by Freud. The term "narcissism" was based on the reference to the classic myth of Narcissus, who is said to have fallen in love with his own reflection in the water of a pool and to have drowned in his attempt to embrace the beloved image (see Figure 10).

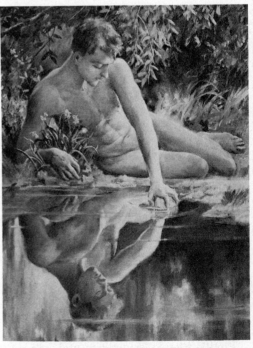

FIGURE 10. Narcissus (Culver Pictures).

Freud observed that in cases of dementia praecox (schizophrenia) libido appeared to have been withdrawn from other persons and objects and turned inward. He concluded that this detachment of libido from external objects may account for the loss of reality contact that was typical of these patients. He speculated that the detached libido had been reinvested and attached to the patient's own ego. This attachment resulted in the megalomanic delusions of these patients; the libidinal investment was reflected in their grandiosity and feelings of omnipotence. Freud also became aware that narcissism was not limited to these psychotic patients. It might also occur in neurotic and to a certain extent even in normal persons under certain conditions. He noted, for example, that, in states of physical illness and hypochondriasis, libidinal cathexis was frequently withdrawn from outside objects and from external activities and interests.

Freud postulated a state of primary narcissism, which he said existed at birth. As Freud saw it, the neonate is entirely narcissistic. His libidinal energies are devoted entirely to the satisfaction of his physiological needs and to the preservation of a state of well-being. Later as the infant gradually comes to recognize the person directly responsible for his care as a source of pleasure or relief from tension, narcissistic libido is released and redirected toward investment in that person, usually the mother.

The development of object relations parallels this shift from primary narcissism to object attachment. But some narcissistic libido is normally present throughout adult life. A healthy and well-integrated narcissism is essential for the maintenance of a sense of well-being and a sense of self-esteem in the developing personality. In a variety of traumatic situations, physical as well as psychological—for example, actual injury or the threat of injury, object loss, or excessive deprivation or frustration—object libido can be withdrawn from its attachment to objects and reinvested in the ego or self.

Autoeroticism refers to eroticism in relationship to the person's own body or its parts. Moreover, autoeroticism implies an absence of any specific object involvement. Secondary narcissism differs in that it refers specifically to the self, rather than to the person's body or its parts.

In adult life a love object may be chosen because the object resembles the person's idealized or fantasied self-image. Or the object may resemble someone who took care of the person during the early years of his life. Freud felt that certain personalities that have a high degree of narcissism, especially certain types of beautiful women, have an appeal over and above their aesthetic attraction. Such women supply for their lovers the lost narcissism that was painfully renounced in the process of turning toward a love object. And in the homosexual object relationship, the person's choice of the object is predicated on the resemblance of the object to the person's own body, with its similarity of sexual organs.

Aggression

In 1915, in *Instincts and Their Vicissitudes*, Freud arrived at a dualistic conception of the instincts as divided into sexual instincts and ego instincts. He recognized a sadistic component of the sexual instincts, but this aspect still lacked a sound theoretical basis.

Increasingly, Freud saw the sadistic component as independent of the libidinal, and he gradually separated it from the libidinal drives. It seemed, too, that there was sadism associated with the ego instincts as well as with the libidinal instincts. The notion of sadism was gradually broadened to include other characteristics under the heading of aggressiveness. At this point in his thinking, Freud attributed aggressiveness to the ego instincts and thus separated the sadistic components from the sexual instincts. Sexual sadism was then explained by the fusion between ego instincts and sexual instincts.

But putting the aggressive instinct in the category of ego instincts had its difficulties. On the basis of clinical evidence of self-destructive tendencies of depressed patients and self-inflicted injuries among his masochistic patients, along with his observations of the wanton destructiveness normally manifested by small children, Freud concluded that in many instances aggression or aggressive impulses did not serve self-preservative purposes.

With the publication of *The Ego and the Id* in 1923, Freud gave aggression a separate status as an instinct with a separate source, which he postulated to be largely the skeletomuscular system, and a separate aim of its own, destruction. The ego was left with its own ego instincts, the nature of which at this point remained unspecified.

Pleasure Principle and Reality Principle

Freud viewed the pleasure principle as an inborn tendency of the organism to avoid pain and seek pleasure through the release of tension by way of energic discharge. The immediate discharge of tension, however, is not always possible. Inevitably, then, the demands of the pleasure principle must be modified to meet the demands of reality. The reality principle modifies the pleasure principle to meet the demands of external reality. The demands of reality necessitate the capacity for delay or postponement of immediate pleasure or release of tension, with the aim of achieving even greater pleasure in the long run. The reality principle is largely a learned function. Consequently, it is closely related to maturation of ego functions and may be impaired in a variety of mental disorders that are the result of impeded ego development.

Life and Death Instincts

Freud postulated that the death instinct was a tendency of all organisms and their component cells to return to a state of total quiescence—that is, to an inanimate state. In opposition to this instinct he set the life instinct, which referred to the tendencies for organic particles to reunite, of parts to bind each other to form greater unities, as in sexual reproduction. As Freud viewed the matter, the ultimate destiny of all biological matter (with the exception of the germ plasm) was to return to an inanimate state. He felt that the dominant force in biological organisms had to be the death instinct. In this final formulation, the life and death instincts were thought to represent abstract biological principles, which transcended the operation of libidinal and aggressive drives. The life and death instincts represented the forces that underlie the sexual and aggressive instincts. Consequently, they represented a general trend in all biological organisms (See Figure 11).

Anxiety Theory

Freud's initial theory of anxiety placed the emphasis on its biological genesis in the sexual instinct. Pathological anxiety was uniformly and unequivocally attributed to disturbances in sexual functioning. Freud distinguished two important groups of pathology in which anxiety played a major role. On the one hand, he classified a group of syndromes that he denominated as the actual neuroses, such as neurosthenia and hypochondriasis. In the actual neuroses, Freud felt that the causative factors had a physical basis. He contrasted these anxiety states to the psychoneuroses, such as hysteria and obsessive-compulsive neurosis, in which the basis of the symptoms was primarily due to psychological factors.

In time, Freud came to realize that anxiety can best be understood in terms of whether it is precipitated by an external or internal danger. His new theory of anxiety was enunciated in *Inhibitions, Symptoms, and Anxiety*, which appeared in 1926. In contrast to the earlier theory, which approached anxiety from the standpoint of the drives, the new theory attacked the problem from the standpoint of the ego. Both real anxiety and neurotic anxiety were viewed as occurring in response to a danger to the organism. In real anxiety, the threat emanated from a known danger outside the person.

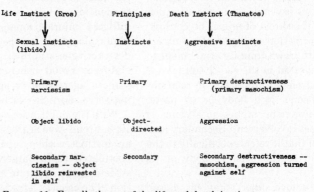

FIGURE 11. Freud's theory of the life and death instincts.

In neurotic anxiety, the danger was precipitated from an unknown source, a source that was not necessarily external.

In his new theory, Freud distinguished two kinds of anxiety-provoking situations. In the first, which took as its prototype the phenomenon of birth, anxiety occurs as a result of excessive instinctual stimulation, which the organism does not have the capacity to bind or handle. The excessive accumulation of instinctual energy overruns the protective barriers of the ego, and a state of panic or trauma results. These traumatic states are most likely to occur in infancy or childhood, when the ego is relatively immature. However, they may also occur in adult life, particularly in states of psychotic turmoil or panic states, when the ego organization is overwhelmed by the threatening danger.

In the more common situation, anxiety rises in anticipation of danger, rather than as its result. But the anxiety that is subjectively experienced may be similar to the anxiety that is caused by a danger that has already occurred. The affect of anxiety serves a protective function by signaling the approach of danger. The signal of danger may arise because the person has learned to recognize, at a preconscious or unconscious level, aspects of a situation that had once proved to be traumatic. Thus, the anxiety serves as a signal for the ego to mobilize protective measures, which can then be directed toward averting the danger and preventing a traumatic situation from arising. The danger may arise from external sources, but it may also arise from internal sources, such as the threatening of the ego or the potential overwhelming of its defenses by instinctual drives. The person may use avoidance mechanisms to escape from a real or imagined danger from without, or the ego may bring to bear psychological defenses to guard against or to reduce the quantity of instinctual excitation.

According to this theory of anxiety, neurotic symptoms, such as phobias, indicate a partial defect in the psychic apparatus. The defensive activity of the ego in phobias has not succeeded in adequately coping with the threatening drive manifestations. Consequently, mental conflict persists, and the danger that actually arose from within is now externalized and treated as though it had its origins in the external world, at least in part. Neurosis can be regarded as a failure in the defensive function of the ego, and this failure results in a distortion of ego's relationship to some aspect of the outside world. In psychotic states, the failure of defensive function is more complete, and the potential threat to the fragile ego and its permeable defenses is all the more overwhelming and annihilating. Greater portions of external reality are perceived as overwhelmingly threatening, and greater distortions of the ego become necessary to accommodate the disortions in the patient's view of the outside world.

Structural Theory

The main deficiency of the topographic model of the psychic apparatus lay in its inability to account for two extremely important characteristics of mental conflict. The first important problem was that many of the defense mechanisms Freud's patients used to avoid pain or unpleasure and that appeared in the form of unconscious resistance during the psychoanalytic treatment were themselves not initially accessible to consciousness. He drew the obvious conclusion that the agency of repression could not be identical with the preconscious, inasmuch as this region of the mind was by definition easily accessible to consciousness. Secondly, he found that his patients frequently exhibited an unconscious need for punishment or an unconscious sense of guilt. However, according to the topographical model, the moral agency making this demand was allied with the anti-instinctual forces available to consciousness in the preconscious level of the mind.

Freud came to realize that what is important is whether mental processes belong to the primary system or to the secondary system. The concepts that were part of this earlier theory and that have retained their usefulness refer to the characteristics of primary and secondary thought processes, the essential importance of wish fulfillment, the tendency toward regression under conditions of frustration or stress, and the existence of a dynamic unconscious and the nature of its operation.

Freud abandoned the topographic model and replaced it with the structural model of the psychic apparatus. The structural model was formulated and presented in *The Ego and the Id*, which appeared in 1923. The structural model of the mind—the tripartite theory, as it is often called—was composed of three distinct entities or organizations within the psychic apparatus: the id. the ego, and the superego. Each refers to a particular aspect of mental functioning, and none of them expresses or represents the sum total of mental functioning at one time. If they often function as quasi-independent systems, they are, nonetheless, ultimately coordinated aspects of the operation of the mental apparatus. Moreover, unlike phenomena such as infantile sexuality and object relations, id, ego, and superego are not empirically demonstrable phenomena in themselves but must be inferred from the observable effects of the operations of specific psychic functions.

In *Inhibitions, Instincts, and Anxiety* in 1926, Freud repudiated the conception of the ego as subservient to the id. Signal anxiety became an autonomous function for the initiating of defense, and the capacity of the ego to turn passively experienced anxiety into active anticipation was underlined. The relatively rudimentary conception of the defensive capacity of the ego was enlarged to include a variety of defenses that the ego had at its disposal and that it could use in the control and direction of id impulses. Moreover, the elaboration of Freud's conception of the reality principle introduced a function of adaptation that allowed the ego to curb instinctual drives when action prompted by them would lead into real danger.

The following survey of the tripartite theory is seen from the contemporary perspective. From a structural viewpoint, the three provinces of the psychic apparatus are distinguished by their different functions. The main distinction lies between the ego and the id. The id is the locus of the instinctual drives and is under the domination of the primary process. It operates according to the dictates of the pleasure principle, without regard for the limiting demands of reality. The ego, on the other hand, represents a coherent organization of functions, the task of which is to avoid unpleasure or pain by opposing or regulating the discharge of instinctual drives to conform to the demands of the external world. The regulation of id discharges is also contributed to by the third structural component of the psychic apparatus, the superego, which contains the internalized moral values, prohibitions, and standards of the parental imagos.

Id

Freud conceived of the id as a completely unorganized, primordial reservoir of energy, derived from the instincts, that is under the domination of the primary process. However, it was not synonymous with the unconscious, since certain functions of the ego—specifically, certain defenses against unconscious instinctual pressures—were unconscious; for the most part, the superego itself also operated on an unconscious level.

Freud postulated that the id was primarily a hereditary given, such that the infant at birth was endowed with an id with instinctual drives seeking gratification. The infant has no capacity to delay, control, or modify these drives. Consequently, in the beginning of life, the infant is completely dependent on the egos of the caretaking persons in his environment to enable him to cope with the external world.

Ego

Those conscious and preconscious functions that are typically associated with the ego—for example, words, ideas, and logic—did not account entirely for its role in mental functioning. The discovery that certain phenomena that emerge most clearly in the psychoanalytic treatment setting—specifically, repression and resistance—could themselves be unconscious pointed up the need for an expanded concept of the ego as an organization that retains its original close relationship to consciousness and to external reality and yet performs a variety of unconscious operations in relation to the drives and their regulation. Once the scope of the ego had been thus broadened, consciousness was redefined as a mental quality that, although exclusive to the ego, constitutes only one of its qualities or functional aspects, rather than a separate mental system itself.

No more comprehensive definition of the ego is available than that Freud gave toward the end of his career in 1938 in *Outline of Psychoanalysis*.

Here are the principal characteristics of the ego. In consequence of the pre-established connection between sense and perception and muscular action, the ego has voluntary movement at its command. It has the task of self-preservation. As regards external events, it performs that task by becoming aware of stimuli by storing up experiences about them (in the memory), by avoiding excessively strong stimuli (through flight), by dealing with moderate stimuli (through adaptation), and finally by learning to bring about expedient changes in the external world to its own advantage (through activity). As regards internal events in relation to the id, it performs that task by gaining control over the demands of the instinct, by deciding whether they are to be allowed satisfaction, by postponing that satisfaction to times and circumstances favorable in the external world, or by suppressing their excitations entirely. It is guided in its activity by consideration of the tension produced by stimuli, whether these tensions are present in it or introduced into it.

Thus, the ego controls the apparatus of motility and perception, contact with reality, and, through the mechanisms of defense, the inhibition of primary instinctual drives.

Origins of the Ego. If one defines the ego as a coherent system of functions for mediating between the instincts and the outside world, one must concede that the newborn infant has no ego or, at best, the most rudimentary of egos. Freud believed that the modification of the id occurs as a result of the impact of the external world on the drives. The pressures of external reality enable the ego to appropriate the energies of the id to do its work. In the process of formation, the ego seeks to bring the influences of the external world to bear on the id, substitute the reality principle for the pleasure principle, and thereby contribute to its own further development. Freud emphasized the role of the instincts in ego development and particularly the role of conflict. At first this conflict is between the id and the outside world, but later it is between the id and the ego itself.

Evolution of the Ego. At first, the infant is unable to differentiate his own body from the rest of the world. The ego begins with the child's ability to perceive his body as distinct from the external world.

Gratification and frustration of drives and needs in the early months of life affect the future state of ego development. Adequate satisfaction of the infant's libidinal needs by the mother or mother surrogate is crucially important. Although it is less clearly understood and appreciated, a certain amount of drive frustration in infancy and early childhood is equally important for the development of a healthy ego. Maternal deprivation at significant stages of development leads to the impairment of ego functions to varying degrees. But overindulgence of the child's instinctual needs interferes with the development of the ego's capacity to tolerate frustration and, consequently, with its ability to regulate the demands of the id in relation to the outside world.

The loss of the loved object or of a particularly gratifying relationship with the object is a painful experience at any stage of life, but it is particularly traumatic in infancy and early childhood, when the ego is not yet strong enough to compensate for the loss. Yet in the early years of life, the child is constantly subjected to such deprivation. In the normal course of events, the young child does not suffer the actual loss of his parents, who are the primary objects at this stage of development, but he must endure constant alterations in his relationships with them. Moreover, at each stage of his development, he must endure the loss of the kind of gratification that was appropriate to the previous phase of his maturation but that must now be given up.

Increasing internalization permits an increasing capacity for delay and detour, increasing independence from the pressure of immediate stimuli, and a more developed capacity for flexibility of response. Internalization, therefore, increases the organism's range of adaptive functions and enlarges its resources for coping with environmental stresses. It includes those processes by which the inner psychic world is built up, including incorporation, introjection, and identification.

Incorporation seems to involve a primitive oral wish for union with an object, which loses all distinction and function as object. The external object is completely assumed into the inner world of the subject. Incorporation is operative in relatively regressive conditions. It can be regarded as the mechanism of primitive, primary internalization and is probably operative in severely regressed psychotic states involving loss of self-object differentiation, permeation of ego boundaries, and psychotic identifications.

Introjection was originally described by Freud in *Mourning and Melancholia* as a process of narcissistic identification, in which the lost object is retained as a part of the internal structure of the psyche. Freud later applied this mechanism to the genesis of the superego, so that introjection became the primary internalizing mechanism by which parental images were internalized at the close of the oedipal phase. The child tries to retain the gratifications derived from these object relationships, at least in fantasy, through the process of introjection. By this mechanism, qualities of the person who was once the center of the gratifying relationship are internalized and re-established as part of the organization of the self.

Since introjects are responsive to and derivative from instinctual drive components, they can serve important defensive functions. Developmentally, their function is, in part, that of binding and mastering and thus modifying the impact of instinctual drives on the emerging ego apparatus. But they can become involved more deeply in the response to and modification of drive pressures, so that they become the foci of internal defensive functions. This defensive function of introjective organizations within the psyche makes them highly susceptible to drive influences and relatively more susceptible to regressive drive pulls. When these defensive pressures predominate in the development of introjects, the result is an impediment to further consolidation and building of internal psychic structure, a susceptibility to regressive pulls, and a liability to projective forms of defense.

The process of introjection can lead not only to the development of a pathological organization within the psyche but also to the development of internal structures that are compatible with the development of healthy object relationships. Identification with the aggressor is a defensive maneuver based on the child's need to protect himself from the severe anxiety experienced in relation to the object. The child protects himself by introjecting the characteristics of the feared person, who is perceived by the child as his attacker and on whom the child is dependent. The perception of the object as attacking is usually due in part to the prior projection of the child's own hostile and destructive impulses onto the object by way of the defensive maneuver of projection. The child defends himself from his own hostile and destructive wishes by allying himself with the aggressor, rather than allowing himself to be the victim. Thus, he can share in the aggressor's power, rather than be helpless and powerless before him.

Such introjections, however, may impoverish the ego by burdening it with negative (aggressive, ambivalent) introjects. These introjects, by reason of the susceptibility to projection, distort and impede the development of object relations and the subsequent capacity for more mature and meaningful relations and also impede the capacity for healthier and more con-structive internalizations by way of identification.

Identification is an active structuralizing process that takes place within the ego, by which the ego constructs the inner constituents of regulatory control on the basis of selected elements derived from the model. What constitutes the model of identification can vary considerably and can include introjects (internalized transitional-like objects), structural aspects of real objects, or even value components of group structures and group cultures.

The lines that differentiate identification from introjection should be kept clear. Introjection operates as a function of instinctual forces—both libidinal and aggressive—so that, in conjunction with projection, it functions intimately in the vicissitudes of instinctual and drive derivatives. Identification, however, functions relatively autonomously from drive derivatives. Introjection is indirectly involved in the transformation and binding of energies. Hence, introjection is much more influenced by drive energies, and its binding permits greater susceptibility to regressive pulls and to primary process forms of organization. The result of binding through identification, however, is more autonomous, more resistant to regressive pulls, and organized more specifically in secondary process terms. Identification, therefore, is specifically the mechanism for the formation of structures of secondary autonomy.

Functions of the Ego. *Control and Regulation of Instinctual Drives.* The development of the capacity to delay immediate discharge of urgent wishes and impulses is essential if the ego is to assure the integrity of the person and to fulfill its role as mediator between the id and the outside world. The development of the capacity to delay or postpone instinctual discharge, like the capacity to test reality, is closely related to the progression in early childhood for the pleasure priniciple to the reality principle.

This progression, parallels the development of secondary process or logical thinking, which aids in the control of drive discharge. The evolution of thought from the initially prelogical primary process thinking to the more logical and deliberate secondary process thinking is one of the means by which the ego learns to postpone the discharge of instinctual drives. For example, the representation in fantasy of instinctual wishes as fulfilled may obviate the need for urgent action that may not always serve the realistic needs of the person. Similarly, the capacity to figure things out or to anticipate consequences represents thought processes that are essential to the realistic functioning of the person. The ego's capacity to control instinctual life and to regulate thinking is closely associated with its defensive functioning.

Relation to Reality. Freud always regarded the ego's capacity for maintaining a relationship to the external world among its principal functions. The character of its relationship to the external world may be divided into three components: the sense of reality, reality testing, and the adaptation to reality.

The sense of reality originates simultaneously with the development of the ego. The infant first becomes aware of the reality of his own bodily sensations. Only gradually does he develop the capacity to distinguish a reality outside of his body.

Reality testing refers to the ego's capacity for objective evaluation and judgment of the external world, which depends on the primary autonomous functions of the ego, such as memory and perception, and on the relative integrity of internal structures of secondary autonomy. Because of the fundamental importance of reality testing for negotiating with the outside world, its impairment may be associated with severe mental disorder. The development of the capacity to test reality, which is closely related to the progression from pleasure principle to reality principle, and to distinguish fantasy from actuality occurs gradually. This capacity, once gained, is subject to regression and temporary deterioration in children, even up to school age, in the face of anxiety, conflict, intense instinctual wishes, or developmental crisis. However, this temporary deterioration is not to be confused with the breakdown of reality testing in adult forms of psychopathology.

Adaptation to reality refers to the capacity of the ego to use the person's resources to form adequate solutions based on previously tested judgments of reality. It is possible for the ego to develop good reality testing in terms of perception and grasp but to develop an inadequate capacity to accommodate the person's resources to the situation thus perceived. Adaptation is closely allied to the concept of mastery in respect to both external tasks and the instincts. It should be distinguished from adjustment, which may entail accommodation to reality at the expense of certain resources of potentialities of the person. The function of adaptation to reality is closely related to the defensive functions of the ego.

Object Relationships. The capacity for mutually satisfying object relationships is one of the fundamental functions of the ego. The child's capacity for relationships with others progresses from narcissism to social relationships within the family and then to relationships within the larger community. The process of the development of object relationship may be disturbed by retarded development, regression, or inherent genetic defects or limitations in the capacity to develop object relationships. The development of object relationships is closely related to the concomitant evolution of drive components and the phase-appropriate defenses that accompany them.

Defense. A systematic and comprehensive study of the defenses used by the ego was first presented by Anna Freud, Sigmund Freud's daughter. In her classic monograph *The Ego and the Mechanisms of Defense*, Ms. Freud maintained that everyone, whether normal or neurotic, uses a characteristic repertoire of defense mechanisms—but to varying degrees.

In the early stages of development, defenses emerge as a result of the ego's struggles to mediate between the pressures of the id and the requirements and strictures of outside reality. At each phase of libidinal development, associated drive components evoke characteristic ego defenses. For example, introjection, denial, and projection are defense mechanisms associated with oral incorporative or oral-sadistic impulses, whereas reaction formations, such as shame and disgust, usually develop in relation to anal impulses and pleasures. Defense mechanisms from earlier phases of development persist side by side with those of later periods. When defenses associated with pregenital phases of development tend to become predominant in adult life over more mature mechanisms, such as sublimation and repression, the personality retains an infantile cast.

Character traits, such as excessive orderliness, are closely related to defenses but are distinguished from them by their greater role both in the over-all functioning of the personality and in situations that are not related to specific conflicts.

Defenses are not of themselves pathological. On the contrary, they may serve an essential function in maintaining normal psychological well-being. Nonetheless, psychopathology may arise as a result of alterations in normal defensive functioning. Table II presents a brief classification and description of some of the basic defense mechanisms.

Synthesis. The synthetic function refers to the ego's capacity to integrate various aspects of its functioning. It involves the capacity of the ego to unite, organize, and bind together various drives, tendencies, and functions within the personality, enabling the person to think, feel, and act in an organized and directed manner. The synthetic function must enlist the cooperation of other ego functions in its operation.

While it subserves the interests of adaptive functioning in the ego, it may also bring together various forces in a way that, although not completely adaptive, is an optimal solution for the person in his particular state at a given time. The formation of a symptom that represents a compromise of opposing tendencies, although somewhat unpleasant, is preferable to yielding to a dangerous instinctual impulse or, conversely, to trying to stifle the impulse completely. Hysterical conversion, for example combines a forbidden wish and the punishment of that wish into a physical symptom. The symptom is often the only possible compromise under the circumstances.

The formation of identifications and introjects and their integration into progressive stages of personality development can be seen, in part, as a function of the ego's capacity for internal synthesis.

Autonomy of the Ego. Although Freud referred to "primal, congenital ego variations" in 1937, the concept of primary autonomy was expanded and clarifed by Hartmann, who advanced a basic formultaion about development—namely, that the ego and the id differentiate from a common matrix, the undifferentiated phase, in which the precursors of the ego are inborn apparatuses of primary autonomy. These apparatuses are rudimentary in nature and present at birth and develop outside the area of conflict with the id. This area Hartmann referred to as a conflict-free area of ego functioning. He included perception, intuition, com-

prehension, thinking, language, certain phases of motor development, learning, and intelligence among the functions in this conflict-free sphere. However, each of these functions may also become secondarily involved in conflict in the course of development. For example, if aggressive, competitive impulses intrude on the impulse to learn, they may evoke inhibitory defensive reactions on the part of the ego, thus interfering with the conflict-free operation of these functions.

Hartmann observed that the conflict-free sphere derived from the structures of primary autonomy can be enlarged and further functions could be withdrawn from the domination of drive influences. This was Hartmann's concept of secondary autonomy. A mechanism that arose originally in the service of defense against instinctual drives may eventually become an independent structure, such that the drive impulse merely triggers the automatized apparatus. The apparatus may come to serve functions other than the original defensive function—for example, adaptation and synthesis. Hartman refers to this removal of specific mechanisms from drive influences as a process of change of function.

Superego

The superego is concerned with moral behavior based on unconscious behavioral patterns learned at early pregenital stages of development. Frequently, the superego allies itself with the ego against the id, imposing demands in the form of conscience or guilt feelings. Occasionally, however, the superego is allied with the id against the ego. This happens in cases of severely regressed reaction, when the functions of the superego may become sexualized once more or may become permeated by aggression, taking on a quality of primitive (usually anal) destructiveness, thus reflecting the quality of the instinctual drives in question.

The superego comes into being with the resolution of the Oedipus complex. The dissolution of the Oedipus complex and the concomitant abandonment of object ties lead to a rapid acceleration of the introjection process. Introjections from both parents become united and form a kind of precipitate within the self, which then confronts the other contents of the psyche as a superego. This identification with the parents is based on the child's struggles to

TABLE II
Defense Mechanisms

Narcissistic Defenses

Denial. Psychotic denial of external reality. Unlike repression, it affects the perception of external reality more than the perception of internal reality. Seeing but refusing to acknowledge what one sees and hearing but negating what is actually heard are examples of denial and exemplify the close relationship of denial to sensory experience. However, not all denial is necessarily psychotic. Like projection, denial may function in the service of neurotic or even adaptive objectives.

Distortion. Grossly reshaping external reality to suit inner needs—including unrealistic megalomanic beliefs, hallucinations, and wish-fulfilling delusions—and using sustained feelings of delusional superiority or entitlement.

Projection. Frank delusions about external reality. usually persecutory; it includes both perception o. one's own feelings in another and subsequent acting on the perception (psychotic paranoid delusions).

Immature Defenses

Acting out. Direct expression of an unconscious wish or impulse to avoid being conscious of the accompanying affect. The unconscious fantasy, involving objects, is lived out impulsively in behavior, thus gratifying the impulse more than the prohibition against it. On a chronic level, acting out involves giving in to impulses to avoid the tension that would result from postponement of expression.

Blocking. Inhibition, usually temporary in nature, of affects (usually), thinking or impulses.

Hypochondriasis. Transformation of reproach toward others—arising from bereavement, loneliness, or unacceptable aggressive impulses—into self-reproach and complaints of pain, somatic illness, and neurasthenia. Existent illness may also be overemphasized or exaggerated for its evasive and regressive possibilities. Thus, responsibility may be avoided, guilt may be circumvented, and instinctual impulses may be warded off.

Introjection. With a loved object, introjection involves the internalization of characteristics of the object with the goal of establishing closeness to and constant presence of the object. Anxiety consequent to separation or tension arising out of ambivalence toward the object is thus diminished. Introjection of a feared object serves to avoid anxiety by internalizing the aggressive characteristics of the object, thereby putting the aggression under one's own control. The aggression is no longer felt as coming from outside but is taken within and used defensively, turning the person's weak, passive position into an active, strong one. Introjection can also arise

out of a sense of guilt, in which the self-punishing introject is attributable to the hostile-destructive component of an ambivalent tie to an object. The self-punitive qualities of the object are taken over and established within one's self as a symptom or character trait, which effectively represents both the destruction and the preservation of the object. This is also called identification with the victim.

Passive-Aggressive behavior. Aggression toward an object expressed indirectly and ineffectively through passivity, masochism, and turning against the self.

Projection. Attributing one's own unacknowledged feelings to others; it includes severe prejudice, rejection of intimacy through suspiciousness, hypervigilance to external danger, and injustice collecting. Projection operates correlatively to introjection; the material of the projection is derived from the internalized configuration of the introjects.

Regression. Return to a previous stage of development or functioning to avoid the anxieties or hostilities involved in later stages; return to earlier points of fixation, embodying modes of behavior previously given up. This defense mechanism is often the result of a disruption of equillibrium at a later phase of development.

Schizoid fantasy. Tendency to use fantasy and to indulge in autistic retreat for the purpose of conflict resolution and gratification.

Somatization. Defensive conversion of psychic derivatives into bodily symptoms.

Neurotic Defenses

Controlling. Excessive attempt to manage or regulate events or objects in the environment in the interest of minimizing anxiety and solving internal conflicts.

Displacement. Purposeful, unconscious shifting from one object to another in the interest of solving a conflict. Although the object is changed, the in-

stinctual nature of the impulse and its aim remain unchanged.

Dissociation. Temporary but drastic modification of character or sense of personal identity to avoid emotional distress; it includes fugue states and hysterical conversion reactions.

Externalization. Tendency to perceive in the external

TABLE II (*continued*)

Neurotic Defenses (*continued*)

world and in external objects components of one's own personality, including instinctual impulses, conflicts, moods, attitudes, and styles of thinking. It is a more general term than projection, which is defined by its derivation from and correlation with specific introjects.

Inhibition. Unconsciously determined limitation or renunciation of specific ego functions, singly or in combination, to avoid anxiety arising out of conflict with instinctual impulses, the superego, or environmental forces or figures.

Intellectualization. Control of affects and impulses by thinking about them instead of experiencing them. It is a systematic excess of thinking, deprived of its affect, to defend against anxiety due to unacceptable impulses.

Isolation. Intrapsychic splitting or separation of affect from content, resulting in represssion of either idea or affect or the displacement of affect to a different or substitute content.

Rationalization. Justification of attitudes, beliefs, or behavior that may otherwise be unacceptable by an incorrect application of justifying reasons or the invention of a convincing fallacy.

Reaction formation. Management of unacceptable impulses by permitting expression of the impulse in antithetical form.

Repression. Expelling and withholding from conscious awareness of an idea or feeling. It may operate by excluding from awareness what was once experienced on a conscious level (secondary repression), or it may curb ideas and feelings before they have reached consciousness (primary repression). The "forgetting" of repression is unique in that it is often accompanied by highly symbolic behavior, which suggests that the repressed is not really forgotten.

Sexualization. Endowing of an object or function with sexual significance that it did not previously have or that it possesses to a lesser degree to ward off anxieties connected with prohibited impulses.

Somatization. Defensive conversion of psychic derivatives into bodily symptoms.

Mature Defenses

Altruism. Vicarious but constructive and instinctually gratifying service to others. This defense mechanism must be distinguished from altruistic surrender, which involves a surrender of direct gratification or of instinctual needs in favor of fulfilling the needs of others to the detriment of the self, with vicarious satisfaction only being gained through introjection.

Anticipation. Realistic anticipation of or planning for furture inner discomfort.

Asceticism. Elimination of directly pleasureable affects attributable to an experience. The moral element is implicit in setting values on specific pleasures. Asceticism is directed against all base pleasures perceived consciously; graftification is derived from the renunciation.

Humor. Overt expression of feelings without personal discomfort or immobilization and without unpleasant effect on others. Humor allows one to bear and yet focus on what is too terrible to be borne; in contrast, wit involves distraction or displacement away from the affective issue.

Sublimation. Gratification of an impulse whose goal is retained but whose aim or object is changed from a socially objectionable one to a socially valued one. Libidinal sublimation involves a desexualization of drive impulses and the placing of a value judgment that substitutes what is valued by the superego or society. Sublimation of aggressive impulses takes place through pleasureable games and sports. Unlike neurotic defenses, sublimation allows instincts to be channeled, rather than dammed or diverted. In sublimation, feelings are acknowledged, modified, and directed toward a relatively significant person or goal, so that modest instinctual satisfaction results.

Suppression. Conscious or semiconscious decision to postpone attention to a conscious impulse or conflict.

---

repress the instinctual aims that were directed toward them, and it is this effort of renunciation that gives the superego its prohibiting character. It is for this reason, too, that the superego results to a great extent from an introjection of the parents' own superegos. Because the superego evolves as a result of repression of the instincts, it has a closer relation to the id than does the ego. The superego's origins are more internal; the ego originates to a greater extent in the external world and is its representative.

Throughout the latency period and thereafter, the child (and later the adult) continues to build on these early identifications through contact with teachers, heroic figures, and admired persons, who form his moral standards, his values, and his ultimate aspirations and ideals. The child's conflicts with his parents continue, but now they are largely internal, between the ego and the superego. The standards, restrictions, commands, and punishments imposed previously by the parents from without are internalized in the child's superego, which now judges and guides his behavior from within, even in the absence of his parents. This initially punitive superego must be modified and softened, so that eventually it can permit adult sexual object choice and fulfillment. The task of adolescence is to modify the oedipal identifications with the parents.

At present, the term "superego" refers primarily to a self-critical, prohibiting agency that bears a close relationship to aggression and aggressive identifications. The ego-ideal, on the other hand, is a kinder agency, based on a transformation of the abandoned perfect state of narcissism, or self-love, that existed in early childhood and has been integrated with positive elements of identification with the parents. Many theorists regard the ego-ideal as an aspect of superego organization derived from good parental images.

Pregenital, especially anal, precursors of the superego are generally thought to provide the very rigid, strict, and aggressive qualities of the superego. These qualities stem from the child's projection of his own sadistic drives and his primitive concept of justice based on retaliation that he attributed to his parents during this period. The harsh emphasis on absolute cleanliness and propriety that is sometimes found in very rigid persons and in obsessional neurotics is based to some extent on this sphincter morality of the anal period.

Character

During the period when Freud was developing his instinctual theory, he noted the relationship between certain character traits and particular psychosexual components. For example, he recognized that obstinancy, orderliness, and parsimoniousness were associated with anality. He noted that ambition was related to urethral eroticism and that generosity was related to orality. He concluded in his paper "Character and Anal Eroticism" that permanent character traits represented "unchanged prolongation of the original instincts, or sublimation of those instincts, or reaction formation against them."

In 1913 Freud made an important distinction between neurotic symptoms and character traits. Neurotic symptoms come into being as a result of the failure of repression; character traits owe their existence to the success of repression or, more accurately, of the defense system, which achieves its aim through a persistent pattern of reaction formation and sublimation. In 1923, Freud observed that the replacement of object attachment by identification (introjection), which set up the lost object inside the ego, also made a significant contribution to character formation. In 1932, Freud emphasized the particular importance of identification (introjection) with the parents for the construction of character, particularly with reference to superego formation.

Psychoanalysis has come to regard character as the pattern of adaptation to instinctual and environmental forces that is typical or habitual for a given person. The character of a person is distinguished from the ego by virtue of the fact that character refers largely to directly observable behavior and styles of defense, as well as of acting, thinking, and feeling.

The formation of character and character traits results from the interplay of multiple factors. Innate biological predisposition plays a role in character formation in both its instinctual and its ego fundaments. Id forces, early ego defenses, and environmental influences, particularly the parents, constitute the major determinants in the development of character. Various early identifications and imitations of objects leave their lasting stamp on character.

The degree to which the ego has developed a capacity to tolerate delay in drive discharge and to neutralize instinctual energies, as a result of early identifications and defense formations, determines the later emergence of such character traits as impulsiveness. The exaggerated development of certain character traits at the expense of others may lead to character disorders in later life. At other times, such distortions in the development of character traits produce a vulnerability in personality organization or a predisposition to psychotic decompensation.

Psychopathology

Neuroses

The fact that, almost invariably, in the course of treatment Freud's patients recalled previously forgotten sexual experiences that had occurred in childhood led him to hypothesize that mental illness was the psychic consequence of a sexual seduction by a child or an adult at an early stage in the patient's development. His assumption that sexual seduction had actually occurred proved incorrect. But the basic proposition that the roots of psychoneuroses lie in a disturbance in early sexual development remains unshaken and is the cornerstone of the psychoanalytic theory of neurotic psychopathology.

Neuroses develop under the following conditions: (1) There is an inner conflict between drives and fear that prevents drive discharge. (2) Sexual drives are involved in these conflicts. (3) Conflict has not been worked through to a realistic solution. Instead, the drives that seek discharge have been expelled from consciousness through repression or another defense mechanism. (4) Repression merely succeeds in rendering the drives unconscious; it does not deprive them of their power and make them innocuous. Consequently, the repressed tendencies fight their way back to consciousness, but they are now disguised as neurotic symptoms. (5) An inner conflict leads to neurosis in adolescence or adulthood only if a neurosis or a rudimentary neurosis based on the same type of conflict existed in early childhood.

Maternal deprivation in the first few months of life may impair ego development. Failure to make necessary introjections and identifications, either because of overindulgence or because of obsessive deprivation and frustration, interferes with the ego's task of mediating between the instincts and the environment. A lack of the capacity for equitable expression of drives, especially the aggressive drive, may lead the person to turn them on himself and to become overtly self-destructive. Inconsistency, excessive harshness, or undue permissiveness on the part of the parent may result in disordered functioning of the superego. Similarly, instinctual conflict may impair the ego's capacity for neutralization or for sublimation, resulting in excessive inhibition of its autonomous functions. Severe conflict that cannot be dealt with through symptom formation may lead to severe restrictions in ego functioning and to impairment of the capacity to learn and to develop new conflict-free skills.

When the ego has been weakened, a shock or a traumatic event later in life that threatens survival (or seems to) may break through the ego's defenses. A large amount of libido is then required to master the resultant excitation. But the libido thus mobilized is withdrawn from the supply normally applied to external objects and from the ego itself, and this withdrawal further diminishes the strength of the ego and produces a sense of inadequacy.

Disappointments, frustrations, and adult strivings can revive infantile longings, which may be dealt with through symptom formation or further regression. Fatigue, intoxication, illness, or overexacting tasks may precipitate a neurotic or even a psychotic illness. As long as the warded-off instinct cannot be tolerated in consciousness, the ego has no choice but to form a symptom or to modify its aims so that the unfulfilled strivings become less urgent. In the movement to any new developmental phase, progression is accompanied by regression.

The reduction of tension and conflict through neurotic illness is the primary purpose or gain of the disorder. The ego, however, may try to gain advantage from the external world by provoking pity to get attention and sympathy, by manipulating others to serve one's own end, or by receiving monetary compensation. These are the secondary gains of neurotic illness.

Each form of neurosis has its own characteristic and predominant form of secondary gain. In the phobias (anxiety hysteria), there is a regression to childhood levels of development, when the patient was still taken care of and protected. Gaining attention through dramatic acting out and deriving material advantages are characteristic of conversion hysteria. In compulsive neurosis there is frequently a narcissistic gain through pride in illness.

Conversion Hysteria. Conversion hysteria is characterized by bodily symptoms that resemble those of physical disease—for example, paralysis, anesthesia, blindness, convulsions, pathological blushing, fainting, and headaches—but that have no somtaic basis. Conversion hysteria provides a defense against overintense libidinal stimulation by means of a transformation or conversion of psychic excitation into physical innervation. As a result, various alterations of motor function or sensations may occur. Fixation at the phallic stage of psychosexual development, a tendency to libidinize thoughts and images, and frustration in external life in relation to strong, unconscious fantasies are causative factors.

The choice of the afflicted region may be

determined by unconscious sexual fantasies and the corresponding erotogenicity of the afflicted part, by physical injury or change in part of the body that increases its susceptibility, by the nature of the situation in which the decisive repression occurred, and by the ability of the organ to express symbolically the unconscious drive in question. Hysteria may imitate a wide variety of diseases.

Phobic Neurosis. Phobias, which are often referred to as forms of anxiety hysteria, are abnormal fear reactions caused by paralyzing conflict due to an increase in sexual excitation attached to an unconscious object. The fear is avoided by displacing the conflict onto an object or situation outside the ego system. After this displacement has occurred, the readiness to develop anxiety is bound to the specific situation that precipitated the first anxiety attack. When situations duplicate or represent the original event symbolically, anxiety becomes manifest. The ego fights off the anxiety through states of inhibition, such as impotence and frigidity, or through the avoidance of objects that have become connected with unconscious conflict, either through historical association or through their symbolic significance.

The patient's history, the nature of the drives warded off, and the mechanisms of defense used determine the clinical symptoms. Phobias about infection and touching often express the need to avoid dirt and show that the patient has to defend himself against anal-erotic temptation. Fear of open streets and stage fright may be defenses against exhibitionistic wishes. Anxieties about high places, closed places, falling, cars, trains, and airplanes are developed to fight pleasurable sensations connected with stimulation involving equilibrium.

Although the object or situation from which the phobic person flees represents primarily the threatening parents, he is also in flight from his own impulses. Even the fear of castration, which is perceived as an external threat, arises primarily as a consequence of the child's own phallic impulses.

In adults, the onset of phobic reaction typically occurs at a time of crisis in the sexual life. Fixation at the phallic stage, sexual frustrations, the presence of an external factor that may weaken the ego, increases in libidinal excitement, and a particular susceptibility to anxiety reactions are the most common causative factors.

Obsessional Neurosis. The obsessional or obsessive-compulsive neurosis is characterized by persistent or urgently recurring thoughts (obsessions) and repetitively performed behavior (compulsion) that bear little relation to the patient's realistic requirements and are experienced by him as foreign or intrusive. This syndrome is characterized by rumination, doubting, and irrational fears. All these symptoms can be accompanied by morbid anxiety when the intruding thoughts or the repetitive acts are prohibited or otherwise interfered with. Other symptoms are a strong tendency to ambivalence, a regression to magical thinking (particularly in relation to the obsessional thoughts), and indications of rigid and destructive superego functioning. The conflicts involved in obsessional neurosis usually lie closer to the prephallic phase of psychosexual development than to the phallic-oedipal phase.

The obsessional neurosis comes about as a result of the separation of affects from ideas or behavior by the defense mechanisms of undoing and isolation, by regression to the anal-sadistic level, or by turning the impulses against the self. As a defense against a painful idea in the unconscious, the affect is displaced onto some other, indirectly associated, more tolerable idea which becomes invested with an inordinate quantity of affect.

Freud described obsessional ideas as self-reproaches that have re-emerged from repression in transmuted form. The onset of obsessive-compulsive neuroses occurs relatively late in childhood because they depend on the formation of the superego. The introjections of the parental imagos into the superego explain the relative predominance of punitive and expiatory symptoms that affect the total personality of the patient.

A phobia may be transformed into an obsession. Certain situations must be avoided by the phobic person, and he exerts greater effort to ensure this avoidance, to the degree that in time these efforts assume an obsessive-compulsive character. Other obsessions may develop that are so remote from the original source of fear that the avoidance is assured.

In the obsessive-compulsive neurosis, fixation of libido at the anal-sadistic stage has taken place. Concomitantly, ego development has been arrested at the accompanying stage of omnipotence of thought. Factors that result in frustration of post-anal-sadistic impulses (usually of a phallic nature) or that impede more mature ego functioning lead to the precipitation of overt symptoms. Defenses are first directed against the phallic-oedipal drives but, as regression occurs, they are directed against the anal-sadistic impulses themselves. External circumstances that remobilize the repressed, infantile sexual conflicts and disturb hitherto effective equilibrium between the repressing and the repressed forces may precipitate acute cases of obsessional neurosis. The more frequently chronic type continues more or less without interruption from adolescence. However, particular external circumstances may precipitate exacerbations from time to time if the defenses become less effective or if the impulses defended against become more intense and unbearable.

Depressive Neurosis. The basic psychoanalytic approach to depressive states was laid down by Freud in *Mourning and Melancholia* in 1917. The basic mechanism he described there is the introjection of a lost object and a turning against the self of the aggressive impulses originally directed against the ambivalent object. A common theme in depressive states is the undermining or diminution of self-esteem.

Neurotic depressions usually involve a reactive component and are to be distinguished from more severe depressive syndromes, such as psychotic depressive states and manic-depressive states, in which the degree of regression is considerably more severe and in which the impairment of reality testing and of interpersonal functioning is much greater.

The patient in a depressive state often complains of disturbances of mood, which are described as involving sadness, unhappiness, and hopelessness. He usually experiences a loss of interest in his usual activities or complains of difficulties in concentration. The patient feels lonely, empty, guilty, worthless, inferior, or inadequate. The depressive symptoms often serve the purpose of eliciting sympathy and support. But at times his complaints are so hostile and demanding that he frustrates his own purpose by irritating or alienating potential sources of affection. Suicidal ideas are frequently a component of depressive syndromes.

Depressive neurosis usually involves reaction to loss or failure. The loss may be the death of a loved person or a disappointment by a love object. A depression can also be triggered by failure to live up to one's own standards or to achieve specific personal or vocational goals.

Important factors affecting self-esteem seem to be the following: First, the patient has a poor self-image, usually based on early pathological development of his concept in an unfavorable or rejecting family atmosphere. Second, the discrepancy between behavior and the values maintained by the superego and the resulting punishment by the superego is experienced as guilt. Third, if the ego-ideal is excessively grandiose, it places excessive demands on the ego. Fourth, the capacity for effective functioning of the ego itself is undermined.

Insufficient parental acceptance and affection, excessive parental devaluation, excessive frustration experienced prematurely, and a sense of ineffectiveness in the early social and independent performance of activities can undetermine self-esteem. Loss of the parent in childhood has long been established as a predisposing factor to depression. During and after childhood, self-esteem can be adversely affected by illness, disfigurement, inattractiveness, or poor social, vocational, or educational performance.

Impulse Disorders

The impulse disorders involve impulsive actions that, although not necessarily overtly sexual, serve the purpose of avoiding or mastering some type of pregenital anxiety that is intolerable to the ego. The strivings for security and for instinctual gratification are characteristically combined in the impulsive actions. Running away, kleptomania, pyromania, gambling, drug addiction, and alcoholism are examples of irresistible impulsive activities.

Psychophysiologic Disorders

These syndromes are characterized by functional and even anatomical alterations. Peptic ulcer, asthma, and ulcerative colitis are typical examples.

Many theories have been advanced to explain the origins of psychophysiologic disorders. The symptoms have been described as affect equivalents, which represent dammed-up emotions or their symbolic representations that cannot be discharged through behavior or speech and that find expression along somatic pathways in the form of structural or functional alterations in organs or organ systems. Anger, sexual excitement, or anxiety may be supplanted by sensations and other changes in the intestinal, respiratory, or circulatory apparatus. For example, cardiac neurosis is thought to be an anxiety equivalent. Although the theory of affect equivalent has some validity, it is generally regarded as an oversimplified explanation of the complex interrelationships between psychological and somatic processes.

Other workers maintain that, given a predisposition or suceptibility to psychophysiologic disorders in particular persons, the inhibition of specific affects may lead to certain hormonal secretions, to changes in physical functions, and, eventually, to alterations in organ tissue. Different unconscious affects, as they occur in specific disorders, probably cause quantitative and qualitative differences in hormonal secretion and thereby bring about a complex combination in the vegetative nervous system of stimulatory (sympathetic) and inhibitory (parasympathetic) responses.

Perversions

Perversions are manifestly sexual in character. When the pathological impulses are released, orgasm is achieved. The sexual aim in adult perversions corresponds to components of sexual drives in children. Factors of anxiety at phallic (castration) and pregenital levels, bisexuality, identifications, structural considerations, and external circumstances—all play a part in determining the genesis of perversions.

The indications for psychoanalytic treatment for patients whose homosexuality is accompanied by neurotic difficulties are much the same as they would be for heterosexual patients with neurotic difficulties. The results of treatment with respect to the neurotic symptoms are quite similar. The alteration of a neurotic preference for one's own sex is by no means assured. The more indications, either conscious or repressed, of some heterosexual interest in the past history of the patient and the less completely the patient has adopted the psychological traits and habits of the other sex, the better is the prognosis. Generally speaking, patients who find their perverse behavior ego-alien and who are relatively well motivated to undertake therapy and to rid themselves of this behavior pattern have the best chance for modification of the perversion and its psychodynamic roots.

Homosexuality may be considered a vicissi-

tude of the Oedipus complex in that the resolution of the oedipal conflict is based on negative oedipal constellations. The child has identified with the parent of the opposite sex and chosen the parent of the same sex as the love object. Narcissistic factors also play an important role in that the choice of an object is based, in part, on its sexual resemblance to the person himself. However, homosexuals have, with justification, resented being labeled as pathological. Much research is needed to determine the extent to which homosexual life choices are alternative sexual orientations that are made maladaptive because of the intolerance of predominantly heterosexual society.

Fetishism refers to the veneration of inanimate objects that symbolize parts of the body of an ambivalently loved person. This mental state involves the fixation of erotic interest on an object or body part that is inappropriate for normal sexual purposes but that is needed by the person for the attainment of sexual gratification.

The transvestite finds dressing in garments characteristic of the opposite sex a source of sexual excitemznt.

Exhibitionism is the deliberate exposure, usually compulsive, of sex organs under inappropriate conditions. Exhibitionism is usually performed by men and is regarded as a defense against castration anxiety because of the shock or fright in the female object at the sight of the penis.

The voyeur achieves sexual gratification by watching the sexual activities of others.

Sadism and masochism often appear early in childhood and represent a tendency to seek out or to inflict physical or mental suffering as a means of achieving sexual arousal or gratification contingent on physical or mental pain, such as beatings, threats, humiliations, or subjugation at the hands of the sexual partner. The sadist gains sexual gratification by inflicting such torment on the sexual partner.

Character Disorders

The psychoanalytic sense of character refers to the person's habitual mode of bringing into harmony the tasks presented by internal demands and the external world. Discrete personality types are rarely found in pure or discrete forms; there is considerable overlap with other character types.

A particular character pattern or type becomes pathological when its manifestations are so exaggerated that behavior destructive to the patient or to others is the result or when the functioning of the person becomes so disturbed or restricted that it becomes a source of distress to himself or to others. Character disorders are also known as personality disorders.

Hysterical characters tend to sexualize all relationships. They tend toward suggestibility, irrational emotional outbreaks, chaotic behavior, dramatization, and histrionic activity.

Phobic characters limit their reactive behavior to the avoidance of the situations they wished for originally. Certain external situations are avoided, as in neurotic phobic behavior. In addition, however, internal reactions, such as rage or love or all intense feelings, may be subjected to phobic avoidance.

Reaction formations are characteristic of compulsive characters. Typically, they attempt to overcome sadism by kindness and politeness, and they conceal pleasure in dirt by rigorous cleanliness. As a result of isolation, there is a lack of adequate affective response and a restriction in the number of available modes of feeling. Object relationships are usually of an anal-sadistic nature.

Depressive characters may show the characteristics of the depressive neurosis on a more enduring and chronic, if more low-keyed, basis. Chronically low self-esteem and feelings of worthlessness are characteristic of this syndrome. Very often there is a history of early object loss or severe deprivation, often involving the loss of a parent. The syndrome of depressive character relates to ego deficiencies and inadequacies.

Cyclical characters exhibit periodic mood swings from the depression to varying degrees of elation. They are particularly concerned with unresolved oral needs and conflicts. They are basically depressive characters who have been able to mobilize manic defenses.

Impulse-ridden characters discharge tension or avoid inner conflict by urgent activity, which is sometimes of a destructive or self-destructive nature.

Narcissistic characters present a pathological picture characterized by an excessive degree of self-reference in interaction with others, an excessive need to be loved and admired by others, and apparently contradictory attitudes of an inflated concept of themselves and an inordinate need for tribute and admiration from others.

Schizoid characters often present a complaint of depression. They complain of feeling cut off, of being isolated and out of touch, of feeling apart or estranged from people and things around them; of feeling that things are somehow unreal, of diminishing interest in things and events around them, of feeling that life is futile and meaningless. Patients often call this state of mind "depression," but it lacks the inner sense of anger and guilt often found in depression. Moreover, depression is essentially object-related. The schizoid character has renounced objects; external relationships have been emptied by a massive withdrawal of libidinal attachment. The schizoid's major defense against anxiety is to keep emotionally out of reach, inaccessible, and isolated. The schizoid condition is based on the internalization of hostile, destructive introjects.

Borderline States

Such patients represent a stable form of personality organization that is intermediate between neurotic levels of integration and the more primitive psychotic forms of personality organization. Anxiety is usually chronic and diffuse. Neurotic symptoms are multiple. Sexuality is frequently promiscuous and often perverse. Personality organization tends to be impulsive and infantile, and the imperative need to gratify impulses breaks through episodically, giving the borderline life-style an acting-out quality. Narcissism is often a predominant element in the character structure. Underlying these elements is often a core of paranoia based on projection of rather primitive oral rage. The underlying character dimensions may also take the form of severe depressive-masochistic pathology.

The inner organization of the borderline personality reveals the weakness in the structure of the ego. The patient shows a marked lack of tolerance for even low degrees of anxiety, has poor capacity for impulse control, lacks suitable channels for sublimation, has a poor capacity for neutralization, and often shows a generalized shift toward primary-process cognitive organization.

It is difficult for the patient to engage in a productive therapeutic relationship. Frustration tolerance is low, and narcissistic expectations are high. The therapeutic interaction is often distorted by attempts to manipulate the therapist in order to gain needed gratification. The manipulation often takes the form of a suicidal gesture aimed at getting the therapist to comply with the patient's wishes.

Psychoses

Freud suggested that psychosis may be best understood as the patient's mode of adapting to his emotional and realistic needs and to the environmental stresses with which he is confronted. He pointed out that both the dream and psychotic thought are representative of a primitive cognitive organization, one characteristic of infantile levels of development and of animistic stages of thinking.

Freud postulated that in paranoia the need to project coincides with an unconscious impulse to homosexual love, which, although of overwhelming intensity, is unconsciously denied by the patient. Paranoid delusions represent sexual conflicts concerning persons of the same sex that have been projected onto some other object or force, which is then perceived as persecuting or threatening.

In his paper "On Narcissism," Freud stated that psychosis is characterized by the patient's incapacity for normal emotional interest in other people and things. He felt that the psychotic process involves a redistribution of the libido that is normally devoted to object love and to self-love. The energy withdrawn from impoverished object relationships produces an abnormally excessive interest in the self. The psychotic patient's use of language indicates a high interest in the verbal symbol, rather than in the object that the word represents. Many of the more obvious symptoms of psychosis can be considered secondary to this primary loss of the capacity for object attachment. As Freud saw it, these symptoms are essentially rudimentary and primitive efforts to re-establish and reconstitute some degree of relationship with external objects. The psychotic regression to earlier levels of mental functioning and development is manifested in prelogical thought patterns and in the fact that the psychotic patient extracts pleasurable experience chiefly from his own sensory experience, without requiring reciprocal relationships between himself and another person.

Subsequent investigations have followed Freud's suggestion that the conflicts that result in psychotic adaptations occur primarily between the person and his environment. In contrast, the conflicts characteristic of the neuroses are primarily within the personality, between unconscious infantile wishes and the constraining or controlling forces that adapt these wishes to the constraints and demands of reality. The psychoses are seen as resulting from defects in the ego's integrative capacities; from a defect in the ego's capacity for fusion and, consequently, from limitations in the ego's capacity to neutralize instinctual energies; from the ineffectiveness of those functions essential to the capacity for establishing real object relations; and from the impairment of functions essential for controlling intense infantile wishes by normal or neurotic mechanisms.

The psychotic, like the neurotic, needs to adapt in a way that enables him to avoid anxiety. However, the psychotic adjustment uses more primitive types of defense, particularly denial, distortion, and projection. The primitive defenses are reflected in flight, social withdrawal, and the simple inhibition of impulses. These defense mechanisms are much less highly organized than the mechanisms of repression and reaction formation. The fear of detection by others, rather than the guilt of later childhood and maturity, is more conspicuous in the social reactions of the psychotic than in the neurotic. Limited patterns of imitation and introjection play important roles in the development of psychosis.

Psychotic Depression. Freud emphasized the fact that the pain in mourning is limited to loss of an external object. By way of contrast, in melancholia it is the ego itself that is impoverished because it has experienced an internal loss. The melancholic suffers a shattering fall in self-esteem. The ego seems poor and empty, and, as such, it is deserving of reproach and attack from the superego.

The basic attributes of depressive states were previously discussed in the consideration of depressive neurosis. Psychotic depressions are marked by their greater intensity and by the degree of fragmentation and helpless vulnerability that characterizes the ego response to the depressive affect. The intensity of the aggression released is more primitive in psychotic states, and psychotic depressions are almost universally accompanied by profound suicidal ideas or serious suicidal attempts. Psychotic depression has also been described as a basic affective state in which the ego feels totally incapable of fulfilling its aims or aspirations, although these aims persist as desired goals. The ego is thus thrown into a state of continuing and total hopelessness. Persons prone to depression often display a pseudoindependence and self-assurance, which is a reaction to early severe deprivation and is intended to serve as a defense against the threat of further deprivation or rejection.

All human beings experience periods of depression in the face of real or fantasied disappointments or disillusionments. However, the orally dependent person who requires constant narcissistic supplies from external sources is most likely to manifest this reaction in its severe form.

With the internalization of the parental images that follows and derives from the resolution of the oedipal situation, the struggle to secure love from the need-satisfying object takes place on the intrapsychic level—that is, the ego now seeks the approval of the superego and seeks to live up to the ideal standards of the ego-ideal. The child experiences this internalized need-satisfying object as initially frustrating and prohibitive, and his attitude toward the object displays a corresponding hostility. The quality of this early, crucial object relationship gives the superego a critical and aggressive dimension. Furthermore, the failure to abandon or modify early narcissistic expectations of the early ego may lead later to intransigent ego-ideal expectations that, when unrealizable, result in depression. The severe self-reproaches of depressed persons are another concomitant of the infant's hostility toward the internalized object and also represent the ego's efforts to win the favor of the superego through devaluation of the self. Once these mechanisms are set into operation by frustration and loss in adult life, they give rise to the depressive response.

Manic-Depressive Psychosis. The manic-depressive psychotic manifests a particular kind of infantile, narcissistic dependency on his love object. To offset his feelings of worthlessness, he requires a constant supply of love and moral support from a highly valued and idealized love object. This object may be a person, an organization, or a cause that he feels he can attach himself to or to which he has a sense of belonging. As long as this object lasts, he is able to function with enthusiasm and effectiveness. But, because of his strong self-punitive tendencies, the manic-depressive's object choice is masochistically determined and is bound to disappoint him. When the patient is disappointed by this idealized love object, his ego functioning is impaired at every level.

The depressive phase of manic-depressive psychosis often resembles paranoia, in so far as the patient's fantasies show a similar desire to incorporate the object. However, hostility in paranoia is directed against a part of the object (breasts, penis, buttocks, hair, feces), rather than the whole, and the patient fantasizes that this incorporated part can be symbolically destroyed and eliminated by defecation.

The depressive phase subsides and gives rise to a state of temporary elation, which is referred to as mania. The transition to mania occurs when the narcissistically important goals and objects appear to be within reach once again, when they have become sufficiently modified or reduced to be realistically attainable, when they are renounced completely, or when the ego recovers from its narcissistic shock and regains its basic self-esteem with the help of various recuperative agencies, with or without a change in the objects and goals.

Mania represents a way of avoiding awareness of inner depression and includes a strong element of denial of painful inner reality and a flight into external reality. Since the manic person does not want to become aware of these inner painful feelings, he cannot permit himself to empathize with others, and he becomes emotionally isolated.

Schizophrenia. Psychoanalytic concepts regarding schizophrenia continue to undergo modification and revision. Originally, Freud postulated that the onset of schizophrenia signified a withdrawal of libido from the outside world. This libido, he thought, was subsequently absorbed into the ego, producing a state of megalomanic grandiosity, or it was returned to the outside world in the form of delusions.

Recent clinical interest in schizophrenia has centered on the intense ambivalence characteristic of schizophrenic patients, their retaliation (persecutory) anxiety, and the infantile ego mechanisms they typically use in their relationship with objects. The failure of these mechanisms results in the patient's decompensation or regressed state. Two stages are particularly conspicuous in the clinical picture of schizophrenic regression: first, the break with reality; second, the attempts to re-establish contact with reality.

One may describe the predisposition to psychosis as due to the tenuous and delicate balance between positive introjections (contributing to the ego-ideal) and the aggressive and destructive introjections (contributing to the punitive superego). The balance between these two is maintained by special ego defenses, by character disorders, or by disorders in psychophysiologic functioning that permit the symbolic expression of the conflict. Special narcissistic defenses used by schizophrenic patients are molded into organized patterns of denial, projection, and distortion. The ego is altered so that it operates in a self-saving manner. To do so, it must deny the presence of the painful sensations, deny any responsibility for the sensations, or lose the ability to distinguish between sensations emanating from internal and external stimuli. Denial, projection, and distortion are themselves methods for altering sensory perceptions so that they can become ego-syntonic. The specialization of the narcissistic defenses becomes necessary because of the inadequacy of positive (ego-ideal) introjections, which impairs the ego's capacity for repression and its ability to use and integrate more mature defenses to varying degrees.

Schizophrenic regression is usually precipitated by loss or frustration of object needs. The effect of loss results in the supremacy of negative affects, thus dislocating the delicate balance between introjective components in the patient's self-organization. There is a loss of equilibrium between the positive good introjects and the negative bad introjects that compose the structure of the self. The inundation with diffused and deneutralized destructive and negative feelings necessitates a regression to a point of deepest fixation—namely, the narcissistic position—where the patient not only is a potential victim but also operates for self-consolidation. At this level, the patient's regressive disorganization is accompanied by a dedifferentiation of boundaries between self and object. Only in this position can the patient achieve release of the internal tension. The path of regression varies according to whether the losses

are acute and overwhelming or slow and cumulative and according to the patient's structural organization.

Admittedly, the preschizophrenic ego is weak in terms of the development of mature defense mechanisms, but, with the onset of psychosis, elements of mature mechanisms that have become established become admixed with infantile patterns. The acute onset of schizophrenia is related to an increased intensity of paranoid (persecutory) anxiety, feelings of omnipotence, and intolerable depressive anxieties—all of which had previously been warded off by narcissistic ego patterns of behavior. In addition, the patient typically demonstrates perceptual distortion, self-hatred, and a reliance on infantile and highly dependent patterns of object relatedness.

Treatment

Early in his approach to therapy, Freud felt that recognition by the physician of the patient's unconscious motivations, the communication of this knowledge to the patient, and its comprehension by the patient would, of itself, effect a cure. Freud found that this approach was insufficient. Such insight might permit clarification of the patient's intellectual appraisal of his problems, but the emotional tensions for which the patients sought treatment were not effectively alleviated. Freud began to see that the success of treatment depended on the patient's ability to understand the emotional significance of an experience on a emotional level and on his capacity to retain and use that insight.

Psychoanalysis tries to bring repressed material back into consciousness, so that the patient, on the basis of his greater understanding of his needs and motives, may find a more realistic solution to his conflict. Freud elaborated a treatment method that attaches minimum importance to the immediate relief of symptoms, to moral support from the therapist, and to guidance. The goal of psychoanalysis is to pull the neurosis out by its roots, rather than to prune off the top. To accomplish this, the analyst must break down the pregenital, deep crystallization of id, ego, and superego and bring the underlying material near enough to the surface of consciousness so that it can be modified and re-evaluated in terms of reality.

The repression of the forces of conflict is

accomplished by design, and the patient is unaware of the psychic mechanisms his mind uses. By isolating his basic problem, the patient has protected himself from what seems to him to be unbearable suffering. No matter how it may impair his functioning, the neurosis is somehow preferable to the emergence of unacceptable wishes and ideas. All the forces that permitted the original repression are mobilized once again in the analysis as a resistance to this threatened encroachment on dangerous territory. No matter how much the patient may cooperate consciously with the therapist and in the analysis and no matter how painful his neurotic symptoms may be, he automatically defends himself against the reopening of old wounds with every subtle resource of defense and resistance available to him.

Patient Selection

The capacity for mature adjustment is limited in some persons, even though they do not have a particularly severe neurosis. Often there is no evidence of strong drive to combat the more infantile aspects of their personalities. Analysis is contraindicated in extreme cases of this kind, since there is no element of personality that will strive to use the treatment for eventual maturity.

Apart from the capacity for logical thought and a certain degree of ego strength, fundamental vigor of personality is a prerequisite. The analytical patient undergoes a difficult experience. From time to time he must be able to accept a temporary increase in unhappiness or anxiety in the expectation of eventual benefit. When there is some question as to the patient's qualifications in this regard, a short period of trial analysis may be recommended to evaluate the problems and potentialities of the patient more completely.

A youthful mind (less in terms of actual years than in terms of elasticity of functioning) is essential. The more mature a person's experience has been, the more apt he will be to use the analysis. In general, however, treatment proceeds more quickly to an effective result when patients are in their twenties and thirties.

Often an important element in patients' lives is that they have been able to preserve and maintain some area of successful ego functioning in a consistent and productive manner. For example, if a person has a consistently good scholastic or work history, the probability of adequate ego capacity is high.

Honest skepticism about analysis is usually a good prognostic sign, as long as it is not extreme. A naive, exuberant conviction at the beginning of treatment that the omnipotent analyst will point the way to existence that will remain forever untroubled, that analysis somehow offers a magic formula that will automatically and painlessly set everything aright, forbodes special difficulties after the treatment is underway.

Borderline personalities often develop a treatment relationship that provides relief of symptoms. By retaining the relationship with the therapist, such patients can avoid serious regression and maintain a reasonable level of adjustment and functioning. A crucial question is the extent to which such patients are capable of internalizing and identifying with the therapist. The capacity for such internalization requires a capacity for tolerating both depressive affects and regressive forms of anxiety that may be experienced in the face of threatened loss. Borderline personalities do not meet the criteria of analyzability.

Potentially analyzable neurotic patients have been able to sustain significant object relations with both parents through the latency years, after the resolution of the oedipal complex. Classical psychoanalysis is the treatment of choice for potentially mature patients in whom the developmental difficulties lie on the level of the mastery of genuine internal conflicts. Patients who are unable to tolerate anxiety or depression are rarely able to work through a transference neurosis. The more significant difficulty for such patients is their inability to terminate any form of therapy successfully.

The most common difficulty in analyzable women is in the area of heterosexual object relations. This difficulty is usually reflected in a hysterical form of personality organization. Hysterical patients are either very good or very difficult patients. For them the development of a tranference neurosis is relatively easy and quick, but it is more difficult for them to engage in and establish the analytical situation.

A common difficulty for analyzable men is likely to be in the area of work inhibitions. Men also predominantly have symptoms of an obsessional nature. Such patients usually have little difficulty in establishing the analytical situation, but few of them are able to develop the overt and analyzable transference neurosis, at least during the first year of analysis.

Analytical Process

The analytical process refers to the regressive emergence, working through, interpretation, and resolution of the transference neurosis. The analytical situation, on the other hand, refers to the setting in which the analytical process takes place—specifically, the positive real relationship between patient and analyst based on the therapeutic alliance. Obsessives can easily establish and participate in the therapeutic alliance, but they experience difficulty in tolerating the regression necessary for establishing and working through the transference neurosis. Hysterics, however, find it relatively easy to regress in the analytical situation and to allow the transference neurosis to form, but they have difficulty in establishing a meaningful and secure one-to-one relationship, which constitutes the therapeutic alliance.

The regression induced by the analytical situation allows for a re-emergence of infantile conflicts and thus induces the formation of a transference neurosis. In the transference neurosis the original infantile conflicts and wishes become focused on the person of the analyst and are re-experienced and relived. In the analytical regression, earlier infantile conflicts are revived and can be seen as a manifestation of the repetition compulsion.

If the analytical regression has a destructive potentiality that must be recognized and guarded against, it also has a progressive potentiality for reopening and reworking infantile conflicts and for achieving a reorganization and consolidation of the personality on a healthier and more mature level. The determining element within the analytical situation against which the regression must be balanced and in terms of which the destructive or constructive potential of the regression can be measured is the therapeutic alliance. A firm and stable alliance offers a buffer against excessive regression and also offers a basis for positive growth.

The analytical process can be usefully divided into three phases. The first phase involves the initiation and consolidation of the analytical situation. The second phase involves the emergence and analysis of the transference neurosis. The third phase involves the carrying through of a successful termination and separation from the analytical process. Each phase requires different capacities in the patient and focuses on different developmental aptitudes. The analyst must determine the relative aptitude of the patient to meet the demands of each phase.

In the first phase the patient must have a capacity to maintain basic trust in the absence of gratification; he must be able to maintain self-object differentiation in the absence of the object; he must retain a capacity to accept the limitations of reality, to tolerate frustrations, and to acknowledge his own limitations and lack of omnipotence. In the second phase the patient must be able to regress sufficiently to allow the transference neurosis to emerge and be analyzed and to work through its various elements. The third phase involves the patient's capacity to tolerate separation and loss and to integrate affects constructively in a pattern of positive identification with the analyst.

Treatment Techniques. The analytical technique is always adapted to the idiosyncrasies of the patient's developmental capacities and needs and defensive constellation, as well as to the stage of the analytical process at which the patient is at any given point.

The cornerstone of the psychoanalytic technique is free association. The primary function of free association, besides the obvious one of providing content for the analysis, is to induce the necessary regression and passive dependence that are connected with establishing and working through the transference neurosis. The use of free association in the analytical process is a relative matter. Although it remains the basic technique and the fundamental rule by which the patient's participation in the analysis is guided, there are frequent occasions in which the process of free association is interrupted or modified, according to the defensive needs or the developmental progression taking place within the analysis.

The most conscientious efforts on the part of the patient to say everything that comes into his mind are never completely successful. No matter how willing and cooperative the patient is in his attempts to free associate, the signs of resistance are apparent throughout the course of every analysis. The sources of the resistance are just as unconscious as the sources of the transference. However, the emotional forces that give rise to resistance are opposed to those that tend to produce the transference neurosis. The role of resistance in the analysis is particularly focused in the second phase, in which the regressive emergence of the transference is a central concern. The resistance offered in the analysis enables the analyst to evaluate and become familiar with the defensive organization of the patient's ego and its functions.

This conflict is a repetition of the sexuality-guilt conflict that originally produced the neurosis itself. The analysis of resistance constitutes a primary function of the analyst.

Interpretation is the chief tool available to the analyst in his efforts to reduce unconscious resistance. The analyst's function as interpreter is not limited to simply paraphrasing the patient's verbal reports; rather, the analyst indicates at appropriate moments what the patient is not reporting. As a general rule, analytical interpretation does not produce immediate symptomatic relief. On the contrary, there may be a heightening of anxiety and an emergence of further resistance.

It is not so much the analyst's insight into the patient's psychodynamics that produces progress in the analysis; rather, it is the analyst's ability to help the patient gain this insight for himself by reducing unconscious resistance to such self-awareness through appropriate, carefully timed interpretations. The most effective interpretation is timed so that it meets the emerging, if hesitant and half-formed, awareness of the patient.

Role of the Analyst. In the initial phase of the analysis, the analyst's task is to facilitate the establishing of the analytical situation and the therapeutic alliance. The quality of the patient's interaction with the analyst is a function of the dimensions of the patient's functioning personality and of the interaction with characteritics of the analyst's personality.

In the transition to the middle phase of analysis, which concerns itself directly with transference neurosis, the analyst uses the approaches and techniques calculated to induce regression in the patient. In the second phase of the analysis, the relative passivity of the analyst implies his avoidance of permissive and authoritative expressions and allows him to limit himself to interpretations of the patient's mental dynamics as heard in his free associations. The analyst's passivity also allows him to clar-ify the way in which the patient's ego defense mechanisms operate to inhibit or preclude free association, preventing insight into unconscious wishes and impulses. The passive role of the analyst reduces the realistic features of the patient-physician relationship, which was the primary focus in the initial phase of the analysis.

Dynamics of the Therapeutic Process. In the course of his analysis, the patient undergoes two processes, remembering and reliving, which constitute the dynamics of the treatment process. Remembering refers to the gradual extension of consciousness back to early childhood, at which time the core of the neurosis was formed, for this stage of development marked the onset of the interference and distortion of the patient's instinctual life. Making the unconscious conscious is accomplished, in part, by the recovery of important childhood experience through the patient's actual memory of these events. More often, however, the recovery is made in other ways—through the use of fantasy, inference, and analogy. In successfully analyzed patients, recovery means more than verbal autobiographical reconstruction. Inevitably, inner convictions and values that were formed in early life are re-evaluated and altered so that they can contribute to, rather than hinder, the patient's optimal functioning. Reliving refers to the actual re-experiencing of these events in the context of the patient's relationship with the analyst.

Through free association, hidden patterns of the patient's mental organization fixated at immature levels are brought to life, comparatively free from disguise. These free associations refer to events or fantasies that are part of the patient's private experience. When they are shared in the analytical setting, the analyst is gradually invested with some of the emotions that accompany them. The patient displaces the feelings he originally directed toward the earlier objects onto the analyst, who then becomes alternately a friend and an enemy, one who is nice to him and one who frustrates his needs and punishes him, one who is loved and hated as the original objects were loved and hated. Moreover, this tendency persists, so that to an increasing extent the patient's feelings toward the analyst replicate his feelings toward the specific people he is talking about or, more accurately, those whom his unconscious is talking about. The special type of object displacement that is an inevitable concomitant of psychoanalytic treatment is referred to as transference.

As unresolved childhood attitudes emerge and begin to function as fantasied projections toward the analyst, he becomes for the patient a phantom composite figure who represents various important persons in the patient's early environment. Gradually, the patient sees himself as he really is, with all his unfulfilled and contradictory needs spread before him.

The transference neurosis usually develops in the second phase of analysis. The patient who at first was eager for improved mental health no longer consistently displays such motivation during the treatment hours. Rather, he is engaged in a continuing battle with the analyst, and it becomes apparent that his most compelling reason for continuing analysis is his desire to attain some kind of emotional satisfaction from the analyst. At this point in the treatment, the transference emotions are more important to the patient than the permanent health he was seeking when he came to analysis. It is at this point that the major, unresolved, unconscious problems of childhood begin to dominate the patient's behavior. They are now reproduced in the transference with all their pent-up emotion. The patient is striving unconsciously to recapture what he was actually deprived of in childhood. The transference neurosis is governed by three outstanding characteristics of instinctual life in early childhood: the pleasure principle, ambivalence, and repetition compulsion.

One situation after another in the life of the patient is analyzed until the original infantile conflict is fully revealed. Only then does the transference neurosis begin to subside. Termination of the analysis begins from that point, but it is a gradual process and is not even complete with the last visit to the analyst. However, at times of emotional crisis the patient may resolve, through association and without assistance, those areas of conflict that were not entirely worked through with the analyst. Part of the patient's capacity to do this depends on his capacity for internalization and effective identification with the strength and objectivity of the analyst. After a variable period, the temporarily accentuated awareness of the unconscious diminishes. Useful repressions are then partially re-established. The patient experiences less need for introspection and self-analysis, and he is gradually able to deal with life on a more mature and satisfactory basis than was previously possible.

The therapeutic alliance is based on the real, one-to-one relationship that the patient established in the interaction with the analyst. This interaction is contributed to by the real personality characteristics of both the patient and the analyst. The therapeutic alliance provides the stable and positive relationship between analyst and patient that enables them both to engage productively in the work of analysis. The therapeutic alliance allows a split to take place in the patient's ego; the observing part of the patient's ego can ally itself with the analyst in a working relationship, which gradually allows it to identify positively with the analyst in analyzing and modifying the pathological defenses put up by the defensive ego against internal danger situations. The maintenance of this therapeutic split and the real relationship to the analyst involved in the therapeutic alliance require the maintenance of self-object differentiation, tolerance and mastery of ambivalence, and the capacity to distinguish fantasy from reality in the relationship.

The therapeutic alliance serves a double function: It acts, on one hand, as a significant barrier to regression of the ego in the analytical process, and it serves, on the other hand, as a fundamental aspect of the analytical situation against which the wishes, feelings, and fantasies evoked by the transference neurosis can be evaluated and measured. In many pathological conditions—some character neuroses, borderline personalities, and the more severe neurotic disorders—it may be impossible to maintain a clinical distinction between the transference neurosis and the therapeutic alliance as a real object relationship.

Results of Treatment. No analyst can ever eliminate all the personality defects and neurotic factors in a given patient, no matter how thorough or successful the treatment. On the other hand, mitigation of the rigors of a punitive superego is an essential criterion of the effectiveness of treatment. Psychoanalysts do not usually regard alleviation of symptoms as the most significant aspect in evaluating therapeutic change. The absence of a recurrence or of a further need for psychotherapy is perhaps a more important index of the value of psychoanalysis. However, the chief basis of evaluation remains the patient's general adjustment to life—his capacity for attaining reasonable happiness and for contributing to the happiness of others, his ability to deal adequately with the normal vicissitudes and stresses of life, and his capacity to enter into and sustain mutually gratifying and rewarding relationships with other people in his life.

More specific criteria of the effectiveness of treatment include the reduction of the patient's unconscious and neurotic need for suffering, reduction of neurotic inhibitions, decrease of infantile dependency needs, and increased capacity for responsibility and for successful relationships in marriage, work, and social relations. Another important criterion is the patient's capacity for pleasurable and rewarding sublimation and for creative and adaptive application of his own potentialities. However, the most important criterion of the success of treatment is the release of the patient's normal potentiality, which had been blocked by neurotic conflicts, for further internal growth, development, and maturation to mature personality function.

REFERENCES

Fenichel, O. *The Psychoanalytic Theory of Neurosis.* W. W. Norton, New York, 1945.

Freud, A. *The Ego and the Mechanisms of Defense.* International Universities Press, New York, 1946.

Freud, S. *Standard Edition of the Complete Psychological Works of Sigmund Freud.* Hogarth Press, London, 1953–1966.

Hartmann, H. *Essays on Ego Psychology.* International Universities Press, New York, 1964.

Jones, E. *The Life and Work of Sigmund Freud,* 3 volumes. Basic Books, New York, 1953–1957.

Rocklin, G. *Man's Aggression: The Defense of the Self.* Gambit, Boston, 1973.

Weisman, A. D. *The Existential Core of Psychoanalysis.* Little, Brown, Boston, 1965.

Zetzel, E. R. *The Capacity for Emotional Growth.* International Universities Press, New York, 1970.

Zetzel, E. R., and Meissner, W. W. *Basic Concepts of Psychoanalytic Psychiatry.* Basic Books, New York, 1973.

6.2.   ERIK ERIKSON

Introduction

Erik Homburger Erikson (see Figure 1) was born in Frankfurt, Germany, the son of Danish parents. His father abandoned his mother before he was born, and he was brought up in

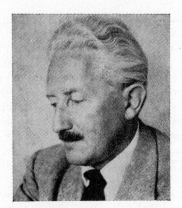

FIGURE 1. Erik Erikson. (Courtesy New York Academy of Medicine.)

Karlsruhe in Baden by his mother and stepfather, Theodor Homburger, a German-Jewish pediatrician. Erikson's parents chose to keep his real parentage a secret from him, and for many years he was known as Erik Homburger.

The concepts of identity, identity crisis, and identity confusion are central to Erikson's thought. By identity, Erikson means a sense of sameness and continuity in the person's inner core maintained amid external change. A sense of identity, emerging at the end of adolescence, is a pyschosocial phenomenon preceded in one form or another by an identity crisis.

In 1927, Peter Blos, a high school friend, invited Erikson to join him in Vienna. Blos, not yet a psychoanalyst, was looking for a fellow teacher in his new school for the children of English and American patients and students of the new discipline of psychoanalysis. Blos and Erikson organized their school in an informal manner—much in the style of the progressive or experimental schools. Children were encouraged to participate in curriculum planning and to express themselves freely.

During this period Erikson became involved with the Freud family, particularly Anna Freud, with whom he began psychoanalysis. Under her tutelage Erikson began more and more to turn his attention to childhood, both his own and that of the children whom he saw in the classroom. Still undecided about his future, Erikson continued to teach school, at the same time studying psychoanalysis at the Vienna Psychoanalytic Institute.

In 1929, he married Joan Mowast Serson, an American of Canadian birth, and was hastily made a full member of the Vienna Psychoanalytic Society—unorthodoxy that allowed him to leave a Vienna threatened by Fascism immediately after his graduation in 1933. After a brief stay in Denmark, the Eriksons moved to Boston, where he became the city's only child analyst.

Erikson was much influenced by Cambridge's circle of young social scientists, including anthropologists Margaret Mead and Ruth Benedict. He found himself more and more interested in the normal personality and in applying his own observations about how young people function and how childhood play affects character formation. His observations about how communal and historical forces influence childrearing became an important contribution to psychology and to the study of man in society.

Theory of Personality

The Healthy Personality

Erikson brought Freud's psychoanalytic theory out of the bounds of the nuclear family, focusing his interest on the wider milieu of the social world, where children interact with peers, teachers, national ethics, and expectations. He added to Freud's theory of infantile sexuality by concentrating on the child's development beyond puberty. Erikson also took the focus of psychoanalysis from pathology to health, providing a picture of how the ego can usually develop in a healthy way if it is given the right environment.

Erikson selected the ego as the tool by which a person organizes outside information, tests perception, selects memories, governs action adaptively, and integrates the capacities of orientation and planning. This is the positive ego, whose functioning produces a sense of self in a state of heightened well-being. One is in this state of well-being when one is and does pretty much what one wishes and feels he ought to be and do.

The wishing and the "oughtness" form polarities in Erikson's scheme. Excessive and barbaric wishes pull from one end of the horizontal axis, and the internalized restrictions of parents and society pull at the other end. Erikson's superego is as barbaric as the id. The strong ego acquires its strength gradually through the expansive process of living, in stages during which the person meets a new situation with his accumulated make-up.

Erikson is probably best known for his positing of eight stages of ego development, which cover the entire life span from birth to death. These stages have both positive and negative aspects, are marked by emotional crises, and are affected by the person's particular culture and by his interaction with the society of which he is a part. Most important is Erikson's contention that personality continues to be molded throughout these eight stages.

Sensory-Oral Stage: Trust versus Mistrust. This first stage covers the first year of life. The infant learns whether he can trust both his own self and the world about him or whether his dominant feeling must be mistrust. Where a person comes to stand on the continuum of trust-mistrust has to do with how well he is cared for.

During the first months the mouth is the most sensitive zone of the body. The infant takes in food, a nipple, a finder. There is hunger for nourishment and for stimulation of the sense organs and the whole surface of the skin. Depending on what happens between the baby and the mother, who is also a bearer of the values of society, the baby develops a basic feeling of trust that his wants will be frequently satisfied or a sense that he is going to lose most of what he wants.

During the second 6 months of life, the dominant social mode moves from getting to taking, which manifests itself orally in biting. However, the nursing child finds the nipple removed if he bites. Weaning begins. Sorrow or nostalgia begins, too. But if his basic trust is strong, he has an in-built and lifelong spring of hope, instead of a well of doom.

Muscular-Anal Stage: Autonomy versus Shame and Doubt. In the second and third years of life, the child learns to walk by himself, to feed himself, to talk, and to control his anal sphincter muscles. He then has a choice of social modes—to keep or to let go. Whether or not this choice becomes fraught with anxiety in the area of bowel and bladder retention or elimination depends on where on the spectrum of indoor, hygienic intolerance and outdoor informality the society is placed.

If the parents allow him to function with some autonomy and if they are supportive without being overprotective, he gains a certain confidence in his autonomy by age 3. He feels a balance of love over hate, of cooperation over willfulness, of self-expression over suppression. Autonomy overbalances shame and doubt, and the child feels not only that he can control himself but also that he has some control over his world. But if his feces are called bad and if he is overrestrained, he feels enraged, foolish, and shamed. Once shamed, he mistrusts his own rightness and comes to doubt himself.

Locomotor-Genital Stage: Initiative versus Guilt. This stage goes through the fifth year. The child now moves among peers and out to the world itself. He is able to initiate activity on his own, both motor and intellectual. Whether or not this initiative is reinforced depends on how much physical freedom the child is given and how well his intellectual curiosity is satisfied. If he is made to feel bad about his behavior or his interests, he may emerge from this period with a sense of guilt about self-initiated activity.

The child takes the first initiative at home, where he involves himself in the family romance by expressing passionate interest in his parent of the opposite sex. Of course, he is disappointed. He may simultaneously be trying to wrest a place for himself in the affection of parents against siblings. He develops a division between what he wants and what he is told he should do. The division increases until a gap grows between the infant's set of expanded desires and his parents' set of restrictions. He gradually turns these parental values into self-punishment. Gradually, the child extracts more initiative than guilt from the conflict and turns happily outward from the home.

Stage of Latency: Industry versus Inferiority. This is the school-age period, the years from 6 to 11. For the first time the child can really reason deductively and can use the tools that adults use. Industry is the keynote of this period. He can become confident of his ability to use adult materials, or he can forsake industry itself and come to the conclusion that he is inferior and cannot operate the things of the world.

Stage of Puberty and Adolescence: Ego Identity versus Role Confusion. During the adolescent years, the teen-ager struggles to develop a personal identity. In the search for identity, the youth falls in love with heroes, ideologies, and members of the opposite sex. Indecision and confusion often cause young people to cling to each other in a clannish manner. The adolescent is in suspension between the morality learned by the child and the

ethics to be developed by the adult. This suspension Erikson calls a moratorium.

How well the youth has fared in the psychosocial conflicts of the earlier stages has much to do with his developing a sense of personal identity. His particular position in his society also helps determine whether he will emerge with a strong sense of ego identity, rather than role confusion.

Stage of Young Adulthood: Intimacy versus Isolation. If the young adult has successfully resolved his identity crisis, he can involve himself with other people without having to fear losing his own identity. If a young adult is not able to share himself in intense and long-term relationships, he may become self-interested and self-indulgent. Without a partner in marriage or a friend, a sense of isolation grows to dangerous proportions.

In true intimacy, there is mutuality. If love and sex become united, rather than separated, the young adult is able to make love that can be shared with another person and that goes back to the world through children.

Stage of Adulthood: Generativity versus Stagnation. During the middle years of life, the adult chooses between generativity and stagnation. Generativity means not a person's bearing or raising children but a vital interest outside the home in establishing and guiding the oncoming generation or in bettering society. The childless can be generative; the adults living only to satisfy personal needs and to acquire comforts and entertainment for themselves are engaged in the self-absorption that is stagnation.

Stage of Maturity: Ego Integrity versus Despair. In Erikson's eighth stage of the life cycle, the conflict is between integrity, the sense of satisfaction one feels when reflecting on a life productively lived, and despair, for one who looks back on a life of little purpose and meaning and can only look ahead to the end of that life. There is no peace in old age, no contented backward look, Erikson says, unless one has lived beyond narcissism, into intimacy and generativity.

Abnormal Development and Functioning

Erikson speaks of five physical modes—passive and active, incorporation, retention, elimination, and intrusion—which underlie the social modes of getting, taking, holding, letting go, and being on the make or making. These modes operate sequentially and relate to the zones of the body. If the mode and the zone are not matched correctly, a neurotic pattern can develop.

In the first zone, the oral, simple incorporation should be dominant. In the second part of the oral stage, once the teeth develop, the dominant mode should be biting. In the muscular-anal stage, the dominant modes should be an alternating retention and elimination. In the locomotor-genital stage, the dominant mode for boys should be intrusive and for girls a return to the two incorporative modes.

Lying and Sitting Stage. If the child is not fed when he is hungry—if, for instance, the mother withdraws the nipple because she is afraid of being bitten—the child may hang on and bite, thus moving into the mode of biting too soon. The mother naturally withdraws further, and the child acquires a frustrating sense that he cannot get what he wants. His resentment at being manipulated can make him compulsive and obsessive, and he may later turn his willfulness toward the manipulation of others.

If trust does not develop and mistrust does, fertile ground for schizophrenia exists. Trust involves mutuality. If either partner is withdrawn, the gap between them widens. In the absence of mutual affect, the infant may begin a flight into a schizophrenic withdrawal.

At the weaning or biting stage, the infant is enraged with his painful teeth, with his mother when she withdraws, and with himself for his powerlessness, developing a sadistic and masochistic confusion. A drastic, sudden weaning and loss of mother without a close substitute can lead to infantile and lifelong depression.

The infant's fear of manipulation becomes the baby's fear of loss of autonomy. At the time of bowel and bladder control, this fear becomes a fear of being robbed by outsiders or by inner saboteurs. A paranoid fear that evil lurks nearby or even within the body can originate at this time. If bowel and bladder training cannot be accomplished in an atmosphere of mutual regulation, the child may become so enraged against manipulation that he tries to control everyone and every event in a compulsion neurosis.

The crawling baby fears not only too much restraint but also too little. Without boundaries, he has trouble in delineating autonomy.

Standing Stage. When the child becomes upright, he experiences in a new way his sense of smallness. He is now vertically measurable and smaller than anyone else. He worries if he will grow.

He looks forward to see the eyes of others examining him. Feeling small, he may not be ready for that exposure. If he has been shamed and made to feel he is bad, he can ultimately develop extreme and sustained defiance after realizing that he cannot be all bad.

The child cannot see his own buttocks, but others can. A feeling develops that others can dominate the backside, even invade and lay low one's autonomy. Paranoid fears of unseen and hostile people can come into being. If others condemn the feces that seemed acceptable when leaving the body, a doubt begins that what one produces and leaves behind is inadequate, bad. Paranoid fears of threats from within are based on this sense.

When the child finally walks, he fears losing that ability or becoming imprisoned or immobile. He also fears having no guidance. Without being told when familiar ground ends, the child does not know against whom he must arm himself or when he can relax.

The child learns he cannot fulfill his sexual fantasies; he may punish himself for those fantasies by fearing harm to his genitals. Under the brutal assault of the developing superego, he may so repress his wishes that he cannot accept even having had them, thus engaging in hysterical denial. If this pattern is carried into late stages, paralysis, inhibition, or impotence can result. Or the child may turn to psychosomatic disease.

School Stage. Erikson talks of two dangers during the elementary school years. One is that of considering oneself less of a workman and provider than the next person. A child who acquired trust, autonomy, and initiative at home can come to school and find himself discriminated against or told that he is inferior. This treatment can cause him to draw away from identification with peers and go back to the personal scene in the home, where he will always remain small. The other danger is that of making work the whole of life.

Adulthood. If adult identity is not secure, a

person may avoid intimacy and retreat into self-aborption or isolation. Fearing the loss of what little ego identity he has managed to develop, he avoids intimacy, shunning friendship and all close associations.

The adult who has no interest in guiding or establishing the oncoming generation is likely to look obsessively for intimacy that is not truly intimate. Such people may marry and even produce children but all within a cocoon of self-concern and isolation. These persons pamper themselves as if they were the children, becoming prey to psychosomatic invalidism. If, looking back on his life, a person feels he never acquired the things he wanted, did not do anything meaningful, never found a sense that his life was integrated into a world order, he is open to a panic at seeing his time run out, his chances used up.

Treatment

One of the primary tasks for the therapist is to help the patient build the trust and confidence that he has failed to acquire in infancy and childhood. Mutuality, so important in Erikson's system of health, is also vital to the cure. He urges that the relationship of the healer to the sick person be one of equals.

Erikson discusses four dimensions of the psychoanalyst's job. The patient's desire to be cured and the analyst's desire to cure him run along an axis of cure research. There is mutuality in that patient and therapist are motivated by cure, and there is a division of labor. The goal is always to help the patient's ego get stronger and cure itself.

The second dimension Erikson calls objectivity-participation. The therapist must keep his mind open. New generalizations must be made and arranged in new configurations that must be abstracted into new models.

The third dimension runs along the axis of knowledge-participation. The therapist applies selected insights to more strictly experimental approaches.

The fourth dimension is tolerance-indignation. The expression of indignation by a controlling therapist is harmful. It widens the gap of inequality that makes more difficult the realization of mutuality.

REFERENCES

Coles, R. *Erik H. Erikson: The Growth of His Work*. Little, Brown, Boston, 1970.

Erikson, E. *Childhood and Society*, W. W. Norton, New York, 1950.

Erikson, E. Identity and the psychosocial development of the child. In *Discussion on Child Development*, vol. 30, International Universities Press, New York, 1958.

Erikson, E. *Young Man Luther: A Study in Psychoanalysis and History*. W. W. Norton, New York, 1958.

Erikson, E. *Insight and Responsibility*. W. W. Norton, New York, 1964.

Erikson, E. *Identity: Youth and Crisis*. W. W. Norton, New York, 1968.

Erikson, E. *Gandhi's Truth*. W. W. Norton, New York, 1969.

Evans, R. I. *Dialogue with Erik Erikson*. E. P. Dutton, New York, 1967.

7

Theories of Personality and Psychopathology: Cultural and Interpersonal Psychoanalytic Schools

7.1. ALFRED ADLER

Introduction

In Alfred Adler's (see Figure 1) first publication, a pamphlet on the health hazards of tailors, he described two concepts that remained basic to all his later teachings: the relationship of the individual to his social environment and the interrelatedness of body and mind.

Relationship with Freud

Adler was invited to join Freud's weekly discussion circle in 1902. For a period of 9 years thereafter, Adler was Freud's co-worker, but his role was that of critic, rather than disciple. In 1907 Adler published *Study of Organ Inferiority*, which received Freud's enthusiastic endorsement, and in 1910 Adler became president of the Vienna Psychoanalytic Society and co-editor of the *Zentralblatt für Psychoanalyse*. Freud and Adler agreed that the meaning of neurotic and psychotic symptoms must be understood by the physician, and that the physician's knowledge of the patient's experiences in early childhood and his dreams might help to clarify the hidden meaning of these symptoms, and that the patient's understanding of the connection between these early experiences and his current dream content and symptoms could result in significant improvement or cure of his mental illness.

Fundamental differences in the thinking of Adler and Freud began to emerge in 1908. Initially, these differences stemmed from Freud's focus on the pathogenesis of neurotic symptoms, as opposed to Adler's interest in their purpose. The final break occurred in 1911, when Adler developed his own theory of personality. He redefined the unconscious and challenged the validity of Freud's concepts of basic drives and the phenomenon of repression as an essential prerequisite for the development of neurotic symptoms. In 1912 Adler coined the term "individual psychology" to describe his school of thought. Ansbacher noted that Freud "firmly believed that the patient's inner psychological world was ultimately determined by objective causes that rested in his past. It was scientifically more revolutionary to proclaim, as did Adler, that the inner psychological world of the individual, which has such far-reaching consequences, was not objectively caused but was ultimately the individual's own creation."

Theory of Personality

Unity of the Individual

Adler was the first theoretician to describe man as an organic purposeful system with the goal of self-realization and social survival. Thus, the unity of personality is emphasized from both an objective and subjective viewpoint. The individual and his behavior are the result of interwoven dynamic, somatic, psychological, and social processes. He also has a need to perceive himself as a unit subjectively. This sense of unity and continuity is the basis for his sense of identity, self-esteem, and self-acceptance.

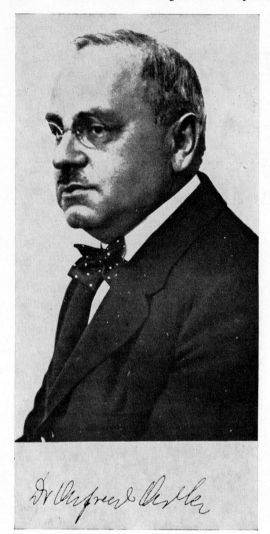

FIGURE 1. Alfred Adler (print includes signature.) (From The Bettmann Archive, New York, N.Y.)

Unified Concept of Motivation

The helplessness of the infant gives rise to universal feelings of inferiority, which supply the motivation for a compensatory striving for superiority. The child wants to overcome his smallness and dependency in his desire for security, mastery, and self-esteem. This striving for self-realization is an integral aspect of life.

Self-determination and Life Goal

The striving for superiority and success is subjective, in that it is based on man's awareness of himself, on his ability to remember past experiences and to project himself into the future. The individual's life goal is determined by his inventive and creative power; it is an expression of his uniqueness. His perception of objective realities influences the formation of his future subjective goals.

The specific kind of superiority the individual wants to attain and the methods he adopts toward its achievement derive from the particular circumstances of his own life, particularly his biological endowment and his early environment.

Life Style

Life style is the individual's active adaptation to the social milieu, which develops as a unique, personal product of his need for integration into that social milieu and for differentiation from it. The growing child selects from among his experiences, especially from his own interactions within his family and his observations of their social relations with others, events that can fit into a consistent, coherent pattern. Events that do not fit into a coherent pattern are considered unimportant and are forgotten, as are thoughts and feelings that would painfully contradict his self-concept. Thus, conscious and unconscious processes are not in conflict but represent dual aspects of a unified relational system.

The life style develops in a step-by-step maturational process. Children concentrate on and seem singularly preoccupied with the behavior of the adults who surround them. These primary experiences constitute the minute pieces of the mosaic created by the child in the first 5 years of his life to form a relatively stable scheme of apperceptions. This individual, creative, goal-directed structuring of memory, perception, and cognition is the basis for the person's life style. The creative interpretation given to experiences in childhood, the meaning found in them, makes for mature freedom of choice and self-determination in later life.

Social Context and Social Feeling

The total person must be considered within the broader context of society. If the child grows up under favorable circumstances, his early self-interest is transformed into the desire for a socially meaningful life, and this goal is attained in accordance with social reality.

Adler conceptualized social feelings as a criterion for mental health. A healthy life style is directed toward achieving competence and social success by working toward the goal of social usefulness. Adler also pointed out that increased social feeling enhances man's intelligence, heightens his self-esteem, and enables him to adjust to unexpected misfortunes.

Theory of Psychopathology

Neurosis

A neurotic disposition stems from childhood experiences that are characterized by overprotection or neglect or by a confusing, alternating mixture of both. Out of these experiences, the growing child creates a negative self-image of helplessness, a conviction of his inability to develop mastery or to cope with the tasks of life. This distorted image of the helpless self is supplemented by his apperception of a social environment that is overly hostile, punishing, and depriving or subtly demanding and frustrating.

These early experiences provide misleading cues, which prevent the child from constructing an apperceptive scheme, a cognitive map, adapted to the tasks of social life. Self-protection becomes his primary objective. Moreover, his self-centeredness and his uncooperative struggle for personal superiority to compensate for his exaggerated feelings of insecurity are substituted for the socially directed goal of a meaningful and useful life. Accordingly, problems are solved in a self-centered private sense, rather than a task-centered common-sense fashion.

Once his cognitive organization or inner psychological world has developed, it is difficult for such an individual to give up even the smallest segment of his distorted subjective creation. All the pieces fit together, and any change would disrupt the only adaptive pattern he has been able to construct from what appeared to be the crucial cues in his early environment.

Psychosis

From Adler's viewpoint, psychosis, whether schizophrenic or manic-depressive, is due to a combination of somatic and psychological factors. Importance is placed on understanding the psychotic's private logic, recognizing its coherence in either grandiose or depressing fantasies, despite a lack of reason or common sense.

The neurotic may suffer from a sense of failure, whether real or imagined, but the psychotic does not accept the ultimate criterion of social validity, and his fantasies compensate for his sense of utter hopelessness and despair of ever achieving significance in the real world.

Treatment

Child Guidance

Adler was convinced that the experiences in early life are the first training and testing ground in social behavior. The mother-child relationship is of crucial importance. Nursery school, kindergarten, and elementary school, with their opportunities for companionship and friendship continue the training in social feeling and provide a testing ground for self-assertion and interaction. Adler also emphasized the influence of the family constellation, the totality of interactions among all the members of the family and, in particular, the significance of the child's ordinal position in relation to his siblings.

Adler maintained that close cooperation between family and school was an important principle in the treatment of disturbed youngsters. Not only the child but also his family and teachers were interviewed and counseled with various professionals present. These techniques were especially helpful in alleviating the child's feeling of isolation and in clarifying for the patient, his siblings, and the adults in his immediate environment the interaction among all the people involved and the impact each had on the other. An atmosphere of optimism prevailed, which derived from the knowledge that others had experienced and solved similar problems, and this optimism was reinforced by attitudes of helpfulness and acceptance. Adler's method—diagnostic exploration of the child's familial and educational situation by questionnaires, family interviews and family treatment, the combined efforts of a therapeutic team—are still in use in child guidance clinics.

Psychotherapy

Adler conceived of psychotherapy as an attempt to mobilize the patient's creative resources and to help him achieve cognitive reorganization. The goal of Adlerian psychotherapy is the reorganization of the patient's life style, leading to a less rigid and more accurate appraisal of reality, to better relationships with others, and to the fulfillment of the patient's creative potentialities.

Therapeutic Process. Therapeutic change is accomplished in several steps, which partly overlap and always dovetail.

In the initial phase of therapy, a relationship is established between therapist and patient that enables the patient to experience contact with a fellow man. The patient's mother may have failed to fulfill her duty to interpret society to the patient in childhood. In that event, the therapist must assume this responsibility as the first step in the therapeutic process, although he is heavily handicapped in his attempt to convince the adult patient to correct a scheme of apperceptions he developed in childhood.

In the second phase, the therapist and then the patient learn to understand the patient's life style and goal. The therapist's understanding of the patient is essential if a reconstructive relationship is to develop and persist throughout therapy. On the other hand, the patient's increased insight into his motivations, intentions, and goals contributes to but is not a prerequisite for therapeutic change; his insight may follow rather than precede changes in behavior.

In the third phase, the patient's inferiority feelings and fears diminish. He develops a positive self-image, and his social feeling is strengthened.

In the fourth phase, the patient is encouraged to select and try out new ways of relating to people and enjoy new methods for coping with the tasks of life. The third and fourth steps in the therapeutic process may occur with or without insight.

Psychotherapeutic Techniques. Encouragement was Adler's main weapon in combating the patient's life style. The patient's exaggerated sensitivity can be overcome by the therapist's kindly and consistent interest in him. As a result of this experience in human relatedless, the patient becomes more hopeful that he will achieve some of his goals, and he learns to feel less isolated and begins to feel that he is part of society.

The therapist must be attentive to details and sensitive to the clues offered by the patient's verbal and nonverbal communications. These must be combined into a meaningful whole, which forms the image of the patient's life style. Four types of observation are generally regarded as particularly important in the

creative reweaving of the fabric that constitutes the patient's life style—early recollections, the family constellation, dreams, and behavior in the therapeutic situation.

Adler considered the Freudian concept of transference misleading. He maintained that the patient's sexual involvement with the therapist was an unnecessary obstacle to therapeutic progress. The patient expects his therapist to be trustworthy, reliable, warm, able, and interested in his welfare in the here-and-now situation.

The therapist understands the patient's resistance to change as a fear of giving up the attitudes he developed in childhood. An active approach, based on the therapist's empathy and expressed awareness of how much courage the neurotic patient requires to seek creatively an alternate choice for his life goal, will restore the patient's faith in himself, help him to realize his strength and ability, and foster his belief in his own dignity and worth. Without encouragement, neither insight nor change is possible.

During this process of re-education, therapeutic neutrality is replaced by the therapist's firm insistence on his right to his own values and his respect for the patient's right to be different. If the patient's uncertainty regarding ethical values arouses guilt feelings, the therapist must discuss the question of right and wrong from his own viewpoint, as well as from that of the patient. Once the problem of values has been resolved through such therapeutic cooperation, the next step is to encourage the patient to use his guilt feelings as a motivation for change. Neurotic guilt is destructive; active remorse is purposeful and constructive.

The therapist's rapport and empathy with the patient, his optimistic attitude with regard to the possibility of change, and his responsive and responsible actions increase the patient's belief in his own worth. Emphasis on the past may perpetuate and strengthen neurotic attitudes. An explanation of persistent neurotic symptoms that focuses on the purpose they serve is a useful therapeutic aid.

Conclusions

As a physician and psychiatrist interested in the cure and prevention of mental disorders, Adler's efforts were directed to the kind of social action that would be described as community psychiatry today. He established child guidance clinics, trained teachers in the dynamics of classroom mental hygiene, discovered methods to re-educate juvenile delinquents, and demonstrated methods of family diagnosis and treatment to workers in the helping professions.

Adler contributed to the field of psychotherapy by stressing the methods and success of short-term therapy. The techniques he advocated for this purpose were confrontation of the patient with the self-defeating and self-deceptive attitudes that made him cling to his symptoms; the purposeful use of interviews and explanations; the therapist's active engagement with the patient; and his hopeful outlook toward the possibility of cure, based on the conviction that every human being, even the psychotic and psychopathic, prefers to be socially useful and accepted.

REFERENCES

Adler, A. *What Life Should Mean To You*. Capricorn, New York, 1958.

Adler, A. *The Problem Child*. G. P. Putnam's Sons, New York, 1963.

Adler, A. *Problems of Neurosis*. Harper & Row, New York, 1964.

Adler, A. *Superiority and Social Interest*. H. L. Ansbacher and R. R. Ansbacher, eds. Northwestern University Press, Evanston, Ill. 1964.

Adler, K. A. Life style in schizophrenia. J. Individ. Psychol., *14:* 68, 1958.

Papanek, H. Psychotherapy without insight: Group therapy as milieu therapy. J. Individ. Psychol., *17:* 184, 1961.

Papanek, H. Adler's psychology and group psychotherapy. Am. J. Psychiatry, *127:* 783, 1970.

7.2. KAREN HORNEY

Introduction

Karen Horney (1885–1952) (see Figure 1) was born in Hamburg, Germany, of a Dutch mother and a Norwegian sea captain father. After completing her early education in Hamburg in 1906, Horney received her medical degree from Berlin University in 1911. When the Berlin Analytic Institute was founded in 1920, Horney became a member and was associated with the leading proponents of classical psychoanalysis. Franz Alexander invited Horney to join him at the Chicago Psychoanalytic Institute in 1932 as associate director. After 2 years, she moved to New York. She was dean of the American Institute for Psychoanalysis, which she helped to found in 1941.

Horney's theory emerged from a unique combination of emotional and intellectual currents, including the German philosophical tradition, modern developments in scientific understanding, and Freud's theories. She said that, if a theory assumes that man is by nature sinful or ridden by primitive instincts, as Freud contended, then there must be superimposed checks and controls. If, however, a theory assumes that there is inherent in human nature both something good and something bad, the emphasis is not exclusively on combatting and suppressing evil. A positive program is required. A third group of theories regarding the nature of man assumes inherent constructive forces, which urge him to realize his given potentialities. He strives toward self-realization. Horney's theory fits into this last group. For her, distortions of equilibrium and balance are not constitutionally built-in-oppositions; they are developments that block the functioning of the flexible and plastic organism.

Theory of Personality

Horney postulated that there is a central inner force she called the real self. It is not an object or a thing but a deep source of growth. A person who is moving with his real-self capacities is one who meets challenges, inner and outer, by using his capacities. He is organized around the fulfilling of goals beneficial to the further development of these capacities, and he has the power to will his own interest. He is able to connect his gifts and capacities to the environment in a way that extends himself.

The growing child needs healthy friction with the wishes and wills of others if he is to evolve his capacities and grow in accordance with his potentials. Given the condition of respect and challenge, trial and error, and a working with the frictions, the basic biological unfolding of a separated and connected unity occurs.

Horney felt that a neurotic person is a collection of parts that are uncoordinated but seeking order. One part fits the concept ego or subject; another part is similar to what is called id or self as object to be worked on; still another part is clearly a set of standards around which the subject programs itself, called by Freud the superego.

Freud saw the ego ideal as an aspect of the self by which the ego measures itself, which it emulates, and whose demand for ever-greater

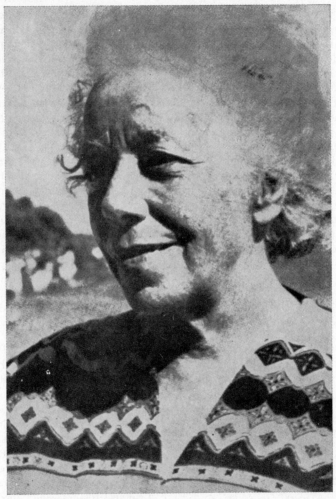

FIGURE 1. Karen Horney. (From the National Library of Medicine, Bethesda, Md.)

perfection it strives to fulfill. This ego ideal is enforced by an agency that measures and pushes for the realization of such an ideal. However, Horney considered the process of idealization to be a secondary result of anxiety and conflict in the evolution of the neurotic process.

Horney also differed from Freud in her view of narcissism. He saw narcissism as an instinctually based given part of human nature. She saw in it an excess of self-love, the sick person's egocentricity that is a secondary result of severe anxiety. The person who is unsure of himself must focus and hold on to himself and block the flow of his participation in the world.

For Horney, a child's experience of immediacy leads him to organize his behavior in every moment by moving toward others, moving away from others, or moving against others. How these functions are used depends on the way a person feels about himself.

A healthy child who feels accepted and loved is able to move flexibly toward another person when he wants support or contact. He is able to oppose the positions of parents and peers when he feels his attitudes are respected. He can move away to be alone with himself, but he will not be lonely. He can do this when he feels that he can depend on himself while alone and that he can depend on others to be there for him when he returns.

The neurotic child feels he is rejected and rejectable, rather than accepted or acceptable. The repertoire of his moves are used in the service of finding safety. Because the self is pervaded by a sense of inadequacy, protection must be found; the actions taken are not for pleasure, they are a necessity; they are driven, rigid, and indiscriminate. The child no longer feels he has a dependable and supporting self in himself or in others and hence is constantly suffused by a feeling of loneliness and helplessness.

Horney operated with the idea that the personality is a problem-solving system. In the everyday process of living, one is constantly facing conflict. It is necessary to be aware of wishes and values because conflicts involve differences and demand comparisons. One must be willing and able to choose and take responsibility for decisions. Out of these tensions in living comes an increased freedom to effect choices through a willingness to engage in a struggle for what one wants.

Theory of Psychopathology

Horney considered anxiety to be the central emotion determining neurotic conflicts. She envisaged several levels of anxiety that lead to neurotic solutions and further anxiety as a result of these solutions.

Horney felt that most anxiety processes have a common denominator relationship to hostility. Usually, some sensitivity is hurt, and this infringement arouses hostility. Under normal conditions, when this hostility is expressed and recognized, it is integrated into the total life process of the person. However, in neurosis, hostility is repressed, intensified, and closed off from moderating influences. It tends to expand in the domain of fantasy.

To avoid the uncertainty of anxiety, human beings immediately shift toward solutions that organize their needs. They deny the anxiety, rationalize it, or narcotize themselves so that they will not know that it is happening. Some people avoid all situations, thoughts, and feelings that arouse hostility.

In neurotic character processes, Horney saw a more deep-seated basic anxiety as the main source of difficulties. She noted that in most neurotics, the family situation lacks genuine warmth and affections, and the parents arouse hostility. This situation encourages the evolution of an increasing, all-pervading feeling of being lonely and helpless in a hostile world.

Basic anxiety and basic hostility are present and unconscious and lie at the core of the personality. Suppression and repression of hostility lead to further anxiety in what Horney called the "neurotic process."

To protect himself from the uncertainties of his orientation in the world, a neurotic person is driven to find safety. He may seek affection, submit to supposedly protective authority, withdraw from contact with reality, or seek power. These moves are effective if life situations do not bring about conflict.

Horney stressed the need to explore three questions in the event of anxiety. What is endangered? What is the source of danger? What accounts for the helplessness of the person feeling the danger? What is endangered is the position, neurotic or healthy, that has vital value. The source of the danger is anything internal or external that jeopardizes any protective structure. Hostility is such a danger. Helplessness is part of the person's connection with his inherent sense of self-weakness. In neurosis there is a feeling of being unable to handle the processes that hostility presents and predicts.

In the neurotic process, a disequilibrium is followed by solutions, which are attempts to reduce tension. These attempts lead to more anxiety, more hostility, and more anxiety because these solutions do not relate the hostility to the person's place in the world. They call for further organizations of personality to balance the pain that emerges from the solutions that do not work. The neurotic process is characterized by seeking ways of disposing of the problems, rather than ways of resolving them.

Horney distinguished the real suffering of a person who is caught in a web of conflicts from the secondary suffering that is a function of the self-protecting or solving mechanisms of the neurotic solutions. The guilt feelings that accompany the neurotic process are solutions that protect the suffering person from assuming responsibility for his life and for his real pain. Suffering may be a way of expressing accusations or a technique for manipulating another person. Pain becomes an opiate.

Attitudes of compliance, aggressiveness, and detachment are mutually exclusive and contradictory. Horney concluded that the conflict born of imcompatible attitudes constitutes the core of neurosis and deserves to be called basic. A person often attempts to repress one set of attitudes and bring the opposite to the fore. The neurotic process presses a person into becoming a type: aggressive, compliant, or detached. This entails radical changes in personality and means the development of a life gestalt. However, the initial transformation around one neurotic trend is not consolidated completely. Further pressure demands that a person assume some identity.

This need is met by what Horney calls the comprehensive solution of the search for glory. There is an idealized image of self. The person feels he must actualize his most deeply embedded and predominant need. He also feels he has attained it.

To make actual what is experienced as a *fait accompli*, the neurotic is involved in what Horney delineated as the pride system, which includes a series of subplans of action—claims, shoulds, self-hate, and pride—that are employed in realizing the search for glory. Although in his imagination the neurotic is his idealized image, he desparately needs, expects, and demands affirmation of this from the environment. The tyranny of the should is the pride system's operational mode by which the self is molded into perfection. Data that contrast with the neurotic's imagined perfection are met with "I should have done it better" or "I should not have bothered." While pursuing the phantom of his glorified self, the neurotic finds his actuality a constant threat. Self-hate is evident in relentless demands on self, self-accusations, self-contempt, self-frustration, self-torment, and self-destructiveness.

The evolution of the comprehensive solution results in a diversity of conflicts. A person identifies with either his idealized self or his despised self in an effort to unify the whole of his personality. But, whichever way he goes, conflicts between the two are always present and painful. Horney defined this process as an aspect of the basic conflict.

In addition, there is central inner conflict, the confrontation between the real self and the pride system oriented toward the search for glory. Other conflicts appear between various shoulds, claims, and forms of self-hate.

For a human system caught up in the neurotic process, the state of alienation from self is a consequence. In its more extreme form, it appears as depersonalization.

Another of the general measures to relieve tension is externalization. Inner processes are experienced in outside forms. Self-hate, for example, is actively experienced as "I hate X" (active externalization) or "X hates me (passive externalization). Psychic fragmentation of compartmentalization attempts to separate difficulties and conflicts from the flow of life. Because of his need to protect his pride, a person may also avoid dealing with members of the opposite sex and thus be led into homosexuality as a general measure to relieve tension. When the tension of self-hate becomes extreme and the person cannot externalize these inner pressures, psychosomatic illness may be generated.

While still evolving as a person meeting new aspects of reality, the neurotic is faced with disparities in his pride system. He needs further organizing solutions if he is to repair the inevitable distorted results of his desperate and continuing attempts to find peace. The major solutions that Horney observed were expansiveness, self-effacement, and resignation.

In the expansive solution, a person's primary inner experience is of being his glorified self. The goal and expectation he has of himself is one of mastery. Horney described three subdivisions of this solution. The narcissistic person believes he is his idealized self and adores what he believes he is. The perfectionistic type is what his standards say he should be. The arrogant, vindictive type lives out what is present in all aspects of the search for glory and revenges himself on any person or thing that interferes.

In the self-effacing solution, the person's basic experience is of being the inadequate, despised self. He is convinced that, to live, he must be loved. He must not allow any self-assertion. The process of morbid dependency is an extension of the self-effacing solution. Intertwined with self-effacement and morbid dependency is the phenomenon of masochism; the suffering present in all three processes serves the function of self-obliteration.

The third major solution is resignation, a move to find freedom from all the conflicts. The primary goal in this solution is the avoidance of any active feelings, wishes, or desires that would highlight such problems. The person restricts his life and is hypersensitive to coercion. Horney defined three categories of the resigned solution. There is persistent resignation, in which the commitment is to withdrawal and turning away from life. Rebellious resignation involves turning against that which provokes conflicts. Or the whole process can end in shallow living. Such a person moves away from his conflicts and may become a well-adapted automaton who lives opportunistically or for prestige.

Therapy

Horney's goals of therapy were to bring about a change in her patient's mode of being and existence. Her efforts were directed toward helping the patient retrieve himself, become aware of his real feelings and wants, evolve his own set of values. The patient can then relate to others more truthfully.

Only as a patient begins to engage and understand the solutions he uses to avoid dealing with conflicts does he make the first steps toward accomplishing the task of therapy. The understanding that came with analysis and self-comprehension was a way of liberating the spontaneous growth forces in the organism that were blocked by these solutions and conflicts.

Horney never denied the past or its influence on the patient. What she emphasized was that the present is where the action is.

Horney revised Freud's notions of transference and repetition to show that in the doctor-patient relationship all the ways of organizing intimacy with self and others and the defenses against it were available to be studied. Analysis is seen neither as a friendship nor as a detached-observer process. It is a functional human event that helps illuminate through the active participation of each person.

The analytical process involves a real relationship between two human beings. The analytical situation is different; for the patient it is being with someone who understands and sanctions his moving into compulsive patterns while helping him find more constructive ways of dealing with his anxiety. In this real context, the analyst is providing assurance that it is possible for the patient to work with his resources.

As Horney's theory became more holistic, she developed the concept of blocking. Whereas the concept of resistance tends to foster the placing of onus on the patient and a halo around the therapist, blocking focuses on the mutual participation in and responsibility for the obstructing process. Blocking refers to any aspect of the process in the analyst or patient or both that

prevents movement in the self-realizing direction. The blockages function specifically to maintain the most deeply embedded solutions.

At first, the analyst may go along with the patient's need to delay confronting his conflicts by meeting his need for relief, by building up his pride, or by helping him avoid his self-hate. At the appropriate time, the analyst must confront the patient with his avoidances and help him move into the experiencing-of-being processes that are obscured.

Followers of Horney do not see the analytical situation as one of doing—the analyst doing to a patient—nor do they think of technique in terms of an agent working on or administering therapy. The two people are one; they are helping the situation unfold toward more opening, connecting with the reality of the uncertainties of the present.

Therapy should be a process in which the patient is always discovering himself, learning more about the ways of his being in the world. The analyst's goal is to help call attention to the aspect of being that will free more spontaneous processes. The analyst almost never asks a patient why this is so or what such and such means. These questions contribute to the neurotic process, which by its very nature involves excessive, compulsive intellectualizing.

Horney emphasized that in dreams people are closer to their reality. Dreams represent attempts to deal with conflicts in a healthy or a neurotic way. Early in analysis, a patient may see in his dreams constructive forces of which he is unaware in his waking life. The analyst helps the patient understand the language of the dream. But he also raises the issue of discrepancy between the self-hate in waking life and the kindness the patient feels in the dream.

The unfolding of the patient's experience of his solutions reveals how they operate. It reveals how compulsive he is and how he shuttles between extremes. It delineates how he wavers and points up his direct relationship to anxiety. As this happens, the patterns of compulsivity give way to the emergence of basic anxiety and of conflicts. The analyst constantly urges the patient to identify and expose the sources of his anxiety, its functions, and his attitudes toward it. The analyst then helps the patient resolve his conflicts.

As the patient becomes more deeply involved in the analytical relationship, he challenges his major defenses, such as dependency, expansiveness, and detachment. As he does so, he begins to have associations, suggesting that the situation now is like that with his parents. This makes the patient feel afraid. He may react by resorting to the old solutions of dependency, by massive withdrawal, or by displaying assaultive behavior and vicious vindictiveness toward the analyst.

In the midst of these repercussions, the enduring work that has built basic trust is the best asset to sustain the patient in the therapeutic process. Through the solid connection between analyst and therapist there develops a partnership that works for self-realization in both. The intensity, extensity, and embeddedness of the patient's formed, less plastic ways of being become somewhat resolved and more flexible. He is more available for creative living.

REFERENCES

Horney, K. *The Neurotic Personality of Our Time.* W. W. Norton, New York, 1937.

Horney, K. *New Ways in Psychoanalysis.* W. W. Norton, New York, 1939.

Horney, K. *Self-Analysis.* W. W. Norton, New York, 1942.

Horney, K. *Our Inner Conflicts.* W. W. Norton, New York, 1945.

Horney, K. *Neurosis and Human Growth.* W. W. Norton, 1950.

Horney, K. *Feminine Psychology*, H. Kelman, editor. W. W. Norton, New York, 1967.

Kelman, H. *Helping People: Karen Horney's Psychoanalytic Approach.* Science House, New York, 1971.

Kelman, H. Chronic analysts and chronic patients: The person of the therapist as instrument. J. Am. Acad. Psychoanal., *1:* 93, 1973.

Kelman, H. Irrational feelings: A therapeutic approach. Compr. Psychiatry, *14:* 217, 1973.

Shainberg, D. *The Transforming Self.* Intercontinental Medical Book Corporation, New York, 1973.

Shainberg, D. The dilemma and challenge of being schizophrenic. J. Am. Acad. Psychoanal., *1:* 271, 1973.

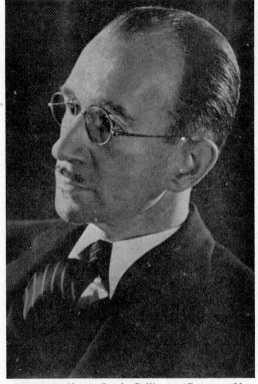

FIGURE 1. Harry Stack Sullivan. (Courtesy New York Academy of Medicine.)

7.3.   HARRY STACK SULLIVAN

Introduction

Harry Stack Sullivan (see Figure 1) was the first major theorist of the cultural school of psychoanalysis. For him, psychiatry was the study of interpersonal relations, real or symbolic or a blend of both. Hence, the unit of study is not the individual but an interpersonal situation. Through the processes of maturation and learning during the long period of time from infancy to adulthood in which a limited number of capacities are developed, one becomes a human, more or less mature individual. This progression occurs in some given cultural context, which is always a network of interpersonal arrangements, organized in numerous and subtle ways into the institutions of a society. Sullivan stressed the interdisciplinary approach for a deep and comprehensive understanding of interpersonal relationships.

At the outset of his career, Sullivan underwent a brief classical analysis. He began his psychiatric career working with psychotics, chiefly schizophrenics. Apart from Adolf Meyer, virtually no psychiatrist in the United States regarded schizophrenics as either curable or treatable until Sullivan came along. This was in 1922 when he became, at the age of 30, United States Veterans Bureau liaison officer at St. Elizabeth's Hospital in Washington, D. C.

In 1923 Sullivan went to Sheppard and Enoch Pratt Hospital, in Baltimore, with the title of assistant physician. Two years later, he was made director of clinical research. Concurrently, he attended Johns Hopkins University's

Phipps Clinic. While there he came under the influence of Adolf Meyer, who conceived of mental disorders as reaction patterns to life situations confronting the sufferers.

At Sheppard, Sullivan set up his special ward for adolescent male schizophrenics. Everyone connected with the work of the special ward was trained by Sullivan to regard the patient as a person, rather than a case, and to be at all times aware of and sensitive to the patient's fragile self-esteem. Their purpose was to assist in the development of the patient's self-esteem. Sullivan practiced a variant of psychoanalysis in which free association was subordinated to direct communication between patient and therapist. Interpretation according to the rules of classical psychoanalysis was modified and subordinated to timely occasions, as was free association. Interpretation when offered, was framed in an indirect hypothetical fashion.

Theory of Personality

Early in his career, Sullivan abandoned Freud's pleasure principle and most of Freud's ideas on psychosexual development. Sullivan, like Freud, believed that a person's past history enters into his present behavior. And, like Freud, he looked for fixation points or what he preferred to call arrests of development. Every patient who suffers a functional mental disorder manifests striking failure in development at some stage or stages because of the inadequacies of his personal relations in the home, school environment, or other milieu. Apart from the idiosyncrasies of the person's family relationships, his inadequacies embody some of the limitations of institutional arrangements.

Four generic factors enter into or influence any experience: biological potentiality, the level of maturation, the results of previous experience, and foresight.

Sullivan did not agree with Freud that the basic structure of personality is established during the first 5 years of a person's life, although he admitted that these years are critical. He held that the organization of personality takes 15, 20, or more than 20 years for its essential development. This development is primarily the ever-increasing elaboration and modification of the person's social relations in connection with the demands, limitations, and opportunities of his society or community. However, the given constitution of every person interacts with environmental conditions. At any era or stage of development, favorable or unfavorable influences may significantly modify personality development.

Self

The self is not synonymous with personality. The personality includes not only the self but those things that, in the course of development, failed to become meaningful or significant to the person or had to be excluded from conscious awareness because of their great anxiety-provoking power. The part or set of processes that is not of the self is said to be dissociated, functionally split off from the self and all meaningful life experience. The self may be described as the person's dynamic organization of relatively enduring and meaningful patterns of interpersonal situations that characterize his life. The distinction between personality and self is chiefly characterized by the degree to which one's experiences are accessible to consciousness.

Eurphoria and Tension

There seems to be built into the human organism a striving or goal-directed process aimed at euphoria, which is simply an objective state of utter well-being. Euphoria is the outcome of the fulfillment of the needs for satisfaction and security. Although certain agents such as narcotics, may provide a temporary subjective feeling of euphoria, they do not fulfill the ongoing requirements of the person. Food and water, the approval of significant others, and a worthwhile, interesting job that one is capable of performing do provide eurphoria.

Sullivan postulated two polar opposites: absolute euphoria and absolute tension. These are ideal constructs and are never reached by any person. In fact, some degree of tension is both normal and biologically necessary. Because of the necessities of daily existence, the level of tensions fluctuates. When a bodily need is not satisfied, the level of tension ordinarily rises until satisfaction is obtained.

Analogously, when one's interpersonal security is decreased, usually as a result of the disapproval of significant others, the level of tension rises and is designated as anxiety tension. When a person experiences anxiety tension, he tends, wittingly or unwittingly, to modify his behavior in a given situation to regain approval. As the self develops, the person may experience anxiety when he does something or perhaps even thinks about something of which he himself disapproves because the self embodies certain standards, values, and ideals that he has acquired. A lowering of interpersonal security or self-esteem is called anxiety tension, which, by definition, entails a loss of euphoria.

Fear and Anxiety

Sullivan asserted that there are two generic causes of fear: (1) any threat to the biological integrity of the human organism, such as disease, injury, the loss of one's livelihood, war, or revolution; (2) a sufficient degree of novelty. The threat of too-great novelty varies considerably among people in a given culture, and probably varies with a person's age and life circumstances.

Anxiety, according to Sullivan, always pertains to interpersonal relations. Moreover, fear and anxiety may combine in given situations. The tension of anxiety, when present in the mothering one, is said to induce anxiety in the infant. As the self-dynamism develops, anxiety becomes a force by means of which the person focuses and restricts awareness to social experiences that meet with approval or tolerance. To a large extent, the self grows in relation to approved or tolerated social norms and behavior patterns. In this connection, significant others serve as intermediaries between the person and the culture.

Stages of Development

Infancy. Normally, the infant experiences the mothering one's tenderness and then gradually develops a generic need for tenderness and, still later, a need to act tenderly. When this generic need is satisfied, the infant's euphoria remains high, apart from periodic discomforts due to such needs as hunger and thirst. Anxiety tension is induced when the mothering one is anxious, upset, disturbed, or disapproving. Sullivan believed that the roots of anxiety states can be traced to this period of life. The infant's experiences of anxiety and his gradually developing power to distinguish between increasing and diminishing anxiety canalize his behavior in various ways as he strives to avoid anxiety.

The person who satisfies the infant's needs is the good mother, who symbolizes forthcoming satisfactions. But she is not the real mother. Nor is the mothering one's personification of the infant the real infant. The mothering one perceives her infant in terms of her previous experience, her current experiences with the infant, and what the baby symbolizes in relation to her social responsibilities. Moreover, the infant also perceives a different sort of mother, who under some circumstances fails to provide satisfactions or induces anxiety tension. In these situations the mothering one is perceived as the bad mother, the bearer of frustrating and anxiety-provoking experiences. Perhaps in late infancy but more definitely in childhood, there is a fusion of the good and bad mother personifications into an approximation of the mothering one as she actually is.

The beginnings of the self are characterized by three personifications: good me, bad me, and not me (not of me). Good me is the beginning personification, it organizes experience in which satisfactions have been enhanced by rewarding increments of tenderness when the mothering one is pleased with her offspring and his behavior. Increasing degrees of anxiety associated with the mothering one's behavior are gradually organized into the personification bad me. The increasing differentiation of tenderness, which induces euphoria, from the increasing differentiation of anxiety-laden attitudes and disapproving behavior, which arouse interpersonal insecurity or anxiety tension, are the source of bad me. The personification not me evolves gradually because it arises from experiences of ineffably intense anxiety. This personification is always of a relatively primitive (infantile) character. Not me embodies poorly grasped aspects of living that gradually become regarded as dreadful and that still later are differentiated into incidents attended by awe, horror, loathing, or the dread experiences that often bedevil schizophrenics.

In the later part of infancy, good me and bad me become fused or assimilated in a rudimentary fashion into the unitary dynamism of the self. Its purpose or function is directed at how to live with the significant other person while avoiding or minimizing incidents of anxiety. Since the mothering one is a product of her community, society and social class, she embodies their irrational as well as rational—that is intelligent and humane—elements. Hence, the origin of the self-system rests on the character of her social environment, particularly its irrational aspects.

Childhood. Childhood is roughly distinguished from infancy by the maturation of the capacity for language behavior. The child also starts to acquire various habits and elaborates numerous individual-social skills that can be grouped under perception, manipulation and motor coordination, and cognition. During this time, there is also emotional development and an increasing elaboration of the self, chiefly from the child's experiences of reflected appraisals. If the child is valued and treated with tenderness, he experiences himself as someone who is valuable, capable, and good. He learns to regard himself as good me, with its accompanying experiences of ever-growing self-confidence and self-respect. If he is subjected to frequent or indiscriminate disapproval, he tends to regard himself as bad and unworthy, with accompanying experiences of anxiety and lack of self-confidence and self-esteem.

Juvenile Era. The juvenile era is ushered in by a need for peers. During this stage, the juvenile enters a new dimension of social experience—the world outside the home. Apart from scholastic skills, the youngster normally learns or enhances the learning of numerous social skills and attitudes, including competition, cooperation, compromise, and social accommodation. The juvenile tends to learn that he no longer has a special place in the universe and must adjust to the limitations and opportunities of the world outside the home. If he fails, his chances for a normal life are gravely diminished. If he belongs to a special racial, ethnic, or religious group, he may encounter crippling experiences, causing his faith in himself and the world to be undermined forever.

In the school society, consensual validation is vigorously enforced. Many of the ideas and behaviors that were accepted in the home must be abandoned if one is to escape punishment. The learning of successful ways of expression and successful types of performance tend to earn one encouragement and rewards. The self usually learns to control focal awareness so that what does not make sense in the juvenile world tends to get less and less attention. However,

the misuse of selective inattention is a stumbling block on the road toward self-understanding, insight, and the learning of healthy interpersonal relations.

Supervisory patterns, complex processes and subpersonifications of the self-system, embody value judgments. Freud's supergo is one form of supervisory pattern, but there are many others. Ideally, these supervisory patterns function suavely and skillfully so that one is barely conscious of them. They are necessary for successful living, since they help maintain a conviction of personal worth.

A striking aspect of good orientation in living is the extent to which foresight governs the handling of intercurrent opportunities. A devotion to instant gratification is a sure sign of immaturity and perhaps a degree of demoralization. If the juvenile has been denied an opportunity to acquire a good orientation in living, he will henceforth be so anxious for the approval and unthinking regard of others that he may seem to live merely to be liked or to amuse.

Preadolescence. A new type of interest in another person normally appears at about 8 or 9 years of age. This interest is focused on a particular member of the same sex who becomes a close friend or chum. When fully developed, chumship is always a reciprocal relationship. The satisfactions and security of the other person become as important as one's own satisfactions and security. In the course of a good, successful preadolescence, one learns to relate to another without fear or anxiety. However, if a preadolescent has been warped by previous experience, the ability for intimacy may be gravely limited and transitory. Loneliness, which appears in full force at preadolescence, may become an everyday companion.

Early Adolescence. Sullivan distinguishes two phases of adolescence. The early phase extends from the eruption of true genital interest to the patterning of sexual behavior. To make sense of the complexities and difficulties that are experienced in adolescence and subsequent phases of life, one must be able to distinguish three generic needs, often intricately related and at the same time contradictory: personal security, intimacy, and sexual genital satisfaction.

During early adolescence, there is normally a

shift in the intimacy need. The boy begins to wonder how he can get to be on as friendly terms with a girl as he has been with his chum. This interest is usually ushered in by changes in his fantasy life and in covert processes generally. There may also be a spread in the area of overt communication between the chums to include ideas, attitudes, and information about the opposite sex.

Collisions of lust, security, and the need for intimacy may occur. Many people in early adolescence suffer much anxiety in connection with their newly developed motivation for sexual activity. Depending on previous learning, one may regard genital activity of any sort as disgraceful, disgusting, and damned. Perhaps because of jealousy, the parents may ridicule the young adolescent's reaching out toward a member of the other sex. Previous experience with the mother may make any promise of intimacy with the other sex too threatening and anxiety-provoking for male adolescents. Establishing collaborative intimacy with anyone, regardless of gender, may turn out to be an impossible task if social institutions are poisoned with an array of irrational elements.

Late Adolescence and Maturity. Late adolescence extends from the patterning of preferred genital activity to the establishment of a fully human or mature repertory of interpersonal relations. The long stretch of late adolescence, if successful, gradually evolves into maturity, which may extend and grow for at least another generation. The person who can attend a university and has the ability and motivation to profit from its educational resources can observe his fellows in various situations, learn about people in various parts of the world, and discuss what he and his fellows have observed within and outside the framework of university life. How to make a living and how to get on with people in the same line of work are similarly a source of observational data.

Theory of Psychopathology

A therapist must be alert to his patient's inadequate and inappropriate personifications of the self and others. Whether the therapist is dealing with hysteria, obsessive-compulsive neurosis, character disorders, schizophrenia, manic-depressive psychosis, or any other functional disorder, grasp of the limitations and distortions of the self-system provides the key to a revelation of the patient's disorder.

As a result of unfortunate past experiences, people develop views, attitudes, and beliefs about themselves that differ widely from the valid picture seen by an expert observer. These distorted views are forever trapping them or impelling them into incongruous and inappropriate situations. Then the person suffers the interference of anxiety, which hinders clear thought, accurate perception, and appropriate behavior. The person may sometimes blindly stumble into destructive situations from which he can extricate himself only with great difficulty, if at all.

With the exception of those who are badly crippled by hereditary or birth injuries, persons suffering from mental disorder are not really very different from most other human beings. Morbid processes are dynamisms pertaining to difficulties in living.

Dynamisms of difficulty are processes of social interaction or transaction that hinder or undermine healthy, satisfactory interpersonal relations. They are the processes of living, the particular parts of everyone's personal equipment, that are often so wrongly applied that they become self-defeating. They are functions of the self-system, and they are always related to arrests of development or regressions to an earlier stage.

Dynamisms of difficulty, thus, are functions of the personality that are often misused. They go into action in fashions that do not achieve a goal or achieve only an unsatisfactory goal. Their frequent recurrence or their tendency to occupy long stretches of time distinguishes the mentally disordered from the comparatively well. The extraordinary dependence of a person on a particular dynamism appears to be fundamental to mental disorder.

For example, a schizophrenic patient is one who, in the course of his life, has persistently manifested the dynamism of dissociation as a means of resolving the conflict between powerful needs, such as lust, and the restrictions that the self imposes on the satisfaction of these needs. Failure to resolve such a conflict may be the last blow to the person's fragile self-esteem and may precipitate the appearance of psychosis.

The obsessional person regresses in certain cognitive operations to early childhood. His magical thinking and ritualistic behavior grow and proliferate. In times of stress, the self-system becomes preoccupied with stratagems to preserve what little security the person has. The obsessional dynamism has relatively little to do with the satisfaction of somatic impulses; it has to do with interpersonal security.

Treatment

The psychiatric interview is a situation or series of situations in a two-member group composed of interviewer (the therapist) and interviewee (the patient or client). The two people are voluntarily more or less integrated in a progressively unfolding expert-client relationship for the purpose of elucidating and clarifying characteristic patterns of living that are experienced by the patient as particularly troublesome or especially valuable.

Any striking emotion on the part of the interviewer may.impede therapy by interfering with the therapist's objectively and by encouraging the patient to act out. Sullivan also took a dim view of the Peeping Tom attitude. Intense curiosity about the details of another person's life, particularly his sexual life, does not belong in a psychiatric interview. In due course, the patient's sexual life may emerge as a significant factor in therapy, but an intense curiosity about the intimate details may be entirely uncalled for and unnecessarily embarrassing to the patient. On the other hand, an attitude of disdainful indifference about what the patient has to offer is equally inappropriate.

Social interaction—interpersonal relations—is a form of mutual participation. The therapist must participate and observe at the same time. The patient's productions are within limits, meaningful to the therapist because they share a large body of similar experiences that have a public, conventional meaning. The more the therapist is conscious of his participation, the more he can control the therapeutic situation.

Perhaps the greatest stumbling block to communication in the two-member group is parataxic distortion, an illusory me-you pattern. In therapy the parataxic mode—operating primarily as a result of immaturity, anxiety, and perhaps regression—facilitates illusory personifications of the therapist. The patient substitutes for the psychiatrist an illusory person or persons strikingly different from the actual interviewer. He addresses his actions and attitudes to this imaginary person and interprets the psychiatrist's statements, questions, and behavior on the basis of the illusory personification. Through parataxic distortion the patient displays some of his gravest problems.

The psychiatrist involved with prolonged, intensive psychotherapy must know how to make transitions, so that the patient can follow the course of the interview and understand what his therapist is driving at. Sometimes the therapist needs to vary from this ideal. Frequently, he must change directions when, for example, the patient is on the verge of bringing up material that would be intolerably anxiety-provoking at that time. Sometimes the interview must proceed from one obscure situation to another when the patient skillfully eludes particular topics, perhaps unwittingly.

The interviewer has the task of discovering the major handicaps and major advantages in the patient's life. This discovery, if it occurs, does so when the psychiatrist experiences the ways interpersonal occurrences follow each other during the interview situation, how those interpersonal events relate to each other, what striking inconsistencies occur. The data of the interview are elicited not so much from the answers to questions as from the timing and stress of what the patient has said, the slight misunderstanding here and there, the omission of important facts, the occasions when the patient got off the subject while volunteering important information.

Sullivan mapped out four overlapping phases of the interview that serve as a guide, especially in prolonged, intensive psychotherapy. They are not meant to be employed rigidly.

Formal Inception

Usually, at the first physical encounter, the interviewee is a stranger and should be greeted accordingly. The psychiatrist immediately takes a good look at the patient—but he will perhaps never stare at him again. Then the interviewer tells the client what he learned about him when he was contacted for an appointment and gives the client an opportunity to revise the information if it is wrong.

The interviewer must be aware that the patient's behavior and what he says are adjusted to what he guesses about the therapist. The interviewer must also be conscious of the immediate impressions he has gained from his observations of the client and what these impressions are contributing to the interpersonal situation. The psychiatrist must also have some notion of how he facilitates or retards various things the patient may have thought of doing. However, the psychiatrist cannot immediately know whether he is right or wrong.

Reconnaissance

During the reconnaissance, the interviewer secures a rough social sketch of the patient's life, not an extensive life history. Sullivan asserted that in intensive psychotherapy he needed 7½ to 15 hours to complete the reconnaissance. During a single interview, when he would never see the patient again, Sullivan devoted about 20 minutes of a 1½-hour consultation to the reconnaissance. Sullivan would engage in hurried picking up of clues useful in assessing personality and habits, although he did not ask anything directly about the person's personality.

During the reconnaissance, a great many topics are covered, including the number of siblings in the family, the client's place in the time order of the siblings, who the family wage earner was, what sort of person the father was, whether the patient's family was happy, and whether his parents were happily married. The interviewer wants to know about the client's educational and occupational history, for these may reveal how well the patient gets along with others and how successful he is in his life and career. At this point, Sullivan would ask about the patient's marital status and, if married, whether he was happily married. By such questions, Sullivan would try to get clues about the client's relationships with the other sex, whether he was married more than once, why, and so on.

At the end of the reconnaissance, Sullivan would review what he had heard and learned. Then he would ask the patient to amend and correct those points the interviewer had misunderstood and to mention any important information he had missed. In his summary, Sullivan always strove to outline what he thought was a major problem in the patient's interpersonal relations.

Detailed Inquiry

The detailed inquiry improves on earlier approximations of understanding. On the basis of data obtained in the detailed inquiry, the therapist must often revise his early impressions of the client. One reason for this is that the patient may have given the psychiatrist information he believes will impress him.

The data the psychiatrist requires during the detailed inquiry pertain to information about the serious deficiencies and assets in the development of the client's personality, along with concomitant signs and symptoms. The deficiencies make up the principal business of the interview. Therefore, in the detailed inquiry Sullivan adhered to an outline that hit the high spots of the patient's developmental history while leaving room for additional details to be filled in as the interview progressed.

Starting with the childhood era—for the patient cannot recall infantile experience—the psychiatrist seeks information about such matters as disorders in learning toilet habits and speech habits. He can ask pointed and ordinarily prohibited questions, but he also looks for less direct clues to such information.

In the juvenile era, children are inducted into games. Games require cooperation, competition, and often a large element of compromise. The psychiatrist may ask direct questions about games and, in the interview itself, he may discover that some patients are manifestly competitive or conciliatory. After the discussion of competition, questions are asked about the client's experiences in grammar school. Did he like school? Did he learn a lot?

The interviewer must not proceed from one developmental era to the next too closely and clearly. To do so would be to risk suggesting to the client what answers or responses are expected of him. After asking something significant about the juvenile era, Sullivan would abruptly leap to college. If the patient attended college, the interviewer would ask how he got along there, both scholastically and socially. Then he would return to the preadolescent era and inquire whether the patient had a chum or close friend then. Questions relating to puberty would follow.

Sullivan inquired extensively about the patient's use of alcohol. Next he would ask about the client's eating habits, since they are occasions for social intercourse.

Sullivan would ask about the patient's sex life—although he rejected the idea that it is a mirror of personality—because it provides clues about the patient's development and important information about his relationships and attitudes toward both sexes. Questions about courtship, marriage, and parenthood logically follow.

The patient's vocational history pertains to his past, but it touches on current events indirectly. The psychiatrist finds out what jobs the client has held, his reasons for taking the jobs, his attitudes toward them, how successfully he performed them, and whether he has moved up or down the socio-economic scale during his occupational career. The psychiatrist tries to discover whether or not the patient's jobs enhanced his self-respect, as reflected by members of society.

An inquiry into the avocational and recreational histories of the patient follows next. Avocational and recreational fields are valuable and self-satisfying, but they also provide opportunities for meeting others and for establishing close relationships or casual acquaintances or for remaining remote.

Sullivan formulated a schematization of the personified self that is useful to the psychiatrist in the detailed inquiry. He suggested an inquiry into the following four types of information:

1. What does the interviewee esteem, and what does he disparge about himself?
2. To what experiences is the patient's self-esteem particularly, unreasonably vulnerable?
3. What characteristic security operations appear after the patient has been made anxious?
4. How great are the interviewee's reserves of security?

Termination or Interruption

In terminating the interview or in interrupting it for any length of time, the therapist must consider what progress has been made and consolidate whatever durable gain has been achieved. Sullivan suggested that the psychiatrist adopt the following four steps: (1) Give the patient a final statement, summarizing what has been learned. However, if the prognosis is unfavorable, the therapist almost never reveals this, since he must not leave the patient deeply disturbed or hopeless about his future. (2) Offer a prescription for action, a course of events in which the patient can engage to improve his chances of success in life. (3) Give the patient an assessment of the final statement and prescription for action, so that he gets a constructive picture of what he has been offered and its probable effects on his life course. (4) Take

formal leave without awkwardness and without prejudicing the benefits that have been accomplished.

REFERENCES

Mullahy, P. *Psychoanalysis and Interpersonal Psychiatry: The Contributions of Harry Stack Sullivan.* Science House, New York, 1970.

Sullivan, H. S. *Conceptions of Modern Psychiatry.* W. W. Norton, New York, 1953.

Sullivan, H. S. *The Interpersonal Theory of Psychiatry.* W. W. Norton, New York, 1953.

Sullivan, H. S. *The Psychiatric Interview.* W. W. Norton, New York, 1954.

Sullivan, H. S. *Clinical Studies in Psychiatry.* W. W. Norton, New York, 1956.

Sullivan, H. S. *Schizophrenia as a Human Process.* W. W. Norton, New York, 1962.

Sullivan, H. S. *The Fusion of Psychiatry and Social Science.* W. W. Norton, New York, 1964.

Sullivan, H. S. *Personal Psychopathology.* W. W. Norton, New York, 1972.

7.4.   SANDOR RADO

Introduction

Sandor Rado, born in Hungary in 1890, was an undergraduate studying law and political science when he made his first contact with Freud and psychoanalysis through reading a pamphlet by Sandor Ferenczi, who encouraged him to study medicine and pursue a career in psychiatry and psychoanalysis. Rado later helped Ferenczi organize the Hungarian Psychoanalytic Society and, while serving as its secretary, made the acquaintance of Freud.

In 1922, Rado joined the faculty of the Berlin Psychoanalytic Institute after he had moved to that city to be analyzed by Karl Abraham. In 1924, Freud appointed Rado managing editor of *Internationale Zeitschrift für Psychoanalyse*, and, several years later, Rado was appointed to the same post on *Imago*. In 1931, the New York Psychoanalytic Society invited him to come to New York to assist in the establishment of a new psychoanalytic institute.

In 1945, Rado was appointed a professor of psychiatry at Columbia University and became director of the first psychoanalytic institute established within a university medical school. After his retirement from Columbia in 1955, Rado founded the New York School of Psychiatry, which was devoted chiefly to training psychiatrists in the New York State hospital system.

Theory of Personality

Rado referred to his theory of adaptational psychodynamics as "based on the Freudian methods of free association and interpretations of unconscious processes by contextual inference." Rado sees his theory as continuing the schema of motivational dynamics and, in accord with Freud's pleasure-pain principle, views the organism as a biological system operating under hedonic control. At other times, however, instead of stressing continuity, Rado speaks of retransforming psychoanalysis into a medical science. There was never any question in Rado's mind that psychoanalysis, despite various methodological differences, should remain an integral part of general psychiatry, medicine, and biological science.

In adaptational terms, the psychologically healthy person is one whose psychic apparatus is performing its adaptive functions effectively. Psychological illness or disordered behavior is defined as a failure of the organism's psychological equipment to perform its adaptive function, the severity of the disorder being measured in terms of the threat to the person's physical and psychosocial survival and well-being.

Levels of Integration

Rado saw the psychological blue print of the human being as consisting of four hierarchically arranged levels of integration—hedonic self-regulation, preverbal brute emotion, emotional thought, and unemotional thought.

At the hedonic level, pain signals to the organism that it is in the presence of damage and motivates it to move away; pleasure indicates to the organism that it is in the presence of a benefit and elicits moving-toward or clinging-to behavior. Pain, as well as having a disorganizing effect if persistent, seems to indicate to the organism that it is failing and hence has a reductive effect on the self-esteem. Pleasure, on the other hand, is viewed as indicating to the organism that it is successful, thereby having the effect of raising self-esteem. Disturbances in the pleasure mechanism are viewed by Rado as playing a primary role in the pathogenesis of certain forms of disordered behavior, particularly drug dependence and schizophrenia.

Rado divided the emotions into two groups—the emergency emotions and the welfare or tender emotions. The emergency emotions, fear and rage, are defined as responses to actual or anticipated pain or damage; they prepare the organism psychologically and physiologically for flight or fight. The welfare emotions are responses to actual or anticipated pleasure or benefit; they prepare the organism psychologically or physiologically to cling to or to possess the pleasurable stimulus. Emotions may be pleasant or painful, have little or considerable thought content, and be expressed through either voluntary motor activity or the autonomic nervous system. The fact that emotional responses are frequently stimulated by symbolic or unconscious impulses is a key factor in the development of emotional illness.

Emotional thought is primarily an intellectual expression of underlying feelings and has little to do with objective reality. Fantasies of all kinds, dreams, prejudices, biases, and a good deal of everyday thinking are largely manifestations of emotional thought. Illusions, delusions, and hallucinations are particularly pure examples of emotional thought. The principal characteristic of emotional thought is that it is selective and tends to justify and feed the emotion from which it springs.

The unemotional thought level acknowledges the human being's capacity to be rational and objective, to see things as they are. However, the motivating and integrating influence of unemotional thought in controlling everyday behavior is relatively weak. Insofar as this level makes it possible for the human being to delay action and gratification, tolerate pain, forego present pleasure for future gain, and control his emotional responses, it is the equivalent of Freud's reality principle. But since man is essentially a hedonic and emotionally organized animal, his behavior is always limited, modified, and controlled to some extent by nonobjective influences. To Rado, man's emotional needs—trust, friendship, love, affectionate exchange—must be met if he is to function in a state of health.

Conscience

The conscience facilitates cooperation and curbs murderous competition by internal controls, rather than by external restraints. The development of conscience is based essentially on the dependent child's need and desire to remain in his parents'—usually his mother's—good graces or, conversely, on his fear of losing her loving approval and support. The child believes that his parents see and know all, and this belief produces in the child a fear of inescapable punishment, the component of guilt that makes the conscience mechanism a powerful influence on behavior. The fully mature conscience operates unconsciously and automatically; it should facilitate and reward good behavior, thereby raising self-esteem, and should restrain and punish bad behavior, which lowers self-esteem.

Pain-dependent behavior—Rado's term for masochistic behavior, sexual or otherwise—is a maladaptive form of expiatory behavior based on strong guilty fears. These fears motivate the person to seek punishment in advance, so that he is then permitted to satisfy the prohibited pleasurable desire.

A complication of discipline and the development of conscience is the inevitable build-up of rage that occurs when a child obeys or submits to parental prohibitions. This repressed rage constantly seeks discharge. Conscience plays a crucial role in determining how much rage is built up and whether it is discharged and used constructively or destructively. Guilty rage externalizes the blame and is temporarily less painful to the person's self-esteem than is guilty fear. However, bouts of guilty rage either elicit quick retaliation or, if sustained, give rise to painful feelings of persecution that may develop into full-blown delusions.

Self

The term Rado substituted for ego is "action-self" (see Figure 1). The action-self integrates the conscious organism into a self-aware and intentionally acting whole. The integral action-self system also functions unconsciously.

Rado saw the action-self originating in the proprioceptive sensations that the infant derives from vigorous sucking at the mother's breast. The child's first or primordial concept of self is that of an omnipotent, magical being. When the child discovers that his actual powers are limited, he is forced to give up or repress this picture of self. On the way to developing a more realistic concept of self, the child delegates his omnipotence and magical powers to his parents, who are then supposed to use these powers for his benefit.

Rado conceives of the organism as appreciating itself as a proved provider of pleasure. This emotional appreciation of self is the basis of self-esteem or pride.

Theory of Psychopathology

The failure of emergency adjustment, fundamentally an overproduction of fear and rage, is at the basis of all disordered behavior, the

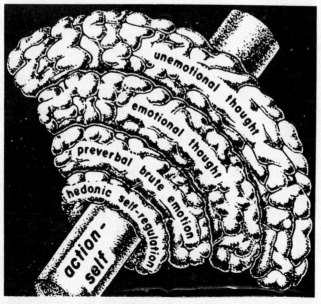

FIGURE 1. Integrative apparatus of the psychodynamic cerebral system. (From Rado, S., *Psychoanalysis of Behavior*, vol. II, p. 46, Grune & Stratton, New York, 1962. By permission of Grune & Stratton.)

severity of the particular disorder being determined by the intensity, extent, and duration of the resulting adaptive failure. When the initial excessive emergency responses either persist or recur, the organism has only limited equipment with which to cope or adapt to the painful and threatening situation (see Table I).

Miscarried Prevention

In its simplest form, miscarried prevention is a reparative response after an attack of fear. This response leads to (1) avoidance of the place in which the attack occurred, in which case it is called phobic avoidance, (2) avoidance of the activity being engaged in when the attack of fear occurred, in which case it is likely to be called an inhibition, or (3) some combination of the two.

Miscarried Repair

Miscarried repair means essentially the maintenance of or revival of patterns of behavior of the helpless, dependent child. The forms most prominent in the production of pathological behavior are (1) further regression to helpless behavior, (2) attempts to break the inhibition by defiant, coercive rage or by ingratiating behavior to obtain permission or regain approval or a combination of the two, as often seen in obsessional behavior, and (3) reliance on magical or illusory fulfillment through wishful

TABLE I
*Rado's Concept of the Development of
Disordered Behavior*

An array of fears of various forms of retaliation or punishment for assertive, angry, defiant, or sexual behavior or feelings lead to:

Inhibitions and losses of healthy function. These are essentially losses of adaptive utility, especially the capacity to work and the ability to obtain the minimal requirement of pleasure and to maintain healthy pride or self-esteem. Since these losses result in damage to functional capacity and to the child's pride and concept of self, they elicit:

Automatic mechanisms of repair:
1. Healthy repair. If successful, the child outgrows the infantile neurosis.
2. Miscarried prevention and repair. Reparative efforts often miscarry for the obvious reason that the behaviorally causative factor, the excessive emergency responses, is usually repressed to some degree, if not entirely.

---

thinking, fantasy, or stature cosmetics, characteristic of hysterical behavior.

The two factors that Rado most strongly emphasized in the production of disordered behavior are the prolonged total helplessness and dependency of the child and the inevitable battle for power that takes place between the mother and the child. The child's fear of loss of approval or other punishment if he asserts himself is viewed as the fundamental problem. These fears of self-assertion manifest themselves most damagingly in the areas of work (capacity to cooperate and compete) and of social and sexual behavior.

Overreactive Behavior

The essence of overreactive or neurotic behavior is emergency dyscontrol, characterized by uncomplicated attacks of fear or rage that, depending on the degree of repression, may be expressed in dreams, phobias, inhibitions of motor behavior, or simple hypochondriac patterns in which the fear of punishment is expressed as a fear of illness.

Neurotic behavior, whatever its final form, is viewed as developing or occurring in persons whose basic pattern of behavior is characterized by some degree of social and familial overdependence and by significant inhibitions in self-assertiveness that interfere with performance in the social, sexual, and work areas in particular. What form the neurotic elaboration takes depends on the family constellation, socio-economic status, and cultural factors. The type of symptomatic behavior depends also on the severity and extent of the early inhibitions in adaptive capacity, the degree of damage to self-esteem, and the degree to which reparative attempts were successful or failed.

Schizotypal Behavior

Rado hypothesizes the presence of an innate integrative pleasure deficiency, as well as a proprioceptive diathesis, probably also innate, as being characteristic of what he called schizotypal organization. One of the most significant ways the integrative pleasure deficiency manifest itself is in a weakness in the motivating and organizing action of pleasure, resulting in a reduction in the welfare or tender emotions—affection, love, joy, pride, and pleasurable desire—which leads to a diminished capacity to deal with people on a warm, spontaneous, emotional level. The proprioceptive diathesis seems to manifest itself most directly in a profound disturbance of self-confidence and extreme self-consciousness.

Among the many clinical traits that may be seen, three stand out: overdependence on others to an extreme degree, compensatory use of intellect (the patient attempts to think his way through life because of a lack of confidence in feelings), and a scarcity economy of pleasure (the patient clings to scarce pleasure resources, even if self-damaging, and experiences any loss of pleasure as a severe blow). A failure or loss in any of these three compensatory areas may precipitate an episode of decompensation or disorganization.

Treatment

Rado tends to define psychological health in terms of the relative predominance of the welfare emotions and the person's capacity to be reasonably independent and self-reliant. The emergency responses are still active but find nondestructive outlets and are not of sufficient intensity or duration to cause maladaptive behavior.

The two primary goals of psychotherapeutic technique are an alteration in the patient's emotional organization and an increase in the patient's self-reliance. Emotional re-education is designed to increase the motivating influence of the welfare emotions and to reduce the influence of the emergency responses. Although it does not neglect the past, the adaptational approach strongly stresses the fact that the main reason for exploring the past is to increase understanding of the present.

In Rado's opinion, the classical method infantilized the patient, instead of achieving Freud's stated goal of helping him achieve the highest level of maturity attainable. Preventing the patient, as much as possible, from developing a transference neurosis and frankly encouraging greater educational activity on the part of the therapist are two of the main points of difference between the two techniques.

The nature and extent of the patient's ability to cooperate is the crucial element in the adaptational technique. A particular psychotherapeutic approach is selected not on the basis of a diagnostic label but, rather, because the particular method is best suited to the patient's capacity to work or cooperate with the therapist. The main purpose of what Rado called interceptive interpretation was essentially the prevention of regressions.

In his treatment approach Rado made a sharp distinction between treatment behavior and life performance. Not only did he stress the role of the therapist as educator, but he also emphasized the importance of successful doing on the part of the patient in the area of everyday practical living.

REFERENCES

Rado, S. *Psychoanalysis of Behavior*, 2 vols. Grune & Stratton, New York, 1956, 1962.
Rado, S. On the retransformation of psychoanalysis into a medical science. Compr. Psychiatry, *3:* 317, 1962.

7.5.   ERIC BERNE

Introduction

Eric Berne (see Figure 1), the founder of transactional analysis, was trained in classical psychoanalysis. He set aside the Freudian treatment modality in favor of more rapidly effective techniques. Transactional analysis was formally developed by Berne from the mid-1950's until his death in 1970, and it was originally used as a specific adjunct in group psychotherapy. Berne was influenced by the innovative California group therapy milieu, including encounter, marathon, the Synanon approach, and, most important, the gestalt techniques of Frederick Perls.

Intuition

Berne initially defined intuition as "knowledge based upon experience and acquired through sensory contact with the subject without the 'intuitor' being able to formulate for himself or others exactly how he came to his conclusion." This knowledge was on a preverbal level. He also noted that intuition is facilitated by a state of awareness that requires intense concentration on the object of intuition. He distinguished intuition from the passive-alert state used by many psychotherapists. He discovered that the intuitive process can be improved on with practice and that accuracy increases with experience. Fatigue tends to decrease intuitive powers; so does being put on the spot. He surmised that the intellect alone is

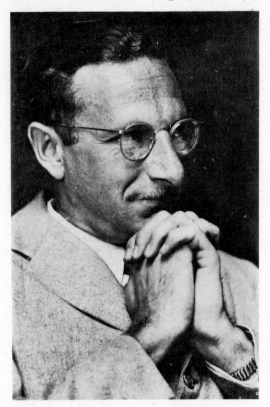

FIGURE 1. Eric Berne (Wide World Photos).

not the dominant force in correct guessing or in understanding life. He challenged the notion that logical and verbal abilities constitute knowledge.

Berne became interested in nonvocal indicators, such as facial expressions, voluntary and involuntary movements, tics, and gazes. He paid particular attention to people's responses to different types of stimuli. Berne was impressed by the ability of small children, even at a preverbal age, to distinguish between friendly and unfriendly people. He also observed that people diagnosed as schizophrenic seem to have this facility from time to time. He further observed this ability in artists, poets, actors, and other creative persons who occasionally operate on nonverbal levels.

Berne distinguished between primal images and ordinary memory images. Primal images have a pseudoperceptual quality and a superior clearness, richness, and accuracy of detail, with brilliant coloration.

Ego States

An ego state is a cohesive system of feelings and thoughts, with a related set of behavior patterns. Each person has a repertoire of ego states that can be broken down into the child ego state, which represents archaic elements that become fixed in early childhood but remain active throughout life; the adult ego state, which is computerlike and is autonomously directed toward objective appraisals of reality; and the parent ego state, which is derived from the person's parental figures.

Berne ascertained that the child ego state is not a direct manifestation of the id. To Berne, the child ego state is a dynamic and functioning part of the personality, conscious and readily observable and involved as a determinant in behavior.

Berne emphasized that the intuitive faculty, which is archaic and lodged in the child ego state, can be cultivated by the successful therapist. A potent therapist resurrects the dormant aspect of the imaginative child. Too much adult ego state, with its rational thinking, decreases the efficiency of the intuitive child ego state. The same holds true for ethical, moral, or prejudicial parental thinking. A see-no-evil type of value, dwelling in the therapist's parent ego state, hinders his intuitive powers.

Intuition works best when the child predominates and when the adult and the parent are decathected and decommissioned. A person uses intuitive faculties as he chooses his playmates at any age in life, and it becomes the most valuable tool of the therapist when diagnosing and treating patients. To Berne, creativity was the child knowing and the adult confirming.

The structure of delusional thinking is exemplified by the breakdown of the functional barriers between the adult and the child, in which fantasy and archaic imagery in the child become mixed with the adult. Another major type of ego state pathology is exclusion, which occurs when a person cannot freely cathect the different ego states. The fixed parent of a prejudiced country preacher, who finds evil and sin under every bush, is an example.

Transactions

Berne defined a transaction as a stimulus from an ego state of one person and the corresponding response from an ego state of another person. He distinguished between two different types of communication—the manifest and the latent. In a *complementary* transaction, the vectors—the stimulus and the response—are parallel. The first rule of communication is: Whenever the vectors are parallel, communication can proceed indefinitely. In a crossed transaction, the corresponding rule is: Whenever the vectors cross, communication on that subject ceases immediately. An ulterior transaction shows a complex use of both the manifest transaction, which Berne called the social level, and the latent transaction, which he called the psychological level, and leads to a third rule of communication: Behavior cannot be predicted by the social level alone. Attention to the psychological message is the key to predicting behavior and is necessary for the understanding of games.

Games

Certain types of human behavior—predictable, stereotyped, usually destructive, and motivated by hidden desires—are clarified by Berne in his definition of psychological *games* (see Figure 2). People learn game patterns in childhood and play them throughout their lives. People are inclined to have a small repertoire of games and base their social relationships on finding suitable people to share them. Berne devised a game formula to which all games conform:

Con + Gimmick = Response → Switch → Payoff

All behavior adhering to this formula is a game; other behavior is not. The switch is represented by the drama triangle. The three positions of the drama triangle are pursecutor, rescuer, and victim.

Games contain ulterior transactions, conform to the game formula, and contain a dramatic switch that leads to the payoff. Game phenomena have predictive value for both the therapist and the patient, foretelling the outcome of treatment and perhaps the life course. The therapist proposes antithetical moves to block the games, disrupting the patient's pathological pattern. Awareness of these patterns allows a patient the opportunity to redecide whether to continue the game or to explore alternative growth possibilities and options.

Strokes

Berne used the term "strokes" to describe what he considered the basic motivating factor of human behavior. Infants need touching or strokes for survival; they gradually learn to obtain stroking in more symbolic or substitute ways as they grow older. Words, glances, and other human recognitions are symbolic strokes, and the developing child learns ways to maximize the number of strokes received from mother, father, and siblings. Ideally, strokes are obtained in a loving and positive way, but in certain families negative strokes are exchanged. Even negative strokes can be important for survival, at least on a temporary basis, because they are better than none at all. A stroke deficit leads to increased game playing and sometimes bizarre behavior.

Scripts

One's success or psychopathology is determined by the degree of conformity to important early transactions. These are symbolized by the script matrix (see Figure 3). A script becomes lodged in the child ego state and is carried into fantasy life. Berne differed from Jung and his theory of the collective unconscious because he felt that these influences and forces are passed

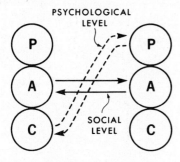

A GAME DIAGRAM

FIGURE 2. Typical game.

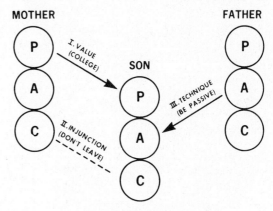

A TYPICAL SCRIPT MATRIX

FIGURE 3. Matrix.

on directly and transactionally from parent to child, from generation to generation.

Contracts

Berne used certain unique techniques in his groups. One consisted of the doctor and the patient forming a distinct contract with a clear and precise end point, colloquially called the "cure." Berne would not accept a contract from a patient unless it was antithetical to that person's usual game playing and script-influenced behavior. He felt that the contractual nature of treatment served to break up games and that it gave both the therapist and the patient the necessary permission to be potent.

Berne encouraged active participation by therapists and focused on the transaction between the therapist and the patient.

The success of transactional analysis is, in part, due to the reduction of the complex maze surrounding human problems and distilling them to their simplest forms. Berne admonished his colleagues to use readily understandable words of two syllables or less. A simple vocabulary of easily defined words evolved in his treatment groups and eliminate the mysterious aura. This simplification helped the therapist and patients talk straight to each other.

REFERENCES

Berne, E. *Transactional Analysis in Psychotherapy.* Grove Press, New York, 1961.
Berne, E. *The Structure and Dynamics of Organizations and Groups.* J. B. Lippincott, Philadelphia, 1963.
Berne, E. *Games People Play.* Grove Press, New York, 1964.
Berne, E. *Principles of Group Treatment.* Oxford University Press, New York, 1966.
Berne, E. *Sex in Human Loving.* Simon and Schuster, New York, 1970.
Berne, E. *What Do You Say after You Say Hello?* Grove Press, New York, 1972.
Dusay, J. Eric Berne's studies of intuition, 1949–1962. Trans. Anal. J., *1:* 1, 1970.
Dusay, J. Egograms and the constancy hypothesis. Trans. Anal. J., *2:* 3, 1972.

8

Theories of Personality and Psychopathology: Other Psychoanalytic and Related Schools

8.1. ADOLF MEYER

Introduction

Adolf Meyer (see Figure 1) was born in Niederwenigen, in the outskirts of Zurich, on November 3, 1866, the son of a Zwinglian minister. In medical school he came under the influence of August Forel, director of the Burghölzli Hospital for the Insane. After he passed the state examination in 1890, Meyer spent a year in Paris, London, and Edinburgh. In Paris, he attended Charcot's lectures and, a year later, studied under the neurologist J. J. Déjérine. In England, he was strongly influence by the Darwinian, ecological orientation of Thomas Huxley and by the teaching of Hughlings Jackson, who posited the functioning of the individual person on progressive levels of integration viewed in the context of the evolution and dissolution of the central nervous system. Unable to find a university position, Meyer emigrated to the United States, where he accepted a position as pathologist at the State Hospital in Kankakee, Illinois.

In 1895 Meyer opposed the emphasis on heredity in psychiatry and stressed, instead, the moral and intellectual characteristics that could be traced back to childhood years. That same year he accepted a position as pathologist at the Worcester State Hospital and secured an academic appointment at the nearby Clark University. In 1902 he was called as director of the Pathological Institute of New York State, later renamed the Psychiatric Institute. From 1904 to 1907, as professor of psychiatry at the Cornell University Medical College, he organized the first psychiatric outpatient clinic in New York City.

In 1903, Meyer postulated that mental disorder often had its roots in a personality imbalance caused by the disorganization of habits. He viewed the incomprehensible symptoms of mental illness as crude and inadequate attempts by the patient to cure himself, attempts that had to be guided, rather than suppressed. Kraepelin stressed deterioration as the eventual outcome in dementia precox, but Meyer believed that personality traits, such as withdrawal, preceded the appearance of the disease, and he suggested that prevention and recovery were possible.

In 1906, Meyer argued that it was possible to classify patients according to a new system of reaction types—that is, typical ways of behaving in difficult or emergency situations. He recommended that the patient's school, family, and community make an attempt to intervene early in the development of mental illness. The first applications of the principles of social work to occupational and recreational therapy with convalescent patients and the organization of aftercare programs were inspired by Meyer's work during this period.

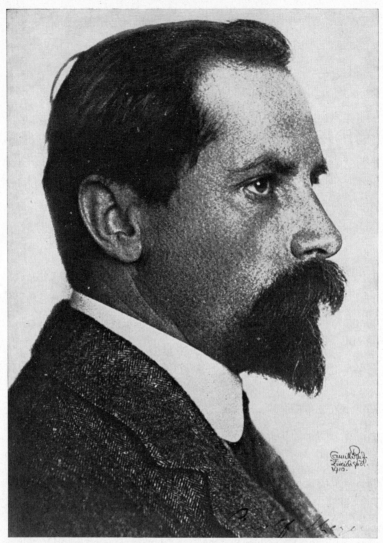

FIGURE 1. Adolf Meyer, 1866–1950. (Courtesy National Library of Medicine, Bethesda, Md.)

Meyer accepted the importance of unconscious factors in psychopathology. In New York, he came in personal contact with some of the earliest adherents of the psychoanalytic movement, notably Brill and Jones. Meyer warned against premature rejection of psychoanalysis, although he objected to Freud's emphasis on the pathological and hypothetical, rather than on the healthy and verifiable aspects of mental functioning. In 1909, he introduced the term "psychobiological interpretation."

Meyer was appointed professor of psychiatry at Johns Hopkins Medical School in 1909, and in 1913 the Phipps Clinic was opened, with Meyer as its director.

Theory of Psychobiology

Psychobiology emphasized the importance of biographical study in understanding the whole person in the whole situation–the biology of the whole personality. The object of such study is the individual person, whom Meyer defined as a biological unit that always functions as a person, whether alone or in groups. Although the person's experiential continuum changes constantly, it enables him to maintain an internal and external homeostatic equilibrium in coping with new situations. In addition, the person's plasticity allows him a wide spectum of differentiation in capacity and function and a relatively high degree of spontaneity and responsiveness. Because of the complexity of human functioning, the psychiatrist who attempts to acquire a scientific understanding of his patients must have a combination of attributes: He must be a methodical investigator, a biographer, an artist, and an educator.

Objective psychobiology consisted of the observation of objective facts, the formulation of predictable conditions in which these facts may occur, and the testing and validation of methods for their controlled modification. Instead of accepting predetermined hypothetical psychological or metapsychological constructs to account for these facts, Meyer emphasized the soundness of common sense, a fact that justified involving all kinds of laymen in working for community mental health.

Although an analysis of psychobiological assets may reveal the presence of a variety of factors in each person, Meyer emphasized the basic tendency toward integration that takes place. Because Meyer believed that multiple biological, social, and psychological forces contribute to the growth and development of the personality, he concluded that psychiatrists must study normal and abnormal behavior from many viewpoints.

Meyer conceived of the clinical value of the biographical approach to personality study as follows: It provides a practical and specific guide for eliciting individual data, a means of organizing that data, and a method for checking and reevaluating data elicited under varying conditions.

Treatment

For Meyer, the clinical psychiatric examination included the following components: (1) identifying the motives or indications for the examination, with particular focus on presenting pertinent details in the patient's life history, elicited through biographical study, (2) listing the obviously related personality items, factors, and reactions, (3) careful study of the physical, neurological, genetic, and social status and of the correlation between these variables and personality factors, (4) differential diagnosis, and (5) formulation of a therapeutic plan geared to each case. Symptoms were viewed as compensatory phenomena.

In interviewing a patient, Meyer considered it better to begin by focusing on his chief complaint, which directed attention to the situation that required immediate therapeutic intervention. Later, the psychiatrist determined the nature and extent of the disturbance in the context of the patient's over-all functioning, his previous medical history, and the role played by such factors as constitution, development, and environment. Unconscious material elicited from the patient, as well as information supplied by his family, supplemented the psychiatrist's efforts and facilitated his understanding of the situation.

Meyer believed that the psychiatrist began to treat the patient at the time of their initial contact, with the patient's exposition of his problem. This did not mean that diagnosis was not essential. However, the first step was the evaluation of the patient's assets and liabilities. This evaluation was best accomplished through the study of his life history, on the basis of current data initially provided by the patient and supplemented by his subsequent reconstruction of past experiences.

The cooperation of the patient's better self—that is, of the healthier part of the patient's ego—was considered essential. Therapy was thought of as a service performed on behalf of the patient. The basic aim of psychobiological therapy was to help an organism, hampered by abnormal conditions, to make the best adaptation possible to life and change.

In the initial stage of treatment, the therapist's concern focused on the patient's sleep habits, his nutrition, and the regulation of his daily routines. It was also important at this stage to induce the patient to describe his difficulties in a concrete way and for the therapist to use the patient's ideation and language to communicate his offer of help and advice.

Problems were approached on a conscious, rather than an unconscious, level. Therapy was administered in the course of ordinary, face-to-face conversation. At the beginning of each therapeutic session, the patient was encouraged to discuss his experiences in the interval since the last interview, beginning with obvious and immediate problems. Eventually, when deeper relevant material had been elicited from the patient, these problems were explored in greater detail. This exploration was accomplished through the use of spontaneous association, a term used by Meyer in preference to "free association" to describe the overcoming of the patient's resistance to verbalizing his basic problems in the unbiased atmosphere of the psychiatrist's office.

The intensity and frequency of the treatment sessions depended on the need of the individual patient. The psychiatrist permitted the patient to arrange his treatment schedule or asked him to agree to a specific therapeutic program. It was the psychiatrist's responsibility to reassure the patient so that he could function adequately between interviews. This reassurance was conveyed through casual comments and sensitive questioning.

Under the guidance of the psychiatrist, the patient analyzed his personality problems and their relative importance and then reconstructed the origin of his conflicts and devised healthier behavioral patterns. The psychobiological therapist asked the patient to formulate his life story by means of a life chart to demonstrate his understanding of the origin of his difficulties and the means he might use to ensure their resolution and to prevent their repetition.

Meyer believed that the essential goal of therapy was to aid the patient's adjustment by helping him to modify unhealthy adaptations; these modifications would lead to personal satisfaction and proper environmental readjustment. He called this "habit training." In the process of habit training, the psychiatrist used a variety of techniques—for example, guidance, suggestion, re-education, and direction—always with emphasis on the current life situation. Psychobiological therapy was especially valuable with psychotics, although it was also recommended for neurotic reactions. To evaluate a patient's progress and his return to normality, Meyer preferred the criteria of the capacity of the person to follow a constructive regimen of work, rest, and play.

Conclusion

Meyer's major contributions to psychiatry include his emphasis on the interactive nature of symptoms and the unity of the individual person's psychological and biological functioning, so that psychoses are described as reactions, a definition that was reflected in the 1952 edition of the American Psychiatric Association's *Diagnostic and Statistical Manual, Mental Disorders*, his pioneering biographical and historical approach to the study of personality, his support of the psychotherapeutic treatment

of schizophrenia, and his enthusiasm for social action, especially for community psychiatry.

However, Meyer shied away from any systematization of his thinking. In particular, he never outlined developmental stages and their critical tasks and, in contrast with Freud and his followers, never presented clear and comprehensive clinical histories of patients and thorough discussions of the therapeutic programs and techniques used. It is likely that his common-sense philosophy, being concrete and understandable to many, was incorporated into the mainstream of psychiatry without any mention of its originator. Moreover, psychobiology focused almost exclusively on the individual and on the community at large but hardly at all on the family as the transmitter of symbolic functioning and communication.

The importance of Meyer's psychobiology lies in its being a trend of thought that paved the way for the acceptance of psychodynamic concepts and in its representing a typical expression of American pluralistic thinking that is relevant today to community mental health.

REFERENCES

Deutsch, A. *The Mentally Ill in America.* Columbia University Press, New York, 1967.
Diethelm, O. Adolf Meyer (1866–1950). In *Grosse Nervenärtze,* K. Kolle, editor, vol. 2, p. 129. Thieme, Stuttgart, 1959.
Hale, N. G. *Freud and the Americans: The Beginning of Psychoanalysis in the United States, 1876–1917.* Oxford University Press, New York, 1971.
Lidz, T. Adolf Meyer and the development of American psychiatry. Am. J. Psychiatry, *123:* 320, 1966.
Lief, A., ed. *The Commonsense Psychiatry of Adolf Meyer.* McGraw-Hill, N. Y., 1948.
Meyer, A. *Collected Papers of Adolf Meyer,* 4 vols. Johns Hopkins Press, Baltimore, 1948–1952.
Meyer, A. *Psychobiology: A Science of Man.* Charles C Thomas, Springfield, Ill., 1957.

8.2. CARL JUNG

Introduction

Carl Gustav Jung (see Figure 1) was born on July 26, 1875, in the Swiss canton Thurgau. His father was a Lutheran minister who was well-intentioned but somewhat strict and puritanical. Jung studied medicine. In 1900, he went to the Psychiatric Clinic of Bürgholzli in Zürich to work as an assistant under Eugen Bleuler.

While at the Burgholzli, Jung undertook studies of word association, wrote a classic

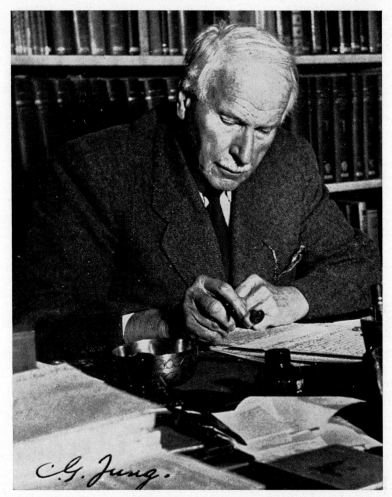

FIGURE 1. Carl Gustav Jung, 1875–1961. (Courtesy National Library of Medicine, Bethesda, Md.)

textbook on schizophrenia, and became an advocate of Sigmund Freud. Jung met Freud for the first time in 1907. When Jung was writing "Transformations and Symbols of the Libido," he knew it would alienate Freud because he suggested that a large part of the unconscious was objective or collective and had nothing to do with the sexual instincts. The publication of the book ended Jung's association with Freud and with the psychoanalytic movement.

After his break with Freud, Jung went into private practice and began a long and arduous exploration of his own unconscious to discover as much as he could about the objective psyche. Analytical psychology centered on the analysis of the symbols of the objective psyche and the realization of the self. Jung died in 1961 at the age of 85.

Symbol

At the heart of Jungian theory lies the concept of the symbol. Within Freudian psychology, symbols, particularly dream symbols, were assumed to reflect wishes and impulses that were repressed from conscious experience but then sought outlet in a disguised, symbolic form. Freud believed that all symbols were related to some hostile or sexual motivation. In the Freudian view, symbols allowed forbidden impulses to gain entry into consciousness, where they agitated the ego to work toward their satisfaction and fulfillment.

Jung agreed with Freud that many symbols did represent what he called the personal unconscious. Symbols in the personal unconscious derived from the person's own life experiences and were memory traces taken over and activated by socially prohibited thoughts and impulses. But Jung argued that such symbols were not the only ones that presented themselves to consciousness in dreams and reverie states. Some symbols originated from a deeper level of the unconscious, which Jung once called the "collective unconscious" but later called the "objective psyche." The symbols in this objective psyche do not derive from individual experience but, rather, from the collective experience of the race. They are archetypical modes of thought.

Not only are the symbols of the objective psyche different in origin from those of the personal unconscious, but they are different in their functions. The function of symbols derived from the personal unconscious is to satisfy some unacceptable instinctual wish or impulse. But the symbols of the objective unconscious are much more closely tied to the total personality. Such symbols provide clues to hidden potentialities and qualities that the conscious mind would not otherwise be aware of. In addition, the symbols of the objective unconscious point toward the future and suggest the direction in which the person is moving in his own development.

In a Jungian analysis, the realization of one's potentials comes about gradually through a laborious process of getting to know various facets of one's objective psyche. Ordinarily, this voyage of personal discovery goes through predictable stages, wherein more or less universal facets of the objective psyche come to the fore in many different guises. Only after these various facets have been confronted is the person free to realize the innermost part of himself that Jung calls the self.

Shadow

In many ways, the shadow is the objective counterpart of the personal unconscious in the sense that it represents some of the unacceptable aspects and components of the objective psyche. Indeed, the shadow can also include aspects of the personal unconscious. The person who rejects the shadow parts of himself can never be totally honest with himself and never reach true integration as a whole personality.

The shadow consists, in part, of all the little sins and faults that one tends to ignore or forget about oneself because they do not fit with one's more flattering self-conceptions. Coming to

grips with this aspect of the shadow requires a certain level of maturity and of perspective, which does not usually emerge until the second half of life. But the other parts of the shadow also begin to emerge in the second half of life, not because they were repressed or denied but because they were never given the opportunity to be realized. These objective psyche components of the shadow can appear in dreams, in a person's artistic productions, or in his actions when he projects the contents of his shadow onto the external world.

Anima and Animus

After a person has come to grips with his shadow, in both its personal and its objective unconscious guises, he next meets his feminine side in the case of a man and her masculine side in the case of the woman. The anima and the animus are combinations of personal and objective unconscious elements. The anima and animus elements can have negative effects if they are ignored and repressed or positive effects if they are integrated within the personality and regarded as symbols of directions to be taken for further development of the personality.

The anima in man involves many different psychological tendencies, such as moods, feelings, and intuitions that are usually characteristic of the opposite sex. Jung argues that the anima in man often appears as receptivity to the irrational, openness to romantic love, and a feeling for nature. Aspects of the anima that derive from personal experience with the mother are colored by her qualities as a person.

Jung suggested that the anima as it is constructed in the individual psyche has four stages. The earliest form of the anima is an Evelike figure who is an earth-mother type and who represents primitive reproductive and sexual functions and pleasures. At the next stage, the anima is personified in a romantic ideal, such as Helen in the story of Faust. Helen represents purity and sexuality at a high and romantic plane. The next stage raises femininity to an even higher level and is embodied in the figure of the Virgin Mary. In Mary the sexual and maternal functions are no longer worldly; they have become spiritual. At the final stage, the anima transcends even the heights of spiritual purity and holiness and exists as a form of pure wisdom.

In dealing with these objective unconscious anima figures, the individual man must avoid two persistent dangers. One of these dangers is to think of the emergent anima figure as a fantasy, a made-up figure with no real meaning and no real function. In treating the anima in this way, the man fails to recognize the message that the anima carries and misses a chance for further personal growth. The opposite danger is to project the anima and to deal with it as real. The man who deals with the anima as the representation of some external verity, institution, or belief loses the personal value that the anima figure may have for him. Likewise, if the anima figure is projected onto a real woman, the man can never deal with her as the person she is but only as the anima that he wants her to be. The result is, at best, disappointment and, at worst, a disaster for both.

In Jung's view, the best way for a man to deal with his anima figures is to accept them as realities of his own psychic existence and to try to understand them as such. Once the man grasps the meaning of these animas for himself, they can be integrated within his personality and become functioning parts of it, under the control of the conscious personality, which can use them for creative and constructive purposes.

The animus of woman has its personal and objective components. On the personal side, the animus contains elements derived from experience with the woman's father. In contrast to the anima, which often appears in the form of an erotic fantasy, the animus most often emerges as an unchallengeable conviction of great personal importance.

The animus also has both negative and positive propensities. When a woman, for example, feels guilty about not having met some obligation, she may dream of negative, destructive, murdering men. When, in addition, she begins to harbor the aggressive, destructive fantasies of the animus and project them onto her family, she can cause everyone involved untold anguish with her hawkish bitchiness. On the other hand, the animus can be of positive value because it embodies the positive masculine qualities of initiative, objectivity, and courage. If the woman can accept and work with the symbols of her animus, she can incorporate these positive qualities and subordinate the negative ones within her own personality and, paradoxically,

become more completely feminine because of having integrated her masculine potentials.

The development of the animus has four stages comparable to those found in the development of the anima. At the earliest stage, the animus is represented by athletic prowess, physical power, and strength, as embodied in a Samson or an Atlas. At the next stage, the animus figure displays qualities of initiative and efficiency and shows the ability to plan and carry out actions. At the third stage, the animus is embodied in the representatives of logos and mind, such as the scholar, the scientist, and the theologian. At the final stage, the animus takes the form of the wise old man and signifies the path through which a woman can renew herself and find new meaning in and for her life.

Self

Within Jungian psychology, the term "self" is used quite differently from the way it is used in other personality theories. For Freud, the self is the conscious part of the personality. For Jung, the self is at the very heart of the psyche and does not come into awareness until the person has succeeded in dealing with his shadow and his anima or animus. In many ways, the self, when it emerges, is experienced as a kind of rebirth, a renewal of life in a new, more integrated, and wise form. In Jung's view, the person who begins to realize the core of his psyche, his self, comes into posession of special psychic powers.

One manifestation of this new psychic power that emerges during the process of individualization or self-realization is synchronization. Synchronicity means that events occur together in a person's life in a way that seems to be accidental, but the events are, in fact, related to each other. Thematic linkage of events become more frequent as the person begins to realize himself and to make progress in the process of individualization.

Persona

The persona is the official social mask or pattern of behavior that the person uses in social situations. The role of doctor, teacher, or minister is defined socially and has prescribed values, orientations, and behaviors. The persona becomes a problem when the person either identifies too closely with it or becomes too distant from it. Personas are useful insofar as they are recognized as patterns that are necessary to but not identical with the true personality.

Introversion-Extroversion

Introversion and extroversion are general human propensities, both of which are embodied in every person. Some persons emphasize their introversion more, and others their extroversion. Extroverts are most concerned with the outer word; introverts are most concerned with the inner world. When a person goes too far in one or the other direction, the opposite pole of his personality begins to assert itself and to seek realization.

Psychological Functions

Jung distinguished four basic psychological functions that are orthogonal to extroversion and to introversion. Two of these functions are rational, thinking and feeling, whereas the other two, sensation and intuition, are irrational. A person may be characterized by a particular function, although he possess all four. Since there is no direct connection with introversion-extroversion, there are eight possible combinations of functions and types. A thinking introvert may be exemplified in the absent-minded professor; the thinking extrovert may be exemplified in the politician or clergyman.

All the psychological functions have archetypal components and so obey the law of opposites. The overemphasis on the realization of thinking leads, at a certain point in life, to an eruption of intuition and sensation; the person who realizes mostly his intuition and sensation finds that the rational functions of thinking and feeling eventually seek their due. These various functions are represented by universal and characteristic symbols that can be found in art, mythology, and dreams. If the person heeds the symbolic cues and works toward the total realization of his personality, these symbols can be helpful. But if he ignores them, if he continues to use the functions that worked for him in the first half of life in the hope that they will work for him during the second, the result will be negative. The denial of one's opposites is a rejection of continued growth of self and personality.

REFERENCES

Jung, C. G. *Memories, Dreams, Reflections*. Vintage Books, New York, 1961.
Jung, C. G. *Two Essays on Analytical Psychology*. Princeton University Press, Princeton, 1966.
Jung, C. G. *Symbols of Transformation*, ed. 2. Princeton University Press, Princeton, 1967.
Jung, C. G. *Archetypes of the Collective Unconscious*. Princeton University Press, Princeton, 1968.
Jung, C. G. *Psychological Reflections*. Princeton University Press, Princeton, 1970.
Jung C. G. *Psychological Types*. Princeton University Press, Princeton, 1971.

8.3.   OTTO RANK

Introduction

His relationship to Freud was the real-life drama of Rank's system of personality development and his method of psychotherapy. In Freud he discovered the meaning of a union with another person, which facilitated his discovery of his own self-worth as a person and as a therapist. To be a member of the prestigious inner circle at the beginning of the psychoanalytic movement gave him the experience of being at one with a developing ideology. Freud

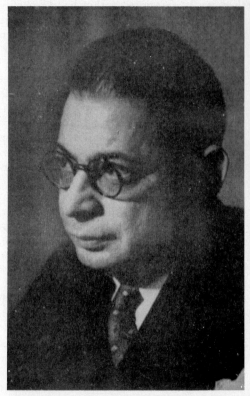

FIGURE 1. Otto Rank. (Courtesy of New York Academy of Medicine.)

took on a father role as Rank matured as therapist, editor of psychoanalytic journals, and researcher of theoretical material. (See Figure 1.)

Rank soon learned that to remain in that circle as the doctrine of psychoanalysis hardened into a fixed system meant the death of his own uniqueness. The fear he now experienced he later defined as the death fear that, he postulated, all people experience as they enter any relationship, especially the therapeutic one.

It was his own fear of death of the creative self by suffocation in the Vienna circle that helped him to formulate and experience the fact of rebirth psychology, which he published in his most scholarly work, *The Trauma of Birth*. This book although dedicated to Freud, led to his immediate expulsion from the group. The intensity of his own agony he now called the life fear—the price that the developing organism must pay for self-affirmation and self-discovery. It is also the price paid in therapy as the new self is born and treatment ends.

Union-Separation

In union with another person or persons or with humanity, one discovers and affirms one's likeness. In the experience of separation one discovers and affirms one's own and another uniqueness or difference. In union, one discovers one's identity. This discovery is often experienced most abruptly, as one is suddenly cut off from someone else because of an error or an impulsive act. Then one stands alone and has a chance to see oneself in clear relief and to discover and affirm one's uniqueness.

Rank's theory is often described in terms of a duality: he plays opposites against each other. The very existence of the one depends on its dialectic opposite. The degree to which any human being moves in any direction depends entirely on the degree to which he is certain of the opposite direction. One can move toward another human being only as one is certain of one's identity, discovered in separation. One can move away from people only as one is internally certain of one's belonging.

Rank believed that this movement back and forth was an act of the will. There are several inhibiting forces that the will must overcome to move toward and away from people. The first inhibiting force is the problem of guilt. To move toward someone in union is laden with guilt for needing someone else or even needing to use someone for one's own growth. To move away evokes greater guilt for having to abandon someone whom one has used and may need again.

A greater risk is that of one's going too far, thus moving beyond the gravitational pull of the dialectic opposite. Because of one's desperate need for union or the other's need for too great a union, one can get lost in the union. It is then a smothering, engulfing encounter, which Rank calls the death fear—fear of dying by smothering. The more unsure one is of one's identity, the greater is the fear. To move away from humanity carries the opposite danger and the concomitant fear. Separation carries with it the danger of moving so far that one overshoots one's orbit, and the pull of the union no longer takes hold. Rank calls this the life fear.

The greatest trauma is that, with each union, a person has to abandon his own will to another's strange will to enjoy brief happiness, unaware of his difference. Each of these experiences must then be abandoned. The fear of the unknown outcome of each movement must be borne as the price paid for growth.

Growth Pattern

Rank's growth process of personality is a continuous movement into and out of relationships. Although one is continuously experiencing unions and separations, there are phases when major leaps forward occur in the growth process. Each phase begins with a major need for union and then moves toward a rebirth in the form of a separation. These movements are not repeated aimlessly; rather, they are direction-oriented toward the ultimate goal of becoming the creative artist.

Familial Phase

Life begins with union. In the intrauterine experience, the organism experiences both physiological and psychological union. Deep into the unconscious is written the meaning and the need for intimacy.

The nirvana of perfect belonging must come to an end. To stay to die, to leave is to take a chance to live. Birth is a traumatic experience for the infant.

The dialectic process moves on as both mother and infant choose to unite again. At the mother's breast, the deepest elected union is dramatically acted out between two people. Inscribed deeply in the infant's being is the message. "I belong. I must be worthy because I am precious to someone."

The body develops, and the child discovers his autonomous anatomy and will. During the next 10 or more years, he makes many small trips to discover his separateness, but the predominant theme is closeness. The child stays close to his family as he learns the family's skills. He is now establishing his self-worth as he identifies with the values, habits, and ideals of his family, clan, community, and culture.

The primary task of adolescence is to affirm for life one's psychological identity, and this affirmation can be done only in separation. While on this venture for selfhood, the adolescent discovers his peer group, which is on the same trip. The mutuality of the experience develops into a new union with a partner of his own choosing.

Societal Phase

A union comes as the young adult internalizes the norms of universal humanity and civilization as his own. A rebirth occurs as he steps out from the crowd to declare his own individual self as separate from the mass. He now claims his psychic-ideal. The neurotic is unable to make this affirmation, since he perceives the norms of society as external commands and wastes his life fighting them, so as to make them correspond to his own self. The artistic type focuses his energy on the creation of his psychic self and thus rises above the mass.

Artistic Phase

The creative person is in close kinship with the outer world of the people to whom he belongs. He is in union with the cosmic reality, with nature, and with human nature about him. In the artistic act, he is listening to the voiceless voice of this reality and then articulating it through his word and deed. He hears clearly what others have felt vaguely, although no less strongly, and their potential experiences are actualized by means of his work. Because of this, the artist is often regarded as a hero, for he is living prototype of man's creative will. He experiences creatively what is dormant or suppressed in others. They are thereby enabled to experience their own latent creativity through him.

Spiritual Phase

This phase begins with a deep identification with an ideological, philosophical, or spiritual union. To claim it as one's own is a commitment of faith and thus a spiritual rebirth, since one is now in touch with the eternal, the universal, or, for some, the personified God. This, then, is a deeply religious rebirth.

To claim one's ethical ideal in its final form, one makes peace with the totality of existence, with one's life, with one's fate, and with death. Even the final separation by death has lost its pangs of fear; one has overcome the guilt for having lived because life was lived to its fullest. The fear of death is primarily the fear of failing to live.

Unions and separations are no longer in tension with each other. Man is in union with the ultimate, even as he experiences himself as distinctively separate.

Therapy

To Rank, the successful therapeutic process was a rebirth experience in which the patient made drastic leaps forward in healing, rather than a slow process of gaining insight followed by adjustment or behavior modification. In the treatment experience, the patient moves into a relationship experience with the therapist that is a re-enactment of all the past struggles with relationship, especially the problem of intimacy. In the actual encounter with the therapist, the patient experientially works through these feelings, especially the death fear, which is the innate fear of losing one's identity because of suffocation in relationship. The rebirth occurs after the relationship between the patient and the therapist has affirmed the patient's innate self-worth. Then the patient has the inner strength to launch out in self-affirmation, separating himself from dependency on the therapist and claiming his own uniqueness. In this process, the patient overcomes the life fear as he dares to face up to his fullest potential and own it for himself.

In the process of therapy, the patient moves through phases that are identical to the phases of the growth process of personality. He first moves into a relationship with the therapist as a person who is a prototype of a particular person in the patient's life and also of universal humanity with whom he must unite. The first rebirth occurs as he claims his own individuality as a person and as a unique part of universal mankind. The second phase begins as he discovers the physical universe and his likeness to it. After this phase, he claims his distinctiveness as a creator within the cosmic reality as the creative artist is born. In the emergence of the self, he moves to the final phase of growth as he unites with the ideological, philosophical, and spiritual reality. This phase is followed by the final birth of the ethical ideal—a self-fulfilled human being who no longer needs to create in order to prove his right to existence.

REFERENCES

Journal of the Otto Rank Association, vols. 1–8, June 1966 to December 1973.

Karpf, F. B. *The Psychology and Psychotherapy of Otto Rank*. Philosophical Library, New York, 1953.

Progoff, I. *The Death and the Rebirth of Psychology*. Julian Press, New York, 1956.

Rank, O. *Beyond Psychology*. Haddon Craftsmen, Camden, N. J., 1941.

Rank, O. *Will Therapy and Truth and Reality*. Alfred A. Knopf, New York, 1952.

Rank, O. *The Trauma of Birth*. Robert Brunner, New York, 1952.

8.4. MELANIE KLEIN

Introduction

Within the broad spectrum of classical and modified psychoanalytic theories and related clinical techniques, the approach of Melanie Klein (1882–1960) is closest to the constitutionalist, instinct-oriented pole; the culturalist approaches represent the opposite pole of stress on the psychosocial determinants of intrapsychic conflict. Between these poles, contemporary ego psychology occupies an intermediate position. Klein's theory of instincts, however, is rooted in traditional psychoanalytic metapsychology, rather than in contemporary neurobiological approaches. And, from the viewpoint of psychoanalytic object-relations theory, the Kleinian approach has important links with the culturalist approaches.

From a technical viewpoint, the Kleinian approach is very close to traditional psychoanalysis, with a heavy emphasis on the psychology of the id and on preserving a classical, nonmodified psychoanalytic technique for all patients.

Instinct Theory

Klein accepted Freud's dual-instinct theory involving the life instinct and the death instinct and particularly stressed the importance of inborn aggression as a reflection of the death instinct. The first manifestation of the death instinct is oral sadism. Both the death instinct and the life instinct express themselves mentally in the form of unconscious fantasies. The contents of these fantasies represent the self and objects under the influence of crude, primitive emotions. The equation of various objects under the influence of the same instinctual drive derivative constitutes the origin of the capacity for symbol formation. Envy, greed, and jealousy are specific emotions derived from oral aggression.

The death instinct, active from birth on and expressed in primitive emotions, is projected outward in the form of fears of persecution and annihilation. Klein postulated the existence of a functional ego from birth on, and the fear of persecution and annihilation refers to annihilation of the ego.

The life instinct or libido is expressed from birth on in pleasurable contacts with gratifying objects, primarily the good breast. These objects are invested with libido and introjected as internal objects infused with emotions representing libido. The projection of the good inner object on new objects emerging in the perceptual field is the basis of trust, of the wish to explore reality, and of learning and knowledge. Gratifying experiences reinforce basic trust, shape the expression of libido, and influence the relative balance of life and death instincts. Cycles of projection and reintrojection of good objects foster growth, and good inner objects promote ego synthesis. The predominant emotion linked with the expression of libido is gratitude.

Klein criticized the sequence postulated by Freud of an autoerotic phase, a narcissistic phase, and finally a phase of object investment. She thought that autoeroticism is based on gratifying experiences with the mother and that narcissism represents an identification with the good object. What Freud called the hallucinatory wish fulfillment is represented by introjective fantasies of the good inner object (breast).

For Klein, both life and death instincts were intimately linked with object relations. Although most of the death instinct is originally projected in terms of paranoid fears, part of it fused with libido, giving rise to the development of masochistic tendencies.

Ego Theory

Klein agreed with Freud that the ego originates from the common matrix of the ego and the id in an effort to deal with reality, and she stated that the ego starts with the beginning of life. She described four basic functions of the ego, all of which start with the beginning of life: the experience of and defenses against anxiety, processes of introjection and projection, object relations, and functions of integration and synthesis.

Anxiety

Anxiety constitutes the ego's response to the expression of the death instinct. Constitutional factors determine the degree of anxiety tolerance. Anxiety is also reinforced by the separation caused by birth and by the frustration of bodily needs. Anxiety becomes fear of persecutory objects and later, through reintrojection of aggression in the form of internalized bad objects, becomes the fear of outer and inner persecutors. Inner persecutors constitute the origin of primitive superego anxiety. The content of paranoid fears varies according to the level of psychosexual development.

Introjection and Projection

These are primary processes of growth, as well as defensive operations of the ego, and they constitute the basic defenses against anxiety. They foster the integration of the ego and the neutralization of the death instinct. Both good and bad experiences are projected. The projection of inner tension states (reflecting basically the death instinct) and of external stimuli that are painful constitutes the origin of paranoid fears, but the projection of pleasurable states (reflecting basically the life instinct) gives rise to basic trust. The introjection of good experiences gives rise to good internal objects, which constitute basic stimuli for ego growth. In the earliest stages of development, all aggression is projected outside. In a later stage of development, projection of aggression is only partially successful; there is a reintrojection and tolerance of bad external objects as internal persecutors that now constitute the early superego.

Object Relations

External stimuli invested with libido or aggression become primitive objects. Objects are at first part objects and only later become total or whole objects.

The tendency to perceive objects as either ideal (all-good) or persecutory (all-bad) is the consequence of the operation of another early defensive operation, splitting. Splitting consists in the active separation of good from bad experiences, perceptions, and emotions linked to object. The predominance of part-object relationships in earliest life is a consequence of the maximal operation of splitting mechanisms. Only later, when splitting mechanisms decrease, is synthesis of good and bad aspects of objects possible and an ambivalence toward whole objects acknowledged.

Integration and Synthesis

The internalization of the good internal object constitutes the basis for growth of an integrative ego; the total projection of bad objects preserves a purified pleasure ego. Later, however, the synthesis of good and bad part objects into total or whole objects further contributes to ego growth and synthesis and to the integration of the experience of reality. A predominance of aggression over libido interferes with ego integration and synthesis; under these circumstances, there occurs an excessive development of idealization—a primitive defensive operation tending to preserve all-good internal and external objects. Excessive aggression also determines an excessive development of splitting mechanisms to protect the good internal and external objects from contamination with badness. Since splitting interferes with the accurate perception of reality, splitting fosters denial of reality.

Paranoid-Schizoid and Depressive Positions

Klein stressed early internalized object relations in the vicissitudes of instincts, intrapsychic conflicts, and psychic structures and stressed pregenital aggression, especially oral sadism, the quality of primitive internal objects.

Paranoid-Schizoid Position

This is the earliest developmental stage, characterized by the predominance of splitting and other related mechanisms, by part-object relationships, and by a basic fear about the preservation or survival of the ego; this fear takes the form of persecutory anxiety. Excessive persecutory fears underlie the development of schizophrenia and paranoid psychoses. If persecutory fears are not excessive, this phase evolves into the next developmental phase, the depressive position, in the second half of the first year. The following defensive mechanisms, specifically directed against persecutory fears, are prevalent in the paranoid-schizoid position: splitting, idealization, denial of inner and external reality, stifling and artificiality of emotions, and projective identification.

The psychoses present a combination of denial of reality, excessive projective identification, and pathological splitting, leading to fragmentation, according to Kleinian theory. Escape into an idealized inner object leads to autistic exalted states; generalized splitting and reintrojection of multiple, fragmented objects lead to confusional states. The predominance of fear of external persecutors, derived from projective identification, is characteristic of paranoia; the projection of persecutors onto the patient's own bodily zones, organs, and functions determines hypochondriacal syndromes.

Schizoid object relationships (characteristic of schizoid personalities) are characterized by shallowness of emotions, incapacity to tolerate guilt feelings in depth, a tendency to experience objects as hostile, and a combination of internal withdrawal from object relations and artificiality in surface social adaptation. Klein suggested that obsessive traits reflect a secondary defense against fears of external control by taking over such excessive control in dealing with external reality. The efforts to escape from feared persecutors by flights into excessive dependency on idealized external objects may give rise to pathological dependency, narcissitic object relations, and sexual promiscuity. Klein stressed the consequences of excessive predominance of envy in terms of projection of such envy onto others, with consequent fear of success.

Depressive Position

At about 6 months of age, splitting processes begin to decrease, and the child's increasing sense of reality brings about a growing awareness that the good and bad external objects are really one and that the mother as a whole object

has good and bad parts. At this point, the infant begins to be able to acknowledge his own aggression toward the good object or to recognize the good aspects of the object he attacks and perceives at such times as bad. Projection is only partially successful now. The infant's attack on the whole object brings about an awareness of his own bad internal parts. In contrast to the persecutory fears characteristic of the paranoid-schizoid position, the predominant fear in the depressive position is of harming the good internal and external objects.

This basic fear about the survival of good inner and external objects constitutes depressive anxiety or guilt, the predominant emotional reaction of the depressive position. Preservation of good objects is more important now than preservation of the ego.

Under normal conditions, certain mechanisms characteristic of the depressive position permit the working through of this position—reparation, increase in reality testing, ambivalence, and gratitude.

Two additional mechanisms are activated in the course of the depressive position—idealization and a sense of triumph over the lost object. However, excessive development of these mechanisms may take the form of pathological constellations.

Pathological mourning is characterized by the loss of the good external and internal objects caused by their fantasied destruction by the hatred directed toward them. The bad internal objects constitute a primitive and sadistic superego, evoke excessive guilt, and determine the feeling that all good objects are dead and that the world is empty of love. Efforts at compensation fail; the idealization of the object only increases guilt and despair. The self-reproaches of the depressed patient are reproaches not against the object but against the self and the internal impulses. Neurotic depression and, particularly, psychotic depression are the clinical manifestations of pathological development of all these defensive operations and the inability to work through the depressive position.

Hypomanic and manic syndromes reflect the pathological predominance of the constellation of manic defenses. Manic defenses, in addition to idealization and manic triumph over the lost object, include, omnipotence, identification with the superego, and compulsive introjection. Patients suffering from manic-depressive symptoms were unable in infancy to establish a good inner object; they were not able to work through the infantile depressive position. Klein believed that normal mourning always implies guilt, reactivating the guilt of the depressive position; involves not only the introjection of the external object but also the internal good object, which is felt threatened and is reinstated; and is characterized by a gratification over being alive, which includes the activation of manic triumph and secondary guilt. In addition, there is also activation of idealization, and, above all, of the normal processes that permit the working through of the depressive position.

Superego Theory

Klein stressed the very early development of the superego and the fundamental contribution of such a primitive superego to psychopathology. The superego starts out in the first year of life as part of the depressive position. Excessive pathological superego pressures bring about a regression to the early paranoid-schizoid constellation. The superego derives from the reintrojected bad objects that earlier had been split off and projected outside, a reintrojection made possible by the mitigation of bad objects because of the introjection of whole or total objects as part of the depressive position. Normally, the predominance of love over hate and the subsequent internalization of predominantly good, demanding whole objects into the superego neutralize the bad inner objects; however, even under ideal circumstances, there is a certain contamination of the predominantly good objects in the superego by the bad objects.

Superego pressures have a persecuting and demanding quality; the superego exerts strong demands to placate and preserve the good objects in the ego with the quality of cruel demands for perfection. Under pathological circumstances, these pressures are expressed as the unremitting harshness of infantile and childhood unconscious morality.

Under normal circumstances, the superego brings about a certain degree of idealization of good inner objects, and realistic demands for improvement and reinforcement of the reparative and sublimatory trends of the ego. Regression to the paranoid-schizoid position when the depressive position cannot be worked through may bring about a reprojection of the sadistic superego as part of an effort to deflect intolerable guilt outside. This reinforces persecutory—in contrast to depressive—fears, decreases the capacity to perceive reality and learning because of the fear of and rebellion against the projected superego, and produces intellectual inhibition and omnipotent denial of reality.

Klein agreed with Freud about the important contribution of oedipal fears and prohibitions to superego development. But she stated that oedipal problems were already active, molded under the primacy of oral drives, from the first year of life on and that such early stages of oedipal development were the basis of the later, classical oedipal constellation.

Psychoanalytic Technique

Kleinians adhere strictly to the classical psychoanalytic setting and deal with the patient's material by means of interpretation exclusively. Interpretations are predominantly transference interpretations, and the same nonmodified psychoanalytic technique is used with patients along the entire spectrum, from neurotic to psychotic or psychopathic disorders. The analysis focuses on the interpretation of unconscious fantasies representing both the content and the defensive operations at primitive levels of the mind. Material is interpeted at very deep levels from the earliest stages of treatment on. The interpretation of primitive fantasies and defenses related to the paranoid-schizoid and the depressive positions is a major focus of Kleinian analysts. Kleinian authors have been particularly interested in the analysis of patients with severe types of character pathology, borderline cases, and psychoses in whom primitive levels of conflicts and defenses predominate.

REFERENCES

Guntrip, H. *Personality Structure and Human Interaction.* International Universities Press, New York, 1961.
Klein, M. The Oedipus complex in the light of early anxieties. In *Contributions to Psycho-Analysis, 1921–1945*, p. 377. Hogarth Press, London, 1948.
Klein, M. Notes on some schizoid mechanisms. In *Developments in Psycho-Analysis*, M. Klein, P. Heimann, S. Isaacs, and J. Riviere, editors, p. 292. Hogarth Press, London, 1952.
Klein, M. *Envy and Gratitude.* Tavistock, London, 1957.
Rosenfeld, H. *Psychotic States: A Psycho-Analytical Approach.* International Universities Press, New York, 1965.
Segal, H. *Introduction to the Work of Melanie Klein.* Basic Books, New York, 1964.

8.5. WILHELM REICH

Introduction

Wilhelm Reich (see Figure 1) was born on March 24, 1897, in Dobrzynia, a part of Galicia that then belonged to the Austrian Empire. His father was a rather stern, taciturn, dictatorial, and jealous man who completely dominated his wife and sons. After World War I, Reich took up his medical studies in Vienna and became affiliated with the psychoanalytic group. Between 1932 and 1939, Reich moved to several Scandinavian countries but settled in Oslo. In Norway, he continued his efforts on behalf of sexual liberation. In 1939, Reich moved to New York. He bought some land in Maine, where he established a summer training workshop, and moved his family and laboratories to Maine in the early 1950's. His claims that his orgone accumulators helped to cure cancer patients brought him under the scrutiny of the Food and Drug Administration. He was convicted and sent to prison, where he suffered the last of a series of heart attacks and died on November 3, 1957.

Theory of Neurosis

Reich argued that every neurosis results from the damming up of sexual energy. This dam-ming-up has three possible outcomes—the development of neurotic symptoms and character traits that are, in effect, maladaptive behavioral channels into which sexual energy flows when the normal outlet, orgasm, is blocked; conversion into anxiety; and release as sadism or aggression.

Reich held that orgasms, in sufficient numbers, would solve individual and social problems but that ejaculation is not a measure of true orgastic potency. A truly orgastically potent person is totally involved with the other person and achieves total release of tension and pressure in the course of the orgasm. The orgastically potent person is moral in the highest sense because of his genuine regard and love for other people.

Theory of Character

Character Formation

Reich accepted Freud's conception of character formation, but suggested that society, through its values and mores, can impose patterns of child-rearing and, hence, affect character formation. Commonality of character in a given society thus reflects commonality of child-rearing practices.

Reich suggested that the bourgeoisie set the standards for child-rearing. In a paternalistic

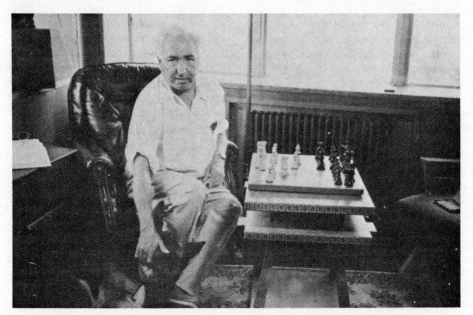

FIGURE 1. Wilhelm Reich at home. (Photo courtesy of Farrar, Straus & Giroux, Inc.)

society, the seeds are sown for producing persons with an authoritarian character structure who are subservient to those in a higher station than themselves but callous toward those of lesser position. Oppressed workers do not revolt because their character structure renders them submissive to authority. Reich believed that children reared in freedom and openness would resist exploitation and oppression.

Character Types

Hysterical Character. Reich said that the hysterical character shows the least character armoring and the most lability of function. One type of behavior most typical of the hysterical character is sexual or seductive behavior. There is, however, a characteristic fearfulness and skittishness, together with high suggestibility and a tendency to disappointment reactions.

Basically, the hysterical person is frightened of his or her genital impulses, which are easily aroused by external stimuli that become a threat and a danger. The hysterical person's seductive behavior is, in reality, an attempt to flush out the danger stimuli, which can then be avoided. Such persons are seldom aware of their provocative behavior and vehemently deny it when it is brought to their attention. Rather, they project their sexual desires and accuse those who respond to their overtures of having initiated them.

Persons with a hysterical character structure do not sublimate very well and are not motivated toward intellectual achievement or toward sustained endeavors in any domain. Such people are generally so apprehensive that most of their time and energy are taken up with avoiding dangerous situations and people.

Compulsive Character. Persons of this character type most often show an inordinate concern for orderliness in all aspects of their lives, circumstantial thinking, thriftiness, indecision, doubt, distrust, restraint, and control. In the emotional domain there is a more or less complete affect block. The compulsive gives the impression of tension and restraint.

The basic dynamic in the compulsive character is anxiety about loss of control over instinctual impulses. All the compulsive person's behaviors are designed to eliminate the unexpected, the unforeseen, and, hence, the uncontrolled. The impulses that the compulsive character is desperately trying to control are power-

ful, sadistic, and angry impulses, and he fears the punishment and guilt that their expression would entail.

Phallic-Narcissistic Character. Persons who fall into this category are self-confident, arrogant, elastic, vigorous, and often impressive. Outwardly, phallic-narcissistic people frequently appear cold, reserved, and defensively aggressive. They are often high achievers and usually hold positions of power and authority in society.

Phallic-narcissistic persons have a more or less total identification with the phallus (in women, with the fantasy of having a penis). Men of this type have strong erective potency but are unable to experience orgasm. Such men are frustrated at the genital exhibitionistic level of development, with a consequent negative, hostile attitude toward women. Many men of this character type become homosexual as a consequence of their negative attitudes toward the mother in particular and women in general. Women who as children were frustrated in their exhibitionistic activities in relation to the father develop negative attitudes toward men and a propensity toward lesbianism.

Masochistic Character. Unlike Freud, Reich demonstrated convincingly that the pleasure principle is sufficient to account for masochism and that postulation of a death instinct is unnecessary. Persons of a masochistic bent report a subjective sense of chronic suffering and have a chronic tendency to complain and to manifest self-damaging and self-deprecating words and actions. Such persons often tend to provoke and torture others and may assume a stance of stupidity and ignorance about matters in the real world and regarding their own behavior.

Reich argued that the masochistic person experiences pleasure as painful. In this formulation, the masochist avoids the build-up of pleasure in anticipation of the pain it causes. The masochist would rather have someone beat him than love him because the beating is less painful than love. Indeed, Reich argued that the masochistic character has an inordinate craving for love but a low tolerance for accepting love.

Treatment

Character Analysis

Reich pointed out that, before a patient can follow the basic rule of free association to say everything that comes to mind, interpersonal issues between patient and therapist have to be resolved. Reich's discussion of character analysis was a detailed exposition with clinical examples, of how to cope with the character resistances manifested by patients in their attempts to prevent treatment from getting underway. Reich argued that the character armor of the patient appears not so much in what the patient says and does but, rather, in how the words are said and the actions done. Reich suggested that a kind of face-to-face therapy is an important prerequisite to the faceless therapy in which the patient lies on the couch and free-associates.

Vegetotherapy

Reich's therapeutic innovations were a direct outgrowth of his theories of character armor as reflecting muscular tension. He attempted to deal directly with this muscular tension and sought to relax the patient by interpreting the patient's muscular patterns and by actual massage. Reich called this type of therapy "vegetotherapy." The need to relax the patient as part of the therapeutic process has been elaborated by others into relaxation therapy. And the use of actual physical encounters with patients was the forerunner of the many contemporary action therapies.

Orgonomy

Reich wanted to find a form of energy that was at once biological and physical. By means of a series of rather strange experiments and shaky theorizing, he arrived at the sought-for energy in the pulsating radiation he produced from inert coal dust. He called it orgone. He then devised an orgone accumulator, a box covered with alternating layers of rock wool and steel wool, that supposedly traps orgone energy from the atmosphere. Reich believed that people with various diseases, including cancer, could be cured by being placed in the orgone box.

REFERENCES

Reich, W. *Character Analysis.* Farrar, Straus & Young, New York, 1949.
Reich, W. *The Function of the Orgasm.* Noonday Press, New York, 1942.
Reich, W. *The Sexual Revolution.* Farrar, Straus & Giroux, New York, 1969.
Reich, W. and Ollendorf, I. *Wilhelm Reich: A Personal Biography.* St. Martins Press, New York, 1969.
Rycroft, C. *Wilhelm Reich.* Viking, New York, 1969.

8.6. BIODYNAMICS

Introduction

Biodynamics is not a separate school of psychiatry; instead, biodynamics connotes an integration of the biological and dynamic vectors of all animate behavior, including its adaptations or vicissitudes in various environments. It encompasses data from evolution, ethology, comparative animal research, anthropology, history, philology, sociology, and other sciences of behavior as well as from clinical evaluations (diagnoses) and salutary transactions (therapy).

Research Studies

Four basic biodynamic principles have been formulated: motivational development (all behavior originates in variably emergent physiological needs for nutrition, fluids, environmental manipulation, sexual and parental conduct, and other conations toward individual and social survival), learned individuation (each organism's evolving patterns of adaptation are the result of its innate potentialities, their various modes and rates of maturation, and its unique experiences), versatile adaptability (most dissatisfactions and frustrations are adequately met by a flexible repertoire of readjusted techniques and substituted goals), and conflict and uncertainty in neurotigenesis (if any animal is stressed by mutually incompatible responses beyond the point at which adequate adaptations become subliminally predictable or satisfactory, severe and persistent deviations of behavior are induced).

Young animals provided with the necessary nutritive, protective, and guiding presence of adults, supplemented by play and other contacts with peers, acquire self-confidence, motor skills, and effective social acculturations. Those deprived of appropriate parental or surrogate comfort or peer interactions, although otherwise physically well cared for, do not develop normal initiative, physical stamina, or appropriate group behavior, apparently because of inadequate physical and social stimuli during critical periods of growth and receptivity.

Animal societies in the laboratory, as well as in the wild, organize themselves in hierarchies of relatively dominant and submissive members. Privileges are generally pre-empted not by size or strength alone but in accordance with

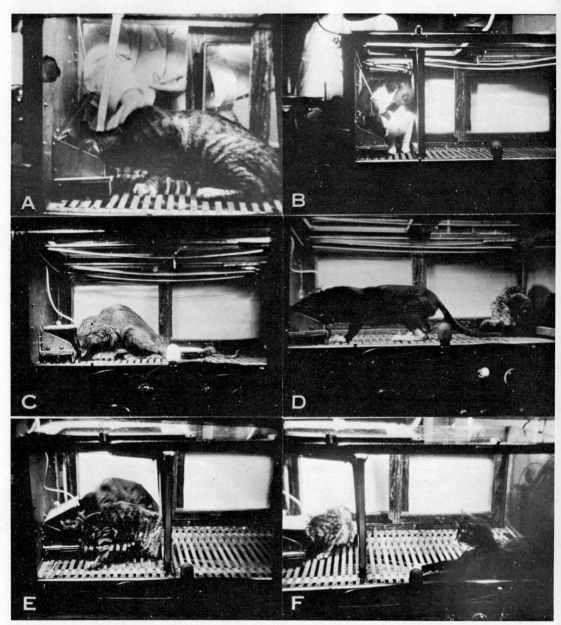

FIGURE 1. Experimental neuroses and therapy in cats. *A*, Control observations: A cat has been trained to pass a barrier at a signal light (upper right flash) and to open the food box for a pellet of food. The animal's behavior is goal-directed and efficiently adaptive. *B*, Conflictful experience: At a later feeding signal, the cat is subjected to a mild air blast at the moment of food-taking. The animal is shown recoiling from the traumatic situation. *C*, Neurotic behavior: After five such experiences at irregular intervals, the cat refuses to feed or approach the box and develops other neurotic aberrations of behavior. The animal, although starved for 48 hours, is here shown in a typical phobic response to a feeding signal—crouched away from the food in cataleptic immobility against an impassable barrier. *D*, Transference retraining: After 4 months of neurosis, the cat is retrained by manual feeding and gentle guidance once again to feed from the box. At first, the animal does so only when being stroked by the experimenter; later, feeding responses may be reconstituted in response not only to the light but even to the air blast (nozzle shown in deep left corner). *E*, Therapeutic result: After 18 days of such retraining, the cat's neurotic reactions largely disappear, and it once again passes barriers for food at the light or air blast signal. *F*, Masochistic patterns: Another cat, trained to depress an electric switch for its feeding signals, was made experimentally neurotic by a mild electric shock at food-taking and then retrained as above to take the food despite the trauma. The animal is here shown once again manipulating the switch with spontaneous avidity to experience the shock with or without the food reward.

special aptitudes, skills, and other personality characteristics. Various relationships seen in animal societies help to trace the biodynamic roots of collaboration, sit-down strikes, division of labor, automation, altruism, and hostilities, as expressed with far greater complexity in human society.

Aberrations of conduct analogous to human neuroses can be induced by training an animal to work a switch that opens a food box and then subjecting it to an unpredictably timed electric shock or air blast during feeding (see Figure 1) or by teaching a monkey to feed at a food box and later confronting it with the unexpected appearance in the food box of a toy rubber snake—an object as representationally dangerous to the monkey as a live snake, harmful or not, would be. Yet, counter to classical Freudian and recent Wolpean doctrines, fear, in the sense of dread of injury, need not be involved. Equally serious and lasting disorganizations of behavior can be induced by requiring difficult choices among mutually exclusive satisfactions, by subjecting the animal to variably delayed feedbacks of its vocalizations, or by subjecting it to irregularly timed or sensorially confused cues that render its milieu seemingly beyond adequate control. Any of these stresses, when it exceeds the organism's predictive and adaptive capacities, can induce physiological and mimetic manifestations of anxiety, spreading inhibitions, generalizing phobias, stereotyped rituals, somatic dysfunctions, addictions to alcohol or other drugs, impaired sexual and social interactions, regressions to immature patterns, cataleptic stupors, and, in monkeys, manifestations of hallucinatory and delusional behavior. Animals closest to man show symptoms most nearly resembling those in human neuroses and psychoses, but the syndromes manifested depend less on the nature of the conflict than on the constitutional predisposition of the animal.

Therapy with Animals

Some animals retest the use of the switch and feeding mechanism and concurrently dispel associated neurotic inhibitions and deviations at their own pace. So, also, most human beings spontaneously and providentially re-explore and reassert their mastery over the residues of traumatic physical or social experiences without direct compulsion, benefit of clergy, or need for treatment.

If autonomous readaptations do not occur, the hungry animal can be mechanically restricted ever closer to highly attractive food in the opened reward box until its feeding and related inhibitions are, in most instances, impulsively overwhelmed by an imperative need for nutrition. In some animals, however, the situationally increased conflicts between attraction and aversion induce a state of agitation and panic paralleling the adverse results of excessively stringent or compulsive behavior therapy in patients with coping capacities (ego strengths) inadequate to the rapid readaptations required.

An inhibited, phobic animal placed with others that respond normally to the experimental situation shows more expeditious amelioration of its neurotic patterns, as in exemplary group guidance in human beings.

The experimenter can retrain the animal by gentle steps: first, to take food from his hand; next, to accept food in the apparatus; then, to open the box while the experimenter merely hovers protectively; and, finally to work the switch and feed without further guidance. This procedure may be the basic paradigm for much dyadic psychotherapy.

In general, alcohol, bromides, barbiturates, opiates, and, less efficiently, various meprobamate or phenothiazine tranquilizers disorganize complex behavior patterns while leaving simple ones relatively intact. The administration of opiates and especially alcohol so lulls the perceptive and mnemonic capacities of animals that they are, while thus inebriated, relatively immune to the neurotigenic effects of experiential traumata. Similarly, many human beings are tempted to take a bracer before facing presumed dangers, including those of imposed social conviviality and the mystique of religious rituals.

When a 35-volt, 60-cycle alternating current (equivalent to that usually employed in clinical convulsive therapy) is passed through the brain of a cat or monkey for 2 seconds, the resultant cortical diaschisis disorganizes recently acquired neurotic patterns more than older and relatively simpler ones, thus restoring approach and feeding responses. However, electroshock also produces permanent impairment, however subtle, of more complex behavioral efficiencies, even when these defects cannot be correlated with detectable pathological changes in the brain.

Circumscribed lesions in the thalamus,

amygdalae, or cingulate gyri disintegrate experimentally induced neurotic patterns and overbalance the corresponding organic loss in adaptive skills by a sufficiently wide margin so that, from the standpoint of survival, the animal is manifestly benefited. However, the effects of apparently identical lesions in different animals vary widely with the animals' previous experiences.

Clinical Applications

The most clinically productive exchanges of views occur when the patient is led by every ethical means available—such as reputation, office setting, manifest interest, and competence—to trust the therapist not only as a physician but also a sincere friend and seraphic counselor. With rapport thus triply established, the initial survey should, by tactfully directed inquiry, elicit the patient's current physical, social, or existential decompensations, especially those requiring the most immediate care. The past history can then survey the patient's genetic proclivities and the later vicissitudes of familial, sexual, and social experiences that induced the vulnerabilities to the special stresses that precipitated his present illness; also, the assets and potentialities can be constructively used in therapy.

Prognosis depends on an evaluation of the origin, tenacity, and influenceability of all the patient's behavior tendencies and on the probability of modifying and channeling them into new and more favorable patterns of adaptation by therapeutic means.

Biodynamic theorists propose that, insofar as any method alleviates the pathogenic anxieties of any patient, it is correspondingly effective; insofar as it does not, it fails. The fundamental parameters of all therapies are to use every physical, social, and psychological modality to help the patient realize that his former fears, escapisms, aggressions, and other deviant patterns are no longer necessary and to guide him by every form of influence, including personal example, into new modes of conduct that he will ultimately adopt as more satisfactory and profitable.

To accomplish this end, the therapist will find the following procedures expeditious:

Explicit assurances of complete confidentiality and, implicitly, of friendly and competent guidance.

A flexible schedule of therapeutic sessions that realistically fits the patient's needs.

Judicious combinations of all modes of therapy, including the ancillary use of drugs and physical modalities when indicated.

Prime concentration on the patient's physical, social, and attitudinal problems in the here and now, with anamnestic tracings only sufficient to clarify retained but outmoded and inept childhood or adolescent behavior.

Pragmatic understanding that the patient will be held responsible for his conduct by society and in one way or another be punished or rewarded accordingly.

Mutually acceptable sessions with family, friends, and employers to help clarify and improve interpersonal relationships.

Emphasis on salutary and realistic behavioral changes as the only valid indication of progress.

Open-end suspensions of treatment at optimum levels, the patients remaining free to communicate or to resume therapy should the need arise.

REFERENCES

Berne, E. *Games People Play*. Grove Press, New York, 1964.
Caplan, G. *An Approach to Community Mental Health*. Grune & Stratton, New York, 1961.
Dubois, P. *The Psychological Origin of Mental Disorders*. Funk and Wagnalls, New York, 1913.
Masserman, J. H. *Practice of Dynamic Psychiatry*. W. B. Saunders, Philadelphia, 1955.
Masserman, J. H. *Behavior and Neurosis*. Hafner Press, New York, 1963.
Masserman, J. H. *Biodynamic Roots of Human Behavior*. Charles C Thomas. Springfield, Ill., 1968.
Masserman, J. H. *A Psychiatric Odyssey*. Science House, New York, 1971.
Masserman, J. H. *Theories and Therapies of Dynamic Psychiatry*. Science House, New York, 1973.
Perls, F. S. *Gestalt Therapy and Human Potentialities*. Charles C Thomas, Springfield, Ill., 1966.
Sullivan, H. S. *Fusion of Psychiatry and Social Science*. W. W. Norton, New York, 1964.

8.7.   EXISTENTIAL PSYCHOANALYSIS

Introduction

Existential psychoanalysis is based on the findings of modern philosophy and on the understandings of psychoanalysis. Both fields share the common aim of dealing with and interpreting people's condition in their world and their possibilities for openness to human development and potential freedom.

There are as many existential philosophies as there are existential philosophers. They show radical differences of opinion among themselves. There seems to be not a common doctrine but a common methodology and elucidation of shared problems.

Existential clinicians are primarily interested in three themes: man and himself, man and his fellow man, and man and his world. This personalistic approach serves to counteract the tendency to objectify falsely man's view of himself and his world because of the reductionist fallacy. Knowledge about one's existence is the basis on which one becomes aware of the existence of others, and its affirmation is the starting point for the analysis of self. Thus, one becomes aware of oneself as a self only by becoming aware of the other as distinct from oneself.

Existential psychoanalysis is a necessary complement in modern times to scientific psychoanalysis, rather than an alternative. It tries to correct human experience as postulated by psychoanalysis today and underpins experience in practical, clinical evaluations. Existential psychoanalysis claims that man is reduced by the scientific attitude to an instinctual model, when actually he has a larger gestalt in which instincts are only the background, operating in dialectical tension with consciousness and a need for greater awareness and freedom of self, fellow man, and one's world. Existential psychoanalysis addresses itself to the problems of modern man and to the possibility that technological progress can lead to an enhancement of man's subjectivity, both as an individual and in community, and does not have to lead to alienation and dehumanization.

History

Brentano

Franz Brentano (1838–1917) was the teacher of Freud and of Edmund Husserl. Brentano was primarily a psychologist who tried to distinguish physical from mental phenomena. He felt that mental phenomena are directed toward objects and are an expression of an intentional existence within consciousness. Phenomenology is the study of the way that consciousness perceives objects.

Husserl

Edmund Husserl (1859–1938) wanted phenomenology to serve as a foundation for an exact science, and he hoped that the world of experience and the world of the mind could be bracketed to arrive at a descriptive analysis of the essential structures and the subjective processes of the mind. He developed Brentano's idea of intentionality, meaning that one cannot in consciousness conceive of anything without thinking of an object, real or imaginary.

Husserl's guiding direction was that one must describe things as they are experienced, and he tried to clear up the confusion between the psychological and the logical orders. His philosophy implies and posits an existing world, a world of space and time.

Freud

Classical psychoanalysis tried to create a model of the mind consisting of imaginary structures, which in reality do not correspond to morphological entities. Freud's orientation toward neurology led him to a materialistic view. He shared with German psychiatrists the concept that mental disorders are disorders of the brain. The psyche was but the epiphenomenon and was determined by the underlying anatomy. Freudian interpretation was based on the use of a biological model of disease, assuming that reality is a given entity that can be tested and measured.

Psychoanalysis maintains a basic therapeutic optimism that behavior often changes significantly and permanently as a result of new experiences in a therapeutic situation. The purely mechanistic and functional concepts of Freud could not really be used to explain the relationship between man and his fellow man. Transference and resistence are phenomenological categories, not naturalistic ones. Freud's greatest contribution was his focus on the inner life history of man, the systematic reconstruction of these intimate experiences, and the sharing of them with the therapist. In this he overcame the focusing on the external events in a person's life that preoccupied psychiatric practice in his time.

Jaspers

Karl Jaspers (1883–1969) was not only a psychiatrist but a prominent philosopher as well. For him, philosophizing was an activity and not a position that one holds, defends, or teaches. It was a search for Being and an understanding of the nature of this Being. Each individual is situated in a concrete and historical environment and must start anew for himself. There can never be a universally and eternally valid doctrine. Jaspers viewed philosophizing as consisting of two dimensions: the dimension of reason and the dimension of existence. Logical means cannot reach Being because the reality of Being can only be grasped existentially. Existence can only be illuminated and not conceptually grasped, since it can never fully be made an object of thought.

Jaspers rejected positivism as taking the methodologically false step from the particular to the general, from the part to the whole, and he rejected idealism because it also subjugates the unique and the particular to the whole and the general. Both leave unique human reality out of account and make the concrete individual into an empirical object or an empty idea, and both falsely pretend that Being is knowable.

Weizsaecker

Viktor von Weizsaecker maintained that every patient-doctor relationship is a single, unified act, an ongoing process between two people that he called "personal intercourse." He hoped to establish an existential basis for the doctor-patient relationship and so to avoid the error of conceiving of every human relationship as a transference or object relationship. He felt that psychic disturbances are factors in the development of illness. The object does not stand in counterdistinction to the subject as an object of knowledge but enters into a relationship with the subject as a subject. Personality is determined by interplay with others in meetings that often may be antilogical and may lead to crises in which responsible decisions have to be made. Personality must create itself and renew itself constantly.

Binswanger

Ludwig Binswanger (1881–1966) maintained that there are two kinds of concrete scientific knowledge. One describes, explains, and controls natural events; it achieves understanding by analysis, classification, and conceptualization. The other seeks to express the experience of what is given to human observation, rather than to explain the processes that give rise to the phenomena. Binswanger recognized the indispensable role of mechanistic explanation as a

forerunner of anthropology as he understood it, as a bearer of an initial order and system. But he felt that such order and knowledge revealed the presence of freedom in human experience. The only answer to a mechanistic view lay for him on the side of freedom, on the side of existence. What was required was a necessary kind of knowledge which showed its own limitations, which explained so well what it wanted to explain that one was unmistakably aware of what was left over, of what else man's wholeness consisted of. Human existence could only be understood, Binswanger concluded, by the empiricism of a phenomenological method.

The attention of the analyst was properly focused not on causation, on what had happened that would account for the aberration, but on the kind of world experienced by the suffering person. Binswanger left it to others to elaborate a taxonomy of mental illness and to try to specify cures for different forms of it. His was a therapy for individual patients.

Binswanger brought into the practice of psychoanalysis Heidegger's philosophical insight that man's existence is defined not by generalities about his nature but by the particularity of his individual limits of time and space. In Binswanger's hands the stress was always on the need for a therapeutic relationship between analyst and patient, and this meant, for him, maintaining to a sufficient degree the critical detachment of the physician. This detachment was part of his recognition that both the therapist and his patient come to the situation with their own experiences, each as a Being-in-the-world. It is the initial task of the therapist to set aside his preconceptions, so far as he is able, in order to enter as fully as possible into his patient's experience, to share it, and to demonstrate by this sharing that a private world may be broken open, its boundaries extended, and a new one chosen.

Boss

Medard Boss is a contemporary Swiss psychiatrist who was a pupil of Sigmund Freud and Martin Heidegger. He accepts the clinical descriptions and therapeutic techniques of Freudian psychoanalysis but rejects Freudian theories, claiming that these theories interfere with the immediacy of the therapeutic experience. Boss hopes to overcome false individualism by positing that every human existence can only be conceived as existence with/over/against other human beings and that the interpersonal relationship is the only primary authentic reality.

Heidegger posited five modes of inauthentic relationships to one's fellow man: subjective, egotistical, idealistic, platonic, and allegorical. All these words confuse conceptual ways of Being-in-the-world with actual, experiential Being-in-the-world. These false modes of existence are described clinically by Medard Boss.

Boss feels that the concept of immediately perceivable phenomena is closer to reality than Freud's descriptions of clinical entities. He has made great contributions by interpreting dreams from an existential point of view and by showing that man in his neurotic or psychotic ways of being can be understood as a unique human being living out his own intentionality, often without awareness, but still relating, even in a distorted way, to his fellow man.

Laing

R. D. Laing, the contemporary European psychiatrist, describes in great detail the thoughts, feelings, and experiences of persons who suffer from delusions and hallucinations and who have compulsive needs for verification of their being by the verbal statements and actions of others. He proposes that the behavior of these disturbed persons may be a sane response to a disturbed world. He claims that schizophrenia is not a disease but a condition appearing only in special social contexts in which there is a dissociation between what people say, do, and feel in their social and private roles. He implies that the cause of mental illness is social, political, economic, and ethical, and he blames our social order for causing this state of Being. He feels that people cannot be evaluated as clinical objects but as persons reacting to a disturbed, psychologically conflicting environment. He takes a position over and against any convention of the established order and against authority within the family, claiming that parents control their young children by not accepting them as persons to be loved and respected and by changing them into living objects to be manipulated. This manipulation puts children in a double bind, creating a logical dilemma from which they cannot escape without living in fantasy.

The children are unable to avoid the responsibility of standing up against the patients' demands while remaining true to their own feelings.

Existential Research

The parameters of existential research are clinical in nature and are based on subjective data collected by psychiatrists and psychotherapists in their daily practice. They stem from the subjective experience of the participants in the meeting between two or more people and do not fulfill the requirements of objective psychological criteria. Objective science will only describe shared behavior and will lose the uniqueness of individual experience, which is the ground on which existential therapy is built.

Every therapist has a unique style and a personal way of relating to disturbed persons. The relationship is a shared, creative encounter between two people as one person tries to help another experience himself more fully and more truthfully and open up his possibilities for living a more authentic life according to his own value system.

The preconditions for existential therapy are the therapist's awareness of his own unique identity and the ability, while working with disturbed people, to maintain it in interpersonal reality, without being overcome by his own fears, wishes, desires, and value systems. He must have the ability to maintain a friendly and genuine relationship with his patients without projecting or displacing his own needs upon the meeting. Thus he is able to recognize the disturbed person as unique, as a true other, and to help him not to project his feelings, thoughts, ideas, impulses, and wishes in the situation onto the doctor.

The existential therapist is relatively uninterested in diagnostic categories, except insofar as these categories can be applied to the question of how rapidly he can help his patient proceed to an understanding of the full meaning of his Being-in-the-world.

The existential therapist is committed to a style of communication that results in attaining a common ground for the expression of the reality that both he and the patient see in the therapeutic situation. The rules for the conduct of therapy are provided, first, by the clinical application of the phenomenological method and, second, by existential illumination of the essential realities and intentions as manifested in a human situation.

Any genuine phenomenological approach must satisfy three minimal conditions: (1) It must start from direct explorations of what is experienced and of the manner in which it presents itself to consciousness. (2) It must seek out the structures behind what is experienced and the relationship between the various elements. (3) It must try to see how these structures develop an image of the phenomena as they are taking shape.

For Husserl, there were three stages in the process of bracketing that must be applied clinically. The first stage is the phenomenological or psychological reduction in which the person is taught to separate himself from his feelings, thoughts, ideas, body sensations, and wishes, which make up his private world. The second reduction teaches the disturbed person to separate himself out as a unique human being who cannot be conceptualized by himself or others without distortion of his unique reality. The third clinical application of Husserlian reduction teaches people not to identify with the value system of their parents, family, schoolmates, or other people.

With the help of these three reductions, the person becomes aware that he is living in a unique world, which may be unconcerned, unfair, and unfeeling in relation to his needs. This awareness of his Being and separating out from his conceptual and perceptual world view lead temporarily to a state of basic anxiety, which the person experiences as a stage of helpless rage until he is taught to develop his own unique value system and point of view.

Many of these people need to learn that they live in a concrete time and place, related to specific people who have unique character structures that they cannot change at will. They must gradually learn that people are not living for or against them but with or without them. Every human being has to live and die in his own skin, experiencing his own feelings and thoughts.

For the existential therapist, a dream is as genuine an experience as a waking experience. He is not trying to see if the dream contains a hidden meaning, has a libidinal or aggressive base, or is caused by the remnants of the day; nor is he concerned with connecting the dream content with interpersonal reality, since he assumes that dreams are intended and, therefore, have experiential value for the patient.

Conclusion

Existential psychoanalysis lends itself primarily to the treatment of neurosis and ambulatory schizophrenia. Group application is possible and can be successful in helping people to live predominantly in interpersonal reality. Existential illumination is a precondition for working through, in the therapeutic relationship, the tendencies of the patient to hide himself and his feelings from himself and his therapist. Existential psychoanalysis is interested in the individual man and tries to help him become self-knowledgeable, aware of his position in time and space and his relation to his fellow man.

REFERENCES

Binswanger, L. *Being-in-the-World*. Basic Books, New York, 1963.

Boss, M. *Psychoanalysis and Daseinsanalysis*. Basic Books, New York, 1963.

Holt, H. The problems of interpretation from the point of view of existential psychoanalysis. In *Use of Interpretation in Treatment*, E. E. Hammer, editor, p. 102. Grune & Stratton, New York, 1968.

Husserl, E. *Ideas*. Macmillan, New York, 1931.

Laing, R. D. *The Politics of Experience*. Ballantine Books, New York, 1967.

Straus, E. W., Nathanson, M., and Ey, H. *Psychiatry and Philosophy*. Springer-Verlag, New York, 1969.

9

Theories of Personality and Psychopathology: Schools Derived from Psychology

9.1. PERSONALITY THEORY DERIVED FROM QUANTITATIVE EXPERIMENT

Introduction

That psychiatry lacks the stability of concepts, the maturity, and the practical effectiveness that are characteristic of a developed science based on quantitative laws and experiment is evidenced by the considerable divergences of theoretical viewpoints represented in this book. This lack is even more apparent in the excessive swings of emphasis in approved practice—for example, the recent change from psychoanalytic therapy to behavior therapy and from the predominance of psychoanalytic treatment in private practice to chemotherapy in mental hospitals. And there is little evidence of objectively measured gain from psychotherapy.

Psychiatry is an applied science. As such, it has elements of artistic skill; but in its essentials it must be based on what the sciences of psychology, physiology, and sociology offer. Among the most recent developments in psychology, those that are most relevant concern the concepts, laws, and predictive powers arising out of the experimental and, especially, the sophisticated quantitative studies conducted in the past 20 years.

The twin pillars that psychology offers in its support of the development of psychiatry are personality theory and learning theory. Until 50 years ago, personality theory developed mainly as a result of clinical observation or was based on what might be called literary and general human observation. The subsequent quantitative and experimental phase initially framed its questions in terms of the theories inherited from the earlier clinical and literary phase. More recently, however, the quantitative phase has built on a theoretical structure of its own. To date, it has failed to produce scientific laws that can aspire to the scope and elaborateness of the scientific speculations derived from the earlier phase. On the other hand, there is every indication that it has constructed a sound foundation. It is the kind of foundation that will produce definite results, expressed as basic laws and having predictive powers.

One reason why the message from the quantitative, experimental approach has not yet come through as clearly as it might is that the dust of conflict hangs over the area, sustained by a battle between the bivariate and the multivariate schools of experimental design. The bivariate school follows the classical plan of experiments in physical science; typically, it deals with one independent and one dependent variable. For example, it manipulates a stimulus and measures a response, trying and often claiming to hold all else constant while doing so. Wundt, Pavlov, and Skinner are among the advocates of this method, which has been inherited in its entirety by the reflexological school of learning.

The second school of experimental design, favoring the multivariate method, springs from Galton, Spearman, and Thurstone, and it is more concerned with correlational methods and the simultaneous study of measurement of many variables. The multivariate method has two major claims to superiority over the classical bivariate experimental design. First, the multivariate experimentalist can grasp wholes —that is, complex pattern entities, like those the clinician deals with—whereas the classical experimentalist usually deals with a single atomistic variable, which is often of minor importance and incapable of representing a complex concept. Second, the multivariate method can claim to uncover complex causal relationships without the actual manipulation of people and circumstances than has always been considered essential to classical experiment.

Structural Measurement

The quantitative approach to psychological theory involves much more than psychological testing. Methods now exist, particularly in factor analysis, that are capable of reducing the multitudes of variables to a limited set of underlying functional unities capable of predicting those variables. However, correlational methods and factor analysis must be used with the added restrictions of a scientific method, rather than the bare postulates of a purely mathematical method.

Surface and Source Traits

A surface trait is a set of behaviors that are observed to go together, to appear together, and to disappear together. A syndrome is one form of surface trait. Computer programs are capable of rapidly finding such clusters. In contrast, a source trait is one of the underlying influences that may be located by factor analysis. Examples of source traits generally include intelligence, anxiety, surgency, ego strength, superego strength, and a number of drive patterns, technically called "ergs." Essentially, the surface traits are heapings up of behavior that derive from intractions of underlying source traits.

Typically, the multivariate experimentalist measures about 300 people with regard to 80 different manifestations in behavior. He then produces a correlation matrix among these 80 variables and by factor analysis finds the factors—that is, the source traits—underlying the variables. When he finds, say, a dozen source traits, he is reasonably sure that he is finding patterns with a high likelihood of replication and with psychological predictive value.

Herein lies the vast difference between ordinary psychological testing and what may be called functional psychological testing. In psychological testing, one simply constructs scales for a priori notions or for quite specific bits of behavior; in functional psychological testing, one discovers the structures to be measured first. That is, one unearths the inherent dynamic, temperamental, or ability structures—the source traits—in the human personality and then sets out to devise functional factor tests that permit the precise measurement of these structures and nothing else.

For the most part, factor analytical work is based on observations on normal subjects. Some of the most important source traits are set out in bipolar form in Table I.

The most convenient way to assess source trait levels is by a questionnaire. The Sixteen Personality Factor Test has been used widely in both clinical and occupational situations to evaluate the level of the person on 16 of the 20 factors that have proved most relevant and most reliable. The test yields 16 scores, each on a 10-point scale. When life circumstances remain fairly stable, most of these traits demonstrate considerable stability from the age of 10 on.

Advances in factorial research in the past decade have not only added seven more normal factors but have shown that patients are distinguishable by more than deviancy on the now 23 normal primaries. Some 12 disease dimensions can be picked up only in pathology items, such as the six depression factors, schizoid tendency, hypochondria, and psychopathic tendencies.

Theoretical Model

The intersection model treats any behavioral event as something that can be accounted for only in terms of concepts of personality, of situation, and of ongoing process. Each of these variables is clearly represented by a specific formula.

Any act is thought, as far as personality is concerned, to involve the total personality— that is, the whole profile of source trait scores. The simplest mathematical way of handling this totality is to assign various appropriate and experimentally obtained weights to the action of specific traits in each given situation and then add these contributions together to get the total strength of the final response. Intersection theory considers the act as the intersection of a multidimensional personality with a multidimensional situation (see Table I).

If the source traits are the natural structures of personality or if they correspond to functional states—such as anxiety, stress, and elation-depression—one can project the prediction beyond what is possible actuarially. One can reason and predict to future dates and different occasions by adding to the formal calculation what one knows about the way in which these source traits will change with time and situation and as a result of other influences.

TABLE I

Brief Descriptions of Some Primary Source Traits Found by Factor Analysis*

Low-Score Description	Technical Labels		Standard Symbol	High-Score Description
	Low Pole	High Pole		
Reserved, detached, critical, cool	Sizothymia	Affectothymia	A	Outgoing, warmhearted, easygoing, participating
Less intelligent, concrete thinking	Low general mental capacity	Intelligence	B	More intelligent, abstract thinking, bright
Affected by feelings, emotionally less stable, easily upset	Lower ego strength	Higher ego strength	C	Emotionally stable, faces reality, calm
Phlegmatic, relaxed	Low excitability	High excitability	D	Excitable, strident, attention seeking
Humble, mild, obedient, conforming	Submissiveness	Dominance	E	Assertive, independent, aggressive, stubborn
Sober, prudent, serious, taciturn	Desurgency	Surgency	F	Happy-go-lucky, heedless, gay, enthusiastic
Expedient, a law to himself, bypasses obligations	Low superego strength	Superego strength	G	Conscientious, persevering, staid, rule-bound
Shy, restrained, diffident, timid	Threctia	Parmia	H	Venturesome, socially bold, uninhibited, spontaneous
Tough minded, self-reliant, realistic, no nonsense	Harria	Premsia	I	Tender minded, dependent, overprotected, sensitive
Trusting, adaptable, free of jealousy, easy to get on with	Alaxia	Protension	L	Suspicious, self-opinionated, hard to fool
Practical, careful, conventional, regulated by external realities, proper	Praxernia	Autia	M	Imaginative, preoccupied with inner urgencies, careless of practical matters, Bohemian
Forthright, natural, artless, sentimental	Artlessness	Shrewdness	N	Shrewd, calculating, worldly, penetrating
Placid, self-assured, confident, serene	Untroubled adequacy	Guilt proneness	O	Apprehensive, worried, depressive, troubled
Conservative, respecting established ideas, tolerant of traditional difficulties	Conservatism	Radicalism	Q_1	Experimental, critical, liberal, analytical, free thinking
Group dependent, a joiner and sound follower	Group adherence	Self-sufficiency	Q_2	Self-sufficient, prefers to make decisions, resourceful
Casual, careless of protocol, untidy, follows own urges	Weak self-sentiment	Strong self-sentiment	Q_3	Controlled, socially precise, self-disciplined, compulsive
Relaxed, tranquil, torpid, unfrustrated	Low ergic tension	High ergic tension	Q_4	Tense, driven, overwrought, fretful

* In ratings and questionnaires and now embodied in the Sixteen Personality Factor Test.

Although the 16 personality factors function well in diagnosing the various forms of neurosis, behavior disorders, homosexuality, and drug addiction, they are not sufficient to give full separation of the psychoses. For this purpose the Clinical Analysis Questionnaire or the Minnesota Multiphasic Personality Inventory is necessary.

Therapeutic Guidelines

A certain correlation cluster or surface traits may be created by several different patterns of source traits. On the other hand, experimental examination of the personality factor profiles of psychiatric patients assigned to a given syndrome group does reveal a certain similarity of profiles. Scores expressed simultaneously in surface and source trait structures should be of great value to the therapist in planning his campaign of therapy for the individual patient.

When the factor analyst studies individual differences and correlates behavior measures, he is, essentially, developing concepts of common traits. However, the peculiarity of expression visible in one source trait is due to the fact that it is combined in particular measures with some other source trait.

On the other hand, one must also recognize unique traits. The psychometrician is rarely concerned with unique traits, and the psychiatrist has usually not grasped the conceptual distinction between a common trait and a unique trait. A good deal of clinical work is concerned with the immediate observation of unique traits, and this concern is apt to obscure the fact that in the long run the psychiatrist may have to give more attention to common traits. For example, initially, the clinician may be interested in specific dynamic conflicts and personal history fixations, but his ultimate objective is to raise, say, the level of the common trait of ego strength and to reduce, say, the level of the common trait of anxiety.

The two main devices for dynamics analysis that were developed primarily in the clinical field—free association and hypnotism—have been based mainly on the verbal report of the patient. This is true of the early contributions of the psychometrists as well. Tests of interest and the questionnaire have also depended on the patient's verbal self-evaluation.

In projective tests the psychologist has offered the psychiatrist an avenue to dynamic trait measurement that is somewhat more sophisticated. Unfortunately, it has also proved very unreliable, as numerous studies of the Thematic Apperception Test (TAT) and other projective tests have shown. A fundamentally different approach from all of these began when some 90 different objective devices for measuring motivational strength were subjected to factor analysis to identify their components. The results show seven types of motivation components that appear regularly, no matter how diverse the content of interest may be. This finding has permitted the measurement of motivational factors by tests that can themselves be construct-validated against the factors. From such objective measures the generalizations that are commonly called the dynamic calculus have emerged.

Being able to measure interest strength by objective tests is only a beginning. The next step is to apply such a battery over a wide array of the typical person's life interests to correlate the grouping and structuring of action-interests. The motivational component factors are groupings within measurement devices, which hold over all areas of interest, whereas the dynamic structure factors are statements about the way in which interests fall into some functional unities.

The main result of the dynamic calculus research, as applied to dynamic structure factors, has been the finding that interest factors are essentially biological drives, on the one hand, and sentiments or aggregates of interests, acquired by education, about certain objects and institutions, on the other hand. This work appears to have verified the psychoanalytic, rather than the biological, position that there are two distinct sexual needs, which Freud described. One, which is directed toward object love, is mainly heterosexual in character; the other is narcissistic in character.

The multivariate experimentalist does something similar to what the clinician does. The main differences between them are that the experimenter actually measures the changing strength of the symptoms from day to day and calculates covariation to see what is connected with what, instead of forming his judgments about connections on the basis of chance observation and mere intuition. Fortunately, the difficulty of extensive calculation has now been overcome by the computer, so that it is now possible for a psychiatrist to hand his measurements to a technician, who then translates the dynamic structure of an individual patient into quantitative form within the hour. The difficulty lies in collecting the data; it has not proved possible statistically to get clear results after fewer than 100 days of repeated measurements.

It is not enough for the psychiatrist to identify the areas of conflict. The patient must also achieve insight and awareness of his conflicts and their origins. But if the therapist can from an early stage in treatment see more exactly where the tensions lie, this insight will be a great aid to him in bringing the patient to the point of achieving such awareness by the best chosen routes.

Dynamic calculus theory and measurement have certain potential advantages. First, they equip the psychiatrist with a set of objective measurements in a field in which the psychologist and the psychometrist previously had little but loose, projective devices to offer. Second, they offer a theoretical foundation for calculations based on these measurements to guide diagnostic and therapeutic decisions. Third, the findings derived from application of the dynamic calculus theory leave less doubt about the number and nature of ergs (constitutional drives).

Most clinicians are familiar with the phenomenon of one symptom disappearing and another appearing when there has not been a fundamental change in personality structure. Whole source traits must be modified if therapy is to be considered successful. This position does not rule out the possibility that the amelioration of a weak ego structure, for example, may be effected by the cumulative effect of a number of highly specific readjustments. But any general personality learning theory must operate on the basis of the measurement of source traits as a whole.

There is a widespread illusion on the part of both psychiatrist and psychometrist that the increasingly liberal use of psychological testing by psychiatrists implies a real use of true quantitatively based theory. Useful though psychological testing practices have been, their application has often had a nonorganic and even patchwork quality because psychiatric theory originates from quite different sources from that of test theory. Consequently, tests

have tended to be extraneous gadgets—for example, special-purpose tests, like the Rorschach—subordinated as diagnostic instruments to concepts that originated within a different frame of reference.

Effective use of the proposed measures of anxiety, ego strength, surgency, intelligence, and schizothymia does require that the psychiatrist comprehend the logical properties of the source trait concepts with which he is dealing and the theoretical setting in which they are embedded. He needs to understand that these source traits derive from factors obtained by correlational methods; that they have a demonstrated functional independence; that they can be considered to interact additively according to weightings decided by the situation in which the action takes place. It would help, too, if he had some idea of second-order factors as influences that modify first-order factors and if he would undertake to become as thoroughly familiar with the nature of 20 or so factors and their typical nature-nurture origins and life history as he is with anatomy.

The intersection model and the dynamic calculus theory that forms part of it are in accord with the view of psychopathology as a problem of disequilibrium and loss of adjustment, rather than the appearance of specifically malignant disease processes. Theoretically, pathology is either an extreme deviation in particular source traits on a normal continuum or, probably with greater frequency, an extreme combination of malfunctioning source traits that are not so deviate individually.

If a theory properly consists of a model plus a set of laws about its operation, the intersection therapy and the dynamic calculus concepts represent only the beginnings of a theory. It is true that the model is clear and that it fits the facts closely enough to permit a great deal of effective research to be done. But the body of laws about the way in which these factors behave is quite fragmentary. Compared with many other theories discussed in this book, the present structure inevitably lacks several necessary floors. What the theoretical development most needs at the present moment are a clear grasp of the particular source trait concepts (temperamental and dynamic) by psychiatrists and an application of these concepts in relation to the rich clinical criteria to which they alone have ready access and in relation to which new intuitive leads for confirmatory research are needed.

The psychiatrist may advantageously be using his art and intuition at a very different level from that of direct observation and interaction with the patient. Effective interaction at the human level with the patient is, of course, absolutely necessary. But the psychiatrist can be presented with an array of quantitative evidence of a hitherto unprecedented richness and precision. He will need to develop his artistic judgment in inferring from this evidence what steps are to be taken in his immediate relation with the patient. He is being asked to stand off for a moment from immediate impressions about the patient and to view the patient's makeup and his environmental problem in the perspective of a complex quantitative model.

REFERENCES

Cattell, R. B. *Personality and Motivation Structure and Measurement.* Harcourt, Brace & World, New York, 1957.
Cattell, R. B. *Personality and Mood by Questionnaire: A Handbook of Questionnaire Theory and Use.* Jossey-Bass, San Francisco, 1973.
Cattell, R. B., and Delhees, K. H. Seven missing normal personality factors in the questionnaire primaries. Mult. Behav. Res., 8: 173, 1973.
Cattell, R. B., Eber, H. J., and Tatsuokas, M. *The Sixteen Personality Factor Questionnaire,* ed. 3. Institute for Personality and Ability Testing, Champaign, Ill., 1970.
Cattell, R. B., and Scheier, I. H. *The Meaning and Measurement of Neuroticism and Anxiety.* Ronald Press, New York, 1961.
Cattell, R. B., and Sells, S. B. *The Clinical Analysis Questionnaire.* Institute for Personality and Ability Testing, Champaign, Ill., 1973.
Eysenck, H. J. *The Dynamics of Anxiety and Hysteria.* Rutledge and Kegan Paul, London, 1957.
Rickels, K., and Cattell, R. B. The clinical factor validity and trueness of the IPAT verbal and objective batteries for anxiety and regression. J. Clin. Psychol., 21: 257, 1965.

9.2.   OTHER PSYCHOLOGICAL PERSONALITY THEORIES

Introduction

Erich Fromm, Gordon W. Allport, Henry A. Murray, Kurt Goldstein, Andras Angyal, Abraham Maslow, Gardner Murphy, Kurt Lewin, and Frederick S. Perls are a highly diversified group of theorists, but they have certain broad areas of general agreement. Most notably, their orientations are essentially consistent with the humanistic point of view.

Goldstein was the first leading exponent of the organismic approach, an extension of Gestalt psychology that the humanistic orientation favors because of its emphasis on the individual person as an integrated, holistic unit. Perhaps the one technical exception to this generalization is Lewin, who emphasizes the psychological or phenomenological field but who is not concerned with the biological aspects of the organism. Some of these theorists, especially Murray and Murphy, stress the importance of developmental history, but many others focus on contemporary experience and conscious awareness in the present. In fact, this group in some ways resembles the ego psychologists in emphasizing the more conscious areas of personality structure and function.

These writers also believe that the betterment of the human condition is at least theoretically possible. They hold a fundamentally optimistic view of human potentialities, maintaining that the limited and fragmented view of the human being that characterizes traditional scientific approaches obscures the actual range of his capabilities. In their attempts to reach a more inclusive view of the potential ranges of human experience, some members of this group are interested in Eastern philosophy and in higher states of consciousness. Areas such as self-actualization, creativity, love, joy, and levels of transpersonal experience become for them legitimate areas of psychological investigation, as well as major goals of psychotherapy, education, and day-to-day living.

Erich Fromm

Erich Fromm (see Figure 1) was born in Germany in 1900. He has been labelled neo-Freudian and a humanistic psychoanalyst. He has retained a strong interest in the role of social factors in determining personality development, and his early writings show a definite Marxist influence. His later publications place increasing emphasis on Eastern and Western philosophy and religion.

Man, according to Fromm has been confronted with one basic problem throughout all ages and in all cultures: "How to overcome separateness, how to achieve union, how to transcend one's individual life and find at-onement." The terrible sense of isolation that no one can escape as he begins to experience himself as a separate being gives rise to intense anxiety and a deep need to reunite with himself, his fellow men, and the world. The whole process of his development depends on how he reacts to this fundamental problem.

Man is in the unique situation of being partly animal and partly human, aspects of his being that Fromm maintains must be recognized and unified. As a separate person, the human being must accept many bitter facts of which animals living in nature are not aware. Historical dichotomies are the many social and cultural tragedies that, being man-made, can at least theroetically be overcome by him. Existential dichotomies, on the other hand, are immutable. Man is subject to disease, loss, and death.

Although the individual cannot change the essential paradox inherent in the human situation, there are many different ways in which he can deal with it. He may, for example, choose to halt the process of individuation, attempting to regress by throwing away his frightening freedom and putting himself into a new kind of bondage. He will, however, only defeat himself. The only constructive synthesis

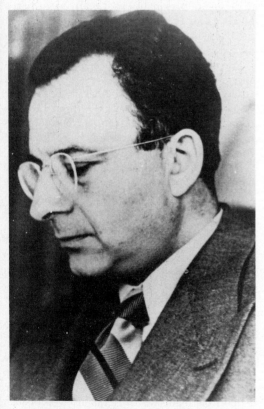

FIGURE 1. Dr. Eric Fromm (Wide World Photos).

for him is to regain his shattered sense of unity on a new and higher level. He can do this, says Fromm, only by accepting his separateness, going through the attendant anxiety, and becoming fully born as a productive being, finding a fair share of happiness and contributing what he can to his society and culture.

Fromm identifies five intrinsic human needs that must be met if a person is to continue to grow. He needs relatedness, a deep feeling of unity with himself and others. He needs transcendence, a sense of rising above the animal in him and becoming genuinely creative. He needs rootedness and identity, through which he feels he belongs and can accept his personal uniqueness accordingly. And, finally, he needs a frame of orientation, a reference point for establishing and maintaining a meaningful and stable perception of himself and his world. To fulfill these needs, a person must have a kind early environment and a beneficent society in which his progress continues.

Unless a person is willing and able to win through to freedom, his fear of separation and aloneness may be so intense that he resorts to mechanisms of escape. Fromm conceives of many such escapes, including withdrawal from the world and engaging in grandiose fantasies at the expense of reality. He lays great emphasis on three major escape routes that he sees as prominent factors in the context of society: (1) The person may seek an authoritarian solution, in which he hopes to live through someone or something external to himself. (2) Destructiveness, as a generalized attitude toward life, is an attempt to eliminate the source of perceived stress. (3) In automaton conformity, the person tries to escape from being himself by becoming as like those around him as possible.

Once a person has turned away from freedom, he is headed toward an unproductive adjustment of life, the nature of which depends on the dominant mechanism of escape he has chosen. Fromm identifies four unproductive orientations on this basis: (1) The receptive character seeks a magic helper to solve his problems for him. (2) The exploitative character is also concerned with getting things from outside, but he tries to take them away from others. (3) The hoarding character saves, stores and puts away. (4) The marketing character is the conformer who, feeling empty and anxious, tries to compensate for his uncertainty by gaining material success. Fromm regards all such unproductive adjustments as evil, since they lead to the loss of the person's good and ultimately to a corrupt and vicious society.

As Fromm believes there is only one basic human problem, so he also sees only one constructive resolution to that problem. This resolution is achieved by the productive character.

Fromm sees a fairly consistent pattern in the development of the ability to love as the person proceeds from the narcissism of the infant to a sense of unity that is universal in its potential application. He also speaks of different kinds or levels of love that are possible in human relationships.

Brotherly love is perhaps the most fundamental form, since it entails a deep sense of caring, respect, responsibility, and knowledge of someone else and is at least potentially reciprocal. Motherly love, on the other hand, is necessarily unequal in nature, since the child needs and the mother gives. Motherly love is not, however, entirely exclusive, since it can be made available to more than one of the mother's children. Fromm regards erotic love as perhaps the most deceptive form, being based by definition on exclusion, rather than on universality. Self-love can be either destructive or constructive, depending on whether it is false or genuine. If it is selfish, Fromm sees it as actually self-hatred, for it is merely uncaring and self-centered vanity. In the truer sense, self-love and love of others become one. The love of God is the highest form of love that Fromm recognizes. This love need not be theistic; it is an individual matter and is as diversified as is the love of man. At the highest level, love of God and love of man become unified, just as love for others and for the self become indistinguishable. The attainment of this all-inclusive love is, for Fromm, the final answer to the human dilemma.

Gordon W. Allport

Gordon W. Allport (1897–1967) was born in Indiana. His theories are based primarily on academic psychology, rather than on clinical experience. His views have been described as humanistic and personalistic, but he preferred to consider his personality theory as an eclecticism that conceives of personality as a unique and open system.

Allport held that, above all, psychology should study a real person and not be satisfied with constructing an artificial person. No area of possible contribution to a better understanding of human behavior should be discouraged or neglected. His own broad interests included work in such diverse areas as values, motivation, morale, prejudice, communication, expressive movement, handwriting, and practical questions in guidance, teaching, and mental health.

Uniqueness is the essence of Allport's theoretical approach to personality, but he recognized the anomalous position of science in relation to the individual person. Science, as presently constituted, is able to investigate primarily groups, common areas, broad generalizations, and common laws. This methodological weakness restricts scientific study largely to nomothetic procedures that, at best, can construct an artificial man and must thus violate personality as it really is. Allport's plea was for the development of more suitable methods for studying the individual person by morphogenic or idiographic techniques.

Personality is what the person really is, the special way in which he works out his own survival. This personal formula is never static or complete; it remains a *becoming* throughout his life. Allport regarded the self as a central focus in the psychology of personality. Selfhood, in Allport's view, develops in a series of stages.

Traits, in Allport's system, are not only the chief unit of personality structure but also the major dynamic source of human motivation. A trait has actual existence. It is more generalized than a habit and is dynamic or, at least, determinative in behavior. It is neither independent of other traits nor synonymous with moral or social judgments. It can be seen within a person or distributed in a population. And, finally, it cannot be disproved by acts or habits that are inconsistent with it.

As his theories developed, the term "traits" was reserved for what he later called "common traits," those that characterize people in the same culture. "Personal dispositions" came to be the term used for individual characteristics. Allport distinguished three major levels of such dispositions. Cardinal dispositions are master sentiments or ruling passions, which are outstanding, dominant, and quite rare. More characteristic of most people are the relatively few but easily recognized central dispositions, which tend to govern their lives. Secondary dispositions are less clear-cut, more diffuse in expression, and less often manifested.

Functional autonomy is "any acquired system of motivation in which the tensions involved are not of the same kind as the antecedent tensions from which the acquired system developed." This concept brings motivation out of the past and into the framework of the contemporary. For Allport, whatever makes a person act must be operating now. Therefore, the adult cannot be said to act as he did when he was a child.

Allport recognized a wide range of motives, including interests, abilities, intentions, plans, habits, and attitudes. He further accepted certain lower-order self-sustaining systems, such as addictions, routines, and various other types of essentially repetitive behavior patterns. He maintained that a maladaptive state of adjustment may sometimes become so tightly structured and firmly entrenched that it actually represents the person's style of life. Such a system, in Allport's view, is probably not amenable to depth analysis.

The mature person in Allport's view has a greatly extended sense of self and can relate warmly to others in both intimate and casual relationships. He is emotionally secure, accepting of others, and aware of outer reality in his thinking, perceiving, and acting. He has zest, enthusiasm, insight, and humor and has achieved a sufficiently unified philosophy of life to use it in directing his living harmoniously. It is the proper function of psychology, psychotherapy, and education to foster the kind of human progress that enables people to work cooperatively rather than competitively with each other.

Henry A. Murray

Henry A. Murray was born in New York City in 1893. He proposes the term "personology" for the study of personality, defining it as "the branch of psychology which principally concerns itself with the study of human lives and the factors that influence their course." The ultimate aim of the personologist is regarded as threefold: to construct a theory of personality,

to devise suitable techniques for studying its important attributes, and to discover its basic facts through careful and extensive investigations of actual human lives. Murray has always been an advocate of interdisciplinary personality studies and accepts a wide range of approaches as useful in personology.

Murray defines personality as "the hypothetical structure of the mind, the consistent establishments and processes of which are manifested over and over again . . . in the internal and external proceedings which constitute a person's life." Personality is hypothetical because it can perhaps be inferred from the facts of a person's life but still transcends them all. It is manifested repeatedly because, although it is constantly changing, it also has recognizable features that persist over time. The term "proceedings" refers to the units of time during which a person attends to either internal or external circumstances of his life. Serials are series of proceedings, related to each other but separate in time, that permit pursuit of long-range goals. Murray sees the person as continually planning and arranging schedules for achieving these goals and setting up serial programs, sequences of subgoals, which serve as steps along the way. Proceedings, serials, schedules, and serial programs constantly arise, shift, and give way to others as circumstances change, and personality inevitably changes with them.

Murray also sees the person as constantly pressured by conflicting internal and external demands, so that throughout his life he must give up as well as take for himself. Personality is made up of integrated and interdependent processes, functionally inseparable and always operating as a whole. This unity, Murray maintains, is possible only because the processes of personality refer to organizations in the brain, without which personality could not exist at all.

Murray holds an essentially Freudian picture of personality development. The id, as he conceives of it, remains the source of energy and the reservoir of unacceptable impulses, as it was for Freud. In Murray's view, however, the id also contains some acceptable and constructive impulses. The ego is not merely a repressor and inhibitor but also has energy of its own and helps some of the id drives find suitable expression. The superego, although still the internal regulator of behavior derived from early experiences, can be significantly changed later by peer-group and other influences, including those associated with literary, historical, and mythological characters with whom the person identifies. Murray's ego ideal, which is associated with the superego, consists of all the various self-images that represent the person at his very best. These ideals help the person maintain goal-directed living and, if they are reasonably in accord with the requirements of his society and culture, enable him to cope with the environment without relinquishing too many desires of his own. In a healthy development Murray sees these three structures changing in relative dominance as the personality unfolds, the id losing its original pre-eminence first to the superego and later to the ego.

Murray also identifies certain relatively specific temporal sequences in childhood that in many ways resemble the Freudian view of psychosexual development. Murray's oral, anal, and phallic states closely resemble their Freudian counterparts, although Murray's are somewhat more broadly interpreted. Murray also introduces two further stages into his own scheme, the claustral and the urethral, the claustral being the tranquil state of prenatal existence and the urethral, which falls between the oral and the anal stages developmentally, involving the pleasurable sensations associated with urethral erotism. If a child is too deprived at any particular stage or lacks sufficient impetus to go ahead, Murray sees the possibility of a fixation in much the Freudian sense. Although some amount of fixation is considered normal and even inevitable, overly strong fixations may lead to complexes, later inducing the adult to strive for enjoyments more suited to earlier period of his life. Murray evolves a character typology based on the predominant developmental influence in the person's life, again following Freud. He does, however, include two further character types, associated with the additional stages he introduces. The claustral complex tends to produce a passive, dependent personality development, with prominent withdrawal tendencies. The urethral complex, on the other hand, results in an overly ambitious, strongly narcissistic adult.

A primary concept in Murray's theory of motivation is the need. To Murray the need represents a force in the brain that can be aroused by either internal or external stimula-

tion. Once aroused, it produces continued activity until it is reduced or satisfied. Murray does not, however, believe that need-tension reduction is the chief purpose of living except, perhaps, in the case of the excessively conflict-ridden or overly anxious. Under normal circumstances, Murray feels that it is the process of tension reduction that is the most satisfying condition. A major goal of personality functioning is, therefore, to reach states in which reducing tension is possible. The person may actually seek out arousal in order to experience this tension reduction.

Murray later attempted to retain the essentials of his need concept through the use of a value-vector schema. The purpose of this approach was to portray simultaneously what a person sees as important in a situation together with what he does to achieve it. The vectors are used to show the direction of his behavior, and the values represent what he holds in esteem.

Needs must be triggered, and Murray finds the source of need arousal in his concept of press. A press is seen as a force in the environment that, whether real or perceived, has the capacity to arouse need-tension in the person. He distinguishes between α press, those aspects of an object or situation that reflect what it really is, and β press, which is the force of the object or situation as the person interprets it. Dominant needs and press are linked in early childhood through repeated associations that may be either satisfying or traumatic.

The thema, the need-press combination, is Murray's unit for psychological study. A method he developed for uncovering dominant themas in the life of a person is the Thematic Apperception Test (TAT), a projective technique widely used in clinical practice.

Kurt Goldstein

Kurt Goldstein (1878–1965) was born in Germany. His early involvement with Gestalt psychology, phenomenology, and existentialism reflects a pervasive interest in philosophical issues that he retained throughout his career. Two of his major constructs were the organismic viewpoint and self-actualization, around which his personality theory is built.

In Goldstein's organismic framework, a person's interrelations with his society, the similarities and differences that exist between him and other members of that society, and even his broader relationships to his culture and to other cultures must all be taken into consideration. Because of the vast amount of information that Goldstein considered necessary to understand the person, he strongly favored intensive, long-term studies of single persons in preference to more superficial investigations of groups.

Goldstein did not hesitate to assume that a living organism has genuinely creative power. This power is inherent in his concept of self-actualization, the single need that he believed to underlie all human behavior, although its outlets and expressions vary from one person to another and from society to society. The specific potentialities of a person, Goldstein maintained, can be inferred from two factors: what the person himself prefers to do and what he does best.

To function reasonably well, the organism must somehow come to terms with the environment in fairly comfortable interaction, since the environment encroaches on the organism, disturbing its equilibrium but also acting as its source of supply. As the person's coping methods become more effective, his chances of self-actualization increase. The undisturbed organism, according to Goldstein, remains in a more or less equal state of tension distribution and normally strives to regain that state when it is upset.

In Goldstein's view of the person's organismic strivings toward self-actualization, there are constant shifts between a central figure and the background from which it emerges. "The capacity that is particularly important for the task is the foreground; the others are in the background." Impairments in the ability to shift figure and ground rapidly and appropriately represent a serious handicap in functioning efficiency.

The ability to react abstractly or concretely as the situation demands is another cardinal requirement for self-actualization in Goldstein's interpretation. Action is thought of as in the realm of the concrete. The abstract attitude may lead to action but does not in itself include it. In the concrete situation, the response aroused is triggered directly by the actual stimulus. In the abstract attitude, the person prepares himself to act by such processes as considering, evaluating, and deciding. Goldstein regarded the abstract attitude as the human organism's highest and essential ability,

but he also insisted that concrete behavior is imperative at times. Smooth functioning depends on the person's skill in shifting appropriately from concrete to abstract responses as the situation requires.

Goldstein saw self-actualization as involving somewhat different goals in sickness and in health. The person in a pathological state may, for example, be forced to limit his expressions of self-actualization to maintenance of the status quo, discharging tension as best he can and perhaps concentrating merely on survival. Goldstein regarded pathology as always associated with isolation, so that the organism's whole integrity is threatened. In response to this threat, the sick person may respond rigidly and compulsively, fall back to more primitive levels of behavior, constrict his interests and activity, or withdraw into routines.

Goldstein saw the healthy person's drive to actualize himself as inducing spontaneity, creativeness, and genuine self-expression. The self-actualizing drive, in health, is capable of enabling the person to accept some amount of risk without retreating into fear because he has retained the spirit of adventure and confidence that Goldstein found inherent in the self-actualization principle. The healthy person is able to reach what Goldstein referred to as the sphere of immediacy, the level at which the human being becomes truly dynamic and finds the source of genuine wholeness and creativity.

Andras Angyal

Andras Angyal (1902–1960) was born in Hungary. His holistic approach is inherent in his concept of the biosphere, which he considered the actual realm of life itself. Person and environment are both included within it—not as separate parts but as different aspects of one reality. Angyal believed that living itself results from the differences in the factors involved in self-regulation on the one hand and those related to external or environmental government on the other. When a special function is required for a particular purpose, a part is thought to differentiate out of the whole in order to meet that need. Once it has arisen, the part may then serve a variety of related activities, thus serving the larger biospheric economy.

Life, according to Angyal, can be regarded as a process of self-expansion. It can be thought of as a circle open at both ends or poles, one pole allowing assimilation or intake and the other facilitating production or output. The assimilating aspect is the source of what is termed autonomy. Autonomous functions include all the self-governing and self-regulating drives, such as choosing, adapting, impulses to action, and urges to master. If these functions are properly directed and appropriately expressed, they result in useful and constructive characteristics, such as competence and ingenuity. Under less fortunate circumstances, however, they may lead to competitive behavior and to drives to dominate and to suppress. The output phase of living becomes the basis for homonomy, the processes by which he also gives out, making his own unique contribution to life. Such homonomous drives represented the essential aspects of humanity to Angyal and were virtually equated with love. Angyal believed that homonomous tendencies, like autonomous drives, can find neurotic as well as healthy avenues of expression.

According to Angyal's concept of universal ambiguity, personality inevitably represents a dual organization. Everyone meets with both fortuitous and traumatic experiences and situations as he develops, so that personality begins to organize around two different nuclei. In time, two different patterns within the personality evolve. One arises from feelings of isolation, failure, helplessness, and doubt. The other springs from a sense of personal adequacy, a reasonable degree of optimism, and sufficient certainty to permit decisive action.

In Angyal's view, mental health and mental illness derive essentially from whichever of the two systems predominates in any particular person. The well-functioning person, in whom the healthy system is stronger and better developed, is capable of acting and thinking on the basis of what he is, rather than on the basis of what others think he should be. When the neurotic system is dominant, the person is primarily concerned with appearances, having lost contact with his own real feelings, thoughts, and desires.

Anxiety, for Angyal, was the person's reaction to the nondominant pattern in his dual personality organization. In the healthy person it is a response to impulses arising from his underlying neurotic pattern. In the neurotic it is a reaction to the threat of his own healthy inclinations. In either case, anxiety is engendered by a sense of

jeopardy to the realization of the person's dominant tendencies, be they healthy or neurotic.

Angyal rested his psychotherapeutic hopes on his conviction that the healthy core of the patient, his real self, his potentialities for self-expansion, can never be completely extinguished. However, the patient cannot recognize the dual nature of his personality while the neurotic pattern retains dominance. He can begin to accept the other side of himself only as the submerged healthy aspect becomes better organized and more developed. At this stage in the therapeutic process, Angyal believed, the patient must become increasingly anxious, his discomfort being greatest when the two systems operating in him reach approximately equal strength. Thereafter, the anxiety subsides as the healthy system begins to gain dominance over the neurotic and as guilt becomes less intense.

Abraham Maslow

Abraham Maslow (1908–1970) was born in Brooklyn, New York. He felt strongly that the rigid application of the scientific model of the physical sciences to psychology merely allowed for a partial picture of the human being. Believing in the need to understand the totality in order to understand at all, Maslow appealed for considerable broadening of psychology both in content and in method. Such a psychology should be firmly based in the humanistic approach and willing to accept and understand the human being as he is. Maslow regarded the overconcern of many personality theorists with psychopathology as a further limit on understanding human behavior.

Maslow saw the impulse to grow and actualize one's potentialities already present in the human baby. The inherent tendencies of the infant are good or, at least, neutral, making up the inner human nature, which Maslow described as "instinctoid." In this inner nature, Maslow identified certain inherent needs that, although differing in expression from person to person and from society to society, are in themselves intrinsic and species-wide. They are, therefore, regarded as basic needs. Maslow subdivided these needs into two groups, the first being called deficiency or D-needs. Needs in this category range in order of importance from such essentials for sustaining life as hunger and thirst to gratification of the drives for affection and self-esteem. Beyond the D-needs are the growth or B-needs, which Maslow also calls "metaneeds." These needs propel the person toward wholeness, uniqueness, and self-fulfilment. To this second group Maslow assigns such human urges as impulses to freedom, beauty, goodness, unity, and justice.

Maslow saw D-needs and B-needs as generating a fundamental and inherent conflict. D-needs induce behavior aimed at supplying deficiencies, and the person must depend on other people and external things. The resulting dependence tends to make him fearful, since the source of supply may fail. The pressure of D-needs is, therefore, apt to induce regressive behavior and lead to defensiveness, clinging to the past, and fear of growth and independence. B-needs, on the other hand, impel the person toward confidence in the world and in himself. They minimize the sense of threat, reducing hostility and allowing the person to become more self-directed, self-sufficient, and self-contained.

The thwarting of basic needs leads to the development of neurotic needs that, being impossible to satisfy, result in wasted human potentiality and depletion of human energy. Basic needs, on the other hand, can be gratified to a reasonable extent, since they entail comparatively free choices and foster a growth process.

All forms of human behavior, in Maslow's theoretical framework, can be thought of in terms of the joint operation of D-needs and B-needs. The particular form of the behavior depends on the ratio of regressive to progressive motivation involved.

Maslow's chief way of approaching health was through studies of its best examples: those persons who are the most fully developed and creative. They are characterized by what Maslow called "self-actualizing creativeness," which he considered a generalized orientation that leads to health and growth, regardless of what the person who possesses it does. Special talents may or may not be involved. The truly creative actualize themselves in everything they do.

He found them all, for example, to be realistically oriented, problem-centered, and generally accepting of themselves and others. They were also spontaneous, independent, and creative; they identified with mankind and were able to transcend their environments. Their values were democratic and their sense of humor genuine, and most of them reported having had mystical or ego-transcending or peak experiences at some level.

The peak experience is an episodic, usually quite brief occurrence, in which the person is suddenly and unexpectedly transformed into full and transcending humanness. He is thought to achieve an orientation that Maslow regarded as "unmotivated, non-striving, non-self-centered, purposeless, self-validating." In this state the person becomes aware of ultimate values that cannot be further analyzed but that do not require further analysis to establish their reality for him.

Gardner Murphy

Gardner Murphy was born in Ohio in 1895. All the theorists discussed here are eclectic to some extent, but Murphy is perhaps the most thoroughgoing in this respect. He consistently argues for increasing interaction of all relevant approaches to the investigation of man and for inclusion of as many vantage points as possible from which to study him.

From psychology Murphy accepts virtually all the major concepts, principles, and methods used in its various branches. Further, he is unwilling merely to pick out an idea here or a principle there without considering the whole context in which it is embedded. His firm belief in the lifelong capacity of personality to change and grow has led him to envision almost unlimited human potentialities. Nor does he remain comfortably within the scientifically safer areas of investigation in considering what these potentialities may be. Murphy has long been interested in psychic paranormal phenomena, considering them part of the total reality of man.

Murphy accepts no real distinction between the biological and social aspects of personality. Biological being is seen as the bedrock of personality, but personality is by no means regarded as what is limited to inside the skin. Personality is seen as a structured organism-environment field that is part of a still larger field, the two aspects being engaged in constant reciprocal interaction.

Murphy describes three essential stages in personality development. The person begins in the stage of undifferentiated wholeness, progresses to the stage of differentiation of function, and proceeds on to the stage of integration. Regression as well as progression is possible along the way, and the process is frequently quite uneven. Each developmental stage is thought to involve functions peculiar to itself, so that adult personality is by no means merely an extension of earlier characteristics. The range of individual differences broadens steadily as development continues.

The most basic structural units in Murphy's schema are psychological dispositions or organic traits. These are tissue tensions that are gradually reconstituted into symbolic traits in the course of development. Personality characteristics derive from organic traits that have either channeled into specific forms of behavior or redirected by conditioning as the person develops.

He identifies four broad categories of inborn human needs: visceral, motor, sensory, and emergency-related. These are thought to become increasingly specific in time, as they are molded by the person's experiences in various social and environmental contexts. A major factor in bringing these changes about is canalization, the process by which a connection is established between a need and a specific way of satisfying it. Early canalizations are particularly important in Murphy's view of personality development, for these are the basis for later canalizations, and they also retain the power to induce regressive behavior under stress in the adult.

Unlike canalizations, which produce actual changes in tension levels, conditioning is seen as a preparatory process that readies the organism for tension reduction but does not affect the tension changes themselves. Also unlike canalization, conditioned responses can be readily generalized and easily shifted, extinguished, and replaced.

Murphy's contributions to parapsychology are both theoretical and experimental. He suggests that, since parapsychological or paranormal experiences may reflect essential aspects of personality, to disregard them may impose arbitrary restrictions on actual human potentialities. However, Murphy urges applying a genuinely experimental method to the area.

Kurt Lewin

Kurt Lewin (1890–1947) was born in the Prussian village of Mongilno, now a part of Poland. His professional career began with studies of learning and perception, from which he turned his attention to the dynamics of conflict, frustration, and the problems of individual motivation, becoming increasingly concerned in later years with social issues and group processes.

Lewin regarded the person and the environment as parts or regions of the same psychological field. He defined a field as the "totality of coexisting facts which are conceived of as mutually interdependent." Behavior thus becomes a function of the person and the environment or, in Lewin's formula, $B = F (P,E)$.

Lewin used topology, a nonmetric branch of mathematics, to present his structural field concepts in mathematical terms and to depict them in diagrammatic form. Person and environment together make up what Lewin called the life space. Within this area, which represents a field in constant flux, Lewin placed everything that influences behavior at a given time. In his topological diagrams, person and environment are depicted as two separate areas that together constitute the life space and that are enclosed within it. This whole area is bounded off from the nonpsychological environment or foreign hull, much as the person and the environment are separated from each other. The environment as Lewin regarded it does not necessarily correspond to external reality. The term refers to the psychological environment, the environment as the person interprets it. Group and individual behavior are thought of in terms of the interactions of regions within the life space, along with those between the life space and adjacent areas of the nonpsychological environment that lie outside.

A single area of the field cannot induce behavior by itself. At least two regions must be involved. Another influencing principle is concreteness, which implies that only facts already present in the field can promote behavior. A related principle is that of contemporaneity, which emphasizes Lewin's strong belief that only present facts are relevant.

Lewin used the term "dynamic" to refer to conditions of change. A primary dynamic concept in the person is the need, which was Lewin's chief motivational construct. A need arouses tension, which is then reduced or equalized as the need is met through either action or ideation. Lewin identified three stages through which needs typically proceed: hunger, satiation, and oversatiation. These states are associated with another dynamic concept, that of valence. A valence is defined as the value with which a person invests a particular environmental region in terms of its potential for need satisfaction. A positive valence is associated with the hunger stage of need arousal, a neutral valence with satiation, and a negative valence with oversatiation.

The motive power for restoring equilibrium is reserved in Lewin's system for the concept of force. The need arises in the person, but the force exists in the environment. A force of sufficient strength pressures the person toward tension reduction, and he selects a path into the environment by which to accomplish this reduction. He may also respond by restructuring the environment or simply by changing his perception of the situation so that it no longer arouses tension in him. His reactions are largely influenced by what Lewin calls his level of aspiration, the degree of difficulty presented by the goal toward which he is striving. His level of aspiration establishes the goal he invests with the highest positive valence or perceived reward, and this is influenced by a number of subjectively determined factors, as well as social pressures and group evaluations. More difficult goals carry greater positive valence than easier ones.

Seen as a dynamic whole, the group must be studied through the interrelationships of its parts. The individual cannot be neglected as a part of the larger field, but the social scientists must also take into consideration the structure of the group as a whole—its cultural values, its ideologies, and the economic factors operating within it.

The now popular term "group dynamics" was introduced by Lewin, and it is probably in this area that his influence is still most strongly felt. Many contemporary techniques originated here, such as action research programs for altering undesirable social conditions and T-groups for facilitating insight into group processes as a means for re-education. Changing group standards were of major concern to Lewin, largely because he believed that persons resist change unless or until group values change.

Lewin broke the process of group change down into three phases, which he called unfreezing, restructuring, and refreezing. Rigid attitudes and beliefs must first be unfrozen, raised to critical consideration and evaluation. A restructuring of perspective, a change in viewpoint, then becomes possible, Thereafter, shifts in attitude and behavior can occur, to be refrozen at more constructive levels.

Gestalt Therapy

The influence of Einstein's field theory on psychological thought led to the development of Gestalt psychology in Germany some 60 years ago. Its chief exponents were Max Wertheimer, Wolfgang Kohler, and Kurt Koffka. Frederick S. Perls (1893–1970), who was born in Berlin, extended some of the principles of Gestalt psychology into the special form of psychotherapy that bears its name.

Gestalt therapy is not an outgrowth of Gestalt psychology exclusively. It is heavily indebted to Freudian theory, to the concepts of Wilhelm Reich and Otto Rank, and to existential thought. Gestalt therapy accepts the humanistic, holistic, and essentially positive view of the human being and his potentialities. It is concerned with such areas of experience as self-enhancement, creativity, and even transcendence. It regards the mere absence of misery and pain as an insufficient goal for living, looking at the person as at least potentially capable of achieving real joy.

A Gestalt, a whole, is defined by Asch as "an extended event, whether an experience or an action, that cannot be adequately described as a sum of smaller, independent events." According to the Gestalt point of view, any atomistic approach omits essential characteristics of actual experience, such as value, meaning, and form. Gestalts are thought of as unified wholes that reflect a balanced distribution of the forces underlying their organization. When this balance is disturbed the organism exerts efforts to restore it. Gestalts need not correspond to external properties, since the person putting the Gestalt together selects the perception out of a larger field and thus puts something of himself into it.

The phenomenal world is seen as organized around needs, and these needs both integrate and energize behavior. Needs are hierarchical and shifting, the central figure in the field being the most dominant or pressing need that the person is experiencing at that moment. As that need is met, it recedes into the background, making room for the next most pressing need to assume the dominant position. This process allows need gratification to proceed in appropriate and orderly sequence. The environment is an essential part of the field because the person must look to it for need satisfaction.

The marked emphasis on the here and now, perhaps the most outstanding characteristic of Gestalt therapy, is in accord with the importance that Gestalt psychology places on data from immediate experience. Gestalt thinking also stresses the relations between processes in the perceiver and the form of what is perceived in the making of a Gestalt.

The person must be able to make sharp differentiations between figure and ground. In terms of motivation, he must recognize what he needs most at a given time, see it clearly as the central figure in the field, and thus put himself in a position where need satisfaction is possible. Well-organized motor responsiveness and goal-directed behavior result.

Perls sees the person as engaged in a constant struggle for balance, since his equilibrium is continually being disturbed by the pressures of internal needs or by environmental demands. The result is increased tension, which is reduced as balance is restored. This process, which is called organismic self-regulation, is considered basic to all motivation.

Disturbances in organismic balance are thought to engender fear and avoidance of actual awareness, so that the genuine reactivity and excitement that characterize healthy experience are not available. Awareness is thought of as the crucial factor in restoring balance.

In the Gestalt view, the neurotic and, still more, the psychotic cannot deal constructively with the many polarizations or splits that characterize living. These polarizations include the dichotomies of body and mind, self and nonself, biological and cultural, unconscious and conscious, and love and aggression. Such dichotomies pose threats to integration that everyone must meet and overcome. In neurotic splitting, however, the attempted resolutions are faulty and damaging to the wholeness of the personality. One part of the split may be held out of awareness, separated from overt concern, or isolated from the other part. Therapy must attempt to restore the personality to wholeness, to its true Gestalt.

The immediate goal of Gestalt therapy is restoration of full awareness to the patient. From a more long-range point of view, the purpose is to restore to him all his previously crippled personality functions so that he can release his inherent potentialities. Healthy contact with himself and with the environment must be established.

The ego is considered as an organismic function with major integrative responsibility. Its basic purpose is to structure the environment. If this structuring can take place easily and consistently, the person is free to continue smooth psychological growth.

The techniques used are largely directed toward opening up the patient's direct, immediate experience—what he is feeling, doing, and thinking right now. Interpretation and intellectual activity in general are discouraged. Efforts are not directed toward finding out why he experiences what he does but how he does it. The therapist is alert to signs of feelings that are being denied awareness, whether in facial expression, vocal tone, posture, or body movements. It is the therapist's chief function to bring the patient's attention back to his immediate experience whenever it wanders, helping him to use the continuum of awareness as a means to return to health.

The therapist, as well as the patient, plays an extremely active role in the therapeutic process. The patient attempts to avoid his problems and to defend himself against pain. The therapist serves to counteract such attempts. He draws the patient's attention to his avoidance mechanisms, to signs of phobic behavior, and to other defensive and unproductive attitudes and feelings. The Gestalt viewpoint emphasizes the value of frustration in fostering growth. The therapist may, therefore, deliberately frustrate the patient to help him increase his frustration tolerance and break through his impasse by finding his own way out. Above all, the patient must come to place his confidence in himself, and for this he must recognize the fantasy nature of the impasse he experiences. He must come to grips with all that he is resisting in himself.

The role of dreams is considered particularly important in the process. The therapist does not approach the dream through interpretation. Instead, he urges the patient to relive it in the immediate situation. He is to act it out like a drama, playing the roles of the people and even the objects that the dream contains.

Gestalt therapy implies a prescription for the

good life that is quite similar to its therapeutic procedures. The elements of this prescription, as suggested by Naranjo, include the following: Live now. Live here. Stop imagining and needless thinking. Express rather than manipulate, justify, and judge. Do not restrict awareness. Accept only your own "shoulds." Take responsibility for your own feelings, thoughts, and actions. And, finally, surrender to being what you are.

REFERENCES

Bischof, L. J. *Interpreting Personality Theories*, ed. 2. Harper & Row, New York, 1970.

Boring, E. G., and Lindzey, G. *A History of Psychology in Autobiography*, vol. 5. Appleton-Century-Crofts, New York, 1967.

Fromm, E. *The Anatomy of Human Destructiveness*. Holt, Rinehart and Winston, New York, 1973.

Hall, C., and Lindzey, G. *Theories of Personality*, ed 2. p. 291. John Wiley, New York, 1970.

Maddi, S. R. *Personality Theories: A Comparative Analysis*. Dorsey, Homewood, Ill., 1968.

Murphy, G. A. Caringtonian approach to reincarnation cases. J. Am. Soc. Psych. Res., *67:* 126, 1973.

Naranjo, C. *The Techniques of Gestalt Therapy*. SAT Press, Berkeley, 1973.

Patterson, C. H. *Theories of Counseling and Psychotherapy*, ed. 2. Harper & Row, New York, 1973.

Riecken, H. Gold Medal Award to Gardner Murphy. Am. Psychol., *28:* 75, 1973.

Sahakian, W. S. *Psychology of Personality: Readings in Theory*. Rand-McNally, Chicago, 1965.

Wepman, J. M., and Heine, R. *Concepts of Personality*. Aldine Publishing Company, Chicago, 1963.

10

Application of Psychoanalytic
Theory to Philosophy

10.1. HERBERT MARCUSE

Introduction

Herbert Marcuse (see Figure 1) comes from
the German academic and philosophical tradition. Born in 1898 in Berlin he has come to be
associated with radical causes and Marxist
philosophy. In Marcuse's view, the unresolved
conflict between man's life instincts and the
demands of the oppressive, irrational social
structure is the basic neurosis of modern society.

Marcuse and Freudian Theory

According to Freud, repression is the founding stone of civilization. The renunciation of
instinctual pleasure frees sexual energy, which
is sublimated and turned to the task of formulating culture. Freud saw civilization as
being founded on the two contrasts of freedom
versus happiness and sexuality versus civilization.

Freedom versus happiness is based on the
contrast between the reality principle, governed
by the ego, and the pleasure principle, governed
by the id. Marcuse, on the other hand, sees a
close connection between freedom and happiness. "Happiness, as the fullfillment of all
potentialities of the individual, presupposes
freedom...at root, it is freedom." Freud also
saw happiness as a goal, but he felt that the
search for it was always doomed to frustration
and failure.

As for the contrast between sexuality and
civilization, Freud saw all social orders as based
on the renunciation of sexual life, but Marcuse

envisions a social order in which libidinal energy and gratification are at the heart of all
human relations. Rather than negating Freud's
contrasts, Marcuse insists that they are a result
of external societal factors and are not intrinsic
to human nature.

To enlarge on Freud's constructs while retaining his theory, Marcuse introduces two concepts. The first, the notion of surplus repression, he distinguishes from basic repression, the
restrictions on instinctual drives that, as Freud
pointed out, are necessary for the existence of
any civilization. Surplus repression refers to

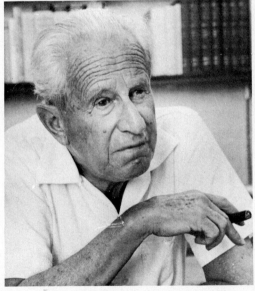

FIGURE 1. Herbert Marcuse (Wide World Photos).

340

those restrictions associated with social domination. Marcuse argues that, although affluent societies have reached a point in technological development at which people should be able to give freer rein to their instinctual lives, they continue to impose unnecessary controls, surplus repression. As technology and industry continue to be refined and improved, the economic scarcity that originally justified repression becomes less and less of a reality, and the repression thus becomes more surplus.

Marcuse's second concept is that of the performance principle. Freud claimed that the reality principle calls for repression because of society's demand for control and order. He believed that progress requires ever-increasing control of the instincts, and he claimed that one of the functions of psychoanalysis is to help soften the effects of psychic repression and frustration. Marcuse, however, argues that the demands of the reality principle are really the demands of society, which sets up an order and hierarchy of performance—a performance principle.

For Marcuse, Freud's death instinct is at the root of the destructiveness of modern technology.

Central to Marcuse's philosophy is the notion that the system must create artificial consumer needs to maintain its cycle of production-consumption-production. To create these needs, the system must involve itself with the consumers' psychic processes, in particular their sexual fantasies, by continuously stimulating their desires and expectations. However, the desired goods are never capable of supplying complete fulfillment; thus, the consumer is left with frustration. This sense of frustration is directed at the self in the form of internalized aggression. The consumer is then forced to turn against falsely created enemies, as in war, or against scapegoat groups or himself with drugs and other self-destructive devices. Because unhappiness, resentment, and aggression must result from working only to sustain needless consumption, Marcuse sees the creation of a new society liberated from the old principles as the only solution to the mass neurosis of modern man.

REFERENCES

Marcuse, H. *Eros and Civilization: A Philosophical Inquiry into Freud*. Beacon Press, Boston, 1955.
Marcuse, H. *One-Dimensional Man*. Beacon Press, Boston, 1964.

10.2.   NORMAN O. BROWN

Introduction

Norman O. Brown was born in El Oro, Mexico. Mankind, says Brown, is mostly unaware of its own needs and desires, is basically hostile to life, and is bent on self-destruction. The frenetic and repressive twentieth century civilization, he says, works against freedom, particularly sexual freedom, the uninhibited, innocent sexuality that, as Freudians believe, motivates behavior throughout life.

Brown and Freudian Theory

Brown displays an almost worshipful reverence for Freud, especially his more mystical and poetic aspects, and applies Freudian principles to areas that Freud himself never touched. Brown claims that viewing the world symbolically will ultimately lead to a new system that will liberate mankind. Body mysticism sees everything as part of a brotherhood in which each body is one great human body. This notion of body mysticism probably expresses, in a metaphysical sense, man's real needs and desires, but it is incompatible with contemporary political institutions, such as the state and private ownership, all of which Brown sees as antihuman and evil.

Selfhood and a strong sense of identity are not goals to be sought, says Brown. "The solution to the problem of identity is, get lost," he comments drily. The ego imposes a division and destructive sense of reality, breaking up the human body into individual entities. Likewise, the supergo sets up excessive prohibitions that further confirm the divisions between us.

Brown believes that sexual repression is the greatest enemy of human beings and is the cause of a universal human neurosis. Social repression derives from self-repression and is created by the disunifying experience of anxiety.

Freud's two instincts, eros and death, though repressed and unrecognized, are the energies that create human culture. To recognize their existence is to reinterpret human culture. Brown seems to equate Freud's two basic instincts with good and evil. Whereas Freud saw life as an integration of the two, Brown asks that the death instinct be discarded entirely.

Brown considers sublimation the link between psychoanalysis and culture analysis. The idea of sublimation presupposes paradoxes, all having to do with high-level cultural life on the one hand and lower bodily regions on the other.

Brown is interested not in social growth and progress but in social archetypes, the basic patterns that underlie all social organization. Archetypes, as Freud knew, are the unconscious themes in which buried hopes and needs are reflected. Brown attempts to codify these archetypes and to apply them to diverse historical and anthropological data. His view of human history is gloomy. He sees the course of human development as a series of catastrophic events, from the divisive act of separating people into men and women to the continuing inventions of new social forms that divide humanity into classes, nations, and the like.

Brown takes an essentially apocalyptic view of life. He points out that "all Freud's work demonstrates that the allegiance of the human psyche to the pleasure principle is indestructi-

ble and that the path of instinctual renunciation is the path of sickness and self-destruction. Brown exhorts his followers to discard the rationalizations that have brought society to such bleak conditions. The only salvation, Brown claims, lies in the total destruction of the present order and in total abolition of repression by affirming the body's instinctual drives. A reconciliation between the pleasure principle and the reality principle is impossible. The only hope is to change reality so that it conforms to the pleasure principle.

In one's unconscious, the same unconscious delineated by Freud, lie the instinctive drives toward unity, a feeling of cosmic oneness that can negate aggressions and fragmentations.

REFERENCES

Brown, N. O. *Life against Death: The Psychoanalytic Meaning of History.* Wesleyan University Press, Middletown, Conn., 1959.

Brown, N. O. Apocalypse: The place of mystery in the life of the mind. Harper's Magazine, *222:* 1961.

Brown, N. O. *Love's Body.* Random House, New York, 1966.

11

Diagnosis: Examination of the Psychiatric Patient

11.1. PSYCHIATRIC INTERVIEW

Introduction

The interview is the main tool used by the psychiatrist to gain a knowledge of the patient and the nature of his problem. An understanding of the patient in health and in sickness comes chiefly from his account of his life events, attitudes, and emotions and of the development of his symptoms. Great emphasis is placed on encouraging the patient to tell his story in his own words. The diagnosis and prognosis are based on these data and the additional information obtained from the patient's relatives, the physical examination, psychological tests, and any other special examinations. With this knowledge, treatment objectives can be formulated, and a plan of therapy that is realistic for the patient can be instituted.

Physician-Patient Relationship

The physician-patient relationship is the keystone of the practice of medicine. The relationship implies that there is an understanding and trust between the psychiatrist and his patient. With rapport, the patient feels that the psychiatrist accepts him and recognizes his assets, even though they may be outnumbered by his liabilities.

Failure of the physician to establish good rapport accounts for much of his ineffectiveness in the care of his patients. If a doctor dislikes a patient he is prone to be ineffective in dealing with him. If, on the other hand, the physician can handle the resentful patient with equanim-

ity, the patient may become loyal and cooperative.

The reaction of the patient toward the psychiatrist is apt to be a repetition of the attitude he has had toward previous physicians or toward parents, teachers, or other authoritative persons who have figured importantly in his life. Not only individual experiences but broad cultural attitudes of patients affect their reactions. It is desirable for the physician to have as much understanding as possible of the subculture of the patient.

As a protective defensive pattern, the psychiatrist may assume a habitual attitude toward all patients. Such rigidity is frequently inappropriate to the particular patient and situation. The psychiatrist must avoid side-stepping issues that are important to the patient but that he finds boring or difficult to deal with.

When the psychiatrist can convey to the patient that he is receptive to hearing about any subject, discussion is facilitated. It is then easier for the patient to talk about topics that are commonly embarrassing or disturbing.

Technique

The patient comes to the psychiatrist for expert assistance. He may have a relatively realistic attitude, or he may yearn for a parental type of guidance and expect magic from the psychiatrist. The psychiatrist may either reinforce this illusion of magic by using a suggestive type of approach or try to dissipate these beliefs through an analysis of the problem.

When the patient shows marked inhibitions, the examiner should aim to put him at ease and allow him to talk freely. If the patient has questions, they should be answered frankly. Explanations should be given in keeping with the patient's capacity to understand. If a patient does not wish to talk to the psychiatrist, it is advisable to discontinue the interview and resume contact at a later time.

If the patient is overbearing, it is likely that he is frightened. The interviewer needs to cope with this underlying fear to dissipate the over-compensatory anger. If the patient feels that the psychiatrist has empathy, he is likely to talk more freely. It is frequently possible to capitalize on the patient's sense of humor in getting him to talk more easily. Smiling with him helps him feel a sense of rapport.

In guiding the interview, the examiner should allow the patient free expression of thoughts and feelings, and he should let the patient tell his story. Gaps can be filled in later. Listening is a major tool. Minimum activity encourages the patient to expand on his thoughts and enables him to bring up relevant topics. Attention must be paid to what the patient omits as well as to what he says. Undue emphasis or exaggeration, overt signs of emotion, and changes in manner and tone of voice may give clues to a distortion.

Interviews should be conducted in privacy. Usually, they should not last longer than an hour, although with some alert, receptive patients the initial interview may be prolonged to an hour and a half. Longer subsequent interviews may also be scheduled, especially if it is not possible or appropriate to see the patient frequently. Fatigue and limited productivity indicate that the interview should be shortened.

Question Techniques

Questions can be injected when the patient gives appropriate leads. Leading questions and interpretive comments should be avoided. The perceptive examiner asks questions that will help the patient develop understanding of himself as a person. The examiner avoids influencing the patient to comply with preconceived theories.

Note-taking and Recording

It is usually desirable to record some verbatim statements. Notes should be taken as unobtrusively as possible and should not be so extensive as to interfere with the free flow of the patient's talk or the interviewer's capacity to listen to the patient. Reassurance that the notes are confidential should be given.

Psychiatrists should be alert to the reaction of the patient. If the patient objects to note-taking, it is best to discontinue it. On the other hand, many patients consider note-taking as a sign of the physician's interest and appreciation of the importance of what is being said.

When notes are not taken during the interview, the physician should take the time to record the data immediately after the patient leaves, or he might consider audio or videotape recordings, which are more complete and interfere less with spontaneous, easy communication. The patient's permission should be given before a recorder is used.

Attitudes of the Psychiatrist

The psychiatrist needs to listen without showing strong reactions, even though he may be reminded of his own disturbing problems or experiences.

However, complete passivity on the part of the psychiatrist leaves the patient feeling helpless. An authoritarian attitude on the part of the psychiatrist is uncalled for and interferes with the patient's ability to talk easily. Indeed, it is likely to constitute a traumatic repetition of a cultural or parental pattern.

Initial Interview

Since patients are usually anxious and may find it difficult to talk, the setting should be quiet, private, and free from interruption. A comfortable chair should be provided for the patient. The psychiatrist should introduce himself and invite the patient to be seated. A courteous, interested, respectful, considerate, and tolerant attitude on the part of the psychiatrist helps put the patient at ease.

The psychiatrist should avoid seeming to be in a hurry, since such an attitude inhibits the patient. A stilted, detached, or cold attitude and evidences of anxiety, anger, or indifference alienate the patient. The psychiatrist may develop empathy by trying consciously to put himself in the patient's place.

Asking the patient about the chief problems that brought him to the psychiatrist or hospital is usually the best way to start the interview. The patient can then be encouraged to tell the story of his present illness in his own words.

The conversation should be guided, rather than pursued in the manner of a prosecuting attorney. Simple explanations, reassurance, and praise may be used to obtain information when the patient needs to have his anxiety alleviated. The use of simple English, rather than technical terms, helps overcome barriers in communication. The psychiatrist should avoid being moralistic, prejudicial, dictatorial, or punitive.

The patient is frequently more able to talk about himself during the first interview than later, when he has mobilized defenses and resistances. Quiet attentiveness on the part of the physician lessens the development of anxiety, which leads to blocking and silences. When the patient does stop talking, the psychiatrist should ask a question or two; prolonged silences are apt to be disconcerting. In asking questions, the psychiatrist should repeat the patient's phrases as much as possible to minimize distortions.

There should be follow-through on the leads the patient gives. When the meaning is not clear to the psychiatrist, tactful inquiry is indicated. Intimate topics can be introduced by asking less emotionally charged questions, such as those concerning physical development. If the patient becomes unduly upset, the subject should be dropped and brought up again at a later interview. When the patient belabors a subject, the psychiatrist should change the topic.

Discussion of present problems gives the psychiatrist an opportunity to ask whether there have been similar problems in the past. This approach gives him insight into the origins of sensitivities. In the first contact with the patient, however, interpretations are usually avoided. It is better to let the patient reach his own conclusions. The psychiatrist should also avoid pointing out inconsistencies until later interviews, when rapport is well-established.

Near the end of the interview the psychiatrist may warn the patient that only a few minutes more time is available. Such a statement should be given during an appropriate pause, rather than injected in the middle of a discussion that seems highly meaningful to the patient. The psychiatrist may then ask the patient to raise questions of his own or to mention something else that he feels is particularly significant.

If no further interviews are anticipated, the psychiatrist can give a brief summary and recommendation. If further interviews are contemplated, the psychiatrist may state that there is need for more discussion, express continued interest, and suggest that the patient think over the topics covered and what he may wish to add during the next interview.

Subsequent Interviews

Subsequent interviews should continue the understanding and therapeutic approach initiated in the first contact. If there is a lag in getting started, the psychiatrist may ask the patient what has been on his mind, how he has been feeling, or what has been happening. The patient may be encouraged to expand on topics introduced during the first interview, or inquiry may be made about areas that were insufficiently covered or were not discussed at all.

To avoid giving excessive direction, the psychiatrist should permit pauses so that the patient can organize his thoughts. If the pause becomes awkward, a question can be asked about the previous statement. When the patient is having difficulty bringing out pertinent data, questions that cover his background and clarify his problems are indicated. A play-by-play account of his daily 24-hour pattern is useful.

If the patient shows some asocial behavior, the psychiatrist should continue an attitude of analyzing and understanding; he should not condone or condemn. There should be respect for his defenses and opinions. When rapport has become well-established, some challenging of the patient's ideas may be interjected.

Special Types of Interviews

Interview techniques need to be varied according to the personality reactions of the patient, the type and degree of illness, and the objectives of the interview. Various degrees of permissiveness and directiveness may be used.

Nondirective Interview

This method emphasizes minimal activity on the part of the interviewer. When there are pauses, the interviewer repeats the last words of the patient. However, extreme nondirectiveness leaves the patient feeling abandoned and is likely to create considerable anxiety. Only a limited number of well-oriented, intelligent patients appear to be suitable for a strictly nondirective approach.

Consultation Interview

The consultant psychiatrist should discuss the patient's problems with the referring physician. The consultant must preserve the relationship of the patient to his doctor, use great discretion in answering the patient's questions, and help facilitate the medical or surgical treatment. The psychiatrist should discuss his findings with the referring physician.

When it is necessary to give an opinion after a limited period of interviewing time, a directive approach is required. As much essential information as possible must be obtained. However, such interviews usually lack depth of understanding and therapeutic value.

Stress Interview

Certain patients are monotonously repetitious or show insufficient emotionality for motivation. Apathy, indifference, and emotional blunting are not conducive to a discussion of personality problems. In patients with such reactions, stimulation of emotions can be constructive. These patients may require probing, challenging, or confrontation to arouse feelings that further understanding.

Interview using Drugs

The use of drugs is of value in interviews with some patients who have difficulty in expressing themselves freely. Sodium isoamylethylbarbiturate (sodium amytal) has proved to be the most generally valuable drug. Drugs are also of value in helping to distinguish between psychogenic and structurally determined disease.

Drugs should not be used in this way with reluctant patients or those with severe physical disease. Caution should be used in those patients with paranoid reactions and in those who appear to be on the verge of a psychosis.

Interview using Hypnosis

Hypnosis may be of value in certain patients who are unable to discuss important conflicts easily. During hypnosis, the patient should be encouraged, but not aggressively forced, to talk freely about important conflicts or memories that he may have forgotten or that he finds it difficult to discuss because of feelings of anger, anxiety, or shame. Since premature confrontation is likely to create undue anxiety and resistance, he may be told that after the hyp-notic interview he will recall only those memories he consciously wishes to discuss.

Interview with Anxious Patient

Attention should be paid to what thoughts and environmental strains precipitate or increase the anxiety. When the stresses are not evident, prolonged investigation may be necessary to elucidate the sources of the emotion. Free association, dream analysis, hypnoanalysis, and narcoanalysis may result in definitive insights.

Interview with Patient Displaying Psychophysiologic Symptoms

Study of the correlations among stresses, resultant feelings, and bodily symptoms leads to an understanding of the mechanisms. Enlisting the aid of the patient as a collaborator is helpful.

Interview with Depressed Patient

Depressed patients have short attention spans and should have relatively brief interviews. Their tendency to reiterate in a destructive, self-deprecatory way may require active interruption by the psychiatrist. The possibility of suicidal preoccupation should be investigated. Many patients feel relieved to be able to talk to a confidant about such thoughts. Verbal expression may lessen the need to take action. Words of reassurance, such as a statement that many people frequently consider death as a possible solution to emotional problems, can be helpful.

The hopelessly ill or dying patient may have some degree of depression. The interviewer can ask the patient how he feels about his illness and allow him to talk about death if he wishes to do so, but should not ask prying questions of those who are not ready to discuss death.

Interview with Delusional Patient

The psychiatrist should show interest, understanding, and receptiveness, but, since he should represent to the patient a person soundly based in reality, he must not subscribe to the patient's delusions. He should neither agree with nor contradict the patient. Rather, he should try to find out more about the nature of the delusional thoughts. A skeptical attitude may help raise doubts in the patient's mind and may eventually lead him to an understanding of the delusions.

Interview with Withdrawn Patient

If a patient is absorbed with his inner world of fantasy and is unable to talk spontaneously about his feelings, the psychiatrist must be active in asking questions. He should pay close attention to the patient's verbal and nonverbal reactions and should change the subject when there is difficulty in discussing certain areas of conflict. In extreme withdrawal, there should be frequent, brief visits. When there is no response, the physician may explain in a kindly manner that he will be available when the patient is ready to communicate with him. The mute patient may be acutely aware of what is going on, so care needs to be exercised to avoid saying anything that may antagonize and further alienate him.

Interview with Manic Patient

Good rapport is not possible with a highly excited patient. The examiner should maintain a calm, receptive attitude and note the thought content carefully. Overtalkative, disturbed patients give valuable information about underlying conflicts that they are not likely to bring up when they gain better control of themselves. Sometimes, especially when the patient is treated with tolerance and understanding, an underlying depression may break through the elation.

Interviewing Relatives

It is essential to interview relatives of children, the mentally retarded, psychotic patients who cannot give a clear history, and patients with character disorders who notoriously misconstrue or misrepresent facts. Relatives of patients with other illnesses can give significant supplemental information and express points of view that add to the understanding of the problem. When a patient has marital conflicts, it is necessary to see the spouse.

The patient should usually be told about contemplated interviews with relatives before they are held and should be reassured that his confidences will not be betrayed. When the patient is strongly opposed to the psychiatrist's interviewing his relatives, the interviews should usually be deferred, conducted in the presence of the patient, or not held at all, unless the patient is a child or grossly psychotic. The psychiatrist must keep in mind that an understanding tolerance is due both his patients and their relatives.

A history obtained from relatives may have greater validity than that given by the patient. However, the patient's fantasies may be of greater significance than reality.

REFERENCES

Deutsch, F., and Murphy, W. F. *The Clinical Interview*, vol. I. International Universities Press, New York, 1955.
Gill, M., Newman, R., and Redlich, F. C. *The Initial Interview in Psychiatric Practice*. International Universities Press, New York, 1954.
MacKinnon, R. A., and Michels, R. *The Psychiatric Interview in Clinical Practice*. W. B. Saunders, Philadelphia, 1971.
Menninger, K. *A Manual for Psychiatric Case Study*. Grune & Stratton, New York, 1952.
Stevenson, I. *The Diagnostic Interview*. Harper & Row, New York, 1971.
Sullivan, H. S. *The Psychiatric Interview*. W. W. Norton, New York, 1954.

11.2. PSYCHIATRIC HISTORY AND MENTAL STATUS EXAMINATION

Introduction

A psychiatric history is assembled by formulating questions to elicit the presenting complaints and assess the severity of associated impairments in social competence and neurovegetative functioning; to establish the chronology of changes and the relation of these changes to potentially stressful experiences; to ascertain whether the patient has had experiences that caused him to be concerned with his psychological well-being in the past; to determine whether and what kind of treatment he has received in the course of the current episode and, if there is a past history of psychiatric disorder, what, if any, treatment was helpful; to obtain the patient's medical history and the family history of both psychiatric and nonpsychiatric illnesses; to elicit the patient's personal history; and to explore his attitude, his reactions to various events, and his style of handling stresses.

The patient's mental status should be an evaluative statement, based entirely on the observations made and the responses given to specific questions or tests in the course of the examination, and should not be contaminated with historical data.

Interpretation of the information gathered and the observations made should be postponed until all the necessary evidence has been obtained and the clinician is ready to formulate the diagnosis and make recommendations. Both the clinical history and the mental status examination have time-limited validity. The length and the focus of the interview vary, but it must be sufficiently broad to document all actions that the clinician may take or refrain from taking. The clinician is always responsible for assessing the patient's level of anxiety, social competence, and impulse control.

Psychiatric History

The order in which the various areas are covered depends on the presenting complaint, the patient's way of relating to the clinician, and the clinician's own preferences. Furthermore, the type of questions the clinician asks will change as epidemiological studies and treatment trials provide new information on the natural history of illnesses and their response to treatment.

The history is usually elicited from the patient, his relatives, and his close friends. In exceptional circumstances, persons who have had an opportunity to observe the patient at work may also be questioned. Data obtained from collateral sources should be recorded separately, clearly indicating the relationship of the informant to the patient, and should be judged for reliability by the clinician.

The examiner must make sure that certain basic identifying data about the patient have been collected before the first meeting ends. Such information should include the patient's name, age, place of birth, religion, marital status, education, occupation, ethnic background, and home address, as well as the name, address, and telephone number of the patient's family physician and of his nearest relative or friend.

Although history taking usually begins with the patient's account of his problem, it is best to explore first the circumstances of the referral whenever the clinician knows or the patient's behavior suggests that he had been inadequately prepared for the examination.

The presenting complaints should be re-corded in the patient's own words, even when he denies having any problems at all or makes illogical or bizarre statements. The examiner must establish the last time the patient felt well or reasonably well, the length of time he has experienced his current complaints, whether these complaints have changed in character or severity since they began, and what kind of relationship exists between the patient's complaints and major changes in his life situation.

The inquiry should include an assessment of the patient's social competence and neurovegetative functioning. It is advisable to inquire whether the patient is currently under care for any nonpsychiatric illness and, if so, when he was last seen by his physician, what treatment he is receiving, and whether the state of his general health is at present stable, improving, or worsening.

Once the characteristics of the present illness have been delineated, the patient should be asked whether he had a psychological disorder in the past and whether the current episode is similar to one he experienced previously. The frequency and duration of past episodes, the age at which the patient was first seen in consultation for a psychological disorder, the treatment he received, the setting in which it took place, and, when there is a history of multiple episodes, the longest time interval the patient got along without psychiatric treatment—all provide important clues for the diagnosis and for future management. The patient should also be asked what information he was given about his condition in the past.

Family History

The family history of psychiatric and nonpsychiatric conditions may be obtained by asking first if any friend or family member has or has had a similar condition. Questions about family history should cover any episode of attempted or completed suicide, mood disorder, psychiatric treatment and hospitalization, drinking problems, delinquency, mental retardation, peculiar or eccentric behavior, and history of any illness, psychiatric or nonpsychiatric, that has occurred in more than one member of the family.

Medical History

The extent to which details of early development and childhood illnesses are dealt with varies according to the patient's problem and age and the availability of collateral sources of information or access to medical records. In every instance, the patient's general health history should include a thorough review of his drug intake.

If the patient is of adolescent age or younger, the history of his early development, including the difficulties the patient's mother may have had with pregnancy and delivery, is very important. Medical and developmental data should include early sleep and feeding patterns, how the patient responded to physical discomfort or other stresses, and the approximate time when major developmental landmarks were completed. Information should also be obtained about such indices of subtle neurological dysfunctioning as choreiform movements and other peculiar or stereotyped activities, persistent somatic complaints, speech defects, and the quality of fine motor coordination.

Next, the inquiry should focus on illnesses and operations since infancy and should include the age at which they occurred, their complications and outcomes, and the patient's reactions to these events. The patient should be asked specifically whether he ever had a head injury, lost consciousness, or had symptoms indicative of central nervous dysfunctioning.

Questions about the patient's drug-taking habits may begin by asking him whether he is presently taking any medication and, if so, what kind and how often; whether he has ever had any allergic or idiosyncratic reaction to a drug and, if so, to what kind of drug and what kind of reaction he experienced; whether he has ever taken more medication than was ordered by the prescribing physician; whether he is currently using sedatives, sleeping pills, antianxiety drugs, alcohol, narcotics, pain killers, stimulants, marijuana, hashish and, if so, how frequently and for what reason; whether he ever experienced any symptoms of withdrawal that were severe enough to require medical attention; whether he was ever treated for acute intoxication; and whether he is a multiple-drug user.

Family Environment

The questioning should begin by asking him to describe, in some detail, the environment he was reared in. Were there any major changes or stresses in the family environment? What were the characteristics of the paternal and maternal supervision and discipline? The attitudes of the parents should be explored in relation to the various developmental stages and life events. (See Figure 1.)

It is also important to determine the patient's view of his siblings and to explore whether the patient believes the parents' attitudes toward his siblings and other members of the family were different from their attitudes toward him. The patient's socialization patterns should be delineated in relation to the family environment to establish whether the patient's increasing independence was fostered or hindered by those who cared for him. Questions about the patient's attitude and ability to make and keep friends and handle kindergarten and school experiences are important, since separation anxiety in childhood is one of the chronic anxieties in adults. Equally important and far easier to verify is the patient's school performance. When the records show that the patient did not perform adequately in school, it is

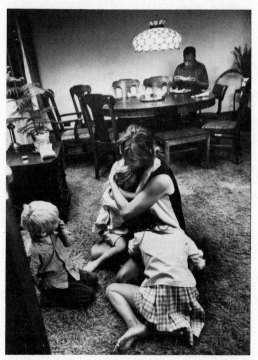

FIGURE 1. Discussion of a patient's relationship to his parents and siblings is a fundamental part of a psychiatric history. And only thereby can the appropriate dynamics be validated. (Courtesy of Abigal Heiman for Magnum Photos, Inc.)

always worthwhile to investigate whether the patient's siblings had similar difficulties.

One should inquire whether the patient ever became a disciplinary problem in school and, if so, for what reason; if the patient showed evidence of antisocial behavior, did he tend to have any accomplices; did he choose playmates who were also unruly or in trouble; and was there any history of antisocial behavior in the siblings or other members of the family?

During adolescence, attitudes toward the family and peers undergo profound changes. Intimate friendships and dating patterns tend to develop, and assertive behavior is practiced on a much larger scale than before. The nature and the extent of the rebelliousness should be carefully delineated. Asking the patient to describe his views and attitudes about adolescent friendships and dating patterns provides a convenient starting point to trace the patient's sexual history and to get an idea of how he handled intimate relationships.

If the patient is married, what was the duration of his courtship; what attracted him to his mate; what was the age of both partners at the time of the marriage; what was the reaction of the respective families to the marriage? What, if any, are some of the major areas of dissatisfaction in the marriage? Has the patient or his spouse engaged in extramarital affairs, and, if so, how were they handled? If the patient has children, what is his relationship to them; do any of them present special problems or stresses for the marriage, and, if so, what are these problems? If the patient is divorced or separated , how many years did the marriage last, and what were the major areas of dissatisfaction that caused the split?

Even if there is nothing in the patient's report to suggest sexual problems, the patient should be tactfully questioned about his sexual preferences, about the possibility of sexual problems; and about how these difficulties affect his relationship with his partner.

A female patient should be asked about her menstrual periods, pregnancies, abortions or miscarriages, and adoptions.

Occupational History

If the patient is still a student, is he currently attending school? If not, when did he drop out, and at what point in his scholastic career did this occur and for what reason? Is the patient's level of education in harmony with his abilities, ambitions, and life goals?

Was the patient ever in military service or in a paramilitary service, and, if so, was there ever any disciplinary action taken against him; what type of discharge did he receive?

What kind of work has the patient done since leaving school? Are the patient's earning capacities and duties and responsibilities the same as they were when he was feeling well? If the patient is no longer employed, when was the last time he held a job, and what was the longest time he ever kept a job? If the patient is a housewife, did her effectiveness in attending to her household tasks change and, if so, in what way?

Who handles the financial responsibilities in the patient's household? Was the patient ever bankrupt? Does he gamble frequently? Is he receiving any financial help and, if so, from whom?

What are the patient's church, community, and leisure time activities? Does he belong to clubs and other organizations and, if so, did his participation in these activities change recently?

Personality Style

The clinician must attempt to obtain enough information to determine whether the behavior patterns displayed represent a lifelong maladaptive style or symptoms of an intercurrent medical or psychiatric illness and what the patient's current and customary responses to stress are.

A few questions asked about the patient's usual way of feeling or behaving will give sufficient information about his level of anxiety, tendencies for phobias and obsessional thinking, social immaturity or excessive dependency needs, aloofness and withdrawal, proneness to cyclothymia, suspiciousness, or outright paranoid attitude. The inquiry should then proceed to determine how the patient handles difficult, frustrating, or otherwise unpleasant events, giving the clinician an opportunity to explore his proneness to suicide or aggressive and antisocial behaviors.

Current Living Conditions

Does the patient live with anyone, or, if he lives alone, does he have any close friends or relatives he can turn to in times of distress?

What is the emotional climate under which the patient is living? Are the significant others in his life able to tell when the patient is not feeling well? Do people close to him approve or disapprove of the patient's being in treatment for psychological problems?

Mental Status Examination

The mental status is a record of current findings. It includes the description of the patient's appearance, general behavior, motor activity, speech, alertness, mood, cognitive functioning, the views he holds about his condition, and the attitudes he displayed throughout the examination, as well as the reactions evoked by the patient in the examiner.

Appearance

The examiner's over-all impression of the patient should be followed by a description of the patient's dress and grooming, unusual features in his physical appearance, expression, and eye contact.

Motor Activity

Is the patient ambulatory? Does he move around restlessly, keep still most of the time, or fluctuate? Movements may be graceful or clumsy. He may appear to have an unusual gait or impairment. He may grimace, have tics, or display waxy flexibility.

Speech Activity

The patient's speech may be unusually fast or slow. There may be sudden interruptions in the flow of speech. The volume of the patient's voice may be loud or scarcely audible. Intonation and modulation may be preserved or altered. His speech may be unusually vivacious, monotonous, or affected. He may have word-finding difficulty or a speech defect. Impairments in hearing or vision may be present or suspected.

If the patient communicates by gestures but does not speak, the clinician must resort to direct examination to determine whether the lack of verbal communication is an isolated event or merely one aspect of an over-all pattern of diminished responsiveness.

Mood

The patient may express feelings of sadness or elation spontaneously or in response to specific questions, or his affect may be so constricted that it remains unaltered or flat, no matter what topics are discussed. The patient's mood may be constant or may fluctuate between elation and sadness throughout the interview. His mood may be appropriate or inappropriate.

Alertness

The patient may be slightly drowsy or somnolent, or he may be watchful or even hyperalert. He may be intermittently alert and drowsy throughout the examination. Changes in alertness are always associated with inattention.

Thought

The patient's thinking may be slowed down or accelerated, resulting in hesitation or blocking. The patient's thinking may be pedantic or incoherent. The content of the patient's thought may include realistic concerns as well as exaggerated ones to an actual life event or concerns that have no discernible connection to reality.

When the patient is invited to describe his nervousness, he may also report somatic symptoms or display observable manifestations of discomfort. The patient may also report having unrealistic fears or phobias, he may show evidence of hypochondriasis, or he may be troubled by obsessive ideas. Compelling ideas may reach delusional proportions.

Perception

Distorted or otherwise altered perceptions may be experienced in reference to self or the environment. Illusions or hallucinations may also be perceived and can occur in any one of the sensory modalities. When the patient does not report abnormal perceptions, but, in the clinician's judgment, his general demeanor suggests that he is having hallucinatory experiences, a notation to this effect should be made.

Intellectual Functioning

The clinician should conduct a formal examination to assess the patient's general fund of knowledge, orientation, memory, ability to perform simple mathematical operations, and capacity for abstract thinking. Questions and tests must be suitable for patients with little or no schooling or with modest intellectual endowment, as well as for patients whose intellectual achievements are considerable.

General fund of knowledge may be determined by asking the patient to name as many items as he can recall in each of the following categories: colors, animals, fruits, towns. Then the following four questions are asked: What are the colors in the American flag? What is a thermometer? How far is it from Los Angeles to New York? What are the names of three countries in the Middle East?

A generally accepted test for immediate recall is the digit span test, which is administered by asking the patient first to repeat three digits after the examiner, then to give them in reverse order; the same operation is then repeated with four, five, six, and seven digits. Recent memory is assessed by asking the patient to describe how he spent the last 24 hours or what he had to eat for his last meal. Memory for the remote past can be evaluated by inquiring about important dates in the patient's life. The answers must be verifiable.

Another simple and practical way of evaluating orientation and memory is to administer Kahn's 10-question mental status examination: (1) What is the name of this place? (2) Where is it located (address)? (3) What day of the week is it? (4) What is the month now? (5) What is the year? (6) How old are you? (7) When were you born (month)? (8) When were you born (year)? (9) Who is the President of the United States? (10) Who was the President before him?

A brief test for calculation consists of asking the patient to subtract 7 from 100; he is asked to repeat this operation until six successive subtractions are obtained.

The capacity for abstract thinking—that is, the ability to make valid generalizations—can be tested by asking the patient to interpret a common proverb. A simpler and probably more reliable test for abstract thinking is an abbreviated object-sorting test, consisting of four toy vehicles, a set of four toy utensils, and four pieces of toy furniture. The patient is asked to group them according to their purpose and utility. The inability to create three distinct sorts is indicative of impaired ability for abstract thinking.

Attitude

The patient may be neutral, displaying little or no feeling in telling his story or in replying to questions, or he may be fearful, perplexed, hostile, evasive, sarcastic, ingratiating, dramatic, seductive, or completely unresponsive, but rarely is any one of these attitudes consist-

ently displayed. The clinician should, therefore, note whether the patient became more comfortable as the interview went on (or vice versa) and whether any of the changes in attitude occurred in relation to specific circumstances or topics discussed.

The patient may regard his condition as psychiatric or nonpsychiatric, he may attribute his condition to a certain cause or causes, or he may fail to acknowledge that he is ill. He may anticipate improvement in his condition or view it as a persistent handicap that will profoundly affect his long-term life plans.

Examiner's Reaction

The clinician may find the patient likable, or he may be angered, irritated, anxious, or frustrated by the patient. If the examiner feels the patient is expressing underlying hostility but displays no overt antagonism, it should be so recorded, along with changes in the clinician's reactions toward the patient during the interview.

This section of the examination report should be concluded with a statement expressing the clinician's judgment regarding the accuracy of the information obtained and pointing out any inconsistencies.

Summary and Recommendations

The clinician should critically examine and summarize his findings. He should state the estimated duration of the current episode and whether in his judgment the patient has improved or deteriorated since he first became ill; describe the course of the illness; summarize all relevant findings; state whether further diagnostic procedures are recommended or additional information is necessary and, if so, from what source.

When the clinician places the patient's illness in a given diagnostic category, he may list all the evidence gathered from the history and examination that is consistent with such a diagnosis, as well as all the evidence that is inconsistent with such a formulation or that points to the necessity of more than one diagnosis. Alternatively, the clinician may choose to defer the diagnosis until he is in a position to obtain and interpret the results of additional studies ordered, or he may conclude that he found no evidence of any psychiatric disorder. The diagnosis should be recorded in accordance with the code provided by the second edition of the American Psychiatric Association's *Diagnostic and Statistical Manual of Mental Disorders* (DSM-II).

In formulating the treatment plan, the clinician should note whether the patient requires psychiatric treatment at this time and, if so, what problems and target symptoms the treatment is aimed at; what kind of treatment or combination of treatments the patient should receive; and what treatment setting seems most appropriate. If hospitalization is recommended, the clinician should specify the reasons for hospitalization, the type of hospitalization indicated, the urgency with which the patient has to be hospitalized, and the anticipated duration of inpatient care.

The clinician should estimate the immediate and long-term prognosis of the patient's illness and the estimated length of treatment.

If either the patient or his family is unwilling to accept the recommendations for treatment and the clinician feels that the refusal of his recommendations may have serious consequences, the patient or a parent or guardian should be invited to sign a statement that the treatment recommended was refused.

REFERENCES

Isaacs, B., and Kennie, A. T. The set test as an aid to the detection of dementia in old people. Br. J. Psychiatry, *123:* 467, 1973.

Kahn, R. L., Goldfarb, A. I., Pollack, M., and Gerber, I. E. The relationship of mental and physical status in institutionalized aged persons. Am. J. Psychiatry, *117:* 120, 1960.

Kupfer, D. J., and Detre, T. P. Development and application of the KDS^{tm}-1 in inpatient and outpatient settings. Psychol. Rep., *29:* 607, 1971.

London University Institute of Psychiatry. *Notes on Eliciting and Recording Clinical Information.* Oxford University Press, London, 1973.

Talland, G. A. *Deranged Memory: A Psychonomic Study of the Amnesic Syndrome.* Academic Press, New York, 1965.

Tumulty, P. A. What is a clinician and what does he do? N. Engl. J. Med., *283:* 20, 1970.

Weed, L. L. Medical records that guide and teach. N. Engl. J. Med., *278:* 593, 1968.

Wogan, M., Amdur, M. J., Kupfer, D. J., and Detre, T. P. The KDS-1: Validity, reliability and independence among symptom clusters for clinical and normal samples. Psychol. Rep., *32:* 503, 1973.

11.3.   PSYCHIATRIC REPORT

I. Psychiatric history

A. *Preliminary identification:* name, age, marital status, sex, occupation, language if other than English, race, nationality, and religion insofar as they are pertinent, previous admissions to a hospital for the same or a different condition

B. *Chief complaint:* exactly why the patient came to the psychiatrist, preferably in the patient's own words; if this information does not come from the patient, note who supplied it

C. *Personal identification:* brief, nontechnical description of the patient's appearance and behavior as a novelist might write it

D. *History of present illness:* background and development of the symptoms or behavioral changes that culminated in the patient's seeking assistance; patient's life circumstances at the time of onset; personality when well; how illness has affected life activities and personal relations—changes in character, interests, mood, attitudes toward others, dress, habits, level of tension, irritability, activity, attention, concentration, memory, or speech; psychophysiological symptoms—nature and details of dysfunction, location, intensity, fluctuation, relationship between physical and psychic symptoms; extent to which illness serves some additional purpose for the patient in his dealings with others—his secondary gain

E. *Previous illness*

　1. Emotional or mental disturbances: extent of incapacity, type of treatment, names of hospitals, length of illness, effect of treatment

　2. Psychophysiologic disorders: hay fever, rheumatoid arthritis, ulcerative colitis, asthma, hyperhyroidism, gastrointestinal upsets, recurrent colds, skin conditions

　3. Medical conditions, following the customary medical review of system, if necessary; lues, use of alcohol or drugs

4. Neurological disorders: history of craniocerebral trauma, convulsions, or tumors
F. *Past personal history:* history (anamnesis) of the patient's life from infancy to the present to the extent it can be recalled; gaps in the history as spontaneously related by the patient, emotions associated with these life periods—painful, stressful conflictual
1. Early childhood (through age 10)
    a. Nature of mother's pregnancy and delivery: length of pregnancy, spontaneity and normality of delivery, birth trauma
    b. Circumstances of teething, walking, talking, etc.; delays or abnormalities associated with these activities
    c. Feeding habits: breast-fed or bottle-fed, eating problems
    d. Toilet training: age, attitude of parents, feelings about it
    e. Symptoms of behavior problems: thumb sucking, temper tantrums, tics, head bumping, night terrors, fears, bed wetting or bed soiling, nail biting
    f. Personality as a child: shy, restless, overactive, withdrawn, studious, outgoing, timid, athletic, friendly
    g. Early or recurrent dreams or fantasies
    h. Early school history: feelings about going to school, early adjustment, scholarship
2. Later childhood (from prepuberty through adolescence)
    a. Social relationships: attitudes toward siblings and playmates, number and closeness of friends, leader or follower, social popularity
    b. School history: how far he went, adjustment to school, relationships with teachers, favorite studies or interests, particular abilities or assets, extracurricular activities, sports, hobbies, relationship of problems or symptoms to any school period
    c. Particular adolescent emotional or physical problems: running away, delinquency, smoking, drug taking, overweight, feeling of inferiority
    d. Psychosexual history
        i. Early curiosity, infantile masturbation, sex play
        ii. Acquiring of sexual knowledge, attitude of parents to sex
        iii. Onset of menses, feelings about it, prepared or not, subsequent feelings about menstruation
        v. Adolescent sexual activity: crushes, parties, petting, masturbation, wet dreams, attitudes toward them
        v. Attitudes toward opposite sex: timid, shy, aggressive, need to impress, seductive, sexual conquests, anxiety
        vi. Sexual practices: sexual problems, homosexual experiences, perversions
    e. Religious background: strict, liberal; mixed (possible conflicts), relationship of background to current religious practices
3. Adulthood
    a. Occupational history: choice of occupation training, ambitions, conflicts, relations with bosses and coworkers; how many jobs and for how long, change to jobs of lesser status, current job, feelings about it
    b. Social activity; does he have friends, is he withdrawn or socializing well; kind of social, intellectual, and physical interests; relationships with opposite sex
    c. Adult sexuality
        i. Premarital sexual relationships
        ii. Feelings about marriage, sexual adjustment, compatibility
        iii. Sexual symptoms: frigidity, impotence
        iv. Attitudes toward pregnancy and having children, contraceptive practices and feelings about them
        v. Sexual perversions
    d. Military history: general adjustment, combat, injuries, referral to psychiatrists, veteran status, draft status

G. *Family history:* elicited from patient and from someone else; ethnic, national, and religious traditions; other people in the home; descriptions of them—personality and intelligence—and what has become of them since patient's childhood; descriptions of different households lived in; present relationships between patient and those who were in family; role of illness in the family; history of mental illness

H. *Martial history:* common-law marriages, legal marriages, length of courtship, age at marriage, family planning and contraception, names and ages of children, attitudes toward children, problems of any family members, housing difficulties if important to the marriage

I. *Current social situation:* where does patient live—slum, project, furnished room, high crime neighborhood, middle-class neighborhood; is home crowded; privacy of family members from each other and from other families; sources of family income; difficulties in obtaining it; public assistance, if any; attitude about it; will patient lose job or apartment by remaining in the hospital; who is caring for children

II. **Mental status:** sum total of the examiner's observations and impressions derived from the initial interviews

A. *General description*
1. Appearance: posture, gait, bearing, cloths, grooming, hair, nails; healthy, sickly, angry, frightened, apathetic, perplexed, contemptuous, ill at ease, poised, old-looking, young-looking, effeminate, masculine
2. Behavior and psychomotor activity; mannerisms, tics, gestures, twitches, stereotypes, picking, touching examiner, echopraxia, clumsy, agile, limp, rigid, retarded, combative, waxy
3. Attitude toward examiner: cooperative, attentive, interested, frank, seductive, defensive, hostile, playful, ingratiating, evasive, guarded

B. *Speech:* rapid, slow, under pressure, hesitant, emotional, monotonous, loud, whispered, slurred, mumbled, stuttering, echolalia; intensity, pitch, ease, spontaneity, productivity, relevance, manner, reaction time, vocabulary

C. *State of consciousness* (note fluctuations)
1. Alertness, clouding of consciousness, responsiveness to environment; does patient respond to examiner, recognize him, understand him, pay attention to what is going on orientation
2. Ability to carry out orders—first simple ones, then complex: putting a specific finger on the nose, then touching another part of the body with the other hand simultaneously

D. *Affective or emotional state*
1. Mood: how does patient say he feels; depth, intensity, duration, and fluctuations of mood—depressed, despairing, irritable, panicky, terrified, angry, enraged, elated, ecstatic, empty, guilty, unreal, awed, futile, self-contemptuous
2. Emotional expression: how examiner evaluates patient's affect—manic, hypomanic, grandiose, agitated, flat, labile
3. Appropriateness: is the emotional expression appropriate to the content, to the culture, to what patient is thinking

E. *Anxiety level*
1. Patient's description: are anxieties generalized and nonspecific (free-floating) or specifically related to particular situations, activities, or objects; how are anxieties handled—avoidance, repetition of feared situation, drugs, use of other activities for distraction
2. Observations: signs of anxiety—moist hand, perspiring forehead, restlessness, tense posture, strained voice, wide eyes; shifts in level of anxiety during interview, abrupt changes of topic

F. *Stream of thought:* quotations from patient if illuminating

1. Productivity: overabundance of ideas, paucity of ideas, flight of ideas, rapid thinking, slow thinking, hesitant thinking; does patient speak spontaneously or only when questions are asked
2. Nature of thoughts: do answers really answer questions; are they relevant or irrelevant; is there a lack of cause-and-effect relationships in patient's explanations; are statements illogical, tangential, circumstantial, rambling, evasive
3. Associative processes: words—coherent or incoherent, incomprehensible, clang associations, neologisms; is patient distractible; is there blocking

G. *Content of thought*
   1. Preoccupations: about the illness, environmental problems; obsessions, compulsions, phobias; obsessions about suicide, homicide, hypochondriacal symptoms, specific antisocial urges
   2. Thought disturbances: ideation and perceptions, patient's attitudes toward them, how they affect his life, compelling force
      a. Delusions: if persecutory, are they systematized, isolated, diffuse, with pervasive suspiciousness
      b. Ideas of reference and ideas of influence
      c. Depersonalization and derealization
   3. Perceptual disturbance: hallucinations and illusions; does patient hear voices or see visions; are there tactile hallucinations

H. *Orientation*
   1. Time: does patient identify the date correctly; can he approximate date, time of day; if he is in a hospital, does he know how long he has been there
   2. Place: does patient know where he is
   3. Person: does patient know who he is; does he know who examiner is

I. *Memory:* impairment, attitude toward impairment, efforts made to cope with impairment—denial, confabulation, catastrophic reaction, circumstantiality
   1. Remote memory: childhood data, important events known to have occurred when patient was younger or free of illness, personal matters, neutral material
   2. Recent past memory: the past few months
   3. Recent memory: the past few days; what did patient do yesterday, the day before; what did he have for breakfast, lunch, dinner
   4. Immediate retention and recall: ability to repeat six figures after examiner dictates them—first forward, then backward, then after a few minutes interruption; other test questions; did same questions, if repeated, call forth different answers at different times

J. *Information and intelligence:* counting, calculation, general knowledge; if patient uses the subway, where is the station, how far is it; subtract 7 from 100 and keep subtracting 7's

K. *Concentration:* if patient cannot subtract 7's can he do easier tasks—4 times 9, 5 times 4

L. *Abstract thinking:* similarities, differences, absurdities, meanings of simple proverbs, such as, "A rolling stone gathers no moss"; answers may be concrete—giving specific examples to illustrate the meaning—or abstract—giving generalized explanation; appropriateness

M. *Judgment*
   1. Social behavior that is harmful to the patient and contrary to accepted behavior in the culture; gross—hitting a policeman, going nude in the street—or a matter of opinion
   2. Test judgment: patient's prediction of what he would do in imaginary situations—what he would do if he found an unstamped, addressed letter in the street

N. *Insight:* degree of awareness and understanding the patient has that he is ill
   1. Complete denial of illness
   2. Slight awareness of being sick and needing help but denying it at the same time

  3. Awareness of being sick but blaming it on others, on external factors, on organic factors
  4. Awareness that illness is due to something unknown in himself
  5. Intellectual insight: admission that he is ill and that his symptoms or failures in social adjustment are due to his own particular irrational feelings of disturbances, without applying this knowledge to future experience
  6. True emotional insight: emotional awareness of the motives and feelings within himself, of underlying symptoms, leading to change in personality and future behavior

 O. *Dreams, fantasies, and value systems*
  1. Dreams: prominent ones, if patient will tell them; nightmares
  2. Fantasies: recurrent, favorite, or unshakable daydreams; hypnagogic phenomena
  3. Value systems: children may be a burden or a joy; work may be seen as a necessary evil, an avoidable chore, or an opportunity for satisfaction; friends may be people to exploit, people to share with, or potential enemies

 P. *Other tests as indicated:* reading comprehension, handwriting, tests for aphasia
 Q. *Reliability:* estimate of examiner's impression of patient's veracity or ability to report his situation accurately

III. **Further diagnostic studies**
 A. *Physical examination*
 B. *Additional psychiatric diagnostic interviews*
 C. *Interviews with family members, friends, or neighbors,* by social worker
 D. *Psychological tests* by psychologist
 E. *Specialized tests:* electroencephalogram, laboratory tests, test of other medical conditions

IV. **Summary of positive findings:** mental symptoms, laboratory findings, psychological tests results, if available; drugs patient has been taking, including dosage and duration of intake

 V. **Diagnosis:** diagnostic classification according to the American Psychiatric Association's *Diagnostic and Statistical Manual of Mental Disorders*—nomenclature, classification number, severity, chronicity; supplemental diagnosis, diagnoses to be ruled out

VI. **Prognosis:** opinion as to the probable future course, extent, and outcome of the illness

VII. **Psychodynamic formulation:** causes of the patient's psychodynamic breakdown—influences in the patient's life that contributed to his present illness; environmental, genetic, and personality factors relevant in determining his symptoms

VIII. **Recommendations:** appropriate treatment, if any, to be followed

---

11.4.   PSYCHOLOGICIAL TESTING OF INTELLIGENCE AND PERSONALITY

Introduction

Standard psychological tests provide a fairly objective means for comparing a relatively controlled sample of the patient's behavior with available normative data representative of a larger reference group. Adequate standardization of tests has probably been achieved most extensively in the area of intelligence testing. Related to the standardization of any test are the available data that presumably demonstrate whether the test is both valid and reliable: Does the test measure what it purports to measure? Does the test yield consistent results over time with different examiners? Consistencies and inconsistencies between tests are helpful in establishing the level of confidence that can be held about any specific inference and in relating surface behavioral characteristics to their motivational origins.

In the test battery a broad range of stimuli on the continuum of structure-ambiguity is available for eliciting a patient's response samples. In contrast to specific or highly structured questions, such as those on an intelligence test, the projective techniques presumably have no right or wrong answers. The person being tested must give meaning to (interpret) the stimulus in accordance with his own inner needs, drives, abilities, defenses, impulses—in short, according to the dictates of his own personality. A basic assumption is that persons who show a certain kind of disturbance in a test situation of a given degree of ambiguity will in all probability show a similar reaction in a social situation of equal ambiguity. The test battery most widely used in clinical practice for evaluation of psychiatric patients generally includes an individual intelligence test, an association technique, a story-telling test, completion methods, and graphomotor tests.

Referral Purposes

Intellectual evaluation can best be accomplished by an individual intelligence test, such as the Wechsler Adult Intelligence Scale. Problems of differential diagnosis can best be answered by recourse to a full test battery in which relationships among tests may offer significant insight into the patient's total pattern of functioning.

Deficiencies that accompany organic brain malfunctioning are frequently highlighted by means of psychological tests. On occasion, they are most apparent in areas ordinarily conceptualized as intellectual. In the other instances, they are most apparent in graphomotor productions. Brain malfunctioning may often be apparent in responses to the projective techniques. Some psychologists have devised special tests and procedures solely for the purpose of detecting brain damage.

Elucidation of personality dynamics usually requires recourse to techniques that vary in the degree to which their stimulus value is obvious and clear. Where weak reality-testing abilities are revealed, supportive treatment is generally considered more advisable than intensive analytical treatments that may precipitate further decompensation of already weakened defenses.

Psychological tests may be helpful in answering specific questions related to a particular patient, such as whether there is evidence of suicidal ideation or whether the patient is likely to be dangerous or homicidal. And many specialized tests are designed to evaluate such issues as educational fitness, occupational interest, and vocational aptitudes.

Classification of Tests

The usual distinctions involve whether the test was devised to evaluate intellectual and cognitive abilities or those other modes of responding assumed to be related to nonintellectual factors, such as personality. However, intellectual functioning may be intimately related to the psychodynamics of personality functioning.

Another traditional distinction involves whether the test is individually administered or given simultaneously to a group. Individual testing has the advantage of providing opportunity for the examiner to evaluate rapport and motivational factors as well as to observe and record the patient's behavior during testing. Careful timing of responses is also possible. Group tests, on the other hand, are usually more easily administered. They have generally been devised for easier scoring and more objective interpretation. But some tests can be administered in either individual or group forms.

Objective personality tests are typically pencil-and-paper tests based on items and questions having obvious meaning and the advantage of yielding numerical scores and profiles easily subjected to mathematical or statistical analysis. Projective tests, on the other hand, present stimuli whose meaning is not immediately obvious—that is, some degree of ambiguity forces the subject to project his own needs into or onto an amorphous, somewhat unstructured situation. Interpretation of the elicited free association data usually requires experience and knowledge of personality theory on the part of the examiner. The philosophy and the interpretative approach of the examiner are important in determining whether the given tool is used as an objective test, a projective technique, or something alternating between them.

Intelligence Testing

General Background

Tremendous individual differences exist in people's ability to assimilate factual knowledge, to recall either recent or remote events, to reason logically, to manipulate concepts (either numbers or words), to translate the abstract to the literal or the literal to the abstract, to analyze and synthesize forms, and, in short, to deal meaningfully and accurately with problems and priorities deemed important in a particular setting.

Present attempts to measure and evaluate intelligence stem from the work of Binet, a French psychologist, and Simon, a French psychiatrist, who were attempting to deal with the practical problem of assessing mental retardates for levels of educability at the turn of the century. A significant breakthrough in mental measurement was achieved through their development of the concept of mental age, representing levels of achievement in children that are found to be characteristic of each age level. Shortly thereafter, W. L. Stern introduced the concept of the I.Q. as the ratio between mental age and chronological age $\times$ 100 (I.Q. $= \frac{M.A.}{C.A.} \times$ 100). When mental age continues to increase in proportion to chronological age, the I.Q. provides an index of relative brightness that can be used to compare children of different ages. As applied to the measurement of adult intelligence, however, the mental age concept becomes less relevant. Proportional increases in developmental intellectual skills decelerate rapidly after the age of 15 years. David Wechsler, in the development of his scales for children and adults, has eliminated dependence on assumptions regarding the relationship between chronological age and mental age by generating separate age norms for the various age groups up to the age of 65, rather than deriving adult norms by a process of statistical extrapolation.

The I.Q., as measured by most intelligence tests, is an interpretation or classification of a total test score in relation to norms established by some group. For this and other reasons, the I.Q. can be misleading, since it is an average of different abilities or levels of ability that themselves may show great variability.

The I.Q. is a measure of present functioning ability, not necessarily of future potential. Although under ordinary circumstances the I.Q. has a surprising stability through life, there is no absolute certainty about its predictive properties. A person's I.Q. must be examined in the light of his past experiences as well as his future opportunities.

The I.Q. itself conveys no meaning as to the origins of its reflected capacities, whether genetic (innate) or environmental. The most useful intelligence test must measure a variety of skills and abilities, including verbal and performance, early learned and recently learned, timed and untimed, culture-free and culture-bound. No intelligence test is totally culture-free, although tests do differ significantly in degree.

Wechsler Adult Intelligence Scale (WAIS)

The WAIS is the best standarized and most widely used intelligence test in clinical practice today. The WAIS comprises 11 subtests (yielding a full-scale I.Q.), including six verbal subtests and five performance subtests (yielding a separate verbal I.Q. and performance I.Q.). Subtest raw scores are weighted so as to be comparable to each other. Intelligence levels are determined statistically, based on the assumption that intellectual abilities are distributed in terms of a normal-curve distribution throughout the population.

The subtests are present in the following order: information, comprehension, arithmetic, similarities, memory for digits, vocabulary, digit symbol, picture completion, block design, picture arrangement, and object assembly. Raw subtest scores are prorated into subtest scores. Verbal and performance I.Q.s, as well as the full-scale I.Q., are determined by the use of separate tables for each of the seven age groups from 16 to 64 years. Variability in functioning is thus revealed through discrepancies between verbal and performance I.Q.s, between scaled subtest scores (intertest variability), and within any subtest, since items in each test are arranged in order of difficulty (intratest variability).

Personality Testing

The tests in the psychological test battery used in most psychiatric settings are usually chosen in terms of how well they serve the purpose of a psychodynamic formulation of personality functioning. Basic to this selection is the assumption that behavior is often motivated by forces that vary as to their degree of accessibility to awareness and behavioral expression. The need for a battery of tests arises not because of the possible invalidity of any single test but because different tests detect different levels of functioning and because the relationships between tests reflect the person's multilevel system of functioning.

Rorschach Test

Surveys over the years suggest that the Rorschach test is the most frequently used individual test, with the possible exception of the WAIS, in clinical settings throughout the United States. The Rorschach was devised by Hermann Rorschach (see Figure 1), a Swiss psychiatrist, who began around 1910 to experiment with ambiguous inkblots (Figure 2). The Rorschach is a standard set of 10 inkblots that serve as the stimuli for associations. In the standard series the blots, administered in order, are reproduced on cards 7 by 9 ½ inches and are numbered from I to X. Five of the blots are in black and white; the remainder include other colors. A verbatim record is kept of the patient's responses, along with initial reaction times and total time spent on each card. After completion of what is called the free association, an inquiry is then conducted by the examiner to determine important aspects of each response that will be crucial to its scoring.

Scoring of responses converts the important aspects of each response into a symbol system related to the following variables: location areas, determinants, and content areas. The location is scored in terms of what portion of the blot was used as the basis for the response. Grossest differentiations involve whether it was the whole blot (W), a large, usual detail of the blot (D), a small detail of the blot (d), or the white space (S). The determinants of each

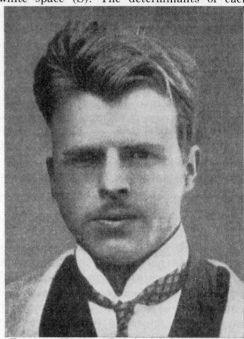

FIGURE 1. Hermann Rorschach. (Courtesy of New York Academy of Medicine.)

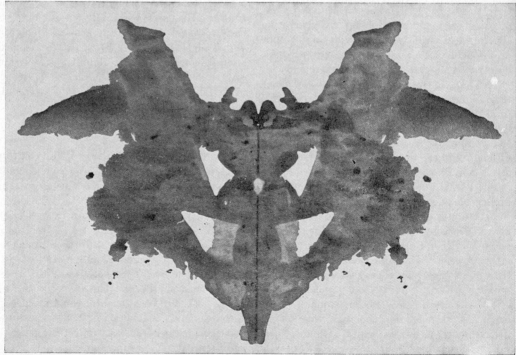

FIGURE 2. Plate I of the Rorschach Test. (Reprinted by permission, Hans Huber Medical Publisher, Berne.)

response reflect what there was about the blot that made it look the way the patient thought it looked. Determinants include form (F), shading (K, t or c), color (C), movement either of humans or animals (M or FM), inanimate movement (m), and various combinations of these determinants with varying emphases. The content areas—human, animal, anatomy, sex, food, nature, and so forth—reflect breadth and range of interests.

The Rorschach is particularly useful as a diagnostic tool (see Table I). The thinking and associational patterns of the patient are highlighted or brought more clearly into focus largely because the ambiguity of the stimulus provides relatively few cues for what may be conventional or standard responses. Recognizing the behavioral differences between hysterical and obsessive-compulsive patients, one could correctly infer that the hysterical patients have fewer and vague responses, are less systematic in approach, and use fewer small detail responses than do the obsessive-compulsive patients. The presumed emotional lability of the hysteric should also dictate that he will probably more freely show uncontrolled color responses (CF and C) on the Rorschach than does the obsessive-compulsive patient. And schizophrenia, which is sometimes difficult to detect through structured interviews only, may be expressed on the Rorschach by poor contact with reality, overgeneralization, unconventionality of thinking, idiosyncrasy of thought, peculiarities of language, suicide indicators, body-image and ego-boundary difficulties, and difficulties in interpersonal relationships.

Other Inkblot Series

In an effort to overcome the psychometric limitations of the Rorschach, in which only 10 cards are used and in which there is no control on the number of responses, Holtzman constructed two parallel forms containing 45 inkblots each. The Holtzman inkblot technique (HIT) presumably offers richer and more varied stimuli while holding the number of responses constant by encouraging the subject to give only one response to a card. The HIT offers substantially great objectivity and precision in analysis, although it has yet to be shown to offer the clinical sensitivity of the Rorschach blots. In spite of its original promise of ultimately replacing the Rorschach, the HIT has not rivaled the Rorschach in clinical usage.

TABLE I

Psychologist's Interpretation of Patient's Responses to Rorschach Card I

1. A bat (Inquiry: It's the whole. Its wings and these are its claws. This is the place where he goes to the bathroom—anus. Rest of body is here: the whole blot.)	Although the popular percept (bat) is given, the elaboration is highly unusual. Introduction of "anus" is idiosyncratic, forewarning of a theme that reaches greater intensity on subsequent cards. Anal responses or the tendency to see figures from the rear are often found in the records of paranoid patients.
2. A lobster (Inquiry: The whole blot. These wings could be claws, too. (?) Just its head is beaked sort of like a lobster. It's hard and stony-like. (?) Shading of the color.)	With its central detail frequently seen as a female figure, card I is sometimes assumed to elicit responses reflecting early attitudes toward the mother-figure. Note the incorporative characteristics attributed to aspects of this card, as well as "beaked" . . . hard and stony-like."
3. Ugh! A monster of some kind. Whatever it is, I don't like it at all. That's just disgusting—horrible. Frightens me somewhat. (Inquiry: Whole. It looks as if they are reaching for something, trying to engulf and eat it up. It looks like a big hand or something trying to engulf all around it. Just an ugly thing. They are all ugly. These are trying to close in on something.)	The theme of incorporation implied in the lobster response breaks through in blatant form in the last response. Loss of distance occurs ("Frightens me somewhat"). Such attributes as "disgusting," "horrible," and "frightens me" connote significant projection, found in phobic if not paranoid patients. The departure from convention ("anus") and the disturbance in ego-boundaries suggest as early as card I that the patient is schizophrenic. In this context, the tendency throughout the test to give responses primarily to the whole blot is consistent with grandiose features.

Harrower offered an inkblot test that can be both self-administered and group-administered. Expendable inkblots permit the subject to mark his responses, which is time-saving and effective. The test was devised as an alternate to the Rorschach and is particularly useful for test-retest purposes.

Thematic Apperception Test (TAT)

The TAT was designed by Henry Murray (Figure 3) and Christiana Morgan as part of a case-study exploration of the normal personality conducted at the Harvard Psychological Clinic in 1943. It consists of a series of 30 pictures (see Figure 4) and one blank card. Only 20 of the cards were originally expected to be used with an individual subject, with the choice of some pictures depending on the subject's sex and age. Today, fewer pictures are usually used, with the selection depending on the examiner's card preference and on what conflict areas he wishes to clarify with a particular patient.

Although most of the pictures obviously depict people, thus making the test stimuli more structured than the inkblots of the Rorschach test, there is ambiguity in all the pictures. Unlike the Rorschach blots, to which the patient is asked to associate, the TAT requires that he construct or create a story.

As the test was originally conceived, an important aspect of each story was the figure (the hero) with whom the storyteller seemed to identify and to whom he was presumably attributing his own wishes, strivings, and conflicts. The characteristics of people other than the hero were considered to represent the subject's view of other people in his environment. But Piotrowski assumes all the figures in a TAT story are equally representative of the subject, with more acceptable and conscious traits and motives being attributed to figures closest to the subject in age, sex, and appearance and the more unacceptable and unconscious traits and motives attributed to figures most unlike the subject.

The stories must be considered from the standpoint of unusualness of theme or plot. Whether the patient is dealing with a common or an uncommon theme, however, his story reflects his own idiosyncratic approach to organization, sequence, vocabulary, style, preconceptions, assumptions, and outcome. TAT cards have different stimulus value and can be assumed to elicit data pertaining to different areas of functioning. Generally, the TAT is most useful as a technique for inferring motivational aspects of behavior.

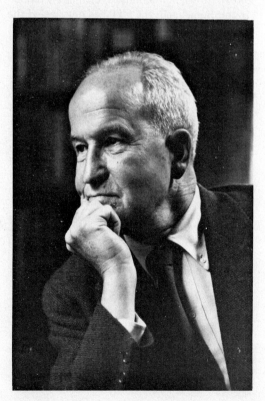

FIGURE 3. Henry A. Murray. (Courtesy of Harvard University News office, Cambridge, Mass.)

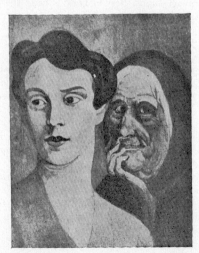

FIGURE 4. Card 12 GF of the Thematic Apperception Test. (Reprinted by permission, Harvard University Press, Cambridge, Mass.)

Sentence Completion Test (SCT)

SCT responses are often most helpful in establishing level of confidence regarding predictions of overt behavior. The SCT is designed to tap the patient's conscious associations to areas of functioning in which the psychologist may be interested. It is composed of series of sentence stems (usually 75 to 100)—such as "I like..." "Sex is..." "Sometimes I wish..." —that the patient is asked to complete in his own words. Since such tests are easily constructed, many psychologists have devised their own form of this test, although copyrighted forms are available.

The patient may be encouraged to take all the time he needs, thus allowing him to consider thoroughly how he wishes to present himself. The test may also be administered verbally by the examiner, similar to the word association technique, in which the patient is told he should reply with the very first thing that comes to his mind. Sentence stems vary in their ambiguity, hence some items serve more as a projective test stimulus ("Sometimes I..."). Others more closely resemble direct-response questionnaires ("My greatest fear is...").

With the individual protocol, most psychologists use an inspection technique, noting particularly those responses that are expressive of strong affects, that tend to be given repetitively, or that are unusual or particularly informative in any way. Areas where denial operates are often revealed through omissions, bland expressions, or factual reports ("My mother *is a woman*). Humor may also reflect an attempt to deny anxiety about a particular issue, person, or event. Important historical material is sometimes revealed directly ("I feel guilty about *the way my sister was drowned*).

With a cooperative patient, sentence completions can usually be taken at face value. More conscious data are directly reported in the SCT than in other projective techniques. Since the SCT usually elicits information the patient is quite willing to give, the level of inference is usually less than in the Rorschach test or TAT interpretations. Less experience and special training are required to make meaningful inferences from sentence completions than from responses to most other tests. Direct quotations from SCT data, when included in the psychologist's report, can illustrate the patient's idiosyncratic characteristics and his major preoccupa-tions, fears, and ambitions in a more meaningful way than can any abstraction or generalization about them made by the psychologist.

The Forer structured sentence completion test (FSSCT) is a copyrighted sentence completion test designed by Bertram Forer that is ideally suited for eliciting data that can be easily integrated with and that complement other tests in the battery. The FSSCT is structured in the sense that a well-planned organization is readily revealed through the use of a check sheet, which can be used to score completions in terms of their expressed characteristics or affect. Alternate forms of the test are used for men, women, adolescent boys, and adolescent girls.

Word-association Technique

The word-association technique consists of presenting stimulus words to the patient and having him respond with the first word that comes to his mind. Frequently used lists have been presented by Jung and by Kent and Rosanoff. Other words can be chosen to tap associations to ideas that may have emotional significance for the particular patient.

Complex indicators include long reaction times, blocking difficulties in making responses, unusual responses, repetition of the stimulus word, apparent misunderstanding of the word, clang associations, perseveration of earlier responses, and ideas or unusual mannerisms or movements accompanying the response. After the initial administration of the list, some clinicians repeat the list, asking the patient to respond with the same words that he used previously; discrepancies between the two administrations may reveal associational difficulties. Because it is easily quantified, the test has continued to be used as a research instrument, although its popularity has diminished greatly over the years.

Bender (Visual Motor) Gestalt Test

The Bender-Gestalt test is a test of visual motor coordination, useful for both children, and adults. It was designed by Lauretta Bender, who used it to evaluate maturational levels in children. Developmentally, a child below the age of 3 is generally unable to reproduce any of the test's designs meaningfully. Around 4 he may be able to copy several, but poorly. At about 6 he should give some recognizable representation of all of the designs, though still unevenly. By 10 and certainly by 12, his copies should be reasonably accurate and well-organized. Bender also presented studies of adults with organic brain defects, mental retardation, aphasias, psychoses, neuroses, and malingering.

The test material consists of nine separate designs, adapted from those used by Wertheimer in his studies in Gesalt psychology. Each design is printed against a white background on a separate card (see Figure 5). Presented with unlined paper, the patient is asked to copy each design with the card in front of him. There is no time limit. This phase of the test is highly structured and does not investigate memory function, since the cards remain in front of the patient while he copies them. Many clinicians include a subsequent recall phase, in which (after an interval of 45 to 60 seconds), the patient is asked to reproduce as many of the designs as he can from memory. This phase not only investigates visual memory but also presents a less structured situation, since the

patient must now rely essentially on his own resources. It is often particularly helpful to compare the patient's functioning under the two conditions.

Probably the most frequent clinical use for the test with adults is as a screening device for detecting signs of organically based interference, especially in grosser forms. Evaluation of the protocol depends on the form of the reproduced figures and on their relationship to each other and to the whole spatial background (see Figures 6 and 7).

Although the test is chiefly an instrument for studying perceptual-motor acuity, a number of other skills and attributes are tapped. To this extent, the patient's productions reflect particular personality traits. Because the test is generally viewed as nonthreatening by the patient, it is an ideal test to introduce the test

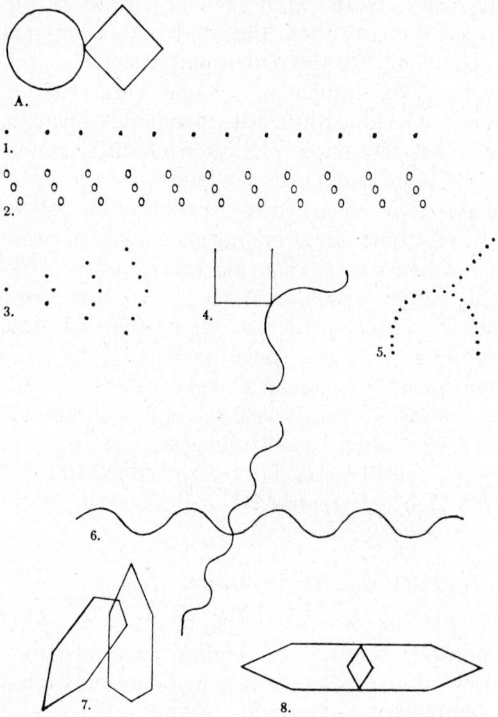

FIGURE 5. Test figures from the Bender Visual Motor Gestalt Test, adapted from Wertheimer. (From Bender, L. *A Visual Motor Gestalt Test and Its Clinical Use.* Research Monograph no. 3, American Orthopsychiatric Association, New York, 1938).

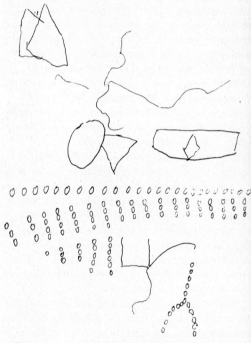

FIGURE 6. Bender-Gestalt drawings of 57-year-old brain-damaged female patient.

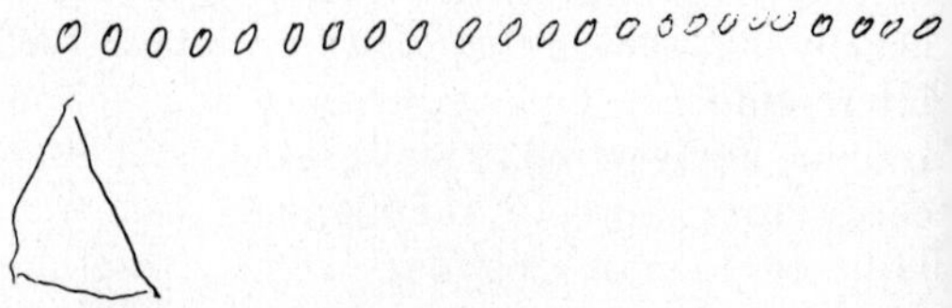

FIGURE 7. Bender-Gestalt "recall" of 57-year-old brain-damaged female patient.

battery, allowing for a discharge of anxiety through motor activity.

Draw a Person Test

The Draw a Person test (DAP) was first used as a measure of intelligence with children. The test is easily administered, usually with the instructions, "I'd like you to draw a picture of a person; draw the best person you can." After the completion of the first drawing, the patient is asked to draw a picture of a person of the opposite sex to that of his first drawing. Some clinicians use an interrogation procedure in which the patient is questioned about his drawings. ("What is he doing? What are his best qualities?") Modifications include asking also for a drawing of a house and a tree (house-tree-person test), of one's family, and of an animal.

A general assumption is that the drawing of a person represents the expression of the self or of the body in the environment (see Figure 8). Interpretive principles rest largely on the assumed functional significance of each body part. Most clinicians use drawings primarily as a screening technique, particularly for the detection of organic brain damage.

Integration of Test Findings

The integration of test findings into a comprehensive, meaningful report is probably the most difficult aspect of psychological evaluations. Inferences from different tests must be related to each other in terms of the confidence

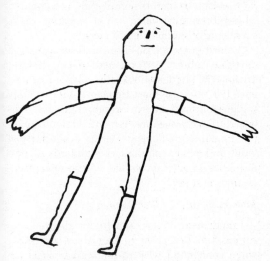

FIGURE 8. "Draw a Person" by 33-year-old brain-damaged male patient.

the psychologist holds about them and of the presumed level of the patient's awareness or consciousness being tapped.

Most psychologists follow some general outline in preparing a psychological report, such as: test behavior, intellectual functioning, personality functioning (reality-testing ability, impulse control, manifest depression and guilt, manifestations of major dysfunction, major defenses, overt symptoms, interpersonal conflicts, self-concept, affects), inferred diagnosis, degree of present overt disturbance, prognosis for social recovery, motivation for personality change, primary assets and weaknesses, recommendations, and summary.

Supplementary Data

Opinions differ among both psychiatrists and psychologists as to whether test results should be interpreted blindly—that is, without knowledge of other clinical data about the patient—or with knowledge of all relevant clinical information. Ideally, it should be the psychologist's function to determine what information he would like and to seek it from appropriate sources. The present author has found it especially valuable to elicit certain reports from the patient through the use of a self-report questionnaire that elicits material of psychodynamic and genetic relevance, material usually not elicited directly by the psychological test battery. In its present form the questionnaire comprises three pages, usually requiring 15 to 25 minutes for completion. As such, it elicits a more complete sample of handwriting and expressive ability than does the standard test battery as usually administered. The clarity of expression and detail varies strikingly between patients, as does the obvious conscientiousness with which the task has been approached.

REFERENCES

Beck, S. J. *Rorschach's Test*, volumes 1, 2, and 3. Grune & Stratton, New York, 1944–1952.

Bender, L. *A Visual Motor Gestalt Test and Its Clinical Use*. American Orthopsychiatric Association. New York, 1938.

Goldberg, P. A. A review of sentence completion methods in personality assessment. J. Proj. Tech. Pers. Assess., *29:* 12, 1965.

Klopfer, B. *Developments in the Rorschach Technique*, 2 vols. World Book, New York, 1954–1956.

Machover, K. *Personality Projection in the Drawing of the Human Figure*. Charles C Thomas, Springfield, Ill., 1949.

Matarazzo, J. D. *Wechsler's Measurement and Appraisal of Adult Intelligence*. Williams & Wilkins, Baltimore, 1972.

Murray, H. A. *Thematic Apperception Test Manual*. Harvard University Press, Cambridge, 1943.

11.5.   PSYCHOLOGICAL TESTS FOR BRAIN DAMAGE

Introduction

Disease or injury at the higher levels of the central nervous system is likely to be reflected in disturbances in mentation, feeling, and conduct. It is this basic fact that makes behavioral assessment an integral part of clinical neurological evaluation, particularly when the question of disease involving the cerebral hemispheres has been raised.

To a considerable degree, the aspects of behavior sampled by clinical observation and by neuropsychological tests are the same—for example, speed of response, level of comprehension, and use of language—but the test procedures assess these aspects of behavior with greater reliability and precision. The tests go on to sample other aspects of behavior, such as visual memory and psychomotor skill, that are not readily elicited in the general examination. Thus, neuropsychological tests both validate the impressionistic findings of the general clinical examination and provide additional information about other aspects of intellect and personality. (See Table I.)

Neuropsychological Tests

General Intelligence and Dementia

Patients with cerebral disease may show an over-all behavioral inefficiency and be unable to meet the diverse intellectual demands associated with the responsibilities of daily life. The normal counterpart of dementia or deterioration is general intelligence.

Dementia implies an over-all impairment in mental capacity with consequent decline in social and economic competence. There are, in fact, clinically distinguishable types of dementia—for example, an aphasic type, an amnesic type, a type showing prominent visuo-perceptual and somatoperceptual defects, and a relatively pure type manifesting impairment in abstract reasoning and problem solving within a setting of fairly intact linguistic and perceptual capacity.

In this country, the Wechsler Adult Intelligence Scale (WAIS) is by far the most widely used test battery to assess general intelligence in adult subjects. In its clinical application, a number of procedures have been used to evaluate the possibility of a decline in general intelligence that may be ascribable to the presence of cerebral disease. The most direct approach is to compare the patient's obtained age-corrected I.Q. score with the age-corrected I.Q. score that might be expected in view of his educational background, cultural level, and occupational history. An obtained I.Q. below the expected I.Q. may be interpreted as raising the question of the presence of cerebral disease. However, many patients with unquestionable cerebral disease do not show an over-all decline in general intelligence of sufficient severity to be reflected in a significant lowering of their WAIS I.Q. score. Consequently, this procedure may be expected to yield a fair proportion of false-negative results.

A variant of this procedure is to compare obtained and expected I.Q. scores on the WAIS performance scale, which consists, for the most part, of nonverbal and relatively novel tasks. This comparison has proved to be practically as useful as the comparison of full scale I.Q. scores.

Since it has been found, at least in nonaphasic patients, that certain types of performance tend to be more seriously affected by cerebral damage than are others, a second approach has been to compare performance level of presumably less sensitive tasks with that on more sensitive tasks. Thus, verbal scale I.Q. is compared to performance scale I.Q., or performance on a set of insensitive tests, such as information or picture completion, is compared with performance on a set of sensitive tests, such as arithmetic or block designs.

A third approach has been to focus attention on those subtest performances (block designs, arithmetic, digit symbol) that clinical experience indicates are most frequently and severely impaired in patients with cerebral disease. This is a rational procedure, but full exploitation of its clinical value depends on the availability of valid and precise normative standards of performance in relation to age, educational background, and sex.

Reasoning and Problem Solving

Impairment of the capacity for abstract reasoning and reduction in behavioral flexibility when confronted with an unfamiliar situation are well-known behavioral characteristics of the brain-damaged patient. But one must rule out

TABLE I

Tests for Assessing Brain Damage

Category	Subcategories	Remarks
General scales	Wechsler scales (WAIS, WISC, WPSSI) Stanford-Binet Halstead-Reitan battery	Given the availability of adequate normative standards in relation to the patient's educational and cultural background, a performance significantly below expectations should raise the question of cerebral damage. This generalization applies to both adults and children.
Reasoning and problem solving	Shipley abstractions Raven progressive matrices Gorham proverbs Elithorn perceptual mazes Porteus mazes Goldstein-Scheerer sorting tests Wisconsin card-sorting test	Performance level is closely related to educational background and premorbid intellectual level. In general, the clinical application of these tests is more useful in the case of educated patients. If specific language and perceptual defects can be ruled out as determinants of defective performance, failure suggests frontal lobe involvement or diffuse cerebral disease.
Memory and orientation	Repetition and reversal of digits Visual memory for designs Auditory memory for words or stories Visual memory for words or pictures Temporal orientation	For complete assessment, a number of memory tasks (auditory versus visual, verbal versus nonverbal, immediate versus recent) should be given. Defects in temporal orientation suggestive of impairment in recent memory may be elicited.
Visuoperceptive and visuoconstructive	Identification of hidden figures Discrimination of complex patterns Facial recognition Inkblot interpretation Block design construction Stick arranging Copying designs Three-dimensional block construction Responsiveness to double visual stimulation	These tasks are useful indicators of the presence of cerebral disease. Analysis of qualitative features of performance and comparison of performance level with the status of language and reasoning abilities often provide indications with regard to locus of the lesion.
Somatoperceptual	Finger recognition Right-left orientation Responsiveness to double tactile stimulation	These are useful indicators of the presence and locus of cerebral disease.
Language	Token test Controlled work association Illinois test of psycholinguistic abilities Diagnostic reading tests	Test performance depends on educational background, and clinical interpretation must allow for this and other possibly significant factors. In adult patients, defective performance (particularly in relation to other abilities) suggests dysfunction of the cerebral hemisphere that is dominant for language. In children, defective performance does not have this localizing significance but does raise the question of the presence of cerebral damage. Performance on verbal reasoning tests, such as Shipley abstractions and Gorham proverbs, may also disclose specific impairment in language function.
Attention, concentration, and motor abilities	Simple and choice reaction time Visual vigilance Imitation of movements Motor impersistence	These are useful behavioral indicators of the presence and sometimes the locus of cerebral disease that deserve more extensive clinical application.

language and perceptual handicaps as determinants of a defective performance before making the inference that the performance indicates impaired reasoning or impaired problem-solving ability.

These tests are valuable for disclosing behavioral deficit in the neurologically negative patient with frontal lobe or beginning diffuse cerebral disease who shows no specific sensory, perceptual, language, or motor impairments and who, on initial encounter, appears to have a functional psychiatric disorder. Conversely, these tests are less useful for the specific purpose of inferring brain disease when applied to unintelligent or uneducated subjects or those suffering from psychosis.

Memory

Impairment of various types of memory, most notably short-term and recent memory, is a prominent behavioral deficit in brain-damaged patients, and it is often the first sign of beginning cerebral disease and of aging.

Memory is a comprehensive term that covers the retention of all types of material over different periods of time and involving diverse forms of response. Consequently, the neuropsychological examiner is more inclined to give specific memory tests and evaluate them separately than to use an omnibus battery that provides for a brief assessment of a large variety of performances and yields a single score in the form of a memory quotient.

Immediate memory may be defined as the reproduction, recognition, or recall of perceived material within a period of not more than 5 seconds after presentation. It is most often assessed by digit repetition and reversal (auditory) and memory-for-designs (visual) tests. Both an auditory-verbal task, such as digit span or memory for words or sentences, and a nonverbal visual task, such as memory for designs or for objects or faces, should be given to assess the patient's immediate memory. Patients with lesions of the right hemisphere are likely to show more severe defect on visual nonverbal tasks than on auditory verbal tasks. Conversely, patients with left hemisphere disease, including those who are not aphasic, are likely to show more severe deficit on the auditory verbal tests with variable performance on the visual nonverbal tasks.

Recent memory refers to the reproduction, recognition, or recall of perceived material after a period of time (10 seconds or longer) has elapsed after the initial presentation. It is typically assessed by measuring the patient's memory for a story read to him, for items in a display of words or pictures or abstract forms, or for material he has learned, such as lists of words or pictures. This type of task provides one of the more sensitive indicators of the presence of cerebral disease. However, quality of performance depends closely on level of effort and attention.

It is commonly believed that remote memory is well-preserved in patients who show pronounced defects in recent memory. This is true only in a relative sense. In fact, the remote memory of senile and amnesic patients is usually significantly inferior to that of normal subjects of comparable age and education. Although events in the remote past are recalled, their placement within a temporal framework is likely to be imprecise, and uncertainty about such items as the dates of Presidential terms or wars or even the birth dates of their children is more the rule than the exception.

Orientation

Orientation for person or place is rarely disturbed in the brain-damaged patient who is not psychotic or severely demented, but defects in temporal orientation, which can be considered to reflect the integrity of recent memory, are common. These defects are often missed by the clinical examiner because of his tendency to regard slight inaccuracy in giving the day of the week or of the month as inconsequential. However, about 25 per cent of nonpsychotic patients with hemispheric cerebral disease are likely to show significant inferiority with respect to precision of temporal orientation (see Table II).

Perceptual and Perceptuomotor Performances

Many patients with brain disease show defective capacity to analyze complex stimulus constellations or inability to translate their perceptions into appropriate motor action. Unless the impairment is of a gross nature, as in visual object agnosia or dressing apraxia, or interferes with a specific occupation skill, these deficits are not likely to be the subject of spontaneous complaint. However, appropriate testing discloses a remarkably high incidence of impaired performance on visuoanalytic, visuospatial, and visuoconstructive tasks in brain-damaged patients, particularly in those with disease involving the right hemisphere. This type of impairment also extends to tactile and auditory perceptual task performances (see Figures 1 and 2).

Although not culture-free (no behavioral performances are), they are generally less dependent on educational level and cultural background than are many of the more intellectual types of task. Many of the perceptual and perceptuomotor tests are relatively sensitive indicators of the presence of cerebral disease. In

TABLE II
Temporal Orientation Schedule

Administration

What is today's date? (The patient is required to give month, day, and year.)
What day of the week is it?
What time is it now? (Examiner makes sure that the patient cannot look at a watch or clock.)

Scoring

Day of week: 1 point off for each day removed from the correct day to a maximum of 3 points.

Day of month: 1 point off for each day removed from the correct day to a maximum of 15 points.

Month: 5 points off for each month removed from the correct month with the qualification that, if the stated date is within 15 days of the correct date, no points are taken off for the incorrect month (for example, May 29 for June 2 = 4 points off).

Year: 10 points off for each year removed from the correct year to a maximum of 60 points with the qualification that, if the stated date is within 15 days of the correct date, no points are taken off for the incorrect year for example, December 26, 1976, for January 2, 1977 = 7 points off).

Time of day: 1 point off for each 30 minutes removed from the correct time to a maximum of 5 points.

The total number of points off for errors is subtracted from 100, and the remainder is considered as the patient's obtained score.

---

addition, they often provide suggestions with regard to the probable locus of the cerebral lesion and thus may help to offer a focus for further neurological exploration.

Language Functions

Gross impairment in language functions in the form of frank aphasia can scarcely be overlooked by the psychiatrist, although the less experienced examiner may sometimes misinterpret paraphasic or jargon speech as a sign of dementia or psychosis. On the other hand, less severe disturbances of language expression and comprehension may go unrecognized for the simple reason that the interview or the application of a few simple tests for aphasia fails to bring them out. But relatively minor defects in the use of language may be valid indicators of the presence of brain disease, particularly if it involves the dominant hemisphere (see Figure 3). Performance on all language tests depends on educational background, and allowance must be made for this variable as well as for

other possibly significant factors, such as age and sex, in clinical interpretation.

Speed and Flexibility of Response

Some brain-damaged patients are quite slow in responding to diverse stimuli and have notable difficulty in modifying their behavior to meet the changing demands of a shifting situation. Reaction time studies have shown that both simple and choice reactions are significantly retarded in 40 to 45 per cent of nonpsychotic brain-damaged patients. Moreover, patients with unilateral cerebral disease show clear retardation even when the hand on the unaffected side of the body is used to effect the response. These results indicate that reaction time is a fairly sensitive indicator of over-all cerebral integrity and that retardation in reaction time reflects the presence of a cerebral lesion, regardless of its locus. Comparison of the reaction times of the right and left hands often provides an indication of the hemisphere locus of the lesion in a patient with unilateral cerebral disease.

Excessive slowness in response to a stimulus that has been preceded by a stimulus in another sense modality (cross-modal retardation effect) is shown both by schizophrenic and by nonpsychotic brain-damaged patients. Neurotic patients do not show this marked susceptibility to the cross-modal retardation effect.

Other measures of behavioral flexibility are provided by tasks in which the patient must

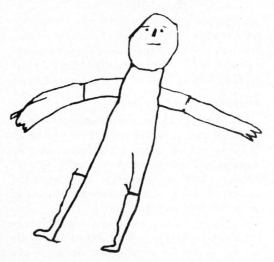

FIGURE 1. "Draw a Person" by a 33-year-old brain-damaged male patient.

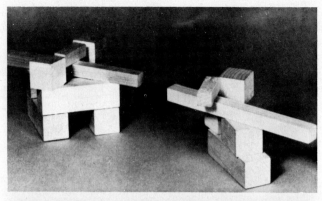

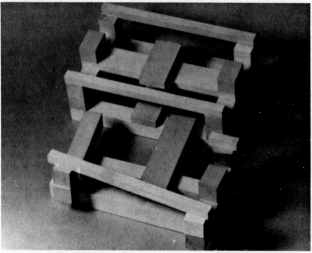

FIGURE 2. Three-dimensional constructional praxis: performances of patients with right hemisphere disease. Upper half shows failure to construct left half of model, indicative of unilateral spatial neglect; lower half illustrates closing-in phenomenon (utilization of part of model in making the construction.

modify his approach to a problem in accordance with changing requirements—color-form sorting tests, object sorting tests, and concept formation tests, which are particularly valuable in identifying patients with frontal lobe disease.

Attention and Concentration

The capacity to sustain a maximal level of attention over a period of time is sometimes impaired in brain-damaged patients, and this impairment is reflected in oscillation in performance level on a continuous or repeated activity. There is some evidence that this instability in performance is related to electroencephalographic abnormality and that the occurrence of inexplicable declines in performance is related temporally to the appearance of certain types of abnormal electrical activity. Simple reaction time provides a convenient measure of variability and speed of simple responses and

possibly is as discriminative and informative as assessments of performance on more complex and lengthy tasks. (See Figure 4.)

Behavioral Indices of Brain Damage in Children

The behavioral consequences, if any, of early brain damage may take many forms, of which the hyperkinetic impulse disorder is only one. Early brain damage may result in little or no behavioral deficit, and, when such deficit does appear, it is usually less severe than that caused by a comparable lesion in adults. Thus, there is reason to believe that many brain-damaged children are not identified by current methods of behavioral assessment.

General Intelligence

As in adults, general intelligence in children is measured by over-all performance level on an

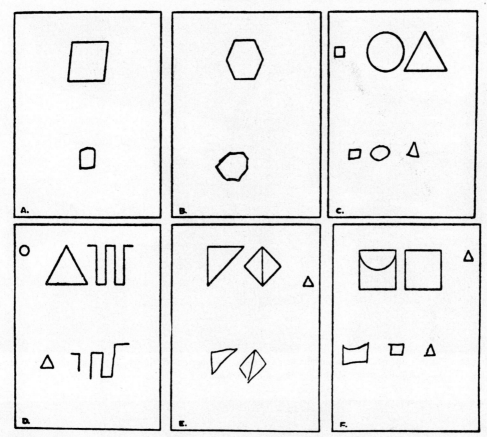

FIGURE 3. Copying of designs by a patient with right hemisphere disease: *A*, Distortion. *B*, Distortion. *C*, Size error in reproduction of left peripheral figure. *D*, Omission of left peripheral figure, size error in reproduction of left major figure, distortion of right major figure. *E*, Omission of right peripheral figure. *F*, Distortion of left major figure, size error in reproduction of right major figure.

omnibus test battery. The most frequently used batteries are the Wechsler Intelligence Scale for Children (WICS), the Stanford-Binet, and the Wechsler Preschool and Primary Scale of Intelligence (WPPSI). A relatively low level of general intelligence is probably the most constant behavioral result of brain damage in children. In contrast to the findings in nonaphasic adults with cerebral disease, the performance scale of the WISC does not seem to be more sensitive than the verbal scale to the effects of brain damage.

Perceptual and Perceptuomotor Performances

Many brain-damaged children with adequate verbal skills show strikingly defective visuoperceptive and visuomotor performances. The test most frequently used is copying of designs, either from a model or from memory. About 25 per cent of brain-damaged school children of adequate verbal intelligence perform defectively—that is, on a level exceeded by 95 per cent of normal children of comparable verbal intelligence. The task discriminates between brain-damaged children and those suffering from presumably psychogenic emotional disturbance.

Tasks involving the recognition of hidden figures and the detection of patterns have disclosed inferior performance in brain-damaged children as compared with normal controls. Defective finger recognition and right-left orientation, often conceptualized as reflecting a disturbance of the body schema, are shown by some nondefective children with brain damage.

Language Functions

Diagnostic evaluation of the child suspected of brain damage has typically depended largely

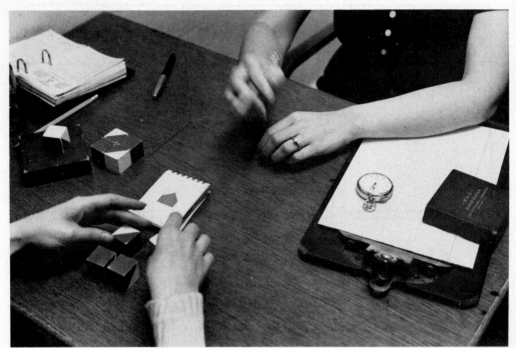

FIGURE 4. In this illustration the patient has a certain time period within which to match blocks to form a design. (Courtesy of Constantine Manos for Magnum Photos, Inc.)

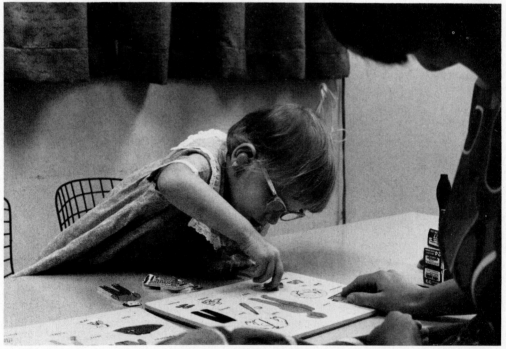

FIGURE 5. The child in this photograph is being tested for manual dexterity as well as for concept formation (Magnum Photos, Inc.).

on assessment of his perceptual and perceptuomotor performances, but the status of his language abilities may be an equally sensitive indicator. There is considerable evidence that aphasic children—those who show a gross maldevelopment of oral language abilities as compared with general mental level—suffer from brain damage. Perinatal brain injury may be a causative factor in at least some cases of developmental dyslexia or more generalized learning disability. The finding of a relatively high incidence of electroencephalographic abnormality in children with learning disabilities points to the same conclusion.

Attention and Concentration

Parents and teachers report that brain-damaged children show inexplicable inconsistency in behavior. This everyday observation has been amply confirmed by analyses of performance on a variety of tests that require sustained attention and concentration. For diagnostic purposes, the continuous performance test of Rosvold and co-workers can be used with older school children as well as adults to probe this capacity. Variability in simple reaction time provides a rational measure in younger children that can be applied clinically if appropriate normative standards are available as a basis for evaluating performance.

Motor Performances

Motor awkwardness and inability to carry out movement sequences on command or by imitation are commonly seen in brain-damaged children. A variety of tests are available for the assessment of manual dexterity—for example, manipulations with tweezers, paper cutting, and peg placing. (See Figure 5.)

Motor impersistence—inability to sustain an action initiated on command, such as keeping the eyes closed or maintaining central fixation during confrontation testing of visual fields—is seen in a relatively small proportion of adult patients with cerebral disease. However, it is shown with remarkably high frequency by nondefective brain-damaged children. Many mental defectives also show excessive motor impersistence, particularly those with frank brain damage.

REFERENCES

Benton, A. L. Disorders of spatial orientation. In *Handbook of Clinical Neurology*, P. J. Vinken and G. W. Bruyn, editors, vol. 3, *Disorders of Higher Nervous Activity*, p. 212. North-Holland Publishing Co., Amsterdam, 1969.

Benton, A. L. Minimal brain dysfunction from a neuropsychological standpoint. Ann. N. Y. Acad. Sci., *205:* 29, 1973.

Hécaen, H. Aphasic, apraxic and agnosic syndromes in right and left hemisphere lesions. In *Handbook of Clinical Neurology*, P. J. Vinken and G. W. Bruyn, editors, vol. 4, *Disorders of Speech, Perception and Symbolic Behaviour*, p. 291. North-Holland Publishing Co., Amsterdam, 1969.

Joynt, R. J., Benton, A. L., and Fogel, M. L. Behavioral and pathological correlates of motor impersistence. Neurology (Minneap)., *12:* 876, 1962.

Matarazzo, J. D. *Wechsler's Measurement and Appraisal of Adult Intelligence*, ed. 5. Williams & Wilkins, Baltimore, 1972.

Rosenhan, D. L. On being sane in insane places. Science, *179:* 250, 1973.

Warrington, E. K. Constructional apraxia. In *Handbook of Clinical Neurology*, P. J. Vinken and G. W. Bruyn, editors, vol. 4, *Disorders of Speech, Perception and Symbolic Behaviour*, p. 67. North-Holland Publishing Co., Amsterdam, 1969.

Zangwill, O. L. The psychopathology of dementia. Proc. R. Soc. Med., *57:* 914, 1964.

11.6.   SOME INSTRUMENTS COMMONLY USED BY CLINICAL PSYCHOLOGISTS

The table below provides a brief reference to the major techniques used by clinical psychologists for psychological evaluation of children and adults. More detailed references to these and other techniques may be found in the *Buros Mental Measurements Yearbooks*.

Name	General Classification	Description	Special Features
Wechsler Adult Intelligence Scale (WAIS)	Individual intelligence test	Eleven subtests tapping different aspects of intellectual functioning. For ages 16 and above.	Yields both verbal and performance I.Q.s and a full-scale I.Q. based on age levels. Scaled subtest scores reflect relative strengths and weaknesses.
Wechsler Intelligence Scale for Children (WISC)	Individual intelligence test	Ten subtests (with two alternates) tapping different aspects of intellectual functioning. For ages 5 through 15.	Yields both verbal and performance I.Q.s and full-scale I.Q.
Wechsler Preschool and Primary Scale of Intelligence (WPPSI)	Individual intelligence test	Overlaps the WISC with similar scales and tests adapted for ages 4 to 6½.	Similar to WAIS and WISC, it yields both verbal and performance I.Q.s and full-scale I.Q.
Stanford-Binet Intelligence Scale (Form L-M)	Individual intelligence test	Variety of tasks at each age level from 2 years, with adult I.Q.s derived by statistical extrapolation.	Age-level concept makes it especially useful with children and for evaluation of mental retardation.
Wechsler Memory Scale (Forms I and II)	Immediate, short-term, and long-term memory scale	Seven memory tests covering current information, orientation, mental control, logical memory, digits forward and backward, visual reproduction, and associate learning.	Yields a memory quotient (M.Q.) useful in comparison with I.Q., especially with senile and brain-damaged patients.
Cattell Infant Intelligence Scale	Individual intelligence test	Downward extension of the Stanford-Binet Scale to cover 3 months to 2½ years.	Yields mental age scores and I.Q.s of questionable predictive value but useful as measure of present functioning.
McCarthy Scales of Children's Abilities	Individual intelligence test	Assesses intellectual and motor abilities of children from 2½ to 8½ years.	In addition to over-all intellectual competence, it yields scores for verbal ability, short-term memory, numerical ability, perceptual performance, motor coordination, and lateral dominance.
Gesell Developmental Schedules	Individual scale of developmental levels	Scale of behavioral observations for study of the mental growth of the preschool child.	Qualitative measure of motor development, adaptive behavior, language development, and personal-social behavior. Of questionable predictive value but useful to evaluate present functioning, such as school readiness.
Raven Progressive Matrices	Group intelligence test	Nonverbal tests involving untimed problems presented in abstract figures and designs. Three forms span ages 5 to 65 years.	Norms based on English populations. Scores correlate highly with comprehensive intelligence tests.
Leiter International Performance Scale	Individual intelligence test	Nonverbal intelligence test for ages 2 years through adult.	Administered without language. Useful for foreign-born, minority groups, and the disadvantaged.

Name	General Classification	Description	Special Features
Columbia Mental Maturity Scale	Individual intelligence test	Developmental age scale; items arranged in a series of eight overlapping scales.	Requires no verbal response and only minimal motor response. For children with impaired verbal or physical functioning.
Vineland Social Maturity Scale, Revised	Individual interview schedule of social competence	Items designed to measure stages of social competence from infancy to adult life.	Useful in evaluating mental retardates in relation to I.Q.
Rorschach Technique	Projective (personality) technique	Ten inkblots used as basis for eliciting associations; most widely used projective technique.	Especially revealing of personality structure. Other inkblot tests include the Holtzman Inkblot Technique (controls for number of responses) and the Harrower Inkblot Technique (self- and group-administrable).
Thematic Apperception Test (TAT)	Projective (personality) technique	Pictures used as stimuli for making up a story. Some pictures are designed specifically for women, men, girls, or boys.	Especially useful for revealing personality dynamics. Similar techniques include Symonds Picture-Story test (for adolescents), Bellak Children's Apperception test (drawings of animals for children), and Schneidman Make a Picture Story technique (pictures created by cutouts and background settings).
Word Association Technique	Projective (personality test)	Stimulus words to which patient responds with first association that comes to mind.	Flexible; may be used to tap associations to different conflict areas. Generally not as revealing as SCT responses.
Sentence Completion Test (SCT)	Personality test; varies from direct-response questionnaire to projective technique	Incomplete sentence stems that vary as to their ambiguity.	Highly flexible; may be used to tap specific conflict areas. Reveals generally more conscious, overt attitudes and feelings.
Blacky Test	Projective (personality) technique	Cartoons about a dog and his/her family used to elicit stories with subsequent interrogation about each.	Systematized approach to different stages of psychosexual development. Designed for both children and adults, it is used more widely with children.
Draw a Person Test	Graphomotor projective (personality) technique	Patient is asked to draw a person, then one of the sex opposite to the first drawing.	Projects body image, how the body is conceived and perceived. Sometimes useful for detecting brain damage. Modifications include: Draw an animal; Draw a house, a tree, and a person (H-T-P); Draw your family; and Draw the most unpleasant concept you can think of.
Bender (Visual Motor)-Gestalt Test	Graphomotor technique	Geometric designs that the patient is asked to draw or copy, with design in view.	Sometimes useful for detecting psychomotor difficulties correlated with brain damage. Also used by some pyschologists as a projective technique.
Benton Revised Visual Retention Test	Graphomotor technique	Geometric designs that the patient is asked to draw; various administrations alter exposure time and delay interval before reproduction.	Less flexible than the Bender-Gestalt test as a projective technique but more objective as a measure of possible brain damage.

Name	General Classification	Description	Special Features
Minnesota Multiphasic Personality Inventory (MMPI) (Forms: Individual, Group, and Shortened "R")	Objective personality test	True-false questionnaire yielding scores for 10 clinical scales in addition to other scales.	Includes scales related to test-taking attitudes. Empirically constructed on basis of clinical criteria. Computer interpretation services available.
Cattell 16 Personality Factor Questionnaire (16 P.F.)	Objective personality test	Questionnaire covering 16 personality factors derived from factor-analytical studies.	Bipolar variables allow for interpretation of scores varying either above or below the norm: reserved versus outgoing, trusting versus suspicious, timid versus venturesome, and so forth.
California Personality Inventory	Objective personality test	Seventeen scales developed presumably for normal populations for use in guidance and selection.	Less emphasis on mental illness than MMPI scales; dominance, responsibility, socialization, and so forth.
Edwards Personal Preference Schedule	Objective personality test	Forced-choice inventory to show relative importance of 15 key needs or motives, such as nurturance, achievement, order, autonomy. For college students and adults.	Related to Murray's needs theory. Format presumably reduces effects of social desirability.

11.7.   PSYCHIATRIC SOCIAL SERVICE INFORMATION

Psychiatric Team

The proliferation of child guidance clinics in the 1920's and 1930's brought the social caseworker firmly into the psychiatric fold and fostered a subspecialty, psychiatric social work. Through the demonstrated usefulness of skilled diagnostic and therapeutic work with the parents of disturbed children and the adoption of the signal contributions of psychometric and projective testing, the formation of the classical tripartite team of psychiatrist, clinical psychologist, and psychiatric social worker eventuated. Application of this team concept in a variety of settings encouraged flexibility, and many other professionals—nurse, occupational therapist, vocational rehabilitation specialist, neurologist, chaplain, neighborhood worker— became established team members.

The team concept implies that a comprehensive evaluation requires more data than the psychiatrist obtains from a patient. A thorough understanding of assets, limitations, and noxious elements in the patient and in his environment must be gained.

Since members of a patient's family are a valuable source of such data, the psychiatrist interviews the patient and the social worker traditionally interviews his family. This arrangement provides the relatives with one particular professional person to relate to, one who, they can feel, cares about their needs and the affliction the patient's illness brings them. And, when an adolescent is the patient, the psychiatrist does not need to communicate directly with the relatives; thus he is able to avoid the appearance and risk of revealing his patient's confidences to anyone.

Diagnostic Social Work

Relatives' observations of changes from preillness functioning in the patient's thinking, mood, verbalizations, and behavior provide valuable information to compare with what the psychiatrist obtains from the patient and to check for concordances, differences, omissions, and distortions from either source. Parents and older siblings can give clues to significant early interpersonal relationships, lags or distortions in growth, early traumata, and factors establishing basic character traits.

The social and cultural mores, taboos, rules, and directives peculiar to the environment within which the patient and his family interact must be investigated. Class, culture, value systems, religion, family economics, child-care practices, and attitudes toward mental illness and psychiatry are among the pertinent realities to be considered.

The social worker can obtain school, military, court, medical, and work records; discover the patient's and family's previous experiences with community agencies; and provide a preliminary evaluation of community resources available and acceptable to the family and possibly to be enlisted in the eventual treatment plan.

It is useful to establish a base line of the patient's preillness functioning for measuring in a rough way the degree of deviance manifested in his present symptoms and for determining a potential therapeutic goal that will signify, when reached, the patient's return to his particular type of normality. Comparison of social worker's and psychiatrist's data should be routine.

Relatives can usually describe much more graphically than can the patient the factors of secondary gain that serve to sustain the patient's symptoms. Conversely, astute observations of the relatives' productions can reveal the family's uses of the patient's illness for secondary advantages. Focus on the sick patient alone may divert attention from a sick family constellation.

Work with Children

The social worker's contributions to the total team effort are more crucial in diagnostic evaluations of children than in evaluations of adults. Children's limitations as reporters are attributable not only to their state of being ill but also to their incompleteness of cognitive, verbal, mnemonic, and experiential development.

The child has few options for independent behavior; his family's intercommunication, mores, style, values, and standards constitute nearly the whole of his social life. Also, those close to him, chiefly his parents, exercise functions in his behalf that he will assume for himself when older. Parents are his auxiliary or supplemental ego and superego. Diagnostic study of the whole young person must encompass scrutiny of environmental structures and functions in a manner qualitatively and quantitatively different from the procedure in evaluating a relatively self-sufficient adult.

In child psychiatry practice the basic team is frequently augmented by a pediatrician, a neurologist, and a speech therapist. As the evaluation proceeds, the social worker must be pre-pared to organize, sort, and relay information from his accumulating data relevant to developmental history, family relationships, onset of symptoms, present functioning, housing, nutritional deficiencies, lead ingestion, family history of hereditary disorders, deviation from growth norms suggesting a degree of mental retardation, learning disabilities, hearing or sight or speech defects, life crises, and such traumata as child abuse.

Ordinarily a child is not presented for diagnostic study until his parents are sufficiently distressed; they provide the motivation. The parents of a child in diagnostic study always need help, particularly at the end of evaluation, when recommendations for treatment are presented. A disturbed child's parents are often expected to play a large role in the implementation of a treatment program.

Two of the most trying experiences for parents occur when recommendations for helping the child include separating him from their home and suggesting needed alterations in the parent's attitudes, behavior, and marital interaction.

The social worker must work through the implications of the needed changes with the parents and, if indicated, maintain an ongoing professional relationship with them during the implementation of the prescribed therapeutic program.

Team Functioning

The patient and relatives must become engaged with the team's members in a diagnostic process. The informants' attitudes and feelings must be discovered, assayed, and understood in the context of their life circumstances. Their resistance, defense, evasion, reticence, and denial must be invalidated sufficiently for the actual state of affairs to emerge and be viewed. The informants must actively participate in the solution of the clinical problem that they brought to the psychiatrist.

To function smoothly, economically, and flexibly, the team needs to become integrated through a process of group growth. Each member needs to contribute to the work of each of the other team members. The significance of integration is that each member identifies himself with the group as a whole; in his professional participation he acts as an agent of the team in accomplishing a team purpose. In such a flexible team, the patient and his relatives are easily admitted as temporary members to contribute to and participate in the team's tasks with as much responsibility as the team considers reasonable to expect.

An initial meeting of the patient and his relatives with the team members should facilitate introducing them to the team concept, to the diagnostic process, and to each other. Such a meeting allows the patient and his relatives to become acquainted with each other's professional associate and thus largely avoids distracting speculation and fantasy about team members.

At termination, the complex task of presenting recommendations for treatment can be facilitated in a joint conference. If the patient and relatives have been successfully drawn into the evolving treatment plan during the diagnostic process, the final team recommendations will hold few surprises for them.

The joint conference offers an opportunity for the therapeutic team, the patient, and the relatives to examine the implications of the recommendations and to gain a shared understanding of what is being proposed, including the fixing of responsibility for implementing various parts of the proposals. The social worker may suggest that he meet again with the relatives to help them digest and assimilate the recommendations. If some aspects of the remedial program need to be communicated to a court, probation office, school, employer, or welfare department, the social worker may be assigned as the team representative to explain the program, enlist the agency's cooperation, and maintain contact until he is assured that the desired program is in operation.

Social Worker Diagnostician

In many psychiatric clinics, hospitals, mental health centers, and service agencies, one of the psychiatric social worker's responsibilities is to interview prospective patients or clients and to determine their suitability for admission to the agency or institution. The social worker must make at least three determinations: (1) the type and severity of the prospective client's problems, (2) the functions and limitations of his agency in handling such problems and (3) the other community resources that may be better qualified to meet the client's needs. The intake social worker's task is to check the referring diagnosis and agree or disagree with it or modify it.

When a person is deemed ready for termination of treatment or a move from one facility to another, the social worker must evaluate the readiness or reluctance of the family, the community at large, or specific helping agencies to accept him.

In community mental health centers the psychiatric social worker fills many roles: administrator, supervisor, teacher, researcher, clinician. Since many centers serve mostly the economically, racially, and socially disadvantaged, the center's staff must learn a kind of psychosocial practice, a coordination of intrapsychic, interpersonal, intrafamilial, and person-environment perspectives. The psychiatrist, the clinical psychologist, and the psychiatric social worker assimilate some of each others' skills and perspectives and interchangeably work to carry out much of the center's program. Storefront operations, satellite clinics, and remote rural centers are commonly manned by social workers, clinical psychologists, and paraprofessional mental health workers. A consulting psychiatrist may visit weekly or simply be on call. In these facilities the social worker functions as an all-purpose clinician.

REFERENCES

Briar, S. Social casework and social group work: Historical and social science foundations. In *Encyclopedia of Social Work*, p. 1237. National Association of Social Workers, New York, 1971.
Group for the Advancement of Psychiatry. *The Diagnostic Process in Child Psychiatry*. Group for the Advancement of Psychiatry, New York, 1957.
Hall, B., and Wheeler, W. The patient and his relatives: Initial joint interview. Soc. Work, 2: 75, 1957.
Menninger Clinic Children's Division. *Disturbed Children: Examination and Assessment through Team Process*. Jossey-Bass, San Francisco, 1969.
Meyers, H. L. The therapeutic functions of the evaluation process. Bull. Menninger Clin., *20:* 9, 1956.
Modlin, H. C., Gardner, R. W., and Faris, M. T. Implications of a therapeutic process in evaluations by psychiatric teams. Am. J. Orthopsychiatry, *28:* 647, 1958.

11.8.   MEDICAL ASSESSMENT

Introduction

Some psychiatrists proclaim that a complete medical work-up is essential for every patient;

others maintain that a complete medical work-up for every patient is both impractical and unnecessary. The medical status of every patient should be considered.

The medical evaluation of the psychiatric patient has a three fold objective: (1) the detection of underlying and perhaps unsuspected organic pathology that may be primarily responsible for the psychiatric symptoms, (2) an understanding of demonstrated disease as a factor in over-all psychiatric debility, and (3) an appreciation of somatic symptoms reflecting primarily psychological disease.

Selection of Patients

The nature of a patient's complaints is a criterion for selecting those who should undergo a complete medical examination and those who need not. The complaints can be divided into three groups, depending on whether they involve the body, the mind, or social interactions.

If symptoms involve the body—as with headache, impotence, or palpitations—a complete medical examination is required to differentiate somatic from psychological processes as the primary cause of the distress. The same approach is indicated for such mental symptoms as depression, anxiety, hallucinations, and paranoid delusions, since they can be expressions of· a somatic process. However, if the patient complains only of being upset because of long-standing difficulties in his interactions with teachers, employers, parents, or spouse, there is no special indication for a medical examination.

Psychiatrist's Role

For practical reasons, most psychiatric patients who require a medical assessment should have it performed by an internist or general practitioner, rather than a psychiatrist. Few psychiatrists see enough patients requiring complete medical evaluations to maintain their skills in performing physical examinations. Moreover, the demands on psychiatrists' time are such that it is impractical for them to do what other physicians regard as their primary responsibility.

Although the psychiatrist may not conduct the medical examination himself, he should make certain that it has been carried out properly, and he should become fully conversant with the results and their implications.

Medical Assessment

History

When patients are seen for psychiatric evaluation, two aspects of medical history-taking should be developed: First, regular inquiries should be made to elicit facts regarding known physical disease and dysfunction. Second, if the patient has specific physical complaints, these should be elucidated.

The first objective can usually be achieved by the routine inquiry about disease or dysfunction affecting the heart and vascular system, lungs, gastrointestinal tract, endocrine glands, genito-urinary system, liver, blood, musculoskeletal and nervous systems. As a rule, it is not necessary to carry out a complete review of systems or to elicit a full medical history. An inquiry should also be made into the present and past use of alcohol, drugs, and medications.

In the development of information regarding specific complaints presented by the patient, the complementary nature of the physician's medical and psychological knowledge comes into full play. For example, the physician must be able to elicit from the patient complaining of headache sufficient information to allow him to predict with considerable certainty that the pain is or is not the result of cranial pathology.

The psychiatrist must be thoroughly familiar with the behavioral, perceptual, cognitive, and affective concomitants of diseases involving specific bodily organs and systems. Psychiatric symptoms are an expected concomitant of disorders involving the central nervous system, the gastrointestinal system, and the endocrine system, whereas in diseases involving the pulmonary, cardiovascular, hematopoietic, and musculoskeletal systems, psychiatric symptoms may be rare, except in the case of advanced disease. In sexual dysfunctions, the patient may complain of specific organ dysfunctions in which structural abnormalities can rarely be established to account for the symptoms.

Few patients arrive for psychiatric evaluation presenting the classical symptoms and signs of organic brain disease. When they do, recognizing organic brain dysfunction is easy, although detecting its cause may be a formidable task. More commonly, the psychiatrist sees the patient with organic brain disease early in the course of illness, when the evidence of organicity is relatively slight. He should then respond to the possibility when only hints are available. Specifically, he should be suspicious of organicity when the patient presents numerous somatic complaints that conform to no recognizable pattern of disease, especially if these complaints are not consonant with his long-standing life style; when the patient presents numerous psychiatric symptoms that conform to no definite psychiatric diagnostic category, especially if similar complaints have been uncommon in the past; and when the patient's history remains vague and unclear even after detailed and precise questioning.

When organic brain dysfunction is suggested, the examiner is likely to use those parts of the mental status examination especially designed to demonstrate defects. Orientation, often taken for granted in the ordinary interview, should be ascertained by direct questions. Specific memory components are evaluated. The level of intellectual function is measured by questions designed to elicit general information, by calculations, and by problems involving discrimination and judgment.

Occasionally, symptoms typical of a psychiatric disorder alert the examiner to the possibility of a medical disorder. Auditory hallucinations in which voices are heard only toward one side and visual hallucinations in which a person or object is seen only in one part of the visual field may be encountered in schizophrenia, but they should first suggest the possibility of a space-occupying cerebral lesion, and neurological studies should be conducted.

Observation

The psychiatrist's scrutiny of his patient begins at their first encounter. As the patient moves from the waiting room to the interview room, his gait is observed for telltale signs of dysfunction. As soon as the patient is seated, the examiner's attention is attracted by his grooming. Although lack of attention to dress and appearance is common in emotional disturbances, it is also a hallmark of organic brain disease. The patient's posture and automatic movements are noted. Next, the psychiatrist scrutinizes the appearance of the patient to assess his general health. The skin frequently manifests evidence of organic disease. The examiner should quickly scan the face and head for evidence of disease (see Figures 1 and 2). Finally, the patient's state of alertness and responsiveness should be carefully evaluated.

The examiner must listen as intently as he looks for evidence of physical disease. Slowness of speech is characteristic not only of depression but of diffuse brain disease; unusually rapid speech is typical not only of mania but also of hyperthyroidism. The psychiatrist pays attention not only to the quality of the speech but to the word production as well. Even occasional mispronunciations or choice of an incorrect word will suggest aphasia to the attentive lis-

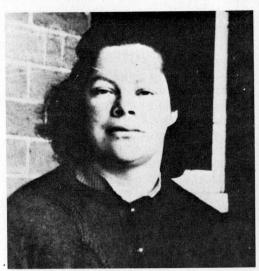

FIGURE 1. Patient with myxedema on admission to hospital. (From Haughton, C. S. Psychosis with myxoedema. Med. J. Aust., 2: 766, 1959.)

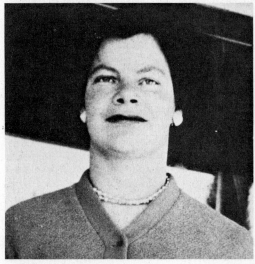

FIGURE 2. Hospitalized patient with myxedema following treatment (2 months later). (From Haughton, C. S. Psychosis with myxoedema. Med. J. Aust., 2: 766, 1959.)

tener and thus the possibility of a lesion of the dominant hemisphere.

The unpleasant odor in a patient who fails to bathe rouses suspicion not only of depression but of inattentivenss to self-care and hygiene secondary to organic brain dysfunction. The odor of alcohol or of substances employed to hide it frequently allows a correct diagnosis in the patient who attempts to conceal his history of drinking. Occasionally, a uriniferous odor calls attention to bladder dysfunction secondary to organic nervous system disease.

Physical Examination

A number of psychological considerations should be borne in mind while performing a physical examination. The physician's instruments and procedures may be strange and frightening to the patient. A simple, running account of what is being done can prevent much needless anxiety.

The physical examination can also stir up sexual feelings. The presence of a nurse or an office assistant is recommended.

The physical examination occasionally serves a psychotherapeutic function. An anxious patient may be relieved to learn that, in spite of his symptoms, he does not have the serious illness he fears. The reassurance, however, takes care only of the acute episode. Unless psychotherapy succeeds in relieving the unconscious determinants of the reaction, recurrent episodes are likely.

During the performance of the physical examination, an observant physician may note indications of emotional distress in his patient. Using his observations, the physician may ask questions that encourage the patient to describe his distress and express his desire for help.

Occasional circumstances make it necessary or desirable to defer a complete medical assessment. An example is the paranoid patient who is combative and resistive. In this instance, a medical history should be elicited, if possible, from a family member; unless their is a pressing reason, the physical examination should be deferred until the patient has been medicated and is more amenable to being examined.

A careful neurological examination should be performed on each patient suspected of having organic brain dysfunction. The examiner, while taking the patient's history, has already noted his level of awareness, attentiveness to details of the examination, understanding, facial expression, speech, posture, and gait. The examiner now turns to the specifically neurological aspects of the examination with two objectives in mind: to elicit signs pointing to focal, circumscribed cerebral dysfunction and to elicit signs pointing to diffuse, bilateral cerebral disease. The first objective is reached during the routine neurological examination, which primarily reveals asymmetries in the motor, perceptual, or reflex functions of the two sides of the body, thus reflecting focal hemispheric disease. The second objective is reached by performing specific maneuvers designed to elicit signs of diffuse brain dysfunction.

The psychiatrist must be able to evaluate the significance of the findings uncovered. Some lesion may be found that accounts for a symptom, but the psychiatrist should make every effort to separate a causative lesion from an incidental one.

Diagnostic Studies

Diagnostic studies should never be performed merely for the sake of completeness. To do so may subject the patient to unwarranted discomfort or expense. In the absence of new signs or symptoms, diagnostic procedures recently performed and reported as negative should not be repeated. Diagnostic procedures likely to produce much discomfort and those entailing some risk should be ordered only if there is reasonable likelihood that the findings will alter the plan of treatment.

If a procedure is pressingly indicated for medical reasons, it should be done, regardless of the patient's emotional or mental state. But every effort should be made to assuage anxiety, reduce pain, and make the timing as favorable as possible.

When the problem is whether the patient's symptoms should be attributed primarily to psychological dysfunction or primarily to disease of the central nervous system, the psychiatrist usually must assume responsibility. Even after a thorough history and neurological examination, the psychiatrist may still be in doubt as to the presence or absence of organic brain dysfunction, and he may have to turn to ancillary testing procedures. Psychological assessment is likely to be the most useful procedure.

In most patients suspected of organic brain disease, skull X-rays and an electroencephalogram are also indicated.

Definite evidence for organic dysfunction

demonstrated by any diagnostic step may result in ordering additional procedures—spinal fluid examination, radioactive brain scan, radioiodinated serum albumin scan, pneumoencephalography. These studies should be reserved, however, for those patients in whom simpler studies have demonstrated unequivocal organic involvement.

Planning for Patient Care

Physical illness is common in patients requiring psychiatric care. The psychiatrist should assess the dangers of a particular medication against its possible benefits. Contraindications to the use of medications vary widely. The chief contraindications are cardiovascular, renal, and hepatic diseases. Clinical experience and judgment often have to serve as the basis for decision making.

Relatively few special medical considerations arise when electroconvulsive therapy is being considered. The regular use of a relaxant, such as succinylcholine, has greatly reduced both the dangers and the complications of electroconvulsive therapy. A chest X-ray and an electrocardiogram are required before instituting therapy.

Occasionally, the psychiatrist treats a patient suffering from both a psychiatric disorder and a medical disorder. The physician must then choose where the patient can best be treated. Generally, if the psychiatric disorder is such that it will not interfere with medical care, the patient should first be hospitalized in a medical facility, then transferred to a psychiatric unit when his medical needs become less pressing. If the patient's psychiatric status threatens to interfere seriously with the administration of medical care, however, hospitalization in a psychiatric unit may be necessary.

REFERENCES

Asher, R. Myxoedematous madness. Br. Med. J., 2: 555, 1949.
Hollender, M. H. The Psychology of Medical Practice. W. B. Saunders, Philadelphia, 1958.
Horenstein, S. The clinical use of psychological testing in dementia. In Dementia, C. E. Wells, editor, p.61. F. A. Davis, Philadelphia, 1971.
Klein, D. F., and Davis, J. M. Diagnosis and Drug Treatment of Psychiatric Disorders. Williams & Wilkins, Baltimore, 1969.
Paulson, G. W. The neurological examination in dementia. In Dementia, C. E. Wells, editor, p. 13, F. A. Davis, Philadelphia, 1971.
Penick, S. B., and Carrier, R. N. Serious medical illness in an acute psychiatric hospital. J. Med. Soc. N. J., 64: 651, 1967.

12

Diagnosis: Symptoms of Psychiatric Disorders

Introduction

The life process in health and disease consists of an ongoing series of adaptations. Thus, a symptom or even a complex disease process in its entirety may be viewed as a reaction pattern having adaptational significance.

The clinical manifestations of all illness, nonpsychiatric as well as psychiatric, are the outcome of complex interacting forces—biological, sociocultural, and psychological (see Figure 1). The weight of the factors differs from case to case and from day to day in a given case. They vary, too, according to the stage of the illness. In every instance the person is challenged by his human environment, and he must adapt. Adaptation is a process of conforming or reacting to the environment in such a way as to fulfill one's wishes and needs. Breakdowns in this process are expressed psychiatrically as abnormalities of thoughts, feelings, and actions. A stressful or a traumatic life situation is one that generates challenges to which the organism cannot competently respond (see Table I). Holmes and Rahe have devised a social readjustment rating scale. This is a list of 43 life events associated with varying amounts of disruption in the average person's life (see Table I).

The scale was constructed by having hundreds of persons of different ages, cultures, and walks of life rank the relative amount of adjustment necessitated by these life events. Holmes and Rahe named these stress values "life change units." They found that an accumulation of 200 or more life change units in a single year was followed by a significantly increased incidence of such disease as myocardial infarction, peptic

ulcer, infection, and a variety of psychiatric disorders. An estimate of the life change unit score may provide a basis for recommending caution before proceeding with further change.

Psychiatric symptoms may be classified into primary and the secondary symptoms. Bleuler believed that the primary symptoms of schizophrenia include disturbances in associations, disturbances of affect, ambivalence, autism, attention defects, disturbances of the will, changes in the personality, disturbances of activity and behavior, and dementia. Bleuler's secondary symptoms include delusions, hallucinations, ideas of reference, and certain types of memory disturbances.

From another point of view, there are two primary symptoms of schizophrenia—an irrational fear of intimate human relationship and an intolerable feeling of loneliness consequent to social withdrawal. All other manifestations of schizophrenia may be regarded as secondary symptoms.

One may also recognize secondary or restitutive symptoms in nonschizophrenic categories. For example, depressed patients in the early stages of their illness are particularly prone to combat primary feelings of emptiness by acting out sexually, developing addictions, reckless behavior, shop-lifting, and self-inflicted injuries.

One may also speak of deficit symptoms and release symptoms. For example, a focal cortical brain injury may result in a circumscribed language disorder, aphasia, which is a deficit symptom. However, if the cortical injury is widespread, there may be generalized personality changes associated with inappropriate social

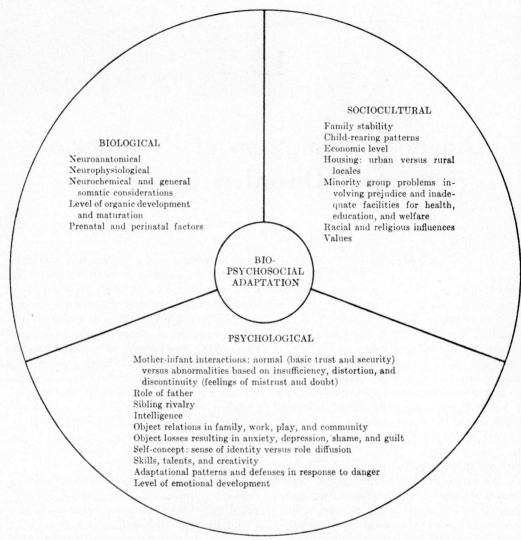

FIG. 1. Biological, sociocultural, and psychological forces. All these forces interact and affect the psychiatric health of the person. (Modified after G. B. Richmond and S. L. Lustman, J. Med. Educ., *29:* 23, 1954.

behavior, which may be interpreted as release symptoms that may result from the the dissolution of higher controlling levels of brain functioning.

Disturbances in Thinking

Normal thought or cognition refers to ideational or informational experience, as contrasted to affects or feelings. It refers to a broad range of psychic phenomena, including abstract and concrete thinking, judgment, orientation, memory, perception, and imagery. Normal rational thinking consists of a goal-directed flow of ideas, symbols, and associations initiated by a problem and leading to reality-oriented con-

clusions. In primary process thinking, there is a tendency to concrete thinking, condensation of separate psychological items into one item, displacement of feelings from one item to another, a disregard for time sequence, and considerable use of metaphor and symbolism. In the loosening of the associations, the flow of thought may seem haphazard, purposeless, illogical, confused, incorrect, abrupt, and bizarre.

Disturbances in Form and Stream of Thought

Dereism or dereistic thinking emphasizes the disconnections from reality. Autism emphasizes the preoccupation with inner thoughts, day-

TABLE I

*The Stress of Adjusting to Change**

Event	Scale of Impact
Death of spouse	100
Divorce	73
Marital separation	65
Jail term	63
Death of close family member	63
Personal injury or illness	53
Marriage	50
Fired at work	47
Marital reconciliation	45
Retirement	45
Change in health of family member	44
Pregnancy	40
Sex difficulties	39
Gain of new family member	39
Business readjustment	39
Change in financial state	38
Death of close friend	37
Change to different line of work	36
Change in number or arguments with spouse	35
Mortgage over $10,000	31
Foreclosure of mortgage or loan	30
Change in responsibilities at work	29
Son or daughter leaving home	29
Trouble with in-laws	29
Outstanding personal achievement	28
Wife begins or stops work	26
Begin or end school	26
Change in living conditions	25
Revision of personal habits	24
Trouble with boss	23
Change in work hours or conditions	20
Change in residence	20
Change in schools	20
Change in recreation	19
Change in church activities	19
Change in social activities	18
Mortgage or loan less than $10,000	17
Change in sleeping habits	16
Change in number of family get-togethers	15
Change in eating habits	15
Vacation	13
Christmas	12
Minor violations of the law	11

* Source: Dr. Thomas J. Holmes. From *The New York Times*, June 10, 1973.

dreams, fantasies, delusions, and hallucinations that occur after disconnection from reality. Autistic thinking is less subject to correction by reality and is much less likely to be followed by action.

Neologism is the coinage of new words, usu-ally by condensing several other words that have special meanings for the patient. In extreme forms of neologism, a word salad ensues that is characterized most of all by its unintelligibility.

Magical thinking refers to the belief that specific thoughts, verbalization, associations, gestures, or postures can in some mystical manner lead to the fulfillment of certain wishes or the warding off of certain evils. Young children are prone to this form of thinking as a consequence of their limited understanding of causality. It is a prominent aspect of obsessive-compulsive thinking. It achieves its most extreme expression in schizophrenia.

Intellectualization is a flight into intellectual concepts and words that are emotionally neutral in order to avoid objectionable feelings or impulses of a sexual or aggressive nature. It may take the form of brooding or anxious pondering about abstract, theoretical, or philosophical issues. It occurs commonly in normal adolescence. It is also seen in obsessive-compulsive neurosis, as a cognitive style in certain character types, and as a mechanism of defense in some schizophrenics.

Circumstantiality is a disorder of association in which too many associated ideas come into consciousness because of too little selective suppression. The circumstantial patient eventually reaches his goal in spite of many digressions. Circumstantiality may thus be distinguished from tangential thinking, in which the goal is never clearly defined or ever reached. In circumstantiality, excessive detail is used to describe simple events, at times to an absurd or bizarre degree. Like intellectualization, it often represents a way of avoiding objectionable impulses and feelings.

Tangential thinking involves verbal interjections that derail the dialogue. By moving at a tangent to the main orbit of the discussion, the patient avoids intimate interactions. A similar effect can result from punning, which is a form of tangential thinking.

Clang associations represent a thought disturbance in which the mere sound of the word, rather than its meaning, touches off a new train of thought. It is thus related to tangential thinking. It occurs most often in manic states with flight of ideas and may result in a series of punning and rhyming nonsensical associations.

Stereotypy is the constant repetition of a speech or action from force of habit or limitations of choice based on irrational fear or chronic mental disorder. When stereotypy expresses itself as the reiteration of a specific word or phrase, it is called verbigeration. It may occur in either spoken or written form. It is most often seen in schizophrenia.

Perseveration is the persisting response to a prior stimulus after a new stimulus has been presented. It is most often associated with organic brain disease.

The capacity for abstract thinking is impaired in many patients with organic brain disease. Schizophrenics, however, are often capable of a higher order of abstract thinking in the context of mathematics or other scientific work. Their difficulties with the interpretation of proverbs are the result of a tendency to bizarre idiosyncratic thinking.

Foreign-language patients who are depressed or frightened fall back on their mother tongue and seem incapable of speaking English. As such patients improve, they often surprise their physicians with the amount they do understand and the degree to which they can make themselves understood.

Blocking consists of sudden suppressions in the flow of thought or speech in the middle of a sentence. Commonly, the patient is unable to explain the reason for the interruption, which is usually the result of an unconscious mental intrusion. When, with conscious effort, the patient endeavors to continue the thought, new thoughts may crop up, which neither the patient nor the observer can bring into connection with the previous stream of thought. Blocking is also known as thought deprivation. It occurs most strikingly in schizophrenia.

In depressed states, the flow of associations is slowed up as an ongoing consequence of sadness. The patient thinks and speaks slowly. He is essentially unresponsive to his environment. In extreme states of slowing due to depression, the clinical picture may resemble the mutism of a catatonic schizophrenic.

As depression lifts, the rate of thought and speech also accelerates. If the condition swings over to a manic state, pressure of speech occurs; this voluble speech is difficult for the listener to interrupt. Pressure of speech may progress to flight of ideas, a nearly continuous high-speed flow of speech. The patient leaps rapidly from one topic to another, each topic being more or less meaningfully related to the preceding topic or to adventitious environmental stimuli, but progression of thought is illogical, and the goal is never reached.

Pressure of speech may occur more or less within the limits of normal conversation, and one then speaks of volubility. In certain neurotic disorders, talkativeness may acquire a compulsive quality that is called logorrhea. Logorrhea occasionally occurs episodically as a manifestation of temporal lobe epilepsy.

Organic brain disease is a major cause of disturbance in the flow of speech. Aphasia is a disturbance of language output, resulting almost always from damage to the left side of the brain. However distorted a patient's speech may sound, if his productions read as correct English sentences when transcribed, he is suffering not from aphasia but from some form of articulatory speech disability. Nonfluent aphasias result from lesions in Broca's area. These lesions generally involve the adjacent motor cortex and cause an associated hemiplegia. By contrast, fluent aphasias result from lesions in Wernicke's area and typically have no associated hemiplegia.

Anomic or amnestic aphasia is manifested by a difficulty in finding the right name for an object or person. In its mildest form it is seen in fatigue, anxiety, acute alcoholic intoxication, diffuse brain disease, and a variety of toxic-metabolic states. When this asphasia occurs acutely as a result of vascular occlusion, the lesion most commonly lies in the region of the angular gyrus.

Every patient who is aphasic in speech is also aphasic in writing, although a few patients are aphasic in writing but not in speech. Therefore, if a patient is able to produce full normal language in a written form but does not speak, one must conclude that he is suffering not from aphasia but from some form of mutism. Mutism may occur in catatonic schizophrenia, severe depressions, hysterical aphonia, and a variety of organic disorders involving the speech apparatus, as contrasted to the language areas of the left cerebral cortex. Patients with organic disorders of the speech apparatus may, on recovery, show dysarthria, difficulty in articulation but not in word-finding or in gammar.

Disturbances in Though Content

Certain types of thought content are essentially nonverbal. The most oustanding example is the mystical experience. This phenomenon can occur fleetingly in normal persons during the induction phase of general anesthesia. It may be chemically induced in addicts. It can occur transiently in schizophrenia and in the experiences of religious mystics.

A fantasy is a mental representation of a scene or occurrence that is recognized as unreal but is either expected or hoped for. Creative fantasy prepares for some later action. Daydreaming fantasy is the refuge for wishes that cannot be fulfilled. In autistic characters and in borderline psychotic states, daydreaming may pre-empt so much time and energy that it seriously impairs the person's capacity for normal relationships and responsibilities. Pseudologia fantastica or pathological lying differs from normal daydreaming in that the person believes in the reality of his fantasies intermittently and for long enough intervals of time to act on them. The impostor is a type of pathological liar who seeks to gain some advantage by imposing on others various lies about his attainments, social position, or worldly possessions.

A phobia is an exaggerated and invariably pathological dread of some specific type of stimulus or situation. Table II lists common phobias.

An obsession is the pathological presence of a persistent and irresistible thought, feeling, or impulse that cannot be eliminated from consciousness by any logical effort. Typically, the patient feels compelled to carry out specific ritualized or stereotyped acts, known as compulsions, in order to minimize their distressing effects—hence, obsessive-compulsive neurosis. Obsessive fears and doubts may overlap the phobias.

When thought content centers around a particular idea and is associated with a strong affective tone, the patient is said to be dominated by a trend or preoccupation.

When a patient ascribes personal significance to neutral remarks or comments, he is said to show referential thinking or to display ideas of reference. These ideas arise when the patient attributes to others thoughts and feelings that he himself has imagined, a process called projection. The associated pattern of oversuspiciousness is called paranoid thinking.

A delusion is a false belief that arises without appropriate external stimulation and that is maintained unshakably in the face of reason. The belief held is not ordinarily shared by other members of the patient's sociocultural and educational group. Delusions are pathognomonic of the psychoses. They occur most frequently in schizophrenia, but they can be observed in all psychotic states, including those of organic origin.

In some delusional states, persecutory feelings become attached to body feelings, such as intestinal movements or the sensation of stool in the rectum. Somatic delusions are characterized by their bizarre quality. In other delusional states, sexual feelings are attributed to a distantly located influencing machine operated by a persecutor.

Pathological jealousy may occur when a spouse has unconscious extramarital sexual impulses, either heterosexual or homosexual, which are then projected onto the marital partner and may emerge clinically as delusions of infidelity.

Litigiousness is a pathological tendency to take legal action because of imagined mistreatment or persecution.

Ecstatic states may be associated with delusions of grandeur or megalomania, a delusionally exaggerated idea of one's importance. Delusions of grandeur may result in identifications with political or military figures of great power.

TABLE II

Phobias*

Phobia	Dread of	Phobia	Dread of
Acro	High places	Nycto-	Darkness, night
Agora-	Open places		
Algo-	Pain	Patho-	Disease, suffering
Astra-	Thunder and lightning	(Noso-)	
(Astrapo-)		Peccato-	Sinning
Claustro-	Closed (confined) places	Phono-	Speaking aloud
		Photo-	Strong light
Copro-	Excreta		
Hemato-	Sight of blood	Sito-	Eating
		Tapho-	Being buried alive
Hydro-	Water		
Lalo-	Speaking		
(Glosso-)		Thanato-	Death
Myso-	Dirt, contamination	Toxo-	Being poisoned
		Xeno-	Strangers
Necro-	Dead bodies	Zoo-	Animals

* Modified from H. C. Warren, *Dictionary of Psychology*. Houghton Mifflin, New York, 1934.

The salvation of the world is the basic delusional goal. Often, this grandiose goal is to compensate for feelings of inadequacy. In manic states, inapporpriate delusions of great wealth may result in crippling financial expenditures.

A shift of mood from elation to depression may result in the self-accusatory delusion of having committed an unpardonable sin. This delusion is associated with intense guilt and remorse. In place of the delusions of saving the world, there may appear the end-of-the-world fantasy, the delusional belief that the world is about to come to an end. The patient may be convinced that the salvation of the world depends on his own death; as a consequence, he may destroy or seriously mutilate himself. In less bizarre terms, the depressed patient may feel that the world would be better off without him and may have suicidal impulses or ideation on an altruistic basis. In contrast to the delusion of great wealth, there may be, in the depressed state, a delusion of poverty. Loss of appetite for food may be the result of delusions of poisoning, as a result of which the patient does not eat, to the point of losing much weight.

Patients with widespread brain injury act like persons in a waking dream. They display the syndrome of anosognosia, the denial that physical illness is present. Some patients deny the major illness and ascribe the need for hospitalization to a trivial illness or to a previous illness from which they have long since recovered. On occasion, a patient admits that he cannot move a paralyzed leg but rationalizes this inability as a result of fatigue or laziness. A patient with a paralyzed limb may disown the incapacitated extremity by saying that it belongs to someone else.

In reduplication the patient acknowledges that he is in a hospital but insists that it is a good hospital, compared with one with the identical name nearby. A patient may acknowledge that a right arm is paralyzed but insist that there is an extra right arm that is not paralyzed.

The anosognosic patient may be mute and unresponsive when questioned by a physician and yet speak freely to a relative. Or the anosognosic patient may show a language disorder called paraphasia, the use of word substitutes. Other language patterns seen in anosognosic patients include intellectualization and the liberal use of clichés. Characteristic of anosognosic patients is the fact that they do not alter their basic errors, in spite of repeated corrections by the examiner. Since the fact of brain damage impairs the availability of language and ideas, anosognosic patients tend to lack verbal and ideational compexity.

Disturbances in Judgment.

Judgment is the mental act of comparing or evaluating alternatives within the framework of a given set of values for the purpose of deciding on a course of action. If the course of action decided on is consonant with reality as measured by mature adult standards, judgment is said to be good, intact, or normal. If, on the other hand, wish fulfilling impulses predominate and lead to impulsive decisions based on the need for immediate infantile gratification, judgment is said to be poor, impaired, or abnormal. Mental states that avoid painful reality are inevitably associated with impairment of judgment. Impaired judgment is a regular accompaniment of all psychotic states. And a significantly higher score in the performance scale over that in the verbal scale in the Wechsler Adult Intelligence Scale suggests a character disorder associated with impairment of judgment.

Disturbances in Intelligence.

Intelligence may be defined as the capacity to meet a novel situation by improvising a novel adaptive response. This capacity is composed of three factors: abstract intelligence, which is the capacity to understand and manage abstract ideas and symbols; mechanical intelligence, which is the capacity to understand, invent, and manage mechanisms; and social intelligence, which is the capacity to act reasonably and wisely in human relations and social affairs.

Mental retardation is a lack of intelligence to a degree in which there is interference with social and vocational performance.

The intelligence quotient (I.Q.) correlates with prognosis in schizophrenia. In a family predisposed to schizophrenia, the child with the lowest I.Q. is the most vulnerable to clinical disease.

Dyslexia—which is a syndrome characterized by a specific difficulty in learning to read, spell, and write—can masquerade as an impairment of intelligence. Frequently, secondary emotional and behavioral disorders confuse the clinical picture even further. The ratio of boys to girls with this disorder is above five to one.

Children and adolescents suffering from depression may surface clinically as academic underachievers and must be differentiated from those with other causes of learning disability.

Disturbances of Consciousness

Consciousness is synonymous with the quality of being aware and of having knowledge. It is a faculty of perception that draws on information from the outer world directly through the sense organs and indirectly through stored memory traces. Implicit in the concept of full consciousness is the capacity to understand information and to use it effectively to influence the relationship of the self to the environment.

Akinetic mutism or coma vigil is a syndrome usually associated with tumors of the third ventricle. Although essentially unresponsive to stimuli, patients in this condition do follow the human face. Sucking and grasping reflexes are also usually present.

Attention is an aspect of consciousness that relates to the amount of effort exerted in focusing on certain portions of an experience so that they become relatively more vivid. Primary attention is passive, involuntary, automatic, instinctive, or reflexive. Secondary attention is active or voluntary.

Attention may fluctuate in intensity from moment to moment in acute brain disorders and toxic metabolic states. In distractibility a person's attention is too easily drawn away from a given focus by extraneous stimuli. In its most extreme form it occurs in manic states. However, in milder forms it characterizes neurotic reactions of anxiety and depression and may play an important role in learning disabilities. Distractions may also be a result of the intrusion of fantasies, and these occur most intensely in schizophrenia. Attention span may be defined as the reciprocal of distractibility. In selective inattention or denial the person blocks out those environmental details that generate unpleasant feelings. An extreme form is seen in childhood schizophrenia as pain anosognosia, in which the child is not only unresponsive to pain but may inflict mutilating wounds on himself.

Self-consciousness is typically associated with lowered self-esteem and the expectation of rejection by others. It occurs in neurotic states of anxiety and depression, as well as in schizo-phrenia and the depressive psychoses. In the psychotic states the consciousness of self may become so extreme that one's own thoughts acquire the vividness of auditory hallucinations.

Suggestibility exists when a person reponds compliantly with unusual readiness. It can occur acutely when the person is overwhelmed by feelings of helplessness and passivity. Suggestibility can occur as an ongoing character trait in certain emotionally immature persons and expresses itself as gullibility. Extreme forms of suggestibility occur in catatonic stupor in the form of automatic obedience as echolalia, echopraxia, and waxy flexibility.

In catatonic stupor the patient is motionless, mute, and more or less nonresponsive to painful stimuli. The patient is aware of his environment with a clarity and intensity that is belied by his superficially stuporous appearance.

Suggestibility also plays an important role in communicated insanity (*folie á deux*), a psychotic reaction in which two or more closely related and associated persons simultaneously show the same symptoms and in which one member seems to have influenced or suggested the clinical picture to the other.

In hypnosis the subject enters into a hyperattentive relationship with the hypnotist during which a trance state occurs, characterized by heightened suggestibility. As a result, a variety of hysterialike sensory and motor abnormalities may be induced, as well as dissociative states and hypermnesia.

Dissociation means a loss of the usual consistency and relatedness between various groups of mental processes. Dissociation and splitting are used more or less synonymously, but dissociative usually refers to hysterical or hypnosis-induced dissociative states, whereas splitting is used with reference to schizophrenia. Dissociation underlies every symptom of hysteria.

Double and multiple personalities are the terms applied when a person at different times appears to be in possession of an entirely different mental content, disposition, and character and when one of the different phases shows complete ignorance of the other.

In trance states, which may occur spontaneously in hysteria or in response to hypnotic suggestion, the apparently sleeping subject may express the dissociative state in the form of automatic writing. The performance of automatic writing and other actions during a trance state in response to a command or a suggestion is called command automatism.

Perhaps the most familiar example of a dissociative state is that experienced during a nightmare. At a particularly terrifying moment in the dream, the dreamer may suddenly reassure himself: "This is only a dream. You are not in real danger. You can wake up any time you want."

An automatism is an activity performed without conscious knowledge on the part of the subject and is usually followed by complete amnesia. It occurs most often after a grand mal seizure, head trauma, or pathological alcoholic intoxication. It may also occur as a posthypnotic suggestion.

Some teenagers display one moral code while at home or in school and a completely dissociated (delinquent) code while with the gang. And students of mob psychology have noted the elation, the impulsivity, the general emotional regression, and the personality dissociation that can occur in a seemingly normal adult when he becomes part of a mob.

Sleep Disturbances.

Sleep is a complex state of altered consciousness consisting of at least four separate stages of varying depth, sensory and motor activity, and responsivity.

Narcolepsy is characterized by a sudden overpowering desire to sleep. The patient goes to sleep anywhere, anytime. The sleep may last from a few seconds to several minutes; only rarely does it last a few hours. The patient can generally be aroused easily, and, when he wakes, he is perfectly fresh and able to go on with his work. He may have several attacks in a day. Associated with narcolepsy is cataplexy, which consists of attacks of sudden weakness, limpness of the arms or legs, or falling of the head to one side. During the cataplectic attack, the patient cannot speak. These attacks are often brought on by strong emotion, such as a sudden burst of laughter, anger, surprise, or pleasure.

Night terror, also known as pavor nocturnus, is in its most severe form, a combination of extreme panic, fight-flight reaction in the form of motility and somnambulism, and sleep utterances in the form of gasps, moans, groans, curses, and blood-curdling, piercing screams. The person may be hallucinating and delusional while he acts out the night-terror. Heart rates

attain levels of 160 to 170 a minute in 15 to 30 seconds. The respiratory rate is increased, but the most striking change is a tremendous increase in respiratory amplitude. The entire episode lasts one to two minutes, and the person returns to sleep rapidly. The content of the episode usually consists of a single, brief, frightening image or thought, such as the idea of an intruder in the room, and contrasts strikingly with the nightmare, which is more complex in content and far less severe in its somatic concomitants.

Insomnia is a pathological inability to sleep. In catatonic or manic excitement the patient may remain uninterruptedly sleepless for 24 to 48 hours at a time. These reactions of extreme excitement may go on to hyperthermia and death due to exhaustion.

Depressed patients usually complain of frequent awakenings during the night but most of all of early-morning insomnia; the patient wakes up too early and is often bathed in anguished perspiration. This sleep pattern is commonly associated with anorexia, weight loss, feelings of sadness, and suicidal ideation.

Inability to fall asleep is a form of insomnia more characteristic of the neuroses. The patient often fears sleep because of nightmares. This phenomenon is particularly common in the traumatic neuroses induced by battlefield experiences.

Hypersomnia or excessive sleeping is often seen in depressive reactions occurring in neurosis. It is commonly associated with other depressive equivalents, such as overeating, and a variety of other addictive states, as well as sexual and aggressive acting out and academic underachievement. It may also occur in the early stage of a psychotic depressive illness.

Reversal of sleep habit is a common accompaniment of hypersomnia. The patient sleeps soundly through the early morning hours, wakes up gradually in the early afternoon, and achieves full wakefulness at a time when most people are going to bed.

Drowsiness is characterized by a general slowing up of the thought processes, with a tendency to concrete thinking and hallucinatory phenomena, auditory and visual, which can occur normally just before sleep (hypnagogic hallucinations) or waking (hypnopompic hallucinations).

Somnolence is abnormal drowsiness. It occurs in a variety of toxic, metabolic, and inflammatory diseases of the brain and with brain tumors that press on the floor of the third ventricle.

Epileptic and Convulsive Disorders

The essence of epilepsy is the periodic recurrence of short-lived disturbances of consciousness. Petit mal and grand mal seizures are characteristically associated with full loss of consciousness in the midst of the attack. In petit mal epilepsy consciousness blinks on and off for intervals lasting between 1 and 40 seconds each. These individual attacks are not associated with a preattack warning and are not followed by characteristic subjective or objective sequelae. The attacks may occur as often as 100 times in a single day or as occasional, isolated attacks days or weeks apart.

In grand mal epilepsy muscular movements are typically preceded by an aura, which may consist of a variety of clouded states of general awareness, including feelings of unreality and depersonalization. Such preconvulsive alterations of consciousness may last for hours or even days before the actual seizure. During the convulsion, loss of consciousness is complete, and amnesia for the events during the actual seizure is also complete. After the grand mal seizure, the patient displays a clouded state of consciousness, which varies in duration from a few minutes to a period of hours. Amnesia for the postseizure period may be complete or interspersed with fragmentary islands of recall.

Twilight states, dreamlike states of consciousness, can occur as independent seizure phenomena apart from grand mal seizures and are called psychomotor epilepsy. If the associated EEG abnormality is confined to the temporal lobe, one may speak of temporal lobe epilepsy; if the twilight states are associated with unpleasant olfactory and gustatory hallucinations, with tasting tongue and lip movements, one may speak of uncinate fits. They are also characterized by circumscribed periods of intellectual dulling, disturbances in consciousness, confusion, and disorientation. Brief auditory and visual hallucinatory symptoms and schizophreniclike psychotic reactions have been described. Generally, there is an amnesia for actions during this period.

Disturbances of Orientation

Orientation may be defined as the ability to recognize one's surroundings and their temporal and spatial relationships to one's self or to appreciate one's relations to the social environment. The capacity for orientation involves time, place, and person.

Disorientation for Time

Hospitalized patients without organic brain disease commonly lose track of the date, the day of the week, and even the month. Correct answers may be expressive of an alert and intact sensorium, but errors in these categories are not diagnostic of organic brain disease. An error in the year, on the other hand, is of diagnostic significance. Errors for the time of day are significant as evidence of organic brain disease if the error crosses a mealtime.

Neurotic problems involving rebellious attitudes or a need to avoid painful reality may result in patterns of persistent tardiness. The affective state also plays a role in temporal orientation. During moods of elation, time seems to move quickly, whereas depressive moods are associated with a feeling that time is dragging.

Disorientation for Place

The brain-injured patient in a general hospital may express the wish to be well by insisting that he is not in a hospital but in his home, a hotel, a restaurant, or a convalescent home. On occasion, the patient gives the name of the hospital correctly but places the hospital close to home or locates himself in another hospital in which he was treated many years ago for a relatively minor illness from which he recovered. Temporal disorientation commonly accompanies this pattern of spatial disorientation. In duplication or reduplicative paramnesia, patients give the name and location of the hospital correctly but insist that another "bad" hospital with the same name is located nearby.

Schizophrenic patients may be disoriented for place in less predictable ways but always meaningfully in terms of their delusions.

Disorientation for Person

A married female patient displaying disorientation for person may give her maiden name and insist that she is not married. Such denials often express elements of marital disharmony from which the patient wishes to take flight. They may also be associated with temporal disorientation representing regression to a time preceding the onset of illness.

Anosognosic patients tend to misidentify to deny illness. The hospital doctor in a white coat may be identified as a fish peddler and the place of their encounter as the Fulton Fish Market. Some physical or characterological trait in a doctor or nurse may be the basis for a persistent misidentification of this person as a friend from the past who has no connection with illness.

Duplication may involve not only the entire person but part of a person. For instance, a hemiplegic patient may insist that he has two left arms, one good left arm and one bad left arm.

In patients without organic brain disease, the concept of self may be so chaotic that the vulnerable patient tends to be highly suggestible and to identify with any dominant person he is with. He may incorporate specific mannerisms of speech and dress and self-destructive patterns of behavior, such as narcotic addiction. This instability of self-concept is particularly conspicuous in teenage girls, who are vulnerable to mass hysterical behavior. The chaotic concept of self most characteristic of adolescents is what Erikson refers to as the identity crisis.

Disturbances of Memory

Memory is based on three essential processes: registration, the ability to establish a record of an experience in the central nervous system; retention, the persistence or permanence of a registered experience; and recall, the ability to arouse and report in consciousness a previously registered experience.

Although a good memory is one of the factors in the complex of mental capacities that make up intelligence, phenomenal feats of memory are occasionally encountered in settings of apparent mental retardation. These feats of memory usually involve rote memory, the capacity to retain and reproduce data verbatim, without reference to meaning.

Some persons are particularly well endowed with visual memory and can recall images with virtual hallucinatory intensity. Such subjects are called eidetic persons, and the reproduced memories are called eidetic images. This eidetic capacity tends to occur in childhood and subside with age. Eidetic mental retardates tend to retain this quality longer than normal subjects.

Memory for music, mathematics, muscular movements such as those involved in the performing arts, spatial relationships, and emotional feelings are examples of nonverbal memory. Verbal memories depend on the development of verbal skills.

Disturbances in Registration

Registration depends on the level of consciousness. Anything that diminishes consciousness, such as alcoholism or concussion, interferes with registration. A circumscribed memory loss occurring during the time after an acute brain injury is called anterograde amnesia. Disturbed states of consciousness lasting for weeks and months associated with encephalitis, subarachnoid hemorrhage, and severe brain trauma may be followed by a permanent inability to recall the events experienced during that period because of defects involving registration and retention. Electroconvulsive therapy (ECT) may be followed by both anterograde amnesia and retrograde amnesia, memory loss for events preceding shock therapy. With cessation of ECT, memory functioning rapidly improves. The term "retrograde amnesia" is also used for a memory pattern found in chronic organic brain disease, such as senile dementia, in which the capacity to recall recent events is primarily impaired, whereas memory for remote events remains relatively intact.

In catatonic schizophrenia and severe panic states, registration seems to be impaired because the patient appears to be totally nonreactive. However, when the brain is intact but perceived experiences are repressed or denied for purely emotional reasons, registration is normal.

Disturbances in Retention

In the establishment of lasting memories, there is a preliminary learning stage during which the memory trace is unstable. For persons with good memories, memory traces are quickly established, and the curve of forgetting is prolonged and may extend over the entire lifetime. In some instances of organic brain disease, the curve of forgetting is accelerated. In Korsakoff's psychosis, memory for recently acquired facts may decay in a matter of seconds.

Disturbances in Recall

Amnesia is the partial or total inability to recall past experiences. Chronic brain disease impairs both registration and recall. This is seen in Korsakoff's syndrome, vascular disease, senile dementia, and tumor. When memories are presumed to have been formed and stored permanently but access to them is somehow prevented, the result is an amnesia that in many cases is temporary and treatable. This is referred to as recall amnesia. Most amnesias seen in relation to organic brain disease are mixed amnesias with both organic deficits and emotional interference with recall.

Hysterical amnesia is a loss of memory for a particular period of past life or for certain situations associated with great fear, rage, or shameful humiliation. This form of amnesia is highly selective and systematized to fulfill the patient's specific emotional needs.

The brain-injured patient who is highly motivated may succeed in overcoming organically determined impairments of recall by a variety of mnemonic devices.

The hysterical fugue state is a form of dissociative reaction that sets in after a severe emotional trauma. Usually, the lost memory is readily recoverable with hypnosis, narcoanalysis, or strong suggestion, particularly when offered in a setting that promises extended relief or physical separation from the traumatic life situation.

Paramnesia is a distortion of recall resulting from the inclusion of false details, meanings, or emotions or wrong temporal relationships. It is also known as *fausee reconnaisance* and retrospective falsification.

Confabulation is the unconscious filling in of memory gaps by imagined experiences. It is characteristic of diffuse organic brain disease. These recollections change from moment to moment and are easily induced by suggestion.

Déjà vu is an illusion of recognition in which a new situation is incorrectly regarded as a repetition of a previous memory. It can occur in normal persons, particularly in settings generating anxiety. It is more common in neurotic states and occurs occasionally in the aura of grand mal epilepsy. In *jamais vu* there is a feeling of unfamiliarity with a situation that one has actually experienced.

Related to *déjà vu* are *déjà entendu*, in which a comment never heard before is incorrectly regarded as a repetition of a previous conversation, and *déjà pensé*, in which a thought never entertained before is incorrectly regarded as a repetition on a previous thought.

Hypermnesia is the capacity for an exaggerated degree of recall. It can be elicited episodically in a hypnotic trance. It is seen as an ongoing state in certain prodigies, obsessive-compulsive neurosis, paranoia, and mania.

Disturbances in Perception

Perception is the awareness of objects, qualities, or relations that follows stimulation of peripheral sense organs, as distinct from the awareness that results from memory. Perception is connected with memory through the process of memory registration. Impairments in perception set the stage for delusions, hallucinations, and a variety of misinterpretations of reality.

A lesion in Wernicke's area gives rise to agnosia, an inability to recognize and interpret the significance of sensory impressions. This inability sets the stage for anosognosia, the delusional denial of physical illness. Clouding of consciousness due to diffuse brain disease gives rise to a variety of perceptual disturbances. Many central nervous system toxins are hallucinogens with differing effects on specific sensory modalities.

Perception begins with a tuning-in process, an act of paying attention. Depressed patients see less because of lack of interest. Schizophrenics are inclined to see less because they fear what they see. Manic patients may seem to take in everything, but their perceptual pattern is primarily in the service of avoiding key issues.

Apperception is conscious awareness of the significance of a percept. It is based on the complex psychological components that determine its total impact.

Emotionally induced fainting eliminates all perception. (See Figure 2.) Circumscribed eliminations of perception may occur as a device for coping with traumatic stimuli and are usually part of the syndrome of hysteria. Any modality of perception may be disordered in hysteria.

In macropsia, objects appear larger than they really are. In micropsia, objects appear smaller than they really are. The condition may alternate with macropsia in hysteria, but it has also been described as an aura in epilepsy.

Frigidity, including all degrees of anesthesia of the vagina and external genitalia, is a common hysterical defense against sexual excitement. In each circumstance, there is a with-

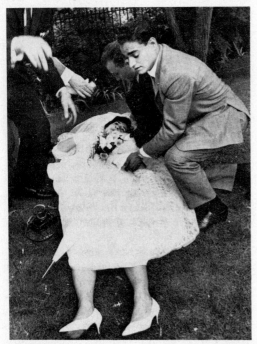

FIG. 2. The marriage ceremony is a stress for some people and in cases of extreme anxiety, fainting eliminates the need to cope with this stressful situation. Emotionally induced fainting is part of the hysterical syndrome (Magnum Photos, Inc.).

drawal of attention from potentially traumatic external events.

Just as withdrawal of attention from a body part can reduce perception to the point of complete anesthesia, so can a sensory end organ be overinvested with attention because of anxiety. There may be areas of hyperalgesia to touch, headaches, and other body pains.

Hypochondriasis

A generalized withdrawal of attention from external objects is almost always followed by an increase in the attention focused on the self as an object. A pathological awareness of body feelings may emerge. This awareness is the basis for hypochondriasis, the unshakable belief that widespread physical disease is present, in the face of all evidence to the contrary. The symptom is most common in the depressions, particularly those of the involutional period. It may take bizarre forms in schizophrenia, in which case one may speak more appropriately of somatic delusions. It may occur in a chronic low-grade form over a period of years as part of a neurotic reaction. An important difference be-

tween the hysteric and the hypochondriac is the degree to which contacts with real objects in the external world have been retained or surrendered.

Illusions

In an illusion there is perceptual misinterpretation of a real external sensory experience. A schizophrenic patient may hear an insulting remark in the chime of a clock or feel the sinister hand of death in a casual handshake. Illusions may occur in certain toxic states. Frightened reactions to ambiguous or neutral stimuli indicate that the patient is projecting and is on the threshold of ideas of reference.

Hallucinations

A hallucination is the apparent perception of an external object when no corresponding real object exists. A dream is a simple example of a hallucination in normal experience. Any modality of perception may be involved. Hypnagogic hallucinations occur in the drowsy state preceding deep sleep. They may contain both auditory and visual elements with great clarity and intensity. Hypnopompic hallucinations occur during the drowsy state after deep sleep and before awakening.

The schizophrenic may experience hallucinations as vivid as those experienced by normal people during dreams. He often acts on these inner perceptions, as though they were more compelling than the external realities that compete for his attention.

Hallucinosis is a psychotic state in which the patient seems to be alert and well-oriented, in spite of the fact that he is hallucinating. Such patients may slip in and out of the hallucinatory state, with intervals of insight and lucidity. A group of hallucinogenic psychotomimetic drugs characteristically elicit hallucinosis. Mescaline and lysergic acid diethylamide (LSD) are well-known representatives of this group of drugs.

In the convulsive disorders, relatively unformed percepts may occur during the aura. Olfactory and gustatory hallucinations occur in temporal lobe lesions in the uncinate fits. Social patients may experience nausea or flashes of light as part of the aura. Less commonly, the aura in uncinate fits is associated with complex hallucinatory experiences involving visual and auditory components and possessing an affective quality of reminiscence.

Generalized organic brain disease of almost any cause can be associated with hallucinatory states that are at times indistinguishable from schizophrenia. Atropine and its derivatives may cause characteristic Lilliputian hallucinations in drug-sensitive patients. In Lilliputian hallucinations the hallucinated objects, usually people, appear greatly reduced in size. They are to be differentiated from micropsia, a hysterical phenomenon in which real objects in the environment appear reduced in size.

Relatively small doses of alcohol or marijuana can produce hallucinations in sensitive subjects. Even the phenothiazines, which are administered to decrease psychotic manifestations, may intensify hallucinations or elicit new ones.

Patients who are chronically habituated to any sedative substance—such as alcohol, barbiturates, meprobamate, or diazepoxide—often experience hallucinations when these drugs are withdrawn. These hallucinatory states are commonly associated with great terror.

Brain tumors, subarachnoid hemmorrhage, uremia, strokes, endocrine abnormalities, and a variety of drugs may help initiate hallucinatory states. Different chemical agents may have the same hallucinatory effect on a given person, and conversely, a given chemical may produce widely varying responses in different persons. In addition, the effect of a chemical agent varies with the mood, social setting, and physical condition of the patient.

Hallucinations and delusions occur on a continuum and are measured by the degree of the patient's conviction of the objective reality of a bizarre experience.

A haptic hallucination is one associated with the sensation of touch. Although it may occur in schizophrenia, it is more common in delirium tremens, in which these cutaneous hallucinations are commonly associated with visual hallucinations of tiny, crawling animals. Creeping sensations under the skin are known as formication. Olfactory and gustatory hallucinations of bad tastes and odors may be encountered as part of the aura of temporal lobe epilepsy (uncinate fit). They may also occur in schizophrenia, with complex delusional elaborations of being poisoned. The auditory sphere is probably the most frequently involved sensory modality in the hallucinations of schizophrenia. Kinesthetic hallucinations may occur in amputees, as part of the phantom limb experience.

As in dreams, memory traces constitute the building blocks of hallucinations. The content reflects the effort to master anxiety and to fulfill various wishes and needs. Whereas patients with organic brain disease tend to express simple ideas related to the wish to be well and to be home, patients with functional psychoses express more complex ideas based on interactions with imagined partners and concern themselves primarily with sexual and aggressive drives that the patient has been unable to master in real life.

Disturbances in Affect

Affect is the feeling tone, pleasurable or unpleasurable, that accompanies an idea. Affect and emotion are used interchangeably and include such feelings as rage, grief, and joy. Affect determines the general attitude, whether rejection, acceptance, flight, fight, or indifference. Affect may be described as shallow or inadequate (emotional flatness), inappropriate (when the emotion does not correspond to the stimulus), or labile (changeable).

Attitude refers to the affective state with which a person habitually confronts his environment. Attitude is determined in early childhood by what Erikson called basic trust.

Disposition refers to the affective state with which a person habitually confronts himself. Whenever what Erikson called basic security has evolved, there is also a clear sense of personal identity. Associated with this sense is a sustaining sense of well-being and optimism. Basic security is part of self-esteem or normal narcissism.

Conscious human behavior is the result, primarily, of certain felt needs and can be divided simply into two main categories, those associated with pleasure, which result in movements toward a goal, and those associated with pain, which result in movements away.

Euphoria refers to the first, moderate level in the scale of pleasurable affects. It is a positive feeling of emotional and physical well-being. When it occurs in a manifestly inappropriate setting, it is indicative of mental disorder. Although it is usually psychogenic, it may be observed in organic brain disease.

Elation, the second level in the scale of pleasurable affects, is characterized by a definite affect of gladness in which there is an air of enjoyment and self-confidence, and motor activity is increased. This affect belongs within the limits of normal life experience, yet it may be indicative of mental disorders when it occurs in a manifestly inappropraite setting.

Various pharmacological agents may induce euphoria or elation. Alcohol, narcotics, and the amphetamines enable the person to repress or deny the existence of painful affects. Brain lesions may have a similar impact on painful affects.

By using the psychological defense mechanism of denial or selective inattention, some patients avoid confrontations with traumatic percepts, and, by means of repression, they avoid confrontations with painful memories. If these mechanisms are sufficiently successful, a psychotic state supervenes. The manic patient feels elated. Often, the manic reaction thinly disguises an underlying depression, by which it may be abruptly replaced. In some instances, a hypomanic reaction may be indefinitely prolonged and may be regarded as a hypomanic character disorder.

Exaltation is extreme elation; it is usually associated with delusions of grandeur. It merges into ecstasy, which represents a peak state of rapture. These affects in inappropriate circumstances are found almost exclusively in relation to psychosis.

Anxiety

Anxiety is a disagreeable emotional state with feelings of impending danger, characterized by uneasiness, tension, or apprehension. The cause is usually unconscious or unrecognized intrapsychic conflict. Anxiety is associated with a characteristic pattern of autonomic nervous system discharge involving altered respiration rate, increased heart rate, pallor, dryness of the mouth, increased sweating, and musculoskeletal disturbances, involving trembling and feelings of weakness. Anxiety is to be differentiated from fear, a reaction to a real, conscious, and external danger that is present or that threatens to materialize. Panic is a state of extreme, acute, intense anxiety accompanied by disorganization of personality and function.

Free-floating anxiety is the nucleus and key symptom of neurosis. It consists of a feeling of dread that the patient cannot logically assign to a specific cause.

Anxiety neurosis is a neurotic state based primarily on free-floating anxiety. It is characterized by irritability, anxious expectation, pangs of conscience, and episodes of panic. There is hypersensitivity to ordinary sights and sounds. Cardiac palpitation, breathlessness, giddiness, nausea, dryness of mouth, diarrhea, compulsive eating, urinary frequency, seminal emissions, blurring of vision, general physical weakness, and other physical manifestations may occur chronically as part of anxiety neurosis. In an effort to reduce the unpleasant feelings associated with anxiety, the person evolves a variety of defensive devices.

Conversion hysteria is a neurosis characterized by sensory and motor deficits without a corresponding structural organic lesion. Often, the patient displays an attitude of calm (*la belle indifference*) that contrasts strangely with the extent of the physical disability.

Anxiety hysteria is a neurosis in which the patient develops fears or phobias in relation to specific situations that may stimulate erotic or aggressive impulses unconsciuosly desired and rejected by the patient.

Depression

The phenomena associated with depression are often indistinguishable from those seen in bereavement, the normal reaction of grief and mourning. What differentiates a depressive neurosis from a normal mourning reaction is the severity of the depression and its persistence beyond a reasonable period of mourning.

Certain medications can precipitate a severe depression. Reserpine and corticosteroids in high dosages and phenothiazines are familiar examples. Retroperitoneal neoplasms, such as carcinoma of the pancreas and lymphoma, can precipitate depression. Depressive illness may set in after certain viral infections, such as hepatitis, infectious mononucleosis, and influenza. In addition, there is evidence for a biologically based hereditary factor in vulnerability to depression, particularly in the recurrent depressions of manic-depressive illness.

Some depressive symptoms are best understood as a cry for help. When depressogenic factors first appear, the victim often displays a reaction of protest.

The somatic complaints commonly seen in depression may have symbolic connections with a loved one from whom separation is dreaded or has already occurred. In these instances one is dealing primarily with conversion hysteria. In other instances the patient may complain of an existing relatively mild physical disorder, in the hope that hospitalization will provide an escape from an unbearable conflict or compel attention that is not otherwise obtainable.

The patient may develop a reaction of detachment associated with feelings of depersonalization, derealization, and long-lasting personality impairments. The entire spectrum of addictive states can be understood as attempts to ward off depression. The patient may seek to overcome feelings of emptiness by various forms of acting out. The patient may retreat into patterns of excessive sleep.

While these defenses against depression operate, the person may seem to be cheerful, on occasion even functioning competently and successfully. Yet close inspection reveals a joylessness in these activities. The patient lives rigidly and compulsively.

When the breakthrough occurs, the very appearance of the victim changes. He looks old and sad. In simple depression, psychological and motor spontaneity are lost. All previous interests are lost. There is anorexia, with weight loss. There is loss of sexual desire and of interest in recreation, work, family, and friends. He complains of an indescribable misery that he sometimes locates in his chest or abdomen. He is filled with self-reproach and is convinced that he is a failure. He expresses feelings of pessimism, poverty, hopelessness, and futility. He is filled with guilt and shame. He expects punishment. He has suicidal thoughts and impulses. Insomnia sets in and is most commonly associated with frequent waking spells during the night and early-morning agitation, with sweating and feelings of anguish. As interest in the outer world is withdrawn, there comes an intensified awareness of the body, with hypochondriasis and somatic delusions.

If a reactive depression is so severe that effective contact with reality is lost and is accompanied by the appearance of delusions and severe suicidal ideation, this is called a psychotic depressive reaction and is seen, for example, in postpartum depression. Many depressions occur without a clearly recognizable connection to external life circumstances. One may then speak of endogenous depression. If there is a history of one or more previous episodes of depression, with intervening normal periods, one speaks of manic-depressive illness, depressed type. When manic as well as depressive episodes occur in the life history, one speaks of manic-depressive illness, circular type. When a patient develops a psychotic depression for the first time during the involutional period, one speaks of involutional melancholia. Some patients show schizophrenic symptoms mixed with depression. These patients often have a history of episodic illness, with intervals of relatively normal functioning, and are classified as having schizophrenia, schizo-affective type. In transient situational disturbance, depression can be a prominent feature. This category is reserved for disorders that occur in persons without any apparent underlying mental disorder and that represent an acute reaction to overwhelming environmental stress.

Anaclitic depression refers to the syndrome shown by infants during the first years of life if they are deprived of the attentions of a suitable mothering figure. On separation from the mother, the infant goes through a characteristic sequence of changes. There is an initial phase of protest, characterized by intense crying and struggling. If this state of deprivation continues, the infant lapses into the phase of despair. At this point, behavior suggests hopelessness. Struggling decreases, and crying is softer and monotonous. The infant may stop eating and then waste away and die, a state called marasmus. Or he may lapse into a phase of detachment in which he withdraws from human relationships and becomes preoccupied with inanimate objects or his own body parts, engaging in masturbation, fecal smearing, head banging, or rocking.

In the aged, loss of love objects presents a universal psychological problem. The loss of an accustomed work role presents a number of social problems. And the loss of general physical health and brain power represents a major loss. Depression is the most common psychiatric symptom in old age.

Depression can appear paradoxically as the aftermath of some great success in those who are destroyed by success. To avoid this kind of depression these patients are characteristically self-defeating.

Suicide is an important consideration in the problems of depression.

Aggression

Aggression is a constellation of specific thoughts, feelings, and actions; it is mobilized by an obstruction to a wish or need; and its goal is to remove the obstruction in order to permit drive discharge. Aggression is inseparable from the complex of wishes and needs that together make up the life drive or the wish to live.

Family quarrels and social situations that threaten self-esteem commonly precipitate acts of violence. Episodes of violence may occur as manifestations of a seizure disorder. Schizophrenics may become violent when unwanted intimacies are forced on them. Violence associated with criminal acts of breaking and entering may be connected with perverse sexual impulses. Sadistic and masochistic fantasies may inadvertently lead to violence.

Irritability is a chronic diffuse state of anger that occurs as an interpersonal distance-regulating device. It may occur in paranoid personality disorder. It is commonly encountered in adolescents who are warding off sexually charged encounters with parents or siblings.

Vandalism is an act of indiscriminate violence that has many qualities in common with the temper tantrum of a child. It represents a displacement from the true target of the rage and is associated with a personal feeling of impotent fury.

Ambivalence refers to the coexistence of antithetical emotions, attitudes, ideas, or wishes toward a given object or situation. Usually, only one attitude emerges into consciousness, the other remaining unconscious. Ambivalence is encountered in all instances of affective instability.

Compound Emotions

Smugness is compounded of self-satisfaction, self-absorption, and a reduced awareness of the environment. With it, there is also greediness and grasping, without associated guilt (see Table III).

Bitterness is a feeling of resentment over what appears to be a justified grievance. It is associated with demands for redress.

Boredom is a state of dissatisfaction and disinclination to act. Time drags in a manner similar to depression, but the feeling is one of emptiness or apathy.

Pathological jealousy is compounded of grief, hatred, loss of self-esteem, and ambivalence. It may have its roots in unconscious homosexual attachments and merge into paranoid delusional thinking.

Vengefulness is a striving toward an object, as in love, but for the purpose of ensuring its destruction. It is associated with a desire to get even and is calculated to assuage guilt and to relieve feelings of fear and hatred.

Curiosity is a feeling state that gives rise to exploratory behavior. It is a drive to generate and increase anticipatory pleasure.

Mechanisms for Maintaining Mood Control

Mood is a sustained and prevailing emotional set. The defense mechanisms include repression, denial, projection, sublimation, intellectualization, rationalization, regression, suppression, reaction formation, undoing, introjection, identification, isolation, and displacement. One may also include depersonalization and derealization.

Depersonalization is a mental phenomenon characterized by a feeling of unreality and strangeness about one's self. Derealization is a mental phenomenon characterized by loss of the sense of reality concerning one's surroundings. Derealization includes distortions of spatial and temporal relationships so that an essentially neutral environment seems strangely familiar (*déjà vu*) or strangely unfamiliar (*jamais vu*) or otherwise strange and distorted. Both depersonalization and derealization can be partial or complete, transient or long-lasting. They may occur in hysteria or as part of the aura of epilepsy but tend to be most complete and persistent in schizophrenic states.

Defense or distance-regulating mechanisms may be established during a developmental period when they fulfill a more or less useful

TABLE III

Catalog of the Emotions

Anger	Envy	Petulance
Anxiety	Faith	Poise
Arrogance	Fear	Querulence
Bitterness	Gloating	Rage
Boredom	Gratitude	Sadism
Cheating	Grief	Sarcasm
Confusion	Guilt	Shame
Curiosity	Gullibility	Shyness
Cynicism	Hate	Smugness
Depression	Homesickness	Teasing
Derision	Hope	Trust
Disillusionment	Jealousy	Uncanny feelings
Elation	Masochism	Vengefulness
Enthusiasm	Nostalgia	

adaptational function. With further maturation, these mechanisms may outlive this function and become counterproductive. The removal of such mechanisms can result in depression or substitute symptom formation or may necessitate alterations in basic relationships.

Disturbances in Motor Aspects of Behavior

Conation or the conative aspect of mental functioning refers to the capacity to initiate action or motor discharge and concerns the basic strivings of a person as expressed through his behavior. The affective component of an idea determines the force and the direction of the action that follows that idea.

The simple schizophrenic has difficulty initiating goal-directed activity. He may in some instances be capable of useful work if it is initiated for him and carried out under supervision, as in a sheltered workshop. Some schizophrenics respond to suggestions automatically and uncritically (command automatism) or by echolalia, the pathological repetition by imitation of the speech of another person. Echopraxia is the pathological repetition by imitation of the movements of another person. Waxy flexibility (cerea flexibilitas) is the maintenance by a patient of imposed postures with increased muscle tone, as when a limb remains passively in the position in which it is placed. Waxy flexibility is most characteristic of catatonic schizophrenia.

Learned sphincter control may be lost during periods of emotional stress. In adult patients, encopresis, loss of anal sphincter control, is usually a result of organic disease of the central nervous system. In the absence of organic disease, encopresis is usually associated with schizophrenia.

A mannerism is a gesture or other form of motor expression peculiar to a given person. It is used interchangeably with stereotypy and posturing, assuming specific physical attitudes.

The startle reaction is a reflex response to an unexpected stimulus of great intensity. It is associated with a sudden increase in the level of consciousness and a diffuse motor response involving flexion movements of the trunk and extremities. It may be elicited in acute anxiety neurosis.

Overactivity

The hyperkinetic child is characterized by overactivity, distractibility, impulsiveness, and excitability. The condition occurs predominantly in boys. It is associated with difficulties in peer relationships, with disciplinary problems, and with severe learning impairments. Children and adolescents suffering from depression often show hyperactivity. Depressed adolescents may be reckless, antisocial, and sexually promiscuous.

Agitation refers to a state of pacing, hand-wringing, and verbalized complaints of suffering, which occurs in agitated depression.

The phenothiazines and other antipsychotic drugs can cause a variety of motor abnormalities that are regarded as extrapyramidal side effects.

Hysterical convulsions usually consist of pantomimic expressions of sexual and aggressive fantansies. Occasionally, a hysteric patient mimics a grand mal seizure.

Sleepwalking, somnambulism, is primarily a motor disturbance of childhood. It is often associated with sleeptalking and enuresis. It seems to be related to nocturnal fears and loneliness and a wish to enter the parental bed. It is also associated with pavor nocturnus.

Neurotic reactions of the obsessive-compulsive type are characterized both by obsessive thoughts and by complex compulsive rituals. Most common are compulsive hand-washing, counting, and repetitive ceremonial rituals. In each instance, the compulsive act simultaneously carries out a forbidden wish and then undoes it.

Other types of compulsive acts are not usually connected with obsessive-compulsive neurosis—for example, alcoholism (dipsomania), compulsive stealing (kleptomania), compulsive fire setting (pyromania), and compulsive sexual acting out in a woman (nymphomania).

The compulsive eating of scaling wall paint in children is called pica. It has been hypothesized that an underlying nutritional deficiency is the cause. However, the missing ingredient is usually an unavailable mother.

A tic is an intermittent spasmodic twitching of the face or other body part, repeated at frequent intervals and without external stimulus.

Manic patients may talk, sing, dance, and joke with apparently inexhaustible energy and good spirits. In agitated depression, there may be crying, pacing, and wringing of hands. In catatonic excitement, the pattern of overactivity is extreme and bewildering. Talking, which may be loud and voluble, is in response to delusions and hallucinations. The excited catatonic patient may execute various gestures that have the intent of influencing the world by means of magic.

Underactivity (Psychomotor Retardation)

Simple depression is characterized by the absence of anxiety and by decreased motor activity. There is a feeling of pronounced fatigue and great difficulty in initiating any activity, including speech. Responses to stimuli are slowed up. The patient's posture is expressive of the underlying affect of hopelessness and futility.

Hysterical motor disturbances can affect any of the voluntary muscle groups in patterns calculated to ward off forbidden sexual and aggressive discharges or to avoid situations of physical danger. They may present clinically as paralysis or muscular weakness (asthenia), abnormal posture, or gait disturbances. The speech apparatus may be affected with aphonia, hoarseness, and stammering. The muscular abnormalities of hysteria are usually associated with an increase in muscular tonus. Hysterical spasm of the muscles of the pelvic floor may cause vaginismus.

Cataplexy, commonly associated with narcolepsy, is characterized by sudden loss of motor tone, with profound weakness of the arms, legs, neck, and speech apparatus. These attacks are brought on by unexpected strong emotional reactions involving laughter, anger, surprise, or pleasure.

In schizophrenic catatonic stupor, the patient is immobile. His face may be masklike. He is unresponsive to questions or commands, except occasionally when he manifests echolalia or echopraxia. Ambivalence may modify the muscle tonus of the patient with catatonic stupor to the extent that he permits bending of his arm but against a resistance, so that a characteristic tonus quality emerges known as waxy flexibility.

Speech disturbances may express themselves as motoric inhibitions—for example, hysterical hoarseness or mutism. Stammering is a disorder characterized by spasmodic, halting, or hesitating speech. Stuttering is a more severe degree of stammering. It tends to have an explosive quality. It usually appears between the ages of 2 and 6 years. It occurs much more frequently in males and is said to be more frequent in those who are left-handed.

In male sexual functioning, motor inhibition may be expressed as impotence, premature ejaculation, or retarded ejaculation. Heroin addicts have a high incidence of sexual inhibition.

Disturbances of Personality

Personality refers to the sum total of the thoughts, feelings, and actions that a person habitually uses in his ongoing adaptations to life. Personality is essentially synonymous with character. These are deeply ingrained behavior patterns clearly recognized by adolescence and occasionally earlier.

The American Psychiatric Association's standard classification of mental disorders lists a number of identifiable personality patterns—paranoid, cyclothymic, schizoid, explosive, obsessive-compulsive, hysterical, asthenic, antisocial, passive-aggressive, and inadequate.

Psychoanalytic literature describes personality types in terms of levels of emotional development. The oral character or personality is a passive-dependent person who tries to recreate in his relationships the pattern of being fed by a loving mother. Such persons may be particularly prone to depressive illness. The anal character's outstanding qualities are excessive orderliness, frugality, and obstinacy, qualities persumably developed in the interactions with the mother during bowel training. The genital character is the emotionally mature ideal with maximally effective adaptability.

Disturbances in Appearance

Excessive fastidiousness may suggest an obsessive-compulsive disorder. Deterioration from a previous normal level of neatness may be an early sign of depression or schizophrenia. When a female patient seeks to arouse sexual desire by her seductive dress and manners, a hysterical character disorder may be an element in the clinical diagnosis. Some male homosexuals are distinguished by their exhibitionistic attire. A sexually fearful woman may deliberately choose neutral or drab clothing to discourage the interest of potential sexual partners. Regressive clinging to childhood may be expressed in childish patterns of dress. Repulsive body odor due to lack of bathing is calculated to keep a frightening world at a safe distance.

Paranoid patients may wear dark glasses so that they can spy on others without themselves being spied on. Transvestites are sometimes acting out complex fantasies involving a wish to recapture a lost parent figure. Schizophrenic patients may first reveal the delusion of body change by complaining that a hat or a pair of eye glasses no longer fits properly.

Disturbances in Patterns of Human Relationships

Family

The family may scapegoat a specific family member. As a consequence, this person may become a battered child (see Figure 3), and later in life grow up to be a battering parent and to display other forms of psychopathology.

Within a family group, one can identify the following roles: spouse, parent, and child. Each of these roles involves a complex of capacities and responsibilities. Potency disturbances can have a severe undermining effect on family happiness. Or, if the wife is frigid and incapable of sexual satisfaction, this incapacity may undermine the husband's self-esteem and have a

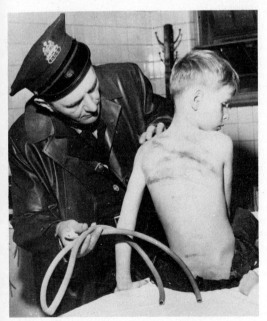

Fig. 3. The battered child is an innocent victim of a parent who cannot control his frustration and rage. Unfortunately, this child is likely to repeat the tragedy when he becomes a parent, unless he is removed from his destructive environment and given psychological help. (Courtesy of UPI.)

destructive impact on his over-all performance. In their studies of human sexuality, Masters and Johnson emphasized that most sexual malfunctioning in marriage is the result of a bilateral communication breakdown. Their focus is on the marital unit.

A reversal of roles is often seen in disturbed households in which an emotionally immature parent makes unrealistic demands on a young child. A schizophrenic or depressed mother may take to her bed and expect her little daughter to mother her. Fathers who refuse to relinquish their primary hold on the mother's attention and who compete actively for her love may seriously impair the emotional development of their children.

Loss of a spouse is a major life stress and may play an etiological role in a wide range of mental and physical disorders. The relative loss of a wife when she has given birth to a child may precipitate various disorders in the husband, including depression, accident-proneness with injury at work, and episodes of sexual deviation. Families without fathers are particularly prone to psychopathology, whatever the cause of his absence.

Children develop basic security and basic trust in their relationships with their parents. When the opportunity for this trust does not exist, attitudes of cynicism and distrust emerge and seriously impair the development process.

The birth of a sibling is universally experienced as a trauma. The displaced youngster has feelings of rage, with which he needs help from his parents. If this help is not forthcoming, the youngster does not internalize his aggression or learn to sublimate it. Instead, he expresses it outwardly.

Work

Work is a major source of self-esteem. It fulfills a need to be needed. Loss of work or the threat of it can be a crushing narcissistic blow, with major mental and physical pathological repercussions.

Job satisfaction is the strongest predictor of longevity. Heart attacks, addictions of all kinds, depression, and suicide all correlate highly with job dissatisfaction. In addition, extraoccupational life changes may alter work attitudes so that a previous steady worker becomes accident-prone.

Many schizophrenic patients shy away from

TABLE IV

Typical Signs and Symptoms of Psychiatric Illness

I. **Consciousness:** state of awareness

Apperception: perception modified by one's own emotions and thoughts

Sensorium: state of functioning of the special senses

A. *Disturbances of consciousness*

  1. Confusion: disturbance of orientation as to time, place, or person
  2. Clouding of consciousness: incomplete clearmindedness with disturbance in perception and attitudes
  3. Stupor: lack of reaction to and unawareness of surroundings
  4. Delirium: bewildered, restless, confused, disoriented reaction associated with fear and hallucinations
  5. Coma: profound degree of unconsciousness
  6. Coma vigil: coma in which eyes remain open
  7. Dreamy state (twilight): disturbed consciousness with hallucinations

B. *Disturbances of attention:* the amount of effort exerted in focusing on certain portions of an experience

  1. Distractability: inability to concentrate attention
  2. Selective inattention: blocking out of things that generate anxiety

C. *Disturbances in suggestibility:* compliant and uncritical response to an idea or influence

  1. *Folie à deux* (or *folie à trois*): communicated emotional illness between two (or three) persons
  2. Hypnosis: artifically induced modification of consciousness

II. **Affect:** emotional feeling tone

Disturbances in affect

A. Inappropriate affect: disharmony of affect and ideation

B. Pleasurable affects

  1. Euphoria: heightened feeling of psychological well-being inappropriate to apparent events
  2. Elation: air of confidence and enjoyment associated with increased motor activity
  3. Exaltation: intense elation with feelings of grandeur
  4. Ecstasy: feeling of intense rapture

C. Unpleasurable affects

  1. Depression: psychopathological feeling of sadness
  2. Grief or mourning: sadness appropriate to a real loss

D. Other affects

  1. Anxiety: feeling of apprehension due to unconscious conflicts
  2. Fear: anxiety due to consciously recognized and realistic danger
  3. Agitation: anxiety associated with severe motor restlessness
  4. Tension with increased motor and psychological activity that is unpleasant
  5. Panic: acute intense attack of anxiety associated with personality disorganization
  6. Free-floating anxiety: pervasive fear not attached to any idea
  7. Apathy: dulled emotional tone associated with detachment or indifference
  8. Ambivalence: coexistence of two opposing impulses toward the same thing in the same person at the same time
  9. Depersonalization: feeling of unreality concerning oneself or one's environment
  10. Derealization: distortion of spatial relationships so that the environment becomes unfamiliar
  11. Aggression: forceful goal-directed action that may be verbal or physical and that is the motor counterpart of the counterpart of the affect of rage, anger, or hostility
  12. Mood swings: oscillations between periods of euphoria and depression or anxiety

III. **Motor behavior (conation):** the capacity to initiate action or motor discharge that concerns the basic strivings of a person as expressed through his behavior

Disturbances of conation

A. Echolalia: psychopathological repeating of words of one person by another

B. Echopraxia: pathological imitation of movements of one person by another

C. Cerea flexibilitas (waxy flexibility): state in which patient maintains body position into which he is placed

D. Catalepsy: state of unconsciousness in which immobile position is constantly maintained

E. Command automatism: automatic following of suggestions

F. Automatism: automatic performance of acts representative of unconscious symbolic activity
G. Cataplexy: temporary loss of muscle tone and weakness precipitated by a variety of emotional states
H. Sterotypy: continuous repetition of speech or physical activities
I. Negativism: frequent opposition to suggestions
J. Mannerisms: sterotyped involuntary movements
K. Verbigeration: meaningless repetitions of speech
L. Overactivity
   1. Hyperactivity (hyperkinesis): restless, aggressive, destructive activity
   2. Tic: spasmodic, repetitive motor movements
   3. Sleepwalking (somnambulism): motor activity during sleep
   4. Compulsion: uncontrollable impulse to perform an act repetitively
      a. Dipsomania: compulsion to drink alcohol
      b. Egomania: pathological self-preoccupation
      c. Erotomania: pathological preoccupation with sex
      d. Kleptomania: Compulsion to steal
      e. Megalomania: pathological sense of power
      f. Monomania: preoccupation with a single subject
      g. Nymphomania: excessive need for coitus in female
      h. Satyriasis: excessive need for coitus in male
      i. Trichotilomania: compulsion to pull out one's hair
      j. Ritual: automatic activity compulsive in nature, emotional in origin
M. Hypoactivity: decreased activity or retardation, as in psychomotor retardation; slowing of psychological and physical functioning
N. Mimicry: simple, imitative motion activity of childhood
IV. **Thinking:** goal-directed flow of ideas, symbols, and associations, initiated by a problem or task and leading toward a reality-oriented conclusion; when a logical sequence occurs, thinking is normal
   A. *Disturbances in form of thinking*
      1. Dereism: mental activity not concordant with logic or experience
      2. Autistic thinking: thinking that gratifies unfulfilled desires but has no regard for reality; term used somewhat synonymously with dereism
   B. *Disturbances in structure of associations*
      1. Neologism: new words created by the patient for psychological reasons
      2. Word salad: incoherent mixture of words and phrases
      3. Circumstantiality: digression of inappropriate thoughts into ideational processes, but patient eventually gets from starting point to desired goal
      4. Tangenitality: inability to have goal-directed associations of thought; patient never gets from starting point to desired goal
      5. Incoherence: running together of thoughts with no logical connection, resulting in disorganization
      6. Perseveration: psychopathological repetition of the same word or idea in response to different questions
      7. Condensation: fusion of various concepts into one
      8. Irrelevant answer: answer that is not in harmony with question asked
   C. *Disturbances in speed of associations*
      1. Flight of ideas: rapid verbalizations so that there is a shifting from one idea to another
      2. Clang associations: words similar in sound but not in meaning call up new thoughts
      3. Blocking: interruption in train of thinking, unconscious in origin
      4. Pressure of speech: voluble speech difficult to interrupt
      5. Volubility (logorrhea): copious, coherent, logical speech
   D. *Disturbances in type of associations*
      1. Motor aphasia: disturbance of speech due to organic brain disorder in which understanding remains but ability to speak is lost
      2. Sensory aphasia: loss of ability to comprehend the meaning of words or use of objects
      3. Nominal aphasia: difficulty in finding right name for an object
      4. Syntactial aphasia: inability to arrange words in proper sequence

Table IV—*Continued*

E. *Disturbances in content of thought*
   1. Delusion: false belief, not consistent with patient's intelligence and cultural background, that cannot be corrected by reasoning
     a. Delusion of grandeur: exaggerated conception of one's importance
     b. Delusion of persecution: false belief that one is being persecuted; often found in litigious patients
     c. Delusion of reference: false belief that the behavior of others refers to oneself; derived from ideas of reference in which patient falsely feels he is being talked about by others
     d. Delusion of self-accusation: false feeling of remorse
     e. Delusion of control: false feeling that one is being controlled by others
     f. Delusion of infidelity: false belief derived from pathological jealousy that one's lover is unfaithful
     g. Paranoid delusions: oversuspiciousness leading to persecutory delusions
   2. Trend or preoccupation of thought: centering of thought content around a particular idea, associated with a strong affective tone
   3. Hypochondria: exaggerated concern over one's health that is not based on real organic pathology
   4. Obsession: pathological persistence of an irristible thought, feeling, or impulse that cannot be eliminated from consciousness by logical effort
   5. Phobia: exaggerated and invariably pathological dread of some specific type of stimulus or situation
     a. Acrophobia: dread of high places
     b. Agoraphobia: dread of open places
     c. Algophobia: dread of pain
     d. Claustrophobia: dread of closed places
     e. Xenophobia: dread of strangers
     f. Zoophobia: dread of animals

V. **Perception:** awareness of objects and relations that follows stimulation of peripheral sense organs
  A. *Disturbances associated with organic brain disease,* such as agnosia—that is, an inability to recognize and interpret the significance of sensory impressions
  B. *Disturbances associated with hysteria:* illnesses characterized by emotional conflict, the use of the defense mechanism of conversion, and the development of physical symptoms involving the voluntary muscles or special sense organs
   1. Hysterical anesthesia: loss of sensory modalities resulting from emotional conflicts
   2. Macropsia: state in which objects appear larger than they are
   3. Micropsia: state in which objects appear smaller than they are
  C. *Hallucinations:* false sensory perceptions not associated with real external stimuli
   1. Hypnagogic hallucination: false sensory perception occuring midway between falling asleep and being awake
   2. Auditory hallucination: false auditory perception
   3. Visual hallucination: false visual perception
   4. Olfactory hallucination: false perception of smell
   5. Gustatory hallucination: false perception of taste, such as unpleasant taste due to an uncinate fit
   6. Tactile haptic hallucination: false perception of touch, such as the feeling of worms under the skin
   7. Kinesthetic hallucination: false perception of movement or sensation, as from an amputated limb (phantom limb)
   8. Lilliputian hallucination: perception of objects as reduced in size
  D. *Illusions:* false sensory perceptions of real external sensory stimuli

VI. **Memory:** function by which information stored in the brain is later recalled to consciousness
Disturbances of memory
  A. Amnesia: partial or total inability to recall past experiences
  B. Paramnesia: falsification of memory by distortion of recall
   1. *Fausse reconnaissance:* false recognition
   2. Retrospective falsification: recollection of a true memory to which the patient adds false details
   3. Confabulation: unconscious filling of gaps in memory by imagined or untrue experiences that patient believes but that have no basis in fact

Table IV—*Continued*

4. *Déjà vu:* illusion of visual recognition in which a new situation is incorrectly regarded as a repetition of a previous memory
5. *Déjà entendu:* illusion of auditory recognition
6. *Jamais vu:* false feeling of unfamiliarity with a real situation one has experienced

C. Hypermnesia: exaggerated degree of retention and recall

VII. **Intelligence:** the ability to understand, recall, mobilize, and integrate constructively previous learning in meeting new situtations

A. *Mental retardation:* organically caused lack of intelligence to such a degree that there is interference with social and vocational performance: mild (I.Q. of 50 to 70), moderate (I.Q. of 35 to 49), severe (I.Q. of 20 to 34), or profound (I.Q. below 20); obsolescent terms are idiot (mental age less than 3 years), imbecile (mental age of 3 to 7 years), and moron (mental age of 8 or more)

B. *Dementia:* organic loss of mental function

---

regular employment, even though they may show considerable occupational aptitude in volunteer or sheltered work settings. The schizophrenic has limited ability to relate to other people and so may have difficulties with superiors, peers, and even passing strangers. If he works at all, he chooses work settings that are highly structured and that permit isolation from other human beings.

Many people work far below their potential because of psychopathological work inhibitions. Some are self-defeating out of a sense of guilt. Others are self-defeating because of a fear of success. Some fall behind because they must rebel in their quest for identity. On a school level, this rebellion expresses itself as an impaired capacity for learning and in the school dropout problem.

Retirement from work may have a severe disruptive impact on the adaptational patterns in a family and may touch off a vicious cycle of psychopathology. Some work addicts are guilt-ridden people who work compulsively. For them, in particular, loss of a job or retirement upsets a delicately balanced adaptational state.

Doctors and nurses are particularly prone to narcotic addiction because of the pressures of their work and their relatively easy access to opiates. The father who commutes a long distance to work may create a family void as traumatic as an absent father. Unskilled jobs associated with danger, monotony, and poor pay are particularly associated with accident neurosis and litigiousness.

Play

Some people in recreational situations are like work addicts: they play compulsively, angrily, and anxiously. They suffer severely if they make errors; if they lose a game, they become depressed. In these instances, the superego remains too much in control, and there is no opportunity for genuine sublimation.

Community

Many people become involved in community work for pathological reasons, such as guilt, exhibitionism, and a need for self-aggrandizement. In such instances the formal goal of the group may clash with the pathological informal goals of the person.

REFERENCES

Bender, M. B. *Disorders of Perception.* Charles C Thomas, Springfield, Ill., 1952.
Burnham, D. L., Gladstone, S. I., and Gibson, R. W. *Schizophrenia and the Need-Fear Dilemma.* International Universities Press, New York, 1969.
Fenichel, O. *Psychoanalytic Theory of the Neuroses.* W. W. Norton, New York, 1945.
Fish, B., and Haggin, R. Visual-motor disorders in infants at risk for schizophrenia. Arch. Gen. Psychiatry. *28:* 900, 1973.
Fisher, C., Kahn, E., Edwards, A., and Davis, D. M. A psychophysiological study of nightmares and night terrors. Arch. Gen. Psychiatry, *28:* 252, 1973.
Geschwind, N. Aphasia. N. Engl. J. Med., *284:* 651, 1971.
Holmes, T. H., and Rahe, R. H. The social readjustment rating scale. J. Psychosom. Res., *11:* 213, 1967.
Parkes, C. M. *Bereavement: Studies of Grief in Adult Life.* International Universities Press, New York, 1972.
Schreiber, F. R. *Sybil.* Henry Regnery, Chicago, 1973.
Spiegel, H. *Manual for the Hypnotic Induction Profile.* Soni Medica, New York, 1973.
Thompson, L. J. Learning disabilities: An overview. Am. J. Psychiatry, *130:* 393, 1973.

13

Classification

13.1. NOSOLOGY AND THE OFFICIAL PSYCHIATRIC NOMENCLATURE

Principles of Classification

Classification is the process by which a person reduces the complexity of phenomena by arranging them into categories according to some established criteria for one or more purposes. Classification is the formal human process analogous to concept formation that occurs in all higher animals as they attempt to master their environments. A classification of disease entities is called a nosology, from the Greek words *nosos* (disease) and *logia* (study). The terms used to identify the categories are called a nomenclature. It includes the names of the disorders and any other technical terms used to describe patients. Whereas the classification system indicates how the various disorders relate to each other, the nomenclature is merely an arbitrary collection of technical terms, independent of any underlying characteristics.

A nosology is reliable to the extent that the rules for categorization are so clear that all users of the system diagnose patients in the same way. A nosology is valid to the extent that it is useful in accomplishing the three purposes of all classification systems—communication, control, and comprehension. In medicine, communication involves using names that function as efficient symbols for summarizing naturally occurring clusters of data that would otherwise require a larger number of descriptive terms. The ability to predict the course and outcome of a disorder provides a limited form of control. The ability to modify the disorder by treatment adds additional control. Comprehension means understanding the cause and pathological process of the disorder. In psychiatry, as in the rest of medicine, there are many disorders that can be treated effectively without understanding either the cause or the pathological process.

Defining Mental Disorder

None of the standard textbooks of psychiatry and neither the first nor the second edition of the American Psychiatric Association's *Diagnostic and Statistical Manual of Mental Disorders* provide a definition of mental disorder. Mental disorders are manifested by deviations in behavior (which includes ideation and affect) from some normative concept. The problem in defining mental disorder is that the widespread consensus that exists regarding the undesirability of specific manifestations of nonpsychiatric medical disorder—pain, disability, death—does not always exist for the behavioral manifestations of what have traditionally been regarded as mental disorders.

The lack of consensus regarding the specific manifestations of psychiatric disorder may take three forms: controversy as to whether a given condition should be regarded as undesirable at all; how undesirable a condition should be to warrant its designation as an illness; and whether the condition, even if markedly undesirable, should be regarded as within the domain of psychiatry or of some other discipline. An example of the first form is the controversy as to whether preferential homosexual behavior should be regarded as undesirable. An example of the second form is disagreement about whether certain mild personality patterns are sufficiently undesirable to warrant designation as a psychiatric disorder or whether they should be viewed purely as descriptive traits. An example of the third form is the controversy as to whether certain forms of serious antisocial behavior should be regarded as sick (manifestations of psychiatric disorders) or bad (the responsibility of the criminal justice system).

As yet, no explicit definition of mental disorder is universally accepted by the psychiatric profession, but, by examining the labeling practices of psychiatrists, one can identify at least two main approaches to the problem. The first, or broad, approach views mental disorder as any significant deviation from an ideal state of positive mental health. Thus, sexual practices, value systems, and personality traits that are deemed less than optimal or a result of intrapsychic conflict are viewed as manifestations of mental disorder. The second, or narrow, approach also accepts the notion of a continuum of conditions from highly desirable (positive mental health) to highly undesirable (mental illness) but places the cutoff point for mental disorder closer to the highly undesirable end of the continuum, so that only conditions clearly associated with suffering and disability are designated as illness or disorder. The broad approach has its strongest adherents among psychoanalytically oriented psychiatrists in the United States. In contrast, the narrow approach seems more characteristic of the approach taken by almost all European psychiatrists and may explain the tendency in epidemiological studies conducted in the United States to report a much higher incidence of mental disorder than is generally reported in European studies.

The definition of a mental disorder proposed here is:

1. The manifestations of the condition are primarily psychological and involve alterations in behavior. However, it includes conditions manifested by somatic changes, such as psychophysiologic reactions, if an understanding of the cause and course of the conditions is largely dependent on the use of psychological concepts, such as personality, motivation, and conflict.

2. The condition in its full-blown state is regularly and intrinsically associated with subjective distress, generalized impairment in social effectiveness or functioning, or voluntary behavior that the subject wishes he could stop because it is regularly associated with physical disability or illness.

3. The condition is distinct from other conditions in terms of the clinical picture and, ideally, follow-up, family studies, and response to treatment.

The criteria for a mental disorder proposed here in no way depend on the cause of the condition, which does not speak to the issue of whether the condition, once it has developed, is inherently undesirable and, therefore, potentially classified as a disorder or illness.

How well do the criteria for a mental disorder proposed here apply to the psychiatric disorders in the traditional nomenclature? All the conditions in the traditional nomenclature satisfy the first criterion, although the exact role of psychological factors in the development and course of the psychosomatic disorders remains unclear. The second criterion seems to apply to virtually all the conditions in the traditional nomenclature with the exception of sexual deviations in mild form. And the second criterion includes such conditions as compulsive cigarette smoking and compulsive eating, which are not now in the standard nomenclature. The greatest discrepancy between the three criteria proposed here and the traditional nomenclature is in the third criterion. Many of the personality disorders and some of the subtypes of neurosis in the standard nomenclature have not been demonstrated to be distinct conditions.

The definition proposed here, because it takes the narrow approach to defining a mental disorder, is helpful in answering the charge that, by defining certain conditions as mental disorders, psychiatry is merely acting as an agent of social control. On the other hand, this definition may need to be changed in future years to correspond with a change in the attitude of society and the psychiatric profession toward certain conditions.

Levels of Psychiatric Diagnosis

At the simplest level, one speaks of a sign or symptom that represents a specific discernible abnormality—anxiety, depressed mood, hallucinations. Signs and symptoms by themselves fulfill the first two criteria of the definition of a mental disorder offered above but not the third, since they do not represent distinct entities. At the next level, recurring groupings or patterns of symptoms are designated as syndromes. Many different specific processes may be involved in producing the disturbance. When the best evidence available suggests a distinct pathogogical process, one then speaks of a mental disorder.

History

According to Menninger, the first specific description of a mental illness appeared about 3,000 B.C. in a depiction of senile deterioration, ascribed to Prince Ptahhotep. The syndromes of melancholia and hysteria appear in the Sumerian and Egyptian literature as far back as 2,600 B.C. In the Ebers papyrus (1,500 B.C.) both senile deterioration and alcoholism are described.

Hippocrates (about 460–377 B.C.) is usually regarded as the one who introduced the concept of psychiatric illness into medicine. His writings describe acute mental disturbances with fever (perhaps acute organic brain syndromes), acute mental disturbances without fever (probably analogous to functional psychoses but called mania), chronic disturbances without fever (called melancholia), hysteria (broader than its later use), and Scythian disease (similar to transvestitism).

Caelius Aurelianus, a 5th century physician living in the Roman Empire, described homosexuality as an affliction of a diseased mind, found in both men and women. Mental deficiency and dementia were noted by Swiss Renaissance physician Felix Platter (1536–1614).

Before the time of the English physician Sydenham (1624–1663), an illness, despite the differences in appearance between the different syndromes, was attributed to a single pathogenic process, either a disturbance of the humoral balance or a disturbance in the tensions of the solid tissues. Sydenham, on the other hand, believed that each illness had a specific cause.

Philippe Pinel (1745–1826), a French physician, simplified the complex diagnostic systems that preceded him by recognizing four fundamental clinical types: mania (conditions with acute excitement or fury), melancholia (depressive disorders and delusions with limited topics), dementia (lack of cohesion in ideas), and idiotism (idiocy and organic dementia). Pinel thus reacted against the specific disease entity tradition of Sydenham and went back to a noncomplex Hippocratic system of classification. All mental illnesses were in a category of physical illnesses called "neuroses," which were defined as "functional diseases of the nervous system"—that is, illnesses that were not accompanied by fever, inflammation, hemorrhage, or anatomic lesion.

By the 19th century, mental disease began to be regarded consistently as the manifestation of physical pathology, and scientists searched for specific lesions, parallel to the investigation of bodily diseases. Benedict-Augustin Morel (1809–1873) was the first to use the course of an illness as a basis for classification. His *démence précoce* was not a disease entity but a particular form of the course of mental disease.

Karl Ludwig Kahlbaum (1828–1899), a German descriptive psychiatrist who foreshadowed Kraepelin, introduced the concepts of temporary symptom complex as opposed to the underlying disease, the distinction between organic and nonorganic mental disease, and considering the patient's age at the time of onset and the characteristic development of the disorder as bases for classification.

The finding made by Bayle (1822) that progressive paresis was a specific organic disease of the brain and the discovery of Paul Broca (1861) that some forms of asphasia were related to definite lesions of the cortex increased attempts to base all classification of mental disorders on demonstrated brain lesions or disturbance in vascular or nutritional physiology. It led Wilhelm Greisinger (1818–1868) to coin the slogan "mental diseases are brain diseases."

In the last two decades of the 19th century, Emil Kraepelin (1856–1926) synthesized three approaches: the clinical-descriptive, the somatic, and the consideration of the course of the disease. He viewed mental illnesses as organic disease entities that could be classified on the basis of knowledge about their cause, course, and outcome. He brought the manic and depressive disturbances together into one illness, manic-depressive psychosis, and distinguished it, on the basis of its period of remission, from the chronic deteriorating illness dementia precox, which Bleuler later renamed schizophrenia. Kraepelin also recognized paranoia as distinct from dementia precox, distinguished the deliria (acute organic brain syndromes) from the dementias (chronic brain syndromes), and included the concepts of psychogenic neuroses and psychopathic personalities.

The basic approach of Karepelin toward classification was to search for that combination of clinical features that would best predict outcome. In contrast, Eugene Bleuler (1857–1937), who expanded the concepts of dementia precox and coined the term schizophrenia, based his classification system on an inferred psychopathological process, such as a disturbance in the associative process in schizophrenia.

The personality disorders were first noted in the psychiatric literature by J. C. Prichard (1835) with his introduction of the concepts of moral insanity and moral imbecility. August Koch (1891) coined the terms "psychopathic personality" and "psychopathic constitutional inferiority." The dynamic concepts of Freud expanded the boundaries of what was considered to be mental illness so that it included the milder forms of personality deviation.

Despite the advances in the understanding of mental disorders in the last 50 years, the major categories in the current *Diagnostic and Statistical Manual of Mental Disorders* (DSM-II) are based primarily on the concepts of Kraepelin (manic-depressive illness), Bleuler (schizophrenia), and Freud (neuroses and personality disorders).

The first official system for tabulating mental illness in the United States was used for the decennial census of 1840. It contained only one category for all mental illness and lumped together the idiotic and the insane. Forty years later, in the census of 1880, the mentally ill were subdivided into separate categories for the first time. Seven categories were recognized: mania, melancholia, monomania, paresis, dementia, dipsomania, and epilepsy.

For a special census of patients in hospitals for mental disease in 1923, the Bureau of the Census used a classification system developed in collaboration with the American Psychiatric Association (then the American Medico-Psychological Association) and the National Committee for Mental Health. This system had been adopted by the American Psychiatric Association in 1917, and it was used until 1934, when it was revised for incorporation into the first edition of the American Medical Association's *Standard Classified Nomenclature of Disease.*

This 1934 classification was designed primarily for chronic in-patients and, therefore, proved inadequate for use with the psychiatric casualties of World War II, who required classifications for acute disturbances, psychosomatic disorders, and personality disorders, which were not represented in the 1934 classification. In addition, the system was considered anachronistic by the increasing number of psychodynamically oriented psychiatrists.

To fill this void, the Veterans Administration and the military services developed competing systems. In addition, in 1948 there appeared the first international classification of mental disorders, a section in the sixth edition of the *International Classification of Diseases* (ICD-6), published by the World Health Organization in Geneva, Switzerland. The lack of provision in ICD-6 for the chronic brain syndromes, many personality disorders, and transient situational reactions rendered it unsatisfactory for use in America. Consequently, in 1951 the United States Public Health Service commissioned a working party, with representation from the American Psychiatric Association, to develop an alternative to the mental disorder section of ICD-6 for use in this country. This document, based heavily on the Veterans Administration classification system, was published in 1952 by the American Psychiatric Association as *Diagnostic and Statistical Manual, Mental Disorders* (DSM-I).

In the definitions of the diagnostic categories, the frequent use of the term "reaction," as in "schizophrenic reaction" and "psychoneurotic reaction," expressed the strong environmental orientation of Adolf Meyer; and the frequent reference to defense mechanisms, particularly as an explanation of the neuroses and personality disorders, reflected the wide acceptance of psychoanalytic concepts. Despite its widespread influence and impact on American psychiatric literature, DSM-I was not universally accepted as the official nomenclature throughout the country.

The World Health Organization sponsored an international effort to develop a classification system for mental disorders that would improve on ICD-6 and be acceptable to all member nations. The mental disorder section of ICD-8 was approved by the World Health Organization in 1966 and became effective in 1968.

In 1965, the American Psychiatric Association assigned its Committee on Nomenclature and Statistics the task of preparing a new diagnostic manual of disorders compatible with the ICD-8 list of mental disorders but defining each disorder for American use. The new manual, *Diagnostic and Statistical Manual of Mental Disorders* (DSM-II), was adopted by the American Psychiatric Association in 1967 and published and officially accepted throughout the country in 1968, although reaction to it was mixed.

DSM-II is the basis for the official diagnostic

manuals used in Canada, India, and several Latin American countries, but other national glossaries have also been prepared, and they have defined the ICD list of terms in their own way. The most influential glossary, other than DSM-II, is *Great Britain's Glossary of Mental Disorders*, prepared in 1968.

The strenghts of the multipurpose synthetic classification system of the type used in DSM-II and in ICD-8 suggest that this type of classification system will probably be around for many years, despite the problems of reliability and validity surrounding many of its categories. At the same time that the social learning theorists are proposing alternative systems, recent work is going a long way toward refining and strengthening the existing system. This work includes refining the criteria for diagnosis so as to improve its predictive validity, genetic studies to validate the diagnostic concepts, and improving methods for gathering clinical data. In addition, there has been work with nonclinical methods, using mathematical models for generating diagnostic types and computer programs for simulating the differential diagnostic process of clinicians. At the present time a committee of the American Psychiatric Association directed by Robert Spitzer, M.D., is working on a revision of the **Diagnostic and Statistical Manual,** to be called DSM-III and scheduled to be published in 1978. DSM-III will be coordinated with a new edition of the **International Classification of Diseases** to be called ICD-9.

Categories and Features of DSM-II

Table I presents the nomenclature and classification of DSM-II. It divides disorders into 10 major categories. The system of classification differs from one section to another. DSM-II, therefore, is actually a collection of classification systems that together attempt to encompass the entire field of mental disorders.

Unlike its predecessor, DSM-II encourages clinicians to diagnose every disorder that is present, even if one is the symptomatic expression of another. Furthermore, DSM-II gives clear principles for determining which of two or more diagnoses should be listed first—the condition that most urgently requires treatment or, when there is no issue of disposition or treatment priority, the more serious condition. Unfortunately, DSM-II does not provide any guidelines as to what combinations of diagnoses are legitimate.

In DSM-I any of four qualifying phrases could be used (except where redundant) with any disorder; in DSM-II there are seven different qualifying phrases, but all except one are limited to specific sections. The qualifying phrases "acute" and "chronic" can be used and coded in section II, organic brain syndrome. The qualifying phrase "not psychotic" can be used and coded in section III, functional psychoses, for patients who are not psychotic at the time of the evaluation but who, nevertheless, have a disorder traditionally classified as psychosis. The qualifying phrases "mild," "moderate," and "severe" are appropriate for disorders in section IV, neuroses, and section IX, behavior disorders of childhood and adolescence. The qualifying phrase "in remission" can be used and coded, at least theoretically, with all disorders. It is most appropriate for conditions that consist of episodes separated by symptom-free intervals, such as the manic-depressive illnesses.

Mental Retardation

This category includes all subnormal general intellecutal functioning that originates during the developmental period (before about age 16) and is associated with impairment of either learning and social adjustment or maturation or both. The primary basis for subclassification is the level of retardation, and each level of retardation is further subdivided by presumed cause.

Because this section of DSM-II was adopted from the *Manual on Terminology and Classification in Mental Retardation* (second edition, 1961), it reflects the most advanced thinking of experts in this field. Not surprisingly, there have been no major criticisms of it.

Organic Brain Syndromes

This category corresponds to the ICD category, "disorders caused by or associated with impairment of brain tissue function," but in DSM-II this condition is defined more restrictively and is limited to conditions that manifest the symptoms of impaired orientation, memory, intellectual functions and judgment, and lability and shallowness of affect. This is the only major category in DSM-II in which the cause of the condition is explicit—namely, impairment of brain tissue function.

The main subclassifications of the organic brain syndromes are the psychotic and the nonpsychotic conditions, which are then further

TABLE I

Diagnostic Nomenclature of the American Psychiatric Association (DSM-II)

I. **Mental Retardation**
- 310. Borderline
- 311. Mild
- 312. Moderate
- 313. Severe
- 314. Profound
- 315. Unspecified

With each: following or associated with
- .0 Infection or intoxication
- .1 Trauma or physical agent
- .2 Disorders of metabolism, growth, or nutrition
- .3 Gross brain disease (postnatal)
- .4 Unknown prenatal influence
- .5 Chromosomal abnormality
- .6 Prematurity
- .7 Major psychiatric disorder
- .8 Psychosocial (environmental) deprivation
- .9 Other condition

II. **Organic Brain Syndrome (OBS)**

A. **Psychoses**

Senile and presenile dementia
- 290.0 Senile dementia
- 290.1 Presenile dementia

Alcoholic psychosis
- 291.0 Delirium tremens
- 291.1 Korsakov's psychosis
- 291.2 Other alcoholic hallucinosis
- 291.3 Alcohol paranoid state
- 291.4* Acute alcohol intoxication*
- 291.5* Alcoholic deterioration*
- 291.6* Pathological intoxication*
- 291.9 Other alcoholic psychosis

Psychosis associated with intracranial infection
- 292.0 General paralysis
- 292.1 Syphilis of central nervous system (CNS)
- 292.2 Epidemic encephalitis
- 292.3 Other and unspecified encephalitis
- 292.9 Other intracranial infection

Psychosis associated with other cerebral condition
- 293.0 Cerebral arteriosclerosis
- 293.1 Other cerebrovascular disturbance
- 293.2 Epilepsy
- 293.3 Intracranial neoplasm
- 293.4 Degenerative disease of the CNS
- 293.5 Brain trauma
- 293.9 Other cerebral condition

Psychosis associated with other physical condition
- 294.0 Endocrine disorder
- 294.1 Metabolic and nutritional disorder
- 294.2 Systemic infection
- 294.3 Drug or poison intoxication (other than alcohol)
- 294.4 Childbirth
- 294.8 Other and undiagnosed physical condition

B. **Nonpsychotic OBS**
- 309.0 Intracranial infection
- 309.13* Alcohol* (simple drunkenness)
- 309.14* Other drug, poison, or systemic intoxication*
- 309.2 Brain trauma
- 309.3 Circulatory disturbance
- 309.4 Epilepsy
- 309.5 Disturbance of metabolism, growth, or nutrition
- 309.6 Senile or presenile brain disease
- 309.7 Intracranial neoplasm
- 309.8 Degenerative disease of the CNS
- 309.9 Other physical condition

III. **Psychoses Not Attributed to Physical Conditions Listed Previously**

Schizophrenia
- 295.0 Simple
- 295.1 Hebephrenic
- 295.2 Catatonic
- 295.23* Catatonic type, excited*
- 295.24* Catatonic type, withdrawn*
- 295.3 Paranoid
- 295.4 Acute schizophrenic episode
- 295.5 Latent
- 295.6 Residual
- 295.7 Schizo-affective
- 295.73* Schizo-affective, excited*
- 295.74* Schizo-affective, depressed*
- 295.8* Childhood*
- 295.90* Chronic undifferentiated*
- 295.99* Other schizophrenia*

Major affective disorders
- 296.0 Involutional melancholia
- 296.1 Manic-depressive illness, manic
- 296.2 Manic-depressive illness, depressed
- 296.3 Manic-depressive illness, circular
- 296.33* Manic-depressive, circular, manic*
- 296.34* Manic-depressive, circular, depressed*
- 296.8 Other major affective disorder

Paranoid states
- 297.0 Paranoia
- 297.1 Involutional paranoid state
- 297.9 Other paranoid state

Other psychoses
- 298.0 Psychotic depressive reaction

IV. **Neuroses**
- 300.0 Anxiety
- 300.1 Hysterical
- 300.13* Hysterical, conversion type*
- 300.14* Hysterical, dissociative type*
- 300.2 Phobic
- 300.3 Obsessive-compulsive
- 300.4 Depressive
- 300.5 Neurasthenic
- 300.6 Depersonalization
- 300.7 Hypochondriacal
- 300.8 Other neurosis

V. **Personality Disorders and Certain Other Nonphychotic Mental Disorders**

Personality disorders
- 301.0 Paranoid
- 301.1 Cyclothymic
- 301.2 Schizoid
- 301.3 Explosive
- 301.4 Obsessive-compulsive
- 301.5 Hysterical
- 301.6 Asthenic
- 301.7 Antisocial
- 301.81* Passive-aggressive*
- 301.82* Inadequate*
- 301.89* Other specified types*

Sexual deviation
- 302.0 Sexual orientation disturbance
- 302.1 Fetishism
- 302.2 Pedophilia
- 302.3 Transvestitism
- 302.4 Exhibitionism
- 302.5* Voyeurism*
- 302.6* Sadism*

TABLE I—*Continued*

302.7*	Masochism*						reaction*
302.8	Other sexual deviation	305.6	Genitourinary			308.2*	Over anxious reaction*
Alcoholism		305.7	Endocrine			308.3*	Runaway reaction*
303.0	Episodic excessive drinking	305.8	Organ or special sense			308.4*	Unsocialized aggressive reaction*
303.1	Habitual excessive drinking	305.9	Other type			308.5*	Group delinquent reaction*
303.2	Alcohol addiction	**VII.**	**Special Symptoms**			308.9*	Other reaction*
303.9	Other alcoholism	306.0	Speech disturbance				
Drug dependence		306.1	Specific learning disturbance	**X.**	**Conditions Without Manifest Psychiatric Disorder and Nonspecific Conditions**		
304.0	Opium, opium alkaloids, and their derivatives	306.2	Tic	**Social maladjustment without manifest psychiatric disorder**			
304.1	Synthetic analgesics with morphinelike effects	306.3	Other psychomotor disorder				
		306.4	Disorders of sleep	316.0*	Marital maladjustment*		
304.2	Barbiturates	306.5	Feeding disturbance	316.1*	Social maladjustment*		
304.3	Other hypnotics and sedatives or tranquilizers	306.6	Enuresis				
		306.7	Encopresis	316.2*	Occupational maladjustment*		
304.4	Cocaine	306.8	Cephalalgia	316.3*	Dyssocial behavior*		
304.5	Cannabis sativa (hashish, marijuana)	306.9	Other special symptom	316.9*	Other social maladjustment*		
304.6	Other psychostimulants	**VIII.**	**Transient Situational Disturbances**	**Nonspecific conditions**			
304.7	Hallucinogens	307.0*	Adjustment reaction of infancy*	317*	Nonspecific conditions*		
304.8	Other drug dependence	307.1*	Adjustment reaction of childhood*	**No mental disorder**			
VI.	**Psychophysiologic Disorders**	307.2*	Adjustment reaction of adolescence*	318*	No mental disorder*		
305.0	Skin	307.3*	Adjustment reaction of adult life*	**XI.**	**Nondiagnostic Terms for Administrative Use**		
305.1	Musculoskeletal	307.4*	Adjustment reaction of late life*				
305.2	Respiratory			319.0*	Diagnosis deferred*		
305.3	Cardiovascular	**IX.**	**Behavior Disorders of Childhood and Adolescence**	319.1*	Boarder*		
305.4	Hemic and lymphatic	308.0*	Hyperkinetic reaction*	319.2*	Experiment only*		
305.5	Gastrointestinal	308.1*	Withdrawing	319.3*	Other*		

* Categories added to ICD-8 for use in United States only.

subdivided into specific etiological subcategories, such as due to alcohol and due to drugs. The distinction between acute (reversible) and chronic (irreversible) brain syndromes is relegated to a qualifying phrase—coded by a fifth digit—for those brain syndromes that can exist in both forms, such as the organic syndromes associated with drug intoxication.

DSM-II defines psychotic as manifesting "mental functioning...sufficiently impaired to interfere grossly with [the] capacity to meet the ordinary demands of life." However, this definition would include many conditions, such as severe obsessional neuroses, that are not thought of as psychotic, and conversely, many patients with impaired reality testing are able to meet the demands of everyday life quite well. Furthermore, the phrase "ordinary demands of life" is too vague to be used as a criterion for such a fundamental distinction as that between psychotic and nonpsychotic.

Psychoses Not Attributed to Physical Conditions Listed Previously

This awkward but precise term corresponds to the clinical term "functional psychoses." It avoids specific etiological explanations for the functional psychoses while acknowledging that specific physical bases for them may one day be discovered. It assumes, however, that whatever physical bases may be discovered in the future will not include such agents as alcohol, drugs, and other toxins responsible for the organic brain syndromes.

The two largest subdivisions of this category reflect the basic distinction between the disorders of mood (major affective disorders, such as manic-depressive illness and involutional melancholia, as delineated by Kraepelin) and the more chronic disorders of thinking (schizophrenia, as described by Bleuler). In addition, there are two other categories, the paranoid states, which are characterized by persecutory delusions not explainable by a disorder of thinking or mood, and disorders of mood presumably due to external stresses (psychotic depressive reaction).

The DSM-II definition of schizophrenia offers no stringent guide to the scope of this term.

DSM-II gave official sanction to the dichotomization between affective illnesses that are caused by a precipitating life experience (the psychotic depressive reactions) and those whose "onset of... mood does not seem to be related directly to a precipitating life experience" (the endogenous depressions), such as manic-depressive illness. This distinction flies in the face of common clinical experience, which suggests that many manic-depressive episodes are seemingly precipitated by life events. Also, research evidence indicates that, even with single episodes of depression, which ordinarily would be considered reactive depressions, the relationship to life stress is by no means well understood.

Recent research in affective illness suggests that there are two distinctions more fundamental than the one based on presence or absence of precipitating stress. These are the distinction between unipolar (always depressed) and bipolar (manic and depressed) depressions and the distinction between depressions with physiological symptoms and autonomous course (endogenous symptoms) and depressions without physiological symptoms whose course is reactive to environmental events.

Neuroses

This cateogry includes disorders characterized by a specific symptom that is usually ego-dystonic and that dominates the clinical picture, such as anxiety, depression, phobia, obsession, or compulsion. The definition in DSM-II is based on the psychoanalytic notion that the neuroses are defenses against anxiety, and so the criterion for classification seems to be based on the presence of a presumed pathological mechanism. Since classical neurotic symptoms are commonly associated with the functional psychoses, the diagnosis of a neurosis is thus actually made by exclusion. A neurosis is considered to be present when a neurotic symptom exists in the absence of a functional psychosis or a transient situational reaction.

Some students of psychiatric classification have challenged the entity status of the neuroses, claiming that they are, in reality, nothing more than symptom complexes. They argue that these conditions are analogous to the special symptoms in that they are diagnosed only in the absence of more fundamental disturbances.

DSM-II implies that anxiety plays a central role in the neuroses but presumably does not play a central role in other mental disorders and that anxiety is involved in the development of all the neuroses. Both suppositions are open to question.

Personality Disorders and Certain Other Nonpsychotic Mental Disorders

Personality Disorders. The personality disorders are characterized by lifelong, generally ego-syntonic maladaptive patterns of behavior. The criterion for classification is the phenomenology (ego-syntonic behavior patterns rather than ego-dystonic symptoms) and the course of the disorder (lifelong rather than episodic). Subdivisions within the personality disorders are based on stereotypes manifesting typical clusters of behavior, such as the obsessive-compulsive personality and the hysterical personality

In defining the personality disorders, DSM-II notes:

This group of disorders is characterized by deeply ingrained maladaptive patterns of behavior that are perceptibly different in quality from psychotic and neurotic symptoms.

The reader is not told what the "perceptible" differences are.

DSM-II interpreted the ICD category "affective personality" to mean cyclothymic personality, which requires "recurring and alternating periods of depression and elation." On the other hand, other countries have interpreted the term to include not only patients who have alternating moods but also patients with persistent depressed mood (depressive character) or elated mood (hypomanic character). The consequence of the DSM-II definition is that a category is provided for the comparatively few truly cyclothymic patients, but no adequate classification is furnished for the much larger number of characterologically depressed patients.

Sexual Deviations. Although DSM-II has an

introductory definition of sexual deviations, the individual disorders are not defined.

In 1972 the American Psychiatric Association's Task Force on Nomenclature and Statistics began consideration of whether homosexuality should be regarded as a mental disorder. A position paper by Spitzer argued that homosexuality does not meet the criteria for a mental disorder but that no inference should be taken that it is normal or as valuable as heterosexuality. The position paper suggested that homosexuality be deleted from subsequent printings of DSM-II and replaced by a new category, sexual orientation disturbance, to apply only to those homosexuals who are disturbed by their sexual orientation. In the seventh and later printings of DSM-II, category 302.0 reads:

Sexual Orientation Disturbance. This is for individuals whose sexual interests are directed primarily toward people of the same sex and who are either disturbed by, in conflict with, or wish to change their sexual orientation. This diagnostic category is distinguished from homosexuality, which by itself does not necessarily constitute a psychiatric disorder. Homosexuality per se is one form of sexual behavior and, with other forms of sexual behavior which are not by themselves psychiatric disorders, is not listed in this nomenclature.

Alcoholism. The subdivision of alcoholism into episodic excessive drinking, habitual excessive drinking, and alcohol addiction is made on the basis of what appears to be a meaningless distinction—the number of times drunk a year—and does not allow for categorizing the various stages in the progression of alcoholism.

Drug Dependence. According to the DSM-I definition, drug addiction could be diagnosed only when the patient was actually addicted. DSM-II provides a more comprehensive diagnosis, drug dependence, which does not require the presence of physiological addiction; "evidence of habitual use or a clear sense of need for the drug" suffices for making the diagnosis.

Psychophysiologic Disorders

This group of disorders is characterized by physical symptoms that are caused by emotional factors and that involve a single organ system, usually under autonomic nervous system innervation. The mere presence of a physical symptom, such as high blood pressure or peptic ulcer, is not sufficient to warrant the diagnosis.

There are many difficulties with this category. First, one could question whether one should classify a condition that manifests itself entirely in a medical (nonbehavioral) way as mental disorder. Second, this category of disorder often looks very similar to some forms of hysterical neurosis. In practice, it is rarely used as a primary diagnosis. Third, one might question whether anyone has ever seen a psychophysiologic hemic and lymphatic disorder.

Special Symptoms

This category is for a small list of symptoms occurring in the absence of any other mental disorder. Most of the symptoms are more likely to be seen in children than in adults. The rules for special symptoms specifically limit their use to situations in which there is no other mental disorder. This section includes anorexia nervosa, which is not merely a symptom but has all of the features of a complete psychiatric disorder.

Transient Situational Disturbances

This category is reserved for more or less transient disorders of any severity, including those of psychotic proportion, that occur as acute reactions to overwhelming environmental stress in patients without any apparent underlying mental disorders.

The diagnostic criteria for these disorders are absence of previous history of psychopathology, overwhelming environmental stress, and brief duration. The category is subdivided according to the patient's developmental stage.

Behavior Disorders of Childhood and Adolescence

This category is reserved for childhood and adolescent disorders that are more stable, internalized, and resistant to treatment than transient situational disturbances but less so than psychoses, neuroses, and personality disorders. This is the only major category in DSM-II that is based on age. The other criterion is severity, excluding disorders that are too mild or too severe. Within this category, as within the personality disorders, the subdivisions are based on stereotypes manifesting typical clusters of behavior. Several child psychiatrists have expressed dissatisfaction with the subgroups chosen.

Conditions without Manifest Psychiatric Disorder and Nonspecific Conditions

This category performs the function of encompassing the "conditions of individuals who are psychiatrically normal but who nevertheless have severe enough problems to warrant examination by a psychiatrists." These conditions are, therefore, not mental disorders. The category is subdivided into three groups: social maladjustment without manifest psychiatric disorder, such as marital and occupational maladjustment; nonspecific conditions, for conditions that cannot be classified under any of the previous categories; and no mental disorder.

REFERENCES

Akiskal, H. S., and McKinney, W. T., Jr. Psychiatry and pseudopsychiatry. Arch. Gen. Psychiatry, *28:* 367, 1973.

American Psychiatric Association. *Diagnostic and Statistical Manual, Mental Disorders* (DSM-I). American Psychiatric Association, Washington, 1952.

American Psychiatric Association. *Diagnostic and Statistical Manual of Mental Disorders* (DSM-II). American Psychiatric Association, Washington, 1968.

Beck, A. T., Ward, C. H., Mendelson, M., et al. Reliability of psychiatric diagnosis. 2. A study of consistency of clinical judgments and ratings. Am. J. Psychiatry, *119:* 351, 1962.

Feighner, J. P., Robins, E., Guze, S. B., et al. Diagnostic criteria for use in psychiatric research. Arch. Gen. Psychiatry. *26:* 57, 1972.

Kanfer, F. H., and Saslow, G. Behavioral diagnosis. In *Behavior Therapy: Appraisal and Status*, C. M. Franks, editor, p. 417. McGraw-Hill, New York, 1969.

Klein, D. F., and Davis. J. M. *Diagnosis and Drug Treatment of Psychiatric Disorders*. Williams & Wilkins, Baltimore, 1969.

Kramer, M. The history of the efforts to agree on an international classification of mental disorders. In *Diagnostic and Statistical Manual of Mental Disorders* (DSM-II). printing 5, p. 135. American Psychiatric Association, Washington, 1973.

Paul, G. L. Experimental-behavioral approaches to "schizophrenia." In *Strategic Intervention in Schizophrenia*, Cancro, R., Fox, E., and Shapiro, J., editors, p. 187. Behavioral Publications, New York, 1974.

Rosenhan, D. L. On being sane in insane places. Science, *179:* 250, 1973.

Spitzer, R. L., A proposal about homosexuality and the APA nomenclature: Homosexuality as an irregular form of sexual development and sexual orientation disturbance as a psychiatric disorder. Am. J. Psychiatry, *1207:* 30, 1973.

Spitzer, R. L., and Endicott, J. Computer diagnosis in an automated record keeping system: A study in clinical acceptability. In *Progress in Psychiatric Information Systems: Computer Applications*, J. L. Crawford, D. W. Morgan and D. T. Giantinco, editors, p. 73. Ballinger, Cambridge, 1974.

Spitzer, R. L., and Endicott, J. Can the computer assist clinicians in diagnosis? Am. J. Psychiatry, *131:* 523, 1974.

13.2.   NEUROSIS, PSYCHOSIS, AND BORDERLINE STATES

Neurosis

It is difficult to classify neuroses. At one time, anyone who evidenced some psychological im-balance was presumed to have a neurosis. Freud's general theory of psychological causes highlighted conflict between sexual drives and inhibiting reality. If one was stronger than the other, anxiety or its defenses would appear. Later, he included aggressive drives derived from a death instinct in opposition to social inhibitions. However, what parents or society condemned became internalized and continued to maintain conflict with internal drives. The ego forces, at the behest of the assimilated conscience or superego, maintain contact with reality, abandoning only a segment of its functions in the service of repression, and ignore only part of reality.

In the process of civilization, the drives can never be fully or directly expressed, always leading to some internal conflict and to conflict among total personalities of others. Therefore, the neurotic process is ubiquitous. Its quantitative degree and its fit for special life situations determine whether the neurosis is healthy or an illness. This discrimination depends not only on the degree of conflict but also on the method of defense used by the ego and the life situation in which the bearer of a lifestyle finds himself.

Anxiety as a signal of danger underlies all neurotic forms that characterize the type of the defenses. Defenses against anxiety are successful in the normal neurotic but, when quantitatively excessive, are associated with discomfort and failure in many life situations and may be associated with free anxiety, dissociations, and low self-esteem.

The classification of neuroses is based on the mode of psychological defense and the degree to which one aspect of the personality dominates internal or external conflict. Since the situational component and the phase of development are important determinants of neuroses, the course is variable, and the degrees of crippling in the end are determined by nonpsychological external elements.

There is no evidence of biogenetic factors in neurotic development, but constitutional differences, not inheritable, may be contributory. Acting on these elements, early life experiences, child care programs, parental personalities, and family dynamics lead to internalization of identifications that prevent the development of an integrated personality. When anxiety breaks through and the neurosis is associated with a deficit in social behavior and a decrease in the feeling of internal security beyond a critical period, only help in reconstituting or creating defenses may be possible.

Since everyone is, to some degree, neurotic, the definition of normality or health is indeed difficult. The estimation of mental health is based on a combination of descriptive and psychogenetic studies concerned with development, anecdotal incidents about reactions to life situations, stress, and critical periods of growth. The greater the repertoire of internalized roles, the better the adaptation.

Psychosis

Psychosis is a behavioral term designating a withdrawal from reality or an active attempt to reconcile reality with an inner world of disorganized thinking and feeling. Restitution is a tempted by means of delusions and hallucinations. Unrealistic behavior, which disrupts most if not all forms of adaptation and seriously disorganizes personality, characterizes psychosis.

There are many types of functional psychoses, including the schizophrenias, mania, depression, and the organic psychoses called senile, arteriosclerotic, alcoholic, toxic, infectious, and traumatic. Neurotic symptoms may overlay the primary disturbance in an attempt to fend off a psychotic breakdown.

Many factors may contribute to the psychoses—biogenetics, child rearing, early physical disease, traumatic experiences, family patterns and systems of communication, life stresses, socio-economics, and culture. Which of them are most significant is not known. Biological, psychological, sociological, and cultural explanations for the changing phenomenology of psychoses are not at hand.

Some serious psychiatrists believe that psychoses and neuroses represent degrees of the same process. But schizophrenic psychoses show a host of behavioral symptoms not seen in the neuroses. For the psychoses, purely psychological approaches are inadequate. At present, schizophrenia is characterized by disorders of thinking, feeling, and sensorimotor function.

Schizophrenia is assumed to be a polyvalent outcome of several variables making up a system or organization that represents a form of functional adaptation. The form is only fixed as an end product, since individual patients show a high degree of variability.

There is not sufficient evidence to determine whether the primary defect is within a part of a developing or functioning psychobiological system or in the organizational processes ordinarily successfully integrating the parts. These processes may be biological, psychological, or environmental. Experiential challenges evoke the vulnerabilities within the parts or the whole system and spontaneous or life challenges are necessary.

Borderline States

Beginning in 1884, borderline or borderland terms have been used to designate conditions lying between schizophrenia and neuroses of various kinds. Often the diagnosis indicated a latent, potential, or transitional phase of schizophrenia. But the borderline diagnosis is not included in the official psychiatric classification.

The borderline represents a defect in psychological development and not a regression. The borderline patient, in general, has a defect in his affectional relationships, angry explosions, lack of consistent self-identity, and depression characterized by loneliness rather than guilt or shame. Borderline patients do not have the thought disorders characteristic of even latent schizophrenia. They do not have the capacity to develop schizophrenia.

The borderline syndrome is caused by some unknown developmental variants. The borderline personality is a lifestyle of vacillating eccentricity. What pushes it into the overt syndrome or back into a remission is not known.

All forms of therapy have been used in the treatment of the borderline states. Few cures have been reported. A milieu characterized by warm and accepting attitudes, with direct advice and experience about social behavior, seems to ready the patients for return to their individual worlds. Certainly, insight therapy of any kind is noneffective and contraindicated. Furthermore, despite the best of approaches —individual, group, or milieu therapy—the borderline patient in follow-up years remains socially inept and awkward.

Treatment of the borderline based on learning theory and encompassed under the rubric of behavior therapy is minimally effective. This suggests that the external influences brought to bear on the child to produce the borderline personality and eventually the overt syndrome happen at an early age, and the critical period, beyond which reversal could be possible, occurs early.

REFERENCES

Grinker, R. R., Sr. Changing styles in psychoses and borderline states. Am. J. Psychiatry, *130:* 151, 1973.

Grinker, R. R., Sr., and Holzman, P. S. Schizophrenic pathology in young adults. Arch. Gen. Psychiatry, *28:* 168, 1973.

Grinker, R. R., Sr., Werble, B., and Drye, R. C. *The Borderline Syndrome*. Basic Books, New York, 1968.

Gruenwald, D. A psychologist's view of the borderline syndrome. Arch. Gen. Psychiatry, *23:* 180, 1970.

Kayton, L. Good outcome in young adult schizophrenia. Arch. Gen. Psychiatry, *29:* 103–111, 1973.

Kernberg, O. Borderline personality organization. J. Am. Psychoanal. Assoc., *15:* 641, 1967.

Knight, R. P. Borderline states, in *Psychoanalytic Psychiatry and Psychology*, R. P. Knight and C. R. Friedman, editors. p. 110. International Universities Press, New York, 1954.

Meehl, P. E. Some ruminations on the validation of clinical procedures. Can. J. Psychol. *13:* 102, 1959.

14

Schizophrenia

14.1 SCHIZOPHRENIA: INTRODUCTION AND HISTORY

Introduction

An estimated 180,000 patients are hospitalized for schizophrenia in the United States each year. When undiagnosed, untreated, and ambulatory cases are added to this number, the total probably rises to about half a million. In 1968, more than 320,000 schizophrenic episodes were diagnosed in the United States. The direct and indirect cost of schizophrenia to the United States is estimated at $14 billion a year. The odds today are one in 100 that a person will be hospitalized as a schizophrenic patient sometime during his life. There may be more than 2 million new cases of schizophrenia in the world every year, and the total world schizophrenic population now numbers close to 10 million.

History

As early as 1400 B.C., a Hindu fragment from the Ayur-Veda described a condition, brought on by devils, in which the afflicted is "gluttonous, filthy, walks naked, has lost his memory, and moves about in an uneasy manner." In the 1st century A.D., the physician Aretaeus of Cappadocia noted the essential qualitative difference between patients suffering from the then traditional catch-all known as mania and those whom he described as "stupid, absent, and musing." Soranus, in the 2nd century, A.D., described delusions of grandeur in patients who "believe themselves to be God" or who "refuse to urinate for fear of causing a new deluge." He also gave careful descriptions of stupor states.

Treatment

The idea of caring for people with mental disorders, rather than simply containing them, did not emerge again until the 18th century. Shock treatment in the 18th and 19th centuries consisted of twirling the patient on a stool until he lost consciousness or dropping him through a trap door into an icy lake (see Figure 1).

Moral treatment, applied widely to hospitalized psychotics in the United States during the middle 19th century, resembled today's milieu therapy and other social therapies and was probably an effective therapeutic approach to schizophrenic patients. With the advent of huge mental hospitals, in which a personal approach was impossible, moral treatment and its therapeutic gains were lost. A therapeutic vacuum persisted for half a century until the development, in the middle 1930's, of Sakel's hypoglycemic coma treatment and Meduna's convulsive therapy.

The neuroleptic drugs in the 1950's brought important further gains, particularly in the sustained control of schizophrenic manifestations. Psychotherapy is frequently effective and can provide new insights into the complex psychopathology of the schizophrenic patient.

Causes

Among the earliest theories were the suggestions that insanity resulted from possession by the devil or evil spirits and that insanity indicated punishment by the gods. Physical factors in the form of vapors and pressure on the brain were held responsible by those who later tried to cure these states by venesection and purging.

In the 18th century Georg Stahl introduced the idea of a vital force. And in the 19th century Heinrich Neumann suggested that insanity was due to a "loosening of the togetherness." During the 19th century a violent controversy developed between those psychiatrists who, like Griesinger, believed that all mental disorders were due to physical brain disease and those who thought that mental disorders were due to a dynamic, psychological struggle. Heredity was also considered by psychiatrists of the early 19th century as a possible cause of psychosis.

The debate between somatogenic and psychogenic schools of thought on the causes of mental disorder continues strong today.

Classification and Diagnosis

In the 1780's Thomas Arnold differentiated ideal and notional insanity from other types of mental disease. In the 19th century Esquirol introduced the term "hallucinations." He also described monomania, which seems to have corresponded to a certain form of paranoid or paraphrenic schizophrenia.

Morel introduced the term dé*mence précoce* in 1856. At that time, the first methodological distinction was made between the terms "idiocy" and "dementia." Idiocy referred to congenital or very early defects, and dementia referred to acquired or reversible defects.

The French concept of *délires*, meaning delusional states, had in Germany been termed *paranoia*. This term was first used by Vogel in 1764. Wilhelm Sander in 1868 described para-

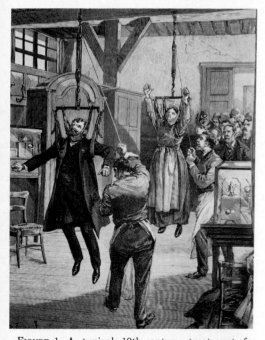

FIGURE 1. A typical 19th-century treatment for mental disorders, in which patients were hoisted from the floor in harnesses and twirled around (Culver Pictures).

noid states much as they are understood today, and Lasêgue in 1871 published a study on the *délire de persécutions*.

Kahlbaum described a pattern characterized by pathologically changed motor tension, to which he gave the name *katatonia* in 1868. Kahlbaum's assistant, Hecker, described the symptomatic picture of hebephrenia and gave it its name in 1870.

In 1887, Kraepelin thought that dementia precox was identical with hebephrenia and that catatonia and dementia paranoides were separate diseases. The 1896 edition of his textbook distinguished dementia precox, which ends in deterioration, and manic-depressive psychosis, which does not end in deterioration. And in 1898, he unified all primary and secondary dementias into one mental disease characterized by the lack of external causes, by its occurrence usually in young and previously healthy persons, and, most important, by ultimate deterioration.

Eugen Bleuler introduced the new term "schizophrenia" for dementia precox in 1911. Translated literally, schizophrenia means split-mindedness, and Bleuler saw the splitting of the personality, rather than the outcome, as the central feature of this disease.

Bleuler's fundamental contribution was the introduction of a hierarchy of symptoms to replace the mere description of unweighted clinical phenomena. To Bleuler, the primary symptoms included disturbances of affect, association, and volition. But virtually the entire clinical picture that Kraepelin had described as typical of schizophrenic pathology was seen by Bleuler as consisting of secondary symptoms— for example, hallucinations, delusions, negativism, and stupor. Ambivalence and the concept that Bleuler first described and that he named "autism" are particularly important features in his clinical picture of schizophrenia.

Carl Jung, influenced by Freud's interpretations of psychopathological phenomena in hysterical patients, applied the new methods and the new insights of psychoanalysis to the symptoms of schizophrenic patients. Jung developed the first experimental method of using associations in the exploration of certain unconscious sets and biases, which he named complexes, and he made the original distinction between introverted and extroverted personalities.

Adolf Meyer, the founder of the psychobiological school of psychiatry, believed that schizophrenic behavior was not brought about by hidden physical or psychic causes but that it was the natural result of a life history that could be clearly traced to various physical, social, and psychological factors in the patient's past. Rather than explaining a patient's symptoms in terms of a number of universal psychodynamic principles or diagnosing disorders on the basis of a few general principles of classification, Meyer insisted on the unique, idiosyncratic nature of every patient's psychiatric disorder.

In 1939 Langfeldt introduced the concept of schizophreniform psychoses and described an additional distinction between process schizophrenia and schizophrenic reaction. The process form of schizophrenia referred back to the old dementia precox concept and was to be diagnosed in schizophrenic patients when final deterioration had either occurred or was to be expected. The schizophrenic reaction, on the other hand, was characterized by schizophreniform symptoms, which are the ones most observers consider typical for acute schizophrenia, and by certain factors in the patient's background: His prepsychotic personality was not characteristically schizoid but was fairly well adjusted to work and to social situations; his psychotic breakdown may have occurred soon after—and probably was caused by—a traumatic event in his life situation. By contrast, in cases of process schizophrenia, the breakdown occurred without any discernible external cause.

Langfeldt's distinction into process and reactive schizophrenia is an attractive device that many clinicians use to make a clinical prognosis—good in the case of schizophrenic reaction, poor in the case of schizophrenic process. A great deal of research has been focused on an objective classification and separation of these two clinical types, either by means of psychological tests or according to some biochemical or other physical factors. However, there is still no decisive evidence to prove that these two types are really of a qualitatively different nature and are not simply different degrees of severity on a psychopathological continuum.

During the past decade, schizophrenic patients have frequently been divided, for research purposes, into paranoid and nonparanoid groups; there is growing evidence that groups selected according to the presence or absence of paranoid symptoms are more homogeneous in their personality structures and their psychological and biological reactions than are randomly selected schizophrenics.

Another system often used today for classifying schizophrenics is that of a well or poorly adjusted premorbid personality—a dichotomy that is almost identical with that of process and reactive (schizophreniform) schizophrenias.

Unlike Kraepelin, Carl Schneider did not see schizophrenia as a single nosological entity but, rather, as the pathological fragmentation of three basic functions that are smoothly integrated in the normal person. The three functions are an undisturbed identity feeling, continuity of psychic processes, and reality contact. When a breakdown of these functions occurs, the following three symptom complexes may occur: may occur:

Thought withdrawal. This complex is associated with the following symptoms: thought stopping, thought insertion, thought hearing, perplexity, experiences of being controlled, and speech disorders.

Derailment. Its related symptoms are lack of affect, inappropriate rage, depression, despair, depersonalization, and hallucinations.

Faselin. This German term lends itself poorly to translation. Its meaning includes rambling and talking in a disconnected manner, with the following symptoms: delusions, looseness of associations, inadequate emotional response, and ego-alien impulses.

Schneider is convinced that only through the systematic analysis of symptom complexes originating in these three functional units will it be possible to reach the underlying causes of the schizophrenic disorder.

In a move toward the pre-Kraepelinian multitude of functional psychoses and in a search for greater homogeneity, Leonhard has spent a major part of his career trying to detach certain so-called atypical schizophrenic syndromes from schizophrenia and to establish them as independent disease entities classified as the nonsystematic schizophrenic psychoses.

Kraepelin described three basic types of dementia precox: catatonic, hebephrenic, and paranoid. Diem and later Bleuler added a fourth type: simple schizophrenia. These four types are still generally accepted today as basic schizophrenic syndromes. Later investigators have added a number of new subtypes, including schizo-affective and pseudoneurotic schizophrenia. The *Diagnostic and Statistical Manual of*

Mental Disorders; prepared by the American Psychiatric Association, includes childhood type and chronic undifferentiated type under schizophrenia but does not list the pseudoneurotic type.

Conceptual Framework

Physical-Biological Models

These models focus on the physical causes of schizophrenia. The physical factors of heredity and pressure of vapors on the brain were at first considered to be the causes of schizophrenic symptoms. Later, autotoxic factors and gonadal (testicular) insufficiency were discussed as possibilities, as was bacterial infection. More recent theories have been focusing on specific toxic factors in the blood, such as an adrenaline derivative and a globulin plasma factor on enzyme abnormalities that may interfere with the normal functioning, production, and degradation of biogenic amines; particularly the catecholamines and indoleamines; on disturbances of nitrogen metabolism; on a disturbance of transmethylation processes in the organism; on the causative role of autoimmune reactions; and on other immunological reactions.

The latest results of research on the hereditary transmission of schizophrenia, using sophisticated methods of twin studies and observations on children of schizophrenic parents raised in adoptive families, have left little doubt that at least 40 per cent of schizophrenia cases are attributable to genetic factors. The experimental production of model psychoses through the action of psychotomimetic drugs may also be regarded as an attempt to introduce possible toxic factors that may simulate schizophrenic symptoms.

Description-Classification Models

These models are oriented primarily toward clinical observation, recording, description, and classification, and they use three main approaches: (1) simple, clinical description of syndromes and reaction patterns, (2) synthesis of nosological entities based mainly on clinical judgment, and (3) computer-derived typology based on factor analysis and cluster analysis of behavioral manifestations.

Psychodynamic-Interaction Models

These models are characterized by empathic understanding and theoretical explanations of the observed psychopathology. The explanations are based not on experiments but on concepts and constructs referring mainly to functional intrapersonal dynamics and interpersonal relationships.

Freud described schizophrenia as a deep, primary disturbance of a person's object relations, a narcissistic psychosis that precluded psychotherapy because the patient was not capable of an effective transference relationship with the therapist. The different symptomatic manifestations of schizophrenia were explained as an interaction of various defense mechanisms against anxiety arising from early psychic traumas, not essentially differing from the dynamics prevailing in neuroses.

Another model postulates that certain stages follow each other in regular sequence during the development of the human infant. According to this theory, which presupposes a primary disturbance of object relations, a paranoid psychosis occurring in adult life may represent a pathological regression to an earlier developmental stage.

The most widely accepted psychodynamic model today—the environmentalist neo-Freudian school—stresses the primary importance of deeply disturbed interpersonal relationships. Disturbed family communications and interactions are considered likely to be the origin of the disorder and effective psychotherapy requires many modifications.

Phenomenological-Existential Models

Here the orientation is toward the understanding of a schizophrenic patient's mode of existing in and experiencing his world. The emphasis in these models is on the immediacy and directness of the patient's lived experiences. These experiences are accepted and appreciated as phenomena in their own right and are analyzed strictly within the limits of their own self-evidence.

Conditioning-Behavioral Models

These models aim at explanations of deviant behavior on the basis of experientially established disturbances of acquired response patterns in primitive signal systems that normally enable the organism to adapt to changes in the perceived environment through neurophysiological and psychophysiological learning. Pavlov saw in schizophrenia the manifestation of generalized inhibition, the result of ultramaximal stimulation. Current models consider schizophrenia a chronic condition of learned, nonadaptive responding, due to disturbed reinforcement patterns of early experiences.

Sociological Model

Sociologists and psychiatrists have debated whether urban ghettos specifically attract schizophrenics (the drift hypothesis) or whether they tend to produce a schizophrenic pathology (the breeder hypothesis). In recent years the evidence has favored the drift hypothesis.

Current Status

Today, etiological research is actively exploring four major factors: (1) the genetic, the role of heredity; (2) the biochemical, searching for a toxic factor that may be the result of an innate metabolic error; (3) the psychodynamic, the effects of early psychic trauma or a psychological deficiency state on defense mechanisms; and (4) the social, focusing on the role of a disturbed family or community structure in the life of a schizophrenic.

The greatest progress has been made in the therapeutic management of schizophrenia. With modern pharmacotherapy it is possible to maintain many schizophrenic patients in symptom-free remission over many years and thus to prevent relapses. Yet the search for a cure goes on and awaits the solution of the etiological riddle.

Is Schizophrenia Universal?

Cultural influences determine, to a significant extent, the manifestations of most mental illnesses, including schizophrenia.

In some parts of Europe, the catatonic form of schizophrenia is the most common form; in the United States, paranoid schizophrenia is the most common. In Brazil and in Africa there is a remarkably low incidence of the paranoid type of schizophrenia and a much higher incidence of hebephrenic schizophrenia than in Europe and the United States. In general, it appears that paranoid reactions prevail among schizophrenics from more differentiated cultures and that catatonic reactions occur more frequently in less developed cultures.

Spitzer and co-workers observed that schizophrenics in Kentucky were more likely to present symptoms of decreased communication,

denial of illness, and impaired grooming; schizophrenics in New York clearly showed more affective symptoms than the less sophisticated sample of schizophrenics in Kentucky.

Recent studies have established clearly that historical changes in philosophical, religious, technical, moral, and political value systems have a significant influence on the relative frequency of individual schizophrenic symptoms. Several investigators have observed, for example, that the catatonic form of schizophrenia is gradually becoming less frequent in the United States. Schizophrenics today are definitely less agressive than they were 50 years ago. Delusions of grandeur increased for a while during World War I and again during World War II but otherwise have been in a general decline over the years. Delusions of witchcraft and other magic have become less frequent, and ideas about being hypnotized or being influenced by radiation and electricity have definitely increased in frequency in recent years. In general, there is apparently a definite tendency for the contents of delusions to become more realistic, sober, plausible, and anonymous.

Most researchers agree that delusions of being controlled or being poisoned have not been influenced by historical or cultural changes. These delusions seem to represent a stable core of schizophrenic pathology that remains the same in various parts of the world and in different periods of time.

General trends include a decrease of catatonic reactions and an increase of paranoid reactions among schizophrenics belonging to sophisticated cultural groups, a decrease of supernatural delusions and an increase of delusions involving modern technical and scientific apparatus.

Is Schizophrenia Increasing?

Hospital records suggest that the incidence of schizophrenia in the United States has probably remained unchanged, at least for the past 100 years and possibly throughout the entire history of the country, despite tremendous socio-economic and population changes. In the past, the reproductivity rate of schizophrenics has always been distinctly lower than that of the general population, and schizophrenics' mortality rate was higher, mainly because of the high incidence of tuberculosis among those who were hospitalized. However, treatment has lowered this mortality rate and has increased the reproductivity rate of schizophrenics. Thus, the selective biological disadvantage that in the past had a braking effect of the incidence of schizophrenia now seems to be gradually disappearing.

Whether one accepts the genetic or the environmental origin of schizophrenia, there is little doubt that more children in families with schizophrenic parents will mean a growing incidence of schizophrenia in the future. And the cost of schizophrenia, not only in dollars spent for medical and social services but also in human suffering and productivity loss, could become even more astronomical than it is today.

REFERENCES

Bleuler, E. *Dementia Praecox or the Group of Schizophrenias.* International Universities Press, New York, 1950.

Kety, S. S., Rosenthal, D., Wender, P. H., and Schulsinger, F. Mental Illness in the biological and adoptive families of adopted schizophrenics. Am. J. Psychiatry, *128:* 302, 1971.

Langfeldt, G. *The Schizophreniform States.* Munksgaard, Copenhagen, 1939.

London, N. J. An Essay on psychoanalytic theory: Two theories of schizophrenia. part I: Review and critical assessment of the development of the two theories. Int. J. Psycho-Anal., *54:* 169, 1973.

Mednick, S. A., and McNeil, T. F. Current methodology in research on the etiology of schizophrenia: Serious difficulties which suggest the use of the high-risk-group method. Psychol. Bull., *70:* 681, 1968.

Szasz, T. S. *The Myth of Mental Illness.* Harper, New York, 1961.

World Health Organization. *Report of the International Pilot Study of Schizophrenia,* vol. 1, World Health Organization, Geneva, 1973.

14.2   SCHIZOPHRENIA: EPIDEMIOLOGY

Diagnosis

Differences in diagnostic techniques prohibit uniform and comparable epidemiological studies of schizophrenia. Recent comparative diagnostic studies of British and American clinicians demonstrated that differences in diagnostic practices, rather than types of patients, were the major contributors to differing rates of schizophrenia between the two countries. The International Pilot Study of Schizophrenia undertaken by the World Health Organization in 1973 and other studies are promoting the development of objective methods for the diagnosis of schizophrenia.

Methods of Study

Treatment Facilities

Most available incidence rates of schizophrenia are based on first admissions to public and private psychiatric hospitals. These studies do not account for patients who are not hospitalized but are treated in other facilities, such as day hospitals and ambulatory clinics. They also ignore those persons suffering from the disease who do not use any of a community's mental health services. Some investigators have relied on surveys of records of all treatment facilities, including most of the private practicing psychiatrists of the community, over a specific period of time. These studies provide incidence and period prevalence rates for the treated or diagnosed segment of the population.

Psychiatric Case Registers

Case registers provide a longitudinal record for every person receiving care in the mental health facilities of a geographically defined community. Each person is registered on his initial experience with any mental health service, and all subsequent episodes of illness and use of different facilities are added to this file. Registers do not solve the problem of untreated persons or those treated only by nonpsychiatric professionals, such as general practitioners and internists. Not all registers receive complete reporting from all the mental health facilities of a community; most commonly missing are reports by psychiatrists in private practice. Another problem with this method is the mobility of the population in the area covered by the register and the number of persons who seek care in facilities outside the area.

Registers, by virtue of their being ongoing data collection systems, can provide period or lifetime prevalence rates, comparative rates for different periods of time, an accurate account of the use of different facilities by groups of patients with schizophrenia and other diagnoses, and a sampling base for more intensive investigations and studies of high-risk groups.

Field Surveys

The survey is the most frequently used method in epidemiological studies. Some surveys take into consideration every person in a community; others rely on representative random samples of the population. Usually, members of households are interviewed by trained interviewers, and a determination is made of whether or not a person is schizophrenic. Some investigators check the diagnosis of interviewers with those of experienced clinicians; others do not. Surveys provide prevalence rates of schizophrenia and identify persons who have not been treated in mental health facilities and add them to those who have a psychiatric history. Most surveys provide lifetime prevalence rates, considering the number of active and inactive cases identified through this specific case-finding method as of the date of the survey. Such surveys do not provide incidence rates.

Incidence

The true incidence rate of schizophrenia is difficult to obtain. In addition to the lack of objective diagnostic methods that complicates the process of identification of cases, complete identification entails the detection of every person afflicted by the disease in a well-defined community and the ability to determine the actual date of onset of the illness. The age groups investigated also vary, with most studies considering the segment of the population aged 15 and over. The incidence rates for schizophrenia from studies that consider all ages in the United States vary from a low of 0.43 per 1,000 population to a high of 0.69 per 1,000. For the age group 15 and over, the rates range from a low of 0.30 per 1,000 to a high of 1.20 per 1,000.

Prevalence

The variation in prevalence rates from studies around the world is much greater than the variation in incidence rates. European and Asiatic investigators record lifetime prevalence rates through surveys. They consider treated and untreated cases and count all persons who have had a schizophrenic episode, whether they are under active treatment or not during the survey period. The lifetime prevalence rates for European studies range from a low of 1.9 per 1,000 to a high of 9.5 per 1,000; the range is much smaller for Asiatic studies, 2.1 to 3.8 per 1,000. Two North American studies of lifetime prevalance provide low rates of 1.0 and 1.9 per 1,000, respectively. Other studies in the United States give period prevalence rates for treated cases, and they range from 2.3 to 3.6 per 1,000. As in the case of incidence rates, age, sex, and race are major variables that affect prevalence rates.

In the United States, between 0.23 per cent and 0.47 per cent of the total population is likely to receive psychiatric treatment for a schizophrenic illness during any particular year, provided that adequate mental health care facilities are available in all communities. This means that a minimum of 460,000 and a maximum of 940,000 persons will need treatment annually for this illness. For 62 per cent of each group, treatment will involve at least one hospitalization during the year. With a lifetime prevalence of about 1 per cent, 2 million Americans may be suffering from a mental disorder that would be classified as schizophrenia today.

Risk of Death

The excess mortality among schizophrenics and other patients with mental illness is not readily explainable. The lower relative risk of death for schizophrenics as compared with the other major mental disorders may be due to the more sheltered and restricted lives that schizophrenics lead. Institutional care, which in the past was one of the major factors involved in the high mortality rates among schizophrenics, does not appear to be a major contributor to death in this population.

Reproduction Rates

Incidence and prevalence rates of schizophrenia are affected by the mortality and reproduction rates of schizophrenic populations. Mortality rates affect mainly prevalence; reproduction rates influence both incidence and prevalence. The expectation of becoming schizophrenic for members of a family increases if one of them is already suffering from schizophrenia. The expected rates of schizophrenia for relatives of schizophrenics are always higher than the expected rate for the general population, which is approximately 1 per cent, considering all age groups. Although a certain percentage of the relationship between family membership and schizophrenia is probably genetic, environmental factors are also thought to play a role. Obviously, then, increases in reproduction rates for schizophrenics and decreases in mortality rates eventually result in an increase in the incidence and prevalence rates of schizophrenia.

The single, separated, divorced, and widowed

are overrepresented among first admissions to hospitals with psychotic diagnoses. Schizophrenic populations are also known to have lower rates of marriage and reproduction than does the general population. However, with the advent of psychoactive drugs, open-door policies, the emphasis on rehabilitation, and community-based care for the schizophrenic, increased rates of marriage and fertility have been observed. Women schizophrenics produce more children than do men schizophrenics. Although the reproduction rates of schizophrenics are increasing, these rates remain lower than the rate for the general population.

Mental Hospital Beds

A significant proportion of mental hospital beds are occupied by schizophrenic patients. Over the past 2 decades, the duration of each hospital experience has diminished, and the number of readmissions has increased. Patients are now being hospitalized more often for shorter periods of time.

Socio-Economic Status

One of the most consistent findings in epidemiological studies of schizophrenia is the presence of a disproportionate number of schizophrenics in the lower socio-economic classes. Two major hypotheses have been proposed to explain the relationship of social class to schizophrenia. The first is generally known as the social causation hypothesis, which assumes that the social and economic stresses experienced by the lower classes are etiologically related to schizophrenic illness. The second is generally known as the social selection or drift hypothesis, which claims that low social class membership rates in schizophrenia are more a function of schizophrenic illness and that schizophrenic patients tend to be downwardly mobile. Neither of these hypotheses has been definitely proved, nor has the extent of contribution of either hypothesis been demonstrated.

Conclusion

Despite major advances in the care and treatment of the mentally ill, schizophrenia continues to be a chronic incapacitating disease. Each year, anywhere between 100,000 and 200,000 Americans are afflicted by the disease. About 1 million schizophrenics would require some psychiatric attention and treatment in the United States annually if adequate mental health facilities were available across the country; 62 per cent of them would need either hospitalization or care in a transitional facility. An estimated total of 2 million Americans suffer from schizophrenia today.

Schizophrenia is an illness of adolescents and young adults and is most prevalent between the ages of 15 and 54, the major productive years of most persons. The total annual direct and indirect cost of schizophrenic illness for society is estimated at $14 billion in the United States. Both incidence and prevalence rates are higher among nonwhites than among whites. The prevalence rates of schizophrenia are highest among the lower socio-economic classes. The expectation of schizophrenia is higher among the relatives of schizophrenics than among the general population. This expectation is 12 per cent for the children of one schizophrenic parent and 35 to 44 per cent for the children of two schizophrenic parents. The marriage and reproduction rates of schizophrenics are lower than those of the general population, although substantial increases have been noted in these rates since the introduction of new methods of treatment. Schizophrenics have a higher mortality rate than does the general population, even though this rate is lower than the rates for those suffering from affective disorders, neuroses, and character disorders.

Epidemiological studies have helped in the formulation of several hypotheses to explain the cause of schizophrenia. These hypotheses have mainly involved genetic, social, and cultural factors. Although most investigators believe that a combination of genetic predisposition and environmental factors is required to precipitate schizophrenic illness, the exact nature of the prerequisites and their interaction has not been explained.

REFERENCES

Dunham, H. W. *Community and Schizophrenia.* Wayne State University Press, Detroit, 1965.
Faris, R. E. L., and Dunham, H. W. *Mental Disorders in Urban Areas.* Chicago University Press, Chicago, 1939.
Hollingshead, A. B., and Redlich, F. C. *Social Class and Mental Illness.* Wiley, New York, 1958.
Jaco, E. G. *Social Epidemiology of Mental Disorders: A Psychiatric Survey of Texas.* Russell Sage Foundation, New York, 1960.
Murphy, H. B. M. Cultural factors in the genesis of schizophrenia. In *The Transmission of Schizophrenia.* D. Rosenthal and S. S. Kety, editors, p. 137. Pergamon Press. London, 1968.
Rosenthal, D. The heredity-environment issue in schizophre-

nia. In *The Transmission of Schizophrenia*. D. Rosenthal and S. S. Kety, editors, p. 413, Pergamon Press, London, 1968.

Torrey, E. F. Is schizophrenia universal?: An open question. Schizophrenia Bull., 7: 53, 1973.

World Health Organization. *Report of the International Pilot Study of Schizophrenia*, vol. I. World Health Organization, Geneva, 1973.

14.3   SCHIZOPHRENIA: ETIOLOGY

Problems

Definition

In any discussion of the causes of schizophrenia, an immediate question arises: What is meant by the term "schizophrenia"? Unfortunately there is no consensus on this point. Frequently, the diagnosis is accorded to anyone who shows serious behavioral disturbances or marked impropriety of behavior or who expresses his thoughts in language and words that have no shared meaning. Misperceptions are frequently ascribed to schizophrenia; asocial and even antisocial ways of life are labeled schizophrenic. Criteria vary from country to country and from hospital to hospital. Similarly, behavior and symptoms in schizophrenia do not remain stable or fixed.

The problem of diagnosis becomes particularly urgent in relation to the selection of subjects for experiments and in framing hypotheses concerning the causes of the illness on the basis of such experiments. Investigations have followed three patterns: (1) Two investigators studying the same or similar functions in different populations of schizophrenic patients either have been unable to confirm each other's findings or have produced two sets of contradictory data. (2) When similar criteria are used in the selection of subjects, different investigators, studying the same functions, have been unable to confirm each other's findings. (3) When normal and schizophrenic subjects are compared for differences in performance or functioning, findings have most frequently stressed the variations within the experimental group. However, the experimental and control groups have not shown distinctive differences in central tendencies. One may justifiably ask whether the schizophrenic group is, in fact, in any way homogeneous and the disease a unitary one.

Purpose

What are the various etiological theories supposed to explain about schizophrenia?

If schizophrenia is thought of as a disease modeled after the usual concepts, such as a viral infection or a neoplasm, it is relevant to investigate metabolic pathways and to do cytogenetic or cellular biochemical studies. Many have argued, however, that there are only schizophrenic persons, that schizophrenia is not a disease per se. If that is so, research in personality development or the testing of personality theories may be more relevant and fruitful.

However, current theories, with very few exceptions, do not attempt to relate one level of organization to another. Genetic theories, for instance, do not usually identify the specific factors believed to be transmitted genetically. The nonspecific nature of these theories seems to prevent their wider application and the construction of an integrated theory of the causes of schizophrenia.

Theory Construction

Theories of the causes of schizophrenia have also been impeded by three major conceptual difficulties. First, these theories are frequently stated in terms of single causes, phrased in biochemical language. However, a single etiological factor does not exist in nature. Its complex effects become manifest only through its interaction with other systems.

The second conceptual difficulty: Speculations about schizophrenia follow on the latest fashion in the biomedical sciences. Yet correlations are mistaken for causal explanations; necessary conditions are mistaken for sufficient ones; the language of causes is confused with the language of purposes; and broad biological concepts of the interaction of the genotype with its environment are forgotten.

The third conceptual difficulty: A functional explanation only indicates how something works, not how it got there.

Genetic Hypotheses

Studies of Relatives

Studies of relatives report, on the basis of hospital records, that, in the general population and in stepsiblings, the morbid risk for schizophrenia is from 0.3 to 2.8 per cent; in parents of schizophrenic probands, it is 0.2 to 12 per cent;

n full siblings, it is 3 to 14 per cent; for children with one schizophrenic parent, it is 8 to 18 per cent. If both parents are schizophrenic, the risk for the children is between 15 and 55 per cent. For second-degree relatives, the median risk value is 2.5 per cent.

Many workers have criticized these statistics on methodological grounds. First, the diagnosis of schizophrenia is notoriously unreliable and may be too inclusive or exclusive. Second, for various reasons, hospital records are not good sources of data. Third, the number of hospitalized cases does not reflect the incidence of a disease but, rather, its prevalence. Fourth, for the most part, the variables of socio-economic class and environmental factors are not controlled.

Ideally, studies of the relatives of schizophrenic persons should identify everyone diagnosed as being schizophrenic in a particular population, whether he has been hospitalized or not, using clearly defined diagnostic criteria. At the same time, these criteria should be applied not only to first-degree but also to second-degree relatives. In addition, a comparison group of nonschizophrenic probands and relatives should be used, properly matched for socio-economic and personal variables.

The incidence or prevalence of schizophrenia in the relatives of patients does not necessarily mean that genetic factors play the exclusive or even the preponderant role in transmitting the predisposition. Much more transpires in families than the vertical passing on of genes.

Studies of Twins

The preferred method for testing genetic theories is the study of concordance rates for schizophrenia in monozygotic and dizygotic twins. These rates have ranged from 0 to 86 per cent and from 2 to 17 per cent, respectively, in 11 published studies. Kallmann pointed out that the concordance rate for monozygotic twins who had not lived together for some years before his study was 77.6 per cent, but the rate for those twins who had not been separated was 91.5 per cent. He also found that many more female than male twins were concordant for schizophrenia, whether they were monozygotic or not.

The studies that produced those statistics have been critically scrutinized on methodological grounds. Discordance for a specific clinical picture in twin pairs is likely to be more striking than is concordance for a broad diagnostic label. There is an almost total absence of schizophrenia in the families of discordant twin pairs and a 60 per cent incidence in the families of concordant twin pairs. In addition, the twin in the male discordant pair who does not become ill tends to have a better premorbid social and sexual history than does his psychotic twin.

One of the major problems in twin research is that concordance studies have customarily been done on hospitalized twins. There is a relationship between a high concordance rate and the severity of illness, as adjudged by length of hospitalization. Also, concordance rates in hospitalized twins are demonstrably higher if one selects samples from a hospital population, rather than from consecutive admissions.

The manner in which zygosity is determined is also important; many of the classical studies of schizophrenic twins were done before the introduction of modern, blood-grouping methods of zygosity determination. When less precise methods are used, there is a greater likelihood that monozygotic twins will be classified as dizygotic and that concordance rates will be higher in monozygotic twins.

The studies of twins provide powerful support for the idea that genetic factors do, indeed, play a role in predisposing to schizophrenia. They also suggest that monozygotic twins may be more frequently concordant for some underlying predisposition that expresses itself in concordance for schizophrenia in some and concordance for psychopathology in a greater number of such twins. One might conclude that the genetic predisposition is for either psychopathology or some as yet unknown functional disturbance underlying psychopathology. If this speculation should prove correct, schizophrenia then becomes one of several phenotypic forms of expressions of that disturbance.

Further evidence on this point is obtained in studies whose main original aim is to separate out the relative contributions of heredity and environment in schizophrenia. Parents and their children separated early in life were studied to ascertain the incidence of schizophrenia in the children and their families. These studies indicate that what is probably inherited is not schizophrenia but a range of psychopathology. These studies lend strong support to the contention that genetic factors play a role in schizophrenia. However, most schizophrenic patients do not have psychotic parents.

Mode of Inheritance

Monogenetic Theories. Current genetic theories state that schizophrenia is a specific inherited disease due to a single mutant, inherited gene that is either recessive, dominant, or intermediate. It is further hypothesized that the genotype is characterized by an undiscovered metabolic error that leads to the schizophrenic illness. The fact that there is less than 100 per cent concordance for schizophrenia in monozygotic twins is explained by some as a constitutional resistance to the disease.

In monogenic theories, environmental influences are considered inconsequential. The natural history of the disease—premorbid state, onset, course, remission, and outcome—is either overlooked or is explained in some way by an error in metabolism. Genetic theories account for the variety and instability of clinical subtypes in schizophrenia either by postulating that there is one specific gene for schizophrenia and that other genes modify the phenotype or by postulating that the subtypes lie outside the sphere of genetic influence. On the other hand, some members of this school believe that schizophrenia is not a single disease but that it consists of several diseases or subtypes, which are caused by different genes. In this hypothesis, the single gene controls a metabolic error. It is implied that an enzymatic defect leads to the production or accumulation of an abnormal metabolite.

Two-Gene Theory. Using family pedigree studies, Karlsson proposed a two-gene theory. Each gene (S and P) is inherited independently and has a mutant counterpart (s and p). In different combinations, these genes and their counterparts may lead to a normal or creative person, a schizophrenic or sociopathic person, or a mentally retarded or autistic child. The schizophrenic genotype may be calculated to occur with a frequency of 1 per cent. Such a genotype does not inevitably lead to a schizophrenic phenotype. This theory involves predisposition and stress.

Polygenic Theories. Those who subscribe to the theory that the mode of transmission of schizophrenia is polygenic point out that the illness does not conform closely to a Mendelian pattern of transmission, in which monozygotic twins are 100 per cent concordant for schizophrenia. However, a polygenic inheritance cannot be established by pedigree methods. Polygenic hypotheses about transmission usually state that a biochemical abnormality is not inherited. Rather, what is inherited is a predisposition to develop the illness. Those predisposed to do so develop the illness only by virtue of the fact that an environment elicits the disposition, especially if that environment is stressful. There exist predisposition-stress and predisposition-learning hypotheses. Such theories account for the fact that schizophrenic manifestations do not occur with the high frequency required by a monogenic theory.

What is Inherited?

A number of hypotheses have addressed themselves to the question of what, other than a biochemical defect, could be inherited. In such hypotheses it is implied that the inheritance is polygenic, but not necessarily so, and that what is inherited acts as a predisposing factor in the illness. This predisposition has been variously described as a characterological deficit, a thought disorder, a defect in the autonomic nervous system, and a defect in neural integration.

Predisposition and Learning

Still another series of theories focuses on both predisposition and learning in schizophrenia. The validation of such theories requires the study of physiological variables. Unfortunately, psychophysiologic studies involving schizophrenic subjects have consistently yielded contradictory results.

Mednick's theoretical proposal, which is based on Hullian learning theory, states that the predisposition to schizophrenia is characterized by excessively strong physiological reactions to mild stress, easy or rapid acquisition of conditioned responses, excessively slow recovery from autonomic imbalance, and excessive stimulus generalization reactiveness. In the acute schizophrenic patient, an increase in anxiety is correlated with an increase in the level and breadth of stimulus generalization. As a result, many new stimuli become potentially capable of arousing anxiety, and a vicious cycle is set up. As generalization widens, atypical and tangential thought sequences intrude, and preceptions are distorted. (See Figure 1.) The chronic

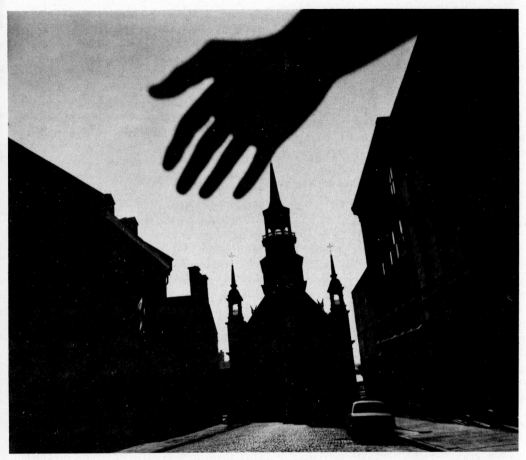

FIGURE 1. In schizophrenia irrational and idiosyncratic ideas create a fearful world that is difficult for others to experience or understand, as symbolized above. (Courtesy of Arthur Tress for Magnum Photos, Inc.)

schizophrenic state is characterized by learning avoidant and irrelevant thoughts that seek to reduce anxiety whenever it occurs. If these thoughts successfully defend against anxiety, they become self-reinforcing.

There is considerable evidence of a high incidence of thought disorder, paranoid behavior and attitudes, or shared delusion in one or the other or both parents of schizophrenic children and adults. The close relationship in the formal aspects of the thought processes of parents and their schizophrenic children could make one believe that the child learns to think illogically, idiosyncratically, delusionally, irrationally, or overinclusively. However, it cannot at present be decided whether this is truly so or whether, in addition, a necessary defect in neural integration must be present before a thought disorder is learned. Alternatively, the formal aspects of the thought disorder could be the direct expression of the neural defect. Nothing known today allows one to decide among these alternatives.

Case Against Genetic Factors

Those who deny the influence of genetic factors point to several pieces of data to support their view. For example, in Kallmann's study more female than male pairs of twins were concordant for schizophrenia. The environmentalist school argues that the concordance rates for schizophrenia in twins may be understood either in terms of the psychology of twins or in more complex ways as a result of the way twins are treated by their families. Those who do not look with favor on a genetic contribution to the illness blame intrauterine, perinatal development and life experiences for the illness.

Developmental and Psychophysiologic Hypotheses

There seems to be some agreement among psychologists and psychiatrists that, because of basic deficits in ego functioning, schizophrenic persons are unable to handle their personal conflicts and to cope with their environment. They find everyday tasks stressful not because the tasks are necessarily stressful but because they perceive the tasks as threats. In addition, their conflicts sensitize them to certain classes of life experiences, such as separation from the home.

Developmental Studies

Some distinguishing diagnostic criteria may be found in the formal disturbances in psychological functioning and in their quality. The recent focus in psychoanalytic hypotheses has shifted to the ego—the organization of functions that is involved in adaptation and the regulation and control of behavior and that includes intellect, language, memory, thinking, perception, attention, intention, reality testing, affectivity, the structure of defenses, object relations, and motility.

Developmental studies do not indicate what other factors play a role in the ultimate disturbances. Although genetic and biochemical factors are acknowledged, they are not deemed appropriate for study by psychological means. Some data suggest that life experiences do modify brain function and that brain function is not only or inevitably the product of genetic factors. In addition, it is possible that intrauterine and perinatal factors may play an important role in impairing brain function.

According to current psychiatric opinion, disturbances of ego functions and of the superego must be attributed to deviations in their development, maturation, and integration in childhood. These disturbances occur as a consequence of genetic, constitutional, or physiological factors or as a result of distortions in the reciprocal relationship between the infant and his mother.

The etiological significance of disturbances in the mother-child relationship is most evident in the autistic and symbiotic psychoses of childhood. The autistic child behaves as though animate objects did not exist, and he seems to be unaware of his mother as a separate and distinct person. In contrast, in the symbiotic psychosis the child is unable to progress beyond the closeness and complete dependence that characterized his relationship to his mother in infancy. The illness is characterized by panic when the mother is not present; rage and violent agitation; outbursts of excitement and pleasure, alternating with periods of destructiveness; symptoms that suggest the child is unable to differentiate between animate and inanimate objects; a tendency to confuse inner experience and external events; an overwhelming need to cling to adults; and magical and dereistic thought processes.

When ego functions are poorly integrated or are not fully differentiated, disturbances in the control and regulation of behavior, personal relationships, and adaptation are evident during the premorbid phase. Characteristically, with the onset of psychosis, further dedifferentiation of ego functions and regressive behavioral phenomena occur. Some postulate that this regressive developmental process occurs because of the intense and terrifying hostility and aggression (and their transformation) mobilized at the beginning of the illness in response to a precipitating event, such as separation. The origins of such hostility and its intensity are not known, but severe deprivation may play a role. Other authors have suggested that there may be some inherent, organismic aspect to this untamed aggression that parallels the inherent disturbances in the rudimentary ego functions. In the course of development, this aggression interacts detrimentally with the maturation and integration of these functions.

Some consensus has been reached that very early in or at the start of personality development—probably as the result of some unspecified genic, polygenic, or congenital influences—serious deviations in the development of higher mental functions occur. Since development is considered to be epigenetic, functions that develop later are adversely influenced by these earlier deviations. As a result of these early functional disturbances, the mother-child relationship is also disturbed, with adverse consequences for future development.

Studies address themselves to the hypothesis that the disturbances in ego function present in childhood and adult schizophrenia are the product of genetic, intrauterine, or perinatal impairment of the brain. This defect may be instigated by a hereditary, congenital, nutritional, metabolic, or structural defect; by an exogenous agent, such as a virus; or by an endogenous source, such as the endocrine glands, occurring during the time that the child is being carried by the mother. As the result of brain damage, development and maturation of neural and psychological functions are impaired. The role of the mothering figure after the child's birth is not necessarily minimized; in responding to such an aberrant child, she may potentiate the existing defects.

Psychophysiologic Hypotheses

Many clinical and experimental psychologists focus on disturbances of one or another psychological function, such as perception, attention, or learning. Others postulate that schizophrenia is a function of a particular kind of social learning process.

In early investigations Kraepelin and Bleuler observed disturbances in attention in schizophrenia. And Jung stated that, to a great extent, formal thought disturbances and symptomatic behavior in schizophrenia could be ascribed to a diminution of attention and apperception. In the years since, many experimental studies of attentional processes in schizophrenia have been performed, but with equivocal results. Some investigators have suggested that schizophrenic persons are more sensitive to external information.

McReynolds formulated the theory that schizophrenic anxiety occurs because the person has been flooded by unassimilable percepts. To defend against this anxiety, he attempts to integrate and reduce these percepts by apathy and withdrawal. A considerable body of evidence suggests that some schizophrenic patients may at first tend to be overly attentive to many or all stimuli, which are often irrelevant, and later exclude, reduce, or avoid these stimuli.

Environmental Factors and Hypotheses

In the past few years, particular emphasis has been placed on the study of the parents and families of schizophrenic patients, with the hope of isolating certain variables—such as some aspects of the behavior, personality, or attitudes of one or both parents—or of specifying modes of family interactions that seem to play an etiological role in schizophrenia. In addition, recent publications have dealt with the relationship between the formal aspects of a parent's cognitive style and the cognitive style of the schizophrenic child.

It is clear that genetic factors predispose to psychopathology, if not to schizophrenia. It is also clear that the inheritance of the gene or genes does not inevitably lead to schizophrenic illness. There must be environmental factors that, in addition to the genotype, produce the schizophrenic phenotype. It is, therefore, entirely legitimate to seek these factors in the family and the cultural, economic, and social environment of the child who becomes schizophrenic sometime in his life.

Characteristics of Parents

In studies of parents, the mother has borne the brunt of the investigative efforts and, regrettably, the blame. The well-documented distortions in the mother's behavior in the reciprocal relationship may, in fact, represent a reaction to the child's behavior, rather than its cause. If a mother consistently fails to elicit a smiling response from her child, she may react with disappointment, exasperation, or whatever.

Sullivan concluded from his clinical investigations that some of his schizophrenic patients had been rendered anxious as infants by their anxious mothers. Others have described the mother of the potential schizophrenic as aggressive, rejecting, domineering, and insecure and have described the father as inadequate, passive, and indifferent. Elsewhere in the literature, these fathers have been depicted as directly threatening, assaultive, or brutal or as overwhelming the child. In contrast to those mothers who are described as either subtly or overtly rejecting, others are said to be fussy and overprotective, perpetuating the symbiotic union. Some mothers are said to assume the role of the martyr to restrict the child's freedom and prevent him from directly expressing hostility.

Several investigators have concluded, on the basis of psychological test findings, that schizophrenic patients perceive one or both parents as authoritarian. But it is not clear from such studies whether the child's perception is distorted or accurate.

Alanen found that the mothers of schizophrenic children tended not to understand their child's needs and feelings, were overpossessive and often hostile to their children, and tied their children to them in an inimical bond, although they were unable to be emotionally or physically close to them. Alanen has also suggested that this type of mother treats her child as she herself was once treated by her own mother.

Characteristics of the Child

Retrospective studies of schizophrenic adults suggest that they have traveled many roads to become schizophrenic. As children, some showed patterns of clinging to the mother, shared her bedroom until late adolescence, had nightmares, were enuretic, and became fearful and panicky when away from home. Others were described as bookish, lonely, friendless, intense, self-conscious, apathetic, listless, shy, disinterested, withdrawn, prone to daydream, seclusive, and oversensitive, with occasional outbursts of temper. A third group was, from an early age, asocial, shameless, and lacking in propriety. The behavior of still another group was overly compliant and conforming; these children were overconcerned with the opinions of peers and parents, prudish, afraid to express themselves, too well-mannered, too anxious to please others, inconspicuous, docile, and dull. Such behavioral traits may be summarized as reflecting deviations in control and regulatory processes and in relationships to other people and a tendency to resort to daydreaming.

Parent-Child Bond

The close bond that exists between some mothers and their children is clinically manifested in the symbiotic psychosis. Some authors have suggested that the longings and close attachment to the mother characteristic of the normal infant persist as part of the psychopathology of adult schizophrenic patients. But it is not known whether such longings have a specific initiating significance or appear in response to anxieties of other origins.

The consequence of early deprivation of maternal care, closeness, and need fulfillment have been discussed at length. Presumably, a child who had been raised in a foster home would be exposed to such deprivation. Yet, in a follow-up study of such foster children, Beres and Obers pointed out that, although the great majority—21 of 38—did manifest some form of personality disturbance, only 4 of the 38 children studied were schizophrenic.

Apparently, these patterns of child-parent interaction lead to a failure or retardation of the child's personality development. This failure or retardation leads to a failure of adaptation in late adolescence and early adulthood and thus to schizophrenia. But it is not known why the failure of adaptation takes the particular form of schizophrenia.

Family Pathology

The study of the family has as its root the concept that the patient's pathology is a symptom of the family pathology and that serious mental disturbances are causally related to mental disease or psychopathology in parents. The child's present maladaptation was once appropriate to the family environment.

The family pathology is conceptualized in such terms as marital schism—that is, a husband and wife stay together despite overt scrapping because one marital partner depends on the other—or marital skew—that is, overt harmony masks covert disagreement. Some investigators of family pathology speak of emotional divorce to characterize marital partnerships in which there are few overt disagreements but no shared feelings or in which husband and wife present a compatible facade to the world but cannot tolerate each other in private. When the inadequate member of such a partnership is the wife, she imparts her feelings of inadequacy to the child and is threatened by the child's growing independence.

Wynne and coworkers conceptualized the pathology in the family of a schizophrenic child in terms of role theory. Wynne called the relationship "pseudomutuality" and described schizophrenia as the breakdown of that pseudomutuality. Family members fit together and interrelate according to assigned formal and conforming roles and at the expense of their individual identity and separateness. In schizophrenic families the number of fixed roles is limited; family members may shift from one role to another within this limited framework. Wynne also stated that certain specific, formal psychological disturbances—for example, the fragmentation of experience, identity diffusion, disturbed modes of perception and of communication—are a result of the internalization of pathological aspects of the family organization.

Another concept, the double bind, focuses on certain ways the mother behaves with her child.

The child cannot win in his relationship with his mother. While his father stands helplessly by, the child is made to feel helpless, enraged, fearful, and exasperated, and he deals with his predicament by withdrawing into psychosis.

At best, these studies suggest that the family interaction of schizophrenic persons is disturbed in one way or another. At the same time, it may be concluded that many of the parents were themselves psychotic, so that the concomitant association of psychosis in the child may be a function of inheritance, rather than a function of family pathology.

Methodological and Conceptual Problems

Most of these studies are clinical and impressionistic, and rater reliability cannot be assessed. To a great extent such studies are retrospective and are based on the assumption that current patterns of interaction were also obtained in the past. Validation of findings is not carried out. Bias is introduced by the foreknowledge that a member of the particular family under investigation is schizophrenic or that the parent under study has a schizophrenic child. With few exceptions, no control groups or control subjects are included in these studies, and no attempt is made to determine whether the same or similar parents or families can also be associated with children who are not schizophrenic. Important variables—such as social class, educational level, ethnic and religious origin—are frequently not controlled.

Sociocultural Theories

The methodological problems inherent in sociocultural research are so considerable that no clear answers have yet been found. The main recurring and confounding problem is the lack of reliable diagnostic criteria. In addition, it is necessary to define and enumerate the population from which the sample is drawn and to be familiar with all the known cases of schizophrenia in that population, as well as the estimated ratio between the known and the undetected cases.

Social Class and Mobility

Investigations of the relationship of social class to schizophrenia have pursued two main themes: the patient's social status at the time he became ill and the ecological characteristics of his community. The highest prevalence of schizophrenia, especially in women, occurs in the lowest social class; the lowest prevalence is found in the managerial classes. Various interpretations have been attached to these findings, ranging from occupational stress to the low prestige associated with certain occupations. Such factors are thought to precipitate the illness. However, it is difficult to determine the validity of these findings, particularly since it is often impossible to determine the precipitating event in schizophrenia.

In ecological studies the highest incidence of schizophrenia is found in the poorest, most disorganized, and often central sections of the city. This observation was made originally by Bleuler, who believed such an environment to be the result rather than a cause of the illness. Others believe that such a social environment is in itself responsible for the illness either indirectly by creating conditions, such as social isolation, that favor the onset of schizophrenia in those who are so predisposed or directly by exposing a child raised in such an area to specific types of family constellations, poor health care, economic deprivation, poor nutrition, criminal behavior, inadequate education, or social and group disruption. A third hypothesis states that persons prone to schizophrenia tend to migrate or drift into such areas, in part because the illness makes them poorly adapted to earn a living or makes them socially incompetent. A subhypothesis describes such persons as socially mobile in a downward direction from generation to generation. Still another hypothesis relates these findings to the relative lack of psychiatric treatment facilities, other than hospitals, for members of the lowest classes.

There is no simple relationship between social class and schizophrenia. Many talented or invulnerable children are born into families in the lowest socio-economic groups. In addition, in the families that harbor schizophrenic children, other children may be talented, creative, and imaginative.

Culture Change

Schizophrenia has also been linked to such stressful processes as urbanization, industrialization, migration, acculturation, and economic change or crisis. The factor of change may be the direct cause of the illness, or change may be a necessary, if not sufficient, precipitating condition in persons predisposed to the illness.

The effects of emigrant status have been studied more extensively than has any other parameter of social change. Odegaard's studies showed that the over-all rate of schizophrenia was higher for emigrant Norwegians in Minnesota than it was for Norwegians in Norway. Malzberg's and Lee's studies concluded that schizophrenia is more prevalent among recent immigrants to New York State and their descendents than it is among persons who were born in New York State.

But for every study that does find a correlation between migration and schizophrenia, there is one that does not. Nor is it understood precisely how migration may lead to schizophrenia, if it does. Studies of other aspects of social change are similarly characterized by a lack of comparable findings.

Cultural Setting and Clinical Subtype

Data concerning relationships between schizophrenic subtypes and membership in a specific subculture are not necessarily of predisposing or initiating significance. To establish the significance of such a relationship, one must show that the two subcultures studied differed in the incidence of schizophrenia. If such a difference was confirmed, it would then be necessary to isolate specific variables prepotent or unique to the subculture with the higher prevalence or to some segment within it. No such evidence has been collected as yet.

One of the most serious problems in this and many other areas of research in schizophrenia is what might be called a Rousseauist bias; that is, the underlying concept is that schizophrenia is a disease of civilization. There is no evidence for this viewpoint.

Initiating Factors

Any comprehensive theory of schizophrenia must explain the onset of the illness at a particular time in the patient's life. It is known that the peak time of onset of schizophrenic illness is at the end of the second and the start of the third decade of life. The illness often begins when young people leave home to marry, to work, to study, to assume responsibility, or to live alone. Divorce or the death of a parent, child, or spouse may also be the setting in which the illness begins.

The meaning of the setting is threatening and therefore, constitutes a stress. But nothing specific about the setting itself is stressful. No one life event by itself is the initiator of the illness. The setting represents a loss or separation.

Sustaining Factors

One factor that may influence the course of the illness is the length of time a child is exposed to a schizophrenic parent, particularly the mother, while that child is growing up.

The course of the illness is influenced by hospitalization. The length of hospitalization is, in turn, influenced by the availability of treatment and by social, economic, and familial factors, not only by the illness itself.

Physiological and Biochemical Factors

The etiological theory most stubbornly clung to over time states that schizophrenia is a physical disease due to a morphological or functional defect in some organ system, perhaps the brain. Recently, the endocrine glands have been held responsible for schizophrenia. The search has been for either an abnormal substance present in body fluids or an aberrant metabolic pathway, both of which are presumably genetic in origin. In other words, schizophrenia is conceived of as an inborn error of metabolism, an error produced by one gene.

It is a well-known clinical fact that the amphetamines induce a paranoid psychosis in persons predisposed to react. It has been suggested that the various central effects of amphetamine are largely to be understood in terms of the release of norepinephrine. Yet the action of amphetamine persists, despite depletion of brain stores of norepinephrine by reserpine. It has also been suggested that amphetamine inhibits monoamine oxidase, despite the fact that inhibitors of this enzyme do not abolish the central effects of amphetamine. It may act on serotonin receptors in the brain or release both dopamine and norepinephrine.

Other questions remain unanswered. If such an inborn metabolic error is present, why does it become manifest only in late adolescence or early adulthood, whereas the effects of various aminoacidurias and phenylketonuria manifest themselves in childhood? If an abnormal metabolite or an aberrant metabolic pathway does exist, how is one to account for different clinical manifestations and subtypes? How can the premorbid personality or the remissions that occur so often be explained metabolically? What accounts for brief or prolonged periods of lucidity and remission? In fact, such periods of lucidity may occur in response to the physician's attempts to understand or his actual understanding of the patient's seemingly incoherent statements. And, if schizophrenia is a chronic delirium, why do fever, surgical operations, and bone fractures produce temporary remissions in some patients?

Despite a marked increase in biochemical and neurochemical research activity in this field, the amount of established, verified factual information accumulated to date is virtually nil. This void may be attributed, in large measure, to the fact that no effort has been made to correct several sources of error that in the past have accounted for positive findings. These errors have resulted from the tendency to report nonspecific findings; and, in several instances, they arose because of the investigators' failure to take certain crucial variables, involving diet and drug intake, into account.

Genetically Inborn Error of Metabolism

This hypothesis is attractive but has not yet been confirmed. As concretized by Heath, it links a whole causal chain, beginning with genetic data and proceeding through biochemistry to deviations in psychological functioning, which interact with family and social factors. Each of these processes is a necessary if not sufficient condition for onset of the illness. The crucial genetic defect is manifested by the presence of a protein, taraxein, which is responsible for an aberration of biogenic amine metabolism.

A variant of this hypothesis is the postulate that epinephrine released by stressful life situations is abnormally metabolized to form hallucinogenic derivatives of epinephrine, adrenochrome, and adrenolutin. However, hallucinosis is not pathognomonic for schizophrenia.

Defect in Energy Metabolism

Defects in oxidative phosphorylation and of the metabolism of phosphorus in erythrocytes have been reported. And schizophrenic patients have been said to have a serum factor producing hyperglycemia, possibly because of an antagonist of insulin present in blood. But it is not clear what such findings are supposed to explain about schizophrenia.

Abnormal Levels of Serum Constituents

The controversy on ceruloplasmin is still unresolved. Taraxein is said to be related to but qualitatively different from ceruloplasmin. Heath reported that, when taraxein is injected into monkeys, behavioral and electroencephalographic changes occur.

There have been reports for many years of the adverse effects of the serum and urine in schizophrenic patients on many dependent variables. The nature of these substances in serum, plasma, or urine has not yet been identified.

It has been proposed that schizophrenia may be an autoimmune disease and that autoimmune autoantibodies may be directed toward cells in organs other than the brain. If so, it is unclear what role such autoantibodies play in the predisposition or initiation of schizophrenic illness.

There have been a number of reports of increased levels of enzymes in the blood of acutely psychotic patients. Most of the research interest has focused on two enzymes, creatine phosphokinase (CPK) and aldolase. But serum levels of CPK are elevated in patients bearing a wide variety of diagnostic labels and in 20 to 40 per cent of the nonpsychotic, first-degree relatives of acutely psychotic patients. Elevated levels of CPK occur mainly at illness onset and have no specificity for schizophrenia.

Intoxication

Some psychotomimetic agents, such as mescaline are methylated congeners of many naturally occurring biogenic amines. In 1962, Friedhoff found that the urine of 70 per cent of his schizophrenic subjects contained the substance 3,4-dimethoxyphenylethylamine(3,4-DMPEA), which is related to dihydroxyphenylethylamine (dopamine) and to mescaline. It is now conceded that the presence of 3,4-DMPEA in urine is not specific to schizophrenia. Its presence may be related to diet. An alternative hypothesis currently under investigation is the search for a metabolic pathway that culminates in the product of another psychotomimetic amine, dimethyltryptamine.

Putative Central Neurotransmitter Agents

That some disturbance in biological transmethylation may occur in schizophrenia is suggested by the research done at the National

Institute of Mental Health. However, it is not known whether the exacerbation of symptoms seen in patients fed *l*-methionine is specific to schizophrenic patients or whether it is due to the nonspecific effects of amino acid intoxication, rather than the suspected mechanism. Other methyldonors, such as betaine, have been shown to produce the same kind of exacerbation but not in all patients. The fact that a drug or drugs rapidly exacerbate symptoms does not prove that it is the cause of the illness. The role of the catecholamines or the products of their methylation in schizophrenia remains enigmatic.

Central Neurohumor

The hypothesis that schizophrenia is due to a deficiency of serotonin is apparently no longer subscribed to. However, this hypothesis is attractive because it shifts attention to the central nervous system and to a substance with known neurobiological activity.

Alternative Theories

Certain kinds of ontogenetic experiences may be reflected in altered brain chemistry. Alternatively, enzyme levels and levels of their biosynthetic products, a genetically determined inborn error of metabolism, or an aberrant metabolic pathway, possibly in the nervous system, may alter the process of personality development in such a manner as to distort or prevent the proper differentiation, integration, maturation, and organization of psychological functions that permit mature adaptation, and such metabolic errors may alter the processing of real life experience.

Obviously, such hypotheses fail to specify the possible metabolic error to be investigated. Furthermore, if such an error were identified, one would also wish to understand the mechanism through which it effected changes in psychological processes.

Conclusion

There are many theories of the causes of schizophrenia, but there are insufficient data to decide which is correct. Despite this conclusion, there can be little doubt that genetic factors play a role in predisposing to schizophrenia. However, the mode of inheritance and the nature of the predisposition are not yet known. Factors in the environment then elicit these tendencies or dispositions.

REFERENCES

Alanen, Y. O. The mothers of schizophrenic patients. Acta Psychiatr. Neurol. Scand., *124:* (Suppl.) 1, 1958.

Armkraut, A., Solomon, G. F., Allansmith, M., McLellan, B., and Rappaport, M. Immunoglobulins and improvement in acute schizophrenic reactions. Arch. Gen. Psychiatry, *28:* 673, 1973.

Boehme, D. H., Cottrell, J. C., Dohan, C. and Hillegass, L. M. Fluorescent antibody studies of immunoglobulin binding by brain tissues: Demonstration of cytoplasmic fluorescense by direct and indirect testing in schizophrenic and nonschizophrenic subjects. Arch. Gen. Psychiatry, *28:* 202, 1973.

Fish, B., and Hagin, R. Visual-motor disorders in infants at risk for schizophrenia. Arch. Gen. Psychiatry, *28:* 900, 1973.

Grinker, R. R., and Holzman, P. S. Schizophrenic pathology in young adults. Arch. Gen. Psychiatry, *28:* 168, 1973.

Harrow, M., Harkavy, K., Bromet, E., and Tucker, G. J. A longitudinal study of schizophrenic thinking. Arch. Gen. Psychiatry, *28:* 179, 1973.

Heston, L. L. The genetics of schizophrenic and schizoid disease. Science, *167:* 249, 1970.

Janowsky, D. S., El-Yousef, K., David, J. M., and Sekerte, N. J. Provocation of schizophrenic systoms by intravenous administration of methylphenidate. Arch. Gen. Psychiatry, *28:* 185, 1973.

Kety, S. S. Biochemical theories of schizophrenia. Int. J. Psychiatry, *1:* 409, 1965.

Mellsop, G., Whittingham, S., and Ungar, B. Schizophrenia and autoimmune serological reactions. Arch. Gen. Psychiatry, *28:* 194, 1973.

Meltzer, H. Y. Muscle enzyme release in the acute psychoses. Arch. Gen. Psychiatry, *21:* 102, 1969.

Rosenthal, D. *The Genetics of Psychopathology.* McGraw-Hill, New York, 1971.

Sullivan, H. S. *Conceptions of Modern Psychiatry.* W. W. Norton, New York, 1947.

Wender, P. H., Rosenthal, D., Kety, S. S., Schulsinger, F., and Weiner, J. Social class and psychopathology in adoptees: A natural experimental method for separating the roles of genetic and experiential factors. Arch. Gen. Psychiatry, *28:* 318, 1973.

Wyatt, R. J., Saavedra, J. M., and Axelrod, J. A dimethyltryptamine-forming enzyme in human blood. Am. J. Psychiatry, *130:* 754, 1973.

14.4   SCHIZOPHRENIA: CLINICAL FEATURES

Key Characteristics

There are no universally accepted objective criteria today for the diagnosis of schizophrenia. On the other hand, a group of symptoms are basic to and characteristic of schizophrenia. Since dementia precox was first described by Kraepelin (see Figure 1) as a nosological entity at the end of the 19th century, many basic features of this disease have come to be generally accepted.

Eugen Bleuler (see Figure 2) described three general primary symptoms of schizophrenia: a disturbance of association, a disturbance of

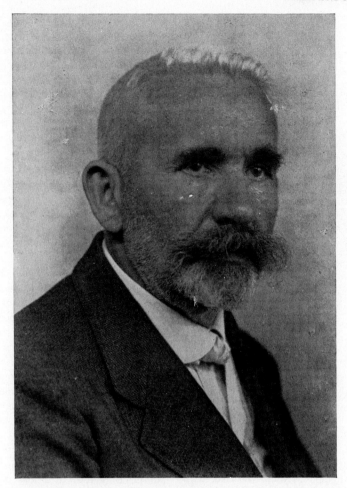

FIGURE 1. Emil Kraepelin, 1856–1926. National Library of Medicine, Bethesda, Maryland.

affect, and a disturbance of activity. Bleuler also stressed the dereistic attitude of the schizophrenic—that is, his detachment from reality and his consequent autism and the ambivalence that expresses itself in his uncertain affectivity and initiative. Thus, Bleuler's system of schizophrenia is often referred to as the four A's: association, affect, autism, and ambivalence.

Bleuler derived the name of the disease from his concept of splitting. The initiative is split into a variety of equivalent potentialities, and the patient is thus split off from reality; thoughts and associations are fragmented and devoid of meaning; the affect is no longer adequate or appropriate to the situation.

Manfred Bleuler describes certain features that exclude a diagnosis of schizophrenia. Psychoses whose primary characteristics are memory and intellectual deficits are not schizophre-

nias. Also excluded are psychoses with rapid recovery after a psychological trauma, psychoses with primary disturbances of consciousness, psychoses with primary quantitative changes in the emotions, and psychoses apparently due to physical illness.

He sees as positive and essential features of schizophrenic psychopathology the strange combination of psychotic and normal mental processes in the same person, changes in associational processes, disturbances of emotionality, and experiences by the patient of having his mind controlled by external, often invisible agents.

Manfred Bleuler points out that nearly all schizophrenic mechanisms can be found in normal people—for example, dereistic thinking in daydreams, hallucinations and bizarre symbolism in dreams during sleep. What is specific

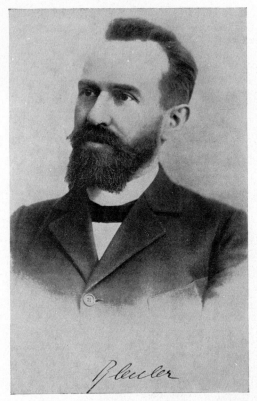

FIGURE 2. Eugene Bleuler, 1857–1939. National Library of Medicine, Bethesda, Maryland.

for the schizophrenic disease is the patient's inability to distinguish between the two realities—that of the internal world and that of the external world.

Symbolism

One of the most characteristic features of schizophrenia is the pronounced symbolism expressed in the patient's often bizarre behavior, ideation, and speech. This symbolism may be impossible to comprehend for anyone but the patient himself, unless the observer takes a great deal of time to analyze it. Schizophrenia consists, particularly in the acute and subacute phases, of a proliferation of psychic productions.

Sensitivity

All schizophrenics are, at least originally, more sensitive than the average person. It is likely that this increased sensitivity and heightened responsiveness to sensory and emotional stimulation is present in schizophrenics from an early age, possibly from birth. In this writer's opinion, schizophrenia is characterized by a genetic hypersensitivity that leaves the patient vulnerable to an overwhelming onslaught of stimuli from without and within. The schizophrenic's withdrawal may be explained as a defensive maneuver designed to reduce excessive stimulus input.

Social Withdrawal

Almost without exception, schizophrenic patients are characterized by social withdrawal, by the emotional distance one experiences in their presence, and by a lack of capacity for establishing rapport with others.

Loss of Ego Boundaries

This symptom may give the patient the delusional conviction that he is reading other people's minds or being controlled by other people's thoughts. It also renders him extremely vulnerable to any kind of external stimulation. His own identity may fuse with that of any object in the universe around him, and he may suffer personally when he becomes aware that some object in his environment is being attacked. The loss of ego boundaries and identity, moreover, produces feelings of depersonalization, followed by experiences of derealization. The resulting loss of contact with reality is the core symptom of any psychosis. One specific symptom related to a loss of identity is the uncertainty many schizophrenics feel about their gender.

Variability

A schizophrenic patient may be incapable at a certain time of carrying on a rational, simple conversation, and yet half an hour later he may write a sensible and remarkably well-composed letter to a relative. He may refuse to change his shirt for weeks and may offend those around him with a deep display of strange behavior, but he may, on the same day, exhibit perfect manners when attending a birthday party. He may be unable to figure the right change for a dollar purchase yet may be able to play a sophisticated game of bridge or chess.

Symptoms

Kurt Schneider's first-rank symptoms include the hearing of one's thoughts spoken aloud, auditory hallucinations that comment on the patient's behavior, somatic hallucinations, the experience of having one's thoughts controlled, the spreading of one's thoughts to others, delusions, and the experience of having one's actions controlled or influenced from the outside. Schizophrenia, Schneider points out, can also be diagnosed exclusively on the basis of second-rank symptoms, along with an otherwise typical clinical appearance. Second-rank symptoms include other forms of hallucinations, perplexity, depressive and euphoric disorders of affect, and emotional blunting.

However, a clear clinical distinction between certain organic psychoses and true schizophrenia is largely illusory. Schneider's system is highly discriminatory for schizophrenia, but his first-rank symptoms should not be regarded as pathognomonic.

Perceptual Disorders

Because of the unpredictable variability of the schizophrenic's experiences, the Gestalt qualities of the visual world are broken into disjointed parts. He frequently sees objects and people change their dimensions, their outline, and their brightness from minute to minute or even from second to second before his eyes (see Figure 3).

Sensory experiences of perceptions without corresponding external stimuli are common

symptoms of schizophrenia. Most common are auditory hallucinations, the hearing of voices. Sometimes the voices are those of God or the devil; sometimes they are the voices of relatives or neighbors. Frequently, the patient can neither recognize nor understand them. Most characteristically, two or more voices talk about the patient, discussing him in the third person. Many schizophrenic patients experience the hearing of their own thoughts.

Visual hallucinations occur less frequently in schizophrenic patients, but they are not rare. Patients suffering from organic or affective psychoses experience visual hallucinations primarily at night or during limited periods of the day, but schizophrenic patients hallucinate as much during the day as they do during the night, sometimes almost continuously. They get relief only in sleep. Visual hallucinations almost always occur in combination with hallucinations in one of the other sensory modalities.

Tactile, olfactory, and gustatory hallucinations are less common.

Schizophrenics often experience kinesthetic hallucinations, sensations of altered states in body organs without any special receptor apparatus to explain the sensations—for example, a burning sensation in the brain, a pushing sensation in the abdominal blood vessels, or a cutting sensation in the heart.

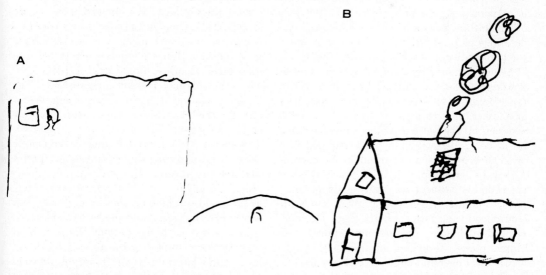

FIGURE 3. Drawings of a house made by a young man during an acute schizophrenic illness. Figure *A* was drawn on admission to the hospital; Figure *B* was drawn after 1 week of phenothiazine treatment. Note the fragmentation of the percept house in the first drawing; the windows are displaced, and the roof is lying on the ground, beside the walls. In the second drawing, the structure and perspective of the house are restored.

The hallucination may absorb much or all of the patient's attention and may control his behavior to a considerable extent. While listening to voices, he may be preoccupied and oblivious to his environment. He may react with laughter or anger or terror, and he may carry on lengthy conversations with the voices.

Modern treatment methods, particularly pharmacotherapy and social therapies that engage the patient in various activities and no longer leave him all day to his own preoccupations, have robbed hallucinations of much of their vividness and persistence. Also, many patients today know what hallucinations are and know that their hearing of voices may be considered pathological or foolish. Thus, the present-day schizophrenic is much less likely to discuss his hallucinations openly than he was only 25 years ago.

Studies of the dream content of schizophrenic patients have shown that their dreams are less coherent and less complex—also less bizarre—than are the dreams of normal persons. Family members appear more often and friends less often. Unpleasant emotions are more common in the dreams of schizophrenics than in the dreams of normals.

Cognitive Disorders

Delusions. Delusions are false ideas that cannot be corrected by reasoning and that are idiosyncratic for the patient—that is, not part of his cultural environment. Most frequent are delusions of persecution, the key symptom in the paranoid type of schizophrenia. The feeling of being controlled by some unseen mysterious power that exercises its influence from a distance occurs in most schizophrenics at one time or another, and for many of them it is a daily experience. The patient who is convinced that he is being persecuted by powerful agencies often harbors delusions of grandeur; he must be a very important person if so much effort is spent on his persecution. Many schizophrenics have elaborate delusions that their minds are controlled by telepathy or hypnotism. The modern schizophrenic may be preoccupied with atomic power, X-rays, or spaceships that take control over his mind and body. Also typical for many schizophrenics are delusional fantasies about the destruction of the world.

Frequently, the schizophrenic's delusions of doom and fears of destruction take the form of a delusional scientific discovery that the patient believes is capable of preventing or counteracting the threat. The patient is driven by an urgent need to get his important message to scientific or government authorities who should be able to put it into action for the protection of mankind. Such patients often use scientific jargon, and the schemes appear almost rational at first glance. Excerpts from a letter sent to this writer by a patient from Australia provide a good illustration of this kind of pseudoscience.

Further to my investigation and research ... I would like to inform you that the TADPOLE in the eyes moves or floats around with the movement of the iris .... The tadpole reveals the photographic and its spirit the parabiological matter. From experience the Spirit is more deadly than the vision—the vision could bring on a person a berserk or manic attitude if he is unaware of its tricks—it could also be a danger to schizoid, alcoholic, and neurotic personalities.

Further to the tadpole, it is luminous in the dark at times and flashes rings of light when both eyes are closed.

Have you any idea if science could produce a solution that could cover the iris and eradicate the tadpole and the luminous matter?

I repeat again, this is a diabolical science deliberately done to destroy human nature.

Disturbances of Thinking. The schizophrenic patient thinks and reasons on his own autistic terms, according to his own intricate private rules of logic. His thought processes are strange and do not lead to conclusions based on reality or universal logic. The schizophrenic may consider things identical merely because they have identical predicates or properties. The schizophrenic patient may reason: "The Virgin Mary was a virgin. I'm a virgin; therefore, I'm the Virgin Mary." The patient loses his ability to generalize correctly (see Figure 4). This defect is often brought out by the simple clinical test of asking the patient to interpret a well-known proverb. One schizophrenic interpreted the saying "A stitch in time saves nine" as "I should sew nine buttons on my coat"—an overly personalized and concrete explanation.

In contrast with the patient whose mental functions are impaired by an organic brain lesion and who tends to omit important items in thought and speech, the schizophrenic tends to include many irrelevant items. This tendency appears to result from a loosening of associations in the schizophrenic patient.

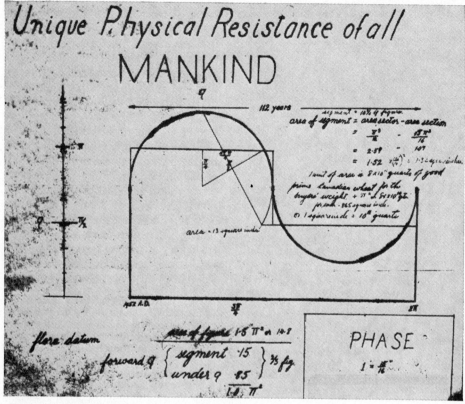

FIGURE 4. Comprehensive graph by a schizophrenic engineer. This shows his retention of engineering information and drafting precision after 10 years of hospitalization, while he attempts to reduce many unrelated matters to one simple mathematical scheme. (Courtesy of Heinz E. Lehmann.)

Schizophrenics generally have an increased arousal level and show greater responsivity to nonrelevant stimuli and less responsivity to relevant stimuli than do normal persons.

Another characteristic symptom of schizophrenia is the abrupt blocking of the stream of thought or sometimes of all psychic activity. After such a blocking episode, which may last seconds or minutes, the patient may be perplexed and have difficulty in coordinating his behavior. When questioned about his experiences, he is likely to report that he had the physical sensation of somebody's taking his thoughts out of his head.

Verbal Disorders

Excessive Concreteness and Symbolism. The one common factor running through the schizophrenic's preoccupation with invisible forces, radiation, witchcraft, religion, philosophy, and psychology is his leaning toward the esoteric, the abstract, the symbolic. Consequently, a schizophrenic's thinking is characterized simultaneously by an overly concrete and an overly symbolic nature (see Figure 5).

Incoherence. For the schizophrenic, language is primarily a means of self-expression, rather than a means of communication. His verbal productions are often either empty or obscure.

Neologisms. Occasionally, the schizophrenic creates a completely new expression, a neologism, when he needs to express a concept for which no ordinary word exists.

A schizophrenic woman who had been hospitalized for several years kept repeating, in an otherwise quite rational conversation, the word "polamolalittersjitterstitttersleelitla." The psychiatrist asked her to spell it out, and she then proceeded to explain to him the meaning of the various components, which she insisted were to be used as one word. "Polamolalitters" was intended to recall the disease poliomyelitis, since the patient wanted to indicate that she felt she was suffering from a serious disease

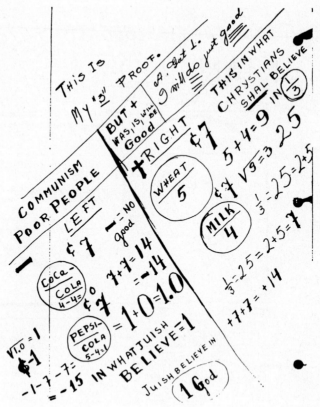

FIGURE 5. Schizophrenic patient's schema. This illustrates his fragmented, abstract, and overly inclusive thinking and preoccupation with religious idiologies and mathematical proofs. (Courtesy Heinz E. Lehmann.)

affecting her nervous system; the component "litters" stood for untidiness or messiness, the way she felt inside; "jitterstitters" reflected her inner nervousness and lack of ease; "leelitla" was a reference to the French *le lit la* (that bed there), meaning that she was both dependent on and feeling handicapped by her illness. This single neologistic production thus enabled the patient to express—in a condensed, autistic manner—information about her preoccupations and apprehensions that otherwise would have taken a whole paragraph to explain in common language.

Mutism. This functional inhibition of speech and vocalization may last for hours or days, but, before the days of modern treatment methods, it commonly used to last for years in chronic schizophrenics of the catatonic type. Many schizophrenics tend to be monosyllabic and to answer questions as briefly as possible. They attempt to restrict contact with the interviewer as much as possible without being altogether uncooperative.

Echolalia. Occasionally, schizophrenic patients exhibit echolalia, repeating in their answers to the interviewer's questions many of the same words the questioner has used. Echolalia seems to signal that the patient is aware of some shortcomings in his ideation and that he is striving to maintain an active rapport with the interviewer.

Verbigeration. This rare symptom is found almost exclusively in chronic and very regressed schizophrenics. It consists of the senseless repetition of the same words or phrases, and it may, at times, go on for days.

Stilted Language. Some schizophrenics make extraordinary efforts to maintain their social relations. But they may betray their rigidity and artificiality in their interpersonal relations by a peculiarly stilted and grotesquely quaint language.

Behavioral Disorders

Changes in a schizophrenic's behavior may be quantitative or qualitative in nature. As an example of quantitative change, the patient usually exhibits a general reduction of energy, spontaneity, and initiative, although in the acute stages he may become excited to the point of threatening his own safety and that of the people around him. Qualitatively, schizophrenic behavior is usually poorly coordinated, unpredictable, eccentric, or inappropriate. Most schizophrenics convey the impression of awkwardness and stiffness.

Mannerisms. Mannerisms of speech and movements are typical for many schizophrenics (see Figure 6). So is grimacing, which can sometimes be noticed only by an experienced observer but is sometimes carried to a grotesque degree. In its more subdued form, grimacing may appear as ticlike movements, particularly in the perioral area.

Stuporous Stages. These states used to be common in the catatonic subtype of schizophrenia (see Figure 7). Until the middle 1930's mental hospitals were filled with stuporous catatonics, many of whom would lie motionless for weeks or months, their eyelids flickering, saliva drooling from their mouths, unresponsive to almost every stimulus. They had to be fed by stomach tube twice a day and sometimes had to

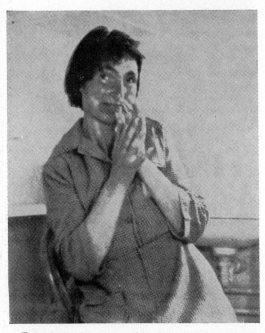

FIGURE 6. A 44-year-old chronic schizophrenic woman showing characteristic mannerism and facial grimacing, (Courtesy New York Academy of Medicine.)

be catheterized regularly. Today modern physical treatment methods permit therapists to interrupt stupors, usually within a few days, either by electroconvulsive treatment or by pharmacotherapy, and the stuporous patient has become a rare phenomenon.

Also rare today is catalepsy, waxy flexibility (flexibilitas cerea), which was present in many patients 40 years ago. It consists of a waxlike yielding of all the movable parts of the body to any efforts made to place them in certain positions. Once placed in position, the arm, leg, or head remains in that position for a long time, sometimes for hours, even if the position is uncomfortable for the patient.

Many chronic schizophrenics still show a pronounced lack of spontaneity and move rarely or only when specifically asked to do certain things. However, a patient who shows almost no response to his environment is capable of perceiving what is going on around him. Even a patient in a complete stupor may, several months later, recall every word of a conversation carried on in front of him while he appeared to be in a state of unconsciousness.

Echopraxia. This motor symptom is the imitation of movements and gestures of a person the schizophrenic is observing.

Automatic Obedience. A catatonic patient may, without hesitation and in a robotlike fashion, carry out most simple commands given to him.

Negativism. A patient may fail to cooperate without any apparent reason. The patient does not appear to be fatigued, depressed, suspicious, or angry. He is obviously capable of physical movement. But he fails to carry out even the simplest requests. Sometimes he may even do the opposite of what he is asked; for instance, he lowers his hand when one asks him to raise it.

Stereotyped Behavior. This behavior is occasionally seen in chronic schizophrenics. It may present itself as repetitive patterns of moving or walking, perhaps pacing in the same circle day in and day out. Or it may be the repetitive performance of strange gestures. Or the patient may again and again, sometimes over a period of years, use the same phrases, ask the same questions, make the same comments. Such stereotyped speech should be distinguished from perseveration of ideas and verbigeration. Most stereotyped behavior can be pre-

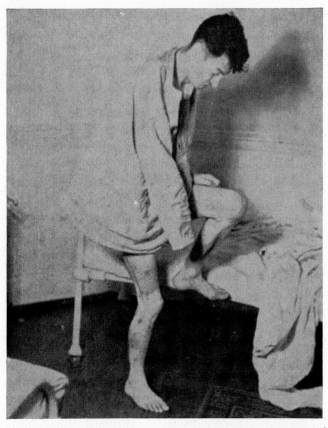

FIGURE 7. A chronic schizophrenic stands in a cataleptic position. He maintained this uncomfortable position for hours. (Courtesy New York Academy of Medicine.)

vented and counteracted effectively by personal attention and social therapies.

Deteriorated Appearance and Manners. Schizophrenic patients tend to deteriorate in their appearance. Their efforts at grooming and self-care may become minimal. In general, schizophrenics show poor regard for the social amenities. They may not return a greeting or a smile, they may not carry their part in a conversation, they may exhibit crude table manners and show, in many other ways, their lack of consideration for the presence and feelings of others.

Affective Disorders

Reduced Emotional Responses. Many schizophrenics appear to be indifferent or, at times, totally apathetic. Others with less marked emotional blunting show some emotional shallowness or a certain lack of depth of feeling. The patient himself often offers information about his own gradual decrease in the ability to experience empathy, which he may have observed introspectively long before it became clinically evident.

Anhedonia. The anhedonic person is incapable of experiencing or even imagining any pleasant emotion. Without being actually depressed, he feels emotionally barren. This hopeless, empty feeling drives some schizophrenics to commit suicide.

Inappropriate Responses. A schizophrenic patient may talk about his child's death with a broad smile, or he may react with rage to a simple question about how he slept last night. This splitting or dissociation of the affective response from the cognitive content is almost pathognomonic for schizophrenia. However, the schizophrenic who expresses an inappropriate emotional reaction does not necessarily experience the particular emotion his behavior conveys. The degree of emotional blunting and the inappropriateness of a schizophrenic's emotional reaction are among the most telling measures of the extent to which the schizophrenic process has invaded his personality.

Abnormal Emotions. Schizophrenia not only alters emotional reactions to external stimuli but may induce strange emotions and moods that are seldom, if ever, experienced under normal conditions. States of exaltation with feelings of omnipotence, oceanic feelings of oneness with the universe, religious ecstasies, terrifying apprehensions about the disintegration of one's own personality or body, anxious moods when the catastrophic destruction of the universe seems to be impending—all are emotional experiences occurring in different stages of schizophrenia, but they are most frequently encountered in the acute phases of the breakdown.

Somatic Symptoms

There are no specific somatic manifestations in schizophrenia. However, in the early stages of the disease, patients often complain of a multitude of symptoms—headache, rheumatic pains in the shoulders, back strain, weakness, and indigestion. Once the disease is fully developed, a schizophrenic patient is, according to some authors, less likely to develop a psychosomatic disease than is the average person. Schizophrenic patients also seem to suffer less frequently than others from various allergies.

Many chronic schizophrenic patients, particularly the severely regressed ones, suffer from chronic constipation. Uncommunicative chronic schizophrenics may remain ambulatory for days with an acutely inflamed appendix, which may be diagnosed only after the uncomplaining patient has collapsed after a rupture of the appendix into the peritoneum. For the same reason, inadequate self-reporting, schizophrenic patients are more likely than others to have silent coronary attacks.

A patient suffering an acute schizophrenic breakdown almost certainly presents the autonomic triad of dilated pupils, moist palms, and moderate tachycardia. He often has a systolic blood pressure 10 to 20 mm. above the norm. These signs of sympathetic excitation may be present even if the patient shows no outward signs of increased emotional tension.

Most schizophrenic patients, unless they are extremely excited, have remarkably little trouble sleeping, even during the acute stage of their illness. However, a schizophrenic's sleep is characterized by a reduction of stage IV (deep) sleep.

Constitutional Characteristics

The relation between body build and personality structure or certain types of mental illness has been intensively studied for many years. Kretschmer showed that schizophrenia occurred more frequently in persons of asthenic (leptosomic), athletic, and dysplastic body types than in the pyknic type. The pyknic type was more likely to develop manic-depressive psychosis than schizophrenia. In Sheldon's classification, schizophrenics tend to be ectomorphics, mesomorphics, and dysplastics.

Syndromes

Kraepelin distinguished and described three basic subtypes of dementia precox: the catatonic, the hebephrenic, and the paranoid. Bleuler later added schizophrenia simplex as a fourth basic type. Since Bleuler, many other types of schizophrenia have been named and described.

Catatonic Schizophrenia

Stuporous Catatonic. The stuporous catatonic may be in a state of complete stupor, or he may show a pronounced decrease of spontaneous movements and activity. He may be mute or nearly so, and he may show distinct negativism, stereotypies, echopraxia, and automatic obedience. However, even after standing or sitting motionless for long periods of time, he may suddenly and without provocation have a brief outburst of destructive violence. Occasionally, catatonic schizophrenics exhibit the phenomenon of catalepsy or waxy flexibility (see Figure 8). A patient in a state of complete catatonic stupor can usually be roused from it in a dramatic manner by the intravenous injection of a short-acting barbiturate. But, spectacular as the immediate results appear to be, the technique has no significant therapeutic value.

A young, unmarried woman, aged 20, was admitted to a psychiatric hospital because she had become violent toward her parents, had been observed gazing into space with a rapt expression, and had been talking to invisible persons. She had been seen to strike odd poses. Her speech had become incoherent.

She had been a good student in high school, then

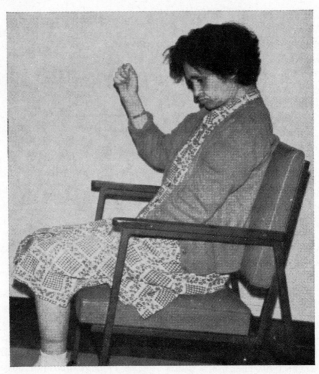

FIGURE 8. Chronic catatonic patient. This patient is immobile, demonstrating waxy flexibility. Note the uncomfortable position of her arm, which is elevated without support, and her stony facial expression with *Schnauzkrampf* or frozen pout. (Courtesy Heinz E. Lehmann.)

went to business school, and, a year before admission to the hospital, started to work in an office as a stenographer. She had always been shy, and, although she was quite attractive, she had not been dating much. Another girl, who worked in the same office, told her about boys and petting and began to exert a great deal of influence over the patient. The second girl could communicate with her from across the room. Even when they went home at night, the patient would get voice messages telling her to do certain things. Then, pictures began to appear on the wall, most of them ugly and sneering. These pictures had names—one was named shyness, another distress, another envy. Her office friend sent her messages to knock at the wall, so as to hit these pictures.

The patient was agitated, noisy, and uncooperative in the hospital for several weeks after she arrived and required sedation. She was given a course of insulin coma therapy, with no significant or sustained improvement. Later, she received several courses of electroconvulsive treatment, which also failed to influence the schizophrenic process to any significant degree. Ten years later, when neuroleptic drugs became available, she received pharmacotherapy.

Despite all these therapeutic efforts, her condition throughout her many years of stay in a mental hospital has remained one of chronic catatonic stupor. She is mute and practically devoid of any spontaneity, but she responds to simple requests. She stays in the same position for hours or sits in a chair in a curled up position. Her facial expression is fixed and stony.

Excited Catatonic. The excited catatonic is in a state of extreme psychomotor agitation. He talks and shouts almost continously. His verbal productions are often incoherent, and his behavior seems to be influenced more by inner stimuli than by responses of his environment. Patients in catatonic excitement urgently require physical and medical control, since they are often destructive and violent to others, and their dangerous excitement can cause them to injure themselves or to collapse from complete exhaustion. Today most patients can be carried safely through the critical period of acute excitement with electroconvulsive treatment and modern pharmacotherapy.

Periodic Catatonic. Motor functions, ideation, and perception in periodic catatonia are closely linked to the patient's changing level of positive or negative nitrogen balance. Patients affected with this rare disease have periodic recurrences of stuporous or excited catatonic states. Relapses in such patients can be prevented by regulating their nitrogen balance through the continuous administration of thyroxin.

Hebephrenic Schizophrenia

The hebephrenic subtype is characterized by a marked regression to primitive, disinhibited, and unorganized behavior. The hebephrenic patient is usually active but in an aimless, nonconstructuve manner. His thought disorder is pronounced, and his contact with reality is extremely poor. His personal appearance and his social behavior are dilapidated. His emotional responses are inappropriate, and he often bursts out laughing without any apparent reason. Incongruous grinning and grimacing are common in this type of patient, whose behavior is best described as silly or fatuous (see Figure 9).

Paranoid Schizophrenia

The paranoid type of schizophrenia is characterized mainly by the presence of delusions of persecution or grandeur. Paranoid schizophrenics are usually older than catatonics or hebephrenics when they break down; that is, they are usually in their late 20's or in their 30's. Patients who have been well up to that age have usually established a place and an identity for themselves in the community. Their ego resources are greater than those of catatonic and hebephrenic patients. Paranoid patients show less regression of mental faculties, emotional response, and behavior than do the other subtypes of schizophrenia.

A typical paranoid patient is tense, suspicious, guarded, and reserved. He is often hostile and aggressive. The paranoid patient usually conducts himself quite well socially. His intelligence in areas not invaded by his delusions may remain high. Repressed homosexuality is, according to psychoanalytic theory, primarily responsible for the need to use the defense of projection, through which the paranoid psychotic elaborates his delusions of persecution (see Figure 10).

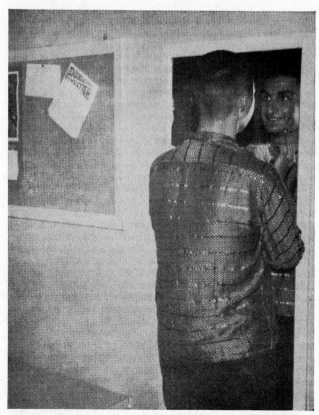

FIGURE 9. Hebephrenic patient. Posturing, grimacing, and mirror gazing are symptomatic of the disease. (Courtesy Heinz E. Lehmann.)

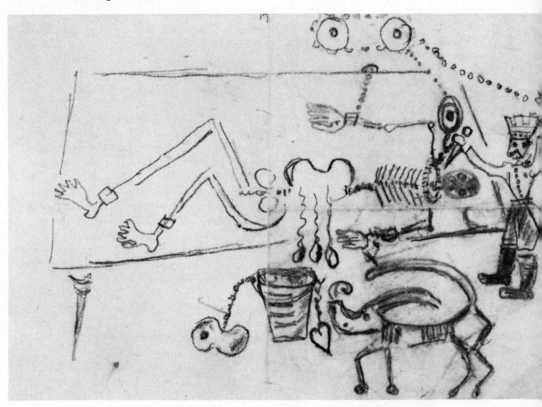

FIGURE 10. A 40-year-old schizophrenic man drew this picture, illustrating his elaborate fantasies of bodily torture and depicting a peculiar mixture of realistic and surrealistic details.

Paraphrenic Schizophrenia

The term "paraphrenia" is often used to describe chronic schizophrenic conditions characterized by the presence of well-systematized delusions that often remain unchanged in content for years. Nonschizophrenic chronic paranoiacs are distinguished by the unrealistic, fantastic, sometimes bizarre, and never plausible nature of their delusions. The personalities of paraphrenic patients, on the other hand, are usually well-preserved, and the patients are often quite happily adjusted to their life situations. In fact, some paraphrenics seem to derive considerable satisfaction from their delusions, which are more often of a grandiose than of a persecutory nature.

Simple Schizophrenia

The simple schizophrenic's principal disorder is a gradual, insidious loss of drive, interest, ambition, and initiative. He is usually not hallucinated or delusional, and, if these symptoms do occur, they do not persist. He withdraws from contact with other people, tends to stay in his room, avoids eating or meeting with other members of the family, and stops seeing his friends. He stops working. If he is still in school, his marks drop to a low level, even if they were consistently high in the past.

The patient avoids going out into the street during the day but may go for long walks by himself at 2:00 and 3:00 in the morning. He tends to sleep until noon or later, after staying up alone most of the night. During the early stages of his illness, a patient may have many somatic complaints, variously diagnosed as fatigue, nervousness, neurosis, psychosomatic disease, or laziness. Later, many simple schizophrenics turn into tramps, hoboes, or pseudohippies. They become increasingly shallow in their emotional responses and are quite content to drift aimlessly through life as long as they are left alone. Although these patients appear to be indifferent to their environment, they may react with sudden rage to persistent nagging by members of their family.

Simple schizophrenics may resemble pathological personalities of the inadequate or schizoid type. The distinguishing feature is that simple schizophrenia makes its appearance at some time during or after puberty and, as a rule, goes on to definite deterioration; personality deviations usually commence earlier and then remain the same over the years.

An unmarried man, 27 years old, was brought to the mental hospital because he had on several occasions become violent toward his father. For a few weeks he had hallucinations and heard voices. The voices eventually ceased, but he then adopted a strange way of life. He would sit up all night, sleep all day, and become very angry when his father tried to get him out of bed. He did not shave or wash for weeks, smoked continuously, ate very irregularly, and drank enormous quantities of tea.

In the hospital he adjusted rapidly to the new environment and was found to be generally cooperative. He showed no marked abnormalities of mental state or behavior, except for his lack of concern for just about everything. He kept to himself as much as possible and conversed little with patients and staff. His personal hygiene had to be supervised by the nursing staff; otherwise, he would quickly become dirty and very untidy.

Sixteen years after his admission to the hospital, he is described as shiftless and careless, sullen and unreasonable. He lies on a couch all day long. Neuroleptic treatment has failed to alter his mental state or behavior. Although many efforts have been made to get the patient to accept therapeutic work assignments, he refuses to consider any kind of regular occupation. In the summer he wanders about the hospital grounds or lies under a tree. In the winter he wanders through the tunnels connecting the various hospital buildings and is often seen stretched out for hours under the warm pipes that carry the steam through the tunnels.

Schizo-Affective Schizophrenia

In the schizo-affective type of schizophrenia, there is a strong element of either depressive or euphoric affect added to an otherwise schizophrenic symptomatology. Schizo-affective patients may be depressed, retarded, and suicidal; at the same time they may express absurd delusions of persecution, complain of being controlled by outside forces, and have a distinct schizophrenic thought disorder. Or patients with similar schizophrenic symptoms may be euphoric, playful, and overactive. In the diagnosis of these cases, the presence of the schizophrenic symptoms is the decisive factor.

The prognosis of patients diagnosed as schizoaffective is generally better than that of other schizophrenics, but it is usually worse than the prognosis for manic-depressive.

Latent and Residual Schizophrenics

Latent schizophrenia is diagnosed in those patients who have a marked schizoid personality and who show occasional behavioral peculiarities or thought disorders, without consistently manifesting any clearly psychotic pathology. This syndrome is also known as borderline schizophrenia.

Residual schizophrenia is similar to latent schizophrenia. But latent schizophrenia is the stage before a schizophrenic breakdown, and residual schizophrenia is the stage after the attack. Residual and latent schizophrenia are also known as ambulatory schizophrenia.

Childhood Schizophrenia

Childhood schizophrenia is diagnosed when schizophrenia makes its appearance before puberty. The prognosis is usually poor. Fortunately, childhood schizophrenia is relatively rare. The male to female ratio is surprisingly high—3.4:1.

Childhood schizophrenia sometimes manifests itself in young children as autism. Autistic children often show certain abnormalities of motor behavior and muscular tone in their first year of life and become arrested in their development during their second or third year. The most pronounced feature of infantile autism is an inability to communicate normally. Eye-to-eye contact is greatly impaired in autistic children and may be replaced by unusual starting. In spite of normal intelligence, autistic children may not learn to speak until they are 5 or 6 years old. Those children who lose their language suddenly at age 2 or 3 seem to have a poorer prognosis than do children in whom the illness has started insidiously.

Autistic children never play normally with other children. They often do not respond normally to their mothers' affections or to any tenderness. They cannot clearly distinguish between animate and inanimate objects and consequently lack the normal childhood interest in pets and other animals. Their behavior is often repetitive and stereotyped. However, the schizophrenic child's behavior in other areas may be more or less appropriate to his actual age. In fact, this phenomenon of being strikingly infantile in some areas of development but normal or precocious in other areas may well be the most characteristic trait of schizophrenic children with a history of infantile autism.

Most schizophrenic children have a disturbed body image; they may, for instance, literally not know where their feet are. They may show poor motor coordination, and many exhibit peculiar motor behavior, such as spinning and twirling.

In childhood schizophrenia, homeostatic mechanisms are deranged to an even greater degree than in adult schizophrenia. In contrast to adult schizophrenics, schizophrenic children frequently have disturbed sleep.

Late Schizophrenia

Although schizophrenia is typically a disease of adolescence or young adulthood, it may, particularly in its paranoid form, make its first appearance in the fifth, sixth, or seventh decade of life. German psychiatrists classify as late schizophrenic many psychotics who, in America, would be diagnosed as suffering from involutional psychosis.

Pseudoneurotic Schizophrenia

Pseudoneurotic schizophrenics are patients who present predominantly neurotic symptoms. But, on close and careful examination, they may reveal schizophrenic abnormalities of thinking and emotional reaction.

The pseudoneurotic schizophrenic is characterized by his lack of response to years of psychiatric treatment that would have produced improvement in most neurotics and by a strange, all-pervading anxiety and a constant preoccupation with sexual problems. The diffuse pananxiety is probably the most specific diagnostic criterion.

Pseudoneurotic schizophrenics may have phobias, but these phobias are not fixed and may amorphously affect all areas of life over a period of time. Unlike patients suffering from anxiety neurosis, the pseudoneurotic schizophrenic's anxiety is always free-floating and hardly ever subsides, even temporarily.

A 34-year-old single man had been hospitalized in a mental hospital for 5 years. His main complaints were: "I feel panicky and very upset inside.... I am afraid something inside me might explode, and I might do something bad .... I feel depressed all the time.... I couldn't hold a job now if I did get one.... My head feels funny inside.... I always feel tense, sometimes I feel like two person, sometimes I feel that everybody's against me...."

He was one of four children born into a family in which all the members had fairly close relationships with each other, and no major problems seemed to exist. Although he was always bright and considered to be the most talented of the four children, he failed his third year of high school and blamed his difficulty on one teacher. He went to a special tutorial school and later earned his Bachelor of Science degree with honors in chemistry at the age of 24. He got along well with his peers and participated actively in boxing, swimming, and singing.

In the 7 years after he graduated from college, he held at least nine different jobs. Several companies where he worked were sufficiently impressed with his ability to offer him special training. Various reasons were offered for the termination of his employment—not getting along with other staff members, poor work, better prospects elsewhere, accidents to company cars, simply leaving the job, and personal difficulties. He was often unemployed. On one occasion he worked as an orderly in a hospital.

In spite of his apparently good social adjustment as a child, he said that he had never really enjoyed life and that he was always anxious with people. However, he never manifested any clearly psychotic symptoms, such as hallucinations, delusions, thought disorders, or irrational behavior.

At the age of 27 he fell acutely ill for the first time after an episode of intense petting with his girl friend. "I was afraid of exploding ... afraid of doing something awful ... just generally tense." He was treated for a few weeks at a psychiatric clinic. Then he went to another city and worked for a short time but soon had to return home and to the psychiatric clinic. He complained of a pulling sensation in the left side of his head.

Since then he has had 2 years of intensive psychotherapy, several courses of continuous sleep treatment, somnolent insulin therapy, several courses of electroconvulsive treatment, and prolonged treatment with a variety of minor and major tranquilizers.

He finally had to remain under close observation because of repeated suicidal threats and a few superficial suicidal attempts. He was convinced that he had some physical brain disease that was responsible for his constant tension, and he insisted that some neurosurgery should be done to correct this. Repeated neurological investigations have not revealed any lesion. His spontaneous activity consisted solely in reading the paper and watching television. He said he was too anxious to remain in any occupational setting for longer than a few days, after which he either asked for a new assignment or claimed he was too weak to work at all. Two years ago he underwent psychosurgery, and, although he still has many of his previous symptoms, he is no longer suicidal and has improved enough to be able to live in the community.

Oneiroid State

In the oneiroid state the patient feels and behaves as though he were in a dream. He may be deeply perplexed and not fully oriented in time and place. During this state of clouded consciousness, he may experience feelings of ecstasy and rapidly shifting hallucinated scenes. Illusionary distortions of his perceptional processes, including disturbances of time perceptional processes, and the symptomatic picture may resemble that of a hysterical twilight state. The patient may be convinced that he is traveling through space on a satellite and, at the same time, conscientiously follow the regular hospital routine. The oneiroid schizophrenic acknowledges everyday realities but gives priority to his world of hallucinatory and delusional experiences. Oneiroid states are usually limited in duration and occur most frequently in acute schizophrenic breakdowns.

Destructive Behavior

Dramatic self-mutilation in schizophrenic patients—for example, the gouging out of an eye or the cutting off of the penis—occurs in probably less than 1 per cent of cases. It may sometimes be the expression of dysmorphobic delusions, the irrational conviction that there exists a serious bodily defect.

More schizophrenics than manic-depressives commit suicide, although the immediate risk of suicide is relatively greater among manic-depressives. A schizophrenic may commit suicide because he is deeply depressed, or he may kill himself in response to the relentless commands he is receiving from hallucinatory voices. Probably the greatest number of schizophrenic suicides occurs among those suffering from incipient schizophrenia.

One schizophrenic, who had jumped to the street from a third floor balcony, sustained several fractures but lived to say that for many days a man's voice had told him persistently to jump out of a window. He did not want to die, and he resisted the voice as long as he could, but he finally had to yield to its demands.

It is exceedingly difficult to prevent most schizophrenic homicides, since usually there is no clear warning. The homicidal schizophrenic patient may appear to be relaxed, even apathetic—then, within a day or two, he kills somebody.

A schizophrenic man who had been going home on weekends for many months was told by his sister that she would not ask for permission any more to take him out of the hospital if he would not do his part with the housework—for instance, help with the dishes. On the weekend visit, the patient killed his sister and his mother. He had shown no signs of disturbance whatsoever during the preceding week, had been sleeping well, and had been attending occupational therapy classes as usual. If anything, he had appeared somewhat more indifferent than usual.

A 19-year-old boy had been discharged from a mental hospital in what appeared to be a residual state of chronic schizophrenia of the undifferentiated type. He stabbed his father to death when the father, during a state of intoxication, told the patient that he was too much of a bother around the house and that he might as well return to the hospital.

Another schizophrenic, whose condition had not yet been diagnosed, complained to a general practitioner about various physical ailments. When the physician finally told him that he should not come anymore because there was nothing else he could do for him, the patient quietly left the office but returned a few hours later and killed the doctor.

The most significant single factor in many suicides and homicides is a traumatic experience of rejection. The schizophrenic's pathological sensitivity makes him extraordinarily vulnerable to all common life stresses. For him, rejection, particularly by members of his own family, seems to be more traumatic than most other stresses. The act of rejection may seem trivial, and it is often not deliberate on the part of those who reject the patient. They are, in fact, practically never aware of it, and the patient may not show any immediate reaction to the rejection at the time.

Diagnosis

In a patient whose personality structure has not been schizoid and whose breakdown occurred in close relation to some traumatic experience, the symptoms should be typical if a diagnosis of schizophrenia is to be made. Since the outcome of the psychosis is not yet known and the prepsychotic personality and endogenous cause are not clearly established, the schizophrenic symptoms must be particularly convincing.

On the other hand, if the history is that of a typical shut-in personality, in whom the psychotic breakdown occurred without any preceding stress situation, the symptoms would not have to be extremely characteristic to defend a diagnosis of schizophrenia. If there is already evidence of personality deterioration after the acute symptoms have subsided and a year or two have passed, the outcome is the overriding parameter in the diagnostic evaluation.

The presence of delusions and hallucinations confirms only the diagnosis of psychosis—not of schizophrenia. There are important qualifications regarding the modality, the time, and the content of the hallucination. Experiences of being controlled by outside forces or of having strange, continuous, somatic (coenesthetic) hallucinations or auditory, verbal hallucinations, particularly if the voices are coming from God or the devil or address the patient in the second person or talk about him, may support a diagnosis of schizophrenia. Perceptual distortions of time or objects in space point toward a diagnosis of schizophrenia, but only if they have been present at least several days; otherwise, they may well be of toxic origin. The time factor applies also to the symptoms of loss of ego boundaries, the experience of being fused with the universe, and the experience of having one's thoughts spread to others. The presence of delusions provides strong presumptive evidence for schizophrenia only if these delusions have strange, magical, esoteric, or bizarre content.

The diagnosis of schizophrenia cannot be made entirely on the basis of observation or logical reasoning or objective measurement. It requires a careful and comprehensive clinical evaluation. Such an evaluation must take into account the presence or absence of certain schizophrenic key symptoms, the patient's prepsychotic personality, the physical findings, the genetic family history, the natural history of the disease, and any possible precipitating factors.

Key Symptoms

The presence of some key symptoms for schizophrenia—for instance, blunting of emotional response or a strikingly inappropriate emotional response—weighs heavily in favor of a diagnosis of schizophrenia. But considerable clinical experience is needed to be certain about the presence of such symptoms.

Loosening of Associations. The loosening of associations is one of the most valuable diagnostic criteria. But a good knowledge of psychopathology is required to be sure of its presence and to avoid confusing it with other forms of disturbed thinking, such as manic flight of ideas, disintegration of thought processes due to clouding of consciousness, and impaired reasoning due to fatigue or distraction. It is not sufficient to ask a patient the meaning of a proverb and then, on the basis of one's personal impression, declare that the patient has a pronounced schizophrenic thinking disturbance.

Bizarre Behavior. Bizarre postures and grimacing are characteristic of schizophrenic conditions, but what constitutes a bizarre posture is not always easy to establish unequivocally. Religious rituals and special positions for meditation or rock-and-roll dancing with which the observer is not familiar may be called bizarre.

True catalepsy may be pathognomonic of schizophrenia, but it is not a common symptom. A stupor is highly suggestive of catatonic schizophrenia, but hysteria or a depressive stupor must be ruled out in the differential diagnosis.

The deterioration of social habits, even the smearing of feces, is not sufficient grounds for the diagnosis of schizophrenia. Such deterioration can occur in various toxic and organic psychoses, temporarily in hysterical twilight states, and even at the peak of a manic attack in manic-depressives.

Pronounced social withdrawal also occurs under many conditions. Sustained passivity and lack of spontaneity should suggest the diagnosis of schizophrenia only if organic and depressive conditions can be definitely ruled out.

Stereotypies and verbigeration strongly suggest schizophrenia. But they occur almost exclusively in chronic institutionalized patients and are rarely seen today. Frequent and lengthy staring into a mirror and other odd mannerisms are also highly suggestive of a diagnosis of schizophrenia.

Prepsychotic Personality

The typical history is that of a schizoid personality: quiet, passive, with few friends as a child; daydreaming, introverted, and shut-in as an adolescent and adult. The child is often reported as having been especially good because he was always obedient and never in any mischief. In school he was good in spelling but poor in arithmetic. He made few friends as a child, and his deficient friendship pattern was particularly noticeable in adolescence.

The typical schizoid adolescent has few dates,

does not learn to dance, and, as a rule, has no close boyfriends or girlfriends. He is not interested in petting or other heterosexual activities but is often disturbed about masturbation. He avoids all competitive sports, but he likes to go to the movies, watch television, or listen to hi-fi music. He may be an avid reader of books on philosophy and psychology.

Typically, schizophrenics have had many different jobs but held none for long. It is usually difficult to ascertain why they did not stay longer in any position. But it appears that everybody was somehow uncomfortable while he was working. It is not unusual for a patient to change jobs 10 or more times in a single year.

Origin and Outcome

Two of the principal criteria that Kraepelin established for his diagnosis of dementia precox—its endogenous origin and the outcome in deterioration—are still valid, although limited in their applicability. An endogenous origin may be obscured if stressful events precipitated but did not cause the final breakdown. Also, in most cases a psychiatrist must make a diagnosis before the patient has deteriorated, and severe regressive deterioration, common around the beginning of the century, has today become a relatively rare phenomenon.

Precox Feeling

Rümke insists that the only valid diagnostic criterion is the precox feeling, an intuitive experience by the examiner that determines whether it is possible to empathize with the patient. Rümke believes that only those patients whose emotional distance makes it impossible to establish an empathic rapport should be diagnosed as schizophrenic; all other conditions should be regarded as schizophreniform. But it appears to be unwise to substitute a single subjective approach for a whole range of clinical skills.

World Health Organization (WHO) Diagnostic Study

A major and successful effort to implement this goal has been made by the World Health Organization which launched in 1965 one of the most ambitious and comprehensive research efforts ever undertaken in the diagnosis of schizophrenia, the international pilot study of schizophrenia. The goal was to discover reliable methods of diagnosing schizophrenia in a standardized and universally acceptable way. The project,

covering 1,202 patients admitted to the participating psychiatric centers, was carried out simultaneously in nine countries: Columbia, Czechoslovakia, Denmark, India, Nigeria, Taiwan, U.S.S.R., United Kingdom, and the United States.

Individual psychiatrists used the present state examination schedule, a standardized interview form, to arrive at their own diagnosis. The interview included 360 detailed items, which were rated by observing and interviewing the patient. The items were then condensed into 129 units of analysis, and these units were further consolidated into 27 groups of units of analysis. As an example, the unit of analysis entitled delusions of persecution is a cluster of several specific questions (items), such as: "Did you notice that someone wanted to harm you?" and "Did you notice that someone was spying on you?" An example of a group of units of analysis is delusions—a category that refers not only to delusions of persecution but also to delusions of grandeur, nihilistic delusions, delusions of guilt, fantastic delusions, sexual delusions, and several other types of delusions.

All data, including psychiatric and social histories of the patients, were computerized and subjected to painstaking statistical evaluation.

Since a major goal of this international pilot study was to make it possible to carry out comparative psychiatric studies in different countries and cultures, it was of primary importance to determine the reliability (intracenter and intercenter consensus) of the data collected and the diagnoses made at the nine centers. It was established that the standardized interview schedule could be satisfactorily administered in each culture, that it was possible to achieve high reliability among interviewers at each center and with several key symptoms across all centers, and that international consensus of the diagnosis of schizophrenia could be reached.

To achieve the highest possible degree of reliability, the investigators took great pains to translate precisely each question into each language. For example, in English one question is: "Does some other force than yourself make you do, feel, or say things that you do not intend? As though you were an automaton, robot (Zombie), marionette, puppet, without a will of your own?" But in zombieless Yoruba, the second part of the same question is posed this way: "As if you were an image without your own will (fairies, image, and others)."

Of the 1,202 patients, 811 were diagnosed as schizophrenic. Three different methods were chosen to arrive at the diagnosis of schizophrenia. The first was the traditional psychiatric diagnosis, using the structured interview, which left the examiner some freedom to expand on the 360 items.

The second method was a computerized diagnosis. The input consisted of raw data, primarily clinical observations, in a program based on the assumption of a hierarchy of weighted symptoms, similar to that accepted by most clinicians today and giving much weight to Schneider's first rank symptoms. The computer then made successive diagnostic decisions based on the presence and relative importance of each symptom of each patient. This computation resulted in a completely objective and uniform classification. Wing's Catego program was used for this study. (A major competitor among computerized programs not used in the WHO Study is Spitzer and Endicott's (1969) DIAGNO.)

The third method of diagnosis used was cluster analysis. This procedure is based on mathematical principles and attaches equal diagnostic weight to all symptoms. It is an empirical method of grouping patients according to the symptoms they have in common. McKeon's method was used to sort the patients into 10 such clusters. Several of these clusters, it turned out, contained a significantly higher number of patients who had been diagnosed as schizophrenic by the computers and by the clinicians than could have been expected purely by chance; thus, these cluster groups were thought to represent most purely schizophrenic patients.

It was found that the present state examination schedule was the principal instrument for arriving at an accurate diagnosis and that in most cases the additional psychiatric and social histories contributed too little to diagnostic accuracy to be included in all three methods.

A concordant group of 306 schizophrenics out of the total of 811 were then separated out and defined as consisting of all those patients who had been diagnosed as schizophrenic by the clinical interview and the computer method and who also belonged to one of the clusters containing a higher than chance number of schizophrenics. The remaining 505 were described as the discrepant group of schizoprenics.

Findings. Any symptom, in order to be most useful for the diagnostician, should possess three qualities: high frequency of occurrence, high reliability, and high discriminatory power (specificity). Tables I and II illustrate some of the key findings on the frequency and reliability of symptoms resulting from the WHO study, as they apply to the least controversial, most clearly schizophrenic, concordant group.

The tables merely hint at the pains the WHO study participants took to categorize and quantify the enormous amount of data collected. They also suggest how circumspect the clinician must be to avoid the diagnostic ruts into which so many have fallen. Many observers may well be surprised, for example, to find ambivalence, visual hallucinations, and a hostile and negativistic attitude among the uncommon symptoms of schizophrenia. Or they may not expect to see "morose mood" on a list of symptoms on which agreement within psychiatric centers was low.

The following are some of the key WHO findings and observations that go beyond the scope of Tables I and II:

Within groups of units of analysis, auditory hallucinations appear to be one of the most valuable symptoms for the diagnosis of schizophrenia; this symptom not only ranks high in discriminatory power but also has a high frequency of occurrence (74 per cent) and a high reliability (0.86). The experience of being controlled rated

highest in reliability. Delusions and qualitative disorders of formal thinking, such as erroneous logic, were rated of medium reliability. Flatness of affect and incongruity of affect were of comparatively low reliability.

A striking finding of this study was that the interrater reliability of the patients' own reports, such as auditory hallucinations and experiences of being controlled, tended to be consistently higher than the reliability of observations of patient behavior—for instance, qualitative disorder of form of thinking or flatness of affect—although the differences were sometimes small. All but one of the top 10 groups of units rated for reliability were symptoms reported by the patients themselves. Most of the symptoms of lowest reliability were observations by the interviewers.

Specificity of symptoms. More significant than sheer statistical frequency of occurrence and even reliability of symptoms is their diagnostic discriminatory power—the specificity of symptoms. For example, a symptom such as the use of neologisms may be rarely observed. However, it is highly specific and almost pathognomonic for schizophrenia. On the other hand, lack of insight is frequently observed in schizophrenics, as it is in all psychotics, but is among the least specific symptoms of schizophrenia. Flatness of affect is frequently reported and also a quite specific symptom; but, unfortunately, its reliability is low; it is often difficult to reach agreement among different examiners as to whether or not this particular symptom is present.

In the area of specificity, the following is a list of six of the most frequently reported symptoms in the concordant schizophrenic group that are not found among the 15 most frequent symptoms in the discrepant schizophrenic group: auditory hallucinations (frequency, 74 per cent), flatness of affect (66 per cent), voices speaking to the patient (65 per cent), thought alienation (52 per cent), thoughts spoken aloud (50 per cent), and delusions of control (48 per cent). These may be considered the core symptoms of schizophrenia, as revealed by the WHO Study.

Conversely, the following are six of the most frequent symptoms that appear in the discrepant group but are not among the 15 most frequently reported symptoms in the concordant group: poor rapport (frequency, 46 per cent), depressed mood (37 per cent), gloomy thoughts

(34 per cent), sleep problems (27 per cent), hopelessness (27 per cent), and hypochondria (23 per cent). These symptoms, although not altogether atypical for schizophrenia, seem to be peripheral symptoms.

The WHO study further determined the probability that patients with specific symptoms would be allocated to three different diagnostic classes. This probability for voices to patient was: 0.91 for schizophrenia and paranoid psychosis, 0.05 for manic psychosis, and 0.03 for depressive psychosis or neurosis. Commentary by voices made the diagnosis of schizophrenia even more probable: 0.97 for schizophrenia, 0.03 for manic psychosis, and 0.01 for depressive psychosis or neurosis. Corresponding values for thought broadcast were: 0.97 probability for schizophrenia, 0.02 for manic psychosis, and 0.01 for depressive psychosis or neurosis; delusions of control: 0.96 for schizophrenia, 0.02 for manic psychosis, and 0.01 for depressive psychosis or neurosis; neologisms: 0.97 for schizophrenia, 0.04 for manic psychosis, and 0.000 for depressive psychosis or neurosis. Therefore, the presence of the single symptom of neologisms gives a 97 per cent probability that the patient would be diagnosed, across the world, as suffering from schizophrenia and a zero probability that he would be diagnosed as depressed or neurotic.

Differential Diagnosis

Neurotic Symptoms in Schizophrenia. Hysterical symptoms are common in acute schizophrenic breakdown. Every schizophrenic breakdown is preceded by a period of marked tension and anxiety. During the acute and subacute stages of a schizophrenic attack, obsessive symptoms are commonly observed in schizophrenic conditions, and an obsessive-compulsive clinical picture can develop into schizophrenia.

Manic-Depressive Disorder Versus Schizophrenia. The behavior of an excited catatonic patient is directed primarily by his own qualitatively disordered mental processes. His actions are unpredictable and appear senseless, his affect is difficult to understand, and his verbal productions may be irrational and incoherent. A manic patient, on the other hand, is always distractible, and most of his actions are determined by his immediate environment. His activity resembles that of an excessively busy person, rushing from one superficial job to another. His affect is clearly one of playful euphoria or angry irritability but always outgoing and expansive. His verbal productions are accelerated and increased in number, and they reveal a quantitative disorder of association processes, rather than the intrinsic, qualitative thought disorder of the schizophrenic.

TABLE I

Frequency of Symptoms in a Pooled Sample of Schizophrenic Patients Examined in Nine International Centers*

Common: Frequency > 30%	Uncommon: Frequency > 4% < 10%	Rare: Frequency < 4%
Loss of interest	Hostile, negativistic	Absence of voluntary movement
Less energy	Outburst of anger in interview	Waxy flexibility
Difficulty in concentration	Fails to respond verbally	Imitation of examiner's movements
Continuous worrying	Ecstatic mood	Automatic obedience
Trouble sleeping	Ambivalence	Lips moving soundlessly
Wants to stay away from people	Suggestibility	Talks to self incoherently
Depressed	Visual hallucinations	Echolalia
Cries	Nihilistic delusions	Neologisms
Variable mood	Confused in interview	Verbigeration
Anxiety	Difficult life situation	
Flattened affect		
Auditory hallucinations		
Delusional		
Behavioral abnormalities		

* Adapted from World Health Organization, *Report of the International Pilot Study of Schizophrenia*, Table 3.1. World Health Organization, Geneva, 1973.

TABLE II

Reliability of Units of Schizophrenic Symptoms Analysis across Nine International Centers*

Units of Analysis		
>0.93, high	0.62–0.60, medium	0.59–0.47, low
Suicidal	Change of interest	Stereotyped behavior
Elated thoughts	Dissociation of speech	Increased libido
Ideas of reference	Perplexity	Negativism
Delusions of grandeur	Lability	Perseveration
Thought-hearing		Body hallucinations
Derealization		Morose mood
Lack of concentration		
Hopelessness		
Delusions of persecution		
Delusions of reference		

* Adapted from World Health Organization, *Report of the International Pilot Study of Schizophrenia*, Table 8.3. World Health Organization, Geneva, 1973.

Depressive conditions should never be diagnosed as schizophrenic unless there are also some unmistakably schizophrenic symptoms present.

Schizophrenia in the Adolescent. Any psychiatric disorder that occurs during adolescence assumes a certain schizophrenic coloring, since many of the features characteristic of non-schizophrenic adolescent turbulence—exaltation, intense preoccupation with abstract ideas, unpredictable variations of mood, daydreaming, introspection, shyness—are often seen in schizophrenia. Therefore, it is not unusual to misdiagnose a manic or depressive phase of manic-depressive psychosis as schizophrenia if the patient's first attack occurs in late adolescence.

Psychological Tests. There are no definitive psychological tests for schizophrenia. There are only psychological tests that are more or less compatible with a diagnosis of schizophrenia, making the diagnosis more or less probable.

In most clinical centers certain psychological test batteries are routinely used to indicate, confirm, or rule out a diagnosis of schizophrenia. These test batteries are usually composed of projective tests, psychometric tests, and personality inventories. The most frequently used projective tests are the Rorschach test, some drawing tests, and the Thematic Apperception Test (TAT). The most commonly used psychometric tests are the Wechsler Adult Intelligence Scale (WAIS) and some tests that probe concept formation and the organization of thought processes. The most widely used personality inventory is the Minnesota Multi-phasic Personality Inventory (MMPI), a self-report questionnaire that renders profiles of psychopathology or response styles.

Some other test instruments, mainly used by psychiatrists, are the Phillips Scale, which is constructed from data gathered from the patient's history and premorbid personality and which yields a prediction of the final outcome in schizophrenic patients, and an ego function appraisal scale, developed by Bellak and associates, which gives a profile of various psychodynamic levels of adaptation of the schizophrenic patient.

As a general rule, projective tests are much less objective than are psychometric tests and, therefore, less reliable. The special value of projective test procedures lies in the richness of the dynamic material they often provide, thus giving the clinician considerable insight into the associations, imagery, preoccupations, conflicts, and defense mechanisms of the tested person.

A diagnosis of schizophrenia is supported by psychological tests if these tests reflect unusual or bizarre perceptual and conceptual processes (Rorschach, TAT, drawing tests, and WAIS, particularly the similarity subtest). Other typical findings are variability and uneven scattering of test scores (WAIS) and disturbances of concept formation—in particular, overinclusive and autistic thought processes (object-sorting and concept formation tests). Self-report personality inventories (MMPI) allow for objective, even automated scoring and can be helpful in the differential diagnosis of doubtful cases.

Drug Factors. Many schizophrenic patients

today have received some form of pharmaco-therapy before they are seen by a psychiatrist. If they were given adequate doses of neuroleptics in the early stages of a schizophrenic attack, important key symptoms—such as the experience of being controlled, thought hearing, delusions, hallucinations, and inappropriate behavior—may have subsided within 2 or 3 days, and the disorder with which the psychiatrist is faced may lack most or all of its more specific distinguishing features.

Many young people who develop psychotic symptoms have a history of having used amphetaminelike stimulants (speed) and hallucinogenic drugs—for instance, LSD (acid) and drugs with similar effects. Amphetamines and amphetaminelike drugs in high doses can produce psychotic, usually paranoid, conditions that mimic schizophrenia in symptoms and course so closely that a differential diagnosis may be impossible in some cases. Fortunately, treatment is the same for amphetamine-induced paranoid psychosis and for paranoid schizophrenia. With hallucinogens, the psychotic symptoms may have more of a toxic character, with vivid nonauditory hallucinations and clouding of consciousness. This type of psychosis is usually of short duration, unless the hallucinogen served only as the trigger for a true schizophrenic attack in an already predisposed person.

The Counterculture. An entirely new set of differential diagnostic problems has been generated by the special life style and philosophy of today's counterculture, with its defiance of conventions, its mistrust of modern science and of analytical thinking generally, and its emphasis on behavior and beliefs borrowed from Eastern cultures.

A diagnosis of schizophrenia can be made only by evaluating specific patterns of behavior and experiences in their cultural context, and psychiatrists in today's society must be fully aware of the differential cultural currents and standards that now exist within the Western cultural sphere and must make allowances for them.

Prognosis

It has been known since Kraepelin and Bleuler that the hebephrenic and simple types of schizophrenia have the poorest prognosis, that paranoid types have an intermediate prog-

nosis, and that acute catatonic types have the best prognosis but that catatonic patients who go on to chronicity usually continue to regress and may become markedly deteriorated.

Modern pharmacotherapy, with neuroleptics has changed many of the old prognostic patterns. Today, a paranoid schizophrenic's chances of making a good recovery are at least equal to those of an acute catatonic. Even hebephrenics often have good remissions after a few months of pharmacotherapy. The simple schizophrenic is still the least responsive to modern physical treatment methods.

The more acute the onset of a schizophrenic attack, the better are the chances for a good remission or complete recovery. If a precipitating event has clearly triggered the breakdown, the chances for a favorable outcome are also relatively better.

The younger a patient is at the onset of his schizophrenic psychosis, the worse is his prognosis, as a rule. Patients who break down in childhood or early puberty seldom recover completely.

A history of good adjustment in the important areas of social, sexual, and occupational functioning before the breakdown also indicates a favorable prognosis. Married schizophrenics have a better prognosis than do single, divorced, or widowed patients. The presence of depression also makes for a better prognosis. Conversely, sustained emotional withdrawal and aloofness or shallow and inappropriate affective responses are ominous prognostic signs. A number of studies in recent years have established the fact that many schizophrenics come from deeply disturbed families. The more often a patient neglects to take his maintenance medication, the more likely he is to suffer a relapse.

Deterioration

The risk of personality deterioration increases with each schizophrenic relapse. This risk of personality deterioration increases rapidly after the second relapse. However, chronic schizophrenia does not inevitably lead to intellectual deterioration. And the schizophrenic process may be reversible over long periods of time.

Final Outcome

A schizophrenia patient's chances for a favorable outcome of his psychosis are estimated today to be about four to five times better than they were only 60 years ago. Today, with good follow-up therapy and well-controlled maintenance drug treatment, only 10 to 15 per cent of patients in remission will relapse within a year, compared with about 35 to 70 per cent who would relapse during the same period without such follow-up treatment.

There are five possible outcomes for the schizophrenic patient: full and permanent recovery; full remission, with one or more future relapses; social remission with personality defect, either capable of self-care and self-support or dependent on protection and supervision; stable chronicity; and deterioration to terminal stage. In the modern mental hospital, it is increasingly difficult to find patients who deteriorate to a terminal stage of schizophrenia. Many schizophrenics, despite all intensive therapeutic efforts, remain in a state of stable chronicity. The majority of schizophrenics today will emerge in the categories of social remission with personality defect or full remission with relapses.

The possibility of full and permanent recovery from a schizophrenic attack is probably considerably brighter today than it was a half century ago, when the chances for such complete recovery were only 2 to 4 per cent.

Present Outlook

About 60 per cent of patients hospitalized for an attack of acute schizophrenia will be socially recovered 5 years later and will have been employed for more than half of that time. About 30 per cent will be handicapped and show some psychopathology but will still be living in the community. Only about 10 per cent will be hospitalized.

By striving for a suitable emotional milieu, good occupational rehabilitation, and adequate pharmacotherapy, psychiatrists today can provide an integrated aftercare approach that may reduce relapse rates and chronicity even further.

REFERENCES

Bleuler, E. Primary and secondary symptoms in schizophrenia. Z. Gen. Neurol. Psychiatry, *124:* 607, 1930.
Bleuler, M. *Die schizophrenen Geistesstörungen im Lichte langjähriger Kranken-und Familiengeschichten. (Schizophrenic Disorders in the Light of Long-term Case and Family Histories).* Thieme, Stuttgart, p. 673, 1972.
Carpenter, W. T., Strauss, J. S., and Muleh, S. Are there pathognomonic symptoms in schizophrenia? An empiric investigation of Schneider's first-rank symptoms. Arch. Gen. Psychiatry, *28:* 847, 1973.
Davison, K., and Bagley, C. R. Schizophrenia-like psychoses associated with organic disorders of the central nervous system: A review of the literature. In *Current Problems in Neuropsychiatry: Schizophrenia, Epilepsy, the Temporal Lobe.* R. N. Herrington, editor, p. 133. Headley, Ashford, Kent, England, 1969.
Finney, J. G., Skeeters, D. E., Anvenshine, C. D., and Smith, D. F. Phases of psychopathology after assassination. Am. J. Psychiatry, *130:* 1379, 1973.
Gross, G., and Huber, G. Prognosis of schizophrenia (Zur prognose der schizophrenien). Psychiatr. Clin. (Basel), *6:* 1, 1973.
Hogarty, G. E., Goldberg, S. C., and Collaborative Study Group. Drug and sociotherapy in the aftercare of schizophrenic patients. Arch. Gen. Psychiatry, *28:* 54, 1973.
Katz, M. M., Cole, J. O., and Lowery, H. A. Studies of the diagnostic process: The influence of symptom perception, past experience, and ethnic background on diagnostic decisions. Am. J. Psychiatry, *125:* 937, 1969.
Langfeldt, G. *The Schizophreniform States.* Oxford University Press, London, 1939.
Marks, A. P., and Seeman, W. *Actuarial Description of Abnormal Personality.* Williams & Wilkins, Baltimore, 1973.
Morrison, J. R. Catatonia: Retarded and excited types. Arch. Gen. Psychiatry, *28:* 39, 1973.
Schneider, L. *Klinische Psychopathologie,* ed. 9. Thieme, Stuttgart, 1971.
Snyder, S. H. Amphetamine psychosis: A "model" schizophrenia mediated by catecholamines. Am. J. Psychiatry, *130:* 61, 1973.
Symonds, M. Parents of schizophrenic children. J. Am. Acad. Psychoanal., *1:* 171, 1973.
World Health Organization. *Report of the International Pilot Study of Schizophrenia.* World Health Organization, Geneva, 1973.
Zimmermann, I. L., and Woo-Sam, J. W. *Clinical Interpretation of the Wechsler Adult Intelligence Scale.* Grune & Stratton, New York, 1973.

14.5   SCHIZOPHRENIA: OVERVIEW OF TREATMENT METHODS

Introduction

The causes of schizophrenia are unclear, and there is, as yet, no universally effective and lasting cure for all patients. With appropriate treatment, acute symptoms may remit with startling rapidity, but, even in these cases, there is usually some residual scarring or vulnerability. When the schizophrenic condition is chronic or severe, the psychiatrist can usually modify symptoms and alleviate suffering, perhaps even reduce the likelihood of relapse and readmission to the hospital, but none of the present forms of treatment can sustain a claim to lasting remission. Many patients have a good prognosis for social remission—that is, restoration of their premorbid level of functioning. Indeed, a number of patients recover rapidly without any special treatment when they are removed from their stress situations. But altering the patient's personality so that he does not continue to react pathologically to the stresses of life is far more difficult; in many cases, it is impossible by the methods currently available.

Three main models of treatment can be distinguished. The concept of a therapeutic milieu is essentially nonspecific, originally based on the mitigating and healing effect of a benign environment and now extended to include more positive corrective interventions that overlap and coordinate with other methods. The various psychoanalytic, psychotherapeutic, and conditioning approaches are based on theoretical formulations of psychic structure and development and of the schizophrenic process. The somatic therapies, such as antipsychotic drugs and electroshock, are primarily empirical.

The patient's schizophrenia has not occurred in isolation, and ivory-tower treatment of the patient alone, apart from his social and family context, is less likely to succeed than is thoughtful, coordinated work with family members, friends, and others who may be significant in his life. In general, the best results are obtained by integrating the various avenues and forms of treatment into a constructive and integrated approach.

A person should not be admitted to the hospital just because he is schizophrenic. Given adequate professional resources and under favorable conditions, many patients can be successfully treated in other settings, such as day hospitals, day-care centers, residential treatment units, halfway houses, foster homes, and outpatient clinics. However, a schizophrenic patient should not be kept in the community merely because such treatment is fashionable. The burden on relatives and the community caused by severely impaired patients is rarely negligible, and, in some cases, it may be intolerable. And there are, almost universally in this country, gross deficiencies in community resources for the treatment and rehabilitation of the schizophrenic patient.

Milieu Therapy

The major portion of the hospital patient's day is spent in the care of nurses and other professionals. Hence the concept of therapeutic milieu, which, originating in the moral treatment of the nineteenth century, has been provided with a degree of direction by the psychoanalytic understanding of Simmel and the differing sociopsychiatric viewpoints of Sullivan and Main.

Observing that the patient's illness was often a collective illness of the patient and those intimately related to him, Simmel concluded that it was necessary to conduct psychoanalysis in more or less strict isolation, to replace the patient's pseudoreality with a new reality, which would act as a kind of extension of the analyst's personality or as a family archetype. This new reality would not only provide the patient with a crutch until he could attain independent existence and enjoyment but would also promote the therapeutic process by limiting his acting out, by refusing to appease unconscious guilts with punitive measures, or by providing substitute oral and maternal gratification.

Sullivan treated young male patients by modification of their personal, social, and cultural environment and by focusing on group relationships. He created an environment in which there was a feeling of therapeutic community, with emphasis on growth by experience of interpersonal relations and on education by communal experience.

Main attacked both the concept of the hospital as a refuge and the traditional hospital authoritarian mixture of charity and discipline that removed the patients' initiative and perpetuated dependency. He substituted the concept of the hospital as a therapeutic institution, with a framework of social reality that provides opportunities for attaining fuller social insight and for expressing and modifying emotional drives according to the demands of real life.

These pioneer efforts and subsequent work led to widespread reforms designed to remove the insidious deculturing and deteriorating effects of custodial authoritarian programs and attitudes. As a result, hospitals now provide varying degrees and mixtures of occupational therapy, attitude therapy, vocational rehabilitation, education, work therapy, recreation, resocialization, remotivation, therapeutic community, and patient government.

Value

The relative value of milieu therapy for the schizophrenic patient has not been conclusively demonstrated by objective research. Recently, there has been serious consideration of the possibility that milieu therapy may have toxic, antitherapeutic effects and so should be used with greater discrimination and more objective monitoring of the patient's response. The trouble with milieu therapy is that techniques and methods highly appropriate for neurotics and patients with character disorders have been indiscriminately applied to overt psychotics.

The introduction of drug therapy also prompts a reappraisal. Drugs are effective at all levels of milieu care, and an intensive milieu program alone is less effective than drug therapy, With current methods, there are still a number of hard-core, treatment-resistant patients, for some of whom long-term hospital care may properly be indicated. But, with the use of modern psychotropic drugs, the hospital can be, for the average schizophrenic patient, essentially a center for relatively brief crisis treatment until he is psychologically ambulatory. The emphasis in hospital milieu care can shift progressively from indiscriminate application of the cumbersome, time-consuming, and expensive methods of today toward specific interventions to expedite the process of restitution and community-oriented techniques, such as preparing the patient and the family for a flexible, integrated, and individually prescribed outpatient program. The hospital professional team should expand into the real world of the community, provide genuine continuity of care, and develop techniques and approaches for extramural milieu therapy, thoughtfully integrated with work and social rehabilitation.

Group Approach

A number of overlapping themes are varyingly embodied in approaches that focus on the group—reality confrontation, democracy, permissiveness, communalism, patient participation in decision-making and in treating other patients, team functioning, communication, freedom, and responsibility. These approaches are implemented by group meetings of patients and staff separately and together, focusing on social functioning, rather than on psychopathology. In general, a therapeutic community encourages self-reliance and rewards the patient progressively for efforts toward social readaptation. He is expected to participate in planning his own treatment program and in helping other

patients and to assume responsibility in ward affairs and the outside world.

At its best, a unit run along those lines has impressively high patient and staff morale. But it is not certain that this high morale is accompanied by a parallel degree of improvement in the patients' schizophrenia. The carefully nurtured communication and feedback can also have a destructive, toxic effect, blowing up trivial disturbances into an explosive collective uproar. And it is a mistake to believe that, left alone, psychotic adults will intuitively and spontaneously make the right decisions for themselves and for others. It is equally a mistake to block, by grandiose domination, patients' attempts to gain mastery. The therapeutic task is to mediate between the two extremes.

Individual Approach

Here the focus is on transactions between the individual patient and individual staff members. Specific staff attitudes and management tactics are prescribed for each patient. The range of possible attitudes is infinite, but those most commonly used are active friendliness, passive friendliness, indulgence, reassurance, praise, tolerance, matter-of-factness, firmness, and insistence. The individual patient's daily program is carefully prescribed and modified to include activities suited to a particular management device.

One difficulty with attitude therapy is that some therapists are never sure what will be therapeutic; a considerable range and variety of responses may be equally effective—or ineffective—at any particular moment. Nor are these therapists comfortable with an artificially prescribed attitude; it is better, they say, to be spontaneous, human, and oneself. Another problem is that an extraordinarily efficient communication system is required to put widely different attitudes into effect for a large number of patients in several different locations and activities throughout the hospital.

Rehabilitation and the Community

Rehabilitation may be loosely defined as a concentrated attempt to order the environment so as to compensate for or at least minimize residual social and psychological difficulties, to take advantage of the patient's assets, and to develop or redevelop his skills. Rehabilitation is a process that must be continuously applied within the hospital and sustained into the community. Unfortunately, rehabilitation efforts are usually poorly organized and commonly fall by the wayside soon after the patient's discharge from the hospital.

A wide range of services are needed to give appropriate domestic and social support—in-hospital living facilities, hostels, halfway houses, communal group living arrangements, family care, foster homes, lodgings, apartments, hotels, ex-patient social clubs, and Schizophrenics Anonymous—and to provide a suitable work setting—vocational counseling, job training, in-hospital work-for-pay programs, sheltered workshops in the hospital or in the community, trial work placement communal and cooperative patient-operated businesses, protected positions in industry. Work and living conditions must be realistic and consistent with the goal of productive participation in the tasks and rewards of society.

Rehabilitation and Drug Therapy

Despite the use of antipsychotic drugs, the general level of schizophrenic patients' performance and social adjustment in the community is disappointingly low. Both drug therapy and rehabilitation are necessary to achieve optimum results, although the precise plan must vary according to the needs of the individual patient. Drug therapy alone may help a few patients to the point where they can find jobs or suitable living arrangements on their own, but, in most cases, they need assistance for adequate social or occupational restoration. Home visits and work with the family may spell the difference between success and failure.

Psychotherapy

Schizophrenic patients can be reached by psychoanalytic psychotherapy, and a relationship can readily be established, although the relationship is intensely charged and quite different from that encountered in the treatment of neurosis. The main distinction between neurotic and psychotic transference is that the psychotic has lost his internal object representations and can no longer differentiate between the self and the object world. He attaches (projects) his delusional complexes to the therapist. Also, patients are never entirely and continuously psychotic. The transference of the schizophrenic patient is at times or in part neurotic;

and there is, as well, a relatively nonneurotic, nonpsychotic, healthy, rational part of the ego that can enter into a working alliance with the therapist. To some extent, the patient is aware of his illness, does want to change, and can work purposefully and cooperatively in a psychotherapeutic relationship.

Value

Confusion between what is good for neurosis and what is appropriate for psychotics has been accompanied by a reluctance to subject hypotheses and techniques to scientific study and controlled comparison, leading to a widespread overestimation of the effectiveness of current methods for psychotherapy of schizophrenia. The result of the relatively few controlled studies have been disappointing.

Psychotherapeutic management—the application of psychodynamic understanding to the management and rehabilitation of the individual patient, establishing a therapeutic relationship, helping him to identify and deal with current life problems, and working with the family and significant others—is practical, realistic, and flexibly usable at any stage of the schizophrenic process. But orthodox, formal psychoanalysis has apparently no place in the treatment of overt psychosis. Even in the outpatient postrestitution phase, when the patient has reintegrated sufficiently and the objective is to work with the damaged personality, major technical modifications of psychoanalytic and psychotherapeutic techniques are probably desirable.

For certain hard-core treatment failures, particularly when antipsychotic drugs have been ineffective, individual psychotherapy in the hospital should be seriously considered; if there are cases that respond specifically to this form of treatment, they would be likely to be concentrated in the group that has failed to respond successfully to other forms of therapy.

Establishing a Relationship

Establishing a relationship is often a peculiarly difficult matter, for the schizophrenic is desperately lonely yet defends against closeness and trust and is likely to become suspicious, anxious, hostile, or regressed when the attempt is made. Simple directness, sincerity, scrupulous observation of distance, and sensitivity to the unspoken significance of social conventions are preferable to premature informality and the condescending use of first names or timid appeasement. Exaggerated warmth or professions of friendship are out of place and likely to be perceived as attempts at bribery, manipulation, or exploitation. Free association and the couch are seldom used.

Within the context of a professional relationship, flexibility is essential. At times, the therapist may have meals with a patient, sit on the floor, go for a walk or out to a restaurant, accept and give gifts, play table tennis, remember his birthday, allow him to telephone the therapist at any hour, or just sit silently with him. More unusual approaches include the use of dream language, immediate and shocking direct interpretation, and entering into the patient's hallucinations and delusions. The main aim is to convey the idea that the therapist wants to understand the patient and will try to do so and that he has faith in the patient's potential as a human being, no matter how disturbed or hostile or bizarre he may be at the moment.

Countertransference

The treatment of schizophrenic patients is always a stressful experience, especially for the therapist who regards primary-process manifestations as alien and frightening and is upset by confusing communication or easily threatened by disturbed behavior. Countertransference can be used constructively if the therapist is able to recognize and accept it without burdening the patient with ill-advised security operations; his reaction may then be used as a signal that he may have the same anxiety as the patient. The therapist must be willing to admit that he may be wrong and to correct his errors but not in an insipid, placating fashion. He should come across as an active person with positive values. Passive acceptance to violence in word or action is inadvisable.

Intervention

Primary-Process Intervention. Primary-process techniques are generally not suitable for the usual therapist, for they require both an extraordinary amount of time and unusual personal qualities. Perhaps the most widely known technique is Rosen's direct analysis. Rosen works in a residential setting with a group of two or more assistants organized as a therapeutic community. The therapist is seen as a nourishing foster parent who provides the kind of care that was lacking in the patient's early maternal environment. The patient is pressed to accept the fact that he is psychotic, dependent, and in need of treatment; to accept the therapist's formulation of the origin and nature of his illness; and to look to him and his assistants to control and cure it. Independent research evaluation of direct analysis does not support the claim that it results in a high degree of recovery.

Schwing, Azima, and Sechehaye re-enact in action or in fantasy the infantile situation so that originally frustrated needs can be gratified. In the first pretransference stage, the objective is to act as a life preserver to which the distressed ego may cling. By understanding the schizophrenic's existential world, the therapist makes him feel secure and no longer alone. The next step is the symbolic realization itself. Oral needs are the most important. The aim is to make the adult ego admit that infantile needs are legitimate. In the next stage, there is an intense schizophrenic transference, in which complete dependency signifies that the patient has progressed from autism to symbiosis. He transfers to the therapist his wishes for a new mother and becomes more capable of formulating his needs. The final goal is reconstruction of the ego; development of identity and worth; reinvestment of reality by means of imitation, introjection, and identification; and differentiation from the therapist.

Secondary-Process Intervention. The first advocacy of this approach may be attributed to Federn, who emphasized the need to rerepress what has broken through into consciousness, to interpret defenses rather than impulses, and to focus on reality rather than unconscious content. There is a cooperative exploration of the patient's internal and external relationships and behavior to examine what he does to reality, education to help him identify sources of danger and anxiety and to react appropriately rather than defensively, and improvement in emotional modulation and frustration tolerance.

The therapeutic process requires that the therapist alternatively and in varying doses look with the patient at his world and give him glimpses of the therapist's world. (See Figure 1.)

and secondary symptoms. There are no great differences in general effectiveness among the currently available phenothiazines, except that mepazine and promazine appear to be somewhat less effective. The main differences lie in side-effects and potency per milligram. Low-dosage (more potent) phenothiazines such as trifluoperazine, perphenazine, and fluphenazine are more likely to induce extrapyramidal side-effects; high-dosage phenothiazines such as chlorpromazine, thioridazine, acetophenazine, and triflupromazine are more likly to have other types of side-effects. However, certain types of patients may do better with different drugs. In general, only one drug should be used at a time.

Dosage

Giving 25 mg. for a short while is poor practice and unlikely to be effective. (Dose examples are given as milligrams of chlorpromazine per day; 25 mg. of chlorpromazine are roughly equivalent to 1.5 to 2.0 mg. of trifluoperazine or 1.0 mg. of fluphenazine.) A few patients do well on relatively low doses (less than 400 mg.), but small doses should not be used unless things are obviously going well. Most hospitalized patients do better on moderate dosage (400 to 1,200 mg.), and acute cases generally need more than 600 mg. A few young patients (under age 40), require doses of 1,300 to 3,000 mg. to achieve a therapeutic effect, but, except in life-threatening situations, dosage above 1,500 mg. daily should generally be avoided unless the patient fails to respond to several weeks or months of more moderate dosage.

Starting low, the therapist should raise the dose gradually to achieve the greatest antipsychotic effect with the least unfavorable side-effects. Except for parenteral medication, the drug may be given as one dose in 24 hours, certainly no more than two. Timing is usually unimportant, unless there are sedative side-effects, in which case it should be given at bedtime. Drowsiness is more frequent with chlorpromazine and may be avoided by using some other drug, such as a low-dosage phenothiazine. If drowsiness does appear, the dose should be maintained until tolerance develops; it will not develop if medication is reduced to an ineffective level. Coffee or caffeine citrate may help, but amphetamines should be avoided, as they may activate psychosis.

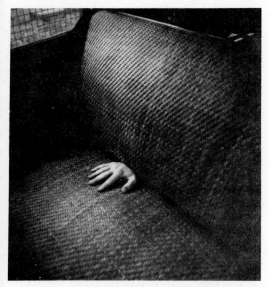

FIGURE 1. This photograph may symbolize the fantasy world of the schizophrenic. Not all psychiatrists are willing or able to attempt to enter that world which is a valuable therapeutic technique.

Group Therapy. Group therapy in the treatment of the schizophrenic has an uncertain status. Some patients feel more open, secure, and trusting in a group, which they find less threatening than the closeness of an individual one-to-one relationship. Group therapy also offers more opportunity for peer confrontation and for testing consensual validation and breaking down isolation.

Family Therapy. The family plays an important role in the treatment of the schizophrenic patient, and his illness is usually accompanied by serious family problems. Appropriate active involvement with the family and significant others is usually essential, both while the patient is in the hospital and after his release.

The intervention is determined by the special circumstances of the individual case. At one extreme, the patient is assisted with the simple problems of everyday life. At the other, there may be deliberate psychotherapeutic work to lessen the degree to which a family participates in and provokes his psychosis or to handle their resistances and anxious interferences.

Drug Therapy

Well-controlled studies have established that the phenothiazines have real value in the treatment of schizophrenia, reducing both primary

Some patients improve only after 3 to 6 months of continuous therapy; accordingly, a trial of 2 to 4 months on high doses should usually be given before deciding that phenothiazine treatment is a failure. The alternative is to change to another type of drug, such as a butyrophenone or a thioxanthene. Before doing this, the therapist should make sure, by urine or blood tests, that the patient is really taking the medication and, if he is taking it, that it is being adequately absorbed and not hypermetabolized away.

Uncooperative Patients

In some acute cases, intramuscular injections may be necessary until the patient becomes sufficiently cooperative to take drugs by mouth. Some patients, however, are a chronic problem. Roughly 20 per cent of patients do not take medication consistently and, despite supervision, may spit out, regurgitate, hide, or discard their pills. Liquid forms make cheating more difficult, but even the best nursing staff can be deceived. In this situation, the use of fluphenazine enanthate or decanoate should be considered; this long-acting, injectable preparation has a duration of action of 2 or more weeks. One of the new, long-acting oral agents might also be considered.

Maintenance Therapy

The aim is to use the lowest dose that is therapeutic. If a patient who requires long-term treatment cannot be maintained on less than 600 mg. of chlorpromazine or thioridazine, the therapist should try a combination to keep dosage below the danger level for chronic side-effects or else switch to another drug. The development of new, long-acting agents may help, for their total dosage is much lower.

Ayd recommends a never-on-Sunday policy for patients on maintenance medication. In some patients this drug holiday may be extended to 2 days or even longer. In many patients, drugs can eventually be discontinued entirely. However, a significant number relapse when phenothiazines are withdrawn, often not until 3 to 6 months later. Withdrawal should be gradual and carefully supervised. As dosage is reduced, special psychotherapeutic and sociotherapeutic efforts are indicated to facilitate cooperation and responsibility and to promote transfer of learning and restitution from the drug to the nondrug condition.

Psychotherapy and Drug Therapy

A fundamental question is whether drug effects interfere with psychotherapy. There is no doubt that toxic reactions and side-effects complicate transactions with the patient, but this complication is readily managed by the competent therapist. In normal subjects, drugs impair speed and coordinated psychomotor and simple perceptual skills, but drugs consistently improve performance under stress or when performance is disrupted by anxiety. Drugs have their greatest use in promoting restitution and contact with reality in the stage of flagrant psychosis. Once restitution has occurred and a more realistic therapeutic alliance has been formed, psychotherapy can be more relevantly directed toward mastery of personality problems and behavior.

It is poor practice to give drugs without establishing a suitable relationship with the patient and without telling the patient what to expect. Discontinuing drugs prescribed by other therapists requires careful evaluation, with thoughtful consideration of the significance of this act in the context of the patient-therapist relationship and with recognition that abrupt withdrawal may precipitate in acute worsening of the patient's condition. It is advisable to review in detail the patient's and the family's prior experience with drugs.

When the physician prescribes an active drug, he will get better results if he potentiates the drug effect by suitably influencing the patient's attitudes and expectations. As much as possible, drug therapy should be structured so that the patient believes that he himself is taking responsibility. Participation in medication decisions can serve as a valuable therapeutic experience in mastery and control, and self-medication is an important part of preparation for discharge.

Other Forms of Therapy

Behavioral Conditioning

Various forms of behavior therapy have been devised, based mostly on the method of operant conditioning first described by Skinner. In this form of learning, actions either lead to reward or prevent a painful stimulus, thus changing behavior by reinforcement or extinction. The simplest application is removing behavior that poses a problem by, for instance, avoidance of a painful electric shock or extinguishing delusional statements by ignoring them and responding only to normal talk. Normal behavior may be rewarded at a simple direct level by positive reinforcement with candy, gum, cigarettes, or approval. More complex experimental programs use generalized reinforcers, such as tokens or points that can be exchanged for money, goods, services, or special privileges.

The precise role of this kind of intervention in the over-all management of the schizophrenic patient has yet to be determined and, for the moment, should be regarded as in the developmental stage. Certainly, conditioning is not a panacea.

Insulin Coma Therapy

A course of insulin treatment, consisting of a series of deep comas produced daily by large doses of insulin, was widely used in the past for the treatment of schizophrenia. It is now virtually obsolete in this country, since drugs apparently produce the same or better results and are less expensive, less dangerous, and more acceptable to patients and to staff.

Electroconvulsive Therapy (ECT)

The status of ECT is unclear. Although it is widely used, its efficacy in schizophrenia has seldom been assessed by controlled investigation, particularly by comparison with drug therapy. The relatively few controlled studies can be taken as establishing that ECT is superior to milieu therapy alone but less effective and more hazardous than drug therapy. Despite the general superiority of drug therapy, ECT has been successfully used in some cases that have failed to respond to drugs.

Reviewers agree that the combination of reserpine and electroshock is dangerous and affords no significant advantage over ECT alone. In the case of phenothiazines combined with ECT, there is some difference of opinion as to the degree of extra risk involved. It is probably more prudent to give the two treatment modalities consecutively, rather than concurrently.

ECT is best given under light intravenous anesthesia, with succinylcholine given to reduce muscular contractions. Unless the therapist is adequately trained in anesthesiology techniques, this phase of treatment should be handled by a qualified anesthetist.

Psychosurgery

Drugs have almost entirely replaced psychosurgery as a treatment method for schizophrenia, although there has been no controlled experimental comparison of the results achieved by the methods.

Nicotinic Acid Megavitamin Therapy

Claims that large doses of niacin (3 mg. or more a day) are effective in the treatment of schizophrenia have yet to be substantiated by acceptable objective evidence, although the rationale rests on a reasonable enough biochemical hypothesis—that schizophrenia results from stress-induced accumulation of adrenochrome, an oxidation product of epinephrine. Major controlled studies indicate that nicotinic acid is no better than a placebo. In fact, if anything, there is some indication that patients treated with phenothiazine alone may do better than those treated with phenothiazine plus nicotinic acid. Large doses of nicotinic acid produce side-effects that, although not major, are sufficiently distressing to merit consideration.

Treatment Failures

About one-third of all schizophrenic patients will do relatively well and return to a reasonable level of functioning. One-third will become hard-core failures, continually more or less severely disabled and spending a great part of their lives in hospitals and under equivalent protection and support. The remainder, the partial treatment failures, will occupy an intermediate status.

The outlook for the nonresponders and the partial responders can be improved considerably by vigorous and intensive rehabilitation efforts, combined with sophisticated management of drug therapy and other therapies. Individual psychotherapy may be of crucial importance in cases of this sort, and serious consideration should be given also to the more radical procedures that are now being used mainly on a research and experimental basis.

Ludwig sees three major phases of treatment: (1) modification of behavior in the hospital, (2) preparation for discharge, and (3) maintenance and rehabilitation in the community. It is, he says, insufficient and negligent to discharge chronic schizophrenic patients without extensive preparation or planning, even if their behavior in the hospital seems adequate. Value systems must be changed, social alienation reversed, deviant and undesirable behavior diminished, coping abilities and social skills developed, and social cost and burdens on the family reduced.

REFERENCES

Bellak, L., and Loeb, L. *The Schizophrenic Syndrome.* Grune & Stratton, New York, 1969.

Bleuler, E. *Dementia Praecox or the Group of Schizophrenias.* International Universities Press, New York, 1950.

Brody, E. B., and Redlich, F. C., editors. *Psychotherapy with Schizophrenics.* International Universities Press, New York, 1952.

Cumming, J., and Cumming, E. *Ego and Milieu: Theory and Practice of Environmental Therapy.* Atherton Press, New York, 1962.

Hogarty, G. E., Goldberg, S. C., and collaborative study group. Drug and sociotherapy in the post-hospital maintenance of schizophrenic patients. One-year relapse rates. Arch. Gen. Psychiatry. *130:* 90, 1973.

Ludwig, A. M. *Treating the Treatment Failures.* Grune & Stratton, New York, 1971.

Marx, A. J., Test, M. H., and Stein, L. I. Prevention of institutionalism through community treatment. Arch. Gen. Psychiatry, *130:* 102, 1973.

May, P. R. A. Psychotherapy and ataraxic drugs. In *Handbook of Psychotherapy and Behavior Change,* A. E. Bergin and S. L. Garfield, editors, p. 495, Wiley, New York, 1971.

May, P. R. A., Wexler, M., Salkin, J., and Schoop. T. Nonverbal techniques in the re-establishment of body image and self identity. Psychiatr. Res. Rep. *16:* 68, 1963.

Schoop, T. *Masque of Madness.* National Press, Palo Alto, 1973.

Van Putten, T. Phenothiazine-induced decompensation. Arch. Gen. Psychiatry, *130:* 52, 1973.

Van Putten, T. Milieu therapy. Contraindications? Arch. Gen. Psychiatry, *130:* 52, 1973.

Wing, J. K. Social treatment, rehabilitation and management. In *Recent Developments in Schizophrenia,* A. Coppen and A. Walk, editors, p. 79, Invicta Press, London, 1967.

Wittenborn, J. R., Weber, E. S. P., and Brown, M. Niacin in the long-term treatment of schizophrenia. Arch. Gen. Psychiatry, *130:* 71, 1973.

14.6   SCHIZOPHRENIA: PSYCHOLOGICAL TREATMENT

Introduction

The psychotherapeutic approach to the schizophrenia problem is designed to facilitate personal growth without restricting individual potential. Psychotherapy is based on the planned use of the human relationship as an agent of change. A factor in that change is understanding of the possible relationship between events of the past and present. Living is thought of as having purpose and goal. Psychotherapeutic intervention should provide a way for further learning, change, and growth. The modification of established patterns of behavior, however, is not accomplished easily or without pain. Desirable though change may seem to be, it will be resisted if the route to it is disagreeable and unpleasant. The psychotherapeutic process does not in itself produce change or cure; it can be used to remove interferences to learning and to open the way to growth. Through this process, each person must find his own way, devise his own style of life, and discover how he can best make use of the abilities and opportunities available to him.

Psychotherapy in Relation to Schizophrenia

Psychotherapy has been questioned as the method of choice in the treatment of schizophrenic patients.

Reasons against Psychotherapy

1. Intensive psychotherapy involves the formation of a human relationship in which the vicissitudes of growing up are recalled and evaluated in the light of current affairs. It is a process of learning and growth and thus takes much time.

2. The cause of schizophrenia is unclear; very likely, multiple factors are involved.

3. If schizophrenia is a representation of organic difficulties, therapy should be in response to their recognition and directed toward their correction. Psychotherapy does not fit such a requirement.

4. The financial costs of psychotherapy are high.

5. The patients in psychotherapy more commonly come from the middle or upper social and economic groups, are above average in intelligence and educational level, and are interesting to the therapist.

6. The schizophrenic patient is, as a rule, poorly motivated for engagement in psychotherapy.

7. The therapist may find that the demands placed on him are excessive or intolerable. These demands include threats of suicide and self-injury, the need for additional sessions, the

appearance of degrees of regression that require hospitalization, physical assault, hostile criticism, and seemingly unyielding despair.

8. Therapists may become discouraged by the repeated questioning of the efficacy and general usefulness of their work.

9. The process of therapy may continue for months or years; it is marked by ups and downs, with the patient appearing at times to be worse, rather than better. Results come slowly and may be difficult to evaluate.

10. The sense of deep personal involvement that is frequently experienced in the psychotherapy of the schizophrenic person may be unwanted.

11. This work must be shared with others, particularly if it is carried on in a hospital setting.

12. In this form of psychotherapy there is no firm guarantee of success.

13. The therapist cannot be dependent for his personal satisfactions on the approval or gratitude of his patient.

14. The therapist who works for long periods of time with a few patients may look back on his life to question what he has accomplished.

15. The indeterminacy of this work may prove to be burdensome.

Reasons for Psychotherapy

1. Patients not otherwise helped do improve.

2. The end result of schizophrenia is not the deterioration secondary to an organic, physiological process; the course is very largely determined by the mode of intervention.

3. Schizophrenic behavior is not different in kind from that of normal experience and thus should not be thought of as unpsychological or completely incomprehensible.

4. Schizophrenia may be looked on as a paradigm of human living.

Aspects of Psychotherapy

Patients

There is no prototypic patient for which a particular treatment can be prescribed. Not all schizophrenic people become patients, many avoid treatment, few seek it out, and for none is the procedure pleasant or without threat. Those patients who have been hospitalized for a long time are wary of efforts that intrude on their isolation and jeopardize their fragile sense of security. Those who have managed to get better are not easily persuaded to risk what gains they have made in order to gain more. The schizoid or schizophrenic person who suffers from feelings of depression, sorrow, and turmoil and who recognizes his failure to make good use of his abilities may, often with hesitancy and little expectation of good results, come to the therapist for help. Others have found life to be a disaster but have kept on fighting; they may protest that nothing useful can be done, but they can be caught up in constructive human relationships, one of which is psychotherapy.

Therapist's View

Common to all definitions of psychotherapy is the notion of change. The procedure—be it individual, group, or whatever—is designed to modify behavior that has been defined as personally or socially painful, troublesome, and undesirable. General agreement about this definition is often lacking; society, family members, a therapist, and a patient may differ in their views of what constitutes good and evil, sick and well, desirable or otherwise. The psychiatrist takes a stand regarding treatment, reveals something of his own system of values, and assumes responsibility for the outcome of his efforts, knowing that he can do harm as well as good.

The psychotherapeutic process is a special instance of an interpersonal relationship and is thus well-suited for intervention in disorders that in themselves have their origins to a large extent in such relationships and reflect current difficulties in them.

The procedure is that of learning in social situations. It is designed to correct misadventures of earlier years through which important aspects of experience have been shut off from awareness, grave misapprehensions of the self and others have developed, and dangerous oversimplifications or complexities of behavior have been formed. The learning and change that are encouraged and made possible are accompanied by increases of anxiety as well as insight, with the result that the treatment process is often unpleasant and resisted by the patient.

The therapeutic relationship is not static; it takes place in a dynamic field, the movement of which may be toward the facilitation of the effectiveness of performance or toward its greater restriction and complexity.

The psychotherapeutic approach embraces the following principles: Past experience is a major factor in determining current behavior. Variants of past experience are continued into the present—usefully or destructively. What a person does is influenced by what has been, by what is, and by what is anticipated of the future. The therapist is the target of motivations developed in the patient's past. Behavior is directed toward a goal, although much of what goes on may be obscure and difficult to comprehend. No matter how deeply seated and fixed behavioral patterns may appear to be, they can be modified through interpersonal experience, and further learning can occur at any period in a person's life.

The treatment process is a discipline about which much can be taught and learned; it is not a catch-as-catch-can procedure in which anything can be said or done. The therapist should be acquainted with the theories of his profession and schooled in its techniques. He will discover, however, that he cannot rely on theory and technique alone. What he does must be carried on in the context of his own personality and thus will not be exactly comparable to that which is done by any of his colleagues. The course of treatment will be influenced by the social field in which it takes place and by the attitudes and beliefs of the therapist and others associated with the task.

The therapist is well-advised if he does not rush in with great enthusiasm to modify rapidly his patient's way of living. If the patient's life is in danger or if his actions seriously jeopardize the welfare of other people, something must be done to resolve a critical situation. However, for the most part, psychotic behavior is not of such a nature that its display must be interrupted immediately. The therapist can assume that his patient's actions are not entirely without merit and that much may be gained from carefully observing them. They have purpose and social as well as personal significance. The therapist who rushes to push the patient toward a state of alleged good health is dealing with a conventional and stereotyped conception of well-being or normality, which may not be suited to the needs and wishes of the particular patient involved. Such energetic emphasis on rapid change may also serve to further convince the patient that everything he does is unsatisfactory and that he himself is of no value; only when he turns into something else will he be acceptable. The first move of a wise therapist is to observe what the patient does and the circumstances in which behavior appears to be normal, psychotic, or otherwise. It may be possible to discover connections between past and present events and the patient's performances.

When the patient is accepted as a person, rather than as a conglomeration of oddities labeled a case of something or other, he may have less need to act in a psychotic manner, with the result that communication improves. The therapist quietly attempts to learn who the patient is at the moment and how he views his world. What does the patient consider to be his ailment? Where does he hurt? What is there about his living that has come to seem unacceptable or overwhelming? What is he trying to do with himself and the people around him? What is all this crazy behavior designed to accomplish? The answers to these questions may not be given quickly or readily, but the questions themselves should be kept in the therapist's awareness. As confidence, trust, and communication increase, the therapist and the patient can learn together what course is desirable and possible for the patient to follow.

Relationship with the Patient

Probably the best advice is for the therapist to try to become a good observer. Spontaneity in itself is often of little value and may be hurtful; the spontaneous act is best derived from knowledge, which is based on observation and careful consideration of the consequences of action. If the therapist can conceive of the disturbed patient as a troubled human being who is fearful, puzzled, and engaged in an effort to resolve a difficult but common human dilemma, he can find ways he can put to use in creating a trusting relationship. He should not set out to cure a disease, as to do so will depersonalize the entire affair; rather, he should enter into a peculiar form of relationship in which he must be an observer and also, to some extent, a participant.

Attachment. All schizophrenic people have difficulties in their attachment to other human beings. To survive, they have become inextricably involved in human relationships, which they need for their existence to continue and which they fear as a source of destruction and evil. The therapist must find ways of engaging in a relationship the patient requires but also dreads. If the therapist is too cautious and diffident, he will always be put off by the rejecting patient. If he is too forward, he may increase the patient's apprehension and withdrawal.

The first requirement for the development of a relationship is that the participants meet with each other. Usually, the meetings take place in the therapist's office, the chief rule being that people and objects are not to be injured—that is, anger is to be controlled and words used, rather than destructive acts. The patient may sit down or walk about, but he is to remain with the therapist. Should the patient find that being in the office makes him too uncomfortable, the meetings may take place in his room or elsewhere, as in a walk. Assaultive behavior may be limited by sitting with the patient while he lies in a wet-sheet pack, which offers not simply restraint but the comfort of extensive bodily contact that cannot at that time be accepted in any other way. Drugs may also be used to control violence but are undesirable if the effect is to dull perception to a great degree and to become a form of chemical restraint. The frequency and length of meetings cannot be specified with precision, but many therapists favor four or more sessions a week, each meeting being long enough to permit the subsidence of anxiety, the carrying on of observations, and the furtherance of communication.

The tie of the schizophrenic person to other people is tenuous and fragile; he is fearful that the tie will become so strong that he will be captured and crippled by it and also that it will be broken, with the result that he will be alone. Should the patient withdraw into silence and evidence psychotic behavior, the therapist may speak up or otherwise act to show that he is present and will not let himself be pushed aside or disappear from the patient's awareness.

The therapist may feel frequently that he is of no importance to the patient and that whatever he does is of no significance. In such instances he should talk to a colleague about his experiences, as his own sense of isolation can best be dealt with by sharing the experience with someone else. In time, it will be found that therapist and patient are becoming tied to each other. This change may go unnoticed in its early stages; on first appearance it may be sensed as discomforting and then denied, resisted, or labeled as dangerous. As security increases, the patient may remain silent or leave the office without becoming disturbed; he is discovering that he can maintain a form of contact with the therapist without looking at him, hearing his voice, or being in his immediate presence. It is not necessary to interfere with such silences, departures, and absences. Attention is paid to the patient's increasing ability to maintain a constancy of the relationship without disrupting increases of anxiety.

As the meetings continue with their emotional accompaniments, the attachment of the participants to each other grows. It may be experienced as desirable or otherwise; it can be described as discomfort, dislike, love, sexuality, hate. As hitherto dissociated aspects of experience are brought into awareness with the integration of increasing intimacy, the patient may experience feelings that are marked by a quality of the uncanny—disgust, horror, loathing, awe, fascination, and dread. These sentiments are ill-defined symbolic representations of events in early life that have been associated with anxiety and have never been fully comprehended or assimilated into the known self. Their experience is unpleasant and disconcerting, leading to increased withdrawal from their apparent source or the person who seems to give rise to them—in this case the therapist. The tendency to withdraw in this instance is evidence of the growing attachment and should not lead the therapist to surrender his task.

The attachment is first developed without words; it cannot be described in language—it can only be experienced. If the therapist seeks to convert all that is happening into logical, easily communicable speech, not only will he fail, but he may interfere with the process itself. Premature insistence on understanding can defeat the eventual organization of ideas that will finally be expressed in communicable language. Attachment, like love, can be discussed, but its true significance cannot be put into words—at least in its early formative stages. It is talked about best when it has become fully established and accepted or when it is a thing of the past—an item of regret, of pleasure, or of no moment. Attachment is the basis of the therapeutic relationship.

Threat of Dissolution. For a person to exist with some sense of comfort, he must have a continuing, dependable identity; in all circumstances he should know who he is, how he will behave, and how others will view him and respond to him. If major aspects of experience are kept out of awareness because of their association with anxiety, care must be taken to avoid engaging in a relationship that might disturb a precarious organization of the personality. This task of keeping oneself unaware of what may easily become obvious requires careful, unending attention to the details of happenings in the environment. In brief, one must become an expert in noticing what not to notice in circumambient events.

An episode that is felt to be a threat to a person's already unstable self-esteem will lead to an increase of anxiety, an activation of behavior designed to reduce this discomfort, and a lessening of the ability to avoid sentiments that have for the most part been kept unrecognized. Such sentiments may become apparent at first in the dream or nightmare; usually, they are not well-understood; they exist without apparent cause, effect, or reason; they are peculiar, fragmented symbols that are difficult to interpret but urgently require understanding; and they are imbued with terror.

To integrate a relationship with another person is to incorporate the two persons into a larger unit, to unite them in such a way that a whole is formed in which emphasis is placed on the "we," rather than on just the "I" and the "you." This increase of social union (the shaping of a two-group) requires the cooperation of the participants, each of whom must accommodate himself to the necessities of the other—a more difficult enterprise than maneuvering figures in a world of fantasy, in which what takes place can be controlled largely by the person who imagines. The growing relationship includes a demand for exposure of personal feelings, desires, hopes, uncertainties, and doubts. At the beginning, the public aspects of the person are acknowledged and accepted. Security in this stage invites and permits the bringing into the open of more private concerns that have been known but hitherto concealed as much as possible from social display. Increasing intimacy tends to bring to the fore many facets of the personality, including some that are autistic and others that are incompletely formulated and not recognized as part of the personality. This process is one of greater coordination of the behaviors of one person with another person and his social and

nonhuman environment, instead of with an accompanying pulling together of previously disparate parts of the self. The shift in the permeability of the previous well-defined boundaries between the person and others—and within himself—may be desirable but, at best, is also experienced as strange and potentially upsetting of equanimity.

For the schizophrenic person, these changes can be terrifying. They may first be manifested in sleep disturbances, the dream becoming a nightmare. Later, the contents of awareness in the waking state can no longer be controlled adequately, and there are intrusions of fragmentary representations of the past that seem to have no referents. In brief, the nightmare occurs outside of sleep, and the state of panic is rapidly approached.

The psychotherapist asks the patient to enter into a situation in which self-revelation is invited, with the possibility of its leading to a sense of disorganization and panic. The patient must have courage and trust to embark on this course. Trust must be formed in the relationship; there is often not much of it at the beginning. One factor in the formation of trust is the therapist's respect for the patient's courage and pain; another is his ability to carry on the work without carelessly or unnecessarily increasing suffering. Intimacy is developed through participation in a multitude of social fields—with the therapist, for example—in which one learns about himself without unacceptable accesses of shame or distress, gains confidence, discovers his abilities as well as his inadequacies, and learns that reality, painful as it often may be, is superior to the nightmare and to fantasy in the service of evasion.

Dependency. Dependency is a state of reliance, in terms of this discussion, on other people. The person who is used for support may also exert influence and power that may be experienced as threatening. The acceptance of support, influence, and power requires trust in the positive regard, motivations, and reliability of another human being. The schizophrenic person does not have the faith that enables him to accept dependency lightly, however much he may need its protective aspects. As the bonds of attachment form in the therapeutic relationship, a quality of dependency becomes apparent, and associated with it are anxiety and a struggle.

With the development of attachment comes

the strange feeling that the boundaries—the sense of separateness between the self and the environment and between the public self, the private self, and the phenomena of the nightmare that are not known or acceptable as part of the self—will be lost (often spoken of as a loss of ego boundaries). There is a fear of fusion of one person with another, in which case there will be a destruction of the personality. In the early stages of the relationship, the participants are not well-known to each other, and each probably treats the other in terms of sterotypes from the past, rather than in response to observations of present happenings. (See Figure 1.) The therapist may then deal more with his concept of the schizophrenic than with his concept of the schizophrenic than with his percept of a human being, and the patient may see only the shrink and not the man or woman. The experience of the relationship as vaguely threatening and inchoate may be defined as psychotic. With the subsidence of anxiety and the increase of perceptual acuity, the object and the subject become more clearly identified, the ego structure improves in organization and stability, and there appear more conventional statements

about the fear of control, domination, and influence.

Regression. Therapists speak of regressive states as being desirable or undesirable and as if these conditions could be prevented or provoked. In general, regressive behavior is a recrudescence of ways of acting that are ordinarily more suitable to earlier developmental stages than to the stage in which they are displayed. The person may be said to behave as a juvenile, child, or infant rather than as an adult; if the actions do not lend themselves to such ready classification, they may be labeled psychotic, in contrast to normal. The concern need not be with what is good or bad. The therapist is interested in the characteristics of a person and a situation that may seem to require the resort to these supposedly outgrown or out-of-date forms of behavior. What makes it necessary to act like a child or to be psychotic?

In general, regressive behavior is invited through the following circumstances: The self-esteem of a person is seriously threatened, and his usual ways of getting along are felt to be inadequate; there is a resort to actions that provided security at earlier and on seemingly

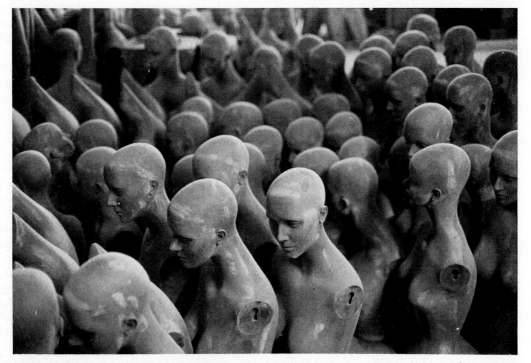

FIGURE 1. A symbolic representation of alienation, increasingly common in our society and most severe in schizophrenia. (Courtesy of Erich Hartmann for Magnum Photos, Inc.)

simpler occasions. Stress is reduced, security is increased, and the more recently acquired and complicated defensive forms of behavior may be temporarily put aside without danger.

Among the uses of regression are the following:

Under stress, behavior from earlier periods of life may be reassuring, since they are less complicated than the thought processes and other acts developed to deal with the struggles to maintain security and self-esteem in adult living.

In a regressive condition the intrusion of external events is held off, and attention is turned to aspects of living that may have been ignored in favor or more immediate and pressing requirements. Ideas and feelings from the past that have not been integrated in the personality may now be considered quietly and become an accepted part of the person.

Some regressive behavior can be dealt with as communicative, symbolic of earlier life events that cannot be expressed adequately in the more refined configurations of speech.

In regressive periods the person has an unusual opportunity to observe what goes on around him, without actually participating in a conventional sense. He may discover how relatives, therapists, and others respond to what he does and how they want to change him, appearing as cruel, stupid, silly, thoughtless, inconsistent, or even observant, considerate, patient, and understanding.

Regression can be a form of remembering. Old ways of acting—put aside as childish or otherwise inappropriate—may be recalled, played with, and perhaps enjoyed. Regression may be a way of escaping for a time from the confinements of adult living and recapturing needed ways of relating—such as being touched, fed, bathed, and comforted—that have been denied as improper for the self-sufficient adult person.

In regressive conditions problem-solving may take place. Matters that have been unclear may be identified and dealt with finally as necessary and acceptable parts of living.

Regression may also serve to modify the environment. The withdrawn or psychotic behavior of the patient may cause the therapist and others to respond as they have not responded previously. For better or worse, they do something different, often revealing hitherto concealed and perhaps significant aspects of themselves about which the patient needed to be informed. In these instances the patient may be said—unfortunately and often inaccurately—to be controlling, demanding, and manipulative.

But prolonged regression interferes with growth, and the cost of a spurious comfort may be the relinquishing of independence and the chance for developing what abilities a person has. Regression is a function of a person's relationship with his environment. Whether such behavior is to be useful or otherwise depends on its purposes, the recognition of these purposes, and the responses made to them. Frequently, the first response to regressive change is to alter it or get rid of it. This can be achieved through the use of such agents as drugs or electroshock. If the behavior is not immediately and seriously threatening to the patient and others, it may prove useful to observe it and learn from it without attempting actively to interfere with it. The therapist who can be forebearing often finds that regressive activities lessen as he becomes for his patient a constant, dependable, identifiable, and stable object.

If regressive behavior is to be put to good use, the patient should not be left alone in the experience. There should be someone with him or constantly available to him who is not afraid of what is occurring and who will not leave.

Forced regression through the use of such agents as electric currents, drugs, or psychological confrontations is not advised. Such attacks on the person may modify behavior but are not usually made with due consideration for the many functions of regression. Regressive processes are not to be taken lightly; unattended or dealt with carelessly, they can at times be disastrous.

Separation. Attachment and dependency are elements of relationships in which can be developed feelings of personal security, self-confidence, trust in others, and a dependable identity. Separation and loss are aspects of all human affiliations. In the course of psychotherapy there is a long preparation for leaving. There are the terminations of sessions, the assurance that other sessions will follow, the use of transitional objects, the increasing ability to hold someone in memory, the making of friendships outside of professional contacts, and the insights regarding previous separations. Change and improved living may be desired, but alterations in the ways to which one has become accustomed are not accepted easily. Each person must discover for himself what is good health for him; it is more than an outward adjustment to the current social scene.

There will be separation not only from the therapist and other people but from the troubles for which some relief has been found. The disordered behaviors have been not only painful and destructive but in some ways comforting and familiar and possibly life-saving. In saying farewell to sickness, the patient is relinquishing a portion of himself.

Conclusion

For some people diagnosed as schizophrenic, psychotherapy can be carried on in an office setting and may deviate little from the generally accepted rules that apply to this procedure. The therapist listens, through his comments helps to open up areas of experience for investigation, prevents increases of anxiety that interfere with communication or provoke seriously destructive behavior, pays particular attention to the therapist-patient relationship (both as distorted and as verifiably real), and helps by his interpretations and his presence in the development of understanding and insight. He attempts to aid the patient find a system of values and a way of living that provide some security and satisfaction but that are not necessarily in accord with the convictions of the therapist or those of the society at large. He knows that reassurance can best come from the revelation and comprehension of data, not simply from the assembling of supposedly cheering phrases.

For the more disturbed patient, hospitalization may be required; his own fragile personality structure may be benefited by living for a time in an environment that has itself a clearly defined and simple structure. Ataractic drugs are of value in reducing extremes of anxiety, controlling grossly destructive behavior, and helping people live in situations that they could not endure without such support. They are, however, not curative of disorder; in excess, they can interfere with learning and social participation, building a form of chemical restraint and a wall between the patient and others.

The psychotherapist may wish to work for the most part without the extensive use of chemical agents, relying on the social group and the interpersonal transaction to allay anxiety and promote learning. The needs of the patient must be evaluated individually when possible. The decision to make use of drugs, hospitalization, a halfway house, home care, and so on can be determined adequately only on the basis of such a personal review of the situation.

The psychotherapeutic process is designed to bring about major and enduring changes in the structure of the personality. It is a process of learning in which the person's development is reviewed and used to illuminate his current ways of living. The patient's behavior in his present environment is considered to be an expression of his past experiences, his immediate predicament, and his anticipations of his future. The therapeutic milieu offers an opportunity for the display of characteristic modes of action, for their observation and control, for the modification of their major inadequacies, and for their understanding. The goals of this treatment method are not always reached, which is true of any enterprise intimately concerned with the intricacies of human relationships.

The psychotherapy of the schizophrenic patient is not carried on by the patient and the therapist alone. Of vital importance to the enterprise is the collaboration of all those significantly associated with the patient. Collaboration is not attained easily or maintained without unremitting effort. The behavior of the patient brings about a wide variety of responses from those who have to do with him. Many of these responses do not appear to be appropriate in a professional setting, and efforts are made to conceal them, in which case they operate covertly and often destructively. There are feelings of anger, hate, contempt, fear, disgust, lust, and so on. These cannot be ignored but should be brought into the open in staff-nursing conferences in which the therapist and sometimes the patient are participants.

The members of the patient's family should be included in the treatment program. They should be acquainted with the goals of therapy, its course, and the vicissitudes that are likely to be encountered in it. If the therapist is to explain what he does, he must himself know what he is about. He should be able to describe his task in nontechnical terms and not find it necessary to hide behind the use of jargon.

Schizophrenia is undesirable but may be more readily accepted than the stresses of change. The patient, his relatives, staff members, and the therapist may desire improvement and work for it but more or less subtly labor to defeat change. All who work in this endeavor should become aware of the fact that growth carries with it pain as well as pleasure. With this recognition, the resistance and reluctance of all concerned can be better understood, shame and guilt reduced, and the work benefited.

The therapist often finds that his task is lonely. He is well-advised to consult frequently with colleagues about what he does; he should speak openly; in so doing, he discovers that he has no great secrets to conceal and that his experiences, as well as those of his patient, are not more or less than simply human. That in itself can be a healing discovery. Personal analysis for the therapist is also recommended. The procedure helps free him from undue influence by processes outside of his awareness and gives him some idea of the difficulties that his patients are invited to face.

In the psychotherapy of the schizophrenic person, there exists a remarkable opportunity for the study of one of the extremes of human living. Schizophrenia reveals with startling clarity characteristics of all people, however classified. All human beings must accept the problems of attachment, dependency loss, and separation, with the attendant phenomena of anxiety, fear, hatred, envy, jealousy, distortions of the body image, identity changes, and love. The therapist can be of help to his patient, and what he is able to observe, learn, and formulate can be of service to others never to be identified as patients. It is his responsibility to make known what knowledge he gains in this enterprise; it has usefulness far beyond the range of psychiatry itself.

REFERENCES

Bowlby, J. *Separation.* Basic Books, New York, 1973.
Fromm-Reichmann, F. *Psychoanalysis and Psychotherapy: Selected Papers of Frieda Fromm-Reichmann,* D. M. Bullard, editor. University of Chicago Press, Chicago, 1959.
Guntrip, H. *Schizoid Phenomena, Object Relations and the Self.* International Universities Press, New York, 1968.
Hill, L. B. *Psychotherapeutic Intervention in Schizophrenia.* University of Chicago Press, Chicago, 1955.
Lazare, A. Hidden conceptual models in clinical psychiatry. N. Engl. J. Med., *288:* 345, 1973.
Lidz, T. *The Origin and Treatment of Schizophrenic Disorders.* Basic Books, New York, 1973.
Mosher, L. R., and Feinsilver, D. A special report: Schizophrenia, publication no. (HSM) 72-9007, National Institute of Mental Health; United States Department of Health, Education, and Welfare, 1973.
Mosher, L. R., and Gunderson, J. G. Special report: Schizophrenia 1972. Schizophrenia Bull., 1973.
Searles, H. D. *Collected Papers on Schizophrenia and Related Subjects.* International Universities Press, New York, 1965.
Sullivan, H. S. Environmental factors in etiology and course under treatment of schizophrenia. In *Schizophrenia as a Human Process,* H. S. Perry, editor. W. W. Norton, New York, 1962.

14.7   SCHIZOPHRENIA: EVALUATION OF TREATMENT METHODS

Introduction

Assessment of the relative value of the different forms of treatment for the schizophrenic condition runs into two major problems. First, with the exception of drug-effect studies, the abundance of opinion and prejudice is equaled only by the dearth of scientific evidence. Second, when scientific studies are attempted, the criteria for success or failure are often questioned.

The two main criteria for evaluation suggested by Kline seem to offer a reasonable beginning: (1) freedom from unusual pain with at least a modicum of enjoyment of life and (2) a degree of productivity and participation in society.

It may also be that multiple outcome criteria could be replaced by simpler and more selective dimensional ordering. For example, Pokorny and Faibish factor-analyzed 27 commonly used clinical and social adjustment variables. Adjustment-hospitalization emerged as the best indicator of outcome, with recurrence, psychotic disturbance, and anxiety-depression as additional factors. The best single indicators were degree of withdrawal, work record, living situation, and hospital stay.

If a treatment is truly powerful, even current crude assessment techniques should demonstrate its effects. If the effects of a treatment elude existing measuring instruments that can demonstrate meaningful change in control groups or with other treatments, then it is unlikely to be very powerful.

This review is confined to studies that meet the following criteria: 1. Published in a recognized scientific or professional journal or in a book that is (or should be) readily available in a university library. 2. A deliberate prospective experiment that systematically compares outcome for a group of patients treated by one particular method with outcome for a comparable group treated in some other way or studied as a formal no-treatment control. 3. Studies in which experimental and control patients were treated in the same hospitals. 4. Reports based on controlled studies.

The important issue is design. The most common defects are nonequivalent control groups, failure to control or measure other treatments, and the inclusion of nonschizophrenic subjects.

The present author has classified individual research reports on a 10-point scale, found in square brackets. The ratings refer to the quality of the design and analysis, not to the investigators' conclusions.

Class I. Sound, solid, substantial, and well-designed. Defects, if any, are minor.

    11. Evaluation is comprehensive and N is adequate (24 or more in each group).

    12. Either N is adequate or evaluation is comprehensive.

    13. Outcome evaluation is limited in scope, and N is small (12 or less).

Class II. May be accepted with some reservations. Definite design defects: acceptable as supporting evidence but not alone.

    21. Subclassified as in class I.

    22. Subclassified as in class I.

    23. Subclassified as in class I.

Class III. Design defects to such an extent that any conclusions drawn should be treated with reserve and regarded as tenuous, uncertain, intangible, and tentative. At best, such studies may be important sources of new leads and hypotheses. At worst, they may be gravely misleading.

    31. Subclassified as in class I.

    32. Subclassified as in class I.

    33. Subclassified as in class I.

Class IV. Uncontrolled experiments, retrospective surveys, etc.

Multiple defects in design may adjust ratings down within a particular class. For example, a study that would otherwise rate as [31] may be classified lower, as [32] or even [33], if there are serious multiple design defects. The ratings also consider relevance to schizophrenia and contamination by nonschizophrenic cases.

For this review, activity therapy was defined, and so distinguished from psychotherapy, as any organized activity in which attention is not deliberately focused on intrapsychic content, personal content, or object relations. The term "active push" has been used to refer to milieu programs in which the main thrust is on more intensive care or on a higher level and diversification of activities.

Object relations therapy is included under psychotherapy. Body-ego technique and remotivation are discussed separately, under milieu therapy and rehabilitation. Discharge planning groups and videotape feedback of patients' behavior have been counted as psychotherapy.

Milieu Therapy and Rehabilitation

The general impression from experimental studies is that vigorous, aggressive outpatient aftercare programs after discharge from the hospital, combined with drug treatment, are effective in maintaining patients in the community and warding off deterioration. There is also good evidence that, for a substantial number of cases, day care or home care is a practical and effective alternative to hospital care. However, two surveys (not controlled experiments) have indicated that the social cost of community care may be higher than that of hospital care in terms of the burden placed on the family and children.

The evidence for enriched inpatient activity programs is more circumscribed and less impressive. It seems that their main usefulness may come from possible prevention of institutionalism and the secondary desocializing and deteriorative effects of a barren environment and from better discharge and employment planning and that their effect on primary psychopathology itself may be relatively small. In some chronic cases, push and intrusive interventions have even been found to aggravate symptoms. More is not necessarily better. Generalized inpatient milieu activity and push programs should be more critically evaluated, with a view to concentrating effort on programs that are specifically tailored to the needs of different types of schizophrenic patients.

Marx and coworkers point out that intensive in-hospital programs have very little effect on future community adjustment of chronic patients and show virtually no relationship to length of community stay after discharge. Readmission rates are as high for chronic patients who have participated in intensive in-hospital experimental programs as they are for control patients who have been involved in less innovative programs.

The failure of in-hospital programs to have an impact on community adjustment and tenure has led to a variety of efforts to provide more intensive aftercare for the discharged chronic patient in order to prevent readmission. Evaluation of such programs leaves little doubt that they are useful in preventing relapse, suggesting that treatment and support *in the community*—precisely where the patient needs help in adjusting—is the appropriate direction for future work with chronic patients.

Psychotherapy

Inpatients: Individual Psychotherapy

Five studies compared individual psychotherapy with no special treatment or with milieu therapy. The only one not contaminated by drug therapy, an [11], found no significant difference except for longer hospital stay with psychotherapy. The other two were contaminated by an unknown or uncertain amount of drug therapy. One [22] found no significant difference; there was, however, some highly questionable evidence that some therapists got better results and some got worse, so, on the average, there was no difference. One [31] found that psychotherapy patients stayed in hospital longer but otherwise found no differences.

One [21] study of individual systematic desensitization plus relaxation (degree of contamination by drugs not known) showed that in younger patients there was no significant difference between this and active push milieu therapy or relaxation alone. However, in older patients there was flimsy evidence that active push was superior to the other two.

One [33] study of individual videotape therapy (viewing oneself on tape without comment by the therapist), degree of contamination by drugs not known, gave results that suggested that this form of treatment might be of value.

Inpatients: Group Therapy

One study, a [33], compared individual and group therapy in patients receiving an unknown amount of drug therapy. There was a nonsignificant trend in favor of individual therapy.

Fourteen studies compared group therapy with no special treatment. Only one of these was uncontaminated by somatic therapy. This [33] study showed no significant change in either controls or patients treated with group therapy and no difference between psychotherapy focusing on insight and psychotherapy focusing on interaction.

In eight studies the amounts of drug therapy are unknown or uncertain. One [23] and one [22] found no significant difference between therapy and control. One [32] found one particular form of group therapy (but not two others) significantly better than control. Two [33]'s found group therapy better, one found equivocal evidence that it was better, and one found no significant difference. One [33] found therapy better than no therapy; however, consultation for an equal amount of time with the ward staff got just as good results.

In three studies, no drugs were given, but the amounts of ECT are unknown and uncertain. In two [33]'s the results were equivocally in favor of therapy. In one [32], there was no significant difference between insight group therapy and control; however, activity group therapy was significantly better than either.

In one [23] study, all patients also received drugs; the results were equivocally in favor of therapy.

In one [33] study, all patients also received ECT. Therapy was better than no therapy.

Outpatients: Group Therapy

There were three studies of therapy in outpatients. One [23], in which all patients were also given drugs, found an advantage in group therapy over no therapy. Another study, [11], in which all patients also received drugs, found group therapy of more benefit than individual therapy. The third, [32], in which patients' drug dosage was unknown or uncertain, found no difference between group and individual therapy.

The number is too small to draw conclusions, but there is a hint that, with schizophrenics, group therapy is more successful with outpatients after discharge than is group or individual therapy with inpatients—two positive results in [11] and [23] studies for outpatients, compared with one no-effect [11], one no-effect [21], two no-effect [22]'s, one no-effect and one negative effect [22], one equivocal [23], and one no-effect [23] for inpatients.

Comparison of Techniques

Four studies (in which the amount of drug therapy is unknown) compared different group techniques, as well as comparing group therapy with control.

One [32] found a rank order of (1) autonomous nonstaff-led patient groups focusing on discharge, (2) staff-led discharge planning groups, (3) control, (4) insight-oriented group therapy.

One [33] found no significant difference between group therapy and an equivalent amount of time consulting with the ward staff as a group; both, however, were better than control.

One [23] and one [33] found activity (interaction) group therapy equal to insight group therapy.

One [12] study in which all patients were given drugs found activity group therapy better than insight therapy. One [32] in which patients may have also been given ECT in unknown amounts showed activity group therapy superior to control and insight group therapy.

Again, the number of studies is small, but there is a definite suggestion that, with schizophrenic patients, groups that focus on real-life plans and on real-life activity and interaction may do better than those that focus on insight and the usual psychotherapy content.

Psychotherapy and Drugs

The controlled studies reviewed by Uhlenhuth et al. and by May indicate that, in general, there is little difference between psychotherapy plus drug and drug therapy alone for hospitalized schizophrenic patients. The combination, however, is quite clearly superior to psychotherapy alone. There are many well-designed studies in which drug therapy has been found to be effective with schizophrenic inpatients. By comparison, there is not a single study that meets the class I or class II standards for this review in which psychotherapy alone, without drugs, has been shown to be more effective than a control in dealing with schizophrenic inpatients. And there are several inpatient studies that show drug therapy alone as more effective than psychotherapy alone.

One [33] study reported no general difference between psychotherapy alone and psychotherapy plus drug; however, some very questionable analyses indicated that, with drug therapy, inexperienced therapists discharged patients rapidly but with worse results both in short-term and long-term reduction of thought disorder, whereas experienced therapists obtained more improvement of thought disorder and less rehospitalization whether or not drugs were used.

Antipsychotic Drugs

In terms of controlled studies and methodological sophistication, drug therapy is the most intensively and scientifically studied method of treatment at the present time. By comparison, there has been little published systematic evaluation of other forms of therapy, and such studies tend to be poorly controlled and relatively primitive in their methodology and statistical treatment of the data.

Early clinical drug evaluation units conduct preliminary trials of promising agents to determine safety, appropriate dosage ranges and side-effects, and indications; they also conduct small, controlled clinical trials and more extensive studies. Computer-generated summaries describing the study and a standard statistical analysis are generated directly from the data and published regularly in the *Psychopharmacology Bulletin* without interpretation. They constitute an early source of information about a given drug, although they do not represent the final conclusions of the study.

Cole and Davis show that 101 out of 127 double-blind, placebo-controlled studies found commonly used phenothiazine drugs more effective than a placebo; in 26 studies the drug and the placebo were equally effective. Most of the latter were early studies conducted before dosages had been properly worked out and in which small fixed doses were used. For example, in the case of chlorpromazine, studies that used less than 400 mg. gave equivocal results (14 more effective than a placebo, nine slightly more effective, and 10 equal). Those with higher doses almost without exception showed a clear therapeutic effect (27 more effective, nine equal to a placebo). Cole and Davis compared also the results of well-designed studies and below-average studies. Those with methodological defects tended to find drugs ineffective, but 12 high-grade, double-blind, placebo-controlled studies with random allocation to treatment showed unequivocally that phenothiazines have substantial therapeutic effect. There is also adequate evidence that some butyrophenones, thioxanthenes, and newer phenothiazines have significant antipsychotic action.

The long-term value of phenothiazines over 10 to 15 years has not been examined in well-controlled, double-blind studies.

Cole and Davis conclude from nine controlled studies that reserpine is less effective than the phenothiazines and that mepazine and promazine are less effective than other phenothiazines. Chlorpromazine, fluphenazine, trifluopromazine, trifluoperazine, acetophenazine, perphenazine, and thiopropazate are approximately equal.

Cole and Davis conclude from nine controlled studies that psychosis recurs in a significant number of patients when phenothiazines are withdrawn, often not until 3 to 6 months after discontinuance. Obviously, the proportion relapsing depends on the type of patient and the skill with which drug treatment has been given previously. Relapse is not likely if the patient does not really need phenothiazine. And, apparently, many chronic hospital patients are given low-dosage maintenance drug therapy without appreciable benefit.

Many long-term failure patients are currently being kept on maintenance medication unnecessarily, and such long-term failures may have the potential for response to organized milieu behavioral programs.

The practical conclusion is that in long-term chronic treatment failures, especially those patients who are withdrawn rather than interactive, maintenance-drug therapy by itself is likely to be less effective than an active milieu program by itself, and, indeed, the drug therapy may slow response to such programs. Hence, in such cases, the ideal is to monitor drug dosage with extreme care, trying to reduce the dosage either to zero or to the minimal level that will alleviate psychotic lack of ego controls and faulty perception, with a minimum of interference with positive ego functions and learning.

The evidence is limited and far from conclusive, but it seems to indicate that powerful phenothiazines with a high incidence of annoying side-effects do well for poor-prognosis patients but should be avoided in good-prognosis patients, where adverse side-effects may be more important. In general, attempts to derive more specific predictors for response to particular drugs have not stood up in cross-validation studies.

Klett and Caffey [11] studied 403 patients who had been taking phenothiazines for at least 6 months plus antiparkinsonism medication for at least 3 months. In 82 per cent, withdrawal by placebo substitution produced no change or, at most, some temporary symptoms. The other 18 per cent developed parkinsonism symptoms.

At first sight it seems reasonable to ask whether drugs are better than milieu therapy. But drug treatment is always given in some sort of milieu, and it would be hard to imagine an experiment that would assay the therapeutic effect of a drug in isolation. It would seem more appropriate to rephrase the question. Are drugs equally effective at all levels of milieu care or in all treatment contexts?

Only a few reports are of major relevance. These were reviewed by May, who concluded that the balance of the evidence indicates that, starting with comparable groups of patients, drug therapy is effective and superior to a placebo at all levels of milieu care from the least to the most intensive.

The evidence is to some extent divided as to whether a more intensive level of milieu care improves the results of drug therapy. It is reasonably well-established that the release rate is increased and that more patients go to work when they leave the hospital, but this finding may be entirely a matter of better discharge planning, rather than any difference in the patients' posttreatment status. Otherwise, there is little effect on level of psychopathology; the results appear to be equally good at all levels of care except under circumstances of virtual neglect or gross deficiency, when a custodial environment is likely to aggravate and even induce withdrawal and social detachment. However, it should not be blandly assumed that drugs and psychosocial measures will always potentiate each other in every type of case.

The conclusions are that (1) drug therapy is advantageous in any hospital setting, (2) the results with drug therapy are likely to be better (at least in terms of employment and release rate) in a more intensive treatment milieu and worse when the level of milieu is grossly deficient, and (3) an intensive treatment milieu by itself (without drug therapy) is not an adequate substitute for treatment with antipsychotic drugs.

There is general agreement in the findings of the various inpatient studies reviewed that inpatients treated with drugs restitute from the acute phase of schizophrenia faster and with better short-term results than those given psychotherapy and social therapy alone and that drug therapy combined with vigorous discharge planning and employment placement gives better results than drugs alone. Nevertheless, these inpatient findings that psychotherapy and milieu therapy add very little in terms of reduction in psychopathology should not be loosely generalized to apply to outpatients or to patients who have restituted sufficiently to be discharged from hospital and followed up in an outpatient treatment. There is evidence from adequately controlled studies that the contributions of psychotherapy, public health nursing, social case work, and rehabilitation may be more relevant and effective in outpatient aftercare.

A reasonable conclusion from the experimental evidence would be that, although drug treatment should in many cases be continued after the acute phase is over to lessen the likelihood of relapse, drugs alone are not sufficient to prevent relapse in all cases or to prevent deterioration in some cases. Hence, in the long term, other additional social, psychotherapeutic, or rehabilitation measures are clearly necessary. At the same time, there is little concrete evidence that these are any more than palliative, rather than curative; they help some persons to make the best use of their resources, rather than actually remedying the primary disorder, whatever that may be.

In general, previous reviews have concluded that drugs produce better results than insulin coma and are less expensive, less dangerous, and more acceptable to patients and to the staff. As in the case of ECT, comparison of the two methods rests to some extent on the unstable ground of personal opinion and historical comparison, most of the reports being retrospective impressions of probably dissimilar groups of patients treated at different periods. Of the few controlled studies, the balance tends to be somewhat in favor of drug therapy.

Behavioral Conditioning

Behavioral therapy of schizophrenia has not yet been adequately evaluated in controlled experiments. As Liberman points out, in behavior modification research the prototypical experiment uses the individual patient as his own control, demonstrating causality in A-B-A or A-B-AB designs or in multiple base line designs in which one target behavior is treated at a time, but measurements are made in many behaviors, hoping to demonstrate a specific effect on the target behavior. This type of experiment is wide open to experimenter bias, expectancy effects, and a number of other confounding elements. There is ample evidence, for instance, that simply monitoring a particular behavior can increase or decrease that behavior compared with the base line.

Although the various behavioral studies may seem to be rigorous controlled experiments, in point of fact, most of them cannot be taken as scientific evidence of the same order as studies that compare groups of patients exposed to different types of interventions. Until such studies are made, confounding factors cannot be entirely ruled out in explaining the apparent effectiveness of behavioral reinforcement. In almost every case the serial assessments of the patient's behavior are susceptible to serious bias. The assessments are not made by independent neutral observers but by staff members who are actively involved in the behavioral treatment and who would, therefore, have high expectations of change. Meltzoff and Kornreich point out that, although specific behaviors may be modified, the question of whether this modification leads to more rapid discharge or generalizes to extramural behavior is not yet answered.

A number of class IV studies suggest that behavioral (operant) conditioning is of value in the treatment of schizophrenic patients, but there are only four studies that meet the formal criteria for inclusion in this review as prospective experiments with an equivalent control group. One [22] found psychotherapy and conditioning to be equal. Two [23]'s found conditioning better than control no-treatment groups, and one of these found it better than group psychotherapy and recreational therapy. One [23] found that older patients did better on milieu therapy than on systematic desensitization and relaxation; younger patients, however, did equally well on all three treatments.

The balance of the evidence, such as it is, indicates that behavioral conditioning may be of value in some cases of schizophrenia, but the indications and relative merits vis-a-vis other forms of treatment remain to be worked out. In particular, the relationship of behavioral conditioning to drug therapy is at this time unknown territory, still at the level of anecdote and case example. The relative values and interactions of drug therapy and behavioral conditioning simply cannot be determined on the basis of the literature available at the present time.

Nicotinic Acid

Three of six controlled studies, two [33]'s and one [23], favored nicotinic acid. Three studies, one [11], one [13], and one [23] showed no significant difference from a placebo. Indeed, two studies, one [11] and one [13], showed a (nonsignificant) trend in favor of a placebo. An appropriate inference is that there is substantive evidence that nicotinic acid is *not* a powerful antipsychotic agent, whether used alone or as an adjuvant to ECT or phenothiazines and that, for the majority of schizophrenic patients, it makes little difference whether nicotinic acid or a placebo is given.

However, it is possible that there may be a relatively small group of patients for whom nicotinic acid may have some beneficial effect. If so, it seems likely that there would be a group of similar size whom it may affect adversely. The crucial experiment to test these two possibilities has yet to be conducted.

Electroconvulsive Therapy

In general, as Riddell points out, the experimental findings and studies are so limited that a firm conclusion cannot be reached, except that ECT is unlikely to be effective in long-term, chronic, hospitalized cases or in those with repeated readmissions. At this point, one cannot make definitive and final statements as to the outcome of ECT in first-admission patients. Nor can one be certain that there may not be a small subgroup of schizophrenic patients who may respond positively or, equally possible, that there may be another small group who get worse on ECT.

The findings of straightforward outcome comparisons with no-treatment controls are to some extent contradictory. On the one hand, five studies—one [11], one [13], one [23], one [32], and one [33]—indicate that ECT was no better than a placebo, and one [33] found ECT less effective than activity push. On the other hand, one [11] found ECT better than milieu therapy

on release rate and a number of other criteria, including length of stay and ratings of clinical status by nurses, therapists, and independent raters. One [33] found no difference in results between four and eight ECT treatments, but one [13] found 20 treatments better than 12.

Drugs are, in general, to be preferred over ECT—and not only because ECT may be more hazardous. The finding the least favorable to drugs among the controlled studies was that, although there was a somewhat higher relapse rate among the drug-treated patients, there was no other significant difference between the two methods. Other controlled studies found that drugs resulted in a shorter stay in the hospital and a higher release rate with an equal amount of clinical improvement, that they had similar release rates but speedier release with drugs; that (regressive) ECT led to deterioration in behavior, but drugs improved it; and that drugs are significantly superior to ECT in terms of a number of criteria, including release rate and ratings of clinical status by nurses, therapists, and independent raters.

Despite this apparent general superiority of drug therapy, there are reports that ECT has been successfully employed in some cases that have failed to respond to drug therapy. There are, however, no controlled data on this subject, and it is perhaps indicative of the state of knowledge that there is still no conclusive controlled evidence regarding the indications for ECT in schizophrenia. Nor have there been any controlled studies investigating the usefulness of ECT in schizo-affective disorders, although the relatively good results in depressive disorders may suggest that schizophrenic patients with depression would be more likely to respond to ECT.

Comparisons with other forms of treatment are scanty and inconclusive. One [22] found ECT better than insulin; one [33] suggested that psychotherapy is more effective than ECT and that the combination may be more effective than either treatment separately. On the other hand, one [11] study found ECT superior to psychotherapy in terms of release rate, length of stay, and clinical outcome ratings by nurses, therapists, and independent raters.

Psychosurgery

Psychosurgery has come a long way since the introduction in 1936 of prefrontal leukotomy, a procedure for which Egas Moniz was awarded a

Nobel Prize in 1939. Psychosurgery has developed into the formation of localized lesions at specific points that are functionally important in emotional activity. The original operation severed the central core of white matter in front of the ventricle, sacrificing an area of importance in relation to personality and intelligence in an attempt to divide unknown pathways subserving emotion that were contained with it. This extensive lesion caused not only damage to intellect and personality but also flattening of emotion with loss of capacity for enjoyment of work or leisure, owing to division of thalamofrontal pathways through which emotion enters consciousness. These defects, together with a high incidence of epilepsy and a variable mortality, led to disenchantment, and by 1948 the use of standard leukotomy was coming to an end.

From 1950, localized operations were designed to isolate cortical areas on the convexity and in the orbital and cingulate regions, leading eventually to the introduction of sterotactic surgery. But by then the gradually increasing use of powerful antipsychotic drugs had virtually eliminated the indications for this type of intervention, except for occasional rare and unusual cases in which affect-laden assaultive, fearful, or depressive symptoms remained treatment-resistant, completely disabling, and distressingly painful.

Controls are a major problem in assessing the design of leukotomy studies. There is, for obvious practical reasons, no study in which a group of patients selected for leukotomy have been randomly assigned to a sham operation or to a real operation. The closest to this ideal control have been studies of patients recommended for the operation but for whom the operation was refused. It is likely that the reasons for rejecting an operation are not independent of psychiatric status or of the family's attitude toward the return of the patient or of the eventual outcome. Severity of illness and symptom remission are not the only criteria on the basis of which a patient is released from the hospital. How he handles his residual symptoms, how readily the family and the community receive him, and a host of other factors enter into the judgment. Other types of control are less satisfactory, even if the patients are matched for age, sex, diagnosis, and duration and severity of illness. When the matching does not include severity of illness, then the control is unacceptable.

Four controlled prospective studies, two [21]'s, one [23], and one [31], showed positive results in terms of variables such as discharge rate, stay in the community, clinical status, and employment. In addition, two studies compared different operations with consistent findings in favor of the bimedial operation, in which only the white matter is severed. One [21] found a definite advantage in favor of bimedial; in the other, [31], bimedial had better results than the original standard procedures and better than undercutting or transorbital leukotomy. Two class IV retrospective surveys that made comparisons with groups that were most unlikely to be comparable showed no beneficial effect. A reasonable conclusion from the literature is that the original operation did have therapeutic value in certain cases but was abandoned because of its adverse secondary effects and because of the introduction of phenothiazines.

It is not possible to formulate an objective scientific judgment as to the value and position of the newer procedures in the treatment of schizophrenia. The newer operations, reported to be more effective and less associated with secondary effects, have simply not been evaluated in any scientific systematic experiment. At most, there has been an attempt to follow up the results of occasional cases without comparison with a control group. In this context, Bridges' formulation is that schizophrenia is not improved by innominate tractotomy, although cingulate operations may modify aggressive or persistently disturbed behavior in those few patients who do not respond to medication.

REFERENCES

Baker, A. A., Game, J. A., and Thorpe, J. G. Physical treatment for schizophrenia. J. Ment. Sci., *104:* 860, 1958.

Borderleau, Jean-Marc. Insulin therapy and psychiatric disorders. L'Union Medicale du Canada, *92:* 208, 1963.

Bridges, P. K. Psychosurgery today: psychiatric aspects. Proc. R. Soc. Med., *65:* 1104, 1972.

Cole, J. O., and Davis, J. M. Antipsychotic drugs. In *The Schizophrenic Syndrome,* L. Bellak and L. Loeb, editors, p. 478. Grune & Stratton, New York, 1969.

Cole, J. O., Klerman, G. L., and Jones, R. T. Drug therapy—1959. In *Progress in Neurology and Psychiatry,* E. J. Spiegel, editor, vol. 15, p. 540. Grune & Stratton, New York, 1960.

Fairweather, G. W., Sanders, D. H., Cressler, D. L., and Maynard, H. *Community Life for the Mentally Ill.* Aldine, Chicago, 1969.

Gilligan, J. Review of literature. In *Drug and Social Therapy in Chronic Schizophrenia.* M. Greenblatt, M. H. Solomon, A. S. Evans, and G. W. Brooks, editors, p. 24. Charles C. Thomas, Springfield, Ill., 1965.

Gonzalez, J. R., and Imahara, J. K. Electroshock therapy with the phenothiazines and reserpines—a survey and report. Am. J. Psychiatry, *121:* 253, 1964.

Grinspoon, L., Ewalt, J. R., and Shader, R. I. *Schizophrenia: Pharmacotherapy and Psychotherapy.* Williams & Wilkins, Baltimore, 1972.

Grinspoon, L., and Greenblatt, M. Pharmacotherapy combined with other treatment methods. Compr. Psychiatry, *4:* 256, 1963.

Klett, C. J., and Caffey, E. Evaluating the long-term need for anti-Parkinson drugs by chronic schizophrenics. Arch. Gen. Psychiatry, *26:* 374, 1972.

Kline, N. S. Brief psychiatric treatment: The selective primacy of pharmacotherapy. Semin. Psychiatry, *1:* 366, 1969.

Liberman, R. P. Behavioral modification of schizophrenia: A review. Schizophrenia Bull., *6:* 37, 1972.

Luborsky, L., Chandler, M., Auerbach, A. N., Cohen, J., and Bachrach, H. M. Factors influencing the outcome of psychotherapy: a review of quantitative research. Psychol. Bull., *75:* 145, 1971.

Ludwig, A. M. *Treating the Treatment Failures.* Grune & Stratton, New York, 1971.

Marx, A. J., Test, M. A., and Stein, L. I. Prevention of institutionalization through "community treatment." Arch. Gen. Psychiatry, *29:* 505–511, 1973.

May, P. R. A. Anti-psychotic drugs and other forms of therapy. In *Psychopharmacology: Review of Progress, 1957–1967,* Publication No. 1836, D. H. Efron, J. O. Cole, J. Levine, and J. R. Wittenborn, editors, p. 1155. U.S. Government Printing Office, Washington, D. C. 1968.

Meltzoff, J., and Kornreich, M. *Research in Psychotherapy.* Atherton, New York, 1970.

Pasamanick, B., Scarpitti, F., and Dinitz, S. *Schizophrenics in the Community.* Appleton-Century-Crofts, New York, 1967.

Riddell, S. A. The therapeutic efficacy of E. C. T. Arch Gen. Psychiatry, *8:* 546, 1963.

Uhlenhuth, E. H., Lipman, R. S., and Covi, L. Combined pharmacotherapy and psychotherapy: Controlled studies. J. Nerv. Ment. Dis., *148:* 52, 1969.

14.8. SCHIZOPHRENIA: RECENT TRENDS

Diagnosis and Description

Traditionally, diagnostic systems have depended on the patient's presenting signs and symptoms; yet their significance to his past life or eventual outcome has been difficult to establish. Moreover, signs and symptoms can vary considerably over time—whether as a function of actual changes in the patient or according to such characteristics of the observer as theoretical stance, depth of knowledge, and relationship to the patient. Recognizing these difficulties, a number of investigators have attempted to develop more objective, standardized, and reliable methods of classifying patients. These instruments use data from structured interview schedules to arrive at both clinical and computer-derived diagnoses. The structured interview format minimizes the amount of intraobserver variability, and the computer diagnosis allows for an evaluation of the patient's state independent of the observer's threshold for making the diagnosis.

A number of investigators have found that patients who exhibited signs of interpersonal competence—for example, having married, dated, or formed friendships—before becoming ill tended to have a more favorable prognosis than did patients who had not exhibited such signs. Dividing schizophrenic patients into good premorbid and poor premorbid subgroups has proved a useful research tool by reducing the amount of within-group variability of response.

Despite its value as a research tool, the good premorbid-poor premorbid classificatory scheme has a number of serious limitations. First, it is based on retrospective assessments and is subject to distortion. Second, the concept seems oversimplified, attempting as it does to divide a complex disorder that affects many aspects of personality and function into only two subgroups. The dichotomy fails to predict outcome accurately with schizophrenic patients who fall, as often happens, in the middle of the good premorbid-poor premorbid continuum.

Schizophrenia is diagnosed twice as frequently in New York as in London, and the converse is true for depression. Two obvious sources of this phenomenon could be (1) actual differences in the occurrence of schizophrenia and depression in the two countries and (2) different diagnostic practices on the part of British and American clinicians. The results reported thus far tend to support the second hypothesis.

Although schizophrenia's universality has for some time been generally accepted, no study thus far conducted has conclusively established the existence of true process schizophrenia, as distinguished from acute psychotic episodes, in preindustrial cultures.

Genetics

Difficulties inherent in the twin studies method led Rosenthal, Kety, and their collaborators to develop a strategy that separated two major variables in the controversy over the cause of schizophrenia—familial genes and familial rearing. The mental health of the adopted-away offspring of one or more schizophrenic parents was compared with that of control adoptees whose biological parents had no history of mental illness. A related strategy compared the prevalence of mental disorder in the biological relatives of two groups of adoptees— one known to be schizophrenic and the other without a history of mental illness. It appears from initial reports that being biologically related to a schizophrenic increases the risk for psychopathology in general and to some extent for schizophrenia, even when the related persons have had no personal contact. This finding, if confirmed and then replicated, would be the first incontrovertible evidence of a genetic factor in schizophrenia.

Another intriguing preliminary finding is a lower-than-expected incidence of schizophrenia in the adopted-away offspring of psychotic parents. Only 4 per cent (based on research criteria) or 1.3 per cent (based on hospital diagnoses) of one sample could be labeled clearly schizophrenic, as compared with a predicted incidence of 10 to 15 per cent derived from previous family studies. This finding suggests that adoptive rearing may be protective, reducing the clinical manifestation of schizophrenia in genetically predisposed persons.

Most investigators, whether their etiological theories emphasize genetic or environmental factors, agree that the children of two schizophrenic parents are at exceptionally high risk for the development of disorder. Four major studies conducted before 1960 found that from 14 to 54 per cent of such offspring became schizophrenic—a mean morbid expectancy rate of about 35 per cent. In a more recent, intensive study, Kringlen found that, of a pool of 70 offspring of schizophrenic couples, 19 per cent were schizophrenic, 38 per cent nonpsychotically mentally ill, and 41 per cent normal. The last group is one that has received little attention in the disorder-oriented psychiatric-genetic literature. How did these high-risk offspring manage to grow up normal, despite the extremely unfavorable genetic and environmental odds against them? Knowledge of these coping skills and their antecedents may be an important aid in developing preventive measures and new treatments.

Gradually, the heredity-versus-environment controversy is beginning to shift ground. Debates increasingly tend to revolve around not whether but how great a role heredity (or environment) plays and in what types of schizophrenia.

Biochemistry and Neurophysiology

The biochemical investigation of schizophrenia has largely been based on the belief that an abnormal substance may be causally related to schizophrenia's occurrence. Wyatt and associates' comprehensive review of work carried out this area during the 1960's concludes: "To date, no biochemical abnormalities have been consistently and exclusively associated with schizophrenia." There remain, however, a number of viable biochemical hypotheses about which the evidence is contradictory or incomplete or both. Tolerance to histamine is one of the few abnormalities that has been consistently found in studies of schizophrenic patients. Elevated plasma creatinine phosphokinase concentrations, although not exclusively associated with schizophrenia, have been a consistently found abnormality in the acute psychoses. The amphetamine psychosis may be a good model for some forms of schizophrenia and may act by producing a hyperactive dopaminergic system. Phenothiazines seem to work by blocking dopaminergic receptors, and there is a recent report of decreased dopamine β-hydroxylase in schizophrenia. Therefore, it is reasonable to hypothesize an imbalance in the dopamine-norepinephrine regulatory system in some forms of schizophrenia. The LSC-dimethyltryptamine hypothesis is viable, and the recent finding of what appears to be genetically determined low platelet monoamine oxidase activity in schizophrenic patients is supportive of this theory.

Recent advances in computer technology have made it possible to define more directly functional central nervous system (CNS) abnormalities. These developments have spawned an entirely new technology and investigatory methodology, the average evoked response (AER) technique. The AER technique allows recovery of relatively specific CNS signals from scalp electroencephalograms. The averaging technique allows the researcher to ferret out an underlying brain response to a stimulus that would otherwise be hidden in the individual electroencephalographic trace. In the past several years, the use of this evoked potential technique as a window to the schizophrenic's brain has permitted the study of populations of patients and nonpatients to determine large-scale differences. It appears that the AER technique, although it has not yet found aberrant electroencephalographic patterns specific to schizophrenia, will be useful in the study of motivation, attention, concentration, and drug effects in schizophrenic and other types of patients.

Experimental Psychology and Psychophysiology

Recent psychological studies have paid special attention to sampling, diagnosis, homogeneous subgroupings, and controls. Particularly important in these investigations has been the attention devoted to confounding variables. Closely related studies began to look at the role of motivation and attention in task performance. Levels of interest, willingness, and distractability of experimental subjects became a legitimate focus of concern. The power of these confounding variables led to the development of research strategies capable of dealing with them more adequately: varying the experimental set, assessing motivation, using appropriate control groups, and developing tasks that require little active performance.

Compared with normal subjects, schizophrenics have a greater tendency toward stimulus avoidance, show a greater inability to maintain attention and set, show a deficit in the appropriateness of their categorizations and generalizations, and are harder to involve in experimental tasks. Schizophrenics, however, seem relatively more motivated in situations in which good performance results in escape from noxious stimuli; they show disturbances in autonomic functioning, the most consistent of which is that they are psychophysiologically less flexible in responding to tasks confronting them; their arousal level is not so directly related to the demands of the situations in which they find themselves as is that of normal subjects; and they are more socially withdrawn and perform more poorly in tasks involving social stimuli as compared with neutral stimuli.

Psychophysiologists have substantially increased their knowledge of the mechanisms underlying the phenomena they attempt to measure, particularly in the field of galvanic skin response. For example, the bulk of the evidence indicates that galvanic skin response arousal in schizophrenia is a measure of level of psychopathology, rather than a trait specific to this disorder, as was held by some earlier investigators.

The computer greatly simplifies the problem of analyzing psychophysiological data. It is now possible to examine reactions not only over extended time periods but also across several different psychophysiological measures during the time period.

The on-line computer, in which there is direct interaction between the computer and the experiment, may remove the contaminating interpersonal effects of the experimenter from the experimental situation. And on-line computers permit the development of experiments in which the nature of a subject's response to a given experimental manipulation can determine which of several alternate experimental manipulations should occur in the immediately succeeding phase of the experiment. With the on-line computer in widespread use, it may become increasingly feasible to ask some of the more complex questions that presently face the researcher of the psychophysiology of mental illness.

Persons at High Risk

It is not possible in any study of already-manifest, diagnosed schizophrenics to determine whether research results reflect a cause or a consequence of the subjects' illness. High-risk studies sidestep this problem by focusing on persons considered vulnerable to psychiatric breakdown before the manifestation of illness. Investigators engaged in high-risk research hope to identify pre-existing characteristics that differentiate between those who later develop schizophrenia and those who do not—a critical step in determining the causes of this disorder. In addition, the identification of persons at risk may eventually make possible preventive intervention.

Although the incidence of schizophrenia in the population at large is only about 1 per cent, 10 to 15 per cent of the offspring of one schizophrenic parent can be expected to develop schizophrenia. Thus, by studying children of schizophrenic parents, the researcher can increase his possible yield of preschizophrenics by 10 or 15 times, as compared with a random sample of the population.

One limitation of ongoing applications of the high-risk strategy is their almost exclusive dependence on the offspring of schizophrenic parents as a pool of vulnerable persons. Since 90 per cent of adult schizophrenics do not have an identified schizophrenic parent, it may be ad-

visable to mount studies focusing on nongeneti-
cally defined groups vulnerable to schizophrenia, such as urban slum dwellers and persons in
cultural transition. Also, since high-risk studies
presently consist almost exclusively of clinic
and laboratory-based studies, studies focusing
on the subject in his natural habitat, such as his
home or school, may be a valuable addition to
the field.

Family Studies

It has become common practice for all members of the family of a schizophrenic patient to
be observed and for reports of their behavior to
be compared and contrasted; for individuals
and groupings of family members to undergo
psychological testing; and for entire families—
psychiatrically normal as well as disordered
members—to be hospitalized for comprehensive
study and treatment. Sophisticated clinicians
are now inclined to consider the impact of the
family on treatment outcome, even if they never
deal with families directly.

Early work in this area focused on content,
such as what persons said about each other.
More recent and much more powerful in its
ability to distinguish varying levels of psychopathology is the use of the analysis of form. That
is, what is said is less important than how it is
said. Analysis of communication styles has
enabled families with a schizophrenic offspring
to be distinguished from those with neurotic or
normal offspring. Methods originally devised
either for the study of individuals—such as the
Rorschach, the Thematic Apperception Test,
the object sorting test—or for the study of small
groups—Bales categories, Strodbeck's revealed
differences—have been modified and applied
with some success to the study of families. In
addition, various new procedures have been
devised, such as the study of experimental
families—for example, parents of normal children interacting with a schizophrenic child.

Spurred by early reports of aberrant child-
rearing patterns in families with schizophrenic
offspring, investigators were prompted to compare child-rearing practices in middle-class and
working-class families. Patterns of child rearing
and value orientation shown by middle-class
families with schizophrenic offspring are similar
to normal working-class patterns, but among
the working class there are no gross differences
in child-rearing patterns between those families
with and those without schizophrenic offspring.

Sociocultural Factors

Rates of occurrence of mental disorders, particularly schizophrenia, are highest at the lowest socio-economic levels. The cause of this
relationship is not certain. One hypothesis advanced, especially in the case of schizophrenia,
is that schizophrenics who may have been born
into higher social class families drift downward
as a result of the incapacitating effects of their
illness. Although no single study is definitive,
the weight of the evidence suggests that the
degree of downward mobility among schizophrenics is insufficient to explain the high concentration of schizophrenia in the lowest socio-
economic strata.

Other sociologically oriented studies have
demonstrated a relationship between the occurrence of stress and depression and schizophrenia. The relationship of class to mental disorders is attributable not merely to differences in
the amount of stress that people endure but also
to social class differences in how effectively
people deal with stress.

A possible explanation of the apparently
inferior ability of persons raised in lower-class
homes to deal satisfactory with stress can be
found in sociological studies on social class
differences in adult orientations and child-rearing values. These studies indicate that, as a
result of the constricted and powerless life
circumstances in which they find themselves,
many lower-class families transmit to their
offspring an orientational system too limited
and too rigid for dealing with complex, changing, and stressful situations. Obviously, since
only a small proportion of lower-class persons
become schizophrenic, the pattern of social
class-related findings cannot in itself explain
either schizophrenia or mental illness in general, but future research must take this pattern
into account.

Treatment

The single most important schizophrenia-
related advance in recent years was the introduction of chlorpromazine during the
mid-1950's. The phenothiazines are generally
given credit for the dramatic decline that has
taken place in the number of resident schizophrenic patients in state and county mental
hospitals. Since this downward trend first became apparent in 1963, eight years after the
phenothiazines first came into widespread use,

there has been an acceleration in the rate of decline of resident schizophrenic patients. This development is somewhat surprising, since the effects of the phenothiazines might logically have been expected to plateau, leaving a hard core of unresponsive and undischargeable patients. For this reason, some authorities believe that the recent, accelerated decreases in patient populations stem from the development of new psychosocial treatment programs and from changes in administrative policies. These new programs and policies are themselves the result of a resurgence of interest in schizophrenia, largely brought about by the phenothiazines' effectiveness.

The phenothiazines have not solved the schizophrenia problem. The probability of readmission within 2 years of discharge for an initial episode of schizophrenia, for example, varies between 40 and 60 per cent, depending on the study. In the United States, between 15 and 25 per cent of discharged schizophrenics are eventually readmitted and receive continued care for a prolonged period of time. Furthermore, only 15 to 40 per cent of schizophrenics living in the community achieve an average level of adjustment. And serious, often irreversible side-effects attendant on the long-term use of these agents have been reported with increasing frequency.

Nonmedical Developments

Whether psychiatry should be responsible for the care of odd and irrational persons in society is a question that is undergoing highly critical examination by a small but vocal group of psychiatrist-philosophers. In the forefront of the questioners are such increasingly well-known figures as Laing, Szasz, Cooper, Scheff, and Goffman. Together, they have helped generate a sociopolitical movement, commonly termed "antipsychiatry," championing the cause of persons labeled schizophrenic. The basic change sought is a redefinition of psychosis as a social-interpersonal situation, rather than as a medical disease or even as a problem falling within the purview of psychiatry.

Particular criticism is directed at the mental hospital, which antipsychiatrists view as a place where deviant persons who have transgressed society's rules and norms are incarcerated and persuaded in various ways to conform. To them, mental illness is not the inexorable unfolding of some disease process within the deviant person but, rather, a label that is applied to those whose actions do not conform to society's definition of socially acceptable behavior.

Their focus on the dehumanizing aspects of hospitalization, treatment, labeling, and stigmatization has sensitized many to the unintended consequences of the medicalization of madness. It has contributed to the patient-rights movement and helped bring about widespread reform of commitment laws.

They have brought into sharper focus a number of the incongruities and contradictions inherent in the mental health system (the doctor as confessor-jailer), in the family (you may be independent so long as you remain dependent on me), and in society (violence and irrationality are to be suppressed, but war and other societal irrationalities are not to be questioned).

REFERENCES

Claridge, G. The schizophrenias as nervous types. Br. J. Psychiatry, *121:* 1, 1972.

Eysenck, H. J. *Handbook of Abnormal Psychology: An Experimental Approach*, ed. 2. Basic Books, New York, 1973.

Garmezy, N. Process and reactive schizophrenia: Some conceptions and issues. In *The Role and Methodology of Classification in Psychiatry and Psychopathology*. M. M. Katz, J. O. Cole, and W. E. Barton, editors, p. 419. United States Government Printing Office, Washington, 1968.

Kety, S. S., Rosenthal, D., Wender, P. H., and Schulsinger, F. Mental Illness in the biological and adoptive families of adopted schizophrenics. Am. J. Psychiatry, *128:* 302, 1971.

Kohn, M. L. Social class and schizophrenia: A critical review and a reformulation. Schizophrenia Bull., *7:* 60, 1973.

Laing, R. D. *The Politics of Experience*. Pantheon, New York, 1967.

Mosher, L. R., Gunderson, J. G., and Buchsbaum, S. Special report: Schizophrenia, 1972. Schizophrenia Bull., *7:* 12, 1973.

Riskin, J. M., and Faunce, E. E. An evaluative review of family interaction research. Fam. Process, *11:* 365, 1973.

Rosenthal, D., Wender, P., Kety, S. S., Welner, J., and Schulsinger, F. The adopted-away offspring of schizophrenics. Am. J. Psychiatry, *128:* 307, 1971.

Torrey, E. F. Is schizophrenia universal? An open question, Schizophrenia Bull., *7:* 53, 1973.

Wise, C. D., and Stein, L. Dopamine-β-hydroxylase deficits in the brains of schizophrenic patients, Science, *181:* 344, 1973.

Wyatt, R. J., Murphy, D. L., Belmaker, R., Cohen, S., Donnelly, C. H., and Pollin, W. Reduced monoamine oxidase activity in platelets: A possible genetic marker for vulnerability to schizophrenia. Science, *179:* 916, 1973.

15

Paranoid States

Definition

Paranoid states are psychotic disturbances characterized by delusions of reference, influence, grandeur, morbid jealousy, or persecution, without any associate hallucinations. The delusions are not scattered or bizarre but are generally well-systematized and developed in a logical progression. There is an appropriate emotional response, and social behavior is well-maintained, with the personality remaining intact or showing minimal deterioration over a prolonged period of time.

Classification and Symptoms

The differences between paranoid states and paranoid schizophrenia are merely matters of degree. Many investigators consider these conditions to be in a continuum. Paranoid schizophrenia occurs early in life, with fairly rapid personality disintegration, whereas the paranoid states occur later in life and show relatively little morbid personality deterioration.

Paranoia

This is a rare paranoid state. There is a gradual development of a well-systematized, chronic delusional state, without hallucinations and usually based on a false belief that is firmly and consistently maintained and logically elaborated in the delusional system. If the original false premise were true, the delusions would be correct and logically fall into place as perfectly normal thought processes with appropriate affective reactions. In spite of a chronic and prolonged course, the personality remains intact and well-preserved.

There are two main elements—first, grandeur or grandiosity with unrealistic feelings of overvaluation of the self (ego inflation); second, irrational and unrealistic ideas of persecution.

Paranoid Reaction or Condition

This state appears to lie somewhere between paranoia and paranoid schizophrenia. It is characterized by paranoid delusions without hallucinations. It lacks the systematized nature of the delusion in paranoia but bears no resemblance to the bizarre fragmentation, deterioration, and hallucinatory phenomena of paranoid schizophrenia. Although generally persistent and chronic, it may be of relatively short duration.

Paranoid Jealousy

Here there is some precipitating factor that the patient often misinterprets because of his feelings of inadequacy, low self-esteem, and ambivalence and because of his malignant ego defense of projection. The patient is constantly watching and thinking that he is finding confirmatory evidence for his jealous delusions in everything that is said, done, and experienced. Denial and projection are prominent characteristics.

Paranoid Eroticism

In this condition the patient's ideas run rampant, and he fancies himself in love with an actual person or someone imagined. He feels that the loved one cannot make a definite avowal of love but indicates it in many silent, indirect, and circuitous ways. Often, the patient, usually a woman, selects a prominent and outstanding figure as the love object.

Paranoid Grandiosity

Here the patient manifests a feeling of grandiosity and omnipotence, simulating the narcissistic feelings of his early childhood. In adult frustration, regression to this omnipotent, grandiose state takes place. The patient feels he possesses remarkable talents as a prophet, scientist, or inventor; that he is extraordinarily attractive and inspired; and that there is nothing in life he cannot accomplish with the greatest success. Although these patients may work zealously and successfully in a legitimate movement or cause for social reform, they generally associate themselves with fanatical fringe activities that they embrace with complete and utter dedication.

Involutional Paranoid State

In the involutional period, the patient for the first time presents frank paranoid delusion formation. There is an absence of conspicuous thought disorders or other evidence of emotional or personality deterioration, as typically occurs in schizophrenia. There is often an associated depression or agitation in conjunction with the florid paranoid delusions. The sensorium is clear, and intellectual function is not affected. The prognosis is less favorable than in involutional melancholia.

Paranoid Litigious State

This is a fairly common form of the paranoid state in which, as a result of some disappointing legal decision, the patient begins brooding about the unfairness of the legal system. He then begins a series of further legal actions that are unrealistic and ill-advised and that result in further negative decisions concerning his case. Every disappointment leads to further grievances and controversies. Because of his underlying insecurity and inadequacy, he must prove at all costs that he is legally right. Often, he feels that everyone is ganging up on him, that there must be a plot against him. Frequently, he had always insisted on his rights, had tended to amplify trivial and inconsequential events, and had been rather stubborn and suspicious.

Symptomatic Paranoid States

In these states, paranoid ideas are grafted onto an organic illness. Patients with cerebral arteriosclerosis, senile brain disease, and other brain diseases may present paranoid ideas. Those with carbon monoxide poisoning, uremia, alcoholic hallucinosis, and other toxic organic states may present paranoid delusions.

Paranoid Personality

The patient may show many paranoid characteristics that are not marked and, therefore, not in the psychotic category. The patient is considered rigid and inflexible, reaching conclusions that cannot be changed, tending to be suspicious and morbidly sensitive, impugning the motives of others concerning even minor and irrelevant matters. He tends to be morose and reserved, watching and observing intently, and is undemonstrative and cold emotionally. He may be insulted easily and fly into outbursts of rage and anger, and he appears to be markedly narcissistic, self-centered, and selfish. If he belongs to groups or organizations, he tends to dominate and control them and is extremely resentful if disagreed with or opposed. He has no close friends, although he may have many acquaintances. Friendships are usually of short duration, since he tends to argue with, resent, and often insult his acquaintances.

Epidemiology

Paranoid states are rare before the age of 30, whereas paranoid schizophrenia may occur much earlier in life. Women are more prone to paranoia than are men. Native Americans appear less susceptible to this disturbance than are immigrants, and the disorder is more frequent in cities than in rural communities.

About 10 per cent of all admissions to mental hospitals are for paranoid states. However most persons with paranoid states have intact personalities, conform to the demands of society, and may never be hospitalized.

Causes

Direct hereditary factors play no discernible role in this disturbance, nor does one find overt and direct neuropathological evidence for the development of paranoid states. Psychological factors do play a large role. The main ego defense mechanisms used are denial and projection. The patient experiences unconscious desires, wishes, or drives, causing tension and guilt. These thoughts are unacceptable to his rather weak ego, so he defends himself by denying that the intolerable ideas and feelings are his. He attributes them to others.

In the paranoid states the ego is not entirely shattered but is capable of multipurposeful and realistic activities. However, the patient denies sex and love altogether and frequently sublimates these needs in religious fervor, grandiose ideas, and paranoid delusions. Some investigators feel that there is some relationship between homosexuality and the paranoid states, but, others indicate that there is not a causal relationship.

Childhood Causes

Basic trust and basic confidence are the keynotes of the child's relationship to parents or parent substitutes. If no trust can be placed in the parents and if unresolved frustrations, disappointments, and humiliations are frequent occurrences, the child develops a feeling that he will constantly be betrayed and that his environment is consistently hostile. (See Figure 1.) Consequently, he attempts to insulate and protect himself from hurt or harm by developing a personality that is secretive, critical, abrasive, hostile, humorless, and insensitive. His relationship with people is characterized by lack of trust because he himself never felt trust and also by a

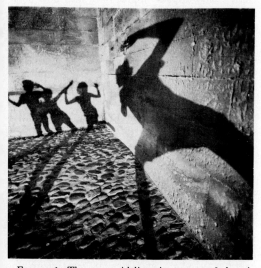

FIGURE 1. The paranoid lives in a state of chronic anxiety and fears the environment which is seen as hostile and threatening as symbolized in this illustration. (Courtesy of Arthur Tress for Magnum Photos, Inc.)

tendency to brood and ruminate about real or imagined slights.

The preparanoid child—never assured of warmth, trust, love, and affection—is nonetheless expected to present almost impossibly high levels of performance. Usually, there is a large element of sadism in the family, with many admonitions, restrictions of normal activity, undeserved and unjustified punishment, or withdrawal of the little love and affection that is occasionally demonstrated.

Cultural Factors

Parnoid states are more common among migratory, immigrant, and minority groups than among the native and permanent population. The adaptational stresses of a new language, a new job, and the feelings of loneliness and isolation may partly explain the appearance of paranoid delusions. If these migratory and immigrant persons return to their native countries, the paranoid ideas frequently disappear.

Paranoid Pseudocommunity

The patient is perplexed and bewildered by the ominous paranoid threats and referential ideas emanating from his surroundings. He cannot explain them, saying merely that he knows the truth and what he believes are the facts in his thinking. He does not know who "they" are or understand the "why" of his persecutions. He searches and speculates and finally comes up with the answer, which leads to the formation of the pseudocommunity—a group of real and imaginary people determined to destroy the patient's reputation or his life. This pseudocommunity is the patient's own formulation. Since he has projected into his fantasy his own rage and hate, the patient may become dangerous and even homicidal, since "they" are after him to ruin or destroy him.

Course and Prognosis

The paranoid person often makes valiant efforts to hide the intensity of his paranoid delusions. At times, he frightens his co-workers or acquaintances by outbursts of hostility, expressions of mistrust toward those with whom he was previously on friendly terms, and a greater tendency to withdrawal and isolation. Since these reactions alienate others, the patient's delusional system is reinforced by an intensification of his feelings that he is surrounded by hostility. To avoid his persecutors, the patient often moves to a new community. Although at first the hostility disappears and the environment seems friendly, within a short time the delusions, suspiciousness, anger, rage, and hostility return; further escape may lead to suicide.

Occasionally, the paranoid person turns his hostility against his persecutors and makes either verbal or physical attacks on others. Eventually, the delusional system becomes more and more obvious, with deeper and deeper conviction on the part of the patient that everyone is plotting against him.

Because of the patient's fairly intact personality, the logical and realistic possibility of his delusional system, his capacity to rationalize and sound convincing, his lack of insight, and his lack of any motivation to seek or accept treatment, the prognosis for the paranoid states is even poorer than the prognosis for paranoid schizophrenia.

Acute paranoid states may be more amenable to therapy, and the prognosis may be more favorable than in the chronic forms of the illness.

Diagnosis

Pertinent clues can be obtained from a careful evaluation of the personality characteristics of the patient. The patient's early life may reveal a complete lack of trust and confidence in the child-parent relationship, with lack of sustained love and affection but with a great deal of hostility and even an active sadistic orientation in the child's development and in his parental interpersonal relationships. The patient tends to be rigid, inflexible, and excessively cautious, often impugning the motives of others or questioning these motives in an unusually intense and unrealistic fashion. There is also a tendency to amplify and elaborate on inconsequential and insignificant details. He leans toward rationalization and feels wronged, slighted, and ignored. He often has difficulty in working with authority figures or with a group.

Physical and Psychiatric Examinations

A physical examination generally reveals no causative factor in relation to paranoid states, nor is there a specific or typical physique associated with this disturbance. There are no consistent physical or laboratory findings to distinguish a paranoid condition.

In the psychiatric examination, one may observe little of significance in the patient's appearance or social behavior. The patient is unusually alert to everything occurring in the office. He weighs every question cautiously; he often asks for the meaning behind the question and asks for specific definitions of what is desired and what he is expected to say.

Occasionally, there may be some pressure of speech and, in the beginning, a guarded defensiveness; later in the interview the patient may manifest continual preoccupation with his delusional ideas. Generally of average or higher than average intelligence, he has an excellent capacity to verbalize, his reasoning and beliefs are so logical and seemingly intact that his expressions appear honest, reasonable, and believable. But the delusional system becomes obvious, with referential ideas, grandiose or erotic, and, finally, active paranoid delusions.

The intellectual function of the patient in a paranoid state remains unimpaired. Orientation is well-maintained, and memory for recent and remote events in not affected.

In the early stages, the affect is well-maintained within normal limits, and the emotional expressions appear appropriate and adequate, although they are often associated with marked tension. Later, as the illness becomes chronic, the delusional ideas may give vent to feelings of rage, anger, and hostility that seem to remain constant. There is little capacity for mirth and humor. Insight is completely lacking. Judgment is generally well-preserved except where the paranoid ideas are involved.

Differential Diagnosis

If the delusional system is consonant with reality factors, is well-systemized, is based on a real event that is misinterpreted and then elaborated, and shows no evidence of hallucinations, the condition is a paranoid state, rather than paranoid schizophrenia. The affect and behavior of paranoid states may be appropriate in every way, even, at times, in relation to the paranoid delusions, whereas in paranoid schizophrenia the general picture is more bizarre and the affect is inappropriate and inconsistent.

Paranoid delusions may occur at the height of

a manic phase of an affective psychosis or even during a severe depression of the manic-depressive variety. But the manic expresses all his feelings spontaneously and with no inhibition, whereas the paranoid patient is reserved, inhibited, and cautious in expressing his true feelings and ideas. The manic frequently changes his paranoid ideas, since he is distractible and influenced by everything that goes on about him. The paranoid state patient has fixed and well-systematized delusions that do not fluctuate. In the intellectual functioning of the manic there is a great deal of expansiveness and productivity, and he may maintain or continue his creativity; in the paranoid state, the intellectuality is restrictive and defensive. The behavior of the manic is determined by outside events and occurrences, whereas the paranoiac's behavior is determined by his thoughts and feelings and, consequently, is markedly subjective. Early in the manic state, judgment is impaired, and the manic patient becomes reckless and impulsive. The paranoid patient, however, is usually cautious and reserved and is able to exert a greater amount of self-control.

In the involutional paranoid state, the onset is much later than in the ordinary paranoid condition. Delusions are usually centered on death, destruction, and persecution, with delusions of grandeur less common than in the other paranoid states, also, there is a much greater hypochondriacal element. In the symptomatic paranoid states, there is marked forgetfulness, impairment of memory, disorientation, and defects in judgment and affect. In the other paranoid states, memory is intact, and no organic defects are observed.

Psychological Tests

Paranoid patients usually cooperate with intelligence tests, so a fairly good appraisal can be made of the patient's intellectual capacity and function. On the Wechsler Adult Intelligence Scale (WAIS), the verbal and information scales are usually higher than the performance scale. The vocabulary performance is fairly good, whereas the similarities and picture arrangement scale may be low in the paranoid states. There are large discrepancies between subtests. In general, the total score is good, although there may be peculiar verbalizations. As the tests become more difficult, the paranoid patient becomes tense and suspicious and at times refuses to cooperate.

Projective technique—such as the Rorschach, the Thematic Apperception Test (TAT), and the Draw a Person Test (DAP)—may be useful. The Rorschach may show little if there is a mild paranoid state but may show a great deal with a frank and open paranoid schizophrenic patient.

The Rorschach may show a total rejection of some of the cards, a prolonged reaction time, or a limited number of total responses. There are more movement than color responses, with a rather high level of form responses. There may also be an excess of whole responses over human movement replies or an excess of animal movement over human movement responses. The patient observes a hostile environment constantly threatening him. There is a confusion of identity between males and females, and homosexual content manifests itself in many of the tests.

In the TAT, there are recurring themes of impugning people's motives, manipulation of main figure by others, sexual distortion of figures, and a tendency to extreme moralizing.

The DAP test is considered the least definitive of the projective techniques. Some characteristics are a large figure, emphasis on the eyes, large head and ears, a rigid posture and speared fingers, and poor differentiation between male and female figures.

Treatment

A difficulty in initiating treatment, especially in early cases, is the lack of motivation on the part of the patient and often on the part of the family. What is necessary is a clear, firm, and unequivocal statement by the most influential member of the family that psychiatric treatment, combined with appropriate medication, is in order.

Unless the patient is a serious threat to himself or others it is more effective therapeutically for the patient to be treated as an outpatient than to be hospitalized, since any effort to restrict freedom of movement or liberty produces an increase of hate and rage and causes the paranoid delusions to be augmented and elaborated.

The treatment of the paranoid patient has two aims: first, to reduce anxiety and, second, to re-establish communication on a realistic level.

Tranquilizing Drugs

The initial aim of attenuating anxiety is accomplished by means of the major tranquilizing drugs, such as chlorpromazine, thioridazine, trifluoperazine, fluphenazine, perphenazine, and promazine.

There appears to be an inverse relationship between the potency and the sedative effects of these drugs. Chlorpromazine is valuable in states or restlessness, excitement, agression, and overactivity. Perphenazine, which is moderately sedative, is used in states of motor restlessness and agitation combined with delusional thinking or perplexed, confused states. Fluphenazine and trifluoperazine, the least sedative drugs, are valuable in manifestations of dullness, apathy, withdrawal, confusion, perplexity, uncommunicative behavior, hallucinations, and delusions.

In patients with an overt depressive element, which often occurs in paranoid involutional patients, a combination with an antidepressant drug is indicated.

Psychotherapy

The initial approach in psychotherapy should be permissive. The therapist should avoid any reference to the patient's delusions and should listen intently without arguing about the delusions, minimizing them, or passing any judgment regarding them. If the therapist reacts with anxiety to the patient's rage, suspiciousness, explosiveness, and aggressiveness, the patient is immediately aware of this reaction, and the therapist's effectiveness is markedly diminished. The therapist must be consistent, firm, and impeccably honest, since any uncertainty, deviation, or evasion is immediately noted by the patient, with consequent impairment in the therapeutic relationship.

One of the essential aims of psychotherapy in the paranoid patient is to obtain his confidence and trust and to cause him to see the therapist as a neutral person who never rejects, deprecates, or condemns the patient's ideas. The patient is thus encouraged to communicate more freely, to break through his isolation, and to describe his frightening experiences. (See Figure 2.) With such a relationship firmly established, the therapist may offer tentative or alter-

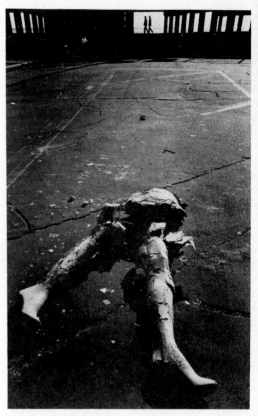

FIGURE 2. Paranoid patients are often unable to separate the thought from the deed and fear that their angry impulses can kill others or themselves. (Courtesy of Arthur Tress for Magnum Photos, Inc.)

native observations or speculations regarding the delusional picture, giving the patient glimpses of his world from another person's point of view. Doubts gradually enter the patient's mind concerning the validity of his assumptions. He may begin to have a more realistic self-appraisal of his position in the reality picture while his ego is beginning to grow and develop. This process evolves very slowly. The therapist may now offer more positive appraisals and suggestions, penetrating deeper into the delusional system and more and more substituting reality for fantasy.

Expressions of unconscious homoerotic fantasies are never interpreted directly or discussed as such. The patient's sexual fears are ventilated in terms of his anxieties regarding the opposite sex. The therapist helps the patient understand that he will sometimes distrust the therapist, but he also suggests strongly that, when such feelings arise, the patient talk about them freely.

Paranoid patients do not do well in group therapy because of their suspiciousness, hypersensitivity, tendencies to misinterpret what is being said, and narcissistic need to apply to themselves whatever is said or done.

REFERENCES

Bleuler, E. *Dementia Praecox or the Group of Schizophrenias.* International Universities Press, New York, 1950.

Cameron, N. A. Paranoid conditions and paranoia. In *American Handbook of Psychiatry.* S. Aricti, editor, 5 vol. 1, p. 508. Basic Books, New York, 1959.

Freud, S. Some neurotic mechanisms in jealousy, paranoia and homosexuality. In *Standard Edition of the Complete Psychological Works of Sigmund Freud,* vol. 18, p. 221. Hogarth Press, London, 1955.

Grunebaum H., and Perlman, M. S. Paranoia and naivete. Arch. Gen. Psychiatry, *28:* 30, 1973.

Haslam, M. T. A case of Capgras syndrome. Am. J. Psychiatry, *130:* 493, 1973.

Kaplan, H. I., and Sadock, B. J. The status of the paranoid today: His diagnosis, prognosis and treatment. Psychiatr. Q., *45:* 528, 1971.

Kolb, L. C. *Modern Clinical Psychiatry.* ed. 8. W. B. Saunders, Philadelphia, 1973.

Polatin. P. *A Guide to Treatment in Psychiatry.* J. B. Lippincott, Philadelphia, 1966.

Snyder, S. H. Amphetamine psychosis: A "model" schizophrenia mediated by catecholamines. Am. J. Psychiatry, *130:* 61, 1973.

Swanson, D. W., Bohnert, P. J., and Smith, J. A. *The Paranoid.* Little, Brown, Boston, 1970.

16

Major Affective Disorders

16.1. OVERVIEW OF DEPRESSION

Introduction

Scientific investigations of depression are only a century or two old, and, although major advances in treatment have been developed, research has yet to clarify fully the nature and causes of this complex disorder. Animal studies, particularly in primates, have established the validity of behavioral models related to separation and loss, which provide a long-needed bridge between clinical observation and experimental psychology. Most dramatic have been the advances in therapy. The neuroleptics, the tricyclic antidepressants, the monoamine oxidase inhibitors, and lithium have entered the armamentarium of the psychiatrist, and the efficacy of these new treatments has greatly improved the prognosis of acute depressive states.

Scope of Depression

For the neurophysiologist, depression refers to any decrease in electrophysiological activity. For the pharmacologist, depression refers to the actions of drugs that decrease the activity of the target organ. For the psychologist, depression refers to any decrement in optimal cognitive, perceptual, or motor performance. For the clinical psychiatrist, however, depression covers a wide range of changes in the affective states. The affective changes may vary in severity from the normal mood swings of everyday life at one extreme to the severe psychotic state called involutional melancholia.

Many clinicians and investigators have postulated that clinical depressive symptoms are the result of reduction of some generalized or specific central nervous system function and, therefore, are best treated with a stimulant drug. This view has been the classic model for the neuropharmacology and pathophysiology of affective states.

Concepts of a bipolar continuum in affective states were correlated with Pavlovian conditioning theory and psychoanalytic libido theory. The early version of the catecholamine hypothesis implied a similar concept, postulating that excessive catecholamines would produce mania and that deficient catecholamines would produce depression. The complexity of actions of the newer psychotropic agents—particularly the phenothiazines, the tricyclic antidepressants, and lithium—makes the traditional stimulant-depressant continuum obsolete and overly simplistic. Until the newer theories of the psychobiology of affective states are validated, the term "depression" is best restricted to clinical phenomena.

Depression as a Normal Mood

Depression is a pervasive feature of normal human experience. The most important insights about normal depressive affect derive from the concepts of Darwin, particularly those related to adaptation. According to the strictest criterion of evolutionary theory, a trait of behavior is adaptive from the phylogenetic viewpoint if it promotes the survival of the species. From the ontogenetic view, a trait is adaptive if it promotes the growth and survival of the individual members of the species.

The genesis of emotion in the child is related to the vicissitudes of the child's attachment bond to mothering figures. With their prolonged state of dependency, human infants are highly vulnerable to the effects of separation and subsequent feelings of helplessness. The infant's depressive behaviors serve to alert the social group, usually the family, to his need for nuturing, assistance, and succor.

When the mammal mother-infant bond is broken by separation or loss, typical behavioral patterns emerge. The initial pattern is characterized by anxiety, agitation and protest. This pattern is followed by withdrawal, decreased social participation, and decreased motor activity. Intensive psychological studies have convinced most observers that these characteristics of animal depression are similar to if not identical with normal emotional states in humans.

One can identify four adaptive functions of affects: social communication, physiological arousal, subjective awareness, and psychodynamic defense.

Normal Depressions versus Clinical Depressive States

Because clinicians and investigators do not fully agree as to the complete range of affective phenomena to be diagnosed as symptomatic, the boundary between normal mood and abnormal depressions remain undefined.

In clinical practice, four criteria are used in the diagnosis of depression: intensity, duration, the precipitating event, and the quality of the psychopathological features. A vaguely defined gradient of intensity exists between normal mood and pathological state, but no clear demarcation has been delineated. And, lacking normative data as to the natural history of normal moods, psychiatrists have only approximations and rough guides as to duration. The presence or absence of an overt life stress (precipitating event) poses multiple dilemmas. Whatever the duration, intensity, or precipitating event, the existence of certain characteristic features—such as hallucinations, delusions, marked weight loss, and suicidal trends—indicate that the boundary between normal and pathological has been passed and that the patient is into the range of psychopathology.

Depression as a Symptom

Affective symptoms seldom occur alone; they are usually combined with somatic and psychosocial impairments, even when associated with other conditions.

Robbins and his associates have proposed a distinction between primary and secondary affective disorders based on two criteria, chronology and the presence of associated illnesses. Primary affective disorders refer to the disorders in patients who have been well or whose only previous episodes of psychiatric disease were mania or depression. Secondary affective disorders occur in mentally ill persons who have had another psychiatric illness. The diagnosis is made regardless of the presence or absence of an apparent life stress (see figure 1).

Although the primary-secondary distinction is conceptually clear-cut, a number of practical problems arise in differentiating those depressive conditions that occur in association with other clinical psychiatric states. In clinical practice, this problem arises in schizophrenia and the schizo-affective states, anxiety neurosis, alcoholism, personality disorders, and hysteria.

The recognition of affective symptoms secondary to systemic disease, drug reactions, and central nervous system states has practical and theoretical significance. Practically, the clinician is always troubled about misdiagnosing depressions that may be associated with tumors or endocrine disorders, especially when appropriate treatment of the disorder is available. Moreover, these secondary depressions often pose difficult therapeutic problems because of the possible interactions between psychotropic drugs and medications that may be used for the systemic disease.

Chemically induced states of depression constitute another group of secondary depressions that have many similarities to primary affective

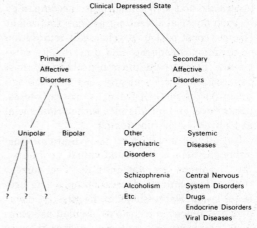

FIGURE 1. Nosology of depression.

disorders. The most significant group of patients are the hypertensives who became depressed when treated with reserpine. Similar reactions have occurred with other antihypertensive drugs. Rebound-depressive reaction may follow the abuse of amphetamine or other addictive substances, such as the barbiturates. Depression may also occur secondary to a wide variety of medical illnesses—for example, viral infections, nutritional deficiencies, endocrine disorders, anemias, and such central nervous system disorders as multiple sclerosis, tumors, and cerebral vascular disease.

The depressions of the elderly are particularly complex because the differential diagnosis often involves organic brain damage and clinical depression. This diagnostic differentiation is complicated by the fact that persons with early signs of senile brain changes, vascular disease, or other neurological diseases associated with age may be more at risk for depressions.

Depression as a Syndrome

In clinical experience the majority of depressions do not occur in clear association with other medical or even psychiatric disorders, and it is on the primary depressions that the greatest attention is focused in both research and clinical practice. In practice, patients present with multiple symptoms, including the abnormal and persisting affective changes associated with feelings of worthlessness, guilt, helplessness and hopelessness, anxiety, crying, suicidal tendencies, loss of interest in work and other activities, impaired capacity to perform everyday social functions, and hypochondriasis, accompanied by such physical alterations as anorexia, weight change, constipation, psychomotor retardation or agitation, headache, and other bodily complaints. Even to the untrained observer, most depressive states are clearly seen as pathological by virtue of their intensity, pervasiveness, persistence, and interference with normal social and physiological functioning.

Not all patients have all the symptoms. But, although there is much individual variability, the variations are not infinite. The current trend is to regard the depressions as a heterogeneous group. Depression and the affective disorders are almost universally classified as symptom complexes or syndromes, rather than as single diseases like anemia, arthritis, or heart failure.

Bipolar-unipolar Distinction

The bipolar-unipolar distinction has achieved considerable rapid acceptance. This distinction separates depressed patients with a history of manic episodes (the bipolar group) from those patients who have had only recurrent episodes of depression (the unipolar group). One concept of unipolar allows for the inclusion of recurrent episodes that may not reach psychotic proportions.

When possible genetic factors were studied, patients with bipolar illness showed a far higher frequency of positive family history than did patients with only depressions. Psychopharmacological studies have also indicated differences in the responses of bipolar and unipolar patients to psychoactive drugs, especially lithium. Patients with bipolar disorders are more likely to develop hypomanic responses to dopa or to imipramine and other tricyclics.

Among the difficulties in applying the unipolar-bipolar affective illness distinction are the varying clinical criteria for the inclusion of depressions within the unipolar group. The criterion for bipolar affective disorders is clear—evidence of a current or past manic episode. It is unclear, however, if all episodes of depression are to be regarded as unipolar.

Psychotic-neurotic Dimension

For many decades, the validity of the distinction between psychotic and neurotic depressions was a major issue, but in recent years this distinction has lost its importance. The frequency with which a truly psychotic depression occurs has decreased greatly. When precise psychopathological criteria are used, psychotic depressions occur in only about 10 per cent of large mixed samples and in perhaps 25 per cent of hospitalized patients.

Furthermore, studies using multivariate statistical techniques have consistently failed to separate a neurotic group from a psychotic group. The neurotic-psychotic distinction appears to form a continuum of grades of severity. There are correlations with age, so that older patients tend to be more severely ill and more likely to show psychotic features than do patients whose psychotic manic-depressive or schizo-affective features occur in late adolescence or in young adulthood.

Endogenous-Reactive Continuum

Interest has revived in the endogenous-reactive continuum as a means of subdividing depressions, particularly those responsive to drug treatment. However, a number of problems have contributed to a shift away from the endogenous-reactive continuum. The criteria for the endogenous diagnosis are uncertain. Some clinicians require the symptom-cluster criteria and minimize the role of life events; others emphasize the history of life events, even if the characteristic symptom complex does not occur. Some require both criteria, and others are flexible in shifting criteria between symptom pattern and reactive events in accordance with clinical judgment.

The endogenous-reactive dichotomy represents a continuum, rather than a means of dividing patients into relatively clear-cut groups. Most patients appear to lie intermediate on the continuum; few are at the extremes.

Stress and Life Events as Precipitating Factors

An extensive literature has developed concerning the relation between stress, separation-loss, and other life events and the various syndromes of depression. In the period immediately before the onset of depression, life events of a variety of types occur with greater frequency among depressed patients than among matched control subjects.

It is not clear, however, whether this research has clearly established an exclusively environmental view of the causation of depression. At best, separation and loss account for only about 25 per cent of a large series of depressed patients. The majority of persons cope quite adequately, and only a small percentage of persons exposed to such stressful events as widowhood and serious illness do, in fact, develop depressions. One is forced to conclude that loss and separation are not universal before all depressions and that not all persons who experience loss and separation subsequently develop depressions. Moreover, loss and separation are not specific to clinical depression; rather, the evidence indicates that they often serve as the precipitating stimuli for a wide variety of clinical conditions, as often medical as

they are psychiatric. The conclusion seems inevitable that the clinical depressive state in adulthood, although it may follow on a life circumstance, has been the consequence of some attempt of coping. One must look for the factors within the persons that account for those who cope as contrasted with those who develop clinical symptomatic states.

Conclusion

The trend of all studies supports the view that the adult clinical state occurs in relation to the balance between the stresses on the person and some important consideration of vulnerability or predisposition. Environmental stress seems to play a role mainly in the timing and precipitation of the acute episode, but a purely environmentalistic view is incomplete. A major if not the most significant factor accounting for adult depression lies in the predisposition or vulnerability of the person. A number of alternative explanations have been proposed to account for these vulnerabilities. The explanations include genetically determined, hereditary predisposition, as supported by the unipolar-bipolar concept; early life experiences predisposing the person to sensitivity and loss, as proposed in a developmental psychodynamic model; and more recent behaviorist attempts to interpret depressive symptoms as failures of coping and rewards for self-esteem and hopelessness.

Although the depressive affect is clearly a part of human adaptation, psychiatrists dealing with adults often see the maladaptive response, rather than the successful one. Therapeutic efforts, therefore, are often directed at altering this balance by providing for increased capacity for persons to cope, whether with drugs or psychotherapeutic techniques or environmental manipulations, or by attempting to modify the impact of various stresses. Depression, then, is a final common pathway, a heterogeneous group of syndromes, with multiple causations.

REFERENCES

Akiskal, H. S., and McKinney, W. T. Depressive disorders: Toward a unified hypothesis. Science, *182:* 20, 1973.
Beck, A. T. Cognition and psychopathology. In *Depression: Clinical, Experimental, and Theoretical Aspects,* A. T. Beck, editor, p. 253, Harper & Row, New York, 1969.
Bibring, E. Mechanism of depression. In *Affective Disorders,*

P. Greenacre, editor, p. 13. International Universities Press, New York, 1953.

Katz, M. M. On the classification of depression: Normal, clinical, and ethnocultural variations. In *Depression in the 1970's*, R. Fieve, editor. p. 1. New York, 1970.

Klerman, G. L. Clinical research in depression. Am. J. Psychiatry, *24:* 305, 1971.

Klerman, G. L., and Barret, J. E. The affective disorders: Clinical and epidemiological aspects. In *Lithium: Its Role in Psychiatric Research and Treatment*, S. Gershon and B. Shopsin, editors, p. 201. Plenum Press, New York, 1973.

Schmale, A. The adaptive role of depression in health and disease. In *Separation and Depression*, J. P. Scott and E. C. Senay, editors, p. 187. George W. King Printing Co., Baltimore. 1973.

Scott, J. P., Stewart, J. M., and DeGhett, V. J. Separation in infant dogs: Emotional response and motivational consequences. In *Separation and Depression*, J. P. Scott and E. C. Senay, editors, p. 3. George W. King Printing Co., Baltimore, 1973.

Whybrow, P., and Parlatore, A. Melancholia, a model in madness: A discussion of recent psychobiologic research into depressive illness. Psychiatry, Med., *4:* 351, 1973.

Winokur, G. Clayton, P., and Reich, T. *Manic Depressive illness.* C. V. Mosby, St. Louis, 1969.

16.2   MANIC-DEPRESSIVE ILLNESS

Definition

Manic-depressive illnesses are fundamentally severe disorders of mood. The diagnosis is usually made in patients who have a history of an earlier affective psychosis or, in the absence thereof, where there has not been an obvious precipitating event or a different type of pre-existing illness. The patient with the manic type of the disorder characteristically displays elation or irritability, pressure of speech, flight of ideas, and increased motor activity. The patient with the depressed type displays the converse: depressed mood, mental and motor retardation, and agitation and feelings of apprehension. Classified as manic-depressive, circular type (either manic or depressed), are those who have at least one attack of both a depressive episode and a manic episode. Patients in whom manic and depressive symptoms appear almost simultaneously are diagnosed as having other major affective disorder. Manic-depressive illnesses of all types have a tendency to remission and recurrence, although a single illness is not rare, and they do not progress to a state of mental deterioration.

Recent research strongly indicates that this traditional grouping of manic-depressive psy-

choses may be in error. Clinical, genetic, drug response, and biochemical studies all suggest that patients who have had both a manic attack and a depressive attack (bipolar) differ significantly from those who have had only depressive episodes (unipolar).

Epidemiology

The incidence of manic-depressive illnesses appears to have decreased markedly in this century. In 1900, 17 per cent of all admissions to the Boston State Hospital and 37 per cent of admissions to the McLean Hospital were so diagnosed; in 1950, the figures were 8 per cent and 16 per cent, respectively. In 1951, there were 5,240 first admissions of manic-depressives to all United States state hospitals, 4,376 to private psychiatric hospitals, and 4,962 to general hospitals with psychiatric facilities. In 1963, the figures were 1,648 for the state and 1,761 for the private hospitals. Only discharge figures are available for the general hospitals; they show an increase to 6,335. The figures for 1970 have been compiled on a different basis. There were 69,339 admissions of manic-depressive patients to all United States inpatient and outpatient psychiatric services; this accounted for 3.5 per cent of all admissions, a rate of 52.5 per 100,000. In all classes of hospitals, women outnumber men; the ratio is roughly 3 to 2 in the state hospitals and 2 to 1 in the private and general hospitals.

The incidence of manic-depressive illnesses the world over has been commonly given as 3 to 4 per 1,000; it is said to be less in Scandinavia and northern Europe and somewhat higher in southern European countries. The Jews and the Irish are said to have a higher than average incidence and to recover from a degree of disorder that in others might be considered malignant. As is true for the United States, women are afflicted more than men, and—in sharp contradistinction to schizophrenia—the upper social classes more that the lower. In Kraepelin's series, 58 per cent of the first attacks occurred between the ages of 20 and 35; 35 per cent between 35 and 60. The manic form occurs primarily in younger persons, the depressed type in older persons. Compared with schizophrenic patients, a larger percentage of manic-depressives are married; and, also unlike schizophrenia, the marital status is not related to prognosis.

Causes

Hereditary Factors

Manic-depressive illness is overrepresented in the parents, siblings, and children of manic-depressive patients. Kraepelin found "taint from the side of the parents" in 36 per cent of his patients; when he considered only those patients who had repeated attacks, the figure rose to 45 per cent. Others give figures of about 10 per cent. Perhaps the most persuasive evidence comes from the studies of monozygotic and dizygotic twins. Kallman assembled his own findings with those of several others and gives an incidence of 20 to 25 per cent in siblings and nonidentical twins (a level much higher than in the general population), whereas identical twins are found to have incidence figures ranging from 66 to 96 per cent. He believed that the data support the concept of dependence on the effect of a single dominant gene with incomplete penetrance. Rosanoff, attempting to account for a higher incidence of the illness in women, suggested that the gene is sex-linked.

It now appears that, in contrast to unipolar patients, bipolar patients usually have an earlier age of onset, a different premorbid personality, and no apparent precipitating events before recurrences after their first illness. Bipolar patients, when depressed, appear less active and anxious and more withdrawn than the unipolar; the course of illness shows a greater tendency to relapse after age 45; their cortical evoked potentials show an augmenting pattern, as compared with a reducing pattern in the unipolar patients. There is also a different in drug response, with lithium being an effective antidepressant only in the bipolar patient.

Constitutional Factors

Folklore has long associated temperament with physique. Kretschmer elevated these notions to a scientific study in 1921 and reported a disproportionately large number of pyknic persons among those with manic-depressive psychosis specifically and more generally among those with a cyclothymic personality.

A wide range of etiological processes has been advanced, including dysfunctions of the endocrine system, diencephalic centers involved in affective expression, and processes that in lower animals are involved in hibernation, since the psychosis seems to occur more frequently in the spring.

Biological Factors

Attention has been directed to the autonomic nervous system, which appears to increase in some depressive states when psychological defenses fail.

Mood is a complex psychobiological state, and changes in mood must reflect changes in both physiological and psychological processes. The antidepressant drugs attracted interest not only because they favorably affect the course of depressive illness but also because they can be used as probes to explore biochemical mechanisms that may accompany or be responsible for the depressed behavior. The indoleamines and catecholamines are the major neurotransmitters in those areas of the brain that are concerned with emotional function. Monoamine oxidase inhibitors were found to exert an antidepressant effect. Therefore, it was proposed that depression is caused or accompanied by a decrease and elation by an increase in brain catecholamines. Lithium enhances the reuptake of amines and lowers the amount available at the synaptic cleft. Electric shock was found to increase norepinephrine levels.

Changes in the metabolism of the adrenal steroids have also been reported in depression. However, such changes occur in almost any condition of emotional arousal. Some changes in electrolyte, water, and carbohydrate metabolism have also been reported in depressed patients. There is suggestive evidence that there may be an impairment of the mechanism that excludes sodium from cells and a decrease in the rate of transfer of sodium from the blood to cerebrospinal fluid during an acute depressive attack. When electroshock therapy is given, only those patients who improve clinically show a return to normal. Lithium, which increases the uptake of norepinephrine into neuronal storages vesicles, also acts to decrease residual sodium.

Psychological and Psychodynamic Factors

Early writers called attention to the fact that most manic-depressive illnesses occurred in persons who were constitutionally of a depressive, manic, or cyclothymic temperament. The disease was believed to be simply an extreme swing in their characteristic behavior.

Freud indicated that, just as the bereaved mourns the loss of the loved one, the melancholic appears to mourn the loss of his own ego. He suggested that the depressed person, in withdrawing his libidinal attachment from the lost object, invests it in his own ego, rather than in another object. Part of this libidinal energy serves to establish an identification of the ego with the abandoned object; the remaining libido is reduced to sadism visited on the ego. This sadism originally would have been directed toward the depriving object with which the ego is now identified. Freud suggested that struggles between the superego and ego take the place of struggles between the ego and its ambivalently loved object. He believed that the reason the melancholic patient is so often arrogant and demanding, instead of ashamed and submissive, as he describes his unforgiveable sins and utter worthlessness is that these self-reproaches are really directed at the supposedly beloved object.

What had originally been considered as a turning away from objects is considered now as an object-relationship that has been impaired by regressive alteration in ego and superego functions. This regressive change serves as a defense against the development of disruptive anxiety in conflict situations. In the psychoanalytic literature generally, mania is viewed as a defense against melancholia.

Clinical Description

Manic-Depressive Illness, Manic Type

Some people are blessed with unquenchable gaiety and energy. They soon become the center of every group they join. They may be somewhat superficial but are nevertheless alert. They are the movers and doers of the world, never seem to doubt themselves, and only redouble their efforts if they are blocked in achieving their desires.

In hypomania these qualities become intensified. There is a classical triad of symptoms: elated but unstable mood, pressure of speech, and increased motor activity. The hypomanic talks easily, winningly, humorously, and endlessly. He is warm, then friendly, and then uninvitedly intimate and unwelcomely personal. He radiates good health. He is constantly on the go and never seems to tire. Only as one stays with him does one become aware of a distracti-

bility, of impatience and intolerance when his wish is not immediately gratified, of impulsive and ill-considered actions, of unseemly self-indulgence, and of his bland disregard of patent difficulties.

In acute mania all the foregoing manifestations are more intense and more disturbing. Propriety, convention, and discretion are painfully absent. The patient demands and attempts to command the center of the stage. He puns, teases, cracks jokes. His excessive good humor is transformed instantly to the most vicious anger if he is crossed or ignored. He is inconsiderate of others and disregards their needs, comfort, and rights. He is constantly on the go, moves quickly from one activity to another, and never finishes what he starts. His speech is like his movement; flight of ideas may proceed to clang associations and actual incoherence. He may burst into tears momentarily when he is faced with a realistic problem, but an instant later he is all smiles and miles away. Every impulse is expressed in words and, unless he is restrained, in action, too. There is loss of contact with reality, an inability to adhere to a line of thought and pursue it to its logical conclusion, and, frequently, what appears to be a delusion of wealth or of great power of both. The manic has no more control over his behavior than the schizophrenic, but he is not alienated to the same degree; it seems to be a case of denial and loss of normal inhibitions, without the deep disturbance of the sense of identity.

Delirious mania, is the most intense state of disturbance. It may develop gradually or may appear full-blown. All the previously mentioned symptoms may be present but in the most extreme form. The patient is totally out of contact, his speech is incoherent, and he is constantly and purposelessly active. Hallucinations and delusions are common; he may be incontinent of urine and feces. It is impossible to develop sustained contact with the patient, and, hence, one cannot gain his cooperation.

ABC, a professional man in his mid-30's, was admitted to the hospital in a state of excitement and hyperactivity that had been precipitated when Z a woman he had met just a week previously, refused to marry him. This was his fifth manic illness in 20 years. It had been preceded by a period of some concern over his relatively unsuccessful practice, but he had not manifested any marked degree of worry or depression.

The patient was the eldest of three sons. His father,

also educated to a profession, had gone instead into a business that he allowed to run down while he gambled and played cards. The mother, who had married at age 16 to get away from her family, was extremely bitter about the father, criticized him constantly in front of the children, and pushed all of them, but especially the patient, to ever higher levels of achievement. As a child, he exceeded the heavy demands placed upon him. At age 4, he could read the foreign language newspaper to his grandparents; at age 5, he knew every street in the large city in which he lived; at age 15, he graduated from high school at the top of his class. He was an outstanding golfer and, as a schoolboy, was invited to play at an exclusive country club where he was praised for his skills but not accepted socially. He was handsome, aggressive, excelled in physical and intellectual games, and was an unusually successful gambler.

His first illness occurred at age 17 in his second year in college. He had felt unaccepted by his classmates and then suddenly became overactive and convinced that he was to be invited to compete in a golf match with Bobby Jones. He was cared for at home for 2 months during which time the excitement subsided. He then returned to finish college and professional school without incident. His next illness was precipitated by his father's sudden death when the patient was 25; this time, he spent 2 months in a small private hospital, where he made a rapid recovery. However, there were two more recurrences, one at age 27, the other at age 29, during both of which he was treated at a local state hospital. On the last occasion, after 3 months of moderately hyperactive behavior, the excitement and aggressivity slowly diminished. One day, he persuaded a new attendant that he had grounds privileges, made his way into town, called his mother, and dared her to get him readmitted if she could. He got in touch with a lawyer friend and enlisted his aid in threatening a suit against the hospital. His mother and siblings made no effort to get him readmitted, and the case was never brought to trial. He improved on the outside and appeared to make a reasonable adjustment until his current attack.

On this admission to the hospital, he was examined by the female doctor serving as admitting officer that day. When he was prepared for the physical examination, his gown was removed and a sheet placed over the lower part of his body. He immediately discarded the sheet, looked at the physician in a sly way, and asked whether it disturbed her to examine him in the nude. Throughout the examination, there was push of speech. He was irritable, sarcastic, and boastful. As the doctor was leaving the room, he asked, "What did you say your name is?" She replied, "Dr. D." He asked three more times and each time she said "D." He then said, "I hope you get the significance and moral of this story. Freud just sent me a message about this. When I was in professional school, one of the professors taught me at least one thing—when someone asks your name, reply "John Jones" not "Mr. Jones." What is your name?" She replied "D" once more and left.

During the first month in the hospital, the patient was extremely overtalkative and irritable. He was frequently threatening toward other patients and hospital personnel; occasionally combative and always grandiose, demanding, and sarcastic. He gradually became more subdued, cooperative, and friendly, and described some of the thoughts and impulses that impelled him during the manic period. When Z refused to marry him, he had been transiently depressed and discouraged, but then suddenly realized that, in some mysterious way, he had undergone a change for the better. He found himself vividly recalling experiences, ideas, and even things he had learned in school that he had not thought of for many years. He seemed to be able to reason more promptly and with greater effect. He made decisions rapidly, felt more at ease in social contacts, and supremely self-confident. He developed energies to a degree he had not thought possible for him; he felt as if he could work for hours on end without a trace of fatigue. Whereas in days gone by he might forget an idea or an errand simply in walking across a room, he now found that if he forgot the original idea, a dozen better ones would come to mind, and he could follow them out without stopping to think of the original thought that had temporarily escaped him—and anyway that thought would return in time so he never actually lost it.

His family insisted on sending him into a hospital, although, at the time, he did not feel that he was ill and would very much have preferred going to the seashore. But since he was being sent to a hospital, he decided he would make a vacation out of the experience, and since he was in a mental hospital, he would act like a mental patient should act. He had recently read a magazine article that explained that mental patients regained their health by reliving infantile experiences, and in that way removed the inhibitions and feelings of inferiority these experiences had formed in their personality structures. His own ability to do this would be facilitated by the fact that his sensory perceptions were so intense that he could feel and experience everything to a degree never before possible.

He had hoped to find quiet and peace in the hospital, but it proved instead to be a place where doors slammed, beds squeaked, keys grated, patients shouted, and all was hubbub and confusion. Even at night he had no peace since the nurses insisted on keeping the green light on in his room. Because of his sensory perceptions, these stimuli seemed to be multiplied 100-fold, and he decided that he might as well begin his experiments in infantile memory. First he worked on the feelings of inferiority that had been ingrained in him by painful childhood experiences. A group of attendants had decided to give him a pack; as they rolled him into the sheets they touched each of the scars on his body. As they touched each scar, he would recall the episode during which that particular injury had been inflicted and he could almost literally feel the fear due to that experience dropping away from him and leaving him more free. By the time the attendants had touched each of the scars, he was quite free of fear of men, and gave a very good account of himself in the struggle that followed.

He was able to give similar accounts of much of his behavior during the period of manic excitement, which he now looked upon as an effort to cope with the disappointment and temporary discouragement about his relative lack of professional and, to a degree, interpersonal success. Eleven weeks after admission, he was discharged to return home and to work.

Manic-Depressive Illness, Depressed Type

Some people almost always appear somber, quiet, and withdrawn. Somehow, one never quite knows what to say to them; they are invariably polite and briefly responsive to overtures, but they never take the lead, and every conversational gambit seems to die. They are good people, sincere and earnest; they are not without compassion but are moved more easily to tears than to laughter. One gains the impression that they are competent and reliable, but they never seek responsibility and would rather be followers than leaders.

In simple retardation, these qualities become intensified, there is a classical triad of symptoms: depressed mood, difficulty in thinking, and psychomotor retardation. The patient appears dejected and cheerless; everything he says and does is with effort. His expression is dull, he is careworn and bent over, his every move is painfully slow. There is no spontaneity. He speaks only in response to questions and even then answers in a word, not a sentence. He says that everything is hopeless, that he is a disgrace to his family. His appetite is poor. His sleep is restless, and he awakens early each morning, feeling worse than he did when he went to bed. He thinks he should end it all, and suicide is a real danger; he may kill his children, too, to spare them disgrace and the agony of life. However, there is no disorientation or intellectual defect.

Some patients have multiple and persistent somatic complaints. They continue to work but find it difficult to get things done. They cannot read or look at television but find their thoughts turning to their continual discomfort. Careful examination reveals no physical basis for the complaints. There may be a history of a similar episode previously for which the patient could get no help, but it finally passed off after several months. The patient may give a history of an earlier frank depressive attack or of depressive illness in the family. Here, too, suicide is a danger, which makes it doubly imperative that the patient be recognized as having a depressive illness and not an episode of neurotic hypochondriasis.

Acute depression may follow either of the two states described above, or it may develop suddenly. All the symptoms already mentioned are present in more intense form. The patient looks utterly hopeless and deeply dejected. He feels that he has committed unforgivable sins, has brought disgrace on the family, and is responsible for every disaster or misfortune that has befallen them. Not only has he been evil in the past, but everything he does now serves only to spread destruction. He falls asleep readily but awakens in a few hours; frightening dreams are common. His appetite is poor, constipation is marked, and there is considerable weight loss. (See Figure 1.) He feels that he has no insides, that he is stopped up with feces and other corruption, that he will rot away, that he is foul and disgusting. Suicide is an ever-present danger.

Manic-Depressive Illness, Circular Type

In this disorder, there is at least one attack of mania and one of depression; there may often be a brief period of normality as the patient passes

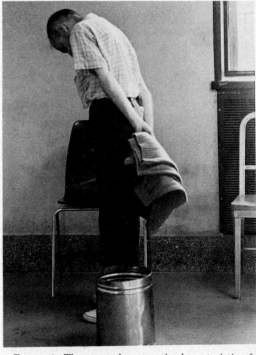

FIGURE 1. The stooped posture is characteristic of this hospitalized depressed patient. (Courtesy of Chris Maynard for Magnum Photos, Inc.)

in either direction from one state to the other, but, in many instances, the transition may occur without such a normal interval.

Other Major Affective Disorders

In some patients the symptoms of mania and depression occur simultaneously. The patient displays a mixture of the signs and symptoms usually present in only one phase of the illness.

Differential Diagnosis

There is no difficulty in establishing the diagnosis of acute mania or acute depression; however, the majority of patients are not so easily placed in a diagnostic pigeonhole. Family history, developmental experiences, temperamental characteristics, and the onset and development of the illness, including all behavioral and physical symptoms, must be thoroughly reviewed.

In recent years, considerable effort has been directed toward the development of criteria that would enable both researchers and clinicians to differentiate manic-depressive illness from other psychiatric disorders more accurately. One noteworthy attempt to create a reliable classification system is the St. Louis diagnostic criteria, first published by Feighner and his associates in 1972. Using formal inclusion and exclusion criteria (see Table I), the diagnostic framework presented by the St. Louis group represents an attempt to increase the reliability and validity of psychiatric differential diagnosis. It has served as a point of departure for other workers, who, like Spitzer and his colleagues, have modified the initial St. Louis criteria. It has also influenced the classification system used in Diagnostic Statistical Manual III.

Somatic Disease

Subclinical or clearly established physical disease may be accompanied by severe depressive symptoms that override the manifestations of the primary process. Depressed mood and apathy or excitement and irritability may be found in hypertensive cardiovascular disease, uremia, various intracranial lesions, psychomotor epilepsy, toxic deliriums, drug intoxications, and drug withdrawal states. Conversely, the first symptoms of depression may be a variety of somatic complaints.

Schizophrenia

This condition may begin with a disorder of mood and continue to present such prominent affective features that the ultimate diagnosis may be schizophrenia, schizo-affective type. However, the manic-depressive usually relates fairly easily to others but in a dependent fashion; he often describes incidents or periods in which there were notable mood swings; he commonly has feelings of guilt and inadequacy; and he shows many of the characterological features of the obsessional neurotic. On the other hand, the schizophrenic has usually been more reserved, remote, and self-contained; his affective responses have appeared to others shallow or even inappropriate; there may have been feelings of strangeness, of bizarre inner alterations, or of sudden enlightenment in which the incomprehensible became clear to him and he became incomprehensible to others. The schizophrenic illness often starts with a period of panic and dissociation, the manic-depressive attack commonly with a depressive mood swing. The therapist often feels fairly close rapport with the manic-depressive in his early interviews and only later begins to experience the patients clinging, wearing, insensitive, limpetlike attachment to him. The schizophrenic patient is more difficult to understand; one may sense a barrier between himself and the patient that cannot be crossed.

Psychotic Depressive Reaction

This disorder is characterized by severely depressed mood, misinterpretation of reality, and, on occasion, delusions and hallucinations. The patient is distinguished from the manic-depressive primarily by the fact that his illness seems to follow immediately a clear-cut precipitating event. He is usually not given to self-reproach but blames others or fate and is quite demanding in attitude. Often, he can be diverted for brief periods but then resumes his depressive complaints. He is not described as having been of a manic-depressive temperament before the illness.

Involutional Melancholia

This disorder has most of the clinical characteristics of acute depression except that instead of displaying psychomotor retardation, the patient is apprehensive, anxious, and agitated. He

Primary affective disorders

Depression: "A" through "C" are required for a diagnosis of depression:

A. Dysphoric mood accompanied by such subjective symptoms as:
   1. Depression
   2. Sadness
   3. The blues
   4. Despondency
   5. Hopelessness
   6. Feeling down in the dumps
   7. Irritability
   8. Fear
   9. Worry
   10. Discouragement
B. At least five of the following criteria are required for a diagnosis of *definite* depression; at least four are required for a diagnosis of *probable* depression:
   1. Poor appetite or weight loss of two pounds in one week, or 10 pounds or more in one year without dieting
   2. Sleep disorder, such as insomnia or hypersomnia
   3. Loss of energy, as noted by fatigability or tiredness
   4. Agitation or retardation
   5. Loss of interest in usual activities or decrease in sexual drive
   6. Feelings of self-reproach or guilt, sometimes of delusional proportions
   7. Complaint of or actual diminished ability to think or concentrate, as shown by slow thinking or mixed-up thoughts
   8. Recurrent thoughts of death or suicide, including thoughts of wishing to be dead
C. A psychiatric illness lasting at least one month with no pre-existing psychiatric conditions, such as:
   1. Schizophrenia
   2. Anxiety neurosis
   3. Phobic neurosis
   4. Obsessive-compulsive neurosis
   5. Hysteria
   6. Alcoholism
   7. Drug dependency
   8. Antisocial personality
   9. Sexual orientation disturbance (homosexuality)
   10. Sexual deviation
   11. Mental retardation
   12. Organic brain syndrome
   The presence of a life-threatening or incapacitating illness preceding and paralleling the depression should preclude the making of a diagnosis of primary depression.

Mania: "A" through "C" are required for a diagnosis of mania:

A. Euphoria or irritability
B. A minimum of three of the following symptom categories must also be present:
   1. Hyperactivity, including motor activity, social activity, and sexual activity
   2. Push of speech—the pressure to keep talking
   3. Flight of ideas—racing thoughts
   4. Grandiosity, sometimes of delusional proportions
   5. Decreased sleep
   6. Distractibility
C. A psychiatric illness lasting at least two weeks with no pre-existing psychiatric conditions, such as:
   1. Schizophrenia

TABLE I—*Continued*

2. Anxiety neurosis
3. Phobic neurosis
4. Obsessive-compulsive neurosis
5. Hysteria
6. Alcoholism
7. Drug dependency
8. Antisocial personality
9. Sexual orientation disturbance (homosexuality)
10. Sexual deviation
11. Mental retardation
12. Organic brain syndrome

Secondary affective disorders

Definite or probable secondary depression is defined in the same way as primary depression, except that it occurs with one of the following:
A pre-existing nonaffective psychiatric illness that may or may not still be present
A life-threatening or incapacitating medical illness that precedes and parallels the symptoms of depression

Schizophrenia

"A" through "C" are required for a diagnosis of schizophrenia:
A. Both of the following must be reported:
   1. A chronic illness with at least six months of symptoms before the initial evaluation without return to the premorbid level of psychosocial adjustment
   2. Absence of a period of depressive or manic symptoms sufficient to qualify for affective disorder or probable affective disorder
B. At least one of the following must be noted:
   1. Delusions or hallucinations *without* significant perplexity or disorientation associated with them
   2. Verbal production that makes communication difficult because of a lack of logical or understandable organization. If a patient is mute, this diagnostic decision must be deferred.
Affect: Patients with schizophrenia have a characteristic blunted or inappropriate affect. When it occurs in mild form, interrater agreement is difficult to achieve. Blunted affect occurs rarely or not at all in the absence of B-1 or B-2.
C. At least three of the following factors must be present for a diagnosis of *probable* schizophrenia:
   1. Unmarried
   2. Poor premorbid social adjustment or work history
   3. Family history of schizophrenia
   4. Absence of alcoholism or drug abuse within one year of onset of psychosis
5. Onset of illness before age 40

---

* Adapted from J. P. Feighner, E. Robins, S. B. Guze, R. A. Woodroff, G. Winokur, and R. Munoz. Diagnostic criteria for use in psychiatric research. Arch. Gen. Psychiat., *26:* 57, 1972.

describes himself as compulsive but gives no history of mood swings. The illness develops during the involutional period. Care must be taken to establish the absence of somatic disease, which is common at this time of life. It is rare for a first true manic-depressive illness to occur in the involutional period.

Neuroses

These disorders are often accompanied by depressive symptoms, and, conversely, depressive attacks may be accompanied by complaints of neurasthenia, anxiety, or obsessive-compulsive manifestations. Neuroses, on the whole, show a variable and irregular course; the clinical features tend to be changeable and are more responsive to external stimuli; phobias, feelings of depersonalization, anxiety, and apprehensiveness may come and go; feelings of extreme guilt and worthlessness are not commonly present. The neurotic patient is more subjectively than objectively depressed, and is easily aroused to action.

Prognosis

Rennie found that the average first manic attack lasted 3½ months, the average first depressive attack 6½ months; the shortest first attack was 3 days, the longest 36 months, except for one case of chronic mania that persisted for 24 years. Up to age 45, recurrent attacks are of approximately the same duration; after 45, they grow definitely longer. The manifest depth of the psychosis was apparently unrelated either to the speed or degree of recovery.

Treatment

There are two important facts to keep in mind regarding the manic-depressive patient. The first is the ever-present danger of suicide, which must always be guarded against, particularly when the patient is going into or apparently coming out of a psychotic episode. The second is that the prognosis for any individual attack is relatively good; hence, an attitude of conservative optimism is warranted.

Hospitalization

If the patient is in a state of acute mania or acute depression, hospitalization is imperative. In simple retardation or hypomania, one may decide to try ambulatory treatment. The items to be considered are the history, the current status, the nature of the patient's interpersonal relations, and the patient-doctor relationship.

Electroconvulsive therapy (ECT)

ECT has been widely used as a specific symptomatic treatment for the depressive attack. Usually, there is dramatic improvement after one or two treatments, and a course of six or nine, given two or three times weekly over a 3- or 4-week period, suffices for most patients who respond favorably. It is used less successfully and less often as a treatment for the manic attack. ECT is most effective in the treatment of involutional melancholia and endogenous depressions, and it is relatively ineffective or may have an adverse effect in anxiety states.

Many psychiatrists believe that ECT should be used with caution and only after other therapeutic approaches have been given a trial. It is, however, the treatment of choice for the middle-aged, agitated patient who is frankly suicidal. In every case it produces transient mental impairment and in rare instances may result in severe memory loss and other defects in intellectual function. Many psychotherapists believe that, when the depressed patient finds himself suddenly relieved of symptoms, he quickly represses conflicts and actively avoids consideration of the situational and experiential factors that may have played a significant role in the development of the illness.

Drug and Electrolyte Therapy

The monoamine oxidase inhibitors (iproniazid, phenelzine, isocarboxazid, tranylcypromine, and pargyline), particularly the tricyclic antidepressants (imipramine, amitriptyline, and doxepine, which are all tertiary amines, and desipramine, nortriptyline, and protriptylene, which are secondary amines), have all been found to be effective in the treatment of depressed patients and to have the additional advantage of maintaining experiential continuity. There is no amnesia or confusion, as there is after ECT.

Lithium salts have proved effective in the treatment of mania and hypomania; there have been dramatic improvements in as few as 4 days, and patients on maintenance therapy have gone for several years without a recurrence. In patients with bipolar disease, it has also proved effective as prophylaxis against the recurrence of depression.

Psychotherapy

For the majority of patients, the psychotherapist aims to offer support and protection during the attack and then to examine customary patterns of interacting with others with a view toward helping the patient make more effective use of his capacities but not to alter his fundamental personality patterns in any essential way. In some patients in whom psychological factors appear to be importantly involved in the genesis or perpetuation of the illness, the patient and physician may decide on a far-reaching effort to bring about a personality change. The major part of the therapeutic work must be done during a period of remission, but it is desirable to lay the groundwork during the psychotic episode.

Establishing and maintaining a therapeutic relationship is difficult with the depressive because he has detached himself from others, has temporarily lost the capacity to relate to them, and is turned in upon himself. The manic, on the other hand, is hyperactive and distractible; he does not stop long enough to do more than barely recognize the existence of another person. The therapist must be active with both depressive and manic patients, and the type of activity—support, reassurance, challenge, annoyance, scolding, uncritical acceptance—must be tailored to the immediate situation and to the stage of the developing relationship.

During the psychotic episode it is important to vary the length of the interview in accordance with the patient's clinical state at the time. Underactive, retarded patients should be seen relatively briefly, so that they are not made to feel that they fall short of an expected standard. Productive depressive and manic patients should be seen regularly for set periods, even though for long intervals it may seem that nothing they say is new or important. A varied program of activity and rest should be prescribed for both manics and depressives.

As the therapeutic relationship develops and the patient improves, he comes to see the physician as a friendly and powerful supportive figure. In this setting, which provides gratification of some of the patient's dependent wishes, one may review with him his relationships and needs with a view to making common-sense alterations in certain poor habit patterns, modifying his compulsiveness, and making more creative use of his assets.

In intensive analytical therapy, the developing dependent relationship to the physician is not used to gratify the patient's desire for love. Rather, it is pointed out to him as an example of how he builds his self-esteem on the approval of others, instead of basing it on the exercise of his own considerable capacity for substantial achievement. The patient gradually comes to an understanding of some of the forces that impel him to this repetitious, self-belittling behavior.

REFERENCES

Baldessarini, R. J., and Lipinski, J. F. Lithium salts, 1970–1975. Ann. Int. Med., *83:* 527, 1975.
Davis, J. M., Janowsky, D. S., and El-Yousef, M. K. The use of lithium in clinical psychiatry. Psychiatr. Ann., *3:* 78, 1973.
Feighner, J. P., Robins, E., Guze, S. B., Woodruff, R. A.,
Winokur, G., and Munoz, R. Diagnostic criteria for use in psychiatric research. Arch. Gen. Psychiat., *26:* 57, 1972.
Goodwin, F. K., and Bunney, W. E., Jr. A psychobiological approach to affective illness. Psychiatr. Ann., *3:* 19, 1973.
Kraepelin, E. *Manic-Depressive Insanity and Paranoia.* G. M. Robertson, editor. E. and S. Livingstone, Edinburgh, 1921.
Murphy, D. L., Goodwin, F. K., and Bunney, W. E., Jr. A reevaluation of biogenic amines in manic and depressive states. Hosp. Prac., *7:* 85, 1972.
Prange, A. J., Jr. The use of drugs in depression: Its theoretical and practical basis. Psychiatr. Ann., *3:* 19, 1973.
Schildkraut, J. J. *Neuropsychopharmacology and the Affective Disorders.* Little, Brown, Boston, 1970.
Spitzer, R. L., Endicott, J., and Robins, E. Clinical criteria for psychiatric diagnosis and DSM-III. Am. J. Psychiat., *132:* 1189, 1975.
Williams, T. A., Katz, M. M., and Shield, J. A., Jr., editors. Recent advances in the psychobiology of depressive illness: Proceedings of a workshop sponsored by the National Institute of Mental Health. Department of Health, Education, and Welfare Publ. No. 70-9053. United States Government Printing Office, Washington, 1972.
Winokur, G. Diagnostic and genetic aspects of affective illness. Psychiatr. Ann., *3:* 6, 1973.

16.3.   INVOLUTIONAL MELANCHOLIA

Introduction

Involutional melancholia is classified in the second edition of the American Psychiatric Association's Diagnostic and Statistical Manual of Mental Disorders (DSM-II) under Major affective disorders, the group of psychoses described as being "characterized by a single disorder of mood, either extreme depression or elation, that dominates the mental life of the patient and is responsible for whatever loss of contact he has with his environment. The onset of the mood does not seem to be related directly to a precipitating life experience and therefore is distinguishable from *Psychotic depressive reaction* and *Depressive neurosis.*"

Involutional melancholia is described this way in DSM-II: "This is a disorder occurring in the involutional period and characterized by worry, anxiety, agitation, and severe insomnia. Feelings of guilt and somatic preoccupations are frequently present and may be of delusional proportions. This disorder is distinguishable from *Manic-depressive illness* (q.v.) by the absence of previous episodes; it is distinguished from *Schizophrenia* (q.v.) in that impaired testing is due to a disorder of mood; and it is distinguished from *Psychotic depressive reac-*

tion (q.v.) in that the depression is not due to some life experience. Opinion is divided as to whether this psychosis can be distinguished from the other affective disorders. It is, therefore, recommended that involutional patients not be given this diagnosis unless all other affective disorders have been ruled out."

Epidemiology

Life expectancy has steadily increased during this century, and it follows that more people are reaching and living through the involutional years. Logically, there should be an increase in the number of cases of involutional melancholia reported. Factually, however, there has been a diminution in incidence, as revealed by statistical studies. It may be that diagnostic criteria are not sufficiently defined to distinguish involutional melancholia from other disorders appearing in that age group. Rosenthal emphasizes that the syndrome has become uncommon because patients receive treatment early in the illness, and the classical involutional patterns that require years to develop never have time to do so.

Kielholz found that women have a higher incidence of involutional melancholia than do men, by a ratio of 3 to 1. It is more prevalent in women between 51 and 60 years of age and in men between 61 and 65 years; the onset in women is usually from 3 to 7 years after menopause.

Frumkin found the incidence of involutional melancholia to be higher in persons from low-income and low-prestige groups than in professional and semiprofessional persons. Formal education was inversely related to occurrence of the condition, as was the degree of family organization, with a higher incidence among widows and divorced persons.

The epidemiological factors that have generally been associated with involutional melancholia are not unique to that diagnosis but are characteristic of the psychiatric population in the involutional age range (see Table I). Minority ethnic groups are relatively less evident in the psychiatric population during the involutional years. This fact suggests that problems of the involutional period may have greater personal significance in the social context of white America, where competition and achievement have been more central concerns.

Causes

Little is known about the cause of involutional melancholia. For many years, hormone replacement therapy was used extensively in treating the female involutional melancholia patient, but research studies have demonstrated that the symptoms and course of involutional melancholia are not influenced by estrogenic preparations. General body decline, changing nutritional requirements, alteration in the neuroendocrine and metabolic activities, a changing way of life, and a different outlook for the future do not precipitate or cause involutional melancholia.

The menopausal years, with the woman's mixed feelings about the cessation of menstruation, have many cultural implications. The phenomenon is associated with loss of the ability to bear children and a threatened loss of personal warmth, sexual desire, and physical attractiveness. Middle age is the period when her children leave home for college, employment, or marriage. An emotional void results for the housewife and mother who has devoted her life to the family and has failed to establish suitable substitutes. Even the presence of a retired husband, if he interferes with her routine, is sufficient to generate poorly controlled aggressiveness and can help precipitate involutional melancholia.

Men equate failing potency with loss of virility, youthful zest, and the best attributes of manhood. Many men approaching the climacteric have a fear of the loss of normal sexual activity. Likewise, the middle-age man is aware of competition by more youthful men. If he is further deflated by retirement, loss of a job and loss of financial independence and prestige may result in an abrupt realization that the social and economic goals of earlier years will never be realized and may constitute enough additional stress to crumble the personality defenses.

The most traumatic experience for both men and women is the death of a spouse, close relative, or dear friend. The separation is doubly important if the lost one fulfilled a supervisory role or gave economic support.

Occasionally, physical trauma, mutilating surgery, or a minor surgical procedure, such as pelvic surgery in women, has precipitated the illness. Chronic and disabling medical disorders may precipitate the illness in a predisposed personality.

TABLE I

Significant Findings Relative to Age Differences in a Psychiatric Population

Demographic and Social History

Age. Primary epidemiological variable defining involutional period.

Race. Increase in relative frequency of white majority ethnic group in involutional period and after.

Sex. Increase in relative frequency of women in the 30 to 39 age decade, with somewhat lower but still increased frequency in the 40 to 59 age range. Greatest relative frequency in men occurred in the youngest and the oldest age groups.

Education. Increased frequency of low educational achievement in the 40 to 59 age range, with relative frequencies of higher educational achievement increased in both younger and older groups.

Work. Increased relative frequency of self-employed and professional or managerial employment in the involutional age range and beyond. Increased relative frequency of skilled occupations in the 30 to 49 age range.

Current marital status. Increased relative frequency of divorced and widowed in the involutional age range, with further increase in widowed in later years.

Divorce history. Increased relative frequency of history of multiple divorces in the involutional age range. Also increased relative frequency of widowed and remarried.

Children. Increased relative frequency of large families among patients in the involutional age range.

Alcohol. Increased relative frequency of alcohol problems in the involutional age range.

Religious involvement. Increased relative frequency of positive and strong positive religious attitudes in the involutional age range and further increase in later years.

Work attitude. Highest relative frequency of excessive involvement with work among involutional-age patients.

Precipitating Factors

Marital conflict. Highest relative frequency in the 30 to 39 decade, decreasing with age.

Separation or divorce (precipitating factor). Highest relative frequency in the 30 to 39 decade, decreasing with age.

Death of loved one. Increased relative frequency in involutional years, further increase in later years.

Social relationships. Decreasing relative frequency with age; highest in youngest age groups.

Work problems. Highest relative frequency in patients of involutional age, considerably lower both earlier and later.

Alcohol (precipitating factor). Highest relative frequency in the 40 to 49 decade, decreasing relative frequency after age 60.

Drug abuse (precipitating factor). Highest relative frequency in youngest age groups, and lowest relative frequency in the involutional age range.

Focal Problem Areas

Marital problems. Highest relative frequency in the 30 to 49 age range, decreasing frequency thereafter.

Socialization problems. Highest relative frequency in the youngest age groups, relatively lower in the involutional period.

Behavior problems. Highest relative frequency in the youngest age groups, relatively lower in the involutional period.

Alcohol problems. Highest relative frequency in the involutional age group, next highest in the 30 to 39 decade.

Drug abuse. Highest relative frequency in the youngest age group, rare in the involutional age range.

Physical problems. Highest relative frequency in the involutional age range.

Sexual problems. Decreasing relative frequency as focal problem in the involutional period.

Phenomenological Characteristics (Outpatients)

Somatic concern. Highest relative frequency in the involutional age group.

Anxiety. Highest relative frequency in the younger involutional age group.

Emotional withdrawal. Highest relative frequency in the youngest age groups, lower in the involutional period.

Conceptual disorganization. Highest relative frequency in the oldest age group.

Guilt feelings. Highest relative frequency in the 20 to 39 age range, lower in involutional period and later.

Tension. Highest relative frequency in the youngest and early involutional age groups, lower relative frequency after age 50.

Depressive mood. Highest relative frequency in the involutional period.

Hostility. Highest relative frequency in the younger age groups, lower in the involutional age range and older.

Suspiciousness. Highest relative frequency in the younger age group.

Motor retardation. Highest relative frequency in the older involutional age group, 50 years and over.

Uncooperativeness. Highest relative frequency in younger age groups, lower in involutional period and later.

TABLE I—*Continued*

Disorientation. Highest relative frequency in the oldest age group, 60 years and over.	*Extrapunitiveness.* More frequent than in psychotic depressive reactions, comparable to schizophrenic reaction, paranoid type.
Phenomenological Characteristics (Inpatients)	*Intropunitiveness.* Slightly less frequent than in psychotic depressive reactions.
Mental disorganization. More frequent than in psychotic depressive reactions.	*Depressive mood.* Comparable to psychotic depressive reactions, and more prominent than in schizophrenic reactions.
Mental distortion. More frequent than in psychotic depressive reactions.	
Bizarre motor behavior. More frequent than in psychotic depressive reactions.	*Anxiety-Tension.* Comparable to psychotic depressive reactions, and more prominent than in schizophrenic reactions.
Motor retardation. Comparable to psychotic depressive reactions.	

Certain types of premorbid personalities are susceptible to the impact of the involutional period—obsessive-compulsive personality, schizoid personality, and hysterical personality. The obsessive-compulsive personality has the greatest predisposition to develop involutional melancholia. Analysis of individual case histories of the obsessive-compulsive personality reveals a childhood filled with unusual anxiety and early insecurity. The home atmosphere was tense, frugality was practiced, and the parents were rigid in discipline. The child had difficulty with interpersonal relations. As an adult, such a person possesses a wealth of strong reaction formations and other personality defense mechanisms to enable him to make a well-concealed, neurotic adjustment to life. This personality has more early life successes than failures; hence, he is more threatened by a decline in ability or possible loss of position.

Psychological hypotheses that attempt to explain the predisposition to psychotic depression in midlife are drawn chiefly from the field of psychoanalysis. The predisposition is related to an alleged inherited capacity to react with intense hate to deprivations in infancy; it is also related to the specific defenses that stabilize the ego up to the point of decompensation. From a psychoanalytic point of view, the significant early deprivations occur during the oral and anal developmental phases. During these periods, the infant experiences the mothering person as both a gratifying and a frustrating object who engenders in him feelings of love and hate. If repeated frustrations overshadow those of gratification, cumulative disappointments and primitive hate felt toward the mother result in the feeling that he is not loved enough or at all. The discharge of tensions associated with

hate through bodily behavior—crying, biting, constipation, or diarrhea—signals the infant's hurt and needfulness. As development proceeds, the nonverbal and verbal mechanisms for the discharge of hate are influenced by the child's perception of the attitudes of the significant others.

In Western culture, forbidding attitudes prevail, permitting only indirect expressions of hostility. These forbidding attitudes are mentally incorporated by the child and serve as internal controls for his destructive impulses. They take the form of what are later noted clinically as premorbid personality traits: schizoid, depressive, obsessive-compulsive, phobic, paranoid and hysterical.

The personal histories of those who present themselves in midlife for the first time in a psychotic depression indicate that their prepsychotic state of equilibrium has been rigidly maintained through the use of one or more of the personality traits. When these traits fail, the patients may be overwhelmed by a sense of irreparable loss or failure to achieve vital personal, social, sexual, and vocational goals.

Clinical Features

Involutional melancholia most often has a prodromal period that varies from a few weeks to 2 or 3 years. Occasionally, there is a sudden or even fulminating onset in response to some major precipitating event. When the onset is gradual, anxiety and apprehension are the core of the prodrome. The patient develops insomnia and feelings of inner tension; he experiences easy mental and physical fatigability, and the waning of biological drives produces loss of sexual desire and loss of appetite for food. Apprehension is followed by worry about personal health. A classical tension headache plagues most patients and is described as constant during the waking hours.

Gradually, the course of illness becomes an extension of apprehension into despondency, with weeping, loss of interest in activities, preoccupation with trifles, inability to make decisions, worsening of the insomnia, weight loss, and multiple somatic complaints. (See Figure 1.) The deepening depression may be intermixed with periods of anger and peevishness, with the early restlessness turning into extreme motor agitation.

Guilt is so prominent that patients berate themselves from unimportant transgressions of the past and believe that they have committed the unpardonable sins. Predictions of some horrible but justified personal fate are accompanied by signs of extreme fearfulness. Self-accusation and self-condemnation progress to the point of desiring relief through death. Suicidal preoccupation, with thoughts of just not waking up in the morning, is common in the prodromal period and become more persistent as the illness progresses. Suicide is a threat at all times. The presence of illusions and hallucinations should raise suspicions of an associated early organic brain disease.

The sensorium is clear, but inattention, difficulty in concentration, and poverty of ideation are seen. Retention and recall, recent and remote memory, and grasp of general information are in keeping with premorbid attainments. There is a loss of abstract thinking ability, and insight is lacking (see Table II).

Mrs. N.M., age 69, a grandmother, was hospitalized in the spring of 1955 at her husband's insistence. The onset of her illness was 4 years before. She was one of seven children; her father lived to be 98 years old; her mother died of cerebrovascular accident at age 68. Neither her parents nor her siblings had ever had a psychiatric illness. Her early home life was happy; she was always ambitious and perfectionistic. She attended college for a year before her marriage at age 21; she had three healthy married daughters. Her general health had been good, with no prior "nerve trouble." Her marriage was happy until the onset of her illness, when she began to worry about her physical health; she was convinced she had stomach trouble and consulted numerous physicians seeking verification. Gradually, she became irascible, demanding, and even whiningly childish. After 4 years, she was referred to a psychiatric service.

On mental status examination, she was tearful and restless; she slept poorly and complained of constant nausea, loss of appetite, and gradual loss of

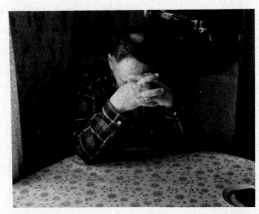

FIGURE 1. Depression is often characterized by feelings that life is no longer worth living. (Courtesy of Roger Malloch for Magnum Photos, Inc.)

weight. She said that her bowels had not moved for months and must be rotten, "and I feel miserable all over," and repetitiously repeated that there was nothing to live for since her grandson whom they cared for, was taken by his mother. She felt hopeless and said, "Nothing can be done for me." Her sensorium was clear. Except for marked weight loss, her physical examination and routine laboratory tests were normal. Her husband said her persistent complaining had driven him to distraction. They lived in a house on the grounds of their floral nursery. Her husband related: "Recently we walked out on our porch as the sun was rising. Our nursery stock was blooming magnificently. I commented about it to her. She replied, 'Everything is dead; it has shriveled.' My prayer was answered, for I knew she was *sick*, not just *mean*." Her response to electroshock was excellent. At Christmas, her psychiatrist received a sack of pecans with a note that she was well and keeping house, and both were contented.

This is a classical case of involutional melancholia as described by Kraepelin and American and British psychiatrists of the 19th and early 20th centuries. Nihilistic delusions (denial of reality) are common and are illustrated by her mistaken beliefs about her body functions and her denial of the beauties of nature. Her premorbid makeup, depression, agitation, hopelessness, insomnia, and weight loss are typical.

Course and Prognosis

In those patients with a long prodromal period, such as a gradually decompensating obsessive-compulsive personality, anxiety presents as the core symptom. If antianxiety and antidepressant therapy are begun at that stage, the illness may be arrested, provided the patient has accompanying adequate physical and emotional support. Once frank depressive symptoms develop, such as insomnia and dis-

TABLE II

Some Psychometric Characteristics of Depression*

Test	Neurotic Depression	Psychotic Depression
General testing behavior	Variable motor retardation Variable associative retardation Frequent expressions of inadequacy Tense, inhibited relationship to examiner Gives up easily Critical of self-help and accepts blame Over-concerned with performance Apologetic and guilty Unable to handle frustration Easily irritated	Severe motor retardation Severe associative retardation Gross irritability and negativism Severe restless agitation or inertia, frequently alternating Constantly despairing and expressing worthlessness Delusional ideas about examiner, purpose of tests, or use of test results Overt impotence Self-condemning Morbid affect, easily evoked Poorly controlled rage reaction in response to failure and frustration
Wechsler intelligence scales	Many performance scales lower than verbal scales Low digit span Difficulty in maintaining concentrated effort Vocabulary and information generally well retained Verbal productions frequently short Concern with accuracy frequently impedes performance	All performance scales grossly lower than verbal scales Unusual verbal scatter Marked fluctuation in quality of performance Comprehension and similarity tests generally low and often psychotic in quality Easily confused on items requiring concentration Excessively low digit span Distorted and morbid picture arrangement stories Distorted picture completion associations
Rorschach	Low R Long reaction times Stereotyped responses High number of F High F+ percentage Occasional inappropriate C responses Hypercritical of responses Irritated by testing Sensitive to shading Many popular or easily seen responses High number of D and low number of W responses Process of inquiry perceived as being critical of productions	Low R Few determinants Many anatomy responses Low F+ percentage Frequent failures Frequent morbid or decaying content Highly variable reaction times Long periods of unproductive handling of cards Many vague D or W responses Frequent rejections Difficult to obtain adequate inquiry
Thematic apperception test	Themes of despair, lack of success, failure, loss of love, and death are frequent Stories usually short and pessi-	Often a paucity of thematic material beyond simple descriptions Themes vary from the morbid, tearful concern with death and punish-

TABLE II—*Continued*

Test	Neurotic Depression	Psychotic Depression
	mistic in attitude Outcomes are bleak Often on verge of tears	ment to highly symbolic variations on themes of happiness versus gloom Frequent tearful responses to stories
Word association test	Generally long reaction times except to very simple stimulus words Concrete or functional associations Considerable difficulty in associating to words involving love, hate, loneliness, or family	Long reaction times or total associative blocking Stimulus-bound associations Frequent multiword associations Excessive number of traumatic words Such stimulus words as suicide evoke unusual responses such as "good" or a specific stated plan of action
Minnesota multiphasic personality inventory	High D scale High PT scale Moderately high F scale Moderately low MA scale Low K scale Difficulty in completing test	Difficulty in being tested Process of decision-making at times impossible Many "cannot say" or refuse to answer Excessive time required in testing High D scale High PT scale Low MA scale In general, high on psychotic triad Low PD scale Excessively high F scale

Rating Scale	Neurotic Depression	Psychotic Depression
Hamilton Depression Scale Hamilton and White (1959) Hamilton (1960)	Initial insomnia Agitation Somatic, G. I. Hypochondriasis Weight loss	Depressed mood (severe) Guilt Suicide Retardation Loss of insight
Brief Psychiatric Rating Scale (BPRS) Overall (1973) Overall and Klett (1972)	Somatic concern Anxiety Guilt feelings Hostility Depressive mood	Depressive mood (severe) Motor retardation Emotional withdrawal Blunted affect Unusual thought content
Present Status Examination (PSE) plus History Stems Kendell and Gourlay (1970)	Suicidal attempt Worse in evenings Annoyed by trivia Frequent weeping Difficulty going to sleep	Hallucinations Marked agitation or slowed body movements Ideas of reference Loss of insight Delusions of guilt
Factor Construct Rating Scale (FCRS) Overall, Henry, and Markette (1972)	Anxiety-tension Passive dependence Neuroticism Depressive mood	Depressive mood (severe) Affective impoverishment Psychomotor retardation

* Prepared by Harold A. Goolishian, Ph.D., Chief of the Division of Psychology, Department of Psychiatry, University of Texas Medical Branch, Galveston, Texas.

turbances in biological functions, the course is almost inevitably downhill. Today, some patients become chronic and never remiss, even after many years of care. However, the recovery rate after current types of treatment is variously reported as 50 per cent to 80 per cent. Wherever electroshock treatment and psychotropic drug therapy are properly and adequately administered, the recovery rate in all types of midlife depressions, in the author's experience, approximates 80 per cent.

The prognosis relies heavily on early detection and adequate and proper treatment. The prognosis is better in the younger, more intelligent patient and whenever treatment is instituted early in the illness. Thus, patients with a rapid onset have a higher recovery rate than do those with a long prodromal stage. Patients with signs of pronounced anxiety, severe depression, and extreme agitation have a higher incidence of recovery.

Diagnosis

The diagnosis of involutional melancholia should be made only after finding the positive criteria that delineate this psychosis. The cardinal features are: (1) personality predisposition—primarily, obsessive-compulsive personality; (2) no history of a prior mental disorder; (3) occurrence within the involutional phase of life; and (4) severe depression with apprehension, agitation, suicidal preoccupation, profound insomnia, appetite and weight loss, extreme feelings of guilt, usually based on exaggerated ideas about minor lifetime transgressions—all culminating in increasing somatic, nihilistic, and, rarely, persecuting delusions.

Routine laboratory studies are always in order. Because of the age group, an electrocardiogram is indicated. A chest X-ray is a must as are special X-rays if the patient is emaciated, because of the high incidence of intraabdominal and other malignancies in this age group. Many chronic physical illnesses also occur at this time of life, so special diagnostic tests may be indicated. If there is a suspicion of an early organic brain syndrome, psychodiagnostic tests—such as the Wechsler Adult Intelligence Scale, the Wechsler Memory Scale, and the Bender-Gestalt—are in order. An electroencephalogram, a brain scan, an echoencephalogram, and possibly a spinal fluid examination may follow. If the

findings justify it, consultation by a neurologist or neurosurgeon is in order.

Psychiatric Examination

The psychiatric interview should be performed in detail and should include collecting historical material from the patient and other available informants and securing information from schools and agencies.

The outline for history-taking covers more or less the following topics; the chief complaint(s) of the patient and of the informant, present illness in a chronological fashion from the onset of the first symptom to the time of examination, and the past personal history of the patient. Included in the past personal history is family history, birth and early development, social and intellectual development, school and occupational history, sexual history, marital and personal family status, the use of alcohol and drugs, past health and medical history.

Differential Diagnosis

Psychoses Associated with Organic Brain Syndromes. People in the involutional ages tend to develop circulatory disturbances, disorders of metabolism and nutrition, metastatic intracranial neoplasms, and senile neurohistological changes. Acute brain disorders—with the picture of altered degrees of consciousness, confusion, delirium, and associated physical and neurological deficits—are well-known.

In obvious chronic brain pathology, intellectual impairment is the chief finding. In the early states, the impairment produces only an alteration of recent memory and easy fatigability. The sensorium needs to be tested repeatedly and the psychodiagnostic tests used. More advanced patients lose all recent memory but have a fair retention of past memory and live in terms of early life experiences. The personality dilapidation is revealed through inattention to personal dress, excreta carelessness, and the habit of either deliberately or unknowingly exposing the genitals. Episodes of gross mental confusion may be associated with transitory fearfulness, which becomes worse at night but is not the sustained, constant fearfulness seen in involutional melancholia; hallucinations and illusions are also episodic, although delusions, especially of the paranoid type, can be persistent.

The existence of more diffuse cerebral pathology produces convulsions and various neurological symptoms and signs. In addition, the physical examination may reveal hypertension, peripheral vascular disease, or other pathology. Consequently, the differential diagnosis requires a thorough medical, neurological, and neurosurgical evaluation.

Functional Psychoses. The patient who develops paranoia during the involutional years has neither symptoms nor signs of a true depression of mood. The affect reveals either veiled or overt hostility, and the patient reacts directly to paranoid delusional content. Such a patient is egocentric rather than guilt-ridden and self-punishing, and his premorbid personality type is either schizoid or paranoid.

The patient with schizophrenia, schizo-affective type, depressed, may exhibit periods of despondency that are secondary to the underlying delusional content. In addition, the patient shows signs of dissociation, mental blocking, some autism, and a global retreat from reality. Introversion, schizoid, and paranoid characteristics are evident in the life adjustments.

The onset of a first psychotic depressive reaction during the involutional period may present diagnostic difficulties. The history reveals that the depressive mood is attributable to some experience in a basically well-adjusted personality structure that finds the environmental situation so overwhelming that it regresses into a depression of psychotic proportions. There are feelings of intense guilt, suicidal rumination, retardation of thought, and psychomotor activity, in contrast to the agitation of the involutional melancholia, with its profound insomnia, delusions of a somatic nature, and occasional hallucinations.

If the depressed type of manic-depressive illness has its first appearance during the involutional period, a careful history may show an early mild depression or an unrecognized episode of hypomania. Often, there is a positive family history, and further analysis of the premorbid personality reveals an outgoing, extroverted person with the mood swings of the cyclothymic personality. Similarly, clinical features of the depressive type of manic-depressive illness show more mental and psychomotor retardation and none of the bizarre delusions of extreme self-condemnation encountered in involutional melancholia.

Neuroses. Depressive neurosis is manifested by an excessive reaction of depression to an internal conflict or to an identifiable event, such as the loss of a love object or a cherished possession. There is no impairment of reality-testing and no severe interference with functional adequacy.

Anxiety is the prevailing emotion in anxiety neurosis and the patient has a lifelong tendency to overreact to stressful situations. The prodromal phase of involutional melancholia can be confused with anxiety neurosis, but there are fluctuations in the prevailing anxiety of the neurosis, in contrast to the continuous apprehensive depression of the psychosis.

Treatment

The first step is to allay the acuteness of the symptoms; second, to assist the patient to a better understanding of his own personality so that he may learn to live amicably with his disability; and third, to modify or alter the patient's environment. Aftercare helps the patient to attain complete rehabilitation and prevent relapse or further complications.

Alleviation of Symptoms

Most psychiatrists prefer to hospitalize all acute or fairly advanced patients to control the ever-present threat of suicide. Patients who are minimally depressed, cooperative, and not a threat to themselves or others may wish to stay home and be treated on an outpatient basis. In this situation, the physician should insist on adequate protection and supervision of the patient.

By the time patients are referred to the psychiatrist, many are severely agitated, even combative, often dehydrated, and in a poor state of nutrition.

Drugs. The acutely agitated, hostile, uncooperative patient may be controlled by one of the injectable neuroleptics. The phenothiazines were the first of the major tranquilizers. Of these, the best known is chlorpromazine. When injectable neuroleptics are used, the blood pressure should be checked before each dose. Prevention of severe postural hypotension is most important in the older age group because of the high risk tendency to hip fractures and other injuries sustained in falls. Other contraindications to the neuroleptics are comatose states; the known presence of large amounts of such central nervous system depressants as alcohol, barbiturates, and narcotics; a known bone marrow depression; and advanced liver disease.

Antidepressant drugs are useful in the early stages when there is no marked agitation, severe depression, pronounced undernutrition, or other serious physical complications and when there is no serious suicidal intent. When the clinical picture is dominated by depressive features, tricyclic derivatives may be considered. When insomnia is severe, amitryptyline hydrochloride is the tricyclic drug of choice for its anxiety-reducing and sedative components.

Contraindications to the tricyclic derivatives are a history of sensitivity to the drugs and a recent myocardial infarction, and tricyclics should not be given concurrently with monoamine oxidase inhibitors. Because of the drugs' atropine like action, glaucoma and sphincter and ureteral spasm, which are common in this age group, may be aggravated. The concurrent ingestion of other potent central nervous system drugs or alcohol may be potentiated. There may be interference with the ability to operate motor vehicles or other dangerous machinery until the desired dosage is attained and the patient is well-regulated on a maintenance dose. Daily blood pressures taken in the upright position are done to detect postural hypotension. The author does not recommend monoamine oxidase inhibitors because of the disadvantages of slow pharmacological action and the probability of a sustained hypotension lasting for many days, even after discontinuation of the drug.

Lithium carbonate has been reported as not helpful in the treatment of acute depressions of manic-depressive illness. Since involutional melancholia is a one-time illness, it is unnecessary to use the drug for prevention.

Electroshock. Electroshock is the treatment of choice for involutional melancholia. Physical contraindications to its use are rare, for even patients with chronic coronary and other forms of heart disease can be treated in consultation with a cardiologist when the cardiovascular condition is stabilized. A recent cerebrovascular accident, advanced emphysema or other severe pulmonary pathology, a major surgical procedure within the preceding month, and a recent fracture of one of the major bones are contraindications. Age alone is not a contraindication.

Treatments should be continued until all presenting symptoms have been relieved. The total number of treatments depends on the patient's response.

Surgery. Lobotomies have been performed on patients suffering from involutional melancholia of long duration who have received several forms of intensive psychiatric treatment without attaining lasting results. Statistical studies are lacking on its application in patients with involutional melancholia, but some successes are known.

According to recent reports by Meyer and colleagues, the most successful psychosurgical procedure to date is stereotactic bilateral cingulum lesioning (cingulotomy). At this time, it is the psychosurgical treatment of choice. Properly accomplished, it produces a precisely positioned and controlled brain lesion, thus eliminating some of the more severe side-effects of other neurosurgical approaches.

Psychotherapy

Supportive psychotherapy should be given during the illness and continued into convalescence, with every effort made to help the patient gain insight into his illness and to better understand his personality problems. Environmental manipulation and maximum rehabilitation should be attempted. Companionship is desirable, especially for recently widowed persons. Retired persons can profit from a hobby or part-time job. The majority of patients with involutional melancholia are inaccessible to depth psychotherapy.

Aftercare

Aftercare may consist only of supportive psychotherapy on a weekly or biweekly basis for the first 2 or 3 months. It is most helpful while the patient is convalescing from somatic therapy. A maintenance dose of psychotropic drugs may be indicated.

Evaluation of Therapy

All writers agree that somatic therapies are of great value, especially electroshock treatment. For resistant patients who are not emaciated, atropine toxicity treatment produces good results. On a last-resort basis, some involutional melancholia patients respond well to lobotomy, although more favorable results are attained from cingulotomy.

Antidepressant drugs, either alone or combined with psychotherapy, produce poor results in patients with severe, chronic symptoms, but they deserve a trial in the prodromal period.

REFERENCES

Angst, J., and Perris, C. Nosology of endogenous depression: Comparison of the findings of two studies. Arch. Psychiatr. Nervenkr. *210:* 373, 1968.

Davis, J. M., Janowsky, D. S., and El-Yousef, M. K. The use of lithium in clinical psychiatry. Psychiatr. Annals. *3:* 78, 1973.

Friedman, E. Sedac electrotherapy. II: Experiences and modifications in paranoid reactions and depression. Dis. Nerv. Syst., *33:* 250, 1972.

Garside, R. F. Depressive illnesses in late life. Br. J. Psychiatry, *122:* 118, 1973.

Kolb, L. C. *Modern Clinical Psychiatry*. W. B. Saunders, Philadelphia, 1973.

Meyer, G. A., McElhaney, M., Martin, W., and McGraw, C. P. Stereotactic cingulotomy with results of acute stimulation and serial psychological testing. In *Surgical Approaches in Psychiatry*. Medical and Technical Publishing, Oxford, 1974.

Overall, J. E. The brief psychiatric rating scale in psychopharmacologic research. In *Psychological Measurements in Pharmacopsychiatry*. P. Pichot and R. O. Martin, editors, S. Karger, Basel, 1973.

Overall, J. E., Henry, B. W., and Markette, J. R. Validity of an empirically derived phenomenological typology. J. Psychiatr. Res., *9:* 87, 1972.

Post, F. The management and nature of depressive illnesses in late life: A follow-through study. Br. J. Psychiatry, *121:* 393, 1972.

Rosenthal, S. H. The involutional depressive syndrome. Am. J. Psychiatry, *124* (Suppl. 21): 1968.

Winokur, G. Depression in the menopause. Am. J. Psychiatry, *130:* 92, 1973.

Winokur, G. Diagnostic and genetic aspects of affective illness. Psychiatr. Annals, *3:* 6, 1973.

17

Other Psychotic Depressive Disorders

17.1 PSYCHOTIC DEPRESSIVE REACTION

Introduction

In the 1968 edition of the *Diagnostic and Statistical Manual of Mental Disorders* (DSM-II) psychotic depressive reaction was removed from "Affective Psychoses" and placed in the group of "Other Psychoses." The definition of psychotic depressive reaction now reads:

This psychosis is distinguished by a depressive mood attributable to some experience. Ordinarily the individual has no history of repeated depressions or cyclothymic mood swings. The differentiation between this condition and *Depressive neurosis* (q.v.) depends on whether the reaction impairs reality testing or functional adequacy enough to be considered as psychosis.

Epidemiology

There are no reliable statistics on the prevalence of psychotic depressive reaction. Indeed, it will be difficult to secure reliable incidence or prevalence figures until there is more knowledge about the parameters of this diagnosis. Cultural, regional, racial, and individual differences attach diverse meanings to possible environmental precipitating factors, such as losses. A person accustomed to making and losing large sums of money gambling in the stock market presumably would not be affected as much by a financial loss as a person whose life savings were swept away by a stock market crash.

According to the United States Public Health Service reports of 1967 for psychotic depressive reaction, the number of admissions to state and county mental hospitals was 1,900, and the number of discharges from general hospital facilities was 11,798. For neurotic depressive reactions, the corresponding figures for 1967 were 10,785 and 80,808.

Causes

Experiences Precipitating Depression

The single unique feature of psychotic depressive reaction is that the depression is attributable to some experience—death of a spouse or close relative, loss of love or property, divorce, demotion, retirement, or other serious loss of status. Sometimes depression follows a promotion or other experience normally attended by increased self-esteem and prestige. The patient may have believed himself incapable of performing his new duties and so suffered an intolerable loss of self-esteem and became depressed. Frequently, a careful history reveals that the patient was gradually developing a depression prior to the alleged loss.

Grief. Probably the most significant human loss is death of a close relative. Lindemann described the symptoms of normal grief: sensations of somatic distress; preoccupation with the image of the deceased; guilt feelings in which the bereaved accuses himself of negligence in relation to the deceased; feelings of hostility toward doctors and others, charging them with not properly caring for the deceased before his death; and a change in conduct patterns, such as restlessness, inability to organize activities or to carry on customary social pleasantries. Normal acute grief lasts 4 to 8 weeks.

Lindemann also listed several varieties of morbid grief reactions—overactivity without a sense of loss; acquisition of symptoms of the last illness of the deceased; marked hostility without showing grief; apathy; and behavior destructive of the patient's interests by uncalled-for generosity, foolish business deals, and agitated depression. Many of the symptoms found in grief are seen in depression, but Lindemann diagnosed depression in only a small fraction of the cases he studied, which raises the possibility that grief is a special reaction and not the antecedent of psychotic depression.

Advanced Age. Levin and Goldfarb have indicated that old people are commonly subject to depression. Other writers have referred to the affective state of the depressed elderly as apathy or disinterest. Still others indicate that psychotic depressions are less common past age 65 and believe that older people are more immune to such depressions and marked grief reactions. Many writers believe that depressive reaction in the elderly is usually a mild syndrome in which neurotic symptoms of earlier life reappear.

Physical Illness and Physical States. Illness may directly affect basic neurochemical mechanisms that regulate mood. For example, depression sometimes follows virus infections or the taking of rauwolfia. In addition, drugs, infection, or metabolic changes may produce greater vulnerability to stresses with which a person could normally cope. Also, if the illness lowers the patient's status, he may experience a deflation of self-esteem. If the prognosis implies a permanent disability, some adjustments are necessary to preserve ego stability.

A wide variety of reactions to illness can occur. Some persons accept their illness with a minimum of difficulty. Others overcompensate by developing new abilities and talents. Still others retreat into helplessness, dependency, or apathy. Possibly more relevant for depression are those persons who refuse to accept the disability and become angry, for the anger may cause their friends to reject them, with consequent further loss of self-esteem. Those who use their physical illness to manipulate and control others may also be rejected, with the subsequent development of feelings of depression.

A 54-year-old widow attempted suicide by slashing her wrists. In the hospital she appeared sad and retarded and gave a history of poor sleep and energy and a hopeless outlook. Because of marked atrophy and flexion contractures of the lower extremities, she required a wheelchair. The depressive features cleared up over 4 weeks, then the patient presented a picture of sweet and smiling dependency. She accepted assistance for her physical care with cheerful gratitude. The main treatment was psychotherapeutic, with physiotherapy to the lower extremities.

The dynamic features of the illness were gradually uncovered. Some 20 years previously she had married following an unhappy love affair. Her marriage was unsuccessful from the start, including a sexual maladjustment, and she soon considered divorce. She complained of vague abdominal distress, irritability, and tension. In this early period the birth of two daughters added to her resentment. Ten years after marriage, her husband was accidentally killed at work where he had gone as a strike breaker at the patient's insistence. She reacted to his death with guilt. There followed a short period of mild depression. She worked as a teacher to support herself and her children. The patient's abdominal complaints occupied much of her attention, and she took to her bed more and more with the gradual development of atrophy and contractures of the lower extremities. Her daughters dutifully kept house and cared for her. Unable to continue teaching school, she managed an insurance and real estate business by mail and telephone. Publicly she presented a picture of a brave woman who rose above all misfortunes. Her presumed strength of character and courage were lauded from the pulpit by her pastor. Two years before admission, the patient's older daughter married. The mother became irritable, exaggerated her physical complaints, and made more demands upon the remaining daughter, who in turn hoped to escape from a relationship more endurable to her. The daughter became secretly engaged and later announced her wedding date. The patient experienced waves of loneliness, hostility, guilt, and depression, and she attempted suicide. Hospital admission followed. After 4 months of treatment, she acquired a healthier attitude and walked out of the hospital without needing the wheelchair.

Mutilating Surgery. Sutherland and Orbach have reported that acute depression can occur in anticipation of surgery. After surgery, depression may occur in relation to the loss of some valued activity. If a substitute activity cannot be found, the depression continues. Breast amputations damage feelings of femininity, facial disfiguration blemishes physical attractiveness, and the loss of a limb cripples productive capacity. A few of the persons suffering these losses may become severely depressed.

Psychological Predisposition

Many writers assume that a predisposition to depression develops in childhood because a loss in that period produced a vulnerability to later losses. But the data, on the whole, strongly suggest that early environmental experiences play an unclear role in predisposing to adult depression.

One analytical writer attributes the predisposition to depression to excessive disappointments before the child has learned to handle his ambivalent feelings toward himself and his love object, at a time when his endopsychic representatives of himself and his objects have not been firmly established or clearly differentiated. Another analyst believes that the infant enters a phase characterized by a complex mixture of feelings of grief and hostility over a feared loss of his love object. Infants who fail to pass beyond this position are likely to succumb to a similar set of depressive feelings in adulthood after a loss of a love object.

Mendelson does not believe, however, that the analytical literature establishes a correlation between infantile experience and adult depression. The theories have been based on too few cases, much of the analytical information is subject to retrospective falsification, and the word depression is not used consistently. Depression is a complex phenomenon, which embraces many affective states and probably results from a combination of inherited, constitutional, and psychological factors.

Clinical Aspects

Clinically, depression is an affective state of sadness or blueness. In mild degree it usually goes unnoticed by relatives and is felt only slightly by the patient; in severe degree everyone remarks on it, and the patient experiences severe suffering. The affective complaint is that of sadness, low spirits, blueness, dullness, failure to enjoy life, not caring to participate in activities, loss of interest or zest, and a gloomy outlook.

Physical Signs

A depressed patient looks sad. Some depressed patients present retardation as a prominent sign, responding and moving slowly. The flow of thinking is sluggish.

Depression depletes the patient's store of energy. His appetite lessens or vanishes, his mouth seems dry, food does not taste right, and he must force himself to eat. Curtailed food intake leads to weight loss. Constipation appears in some patients, infrequently interrupted by short bouts of diarrhea.

Sleep disturbance, considered as almost pathognomonic for depression, often appears as early-morning awakening.

Upon arising, the patient feels blue, anxious, and retarded, but by midafternoon or evening there is partial or complete relief. The perception of the external world may be altered in depression. Colored objects appear dull or gray, although the patients can name colors correctly.

Somatic sensations may exist for months before development of a severe depression. Headache is common. The patient also speaks of heavy or dull feelings, of fullness or bursting sensations, of hazy or dopey feelings in the head. Complaints of blurred vision sometimes lead to the purchase of new glasses.

The skin on any part of the body may be the object of paresthesias. Circulatory symptoms are noted in depressed patients who are also anxious and tense. In such patients, blood pressure is apt to be elevated.

The genitourinary system shows three types of changes: frequency of urination, diminution or disappearance of sex desire, and, in women, reduction or cessation of menstraul flow. Occasionally, an increase in libido appears, related to a strong need for affection.

Involvement of the neuromuscular system includes tremors, muscle twitches, muscular soreness, and shooting pains in the muscles of the face, arms, and legs. These symptoms often localize along the spinal axis and in the back of the neck and the occiput. Associated with muscular complaints are those of fatigue or weakness.

Psychological Signs

Depressed patients, especially in severe cases, may have delusions. Typically the delusions involve ideas of sin or guilt, poverty, and unworthiness. They reflect the patient's cultural background and individual conflicts. Hopelessness easily develops. The patient may conclude that suicide provides the only solution.

One woman felt that she had succumbed to temptation by the devil following an illusion in which she perceived a ray of sunlight as a yellow snake. She believed that the snake had poisoned the well and that she, in turn, was poisoning her own family by cooking with well water. This made the food taste peculiar. God had deserted her, and there was no possible salvation.

A wealthy man of 39 became depressed and insisted he was on the verge of bankruptcy. He could not spend 10 cents for a cigar; he had to walk home rather than ride the bus; medical attention was too expensive and useless.

Mental retardation and indecisiveness make the patient unsure of himself and reduce his self-confidence. He observes in the mirror a change in his appearance, and he suspects that people speculate on his changed appearance. As a consequence, he becomes tense and anxious, perhaps fearful, avoiding people as much as possible. He tries to put up a front and maintain a smiling countenance. All this prepares fertile ground for the growth of ideas of reference and delusions. He comes to view everything pessimistically. He suspects loved ones may desert him and friends turn against him. He feels completely helpless and lost. Some patients seek excessive proofs of affection, presenting a picture of dependent clinging. Others resent the imagined lack of attention and angrily demand it. Both types may make suicidal gestures in an effort to gain affection.

Depressed patients can reveal hostility in varying degrees. In mild depressions, hostility shows by easy irritability and fretting. More severe depressions display hostility by accusing others of slighting or hating the patient, by demanding special consideration, by outbursts of anger, and even by acts of destruction. Hostility may also turn on the self. Suicidal acts may signify an intense anger against the self.

Diagnosis

If a precipitating event precedes the beginning of the depression by only a few weeks, it is easy to think of the event as bearing a causal relationship. As the interval lengthens, however, the relationship between cause and effect becomes tenuous. Events that occur more than 6 to 10 weeks before the onset of a depression should not be regarded as causal.

Some depressions begin acutely and reach severe proportions in a matter of hours or days. Other depressions begin with only one or two symptoms, such as a slight diminution in appetite and a feeling of sluggishness in the morning, then gradually progress to a severe form over a period of weeks or months. A case of rapid onset is justifiably called psychotic. But a case of gradual onset is more apt to be thought of as neurotic in the early stages, especially if there is anxiety and its common somatic signs.

According to the second edition of *Diagnostic and Statistical Manual of Mental Disorders* (DSM II), psychotic depressive reaction is differentiated from manic-depressive psychosis, depressed type, from involutional melancholia,

and from depressive neurosis. All three differentiations present problems. With manic-depressive psychosis, depressed type, no difficulty occurs if a first depression clearly has no precipitating life experience shortly before the appearance of the depression. If a subsequent depression occurs without precipitating stresses, the likelihood increases that the diagnosis is manic-depressive. But if a second depression has a likely cause in experience or if the first depression has a causal experience and the second does not, the experiential event loses much of its diagnostic significance. The case for a diagnosis of manic-depressive psychosis, depressed type, becomes probable if the patient had a prior manic attack and if there is a family history of bipolar affective disorder.

Separation from involutional melancholia arises when a patient has a first depression in the involutional period of life. With no preceding life stress, clinicians tend to favor a diagnosis of involutional melancholia, especially if the depression is severe with delusions, agitation, and a history of obsessional traits.

Depressive neurosis separates itself from psychotic depressive reaction in that the latter shows a break with reality in the form of delusions, hallucinations, or gross functional inadequacy. Both may be precipitated by external stresses, but depressive neurosis should show a positive history of neurotic traits or neurotic depression. A definitive differential diagnosis cannot be made in many cases.

The physical signs of depression may also confuse diagnosis. Poor appetite, weight loss, and constipation suggest bowel disease. Lowered energy and easy fatigability raise a question of thyroid deficiency. For sleep disturbance, sedatives are prescribed without consideration of the presence of depression. Loss of libido calls to the mind of the physician the possibility of hormonal deficiency.

Treatment

Uncovering Unconscious Motivations

Attempts to probe into unconscious factors possibly related to depression are apt to make the patient more introspective, anxious, depressed, and perhaps suicidal. Some psychiatrists urge uncovering psychotherapy for the patient after he has recovered from a depression.

Combating Depressive Ideas

If the patient has ideas of guilt or unworthiness, the psychiatrist attempts to undermine these by minimizing them or by direct denial. If the patient has feelings of hostility for which he blames himself, the importance of these feelings is minimized, rationalized, or denied. At the same time, attempts are made to bolster the patient's feelings of self-esteem by pointing to his achievements and good qualities.

Suicidal ideas and ruminations are a constant concern. Getting these ideas into the open frequently relieves the patient, who then feels that the psychiatrist knows and understands the worst about him. It is often possible to secure a promise that the patient will make no suicidal attempts, a promise the patient rarely breaks.

In all these discussions, hope for recovery is held out to the patient. He will recover, no matter how futile the future seems; thousands of patients with the same kind of trouble do recover. Sometimes a patient feels better about his illness if it is interpreted to him in primarily physical terms.

The more severely depressed the patient, the more transitory are the results in combating depressive ideas. Yet these attempts are often useful in easing the depression until more definitive treatment, with antidepressant drugs or electrotherapy, has had significant effects.

Daily Activities

The patient should be encouraged to continue activities within the limits of his available energy. Activity diverts him from depressive preoccupations and preserves the routine of normal life. Social contacts must be planned.

Environment

Nurses, occupational and recreational therapists, and other hospital personnel who have contact with the patient should be given instruction in the psychopathology of depression so that they can combat depressive ideas without probing into psychodynamic factors. All these persons should pay attention to the patient's physical needs and assist in keeping him active.

With outpatients, relatives should have their roles clarified by giving them information on how depression affects a patient. In general, they should offer support and optimism. Relatives also need instruction in what to expect from electrotherapy and how to reassure the patient who has memory loss associated with this treatment.

Hospitalization

The indications for hospital care are severe depression or serious suicidal preoccupations, inability of relatives to give adequate care, or a seriously depressed patient not responding to treatment.

Drug Therapy

In the experience of some physicians, imipramine has given results nearly as good as electrotherapy. Amitriptyline has also been useful, being slightly more effective than imipramine. Amitriptyline has an additional advantage, a slight sedative effect that calms tension and promotes sleep. The effects of imipramine appear in 7 to 10 days and reach a maximal response in 14 to 18 days. The response to amitriptyline is slightly quicker. Tranylcypromine and monoamine oxidase inhibitors, nialamide and phenelzine sulfate, are worth a trial when other drugs fail. A minimal response to a drug after 4 weeks suggests a trial of another drug or electrotherapy. There is no way to know how long the patient requires a drug.

Electrotherapy

A most effective treatment for depression is electrotherapy, which produces about 80 per cent marked improvement or complete recovery. The technique of unilateral electrotherapy is said to eliminate most postshock confusion and memory loss. Electrotherapy has the great advantage of stopping the depressive attack in 1 to 3 weeks. The average number of treatments for severe depression, is seven to eight, given at the rate of three a week. Mild cases may need only three or four treatments. It has been stated that 50 per cent of patients who fail to improve with antidepressant drugs respond to electrotherapy.

Some patients respond to electrotherapy but relapse after a few weeks and require further treatment. In early stages of relapse, one or two electric treatments may abort a full-blown depression. To prevent relapses after electrotherapy, antidepressant drugs are sometimes tried.

REFERENCES

Brown, G. W., Sklair, F., Harris, T. D., and Birley, J. L. T. Life events and psychiatric disorders. Part I. Some methodological issues. Psychol. Med., *3:* 74, 1973.

Clayton, P. J., Halikas, J. A., and Maurice, W. L. The depression of widowhood. Br. J. Psychiatry, *120:* 71, 1972.

Morrison, J. R., Hudgens, R. A., and Barchha, R. G. Life events and psychiatric illness. Br. J. Psychiatry, *114:* 423, 1968.

Parkes, C. M. *Bereavement, Studies of Grief in Adult Life.* International Universities Press, New York, 1972.

Paykel, E. S., Meyers, J. K., Dienelt, M. N., Klerman, G. L., Lindenthal, J. J., and Pepper, M. P. Life events and depression. Arch. Gen. Psychiatry, *21:* 753, 1969.

Rahe, R. H., and Arthur, R. J. Life change patterns surrounding illness experiences. J. Psychosom. Res., *11:* 341, 1968.

Stewart, M. A., Drake, F., and Winokur, G. Depression among medically ill patients. Dis. Nerv. Syst., *26:* 479, 1965.

Uhlenhuth, E. H., and Paykel, E. S. Symptom intensity and life events. Arch. Gen Psychiatry, *28:* 473, 1973.

17.2.   POSTPARTUM DISORDERS

Introduction

Pregnancy and the postpartum period are generally regarded as maturational crises equal in importance to those of adolescence and the menopause. Stresses undergone during this period include endocrine changes, changes in body image, activation of unconscious psychological conflicts pertaining to pregnancy, and intrapsychic reorganization of becoming a mother. It seems likely that clinically significant interactions of psychosocial and endocrine factors are found in the causes of these disorders.

Epidemiology

Data from studies of normal pregnant women indicate that from 20 to 40 per cent of women report emotional disturbance or cognitive dysfunction in the early postpartum period. Disturbances of psychotic proportions occur much less frequently, with the most often quoted figures being 1 to 2 per 1,000 deliveries. One study indicated that 54 per cent of cases occurred in primipara and 46 per cent in multipara. There was no reported correlation between postpartum disorders and heredity, religion, or sex of the child, and the data were inadequate to reach any conclusions about the influence of the use of anesthesia in delivery, the birth of a dead child, a child with congenital abnormalities, or an illegitimate child or an abortion.

Causes

Biological Factors

Most of the contributions in this area have focused on the possible interaction of thyroid and adrenal function in relation to the high estrogen and progesterone level of pregnancy and the abrupt termination of these high levels of sex hormones at parturition. Protein-bound iodine (PBI) and plasma 17-OH steroid levels are high during pregnancy, largely because of the estrogen-induced elevation of the proteins that bind these hormones, but PBI levels over the first 9 months postpartum are 40 per cent lower than the last pregnancy determination. This change in PBI levels may reflect a corresponding change in the level of production of thyroxine. A recent therapeutic advance in the treatment of depressive illness, unrelated to parturition, involves the use of small amounts of triiodothyronine.

The recurrence of symptoms at the time of the menses also seems to implicate the sex steroid alterations as being related to the precipitation of illness. Menstrual irregularity has frequently been reported in postpartum patients. Treatment with progesterone alone has not been shown to produce a remission of the original illness but has been reported to prevent relapse.

Studies from early pregnancy to the postpartum period revealed that the sleep system is profoundly affected throughout pregnancy and sometimes for several months after delivery. During the third trimester, subnormal levels were the rule. By parturition, there was a marked suppression of total sleep time, which did not reach normal levels again until several weeks postpartum. Stage 4 sleep was considerably depressed in late pregnancy, rebounding 4 to 6 weeks postpartum in most subjects. Investigators questioned whether an excessive drop in the level of stage 4 sleep in late pregnancy or failure or delay in the rebound of this stage in the early postpartum period contributes to increasing one's susceptibility to emotional disturbance.

Research into the vicissitudes of catecholamine metabolism in relation to depressive illness and its treatment has proved fruitful in generating hypotheses concerning the biology of depression. The hormone progesterone is known to affect catecholamine metabolism in animals and has central nervous system-depressant effects in humans.

Psychosocial Factors

Psychodynamic studies of postpartum mental illness point to conflicting feelings within the mother with regard to her mothering experience, her new baby, her husband, and herself. Zilboorg described the patient as ambivalent, with a castration complex, failure of resolution of the oedipal phase of psychosexual development, and sadistic tendencies toward men. He also found that most of his patients had married late in life after prolonged courtships.

Conflicts in assuming the mothering role are seen as leading to an identity diffusion in these women. Although these women were committed to the mothering experience, their own childhood experiences led them to reject their own mothers as models for imitation and identification. Their sense of identity and feelings of competence become fragmented, in that they are mothers without knowing how to act. When the concurrent environment offers little ongoing reinforcement for her mothering activities, as evidenced by a lack of rewards from her husband and the discrepant advice from others, and when there are current stresses—resulting in object loss, frustration, and feelings of entrapment—the woman is prompted to recapture earlier periods of equilibrium—that is, to regress. In this way, her own mother's maternal behavior increasingly becomes a reference or model for her own program of action. If the mothers of these women repudiated the mothering role or were judged as inadequate maternal models, this increased identification entails conflict, since they feel they were rejected. This identification often leads to the new mother's rejection of her own infant.

Clinical Features

Symptoms are almost never noted before the third day postpartum. This latent period is seen as the period during which some kind of chemical or hormonal development related to the childbearing process takes place, leading to later manifestation of illness. Prodromal symptoms include insomnia, restlessness, feelings of fatigue, depression of spirit, irritability, headache, and lability of mood. According to some studies, insomnia is the most distressing symptom. Later symptoms include suspiciousness,

evidence of confusion or incoherence, irrational statements, obsessive concern over trivialities, and refusal of food.

The clinical symptoms center on the patient's relationship to the baby and the maternal role. Depressed patients may manifest excessive concern about the baby's health or welfare or guilt about their lack of love or desire to care for the baby. They may express feelings of inadequacy about taking care of the baby. When psychosis is present, delusional material may involve the idea that the baby is dead or defective in some way. The birth may be denied, and ideas of being unmarried or virginal or ideas of persecution influence or perverse sexuality may be expressed. Hallucinations may contain similar material and may involve voices telling the woman to kill the baby. Behavior toward the baby may be characterized by avoidance or anxious oversolicitude. Infanticide and suicide occasionally occur.

Diagnosis

Most patients who are not hospitalized present with illness that is classified as depressive neurosis, with or without symptoms of anxiety, obsessional thinking, and evidence of cognitive dysfunction in the form of impairment of memory and ability to concentrate. Hospitalized patients are more frequently accorded a diagnosis of psychotic depression, manic-depressive illness, or schizophrenia.

Those with a prior history of schizophrenia or manic-depressive illness are seen as having a recurrence related to the stresses of pregnancy. Because of its clinical similarity to postpartum depression, hypothyroidism should always be considered. Cushing's syndrome is common after a pregnancy and is frequently associated with a depressive state. Drug-induced depression is common, especially in those receiving antihypertensive or other drugs with known central nervous system depressant properties. Those with prominent deleriod phenomena should receive careful evaluation for infection, encephalopathy relating to toxemia, and neoplasm.

Treatment

Electroconvulsive therapy is most often mentioned in the treatment of the psychoses, especially depressive illness. It is probable that there has been a decline in the use of this modality with the advent of the use of tricyclic antidepressants, which are the treatment of choice in all but seriously suicidal patients. Failure of pharmacotherapy is an indication for use of electroconvulsive therapy. For patients who suffer manic illnesses, lithium carbonate therapy alone or in combination with phenothiazines during the first 7 days is the treatment of choice. Phenothiazines in antipsychotic dosages are an effective alternative treatment.

For those with schizophrenictype psychoses, phenothiazine drugs and those with like antipsychotic activity are the treatment of choice. These pharmacological agents are not recommended for use in mothers who are breast feeding.

Psychotherapy is usually indicated for these patients after the period of acute psychosis is past. The therapy is usually directed at the conflictual areas and may involve helping the patient to accept the feminine role. Changes in environmental factors may also be indicated. Increased support from the husband and other persons in the environment may be helpful in reducing stress. Most studies report high rates of recovery from the acute phase of illness.

REFERENCES

Gordon, J. E., Ingals, T. H., and Thomas, C. L. Preventive medicine and epidemiology: psychosis after childbirth: Ecological aspects of a single impact stress. Am. J. Med. Sci., *238:* 363, 1959.

Hamilton, J. A. *Postpartum Psychiatric Problems.* C. V. Mosby, St. Louis, 1962.

Jarrahi-Zadeh, A., Kane, F. J., Jr., Van de Castle, R. L., Lachenbruch, P. A., and Ewing, J. A. Emotional and cognitive changes in pregnancy and early puerperium. Br. J. Psychiatry, *115:* 797, 1969.

Kane, F. J., Jr., and Mohamed, T. Severe emotional disturbance with pentazocrine (Talwin) use. J. La. State Med. Soc., 1973.

Karacan, I., Heine, W., Agnew, H. W., Williams, R. L., Webb, W. B., and Ross, J. J. Characteristics of sleep patterns during late pregnancy and the postpartum periods. Am. J. Obstet. Gynecol., *101:* 570, 1968.

Melges, F. T. Post-partum psychiatric syndromes. In *Psychosomatic Medicine*, M. F. Reiser, editor, Vol. 30, no. 1, pp. 95–108. Hoeber Medical Division, Harper & Row, New York, 1968.

Treadway, C. R., Kane, F. J., Jr., Jarrahi-Zadeh, A., and Lipton, M. A. A psychoendocrine study of pregnancy and puerperium. Am. J. Psychiatry, *125:* 1380, 1969.

18

Organic Brain Syndromes

18.1. INTRODUCTION

Definitions

The standard nomenclature of the American Psychiatric Association defines organic brain syndrome as a "mental condition characteristically resulting from diffuse impairment of brain tissue function from whatever cause." The syndromes are subdivided into psychotic and nonpsychotic, depending on the severity of the functional impairment. The patient who cannot meet the ordinary demands of life is considered psychotic. Acute brain disorders are reversible. In chronic brain disorders, the impairment is permanent and irreversible. The diagnostic nomenclature further subdivides organic brain syndromes according to the presumed causative agent.

Clinical Features

All organic brain syndromes, regardless of their cause and severity, are associated with disturbances of orientation, memory, intellect, judgment, and affect. The specific agent responsible for the impairment of brain tissue function greatly influences the basic syndrome and imparts its own characteristic signature on the clinical picture. As with any somatic illness, the patient reacts to this stress according to his basic personality structure. This reaction is most readily apparent with mild brain disturbances or early in an illness, when the patient perceives the disorder as a threat to his well-being. At this point, the manifestations of organic brain disease may be accompanied by psychological attempts to defend against and to conceal these deficits.

As these attempts fail, symptoms of the classic functional disorders may appear. The clinical expression of the syndrome may also vary with the patient's current emotional conflicts and stresses, his environmental situation, and his interpersonal relationships.

Classification

Patients with similar clinical manifestations may be classified differently, depending on the examiner's discipline, training, and background.

Confronted with a patient who has a mental disturbance, the physician first attempts to decide whether the disturbance represents an organic impairment of brain function or a functional disturbance or both. Once he decides that the patient is, indeed, suffering from an organic disturbance, he may properly classify the disorder as some form of encephalopathy. Only when he is satisfied that a focal disturbance of brain tissue function is absent can he properly use the term "organic brain syndrome" (see Table I).

An acute brain syndrome has four primary characteristics: (1) The onset is often sudden, with the rapid development of impairment of orientation, memory, intellectual function, judgment, and affect. (2) Delirium, stupor, or coma may be present, at times associated with the release of underlying psychotic and neurotic reactions. (3) The syndrome is caused by temporary, reversible, diffuse disturbances of brain function. (4) The clinical course, although usually brief, may persist for a month or longer, but it always ends with some resolution of the organic symptoms.

A chronic brain syndrome also has four primary characteristics. (1) The onset is often but not always slow and insidious, taking several

TABLE I

*Encephalopathy: Clinicopathological Correlation**

Involve-ment of Brain Tissue	Mode of Onset and Temporal Profile		
	Acute (Minutes to Hours)	Subacute (Days)	Chronic (Weeks or Longer)
Focal	Vascular (infarct) Trauma (concussion, contusion)	Inflammation (abscess) Trauma (subdural hematoma)	Neoplasm (mass lesion) Trauma (subdural hematoma)
Diffuse	Vascular (subarachnoid hemorrhage) Toxic-metabolic disorder Anoxia Inflammation (bacterial meningitis)	Inflammation (meningo-encephalitis) Toxic-metabolic disorder	Degenerative disease Toxic-metabolic disorder Inflammation (chronic granulomatous or fungal meningitis)

* These listings are merely general considerations; the exceptions are numerous.

weeks or more and progressively impairing brain tissue function. (2) The clinical expression is often described as a dementia, but sometimes delirium, stupor, and coma supervene, especially in advanced states. As with acute brain syndromes, the symptoms of organic and functional impairment of brain function may coexist. (3) The syndrome is caused by an irreversible, permanent, diffuse alteration of brain function. (4) The clinical course usually progresses over months or years, and the syndrome may end in death. Although the responsible agent is sometimes identified and removed, some permanent alteration in brain function remains. (See Figure 1.)

Delirium

Delirium, a syndrome generally produced by a transient disturbance of brain tissue function, is symptomatic of a wide range of disorders and is characterized by a global impairment of cognitive processes. Although the level of consciousness may be altered, the patient is generally awake and able to answer questions. However, his thinking, memory, perception, and attention are disturbed, reducing his ability to understand and interpret his internal and external environment in accordance with past experiences—that is, his reality testing is defective.

Delirium may be followed by complete recovery, in which case it may properly be defined as an acute brain syndrome. It may progress to an irreversible amnestic syndrome, in which case it may properly be defined as a chronic brain

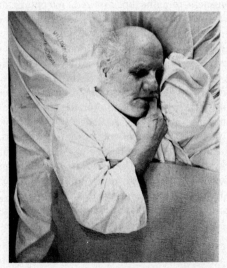

FIGURE 1. The patient with a chronic organic brain syndrome will usually require custodial care in his declining years. Regressive behavior is typical in this state such as finger-sucking. (Courtesy of Bill Stanton for Magnum Photos, Inc.)

syndrome. Or it may progress to irreversible coma and death, in which case the matter of definition seems irrelevant.

Schizophrenia and other functional psychiatric disorders may at times superficially resemble a delirium, but they are not associated with the generalized cognitive defect found with a delirium. In these patients the electroencephalogram may be particularly helpful, with an abnormal record being highly suggestive of an organic disorder.

The search for and removal of the underlying cause is crucial. Drug intake must be carefully reviewed and improper fluid and electrolyte balance corrected because these factors often coexist with and heighten the clinical symptoms produced by the responsible agent. Proper nursing care and the avoidance of sensory deprivation are essential. Sedation, although necessary when the patient is overactive or violent, must be used with extreme caution. Sedatives, especially in mildly delirious patients, may heighten faulty perceptions and deepen the delirium.

Dementia

Dementia is a clinical syndrome caused by brain disease and characterized by failing memory and loss of intellectual functions. Consciousness remains unimpaired, except in extreme and advanced cases. Some cases of dementia are reversible.

Superficially, several functional alterations in mental processes may resemble a dementia, depression being the most common. In depression, impaired concentration, shortened attention span, and psychomotor retardation are sometimes mistakenly regarded by the patient or physician as signs of diminished mental capacity due to organic disease. Patients with focal neurological disorders may appear confused on examination and unable to perform required tasks adequately. In those patients in whom an organic syndrome can be neither confirmed nor denied on the basis of clinical examination, formal psychological testing is indicated (see Table II).

Roentgenograms of the head, electroencephalography, and radioisotope scanning occasionally reveal focal brain lesions not evident after neurological examination. A hematological survey, tests of metabolic function, serological tests, and chest roentgenograms should also be made. Neurological consultation is indicated for the majority of such patients. Examination of the cerebrospinal fluid may prove necessary, but this procedure should not be done routinely in all patients.

Conclusion

An organic brain syndrome is a mental disorder characterized by global or selective impairment of cognitive functions—such as memory, thinking, attention, and perception—due to an impairment of brain tissue function—for example, an encephalopathy. Delirium designates an acute, transient state of impaired cognitive function, often associated with an alteration in consciousness. Dementia refers to a similar but more slowly developing state of impaired mental functioning, at times reversible and likely to be found without alteration in the level of consciousness. Every patient who presents with cognitive impairment—whether classified as an organic brain syndrome (acute or chronic), encephalopathy, delirium, or dementia—requires

TABLE II
*Potentially Treatable Causes of Dementia**

General Cause	Types of Disorders
Neoplastic disorders	Brain tumor (frontal lobe, intraventricular, etc.)
Endocrine disorders	Thyroid, parathyroid, adrenal dysfunction; hypoglycemia
Other metabolic disorders	Hepatic, renal, pulmonary insufficiency; hyponatremia; syndrome of inappropriate antidiuretic hormone secretion; porphyria; Wilson's disease
Exogenous toxins	Drug toxicity (barbiturates, bromides); heavy metal exposure
Deficiency states	Hypovitaminosis B^{12}, Wernicke-Korsakoff syndrome; pellagra
Vascular disorders	Postsubarachnoid hemorrhage with hydrocephalus; secondary to sustained hypertension; systemic lupus erythematosus
Posttraumatic disorders	Subdural hematoma; communicating hydrocephalus
Inflammatory disorders	General paresis; brain abscess; meningoencephalitis, chronic inflammation (various types); postinflammatory arachnoiditis with hydrocephalus
Miscellaneous conditions	Recurrent seizures; hematological disorders (various types); postinflammatory arachnoiditis with hydrocephalus; recurrent seizures; hematological disorders various types; remote effect of carcinoma; occult hydrocephalus

* This list includes some of the more common treatable causes of dementia. Others exist, and the conditions above do not necessarily result in dementia alone.

careful evaluation to exclude potentially treatable causes for his illness. The extent of reversibility of the patient's impairment and, therefore, the use of the diagnoses "acute brain syndrome" and "chronic brain syndrome" may be established only after careful, complete evaluation to eliminate known treatable causes and after long-term observation to validate the accuracy of the original diagnosis.

REFERENCES

Adams, R. D., and Victor, M. Derangements of intellect and behavior including delirium and other confusional states, Korsakoff's amnestic syndrome, and dementia. In *Principles of Internal Medicine*, T. R. Harrision, R. D. Adams, I. L. Bennett, Jr., W. H. Resnik, G. W. Thorn, and M. M. Wintrobe, editors, ed. 5, vol. 1, p. 264. McGraw-Hill, New York, 1966.

American Psychiatric Association. *Diagnostic and Statistical Manual of Mental Disorders*, ed. 2. American Psychiatric Association, Washington, 1968.

Karp, H. Dementias in adults. In *Clinical Neurology*, A. B. Baker and L. H. Baker, editors, vol. 2, chap. 27. Harper & Row, New York, 1973.

Plum, F., and Posner, J. B. *The Diagnosis of Stupor and Coma*. F. A. Davis, Philadelphia, 1966.

Wells, C. E. *Dementia*. F. A. Davis, Philadelphia, 1971.

Wells, C. E. Dementia reconsidered. Arch. Gen Psychiatry, *26*: 385, 1972.

18.2. ORGANIC BRAIN SYNDROMES ASSOCIATED WITH CIRCULATORY DISTURBANCES

Introduction

Circulatory disturbances produce changes in many organ systems that may affect the nervous system, either primarily or secondarily. Circulatory failure may result in ischemia and infarction. The appearance, distribution, and clinical expression of these abnormalities are predicted on certain physiological, pathological, and anatomical principles.

Physiological Principles

The brain needs energy in the form of adenosine triphosphate. This energy is necessary to sustain the life of neural tissue and to allow it to perform its vital functions: maintenance of ionic gradients, establishment of membrane potentials, aid in transmitter synthesis, and production of cellular constituents. The brain can produce adenosine triphosphate efficiently only through the oxidative metabolism of glucose.

The main purpose of the cerebral blood flow is to provide the brain with a continuous supply of glucose and oxygen. The brain receives a preferential proportion of the total blood flow. Although this organ constitutes only 2 per cent of the body weight, it receives 15 per cent of the cardiac output and consumes about 20 per cent of the oxygen used by a resting person. Total cerebral blood flow normally remains quite constant, but regional changes do occur in response to neuronal activity. Blood flow through gray matter is greater than that through white matter.

In the absence of oxygen, brain cell function ceases rapidly. Reversible alteration in cell function because of oxygen lack results in ischemia. Irreversible alteration results in infarction. In general, the perfusion pressure must be high enough to overcome the cerebrovascular resistance, and these must be no hindrance to venous drainage. Vascular resistance can be affected by the vessel diameter and the blood viscosity. It can also be modified by such factors as the elasticity of the vessel walls, intracranial pressure, and structural changes secondary to disease.

The brain has numerous mechanisms available to alter vessel diameter in response to various chemical and physiological stimuli, and it can, except in cases of the widest extremes of blood pressure, keep cerebral blood flow relatively constant in a normal person. This phenomenon is called autoregulation. A reduction in intraluminal pressure causes cerebral vasodilation, as do increased carbon dioxide, increased lactic acid, decreased oxygen, and tissue acidosis. The opposite changes cause vasoconstriction. Because these conditions accompany the ischemic state, their combined effects may increase regional cerebral blood flow enough to prevent infarction. In other situations, these conditions may reduce the size of an infarct. These protective devices reduce the cerebrovascular resistance significantly in regions of ischemia. The single most important factor in maintaining cerebral blood flow to an ischemic zone is the mean arterial blood pressure. When blood pressure is reduced markedly for a prolonged period, the inevitable consequence is infarction.

Pathological Principles

The neuron, being particularly sensitive to ischemia, responds rapidly and distinctively to anoxia with a cytological abnormality commonly called ischemic cell change. The affected nerve cells, stained with hematoxylin and eosin, are seen under the ordinary light microscope as bright, pinkish, shrunken-looking triangular shapes. The nucleus is pyknotic and shrunken, and it stains darkly. Severe infarction is accompained by additional changes, and neuronal loss and tissue necrosis may be extensive. The changes may be distributed diffusely after an episode of cardiac arrest or may be highly localized after a focal cerebral infarction.

Parenchymal infarction may result from occlusion of the adjacent nutrient vessel, either because of disease within the vessel wall or secondary to embolic occlusion of the vessel from a distant vascular lesion. Hemorrhage is the result of extravasation of blood elements from their normal vascular channels, with resultant necrosis of parenchymal tissue or disturbance of neural function.

Anatomical Principles

The brain is supplied with blood by two arterial systems: the internal carotid and the vertebrobasilar. Extensive pathways for collateral flow allow direct and indirect communication between these two arterial systems. The arteries associated with the circle of Willis (see Figure 1), those traveling between various terminal arteries over the parenchyma of the brain, and those running between the extracranial and intracranial arteries provide effective blood flow to the parenchyma when a major vessel is occluded. These collateral channels partly explain the apparent discrepancy between observed disease in major cerebral vessels and normality of brain function.

Clinical Concepts

A disruption of the blood supply to the parenchyma abruptly alters function. Alterations in mental function may be associated with the circulatory disease, may represent a psychological reaction to the patient's perception of failing brain tissue function, or may reflect actual impairment of brain tissue function resulting from circulatory failure. This impairment of parenchymal function may result from ischemia, infarction, or hemorrhage. The resultant changes may be widely distributed over the brain (diffuse), may consist of a discrete localized lesion (focal), or may produce several such lesions (multifocal). The clinical expression of these abnormalities depends on the size, location, nature, and extent of the parenchymal disease.

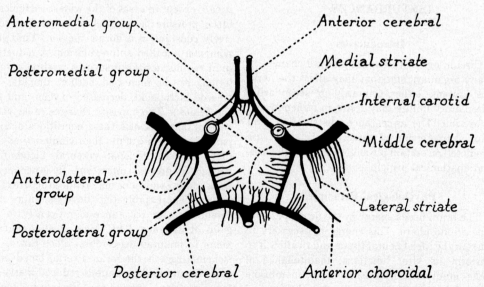

FIGURE 1. This drawing shows the cerebral arterial circle of Willis. (From R. C. Truex, and M. B. Carpenter, *Strong and Elwyn's Human Neuroanatomy*, ed. 5, p. 80. Williams & Wilkins, Baltimore, 1964.)

Small-vessel Cerebrovascular Disease

Disorders affecting small-size and medium-size cerebral vessels generally produce multiple parenchymal lesions spread over wide areas of the brain. The resultant clinical expression represents a summation of the effects of these multiple lesions and consists of a combination of neurological and psychiatric symptoms. Of all disorders involving these small vessels, the most common and most important is the lacunar state.

Lacunae may be defined as ischemic infarcts of restricted size—a few millimeters to 2 cm.—located primarily in the basal ganglia, pons, and subcortical white matter. Although they may be found as isolated lesions, more often they are multiple. Lacunar infarcts are almost exclusively related to arterial hypertension.

The signs and symptoms of lacunar disease are determined by the sites and number of the lesions. An early, prominent feature of this disease is bilateral motor system involvement and signs suggestive of pseudobulbar palsy. Rigidity, akinesia, dysarthria, emotional lability, accentuated deep-tendon reflexes, extensor plantar responses, urinary incontinence, and occasionally a gait disturbance resembling that of parkinsonism may result from multiple lacunae.

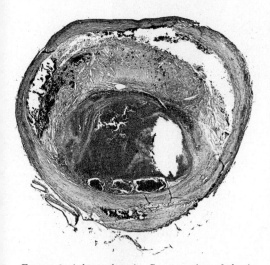

FIGURE 2. Atherosclerosis. Cross-section of the internal carotid artery. Note the narrowed arterial lumen and the destruction of the intima, with some intraluminal thrombus formation. The media shows marked alteration, with prominent cholesterol clefts.

Associated with this syndrome are the typical signs of organic brain disease, including disturbances in judgment, orientation, memory, and cognitive functioning. Careful historical inquiry generally reveals a series of sudden episodes of focal neurological disturbances that clear with variable residue. The appearance of a dementing process is superimposed on the bilateral motor signs. The evolution of the dementia is at times quite slow.

Other disorders may also produce bilateral motor signs, pseudobulbar palsy, and dementia. In the absence of hypertension, this clinical picture may be found in subacute bacterial endocarditis, multiple emboli, and granulomatous angiitis.

No treatment is available to alter the dementia, once it is established. Antihypertensive therapy is effective when started before clinical symptoms develop.

Large-vessel Cerebrovascular Disease

Atherosclerosis. Atherosclerosis is a widespread disorder affecting medium-size and large-size arteries throughout the body. The intima of involved arteries may collect focal deposits of lipids, complex carbohydrates, blood and blood products, fibrous tissue, and calcium (see Figure 2). The clinical complications of atherosclerosis result from ulceration of the arterial plaque, platelet-fibrin aggregation, embolism, thrombosis, stenosis, and arterial occlusion. No effective treatment is available.

Arteriosclerotic Dementia. Cases classified as arteriosclerotic dementia may actually represent the lacunar state, brain syndromes resulting from cerebral infarction, or the senile dementias. Histological examination of brain tissue in cases of arteriosclerotic dementia usually reveals chronic neuronal loss with associated Alzheimer neurofibrillary change and senile plaques. The clinical descriptions of this disorder have included headaches, dizziness, faintness, weakness, transient focal neurological symptoms, memory impairment, sleep disturbance, and such personality changes as emotional lability and hypochondriasis.

If pathological material is used as a basis for differential diagnosis, the cases categorized as arteriosclerotic dementia may be divided into four separate syndromes: the lacunar state, brain syndromes associated with cerebral infarction, degenerative brain disease, and other brain syndromes of unknown cause.

Cerebral Infarction. Little histological difference, other than size, differentiates lacunar lesions from parenchymal infarctions. However, the underlying pathophysiological mechanism and the clinical expression often differ.

Transient cerebral ischemic attacks are not the result of cerebral infarction and do not themselves cause mental deterioration. They are brief episodes of focal neurological dysfunction, lasting less than 24 hours. These episodes are most often the result of microembolization from a proximal, extracranial arterial lesion (see Figure 3) that resolves without significant pathological alteration of the parenchymal tissues.

In general, symptoms of vertebrobasilar disease reflect a transient functional disturbance in either the brainstem or the occipital lobe,

carotid distribution symptoms reflect unilateral hemispheral abnormality. Anticoagulant therapy appears to be effective in cases of symptomatic vertebrobasilar disease, and either anticoagulant therapy or reconstructive extracranial arterial surgery may alleviate the symptoms of carotid system disease.

About one third of untreated patients with transient ischemic attacks later develop a brain infarction, nearly half of them within a few weeks of the transient episodes.

Unilateral cerebral infarction, with its accompanying focal neurological deficit, may be associated with an alteration in mental function. An isolated parenchymal lesion is unlikely to produce the characteristic picture of a dementia, although dysfunction involving specific brain areas can produce symptoms superficially resembling a dementia. Most often confused

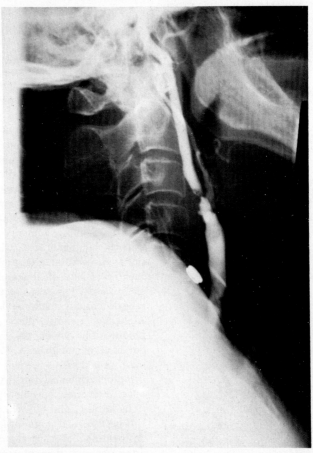

FIGURE 3. Left carotid arteriogram in a 57-year-old patient who had recurrent episodes of right hemiparesis lasting 5 to 15 minutes and a recent episode of sudden, total loss of vision in the left eye lasting 10 minutes (amaurosis fugax). A stenotic ulcerated lesion of the internal carotid artery is visible.

with a dementia are those cases involving patients with unilateral cerebral infarction who have a specific language disorder secondary to dominant hemisphere disease, a visual-spatial orientation defect secondary to nondominant hemisphere disease, and a personality change and emotional lability secondary to frontal lobe disease.

Bilateral or multiple cerebral infarcts are often associated with evidence of mental change. At times, the mental disturbance is severe, overshadowing the concomitant signs of neurological abnormality.

Bilateral lesions of the hippocampus or its connections produce a characteristic syndrome of memory loss, primarily involving recent memory and short-term retention, without other significant mental impairment. This syndrome can be caused by an infarction in the distribution of both posterior cerebral arteries.

Fat embolism may appear in patients who have sustained fractures of the long bones and in patients who develop a syndrome of restlessness, delirium, and confusion associated with fever, tachypnea, and tachycardia 12 to 48 hours after surgery or trauma. Impaired consciousness is the most frequent finding. Bilateral and symmetrical focal neurological signs are also common. Steroid therapy may be effective. The mortality from fat embolism is high, but patients who recover apparently have a low incidence of chronic mental change.

Embolism arising from a cardiac source is commonly associated with chronic atrial fibrillation. The clinician must always consider the possibility of underlying arteriosclerotic or rheumatic heart disease, myocardial infarction, atrial myxoma, and subacute bacterial endocarditis. Cerebral embolism from a cardiac source usually presents as discrete embolic events. Focal neurological signs are apparent, but alterations in consciousness are not generally noted unless bilateral or brainstem embolization has occurred.

When perfusion pressure is reduced, the regions predominantly affected are the overlapping zones between the major cerebral vessels. In patients with significant occlusive disease in the neck or intracranially, the hypotensive effects may be accentuated in these marginally perfused areas along the lateral surfaces of each hemisphere, and infarction can ensue. Mental disturbances suggestive of frontal lobe disease are often associated with signs of motor and sensory disturbance, especially in the arms.

Circulatory Disturbances in the Absence of Significant Cerebrovascular Disease

Neuronal dysfunction and cell death accompany severe anoxia. The distribution of ischemic changes varies widely, although a single, severe hypoxic episode usually produces mainly cortical lesions. Repeated, less severe hypoxic insults cause lesions that are predominantly in the white matter and basal ganglia.

Oxygen lack may result from any of four conditions: (1) Oxygen tension may be reduced in an otherwise normal circulating blood volume (anoxic anoxia), as in carbon monoxide poisoning. (2) The delivery of blood to the tissue may be compromised severely (anemic anoxia), as during cardiac arrest. (3) The circulation may be slowed markedly, so that oxygen consumption exceeds oxygen delivery (stagnant anoxia), as in severe congestive heart failure. (4) There may be interference with the utilization of oxygen by the cells (histotoxic anoxia), generally because a toxic substance, such as cyanide, is circulating in the blood or because not enough substrate is present, as in hypoglycemia.

The clinical symptoms reflect the causative agent, the severity of oxygen deprivation, and its duration of effect. The mental disturbances superimposed on the general neurological picture are remarkably uniform.

In conditions that marginally reduce oxygen perfusion to the central nervous system, extreme restlessness may be seen, often associated with a subjective feeling of air hunger and objective tachypnea. Mental function may be slow and imprecise. Memory is less reliable, and attention span is reduced. Thinking is confused, insight may be lost, and judgment may be impaired. Headache, nausea, and sometimes vomiting may be noted. The predominant feature is acute anxiety. In extreme cases, delirium may be present. This syndrome is seen in many patients with early congestive heart failure or cardiac decompensation. Appropriate therapy can quickly reverse the mental incapacitation.

As oxygen deprivation continues, the delirium becomes less pronounced, and the level of consciousness is altered. Progressive obtundation ensues, leading to stupor and coma. Seizures (both focal and generalized), myoclonic jerking, and decorticate and decerebrate posturing may occur. Pupillary dilatation can be seen; when it occurs, it may be more indicative of circulatory failure than of other causes of hypoxia. Reversibility at this stage depends on the responsible agent.

Patients who recover from the acute stage frequently have widespread neurological and psychiatric sequelae, which are a reflection of the altered brain histology and the causative agent. Mental changes take the form of a dementia, along with features suggestive of Korsakoff's psychosis or of profound psychotic depression. Extrapyramidal syndromes are seen, as are action myoclonus, hyperkinetic states, and focal brain disturbances in the form of apraxias and aphasias. Mental confusion, amnesia, and conceptual difficulties are common. The improvement rate is highly variable, sometimes extending over many weeks or months. A permanent memory defect is common.

In a few patients who recover from a severe anoxic episode, additional neurological and psychiatric signs and symptoms appear spontaneously in 10 to 14 days. Although this deterioration is more common after carbon monoxide poisoning, it may follow other anoxic enceph-

alopathies. The course is one of rapid deterioration. Subcortical demyelination, at times extensive, is found at autopsy examination. The cause is unknown.

Nontraumatic Intracranial Hemorrhage

Nontraumatic intracranial hemorrhage is generally of two types: (1) intracerebral hemorrhage, with focal accumulation of blood in the brain parenchyma (see Figure 4), and (2) subarachnoid hemorrhage, usually the result of a ruptured aneurysm, with extravasation of blood throughout the subarachnoid space. Both are commonly encountered in hypertensive patients. They produce headache of varying severity, altered consciousness, and the cardinal signs of meningeal irritation. Focal neurological deficits may occur in either type but are more common in patients with intracerebral hemorrhage.

Many intracranial events reportedly produce inappropriate secretion of antidiuretic hormone. After a subarachnoid hemorrhage, either the true syndrome is noted or, more often, merely symptomatic hyponatremia is documented. Confusion and agitation or, less frequently, somnolence gradually appears in such

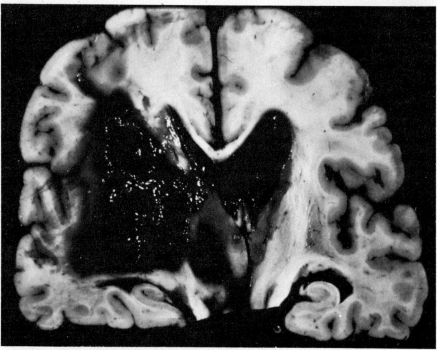

FIGURE 4. Large left intracerebral hemorrhage, with blood extending into the ventricular and subarachnoid spaces.

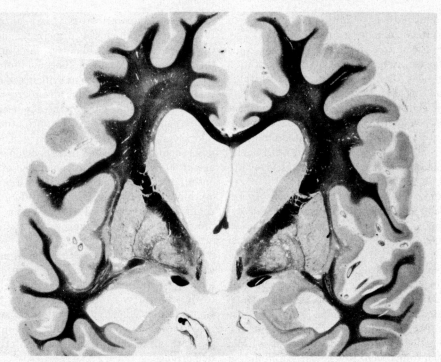

FIGURE 5. Binswanger's disease. The brain is markedly atrophic, with dilatation of the ventricular system. The cortex seems relatively spared, with the most marked loss occurring in the subcortical white matter. The myelin stain used shows areas of patchy demyelination.

patients 1 to 3 days after the primary event. Determinations of serum electrolytes and sometimes urine and serum osmolality confirm the diagnosis. Treatment by simple fluid restriction is often all that is necessary to reverse the condition.

The presence of blood in the subarachnoid pathways can initiate a series of events that lead to decreased circulation and absorption of cerebrospinal fluid over the cerebral hemispheres. This produces the hydrocephalic syndrome of progressive impairment in mentation, akinesia, gait disturbance, and incontinence. This syndrome may occur transiently in many patients after subarachnoid hemorrhage. In a few patients, the defect persists. The presence of mild dementia, impaired memory, slowness of mental and physical activity, lack of spontaneity, easy distractibility, unsteadiness of gait, and urinary incontinence should suggest the presence of this treatable disorder.

Symptoms resembling Korsakoff's syndrome appear to occur primarily in patients with anterior communicating aneurysms, presumably because of ischemic damage to elements of Papez's circuit in the posterior, inferior, and medial frontal areas.

Miscellaneous Syndromes

Binswanger's Disease. The syndrome of progressive dementia and subcortical demyelination, presumably resulting from arteriosclerosis of the small arteries supplying the white matter, was first described by Binswanger (see Figure 5). The disease begins in patients between 50 and 65 years of age, and the dementia is always associated with evidence of focal cerebral disease. The course is described as slowly progressive. Clinical differentiation and antemortem diagnosis do not seem to be possible.

Subacute Bacterial Endocarditis. In a review of the clinical symptoms of this disorder, neuropsychiatric symptoms were found to be either the chief complaint or one of the major presenting complaints in 60 per cent of patients. Severe organic mental disturbances resembling a toxic encephalopathy occurred in nearly one fifth of the cases. Fluctuating confusion, delirium, hallucinations, confusion, and paranoid ideation were common.

Often, the nonspecific findings of a low-grade fever or elevated erythrocyte sedimentation rate, present in nearly 95 per cent of these patients, suggest the possibility of subacute bacterial endocarditis. *Streptococcus viridans* is the most commonly isolated organism, although almost any pathogenic bacteria can produce the disorder. The mortality in patients with bacterial endocarditis and neuropsychiatric symptoms is high.

Systemic Lupus Erythematosus. Abnormalities in mental function in patients with systemic lupus erythematosus may vary between 15 and 50 per cent. The patient may have an acute organic brain syndrome, with disorientation, confusion, inattention, delusions, and hallucinations. A chronic progressive dementia may occur, along with a general deterioration of intellectual function and memory. The disease may produce classical, affective, schizophreniform reactions that are indistinguishable from the usual functional psychoses; catatonic or paranoid behavior is common within this subgroup. Neurotic reactions, including marked anxiety and depression, may occur.

The cause of these mental aberrations is unknown. In many cases, no pathological abnormalities are detected in the brain, and the symptoms are thought to have their genesis in the prepsychotic personality of the patient, the toxic effects of systemic lupus erythematosus on other organ systems, or the side effects of steroid and chloroquine therapy. Pathological changes consisting of hemorrhage, scattered foci of necrosis, arterial wall hyalination, and inflammatory cell infiltration have been seen. The diagnosis can be confirmed by the lupus erythematosus cell test, tissue biopsy, or studies of antinuclear antibodies.

Other Inflammatory Angiopathies. Mental disturbances may accompany the aortic arch syndrome (Takayashu's syndrome), polyarteritis nodosa, cranial arteritis, and noninfectious granulomatous angiitis. The mental changes are neither characteristic nor specific for any of these diseases. Close clinicopathological correlation exists only in cases of granulomatous angiitis with rapid mental deterioration, in which diffuse parenchymal softening is present, along with multiple, widely distributed infarctions.

Cranial (temporal) arteritis is a disorder of the elderly in which the principal manifestations are headache, malaise, lassitude, asthenia, and weight loss. The symptoms are frequently misinterpreted as evidence of depression. When untreated, this disorder produces significant visual loss or blindness in nearly half the patients coming to medical attention. Steroid therapy is remarkably effective. The diagnosis should be suspected in any person over the age of 60 with a persistent headache of recent onset and a systemic reaction. Elevation of the erythrocyte sedimentation rate offers strong confirmatory evidence. Temporal artery biopsy provides histological evidence of the giant cell arteritis.

Hypertensive Crisis. Precise agreement on the specific features of hypertensive encephalopathy is lacking. Some restrict the definition to the clinical syndrome of headache, convulsions, retinal changes, and altered consciousness accompanying an abrupt rise in blood pressure in the absence of cerebral infarction or hemorrhage.

An acute encephalopathic state frequently accompanies an abrupt rise in blood pressure from any cause. Headache, disorientation, and mild mental confusion are common. Agitation and delirium may progress to somnolence, stupor, and coma when the blood pressure remains high. The encephalopathy may be associated with aldosteronism, glomerulonephritis, pheochromocytoma, and eclampsia. A similar syndrome has been noted in patients receiving monoamine oxidase inhibitors who ingest tyramine-containing foods.

One must reduce the patient's blood pressure rapidly and identify the underlying cause to reverse the series of pathological events that may start with reversible arteriolar narrowing and progress to increased capillary permeability, focal cerebral edema, more generalized cerebral edema, neuronal ischemia, necrosis of the vessel wall, and ultimately, intracranial hemorrhage.

Confusional States after Cardiac Surgery. As many as half of the patients undergoing cardiopulmonary bypass and cardiac surgery have neurological and psychiatric symptoms. These symptoms include delayed recovery of consciousness, confusion, disorientation, and focal abnormalities. In most patients, this disorder is transient, although some patients complain of impaired memory and dulled intellect for months after surgery.

Transient Global Amnesia. The precise cause of this disorder is unknown. The patient abruptly loses his ability to recall recent events or to record new memories. Events of the distant past are readily recalled. Although the patient is often aware of some disturbance in function during the episode, he may still perform highly complex mental and physical acts. His behavior may seem relatively normal to all but those closest to him, who often sense some abnormality in mental function. The episode may last 1 to 24 hours and then subside completely. When the episode is over, the patient reports complete amnesia for the events that transpired during the attack and for a variable retrograde period. The attack is most often an isolated event.

REFERENCES

Fisher, C. M. Lacunes: Small, deep cerebral infarcts. Neurology (Minneap.), *15:* 774. 1965.
Fisher, C. M. Dementia and cerebral vascular disease: Dementia in cerebral vascular disease. In *Cerebral Vascular Diseases, Sixth Conference,* J. F. Toole, R. G. Siekert, and J. P. Whisnant, editors, p. 232. Grune & Stratton, New York, 1968.
Karp, H. R. Dementia in cerebrovascular disease and other systemic illnesses. Curr. Concepts Cerebrovasc. Dis. Stroke, 7: 11, 1972.
Patterson, R. H., Brennan, R. W., Kessler, J., and Twichell, J. B. Iatrogenic cerebral ischemia during cardiopulmonary bypass. In *Cerebral Vascular Diseases, Eighth Conference,* F. H. McDowell and R. W. Brennan, editors, p. 181. Grune & Stratton, New York, 1973.
Sandok, B. A. Temporal arteritis. J. A. M. A., *222:* 1405, 1972.
Toole, J. F., and Cole, M. Ischemic cerebrovascular disease. In *Clinical Neurology,* A. B. Baker and L. H. Baker, editors, vol. 1, p. 1. Harper & Row, New York, 1971.
Toole, J. F., and Patel, A. N. *Cerebrovascular Disorders.* McGraw-Hill, New York, 1967.

18.3.   ORGANIC BRAIN SYNDROMES ASSOCIATED WITH DISTURBANCES IN METABOLISM, GROWTH, AND NUTRITION

Introduction

Interference with the normal metabolic processes of the nervous system by endocrine and metabolic diseases, nutritional deficiency, or aberrations due to inborn errors of metabolism can produce neurological and psychological changes. Elderly persons with mild, diffuse neuronal loss due to aging develop changes in mental function more quickly from a metabolic disturbance than do younger persons.

Glucose is the only substrate for the brain, and reserves of glucose and glycogen are minimal in the central nervous system, as compared with other organs. Irreversible neuronal damage results from sustained hypoglycemia. With anoxia, unconsciousness supervenes in 5 to 6 seconds, and irreparable neuronal damage in the cerebral cortex begins after 3 or 4 minutes. After 15 to 20 minutes of anoxia, all nerve cells are destroyed.

The central nervous system also requires vitamins, amino acids, electrolytes, and hormones. These nutrients, as well as glucose and oxygen, depend on an adequate cerebral blood flow. Interference with normal cerebral blood flow leads promptly to neurological dysfunction.

Metabolic and Endocrine Disorders

Metabolic encephalopathy is a common cause of organic brain dysfunction and is capable of producing alterations in mental function, behavior, and neurological function. The earliest signs are likely to be impairment of memory, particularly recent memory, and orientation. Some patients become agitated, anxious, and hyperactive; others become quieter, withdrawn, and inactive. Perceptual errors—such as illusions, delusions, and hallucinations (particularly visual)—often heighten anxiety and agitation. The patient may become tremulous. Postural control of the outstretched arms and hands is impaired. Convulsive seizures, almost always generalized, are common with many severe metabolic disorders, especially hypoglycemic and anoxic encephalopathies. Status epilepticus can develop and is a significant threat to the patient's survival. As metabolic encephalopathies worsen, confusion or delirium gives way to decreased responsiveness, stupor, and coma.

A quiet confusion is more likely to be seen with uremia, pulmonary encephalopathy, and anoxic encephalopathy. An agitated delirium is more likely to be seen with acute liver failure, withdrawal from alcohol or barbiturates, acute intermittent porphyria, and some endocrine disorders. Rapidly developing metabolic derangements of any kind are more likely to produce an agitated delirium.

Most metabolic encephalopathies are potentially responsive to treatment of the underlying disorder, especially if the treatment is begun promptly. If anxiety or agitation is a significant problem, paraldehyde or diazepam may be helpful. Symptoms of withdrawal from barbiturates or tranquilizers require treatment with barbiturates. Convulsions occurring during withdrawal from these medications or from alcohol are best managed with phenobarbital, although the intravenous administration of diazepam may be effective for status epilepticus.

Hepatic Encephalopathy

Severe impairment of liver function may be attended by disturbances of consciousness, mental changes, asterixis, hyperventilation, and electroencephalographic abnormalities. An increase in blood ammonium levels occurs in most of these patients, but other metabolic derangements, poorly understood, are also important. Impairment of the normal detoxification processes in the liver for drugs and other exogenous substances can also contribute to the syndrome when such substances are present.

Associated infection, gastrointestinal bleeding, acid-base imbalance, and electrolyte disturbances, which can complicate hepatic encephalopathy, require specific treatment. In addition, measures to lower blood ammonium levels—such as dietary protein restriction, cathartics, and enemas to clear the intestine of its nitrogenous content—and oral neomycin to reduce the intestinal bacterial flora are required.

Uremic Encephalopathy

Acute or chronic failure of normal renal function leads to serious systemic metabolic changes. Neurological dysfunction—particularly alterations in memory, orientation, and consciousness—is a common accompaniment. Asterixis may be seen. A peripheral neuropathy can develop during chronic uremia. Restlessness and crawling sensations of the limbs, twitching of muscles singly or in groups, and sometimes persistent hiccups can be distressing and exhausting to the patient. In severe uremia, generalized convulsions can occur, sometimes in rapid succession, leading to a greater risk of death. Intravenously administered diazepam may be an effective treatment, but barbiturates or even anesthetics may be required for seizure control.

Hypoglycemic Encephalopathy

Excessive or inappropriate administration of insulin and hyperinsulinism are the two most likely causes of hypoglycemic encephalopathy. Hypoglycemia, if prolonged, can cause irreversible neuronal damage.

Hypoglycemic episodes are more likely to occur in the early morning hours or after exercise. Premonitory symptoms, which do not always occur in every patient, include nausea, sweating, tachycardia, and feelings of hunger, apprehension, and restlessness. With progressive impairment, disorientation, confusion, hallucinations, pallor, and extreme restlesness or agitation develop. Diplopia, and grand mal or focal seizures, myoclonic jerks, and hyperreflexia with clonus and Babinski's responses can be other features. Stupor and then coma may follow quickly.

Many patients with anxiety or other neurotic symptoms are mistakenly thought to have hypoglycemia. Determination of the blood glucose level during an attack is helpful, but, with transient episodes of hypoglycemia, special procedures, such as measurement of blood glucose level after fasting overnight or for as long as 72 hours, are required. The intravenous tolbutamide tolerance test can be useful.

Diabetic Ketoacidosis

Resulting from inadequately treated diabetes mellitus, diabetic ketoacidosis ranges from mild ketonuria to diabetic coma. Ketoacidosis is likely to be precipitated by stress, such as infection, trauma, surgery, or pregnancy.

The condition begins with feelings of weakness, easy fatigability and listlessness, and increasing polyuria and polydipsia. Headache and sometimes nausea and vomiting appear. The situation worsens in hours to several days, with ketonuria, ketonemia, dehydration, metabolic acidosis, and persisting hyperglycemia and glucosuria. Then more rapidly, confusion and stupor lead to coma. With no treatment, circulatory collapse, oliguria, and anuria occur—and ultimately death.

Treatment of diabetic ketoacidosis requires the immediate intravenous administration of regular insulin. If fever is present, an infection requiring treatment should be assumed to exist. Intravenous fluids—0.9 per cent sodium chloride solution initially, followed by 0.45 per cent sodium chloride solution—are also needed. Care should be taken not to give potassium salts until urine volume is adequate and hyperkalemia is absent.

Acute Intermittent Porphyria

This disorder is inherited as an autosomal dominant trait, and its symptoms are most likely to begin after puberty or in the third and fourth decades of life. Women are affected more often than men. A defect in the regulation of the liver enzyme δ-aminolevulinic acid synthetase is important in pyrrole metabolism. Increased quantities are present in the urine during acute episodes of the disease. Certain drugs and hormones—in particular barbiturates, sulfonamides, estrogens, and griseofulvin—appear to enhance the activity of this liver enzyme. The use of barbiturates for any reason is absolutely contraindicated in any person known to have acute intermittent porphyria or to have a relative with this disease.

Symptoms of nervousness and emotional instability are frequently present over a long period. Recurrent abdominal pains, often colicky in nature, are common. Neurological symptoms may become so severe that death results. Peripheral neuropathy involving one or all of the limbs and cranial nerve signs may be seen. Confusion, delirium, convulsions, and coma can develop during acute attacks.

There is, as yet, no satisfactory or specific treatment for acute intermittent porphyria. During acute episodes, only careful symptomatic measures can be used, such as phenothiazines or reserpine for abdominal pains and psychic symptoms, opiates when absolutely necessary to control abdominal pains, and careful nursing for peripheral neuropathy. If bulbar or respiratory muscle involvement appears, mechanical respiratory assistance is required.

Endocrine Disorders

Changes in personality, mental functions, and memory, as well as neurological abnormalities, occur frequently in endocrine disorders. Correction of the underlying endocrine problem usually reverses these changes.

Large tumors arising in or above the sella turcica can compress the overlying hypothalamus and basal portions of the frontal lobes, invade the sphenoid sinus, or involve the cavernous sinus and its related structures. Impair-

ment of memory and intellect can develop with such large lesions. Surgical decompression or removal of the lesion can alleviate these mental changes. The most important neurological problem associated with lesions in or above the sella turcica is visual impairment.

Hypothalamic involvement is associated with behavioral disturbances that are sometimes dramatic—alterations in appetite causing severe inanition or extreme obesity, marked emotional lability, inappropriate rage reactions, aberrations of the normal sleep pattern.

Thyroid Function. These disorders produce hyperthyroidism or myxedema. A sensation of easy fatigability and generalized weakness is felt by most hyperthyroid patients. Insomnia, weight loss in spite of an increased appetite, tremulousness, palpitations, and increased perspiration are all common changes. The patient may appear anxious and restless, and in the early stages a neurotic reaction may be mistakenly considered. Prominent mental disturbances develop in a few patients, with impairment of memory, orientation, and judgment and even manic excitement and schizophreniclike symptoms with delusions and hallucinations. Occasionally, masked hyperthyroidism, characterized by apathy and mental confusion without tremor and overactivity, occurs, especially in old persons.

Treatment of hyperthyroidism in most adults consists of the administration of radioactive iodine. Mental symptoms can be expected to improve with adequate treatment of the hyperthyroidism.

Hypothyroidsm (myxedema) arises because of a deficiency of thyroid hormone. Commonly, it is the result of treatment for hyperthyroidism with radioactive iodine or surgical thyroidectomy.

Easy fatigability, feelings of weakness and sleepiness, increased sensitivity to cold, reduced sweating with dryness and thickening of the skin, brittle and thinning hair, and puffy facies are all common manifestations of myxedema. In some patients, changes in personality, memory, and intellecutal function are prominent and may simulate major psychiatric or organic brain disease. After treatment with thyroid hormone, these changes can be expected to clear, but an occasional patient never does regain normal mental function.

With severe myxedema, the patient may

become obtunded and even comatose. Mortality has always been high—at least 50 per cent even in the best reported series. Stresses such as infection and anesthesia are important precipitating factors. Coma evolves gradually over a period of hours. Rapid replacement of thyroid hormone is mandatory, and antibiotics, fluid restriction, respiratory assistance when indicated, and often steroids are important adjuncts.

Parathyroid Function. Parathyroid dysfunction produces derangements of calcium metabolism. Excessive secretion of parathyroid hormone causes hypercalcemia. Common complaints are lassitude, weakness, increased irritability, and anxiety. Some patients display frank disorders of personality and mental function, such as agitation, paranoid thinking, depression, psychotic reactions, confusion, and stupor. Neuromuscular excitability is reduced, and true muscle weakness may appear.

Hypoparathyroidism may result from the inadvertent removal of the parathyroid glands during thyroidectomy, or it may be idiopathic. Lowered serum calcium levels lead to increased neuromuscular excitability. Mental symptoms such as confusion, agitation or drowsiness, hallucinations, and depression can also develop.

Adrenal Function. These disorders cause changes in the normal secretion of hormones from the adrenal cortex and the adrenal medulla. Patients with chronic adrenocortical insufficiency (Addison's disease) exhibit mild mental symptoms, such as apathy, easy fatigability, irritability, and depression. Occasionally, psychotic reactions or confusion develops. Cortisone or one of its synthetic derivatives is effective in correcting these abnormalities. Acute adrenocortical insufficiency is a life-threatening illness, characterized by vomiting, weakness, dehydration, hypotension, and impairment of consciousness. It is precipitated by a stress in a patient with Addison's disease, or it may follow the abrupt withdrawal of high doses of corticosteroids. Immediate treatment is necessary with administration of cortisol, intravenous injection of isotonic sodium chloride solution, and the correction of any underlying precipitating factor.

Excessive quantities of cortisol are likely to produce euphoria, insomnia, restlesness, and increased motor activity. Some patients become anxious and depressed. Correction of Cushing's syndrome or reduction in the dosage of corticosteroids is followed by improvement, but recovery may take several months.

Primary aldosteronism most often results from excessive secretion of aldosterone. Hypokalemia, hyperkalemia, and alkalosis are characteristic. Recurrent episodes of generalized muscular weakness have been reported. All patients have hypertension.

A pheochromocytoma secretes increased quantities of epinephrine. Sustained or paroxysmal hypertension results. Episodes of sudden paroxysmal hypertension occur in about half of the patients. The paroxysms are characterized by headache, pallor, perspiration, and severe anxiety. If the attack is severe, cerebral hemorrhage and death can occur.

Growth and Nutritional Disorders

In addition to oxygen and glucose, vitamins and minerals are nutrients required by cells of the nervous system for normal functioning. Vitamin deficiencies or inborn errors of metabolism associated with deficient or abnormal enzyme function can result in significant neurological dysfunction. Many of these diseases are amenable to replacement of the deficient substance or to manipulation of the metabolic error through dietary alterations or pharmacological means.

Neurological disorders result particularly from deficiencies of thiamine (vitamin B_1), nicotinic acid, vitamin B_6 (a collective term for pyridoxine, pyridoxal, and pyridoxamine), and vitamin B_{12} (cyanocobalamin). Thiamine (vitamin B_1) deficiency leads to beriberi, characterized chiefly by cardiovascular and neurological changes, and the Wernicke-Korsakoff syndrome, which is most often associated with chronic alcoholism.

Beriberi

This disorder occurs primarily in Asia and in areas of famine or poverty. Subacute or chronic onset is most common. Heart failure with a high cardiac output, cardiac dilation, tachycardia and cardiac arrhythmias, edema, and dyspnea or exertion are the cardiovascular changes. Peripheral neuropathy is common. Paresthesiae and dysesthesiae are experienced. Muscle weakness appears, sometimes severe enough to include wrist-drop and foot-drop. The deep-tendon reflexes are reduced or lost. The peripheral neuropathy of beriberi and that of chronic alcoholism likely represent the same disease process. Mental disturbances such as apathy, depression, irritability, nervousness, and poor concentration are frequently seen.

Wernicke-Korsakoff Syndrome

This syndrome is most often attributable to chronic alcoholism, but nonalcoholic patients have been occasionally described with severe diseases of the gastrointestinal tract. Wernicke's encephalopathy usually develops over a period of days to several weeks, with confusion, occasionally impaired consciousness, ataxia, nystagmus, and ophthalmoplegia. Signs of peripheral neuropathy are common.

Korsakoff's psychosis is a mental disturbance that evolves during and as a sequel to Wernicke's encephalopathy in most instances. Loss of past memories (retrograde amnesia) and an inability to form new permanent memories are characteristic. Confabulation occurs in some patients.

The clinical manifestations of Wernicke's encephalopathy respond promptly to thiamine alone. Improvement begins within hours, and recovery is complete in a week or two. Thiamine given to patients who have not yet developed Korsakoff's psychosis prevents its occurrence.

Central Pontine Myelinolysis

This demyelinizing disorder of the brainstem seems to arise on a nutritional basis. Most patients have been alcoholics. Quadriparesis with bulbar involvement has occurred in some patients; others have shown no clinical changes, the diagnosis being made on postmortem study.

Marchiafava-Bignami Disease

This is another uncommon neurological disorder associated with chronic alcoholism. Focal neurological signs and symptoms—such as hemiparesis, aphasia, apraxias, and grand mal seizures—develop, and mental changes are almost always present, with manic, paranoid, and delusional states, depression, or dementia. It is a progressive disease and ends in death in several years.

Pellagra

Dietary insufficiency of nicotinic acid and its precursor, tryptophan, is associated with pella-gra. Pellagra is characterized by photosensitive erythematous skin rashes on the hands, face, neck, and feet, as well as inflammation and subsequent atrophy of mucous membranes. Because of the latter, stomatitis, glossitis, and enteritis occur. Involvement of the nervous system is important, with headaches, insomnia, apathy, confusional states, delusions, and, eventually, dementia. Cerebellar ataxia can be seen. Peripheral neuropathy is also a frequent feature.

The response of the pellagra patient to treatment with nicotinic acid is rapid, with significant improvement in confusion, abdominal symptoms, and painful swollen tongue being evident in the first 24 hours. However, dementia from prolonged illness may improve slowly and incompletely.

Hartnup's disease is characterized by episodes of cerebellar ataxia, a light-sensitive dermatitis, and mental changes similar to those seen in pellagra. Defective absorption and intracellular transport of tryptophan seem to be present. Aminoaciduria and a large urinary output of indolic compounds can be demonstrated. Nicotinic acid and a good diet with protein seem to be helpful.

Pyridoxine Deficiency

Pyridoxine (vitamin B_6) is required for the formation of a coenzyme active in transamination, the synthesis of serotonin, the metabolism of amino acids containing hydroxyl groups and sulfur, and decarboxylation. The specific metabolic defect is unknown. Patients receiving antituberculosis treatment with isoniazid are prone to develop a peripheral neuropathy. The neuropathy responds to pyridoxine, and the occurrence of the neuropathy can be prevented by giving pyridoxine daily to patients receiving isoniazid therapy.

B_{12} Deficiency

This deficiency state is characterized by the development of a megaloblastic anemia (pernicious anemia) and neurological manifestations due to degenerative changes in the peripheral nerves, the spinal cord, and the brain. About 80 per cent of patients develop neurological changes.

The neurological signs and symptoms are most likely to evolve over a few weeks or months. Paresthesiae of the distal portion of the limbs are the most frequent initial manifestations. These sensations become associated with gait unsteadiness and stiffness as spinal cord involvement begins. The deep-tendon reflexes become depressed or disappear because of the peripheral nerve involvement. Paraplegia and bowel and bladder dysfunction ultimately supervene. Mental changes—such as apathy, depression, irritability, and moodiness—are common. In a few patients, confusion, delusions, hallucinations, and dementia, sometimes with paranoid features, are prominent manifestations.

The neurological manifestations of vitamin B_{12} deficiency can be completely and rapidly arrested by the early and continued administration of parenteral vitamin B_{12} therapy. In patients with symptoms of a few weeks or months, complete or nearly complete recovery can be expected.

Inborn Errors of Metabolism

Metabolic anomalies affecting the normal handling of lipids, and protein are likely to be heredofamillial; many of them are uncommon or rare, and they are particularly prone to appear in infancy or childhood. Involvement of the central nervous system is frequent, causing mental retardation, convulsive disorders, or progressive neurological deterioration and early death.

Inherited as an autosomal recessive defect, Wilson's disease is characterized by abnormal copper metabolism, degenerative changes in the brain, cirrhosis of the liver, and the deposition of brownish copper-containing granules of pigment around the corneal margin in Descemet's membrane of the cornea (Kayser-Fleischer ring). Excessive copper deposition also occurs elsewhere in the body, especially in the liver, brain, and kidneys.

The onset of symptoms is gradual, usually beginning in the second or third decade of life. Mild tremor and incoordination are common early signs. As the disease slowly progresses, chorea, athetosis, muscular rigidity, and ataxia appear. Mild alterations in personality may be present early, with irritability, silliness, difficulty in concentrating, and facile behavior. Impairment of memory and intellect develops in some cases, as do psychotic symptoms, which may include hypomanic or paranoid episodes, irritable outbursts, and hallucinations. Untreated, the disease progresses to a stage of total

disability and confinement to bed over 3 to 10 years.

D-Penicillamine instituted early in the course of the disease and combined with a diet of low copper content, can prevent severe disability and can lead to steady clinical improvement over many months, sometimes to an almost normal contition. Treatment must be continued indefinitely to prevent a return of neurological deterioration.

REFERENCES

Beeson, P. B., and McDermott, W. *Cecil-Loeb Textbook of Medicine*, ed. 13. W. B. Saunders, Phildelphia, 1971.
Bickford, R. G., and Butt, H. R. Hepatic coma: The electroencephalographic pattern. J. Clin. Invest., *34:* 790, 1955.
Garner, R. J., and Koppel, D. M. Hyperparathyroid crisis: Report of a case. Arch. Surg., *98:* 674, 1969.
Goldberg, A. Acute intermittent porphyria: A study of 50 cases. Q. J. Med., *28:* 183, 1959.
Reeves, A. G., and Plum, F. Hyperphagia, rage, and dementia accompanying a ventromedial hypothalamic neoplasm. Arch. Neurol., *20:* 616, 1969.
Victor, M., Adams, R. D., and Collins, G. H. *The Wernicke-Korsakoff Syndrome: A Clinical and Pathological Study of 245 Patients, 82 With Postmortem Examinations.* F. A. Davis, Philadelphia, 1971.
Wilson S. A. K. Progressive lenticular degeneration: A familial nervous disease associated with cirrhosis of the liver. Brain, *34:* 295, 1912.

18.4.   ORGANIC BRAIN SYNDROMES ASSOCIATED WITH DISEASES OF UNKNOWN CAUSE

Senile Dementia and Alzheimer's Disease

Aging is usually associated with brain atrophy and with impairment of the ability to perform well on certain psychological tests. If there is no need to make new decisions and if daily life is simple and structured, patients with intellectual impairment may continue to adapt successfully. If, however, the environment is stressful or if the patient had previously been barely able to adjust, even minor intellectual impairment may precipitate severe problems in adaptation.

In addition to these usual changes with senescence, severe dementia occurs in a significant number of elderly patients. Alois Alzheimer described a similar condition developing in persons under the age of 65, a condition that has been termed presenile dementia.

Senile dementia is a clinical syndrome characterized by a severe loss of intellectual function in an elderly patient for which no other cause is found. The disorder can be differentiated from normal senescence only by considering the degree of dementia.

The cause of senile dementia remains unclear. Although atrophy is most marked in the frontal and temporal lobes, the entire brain is atrophied (see Figure 1). Microscopic examination of the brain reveals a loss of neurons, with a proliferation of glial cells most apparent in the cerebral cortex but also present in the basal ganglia. The specific lesions found in both senile dementia and Alzheimer's disease include senile plaques and Alzheimer's neurofibrillary changes (see Figure 2). These lesions tend to be more severe and widespread in patients who are younger (Alzheimer's disease) than in those who are older (senile dementia). These changes may also be found in older patients who are not demented, but they are less frequent and are not as widely distributed throughout the brain.

The illness begins insidiously. Usually, the patient presents with an impairment of recent memory and then an impairment of judgment. These symptoms are generally associated with some slowing and rigidity of movement and often with a slow and shuffling gait. The illness is progressive and commonly lasts for 1 to 10 years. It may be associated with specific intellectual changes, such as aphasia, apraxia, and agnosia. Late in the illness, myoclonic or generalized seizures may develop, and the patient often becomes helpless. Death is usually from intercurrent illness.

During the disease, the patient's attempts to adapt to his dementia may lead to an exaggeration of any prior psychopathology. The symptoms then often include depression or paranoid responses.

The diagnosis of Alzheimer's disease or senile dementia is made on the basis of a clinical history of progressive dementia in middle or late life. The presumptive diagnosis should be confirmed, when indicated, with appropriate psychological testing and observation. A routine medical and neurological workup is also indicated to exclude other treatable causes of dementia.

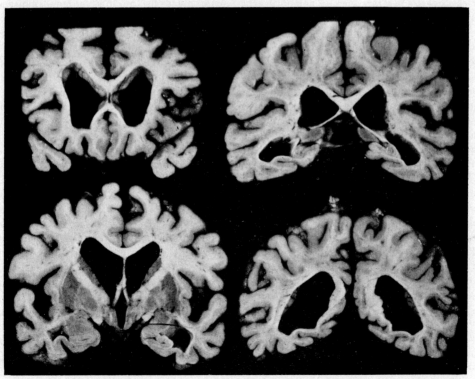

FIGURE 1. Senile dementia (Alzheimer's disease): diffuse cerebral atrophy with dilatation of the ventricles and widening of the cortical sulci. (Courtesy of Dr. Thomas Reagan, Mayo Clinic, Rochester, Minnesota.)

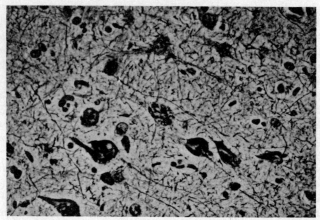

FIGURE 2. Senile dementia (Alzheimer's disease): senile plaques and neurofibrillary degeneration (Bodian stain × 238). (Courtesy of Dr. Thomas Reagan, Mayo Clinic, Rochester, Minnesota.)

The differential diagnosis must include such reversible metabolic diseases as myxedema and pernicious anemia, such infectious diseases as syphilis, and such tumors as fontal lobe meningiomas.

Pick's Disease

Pick's disease is a rare form of dementia that is usually included with Alzheimer's disease as one of the presenile dementias. The cause is unknown, but many familial cases have been reported.

The disorder is distinctive in that it is characterized by lobar atrophy. The frontal and temporal lobes are usually the most seriously affected, the occipital lobes being less affected and the parietal lobes still less so. The line of demarcation between the involved and the noninvolved lobes is usually sharp (see Figure 3). Microscopically, there is neuronal loss (particularly in the outer layers of the cortex), prominent glial proliferation, and, in a large proportion of cases, involvement of the basal ganglia.

The clinical features and course of the disorder are similar to those of senile dementia and Alzheimer's disease. Because the illness is progressive and no causative factors are known, the treatment can only be supportive.

Parkinsonism

In 1817 Parkinson described a clinical syndrome characterized by tremor, apparent paralysis, and abnormal gait. He named this syndrome paralysis agitans. The criteria for this diagnosis have widened to include a peculiar form of rigidity, bradykinesia, impairment of postural stability, facial masking, loss of associated movements, and impairment of speech.

The annual prevalence in the Western hemisphere has been reported to be about 200 per 100,000 people. In most cases, the cause of the syndrome is obscure. It is commonly a disease of middle life and beyond.

Familial occurrence has become increasingly evident.

A study of the brains of patients who die from parkinsonism reveals a decrease in both the amount of the usual dark pigment and the number of cells in the substantia nigra. Another finding is depletion of the dopamine content of the basal ganglia.

Often, the first characteristic sign is a loss of associated movements, with a peculiar immobility of the patient. Tremor may become apparent later; it is most prominent at rest or on assuming a posture and is a characteristic pill-rolling tremor. As with most extrapyramidal disorders, the tremor becomes more prominent with tension and disappears with sleep.

Physical examination reveals an impairment of fine movements and a peculiar, cogwheel kind of rigidity that is most apparent in the neck and in the upper extremities. Sucking reflexes, positive Babinski's signs, and other evidence of pyramidal tract involvement are common.

Intellectual impairment is a common component. Dementia is usually mild, and patients are able to continue their ordinary activities. However, the dementia tends to increase with the duration and severity of the disease and may prevent the patient from participating in his usual occupation. The described incidence of dementia in parkinsonism ranges from 40 per cent to more than 80 per cent.

Depression is frequently associated with parkinsonism, occurring in as many as one third to one half of all such cases. Patients become extremely concerned about their altered physical appearance, and this concern aggravates their symptoms. Patients then often become withdrawn.

The course of parkinsonism is gradually progressive, regardless of therapy. In treating a patient with parkinsonism, one must help him to maintain ordinary activities. Withdrawal from these activities leads to further rigidity, sequelae of disuse, and inevitably, depression. In some instances, motor impairment is an indication for specific exercises to combat these developments. Similarly, speech impairment makes specific speech therapy essential. L-Dopa can benefit most patients with this disease, and in half of the patients the benefit is appreciable. In addition, the previously used anticholinergic drugs may enhance the improvement produced by L-dopa. Amantadine hydrochloride has also proved useful and has the advantages of fewer side effects.

Huntington's Chorea

In 1872 Huntington described a hereditary disorder, characterized by choreiform movements and dementia, that began in adult life. Huntington's chorea is rare; it is estimated that there are about six such patients in 100,000 persons in the Western hemisphere. The disorder is inherited as an autosomal dominant with strong penetrance.

In this disorder the brain is extensively atrophied, particularly in the caudate and putamen. These two nuclei sustain a primary loss of nerve cells. The illness eventually progresses to involve the two facets of the disease. The onset is usually insidious; it is often heralded by a personality change that interferes with the patient's ability to adapt to his environment. The disease may begin at any age but is most

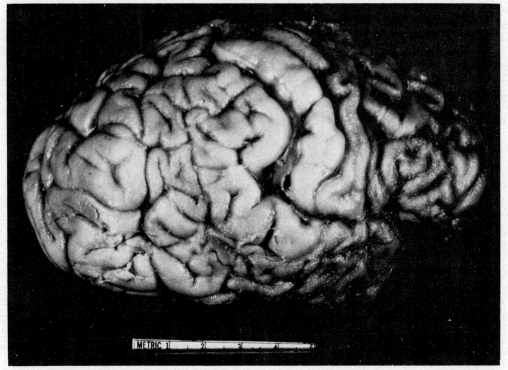

FIGURE 3. Pick's disease: severe frontal and temporal pole cerebral atrophy with sparing of motor and sensory cortex and first temporal convolutions. (Courtesy of Dr. Thomas Reagan, Mayo Clinic, Rochester, Minnesota.)

common in late middle life. When the movements are first noted, they are frequently misinterpreted as inconsequential habit spasms or tics. Eventually, the choreiform movements or the dementia makes chronic hospitalization imperative. The clinical course then is one of gradual progression, death occurring 10 to 20 years after the onset of the disease. Suicide is frequent in patients with this disorder.

The only satisfactory treatment at present is prevention of the transmission of the responsible genes.

Parkinson Dementia of Guam

A syndrome with the features of parkinsonism and dementia has been described among the Chamorro people of Guam, where it accounts for 7 per cent of the deaths in the local population.

The clinical syndrome is characterized by immobility and rigidity. The patient, who is usually in late middle life, gradually withdraws from his usual activities. He no longer engages in spontaneous activity of any sort, and it becomes increasingly difficult to obtain a response, even on stimulation. Dementia is profound and progressive, but it is frequently obscured by the patient's failure to respond. An examination reveals cogwheel rigidity and, often, Babinski's signs and bilateral sucking reflexes. The course is progressive and patients die of the illness 3 to 5 years after onset. There is no effective therapy.

Progressive Supranuclear Palsy (Heterogeneous Systems Disease)

This rare form of neuronal degeneration presents with impairment of eye movement, rigidity, and dementia. The cause of the syndrome is obscure. Histopathological study reveals a loss of nerve cells, gliosis, neurofibrillary tangles, granulovacuolar degeneration, and demyelination in the basal ganglia, brainstem, and nuclei.

The clinical features are a progressive loss of vertical eye movements in middle life, associated with rigidity and dementia. The patient presents with unsteadiness, mild dementia, features of parkinsonism, a minor degree of tremor, and a progressive loss of vertical conjugate gaze. The patient's complaints often include difficulty in walking and frequent stumbling because of difficulty with vertical eye movements. Severe rigidity develops, and the patient often

becomes bedfast. Death usually occurs 5 to 10 years after the onset of the illness. L-Dopa and other drugs used in the treatment of parkinsonism are of little use, if any.

Idiopathic Orthostatic Hypotension

Orthostatic hypotension is commonly associated with peripheral neuropathy, or it may follow the administration of tranquilizers, antidepressants, antihypertensives, and L-dopa. The idiopathic form of orthostatic hypotension is accompanied by signs of central nervous system disease, including dysarthria, pupillary irregularity, tremor, rigidity, and dementia. It often seems to overlap the syndrome of parkinsonism.

The syndrome is rare, and the cause is unknown. Pathological changes in the intermediolateral columns of the spinal cord have been described, and degenerative changes have been reported in the neurons of the cortex and the basal ganglia. The disorder commonly occurs in middle-aged men and is insidious in onset. Fainting on standing usually brings the patient to the attention of the physician. An examination reveals impotence, often incontinence, and dementia. The disorder is progressive and may become so severe that the patient is unable to rise from the recumbent position.

The clinical course is unbroken, and the patient may die from the hypotension or from associated neurological disorders. The treatment is only partially successful; it includes the use of antigravity suits and drugs that improve the circulatory blood volume—for example, flurocortisone.

Normal Pressure Hydrocephalus

A treatable type of dementia is found in patients with enlarged ventricles and normal cerebrospinal fluid pressure. The syndrome is characterized by a progressive dementia. It occurs for the most part in adults of middle or late life. An associated gait disturbance appears to be more of an apraxia of gait than ataxia. There may be some increase in deep reflex activity, and a Babinski's sign may be elicited, although in some patients the reflexes are normal. The patient's relatives frequently state that he has had difficulty in bladder control, attributable more to a lack of concern than to a true loss of control.

The syndrome is thought to be secondary to

an obstruction to the absorption of spinal fluid. In the most common form, it is a sequel of a previous subarachnoid hemorrhage, meningitis, or repeated trauma to the head. In other instances, no cause for the disorder can be elicited. If the diagnosis can be established, the treatment of choice is shunting of the cerebrospinal fluid from the ventricular space to either the atrium or the peritoneal space.

Multiple Sclerosis

Multiple sclerosis is a common neurological disease that may cause severe neurological deficit. It is characterized by remission and exacerbations and by multifocal lesions in the white matter of the central nervous system. It has been estimated that the prevalence of multiple sclerosis in the Western hemisphere is 50 patients per 100,000 population. It is more common in women than in men and is predominantly a disease of young adults.

The cause of multiple sclerosis remains unknown. The two causative factors that are presently fashionable are allergy and infection.

The external surface of the brain appears to be normal. On gross examination, sections of the brain reveal numerous small, grayish patches in the cerebral hemisphere and spinal cord, particularly in the white matter of the paraventricular regions. These patches are the plaques of multiple sclerosis. They vary in size from that of a pinhead to areas involving the majority of the white matter of the frontal lobes.

The disease is characterized by symptoms and signs that are transient and recurrent and that suggest multifocal disease of the central nervous system. Exacerbations tend to be subacute, often reaching their maximum in several days and remitting in weeks to months, although the over-all course tends to be progressive. The clinical course is usually one of decades, although the patient may die of the disease within weeks of onset.

The common presenting complaints of patients with well-established multiple sclerosis usually include a spastic ataxic gait, intention tremor, disorders of ocular movement, and impairment of vision. Features suggesting a psychiatric disorder are frequent. Mental disturbances are present in at least 50 per cent of patients with multiple sclerosis. Hysterical symptoms are often recorded as preceding or being associated with the early signs of the disease. Often, there is a change in emotional tone. The most common initial symptom is anxiety. Impairment of cognition is common as the disease progresses, and this impairment may lead to gross mental deterioration.

The course of the disease is extremely variable, ranging from a matter of weeks from onset to death to more than 60 years. The disease is often very mild.

Since the causative factors have never been established, the treatment remains symptomatic. During an exacerbation of the illness, patients should rest more than usual, and every effort should be made to maintain these patients on an adequate diet.

REFERENCES

Aring, C. D. Observations on multiple sclerosis and conversion hysteria. Brain, *88:* 663, 1965.
Baker, H. L., Jr., Campbell, J. K., Houser, O. W., Reese, D. F. Sheedy, P. F., and Holman, C. B. Computer assisted tomography of the head: An early evaluation. Mayo Clin. Proc., *49:* 17, 1974.
Busse, E. W., and Pfeiffer, E. Mental illness in later life. In *Mental Disorders in Later Life: Organic Brain Syndrome,* p. 107. American Psychiatric Association, Washington, 1973.
Coblentz, J. M., Mattis, S., Zingesser, L. H., Kasoff, S. S., Wisniewski, H. M., and Katzman, R. Presenile dementia: Critical aspects and evaluation of cerebrospinal fluid dynamics. Arch. Neurol. *29:* 299, 1973.
Cotzias, G. C., Papavasiliou, P. S., and Gellene, R. Modification of parkinsonism: Chronic treatment with L-dopa. N. Engl. J. Med., *280:* 337, 1969.
Kurtzke, J. F., and Kurland, L. T. The epidemiology of neurologic disease. In *Clinical Neurology,* A. B. Baker and L. H. Baker, editors, vol. 3, chap. 48. Harper & Row, New York, 1973.
Martin, W. E., Loewenson, R. B., Resch, J. A., and Baker, A. B. Parkinson's disease: Clinical analysis of 100 patients. Neurology (Minneap.), *23:* 783, 1973.
McMenemey, W. H. The dementias and progressive diseases of the basal ganglia. In *Greenfield's Neuropathology,* W. Blackwood, W. H. McMenemey, A. Meyer, R. M. Norman, and D. S. Russel, editors, ed. 2, p. 520. Williams & Wilkins, Baltimore, 1963.
Oakley, G. P., Jr. The neurotoxicity of halogenated hydroxyquinolines: A commentary. J. A. M. A., *225:* 395, 1973.
Wolstenholme, G. E. W., and O'Connor, M., editors. *Alzheimer's Disease and Related Conditions.* J. & A. Churchill, London. 1970.

18.5. ORGANIC BRAIN SYNDROMES ASSOCIATED WITH BRAIN TRAUMA

Introduction

It has been estimated that one person in 200 will require medical care for head injury each year, and on any given day about 1 per cent of the working force is disabled because of head injury. The most serious sequelae of head injury involve severe, disabling mental symptoms resulting from injuries to the brain or neurotic reactions to the injury itself.

Pathophysiology

Traumatic injury of the brain may be produced in three ways: (1) movement of the brain within the skull by sudden acceleration or deceleration, (2) skull fracture and penetration of the brain by a sharp object or bone, and (3) a static loading situation in which the head is subject to pressure of equal intensity from all sides. The first two mechanisms are the most important in producing brain trauma. If the skull collides with a pointed or small object, little mass displacement of the skull itself occurs, and the injury resulting from indentation of the bone or penetration by the object produces local trauma to the brain. Although intracranial pressure rises transiently, there is usually no evidence of trauma other than that caused locally by the penetrating object (see Figure 1). In blunt trauma, the brain rotates within the skull, creating sheer and stress forces on the brain substances. The brain is also compressed near the site of the blow, producing a negative pressure on the opposite side of the brain and causing a contrecoup lesion. Blunt trauma to the head may result in widespread small lesions throughout the brain, presumably because of cavitation phenomena from pressure waves disseminating throughout the brain, vibration effects, or rotational motion, with shearing damage to the brain substance (see Figure 2).

More centrally located damage to the brain can be explained by cavitation phenomena occurring within the ventricles of the brain, particularly in injuries on a sagittal plane. This phenomenon accounts for lesions in the region of the thalamus, corpus callosum, and third ventricle. The location of the brainstem near the mobile craniocervical junction makes it more liable to rotational shearing effects.

Hematomas result from the bursting of small vessels or capillaries secondary to the negative pressure or to tearing secondary to the shearing effects of the blow to the head. Vessels may also be injured directly as a consequence of a penetration of the skull.

Concussion, contusion, hemorrhage, thrombosis, and brain edema are the pathological states usually associated with closed-head injuries. The pathology of concussion is not well understood simply because concussion is not fatal. By classical definition, there should be no demonstrable pathology in the concussed brain.

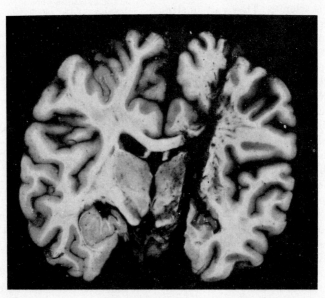

FIG. 1. Brain section, showing penetrating brain trauma in a 32-year-old male alcoholic with depression after recent separation from his wife. He was found dead at home after shooting himself through the roof of the mouth with a 22-caliber revolver.

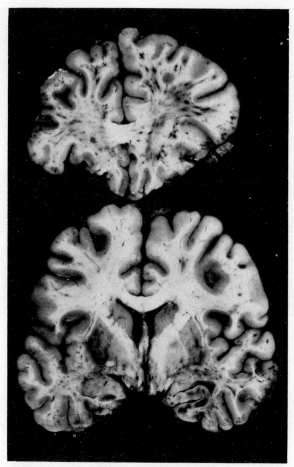

FIG. 2. Brain sections, showing multiple petechial hemorrhages throughout the frontal lobes and contusions of the base. The patient was a 55-year-old man who died after a closed head injury in an automobile accident.

However, experimental studies on animals have shown a loss of cell substance in the thalamic area and reticular formation. Contusion, bruising of the brain substance, may be seen directly under the site of the blow, or it may occur elsewhere in the brain as a contrecoup lesion (see Figure 3). Contusion is usually associated with some degree of subarachnoid hemorrhage. Epidural hemorrhage results from a tearing of the middle meningeal artery or vein, usually resulting from a fracture of the temporal bone. Although these patients are usually lucid immediately after the injury, they rapidly sink into a deep coma and die, unless there is surgical intervention. Subdural hemorrhage may be seen acutely, or it may be discovered later as a chronic process in a patient who appears to have progressive organic brain syndrome. It generally results from a tearing of the veins bridging the subdural space. Intracerebral bleeding may be seen after blunt trauma to the head; in rare cases, it signifies the presence of an arteriovenous vascular malformation. Thromboses of the anterior or middle cerebral arteries may occur, particularly in older people, either because of a tearing of the vessel intima or secondary to a drop in blood pressure and surgical shock at the time of the accident. Brain edema is common after blunt trauma and may be severe enough to cause herniation to the brainstem.

Penetrating wounds from bullets, shell fragments, or pointed objects can have multiple effects: local tissue damage, blast effects, tearing of the brain substance and vessels, and possibly infection. Neurosurgical intervention is often required in this type of injury for debride-

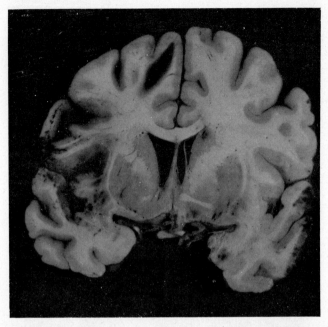

Fig. 3. Brain section, showing coup lesion of the left temporal lobe (smaller contusion) and contrecoup lesion of the right temporal and parietal lobes (larger contusion). This 67-year-old woman died 4 hours after striking the left side of her head and sustaining fractures of the left temporal and parietal bones in an automobile accident.

ment of the damaged tissue, removal of foreign bodies, and elevation of the depressed skull fragments.

Psychopathology

To understand the behavioral changes secondary to head trauma, one must consider the change that a patient's personality undergoes because of the organic damage itself, the changes that result from the ego's attempts to adapt to the organic deficits, and the changes in ego function that represent a reaction to the traumatic event itself, as in the neuroses. Much of the personality change in a brain-damaged person is related to his inability to think in the abstract. Thus, the person lacks many qualities characteristic of the human being: initiative, foresight, inspiration, fantasy, and ability to make plans and decisions. His perceptions, thoughts, and ideas are reduced, and he lacks the capacity for real friendship, love, and social relations. His reactions to the environment are oversimplified, and he is driven to get rid of tensions. His behavior is often abnormally rigid, stereotyped, and compulsive. He is abnormally bound to environmental and internal stimuli.

Initially, he may look completely in con-

trol—happy, collected, and cooperative. However, when confronted with a task that he cannot do, he may suddenly become dazed and agitated, change color, start to fumble, and become unfriendly, evasive, and even aggressive. When the patient's capabilities are insufficient to meet the demands made on him, the discrepancy makes self-realization impossible, and overwhelming anxiety results. To avoid such catastrophic conditions, the brain-injured person may withdraw so that threatening stimuli do not reach him. The patient with organic brain damage cannot bear conflict, anxiety, restriction, or suffering; in this respect, he differs essentially from the neurotic.

The extent of psychiatric disability after a head injury is related more to psychological and sociological factors than to the severity of the injury. Also, the extent of psychiatric disability tends to correlate inversely with the degree of organic brain damage. If the patient has a strong need to feel superior to his environment or to be in absolute control and he then suffers a humiliating failure or accident, he may be overwhelmed and revert to unconscious neurotic defenses.

At first, the neurotic state may change rapidly in intensity and may fluctuate between an anxiety state, conversion hysteria, phobic or compulsive rituals, amnesia, and confusion. Later, the symptoms become more fixed. The final form of the neurotic symptom or personality adaptation depends on the person's background and developmental weaknesses. The patient is often self-centered and preoccupied with his symptoms, and he tries to impress others with their seriousness. This can lead to exaggeration and inconsistencies in his performance. The symptoms also allow the person a good deal of secondary gain.

A complete evaluation of a patient's symptoms after head trauma requires considerations of (1) the organic pathology and the possible behavioral changes resulting from it, (2) the reaction of the patient who attempts to compensate for and adapt to his organic deficits, (3) the premorbid personality of the patient, (4) the circumstances surrounding the trauma itself, (5) the unconscious interpretation of trauma, (6) the strength of the ego in coping with the threat of brain damage, and (7) the special significance that injury to the head may have for a person.

Clinical Syndromes

In general, the clinical syndromes or sequelae that follow head trauma are divided according to the presence or absence of organic brain damage. The following criteria strongly suggest the presence of organic brain damage: roentgenographic evidence of a skull fracture, presence of foreign material within the brain, evidence of focal neurological deficits, bleeding from the ears or nose, bloody spinal fluid, prolonged unconsciousness, distortion or dilatation of the ventricles, posttraumatic seizures, focal abnormalities on the electroencephalogram, abnormal echoencephalogram, continuing symptoms unchanged by suggestion or psychotherapy, psychological testing suggesting organic damage, continuity of the development of symptoms after the injury, and primary interest of the patient in rehabilitation rather than compensation. Table I correlates sites of brain lesions with specific defects and the functional and behavioral changes seen.

Acute Sequelae

The syndrome of coma, delirium, and amnesic confabulation immediately after the injury actually represents the recovery process. The stages may vary greatly in duration, depending on the severity of the injury and the extent of the brain damage. If the injury is mild, the patient may have no coma and may manifest only mild symptoms typical of a simple, posttraumatic syndrome. However, patients with more severe injuries may remain in a deep coma for long periods of time and later have markedly prolonged periods of delirium and amnesia. The recovery of cerebral function from the lowest level (coma) to the highest (normality) occurs in a regular sequence.

Concussion. Concussion may be defined as a symptom complex secondary to head trauma and characterized by a temporary sudden paralysis of cerebral function. The patient loses consciousness briefly and then has traumatic amnesia, but no brain damage is apparent. The lack of visible pathology, the reversibility of the condition, and the absence of mortality distinguish concussion from other head traumas, but the recovery process is similar. Unconsciousness usually lasts less than 5 minutes. A coma exceeding 10 minutes suggests a more severe injury to the brain. Recovery is usually spontaneous and complete, although the patient may have amnesia for the events just preceding the trauma.

Some patients remain conscious but later cannot recall events surrounding the accident. After a more severe injury, the patient is unconscious and has associated flaccid paralysis; then he regains consciousness rapidly. This reaction is usually followed by a brief period of delirium, during which the patient may be confused, restless, and agitated, with associated automatism and subsequent amnesia for events leading up to and including the injury and for the period of automatism. Usually, the patient complains of headache after he recovers from the delirious phase, but otherwise he seems completely normal. In more severe injuries, the patient may develop prolonged delirium or coma.

Patients with concussion receive the same immediate treatment as those with other head traumas. Because the incidence of posttraumatic neuroses is highest after minor head traumas, special attention must be given to the concussed patient's psychological welfare.

Traumatic Coma. The clinical picture of traumatic coma is characterized by a profound loss of consciousness, associated with inability

TABLE I

Correlation of Deficits and Behavior with Area of Brain Damage*

Site of Brain Lesion	Deficits	Behavioral Correlates
Frontal lobe	Inferior quality of thinking, abstraction, and synthesis; failure to inhibit ongoing activity	Perseveration, concreteness, preference for old behavioral patterns, impulsiveness, tactlessness, indifference, incapacity for decision, aggressive behavior, increased libido, euphoria, lack of productive thinking, demanding attitude, childish behavior, lack of foresight and insight, loss of moral, ethical, and social standards
Temporal lobe Bilateral	Retrograde and anterograde amnesia, dementia	Korsakoff's psychosis, dementia
Left	Poor verbal recall, intellectual loss	Memory problems, difficulty with verbal material, atypical schizophreniform psychoses, personality changes
Right	Visual-ideational sequencing problems, difficulty with auditory perception	Difficulty in identifying incongruities in pictures, difficulty in arranging pictures, inability to appreciate musical tone, loudness, timbre, etc.
Brainstem and diencephalon	Alternation of drive states, alteration of mood, diminished alertness	Apathy, sluggishness, depression, hypomania, lability of affect, increased thirst, bulemia, anorexia, changed libido, stupor, coma, sleep alterations
Parietal lobe	Spatial disorientation, body agnosia	Disorientation, ignoring portions or an entire half of the body
Left hemisphere	Ideational and ideomotor apraxia	Inability to express thoughts, blocking, difficulty in initiating action
Right hemisphere	Visual-constructional spatial apraxia	Difficulty in copying designs, difficulty with jigsaw puzzles, spatial disorientation, increased incidence of behavioral changes
	Symptoms showing no correlation with site or degree of injury (therefore, more likely to be psychological in origin)	Headache, giddiness, irritability, sensitivity to sensory stimuli, anxiety, fatigue, difficulty in concentration

* Data are from Piercy (1964), Milner (1969), Lishman (1968), and Zülch (1969)

to respond to the external environment and cessation of voluntary motor activity. A coma lasting more than 2 hours is considered severe. A coma lasting longer than 24 to 48 hours conveys a more dire prognosis, although, even after several weeks of coma, complete recovery is possible. The presence of persistent spasticity, extensor plantar reflexes, nystagmus, or nonreactive, widely dilated pupils may indicate a severe, widespread brain injury. As the coma lightens, the patient may enter a stage of stupor in which he at first cannot speak or respond to commands; later, however, he becomes restless or even violent. At this point, he may respond to a simple command to move a portion of his body. During this period, the patient may show restless confusion alternating with relapses into a stuporous condition. As recovery proceeds, the patient develops the syndrome of traumatic delirium.

Traumatic Delirium. Traumatic delirium may last just a few minutes, or it may persist for weeks. During this phase, the patient, although conscious, is disoriented and confused; has a tendency to relapse into stupor, restlessness, and marked irritability; and is often resistant to examination. He may refuse to take his medications, fight with those who attempt to control him, and try to leave the hospital. In the latter phases of delirium, the patient usually becomes quieter and more cooperative, but he remains confused and has the potential for impulsive and violent behavior, so that he may require constant supervision. Irritability, hostility, panic, and paranoia because of falsely perceived threats from his surroundings make the possibility of injury to himself or others and the danger of suicide important considerations. Delirium lasting longer than several days may indicate more serious brain damage. This phase may last for weeks and may evolve into a stage of automatism in which, although the patient is aware of his environment and responds rationally to external stimuli and inner needs, he behaves as though he had Korsakoff's syndrome.

Korsakoff-like Syndrome (Amnesic Confabulation). During this phase of recovery, the patient may show disturbances of mood. He often seems hypomanic, lacking insight and judgment and having a grossly defective memory for recent events, with consequent disorientation. He usually has a tendency to confabulate in order to cover his recent memory defict. The patient lacks the ability to integrate recent events with previous experience, leaving events detached and disconnected in terms of time, space, and associated affect. This stage progresses to the recovery of recent memory, orientation, and development of insight into the nature of his illness.

Delayed Sequelae

Disorders Primarily Resulting from Brain damage. *Posttraumatic Defect Conditions.* This group of disorders is caused by focal brain damage secondary to loss of brain tissue, gliotic reaction, and meningeal adhesions and scars. Subjective symptoms—including neurosis, personality disorders, and transient psychosis—are absent or minimal. The defect conditions most often occur in patients with penetrating head traumas and are usually associated with focal electroencephalographic or neurological abnormalities. The defect conditions are usually most prominent immediately after the head injury. They may remain static or improve gradually as the brain swelling and tissue damage resolve. The most common defect condition that persists to a disabling degree is dysphasia.

Dementia. Although intellectual deterioration after a head trauma is rare, it may be associated with damage to the left hemisphere, particularly the parietal, temporal, and occipital lobes. It resembles dementia associated with degenerative processes affecting the brain; however, the course is more rapid and usually of abrupt onset.

Subdural Hematoma. Chronic subdural hematoma generally begins with a tearing of small veins in the subdural space. A thin layer of blood beneath the dura mater gradually increases in size secondary to osmosis, with fluid accumulating from the cerebrospinal fluid and blood plasma, associated with additional fresh bleeding within the organized clot (see Figures 4 and 5). The symptoms of chronic subdural hematoma may emerge only days or weeks after the injury. The clinical picture is progressive, with the gradual onset of irritability, inattentiveness, lethargy, and memory difficulty. Later, the gait becomes awkward, with or without focal neurological signs. A common presenting symptom is headache. Papilledema is present in about 20 per cent of the cases. Occasionally, chronic subdural hematoma manifests itself by generalized convulsions and progressive focal neurological deficits.

Posttraumatic Communicating Hydrocephalus. A local injury involving the aqueduct of Sylvius, fourth ventricle, or basal meninges may impede the normal circulation of cerebrospinal fluid and result in posttraumatic hydrocephalus. The symptoms usually begin with episodes of severe headache, associated with drowsiness and occasionally vomiting, ataxia, speech disturbance, and loss of sphincter control. Gradual progression is the rule, with associated loss of intellectual function. Symptoms of hydrocephalus usually begin to develop within several months of the injury.

Traumatic Encephalopathy of Boxers (Punch-Drunk Syndrome). The syndrome consists of slurred speech, ataxic gait, and impaired mental function, simulating alcoholic intoxication. Ataxia of the upper and lower extremities and intention tremor of the head and hands are often the first neurological symptoms. Later, an ataxic or mixed dysarthria and pyramidal and extrapyramidal signs develop in varying degrees. They are characterized by a slowing of muscular action, ataxia, and symptoms resembling parkinsonism. Some patients have progressive dementia associated with progressive neurological deficits.

Many patients have an explosive personality with psychopathic features, often present before the onset of the organic damage. Frequently, the patient is morbidly jealous of his wife, imagining her to be sexually unfaithful. Paranoid psychosis with hallucinations sometimes occurs. The progress of the illness may be slow

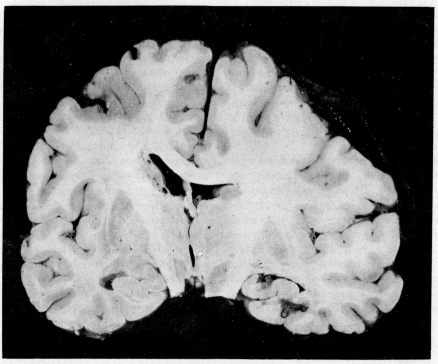

FıG. 4. Chronic subdural hematoma, showing displacement of brain substance and ventricular system with shift of midline structures.

and may even stop temporarily in some cases, or the progress may be rapid.

Posttraumatic Epilepsy. This syndrome is defined by the onset of convulsive seizures a month or more after a brain injury or head trauma. Postraumatic epilepsy must be differentiated from immediate epilepsy with seizures soon after an injury because of anoxia, metabolic disturbance, or local irritation. The extent of the injury correlates directly with the incidence of the posttraumatic epilepsy. The posttraumatic convulsion is classically focal or jacksonian in type, the initial impulse originating in the area of damage. The electroencephalogram shows focal abnormalities in 90 per cent of these patients.

The prognosis for patients with posttraumatic epilepsy is generally good; only 7 or 8 per cent of patients have more than six epileptic attacks a year. In general, the frequency of epileptic seizures is low, decreasing over time; 75 per cent are completely controlled with medication.

Posttraumatic Personality Disorder. This disorder is distinguished from postconcussion syndrome, simple type, and posttraumatic neuroses by evidence that actual organic damage to

the brain has occurred. Many patients develop a concrete attitude, a catastrophic reaction or anxiety reaction to stress, behavior patterns as a defense against the anxiety, and a variety of nonspecific symptoms, including tension headaches, dizziness, irritability, fatigue, insomnia, and anxiety.

Although pleasant, amiable, and conscientious before the head injury, these people may become irritable, impulsive, irascible, and quarrelsome afterward. They may have great difficulty in getting along with their families and may develop sudden outbursts of rage, associated with severe anxiety in the face of threat. Others may become apathetic and uninterested and may lack initiative. They tend to withdraw from people and may show marked emotional lability, with rage, sadness, and laughter following each other in rapid sequence. The withdrawn patient may become selfish, resentful, and petulant and develop paranoid ideation toward the people about him. Many are persistently euphoric, with lack of judgment, reliability, or foresight; their impulses may be discharged crudely and offensively.

The prognosis varies. Some patients improve

gradually over 2 or 3 years and recover completely; others show further deterioration or, at best, lack of improvement and require prolonged institutionalization. Treatment is directed at helping the patient readjust to his situation and at modifying the environment with which he must cope.

Disorders Not Primarily Related to Brain Damage. *Postconcussion Syndrome (Simple Type).* This syndrome is characterized by persistent anxiety associated with headaches, giddiness, irritability, intolerance to such sensory stimuli as light and noise, fatigability, insomnia, reduced tolerance to alcohol, difficulty with concentration and memory, and diminished interest and spontaneity. It differs from posttraumatic personality disorder in that it is less disruptive to the personality makeup of the patient and clear-cut evidence of brain damage is lacking.

Even minimal activity may severely aggravate the anxiety, headache, or dizziness. For this reason, treatment involving graduated physical exercises with gradual return to normal activities has been advocated. Recovery is generally complete within 2 years of the onset of symptoms.

Posttraumatic Neurosis. In general, neurosis after a head trauma is delayed, frequently until all organic sequelae of the head trauma have disappeared. The primary gain achieved through the neurotic symptoms is the reduction of anxiety resulting from the ego's perceived threat of annihilation or loss of autonomy. Secondary gains derived from the neurotic symptoms are related to obtaining attention, sympathy, or financial compensation or to avoiding a difficult job situation or interpersonal conflicts.

Anxiety after a head injury is common. Clinically, the patient appears apprehensive and worried, with fears related to death and possible brain injury. The patient typically overreacts to stress and tends to exaggerate his symptoms. He may display anxiety attacks, with hyperventilation, panic, tachycardia, sweating, and tremor. Complaint of tightness or pressure in the head or chest is common. The patient may have insomnia or feelings of nausea. Frequently, he complains of a vague headache, which tends to be persistent. The patient may complain of dizziness; he may experience numbness of the extremities or fainting spells secondary to hyperventilation.

Hysterical conversion neurosis may begin soon after a head injury and may be the presenting symptom. Characteristically, the patient presents with a lack of affect or concern

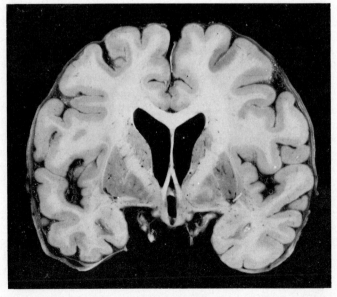

FIG. 5. Brain, showing moderate cerebral atrophy with chornic, organized, bilateral subdural hematomas and dilatation of the ventricles resulting from normal pressure hydrocephalus. This 93-year-old woman had a clinical diagnosis of progressive senile dementia over the preceding 15 years.

about his disability (*la belle indifférence*). He may complain of paralysis or anesthesia affecting an entire half of the body or an entire limb, such peculiar sensations as tingling or bizarre pains in a part of his body, and deafness in one ear or blindness. The results of the neurological examination usually fail to fit a typical organic pattern, and electroencephalograms or other studies show no organic pathology. Hysterical neurosis of the dissociative type is less common, taking the form of amnesic states after a head injury. Obsessive-compulsive neurosis is relatively rare after a head trauma. When it does occur, the patient may have compulsive tics, repetitive spasms of the limbs, obsessive thinking (frequently phobic), counterphobic attitudes, preoccupation with symptoms, or ritualistic behavior patterns. Mixed neurosis is the most common form of neurotic reaction after a head injury, presenting as a complex of symptoms associated with anxiety, conversion symptoms, and hypochondriasis.

Even though the patient's symptoms may be primarily neurotic in character, a combination of organic and psychiatric pathology is often present.

Malingering. Malingering is a patient's willful, deliberate, and fraudulent imitation or exaggeration of illness, with a conscious intent to deceive observers for a specific purpose. The reasons for malingering after a head injury may include the desire for financial compensation or the wish to avoid legal or other responsibilities. The psychiatrist rarely sees malingering, most of his cases actually being the result of conversion neurosis.

Typically, the malingerer exaggerates his manufactured symptoms and seems evasive. He never commits himself to any definite statements about returning to work, financial gain, or other expectations. He often contradicts himself. The neurotic patient is more sincere about his symptoms, but he is often less affectively concerned about them. Neurotic symptoms remain more constant over time, are more sudden in onset, often follow emotional shock, last longer, and tend to be more profound than those of simulated disorders. In hysteria, symptoms characteristically disappear after psychotherapy. This effect is never observed with malingering, unless the malingerer is discovered or the secondary gains that he is seeking are met.

Posttraumatic Psychosis. With the exception of acute psychotic states associated with coma, delirium, and Korsakoff-like syndrome, psychoses are relatively rare after a head injury. The interval between the head injury and the onset of the psychotic symptoms varies, often with a lapse of a year or two. The incidence of delayed psychosis after a head trauma has been reported as between 5 and 9 per cent, most psychoses being schizophreniform, paranoid, affective, or associated with epilepsy. Only about 5 per cent are prolonged acute psychoses associated with a head injury. Before the injury, a significant percentage of these patients were psychically deviant or mentally retarded or had frank psychotic symptoms. The brain injury itself does not cause the psychosis, but weakening of the patient's ego may abet the development of psychoses years afterward.

Clinical Syndromes after Other Forms of Head Trauma

Electrical Injuries

In mild injuries, the patient usually retains consciousness, although mild syncope may be seen for a few minutes. The patient feels tingling, pain, and abnormal sensations of the limbs; he experiences a slight motor weakness, headaches, and deafness and has amnesia for the period of injury. Recovery is rapid, without residual effects. With stronger electrical currents, consciousness is lost; the patient may either recover or deteriorate to deep coma, convulsions, and death. The development of neurotic symptoms after an electric shock injury is common.

Electroconvulsive therapy results in transient confusion and memory loss, although psychotic delirium may develop a few days afterward. No neuropathological changes may be seen in the brain after electroconvulsive therapy. Memory is invariably restored, with no loss of intellectual ability.

Cerebral Blast Syndrome

This syndrome is usually seen during wartime in persons exposed to explosions just outside the lethal range. The shock wave of the blast is thought to be transmitted through the body fluids to the brain itself, causing a syndrome similar to that seen with other types of blunt head trauma. The patients are usually unconscious initially; most of them recover within hours. Most cases resolve completely within 2 years of the injury.

Irradiation Brain Damage

Several cases have been reported of brain damage resulting from irradiation to the scalp for basal cell carcinoma or intracranial tumor. The onset of the symptoms may be delayed for months or years, but, after they do appear, they progress rapidly to death. Apparently, large doses of X-rays produce a vasculitis affecting the arterioles and capillaries of the white matter. In people exposed to atomic irradiation or atomic explosion, pathological changes of the brain may be seen; these changes are characterized by small perivascular hemorrhages.

Ultrasound Brain Damage

Ultrasound may create lesions of the brain tissue, particularly the white matter, if it is applied through a defect in the skull. Apparently, the effects result from the increased temperature of the brain tissue. No clinical or pathological abnormalities have been reported as a result of clinical diagnostic ultrasound (echoencephalography).

Prognosis

The mortality in cases of severe head injury is about 20 per cent, with most deaths occurring within the first 48 hours. Old age, prolonged coma, prolonged posttraumatic amnesia, severe dysphasia, and symptoms suggesting brainstem lesions portend a poor prognosis. The development of the posttraumatic neurotic syndromes depends on the pretraumatic personality makeup of the patient, on how treatment and rehabilitation are carried out, and on factors relating to the patient's primary and secondary gain. Those patients who have extremely severe brain injury and emotional, occupational, or interpersonal problems remain disabled the longest. In general, about 15 per cent of patients with a severe head injury develop psychiatric symptoms; many cases are secondary to some degree of dementia, and the rest are the result of neurotic illness. In contrast, 40 to 50 per cent of patients with minor head injuries develop psychiatric symptoms after injury; most of these symptoms are neurotic in nature.

Treatment

When the medical and neurosurgical aspects of immediate care are paramount, the patient with a head injury should receive his initial treatment at a center equipped and staffed to specialize in the management of such cases. The second phase of recovery—rehabilitation and convalescence—is ideally carried out at a rehabilitation unit or long-term care facility; at times, the patient may remain at home on an ambulatory basis and eventually return to work. It is during this second phase of treatment that the psychological aspects are of most importance.

The patient should be given an opportunity to discuss his concerns and symptoms. Psychiatrists may help the patient regain active function by reliving the traumatic experience and vocalizing current conflicts. Rest is facilitated by satisfying the patient's passive-dependent needs and by helping him to deal with emotional discharges, such as nightmares, hyperactivity, and anxiety. Counseling with the patient's family and employer should be done. If necessary, the patient should be helped to solve compensation and litigation issues.

The use of special therapists is highly recommended to help the patient who has specific neurological defects, such as dysphasias, motor disability, perceptual difficulty, disturbances of the abstract attitude, or intellectual deficits. The final assessment of the patient's ability to function is best delayed until at least 18 months after the injury.

REFERENCES

Brock, S. The neuroses following head (brain) injury. In *Injuries of the Brain and Spinal Cord and Their Coverings*, S. Brock, editor, ed. 4, p. 238. Springer, New York, 1960.

Brosin, H. W. Psychiatric conditions following head injury. In *The American Handbook of Psychiatry*, S. Arieti, editor, vol. 2, p. 1175. Basic Books, New York, 1959.

Dresser, A. C., Meirowsky, A. M., Weiss, G. H., McNeel, M. L., Simon, G. A., and Caveness, W. F. Gainful employment following head injury: Prognostic factors. Arch. Neurol., *29:* 111, 1973.

Goldstein, K. The effect of brain damage on the personality. Psychiatry, *15:* 245, 1952.

Johnson, J. Organic psychosyndromes due to boxing. Br. J. Psychiatry, *115:* 45, 1969.

Lishman, W. A. Brain damage in relation to psychiatric disability after head injury. Br. J. Psychiatry, *114:* 377, 1968.

Miller, H. Problems of medicolegal practice. In *The Late Effects of Head Injury*, A. E. Walker, W. F. Caveness, and M. Critchley, editors, p. 429. Charles C Thomas, Springfield, Ill., 1969.

18.6.   ORGANIC BRAIN SYNDROMES ASSOCIATED WITH DRUG OR POISON INTOXICATION

Sedatives and Hypnotics

Barbiturates

Acute barbiturate intoxication produces depression of central nervous system function. This depression is associated with dizziness and ataxia, occasional excitation, confusion, slurred speech, stupor, and coma. Treatment of acute overdose involves evacuation of the gastric contents and support of the vital functions. Absorbed barbiturate is best eliminated by induction of diuresis. Delirium with agitation and psychosis may be seen as the patient begins to regain consciousness. The patient who is chronically intoxicated with barbiturates develops some drug tolerance, and his behavior is the result of a fluctuating state of consciousness.

Abrupt withdrawal of barbiturates from a patient who is dependent on them produces a definite abstinence syndrome. After about 8 hours, symptoms of central nervous system irritability develop, with anxiety, muscle twitching, tremor, weakness, dizziness, nausea, sweating, hyperactive deep-tendon reflexes, headache, and postural hypotension. These symptoms become increasingly severe, and after 30 to 48 hours grand mal convulsions are likely. Delirium with disorientation and hallucinations may also be seen within 4 to 7 days after administration of the medication is stopped. The delirium may be associated with elevated body temperature. It usually terminates with prolonged sleep within 5 days of onset.

Barbiturates must be withdrawn in a controlled hospital situation. If the daily barbiturate intake is not reliably known, a test dose of 260 mg. of pentobarbital may be given orally, and the patient should be examined after one hour. If the patient is asleep at that time or shows increased signs of intoxication, his chronic ingestion has probably been small. If the patient shows no effect or increased signs of withdrawal, his total daily dose has probably been from 600 to 1,200 mg. In most cases, 200 to 300 mg. of pentobarbital every 6 hours is sufficient to prevent withdrawal symptoms. After the maintenance dose has been stabilized and the necessary medical evaluation completed, the barbiturate is withdrawn at a rate of 10 per cent of the total dose per day. The reduction should not exceed 100 mg. a day. After withdrawal is achieved, the patient should be referred for psychiatric evaluation and psychotherapy.

Minor Tranquilizers

Like the barbiturates, the minor tranquilizers are capable of producing disorientation and toxic confusional states when given in high doses, but the margin of safety is much greater. Toxic states are manifested by hyperactivity, rage, and hostile outbursts. Occasionally, acute maniacal behavior with feelings of depersonalization, hallucinations, and delusions may be seen. As in barbiturate dependence, increasing tolerance and withdrawal symptoms are seen if the drugs are taken in high enough doses. Withdrawal from meprobamate has been associated with grand mal convulsions.

Hypnotics

The hypnotics are generally more potent and hazardous than the minor tranquilizers and produce toxic symptoms similar to those resulting from the barbiturates. Glutethimide may produce chronic clonic convulsions during the period of coma after an overdose. Methaqualone produces marked respiratory depression associated with convulsions, pulmonary edema, and coma. Withdrawal may produce a syndrome of delirium tremens.

Bromides

Acute bromide intoxication is relatively rare because it is difficult to take sufficiently high doses without inducing nausea and emesis. In acute poisoning, symptoms of confusion, weakness, depression, ataxia, and psychosis with delirium and hallucinations have been described.

Chronic bromide intoxication may occur when large doses of bromide preparations have been taken over a long period or are poorly eliminated because of renal failure. A blood bromide level of 150 mg. per 100 ml. is considered necessary to produce symptoms of bromide intoxication. Toxic effects may also depend on the general mental state, personality, duration of ingestion, state of hydration, and electrolyte balance. The reported symptoms of chronic bromide intoxication include coma, headache, irritability, emotional lability, lethargy, delusions, disorientation, hallucinations, loss of memory, cyanosis, vacuous facies, dilated pupils, stupor, blurred vision, fabrication, ataxia, confusion, vertigo, and loss of libido.

Treatment involves the elimination of bromine by the daily administration of sodium chloride. A high fluid intake is mandatory during oral sodium chloride administration, and diuresis may be facilitated with diuretics. The patient may be sedated, if necessary, with small doses of paraldehyde, minor tranquilizers, or chlorpromazine. The reduction of bromides takes 1 to 2 weeks to reduce the level by 50 per cent. In general, recovery is seen within 2 to 3 weeks, but the resolution of symptoms generally lags behind the fall in serum bromide level.

Stimulants

These drugs produce alerting effects on the central nervous system, suppression of appetite, and peripheral effects, including tachycardia, increased blood pressure, dilated pupils, dry mouth, tremor, and sweating.

Amphetamine (Benzedrine), methamphetamine (Desoxyn), and dextroamphetamine (Dexedrine) act primarily on the central nervous system. They produce marked tolerance and a mild withdrawal syndrome characterized by severe fatigue and mental depression, sometimes with suicidal ideation.

The most severe and dangerous side effect of the amphetamines is the production of amphetamine psychosis. Although the psychotic reaction may be seen after a single dose, it is more common after prolonged ingestion in excessive amounts. Symptoms of the psychosis include disorientation; ideas of reference; delusions of persecution; auditory, visual, tactile, and olfactory hallucinations; and feelings of fear and terror. Stereotyped behavior is also seen in chronic amphetamine intoxication.

Acute toxic effects seen with overdosage include restlessness, irritability, hyperactive reflexes, confusion, hallucinations, and disorientation. Palpitation, cardiac arrhythmias, and circulatory collapse may occur. Fatal amphetamine intoxication usually terminates in convulsions and coma.

Amphetamine overdose and the effects of chronic intoxication are best treated with a major tranquilizer, haloperidol (Haldol) being the drug of choice. The effects of an acute overdose usually subside in 36 to 48 hours. However, complete clearing of the psychic effect may be slow, often taking 2 months in cases of chronic amphetamine abuse. If the drugs have been used over a long period, a withdrawal syndrome of marked lethargy and depression must be treated by providing physical rest, emotional support, and supervision to prevent suicide.

The amphetamine derivatives used primarily for appetite suppression are considered less potent than amphetamines, but all are capable of producing the same side effects, including paranoid psychosis.

Methylphenidate (Ritalin) is a cyclic amphetamine derivative that is a mild central nervous system stimulant. Acute toxicity and side effects with prolonged usage are the same as those produced by amphetamines. Aminophylline is commonly used to treat asthmatic attacks; its cumulative effects may produce a delirum characterized by nausea, vomiting, vertigo, anxiety, agitation, confusion, convulsions, and coma.

Hallucinogens

The hallucinogenic agents are capable of markedly altering the normal perceptual, emotional, and cognitive processes. In a sense, they alter the form of consciousness without decreasing alertness; for this reason, they cannot be said to cause classic syndromes of delirium or dementia.

The primary effect of these agents seems to be a marked alteration of sensory perception, leading to profound distortions of visual, auditory, tactile, and proprioceptive sensation. These effects are often associated with hallucinations and emotional states of euphoria, serenity, anxiety, or panic. Cognitive distortions lead to feelings of omnipotence and omniscience. Severe anxiety states and paranoid reactions may be seen acutely; chronic use may be associated with prolonged states of amotivation and behavior resembling simple schizophrenia.

The treatment of acute adverse reactions is psychological support, with calm verbal reassurance to reduce anxiety in the patient. Phenothiazines terminate the reaction; the minor tranquilizers may also be used to reduce associated anxiety.

Psychotropic Agents

Major Tranquilizers

Certain major tranquilizers may produce somnolence to the point of stupor or coma when used in relatively large doses. Acute delirious reactions have also been reported, particularly when these drugs are combined with antiparkinsonian agents or barbiturates. Pre-existing factors, such as advanced age or brain damage, also increase the likelihood of delirium. The use of these drugs sometimes precipitates a depressive illness or aggravates existing depression. Dystonic reactions are common.

An acute overdose may produce confusion, agitation, and disorientation, often associated with marked postural hypotension. In extremely large doses, coma with hypothermia, shock, and rarely, death may result.

Treatment of an overdose involves gastric lavage. If seizures occur after an overdose, they are best treated with intravenous diphenylhydantoin (Dilantin). Barbiturates may deepen the coma and aggravate the hypotension. Acute dystonic reactions are resolved by slow intravenous injection of 50 to 100 mg. of diphenhydramine (Benadryl).

One per cent of nonepileptic patients receiving phenothiazines develop spontaneous convulsions a few days after beginning the medication or after a sudden increase in dosage. Patients with pre-existing organic brain damage or epilepsy show an especially high risk for the development or aggravation of seizures. Chlorpromazine seems somewhat more likely to produce seizures than do the other major tranquilizers.

Antidepressants

Central nervous system side effects include fatigue, weakness, unsteadiness, dizziness, headache, tremor, stimulation, and, rarely, grand mal convulsions at therapeutic doses. Psychotic symptoms may be exacerbated in schizophrenic patients. Other patients, particularly the elderly, may develop typical symptoms of delirium, with disorientation, confusion, paranoia, and hallucinations. In manic-depressive patients, treatment with the antidepressants during the depressive phase may result in a rapid swing to hypomania.

Acute overdoses with the tricyclic antidepressants result in agitation, delirium, and often seizures, followed by central nervous system depression, stupor, and coma associated with hyperpyrexia. Tachycardia, dilated pupils, and cardiac arrhythmias may accompany the central nervous system effects. The tricyclic antidepressants are rapidly detoxified by the liver; the toxic dose is essentially removed from the body within 24 hours. Overdoses with monoamine oxidase inhibitors produce a similar clinical picture, but a lag period of 12 hours precedes the onset of symptoms, and gastric lavage and forced diuresis are of value in treatment.

Lithium

Mild side effects—such as nausea, diarrhea, tremor, and polyuria—are common during lithium therapy. Severe toxic symptoms are characterized by a toxic confusional state, with agitation, nausea, diarrhea, thirst, dizziness, blurred vision, slurred speech, weakness, tremor, and impairment of consciousness, which may proceed to stupor and coma. With high serum lithium concentrations, generalized spasticity and clonic movement of the limbs may be seen, associated with coma and generalized convulsions.

Lithium intoxication is treated by stopping lithium administration and giving sodium chloride with adequate fluids to facilitate lithium excretion. In cases of severe overdose, hemodialysis is indicated.

Anticonvulsants

Anticonvulsants commonly cause a general slowing of mentation. The hydantoin derivatives like the other anticonvulsants, cause a host of side effects, including blood dyscrasias, dermatological disorders, and hepatitis. The central nervous system effects include drowsiness, irritability, mental depression, tremor, dysarthria, diplopia, nystagmus, and choreiform movements. At high doses, delirium may result, with paranoid delusions, confusion, and disorientation. An overdose with hydantoin anticonvulsants initially produces ataxia, dysarthria, and nystagmus proceeding to coma with hypotension. The treatment of an overdose is general support with gastric lavage. Hemodialysis may be particularly useful.

Oxyzolidine derivatives' side effects include ataxia and vertigo at low blood levels. At higher blood levels, nausea, vomiting, nystagmus, diplopia, drowsiness, and emotional lability may be seen. An overdose of these drugs results in marked sedation, associated with nystagmus, dysarthria, and incoordination.

Common side effects of the succinimide derivatives include headache, dizziness, irritability, drowsiness, euphoria, and hyperactivity. Psychiatric changes are common, including nightmares, increased aggressiveness, decreased ability to concentrate, and paranoid psychoses. Of particular note is the precipitation of a depressive syndrome, often associated with suicidal ideation, which may require hospitalization.

Belladonna Alkaloids and Synthetic Anticholinergics

The effects of the belladonna alkaloids on the central nervous system are variable, causing both stimulation and depression. Large doses can produce restlessness, manic behavior, confusion, loss of memory, emotional lability, disorientation, convulsions, and coma.

The piperidine derivatives may produce a delirium that could be interpreted as a worsening of the mental disorder for which the patient is being treated. Treatment of the anticholinergic delirium involves evacuation of the stomach and sedation, if necessary, with a minor tranquilizer or barbiturate. Sedation with one of the major tranquilizers, such as chlorpromazine, should be avoided, as it may aggravate the anticholinergic delirium. Intramuscular injection of physostigmine salicylate (Antilirium) in a dose of 1 mg., followed in 15 to 20 minutes by an additional dose if necessary, has been reported to be beneficial. The dose may have to be repeated after an hour.

L-Dihydroxyphenylalanine

The most common effects of L-dopa include nausea and vomiting in more than half of the treated patients. Dyskinesias in the form of choreoathetosis involving the face, jaw, tongue, shoulders, and trunk or as buccolingual dyskinesia with facial grimacing, lip smacking, and chewing are seen in 50 per cent of treated patients. These symptoms begin with a lessening of parkinsonism symptoms and are usually controlled by a reduction in the dosage. Psychiatric symptoms are reported in 20 to 30 per cent of patients and may occur in association with the dyskinesia. The most common mental side effects are confusion and disorientation associ-

ated with delirium of variable severity. Significant depression, even of suicidal proportion, may be seen in a certain number of patients receiving L-dopa, even though most patients experience an improvement in mood. Psychosis with hallucinations, paranoid delusions, and psychomotor agitation may occur, often associated with delirium but at times in the presence of a clear sensorium. Hypomania may be produced during L-dopa treatment.

Delirium is much more common in patients with Parkinson's disease who have some degree of associated dementia. Psychiatric side effects may not appear until several months after the initiation of treatment and are often controlled by a simple reduction in dosage. It has been reported that administration of L-tryptophan may reverse the psychiatric side effects of L-dopa.

Cardiovascular Agents

The toxic levels of digitalis preparations are very close to the therapeutic serum levels. In addition to the familiar nausea and cardiac dysrhythmia associated with digitalis toxicity, the drug has profound effects on the central nervous system. Delirium secondary to digitalis intoxication is manifested initially by restlessness, nightmares, difficulty in concentration, and apathy. This initial reaction gradually evolves into a full-blown delirium, with marked impairment of cognition, irritability, distractability, delusional thinking, and hallucinations. The toxic effects of digitalis on the central nervous system are greater in persons who are elderly, have cerebrovascular disease, show poor cardiac reserve, or are being treated with other medications. Greater susceptibility is also noted among patients in unfamiliar settings with relative sensory deprivation and sleep disturbance, such as those in an intensive care unit.

Antiarrhythmia agents reduce cardiac irritability. Procainamide (Pronestyl) produces weakness and mild depression in moderate doses. High doses may cause severe depression, with psychotic behavior and hallucinations. Propranolol (Inderal) commonly produces mild central nervous system effects, including drowsiness, lethargy, and headache. In higher doses, propranolol may produce more severe depressions; psychotic reactions have been reported.

Among the antihypertension drugs, the thiocyanates have the most notorious reputation for producing toxic effects on the central nervous system. Thiocyanates cause delirium at blood levels as low as 8 to 12 mg. per 100 ml. Over a time, the drug may accumulate in the body, resulting in sleepiness, weakness, confusion, hallucinations and delirium. Treatment consists of the administration of sodium chloride and hemodialysis in severe cases. Reserpine (Rau-Sed, Serpasil, Ser-Ap-Es) often causes depression. The patient may have distressing nightmares, marked agitation, and a suicidal tendency that may require hospitalization. Methyldopa (Aldomet) commonly causes sedation and may produce mental depression and nightmares, as seen with reserpine, but the reaction is usually less marked and less frequent. Hydralazine (Apresoline) commonly produces headaches, anorexia, and gastrointestinal symptoms. In high doses, hydralazine may produce anxiety, depression, disorientation, confusion, and acute psychotic episodes.

The diuretic agents have a wide margin of safety. The mercurial derivatives and ethacrynic acid may cause rapid loss of fluid and electrolytes, resulting in sodium and potassium depletion and alkalosis secondary to loss of chloride ion. These metabolic abnormalities may produce episodes of weakness, disorientation, confusion, and delirium.

Anesthetics

The volatile anesthetics are virtually never the cause of organic brain syndromes because they are inert and rapidly excreted. Delirium and dementia with associated brain damage may be seen after general anesthesia, but essentially all these cases are secondary to brain anoxia.

Toxic reactions of the central nervous system may result when local anesthetics are injected intravenously to control cardiac arrhythmias, when they are injected into a vein accidentally during local infiltration, or when large amounts are absorbed from a local infiltration site. They act as stimulants to the central nervous system, resulting in initial restlessness, tremor, and convulsions. This reaction may be followed by the depression of vital functions and by death resulting from respiratory failure. Cocaine toxicity rapidly causes the patient to become restless, agitated, anxious, and confused. Headache, hyperpyrexia, dilation of the pupils, nausea, vomiting, and abdominal pain are fre-

quently seen. Delirium, with Cheyne-Stokes respiration and convulsions, occurs terminally. Toxicity with cocaine may occur with extreme rapidity. Procaine (Novocain) is only one fourth as toxic as cocaine, but in toxic doses it may cause central nervous system stimulation and convulsions. Reactions may be avoided by using the smallest effective amount of anesthetic solution in combination with epinephrine to delay absorption.

Hormones

A premorbid personality disturbance or a previous history of psychiatric disorder predisposes the patient to adverse central nervous system reactions. There seems to be no direct correlation between the dose of hormone administered and the severity or duration of psychic changes.

In patients treated with cortisol for Addison's disease, the apathy, depression, irritability, and psychosis commonly associated with this disease are ameliorated by correction of the hormone deficiency. When the glucocorticoids are used, patients commonly display elevation of mood; a certain percentage become euphoric, restless, agitated, and insomnic. High doses of corticosteroids may result in severe psychotic reactions, characterized by manic behavior and paranoid ideation. Confusion, feelings of depersonalization, and a severe depression, with suicidal ideation, may be encountered occasionally. A reduction of the dosage of adrenocorticotropic hormone (ACTH) or cortisone may be necessary for several days if severe psychic changes occur. The dosage may then be gradually increased, or the patient may be maintained at a lower dosage. The substitution of cortisone for ACTH may sometimes relieve the psychiatric symptoms. Electroshock therapy has been of benefit in manic states and in severe depressions associated with corticosteroid therapy.

An overdose of thyroid hormone produces symptoms typical of hyperthyroidism, including fatigue, weakness, tachycardia, tremors, headache, anxiety, agitation, insomnia, and heat intolerance. Overdoses of thyroid preparations result in symptoms of thyroid storm, characterized by severe tachycardia, hyperpyrexia, diarrhea, vomiting, dehydration, and delirium. The antithyroid preparations may precipitate an organic brain syndrome, with confusion, disorientation, delirium, paranoid delusions, and hallucinations—all secondary to the rapid onset of a hypothyroid state. The time of onset after the initiation of therapy varies, often with a delay of days or weeks before the appearance of symptoms. The psychotic state usually responds rapidly to the administration of thyroxine.

Marked changes in psychic function may be produced by insulin and hypoglycemia drugs through the development of hypoglycemia. Initially, the patient may show irritability, intellectual impairment, confusion, headache, and lethargy. This reaction may progress to more full-blown delirium, followed by coma and convulsions. Chronic hypoglycemic states may result in personality changes or eventually cause permanent brain damage, with dementia, epilepsy, or focal neurological symptoms.

Nonnarcotic Analgesics and Antipyretics

The salicylates (aspirin, sodium salicylate) may produce toxic states in high doses, with confusion, agitation, delirium, and hallucinations. Phenacetin may cause depressed mood, lethargy, dizziness, feelings of detachment, impaired concentration, and toxic psychosis with hallucinations. However, phenacetin is invariably found in combination with salicylates, codeine, or barbiturates. It is often difficult to distinguish which of these agents is producing the toxic state.

Carbamazepine (Tegretol) is closely related chemically to the tricyclic antidepressants and produces similar side effects, including the activation of latent psychosis, depression with agitation, and delirium, particularly in older people.

Anti-Inflammatory Drugs

Phenylbutazone (Butazolidin) in large doses may produce a marked delirious state, with hallucinations, coma, and convulsions. Even when lower therapeutic doses are given, particularly if by injection, headaches, psychotic reactions, and depression may result. Indomethacin (Indocin) produces headache in about 50 per cent of patients. More severe effects include depersonalization, ataxia, confusion, nightmares, hallucinations, delirium, and convulsions with coma. Prolonged use of indomethacin may cause severe depression reactions.

Anti-Infection Agents

The sulfonamides have been shown to produce confusion, depression, and acute psychotic reactions. Most commonly, the sulfa drugs produce minor symptoms, such as drowsiness, dizziness, insomnia, irritability, headache, and mild mood changes, particularly in children. Penicillin given intravenously may produce an acute psychotic reaction, characterized by severe anxiety, agitation, hallucinations, and seizures. Antibiotics used in the treatment of gram-negative infections have been associated with depression and delirium, with confusion, excitement, and hallucinations.

Among the various antituberculosis agents, isoniazid, cycloserine, ethionamide, and iproniazid have been shown to produce toxic central nervous system reactions and marked mood changes. Isoniazid, particularly in the high-dose ranges, produces anxiety and restlessness. Prolonged administration may result in irritability, confusion, and paranoid thinking, often with marked belligerence and antagonistic behavior. Schizophrenic symptoms may be reactivated in chronic schizophrenics, or a schizophrenic-like syndrome, with auditory and visual hallucinations, may be induced in apparently normal people. Cycloserine may produce anxiety, irritability, drowsiness, difficulty in concentration, confusion, disorientation, paranoid delusions, hallucinations, and delirium. Cycloserine may also activate schizophrenic symptoms in schizophrenic patients. Ethionamide apparently produces some mental depression, together with lethargy, somnolence, and, at times, suicidal ideation. Iproniazid may produce euphoric states. Manic states and agitated delirium may occur secondary to iproniazid administration.

Toxic doses of amantadine (Symmetrel) produce an agitated delirium, with aggressive behavior and hallucinations.

Chloroquine (Aralen) may produce acute psychotic states with paranoid delusions, aggressive behavior, delirium, and occasionally seizures. Quinacrine (Atabrine) may produce organic brain syndrome—with auditory and visual hallucinations, delusions, and paranoid ideation—or clouding of sensorium, disorientation, amnesia, and confabulation.

Griseofulvin side effects are usually mild, including drowsiness, headache, fatigue, irritability, and insomnia. However, severe depression and states of confusion sometimes occur.

Disulfiram

Minor side effects of fatigue and decreased libido and potency may be seen with disulfiram in the usual dose range of 0.25 gm. daily. In larger doses, toxic psychoses may be produced, with weakness, difficulty with concentration and memory, disorientation, confusion, and somnolence. The drug may also exacerbate psychotic symptoms in schizophrenic patients. The chronic ingestion of excessive amounts of disulfiram results in delirium, depression, parkinsonism, and peripheral neuropathy.

Antineoplastic Agents

The vast majority of antineoplastic agents have few central nervous system effects. The vinca alkaloids have been reported to produce toxic effects, including stupor, hallucinations, and coma when used in extremely high doses. Somnolence and mental depression are common but transient.

Gases

The inhalation of pure oxygen under pressures above one atmosphere may produce pulmonary atelectasis, depression of respiration, retrolental fibroplasia in infants, and irritation of the respiratory tract. Most of these effects can be avoided if the concentration of inhaled oxygen is kept below 50 per cent. When pure oxygen is inhaled at pressures greater than two atmospheres, oxygen intoxication is observed, with dizziness, muscle twitching, paresthesias, irritability, mood changes, loss of consciousness, and generalized convulsions. The intoxication syndrome is reversible if the oxygen pressure is reduced. Oxygen paradox—with symptoms of confusion, incoordination, cardiovascular decompensation, and seizures—may be seen when oxygen is administered after a period of hypoxia.

The effects of carbon dioxide on the brain depend on the concentration breathed. In low concentrations, the cerebral cortex is generally depressed in excitability, and the threshold for the production of seizures is increased. A carbon dioxide mixture of up to 10 per cent produces disagreeable symptoms of dyspnea, restlessness, headache, paresthesias, dizziness, and sweating. Unconsciousness occurs after about

15 minutes of 10 per cent carbon dioxide inhalation. At concentrations of 25 to 30 per cent, subcortical areas are activated, resulting in increased cortical excitability and the possibility of convulsions. At levels above 25 per cent, symptoms of headache, severe mental confusion, and delirium appear. Chronic exposure to low concentrations of around 3 per cent over several days may produce initial excitation, followed by mental depression.

The symptoms of carbon monoxide poisoning depend on the percentage of methoxyhemoglobin in the circulating blood. Below 20 per cent, headache of the throbbing type is the only symptom. Between 20 and 40 per cent, severe headache with dizziness, dimness of vision, nausea, vomiting, weakness, and collapse may occur. Between 40 and 60 per cent, increased respiration and pulse rate are seen, with eventual syncope, coma, convulsions, and Cheyne-Stokes respiration. Respiratory failure and death occur when concentrations reach about 70 to 80 per cent. Generally, if the patient recovers consciousness within an hour after intoxication, the chances of permanent mental or neurological sequelae are small. Acute exposure to large concentrations of carbon monoxide or chronic repeated exposures at lower levels result in permanent brain damage. The most severe neurological symptoms resulting from carbon monoxide poisoning are parkinsonism and seizue disorder. Severe episodic depressions, withdrawal, apathy, and impairment of perception are common psychiatric sequelae. Forgetfulness is common, characterized by marked impairment of orientation. The treatment of carbon monoxide intoxication is the immediate administration of oxygen with 5 per cent carbon dioxide.

Noxious Vapors and Solvents

Acute poisoning may occur when persons ingest or are exposed to high concentrations of vapors in enclosed environments. Table I lists a number of these substances, along with their common uses and the symptoms produced by intoxication.

Heavy Metals

Chronic lead intoxication occurs when the amount of lead ingested exceeds the ability to eliminate it. When the intake exceeds 0.6 mg. of lead a day, chronic intoxication begins. How-

TABLE I

Volatile Agents Producing Intoxication

Class	Substances	Uses	Symptoms of Acute Intoxication	Symptoms of Chronic Intoxication
Aliphatic hydrocarbons	Methane, butane, octane, ethylene, acetylene	Gasoline, heating gas, welding gas, chemical manufacturing, cleaning agents, paint thinners, furniture polish, insecticide vehicle	Headache, vertigo, weakness, excitement, delirium, CNS depression, ventricular fibrillation, death	Fatigue, nausea, abdominal pains, weight loss, episodic confusion, hallucinations
Aromatic hydrocarbons	Benzene, toluene, xylene, naphthalene, styrene	Gasoline, industrial solvents, paint removers, paint and varnish vehicles, airplane glue, dry-cleaning agents, mothballs, plastic manufacturing	CNS depression, muscle spasms, delirium, convulsions	Irritability, headache, vertigo, somnolence
Halogenated hydrocarbons	Methyl chloride, ethylene chloride, carbon tetrachloride, Freon, methyl bromide	Industrial solvents, paint remover, degreasing agents, fire extinguishers, refrigerants, aerosol bases, paint vehicles	Headache, dizziness, nausea, vomiting, CNS depression, stupor, convulsions, coma, liver and kidney toxicity	Nausea, vomiting, anorexia, apathy, episodic confusion, weight loss
Borane hydrogen compounds	Pentaborane	Rocket fuel	CNS excitement, convulsions, memory impairment, tremor	Somnolence, headache, tremor
Ketones	Acetone, butanone, isophorone	Automobile finishes, rubber and plastic industry, paint removers, waterproofing processes, industrial solvents	Mild intoxication with CNS depression, dizziness, incoordination (unconsciousness)	Mild intoxication with CNS depression, dizziness, incoordination
Glycols	Ethylene glycol, propylene glycol, carbitol	Cellulose solvents, printing inks, lacquer and varnish vehicles, automobile antifreeze	CNS depression	Nervousness, tremor, fatigue, ataxia, somnolence, personality change, slurred speech
Alcohols	Methanol, propyl alcohol, butyl alcohol	Rubbing alcohol, solvents, radiator antifreeze, lamp fuel, lacquer and varnish solvents	CNS depression with irritability, delirium, convulsions, visual impairment, acidosis, abdominal pain	
Carbon disulfide	Volatile liquid in pure form	Rayon and rubber industries, plywood adhesive, pesticides	Ataxia, confusion, delirium	Personality changes, memory loss, possible acceleration of cerebral and coronary arteriosclerosis, irritability, episodes of mania and depression, decreased libido, delirium, and dementia

ever, it takes several months for toxic symptoms to appear. The most serious symptoms are produced by lead absorbed through the respiratory tract.

The signs and symptoms of lead intoxication depend on the level of lead in the blood. Chronic anemia is seen when this level exceeds 100 μg. per 100 ml. Levels above 150 μg. per 100 ml. cause loss of appetite, constipation, colicky abdominal pains, and a sweet metallic taste in the mouth. When lead reaches levels above 200 μg. per 100 ml., symptoms of severe lead encephalopathy occur, with dizziness, clumsiness, ataxia, irritability, restlessness, headache, and insomnia. Later, an excited delirium, with associated vomiting and visual disturbances, occurs, progressing to convulsions, lethargy, and coma. The mortality from lead encephalopathy is 25 per cent; among the survivors, 40 per cent have permanent neurological sequelae, including mental retardation, epilepsy, cerebral palsy, and dystonia musculorum deformans.

Treatment of lead encephalopathy should be instituted as rapidly as possible. The symptomatic treatment of lead intoxication is morphine and atropine administration for relief of the abdominal colic and vomiting. Barbiturates help to reduce convulsions and agitation. The treatment of choice to facilitate lead excretion is the daily administration of calcium-disodium edetate (Calcium-Disodium Versenate) intravenously for 5 days. Often, the 5-day courses are repeated every few months. The symptoms of lead poisoning may persist for months after treatment.

In acute mercury intoxication, central nervous system symptoms of lethargy and restlessness may occur, but the primary symptoms are secondary to severe gastrointestinal irritation, with bloody stools, diarrhea, and vomiting leading to circulatory collapse because of dehydration. The delayed effects of acute poisoning may result in stomatitis, kidney and liver damage, lethargy, agitation, and tremor. The early signs of chronic mercury intoxication are gingivitis, tremor, albuminuria, and personality change. Later, the teeth begin to loosen, and colitis, progressive renal damage, anorexia, anemia, hypertension, and peripheral neuritis are seen. Central nervous system symptoms gradually become more obvious, with mental depression, insomnia, fatigue, irritability, lethargy, and hallucinosis. Behavioral changes include excessive embarrassment, timidity, withdrawal, and despondency. Mercury poisoning is best treated with a metal chelating agent, such as penicillamine or dimercaprol.

Early manganese intoxication produces headache, irritability, joint pains, and somnolence. These symptoms become progressively more severe, with an eventual picture of emotional lability, pathological laughter, nightmares, hallucinations, and compulsive and impulsive acts associated with periods of confusion and aggressiveness. Lesions involving the basal ganglia and pyramidal system result in gait impairment, rigidity, monotonous or whispering speech, tremors of the extremities and tongue, masked facies, micrographia, dystonia, dysarthria, and loss of equilibrium. The psychological effects tend to clear 3 or 4 months after the patient's removal from the site of exposure, but the neurological symptoms tend to remain stationary or to progress. There is no specific treatment for manganese intoxication other than removal from the source of poisoning.

Thallium salts intoxication initially causes severe pains in the legs, diarrhea, and vomiting. Within a week, delirium, convulsions, cranial nerve palsies, blindness, choreiform movements, and coma may occur. Behavioral changes include paranoid thinking and depression with suicidal tendencies. Alopecia is a common and important diagnostic clue. Treatment is generally symptomatic.

Severe acute arsenic poisoning results in marked vomiting and diarrhea, followed by dryness of the mucous membranes. Death is the result of shock from fluid loss. Chronic arsenic intoxication has a more insidious onset, with weakness, lethargy, anorexia, diarrhea, nausea, inflammation of the nose and upper respiratory tract, coughing, soreness of the mouth, and dermatitis, with increased pigmentation of the neck, eyelids, nipples, and axillae. Keratosis of the palms and soles is common. Severe liver impairment, edema of the eyelids, face, and ankles, and loss of hair and nails are seen in severe chronic poisoning. The eventual outcome of chronic arsenic intoxication is arsenic encephalopathy, with marked intellectual loss and apathy. Treatment is with a chelating agent, such as dimercaprol.

Organophosphate Insecticides

Mild organophosphate intoxication produces symptoms of headache, fatigue, numbness of the extremities, gastrointestinal upset, dizziness, excessive sweating and salivation, tightness in the chest, and abdominal pain. In severe poisoning, the patient feels extremely weak. Eventually, flaccid paralysis occurs, with decreased respiration, marked myosis, and coma. In severe acute intoxications, a classic picture of delirium is seen, with restlessness, tremulousness, and eventually coma with convulsions and hyperthermia. Chronic effects on the central nervous system include impairment of memory, mental depression, difficulty in concentration, and episodic psychotic behavior. The treatment of organophosphate poisoning is the administration of atropine sulfate, given parenterally in a dose sufficient to produce atropine side effects.

REFERENCES

Agulnik, P. L., DiMascio, A., and Moore, P. Acute brain syndrome associated with lithium therapy. Am. J. Psychiatry, *129:* 621, 1972.

Goodman, L. S., and Gilman. A. *The Pharmacological Basis of Therapeutics: A Textbook of Pharmacology, Toxicology, and Therapeutics for Physicians and Medical Students*, ed. 4. Macmillan, New York, 1970.

Hoff, E. C. Brain syndromes associated with drug or poison intoxication. In *Comprehensive Textbook of Psychiatry*. A. M. Freedman and H. I. Kaplan, editors, p. 759. Williams & Wilkins, Baltimore, 1967.

Meyler, L., and Herxheimer, A. *Side Effects of Drugs: A Survey of Unwanted Effects of Drugs Reported in 1968–1971*, vol. 7. Excerpta Medica, Amsterdam, 1972.

Namba, T. Organophosphate insecticide poisoning. Resident Staff Phys., *19:* 31, June 1973.

Shader, R. I. *Psychiatric Complications of Medical Drugs*. Raven Press, New York, 1972.

Shader, R. I., and DiMascio, A. *Psychotropic Drug Side Effects: Clinical and Theoretical Perspectives*. Williams & Wilkins, Baltimore, 1970.

Singer, I., and Rotenberg, D. Mechanisms of lithium action. N. Engl. J. Med., *289:* 254, 1973.

Swanson, D. W., Weddige, R. L., and Morse, R. M. Abuse of prescription drugs. Mayo Clin. Proc. *48:* 359, 1973.

Swartzburg, M., Lieb, J., and Schwartz, A. H. Methaqualone withdrawal. Arch. Gen. Psychiatry, *29:* 46, 1973.

18.7   ORGANIC BRAIN SYNDROMES ASSOCIATED WITH INFECTIONS

Introduction

Infectious diseases give rise to brain dysfunction either by directly invading brain tissue or by producing toxic, hypoxic, or allergic effects from an infection elsewhere in the body. Mild effects—such as irritability, insomnia, and restlessness—may appear early in the illness but subside completely if the infection is overcome rapidly. With progression of the infection, more severe changes can develop, including combativeness, visual hallucinations, impaired memory, and alterations in consciousness. Ordinarily, these manifestations disappear as the infection is brought under control, but changes of personality and intellect sometimes persist as sequelae of the infection.

Bacterial Infections

Tuberculous Meningitis

All patients with tuberculous meningitis have tuberculous infection elsewhere in the body, but some patients lack clinical evidence of active tuberculosis except in the meninges. The infection is most often seen in patients between the ages of 6 months and 20 years.

The disease develops over a period of several days to several weeks. It is accompanied by fever, headache, vomiting, nuchal stiffness, and lethargy. Infants become increasingly irritable, tend to have a shrill cry, and have bulging of the fontanelles. Stupor may develop and then coma. Papilledema, optic atrophy, convulsive seizures, cranial nerve palsies, and other focal neurological signs may appear as the disease progresses.

Without proper treatment by antituberculosis drugs, this disease is fatal, usually within 3 to 4 weeks of its onset. Relapses are rare in adequately treated patients.

About 25 per cent of the survivors have some neurological sequelae. Cranial nerve abnormalities—such as deafness, blindness, and facial paresis—may be noted, and seizures and hemiparesis are common. Intellectual impairment may occur.

Proper chemotherapy should be instituted promptly. A combination of streptomycin, isoniazid, and p-amino salicylic acid is preferable to any of the three drugs alone, and adminstration of the latter two drugs should be continued for 12 to 18 months. Concomitant daily prophylactic administration of pyridoxine is recommended.

Meningitis from Other Bacteria

Infections with *Neisseria meningitidis, Diplococcus pneumoniae,* and *Haemophilus influenzae* are responsible for the majority of cases in which an organism is identified. Infants and children are frequently stricken. Infection by streptococci and staphylococci, principally *Staphylococcus aureus*, is less frequently encountered but produces the next largest group of cases. A wide variety of bacteria, such as *Escherichia coli* (especially in the newborn), *Pseudomonas aeruginosa,* and *Listeria monocytogenes*, are responsible for occasional cases.

Bacterial meningitis is usually an acute illness. Nonspecific symptoms—such as malaise, headache, fever, nausea, and vomiting—are common. Often, photophobia is present. Lethargy or agitation and confusion with disorientation and hallucinations occur in numerous cases. Stupor or coma may supervene. Seizures frequently occur, particularly in infants.

Nuchal rigidity is found in almost every case. Focal cerebral signs—such as hemiparesis, visual field defect, and aphasia—are noted in some patients. Cranial nerve abnormalities—especially of the oculomotor, abducens, and eight nerves—are common. A petechial skin rash is frequently seen during meningococcal meninigitis. An examination of the cerebrospinal fluid reveals a definite elevation of fluid pressure in many patients. Differential diagnosis can usually be made on the basis of clinical and spinal fluid findings.

Certain factors—such as coma, bacteremia, extremes of age underlying disease, and coexistant trauma—appear to be related to increased mortality. Heightened intracranial pressure is an important cause of death in acute bacterial meningitis. Sequelae occur, especially in infants, as convulsive disorders, deafness, mental retardation, hemiparesis, and hydrocephalus.

Successful treatment rests on early diagnosis, isolation of the causative organism, and prompt antibiotic therapy (see Table I). After some cerebrospinal fluid and blood have been drawn for cultures, empirical therapy with ampicillin or a combination of penicillin, sulfadiazine, and chloramphenicol may be started before the organism has been identified.

Fungal Infection: Mycotic Meningitis

Infection of the meninges and central nervous system results from invasion by pathogenic fungi, most frequently *Cryptococcus neoformans*, *Coccidioides immitis*, or *Histoplasma capsulatum*. The fungi may enter the body through the respiratory tract. They may spread secondarily to the central nervous system or become pathogens in a patient who has an underlying malignant disease or who has been treated extensively with antibacterial agents, steroids, or immunosuppressive agents. Cryptococcal meningitis often occurs in association with lymphoma and leukemia.

Clinically, the patient presents signs and symptoms of meningitis developing over several weeks or months. Repeated cultures of cerebrospinal fluid may be necessary to make the diagnosis.

Formerly, mycotic meningitis was fatal in every instance, but treatment has improved with the development and availability of amphotericin B. However, proper identification of the responsible organism is necessary because not all fungi are best treated with this drug. Toxic side effects are common—for example, fever, elevated blood urea, pain, and phlebitis at the injection site. The treatment must usually be continued for many weeks or months.

Viral Infections

Viral infections of the central nervous system may remain primarily in the leptomeninges (lymphocytic choriomeningitis) or involve the spinal cord (poliomyelitis). More often, though, they involve the brain itself.

Arthropod-borne Encephalitides

Diagnosis is usually made serologically by demonstrating a rise in the complement-fixation antibody for the specific virus. The virus itself is rarely identified.

Western Equine Encephalitis. This acute infectious disease is characterized by involvement of the central nervous system with encephalomyelitis. Diagnosis is confirmed by serum complement-fixation tests or by isolation of the virus.

The clinical syndrome depends partly on the age of the patient. In infants, the illness begins abruptly with high fever and convulsions. After 3 to 7 days the fever and convulsions stop abruptly, and the patient becomes asymptomatic.

Children examined during the acute stage appear gravely ill, with fever and neurological

TABLE I

Chemotherapy of Meningitis

Microorganism	Drugs of Choice
Neisseria meningitidis	Penicillin G or sulfadiazine or both
Diplococcus pneumoniae	Penicillin G
Haemophilus influenzae	Chloramphenicol and sulfadiazine
Staphylococcus aureus	Methicillin or cephalothin first, then adjust according to sensitivities
Streptococcus pyogenes	Penicillin G
Listeria monocytogenes	Penicillin G
Escherichia coli	Streptomycin and tetracycline or colistin
Mycobacterium tuberculosis	Isoniazid, streptomycin, and *p*-aminosalicyclic acid
Treponema pallidum	Penicillin G
Actinomyces bovis	Penicillin G
Nocardia asteroides	Sulfadiazine
Cryptococcus neoformans	Amphotericin B
Coccidioides immitis	Amphotericin B
Unknown	Ampicillin or penicillin G, sulfadiazine, and chloramphenicol

abnormalities. The deep reflexes are more pronounced in the extremity from which the convulsive movements spread. Nuchal rigidity is a prominent finding.

Among adults, the illness begins with fever, chills, and malaise, followed by a severe headache. Often, the headache is accompanied by drowsiness and sometimes by coma. Sometimes, disturbed awareness and perception are accompanied by considerable anxiety and delirium. Less severe symptoms include back pain, nausea, and vomiting. In severe cases, tremor, dysarthria, and paralysis or paresis may ensue.

Death occurs in 5 to 10 per cent of cases, usually in the first 48 to 96 hours. Convalescence is prolonged in adults, requiring 3 to 4 months after severe illness. Infants, if they recover, do so in a few weeks. Sequelae in infants are hemiplegia and focal convulsions. In adults, the sequelae are spasticity, speech problems, weight loss, and organic impairment of psychological functioning. The severity seems directly related to the duration of coma.

Treatment remains symptomatic. Supportive therapy is often lifesaving, especially among stuporous and comatose patients. Preventive measures include the use of a vaccine and mosquito control.

Other Arthropod-borne Encephalitides. Eastern equine encephalitis causes greater morbidity than does the Western type. St. Louis encephalitis has been reported in epidemics in the central United States. In Japanese B encephalitis the human infection is often not apparent. Murray Valley encephalitis is an Australian disease. Russian tick-born encephalitis is a biphasic illness with severe sequelae. Its chronic form may evolve to a chronic progressive disease of the central nervous system with psychiatric symptoms.

Herpes simplex Encephalitis

In this rare encephalitis, mortality is very high and permanent neurological sequelae are common in survivors. The availability of a specific antiviral agent, idoxuridine, may offer the potential of a specific treatment.

Mumps Meningoencephalitis

Meningoencephalitis develops in 0.5 to 10 per cent of patients with mumps. The clinical pattern includes changes in the sensorium, with focal neurological findings, such as hemiplegia. Recovery is usually complete.

Chronic (Slow) Virus Infections

Viral infection of the human nervous system may cause slowly progressive neurological disease over many months or even years after a prolonged inactive or latent phase.

Subacute sclerosing panencephalitis develops primarily in young persons below the age of 20 years, with the gradual appearance of intellecutal impairment, loss of interest in usual activities, restlessness, and behavioral changes. In subsequent weeks and months, periodic myoclonic jerks of muscles of the trunk or limbs or face, incoordination, speech impairment, and paresis of the limbs become evident, eventually culminating in death.

In Creutzfeldt-Jakob disease, mental abnormalities consist of intellectual impairment, behavioral disturbance, apathy, and easy fatigability. Profound, global impairment of intellectual faculties ensues, eventually leading to a mute state associated with spasticity of the limbs, ataxia, choreoathetosis, and myoclonus. Most patients die in 3 to 18 months. The majority of cases have occurred in middle-aged persons.

In progressive multifocal leukoencephalopathy, the clinical course usually progresses to death in 3 to 6 months. Dementia, spasticity of the limbs, visual field defects, nystagmus, aphasia, ataxia, dysarthria, and conjugate gaze palsies are seen.

Spriochetal Infection: Neurosyphilis

Syphilis is a chronic, systemic, infectious disease caused by *Treponema pallidum*, which is usually transmitted by sexual contact.

Meningovascular Syphilis

The invasion of the nervous system is marked by edema, cellular infiltration, increase of connective tissue, and formation of granulomas or gummas. The brain, cord, and nerves may be invaded, causing a profusion of symptoms and signs that come and go. Headache is common.

As the disease progresses, large and small vessels, particularly the arteries of the brain, may undergo perivascular cuffing, intimal changes, and closure, with results dependent on the part of the brain served by the affected vessel. There may be hemiplegia, aphasia, hemianopsia, bulbar symptoms, stupor, or convulsions, often with abrupt onset. The spinal cord, too, may become infarcted, with resultant paraplegia and incontinence. The veins may close, leading to myelomalacia.

General Paralysis of the Insane (Dementia Paralytica)

A psychosis caused by extensive spirochetal invasion of the brain, paresis occurs in about 5 per cent of neurosyphilitic patients usually becoming evident between the ages of 30 and 50 years—some 5 to 15 years after the initial infection. The onset is insidious, evidenced by slight memory defects, deterioration of personal appearance and conduct, increasing irritability, and fits of temper. The illness may follow an acute or a chronic course, but without treatment it ordinarily lasts about 3 years. The final scene is one of intellectual dilapidation, immobility, and filth.

The classic paretic psychosis is manifested by euphoria, overactivity, ideas of grandeur, and megalomania. Delusions of wealth, physical prowess, and the like are common. Most often, the psychosis is intermixed with paranoid ideation, depression, simple dementia, and neurasthenia. Rarely, there may be convulsions and signs of localized brain involvement (Lissauer's general paralysis). The slurred, slovenly speech issuing from the sagging and tremulous lips of a paretic patient at once attracts attention. The pupils may be irregular and small or unequal; they often show the Argyll Robertson response. The tendon reflexes are usually increased; there may be cranial nerve palsy and signs of focal damage to the brain. The Wassermann reaction in the blood and cerebrospinal fluid is almost invariably positive.

Treatment with penicillin has become so effective that the previously favored arsenic, mercury, and fever are rarely used. Response to therapy depends on the amount of brain damage at the time of treatment.

Tabes Dorsalis

A disorder resulting from spinal cord changes caused by syphilis, tabes dorsalis is now rare. One of the early symptoms is lightning pains, most commonly in the lower extremities. Also common is girdle pain, which feels as though a belt has been drawn too tightly around the waistline or chest. Still another type of pain is the gastric crisis, a midline epigastric or abdominal pain. Blindness, caused by simple optic atrophy, may appear early or late in both tabes and paresis. Another common symptom is ataxia. Frequently, the joints are affected by painless swelling, hypermobility, and disintegration, producing the Charcot joint. Trophic ulcers occur frequently, usually on the ball of the foot. Examination also reveals Argyll Robertson pupils and an absence of tendon reflexes, most often in the lower extremities. Appreciation of touch, pain, and temperature may be impaired, lost, or perverted.

Taboparesis

Paresis and tabes are sometimes concurrent. The findings and symptoms are what one might expect in a combination of these two conditions.

Congenital Neurosyphilis

Tabes and paresis, singly or in conjunction, may follow congenitally acquired syphilis. The juvenile variants usually appear between the ages of 9 and 16 years. Treatment is the same as that described for paresis.

Rickettsial Infection: Rocky Mountain Spotted Fever

Rocky Mountain spotted fever is an acute febrile disease caused by infection with *Rickettsia rickettsii*, which is transmitted by various ticks.

Pathological changes are found in the skin, heart, lungs, and central nervous system. Neurological symptoms occur early and include delirium, coma, convulsions, opisthotonos, and mental confusion. Diagnosis is based on the characteristic development of a rash on the extremities first, followed by other symptoms 4 to 6 days after exposure to ticks. The diagnosis depends on neutralization and complement fixation tests.

Without specific antirickettsial therapy, mortality varies from 20 per cent to 80 per cent. Even in patients who recover, residual damage to the central nervous system may be apparent for some months. Chlortetracycline (Aureomycin), chloramphenicol, and oxytetracycline (Terramycin) are effective against rickettsial infections. Sulfonamides enhance the growth of rickettsiae and are contraindicated.

Protozoal Infections

Toxoplasmosis

Infection with the protozoan *Toxoplasma gondii* causes toxoplasmosis. The infection occurs most commonly *in utero* and has a predilection for the brain and the eye. Symptoms in the newborn are inanition, convulsions, spasticity, and chorioretinitis. Most patients die in the first weeks after birth. Mental and neurological deficits persist in those who survive.

Trypanosomiasis

The African form of trypanosomiasis, African sleeping sickness, is an encephalitis due to infection by *Trypanosoma gambiense* or *Trypanosoma rhodesiense*, transmitted by the tsetse fly. A similar disease is present in South America, Chagas' disease.

The first stage of the disease is characterized by remitting fever, chronic adenitis, exanthemata, and asthenia. In the second stage, the involvement of the central nervous system is manifested by tremor, incoordination, convulsions, paralysis, mental disturbance, somnolence, and usually death within a year if treatment is not given. Pentavalent arsenical drugs are the therapeutic agents of choice.

Systemic Infections

Acute Viral Hepatitis

Mental symptoms are frequent and are due to secondary toxic or metabolic changes in the brain from hepatic failure. These changes are frequently characterized by delirium, a flapping tremor, and, if the disease progresses, coma. Treatment is symptomatic.

Malaria

Involvement of the nervous system occurs in a few patients with malaria, most often in the malignant tertiary form caused by *Plasmodium falciparum*. The cerebral symptoms usually appear in the second or third week of the illness and include headache, photophobia, convulsions, delirium, and coma. Psychic symptoms are also common. An examination may reveal nuchal rigidity, paralysis, and cranial nerve palsy. Intravenous administration of specific drugs for malaria is effective if begun at the onset of the mental symptoms.

Acute Disseminated Encephalomyelitis

Cerebral changes occur as sequelae to many of the exanthematous diseases and to vaccination for some of these diseases. Acute disseminated encephalomyelitis more often follows measles (0.5 per cent of cases) than other

diseases. When German measles occurs early in pregnancy, severe cerebral defects may occur in the fetus.

The signs and symptoms begin within a week of the rash. The patient becomes drowsy and stuporous and may have convulsions. Meningeal involvement may be severe, with nuchal rigidity. About 10 per cent of the patients die. Of those who recover, 50 per cent or more have residua, including ataxia, mental deficit, and epilepsy. The treatment is symptomatic.

Infectious Diseases of Undetermined Cause

Epidemic Encephalitis (Encephalitis Lethargica, von Economo's Disease)

The entity known as epidemic encephalitis was pandemic throughout the world from 1915 to 1926 but is not clinically significant now. The many bizarre clinical syndromes that followed the disorder closely resembled the phenothiazine intoxications.

Acute Chorea (Sydenham's Chorea)

This disorder is a kind of convulsion, which chiefly attacks children of both sexes, from 10 to 14 years of age. Patients frequently have or have had manifestations of acute rheumatic fever.

The most common initial manifestation is the gradual development of involuntary movements. The movements are more severe with muscular activity and with excitement. They improve with rest and quiet, and they disappear during sleep. Irritability, fretfulness, and mild insomnia are often seen. Less frequent are severe symptoms, such as marked agitation, excitement, insomnia, confusion, and hallucinations.

Patients usually recover completely in 6 weeks to 3 months, and mortality is low (2 per cent). However, in about a third of the cases, the disorder recurs, especially during pregnancy. No sequelae are seen. Since this disorder is probably a manifestation of rheumatic fever, long-term daily administration of penicillin as prophylaxis against future infection by the β-hemolytic streptococcus is imperative.

Management

The management of brain syndromes accompanying infection is, for the most part, the management of the specific infection. The symptomatic treatment is much like that for other acute and chronic brain syndromes. The preservation of a familiar and simple environment for the patient is important.

Patients with meningitis frequently have severe headaches, which may be relieved partially by 600 mg. (10 grains) of aspirin with 30 mg of codeine. Morphine and similar analgesics must be avoided because of their depressant effect on cerebral function. To control restlessness and delirium, the physician may prescribe sedatives but only as a last resort because sedation often adds to the patient's disorientation and further depresses his respiration. If sedation is necessary, paraldehyde is the drug of choice.

REFERENCES

Beeson, P. B., and McDermott, W. *Cecil-Loeb Textbook of Medicine*, ed. 17. W. B. Saunders, Philadelphia, 1971.
Dodge, P. R., and Swartz, M. N. Bacterial meningitis: A review of selected aspects. II. Special neurologic problems, postmeningitic complications and clinicopathological correlations. N. Engl. J. Med. *272:* 1003, 1965.
Eigler, J. O. C., Wellman, W. E., Rooke, E. D., Keith, H. M., and Svien, H. J. Bacterial meningitis. I. General review (294 cases). Proc. Staff Meet. Mayo Clin., *36:* 357, 1961.
Harrison, T. R., Adams, R. D., Bennett, I. L., Jr., Resnik, W. H., Thorn, G. W., and Wintrobe, M. M. *Principles of Internal Medicine*, ed. 7. McGraw-Hill, New York, 1974.
Horta-Barbosa, L., Fuccillo, D. A., Sever, J. L., and Zeman, W. Subacute sclerosing panencephalitis: Isolation of measles virus from a brain biopsy. Nature (London), *221:* 974, 1969.
Payne, F. E., Baublis, J. V., and Itabashi, H. H. Isolation of measles virus from cell cultures of brain from a patient with subacute sclerosing panencephalitis. N. Engl. J. Med., *281:* 585, 1969.
Sydenham, T. An essay on the rise of a new fever. Med. Classics, *4:* 327, 1939.

18.8.   ORGANIC BRAIN SYNDROMES ASSOCIATED WITH INTRACRANIAL NEOPLASMS

Introduction

The brain is one of the most common tumor sites in the body. The psychiatric or mental symptoms associated with brain tumors depend partly on the nature and location of the tumor and are often the earliest and occasionally the only symptoms of an intracranial tumor. The behavioral changes are due to insidious but relentless alterations of cerebral function and the patient's responses to these changes. The mental symptoms may vary not only in different patients but in the same patient from hour to hour.

Pathology

Glioma

Tumors arising from the glia or supporting tissue of the brain are the largest single group of brain tumors.

The astrocytoma (grades 1 and 2) is an infiltrating tumor. In adults, astrocytomas are most often found in the frontal, parietal, and temporal lobes. In children, they occur most frequently in the cerebellar hemisphere. Generally, these lesions grow slowly. In children, an astrocytoma produces no psychiatric symptoms until late in the illness. In adults, astrocytomas sometimes give rise to no symptoms other than focal convulsive episodes until the illness is far advanced.

Glioblastoma multiforme (astrocytoma, grades 3 and 4) is a rapidly growing tumor of late life. It arises most often in the frontal, parietal, and occipital lobes. Mental symptoms appear early. Often the tumor grows so rapidly that the patient cannot adapt successfully to his ever-constricting mental function, and he may react catastrophically, sometimes before neurological findings are recognizable. If the tumor arises in the temporal lobe, the visual pathways are often involved early in the destructive process. If the tumor arises in the dominant hemisphere, aphasia becomes apparent. Focal epileptic seizures are the classic symptom of temporal lobe tumors.

Medulloblastoma, a rapidly growing tumor of the cerebellum, is one of the common intracranial tumors of childhood; 80 per cent of them appear before the age of 15 years. Medulloblastoma usually gives rise to headache, nausea, vomiting, ataxia, cranial nerve palsies, and increased intracranial pressure.

Meningioma

Meningiomas are benign tumors arising from the meninges of the brain and spinal cord (see Figure 1). Meningiomas grow slowly. Often, function is lost so gradually that the patient can adapt more or less satisfactorily at first. Because of the predilection of these tumors for the anterior basal part of the skull or the parasagittal area, they often become extremely large with no clinical manifestations other than gradually progressive dementia and ever-reduced adaptive capacity. The patient usually reacts to the

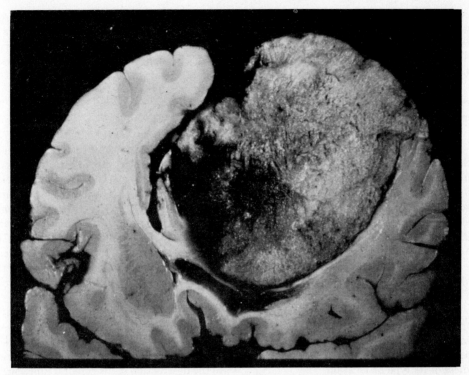

FIGURE 1. Large parasagittal meningioma. The patient with this tumor presented with depression and later developed hemiplegia.

reduction in adaptive capacity with his premorbid defense mechanisms.

Meningiomas arising in the parasagittal areas in the frontal pole of the brain may cause few or no symptoms other than progressive loss of intellectual function. When neurological signs result from parasagittal meningioma, they may be limited to the lower extremities.

Focal convulsive disorders are frequent presenting symptoms of meningiomas. Because early meningiomas can be cured by surgery, prompt diagnosis is of crucial importance.

Pituitary Tumor

Tumors of the pituitary, third ventricle, and hypothalamus give rise to various endocrine and visual disturbances. In addition, tumors in and near the third ventricle can produce serious psychiatric abnormalities. As the tumor expands and compresses the walls of the third ventricle or the frontal lobes of the brain, symptoms become apparent. They include dullness progressing to somnolence, apathy, and difficulty in concentration. Memory may also

be impaired, leading to confusion and sometimes to confabulation. If the patient is aroused, he may be irritable and hyperactive. Poor judgment is common, and delusions and hallucinations may occur.

Metastatic Tumor

Metastatic tumors constitute 5 to 25 per cent of all brain tumors. Usually, brain metastases are multiple; there may be 50 or more nodules of different sizes. The signs and symptoms of such lesions closely resemble those of glioblastoma multiforme, although patients with brain metastases more often have confusion than do patients with a primary brain tumor. This confusion, often associated with apathy, may be secondary to the endocrine and electrolyte changes found in patients with metastatic carcinoma.

Brain Abscess

Since the advent of antibiotic medications, brain abscesses have become rare. Blood-borne infections may result in multiple intracerebral abscesses. Such abscesses often cause symptoms by their mass effect alone, and they must be removed.

The most striking early change is in the patient's mental alertness and emotional tone. His memory is poor, and his attention span is short. He may be apathetic and drowsy. Yet the neurological findings may be minimal.

Clinical Symptoms and Course

The patient with a brain tumor suffers a relentless progression in symptoms. The classic neurological symptoms are headache and impaired motor or sensory function. Even when these disturbances are present, they may be obscured by the patient's mental symptoms at first. The salient features of the patient's history are often the unremitting progression of his symptoms and his attempts to adapt, producing only temporary periods of respite.

Impairments Directly Caused by Brain Tumor

Impaired intellectual functioning often accompanies the presence of a brain tumor, regardless of its type or location.

Disorders of language function, particularly if tumor growth is rapid, may be severe. In fact, defects of language function often obscure all other mental symptoms. Lesions that produce language disorders are usually located in the left hemisphere.

Loss of memory is a frequent symptom of brain tumors. These lesions are usually bilateral and affect the area of the diencephalon and mesencephalon.

Prominent perceptual defects are often associated with behavioral disorders, especially when the problem involves summation of the tactile-auditory-visual perception. The mental disorder then seems proportional to the amount of brain damage. Such disorders are commonly caused by a lesion in the right temporoparietal junction and its underlying white matter. This impaired cerebral function is manifested by a behavioral disorder called amorphosynthesis. This symptom is clinically manifested by an unawareness and neglect of one side of the body—usually the left, since the responsible intracranial lesion most often occurs on the right.

Alterations of consciousness are common late symptoms of increased intracranial pressure due to a brain tumor. Tumors arising in the upper part of the brain stem may produce akinetic mutism or coma vigil. Tumors that give rise to such symptoms include lesions of the third ventricle, craniopharyngiomas, and astrocytomas of the midbrain.

Symptoms Occurring as Epileptic Disorders

Epileptic disorders are the most dramatic psychiatric symptoms in patients with brain tumors. Focal convulsive seizures are often the hallmark of localized pathological lesions of the brain, whether the seizure is motor (Jacksonian) or sensory. This is equally true of paroxysmal seizures consisting of or initiated by mental events. Psychic seizures beginning in patients over 30 years of age are a symptom of brain tumor in one fourth to one fifth of all patients so affected. The symptoms include forced thinking, hallucinations, illusions, disturbances of mood, and automatisms.

Response to Cerebral Loss

Most mental symptoms in patients with brain tumors result from the patient's response to the destruction of his cerebral function. If the patient becomes aware of the destruction only gradually, the earliest psychiatric symptom is often irritability. Later, the patient usually becomes anxious and depressed. He may finally respond to a progressive cerebral impairment by denial of even the most flagrant loss, with a resultant disappearance of his anxiety and depression. Each patient seems to react in accordance with his previous personality, his previous adjustment, and the rapidity of his brain destruction. If the brain tumor grows slowly, the patient may gradually disengage from the more complex aspects of his environment.

Diagnosis

A brain tumor is particularly difficult to diagnose when the presenting symptoms are psychiatric. In all patients with a suspected tumor, a detailed neurological examination should be carried out, including funduscopic examination. In addition, skull roentgenograms should be obtained. Because of the high incidence of metastatic disease to the brain, chest roentgenograms are also indicated.

Psychological tests may help distinguish an organic brain disease from a tumor. They have also been thought to help determine the site of brain tumors. The electroencephalogram is particularly useful when an epileptic syndrome is suspected. The brain scan is particularly valuable when the tumor being sought is highly vascular. The echoencephalogram may demonstrate a shift of midline structures in the brain. The EMIscan may prove to be the most successful noninvasive diagnostic test for brain tumor (see Figure 2). Often, the diagnosis can be confirmed only by biopsy examination.

Treatment

Once the diagnosis is established, treatment of the tumor depends on the cell type. When the tumor arises from the meninges (meningioma), surgical extirpation alleviates the patient's mental symptoms and often cures the disease. When the tumor arises within the brain substance, such as an astrocytoma, surgery may be only palliative, although it can confirm the diagnosis and temporarily relieve some of the patient's symptoms. When the patient has more than one brain lesion, presumably metastatic, surgical intervention, with its resultant edema, can only lead to further disability.

Patients with intrinsic brain tumors are ideal candidates for either radiotherapy or chemotherapy. Many of the patient's symptoms may be related to edema. These symptoms often respond to treatment with dexamethasone.

REFERENCES

Baker, A. B. Intracranial neoplasm. In *Clinical Neurology*, A. B. Baker and H. L. Baker, editors, vol. 1, chap. 9, p. 8, Harper & Row, New York, 1973.
Baker, H. L., Jr., Campbell, J. K., Houser, O. W., Reese, D. F., Sheedy, P. F., and Holman, C. B. Computer assisted tomography of the head: An early evaluation. Mayo Clin. Proc., *49:* 17, 1974.
Critchley, M. *The Parietal Lobes.* Arnold, London, 1953.
Horenstein, S. Effects of cerebrovascular disease on personality and emotionality. In *Behavioral Change in Cerebrovascular Disease*, A. L. Benton, editor, p. 171. Harper & Row, New York, 1970.
Mulder, D. W., and Daly, D. Psychiatric symptoms associated with lesions of temporal lobe. J. A. M. A., *150:* 173, 1952.
Piercy, M. Neurological aspects of intelligence. In *Handbook of Clinical Neurology*. P. J. Vinken and G. W. Bruyn, editors, vol. 3, p. 296. North-Holland, Amsterdam, 1969.
Samson, D. S., and Clark, K. A current review of brain abscess. Am. J. Med., *54:* 201, 1973.
Weinstein, J. D., Toy, F. J., Jaffe, M. E., and Goldberg, H. I. The effect of dexamethasone on brain edema in patients with metastatic brain tumors. Neurology (Minneap.), *23:* 121, 1973.
Zangwill, O. L. The amnesic syndrome. In *Amnesia*, C. W. M. Whitty and O. L. Zangwill, editors, p. 77. Appleton-Century-Crofts, New York, 1966.

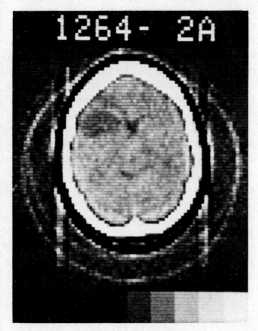

FIGURE 2. An EMIscan, demonstrating a lesion in the left frontal lobe about level with the caudate nucleus. The lesion consisted of an area of decreased density surrounded by an area of increased density. A second, smaller lesion can be seen in the right temporoparietal area. This patient had noted the gradual onset of confusion and difficulty in speaking 2 months before the examination. These symptoms had been progressive. A left carotid angiogram revealed a lesion in the left posterior and frontal regions. Because of the location of the left sided lesion and the presence of multiple lesions, surgery was not advised.

18.9. ORGANIC BRAIN SYNDROMES ASSOCIATED WITH EPILEPSY

Definition

Epilepsy is that state of impaired brain function characterized by a recurrent, paroxysmal disturbance in mental function, with concomitant alterations in behavior or thought processes.

Diagnosis

A seizure is a symptom of brain dysfunction, either localized or general, and should be investigated as only one of a potential complex of signs and symptoms. The occurrence of a fit signals that the neural, humoral, metabolic, and vascular regulatory systems of the brain are in imbalance.

Hypoglycemia, pyridoxine deficiency, eclampsia, uremia, anoxia, hyponatremia, water intoxication, and fever are all states that may lead to convulsions. In the same class should be mentioned seizures after the withdrawal, usually abrupt, of a wide class of pharmacological agents, especially alcohol, barbiturates, meprobamate, diazepoxide, and anticonvulsants.

More common are seizures after cerebrovascular hemorrhage and thrombosis. Cerebral vascular disease is particularly to be suspected with seizures occurring for the first time in adults, particularly those past midlife. Whether the pathology is neoplasm, vascular disease, vascular malformation, abscess, acute or chronic infection, or degenerative disease, fits may be an early symptom and are often important in the localization of the lesion.

A more easily recognized but much abused cause is trauma. The problem is that many patients and families remember all too clearly some recent head injury, to which is attributed all subsequent misfortunes of the patient.

Before one settles down to classify and treat an epileptic, a careful diagnostic work-up is necessary. Minimally, a set of skull X-rays, lumbar puncture, blood serology, fasting blood sugar, brain scan, and electroencephalogram (EEG) should be added to a meticulous physical, neurological, and routine clinical laboratory examination and careful history: particular attention should be paid to recent drug intake. A thorough documentation of mental status by a good psychology laboratory should be done.

The standard shibboleths for seizure diagnosis seem to include unconsciousness, tonic and colonic movement, loss of sphincter control, amnesia, and self-injury, such as bitten tongue and head injury from falling. This set of phenomena describes many grand mal seizures but is not *sine qua non* for all epilepsies. Focal seizures may not be accompanied by loss of consciousness unless the motor symptoms become bilateral. Some psychomotor patients may retain a hazy or distorted memory of the seizure period and may not appear unconscious to an observer. And a number of patients with a real seizure problem have also learned to use the seizure for secondary gain. They may learn ways of precipitating a fit—by hyperventilation, for instance—or they may simulate a fit. Recognition of the simulation by a professional observer may prejudice him against diagnosis of the patient's coexisting epilepsy.

A person reported to have abrupt, self-limited, recurrent alterations of sensation, behavior, or consciousness, especially with motor manifestations, should be suspected of having epilepsy. First, attention is directed to confirming the existence of a seizure. Second, one attempts to recognize pathological conditions to which the seizure is a secondary phenomenon. Having excluded other conditions, one is left with an epileptic patient to be further categorized.

Classification

The categorization of an epileptic patient depends primarily on two data: a description of the seizure and an electroencephalogram. Attention should be paid to precipitating circumstances, periodicity, frequency, warnings, and the first signs of the ictus. The duration and form of termination of the seizure and the subsequent state of the patient should be documented.

The EEG is of considerable assistance in a differential diagnosis, but, expecially in the focal epilepsies, it may be difficult to obtain an abnormal record. A single normal EEG is of no significance in a suspect epileptic. Nearly half of all epileptics have grand mal seizures alone; of these, only about 20 per cent show waking interseizure abnormalities of the EEG. Recording during sleep increases the incidence to 80 per cent. Like other biological measures, brain waves are more likely to betray abnormality under pressure.

More than half of all focal seizures occur in association with grand mal. Therefore, the dramatic presence of grand mal fits should not preclude the careful investigation of any focal signs or symptoms that may point to dangerous pathology, such as a tumor.

Petit mal is extremely rare in adults, and the occurrence of minor seizures with lapse of consciousness is much more often caused by psychomotor or other focal seizures than to true petit mal. Because the drugs of choice are rather different in the two cases, this is an important distinction. The EEG should be definitive on this distinction.

Centrencephalic Seizures

These seizures are characterized by bilateral synchronous EEG abnormality at the time of the seizure or on interictal examination and by clinical unconsciousness at the onset of the seizures. They include grand mal and petit mal seizures.

Grand Mal Seizures. These seizures may have a brief aura and are often initiated by a cry, presumably caused by the forced expiration of air. The cry is followed by or is simultaneous with the loss of consciousness, which is followed by falling to the floor, often with physical injury, and the advent of extreme tonic spasm, the extensor muscles dominating the flexors. This phase is usually followed by a clonic phase, in which there is alternating flexion and extension of the body musculature, which may lead to biting of the tongue or mouth or further injury to the head. Cyanosis is often marked until the seizure terminates with deep, noisy breathing and often with profuse sweating and salivation. There may be relaxation of the sphincters, with loss of urine or feces during the seizure, and the ejaculation of semen, usually with erection, may occur in the male. The EEG during this period is dominated by high-voltage, fast activity in all leads and often terminates with an isoelectric period, during which little or no spontaneous electrical activity is visible. The patient may waken into a confused state described as the postictal automatism or postictal twilight state; he may become perfectly alert and oriented, although somewhat slowed down and dull, or he may lapse into an apparently normal sleep for some minutes or an hour or two. On recovery, he usually complains of muscular aches and often of a severe headache. A marked bulimia may occur on recovery, especially in the twilight state, that leads the patient to ingest copious volumes of food or liquid. With complete and prompt recovery, there may well be feelings of depression and despair, often in reaction to concern and apprehension about the reality aspects of the seizure and social embarrassment.

Petit Mal Seizures. The classic triad of petit mal seizures includes the *absence*, myoclonic seizures or lightning jerks (including salaam seizures), and atonic seizures. The attack is accompanied by bilaterally synchronous EEG wave-and-spike formations at about three per second and is easily brought on by hyperventilation. A characteristic attack is quite brief—10 to 30 seconds—and may pass unnoticed by the patient or by an unskilled observer. It is accompanied by total unconsciousness but of such a brief duration as to make only a transient lapse in conversation and with so little retrograde amnesia that it can easily be concealed.

The myoclonic seizures may or may not include unconsciousness. They are characterized by a very short jerky movement of the body, either a sudden flexion movement of the trunk muscles with raising of the arms, giving rise to the name "salaam," or, particularly in older patients, an abrupt extension movement, notably of the shoulders, arms, and hands.

Atonic seizures are momentary losses of muscle tone, usually with unconsciousness, that cause the patient to slump to the ground but to recover promptly.

Petit mal seizures most often occur in children and may lead to psychiatric referral.

Petit mal seizures are rare in adults. Brief absences are more likely to be focal cortical in origin.

Petit Mal Variant. In petit mal variant, the EEG record is dominated by wave-and-spike complexes of two per second, which is slower than true petit mal. These may be focal abnormalities, and there may be admixtures of slow or other abnormal activity. The clinical picture is one of grand mal or focal seizures. The onset is in infancy or childhood, and more than half of these patients are mentally deficient. The prognosis is quite poor with this diagnosis. These patients, more than any other group, are likely to die in status epilepticus.

Focal Seizures

These seizures have clinical or EEG evidence of a specific, usually cortical, site of origin. They are more likely to be caused by identifiable pathology—a scar, vascular lesion, tumor, brain atrophy—than are the generalized seizures. However, the majority of patients with focal seizures also show characteristic grand mal seizures. Of particular importance in diagnosing and localizing the focal seizure are the events just preceding or initiating the attack.

Jacksonian Seizures. These seizures, first described by Hughlings Jackson, have a focus

TABLE I

Classification of Epilepsies

Type	Common EEG Abnormality	Interseizure EEG Abnormality*	Relative Incidence of Pure Forms*	Peak Age(s) of Onset*	Common Signs and Symptoms	Comment
I. Centrencephalic	Bilaterally synchronous discharge					
Grand mal	High-voltage fast activity	20% awake, 40% asleep	50%	1–15	Fifty % have brief aura, unconsciousness, followed by tonic-clonic seizure	Should be brought readily under drug control
Petit mal *Classic absence* Myoclonic Salaam Akinetic (atonic)	Three-per-second spike and wave; often 4-per-second at beginning of seizure, 2-per-second at end; easily provoked by hyperventilation	85% awake, 90% asleep	3%	5	No aura: 2 to 15 seconds of unconsciousness; may show 3-per-second blinking; lightning twitches, loss of muscle tone, and unconsciousness	Do not confuse minor lapses of adults, usually focal; distinguish psychomotor variant. May be quite frequent, from several to several hundred daily. Often occurs in combination with grand mal. rare in adults
II. Focal						
Jacksonian, focus around central sulcus	Focal slow activity, fast activity, or spiking	30% awake, 60% asleep	5%		Onset most common in thumb or face; motor or sensory march of symptoms	Often posttraumatic
Psychomotor (temporal lobe)	Anterior temporal lobe spike or slow wave; may be bilateral	20% awake, 80% asleep	5% alone, 15% with grand mal	20	May end with grand mal; may have independent grand mal seizures	Phenothiazines useful adjunct to therapy; surgery should be considered
Other focal	Focal spikes spreading with phase reversal to other areas	20% awake, 80% asleep				
Frontal				2.5%	3	Aura common; related to localization; onset with adversive eye movements in grand mal; focal fits	May indicate structural lesion requiring surgery
Midtemporal				6	Facial movements at onset	Commonest focal site other than anterior temporal. Tendency for both EEG abnormality and seizures to disappear in adulthood

Occipital	1	(rare)			Visual (unformed) aura; grand mal seizure; strabismus common	
III. Other						
Petit mal variant	1	3%	Two-per-second wave and spike	85% awake	Fifty % mentally defective; massive myoclonic jerks common; grand mal seizures	An EEG diagnostic entity with poor prognosis
Fourteen- and 6-per-second positive spiking (hypothalamic)	15	6%	Fourteen- and/or 6-per-second spikes; usually unilateral but may appear on either side from time to time	8% show 14 and 6 awake; others show it asleep only	Behavior disorders, especially rage attacks, prominent; may have no seizures or show grand mal or visceral fits; emotional, sensory, and vegetative auras	An EEG, not a clinical, diagnostic entity; atypical seizures are common

* Data from F. Gibbs and E. L. Gibbs, *Atlas of Electroencephalography*, volume 2. Addison-Wesley, Cambridge, Mass., 1951.

around the central sulcus and are introduced by contralateral focal motor or sensory phenomena. Characteristically, the thumb or corner of the mouth is first involved; the involvement then spreads by contiguity. If primarily motor, the manifestation is muscle twitching; if primarily sensory, the manifestation is usually numbness, paresthesia, and tingling. As long as the symptoms remain unilateral, the patient does not lose consciousness, but the motor phenomena may become bilateral, consciousness may be lost, and the patient may show a characteristic generalized seizure. Jacksonian seizures are often posttraumatic in origin, although other pathology should be suspected.

Anterior Temporal Focus. An anterior temporal lobe abnormality is the commonest of the focal phenomena by EEG findings. Most characteristic is the spike or a train of spikes, although slow waves may also be seen in this region. The anterior temporal lobe abnormality is accompanied most commonly by psychomotor seizures, but the abnormality may manifest grand mal seizures. The clinical picture is often characterized by lapses of consciousness, which are sometimes confused by the unwary with petit mal attacks and which frequently begin with head turning, orienting movements of the eyes, lip smacking, swallowing, and salivation.

Other Focal Seizures. Foci in the frontal, midtemporal, and occipital regions of the brain are quite rare. The EEG is usually characterized by focal spikes that may spread to involve other brain regions. Frontal seizures are often initiated with adversive eye movements or occasionally by head movements and may include phenomena of forced thought. Midtemporal foci are more common than the others and show an unusual propensity for the disappearance of both the EEG abnormality and the seizures in late adolescence or adulthood. The clinical phenomena usually include grand mal seizures, and there may be focal facial movements at the onset. Occipital seizures are probably the rarest of the group and usually manifest themselves primarily with a grand mal seizure; there may be an initial visual aura of flashing lights and diplopia. Strabismus is common in these cases (see Figure 1).

Psychic Seizures

Psychic seizures seem to be primarily of temporal lobe origin and may either precede a

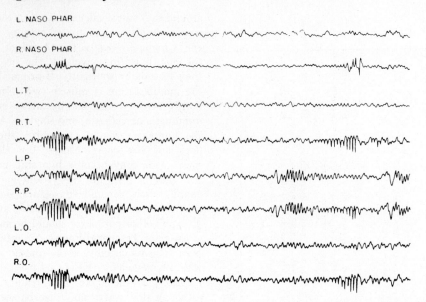

FIGURE 1. Thalamic or hypothalamic epilepsy in a sleeping female adolescent. Onset of grand mal seizures was at the age of 15 years. She has rage attacks with aura of *déjà vu*, and delinquent and severe behavior problems. EEG shows 14-per-second positive spikes of high amplitude, much worse on the right and showing to some extent with reversed polarity in the nasopharyngeal leads, maximal on the right. The 12-per-second sleep spindles are easily distinguished from the 14-per-second positive spikes. Voltage calibration: 7-mm. deflection for 50 microvolts. In two cases reversal of polarity of 14- and 6-per-second positive spikes has been observed in recordings from the nasopharynx, but in four cases no spike activity could be obtained with nasopharyngeal leads. (From F. A. Gibbs and E. L. Gibbs, *Atlas of Electroencephalography*, vol. II. Addison-Wesley, Cambridge, Mass., 1951.)

generalized convulsion or, more commonly, occur without loss of consciousness.

Perceptual Changes. The most common changes are in visual perception, described as changes in the size of an object, as if it were receding or approaching. Everything may look very small and distant or quite large. With auditory phenomena, the voices in a room become very distant or very loud and confused, as if everyone were shouting. Occasionally, distortions occur, as with one patient who described the floor and walls as wavy.

Changes in Self-awareness. Feelings of depersonalization and derealization may last for a matter of seconds or a few minutes and then abruptly disappear or be followed by some further elaboration of the seizure sequences.

Related to these feelings perhaps are the sudden feelings of intense familiarity, the phenomenon of *déjà vu*. The reciprocal experience of *jamais vu* is also seen, in which the person, although in a familiar situation, feels that it is entirely new and strange. In both these situations, there is usually an awareness that the feeling is not reasonable.

Changes in body image may consist of a simple sensation of growing larger or smaller, or one hand or arm may lengthen and enlarge, or one side of the face may become distorted and ugly.

Changes in Thought. Particularly striking is the phenomenon of forced thought, in which a thought, a word, or a sentence may obtrude itself on the consciousness and seem to occupy the whole center of awareness. On occasion, this thought or word may be an obscenity, but it may equally well be an apparent nonsense phrase, a slogan, or a melody. It may be clearly remembered after the attack, or it may be only dimly remembered or forgotten. Disorganization of thought may be another such phenomenon, with the patient complaining that there is a brief period during which he seems to know what he wants to think about but cannot put the ideas together.

Changes in Mood and Affect. Paroxysmal attacks of fear, from anxiety to terror, are frequently accompaniments of this kind of psychic seizure. These attacks are described as different from the apprehension many epileptics feel at the onset of the seizure. The attacks are often described as isolated, free-floating anxiety, far out of proportion to external events.

There are similar occurrences of acute feelings of despair and depression, including the feeling that life is so empty that suicide is called for. Feelings of pleasure, elation, or serenity seem to be somewhat rare.

Complex Hallucinatory Experiences. Although these experiences may include quite complex auditory, visual, and tactile phenomena, they are probably most often auditory hallucinations with simple but well-structured phenomena, such as hearing one's name called or a piece of music played. The patient usually has a clear insight into the hallucinatory nature of the phenomenon and feels it as alien to himself, but he may be quite anxious as to its reflections on his sanity.

Complex Stereotyped Automatisms. Complex acts appear to be purposeful but are inappropriate to the situation and, in general, are stereotyped—that is, repeated almost identically in the same form on each occasion. Most common is fumbling with buttons, perhaps buttoning and unbuttoning a coat, or there may be the simple repetition of a verbal phrase, either lucid or jargon.

In a few patients, a seizure can be precipitated by asking them consciously to begin carrying out their characteristic automatism. In others, carrying out the act under hypnosis gives rise to a rich associative flow, reinforcing the impression that the act has symbolic significance for the patient.

Twilight States

Postictal Twilight State. This state usually follows one or several seizures. At the close of the grand mal seizure or perhaps after a postictal sleep, the patient may be apparently awake but in a confused state. He may mumble incoherently and fumble with his clothing or other objects. Periods of excitement sometimes appear, lasting for minutes to (rarely) several days. This excitement may include extreme agitation, paranoid ideation, hallucinations, and delusions that may lead to aggressive outbursts. There is markedly disturbed consciousness without either motor or speech impairment. There is usually complete amnesia for these periods. Such states usually clear completely and with surprising abruptness.

Throughout this period of confusion, the EEG shows diffuse symmetrical slow activity, not the paroxysmal activity of the seizure state.

Ictal Twilight State. This state may begin with the disturbance of consciousness and no other warning, or, more often, it may be preceded by symptoms of focal disturbance, usually of the temporal lobe. The most common early symptoms are searching movements of the head and eyes, lip smacking, masticatory movements, and swallowing. During the state itself, the patient becomes disoriented and is only partially aware of his surroundings. He may wander around aimlessly, fumble with his clothing, mumble unintelligibly, or say phrases of intelligible words that are inappropriate in context. He may respond to external stimuli, but he does so inappropriately. The period may last for 5 or 10 minutes. If the state is prolonged, there may be more overt agitation, expressions of fear, anxiety, incoherent talk, and aggressive acts, particularly if attempts are made to restrain the patient. Some patients present apparently purposeful and well-coordinated behavior with no recall or only dim memories of the period, which may last hours to days.

Petit Mal Status. The twilight states associated with petit mal status are relatively uncommon. The EEG in these cases is characterized by continuous or nearly continuous bilaterally synchronous spike-and-wave patterns, and the clinical picture is apparently dominated by confusion but frequently with fairly complex confused behavior. An attenuated form of this phenomenon may appear in patients who complain of mental dullness, which may last for several days, characterized by difficulty in concentration and general slowing of the thought processes without a confusional picture. These protracted periods of mental slowing may terminate abruptly or be terminated with adequate treatment.

Mechanism

The mechanism by which certain scars, tumors, ischemia, and inflammations produce a hypersynchronous neuronal discharge is far from obvious, as are the reasons for the varying seizure thresholds throughout the brain. Occasionally, no anatomical lesion exists in the extirpated tissue. The EEG may have limited value in localization.

Pyridoxine deficiency can both lower the

levels of brain γ-aminobutyric acid and cause convulsions in human beings. A state of relative pyridoxine deficiency may exist, and tryptophan loading should be routinely tested in epileptics.

Incidence

Perhaps half the epilepsy cases in this country are preventable in the sense that they are the sequelae of trauma, infections, birth injury, and so on, with clear damage to the brain. These secondary cases are increased when there is poor prenatal and perinatal care and in regions that pay the usual price of poverty and overcrowding in malnutrition, neglect, and violence.

From a world health point of view, epilepsy is a common and disabling condition, particularly in regions where there is high incidence of low virulence central nervous system infections causing secondary cases and where traumas, particularly the subdural hematomas of infancy and early childhood, are neglected. However, in the United States the incidence is about 0.3 to 0.4 per cent or roughly one tenth the incidence of mental deficiency and perhaps one half the incidence of schizophrenia.

Psychiatric Aspects

Most psychiatric difficulties, except for the major psychoses, are quite widespread throughout the epileptic population and can be expected to involve that population by chance.

Personality of the Epileptic

Social Problems. Some 60 per cent of all epileptics and nearly two thirds of the centrencephalic or idiopathic group may have the onset of their seizures in the first decade of life, which means that these persons grow up with a dramatic handicap. A great miasma of social taboos and misapprehensions about the epileptic seizure beclouds the person's adjustment. Many schools do not allow the epileptic in class, and a fair number of classroom teachers are frightened of the child who has a seizure and willing to ridicule him. Parents may be ashamed and apprehensive, guilty and overprotective, or they may feel frightened and impotent with their child's seizures.

In later life, employers and employees discriminate against hiring the epileptic. The ever-present possibility of a major seizure in public, with the attendant helplessness and the inevitable social embarrassment, hang heavily over the epileptic. Under these conditions, it is not surprising that he has difficulty in establishing a sense of personal security and clear ego identity.

The understanding physician can do a great deal for his patient. If he is willing to add to his vigorous attempts at medication control of seizures, he can give personal counsel, intervene in parental misapprehensions, and do occasional battle with the school system, the scout troop, and other social establishments.

Physiological Problems. Abnormal brain function occurs unpredictably and with much greater frequency than is manifest by the overt seizure. Children who have few overt petit mal seizures but many bursts of EEG abnormality are found to have difficulty in school and in making peer adjustments. Many children present themselves as learning problems or behavior problems as they react to the confusing situation in which they find themselves.

Other paroxysmal discharges, such as the grand mal or the temporal lobe discharge, may have similar cumulative effects on the person's ability to integrate life experience. The seizure discharges in the temporal lobe—often widespread and profound in subcortical structures, particularly rhinencephalic structures—must be disruptive of normal functioning of these systems, which are important in the integration and expression of emotion and in learning and memory.

The problem of paroxysmal cerebral dysrhythmia, the complications of poor medical control—leading to frequent falling and self-injury, usually involving the head, with possible attendant secondary brain damage—and the potential problems of chronic drug intake add up to a heavy set of physiological hazards facing the epileptic.

Adjustment to Seizures. Having epilepsy and having seizures become integral parts of the epileptic's life. There is the problem of the patient who uses his seizures for secondary gain, either to attract attention or to avoid uncomfortable situations. Some epileptics consciously precipitate seizures by hyperventilation or similar physiological stress.

Aura

The earliest symptoms in a seizure, particularly the aura, have an important localizing value in cases of focal epilepsy. The aura is perhaps of equal importance to the epileptic himself, for it warns him of the onset of a seizure and allows him a little time to find a safe place to lie down or park his car. The acute phenomenon is frequently described as diffusely visceral—a feeling of butterflies in the stomach, of fullness in the head, of apprehension. This feeling may last for only a few seconds or several minutes before the overt seizure.

Several hours or days of increasing irritability, restlessness, and mild depressive symptoms precede a major seizure. These symptoms usually disappear abruptly after the seizure itself. Some patients under good control develop protracted states of irritability, nervousness, or depression, with gradually mounting tension. Many of them recognize the phenomenon and deliberately skip medication for a day or two in order to precipitate a seizure and clear the air. A number of persons with protracted preictal auras or a continous aura phenomenon turn to alcohol in an attempt to relieve their symptoms.

Epileptic Personality

Does a characteristic epileptic personality exist? Those who insist on a set of common personality traits identify the following: slowness of reactions, perseveration, rigid emotional attitudes, unresponsiveness to external factors, self-centeredness, hypochondriasis, and fixed opinions, particularly concerning religious issues. Most authors, however, agree that personality types and abnormalities show the general broad range noted in the rest of the population. It may well be that many of the traits described are not issues of personality but reflect the underlying cerebral dysfunction.

Acute Psychotic States Related to Epilepsy

Temporal lobe epileptics may show acute psychotic episodes with prominent schizophrenia-like features and little or no EEG abnormality to suggest a relationship to epilepsy. These episodes may last for days or weeks and end abruptly. In addition, it seems likely that some patients not manifesting clinical temporal lobe epilepsy do show temporal lobe EEG abnormalities and do manifest acute or subacute psychotic episodes, which are often misdiagnosed as schizophrenia. These patients may suffer from the same basic pathophysiology as the known epileptics, and vigorous treatment may improve their prognosis considerably.

Chronic Psychotic States and Epileptic Deterioration

One sees in state hospitals a number of chronic epileptic patients in whom recurrent seizures, social neglect, recurrent head injuries, and perhaps overmedication have led to a sad state of deterioration, but it seems unlikely that there is any unique psychotic end point for the epileptic. Even many of the apparently deteriorated patients can be markedly improved by good medical attention. Some epileptic patients face the statistical coincidence of a schizophrenic psychosis in addition to their epilepsy.

Genetics and Marriage

In the United States, 11 states have sterilization laws applying to persons with epilepsy.

The twin pair data of Lennox and other workers indicate a strong inheritable predilection for epilepsy. They find about 85 per cent concordance for cryptogenic epilepsy in monozygotic twins (versus 5 per cent for dizygotic twins); and among monozygotic twins with symptomatic epilepsy, they find about 14 per cent concordance (versus 0 per cent for dizygotic twins). These figures indicate that manifestation of epilepsy is not inevitable, even in identical twins, but sensitivity does seem to be inherited, even to symptomatic epilepsy.

Marriage laws concerning epileptics are antiquated and usually disregarded. In counseling couples, the clinican must inform and reassure both the patient and his future partner. When the couple ask about having children, the first consideration is whether the patient's physical and mental condition allows him to be a good parent; only then can the discussion be directed toward the genetic possibilities. If only one future parent is afflicted with epilepsy and if head injury has been eliminated as the precipitating factor, the current estimate is that each of their children has a probability of between 0.025 and 0.05 of developing overt convulsions—a very slight risk. Evidence shows that this probability is increased if the other future parent has subclinical cerebral dysrhythmia or if both have epilepsy, but accurate figures are unavailable. Meticulous study of pedigrees is of more validity than applying figures from the general population. It appears that the risk of transmitting epilepsy alone is generally too minute to warrant advising strictly against progeny, especially now, when so many convulsions can be completely controlled or cured by drugs or surgery and when the outlook is auspicious for further advances.

Treatment

Medication

Most seizures can be controlled with medication. For petit mal seizures, trimethadione (Tridione) and paramethadione (Paradione) are the drugs of choice. On occasion in petit mal status or in some of the twilight states presented by them, the use of an amphetamine, particularly benzedrine, is effective. All other seizures are best initially treated with diphenylhydantoin (Dilantin), alone or in combination with phenobarbital.

Should this approach not be effective or be precluded by toxic or allergic reactions, a broad spectrum of other drugs may be used. At the present time, particularly useful drugs are methylphenylethylhydantoin (Mesantoin), primidone (Mysoline), chlordiazepoxide (Librium), and methsuximide (Celontin).

The goal should be complete control of seizures. Control at the level of one seizure every 6 weeks may be quite satisfactory to the physician who has seen the patient have three or four a week, but it is not good enough for adequate rehabilitation of the epileptic. One seizure every 6 weeks may be just enough to preclude a normal social life and gainful employment.

All these drugs are potentially toxic and particularly affect the hematopoietic system. Phenacemide (Phenurone) is often quite effective in temporal lobe seizures notoriously resistant to other forms of drug medication. It is, however, an extremely toxic drug with liver complications and with a relatively high incidence of psychotic disorders. Phenurone should be used quite carefully and should probably be initiated under hospital surveillance, with frequent checkups thereafter.

Adjuncts to therapy sometimes include shifting of the acid-base balance, particularly in petit mal patients. Acetazolamide (Diamox) or a similar carbonic anhydrase inhibitor may be useful. Attention should also be paid to maintaining physiological homeostasis for the patient. Seizure threshold may be lowered by fever, fatigue, salt and water retention, and other conditions. Should these conditions occur because of intercurrent illness, it may be desirable to increase medication.

Psychotherapy

Since the epileptic patient has a condition that may persist for life and around which his future must be organized, it is well for him to have a reasonable psychotherapeutic relationship with his physician. The physician may have to intervene in some situations, particularly in those school systems that exclude epileptic children of normal intelligence from classroom activities. Problems of driver's licenses, hazardous work, legal responsibility —all need the thoughtful willingness of a physician to participate in constructive problem solving.

Surgical Intervention

When focal seizures are a manifestation of identifiable structural pathology and good medication control of the seizures is not obtained or the pathological process is itself progressive, surgical ablation is indicated, provided it does not lead to crippling effects, such as aphasia and major hemiparesis.

Temporal lobe epileptics are difficult to control with medication, and a number of them may have disturbed lives as a result of their seizures or their interseizure dysfunction. Ablation of the anterior temporal lobe can be an effective therapeutic measure in curing or at least making amenable to pharmacotherapy a number of temporal lobe epileptics.

REFERENCES

Currie, S., Heathfield, K. W. G., Henson, R. A., and Scott, D. F. Clinical course and prognosis of temporal lobe epilepsy, a survey of 666 patients. Brain, 94: 173, 1971.

Falconer, M. A. Temporal lobe resection for epilepsy and behavioral abnormalities. N. Engl. J. Med., 289: 451, 1973.

Falconer, M. A., Serafetinides, E. A., and Corsellis, J. A. N. Etiology and pathogenesis of temporal lobe epilepsy. Arch. Neurol., 10: 233, 1964.

Flor-Henry. P. Psychosis and temporal lobe epilepsy. A controlled investigation. Epilepsia (Amst.) 10: 363, 1969.

Morrell, F. Interseizure disturbances in focal epilepsy. Neurology, 6: 327, 1956.

Rodin, E. A. Psychomotor epilepsy and aggressive behavior. Arch. Gen. Psychiatry, 28: 210, 1973.

Slater, E., Beard, A. W., and Glithero, E. The schizophrenia-like psychoses of epilepsy. Br. J. Psychiatry, 109: 95, 1963.

Taylor, D. C. The ontogenesis of chronic epileptic psychoses. A reanalysis. Psychol. Med., 1: 247, 1971.

19

Mental Retardation

Introduction

Mental retardation may be viewed as a medical, psychological, or educational problem, but in its final analysis it is primarily a social problem. Throughout history the attitude toward the mentally retarded has often reflected the general social attitudes of a given people or a given culture.

In modern history there have been three distinct junctures characterized by great public interest and professional creative thinking in the field of mental retardation. Characteristically, they all followed crucial periods of great social upheaval, resulting in a popular adoption of gradually more liberal, more truly democratic attitudes toward society's less fortunate members, including the mentally retarded.

The first germinal period in the field of mental retardation coincided with the time of the French and American Revolutions and the ideas of equality and rights for all, which upset the feudal, vertical social structure. The times of Itard and his pioneering labors were also the times of Pinel, who unchained the insane, and the beginning of the popular vote and social legislation.

The second period followed the revolutions that swept Europe in 1848, in the wake of which a further liberalization of public opinion and gradually increasing legislative justice took place. In such a favorable climate, the ideas of Guggenbühl, Séguin, and Howe about special educational opportunities for the mentally retarded spread rapidly throughout Europe and North America.

The third period followed the cataclysm of World War II. The great resurgence of professional and public interest in mental retardation and its sudden respectability are the results of several factors. Probably the most important factor was the radical change in the social climate felt everywhere on the local, national, and international levels. As if to atone for the ravages of World War II, the Western world has been moving toward securing equal rights and opportunities for all human beings. Government involvement in an increasing range of social issues has become accepted, despite some opposition by advocates of laissez-faire.

Definition and Classification

The biomedical and the sociocultural adaptational models represent the two major approaches to the conceptual definition of mental retardation. The adherents of the biomedical model insist on the presence of basic changes in the brain as a *sine qua non* in the diagnosis of mental retardation. The proponents of the sociocultural adaptational model emphasize social functioning and general adaptation to accepted norms.

Brain damage may be viewed as a demonstrable anatomical lesion, an alteration of the basic constituents of the brain tissue, a failure of development, a metabolic disturbance of the nerve cell, a diminished capacity for interneuronal impulse transmission, or a combination of all these factors.

The sociopsychological approach focuses on developmental impairment in infancy and preschool years, on learning difficulties in school age, and on poor social-vocational adjustment in adulthood. The prevailing cultural norms against which a person's performance is judged, rather than his neuropathology, may be decisive in defining the degree of social inadequacy—that is, the inability to learn and adapt to the demands of a society and to be self-sufficient. Persons classified as mentally retarded in this technological, complex society might have been competent and successful in a more primitive and intellectually less demanding environment.

Mental retardation has to be considered as a multidimensional phenomenon that involves overlapping physiological, psychological, medical, educational, and social aspects of human functioning and behavior. This broad view is reflected in the definition of mental retardation adopted by the American Association on Mental Deficiency in 1961: "Mental retardation refers to subaverage general intellectual functioning which originates in the developmental period and is associated with impairment in adaptive behavior." This description circumvents the question of cause, the problem of nature versus nurture, and the clinical course of mental retardation—that is, its treatability or even curability.

The degrees or levels of retardation are expressed in various terms. The American Psychiatric Association uses the terms "borderline mental retardation" (I.Q. 68 to 85), "mild mental retardation" (I.Q. 52 to 67), "moderate mental retardation" (I.Q. 36 to 51), "severe mental retardation" (I.Q. 20 to 35), and "profound mental retardation" (I.Q. below 20). The same terms are used by the World Health Organization. The American Association on Mental Deficiency adopted the terms "border-line" (I.Q. 70 to 84), "mild" (I.Q. 55 to 69), "moderate" (I.Q. 40 to 54), "severe" (I.Q. 25 to 39), and "profound" (I.Q. 24 or less) (see Table I).

Epidemiology

It is estimated that 3 per cent (6,000,000) of the United States population is mentally retarded. In the preschool years, only about 1 per cent of the population is diagnosed as mentally retarded, since only the severe forms of this disorder are recognized on routine examination. The highest incidence is found in school-age children, with the peak at ages 10 to 14, reflecting the close supervision and continuous evaluation of children's intellectual and social performance in a school setting. The figures drop abruptly after school age, when most of those who were identified as mentally retarded blend into the general population. The overwhelming majority of the mentally retarded fall into the borderline and mild categories.

Causes and Syndromes

Prenatal Factors

The known hereditary metabolic defects probably account for only a minority of mental defectives. The success of dietary measures in

TABLE I

*Developmental Characteristics of the Mentally Retarded**

This table integrates chronological age, degree of retardation, and level of intellectual, vocational, and social functioning.

Degree of Mental Retardation	Preschool Age 0–5 (Maturation and Development)	School Age 6–20 (Training and Education)	Adult 21 and Over (Social and Vocational Adequacy)
Profound	Gross retardation; minimal capacity for functioning in sensorimotor areas; needs nursing care	Some motor development present; may respond to minimal or limited training in self-help	Some motor and speech development; may achieve very limited self-care; needs nursing care
Severe	Poor motor development; speech minimal; generally unable to profit from training in self-help; little or no communication skills	Can talk or learn to communicate; can be trained in elemental health habits; profits from systematic habit training	May contribute partially to self-maintenance under complete supervision; can develop self-protection skills to a minimal useful level in controlled environment
Moderate	Can talk or learn to communicate; poor social awareness; fair motor development; profits from training in self-help; can be managed with moderate supervision	Can profit from training in social and occupational skills; unlikely to progress beyond 2nd grade level in academic subjects; may learn to travel alone in familiar places	May achieve self-maintenance in unskilled or semiskilled work under sheltered conditions; needs supervision and guidance when under mild social or economic stress
Mild	Can develop social and communication skills; minimal retardation in sensorimotor areas; often not distinguished from normal until later age	Can learn academic skills up to 6th-grade level by late teens; can be guided toward social conformity	Can usually achieve social and vocational skills adequate to minimum self-support but may need guidance and assistance when under unusual social or economic stress

* Adapted from *Mental Retardation Activities of the U.S. Department of Health, Education, and Welfare*, p. 2. United States Government Printing Office, Washington, 1963.

phenylketonuria (PKU), maple syrup disease, and galactosemia represents a major triumph in the medical treatment of mental retardation. Although the mechanism of injury to the central nervous system in these disorders is not known, it is believed to be a result of an abnormal accumulation of metabolites. The therapy is based on the principle of dietary omission or reduction of a specific dietary ingredient that cannot be properly metabolized because of a specific enzymatic block. Another therapeutic approach consists of the dietary addition of essential metabolites, such as the addition of cystine in homocystinuria.

Disorders of Amino Acid Metabolism. *Phenylketonuria.* PKU is transmitted as a simple recessive autosomal Mendelian trait. Its frequency in the United States and various parts of Europe ranges between one in 10,000 and one in 20,000. The basic metabolic defect is an inability to convert phenylalanine, an essential amino acid, to *para*-tyrosine because of the absence or inactivity of the liver enzyme phenylalanine hydroxylase, which catalyzes this conversion.

The majority of patients with PKU are severely retarded, but some patients are reported to have borderline or normal intelligence. Eczema and convulsions are present in about a third of all cases. The majority of patients are undersized and have light complexions, coarse features, and small heads. Although the clinical picture varies, typical PKU children are hyperactive and exhibit erratic, unpredictable behavior, which makes them difficult to manage. They have frequent temper tantrums and often display bizarre movements of their bodies and upper extremities and twisting hand mannerisms that sometimes resemble the behavior of autistic or schizophrenic children. Verbal and nonverbal communication is usually severely impaired or nonexistent. Coordination is poor, and perceptual difficulties are many.

The best known screening test depends on the reaction of phenylpyruvic acid in the urine with ferric chloride solution to give a vivid green color. Another screening method, the Guthrie test, measures the phenylalanine level in the blood, using a bacteriological procedure. Early diagnosis is of extreme importance, since a low-phenylalanine diet results in significant improvement in both behavior and developmental progress. The attainment of normal or near-normal intelligence is possible if the die-

tary treatment is begun before 3 months of age. In addition, children on this diet become more responsive, less hyperactive, and much easier to manage. There is also an improvement in the EEG pattern and a diminution or cessation of seizures.

Dietary treatment is not without dangers. Phenylalanine is an essential amino acid, and its complete omission from the diet may lead to anemia, hypoglycemia, edema, and even death. Dietary treatment of PKU can often be discontinued at the age of 5 or 6 years. Sometimes, however, withdrawal of the diet results in a deterioration of behavior and a recurrence of seizures.

The parents of PKU children and some of these children's normal siblings are heterozygous carriers and can be detected by a phenylalanine tolerance test, which may be of great importance in genetic counseling of these people.

The exact mechanism of the brain damage in PKU is still unknown.

Maple Syrup Disease (*Menkes Disease*). Maple syrup disease is an inborn error of metabolism transmitted by a rare single autosomal recessive gene. The biochemical defect interferes with the decarboxylation of the branched chain amino acids—leucine, isoleucine, and valine. As a result, these amino acids and their respective keto acids accumulate in the blood and cause overflow amino aciduria. The urine's characteristic odor gave the condition its name.

The diagnosis can be confirmed by the use of ferric chloride or dinitrophenylhydrazine, each of which interacts with the urine to give, respectively, a navy blue color or a yellow precipitate. The pathological changes include a small brain, thin cortex, and poorly myelinated subcortical U fibers.

During the first week of life the infant deteriorates rapidly and develops decerebrate rigidity, seizures, respiratory irregularity, and hypoglycemia. If untreated, most patients die in the first months of life, and the survivors are severely retarded.

Treatment consists of a diet very low in the three involved amino acids. The exact nature of the brain damage is still not clear.

Hartnup Disease. This rare disorder is transmitted by a single recessive autosomal gene. The symptoms include a photosensitive pellagralike rash on extension surfaces, episodic cerebellar ataxia, and mental deficiency. Transient personality changes and psychoses may be the only manifestations of the disease.

The metabolic defect involves defective tryptophan transport, and the biochemical findings consist of a marked amino aciduria and increased excretion of indican and indole derivatives. The diagnosis can be made by paper chromatography of the urine.

Treatment with nicotinic acid and antibiotics such as neomycin may relieve the skin rash and possibly the ataxia, but it does not affect the mental retardation.

Other Disorders of Amino Acid Metabolism. Citrullinuria is a rare disorder involving the urea cycle. The level of citrulline in the blood, cerebrospinal fluid, and urine is elevated. The disorder is accompanied by mental retardation.

Hyperammonemia is another rare defect involving urea synthesis. The serum ammonia is elevated.

Argininosuccinic aciduria is another rare disorder of the urea cycle. The argininosuccinic acid is elevated in the cerebrospinal fluid and to a lesser extent in the blood and urine. The clinical manifestations include mental retardation, grand mal seizures, brittle white hair, and intermittent coma.

Idiopathic hyperglycinemia is a rare condition consisting of a marked elevation of the blood and urine glycine levels. The nature of the metabolic defect is unknown. The clinical picture is characterized by intermittent vomiting and ketosis, severe mental deficiency, and choreoathetosis.

Histidinemia is transmitted by a single autosomal recessive gene and involves a block in the conversion of histidine to urocanic acid resulting from histidase deficiency. This block leads to an elevated histidine level in serum and urine. The urine also contains imidazole pyruvic, imidazole lactic, and imidazole acetic acids in increased amounts, which give a positive ferric chloride test (green). Mild mental retardation and sometimes speech defects are part of the clinical picture.

Homocystinuria consists of a reduction or absence of cystathionine synthetase activity. Homocystine is excreted in the urine. The patients have an odd appearance and are mentally retarded. Subluxation of the lens of the eye is a characteristic clinical feature.

Lowe's oculorenal dystrophy, transmitted by an autosomal recessive gene, presents buph-

thalmos, microphthalmos, cataracts, and corneal opacities. Renal ammonia production is decreased, and a generalized amino aciduria is found.

Cystathionuria consists of a block at the site of cleavage of cysthationine to cysteine and homoserine. Cystathionine is found in the urine, and the patients are mentally retarded. Prolonged administration of pyridoxine may improve intellectual performance.

Hyperprolinemia consists of proline oxidase deficiency in type I and pyrroline-5-carboxylase dehydrogenase deficiency in type II. Both types have elevated serum and urinary proline and are associated with mental retardation.

Tyrosinosis is transmitted by an autosomal recessive gene. *p*-Hydroxyphenylpyruvic acid oxidase deficiency is responsible for the clinical picture, which includes vomiting, steatorrhea, sweet odor, vitamin D-resistant rickets, osteoporosis, hepatosplenomegaly, failure to thrive, and mild mental retardation.

Hyperlysinemia presents elevated blood and urine lysine and elevated urinary homoarginine and homocitrulline. The mental retardation is usually severe, and one finds growth failure, microcephaly, hypotonia, and petit mal seizures.

Disorders of Fat Metabolism. *Cerebromacular Degenerations.* The cerebromacular degenerations represent a group of disturbances in which there is progressive mental deterioration and loss of visual function. They are all transmitted by an autosomal recessive gene. The four types of cerebromacular degeneration differ as to the age of onset. The earliest one, Tay-Sachs disease, occurs chiefly among Jewish infants, particularly those from Eastern Europe; the others are found in members of all races.

The accumulation of gangliosides in the nerve cells throughout the CNS is a characteristic in all forms of this disorder. In the Tay-Sachs variant, there is also an accumulation of gangliosides in the ganglion cells of the retina; in others the ganglioside deposits are found in the outer retinal layer.

Tay-Sachs disease begins in infants 4 to 8 months of age. The infants become hypotonic, slow down in their developmental progress, and become weak and apathetic. In addition, there are spasticity, accompanied by persistent primitive postural reflexes, cherry-red spots in the macula lutea of each retina, convulsions, and progressive physical and mental deterioration leading to death in 2 to 4 years.

The Jansky-Bielschowsky type has its onset at 2 to 4 years of age. There is pigmentary degeneration of the macula and progressive dementia.

The juvenile form, Spielmeyer-Stock-Vogt-Koyanagi, is characterized by a much slower degenerative process and usually starts at the age of 5 or 6 years, when impairment of vision appears as the first symptom. The impairment leads to blindness because of atrophy of the optic nerve and pigmentary degeneration of the macula. Ataxia, convulsions, and mental deterioration complete the picture. The course is protracted over a period of 10 to 15 years.

The late juvenile form, Kuf's disease, is rare and occurs after 15 years of age.

All these variants of cerebromacular degeneration are progressive, and there is no treatment available to date.

Niemann-Pick Disease. This disease is transmitted by an autosomal recessive gene and occurs predominantly in Jewish infants. The biochemical defect involves the storage of sphingomyelins in the neurons, liver, and spleen; the defect can be identified by biopsy of the rectum or the brain. The clinical picture consists of a developmental arrest and mental regression, accompanied by abdominal enlargement due to hepatosplenomegaly, anemia, general emaciation, and occasionally a cherry-red spot in the retina. The onset is usually in infancy, after an initially normal development. No treatment is known, and death occurs in most cases before the age of 4.

Gaucher's Disease. This lipidosis also occurs mostly in Jewish children and has an autosomal recessive mode of genetic transmission. A diminution of enzyme activity leads to an accumulation of cerebroside in the neurons and in the cells of the reticuloendothelial system. Characteristically, there is an accumulation of Gaucher cells—that is, large, pale, round cells filled with cerebroside—first in the reticuloendothelial system and then in other tissues.

The acute form has its onset in infancy, after several months of normal development, and is characterized by progressive mental deterioration and developmental arrest. Hepatosplenomegaly, abdominal and cranial enlargement, hypotonia, and opisthotonus complete the clinical course, which is usually fatal before the end of the first year of life.

The chronic form has an insidious onset, usually before the tenth year of life. There is little or no involvement of the CNS.

Progressive Leukoencephalopathies. These disorders are characterized by a degeneration of the cortical white matter, with the onset varying from infancy to adulthood and even senility. The central pathological feature is the demyelination of the cerebral white matter, followed by a degeneration of the axon cylinders.

The genetic mode of transmission is autosomal recessive, except for Merzbacher-Pelizaeus disease, which is transmitted by a sex-linked recessive gene.

The clinical course often begins with irritability and hypersensitivity to external stimuli but soon progresses to dementia, developmental regression, hypotonia, spasticity, ataxia, cortical blindness and deafness, convulsions, and paroxysmal attacks of laughing. The nature of the clinical symptoms depends on the localization of the degenerative process. The prognosis is usually hopeless, and no treatment is available.

Schilder's disease may begin at any age, but it is more common in older children and adults. There is demyelination of cerebral white matter to sudanophilic neutral fat. Personality and behavioral changes often precede the neurological manifestations. Spastic paraparesis and tetraparesis are usually the first neurological symptoms, followed by cortical blindness and deafness, convulsions and dementia.

In Krabbe's disease the developmental regression begins in the first year of life. There is profound deficiency in the activity of galactocerebroside β-galactosidase.

In Merzbacher-Pelizaeus disease the onset is usually in the first years of life, beginning with ataxia and nystagmus, followed by a progressive dementia, spasticity, and rigidity.

Other Disorders of Fat Metabolism. Metachromatic leukodystrophy is a familial disorder characterized by demyelination and the accumulation of metachromatic lipids in the white matter of the CNS, peripheral nerves, and the viscera. The disorder is transmitted as an autosomal recessive trait and can be diagnosed by demonstration of arylsulfatase deficiency in white blood cells or urine, by the demonstration of excess sulfatides in the urine, by the demonstration of metachromatic lipids in tissue biopsies.

Clinically, the disease is characterized by progressive paralysis and dementia, beginning in the second year of life. The disease is usually fatal in 2 to 10 years. In the rare adult form, psychic disorders and dementia may precede by decades the development of motor dysfunction.

Bigler and Hsia syndrome is transmitted by an autosomal recessive gene. Its biochemical abnormality consists of an elevation of triglycerides in the blood.

Disorders of Carbohydrate Metabolism. *Galactosemia.* Galactosemia is transmitted by an autosomal recessive gene. Its metabolic defect consists of the inability to convert galactose to glucose. The urinary findings include the presence of galactose and general amino aciduria. Heterozygous carriers can be detected by a galactose tolerance test, but the tolerance test may also be abnormal in infants recovering from severe diarrhea and in patients with liver disease or hyperthyroidism.

The clinical manifestations begin after a few days of milk feeding and include jaundice, vomiting, diarrhea, failure to thrive, and hepatomegaly. If untreated, the disease may be fatal within a short time, or it may lead to progressive mental deterioration associated with cataracts, hepatic insufficiency, and occasional hypoglycemic convulsions. A galactose-free diet, instituted early, prevents all clinical manifestations and allows normal physical and mental development.

Glycogen Storage Disease (von Gierke's Disease). There are several forms of this autosomal recessive metabolic disorder of glycogen metabolism. The variant most frequently associated with mental retardation is the neuromuscular form of glycogenosis, characterized by glycogen storage in the nerve cells, muscles, and tissues of the liver, heart, kidneys, adrenals, and reticuloendothelial system.

The clinical manifestations usually begin in the neonatal period and include hepatomegaly, failure to thrive, acidosis, frequent hypoglycemic convulsions, and mental retardation. Hypotonia and heart involvement leading to cardiac failure are often encountered. Only symptomatic treatment is available.

Other Disorders of Carbohydrate Metabolism. McQuarrie type of hypoglycemia is autosomal recessive. The major feature is a recurrent hypoglycemia associated with convulsions and coma, caused by a deficiency of α cells in the pancreas. The symptoms appear early in life, often shortly after birth, and lead to progressive mental retardation. Therapy with adrenocorticotropic hormone or glucagon is effective and prevents mental retardation.

Leucine-sensitive hypoglycemia is characterized by episodic hypoglycemia, associated with coma and convulsions, after the ingestion of leucine. Mental retardation develops if the condition is not recognized and treated. Hypoglycemia after a leucine tolerance test is diagnostic for this disease. Treatment consists of a low-protein diet or a leucine-deficient diet.

Fructose intolerance is characterized by episodes of hypoglycemia after the intake of fructose or sucrose. Mental retardation may be prevented by the replacement of sucrose and fructose with other sugars.

In sucrosuria and hiatus hernia the characteristic findings include sucrosuria after a normal diet, esophageal hernia, and mental retardation.

Miscellaneous Metabolic Disorders. Idiopathic hypercalcemia is autosomal recessive, and hypersensitivity to vitamin D probably represents the metabolic aberration. The clinical features include irritability, mental retardation, a peculiar elfin facial appearance, short stature, hypotonia, hypertension, strabismus, and nephrocalcinosis. The maintenance of patients on cortisone is the most common therapy in this country. The more severe form of the illness does not respond to therapy and often leads to early death or progressive mental deterioration.

Hypoparathyroidism consists of a deficient production of parathyroid hormone by the parathyroid gland. The clinical picture is dominated by episodic tetany and tonic convulsions. X-rays may reveal calcifications in the brain with a predilection for the basal ganglia. Symptoms of hypocalcemia and mental deterioration often develop in protracted cases. Treatment in early recognized cases consists of administration of calcium and vitamin D or A T 10. In untreated cases of long standing, the mental deterioration is irreversible.

Pseudohypoparathyroidism is an autosomal recessive disorder. The renal tubules fail to inhibit resorption of phosphorus in response to parathormone. The illness is characterized by tetany, convulsions, intracranial calcifications, a peculiar round face, and many skeletal abnormalities, particularly of the hands. Mental retardation follows the repeated seizures. Treatment includes vitamin D and calcium.

Pseudopseudohypoparathyroidism, an autosomal recessive metabolic abnormality, produces signs similar to pseudohypoparathyroidism, including mental retardation, despite a normal blood level of both calcium and phosphorus. No treatment is available.

Goitrous cretinism occurs in certain regions as a result of iodine deficiency in the diet. Sporadic athyreosis, congenital absence of the thyroid gland, is the common variety in this country and may be caused by transplacental transmission of immune bodies against thyroid from the mother. Other varieties of sporadic cretinism occur in persons with adequate iodine intake. Several variants result in faulty synthesis of thyroid hormone but associated with varying metabolic defects determined by autosomal recessive genes.

The clinical signs in all varieties include hypothyroidism, goiter (except in athyreosis), dwarfism, coarse skin, disturbances in ossification, hypertelorism, and a large tongue. Mental retardation becomes a part of the clinical picture if the disease is unrecognized and untreated in infancy. The children are sluggish, their voices are hoarse, and speech does not develop.

Treatment with thyroid extract may avert most of the symptoms if instituted early in life. It is not effective in adult cretins.

Crigler-Najjar disease (familial nonhemolytic jaundice) represents an autosomal recessive trait. The indirect bilirubin in the serum is elevated, which leads to a gradual development of brain damage (kernicterus) and mental deterioration.

Pyridoxine dependency is an autosomal recessive disorder. Affected infants have abnormally high pyridoxine requirements. The clinical symptoms consist of seizures, accompanied by EEG changes, beginning toward the end of the first week of life. If the condition remains untreated, it results in spasticity and mental deficiency. The addition of 10 mg. of pyridoxine to the daily diet is required to keep the patient symptom-free.

Wilson's disease (hepatolenticular degeneration), a disorder of copper metabolism, has a recessive mode of inheritance. The juvenile and the adult forms are inherited independently. The biochemical changes in both forms consist of a diminished blood level of copper-containing ceruloplasmin. This low blood level is accompanied by excessive copper deposits in various tissues, chiefly in the liver and the brain. Heterozygous carriers are asymptomatic but often manifest abnormal levels of ceruloplasmin in the blood and a tendency to various hepatic difficulties.

Clinical manifestations include cirrhosis of the liver, progressive emotional and mental deterioration, pseudobulbar palsy, fatuous facial expression, spasticity, and a greenish-brown ring in the iris (Kayser-Fleisher ring).

The juvenile form begins between the ages of 7 and 15. Inattentiveness in school and dystonia, often with bizarre wing-flapping movements, are usually the first signs. This form is usually unresponsive to treatment, since the dystonia is related to hepatic dysfunction, which causes brain damage to the basal ganglia.

The adult form usually begins with tremors and dysarthria but may begin with psychiatric symptoms. It has a good prognosis. Treatment aims at lowering the serum copper level and increasing the urinary copper excretion. Penicillamine is the most effective therapeutic agent.

Mucopolysaccharidoses include a number of heritable diseases characterized by the storage of dermatan sulfate and heparan sulfate. Hurler's syndrome—mucopolysaccharidosis I (gargoylism)—is transmitted by an autosomal recessive trait. The clinical course starts at a very early age, leading to death before adolescence. Hepatosplenomegaly causes abdominal enlargement. The stature is dwarfed, and the facial characteristics include bushy confluent eyebrows, thick lips, large tongue, and coarse features. Spade-like hands and sometimes hypertelorism and hydrocephalus complete the picture. No treatment is available.

Hunter's syndrome—mucopolysaccharidosis II—affects only males and is transmitted as an X-linked recessive trait. The clinical picture is milder than in Hurler's syndrome, with only moderate mental retardation and no corneal opacities. The children have gargoyle features, dwarfism, and marked skeletal abnormalities.

Sanfilippo's syndrome—mucopolysaccharidosis III—is transmitted as an autosomal recessive trait. There is severe mental retardation, mild skeletal changes, seizures, and athetosis.

Morquio's syndrome—mucopolysaccharidosis IV—is an autosomal recessive disorder. The children are dwarfed and have severe skeletal deformities, marked spondylepiphyseal dysplasia, and no mental retardation.

Scheie's syndrome—mucopolysaccharidosis V—presents no mental retardation. The mode of transmission is autosomal recessive.

Maroteaux-Lamy's syndrome—mucopolysaccharidosis VI—is characterized by dwarfism, corneal opacities, skeletal changes, and dermatan sulfate in the urine. There is no mental retardation.

Lesch-Nyhan syndrome occurs mainly in boys and is thought to be X-linked recessive. There is an elevation of uric acid in the blood. In addition to severe mental retardation, there is self-mutilating behavior, such as biting of the fingers and lips, often leading to permanent tissue destruction. Allopurinal lowers the level of uric acid, leading to some improvement of behavior but not of the mental retardation.

Chromosomal Aberrations. The degree of mental retardation is severe in autosomal aberrations and milder in sex-chromosome aberrations. With the exception of Down's syndrome,

the reported number of patients with chromosomal disorders is rather small.

Autosomal disorders. DOWN'S SYNDROME (MONGOLISM). There are three distinct types of chromosomal aberrations in Down's syndrome:

1. Patients with trisomy 21 (three of chromosome 21, instead of the usual two), who represent the overwhelming majority of mongoloid patients, have 47 chromosomes, with an extra chromosome 21. The karyotypes of the mothers are normal. A nondisjunction during miosis is held responsible for this disorder (see Figure 1).

2. Nondisjunction occurring after fertilization in any cell division results in mosaicism, a condition in which both normal and trisomic cells are found in various tissues.

3. In translocation, there is a fusion of two chromosomes, usually 21 and 15, resulting in a total of 46 chromosomes in affected patients, despite the extra chromosomal material. This disorder, unlike trisomy 21, is usually inherited, and the translocation chromosome may be found in unaffected parents and siblings. These asymptomatic carriers have only 45 chromosomes.

The incidence of Down's syndrome in the United States is about one in every 700 births. In a middle-aged mother (over 32 years), the

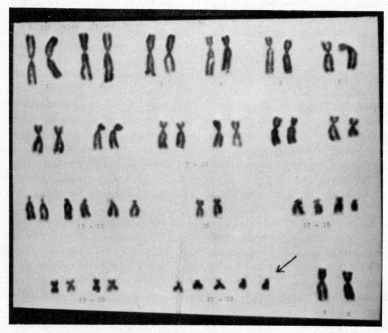

FIGURE 1. Karyogram in a child with Down's syndrome (trisomy 21). Note the three chromosomes 21 instead of the usual two. (Courtesy of Dr. Cecil Jacobson, George Washington University Medical School.)

risk of having a mongoloid child with trisomy 21 is about one in 100, but when translocation is present, the risk is about one in three.

Mental retardation is the overriding feature of Down's syndrome. The majority of patients belong to the moderately and severely retarded groups, with only a minority having an I.Q. above 50. According to many sources, patients with Down's syndrome are placid, cheerful, and cooperative. The picture, however, changes in adolescence, especially in institutions, where a variety of emotional difficulties, behavior disorders, and (rarely) psychotic illnesses may be seen.

The most important signs in newborns include general hypotonia, oblique palpebral fissures, abundant neck skin, small flattened skull, high cheek bones, and a protruding tongue. The hands are broad and thick, with a single palmar transversal crease, and the little fingers are short and curved inward (see Figure 2). Moro's reflex is weak or absent.

With the advent of antibiotics, few young patients succumb to infections, but most of them do not live beyond the age of 40. No treatment has proved to be effective.

OTHER AUTOSOMAL DISORDERS. Cat-cry syndrome (cri du chat) consists of a missing part of the fifth chromosome. The affected children are severely retarded and show many stigmata often associated with chromosomal aberrations, such as microcephaly, low-set ears, oblique palpebral fissures, hypertelorism, and micrognathia. The characteristic cat-like cry—due to laryngeal abnormalities—gradually changes and disappears with increasing age.

Trisomy 13 is characterized by rudimentary olfactory lobes. Among the clinical signs are low-set ears, cleft palate, cleft lip, sloping forehead, single transversal palmar crease, polydactyly, and abnormal dermal patterns. The patients are mentally retarded and often have minor motor seizures and apneic spells.

Trisomy 18 occurs with a frequency of 1 in 500 live births. The cases reported to date show a preponderance of females (80 per cent). The clinical picture includes mental retardation, low-set ears, micrognathia, cardiac anomalies, prominent occiput, hypotonicity at birth followed by hypertonicity, short stature, equinovarus, and overriding fingers and toes.

Trisomy 22 is characterized by mental retardation, microcephaly, slanted eyes, growth re-

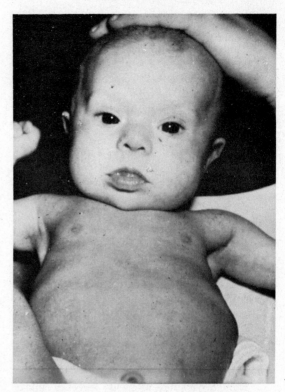

FIGURE 2. Infant with Down's syndrome (mongolism). Note the slanted eyes and protruding tongue. (Courtesy of Dr. Michael Malone, Children's Hospital, Washington, D.C.)

tardation, micrognathia, and congenital heart disease.

Anomalies of the Sex Chromosomes. Klinefelter's syndrome affects male patients, with testicular atrophy evident at puberty and signs of feminization, such as gynecomastia. Their karyotypes usually show an XXY pattern. Other variants with similar physical characteristics, mostly among the institutionalized mentally retarded, show a wide range of aberrations, such as XXXY, XXXXY, and XXYY. The degree of mental retardation in all these patients may vary from mild to severe, but many of them have normal intelligence. The patients are generally cooperative, but many develop serious social and body image difficulties, sometimes leading to social withdrawal, serious difficulties in adjustment, and paranoid tendencies.

Ovarian dysgenesis (Turner's syndrome) presents small stature, webbed neck, and cubitus valgus. The chromosomal pattern is usually XO, and only a minority of the patients are mentally retarded. A greater preponderance of mental retardation of mild to moderate degree is found among those who have three X chromosomes, giving them a total of 47.

Neuropathological Aspects of Prenatal Developmental Anomalies. The time of the insult to the CNS, the nature of the injurious agent, and the extent of tissue recovery are the decisive factors in determining the ultimate extent and effect of the CNS damage.

Autosomal Dominant Disorders. These anomalies are determined by single dominant genes of variable expressivity and penetrance and are rare, since many of those afflicted are infertile. The clinical picture varies greatly. In addition to cerebral defects, these disorders involve ectodermal, visceral, and skeletal anomalies.

Dystrophia myotonica is characterized by wasting and weakness of muscles of the extremities, face, jaw and neck. Cataracts, alopecia, and testicular atrophy are found in some cases. All symptoms usually appear in young adults and are often accompanied by moderate to severe mental retardation.

Epiloia (tuberous sclerosis) presents skin lesions. Throughout the cerebral cortex in the lateral ventricles and in the cerebellum, multiple nodules are found. These tumors may cause hydrocephalus owing to obstruction. In addition, tumors are found in various parts of the body.

The clinical picture is often complicated by systemic manifestations, such as cardiac failure, respiratory disease due to pulmonary cysts, and retinal involvement. The degree of mental retardation may vary from mild to very severe. Some patients have psychotic symptoms, often with only moderate retardation.

The prognosis varies with the degree and location of the systemic involvement. Treatment is limited to anticonvulsant medication.

Neurofibromatosis (von Recklinghausen disease) presents small brown patches distributed over the entire body along the course of subcutaneous nerves, autonomic nerves, and nerve trunks. Astrocytomas, ependymomas, and meningiomas may be found in the brain. The skin manifestations usually begins in childhood and may include large skin polyps and *café au lait* spots over the trunk and extremities. Bilateral acoustic neurinomas are almost diagnostic of this disease. The clinical picture includes epilepsy and, in about 10 per cent of cases, mental retardation. Anticonvulsant medication and neurosurgery may sometimes be effective.

Encephalofacial angiomatosis (Sturge-Weber disease) includes a facial nevus in the distribution of the fifth cranial nerve, buphthalmos, hemiparesis of the contralateral extremities, convulsions, and mental retardation.

Retinocerebellar angiomatosis (Hippel-Lindau disease) presents angiomata in the cerebellum and the retina. The clinical picture includes mental retardation and cerebellar signs.

Arachnodactyly (Marfan's syndrome) is an inheritable disorder, probably transmitted by a single, dominant gene of variable expressivity. It involves changes in the skeletal, cardiovascular, and ocular structures. The patients are tall, have long extremities, coloboma, bilateral lens dislocation, and cardiac anomalies. The accompanying mental retardation is usually mild.

Sjögren's disease is transmitted by a dominant autosomal gene. Its clinical features include mental retardation, congenital cataracts, and ataxia.

Congenital ichthyosis (Sjögren-Larsson syndrome) is characterized by generalized scaliness, associated with spastic diplegia or epilepsy in the form of generalized motor seizures. The mental retardation varies from moderate in patients with epilepsy to severe in patients with spastic diplegia.

Chondrodystrophy (achondroplasia) is characterized by very short limbs due to a disturbed ossification of the cartilage. The head is often large and the accompanying mental retardation mild.

Craniosynostosis includes several conditions characterized by premature closure of cranial sutures, skull deformities, and brain damage due to increased intracranial pressure. The shape of the skull may vary greatly. Its normal growth is inhibited in a direction perpendicular to the obliterated suture line, and compensatory growth takes place in other directions (see Figure 3). Mental retardation often follows. The severity of the clinical picture rises in inverse proportion to the time of the fusion.

Hypertelorism is characterized by a wide distance between the eyes. Familial occurrence of this disorder indicates a dominant mode of inheritance in most cases. Patients manifest a flat nasal bridge, external strabismus, and sometimes a vertical midline groove in the

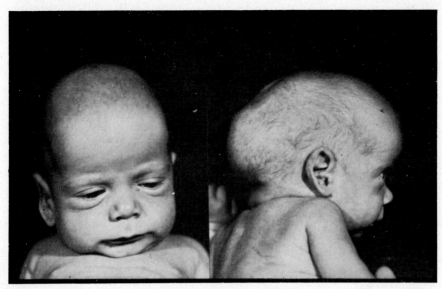

FIGURE 3. Infant with sagittal synostosis. Note the elongated cranium. (Courtesy of Dr. Michael Malone, Children's Hospital, Washington, D.C.)

forehead. The mentality ranges from normal to moderate retardation. Some retarded patients with this anomaly have hyperamino aciduria. Convulsions may occur.

Nephrogenic diabetes insipidus is usually restricted to males. The defect lies in the renal tubules and leads to periodic dehydration. Mental retardation and delay in growth are frequent.

Developmental Anomalies Due to Recessive or Unknown Genetic Mechanism. Anencephaly is believed by some to be an autosomal recessive disorder. Its incidence ranges between 0.5 and 3.7 per 1,000. The anencephalic fetus usually succumbs during delivery or shortly thereafter. The pathological findings include an absence of the cranial vault and most of the central nervous system or at least the absence of both cerebral hemispheres.

Hydranencephaly is characterized by the absence of the cerebral cortex but intact meninges and cranium, the latter filled with clear fluid. The infant may appear normal at birth. Shortly thereafter, however, he develops spasticity, convulsions, and rigidity of the extremities, and the head enlarges rapidly.

Porencephaly is characterized by cystic formations in the cerebral hemisphere. The clinical picture depends on the amount of remaining functional cortical tissue. The patients who

survive early childhood are usually bedridden, have bilateral hemiplegia or tetraplegia, and are either severely or moderately retarded.

Microcephaly is a purely descriptive term, covering a variety of disorders whose main clinical feature is a small, peculiarly shaped head and mental retardation (see Figure 4).

The hereditary group is relatively uncommon. The clinical picture is milder than in acquired microcephaly. Only a minority of patients in this group have disturbance in motor functions, and they are usually severely retarded. The rest fit into the moderately retarded group.

Microcephaly due to intrauterine influences is found in a far larger group of patients. The causes include X-radiation during pregnancy, maternal rubella, toxoplasmosis, maternal diabetes, and cytomegalic inclusion body disease. These variants often have severe neurological abnormalities in the motor and sensory areas that range from mild spastic paralysis with general delay in development to a spastic tetraplegia or blindness associated with profound mental retardation. Convulsions occur in this group of patients with great frequency.

Macrocephaly is due primarily to the proliferation of the glial tissue in the white matter of the hemispheres. The clinical features include mental retardation, epilepsy, and disturbances of vision.

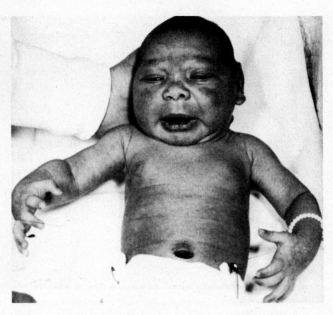

Figure 4. Infant with microcephaly. (Courtesy of Dr. Michael Malone, Children's Hospital, Washington, D.C.)

Hydrocephalus covers a number of conditions having in common an increase in the cerebrospinal fluid, resulting in the enlargement of the head or the ventricles. The abnormality is seldom noted until the second or third month of life, when a rapid enlargement of the head circumference makes its first clinical appearance. Symptoms of increased intracranial pressure—vomiting, papilledema, rigidity—soon follow. Progressive hydrocephalus often ends in complete mental and physical deterioration. In milder cases the condition may become spontaneously arrested, and the afflicted child may be only mildly retarded or have normal intelligence.

Agenesis of the corpus callosum is characterized by the partial or total absence of the great commissure connecting the cerebral hemispheres. The clinical picture varies with the extent of the associated brain anomalies. Mental retardation of varying severity and major, minor, or focal seizures are common.

Laurence-Moon-Bidel syndrome usually follows an autosomal recessive mode of transmission, but some sex-linked tendency may be suspected from a higher frequency in males. The main features include mental retardation, retinitis pigmentosa, obesity, hypogenitalism, polydactyly, and deaf-mutism.

Prader-Willi syndrome is characterized by mental retardation, muscular hypotonia, obesity, short stature, and hypogonadism. The children often develop insulin-resistant diabetes.

Ataxia-telangiectasia is often diagnosed initially as cerebral palsy. Cerebellar ataxia may be the first manifestation, and cutaneous telangiectasia and progressive mental retardation appear later. The mode of transmission is autosomal recessive.

Norrie's disease, an X-linked recessive syndrome, is characterized by retinal malformations, mental retardation, and progressive deafness.

Maternal Infections during Pregnancy. Syphilis in pregnant women used to be a major cause of a variety of neuropathological changes in their offspring, including mental retardation.

Rubella (German measles) has replaced syphilis as the major cause of congenital malformations and mental retardation due to maternal infection. The children of affected mothers may present congenital heart disease, mental retardation, cataracts, deafness, microcephaly, and microphthalmia. When mothers are infected in the first trimester of pregnancy, 10 to 15 per cent of the children are affected, and the incidence rises to almost 50 per cent when the infection occurs in the first month of pregnancy.

Brain damage due to toxoplasmosis and cytomegalic inclusion body disease transmitted from the pregnant mother to the fetus is a relatively rare complication of pregnancy that often results in mental retardation and a variety of brain malformations. Damage to the fetus from maternal hepatitis has also been reported.

Complications of Pregnancy. Toxemia of pregnancy and uncontrolled maternal diabetes present hazards to the fetus and may sometimes result in mental retardation. Maternal malnutrition during pregnancy often results in prematurity and other obstetrical complications. Vaginal hemorrhage, placenta previa, premature separation of the placenta, and prolapse of the cord may damage the fetal brain by causing anoxia.

Perinatal Factors

Prematurity may result in intellectual deficits, sensory and motor handicaps, convulsive disorders, and learning and emotional difficulties. Only a minority of infants weighing less than 1,500 gm. (3 lb. 4 oz.) escape these sequelae. Prematurity is more prevalent in low socio-economic segments of the population. Its causes are many and include inadequate prenatal care, with resulting obstetrical complications, such as toxemia, pretoxemic states, and multiple births; illegitimate pregnancy; poor maternal nutritional status; the mother's smoking habits; and urinary infections.

About a third of all low-birth-weight infants are born at term and suffer from intrauterine growth retardation. Problems associated with this condition include congenital anomalies, CNS depression, meconium aspiration pneumonia, pulmonary hemorrhage, and transient hypoglycemia. There is a considerable risk of early death or brain damage.

Traumatic cerebral insults include cephalopelvic disproportion, breech delivery, abnormal presentations, and prolonged labor. They may result in subarachnoid and intraventricular hemorrhage.

Anoxemia may occur before, during, and after delivery. Cesarean section and some obstetrical complications may result in fetal anoxia due to a fall in systemic blood pressure. Changes in fetal heart rate, especially bradycardia, are the best indicators of fetal distress. Respiratory difficulties may be caused by mechanical factors, such as intratracheal mucus plug, or by

fetal respiratory depression due to analgesic and anesthetic drugs administered to the mother during labor.

Kernicterus refers to yellow staining of the basal ganglia, cerebellum, and brain stem, frequently resulting in cerebral palsy, mental retardation, and hearing deficit. The pigmentation is caused by the excess of nonconjugated (indirect) bilirubin, which is neurotropic, while, for still unexplained reasons, the conjugated (direct) bilirubin does not enter the nerve cell. Kernicterus follows some cases of neonatal jaundice. The jaundice usually begins shortly after birth and becomes progressively more extensive, leading to hepatosplenomegaly, apathy, and neurological signs, usually on the third to fifth day after birth.

Erythroblastosis fetalis is the most common cause of nonphysiological jaundice and is due to mother-child imcompatability regarding the Rh factor, A or B, or (rarely) Kell, Kidd, and Duffy factors in the blood. The resulting breakdown of the infant's red cells causes bilirubinemia and anemia. Stillbirth due to a generalized edema occurs in some cases.

Postnatal Factors

Purulent meningitis may be successfully treated in most cases if recognized early, but drug-resistant cases may lead to extensive destruction of brain tissue. Subdural effusion is one of many complications that may cause brain damage if unrecognized and untreated. Meningitis caused by pneumococcus usually results in the highest frequency of brain damage; meningococcus meningitis is the most benign. Tuberculous meningitis also leaves many survivors with extensive chronic encephalopathy.

Viral meningoencephalitis includes poliomyelitis, ECHO virus, Coxsackie virus, herpes simplex, and anthropod-borne encephalitis. The clinical course varies a great deal, as does the extent of damage to the CNS. Infants run the greatest risk of permanent sequelae, but recovery in even severe cases is spectacular at times.

Aseptic meningitis is seen with the Coxsackie and ECHO viruses, mumps, and herpes simplex. It is usually benign and without residue. An exception is that due to the herpes simplex virus in the newborn, which produces encephalohepatomyocarditis, with a high fatality rate and usually damaged survivors. Parainfectious encephalomyelitis involves small areas of perivenous demyelination but has a lesser inflammatory reaction and does not involve a direct viral invasion of the central nervous system. The sequelae of these complications may include sensory and motor disabilities, convulsive disorders, and mental retardation.

Lead poisoning, most often resulting from pica, frequently leads to chronic encephalopathy and mental retardation. Treatment with chelating agents, such as Versene, followed by removal of the source of lead, may prevent residual damage. Many other toxic substances accidentally ingested by infants and children may cause brain damage and are seen most frequently in chaotic households where children lack supervision and mothers are overwhelmed by their family obligations.

Although most convulsive disorders probably result from prenatal or perinatal influences, they make their appearance in the postnatal period, and their causes often remain unclear. Failure to treat status epilepticus promptly and vigorously may lead to progressive mental deterioration. Major motor and mixed or unclassifiable seizures account for the majority of convulsive disorders among the mentally retarded.

Infantile spasms usually affect infants between 3 and 12 months of age. The illness is characterized by brief lapses of consciousness, with abrupt symmetrical flexion of the head, trunk, or extremities. The condition leads to progressive mental deterioration, and mental retardation has been reported in close to 90 per cent of the cases. The causes are unclear and probably include a variety of mechanical (birth) and biochemical insults to the central nervous system. The majority of cases occur suddenly and for no apparent reason in a previously normal child.

Patients with cerebral palsy have a high incidence of mental retardation. The patients in the spastic tetraplegic group are most affected, and less than 15 per cent possess normal intelligence. In the hemiplegic category, the patients who acquire the handicap postnatally, especially in infancy, do worse than patients with hemiplegia due to prenatal or perinatal causes. The incidence of mental defect in the hemiplegic group ranges from 40 to 50 per cent. Of the remainder, about half are of borderline intelligence. Patients with the extrapyramidal type of cerebral palsy are more intelligent than the spastic group, and as many as 50 per cent may fall in the normal or superior range of intelligence.

Heller's disease has been the subject of a heated controversy. Some accept it as a legitimate disease entity, and some regard it as a meaningless label covering a variety of neuropathological and psychotic conditions. In his original report, Heller described children who developed normally in all respects until their third or fourth year, when, without any apparent reason, they began to show signs of progressive deterioration. The changes began with restlessness, sterotyped and anxious behavior, and loss of already learned speech and led to complete dementia.

Early caloric and protein deficiencies affect growth and may produce irreversible mental changes.

Sociocultural Factors

The overwhelming majority of the mentally retarded in the United States come from the lowest socio-economic group. Estimates of the frequency of mental retardation in this segment of the population range from 10 to 30 per cent, as contrasted with about 3 per cent in the total population.

Medical Problems. The prospective mother is frequently malnourished and shorter than average. She is likely to have poor, little, or no prenatal care. Consequently, pretoxemic and toxemic states are seen in the disadvantaged in much higher proportions than in the general population. Maternal infections during pregnancy, including lues, are treated with delay or not at all. Infant mortality is higher than usual, and so is the rate of prematurity. Diabetes in the mother is often uncontrolled. Each of the many fetal risks may result in brain damage and mental retardation.

The baby may never have regular postnatal care. As a result, he is more likely to have serious bacterial and viral infections. He is treated relatively late in the course of illness for conditions such as meningitis and dehydration, often when permanent damage has already been done. When there is mild brain damage, it often persists because of under- or overstimulation. The infant's nutrition is often inadequate. Chronic protein depletion may produce irreversible mental retardation of mild to moderate degree.

Pica often ends in lead poisoning, encephalopathy, and mental retardation. The frequency of the battered-child syndrome, burns, serious accidents, and ingestion of toxic substances, with inherent risks to the central nervous system, is disproportionately high in this group.

Emotional and Social Problems. The lowest 15 to 20 per cent of the severely disadvantaged produce the majority of functionally based retardation. Family cohesion is often missing; the children are often illegitimate and reared by a variety of caretakers. Often, the roles of the family members are ill-defined, resulting in a chaotic, disorganized household. The dependency needs of the growing child may not be met, and he is forced to fend for himself long before he is ready. The children may identify themselves with patterns of poor impulse control and are apt to act out, rather than sublimate, their aggressive and sexual drives. The child's self-concept may be faulty. The fatalistic, hopeless attitudes of the slum environment can stifle initiative and motivation. The defenses necessary to survive in this environment may interfere with intellectual progress.

Environmental Deprivation. Young children need routine and predictability in their environment, as well as variety, offered in proper balance. In a disadvantaged environment the level of sensory stimulation may be too low or too high, or it may vacillate between the two extremes. The verbal stimulation is frequently deficient, resulting in a meager vocabulary, poor sentence structure, and concrete reasoning. The caretaking figure may satisfy the child's physical wants but have little or no opportunity for playing with the child or providing him with new pleasurable experiences. In the institutional setting for infants and young children, the greatest hazards exist for environmental deprivation.

Familial Mental Retardation. Children in this category make up about 75 per cent of all the mentally retarded in this country and usually come from the lowest socio-economic group. They have no neurological signs, neuropathological abnormalities, chromosomal or known biochemical characteristics to distinguish them from the rest of the population. In borderline to mild retardation there is usually a consistency in I.Q. among members of the same family. However, children of retarded parents can develop intellectually along normal lines if given an intensive enrichment program.

Effects of Retardation

Psychiatric Factors

Personality Development. Given an accepting and adequately stimulating family environment and appropriate educational and vocational training facilities, the majority of retarded children can develop good social and vocational adjustment and capacity for appropriate interpersonal interactions and attachments. However, they face hazards along the way that exceed the ones facing the normal population. Such hazards seem to increase in direct proportion to the degree of retardation.

Emotional Vulnerability. *Constitutional Factors.* Many mentally retarded children are unable to process and adapt to levels of sensory stimuli of more than low intensity. A rising intensity of such stimuli is perceived by the child as disturbing or even painful and can lead to behavioral disorganization.

Sensory hypersensitivity can be blamed for hyperactivity in some cases. Many other mentally retarded children seem to be hyperactive on a constitutional basis without a history of a clear-cut sensory handicap. The hyperactive mentally retarded child finds it particularly difficult to adapt to the already handicapped process of learning and socialization. The reaction of others to disruption may be one of rejection, exclusion, punishment, or the disorganization of the group itself.

Irritability may be pervasive, always present, or it may appear only in sporadic bursts at times of increased environmental or inner stimulation, related to the low frustration tolerance exhibited by such children. The response of the environment to such an irritable, easily frustrated child may be one of annoyance, anger, punitiveness or exclusion. On the other hand, there may be efforts of constant appeasement, avoidance of any frustration, and, in effect, subordination of the behavior and needs of the group to every whim and mood change of the child. Both types of response tend to perpetuate and accentuate the child's low frustration threshold.

Some children with hypersensitivity to environmental stimuli resort to a screening-out behavior. Such children either avoid situations involving intense stimulation, anxiety, and frustration or develop a capacity to tune out the environment and remain unresponsive.

A smaller proportion of mentally retarded

children have an innate reduced sensitivity to incoming environment signals. In mild cases, such a stimulus barrier may shield the child from stressful situations. However, a too-high response threshold may lead to lack of contact with the environment and to withdrawal, resulting in impairment of social responsiveness and inability to learn.

Aggressive behavior is often seen in moderately and severely retarded children. It often takes the form of panaggression, directed indiscriminately toward anybody approaching the child and intruding on his private world. In other children, the aggression is directed only toward certain people. The aggressive behavior may be totally unprovoked and unpredictable, and it is often coupled with the destruction of toys and furniture.

Many mentally retarded children seem unable to tolerate any change. A change in the environment may make the child tense and upset. Any breaks or changes in the daily routine may have the same disruptive effects. The reaction of the child may range from mild irritability to a total behavioral disorganization.

Socialization. The early child-mother emotional bond affects all future interactions with human beings. The development of this crucial bond occurs in infancy, passing through an orderly sequence.

Also, a certain minimum level of intellectual activity and comprehension is necessary for the development of meaningful human ties. The infant's recognition of his mother as an entity, separate from himself and clearly distinguishable from others, is an intellectual process that depends on intact sensory and perceptual mechanisms, memory, and the ability to organize bits and pieces of information into a meaningful whole. The mentally retarded infant's failure or delay in the recognition of his mother retards development of these vital early attachments, thus disrupting the timetable of emotional development. One such distortion is the longer duration and greater intensity of the child's dependency needs, causing a delay in developing independence and autonomy. The phase of negativism often starts later in infancy in the retarded and lasts longer than usual, which may interfere with the process of learning and social cooperation.

Low Self-Esteem. The growing mentally retarded child becomes progressively aware of being different from normal people. The feeling of inadequacy and low self-esteem may lead to overt depression, with attendant psychomotor retardation and social withdrawal. The mentally retarded adolescent is particularly vulnerable to feelings of inadequacy and poor self-image. His developing intellect permits more accurate self-evaluation, and his progressive loneliness makes denial of his inferiority difficult or impossible.

The mentally retarded child may lack originality in his play. He may lean toward repetition and stereotype, particularly if there are organic bases for his difficulty. Such children use a minimum of toys and are often unable to play in larger groups or to initiate play without help.

Role of the Family. Delay in the child's responses and knowledge of his mental retardation often induce parental inner turmoil, grief, a sense of disappointment, shattered hopes, and sometimes feelings of guilt and failure. These feelings, if unresolved, make it difficult for many parents to accept the child, to be proud of him, and to give him affection and recognition.

Ignorance of the fact that the child is mentally retarded is equally hazardous, since parental expectation of normal behavior may be frustrated, leading to tension, confusion, and often estrangement between parent and child. The parents sometimes respond by vacillating among denial, overprotection, infantilization, and overt or covert rejection. Rejection is probably the most damaging but most common reaction of family members to the mentally retarded child.

Influence of the Community. The prevailing general attitudes toward mental retardation profoundly influence the parents' reaction to having a retarded child. Technologically advanced, sophisticated communities, which put a premium on education and intellectual achievement, have been less accepting and less tolerant than more primitive, underdeveloped communities.

As the child grows older and his social world widens, he comes to depend more on his peers for emotional support and stimulation. His acceptance by other children depends largely on the personal attitudes, tolerance, and compassion of their parents.

Maternal Deprivation. The retarded child needs more than the usual amount of mothering, affection, and stimulation. Denial of this attention results in an often irretrievable loss of whatever inner resources the child possesses. A subtle form of maternal deprivation may result from the child's inability to respond to normal mothering because of sensory or perceptual difficulties. The mother's depression, self-preoccupation, or rejection may lead her to neglect the child's emotional needs.

Impact of Retarded Children on the Family. Most parents experience considerable tension and anguish at the time of initial diagnosis, causing a weakening of the habitual defense system and a temporary breakdown of adjustment patterns. The ultimate impact of the retarded child on the family depends on the degree of retardation, personality development, life adjustment of each parent preceding the arrival of the retarded child, the degree of their professional and social success, the adequacy of the marital adjustment, other children in the family and their intellectual progress, and the parental socio-economic status.

Reasonably well-adjusted parents with a positive self-image are usually able to absorb the retarded child without upsetting the family balance or jeopardizing the well-being of other family members. If, however, the parents are emotionally immature and beset by neurotic conflicts, the arrival of a defective child may precipitate a crisis that sometimes leads to family breakdown. The child may be cast in the role of the family scapegoat, destined to drain off family tensions. The siblings' acceptance of the retarded child depends largely on parental attitudes and on gratification of their own dependency needs. The degree of family turmoil rises in direct proportion to the parents' social status.

The predominant defenses of the family may help or hinder their adjustment to the presence and handling of their retarded child. Denial may allow the family to work usefully with the child. The danger is in overprotection and unrealistic pressure on the child for achievement. Projection, with the parents concentrating on blaming others for the child's situation, can lead to losing sight of the child's needs. Displacement can involve the parents in community action on behalf of the retarded. Withdrawal can lead to the whole family's isolating itself or concentrating on the retarded child to the neglect of the other children in the family.

Role of the Physician. An informed and interested physician can clarify, support and reassure. The physician's empathy and flexibility help to bring the parents' feelings and attitudes to the surface. Many parents profit greatly from counseling by an experienced social worker, and some may need psychiatric treatment. Group therapy for parents of retarded children has also been useful. Above all, the physician should relieve the parents' helplessness. He needs to give them appropriate things to do.

Psychopathology of the Mentally Retarded. The most frequently seen disorders are adjustment reactions, chronic brain syndrome with behavior disturbance, and psychotic reactions. The delay and deficits in the development of human attachment patterns are a function of the intellectual deficit. The distortion of attachment patterns is bound to contribute to a shallowness in object relations. Mental retardation constitutes a definite hazard to personality development. Whether or not such a hazard results in a specific psychopathology depends on the child's life experiences and their modifying or aggravating environmental influences.

Psychological Factors

There is general agreement about the reduced ability of the mental retardate to learn, to acquire knowledge at the same rate and in the same quantity as normal children do. The differences are small in the simple forms of learning, but the gap widens in direct proportion to the complexity of the learning process. Short-term retention seems deficient in the mentally retarded, but long-term retention is not disturbed.

The sensory and perceptual handicaps found in many of the mentally retarded may significantly contribute to their learning difficulties. The inability to inhibit already-learned responses hinders the broadening of the available repertoire of responses. The main handicap is represented by the diminished capacity in abstracting and generalizing from experience, owing to the deficit in verbal ability.

The major periods of Jean Piaget's model of intelligence development are (1) the sensorimotor stage (birth to 18 months), (2) the preoperational stage, subdivided into the preconceptual stage (18 months to 4 years) and the intuitive stage (4 to 7 years), (3) the stage of concrete operations (7 to 11 years), and (4) the stage of abstract operations (11 years onward). Rather than describe a retarded person in terms of an I.Q. number, one may find it more useful to describe his functioning in terms of his arriving at a certain stage of his intellectual development, characterized by a specific behavior and resoning process. Thus, the profoundly retarded person may be viewed as arrested or fixated at the sensorimotor stage of development; the moderately retarded person is capable of reaching only the intuitive and preconceptual stages; the mildly retarded person does not advance beyond the stage of concrete operations; and the borderline retarded person stops at the simpler levels of abstract thinking.

Diagnosis

History

Although caution is indicated in taking history from a parent, it often remains the only source of information. The history of the pregnancy delivery, the consanguinity of the parents, and the presence of hereditary disorders in their families deserve particular attention. The parents may also provide information about the child's developmental milestones. A history is particularly helpful in assessing the emotional climate of the family and the sociocultural background.

Physical Examination

This examination has to include a careful observation of the child's level of activity and the quality of his interaction with his parents, strangers, and inanimate objects. Various parts of the body may have certain characteristics commonly found in the mentally retarded. The configuration and size of the head offer clues to a variety of conditions. The patient's face may have some of the stigmata of mental retardation—hypertelorism, flat nasal bridge, prominent eyebrows, epicanthal folds, corneal opacities, retinal changes, low-set and small or misshapen ears, protruding tongue, and disturbance in dentition. The color and texture of the skin and hair, a high arched palate, the size of the thyroid gland, the size of the child, and his trunk and extremities are additional areas to be explored. Measurement of the head circumference is an essential part of the clinical investigation. Handprinting patterns may offer another diagnostic tool, since uncommon ridge patterns and flexion creases are often found in retarded children.

Neurological Examination

Disturbances in motor areas manifest themselves in abnormalities of muscle tone, reflexes, and involuntary movements. A lesser degree of disability manifests itself in clumsiness and poor coordination. Sensory disturbances may include hearing difficulties and disturbances.

Hyperirritable infants, jittery or convulsing with asymmetrical neurological signs, need careful attention, since about half of them may be brain-damaged in later life. The infants with the poorest prognosis are those who manifest a combination of inactivity, general depression, and exaggerated response to stimuli. In older children, hyperactivity, short attention span, distractibility, and a low frustration tolerance are further hallmarks of brain damage.

Skull X-rays illuminating only in a relatively few conditions, such as craniosynostosis, hydrocephalus, and several others that result in intracranial calcifications. In patients with hypsarrhythmia or grand mal seizures, the EEG may help establish the diagnosis and suggest treatment. In most other conditions, one deals with a diffuse cerebral disorder that produces nonspecific EEG changes.

Laboratory Procedures

These procedures include examination of the urine and blood for metabolic disorders. Enzymatic abnormalities in chromosomal disorders, notably Down's syndrome, promise to become useful diagnostic tools. Determination of the karyotype is indicated whenever a chromosomal disorder is suspected.

Hearing and Speech Evaluations

The development of speech may be the most reliable criterion in the investigation of mental retardation. Various hearing impairments are often present in the mentally retarded.

Psychiatric Examination

Nonverbal communication and careful observation of the patient and his activity are of great importance. The way the retarded patient reacts to human and inanimate objects and how he relates to the examiner and to his mother or caretakers may tell most about his social maturity. It may be useful to examine even the older retarded patient with and without a parent or a parent substitute in evaluating dependency status and response to separation.

The child's control over motility patterns should be ascertained, and clinical evidences of distractibility and distortions in perception and memory may be evaluated. The use of speech, reality testing, and the ability to generalize from experiences are important to note.

The nature and maturity of the child's defenses—particularly the exaggerated or self-defeating uses of avoidance, repression, denial, introjection, and isolation—should be observed. Sublimation potential, frustration tolerance, and impulse control should be assessed. Also important is self-image and its role in the development of self-confidence.

In general, there should be a picture of how the child has solved the stages of personality development. From the areas of failure or regression, it is possible to develop a personality profile of a type that allows for more logical planning of management and remedial approaches.

Psychological Examination

The Gesell, Bayley, and Cattell tests are most commonly applied in infants. For children, the Stanford-Binet and the Wechsler Intelligence Scale for Children are the most widely used tests in this country. Some people have tried to overcome the language barrier of the mentally retarded by devising picture vocabulary tests, of which the Peabody Vocabulary Test is the most widely used.

The tests often found useful in detecting brain damage are the Bender-Gestalt and the Benton Visual Retention Tests. These tests are also applicable in mildly retarded children. In addition, a psychological evaluation should assess perceptual, motor, linguistic, and connitive abilities. Of extreme importance is information on motivational, emotional, and interpersonal factors.

The Illinois Test of Psycholinguistic Abilities tests auditory, vocal, and motor responses, both alone and in combination. The most popular test that measures social functioning is the Vineland Social Maturity Scale.

Differential Diagnostic Problems

A variety of conditions may stimulate mental retardation. Children who come from deprived homes that provide inadequate stimulation may manifest motor and mental retardation that is reversible if an enriched, stimulating environment is provided in early childhood. A number of sensory handicaps, especially deafness and blindness, may be mistaken for mental retardation if, during testing, no compensation for the handicap is provided. Speech deficits and cerebral palsy often make a child appear retarded, even in the presence of normal intelligence.

Chronic, debilitating diseases may depress the child's functioning in all areas. Convulsive disorders may give an impression of mental retardation, especially in the presence of uncontrolled seizures. Chronic brain syndromes may result in isolated handicaps—failure to read, failure to write and failure to communicate—that may exist in a person of normal and even superior intelligence.

Emotional difficulties often lead to an apparent retardation. Emotionally disturbed children do poorly in school and often perform far below their actual mental level.

The most controversial differential diagnostic problem concerns children with severe retardation, brain damage, early infantile autism, childhood schizophrenia, and, according to some, Heller's disease. The confusion stems from the fact that details of early history are often unavailable or unreliable, and, by the time they are evaluated, many children with these conditions manifest similar bizarre and stereotyped behavior, mutism, or echolalia and function on a retarded level.

Prevention

Primary Prevention

Public Education. A preventive approach to mental retardation can only succeed in an educated, enlightened community. The public has to be taught that mental retardation is a handicap and not a curse or visitation; that its causes can be studied, treatment found for some of its variants, and amelioration found for most; that mentally retarded people have feelings of love and hate, anger and compassion, and have a need for affection, comradeship, and a sense of belonging, like all of us; and that, as citizens, they have inalienable rights, which include the best that medicine and education have to offer and the right to the pursuit of happiness, which, in the case of the mentally retarded, means a right, inasmuch as possible, to a productive existence and humane treatment.

Public education must proceed on several levels—impressing school children with basic facts about mental retardation, reaching their parents through communication media and through personal efforts of interested professionals, going out among those of the underprivileged who are at greatest risk and trying to win their cooperation.

Improvement of Socio-Ecomonic Standards. Basic to any real improvement is the raising of the standards of living and education among disadvantaged citizens. One has to attack the basic social and economic conditions that give rise to all the secondary phenomena, such as malnutrition, prematurity, obstetrical hazards, understimulation, and overstimulation. People who are given good vocational training that permits them to compete successfully in the labor market and to be economically secure are much more inclined to think in terms of securing good health and education for themselves and their families.

Medical Measures. Restricting the number of pregnancies in adolescence and after the age of 40 would reduce the risk of chromosomal aberrations and obstetrical complications. Prevention of prematurity; detection of Rh and other blood incompatibilities; adequate nutrition during pregnancy, including vitamin and mineral supplements; control of maternal diabetes, pretoxemic states, syphilis, and other infections by appropriate medication and diet —all these would help reduce the number of reproductive casualties.

Preventive obstetrical measures include good technical preparation of the delivering physician, reduction of the amounts of anesthetic and analgesic drugs given to women in labor, more attention to neonatal transient apnea, better monitoring of the vital fetal signs during labor, caution in the use of drugs during pregnancy, and standardization of delivery records by the universal adoption of the Apgar scoring system.

Pediatric preventive measures covering acute problems include improvements in infant resuscitation techniques and early recognition and treatment of hemolytic diseases and transient convulsive disorders. Long-range pediatric measures involve prevention of acute illness potentially dangerous to the central nervous system,

and improvement in the infant's nutritional status.

Genetic Counseling. Genetic counseling must be preceded by an exact diagnosis, which may require biochemical and cytogenetic studies. With some exceptions, conditions known to be caused by a dominant recessive gene are quite predictable, in that the children of affected persons have a one-in-two chance of inheriting the same disorder, but the asymptomatic relatives do not carry the deleterious gene. In cases of autosomal recessive genes, the prognosis is more complicated. The parents of one child with such a condition run a one-in-four risk of having a second affected child. This is true in PKU and galactosemia. The siblings of PKU patients are heterozygous carriers in two thirds of all the cases that can be confirmed or ruled out by a phenylalanine-tolerance test, but their chance of having a PKU child is only 1 in 250, provided that they marry outside their own family. In the sex-linked diseases, half the sons of a carrier mother are affected, and half the daughters are carriers.

The physician's role is to present the known facts and also the uncertainties to the parents frankly and openly, to tell them what the chances are insofar as these are known, but to recognize that what to do in the presence of any particular set of odds is a parental, rather than a medical decision.

Direct measurement and study of enzyme activity and karyotypes of cultured fetal cells enables the geneticist to diagnose in utero many metabolic and chromosomal disorders. The use of therapeutic abortions in such cases is gaining wide acceptance.

Secondary Prevention

Early Identification and Treatment of Hereditary Disorders. Mass screening for inborn errors of metabolism is recommended at present only for PKU, galactosemia, and possibly maple syrup disease. In PKU, dietary treatment with a low-phenylalanine diet is effective in preventing at least the severe degrees of retardation and the behavioral manifestations if the diet is started in the first 6 months of life. In galactosemia, treatment requires the omission of milk from the diet. Early detection and institution of treatment is effective in preventing mental retardation and other manifestations of this disease. Milk may be reintroduced into the diet in moderate quantities at the age of 4 or 5 years. In hypothyroidism, treatment with thyroid extract, preferably during the first 6 months of life, is essential. Treatment started after that time seldom prevents mental retardation, although it may mitigate the results of thyroid deficiency.

Medical and Surgical Treatment of Other Conditions. Prompt diagnosis and treatment of bacterial meningitis with antibiotics and occasionally with steroids may prevent neurological sequelae, including mental retardation. The sequelae of viral meningoencephalitis are best prevented by immunizations.

Lead poisoning, caused by the chronic ingestion of lead, should be suspected, especially in indigent populations, in cases of unexplained vomiting, abdominal pain, irritability, failure to thrive, and encephalitic signs. Prompt deleading with Versene is usually effective, but relapses are frequent, owing to personality difficulties of the mothers and the continued availability of lead paint in dilapidated slum dwellings. Effective prevention must include the provision of decent, lead-free housing and intensive parental counseling.

Evacuation of a subdural hematoma after a trauma or meningitis must be supplemented in some cases by the excision of the membrane from the subdural space. If untreated, the condition may result in irreversible brain damage and mental retardation.

Craniosynostosis, premature closure of the suture lines, may be corrected by a craniectomy. However, the results of surgical intervention are often disappointing because of the associated primary abnormality of the brain. Excision of the epileptogenic focus in temporal lobe epilepsy may be effective in cases that fail to respond to anticonvulsant medication.

Early Recognition and Handling of Children with Isolated Handicaps. Perceptual difficulties may manifest themselves in disturbances of body image, spatial relationships, and design recognition. These disturbances are often accompanied by EEG changes and give rise to many learning problems. In sensory deficits such as deafness and blindness, the child can be helped by intensive use of the remaining normal sensory pathways. Failure to recognize these handicaps early and to use compensatory avenues of sensory imput often results in preventable mental retardation and withdrawal.

Deficiency in the motor area may manifest itself as general clumsiness and poor coordination. Making allowances for this deficiency prevents penalizing the child and holding him back in school.

Isolated scholastic difficulties may involve reading, handwriting, and abstract thinking. Help in these areas, by way of small groups or individual tutoring, may make it possible for the child to keep up with his agemates.

Distractibility and hyperactivity due to mild brain damage or to unspecified constitutional factors present stumbling blocks to learning and are starting points to child-parent and child-teacher conflict. Medical measures include the use of amphetamines, phenothiazines, and some antihistamines. Small classes for such children allow the teacher more flexibility and a more liberal behavior policy than is possible in a regular classroom.

The difficulty in aphasia in children is primarily on the receptive level and may occur at any point of the central auditory pathways. If not recognized and treated early, aphasias may result in mental retardation or autistic withdrawal. Training is best done under the aegis of a hearing and speech department in an academic center.

Psychotherapy is required only for those few patients who have already developed serious school difficulties. Environmental adjustments—such as the appropriate regulation of the sensory input and the opportunity to burn excess energy—often result in a rapid, striking improvement, particularly in infants and young children.

Prevention of Emotional and Behavioral Disturbances. In the first five years of life, it is particularly important to ensure proper resolution of dependency needs. This phase of development is best handled in the child's home.

Early Recognition of Mental Retardation. Mental retardation is unrecognized in many children until their second or third year of life. The parents vividly describe their feelings of frustration, anger, guilt, and dashed hopes during the time preceding the definitive diagnosis. In contrast, an early diagnosis forces the parents to come to grips with the problem in a realistic manner and to gear their expectations to the child's true potential. This realistic attitude fosters adjustment and reduces frustration and tension. Thus, an early diagnosis could improve the chances for a harmonious parent-child relationship. Developmental evaluations routinely included in periodic health checkups would sharpen the physician's diagnostic acumen and heighten his index of suspicion.

Enhancing the Self-Image of the Mentally Retarded Child. Acceptance by his parents despite his handicap is the best assurance of an adequate self-image in the mentally retarded child. An opportunity for learning and developing social, academic, vocational, and motor skills in a good school setting is also essential. As the child grows older, a steady job, however simple, and regularly scheduled tasks contribute to feelings of dignity, belonging, and identity. The social isolation of the mentally retarded adolescent and young adult is best prevented by the provision of appropriate social outlets.

Physician's Guidance in Handling the Child's Vulnerabilities. If the child exhibits hypersensitivity to external stimuli, the parents are advised to lower the intensity of such stimuli in the child's environment and to strive toward a calm atmosphere. On the other hand, parents of a child with hyposensitivity are advised to intensify sensory stimulation. The child's inability to handle frustration and anxiety is explained as an innate handicap, rather than as willful misbehavior, and parents should be directed toward efforts to minimize anxiety-producing situations as much as possible.

Preparation of a mother for a delay in the child's responses to her social overtures reduces her disappointment, guilt, and pain and ensures her continuous involvement with the child. The primary emphases must be on helping the child to emerge from the primitive state of primary autism and on establishing a bond of closeness between mother and child. The delayed onset and prolonged duration of the phase of negativism in the mentally retarded child may give rise to strong parent-child conflicts. Parents have to be guided to avoid head-on collisions and to be selective in placing emphasis on disciplinary matters. The parents must realize that it is risky to leave things to chance in hopes that the mentally retarded child will amuse himself and keep busy.

Early Identification and Treatment of the Culturally Deprived Child. Periodic developmental examinations or screenings are the best guarantee of early detection of environmental deprivation. Providing more sensory, verbal, and emotional stimulation and introducing new, pleasurable experiences and useful skills can widen the child's intellectual horizon. A well-staffed childcare day center provides the most appropriate setting for the mental rehabilitation of these children.

Tertiary Prevention

Treatment of Behavioral and Personality Difficulties. The chief obstacle to effective psychotherapy is the difficulty in establishing communication with the child, owing to faulty language development and impairment of concept formation. The therapist must operate on a very concrete level to reach the child and, above all, must be flexible and pragmatic. Engaging the child in shared activities is probably the most effective way to establish a meaningful relationship. Firm limits have to be established and adhered to consistently, particularly in children with difficulty in impulse control. Verbal and nonverbal reassurance and praise should be used generously, and situations should be set up that permit the patient to succeed. In addition, concrete evidence of affection in the form of small gifts, toys, and candy is very helpful, as are such pleasurable activities as trips to the drugstore, park, and playground.

Individual and group psychotherapy may be effective only if they are integral parts of a structured program involving the total milieu of the child. Establishing an appropriate school program, matching the child with suitable teachers and child care workers, establishing order and consistency at home, and building an appropriate recreational program are all essential components of such a total program. The psychiatrist's role is primarily that of coordinator and guide of such programs.

Drugs play an important role in the psychiatric treatment of the mentally retarded. Since most of the ataractic drugs are not without hazards, caution is indicated, and excessive dosage should be discouraged. Phenothiazines are the most widely used and probably the most effective drugs. Hyperactive children often profit from amphetamines. Antihistamines have also been used with good results. Barbiturates are usually contraindicated, since they often increase the hyperactive child's restlessness and tension.

Behavior Modification. Behaviorists stress

environmental factors that demonstrably influence behavior and pay little attention to intrapsychic factors. Behavior modification includes pinpointing the observable behavior to be changed, recording the frequency of that behavior, and reinforcing either positively or negatively (extinction) the target behavior. Behavior shaping involves breaking the target tasks into small parts, teaching one part at a time, and rewarding each change in the direction of the desired behavior.

Positive reinforcement involves a system of rewards that may be tangible, such as food or candy, or intangible, such as praise. As a rule, tangible rewards are preferred by the more severely retarded. Negative reinforcement seeks the extinction of undesirable behavior. The techniques used include purposeful ignoring of a behavior, punishment, primary aversive stimulation, time-out periods, and the introduction of behaviors incompatible with those to be eliminated.

Parent Counseling. The parents' helplessness is best handled by giving them specific things to do and by stressing their crucial role in helping the child to develop as normal a personality as possible. The parents' tension may also be usefully channeled into community efforts on behalf of the retarded.

The approach to parents must be flexible and pragmatic. Some parents need help only in coming to grips with their feelings about the child and require a conventional dynamic casework approach. Judiciously used support, reassurance, guidance, and practical advice as to the management of the child are often indicated. Homemaking services and temporary placement of the child in an institution increase the parents' effectiveness by giving them periodic relief. Group therapy permits the sharing of burdens and the getting of reassurance from similarly afflicted parents.

Institutionalization before age 6 is seldom indicated and takes a heavy toll in the social and intellectual development of the child. Many parents might keep the retarded child at home, at least for the first few formative years, if they had the appropriate guidance, support, and interest of the physician. Effective parent counseling by the physician requires his thorough knowledge of the appropriate community agencies and resources in his area.

Institutional Care. Training, education,

treatment, and rehabilitation are the primary goals. A homelike setting is advocated. Dealing with a relatively small, stable group of children and adults helps the retarded child in the areas of impulse control and the development of meaningful human relationships. Children are grouped according to age, degree of retardation, and type of handicap. Contact with the child's family should be maintained primarily by locating residential care centers within the community, by liberal visting hours, and by the encouragement of regular, frequent home visits whenever feasible.

A number of other facilities may serve the needs of mildly retarded persons who cannot be cared for at home and yet do not require a full-time residential center. These facilities are best located in the vicinity of a large institution or health care center, where needed services may be obtained without delay. (See Figure 5.)

Vocational Rehabilitation. To be effective,

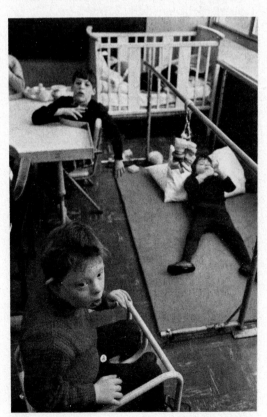

FIGURE 5. Institutions for the mentally retarded should be well equipped to deal with the special needs of the patients. (Courtesy of Ian Berry for Magnum Photos, Inc.)

vocational programs must include a variety of training possibilities tailored to the patient's skills and previous experiences. A detailed assessment of the patient's strengths and defects in functioning must precede program planning. The success of such programs depends largely on a low instructor-to-trainee ratio, on the amount of individual attention available, and on the support of the community. Vocational services should include counseling of the trainees and their families and an employment placement service.

Physical Rehabilitation. Sensory deficits, especially of vision and hearing, require correction whenever possible and special training if the damage is irreversible. As a rule, blind, deaf, or aphasic children do better in specialized centers, with special training and educational facilities. Children with motor difficulties often require orthopedic services and physical therapy. Plastic surgery can correct some of the stigmata of the mentally retarded.

Special Education. The present system of special education uses the division between the educable—those capable of grasping the rudiments of academic skills—and the trainable—those capable of acquiring only basic social habits. The general characteristics of the retarded, particularly when there is also brain damage, include rigidity and concreteness of thinking, distractibility, and poor motivation. The methods applied to overcome these handicaps limit the number of available stimuli, gradually introduce new, more complex experiences, emphasize success to bolster motivation, and use several mutually reinforcing approaches—visual, auditory, tactile, kinesthetic, and verbal—in the teaching of a single concept.

New trends in special education include (1) lessened emphasis on academic performance and greater stress on prevocational and vocational training and on practical life experiences, (2) the attempt to recognize small rather than global units of the child's functioning, permitting the precise identification of his assets and building an individual program around these assets, (3) the introduction of operant conditioning techniques, based on the principles of reinforcement of desired behavior by reward, and (4) the recognition of the value of psychiatric guidance and consultation by teachers and instructors.

The current emphasis on preschool education may be considered the most important innovation in the field of special education. Early intervention may accelerate mental and social development and break up or correct faulty learning habits.

Legal Aspects

The most expedient and just approach to the definition of mental retardation for legal purposes must include the person's level of present functioning and his intellectual potential as measured by various standardized tests.

Civil Law

Whenever possible, one prefers a voluntary admission to an involuntary commitment. In the case of a minor, the parents usually assume responsibility for the decision, and, in cases of parental neglect or absence, the child falls under the general jurisdiction of the juvenile court and other official protective services. In the case of an adult patient, a legal procedure to determine his incompetency is often necessary before an involuntary commitment takes place. Since permanent institutionalization is no longer considered beneficial or necessary for most mentally retarded persons, it is important to retest the mentally retarded patients in institutions at regular intervals to guarantee their basic right to live in a normal community if their general level of functioning improves sufficiently to permit it.

A flexible plan of guardianship may prevent the mentally retarded person from administering his property but not restrain him from making decisions concerning his person. In such matters as the signing of legal documents, voting, driving, marriage, adoption, and eugenic sterilization, the court has to rely on professional opinion. The role of the psychiatrist as an expert in the area of human behavior is of crucial importance in helping the legal authorities arrive at a just solution.

Criminal Law

The paramount issue is that of competency to stand trial. The court must rely on professional, expert opinion. The psychiatrist's testimony can help the court determine the defendant's capacity to exercise sound judgment, highlight the circumstances leading to and surrounding the crime, and decide on appropriate measures designed to be therapeutic. The psychiatrist may also be called on to help determine what degree and extent of isolation of a mentally retarded criminal is necessary for the protection of the community.

Role of the Psychiatrist

The psychiatrist must be a consultant to other physicians, educators, and rehabilitation programs and a direct participant, when indicated, in the treatment, care, and rehabilitation of the retarded. By timely intervention, he may direct the handling of distorted personality patterns so as to identify and help to interrupt patterns of pathological interaction between the retarded patient and his family or his caretakers.

The psychiatrist's role as an interdisciplinary coordinator seems especially applicable to the field of mental retardation, because of his knowledge of group dynamics and his training in recognizing and dealing with the interaction of social, biological, and psychological factors. Furthermore, as an expert in human personality development, he should play an important role in the training and education of physicians, psychologists, social workers, and educators in the field of mental retardation. Psychiatric guidance and supervision may increase volunteers' competence and permit the maximum use of their services, particularly in the process of social rehabilitation.

REFERENCES

Katz, E., editor. *Mental Health Services for the Mentally Retarded*. Charles C Thomas, Springfield, Ill., 1972.

Koch, R., and Dobson, J. C., editors. *The Mentally Retarded Child and His Family*. Brunner/Mazel, New York, 1970.

Lourie, R. S., and Rieger, R. Psychiatric and psychological examination of children. In *American Handbook of Psychiatry*, ed. 2, S. Arieti, editor. Basic Books, New York, 1974.

Menolascino, F. J., editor. *Psychiatric Aspects of the Diagnosis and Treatment of Mental Retardation*. Washington Special Child Publications, Seattle, 1971.

National Clearinghouse for Mental Health Information. *Mental Retardation Abstracts*. National Institutes of Health, Bethesda, Md., 1961–1973.

Philips, I., editor. *Prevention and Treatment of Mental Retardation*. Basic Books, New York, 1966.

President's Panel on Mental Retardation. *National Action to Combat Mental Retardation*. United States Government Printing Office, Washington, 1962.

Stanbury, J. B., Wyngaarden, J. B., and Friedrickson, D. S., editors. *The Metabolic Basis of Inherited Disease*. McGraw-Hill, New York, 1972.

Tarjan, G., Wright, S. W., Eyman, R. J., and Keeran, C. V. National history of mental retardation: Some aspects of epidemiology. Am. J. Ment. Defic., *77:* 369, 1973.

Wortis, J., editor. *Mental Retardation and Developmental Disabilities: An Annual Review*, vol. 5. Brunner/Mazel, New York, 1973.

20

Neuroses

20.1. ANXIETY NEUROSIS

Definition

According to the second edition of the American Psychiatric Association's *Diagnostic and Statistical Manual of Mental Disorders* (DSM-II), anxiety neurosis "is characterized by anxious over-concern extending to panic and frequently associated with somatic symptoms. Unlike *Phobic neurosis*, anxiety may occur under any circumstances and is not restricted to specific situations or objects. This disorder must be distinguished from normal apprehension or fear, which occurs in realistically dangerous situations."

Epidemiology

Anxiety as a symptom is a component of almost every psychiatric disorder, and anxiety neurosis is widespread. It is hard, however, to give exact figures concerning its occurrence, since hospitalization is rarely required for patients with the milder, chronic forms of anxiety neurosis, and statistics are unavailable concerning the multitude who seek help for their discomfort from private physicians. Clinical surveys indicate that some 10 per cent of patients with cardiac illness are suffering from this disorder, women outnumbering men in a ratio of 3 to 2.

Clinical Description

Onset

Anxiety neurosis may begin slowly and insidiously with general feelings of tension and nervous discomfort, or its onset may be sudden, heralded by the abrupt outbreak of attacks of acute anxiety. Although it is characteristically a disorder of young adults, the initial anxiety attack occurs at any age.

Usually, the symptoms of anxiety are unrelated to other neurotic manifestations. But, if the patient associates freely about his anxiety and the circumstances under which it has appeared, the interviewer can uncover the environmental events that have contributed to stimulating the internal conflict. One precipitant found frequently is the death of a near relative from a myocardial infarction. The survivor develops the cardiac and respiratory symptoms of an acute anxiety neurosis, along with the apprehensive conviction that he has the same disease as the departed.

Symptoms

Although there are numerous somatic manifestations of anxiety neurosis, the central, intensely painful affect—often reaching a degree of panic and terror—predominates in the minds of most patients. The most common symptoms, in addition to panic, are palpitations, pains in the chest, respiratory difficulties, and a sense of dizziness, weakness, or faintness.

The feeling of panic often has a peculiar quality that differentiates it from simple fear of a real external danger—a quality that patients describe as weird, eerie, or strangely and dreadfully awesome. The patient is overwhelmed with a sense of some imminent catastrophe about to engulf him. Often, the patient's awareness of his heart action forces on him the dreadful anticipation of dropping dead of a heart attack. Quite as commonly he fears only fainting, but the fear is compounded by a terror of being seen by others in this weak and helpless state. Sometimes the patient cannot specify what he dreads, and the mystery about what lies ahead and about what is causing his panic only adds to his desperation. The anxiety often has an impelling quality; the patient feels that he must do something—run, hide, scream, or get away—although just what he is to do or where he is to go is as undefined as the reason for his terror.

The cardiac symptoms result from the patient's awareness of an actual change in function as the heart beats more rapidly and forcefully. The symptom of palpitation is the result of an increased action of the heart that is regular and normally rhythmical. Chest pains are usually sharp and sticking in quality. Unlike the pains of coronary artery disease, those associated with anxiety last only a few seconds at a time, and they are unrelated to exertion, are not relieved by a cessation of activity, and may come on while the patient is resting in bed.

Nearly as common as the cardiac manifestations are feelings of respiratory discomfort, usually described by the patient as a sense of not being able to get enough air into the lungs, accompanied by a feeling of fullness in the chest and of inadequate respiration. Patients often breathe more rapidly and more deeply and may feel impelled to run out of doors to get more air. In patients with prolonged hyperventilation because of respiratory discomfort, sufficient carbon dioxide may be blown off to bring on a respiratory alkalosis.

Dizziness is described as an awareness of an irregular, blurring, and swimming motion of the surroundings. There is usually a sense of light-headedness and faintness.

Gastrointestinal symptoms are either epigastric pains or a feeling of a jittery, hollow fluttering in the epigastric region.

The individual episodes of acute anxiety vary in intensity and duration. They may range from a sudden rising of affect that the patient manages to control and dispel to a siege lasting hours, during which the victim cowers in a state of persistent, intensely painful anxiety, punctuated by waves of utter panic and terror.

Acute anxiety attacks may appear suddenly with no forewarning in a person who, until their onset, has been reasonably calm and untroubled. More commonly, they occur against a background of chronic anxiety, in which many of the symptoms of the acute phase have been present in a minor key over long periods of time.

Furthermore, many patients experience only chronic anxiety without being subject to eruptions of the acute form. The patient with chronic anxiety may not be able to state what is making him anxious, but some can relate their chronic tension to environmental troubles, such as marital discord and pressures at work.

The chronic anxiety patient commonly complains of feeling nervous, tense, jumpy, and irritable. He may have difficulty in falling asleep at night and fatigues easily during the day. Gastrointestinal symptoms and headaches are common. The patient may complain of muscular tension or pain, especially in his neck and back. He sweats easily, particularly on the palms of his hands, often senses a flushing in his face, is troubled by dryness of the mouth, and frequently feels shaky and tremulous. Particularly troubling to those whose occupation requires mental work is the difficulty patients frequently experience in concentration, in marshaling their thoughts, and in thinking problems through.

Physical Signs and Behavior

The characteristic signs and behavior of the patient suffering from the extremes of acute anxiety are hard to miss. The patient often paces anxiously or, if he remains seated, moves his arms and legs restlessly, complains loudly of his inner turmoil, and vociferously demands help. He may be visibly perspiring, may sigh frequently, and is often hyperventilating. Physical examination discloses no structural abnormalities. The heartbeat is forceful and regular. Elevations of blood pressure, when present, are slight and transient. A fine tremor of the outstretched hands is often observed.

Patients with chronic and lesser degrees of anxiety show many of the same signs as those with the acute variety, but they are of smaller magnitude. A cold, clammy handshake is practically diagnostic. Patients with chronic anxiety do not usually give physical evidence of respiratory alkalosis, but one may find them to be unusually sensitive to hyperventilation.

Course and Prognosis

The paucity of studies concerning the natural history and evolution of anxiety neurosis makes it difficult to speak authoritatively about either its course or its prognosis. Perhaps one-third either recover completely or make a significant improvement. The majority continue to manifest symptoms and incapacitation of varying degrees of severity. The chronically anxious young adult tends to become less so as he grows older, especially if he has achieved a degree of success and stability in his personal life. The nature of the symptoms does not usually help in forecasting the outcome. Prognosis is guided by the degree of environmental stress involved, the maturity of the patient's ego, the stability of his personal relationships, his work performance, and the duration of the symptoms.

Causes

Psychological Aspects

Anxiety is a universal human experience, characterized by fearful anticipation of an unpleasant event in the future. In psychoanalytic theory, anxiety is differentiated from fear. Anxiety is the response to a danger that threatens from *within*, in the form of a forbidden instinctual drive that is about to escape from the person's control. Fear, on the other hand, is the reaction to a real *external* danger that threatens the person with possible injury or death.

As the ego's reaction to an internal threat arising from forbidden instinctual drives, anxiety is experienced in consciousness as mental pain. The pain motivates the ego to defensive maneuvers aimed at controlling the drives in order to avoid the mental suffering. Anxiety, in other words, is viewed as a signal to the ego of the need to erect psychological defenses and of the successfulness of their functioning.

Anxiety is found as a symptom in all forms of emotional illness. When it occurs, it is an indication that something is disturbing the internal psychological equilibrium. If the person's defenses—typically, repression—are successful, the anxiety is dispelled or safely contained, but, more often than not, repression is not entirely effective, and it is necessary to call into play auxiliary defenses, such as conversion or displacement or regression, through which the repressed drives achieve a partial, though disguised, expression in the symptoms of hysteria or phobic neurosis or obsessive-compulsive disorder, depending on the defense that predominates.

If repression fails to function adequately and if other defenses are not called into play, anxiety is the only symptom. When it rises above the low level of intensity characteristic of its function as a signal, it may emerge in all the fury of an anxiety attack. This internal state of affairs is manifested as anxiety neurosis. Stimuli from the patient's adult environment activate the conflicts that he carries with him, disturb his psychic equilibrium, and mobilize the signal anxiety that calls the various ego defenses into play.

When faced with a patient with anxiety neurosis, the therapist must ask himself two questions: What inner drive is the patient afraid of? What are the consequences he fears from its expression?

In neurotic conflicts, the drives are either sexual or aggressive in nature. The consequences the patient fears determines the quality of the anxiety that he experiences. Anxiety falls into four major categories; superego anxiety, castration anxiety, separation anxiety, and id or impulse anxiety.

The varieties of anxiety have their source and take their coloring from the various points along the continuum of early growth and development. Id or impulse anxiety is related to the primitive, diffuse discomfort of the infant when he feels himself overwhelmed by needs and stimuli over which he has no control. Separation anxiety refers to the stage of the somewhat older but still preoedipal child who fears the loss of love or even abandonment by his parents if he fails to control his impulses in conformity with their standards and demands. The fantasies of castration that characterize the oedipal child, particularly in relation to his developing sexual impulses, are reflected in the adult's castration anxiety. And superego anxiety is the direct result of the development of the superego, which marks the passing of the Oedipus complex and the advent of the prepubertal period of latency.

A married man of 32, for example, was referred for therapy for a severe and incapacitating anxiety neurosis, which was clinically manifested as repeated outbreaks of acute attacks of panic arising from a background of chronically distressing nervous tension. Initially, he had absolutely no idea what had precipitated his attacks, nor were they associated with any conscious mental content. In the early weeks of treatment he spent most of his time trying to impress the doctor with how hard he had worked and how effectively he had functioned before he was taken ill. At the same time he described how fearful he was that he would fail at a new business venture he had embarked on. One day, with obvious acute anxiety that practically prevented him from talking, he revealed a fantasy that had suddenly popped into his mind a day or two before and had had led to the outbreak of a severe anxiety attack. He had had the image of a large spike being driven through his penis. Over the next few days he recalled that, as a child of 7, he was fascinated by his mother's clothing and that, on occasion, when she was out of the house, he had dressed himself up in them. From there his associations led to a confession that, as an adult, he was fascinated by female lingerie and would sometimes find himself impelled by a desire to wear women's clothing. He had never yielded to the impulse, and indeed on those few occasions when the idea had entered his consciousness, he had been so overwhelmed by acute anxiety that he could think of it no further.

Physiological Aspects

Clinical and experimental evidence point to the metabolism of the monamines and the function of the limbic system as central to the normal and abnormal expression of emotions, including anxiety, but more detailed information about this complex aspect of brain functioning must be forthcoming before the specific pathways and pathology can be incriminated.

Peripherally, the autonomic nervous system is the mediator of many of the bodily changes experienced by anxious patients. Both sympathetic and parasympathetic effects are observed, and the pattern of the somatic manifestations is determined by the balance in autonomic functioning specifically characteristic for a given patient. A number of recent investigations concern the neurohormonal processes occurring at autonomic nerve endings and the effect of adrenergic reaction blocking agents, such as propranolol, on the autonomic symptoms of anxiety.

Several investigators have shown that patients suffering from anxiety manifest an excessive production of lactate after exercise. Anything causing an increase in lactate production—from chronic centrally determined overproduction of epinephrine, which raises lactate levels, to a disturbance in peripheral metabolic pathways—could lead to the symptoms of anxiety seen in anxiety neurosis.

Differential Diagnosis

Anxiety as a symptom is found in almost all patients suffering from psychiatric illness. What characterizes anxiety neurosis as a syndrome is the fact that it manifests the symptoms of acute and chronic anxiety alone.

The prominence of cardiac symptoms, chest pain, and respiratory distress in acute anxiety attacks occasionally lead even sophisticated physicians to mistake them for coronary artery disease. But when objective evidence for the diagnosis is missing, anxiety neurosis should be suspected, and further positive indications for its existence should be looked for.

Because of the similarity of many of the symptoms of anxiety neurosis and hyperthyroidism, the latter should be considered in patients who complain of anxiety. The diagnosis of thyroid disease is made on the basis of the characteristic physical and laboratory findings, but patients with hyperthyroidism who have become euthyroid after treatment frequently have persisting anxiety that is clearly psychogenic and may require psychotherapy.

The episodic outpouring of epinephrine and norepinephrine in patients with pheochromocytoma causes sudden attacks of tachycardia, palpitations, chest pain, sweating, tremor, apprehension, and elevated blood pressure that may be clinically indistinguishable from acute anxiety attacks. But pheochromocytoma is a rare disorder, occurring in 0.1 per cent of patients with hypertension, and can usually be differentiated from anxiety neurosis by the history of past emotional problems and the evidence of emotional conflict in patients with anxiety and by the presence of positive findings associated with pheochromocytoma, including a palpable suprarenal mass that may, on being squeezed, produce a typical attack and pyelographic evidence of kidney displacement by the adrenal tumor.

The sudden attacks of dizziness in Ménière's disease may occasionally be confused with acute anxiety. Characteristically, the dizziness of Ménière's disease is a true vertigo and is associated with nystagmus, deafness, and other signs of middle ear disease that are not found in anxiety neurosis.

Treatment

The stability of human relationships and of work situations, the ability to bear painful affects and to relate to the therapist, intelligence, motivation for treatment, the capacity for introspection and insight—all must be assessed in determining the chances for a good response to insight psychotherapy. Once the patient's suitability for such therapy has been determined, the approach depends on the nature of the problem underlying the anxiety. As a general rule, neurotic difficulties that involve characterological difficulties require psychoanalysis or one of the more prolonged forms of treatment. If the psychological problem is circumscribed and is related to specific external circumstances, briefer forms of uncovering therapy may be quite effective in freeing the patient of his symptoms.

Reassurance about unrealistic fears, encouragement to face anxiety-provoking situations, and the continued opportunity to talk regularly to the psychiatrist about problems are all helpful to the patient, even if they are not definitively curative. If the therapist discovers external situations that are anxiety-provoking, he may be able himself or with the help of the patient and his family to change the environment so as to reduce the stressful pressures. A reduction in symptoms often allows the patient to function more effectively in his daily work and relationships, which provides new rewards and gratifications that are in themselves therapeutic.

The relaxing techniques used by hypnotists and behavior therapists may prove helpful to many patients, especially those who are suggestible. In the initial stages, after the psychiatrist has instructed the patient in the various methods of relaxation, he should allow the patient to practice them in the office, so that the psychiatrist can add his encouragement and positive suggestion to the patient's efforts. The ultimate goal is to enable the patient to use the techniques alone in the course of his daily life. He should follow a regular daily schedule of exercises and use them whenever he is facing an anxiety-provoking situation or feels his inner tension rising.

Drugs, particularly tranquilizers, may play an important part in symptom control. Generally speaking, the phenothiazines should be reserved for the anxiety associated with schizophrenia and other forms of psychotic illness. Most patients respond adequately to therapeutic doses of the minor tranquilizers. Barbiturates, especially the shorter-acting forms are helpful when the patient has trouble falling asleep, but the dangers of addiction in the chronically anxious, dependent patient often make one prefer the use of a nightime dose of one of the tranquilizers, which are frequently highly effective sedatives.

Medication is only an adjunct to, not a substitute for, the doctor-patient relationship. But the effect of the various forms of psycho-

therapy may be enchanced if the chemical control of painful symptoms allows the patient to direct his attention more freely to the conflicts underlying his anxiety.

REFERENCES

DaCosta, J. M. On irritable heart: A clinical study of a form of functional cardiac disorder and its consequences. Am. J. Med. Sci., *61:* 17, 1871.

Engel, G. L., Ferris, E. B., and Logan, M. Hyperventilation: Analysis of clinical symptomatology. Ann. Intern. Med., *27:* 683, 1947.

Freud, S., Inhibitions, symptoms, and anxiety. In *Standard Edition of the Complete Psychological Works of Sigmund Freud*, vol. 20, p. 87. Hogarth Press, London, 1959.

Freud, S. On the grounds for detaching a particular syndrome from neurasthenia under the description "anxiety neurosis." In *Standard Edition of the Complete Psychological Works of Sigmund Freud*, vol. 3, p. 90. Hogarth Press, London, 1962.

Janet, P. *Les Obsessions et la Psychasthénie.* 2 vols. Félix Alcan, Paris, 1903.

May, R. *The Meaning of Anxiety.* Ronald Press, New York, 1950.

20.2.   HYSTERICAL NEUROSIS, CONVERSION TYPE

Definition

In the second edition of the American Psychiatric Association's *Diagnostic and Statistical Manual of Mental Disorders* (DMS-II), hysterical neurosis, conversion type, is defined as a disorder in which "the special senses or voluntary nervous system are affected, causing such symptoms as blindness, deafness, anosmia, anaesthesias, paraethesias, paralyses, ataxias, akinesias, and dyskinesias. Often the patient shows an inappropriate lack of concern or *belle indifférence* about these symptoms, which may actually provide secondary gains by winning him sympathy or relieving him of unpleasant responsibilities. This type of hysterical neurosis must be distinguished from psychophysiologic disorders, which are mediated by the automatic nervous system; from malingering, which is done consciously; and from neurological lesions, which cause anatomically circumscribed symptoms."

Epidemiology

It is often stated that conversion hysteria is less frequently seen in contemporary psychiatric practice than it was 70 years ago. If by conversion hysteria one means the classically described major sensorimotor symptoms of paralyses, anesthesias, convulsions, and so on, there are possibly some grounds for the statement. However, this does not necessarily mean that conversion hysteria is any less frequent. It is possible that there has merely been a shift from the predominance of one type of conversion hysteria to another, the total number remaining the same. Indeed, evidence from contemporary clinical experience suggests that pain and the simulation of bodily disease are the predominant forms of hysteria now manifested by patients.

Pathology

There are no known neuropathological lesions underlying the symptoms, and the pathology associated with the condition is purely secondary to the hysterical paralyses and contractures. If these are of long duration, muscle atrophy, stiffening, and limitation of motion of the affected limb or limbs may occur as a result of the prolonged disuse.

Causes

A fixation in early psychosexual development at the level of the Oedipus complex, with a failure to relinquish the incestuous tie to the loved parent, leads to a conflict in adult life over the sexual drive because it retains its forbidden incestuous quality. The drive is, therefore, subjected to the defensive psychological maneuver of repression. The energy deriving from the drive is converted into the hysterical symptom, which not only protects the patient from a conscious awareness of the drive but often provides a symbolic expression of it. Hysteria is conceived of as a specific clinical entity arising from specific sexual conflicts originating in the oedipal period of psychosexual development.

It is difficult for patients with hysterical reactions to relinquish their symptoms, partly because to do so subjects them to the mental discomfort associated with being aware of the forbidden impulse. In addition, the symptom itself can bring certain advantages to the patient. It defines him as a sick and disabled person, and the people in his environment act accordingly. Attention, sympathy, and help are focused on him because he is ill, and he is not required to carry out the duties and responsibilities expected of a healthy adult. Such advantages gratify the dependency needs of the

patient and tend to reinforce the perpetuation of hysterical symptoms.

Hysterical symptoms do not always occur in a circumscribed clinical syndrome. In the mixed neuroses the hysterical symptom is only one of a repertoire of clinical manifestations that may include phobias, obsessions, compulsions, and neurotic depression, in which, according to psychoanalytic theory, the psychogenetic factors are primarily preoedipal and pregenital. Hysterical symptoms are found in a variety of personality types—such as the passive-aggressive, the schizoid, and the paranoid personality—in which, according to Freudian theory, pregenital conflicts play a predominant role.

It has long been known that hysterical symptoms may result from a frightening physical accident that has produced no bodily injuries. The primary motivation for these symptoms is self-preservation, rather than oedipal genital drives; the symptoms enable the patient to escape a dangerous situation, to be relieved of onerous responsibilities, and to receive protection, help, and attention. These unconscious dependency needs are a source of conflict for the patient, since they run counter to the image of himself as a strong, self-sufficient person, which he must preserve to maintain his self-esteem. Because his symptoms appear to the patient to be the result of a bodily illness that has afflicted him without his consent or participation, he can allow himself to become an incapacitated invalid, dependent on others for help and attention.

For learning theorists, psychiatric symptoms are not only pathological adaptations to external stimuli but learned responses. The learning is reinforced and facilitated by the reduction of the intensity of an inner, painful psychological drive that follows the response.

In the case of hysterical paralysis, for example, the initial episode of paralysis results in a reduction of the painful drive of fear or anxiety. The psychological relief thus obtained reinforces the hysterical response that has produced it and predisposes to a repetition of the same palliative response each time the anxiety occurs. In this way, a pattern of behavior is evolved that may become chronic.

Another approach to conversion hysteria is based on the study of communication in the interpersonal situation. In this framework, the hysterical symptom is looked on as nonverbal communication intended to coerce another person to some action, such as helping or paying attention.

Clinical Description

Although it does occur in men especially when financial compensation is a factor, conversion hysteria is predominantly a disorder of women. It frequently begins in adolescence or early adulthood, but the symptoms may appear for the first time during middle age or even in the later decades of life. The manifestations may be sporadic and episodic, often arising at times of emotional distress resulting from external crises. The site and nature of the symptoms may vary within a person from time to time, or a single symptom may become rigidly fixed and persist intractably for years.

Physical Characteristics

Motor Disturbances. There are two kinds of motor disturbances; abnormal movements and paralyses.

Abnormal movements may take many forms. Gross, rhythmical tremors of the head, arms, and legs are seen. A variety of choreiform tics and jerks may be observed; these are usually more organized and stereotyped than the movements of true neurogenic chorea. Convulsive movements of the entire body are sometimes found. Unlike true neurogenic epilepsy, hysterical seizures are characterized by a wild, disorganized, seemingly unpatterned thrashing and writhing of the body. But the patient does react to stimuli. When the patient recovers from his seizure, he can often remember what was going on around him during his convulsion. Astasia abasia is also seen.

Paralysis and paresis most commonly affect the extremities as monoplegia, hemiplegia, or paraplegia. The affected parts are flaccid in character or show the result of sustained contractures in antagonistic muscle groups. The paralysis does not conform to the pattern resulting from damage to the peripheral or central nervous system; rather, it follows a distribution conforming to the conventional idea of the part affected. The hand is paralyzed from the wrist down, the forearm from the elbow, and the whole arm from the shoulder down. If the problem is one of paresis, the weakness may be most severe at the proximal portion of the limb, rather than distally—the opposite of what occurs in central nervous system disease. When

the paralyzed or paretic part is examined carefully, it readily becomes apparent that there is no genuine deficit in muscle function. A special and localized form of paralysis may also occur in the muscles affecting the vocal cords, leading to hysterical aphonia. In this condition, the patient is usually able to whisper with no difficulty but can make no vocalized sound whatsoever. Examination reveals normal movement of the lips, tongue, and pharynx and the vocal cords during respiration.

Sensory Disturbances. Hysterical disturbances of sensation, especially anesthesias, may go unnoticed unless they are specifically looked for, since patients do not often complain of them.

Disturbances of skin sensation may occur in any location, shape, and pattern. Most commonly, the sensory disturbances are found in the extremities. When disorders of motor function occur, these are generally accompanied by diminished or totally absent sensation. As with the motor disorders, the distribution of the sensory disturbance follows a pattern determined by the patient's idea of the limb affected, rather than by the neural structures innervating it.

The special organs of sense may also exhibit a loss of function, the patient manifesting varying degrees of deafness and loss of vision. The disturbance may be unilateral or bilateral. A peculiar feature of the visual disorder is a regular, concentric diminution of the visual field that, in its extreme form, leaves only central vision intact. Certain observations indicate that peripheral stimuli are being received, transmitted, registered centrally, and used in integrated actions but that at the highest levels of mental function the patient remains totally unaware of them.

There may also be sensory hallucinations. The most frequently affected modality is vision. Characteristically, visual hallucinations are of complex scenes or fragments of action that appear repeatedly and with sterotyped repetition, often reproducing the scenes of a real past event of emotional significance to the patient.

Hysterical pain may be based on a heightened awareness of the myriad little stimuli normally arising from all parts of the body that are ordinarily ignored but may be perceived and even felt as uncomfortable if attention is focused on them. Whatever its origin, hysterical pain is common and may affect any part of the body. A common site is the abdomen, which has led to frequent misdiagnoses and much unnecessary surgery.

Symptoms Simulating Physical Illness. Identification with the symptoms of a person with whom the patient has a close relationship is a key mechanism. This identification is commonly with a person who has recently died, and it is often accompanied by the signs and symptoms of pathological grief. But Freud's patient Dora developed a hysterical cough through identification with the same symptom in an older woman she felt to be a rival. On occasion, one may find rhythmical, hard abdominal pains in a man whose wife is in labor.

A young man consulted his physician for severe precordial chest pains, which, he was convinced, were evidence that he had a fatal heart disease. Careful and repeated physical, laboratory, and electrocardiographic examinations disclosed no indication of cardiac difficulty, but a careful history revealed that the patient's father had died suddenly of a second episode of myocardial infarction several months before. Neither at the time nor since then had the patient experienced any conscious grief for his father; instead, he developed symptoms like those of his father's fatal illness and, to his own amazement, adopted a number of his father's characteristic behavior patterns.

Symptoms Complicating Physical Illness. Pain that begins as a result of a local disease process may be prolonged as a hysterical symptom long after the physical lesion has healed. Occasionally, one sees patients who, after a true epileptic seizure, continue to have hysterical seizures that closely imitate the initial spells. More perplexing are those patients who manifest symptoms resulting from a local bodily lesion but in whom the severity of the complaints and the magnitude of the disability are far greater than would be expected from the nature and extent of the local lesion alone.

Behavioral Characteristics

The patient with conversion hysteria does not show major abnormalities in his mental status. The patient's mental status reveals no indications of a psychosis or of a gross physiological disturbance of brain function.

The most characteristic behavioral feature in patients with conversion hysteria is *la belle indifference*. Despite what appear to be the most extensive and crippling disturbances in function, the patient is completely unconcerned

and, indeed, may not spontaneously mention such disturbances, which often results in their being overlooked unless specifically searched for. The lack of concern applies to the hysterical symptom or symptoms alone; it is not a general indifference or absence of anxiety.

Although hysterical patients do not show the major abnormalities of mood, thought, and behavior listed in the formal mental status examination checklist, they often tend to exhibit subtler forms of behavior patterns that make up the hysterical personality. These patients are often described as having the following behavior: dramatic, exhibitionistic, narcissistic, emotional, seductive, dependent, and manipulative.

Diagnosis

Generally speaking, the phenomena of abnormal movements, paralyses, and anesthesias present few diagnostic problems. It is when one is dealing with pain and other symptoms simulating bodily disease that difficulties arise.

That pain or other local symptoms are wholly or in part the manifestation of conversion hysteria is strongly suggested by a history or the presence of many of the following additional factors: (1) such symptoms as paralyses and anesthesias, (2) such overtly neurotic symptoms as anxiety, depression, obsessions, and phobias, (3) multiple illnesses, possibly resulting in surgery, for which no clear-cut physical origins have been found, (4) sexual disturbances, with frigidity and a distaste for sexuality playing a prominent role, (5) the behavioral characteristics of the hysterical personality, (6) *la belle indifférence*, (7) the recent death of a person important to the patient or other disturbances in personal relationships temporally related to the onset of the symptoms.

In establishing the diagnosis, one's approach to the patient is of central importance. Confronting him with direct questions requiring direct answers frequently elicits no information or misinformation. Only by allowing the patient to talk in his own way about his illness and by using nondirective forms of interviewing techniques will the physician elicit clues to the presence of hysterical mechanisms.

Psychological tests may confirm the clinical findings. As compared with patients suffering from other neurotic syndromes, those with conversion hysteria give test responses that are freer and more imaginative, accompanied by a more labile affect and a tendency toward impulsiveness.

The earliest manifestations of central nervous system disease may be confused with conversion hysteria. A transitory disturbance of vision in one eye or a passing weakness of an arm or leg that heralds the onset of multiple sclerosis may lead the unwary to dismiss the complaints as hysterical symptoms. It is important to follow the patient carefully for subsequent episodes in which the emergence of neurological signs or the lack of them, along with emerging positive indications of hysteria, aids in making a definite diagnosis.

The fact that hysterical patients sometimes present with hallucinations leads to a diagnostic confusion with schizophrenia. In general, schizophrenic hallucinations are auditory and are often bizarre and vague in content and form. Hysterical hallucinations, on the other hand, are usually visual and represent complex, elaborate scenes that are repeated in a sterotyped fashion. The hysterical patient does not show the gross disturbances of thought and affect that characterize schizophrenia.

A distinction that is sometimes difficult to make is that between conversion hysteria and malingering. The tendency of many hysterical patients to be histrionic and to use their symptoms as a vehicle of communication and of coercion of others, plus the often obvious secondary gain to be derived from symptoms, convince the observer that the patient is consciously simulating illness to obtain his own ends. Patients with true, conscious malingering appear to be rare; there are more inconsistencies in their histories as they are repeated to various people, and the patient consciously simulating a disease often deliberately produces physical signs and findings, which is a rare pattern of behavior in hysterical patients.

Prognosis

Some patients develop transitory hysterical symptoms that clear without any treatment at all, whereas others have clinical manifestations that remain fixed and totally intractable to therapeutic measures for years. The rare systematic studies of prognosis indicate that, although 50 per cent of patients lose their symptoms within a year, 30 per cent still have symptoms at the end of 5 years, and 20 per cent retain them for 15 years or longer. Hysterical symptoms tend to come and go in response to environmental stresses.

Factors that make for a good prognosis, especially when skilled psychotherapy is available, are: (1) a psychological conflict that centers primarily around genital, oedipal sexuality, (2) evidence of stability in relationships, as indicated by generally good relationships with family and friends and a stable work history, (3) the ability to relate to the physician and to develop a therapeutic alliance, (4) the capacity to feel and to express emotions without developing incapacitating anxiety or depressions, (5) the ability to retain psychological distance from consciously experienced emotions, (6) the capacity for introspection, and (7) symptoms that are fairly well circumscribed and are related to definite environmental stresses.

Treatment

The choice of therapy rests not on the nature of the symptoms but on the patient's personality structure. The factors pointing to a good prognosis also indicate which patients will do well with treatment methods that aim to develop insight. Psychoanalysis, the most extensive and profound of the therapeutic measures, is most likely to make permanent changes for the better in both the symptoms and the personality structure of patients who need techniques involving insight. But good and lasting results may be effected with less protracted methods, and success has been reported with the techniques of hypnoanalysis.

Only a portion of the total number of patients with hysterical phenomena are candidates for psychoanalysis or modified techniques based on achieving insight. The remainder require some form of supportive psychotherapy.

Those patients who are not candidates for one of the insight psychotherapies are generally suffering from narcissistic character problems in addition to their hysterical symptoms, with predominantly pregenital conflicts, particularly those centering on dependency needs. For such patients, supportive therapy is indicated in a one-to-one relationship, a group therapy setting, or a combination of the two therapeutic approaches. Environmental manipulation is often an important and helpful measure and includes working with the patient's immediate family and other people close to him.

A number of physical treatment measures have been attempted and advocated, such as electroconvulsive therapy, various forms of leukotomies, and carbon dioxide inhalation, but there is little or no evidence to indicate that they have any lasting or basic effect on the disorder. Recently, conditioning therapy has been used. Drug therapy is sometimes a useful adjunct to psychotherapy, especially if disabling anxiety is present, but no drug in current use affects the hysterical symptom itself.

Prevention

Patients who develop hysterical symptoms that complicate physical illnesses and lead to psychogenic prolongation of their disabilities have frequently been hardworking, conscientious, self-sufficient, and independent people before their illness. The behavior pattern before the onset of the illness represented, in part at least, a reaction formation that kept underlying dependency needs out of the patient's awareness and under control. However, his personality organization made him vulnerable to serious psychological complications when he developed a physical illness. The dependency needs emerged in the patient's overt behavior, using the symptoms as a vehicle of expression. A new psychological equilibrium was established, and, even though the physical lesion initially underlying the symptoms of the illness was healed or much improved, the symptoms remained in full force as a means of gratifying the dependency needs that have been grafted into them. Psychological invalidism replaced a physical illness.

This shift in equilibrium takes time. The behavior of the people in the patient's environment can often play a large part in determining whether the shift will occur. If the professional personnel caring for the patient and his family force him into passivity and dependency by being overly solicitous and overly helpful, by unnecessarily restricting his activities, and by emphasizing the disability caused by his symptoms, they can often bring about or hasten the march to chronic psychological invalidism. If, however, from the start of the illness, they allow the patient as much freedom of action, autonomy, and independent self-sufficiency as the nature of the illness permits; if they emphasize the positive capabilities that remain to the patient, despite his sickness; if, from the beginning, they help him to focus his attention ahead

to a return to self-sufficiency and encourage him to increased independence as his physical disorder improves, there is a good chance that the patient will avoid a major and catastrophic regression. Once the equilibrium has shifted to produce psychological invalidism, it is often impossible to effect a change, and the condition becomes chronic.

REFERENCES

Bernheim, H. *Suggestive Therapeutics.* G. P. Putnam's Sons, New York, 1897.
Breuer, J., and Freud, S. Studies on hysteria. In *Standard Edition of the Complete Psychological Works of Sigmund Freud,* vol. 2, p. 3. Hogarth Press, London, 1955.
Chodoff, P., and Lyons, H. Hysteria, the hysterical personality and "hysterical" conversion. Am. J. Psychiatry. *114:* 734, 1958.
Freud, S. The neuropsychoses of defence. In *Standard Edition of the Complete Psychological Works of Sigmund Freud,* vol. 3, p. 45. Hogarth Press, London, 1962.
Janet, P. *The Major Symptoms of Hysteria.* Macmillan, New York, 1907.
Rangell, L. The nature of conversion. J. Am. Psychoanal. Assoc. *7:* 632, 1959.

20.3. HYSTERICAL NEUROSIS, DISSOCIATIVE TYPE

Definition

In the second edition of the American Psychiatric Association's *Diagnostic and Statistical Manual of Mental Disorders* (DSM-II), hysterical neurosis, dissociative type, is defined as that form of hysterical neurosis in which "alterations may occur in the patient's state of consciousness or in his identity, to produce such symptoms as amnesia, somnambulism, fugue, and multiple personality."

Epidemiology

No evidence suggests that there has been a diminution in the incidence of dissociative hysteria. The one exception to this statement is that form manifested as multiple personality. This condition appears to be relatively rare, as compared with the situation 80 years ago.

Clinical Description

Onset

The various forms of dissociative hysteria begin and end abruptly. The patient slips rapidly into a somnambulistic state, or he is suddenly aware that he has lost his memory for a period of time in his immediate past. Or he may wake up to find himself in a strange place with no knowledge of how he got there or what he has been doing in the time that has elapsed from the last thing that he can remember.

Although many episodes apparently occur spontaneously, there may be a history of a specific emotional trauma or a situation charged with painful emotions and psychological conflict. Amnesia is, at times, preceded by a physical head trauma. In susceptible persons, treatment with electroshock may lead to hysterical amnesia. On occasion, hypnosis may precipitate a self-limited but sometimes prolonged somnambulistic episode in the hypnotic subject. And intense concentration tends to induce somnambulistic states in some persons.

Symptoms

The manifestations of dissociative hysteria are varied, often complex, and frequently hard to distinguish sharply from one another. One characteristic links them together. A cluster of recent, related mental events is beyond the patient's power of conscious recall but remains capable, under given circumstances, of returning to his conscious awareness. At least three factors determine the separate natures of the various forms: the state of consciousness during an episode of hysterical dissociation, the pattern of the amnesia, and the quality of changes in personality and behavior that may accompany the episode.

Forms

Somnambulism. In somnambulism the patient exhibits an altered state of conscious awareness of his surroundings and often has vivid hallucinatory recollections of an emotionally traumatic event in his past of which he may have no memory during his usual waking state. Somnambulistic episodes may arise either during sleep or during the patient's waking hours and should not be confused with the episodes of sleepwalking commonly seen in children. In somnambulism, the patient is out of contact with his environment, appears preoccupied with a private world and stares into space if his eyes are open. (See Figure 1.) He may seem emotionally upset, speak excitedly in words and sentences that are frequently hard to understand, or engage in a pattern of seemingly meaningful

activities that is repeated every time an episode occurs. This behavior often represents the external manifestations of a hallucinatory re-experiencing of a traumatic event, the memories of which are normally repressed. There is amnesia for the somnambulistic episode once it is terminated.

Amnesia. In localized and general amnesia the patient suddenly becomes aware that he has a total loss of memory for the events of a period of time covering anything from a few hours (localized form) to a whole lifetime of experience (general form). The amnesic patient usually gives no indication that there is anything amiss and seems entirely alert both before and after the amnesia occurs.

In systematized amnesia the patient loses memory only for specific and related past events. The patient with continuous amnesia forgets each successive event as it occurs, although he is clearly alert and aware of what is going on around him.

Fugue. In the fugue the patient wanders, usually far from home and for days at a time. During this period, he is completely forgetful of his past life and associations, but, unlike the patient with amnesia, he is unaware that he has forgotten anything. When he suddenly comes

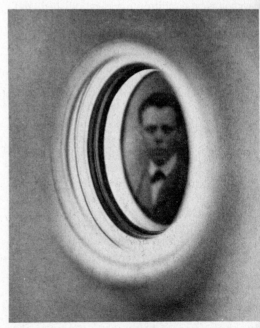

FIGURE 1. Dissociative states are characterized by feelings of unreality, as evoked in this photograph. (Courtesy of Arthur Tress for Magnum Photos, Inc.)

back to his former self, he recalls the time antedating the onset of the fugue but is amnesic for the period covered by the fugue itself. Unlike those in a somnambulistic state, the patient in a fugue does not appear to be behaving in any way that is out of the ordinary, nor does he give evidence of acting out any specific memory of a traumatic event. On the contrary, he generally leads a quiet, prosaic, somewhat seclusive existence, works at simple occupations, lives modestly, and does nothing to draw the attention or suspicion of his neighbors and acquaintances.

Multiple Personality. In this disorder the patient is dominated by one of two or more distinct personalities, each of which determines the nature of his behavior and attitudes during the period that it is upper most in consciousness. The transition from one personality state to another is sudden, often dramatic in occurrence. There is generally amnesia during each state for the existence of the others and for the events that took place when another personality was in the ascendancy. Often, however, one personality state is not bound by such amnesia and retains complete awareness of the existence, qualities, and activities of the other personalities. Each personality is a fully integrated, highly complex set of associated memories with characteristic attitudes, personal relationships, and behavior patterns. The patient generally shows nothing unusual in his mental status. The first appearance of the secondary personality or personalities may be spontaneous, or it may emerge in relation to what appears to be a precipitant.

Morton Prince's "Sally Beauchamp" ("The Saint, the Devil, the Woman," as he hesitantly christens her) is the most renowned of the some 200 patients known to have developed multiple personalities. In *The Dissociation of a Personality* (1906), the volume devoted to her biography, Prince has summarized the essence of her clinical problem in a brief paragraph that illustrates most of the characteristic features of the disorder.

In addition to the real, original or normal self, the self that was born and which she was intended by nature to be, she may be any one of three different persons. I say three different, because although making use of the same body, each, nevertheless, has a distinctly different character; a difference manifested by different trains of thought, by different views, beliefs, ideals, and temperament, and by different acquisitions, tastes, habits, experiences, and memories. Each varies in these respects from the other two, and from the original Miss Beauchamp. Two of these personalities have no knowledge of each other or of the third, excepting such information as may be obtained by inference or second hand, so that in the memory of each of these two there are blanks which correspond to the times when the others are in the flesh. Of a sudden one or the other wakes up to find herself, she knows not where, and ignorant of what she has said or done a moment before. Only one of the three has knowledge of the lives of the others, and this one presents such a bizarre character, so far removed from the others in individuality, that the transformation from one of the other personalities to herself is one of the most striking and dramatic features of the case. The personalities come and go in kaleidoscopic succession, many changes often being made in the course of twenty-four hours. And so it happens that Miss Beauchamp, if I may use the name to designate several distinct people, at one moment says and does and plans and arranges something to which a short time before she most strongly objected, indulges in tastes which a moment before would have been abhorrent to her ideals, and undoes what she had just laboriously planned and arranged.

Other Dissociative States. A curious form of dissociation is that manifested as the trance states of spirit mediums who preside over spiritual seances. Typically, the medium enters a somnambulistic state, during which the so-called control takes over much of her conscious awareness and influences her thoughts and speech. In automatic writing there is not necessarily an alteration of consciousness, the dissociation affecting only the arm and the hand, producing a written message that often discloses mental contents of which the writer is unaware. Crystal gazing, on the other hand, results in a somnambulistic state in which visual hallucinations are prominent. Phenomena related to crystal gazing are the condition of highway hypnosis and the similar mental states experienced by airplane pilots. In both, the monotony of movement at high speeds through environments that provide little in the way of distractions to the operator of the vehicle leads to a fixation of his attention on a single object. There results a trancelike state of consciousness in which visual hallucinations may occur. Possibly in the same order of phenomena are the hallucinations and dissociated mental states described in patients who have been confined to respirators for long periods of time without adequate environmental distractions.

Ganser's syndrome, occasionally seen in prisoners in penal institutions, is characterized by behavior that appears so nonsensical that the patient is often thought to be consciously pretending to be psychotic. For example, when asked to add simple digits, he gives an answer that is wrong by one or two figures. It is probably that the patient, although aware of what he is doing, is responding automatically with a dissociated portion of his mental apparatus.

Mystical experiences have been reported by religious geniuses of all ages throughout the world. The volumes of autobiography and instruction produced by men and women like St. Teresa of Avila and St. John of the Cross make it evident that conscious, voluntary concentration of attention is the starting point of these states. The adept is able to venture to a higher stage of meditation, in which the mind is emptied of all mental contents and the person experiences pure, conscious awareness alone, devoid of thoughts, fantasies, and concepts. At this point he may be filled with the sense of mystical oneness with the universe, a profoundly moving experience, the essence of which, as the saints invariably insist, is ineffable and impossible to communicate to others, except by showing them the steps by which they may find it for themselves.

Causes

Current explanations of dissociative hysteria are based on Freud's dynamic concepts. The repression of mental contents that leads to amnesia and other manifestations of the resulting dissociation is conceived of as being a mechanism for protecting the patient from emotional pain that has arisen either from disturbing external circumstances—or from anxiety-provoking inner drives and effects.

Some patients—when faced with a situation that arouse overwhelming grief, despair, or anxiety—may respond by a total repression of the memories of the disturbing events, accompanied by a disappearance of the painful effect. Most patients with amnesia who are seen in modern-day hospitals have developed their symptoms in response to a difficult life situation. Furthermore, the majority of patients manifesting somnambulism are re-enacting a traumatic event that has actually occurred at some time in their past.

In patients with multiple personalities and in those with fugue states, however, a drive that is usually repressed or patterns of behavior that are normally under control may emerge into open expression in a dissociative state. In many patients exhibiting multiple personalities, the primary personality—that is, the one that has characterized the patient during the greater part of his life—is a somewhat emotionally constricted, restrained, moralistic, and proper one. A secondary personality on the other hand, exhibits attitudes and behavior patterns of quite the opposite sort. The primary personality remains unaware of the existence of the secondary personality, but the secondary personality is usually fully aware of all the thoughts and activities of the first, often being quite scornful of the priggishness of his better half.

The psychological conflicts in the adult patient that lead to dissociative symptoms are the result of earlier disturbances in the course of growth and development. Both oedipal and preoedipal elements contribute to the psychogenesis of dissociative hysteria, but these are in no way different from what is found in the conversion type of the disorder.

Course and Prognosis

The outlook for individual episodes of dissociative states, such as amnesias and fugues, is good, particularly if energetic therapeutic measures are applied. On the other hand, the tendency of a person to resort to dissociative mechanisms when he is under instinctual or environmental pressures can be a continuing liability for him over long periods of time.

The rare condition of multiple personality is probably a more serious phenomenon, involving major disturbances of ego function. Partial success in its treatment has been reported in the literature.

Differential Diagnosis

Schizophrenia

A dissociative trance state frequently resembles catatonic stupor, and it may be difficult to distinguish between them, especially if the hysterical patient is negativistic or if it is impossible to establish communication with him while the dissociative mechanisms are at work. The patient in a somnambulistic episode usually gives evidence to indicate that he is engaged in the reliving of a traumatic event, and most dissociative trance states, as contrasted with catatonia, are self-limited and of short duration. Furthermore, when contact can be established with the hysterical patient, the disorders of thought and affect characteristic of schizophrenia are not present.

Sleepwalking

Very commonly in childhood and less frequently in adulthood, a person may get out of bed and wander around while still asleep. Such behavior is not necessarily pathological, especially in children, and it differs from hysterical somnambulism in that sleepwalking occurs during deep sleep unassociated with dreams, is poorly integrated and nonpurposive in nature, and is characterized by actions that are awkward and fumbling and show a lack of dexterity. Dissociative somnambulistic episodes may occur at night, but they are as different from normal sleepwalking as hypnosis is from true sleep.

Postconcussional Amnesia

Dissociative amnesia may be associated with head injury, and in such cases there may be a combination of hysterical and postconcussional amnesia. In general, the retrograde amnesia after concussion does not extend beyond a period of one week. Postconcussional amnesia, furthermore, disappears slowly, and memory is usually not completely restored for the events that have occurred during the amnesic period, whereas a patient recovers from hysterical amnesia suddenly and with a total restoration of memory.

Temporal Lobe Epilepsy

In temporal lobe epilepsy, the patient, like the patient in a hysterical fugue, may appear to be entirely alert as he skillfully carries out a highly complex pattern of behavior. In some patients with electroencephalographic evidence of temporal lobe dysfunction, their seizural behavior patterns have reference to a memory of a significant past event in their lives, as is often the case in patients with hysterical somnambulism. In general, when trance like episodes occur in conjunction with evidence of other typical hysterical symptoms and stigmata and when they are unaccompanied by positive electroencephalographic indications of temporal lobe dysfunction, the episodes are a form of dissociative hysteria. On the other hand, when there is brain wave evidence of a temporal lobe dys-

rhythmia, even if a clinical episode has features characteristic of hysterical dissociation, it should be considered, in part at least, the result of a gross brain lesion.

Treatment

Amnesia is the most common form of dissociative hysteria. In patients with this disorder, as well as in those with the less commonly seen fugue states, it is important to restore the lost memories to consciousness as soon as possible. Otherwise, it is likely that the mental contents remaining in an unconscious state will form a nucleus for the production of a future episode of amnesia or fugue.

It is usually possible to recover the lost memories by various therapeutic interventions. In some patients, one can get at the unconscious mental contents within the span of one or two interviews by allowing the patient to free associate or by encouraging him to give his associations to a specific fragment of the repressed material that has returned in the form of a conscious image, dream, or hallucination. At other times, more active measures, such as hypnosis and intravenous pentothal, may be required to mobilize the memories. Once the memories are obtained, the suggestion must be made to the patient that he will retain them in consciousness after awakening.

If there is a significant degree of secondary gain resulting from the presence of the amnesia itself, it may be very difficult for the therapist to persuade the patient to abandon his symptoms. When the amnesia is firmly fixed, one must consider the possibility that it is protecting the patient from a continuing difficult situation. At times, there may be an element of malingering in the patient's preservation of symptoms, but one should be careful of assuming that the patient is consciously pretending unless there is strong evidence to support the supposition.

The treatment measures aimed at the immediate symptoms of dissociative neurosis should ideally be combined with a therapeutic plan designed to help the patient with the basic conflicts that have resulted in symptom formation. The type of treatment used depends on the nature of the illness and of the circumstances in which it occurs. In patients who are responding to severe environmental stress through the use of dissociative mechanisms, it is often useful to provide a supportive relationship in combination with evironmental manipulation aimed at ameliorating the stressful situation, a therapeutic strategy that may also prevent further episodes of dissociation. In those patients in whom the dissociative phenomena arise against a background of intrapsychic conflict, a more radical approach aimed at developing insight may be attempted, combined with attempts to modulate the severity of the patient's superego demands when their excessiveness is a causative factor.

REFERENCES

Flournoy, T. *From India to the Planet Mars.* Harper & Brothers, New York, 1900.
Flournoy, T. Une mystique moderne. Arch. Psychol. (Génève), *15:* 1, 1915.
Janet, P. *L'automatisme psychologique.* Fèlix Alcan, Paris, 1889.
Kiersch, T. A. Amnesia: A clinical study of ninety-eight cases. Am. J. Psychiatry, *119:* 57, 1962.
Prince, M. *The Dissociation of a Personality.* Longmans, Green, New York, 1906.
Prince, M. *The Unconscious.* Macmillan, New York, 1924.

20.4 PHOBIC NEUROSIS

Definition

The second edition of the American Psychiatric Association's *Diagnostic and Statistical Manual of Mental Disorders* (DSM-II) says that phobic neurosis "is characterized by intense fear of an object or situation which the patient consciously recognizes as no real danger to him. . . . A wide range of phobias has been described".

In phobic neurosis, anxiety is a central component—no longer free-floating., as in anxiety neurosis, but attached to a specific idea, object, or situation. The anxiety is not justified by the stimulus that provokes it or is out of proportion to the real situation. The sufferer is completely aware of the irrationality of his reaction.

Epidemiology

Observations of children indicate that mild phobic manifestations are widespread during the early oedipal phase of growth and development; around the age of 3 or 4, most youngsters normally have occasional nightmares and sporadic, irrational fears of animals or common objects. There are, no doubt, many adults with circumscribed phobias that cause little in the way of disability and do not lead them to seek psychiatric help. Unless a phobic neurosis causes a marked impairment in function, such as results from a severe agoraphobia, it rarely requires hospitalization, and patients suffering from the disorder are frequently treated by private physicians. Estimates derived from outpatient clinic figures suggest that phobic neurosis constitutes less than 5 per cent of all neurotic disorders seen in patients over 18, occurring slightly more frequently in men than in women.

Clinical Description

Onset

With the exception of the school phobias of childhood, phobic neurosis usually begins in the late teens or early adulthood and is generally sudden in onset, heralded by the outburst of an attack of anxiety in the face of what is destined, from that time on, to be the phobic object or situation. More often than not, the reason for the appearance of symptoms is not immediately apparent.

Symptoms

The central and diagnostic symptom of phobic neurosis is the phobia. Phobias are characterized by the arousal in the patient of severe anxiety, often mounting to panic, in circumstances specific to each person—circumstances that do not warrant the emotional reactions evoked. In many patients, the anxiety may be compounded by a feeling of depersonalization. As a secondary response to his intense discomfort, the patient does everything in his power to avoid the situation that stimulates his phobic anxiety.

The kinds of phobic circumstances are legion, but a few are found with great regularity and probably account for the majority of the clinically significant phobic neuroses. Fears of streets and open spaces, of crowded and enclosed places (such as churches and theaters), and of vehicles of transporation (most notably, the airplane) are the most common. The severity of the syndrome and the incapacity resulting from it depend on the practical significance for the patient of the phobic circumstances. A phobia of planes that is a mere unpleasant curiosity to the person who does not have to fly can be a source of great discomfort, if not outright incapacity, to the person whose work requires him to make frequent long trips that necessitate air travel.

The characteristic irrationality of the fear that constitutes the central emotion of the phobia is well demonstrated in the following autobiographical fragment from a psychiatrist with a phobia of planes:

I was pampering my neurosis by taking the train to a meeting in Philadelphia. It was a nasty day out, the fog so thick you could see only a few feet ahead of your face, and the train, which had been late in leaving New York, was making up time by hurtling at a great rate across the flat land of New Jersey. As I sat there comfortably enjoying the ride, I happened to glance at the headlines of a late edition which one of the passengers who had boarded in New York was reading. "TRAINS CRASH IN FOG," ran the banner headlines, "10 DEAD, MANY INJURED." I reflected on our speed, the dense fog outside, and had a mild, transitory moment of concern that the fog might claim us victim, too, and then relaxed as I picked up the novel I had been reading. Some minutes later the thought suddenly entered my mind that had I not "chickened out" about flying, I might at that moment be overhead in a plane. At the mere image of sitting up there strapped in by a seat belt, my hands began to sweat, my heart to beat perceptibly faster, and I felt a kind of nervous uneasiness in my gut. The sensation lasted until I forced myself back to my book and forgot about the imagery.

I must say I found this experience a vivid lesson in the nature of phobias. Here I had reacted with hardly a flicker to an admittedly small, but real danger of accident, as evidence by the fog-caused train crash an hour or two earlier; and at the same time had responded to a purely imaginary situation with an unpleasant start of nervousness, experienced both as somatic symptoms, and as an inner sense of indescribable dread so characteristic of anxiety. The unreasonableness of the latter was highlighted for me by its contrast with the absence of concern about the speeding train, which if I had worried about it, would have been an apprehension grounded on real, external circumstances.

It is characteristic of the patient with an agoraphobic neurosis that he singles out one of two people in whose presence he has relative freedom of movement. He may become extremely dependent on and demanding of this obligatory companion. The person chosen is usually one with whom the patient has an ambivalent relationship, and the patient's can become a source of considerable inconvenience and exasperation for the person on whom the patient depends.

Erythrophobia (fear of blushing) can be a particularly painful and stubborn symptom. The symptom is restricted to situations in which other people are present. A change in color may not be at all evident to the observer, despite the fact that the patient, commonly a woman, insists that she feels bright red; the force of her fear often leads the patient to a severe restriction of her social life.

Fear of eating is another uncommon but troublesome kind of phobia. It may be limited to a dread of eating in the company of others, but in some patients the restriction applies to the intake of food under any circumstances. Patients frequently complain of severe anxiety mounting to panic if they are forced to eat and are able to gain relief only by vomiting or by taking large doses of cathartics in order to get the food out of their bodies. The avoidance of eating to prevent such anxiety is a true phobic mechanism.

Phobic anxiety can be hidden behind attitudes and behavior patterns that represent a denial that the dreaded object or situation is dangerous or that one is afraid of it. The counterphobic person, at times with a persistence that is almost obsessional, seeks out situations of danger and rushes enthusiastically toward them.

Causes

In *Inhibitions, Symptoms, and Anxiety*, published in 1926, Freud reached his final formulation of the phobic neurosis. This formulation has remained the analytical explanation of the disorder.

Freud viewed anxiety as the ego's reaction to danger. Anxiety had, as its major function, the task of signaling to the ego the fact that a forbidden unconscious drive was pushing for conscious expression, thus altering the ego to strengthen and marshal its defenses against the threatening instinctual force. In this new view, anxiety was seen not as the *result* of repression, which set in motion the transformation of affects and drives, but as the *cause* of repression through its stimulation of the ego to take defensive action.

In this new theoretical framework, Freud viewed the phobic neurosis as resulting from conflicts centered on an unresolved childhood oedipal situation. In the adult, the sexual drive continues to have a strong incestuous coloring, and its arousal tends to arouse anxiety. The anxiety then alerts the ego to exert repression to keep the drive away from conscious representation and discharge. When repression fails to be entirely successful in its function, the ego must call on auxiliary defenses. In phobic patients, these defenses involve primarily the use of displacement. The sexual conflict is displaced from the person who evokes the conflict to a seemingly unimportant, irrelevant object or situation, which now has the power to arouse the entire constellation of affects, including signal anxiety. The phobic object or situation selected usually has a direct associative connection with the primary source of the conflict. Furthermore, the situation or object is usually such that the patient is able to keep out of its way.

Writers like Lewin have developed the theory of the processes by which the phobic facade is created, pointing out the similarity between the manifest content of dreams and the associative links that tie the phobic object or situation to the basic conflict. In addition to castration anxiety, other forms of that affect, notably separation anxiety, are prominent in many phobias. And clinical observations indicate that aggression and pregenital sexual drives, as well as oedipal sexuality, may contribute to the formation of phobic symptoms.

In the classical stimulus-response theory, the conditioned stimulus is seen as gradually losing its potency to arouse a response if it is not reinforced by a periodic repetition of the unconditioned stimulus. In the phobic symptom, this attenuation of the response to the phobic (conditioned) stimulus does not occur, and the symptom may last for years without any apparent external reinforcement. In operant conditioning theory, however, anxiety is viewed as a drive that motivates the organism suffering from it to do what it can to obviate the painful affect. In the course of its random behavior, the animal soon learns that certain actions enable it to avoid the stimulus to anxiety and the consequent experience of pain. The avoidance patterns thus set up remain stable for long periods of time as a result of the reinforcement they receive from their success in drive reduction—that is, their capacity to diminish anxiety. This model is readily applicable to the phobia in which avoidance of the anxiety-provoking object or situation plays a central part. Such avoidance behavior becomes fixed as a stable symptom because of its effectiveness in protecting the patient from the phobic anxiety.

Course and Prognosis

Clinical experience suggests that phobic neurosis is a chronic disorder, with a frequent recurrence of symptoms that are resistant to most therapeutic measures. Some forms of phobic symptoms, particularly agoraphobia, are notoriously hard to manage and may cause the patient to lead a severely constricted life of psychologically induced incapacitation for years on end.

Differential Diagnosis

A clear-cut phobia is not difficult to recognize. When it constitutes the main clinical manifestation of an emotional disorder, it places the patient in the diagnostic category of phobic neurosis.

Occasionally, however, phobias are found in patients whose illness is primarily schizophrenic. At times, the onset of an acute schizophrenic episode is heralded by the sudden onset of phobic symptoms (along with other clinical manifestations usually thought of as neurotic, such as obsessions and compulsions), and they may also form part of the syndrome of pseudoneurotic schizophrenia. In other cases, the phobia coexists with other mental disturbances characteristic of chronic schizophrenia.

Treatment

A measure of activity on the part of the therapist is often required to get at the phobic anxiety. A growing body of clinical experience has made it evident that many phobic patients are not readily helped by analytical techniques, especially those suffering from phobias rooted in serious preoedipal conflicts. The decision to apply the techniques of psychodynamic insight therapy should be based on positive indications from the patient's ego structure and life patterns for the use of this treatment method.

The support afforded the patient by a positive relationship with his physician has a beneficial effect. The psychiatrist usually has to use active measures of encouragement, exhortation, instruction, and suggestion as he tries to help his patient overcome the dread of the phobic situation. The more the patient avoids what he fears, the more he is liable to fear it and to become discouraged and downhearted at his pusillanimity. If he can be persuaded to face the phobic situation and come through the experience with a measure of success, the increase in his self-esteem and self-confidence will make it easier for him to try it again. Each successful attempt makes the next less of an ordeal, and the vicious downward cycle of avoidance can, at times, be reversed so that the patient either loses his symptoms or so masters them that his life is no longer seriously constricted by the limitations they had previously imposed on his actions.

Hypnosis is useful not only in enhancing the suggestion that is a part of the therapist's generally supportive approach but in directly combating the anxiety arising from the phobic situation. The patient can be taught the techniques of autohypnosis, through which he can achieve a degree of relaxation when he is facing the phobic situation that will enable him to tolerate it.

Those patients who cannot be hypnotized may be taught techniques of muscular relaxation. In addition, the minor tranquilizers have a particularly important place in this aspect of the treatment of the phobic neurosis. Chlordiazepoxide hydrochloride and diazepam are both effective aids to the patient in his struggle with the phobic situation if they are taken in sufficient doses to produce relaxation.

In recent years, a number of dramatic cures of patients with phobic neurosis have been reported through the use of techniques derived from the concepts of learning theory. Various behavioral treatment techniques have been employed, the most common being a combination of desensitization and reciprocal inhibition. In desensitization, the patient is exposed serially to a predetermined list of anxiety-provoking stimuli graded in a heirarchy from the least to the most frightening. As he becomes desensitized to each stimulus in the scale, through techniques of progressive relaxation at each stage, the patient moves up to the next until what was the most productive of anxiety is no longer capable of eliciting the painful affect. Reciprocal inhibition refers to the principle of pairing the anxiety-provoking stimulus with another affect of an opposite quality strong enough to suppress the anxiety. Through the use of tranquilizing drugs, hypnosis, and instruction in the art of muscle relaxation, the patient is taught how to induce in himself both mental and physical repose. Once he has mastered these techniques, he is instructed to use them in the face of each anxiety-provoking stimulus in the hierarchy as these are presented to him seriatim, from the least to the most potent. This technique has proved successful in enabling patients to overcome their fearful reactions not only to phobic objects and situations but also to those stimuli that are naturally and inherently frightening. Recent studies suggest, however, that combining exposure to the phobic situation with relaxation procedures is no more effective than merely requiring the patient to face the anxiety-producing object or situation without relaxation.

Current interest in the area of behavior therapy is focused on the techniques of flooding and implosion. In flooding, the patient is required, usually in the presence of a supportive therapist, to face the phobic situation and experience the full storm of his anxiety for periods of time extending up to several hours a session. Implosion involves a similar lengthy experiencing of the extremes of anxiety as a response to the fantasy of the phobic object or situation, not to its actual presence. Long-lasting relief of symptoms has been reported after 10 to 20 flooding or implosion sessions, with results that are significantly better than those achieved by relaxation or other techniques.

REFERENCES

Fenichel, O. The counterphobic attitude. Int. J. Psychoanal., *20:* 263, 1939.

Ferenczi, S. The further development of an active therapy in psychoanalysis. In *Further Contributions to the Theory and Technique of Psycho-analysis*, S. Ferenczi, editor, p. 178. Hogarth Press, London, 1950.

Freud, S. Analysis of a phobia in a five-year-old boy. In *Standard Edition of the Complete Psychological Works of Sigmund Freud*, vol. 10, p. 5, Hogarth Press, London, 1955.

Janet, P. *Les Obsessions et al Psychasthenie*, 2 vols. Félix Alcan, Paris, 1903.

Marks, I. M. Flooding (implosion) and allied treatments. In *Behavior Modification, Principles and Clinical Applications*, W. S. Agras, editor. Little, Brown, Boston, 1972.

Roth, M. The phobic anxiety-depersonalization syndrome. Proc. R. Soc. Med., *52:* 587, 1959.

20.5.   OBSESSIVE-COMPULSIVE NEUROSIS

Introduction

Freud's first psychodynamic formulations were created to account for the formation of the symptoms of conversion hysteria. When an idea is incompatible with a person's ego (so ran his theory), the affect associated with the idea is rendered unconscious by repression and is converted into a sensorimotor disturbance that symbolically represents the unacceptable idea. The formulation was satisfactory, for it adequately explained the observed clinical manifestations of conversion hysteria.

It soon became apparent, however, that the theory was not adequate to explain other forms of neurotic symptoms. In patients suffering from obsessions and phobias, for example, the predominant clinical manifestations are not somatic but psychic; instead of being disabled by disturbances in his sensations or motor functions, the patient is afflicted by distressing, consciously experienced ideas. Furthermore, in contrast to hysterical symptoms, these ideas are accompanied by an acute, conscious awareness of such painful emotions as anxiety and shame. Freud separated off from the somatosensory symptoms of hysteria a group of symptoms characterized by thier psychical nature.

Definition

The word "obsessive" (or "obsession") refers to an intrusive idea or thought. The word "compulsive" (or "compulsion") refers to an urge or impulse to action that, when put into operation, leads to a compulsive act.

Obsessions and compulsions have certain features in common: (1) An idea or an impulse obtrudes itself insistently, persistently, and impellingly into the person's conscious awareness. (2) A feeling of anxious dread accompanies the central manifestation and frequently leads the person to take countermeasures against the initial idea or impulse. (3) The obsession or compulsion is ego-alien—that is, it is experienced as being foreign to and not a usual part of one's experience of oneself as a psychological being; it is undesired, unacceptable, and uncontrollable. (4) No matter how vivid and compelling the obsession or compulsion, the person recognizes it as absurd and irrational; he retains his insight. (5) Finally, the person suffering from these manifestations feels a strong need to resist them.

Most of these characteristics are embodied in the official definition of the disorder given in the second edition of The American Psychiatric Association's *Diagnostic and Statistical Manual of Mental Disorders* (DSM-II). Obsessive-compulsive neurosis "is characterized by the persistent intrusion of unwanted thoughts, urges, or actions that the patient is unable to stop. The

thoughts may consist of single words or ideas, ruminations, or trains of thought often perceived by the patient as nonsensical. The actions vary from simple movements to complex rituals such as repeated handwashing. Anxiety and distress are often present either if the patient is prevented from completing his compulsive ritual or if he is concerned about being unable to control it himself."

Epidemiology

Scattered anecdotal evidence indicates that obsessive-compulsive neurosis has occurred throughout history. Those who have studied the natural history of the disorder have found an incidence that is never higher than 5 per cent of all neurotic patients.

There appears to be no significant sexual difference in the disorder. A large proportion of obsessive-compulsive patients remain unmarried, up to 50 per cent in some surveys. Recent studies indicate that the frequency of the disorder is higher in upper-class persons and in those with high intelligence.

Clinical Description

Onset

The onset of the disorder occurs predominantly in adolescence or early adulthood. The symptoms first appear in more than two thirds of the patients by the time they are 25 and frequently before the age of 10. In less than 5 per cent do the symptoms begin for the first time after the fourth decade of life. As compared with patients suffering from hysterical symptoms or anxiety, those with obsessions and compulsions seek professional help at an earlier age. In more than half of the patients a clear environmental precipitating event can be found.

Symptoms

The phenomena may be manifested psychically or behaviorally; they may be experienced as ideas or as impulses; they may refer to events anticipated in the future or actions already completed; they may express desires and wishes or protective measures against such desires; they may be simple, uncomplicated acts and ideas or elaborate, ritualized patterns of thinking and behavior; their meaning may be obvious to the most unsophisticated observer, or they may be the end result of highly complicated psychological condensations and distortions that yield their secret only to the skilled investigator.

Psychic Manifestations. *Obsessional Thoughts.* Perhaps the simplest of the psychic symptoms are those in which thoughts, words, or mental images are obtruded against the patient's will into his conscious awareness.

A special form of forced preoccupation with thoughts is designated by the term "obsessive-ruminative states." The central feature is rumination about a topic or problem, often of a religious or abstrusely philosophical nature. The pros and cons of the questions are repetitively considered, and imponderables are weighed in a prolonged, fruitless, and inconclusive inner dialogue filled with doubting and despair.

Compulsions. In another form of the psychic phenomena, ideas and images may be present, but the central feature is an irrational impulse to some form of action. The impulse, however, remains merely an impulse and is not acted on by the patient, no matter how fearful he may be that he will lose control of his behavior.

The patient may feel the impulse to jump out of a window of a high building or to throw himself in the path of a moving train or car, or his aggressions may be aimed at others, rather than himself. The aggressive compulsion need not be physical but may be an urge toward an act of defiance or one that is socially inappropriate or shocking, such as shouting obscenities in church. Although these impulses do not lead to action, they frequently arouse strong anxiety in the patient and cause him to avoid the situation or object that evokes the impulse.

Behavioral Manifestations. When these obsessive-compulsive phenomena are psychic, no one knows that there is anything unusual going on in the patient unless he chooses to divulge his purely private experiences. In the case of compulsive acts, the phenomena are behavioral and usually visible to anyone who is there to see them. Often, out of shame or embarrassment, the patient tries to restrict his actions to those times when he is alone. There are two principal types of compulsive acts: those that give expression to the primary urges or impulses that underlie them and those that are a reaction to or an attempt to control the primary impulse.

Compulsive acts that simply and directly express the underlying urges are rare. In most instances the compulsion expressing an urge remains in the psychic sphere and is not visible in action, except when it contaminates a compulsive act that began as a controlling maneuver.

In general, compulsive acts are or, at least, begin as attempts to control or modify a primary obsession or compulsion, either because the patient fears the consequences of his obsession or because he is afraid that he will not be able to control his impulse. Such defensive compulsive acts are used to contain, neutralize, or ward off the feared results of concurrent obsessions and compulsions, or they may represent a desire to make sure that some action in the past has not led to disaster.

At times, the patient's compulsive behavior becomes highly elaborate and repetitively sterotyped in the form of compulsive rituals. On going to bed, for example, the process of undressing must conform to an exact pattern. Any deviation in the pattern arouses anxiety in the patient, and he must be certain that all has been done properly before he can drop off to sleep.

The element of doubt is often found in connection with compulsive acts performed to ward off the feared consequences of obsessional ideas and compulsive urges. The patient is never sure that he has contained his ever-pressing impulses, that they have not somehow leaked out inadvertently into his behavior or in some other way created the trouble he is at such pains to avoid. And often the patient's concerns are justified. Despite the best of his cautious intentions, the underlying impulse may manifest itself in the very process of carrying out defensive compulsive acts and may distort these actions so that they achieve or, at least, seem to the patient to achieve exactly the effect they are designed to prevent. One of Freud's patients, for example, spent hours saying simple prayers designed to combat obsessional ideas of harm coming to others, but when he wished to say, "May God protect him," he would find the words coming out, "May God *not* protect him."

Character Traits. The person who exhibits obsessive-compulsive character traits has been described as having an obsessional character, an anal personality, or an anancastic personality. All these terms refer to a group of behavioral phenomena characterized by control, in contrast to the hysterical personality, in which a tendency toward a flamboyant expression of fantasies and feelings predominates.

The person with obsessional personality traits is cautious, deliberate, thoughtful, and rational in his approach to life and its problems and may appear dry and pedantic when these traits are carried to an extreme. He emphasizes reason and logic at the expense of feeling and intuition, and he does his best to be objective and to avoid being carried away by subjective enthusiasms. As a result, he often appears sober and emotionally distant, but at the same time he is a person with great steadiness of purpose, reliability, and ernest conscientiousness. What he lacks in flexibility, imagination, and inventiveness, he makes up for in a conservative cautiousness about change that provides a salutary balance to the transient but violent enthusiasms of others.

In addition, he likes to feel that he has control of his environment. Neatness, orderliness, and tidiness characterize his arrangement of space, as does punctuality his management of time. He likes people and institutions that behave predictably and conform to his predilections. He can be surprisingly obstinate and stubborn when challenged or contradicted. He sets great store by justice and honesty, has a strong sense of property rights, manages his own resources with frugality, and does not easily part with his possessions.

The presence of obsessional character traits is not in itself an indication of abnormality. On the contrary, they may be a great asset to their owners, and society owes much of its stability and its efficiency to its more obsessional members. It is only when such traits are carried to an extreme or when the balance between control and impulse expression leads to paralysis that they became a liability. Furthermore, there is no necessary connection between obsessional character traits and obsessive-compulsive symptoms. The obsessional personality in the population is far more common than obsessive-compulsive neurosis, which is relatively infrequent.

Mental Status

The patient retains full insight. He recognizes that his pathological thoughts and impulses are unreasonable and alien to the mainstream of his personality.

The patient is often neatly dressed and groomed, sometimes with almost fussy tidiness. Reserved and formal in manner, he sits before the examiner stiff and prim, showing little in the way of gestures or facial expression, and his movements are careful and precise without spontaneity or easy grace. The controlled quality of his posture and movement is matched in his speech. His sentences may be long and involved and full of stilted phraseology or sterotyped expressions. He characteristically balances one clause against another. He says the same thing several times in succession. He qualifies any direct statement with words like "maybe," "perhaps," or "possibly" to avoid sounding dogmatic or to escape being caught in an error. He relies heavily on rational argument and talks in highly intellectual and intellectualized terms about the simplest matters. He recounts events in infinite detail, with a painful attention to accuracy and completeness, sometimes referring to written notes he has brought with him. Often, it turns out that he has rehearsed what he plans to say in the interview for hours before it takes place and has tried to anticipate every move and question the interviewer may introduce. Any attempt to hurry him along, to cut him short, to switch to another topic is met by the patient's resistance and rigid adherence to his preconceived program of action. Evidence or expression of emotion, save possibly controlled anxiety, is at a minimum or entirely absent. If he is sophisticated about psychiatric theory, and such patients ofter are, he will discourse at length about his conflicts, his defenses, his aggression, or his libido. But in answer to direct questioning, he denies having any of the feelings related to these words.

Despite the psychiatrist's attempts to focus on and to promote the expression of emotion, the patient maintains his formality and his distance. A meaningful, warm, affective relationship appears to develop very slowly, if it develops at all. And yet in many patients evidence of a strong dependence on the doctor can be found early in the relationship, despite their attempts to control their emotions.

Course and Prognosis

On first consulting a physician for their difficulty, two thirds of the patients give a history of prior episodes of obsessive-compulsive symptoms, some 10 to 15 per cent having first experienced them before the age of 10. The large majority of patients have had only one such prior attack, although a good number, roughly 30 per cent, have experienced two or three episodes. In 85 per cent of these attacks the duration was less than a year, although some attacks may have lasted 4 to 5 years.

One to 10 years after treatment, some 15 per cent are well, 45 per cent are improved, and 40 per cent are unchanged or worse. Those considered improved fall into two groups: patients whose symptoms have lessened to a point at which they are able to work and function socially and those who run a fluctuating course, often with long periods of complete remission of symptoms.

In general, obsessive-compulsive neurosis is a chronic disorder, often following a remitting course. The prognosis is better (1) the shorter the duration of symptoms before the patient is first seen, (2) the greater the element of environmental stress associated with the onset of the disorder, (3) the better the environment to which the patient must return after treatment, and (4) the better his general social adjustment and relationship.

Causes

Psychoanalytic Theories

Psychodynamic Factors. *Isolation.* Isolation is a defense mechanism that protects a person from anxiety-provoking affects and impulses by separating them from their ideational components and pushing them out of consciousness. If isolation is completely successful, the impulse and its associated affect are totally repressed, and the patient is consciously aware only of the affectless idea that is related to it. If isolation is less effective, the impulse and its associated affect cannot be completely restrained from entering the patient's consciousness. He experiences a partial awareness of the impulse without fully recognizing its meaning or significance. He may, for example, have frightening and compelling murderous impulses toward strangers or casual acquaintances; here, the impulse makes itself felt as an urge to violent action, but the direction of the urge is displaced from the true object of the patient's aggression to other people in his environment. At the same time, isolation exerts a partial effect by rendering the patient unaware that he is angry, so that he is puzzled, mystified, and disturbed by his compulsions.

Undoing. In the face of the constant threat of the impulse to escape the primary defense of isolation and break free, further secondary defensive operations are required to combat it and to quiet the anxiety that the imminent eruption of the impulse into consciousness arouses in the patient. A particularly important secondary defensive operation is the mechanism of undoing, a compulsive act that is performed in an attempt to prevent or undo the consequences that the patient irrationally anticipates from a frightening obsessional thought or impulse.

Reaction Formation. Reaction formation results in the formation of character traits, rather than symptoms. It involves manifest patterns of behavior and consciously experienced attitudes that are exactly the opposite of the underlying impulses. Often these patterns appear to an observer to be highly exaggerated and at times quite inappropriate.

Psychogenetic Factors. Among the striking features of patients with obsessive-compulsive neurosis is the degree to which they are preoccupied with aggression or dirt, either overtly in the content of their symptoms or in the associations that lie behind them. This and other observations have led to the proposition that the psychogenesis of the obsessive-compulsive disorder lies in disturbances in normal growth and development related to the anal-sadistic phase. Normally, the impulses associated with the anal-sadistic phase are modified in the oedipal and succeeding stages of development. If, however, disturbances occur in this developmental process, unmodified anal-sadistic impulses remain as components of the person's psychological make-up.

Regression. In the classic analytical formulation, regression is the central mechanism in the formation of obsessive-compulsive neurosis and determines that a person will develop that disorder rather than conversion hysteria. According to psychoanalytic theory, in conversion hysteria the patient represses oedipal genital libido, the energy from this undischarged impulse being then converted into somatic symptoms. The obsessive-compulsive patient may begin with a conflict over the oedipal genital impulse. However, instead of a repressing and converting this impulse; he abandons the genital impulses and regresses to the earlier anal-sadistic phase of psychosexual development. The return to that earlier stage is facilitated by the fixation points that have remained from the distortions that occurred during his childhood development.

As a result of the regressive movement of psychic energies, all the anal-sadistic impulses from the earlier phase of development are reinforced, augmented, and strengthened. The pressure of reactivated anal and aggressive impulses arouses new anxieties and new conflicts and requires new defensive operations. Prominent among these emergency measures are isolation, undoing, and displacement. These defenses, in conjunction with the constantly pressing impulses, lead to the appearance of obsessive-compulsive symptoms.

Ambivalence. Ambivalence is the direct result of a change in the characteristics of the impulse life. It is an important feature of the normal child during the anal-sadistic developmental phase—that is, he feels both love and murderous hate toward an object. In the normal course of development, much of the aggression is neutralized, and what remains becomes a desire to win out over the other person rather than to destroy him. When regression occurs, ambivalence is a characteristic mode of feeling. This conflict of opposing emotions may be seen in the doing-undoing patterns of behavior and paralyzing doubt in the face of choices that are frequently found in patients with this emotional disorder.

Magical Thinking. In the phenomenon of magical thinking, the regression uncovers earlier modes of thought, rather than impulses. Inherent in magical thinking is omnipotence of thought. The patient feels that, merely by thinking about an event in the external world, he can cause that event to occur without intermediate physical actions.

Changes in the Superego. The standards and ideals of the mature person are generally within the limits of potential achievement, and for the most part he lives at peace with his conscience, which pricks him only when he has clearly violated his ethical principles. In the patient with obsessive-compulsive neurosis, the number and range of mental and behavioral activities that are taboo are markedly increased, the patient has a heightened self-awareness and self-criticalness, and he becomes harsher in his self-judgments. There has been a regression to developmentally earlier stages of the infantile superego—the harsh, exacting, punitive characteristics of which now reappear in the mental functioning of the neurotically ill adult.

Learning Theory

According to learning theory, the obsession represents a conditioned stimulus to anxiety. Because of an association with an unconditioned anxiety-provoking stimulus, the originally neutral obsessional thought gains the capacity to arouse anxiety; that is, a new mode of behavior has been learned. The compulsion is established when the person discovers that a certain action reduces the anxiety attached to the obsessional thought. The relief brought about when the anxiety, which operates as a negative drive state, is reduced by the performance of the compulsive act reinforces that act. Gradually, because of its usefulness in reducing a painful secondary drive (the anxiety), the act becomes fixed in a learned pattern of behavior.

But in its present form, learning theory leaves many questions unanswered, such as the reason for the obsessional preoccupation with ideas that provoke anxiety (one would expect an avoidance of them), the magical quality of the thought processes in the obsessive-compulsive phenomena, and the special prominence of ideas concerning dirt and aggression.

Differential Diagnosis

Phobic Neurosis

In general, phobic neurosis is characterized by anxiety that harm will come to the phobic person from an external object or situation, and the patient controls his anxiety by avoiding the object. The important mechanisms in phobia formation are displacement and projection, and the underlying conflicts are often oedipal in nature. In obsessive-compulsive neurosis, the patient fears that he will hurt others, his anxiety is controlled by compulsive acts and by the mechanisms of undoing and isolation, and the underlying conflicts are predominantly pre-oedipal in nature. However, it is not possible in every instance to make a sharp distinction between phobic and obsessive-compulsive neuroses.

Depression

In obsessive-compulsive neurosis, hope still exists. Although evil impulses are attacking with all their forces, the patient still resists. In depression, the patient has surrendered to the besiegers. He acknowledges his wickedness in guilty despair and, utterly alone, hopelessly anticipates the punishment of the damned.

The depressed patient tends to retreat from his relationships with others. In the obsessive-compulsive patient, the emotional tie to other people remains intact, but it has the coloring of ambivalence.

Schizophrenia

No matter how bizarre the content of the obsessive-compulsive patient's thoughts or how strange his acts, he usually maintains full contact with reality and is painfully aware of the absurdity of his thinking and behavior. No matter how preoccupied he may appear to be with his symptoms, he does not retreat from his relationships with the people around him, and his affect remains appropriate.

Treatment

Psychotherapy

It is possible to effect a complete disappearance of compulsive behavior in some patients by the simple device of informing them that the doctor will assume complete responsibility for anything that may happen as a result of their impulses. With this reassurance an occasional patient may abruptly give up a chronic compulsive ritual. Unfortunately, the improvement usually lasts for only a few hours. The patient begins to doubt the doctor's capacity to assume responsibility and soon returns to his compulsive acts.

In general, the more chronic and fixed the sympton pattern, the less liable the disorder is to modification by psychotherapy or, in fact, any treatment measure. The criteria in choosing patients for insight psychotherapy depend primarily on factors other than symptoms: (1) the prominence of situational precipitating events, (2) capacity to relate to the physician, (3) evidence of good relationships with others, (4) stable work patterns, (5) capacity to tolerate anxiety and depression, (6) ability to express emotion, (7) intelligence, (8) ability to be introspective, and (9) flexibility in thinking and behavior.

Occasionally when obsessional rituals and anxiety reach an intolerable intensity, it may be necessary to hospitalize the patient until the shelter of an institution and the removal from external environmental stresses bring the symptoms to a more tolerable level. And any psychotherapeutic endeavors must include attention to family members through the provision of emotional support, reassurance, explanation, and advice on how to manage and respond to the patient.

Behavior Therapy

Behavior therapists ignore the complexities of the conflicts and personality disturbances that underlie the clinical phenomena and focus almost entirely on the removal of symptoms. Behavior therapy has been applied primarily to patients with phobias, but a few cases of obsessive-compulsive neurosis appear to have responded to the technique of flooding by forcing the patient to face the obsession-producing situation and preventing him from carrying out his defensive compulsive rituals. Flooding may be combined with modeling, in which the therapist first carries out the anxiety-producing actions he wants the patient to imitate.

Physical Therapies

No drugs have a specific action on the obsessive-compulsive symptoms themselves, but the use of sedatives and tranquilizers as an adjunct to psychotherapy may be helpful when anxiety is excessive. Likewise, electric shock treatment and antidepressant medication appear to have no direct effect on obsessions and compulsions. But if these symptoms are secondary phenomena to a primary mood disorder, physical treatment may improve them, along with the affective distrubance.

Leukotomy has been recommended by some authors. As a general rule, one wishes to avoid irreversible surgical procedures on the brain in patients with psychogenic disorders, particularly when these disorders run an intermittent course. However, leukotomy can lessen the intensity of obsessions and compulsions and can diminish the suffering they engender. On this basis, it should be considered when a chronic, severe, unremitting obsessive-compulsive neurosis has not responded to any of the less drastic forms of treatment.

REFERENCES

Abraham, K. Contributions to the theory of the anal character. In *Selected Papers*, p. 370.. Hogarth Press, London, 1942.

Fenichel, O. *Outline of Clinical Psychoanalysis*. W. W. Norton, New York, 1934.

Freud, S. Notes upon a case of obsessional neurosis. In *Standard Edition of the Complete Psychological Works of Sigmund Freud*, vol. 10, p. 153. Hogarth Press, London, 1955.

Janet, P., and Raymond, F. *Les obsessions et la psychasthénie*, 2 vols. Félix Alcan, Paris, 1903.

Pollitt, J. D. Natural history studies in mental illness: A discussion based on a pilot study of obsessional states. J. Ment. Sci., *106:* 93, 1960.

Salzman, L. *The Obsessive Personality.* Science House, New York, 1968.

20.6.   DEPRESSIVE NEUROSIS

Definition

According to the second edition of the American Psychiatric Association's *Diagnostic and Statistical Manual of Mental Disorders* (DSM-II), depressive neurosis "is manifested by an excessive reaction of depression to an internal conflict or to an identifiable event such as the loss of a love object or cherished possession. It is to be distinguished from *Involutional Melancholia* and *Manic-depressive* illness. *Reactive depressions* or *Depressive reactions* are to be classified here."

Epidemiology

The person with depressive neurosis usually remains an outpatient. Estimates from outpatient clinics indicate that roughly 5 to 10 per cent of all patients evaluated in such settings are suffering from depressive neurosis as the primary disorder. Those patients who visit a private psychiatrist or are treated by their medical physician are not included in these statistics, but they must be legion. Suffice it to say that the disorder is ubiquitous.

Clinical Description

Onset

A precipitant can almost invariably be found to have set in motion the processes leading to the appearance of depressive neurosis. The loss of a valued person or possession or a situation resulting in a lowering of self-esteem may trigger depression. The more sensitive a person is to such events, the less it takes to bring on the symptoms of the illness. The most common precipitants are separations from loved ones by death, departure, or rejection. Persons whose self-esteem is based on being active, vigorous, independent and self-sufficient often become profoundly depressed when faced with a chronically disabling physical illness. The resulting mood disorder may secondarily complicate and intensify the symptoms of the primary illness.

In general, the onset of depression after a discrete triggering event is abrupt, and the symptoms develop rapidly. Depressions may, however, evolve more slowly, especially when the person is exposed to a chronically troubling situation, such as marital difficulties, unsatisfactory working conditions, or financial worries that gradually reduce his psychological resiliency.

Symptoms

Central to depressive neurosis is the symptom of depressive affect. Associated with the patient's feeling of loneliness, desolation, and melancholy is a sense of inner deadness, apathy, and unresponsiveness to the world around him, accompanied by a loss of interest in human relationships that creates in him an emotional isolation from his friends and relatives. He experiences a certain irritability and anger at people in his surroundings. Throughout is a sense of loss, of change, of something missing in the world, and his perceptions of that world are colored by the bleakness of his inner state. His language, moreover, reflects and evokes gloom and depression. One finds, too, suggestions of somatic sensations: suffocation, nausea, and weariness. But he maintains a certain degree of insight.

A closely related phenomenon is the tendency of the depressed patient to varying degrees of harsh self-criticism. The central thread is a sense of lessened self-worth, of lowered self-esteem, as he measures himself against the standards of his ideals and decides that he has fallen short of the mark.

In some patients, physical symptoms may play a leading role and on occasion may be all that appears on the surface. Fatigue, headaches, insomnia, back pain, poorly localized discomfort in the limbs, and undiagnostic gastrointestinal symptoms may initially mask an underlying depression.

The patient's facial expression is glum and dispirited, his voice flat and colorless, his posture slumped and lifeless, and he often appears pale, wan, and fatigued. He may sigh, tear, or openly cry as he talks about his troubles, but he remains in contact with the examiner. His mood may vary during the course of an interview, the sadness deepening as one touches on troubling topics but giving way to a smile, even a laugh, if the subject warrants it. Many patients exhibit a passive, clinging, dependent, beseeching, at times demanding quality in their relationship with the doctor. In some an irritability and a biting, sarcastic aggressiveness of speech and manner may be more prominent than the depressive features.

Personality Features

Pessimism, a looking on the darker side of life, a confident expectation that things will turn out wrong, a dissatisfaction with oneself and one's lot, a lack of self-confidence and diffidence, a tendency to have one's feelings easily hurt, a penchant for sadness, loneliness and *Weltschmerz*, a degree of chronic irritability, a subtle passivity and demandingness—all the qualities that characterize depressive illness may, if woven into the fabric of the personality, determine a persistent view of the world and a habitual response to life that appear on the surface as depressive character traits. However, the person with a depressive personality structure does not invariably develop a depressive illness.

The emotionality, the tendency to dramatize, and the exhibitionism of those with hysterical personalities may make a depression from which they are suffering appear to be more serious than it really is. They cry easily and copiously, complain loudly of their misery and despair, make vigorous demands for attention and medication, and generally dramatize their depressed state. The manipulative aspect of hysterical character traits may give cause for concern about a coincident depression, especially when it leads the patient to threaten and often to attempt suicide. Suicide itself is generally not a feature of depressive neurosis, but the gestural suicide attempt is a frequent occurrence. On occasion, a gestural suicide attempt leads to serious physical consequences, even death.

Depression in those with obsessional personalities is often muted and underplayed. Depressive affect may be largely or totally absent, and the patient may appear merely dull and apathetic.

Causes

Four basic factors are involved in the production of depressive neurosis: (1) the immediate changes in mood as a response to an environmental loss, disappointment, or deprivation, (2) changes in the level of self-esteem, (3) conflicts over the aggressive drive, and (4) a pre-existing personality structure—characterized by narcissism, dependency, and ambivalence—that helps to determine the quality and quantity of the first three factors listed.

Mood

The sadness, loneliness, and despair of grief normally follow on the loss of a treasured person or object. Environmental events may bring about profound alterations in mood and accompanying somatic functions, and normal grief and depressive illness have many features in common. But there are differences. When the severity of the reaction is such that the person cannot function outside a hospital, this quantitative fact in itself tends to place the response in the category of depressive neurosis. In addition, dependency, self-criticism, and aggression are important factors in the development of pathological depressive reactions.

Self-Esteem and Personality Structure

Lowered self-esteem is so intimately associated with depression that it is in many instances a *sine qua non*. The normal person—although usually enjoying a reasonable degree of autonomy, self-confidence, and self-assurance—frequently finds his self-esteem assaulted and diminished by a variety of situations and events. But his bouts of despondency are neither long in duration nor incapacitating in degree, and he has a variety of ways of restoring his emotional equilibrium. The person who is abnormally dependent on other people usually finds himself in difficulties when faced by a situation that lowers his self-esteem. His self-assessment tends to be more harshly critical, and his confidence in his capabilities and his basic worth is generally shaky. Faced with an event that hits at his self-esteem, he has little in the way of resources to combat its diminution, and his consequent despondency may be prolonged and severe. In the relative absence of inner resources, he turns to other people for emotional support and reassurance and frequently needs a constant supply of these externally derived strengths to maintain his unstable equilibrium. The number of people on whom he feels he can depend is often extremely restricted, frequently being limited to a singly highly important person. If his self-esteem is lowered as the result of failing to achieve a goal, he may feel that others are critical and rejecting of him. The resulting despair and depression at this imagined loss compound the original feeling of worthlessness. If he suffers the actual loss of a needed person, the consequences can be profoundly disturbing, since he has lost the source of his desperately needed emotional support, and the depression that results may be of severely pathological proportions.

Aggression

Highly dependent relationships are usually ambivalent in nature. Within such a relationship the potential for anger remains strong, and a major source of stimuli to its arousal lies in the failure to receive satisfaction for dependency needs.

Course and Prognosis

Empirical clinical experience suggests that the course is of shorter duration and the outlook for recovery is better in those cases in which the precipitating factor is a single event or set of events circumscribed in time, the precipitating event is a more significant factor in the appearance of depression than the personality structure, and the complications resulting from conflicts over aggression are absent or minimal.

A psychologically healthy person may be overwhelmed and temporarily incapacitated if the precipitating event is realistically catastrophic, but he ordinarily recovers completely, given time and protection from further environmental buffets. But a person with severe personality conflicts concerning dependency and aggression may develop a moderately severe depressive neurosis as the result of a minor environmental insult, and his illness is liable to be longer and more incapacitating.

There is a point at which the person ceases merely to respond directly to an external stimulus; the process set in motion by the environmental precipitant is carried on independently.

Diagnosis

Quantitatively, one considers a depression to be pathological if it is too severe a response to the magnitude of the precipitating event or if a response to a serious loss is too prolonged. The acute manifestations of normal grief should ordinarily no longer be in evidence by the end of 6 months; if they are more protracted, neurotic mechanisms should be suspected. Conversely, the absence of grief in the face of a significant loss should lead one to consider the possibility

that pathological intrapsychic forces are at work.

From a qualitative standpoint, the case for making the diagnosis of depressive neurosis is strengthened if the manifestations of depressive affect and lowered self-esteem are found in patients with a prior history of neurotic symptoms or of personality traits involving conflicts over dependency and aggression. Furthermore, evidence of the presence of specific psychological conflicts in patients manifesting depression, such as those associated with debilitating illness or with chronic dissatisfaction over one's sexual role, lends support to the diagnosis of pathological depression.

Differential Diagnosis

Depressive affect may be observed in patients with a variety of neurotic conditions, but generally the presence of specific symptoms determine the appropriate diagnostic category. Anxiety and depression often coexist in the same patient, and the ultimate diagnosis must rest on the judgment of the clinician as to which affect is the more significant.

The presence of marked changes in bodily function—such as severe anorexia, weight loss, constipation, insomnia, and psychomotor retardation—as well as depressive delusions and serious suicidal preoccupations, place the depressive illness at the psychotic end of the spectrum. In disorders that fall in the middle range, the clinician has few differentiating diagnostic aids.

Schizophrenic patients may show depressive affect or may exhibit an apathy that appears superficially like depression. On closer examination, however, the apathy usually proves to be an emptiness or dulling of affective tone, rather than the more positively painful experience that constitutes true depression. Furthermore, the typical manifestations of schizophrenic thought disturbances readily distinguish the two disorders in most cases.

The fatigue and enervation associated with subacute infectious illnesses and with infectious mononucleosis may somtimes be confused with depressive neurosis, and hypothyroidism has occasionally been similarly mistaken for a depressive illness. The absence of any clear-cut precipitating emotional trauma and the presence of diagnostic laboratory findings in patients with somatic illnesses ordinarily make the differentiation clear.

In the elderly, depression may be associated with early degenerative disease of the brain. Such tissue changes should be suspected in older patients complaining of depression. In all such instances a careful mental status and evaluation of cognitive functions, as well as appropriate neurological studies, should be undertaken.

Treatment

Psychotherapeutic Measures

One of the most immediately helpful things for the patient in the midst of an acute depression is the supportive relationship provided by the physician, and the opportunity to talk about his troubles is often all that a patient needs to see him through a bad period. Since environmental circumstances are usually a significant factor in depressive neuroses, the psychiatrist may often find it useful to help the patient with practical suggestions toward altering those environmental elements that can be changed. Furthermore, since dependency needs are often closely related to the depressed state, the physician may wish to help the patient find other appropriate relationships in his environment. Nor should the physician hesitate to consult with the patient's relatives, not only to help them understand what the patient is experiencing but also to aid and encourage them in providing support to the patient in their relationships with him.

The decision to use insight psychotherapy for patients with depressive neuroses should be based not primarily on the nature of their symptoms but on the presence of those criteria referable to ego functions that indicate the likelihood of a good response to such therapy. Often enough, insight therapy is not necessary, especially in those patients whose depression is the result of severe external traumata temporarily overwhelming a relatively mature personality. Furthermore, practical clinical experience indicates that the sensitive, dependent, ambivalent patient often does not have the capacity to respond to insight therapy and can best be helped by supportive measures.

In patients with pathological grief reactions whose grief work has been blocked by unresolved aggression toward the lost person, careful uncovering of the unconscious anger in the course of insight psychotherapy can thaw out the emotional freeze and enable the patient to express both his anger and his grief and thus lose the depressive symptoms.

When the depressive neurosis arises from marital difficulties, recourse to marital therapy should be considered.

Chemotherapy

The use of chemical agents often has a central place in the treatment of patients with depressive neuroses, the tricyclic antidepressants, especially imipramine and amitryptiline, being the drugs of choice. To reduce the incidence of common side effects, such as hypotension and blurring of vision (about which the patient should be informed), one generally starts the medication at lower than optimal doses, beginning with 25 mg t.i.d. and increasing the dosage 25 mg every 4 or 5 days until a maximum of 250 to 300 mg daily has been reached. One should not consider drug treatment to be ineffective until the patient has been continued on full doses for 3 to 4 weeks without therapeutic results.

The MAO inhibitors are generally reserved for patients with psychotic depressions who have not responded to a trial of tricyclic drugs, and there is a growing trend against using the MAO inhibitors at all because of the frequent serious side effects. In addition, amphetamines in various forms and combined with barbiturates (Dexamyl) are often useful in mild depressive states. They can be used for short periods of time to combat lethargy, withdrawal, and depressed moods in these patients. For night-time sedation, chlorol hydrate, diazepam, or barbiturates are of use. It is best to prescribe all medications in small amounts if the clinician suspects a suicidal risk. Drugs should never be allowed to become a substitute for a relationship with the doctor.

REFERENCES

Bibring, E. The Mechanism of Depression. In *Affective Disorders*, P. Greenacre, editor, p. 13. International Universities Press, New York, 1953.

Freud, S. Mourning and melancholia. In *Standard Edition of the Complete Psychological Works of Sigmund Freud*, vol. 14, p. 243. Hogarth Press, London, 1957.

Hill, D. Depression: Disease, reaction, or posture? Am. J. Psychiatry, *125*: 445, 1968.

Lewis, A. J. Melancholia: A clinical survey of depressive states. J. Ment. Sci., *80*: 277, 1934.

Lindemann, E. Symptomatology and management of acute grief. Am. J. Psychiatry, *101*: 141, 1944.

Rochlin, G. *Griefs and Discontents*. Little, Brown, Boston, 1965.

Schidkraut, J. J. Neuropharmacology of the affective disorders. Ann. Res. Pharmacol., *13*: 427, 1973.

20.7.   NEURASTHENIC NEUROSIS

Definition

According to the second edition of the American Psychiatric Association's *Diagnostic and Statistical Manual of Mental Disorders* (DSM-II) neurasthenic neurosis "is characterized by complaints of chronic weakness, easy fatigability, and sometimes exhaustion. Unlike hysterical neurosis the patient's complaints are genuinely distressing to him and there is no evidence of secondary gain. It differs from *Anxiety neurosis* and from the *Psychophysiologic disorders* in the nature of the predominant complaint. It differs from *Depressive neurosis* in the moderateness of the depression and in the chronicity of its course."

Clinical Description

In the older literature, various precipitating factors were described, the emphasis generally being placed on mental and physical overwork, especially in situations conducive to emotional tension. Other events—such as the death of a loved one, the excessive use of stimulants or narcotics, infective fevers, and the "abuse of the sexual organs"—were found to produce symptoms in specific individual cases. The onset of the disorder might be gradual or sudden, and the symptoms themselves might either be episodic in nature or persist unremittingly over long periods of time. The central characteristics of the syndrome as a whole were its tendency to chronicity and the frequently severe incapacitation to which it subjected its victims.

Overwhelming weakness, weariness, and exhaustion constitute the whole of neurasthenia as defined in DSM-II. However, earlier patients complained of many other difficulties as well—depression, anxiety, insomnia, digestive disturbances, headaches, arthralgias, colitis, inability to make decisions.

There are no major distortions of thinking and behavior in patients with neurasthenia. What is perhaps most characteristic is the appearance of listlessness, apathy, and enervation that accompanies the inner sense of exhaustion. The patient complains of his utter fatigue, drops limp and lifeless into a chair or bed whenever he sits or lies down, and does whatever he has to do as if every movement required the greatest effort. The patient finds his symptoms unpleasant, distasteful, even painful.

Causes

In Freud's scheme, neurasthenic symptoms were the result of the excessive dissipation of libido through masturbation or nocturnal emissions. Later analytical investigators, like Fenichel, introduced psychodynamic notions into their theoretical formulations. A lowering of libidinal energy was still the phenomenon to be explained, but it was considered to be the result not so much of a direct, physiological loss through sexual discharge as of the expenditure of energy involved in intrapsychic conflict. The energy required by repression and other defensive measures to keep forbidden impulses under control diminished the amount available for other psychic functions. As analytical theory became more cognizant of the significance of human aggression, conflicts over this impulse were viewed as having particular relevance to neurasthenic symptoms. In general, however, psychoanalytic investigators have paid little attention to the clinical problems of neurotic weakness and fatigue.

Differential Diagnosis

Feelings of fatigue and loss of energy are among the cardinal symptoms of depressive illness, and they may be the major presenting complaints.

Certain chronic and subacute infectious diseases, such as brucellosis and infectious mononucleosis, may produce symptoms of fatigue and lassitude. These diseases are to be distinguished from neurasthenia by positive laboratory tests specific for each infection and by other signs and symptoms of systemic disease.

Fatigue is common in both hypothyroidism and hyperthyroidism and in Addison's disease and panhypopituitarism (Simmond's disease). In each instance the differential diagnosis from neurasthenia is to be made by positive laboratory tests and the signs and symptoms pathognomonic of each of the endocrine disorders.

The rare disorder of periodic familial paralysis is characterized by episodes of almost overwhelming weakness, related to a disturbance in potassium metabolism. Such symptoms may initially be confused with neurasthenia, but the familial nature of the disorder, the pattern of the symptoms, and laboratory evidence of faulty potassium metabolism enable the clinician to make a correct diagnosis.

Certain diuretics, such as chlorothiazide (Diuril), may lower body potassium to a point at which symptoms of marked lassitude and weakness occur. Removal of the drug or replacement of potassium ion suffice to bring about a cure.

Treatment

No psychological treatment methods are specific for neurasthenia. The form of treatment and the need for environmental manipulation are determined by the diagnostic assessment.

Medication is frequently helpful in patients with neurasthenic complaints. Psycholeptics, such as Dexedrine, 5 to 10 mg orally morning and noon, may bring about symptomatic improvement and restore the patient's energy for his daily tasks. If insomnia becomes a problem, the short-acting barbiturates may be taken at bedtime, or chloral hydrate may be prescribed if the patients's age makes the use of barbiturates inadvisable.

When the neurasthenic symptoms are part of a depressive illness, one may wish to use the psycholeptic drugs for symptom relief, but one should use the more specific treatment measures for depression, antidepressant medication and electroshock treatment, as these are indicated by the nature of the depression itself.

REFERENCES

Beard, G. M. *A Practical Treatise on Nervous Exhaustion* (*Neurasthenia*). Wm. Wood, New York, 1880.
Fenichel, O. *The Psychoanalytic Theory of Neurosis*. W. W. Norton, New York, 1945.
Ferenczi, S. Actual- and psycho-neuroses in the light of Freud's investigations and psychoanalysis. In *Further Contributions to the Theory and Technique of Psycho-analysis*. Hogarth Press, London, 1950.
Freud, S. On the grounds for detaching a particular syndrome from nehrastenia under the description "anxiety neurosis." In *Standard Edition of the Complete Psychological Works of Sigmund Freud*, vol. 3, p. 90. Hogarth Press, London, 1962.
Janet, P. *Les Obsessions et la Psychasthénie*, 2 vols. Félix Alcan, Paris, 1903.
Schilder, P. *The Image and Appearance of the Human Body*. International Universities Press, New York, 1950.

20.8.   DEPERSONALIZATION NEUROSIS

Definition

According to the second edition of the American Psychiatric Association's *Diagnostic and Statistical Manual of Mental Disorders* (DSM-II), depersonalization neurosis "is dominated by a feeling of unreality and of estrangement from the self, body, or surroundings. This diagnosis should not be used if the condition is part of some other mental disorder, such as an acute situational reaction. A brief experience of depersonalization is not necessarily a symptom of illness."

Some clinicians distinguish between depersonalization and derealization. They apply the former term to the feeling that one's body or one's personal self is strange and unreal, the latter to the experience of perceiving objects in the external world as having the same quality of unreality and estrangement. Clinical investigators have also included *déjà vu* and related phenomena in the same category as those of depersonalization. In *déjà vu*, however, what is new, alien, and previously unexperienced is felt as being familiar and as having been perceived before, whereas in depersonalization what is familiar is sensed as strange, novel, and unreal. In this discussion, depersonalization conforms to the DSM-II definition of the term.

Epidemiology

As an occasional isolated experience, depersonalization is a common phenomenon and not necessarily pathological. Studies of its incidence in normal college students indicate that transient depersonalization may occur in as many as 50 per cent of a given population, without any significant difference in incidence between men and women. It is a frequent event in children as they develop the capacity for self-awareness, and adults often undergo a temporary sense of unreality when they travel to new and strange places.

Information about the epidemiology of depersonalization of pathological proportions is more scanty. Frequently found as a symptom in association with anxiety neurosis, depression, and schizophrenia, it is apparently rare as a pure syndrome. In the few studies recently made of the condition, it occurs twice as frequently in women as in men and is a disorder of young people, rarely being found in those over 40.

Clinical Description

Onset and Course

In the large majority of patients, the symptoms first appear suddenly. The disorder starts most commonly between the ages of 15 and 30, but it has been seen in patients as young as 10;

it occurs less frequently after 30 and almost never in the later decades of life. In more than half the cases it tends to be a long-lasting, chronic condition. In many patients the symptoms run a steady course, without a significant fluctuation in intensity, but they may occur in a series of attacks interspersed with symptom-free intervals. Little is known about precipitating factors, although the disorder has been observed to begin during a period of relaxation after a time of fatiguing psychological stress. It is sometimes ushered in by an attack of acute anxiety, frequently accompanied by hyperventilation.

Clinical Symptoms and Signs

The central characteristic of depersonalization is the quality of unreality and estrangement attached to conscious experience. Inner mental processes and external events go on seemingly exactly as before, yet everything is different and seems no longer to have any personal relation or meaning to the person who is aware of them. The feeling of unreality affects the person's perception of his physical and psychological self and of the world around him. Parts of one's body or one's entire physical being may appear foreign. In the same way, all mental operations and behavior may feel alien. A common manifestation is a loss of the capacity to experience emotions, even though the patient may appear to express them. Similar feelings of unreality and strangeness may invade the patient's perceptions of the objects and people in the world around him.

Dizziness frequently appears as a symptom. Anxiety is commonly found as an accompaniment of the disorder, and many patients complain of distortions in their sense of time and space. Especially common is the experience of a change in the patient's body; in addition to his general sense of estrangement from his bodily self, he may feel that his extremities are bigger or smaller than usual. An occasional phenomenon is that of doubling; the patient feels that his point of conscious I-ness is outside of his body, commonly a few feet overhead, whence he observes himself as if he were another person.

The experience of depersonalization is often accompanied by considerable secondary anxiety, and frequently the patient fears that his symptoms are a sign that he is going insane. The patient's keen and unfailing awareness of the disturbances in his sense of reality is considered to be one of the salient characteristics of the syndrome.

Mental Status

Little is remarkable about the appearance of the patient suffering from depersonalization. Although he may complain about feelings of estrangement and absence of emotions, he shows genuine concern about his symptoms and may manifest considerable anxiety. He remains in contact with the examiner and gives no evidence of a major disturbance in affect or of disorganized thought processes.

Causes

Physiological Theories

Among the distortions of perception that follow the use of psychotomimetic drugs, such as mescaline and lysergic acid diethylamide, alterations in the sense of reality may be prominent. Diseases of the central nervous system may have the same effect. Depersonalization phenomena have been associated with electrical stimulation of the cortex of the temporal lobes. And persons subjected to sensory deprivation occasionally experience the phenomena of depersonalization.

Psychological Theories

From the earliest development of psychoanalytic concepts, the experience of estrangement has been viewed as a psychological defense. Some analytical investigators saw depersonalization and derealization as the result of changes in libidinal cathexes. Recently, attention has been paid to the role of disturbances in ego identifications. The majority of recent authors, furthermore, emphasize the fact that depersonalization is a primitive, highly pathological defense, allied to denial and used as an emergency measure when the more usual mechanism of repression fails to control unacceptable impulses.

Little is known about the psychogenetic origins of depersonalization phenomena.

Differential Diagnosis

Depersonalization may occur as a symptom in many psychiatric syndromes. Indeed, some clinicians consider it an integral part of all psychological illness. The common occurrence of depersonalization in patients with depression and schizophrenia should alert the clinician to the possibility that the patient who initially complains of feelings of unreality and estrangement is actually suffering from these more common disorders.

Because of the frequency with which psychotomimetic drugs induce long-lasting changes in the experience of the reality of one's self and one's environment, it is important to inquire about the use of these substances.

The fact that depersonalization phenomena may result from gross distrubances in brain function underlines the necessity for a careful neurological evaluation, especially when the depersonalization is not accompanied by other more common and obvious psychiatric symptoms. In particular, the possibility of brain tumor and epilepsy should be entertained.

Treatment

Phenothiazines may be of use in some patients and supportive psychotherapy for others; however, little attention has been focused on the treatment of patients with depersonalization neurosis.

REFERENCES

Ackner, B. Depersonalization. II. Clinical syndromes. J. Ment. Sci., *100*: 854, 1954.
Dugas, L., and Moutier, F. *Lodépersonnalisation*. Félix Alcan, Paris, 1911.
Federn, P. *Ego Psychology and the Psychoses*. Imago, London, 1953.
Krishaber, M. *De la néuropathie cérèbro-cardiaque*. Masson, Paris, 1873.
Roth, M. The phobic anxiety-depersonalization syndrome. Proc. R. Soc. Med., *52:* 587, 1959.
Shorvon, H. J. The depersonalization syndrome. Proc. R. Soc. Med., *39:* 779, 1946.

20.9. HYPOCHONDRIACAL NEUROSIS

Definition

According to the second edition of the American Psychiatric Association's *Diagnostic and Statistical Manual of Mental Disorders* (DSM-II), hypochondriacal neurosis "is dominated by preoccupation with the body and with fear of presumed diseases of various organs. Though the fears are not of delusional quality as in psychotic depressions, they persist despite reassurance. The condition differs from hysterical neurosis in that there are no actual losses or distortions of function."

Epidemiology

Kenyon studied hypochondriacal patients at the Maudsley-Bethlem Royal Hospital from 1951 to 1960. Of the 500-odd patients with hypochondriacal symptoms, these symptoms formed the primary disturbance in 60 per cent, and the total number represented 1 per cent of all patients diagnosed during that period in both outpatient and inpatient facilities. The incidence in the population at large is unknown, but it is presumably larger than that among psychiatric patients. There was no difference in incidence between the sexes. More than 60 per cent of the patients were married, a quarter were single, and the remainder were widowed or divorced.

Clinical Description

Onset

Hypochondriacal symptoms may first appear at any age from early childhood on. In Kenyon's series the peak incidence in men was during the fourth decade, in women during the fifth. In a little more than half of Kenyon's patients, no precipitating factors could be found. In nearly a third, the hypochondriacal concerns appeared to arise from a substrate of symptoms referable to bodily disease. Among the remainder a variety of psychological stresses preceded their onset.

Symptoms

The symptoms are diffuse and variegated, involving many different areas of the body. The most common sites are the abdominal viscera, the chest, and the head and neck. There is often a mixture of the minutely specific and the diffusely vague in the quality of his complaints. The symptoms often arise from the patient's heightened awareness of a bodily sensation, of a normal bodily function, or of a minor somatic abnormality. The symptoms have little pathological significance.

The patient presents his complaints at length, in detail, and with an urgent, insistent pressure of speech that rarely allows the physician to get a word in edgewise. The patient frequently punctuates his recitation of symptoms by showing the doctor the parts affected, by demonstrating what he considers a disorder of function, or by pointing out the small, usually insignificant structural lesion that is his major source of concern.

The content of the patient's thought and speech is entirely centered on his bodily complaints, on how they have affected him, and on the saga of his unsuccessful attempts to find help or relief. He rarely speaks spontaneously of human relationships, activities, feelings, or fantasies that are unconnected with his somatic preoccupations. He often uses medical terms or jargon acquired from his previous contacts with physicians or from his reading of medical texts and articles.

The hypochondriacal patient is characteristically worried, anxious, and concerned about his symptoms—an affective state of mind and behavior that is in contrast to the bland *belle indifférence* of the patient with hysterical neurosis. The hypochondriacal concern may be based on physiological sensations overlooked or unobserved by the normal person or on symptoms arising from minor physical conditions that the patient exaggerates out of all proportion to their medical significance.

Many patients develop a pattern of visiting doctors and clinics that becomes almost a way of life. Some become attached to a single physician whom they consult repeatedly on the smallest pretext. Others, more fickle in their medical attachments, wander from doctor to doctor and clinic to clinic, undergoing endless examinations and evaluations.

The patient's fear of and preoccupation with illness do not attain the level of delusional conviction that he has this or that disease, and mental examination reveals no evidence of psychotic disturbances of thought or affect. However, in many patients the fixity and intensity of their somatic preoccupation make the line between anxious concern and delusional conviction seem very thin.

Many hypochondriacal patients arouse in their physicians feelings of frustration and resentment that frequently make it difficult to care for them with compassionate objectivity. The tendency to refer such patients to a colleague or to another clinic no doubt enhances their own natural proclivity for multiple consultations.

No personality pattern is specifically charac-

teristic of the patient with hypochondriacal neurosis or sets him apart from patients with other emotional disorders. However, many show obsessive-compulsive traits—in particular, obstinacy, defiance, miserliness, and conscientiousness—and narcissism is a prominent feature. Patients with the disorder focus their interest, attention, and psychic energy on their bodily function to the almost complete exclusion of a concern for people and objects in the world around them.

Course and Prognosis

Clinical experience has led to the empirical generalization that depressed patients in whom hypochondriacal symptoms are prominent have a much poorer prognosis for recovery than do those whose symptoms are predominatly affective in nature. Hypochondriasis must be considered a chronic disorder with a poor prognosis for cure.

Causes

When Freud developed his concept of narcissistic libido, he had a framework for the explanation of hypochondriacal symptoms. Libido withdrawn from external objects is invested as narcissistic libido in the self. The initial increase in narcissistic libido can at first be kept within tolerable limits by its being mentally worked over in the form of megalomanic fantasies. The eventual failure of this mechanism to dissipate sufficient narcissistic libido, however, results in a further process by which the libido is transformed into somatic changes that are experienced as the anxiety-provoking sensations of hypochondriacal symptoms.

An early group of theoreticians developed Freud's concept of narcissistic libido along psychological lines. In their views, sexual object libido, through the psychological mechanism of regression, is withdrawn from the object and redirected onward to the self as narcissistic libido. Other clinical investigators see hypochondriacal symptoms as playing primarily a defensive role in the psychic economy.

Differential Diagnosis

Hypochondriacal symptoms may mask or point to other psychiatric disorders requiring specific forms of treatment. In particular, the signs and symptoms of depression and schizophrenia should be looked for in patients who present hypochondriacal complaints. There should be little difficulty in distinguishing between the classical sensorimotor phenomena of hysterical neurosis and the visceral somatic symptoms of hypochondriasis, but, when hysteria takes the form of pain, especially in the abdomen, the differential diagnosis may be difficult and must rest on a careful assessment of the patient's psychological conflicts, personality structure, and human relationships. Finally, hypochondriacal patients may develop serious bodily illnesses. But, because of their tendancy to cry wolf about somatic sensation, their physicians may be lulled into a false sense that any complaint is psychogenic.

Treatment

Hypochondriasis is notoriously refractory to treatment. Clinical evidence suggests that, unless hypochondriasis is a part of a depressive disorder with an overt affective disturbance, medications and electroconvulsive therapy are without effect.

Generally, the best that one can offer a hypochondriacal patient is an understanding and supportive relationship in which one listens sympathetically to complaints but refrains from challenging symptoms or depriving him of the status of an invalid. It is important to work with the patient's relatives to aid them in understanding the nature of the patient's complaints, to guide them in providing him with a properly supportive relationship, and to give them the emotional strength to do so.

Although the character structure of hypochondriacal patients usually precludes the use of insight psychotherapy, on rare occasions it is possible to penetrate the almost impregnable wall of somatic complaints and to bring the underlying affects—commonly, anger and depression—into conscious awareness and expression. In such cases the diminution in somatic symptoms and the general improvement in the patient's functioning can be surprising and gratifying.

REFERENCES

Burton, R. *The Anatomy of Melancholy*. Dent, London, 1964.
Freud, S. On narcissism: An introduction. In *Standard Edition of the Complete Psychological Works of Sigmund Freud*, vol. 14, p. 67. Hogarth Press, London, 1957.
Gillespie, R. D. Hypochondria: It definition, nosology and psychopathology. Guys Hosp. Rep., 78: 408, 1928.
Kenyon, F. E. Hypochondriasis: A clinical study. Br. J. Psychiatry, *110:* 478. 1964.
Ladee, G. A. *Hypochondriacal Syndromes*. Elsevier, Amsterdam, 1966.
Veith, I. On hysterical and hypochondriacal afflictions. Bull. Hist. Med., *30:* 233, 1956.

21

Personality Disorders

Introduction

Webster's Third New International Dictionary defines personality as "the totality of an individual's emergent tendencies to act or behave" and "the organization of the individual's distinguishing character traits, attitudes, or habits." A patient may appear at a psychiatrist's office because his personality attributes make it difficult for him to get along with other people; he finds that his behavior leads to ineffectual functioning or that it gets him into trouble with his peers, teachers, parents, or friends. He may seek help because other people have complained about him. On the other hand, a person may want help because his difficulties in coping with problems lead to discomfort and unhappiness.

Diagnosis

A collection of symptoms or traits should be definable on the basis of specified criteria. This syndrome should have a reasonably predictable course or outcome. The diagnosis should not change to another one in the course of time. Further, a specific family history and causes should be evident. The pathophysiology should be clear, and a specific treatment should be relevant to all the previously stated findings. In the personality disorders, (except for antisocial personality), such data do not exist.

However, some personality disorders are related to brain damage or clear neurological diagnoses, and other personality disorders exist in the absence of gross malfunction of the brain. In those disorders associated with neurological disease, the onsets of the personality difficulties are associated with sensorium difficulties, positive findings on neurological examination, or laboratory evidence of gross brain dysfunction.

In the disorders that exist in the absence of a known organic neurological illness, the onsets are difficult to date. They start early in life, perhaps in adolescence or even earlier. All personality disorders need some kind of interpersonal situations to make them apparent. Thus, life stresses are related to personality characteristics but are not necessarily the cause of deviant behavior.

Classification

The second edition of the American Psychiatric Association's *Diagnostic and Statistical Manual of Mental Disorders* (DSM-II) notes that personality disorders are frequently seen with gross neurological disease, but it places these disorders under the specific organic brain illnesses. A number of descriptions are given of specific personality disorders, including paranoid personality, cyclothymic personality, schizoid personality, explosive personality, obsessive-compulsive personality, hysterical personality, asthenic personality, antisocial personality, passive-aggressive personality, inadequate personality, and other personality disorders of specified types, such as immature personality and passive-dependent personality.

Personality disorders may be associated with known brain damage or dysfunction or neurological disease, bear some relationship to major psychiatric diagnoses, or exist as independent entities.

Associated with Brain Dysfunction or Damage

Almost any of the major illnesses that affect the central nervous system can cause or be related to personality disorders. These illnesses include encephalitis, arteriosclerotic brain disease, senile dementia, Alzheimer's disease,

Pick's disease, thyrotoxicosis, chorea, and alcoholism. The bases for personality impairment in brain damage include an impairment of the capacity to abstract and difficulties in memory and attention. Further, there is an impairment of emotional response, and the patient often appears dull under some conditions and inappropriately excited under others. Impulsivity is seen because of a need to release tension. Witticisms produced by the brain-damaged person are frequently inappropriate to the situation. Language is impaired and words frequently lose their commonly accepted meaning. Severe anxiety is seen. The brain-damaged person may be withdrawn, and he may show extreme orderliness.

Epileptic Personality Deterioration. No personality disorder leads to epilepsy. If personality changes have occurred before the epileptic phenomena have been noted, they may be evidence of brain pathology that did not present a clear picture up to the time of the seizure formation.

An obvious personality change in epilepsy is easily recognized. One sees intellectual retardation and perseveration and a great deal of circumstantiality. The patient with epileptic personality is heavy-handed and pompous, lacks wit, has tremendous egotism, perseverates on one or another topic, has sanctimonious attitude toward religion, is quick to take offense, and bears malice for long periods of time. He is frequently mulish, morose, rancorous, and given to explosions of affect.

Not all epileptics have this kind of personality, and this kind of personality is seen in patients who do not have epilepsy.

Personality Disorder in Multiple Sclerosis. In one study, about two thirds of multiple sclerosis patients had some intellectual deterioration. About one fourth of the patients had a depression that was reactive in nature, and another one fourth were euphoric, with the euphoria associated with intellectual deterioration and denial of disability. There was some exaggeration of emotional expression in about 10 per cent of the patients.

Associated with Major Psychiatric Illness

A number of personality disorders listed in DSM-II may be significantly related to major psychiatric illnesses. Thus, paranoid personal-ity may be related to paranoid schizophrenia or paranoia, cyclothymic personality may be related to bipolar manic-depressive illness, schizoid personality may be associated with schizophrenia, and obsessive-compulsive personality may be associated with obsessive compulsive neurosis and depressive illness.

Paranoid Personality. The words used to describe this kind of personality in DSM-II are "hypersensitivity, rigidity, unwarranted suspicion, jealousy, envy, and excessive self-importance." There is a tendency to place blame on others and to consider them as having malignant intent. The interpersonal relations of the patient with paranoid personality are extremely disturbed, and he is in constant conflict with his spouse, friends, or legal authorities. He feels mistreated and misjudged.

Paranoid personality may well be related to schizophrenia—in particular, paranoid schizophrenia.

Cyclothymic Personality. This personality is marked by recurring episodes of high and low moods. The periods of elation or high moods are characterized by ambition, warmth, enthusiasm, optimism, and high energy. The low or depressive periods are manifested by pessimism, low energy, the feeling that the future is not worthwhile, and general despair. These fluctuations are not related specifically to external circumstances. Sometimes the fluctuations are rapid, and sometimes they occur over the course of weeks or months. Within this category of cyclothymic personality, one may place the person with a hypomanic personality which shows persistent euphoria. There is also the opposite, a depressive personality in which the characteristics of the low side of the swing are constantly manifest.

The cyclothymic personality seems to be related to manic-depressive illness.

Schizoid Personality. The person who may be diagnosed as schizoid personality is withdrawn, oversensitive, and shy. He frequently lives by himself, has few or no close friends, interacts rarely in the community, and perhaps shows some eccentricities. Such a person is prone to daydreaming. He lacks the ability to express himself or to show anger. He responds to conflictual situations with relative detachment. Many of these characteristics are also seen in the paranoid personality, particularly the oversensitivity and seclusiveness. However, schizoid personality, unlike the paranoid personality, is poorly integrated and unable to express overt aggression or hostility.

Schizoid personality has a considerable relationship to schizophrenia.

Obsessive-Compulsive Personality. This term is synonymous with that of anankastic personality. It is a term or a diagnosis that describes an overly conscientious, overly meticulous, perfectionistic kind of person. The obsessive-compulsive personality is described in DSM-II as having "an excessive concern with conformity and adherence to standards of conscience." A person exhibiting this pattern is rigid in his viewpoint and sometimes quite inhibited in his behavior and tends toward considerable anxiety and tension in order to adhere to his rather strict standards. He may be involved in constant checking. He is prone to ruminative self-doubt and may be stubborn and overly cautious.

In general, the person with the obsessive-compulsive personality is a problem to his community and family because of his insistence on performing up to unrealistic standards. His concerns are frequently enough to drive a spouse or a child to distraction. Because the obsessive-compulsive character is beset by doubt about himself and the world, he is constantly unhappy and chronically anxious.

The obsessive-compulsive personality is related to two kinds of major psychiatric illnesses. One of these is obsessive-compulsive neurosis, and the other is depressive disease. To differentiate the obsessive-compulsive personality from obsessive-compulsive neurosis is frequently a matter of judgment. The presence of incapacitating obsessions or compulsions pushes the diagnosis toward the neurosis. And it has been said that patients with involutional melancholia develop their depressions on top of an obsessive-compulsive personality.

The obsessive-compulsive personality does not necessarily bode ill for the person. A physician who is overly meticulous and overly conscientious is in considerable favor with his patient. On the other hand, a physician in academic medicine who is prone to demanding perfection from himself may have difficulty producing research and consequently, not be promoted. The few papers he does publish, however, may well be first-rate.

Separate Entities

Explosive Personality. The definition in DSM-II states that this pattern is characterized by gross outbursts of rage and of verbal or physical aggressiveness. In between these episodes the person may be quite ordinary, and after an outburst he may feel extremely repentant. These aggressive episodes are usually in response to social and psychological stimuli. The explosive episodes are extremely intense and, therefore, are at the end of a continuum of irritability and hostile behavior. A person who experiences them appears to be out of control. Explosive behavior may be related to epilepsy or to excessive alcohol intake, but those circumstances should preclude making a diagnosis of explosive personality, which should be made on the basis of totally unexplained, precipitous, grossly destructive behavior.

A logical way to document the existence of this personality type is to search for some consequence that is a result of explosive behavior, such as a sudden murder.

Hysterical Personality. DSM-II considers the hysterical personality as one characterized by "excitability, emotional instability, over-reactivity, and self-dramatization." Sometimes the patient is attention-seeking, and frequently he is seductive toward the physician or other meaningful people. The patient is not always aware of these last characteristics. As part of the definition, such words as "immature, self-centered, often vain, and usually dependent on others" are used.

The hysterical personality is frequently seen in the person who may be diagnosed as having hysterical neurosis. Patients who suffer from hysterical neurosis have been noted to be outgoing, histrionic, and given to exaggeration. However, the diagnosis of hysterical neurosis is made considerably less frequently than the diagnosis of hysterical personality, and one must assume that most of the time hysterical personality bears no relationship to the full-blown picture of the hysterical neurosis.

Little is known about the psychophysiology of the hysterical personality.

Asthenic Personality. The defining characteristics of the asthenic personality are fatigability, low energy level, lack of enthusiasm, and anhedonia. Further, such patients are considered oversensitive to both physically and emotionally taxing situations.

The difficulty with this diagnosis is that a number of these traits are seen in patients who develop anxiety neurosis. Thus, it is possible that this personality disorder diagnosis belongs with the group of personality disorders related to other major psychiatric illnesses.

The asthenic personality probably exists, but it is extremely difficult to differentiate it from the neurasthenic neurosis. No doubt there are people who show excessive tiredness and lack of drive and are very unhappy about this. Presumably these are the people who would be considered to have an asthenic personality, if, in fact, they did not develop such symptoms as shortness of breath, panic attacks, phobias, obsessions, and compulsions, in which case they should be diagnosed as having either anxiety neurosis or obsessive-compulsive neurosis.

Passive-Aggressive Personality. In this disorder the patient's behavior is passive, but he uses this behavior to express hostility. Such symptoms as obstructionism, pouting, procrastination, stubbornness, and intentional inefficiency are seen. The patient is resentful at failing to find his emotional needs met by significant people or institutions. This diagnosis is made on the basis of interpreting a person's motivation. Clearly then, judgment on the part of the examiner comes into play, and the way is open for overinterpretation.

Inadequate Personality. This personality disorder is defined in DMS-II as belonging to a person who makes ineffectual responses to social, psychological, and physical demands. Such a person is not physically or mentally incapacitated, or retarded, but he does respond with ineptness and social instability. He may lack stamina, both physically and emotionally, and he responds with poor judgment. He adapts poorly to ordinary situations.

Antisocial Personality. Antisocial personality is one of the less frequent disorders psychiatrists are called on to deal with. The antisocial person does not often consult psychiatrists on his own initiative. However, this small segment of society demands a disproportionate amount of time and money from the rest of society. A substantial number of criminal and violent people are antisocial personalities.

According to the second edition of the American Psychiatric Association's *Diagnostic and Statistical Manual of Mental Disorders* (DSM-II), the term antisocial personality "is reserved for individuals who are basically unsocialized and whose behavior pattern brings them repeatedly into conflict with society. They are incapable of significant loyalty to individuals, groups, or social values. They are grossly selfish, callous, irresponsible, impulsive, and unable to feel guilt or to learn from experience and punishment. Frustration tolerance is low. They tend to blame others or offer plausible rationalizations for their behavior. A mere history of repeated legal or social offenses is not sufficient to justify this diagnosis." (See Table I.)

Causes. *Environment.* The antisocial personality may be viewed as a failure of the process of socialization. The disorder frequently arises amid a chaotic home environment. A number of early studies suggested a relationship between maternal deprivation in early life and severe personality disorder later. However, more recent work has yielded contradictory results and casts some doubt on the universality of this relationship between early deprivation and affectionless psychopathy. Although deprivation is clearly related to later emotional disorder, the disorder is neither as severe nor as specific as

TABLE I

Clinical Profile of the Antisocial Personality*

Superficial charm and good intelligence
Absence of delusions and other signs of irrational thinking
Absence of nervousness or psychoneurotic manifestations
Unreliability
Untruthfulness and insincerity
Lack of remorse or shame
Inadequately motivated antisocial behavior
Poor judgment and failure to learn by experience
Pathological egocentricity and incapacity for love
General poverty in major affective reactions
Specific loss of insight
Unresponsiveness in general interpersonal relations
Fantastic and uninviting behavior with drink and sometimes without
Suicide rarely carried out
Sex life impersonal, trivial, and poorly integrated
Failure to follow any life plan

* Data from *The Mask of Sanity*, Cleckley, H. ed. 4. C. V. Mosby, St. Louis, 1964.

the early work suggested. The critical factor responsible for affectionless psychopathy is probably deprivation of emotional ties with any significant person, rather than specifically maternal or even parental deprivation.

The term "parental deprivation" has referred to separation from the parents in the first years of life. There is evidence for an association between antisocial behavior and parental separation during later childhood. The effect of temporary separation is entirely dependent on the quality of the marriage before the separation. Separation occurring in poor marriages results in increased rates of antisocial behavior in the children. However, if the marital relationship is reasonably good before the separation, antisocial behavior does not occur. Antisocial behavior is also strongly related to the reason for the separation. Separations due to family discord or psychiatric illness result in a much higher rate of antisocial behavior in the children than separations due to physical illness or vacations. This same finding also holds true for homes that are permanently broken. Homes broken by divorce or separation consistently result in higher rates of delinquency and antisocial behavior in the children than do homes broken by death. This finding suggests that the important factor in predicting antisocial behavior is the parental pathology underlying the separation, rather than the separation itself.

One attitude that has frequently been found in parents of unsocialized children is rejection. The unsocialized aggressive child is likely to be the product of a home in which he is unwanted or illegitimate and has met with open rejection from the mother. By contrast, the socialized delinquent comes from a home in which he is wanted and accepted but has been neglected by the parents or has an absent father figure. Thus, rejection correlates more strongly with unsocialized aggressive behavior than with other forms of childhood delinquent behavior.

Having a sociopathic or alcoholic father is a significant predictor of antisocal personality in adult life. But the effect of having a sociopathic or alcoholic father on antisocial outcome is unrelated to whether the child was reared with the father in the home. If the father is sociopathic, a harmonious marriage does not protect the child from an increased risk of developing an antisocial personality. Therefore, exposure to marital disharmony appears to be a product of parental psychopathology, rather than an independent factor predisposing the child to an antisocial personality. Discipline, when adequate or strict, militates against the development of antisocial personality. Leniency, particularly on the part of both parents, is associated with higher rates of antisocial personality in the children.

The children of deviant parents are likely to be separated from their parents during infancy and subjected to emotionally depriving circumstances. Those who remain with their parents are likely to encounter open hostility and rejection on the part of their parents. If one prerequisite to socialization is emotional bond formation in the first years of life—and this could be the case—the environment that the antisocial often encounters in infancy is enough to thwart any attempt at bond formation. As he grows older, socialization may be further retarded by the absence of adequate or consistent discipline.

Heredity. Although psychopathy and criminality run in families, this fact alone does not speak for the role of either heredity or environment as an etiological factor. Twin studies have found a higher concordance between monozygotic than between dizygotic twins, a finding suggesting a genetic influence. But the rates of dizygotic twins are still high, and concordance rates for same—sex dizygotic twins are higher than for opposite-sex twins, which supports environmental influences. The greater similarity of the identical twins could be due to the effects of the environment and not heredity. Adoption studies, however, support the presence of a significant genetic factor.

The greatest likelihood of a criminal outcome occurs when both biological and foster parents are criminals. The second greatest likelihood occurs when the biological parent is criminal but foster parents are not. And the lowest likelihood occurs when the biological parent is noncriminal, regardless of the criminal status of the foster parent.

Psychophysiology. Electroencephalographic (EEG) studies have repeatedly shown that criminals and antisocials have more frequent EEG abnormalities than does the general population. The most frequent abnormal finding is an excess of bilateral rhythmical slow-wave activity. This slow wave activity has been cited as evidence for delayed cortical maturation in antisocials, which, if true, might account for some antisocial behavior, such as their difficulty in gaining impulse control and developing social maturity, and is consistent with the tendency for the disorder to abate as the person grows older. However, it does not account for many other antisocial symptoms.

Evidence suggests that antisocials have a lower base-line anxiety level in nonstressful situations, perhaps react to stress with less anxiety, and recover from stressful situations more readily than do nonantisocials. Antisocials do not learn conditioned fear responses as readily as nonantisocials and, therefore, have more difficulty learning responses that are motivated by fear of anxiety.

Clinical Features

The antisocial often has a charming or ingratiating quality about him and impresses the observer as being of good intelligence. Despite the seemingly irrational nature of much of his antisocial behavior, it cannot be attributed to a lack of intelligence or to irrational or psychotic thinking. He often demonstrates a lack of anxiety or tension that can be grossly incongruous with the situation. Unreliability, untruthfulness, and insincerity are further traits of the disorder. The most frustrating aspects of this behavior is its unpredictability. The antisocial typically shows no remorse or guilt over his misbehavior, even when directly confronted with it. When confronted, he is skillful at projecting the blame on others or justifying his behavior through some rationalization. He is well-known for his ability to talk his way out of punishment. Another characteristic is the apparent lack of motivation for much of the antisocial behavior.

The antisocial is a highly narcissistic, hedonistic person whose interests rarely go beyond satisfying his own immediate needs. He is generally incapable of meaningful interpersonal relationships. He appears not to experience any deep emotion, although he may be skillful at dissimilating feelings. Although he may show clear insight into why he is in a particular jam, he can show a striking lack of insight into the fact that he has done anything wrong and may even seem surprised that others are angry at him. The antisocial typically fails to follow any life plan. His behavior often has the appearance of being randomly determined, rather than guided by adherence to any direction or goal in life. His behavior may be self-defeating in that it is directly contrary to his own self-interest.

Antisocial personality is a disorder that begins in childhood or early adolescence and affects the person in multiple life areas of social functioning. For this reason, the clinical picture varies considerably, depending on the age at which it is viewed. In childhood, the person's life is centered primarily on home and school, and this is where antisocial symptoms are found in this age group. As the person matures and his areas of social involvement expand, so does the clinical picture of the disorder.

Childhood Symptoms. The symptoms most typical of the young antisocial are theft, incorrigibility, truancy, running away from home, associating with bad companions, staying out late at night, physical aggression, poor employment record in those old enough to work, impulsivity, recklessness and irresponsibility, slovenly appearance, enuresis, lack of guilt, premarital intercourse, sexual perversion, and pathological lying. The three best predictors of adult antisocial personality are number, frequency, and seriousness of juvenile antisocial symptoms. (See Table II.)

Adult Symptoms. Typical problems are frequent job changes, lengthy periods of unemployment, and interpersonal problems with bosses or peers. Financial dependency includes partial or total support by relatives, social agencies, or institutions. An arrest record is a more common finding among men than among women and refers to repeated nontraffic arrests. Their marriages often reveal verbal and physical fighting, separations, and divorces. Spouses themselves are likely to be deviant, and problems such as desertion and nonsupport are frequent findings. Alcohol and drug abuse are seen with increased frequency among antisocials.

A history of impulsive behavior, such as a precipitous decision to marry, is often found. Sexual promiscuity is reported more frequently in women than in men. Many antisocials report a wild adolescence. Vagrancy or a period of wanderlust, traveling about the country without ties to any person or place, is frequently seen. Belligerency refers to frequent fighting, especially after the age of 18, or the use of weapons or other lethal objects in a fight. The antisocial is frequently socially isolated, without any true friends, although casual acquaintances are com-

TABLE II

*Childhood Symptoms Predictive of Antisocial Personality**

Symptom	Percentage of Adult Antisocials Who Had Symptom	Percentage of children with Symptom Who Became Antisocial
Theft	83	31
Incorrigibility	80	30
Truancy	66	34
Running away	65	33
Bad companions	56	30
Staying out late	54	30
Physical aggression	45	32
Poor employment record	44	32
Impulsivity	38	35
Reckless, irresponsible	35	29
Slovenly appearance	32	34
Enuresis	32	29
Lack of guilt	32	38
Premarital intercourse	28	31
Pathological lying	26	39
Sexual perversion	18	37

* Data from L. N. Robins, *Deviant Children Grown Up; A Sociological and Psychiatric Study of Sociopathic Personality*. Williams & Wilkins, Baltimore, 1966.

mon. Lack of guilt is a clinical judgment often described. Military records are characterized by absences without leave, desertions, nonjudicial punishment, and courts-martial. The final discharge is likely to be less than honorable. Such symptoms as pathological lying, suicide attempts, and the use of aliases are seen in a minority of cases (See Table III.)

Family History. Four psychiatric illnesses are found with greater frequency among first-degree relatives of antisocials than in the general population—antisocial personality, hysteria, alcoholism, and drug addiction. The parental behaviors most predictive of an antisocial outcome in the child are arrests, chronic unemployment, desertion, excessive drinking, and failure to support.

Course and Prognosis. The disorder invariably begins in childhood or early adolescence, and symptoms are present before the age of 15. It tends to develop earlier in boys than in girls; boys are likely to show symptoms before the age of 12. Once the disorder develops, it runs an unremitting course, with the height of the

antisocial behavior usually occurring during late adolescence and early adult life. The prognosis is variable. If improvement does occur, it tends to occur in the fourth decade of life. However, there is no age beyond which improvement does not occur. Those who improve are still not entirely normal, as they continue to have problems with interpersonal relations. Nevertheless, the disorder may abate sufficiently to allow a more stable life than they had before.

Diagnosis

For a diagnosis, three conditions should be met. First, the disorder should begin before the age of 15. Second, the clinical picture should be of antisocial behavior involving multiple areas of social functioning. Third, there should be no other psychiatric illness that could explain the symptoms.

The interviewer should always inquire about childhood and adolescent problems. The adult

TABLE III

*Adult Symptoms of Antisocial Personality**

Life Area	Percentage of Antisocials with Significant Problems in This Area
Work problems	85
Marital problems	81
Financial dependency	79
Arrests	75
Alcohol abuse	72
School problems	71
Impulsiveness	67
Sexual behavior	64
Wild adolescence	62
Vagrancy	60
Belligerency	58
Social isolation	56
Military record (of those serving)	53
Lack of guilt	40
Somatic complaints	31
Use of aliases	29
Pathological lying	16
Drug abuse	15
Suicide attempts	11

* Data from L. N. Robins, *Deviant Children Grown Up; A Sociological and Psychiatric Study of Sociopathic Personality*. Willims & Wilkins, Baltimore, 1966.

adjustment is assessed by inquiring in some detail into the various areas of the person's life that are most often affected—employment, military service, financial dependency. The examiner should always look for typically antisocial symptoms, such as vagrancy, repeated arrests, drug and alcohol abuse, and physical aggression as an adult. In taking a family history, antisocial behavior on the part of the parents and siblings should be evaluated.

The mental status examination is of more value in ruling out others disorders than it is in establishing a diagnosis of antisocial personality. The antisocial demonstrates no evidence of thought disorder, and there are no typically psychotic symptoms, although his tendency to blame others may be mistaken for paranoid thinking.

Alcoholism and drug dependence are the two disorders most difficult to distinguish from antisocial personality. Both are common among antisocials, and alcoholics and drug users often show antisocial behavior that is secondary to their basic problem. The disorders can be distinguished if a clear history of antisocial behavior can be obtained that either antedated or occurred in the absence of the drug involvement. In this case, the drug or alcohol dependency is considered secondary, and the primary diagnosis is antisocial personality.

A manic patient may become involved in a certain amount of antisocial behavior during the hypomanic phase. Such problems as wanderlust, sexual promiscuity, and financial difficulty may superficially resemble antisocial personality. However, manic-depressive illness, unlike antisocial personality, typically has an onset after the age of 15 and is characterized by discrete attacks, with clear periods of remission, during which the person returns to normal. The manic phase is characterized by euphoria or irritability and the usual symptoms of flight of ideas, pressure of speech, and hyperactivity, which are helpful in distinguishing it from antisocial personality.

Schizophrenia may present with antisocial behavior, but, when the symptom picture of the disease develops, it is not difficult to distinguish from antisocial personality. The antisocial is free of typical schizophrenic symptoms, such as thought disorder, delusions, hallucinations, and flattening of affect.

Chronic brain syndrome may mimic antiso-cial personality because of the poor judgment, aggressive behavior, and antisocial acts that may accompany the syndrome. It can be distinguished on the basis of mental status examination or psychological testing. The antisocial shows no impairment or deterioration of cognitive ability.

Dyssocial behavior may be mistaken for antisocial personality because dyssocial behavior is regarded as antisocial by society's standards. The person with dyssocial behavior, however, is a socialized person who belongs to a deviant subculture and, within the standards of his subculture, shows no antisocial behavior. The dyssocial person may be involved in criminal activity, but other life areas are free of antisocial problems.

The psychological examinations most likely to be of value in evaluating the antisocial personality are the Minnesota Multiphasic Personality Inventory, the Bender-Gestalt, and the Wechsler Adult Intelligence Scale. The MMPI is useful in providing supporting evidence, and the latter two tests are sometimes necessary to rule out other disorders.

Treatment. The usefulness of outpatient psychotherapy along traditional lines for the offender is highly questionable. The results of treatment within an adolescent institution using such modalities as therapeutic community and group therapy all show positive results. This finding suggests that well-planned institutional treatment programs may be effective in modifying adolescent delinquent behavior. At this time, the evidence is insufficient to support any conclusions about treatment of the adult antisocial.

The treatment of the antisocial is aimed at helping him establish internal controls over his behavior. This end is accomplished by maintaining a firm but accepting attitude toward the patient while imposing external limitations on his actions. An inpatient setting may be necessary to provide the necessary external controls. This implies the use of authority and at times punishment.

REFERENCES

Cleckley, H. *The Mask of Sanity*, ed. 4. C. V. Mosby, St. Louis, 1964.
Cloninger, C. R., and Guze, S. B. Psychiatric illness in the families of female criminals: A study of 288 first-degree relatives. Br. J. Psychiatry, *122:* 697, 1973.
Hutchings, B., and Mednick, S. A. Registered criminality in

the adoptive and biological parents of registered male adoptees. In *Genetic Research in Psychiatry*, R. R. Fieve, H. Brill, and D. Rosenthal, editors. University Press, New York, 1974.

Jenkins, R. L. The psychopathic or antisocial personality. J. Nerv. Ment. Dis., *131*: 318, 1960.

Knott, J. R., Platt, E. B., Ashby M. C., and Gottlieb, J. S. A familial evaluation of the electro-encephalogram of patients with primary behavior disorder and psychopathic personality. Electroencephalogr. Clin. Neurophysiol., *5:* 363, 1953.

Liss, J., Welner, A., and Robins, E. Personality disorder. I. Record study. Br. J. Psychiatry, *123:* 685, 1973.

Robins, L. R. *Deviant Children Grown Up: A Sociological and Psychiatric Study of Sociopathic Personality.* Williams & Wilkins, Baltimore, 1966.

Schulsinger, F. Psychopathy: Heredity and environment. Int. J. Ment. Health, *1:* 190, 1972.

Tolle, R. The mastery of life by psychopathic personalities. Psychiatr. Clin., *1:* 1, 1968.

22

Drug Dependence

22.1. OPIATE DEPENDENCE

Definition

In the American Psychiatric Association's second edition of *Diagnostic and Statistical Manual of Mental Disorders* (DSM-II), "drug dependence" is substituted for the term "drug addiction," which was used in the first edition. This change reflects the attempt by the World Health Organization (WHO) Expert Committee on Addiction-producing Drugs to resolve the confusion about terminology. WHO defined drug dependence as a "state arising from repeated administration of a drug on a periodic or continuous basis." The characteristics of the drug-dependent state vary, depending on the drug involved.

DSM-II categorizes drug dependence under "Personality disorders and certain other non-psychiatric mental disorders." Drug dependence is defined as covering, "patients who are addicted to or dependent on drugs other than alcohol, tobacco, and ordinary caffeine-containing beverages." This definition of dependence does not apply if the drug is medically prescribed and the intake conforms to the medical need. To make a diagnosis, the therapist must have evidence of habitual use or a clear sense of need in the patient. The presence of the abstinence syndrome is not the only evidence of dependence, even though it is invariably present on abrupt withdrawal of opium derivatives. The diagnosis may stand alone, or it may be joined with another diagnosis.

Although the use of the term "drug dependence" is a distinct improvement over the earlier term in DSM-I, ambiguities remain. In the WHO definition is the implication that the use of the drug has harmful effects on a person or society or both. The WHO Committee stated: "With morphine, the harm to the individual is mainly indirect, arising from preoccupation with drug taking; personal neglect, malnutrition, and infection are frequent consequences. For society also, the harm may be related to the preoccupation of the individual with drug taking; disruption of interpersonal relationships, economic loss, and crimes against property are frequent consequences."

Prevalence

The National Institute of Mental Health, in its evaluation of the mental health in urban America, stated that "there were 62,045 active narcotic addicts as of December 31, 1967." More than half the known addicts were in New York City. Most of the others were in other large cities. Almost 98 per cent of the addicts admitted in 1966 to the Lexington and Fort Worth Public Health Service hospitals were urban residents. Men were primarily affected; the male-to-female addict ratio has been five to one or four to one. The bulk of the addict population consisted of members of the black and Spanish-speaking minorities.

New York City's Addiction Services Agency in 1973 estimated 100,000 to 150,000 New York City addicts, as did the 1972 Ford Foundation's report. Since only about half of the persons who died of causes related to heroin abuse are believed to be included in the New York City Narcotics Register, the total number of New York City addicts may be 200,000 to 300,000. Estimates suggest that there are between 250,000 and 300,000 addicts nationwide; the actual number may be two or three times that.

Outside of New York, one of the most thoroughgoing studies of the number of addicts has been done in Washington, D. C. Of the 17,000 to 18,000 addicts, two thirds were under 26 years of age, 91 per cent were black, 74 per cent were male, and 52 per cent began heroin use during the 4 years before the study. In one part of central Washington, 20 per cent of the boys from 15 to 19 and 38 per cent of the young men between 20 and 24 were heroin addicts.

Around 1950 the typical heroin addict was urban, a member of a minority group, male, and in his late twenties or early thirties. Since then, there has been a distinct shift toward younger and younger addicts. In New York City the average age of youngsters in drug-free programs appears to be just over 17 years; the average age of those in hospital methadone maintenance and antagonist therapy programs is in the low twenties. The Board of Education of New York City estimates that 8 per cent of the high school-age youngsters in the city use heroin. At first, most adolescent heroin addicts were black or Puerto Rican, but more and more new recruits are white. The January 1972 census taken by New York City's Addiction Services Agency found 41.8 per cent of the participants in its drug programs were black, 20.8 per cent Puerto Rican, and the rest Caucasian. According to the Bureau of Narcotics and Dangerous Drugs, 51 per cent of addicts in the United States were white in 1971, compared with 44 per cent in 1959. Their average age had dropped from 35 in 1950 to 23 in 1971.

Within the medical profession, the narcotic addiction rate is estimated at between 1 and 2 per cent, in contrast to the United States population rate of 0.3 per cent and the central Harlem rate of 6 per cent.

Causes

There seems to be no unitary theory to explain opiate addiction.

Interpersonal

In the older psychoanalytic literature the behavior of narcotic addicts was described in terms of regression and fixation at pregenital, oral, or even more archaic levels of psychosexual development. More recently, it has been stated that severe emotional pathology and its manifestations invariably precede, accompany, and follow the compulsive use of drugs.

One family constellation frequently described consists of vacillation between seduction and vindictiveness. In other families the conflict may be between an intrusive form of pseudolove and overprotective care on the one hand and a complete disregard for the individuality of the child and his real emotional needs on the other hand. In still other families the parents' self-centered preoccupation with success and prestige gives rise to the child's self-centered retreat into a drug-induced dream world.

It appears that the parents themselves are often deeply involved in using prescribed or nonprescription drugs or alcohol. By and large, the symptom of drug taking by the child is derivative or a reflection of the whole family's attitude of inconsistency, self-centeredness, and, very often, inner dishonesty.

Addicts appear to take advantage of the powerful action of the drug to mute and extinguish their emotions and to solve, at least in the short run, problems associated with interpersonal relations. Practices of the pseudoculture in which the addict immerses himself also play a part in filling the social vacuum and provide an alternative to the establishment of meaningful attachments to other people.

Socio-economic

In the early 1950's there was thought to be a direct relation between socio-economic deprivation and heroin addiction. Unfortunately, the steady increase in the number of middle-class addicts from privileged homes has cast doubt on any exclusive relation between addiction and socio-economic status.

Cultural and Ethnic

Many observers have been persuaded that United States minorities—such as blacks, Spanish-speaking, and native Indians—have a higher risk for drug dependence in the sense that they are disproportionately poor. Since social and economic forces restrict the upward mobility of these groups, particularly the young men, they remain at high risk of developing drug dependence because of their intense frustration. Drugs not only afford surcease but become a symbol of importance. Studies of slum youth indicate that their model may often be the drug pusher, with his fancy clothes and custom car.

As with the socio-economic factors, a broader explanation must be sought in light of the fact that black, Puerto Rican, and chicano addicts have been joined by their white brothers from the suburbs and the middle-class sections of the city.

Youth Culture

As one examines adolescent heroin abusers, certain consistent behavior patterns seem especially pronounced in the younger addicts: underlying depression, often of an agitated type and frequently accompanied by anxiety symptoms; impulsiveness expressed by a passive-aggressive orientation; fear of failure; use of heroin as an antianxiety agent to mask feelings of low self-esteem, hopelessness, and aggression; cognitive restrictions—that is, limited coping strategies and low frustration tolerance —accompanied by the need for immediate gratification; sensitivity to drug contingencies, with a keen awareness of the relation between good feelings and the act of drug taking; feelings of behavioral impotence counteracted by momentary control over the life situation by means of drugs, with the injection ritual a valued life event; and disturbances in social and interpersonal relations, with peer relations maintained by mutual drug experiences.

But what is there about society that makes it necessary for significant sectors of the youth culture to experiment and use drugs? This crucial question involves a confrontation between the adult world and the youth world. With the past failing to provide models and with the future gloomy and uncertain, the only certainty is the present. Any action that will intensify and give more meaning to the present moment is worthwhile. With authentic engagement not attractive or feasible for many, drug abuse becomes, for a small but growing minority, a form of identification and engagement.

Pharmacological

Some substances are more likely to become abused than are others. The capacity of opioids to produce tolerance and physical dependence is certainly a major contributing factor. The constant reinforcement and development of the conditioned abstinence syndrome also ensures the steady progress of experimenters to addiction. Yet many experimenters do not become addicts.

Ecological

This model suggests that people and their drug environment are inextricably interwoven in a complex system that includes all social systems. Each part of the system affects all others, and the introduction of one drug may alter the balance and the relations existing between people, the drug environment, and many social systems. Likewise, a change in the social system may influence people and the drug environment—increasing, decreasing, or changing drug use.

Pharmacology

Opium

Opium is produced from the milky exudate of the unripe seed capsules of the poppy plant, *Papaver somniferum*. Only a few alkaloids—morphine, codeine, papaverine, and noscapine—have clinical usefulness. A dose of 0.06 gm. of opium is equivalent to 6 mg. of morphine. (See Table I.)

Morphine

Morphine is by far the most important phenanthrene alkaloid of opium, and it gives to opium its predominant pharmacological characteristics. Morphine has the ability to produce analgesia, respiratory depression, gastrointestinal spasm, and physical dependence. Toxic doses may produce convulsions. Nalorphine and related antagonists to morphine counteract the analgesic, gastrointestinal, and depressant effects and also the convulsions.

The mechansims whereby morphine and the opiates generally exert their effects remain unknown, but their major areas of activity are in the central nervous system and the bowel. Flushing and itching of the skin result from a release of histamine, constipation by a decrease of peristalsis. Most of an injected single dose of morphine appears in the urine within 24 hours, with the remainder appearing in the feces later.

Analgesia, drowsiness, changes in mood, and mental clouding are among the central nervous system effects exerted by morphine. Small to moderate amounts (5 to 10 mg.) produce such analgesia, often without sleep. Other manifestations include drowsiness and a feeling of warmth, with the extremities feeling heavy; the face, particularly the nose, may itch, and the

TABLE I

Chemical Structures of Opiates

Opium alkaloids that occur in nature

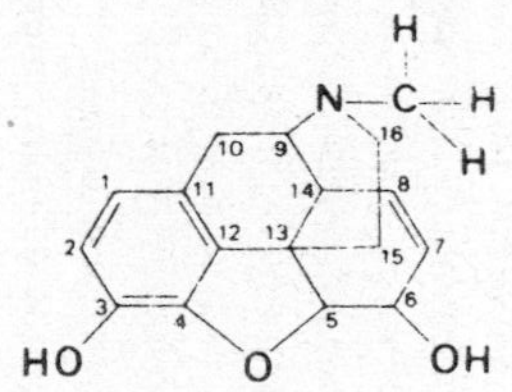

Morphine†

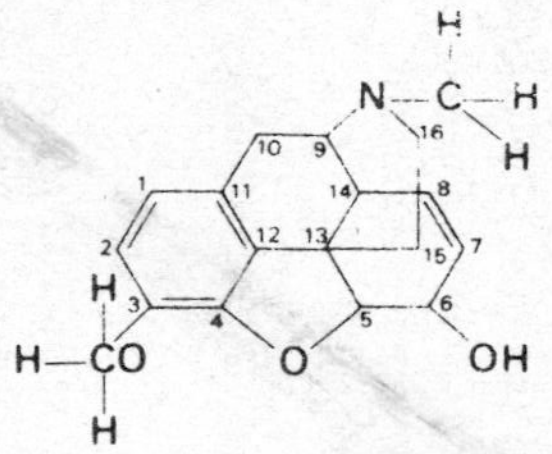

Codeine†

Semisynthetic derivatives of morphine

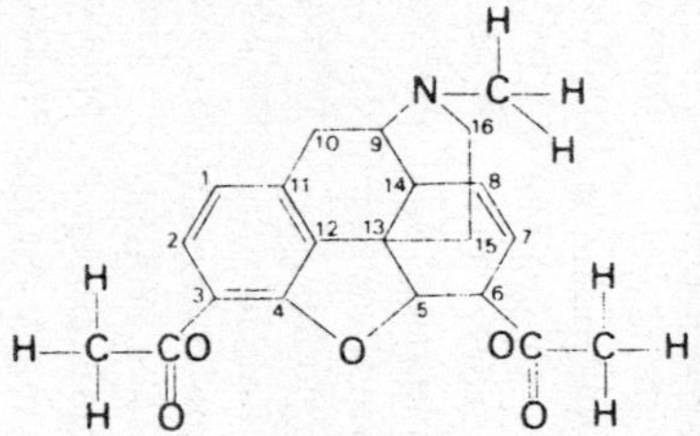

Heroin†

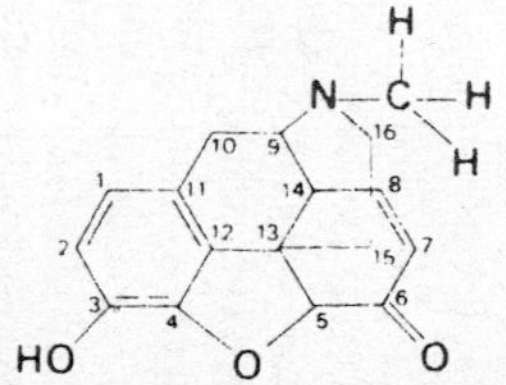

Hydromorphone (Dilaudid®)†

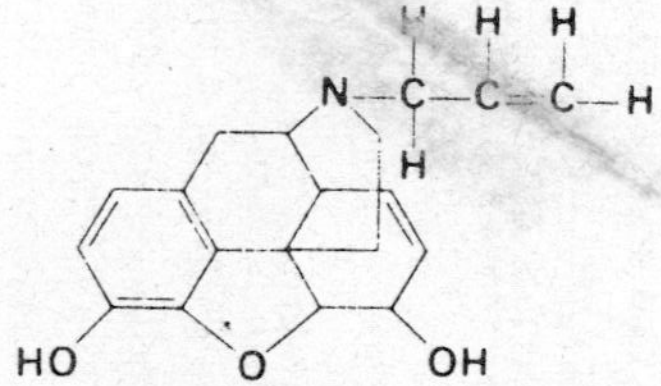

Nalorphine (Nalline®)*

Synthetic compounds (morphinans)

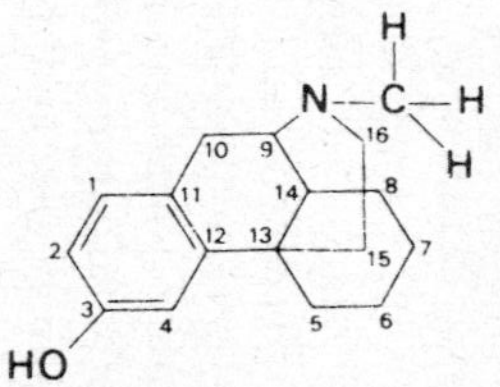

Levorphanol (Levo-Dromoran®)†

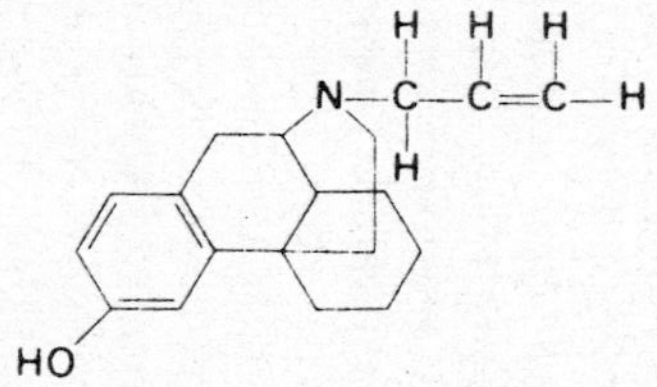

Levallorphan (Lorfan®)

Methadones

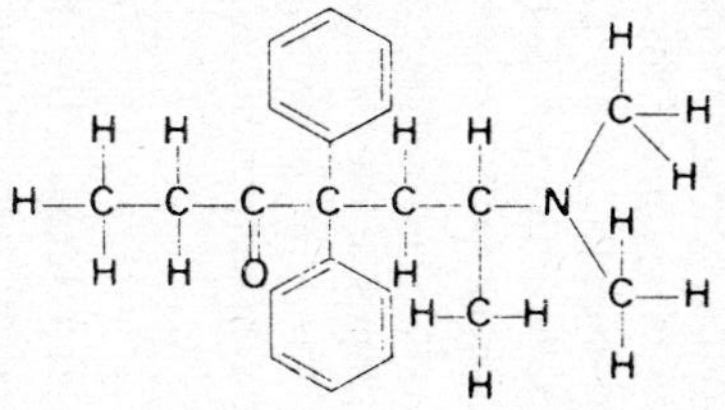

Methadone (Dolophine®)

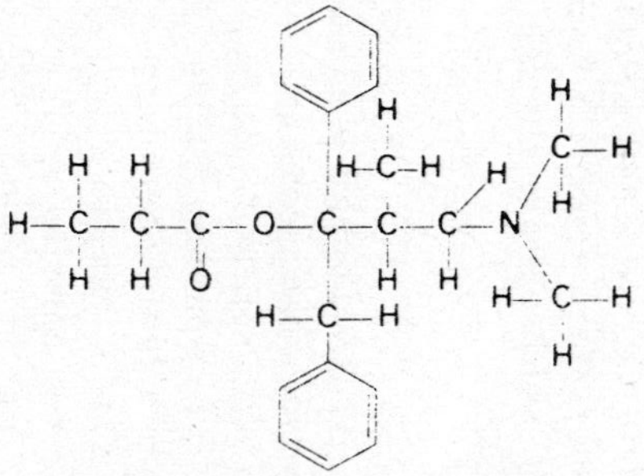

Dextropropoxyphene (Darvon®)

Piperidines

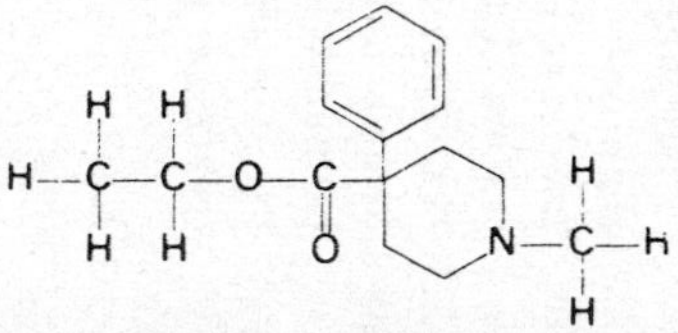

Meperidine (Demerol®)

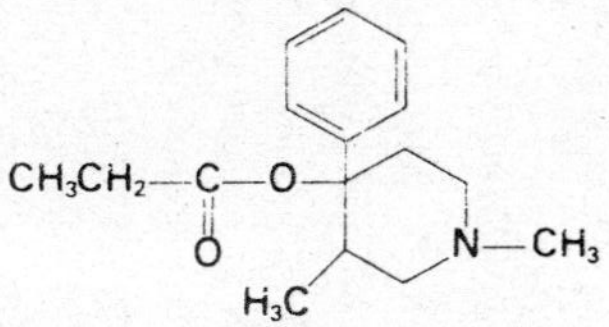

Alphaprodine

Miscellaneous

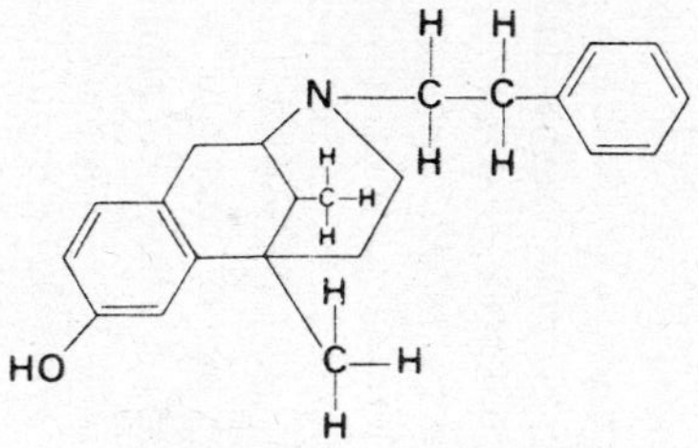

Phenazocine (Prinadol®)*

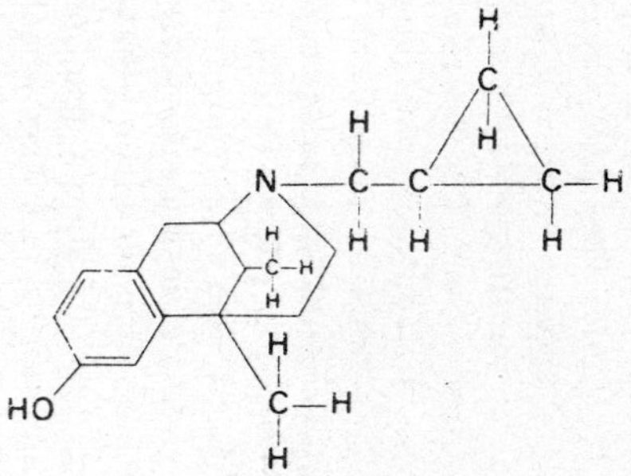

Cyclazocine*

* Opiate antagonists.
† Opiates with intact phenanthrene nucleus.

mouth becomes dry. In addition to relief of distress, some patients experience euphoria, an unrealistic sense of well-being. If the external situation is favorable, sleep and dreaming ensue. However, dysphoria—with mild anxiety or fear, nausea or vomiting—may occur in the normal, pain-free person. The further psychological effects of morphine may be mental clouding, with drowsiness, inability to concentrate, difficulty in thinking, apathy, and lethargy. These subjective effects tend to become more pronounced with larger doses (15 to 20 mg.). Idiosyncratic responses—such as insomnia, rather than sedation—have been widely reported, as are allergic reactions, such as urticaria and other skin rashes, wheals at the site of injection, and even anaphylactoid shock, which may be responsible for many of the sudden deaths and episodes of pulmonary edema that occur among heroin addicts.

Morphine analgesia is relatively selective in that touch, vision, and hearing are not blunted. Morphine and other opioid analgesics do not alter the responsivity or threshold of nerve endings to noxious stimuli. Neither do they alter the conduction of the nerve impulse along the peripheral nerves. In the clinical situation, morphine and other opioid analgesics are said to act on systems responsible for affective responses to painful stimuli, thus increasing a patient's tolerance to pain, even though his capacity to perceive the situation may be unchanged. Continuous, dull pain is relieved more effectively than is sharp, intermittent pain, but sufficient amounts of morphine alleviate the intense pain of renal and biliary colic. Morphine is a primary and continuous depressant of respiration because of its direct effect on the brain stem respiratory centers. In human beings, death is nearly always due to respiratory arrest. Peripheral vasodilation, blood pressure, heart rate, and the cerebral circulation do not appear to be prominent effects of the drug. The depressant effects of morphine and related narcotics may be exaggerated and prolonged by phenothiazines, monoamine oxidase inhibitors, and imipraminelike drugs.

Heroin

The most widely abused opiate, heroin (diacetylmorphine) is a simple derivative of morphine. Heroin acts like morphine, inducing analgesia, drowsiness, and changes in mood. An initial dose may produce an unpleasant sensation, dysphoria, nausea, often even vomiting. In the normal person, this effect is brief: the pleasurable and therapeutic actions of heroin persist for many hours. In equipotent injectable doses, 1 mg of heroin is equal to 1.80 to 2.66 mg. of morphine sulfate. Compared with morphine, heroin has greater potency, apparently because of its relatively easier passage through the blood-brain barrier.

Methadone

Methadone is not like morphine in its chemical structure, but its pharmacological properties are qualitatively identical. Methadone also causes sedation and respiratory depression: its effect on smooth muscle and the cardiovascular system is like that of morphine. In human beings, methadone is constipating but less so than morphine, and it causes biliary tract spasm. The side effects of methadone are similar to those of morphine. The principal danger in overdosage is diminished pulmonary ventilation.

Tolerance to methadone develops more slowly than does tolerance to morphine: Physical dependence is developed during chronic administration. The subcutaneous injection of 10 to 20 mg. of methadone produces definite euphoria in former narcotic addicts. Methadone is used primarily in the treatment of narcotic addicts, but it is also used for the relief of pain and the treatment of narcotic abstinence syndromes.

Narcotic Antagonists

N-Allylnorcodeine counteracts the respiratory depression induced by morphine or heroin. Nalorphine can precipitate acute abstinence syndromes in withdrawn addicts after the administration of morphine, methadone, or heroin for a brief period. In the majority of nonaddicted subjects, large doses of nalorphine produce dysphoria and anxiety, rather than euphoria. Nalorphine has strong analgesic properties, even though it counteracts the analgesic effect of morphine. The dysphoric effects of nalorphine make it unsuitable for clinical use.

As a group, the narcotic antagonists are presently believed to be relatively free of abuse potential. For their compounds to be useful in either the treatment or prevention of addiction, they need to possess a structural similarity to narcotics, so that they are able to occupy the same central nervous system receptor sites as the narcotic drugs, thereby producing competitive inhibition. Also, these narcotic antagonists must have little or no morphinelike or agonistic action at the receptor site, so that by their occupation they prevent or reverse the action of the opiates. They must also have the ability to antagonize the euphoric high of opiates, none or few pharmacological effects of their own, the inability to cause physical dependence, no evidence of increasing tolerance to their antagonistic actions, the absence of serious side effects and toxicity even in chronic use, ease of administration, long-lasting or moderate-lasting antagonistic effects, an abuse potential that is low or absent, reversible effects in case of medical emergency, high potency to permit the administration of small amounts in a depot preparation, easy availability, and low cost.

As yet, none of the antagonists completely meets all these criteria. Cyclazocine, a benzomorphan compound, and naloxone (*N*-allyl-noroxymorphine) (Narcan) are the two narcotic antagonists that have been most widely used experimentally. Naltrexone, a recently introduced antagonist, is still in early study and appears promising.

In maintenance doses of 4 to 5 mg., cyclazocine, the more widely used antagonist, blocks heroin's habituating effects and euphoria for 24 hours or more. Higher doses of up to 20 mg. can extend this blocking action to 48 to 72 hours. Patients in early treatment may experience some unpleasant side effects, unless their doses are built up gradually, but these side effects are transient and do not necessarily interfere with treatment.

Pharmacologically, naloxone seems to be an almost perfect antagonist, causing far fewer side effects than cyclazocine. Naloxone (Narcon) is used primarily to treat a heroin overdose. For the treatment and prevention of addiction, it is not ideal, since its antagonist effects at maintenance doses last only 4 to 10 hours.

Dependence

If physiological disturbances follow withdrawal of a drug, the dependence may be called physical; if the disturbance is psychological, the dependence may be called psychic. Many dependences, such as that on morphine, are both.

The predominantly depressant effect of morphine, according to one hypothesis, induces a compensating homeostatic mechanism in the autonomic nervous system with a greater excitability or reactivity that is checked by the presence of a drug. When the morphine is withdrawn, this compensating mechanism is freed to express itself as the abstinence syndrome. Research findings have failed to confirm this proposal. But the finding that inhibitors of nucleic acid or protein synthesis block the induction of tolerance and dependence supports the general proposition that some kind of receptor multiplication is involved. Psychic and physical dependence can be regarded as subjective and objective manifestations of the same state. The liability to induce physical dependence in determining the danger of abuse. And the essential psychopharmacological action of a drug that leads to its abuse is that of enhancing pleasurable excitement, escape, or relaxation and of lessening painful boredom, anxiety, or defensiveness. In short, all drugs of abuse induce a sense of reward without exacting the natural labor of achieving it.

Tolerance

Defined as the increased amount of drug required to produce the effect obtained with the initial dose of the drug, tolerance is a shift in the dose-response curve to the right. Unlike tolerance to any other class of sedative drugs, tolerance to heroin can be increased to levels more than 100 times the initial effective dose.

In heroin use, tolerance occurs fairly rapidly and can be shown to occur within a matter of days after the periodic administration of the drug. If the tolerant person is challenged with an antagonist such as naloxone, a precipitated withdrawal syndrome follows. Withdrawal signs include rhinorrhea, tearing, gooseflesh, abdominal and muscular cramps, tachycardia, and a rise in temperature, with dilation of the pupils.

Clinical Effects

The clinical effects of morphine may be used as the model for all opiates. The particular setting in which the drug is administered, the person's history of receiving opiates, his personality, and the presence or absence of pain contribute to the effects. For the naive subject without pain, morphine generally produces dysphoria brought about by nausea, giddiness, and a subjective sense of mental clouding. There is no impairment of psychomotor performance, except under stress or demand for speed. Since morphine relieves pain, a person who is in pain displays a negative euphoria on injection of morphine, with the pain relieved. Likewise, apprehension and similar emotional states are assuaged.

For the narcotic addict who is nontolerant to morphine and for certain other persons who are not suffering pain, a single injection usually produces a pleasant state of positive euphoria. But some persons may vomit or exhibit an extreme state of pallor. Further, a state of easily aroused semisomnolence (nodding) may be observed. Unaccustomed energy may be displayed in carrying out assigned duties. The sensorium remains intact, and skilled acts are not grossly impaired. Morphine appears to reduce or change the incentive level. Although most addicts do not report an enrichment of their fantasy life, increased fantasy and inner living has been recorded by means of Rorschach tests after parenteral administration of morphine under experimental conditions.

Intravenous injection produces some particular phenomena. Noteworthy is the reported sensation, similar to orgasm, localized in the abdomen. Although opiates decrease sexual activity and potency, addicts occasionally report improved sexual performance very early in their addiction; this improvement can be ascribed to the reduction of anxiety and some delay in orgasm. However, the continued use of opiates produces a diminution of function.

Flushing and itching of the skin are also common after the intravenous injection of morphine. Pupillary constriction, depression of the respiratory rate, slowing of the cardiac rate, a slight lowering of the body temperature, and spasms of smooth muscle sphincters are also seen after single doses of morphine.

In general, the effects of a single dose of morphine reach peak intensity about 20 minutes after an intravenous injection and about 1 hour after a subcutaneous injection. These effects persist in declining intensity for 4 to 6 hours and are followed by a let-down feeling.

Acute Intoxication

Opiate poisoning causes marked unresponsiveness, slow and periodic respiration, pinpoint pupils, bradycardia, hypotension, and hypothermia. The pupils may be dilated in cases of severe poisoning; reflexes may be absent, cyanosis marked, and the pulse rapid, weak, and thready. Mild opiate poisoning should be treated vigorously by gastric lavage if the drug has been taken orally. If necessary, the air passages should be cleared, an airway or trachea cannula inserted, and artificial respiration instituted.

Narcotic addicts have a reportedly high mortality rate due to acute illness associated with drug abuse. Tetanus, acute viral hepatitis, malaria, and opiate overdose—diseases believed to be caused by addiction—accounted for less than 2 per cent of the 385 deaths of hospitalized narcotic addicts at the Lexington Clinical Research Center during the years 1935 to 1966. Heart disease (including infective endocarditis), tuberculosis, and carcinoma of the lung accounted for more than half of the deaths. Tuberculosis and nephritis were more frequent causes of addict death than one might expect in random samples of the United States population.

If a patient is brought unconscious into a hospital as a result of taking a drug overdose, immediate conservative treatment should be instituted. If heroin overdosage is suspected, naloxone (Narcan), given intravenously (0.4 to 0.8 mg.), may be lifesaving and diagnostic. This therapy may lead to immediate recovery of consciousness. A patient who continues to have relapses after single ampule doses of the antagonist drug should be given an intravenous drip of naloxone. The dosage must be established according to the individual response. No significant side effects of naloxone treatment are known.

Chronic Intoxication

Among the effects of chronic intoxication with opiates are decreases at a relatively rapid rate of euphoria, relief of pain, anxiety, and rates of respiration, as well as nausea and vomiting. However, the constrictions of pupils, smooth muscle spasms, constipation, impotence, and failure to menstruate may be permanent. Increasing the dosage of the opiate may restore the original effects of the drug, but even enormous doses may not recaputre the previous euphoria. Instead, after high degrees of tolerance and physical dependence have occurred, there is the overwhelming feeling of dysphoria, anxiety, and guilt feelings; and, supposedly, the addicted person's predominant motivation is to avoid the suppression of the abstinence phenomenon.

The abstinence phenomenon consists of a constellation of signs that are believed to reach peak intensity on the second or third day after the last dose of the opiate. These signs subside rapidly during the next 7 days. However, a stable state may not be approached for 6 months or longer. During the abstinence period a single dose of an opiate abolishes the abstinence phenomenon, which reappears after the effects of the new drug have worn off. The abstinence syndrome is dangerous to a person with heart disease, tuberculosis, or other chronic debilitating conditions. The yawning, rhinorrhea, lacrimation, pupillary dilation, sweating, piloerection, and restlessness are observed from 12 to 16 hours after the last dose of an opiate. Later muscular aches and twitching, abdominal cramps, vomiting, diarrhea hypertension, insomnia, anorexis, agitation, profuse sweating, weight loss, hyperglycemia, increased output of 17 ketosteroids, and spontaneous ejaculation or profuse menstrual bleeding have been observed as part of the abstinence phenomenon. But there are marked individual differences.

Diagnosis

The typical abstinence syndrome is perhaps the best clue to the diagnosis of an addiction. The syndrome can be observed over a period of 14 to 48 hours in a drug-controlled setting. A more rapid method of diagnosis is the subcutaneous administration of 3 mg. of Nalline. If mydriasis, tachypnea, sweating, yawning, and gooseflesh are not displayed within 20 minutes after the first injection, a second dose of 5 mg. may be given; if no signs are elicited within 20 minutes after the second injection, a third and final dose of 7 mg. may be administered. If this dose fails to elicit abstinence syndromes, the findings should be considered negative. The result of the Nalline test must not be considered positive unless the pattern of elicited signs is characteristic.

Naloxone (Narcan) may be substituted, starting with an intramuscular dose of 0.16 mg.

If there are no signs of abstinence, a second dose of 0.24 mg. is given intravenously. Observations are repeated in 15 minutes.

The more usual diagnostic signs of addiction are needle marks and bluish phlebitis scars, the presence of myosis, and some drowsiness. If opiates have been used in the past 24 hours, they may be detected in the urine.

Treatment

The first step in drug-free and antagonist treatment programs is the withdrawal of the drug user from the drug of abuse. In some methadone maintenance programs, the direct substitution of methadone for heroin is made, and the maintenance dose is increased from that point. More commonly, the user is withdrawn from heroin or another opiate and is stabilized. Then the methadone, antagonist, or other drug is slowly increased in dosage.

The most widely used method is methadone substitution, either in an inpatient setting or on an ambulatory basis. In either case, the necessary prerequisites are a complete medical and psychiatric history and a thorough physical examination. Since many heroin addicts are multiple drug users, a careful and detailed history of drug use must be obtained.

An initial dose of methadone syndrome is administered orally in an orange solution. Generally, an initial dose of 30 mg. to 40 mg. is sufficient. After the satisfactory initial suppression of the abstinence syndrome, the methadone is withdrawn progressively over a period of 3 to 7 days. Generally, the rate of withdrawal is 5 mg. a day.

If there is a history of dependence on barbiturates, alcohol, or other sedatives, appropriate measures for detoxification from these substances must also be taken to prevent the emergence of seizures or delirium tremens.

If therapeutic communities that are crusadingly drug-free, it is the practice to use drug-free detoxification. Withdrawal symptoms are influenced by fear of peer alienation; therefore, they are suppressed. Other unusual drug-free methods have also been used for detoxification, including transcendental meditation and acupuncture.

Present treatment approaches appear to stress either nonbiological or biological models. Among the nonbiological models are various psychotherapeutic attempts, including group psychotherapy; residential treatment centers, such as Synanon and Daytop; therapeutic communities, such as Odyssey House and Phoenix House; religious, political, and social pressures exerted by Black Muslims and Black Panthers; and strict, harsh, punitive legal enforcements. Five biological models have been proposed for the treatment of narcotic addiction—maintenance, narcotic antagonists, biochemical blockade, receptor blockade, and immune therapy.

Therapeutic Communities

The therapeutic communities are psychologically oriented and drug-free and favor the residential treatment modality. Synanon's rehabilitation efforts rely on harsh group encounters, re-education, and hard work. The major tenet of Synanon and the other programs is that addicts are immature people in flight from reality and responsibility, and, therefore, they must be given a second chance to grow up. The therapeutic communities adhere to the concept that the abuse of drugs is symptomatic of underlying antisocial personality problems and behavior patterns.

The largest therapeutic community, Phoenix House in New York City, consisted of 15 houses and more than 1,000 residents in 1970. From 1967 to 1970, during the first 3 years of its existence, only 148 Phoenix House residents completed a 2½-year program and returned to a drug-free life in the world outside. A study of 2,110 admissions to Phoenix House between 1967 and 1970 revealed that 53 per cent of the addicts admitted to the program withdrew from it. At the time of the study, in 1971, only 4 per cent of those admitted had completed the course of treatment, and most of them were employed by Phoenix House.

Methadone Maintenance

This approach is based on the assumption that heroin addiction is a metabolic disease—a concept that has not gained general acceptance—on the principle of cross-tolerance between methadone and opiates, and on gradual accumulation of the drug followed by slow excretion. Further, it is assumed that, if the addict is supplied with adequate quantities of opiate, he will not find it necessary to resort to criminal activity. Orally administered methadone at a certain dosage level does not appear to have a euphorigenic effect, but it induces a marked, slowly developing tolerance to all opiate-like drugs, including methadone itself. As a result, the patient cannot feel the euphoric effect of ordinary doses of other narcotics, such as heroin and morphine.

Although methadone maintenance has achieved a certain amount of success in moving the addict toward socially productive behavior, it has, since it is an agonist narcotic, also created a wide variety of medical, social, and legal problems, such as the diversion of methadone to illegal channels and overdose-related deaths. These problems have been attributed to the exclusive focus of unsupported drug therapy devoid of adjunctive services. There are also major problems with methadone itself that have led to investigations of longer-lasting methadonelike drugs, such as l-alpha-acetylmethadol (LAAM) and the opiate antagonists.

Methadone maintenance, as used in the United States, is an oral method, in contrast to the intravenous use of methadone in the British Isles.

One of the problems in methadone maintenance programs is whether to aim for a therapeutic goal of attaining drug abstinence of some appropriate time or to opt for the indeterminate administration of methadone, possibly for life.

The National Research Council and The American Medical Association oppose methadone maintenance in the office practice of private physicians, since the individual physician cannot provide all the services for the various therapeutic needs of the patient. Also, the individual physician is not in a position to ensure control against the redistribution of the drug into illicit channels, to maintain control of doses, and to establish the elements for proper evaluation of the treatment.

Heroin Maintenance

Among the proponents of methadone maintenance, a subgroup urges the expansion of the concept of maintenance to include heroin. The reasons given are that heroin is the drug of choice for most addicts and that methadone maintenance treatment attracts the older addicts, whose average age in New York is 33.7 years, rather than the younger addicts. Furthermore, heroin maintenance proponents suggest that the dwindling size of waiting lists at methadone maintenance clinics indicates that this approach has reached all those it is likely to help and, thus, has a finite appeal.

The suggestion that addicts be maintained on heroin is opposed by many on the ground that this treatment approach would create more problems than it is likely to solve. Opponents of heroin maintenance state that establishing heroin maintenance in the United States would (1) render addiction less costly, more attractive, and more socially acceptable, (2) free additional supplies of heroin to further feed newcomers to the drug without the compensating benefit of having cured any heroin addicts, (3) establish a so-called legitimate use for heroin that would make the international goal of eliminating opium cultivation contradictory and unrealistic, (4) discourage bona fide treatment efforts that would be unable to compete with free heroin, and (5) reduce by an unknown number some property crimes but make it unlikely that these crimes would be of significance, since a heroin-maintained addict would continue in his usual incapacitated state of euphoria and be unable to earn a normal working wage.

Narcotic Antagonists

Narcotic antagonists are useful in heroin and other narcotic addictions, since they block or antagonize the opiates, preventing them from acting. Unlike methadone, the narcotic antagonists do not in themselves exert narcotic effects, nor are they addictive.

The conditioning hypothesis suggests that the extinction of drug-seeking behavior could provide a means to reverse the pathophysiology of addiction. If the relief afforded by narcotics during the period of conditioned abstinence were blocked, the extinction of physical and psychic dependence could occur. This extinction could be accomplished by a substance without narcotic effects that would block the ability of administered opiates to affect the central nervous system. Narcotic antagonists are such substances.

Molecular alterations of narcotic analgesics have yielded compounds that antagonize the respiratory effects of narcotics. N-Allylnormorphine or nalorphine (Nalline) has been used in the treatment of opiate overdose. Similar chemical substitutions have yielded cyclazocine, na-loxone, and naltrexone—three antagonists used for the treatment of opiate dependence.

The major weakness of the antagonist model is the lack of any mechanism compelling the addict receiving the antagonist to continue. Thus, the addict on cyclazocine may, under personal stress, decide not to take the cyclazocine on a Saturday morning. By Sunday morning, he can experience a high from heroin. There is no significant withdrawal from cyclazocine. He can then return to cyclazocine on Monday morning and continue on the program, or he may decide to abandon the whole program.

Community Approach

The treatment of opioid addiction is characterized by fragmentation, with proponents of various modalities competing with each other. The existing variability among addicts requires a wide range of goals to achieve the highest level of social rehabilitation feasible for a particular addict. These varied goals require differential diagnosis and differential treatment consisting of a variety of modalities based on criteria developed for judging the appropriateness of these modalities for any particular patient.

In addition to such individual multimodality approaches, intervention in the important institutions of society must be considered. These institutions include housing, schools, employment, and the law—all of which contribute to the causes of addiction. Of special importance are the implications of growing up in a highly industrialized, technically advanced society. The spread of addiction to young people around the world indicates common factors in the youth culture that must be understood if one is to work with adolescent addicts. An approach based on both individual and institutional interventions requires that programs be based in a community with the full participation of community representatives as partners.

Prevention

A wise prevention course appears to be the integration of drug and drug-use information into broad hygiene and problem-solving courses in the schools, rather than the use of exclusive drug courses. The participation of students, faculty, and school administrators in the planning and implementation of these courses, with particular emphasis on students' playing a major and active role, is crucial for success.

Effective prevention also depends on active intervention in those institutions of society that contribute to the genesis of drug abuse. The correction of gross inequities in society in regard to housing, race, youth, law, and personal values can only benefit the target population.

REFERENCES

Brill, H. History of the medical treatment of drug dependence. In *Drug Use in America: Problem in Perspective: The Technical Papers of the Second Report of the National Commission on Marihuana and Drug Abuse*, vol 4, p. 109. United States Government Printing Office, Washington, 1973.

Brotman, R. E., and Suffet, F. Illicit Drug use: Preventive education in the schools, Psychiatr. Ann., *3:* 48, 1973.

Brown, B. S. The treatment and rehabilitation of narcotic addicts in the United States. In *Drug Use in America: Problem in Perspective: The Technical Papers of the Second Report of the National Commission on Marihuana and Drug Abuse*, vol. 9, p. 127. United States Government Printing Office, Washington, 1973.

Chein, I., Gerard, D. L., Lee, R. S., and Rosenfeld, E. *The Road to H: Narcotics, Delinquency, and Social Policy.* Basic Books, New York, 1964.

Colburn, D., and Colburn, K. Integrity House: The addict as a total institution. Society. *10*, 39, 1973.

Cushman, P., and Dole. V. P. Detoxification of methadone maintained patients. J. A. M. A., *226*, 747, 1973.

Densen-Gerber, J. *We Mainline Dreams: The Odyssey House Story.* Doubleday. New York, 1973.

Dole, V. P. Editorial: Detoxification of methadone patients and public policy. J. A. M. A., *226:* 780, 1973.

Dole, V. P., and Nyswander, M. A medical treatment for diacetylmorphine (heroin) addiction: A clinical trial with methadone hydrochloride. J. A. M. A., *193:* 646, 1965.

Drug Use in America: Problem in Perspective: Second Report of the National Commission on Marihuana and Drug Abuse, p. 347. United States Government Printing Office, Washington, 1973.

Dumont, M. P. Technology and the treatment of addiction. In *Opiate Addiction: Origins and Treatments*, S. Fisher and A. M. Freedman, editors, p. 163. V. H. Winston, Washington, 1973.

Federal Register. vol. 38(90), sect. 130.44(8), May 10, 1973.

Ferretti, F. Narcotics: Hard drugs face hard new law. *The New York Times*, sect. 4. p. 3 Aug. 26, 1973.

Freedman, A. M. Drugs and society: An ecological approach. Comp. Psychiatry. *13:* 411, 1972.

Freedman, A. M. The adolescent heroin abuse epidemic in New York City, 1949. Excerpta Medica, series 274. Psychiatry (Part II) Symposium 36, Amsterdam, 1974.

Friedman, C. J., and Friedman, A. S. Drug abuse and delinquency. In *Drug Abuse in America: Problem in Perspective: The Technical Papers of the Second Report of the National Commission on Marihuana and Drug Abuse*, vol. 1. p. 398. United States Government Printing Office, Washington, 1973.

Levine, R., Zaks, A., Fink, M., and Freedman, A. M. Levomethadyl acetate. J. A. M. A., *226:* 316, 1973.

Lewis, E., Jr. A Heroin maintenance program in the United States? J. A. M. A., *223:* 539, 1973.

Lowney, L., Schulz, K., Lowery, P., and Goldstein. A. Partial purification of an opiate receptor from mouse brain. Science, *183:* 749, 1974.

Martin, W. R., Jasinski, O. R., Haertzen, C. A., Kay, D. C. Jones, B., Mansky, P. A., and Carpenter. R. W. Methadone: A reevaluation. Arch. Gen. Psychiatry. *28:* 286, 1973.

Musto, D. F. The great American dilemma. Drugs and Society, *2:* 13, 1973.

New York Addiction Services Agency. *Comprehensive Plan for the Control of Drug Abuse and Addiction.* New York, 1973.

Pert, C. B., and Snyder, S. H. Opiate receptor: Demonstration in nervous tissue. Science. *179:* 1011, 1973.

Powell, D. H. A pilot study of occasional heroin users. Arch. Gen. Psychiatry, *28:* 586, 1973.

Raynes, A. E., and Patch, V. D. An improved detoxification technique for heroin addicts. Arch. Gen. Psychiatry, *29:* 417, 1973.

Resnick, R., Fink, M., and Freedman, A. M. High dose cyclazocine therapy of opiate dependence. Am. J. Psychiatry, *131:* 595, 1974.

Resnick, R., Volavka, J. Freedman, A. M. and Thomas, M. Studies of EN-1639A (naltrexone): A new narcotic antagonist. Am. J. Psyciatry, *131:* 646, 1974.

Robins, L. N., Davis, D. H., and Goodwin, D. W. Drug use by U. S. Army enlisted men in Vietnam: A follow-up on their return home. Am. J. Epidemiol., *99:* 235, 1974.

Siegel, A. J. The heroin crisis among U. S. forces in Southeast Asia. J. A. M. A., *223:* 1258, 1973.

Szara, S., and Bunney, W. E., Jr. Recent research on opiate addiction: Review of a national program. In *Opiate Addiction: Origins and Treatment*, S. Fisher and A. M. Freedman, editors, p. 43. V. H. Winston, Washington, 1973.

Vaillant, G. E. A 20-year follow-up of New York narcotic addicts. Arch. Gen. Psychiatry, *29:* 237, 1973.

Wald, P. M., and Hutt, P. B. The drug abuse survey project: Summary of findings, conclusions, and recommendations. In *Dealing with Drug Abuse: A Report to the Ford Foundation*, p. 3. Praeger, New York, 1972.

Waldron, V. D., Klimt, C. R., and Seibel, J. E. Methadone overdose treated with naloxone infusion. J. A. M. A., *225:* 53, 1973.

Way, E. L. Some biochemical aspects of morphine tolerance and physical dependence. In *Opiate Addiction: Origins and Treatments*, S. Fisher and A. M. Freedman, editors, p. 99. V. H. Winston, Washington, 1973.

Wikler, A. Dynamics of drug dependence: Implications of a conditioning theory for research and treatment. In *Opiate Addiction: Origins and Treatment.* S. Fisher and A. M. Freedman, editors, p. 7. V. H. Winston, Washington, 1973.

Woodson, D. SAODAP chief resigns after "bitter struggle." J. Addiction Res. Foundation. *2:* 1, 1973.

22.2.   DEPENDENCE ON NONNARCOTIC AGENTS

Introduction

Drug abuse means the taking of drugs at dose levels and under circumstances and in settings that significantly augment the potential for harm, whether or not such use is legal and whether it is intended to be therapeutic, pleasurable, consciousness-expanding, or physician-prescribed.

Psychological dependence is defined as the development of a craving for the drug because its effects are perceived as pleasurable. Physical dependence implies some kind of biochemical or physiological change wherein the body requires the continued presence of the drug if a withdrawal syndrome is to be avoided after discontinuation of the drug. Tolerance refers to the fact that, on repeated administration of the same dose of the drug, there is a declining effect of the drug or, conversely, the necessity to increase the dose on repeated administrations in order to obtain the initial degree of effect.

Marijuana

Marijuana is the dried and chopped-up flowering pistillate and staminate tops and leaves of the hemp plant, *Cannabis sativa*. (See Figure 1.) It has analgesic, anticonvulsant, and muscle-relaxant properties. Throughout history the principal interest in the hemp plant has been in its properties as an agent for achieving euphoria. In this country, it is almost invariably smoked, usually as a cigarette, but elsewhere the drug is often taken in the form of a drink or in foods such as sweetmeats.

Drug preparations from the hemp plant vary widely in quality and potency, depending on the seeds, climate, soil, cultivation, and method of preparation. When the cultivated plant is fully ripe, a sticky, golden yellow resin with a minty fragrance covers its flower clusters and top leaves. The plant's resin contains the active substances. Preparations of the drug come in three grades, identified by Indian names. The cheapest and least potent, called bhang, is derived from the cut tops of uncultivated plants and has a low resin content. Most of the marijuana smoked in the United States is of this grade. Ganja is obtained from the flowering tops and leaves of carefully selected cultivated plants, and it has a higher quality and quantity of resin. The third and highest grade of the drug, called charas in India, is largely made from the resin itself, obtained from the tops of mature plants; only this version of the drug is properly called hashish. Hashish is roughly 5 to 8 times more potent than most of the marijuana regularly available in the United States.

The effects of cannabis (a general term for the various forms of the psychoactive products of the plant) in animals are confined to the central nervous system. The drug does not noticeably affect the gross behavior of rats or mice or simple learning in rats; it does, however, calm mice that have been made aggressive by isolation, and in dogs it induces a dreamy, somnolent state reminiscent of the last stage of a human high. In large doses, cannabis produces in animals symptoms such as vomiting, diarrhea, fibrillary tremors, and failure of muscular coordination.

The psychic effects from smoking marijuana last for 2 to 4 hours; from ingestion of the drug, the effects last for 5 to 12 hours. For a new user, the initial anxiety that sometimes occurs is alleviated if supportive friends are present. It is contended that the intoxication heightens sensitivity to external stimuli, reveals details that would ordinarily be overlooked, makes colors seem brighter and richer, brings out values in works of art that previously had little or no meaning to the viewer, and enhances the appreciation of music.

The sense of time is distorted: 10 minutes may seem like an hour. There is often a splitting of consciousness, so that the smoker, while experiencing the high, is at the same time an objective observer of his own intoxication.

Marijuana is commonly referred to as a hallucinogen. As with LSD, the wavelike aspect of the experience is often reported, as is the distorted perception of various parts of the body, spatial and temporal distortion, and depersonalization. Other phenomena commonly associated with both types of drugs are increased sensitivity to sound, synesthesia, heightened suggestibility, and a sense of thinking more clearly and having deeper awareness of the meaning of things. Anxiety and paranoid reactions are sometimes seen as consequences of either drug. However, the agonizingly nightmarish reactions that even the experienced LSD user may endure are quite rare to the experienced marijuana smoker. Furthermore, cannabis has a tendency to produce sedation, whereas LSD and the LSD-type drugs may induce long periods of wakefulness and even restlessness. Unlike LSD, marijuana does not dilate the pupils or materially heighten blood pressure, reflexes, and body temperature. On the other hand, it does increase the pulse rate. However, it is questionable whether marijuana in doses ordinarily used in this country can produce true hallucinations. An important difference is the fact that tolerance rapidly develops with the LSD-type drugs but not at all with cannabis. Finally, there is the fact that marijuana lacks the potent consciousness-altering qualities of LSD, peyote, mescaline, psilocybin, and so on. These differences, particularly the

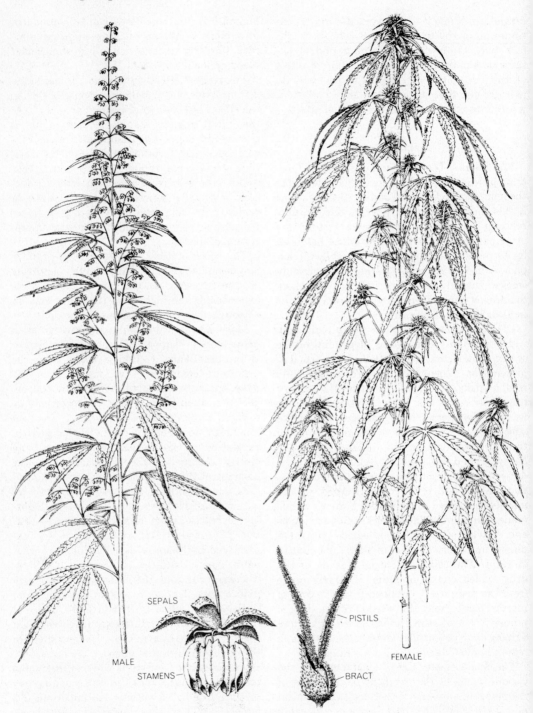

SEPALS

PISTILS

MALE

STAMENS

BRACT

FEMALE

Fig. 1. Hemp plant (*Cannabis sativa*) is a common weed growing freely in many parts of the world, where it is used as a medicine, an intoxicant, and a source of fiber. It is classified as a dioecious plant—that is, the male reproductive parts are on one plant (left) and the female parts are on another (right). Details of the two types of flower are show at bottom.

last, cast considerable doubt on marijuana's credentials for inclusion in this group.

There is an abundance of evidence that marijuana is not a drug that produces physical dependence; cessation of its use produces no withdrawal symptoms, nor does a user feel any need to increase the dosage as he becomes accustomed to the drug. Furthermore, its capacity to lead to psychological dependence is not as strong as that of either tobacco or alcohol.

Only the unsophisticated continued to believe that cannabis leads to violence and crime. Indeed, instead of inciting criminal behavior, cannabis may tend to suppress it. The intoxication induces a lethargy that is not conducive to any physical activity, let alone the committing of crimes. The release of inhibitions results in fantasy and verbal rather than behavioral expression.

There is little evidence that cannabis stimulates sexual desire or power. Many marijuana users report that the high enhances the enjoyment of sexual intercourse. This may be true in the same sense that the enjoyment of art and music is apparently enhanced. It is questionable, however, that the intoxication breaks down moral barriers that are not already broken.

Reports from many investigators indicate that long-term users of the potent versions of cannabis are typically passive, nonproductive, slothful, and totally lacking in ambition. It is possible that chronic use of the drug in its stronger forms may have debilitating effects, as prolonged heavy drinking does. However, many of those who take up cannabis in the Orient are people who are hungry, sick, hopeless, or defeated, seeking through this inexpensive drug to soften the impact of an otherwise unbearable reality. There is a substantial body of evidence that moderate use of marijuana does not produce physical or mental deterioration.

Although it has not been conclusively established that marijuana may precipitate a psychosis, it stands to reason that a person maintaining a delicate balance of ego functioning—so that, for instance, the ego is threatened by a severe loss or a surgical assault or even an alcoholic debauch—may also be overwhelmed or precipitated into a schizophrenic reaction by a drug that alters, however mildly, his state of consciousness. Among heavy users of the drug, the proportion of people with neuroses or personality disorders is usually higher than in the general population; one may, therefore, expect the incidence of psychoses also to be higher in this group. The fact that it is not suggests that for some mentally disturbed people the escape provided by the drug may serve to prevent a psychotic breakdown.

However, it seems clear that the drug may precipitate in susceptible people one of several types of mental dysfunction. The most serious and disturbing is the toxic psychosis, an acute state that resembles the delirium of a high fever and is caused by the presence in the brain of toxic substances that interfere with a variety of cerebral functions. Generally speaking, as the toxins disappear, so do the symptoms of toxin psychosis. The syndrome often includes clouding of consciousness, restlessness, confusion, bewilderment, disorientation, dreamlike thinking, apprehension, fear, illusions, and hallucinations. Cannabis can induce a toxic psychosis, but it generally requires a large ingested dose. Such a reaction is apparently much less likely to occur when cannabis is smoked.

Some people may suffer short-lived, acute anxiety states, sometimes with and sometimes without accompanying paranoid thoughts. The anxiety may reach such proportion as to be called panic. Panic reactions, although uncommon, probably constitute the most frequent adverse reaction to the moderate use of smoked marijuana. During this reaction, the sufferer may believe that the various distortions of his perception of his body mean that he is dying or that he is undergoing some great physical catastrophe, and similarly he may interpret the psychological distortions induced by the drug as an indication that he is losing his sanity. Set and setting undoubtedly contribute to this type of reaction.

If this panic reaction is accompanied by paranoid ideation, the user may, for example, believe that the others in the room, especially if they are not well known to him, have some hostile intentions toward him or that someone is going to inform on him for smoking marijuana. Generally speaking, these paranoid ideas are not strongly held, and simple reassurance dispels them. Set and setting are, again, very important.

Some rare reactions occur in people who have previously taken hallucinogenic drugs. One reaction is the recurrence of hallucinogenic symptoms, the so-called flashbacks. For some this is an enjoyable experience; for others it is distressing. Generally, this type of reaction fades with the passage of time.

Rarely, but especially among new users of marijuana, there occurs an acute depressive reaction. It is generally rather mild and transient but may sometimes require psychiatric intervention. This type of reaction is most likely to occur in a user who has some degree of underlying depression.

Amphetamines

Recent surveys among student populations have revealed that in some cities significant amphetamine abuse is occurring as early as the fifth and sixth grades and that between 15 and 25 per cent of all high school students are regular "speed" users.

Today, even though the Food and Drug Administration officially recognizes only short-term appetite reduction, narcolepsy, some types of parkinsonism, and certain behavioral disorders in hyperkinetic young children as valid therapeutic indications for the amphetamines, these drugs continue to be prescribed by many physicians.

By 1958, the annual legal United States production of amphetamines has risen to 75,000 pounds, or 3.5 billion tablets—enough to supply every man, women, and child with about 20 standard (5 mg.) doses. Less than 10 years later, the drug industry was pouring out 160,000 pounds—about 8 billion tablets—a year, enough for 35 to 50 pills for every living American. By 1970, reported legal amphetamine production has risen to more than 10 billion tablets. And since the mid-1960's there has been a considerable growth of both black market diversion of legitimately produced amphetamine and illicit bathroom laboratories that synthesize high concentrations of injectable methamphetamine.

Characteristics

The amphetamines produce definite physical dependence. Withdrawal from amphetamines can be most distressing. Extreme lethargy, fatigue, anxiety, terrifying nightmares, and suicidally severe depression are common. The person is often disoriented, bewildered, and confused. He is apt to be extremely irritable and demanding, which drives people away just when he most needs their help. His psychic disruption and loss of self-control may lead to violent acting-out of aggressive impulses. His head aches, he sweats profusely, and his body is racked with alternating sensations of extreme heat and extreme cold and with excruciating muscle cramps. He characteristically suffers painful gastrointestinal cramps. Especially if he is alone and despite his sometimes incredible hunger, he often lacks the strength to eat at all, aggravating his condition through malnutrition.

From 1939 to the present, there have been reported several hundred cases of acute physical amphetamine poisoning and a like number from chronic use. The signs and symptoms reported include flushing, pallor, cyanosis, fever, tachycardia, serious cardiac problems, markedly elevated blood pressure, hemorrhage or other vascular accidents, nausea, vomiting, difficulty in breathing, tremor, ataxia, loss of sensory abilities, twitchings, tetany, convulsions, loss of consciousness, and coma. Death from overdose is usually associated with hyperpyrexia, convulsions, and cardiovascular shock. By 1966, cases of severe serum hepatitis, lung abscess, and endocarditis resulting from intravenous abuse of amphetamines were being regarded as fairly common occurrences, and, by 1970, the first clinical evidence that intravenous "speed" may cause necrotizing angiitis was presented.

Although restlessness, dysphoria, logorrhea, insomnia, some degree of confusion, dizziness, transient nausea, tension, anxiety, and fear to the point of acute panic have been reported by a large number of authors, these effects are probably best considered as inseparable components of the amphetamines' alerting, stimulating, and euphoric properties.

That a psychosis may be induced in essentially normal people by amphetamines has been substantiated by at least two clinical experiments using human volunteers. Like paranoid schizophrenics, patients with amphetamine psychosis are often markedly paranoid, with delusions of persecution and ideas of reference. The paranoid state is often preceded by a state of restlessness, increased irritability, and increased perceptual sensitivity. The patients often experience visual and auditory hallucinations, frequently of a bizarre nature. The most reliable means of establishing the diagnosis of amphetamine psychosis is to use the methyl orange test or other laboratory tests more specific for amphetamine to detect its presence in the urine. With few exceptions the symptoms of amphetamine psychosis disappear within a matter of days or, at the most, weeks after the drug has been withdrawn. However, in some patients a degree of suspiciousness and tendencies toward misinterpretation and ideas of reference may remain for months after the manifest, overt psychosis has disappeared.

Treatment

Since amphetamine psychosis is generally self-limiting, treatment usually requires little more than supportive measures. The elimination of the amphetamines may be facilitated by acidifying the urine through the use of ammonium chloride. Antipsychotics, either a phenothiazine or haloperidol, may be prescribed for the first few days of the psychosis; beyond that time there is usually little need for drug treatment. Because the amphetamine psychotic may be assaultive, it may be necessary to treat him in a hospital setting. The withdrawal depression may be treated with tricyclic antidepressants; however, symptomatic treatment may require weeks or even a month or so. Ultimately more important than these aspects of treatment is the need to establish the beginnings of a therapeutic alliance during this phase and to make good use of this psychotherapeutic relationship in the treatment of the underlying depression or character disorder or both. However, inasmuch as many of these patients have become dependent on the drug, one can anticipate that psychotherapy will be especially difficult.

In spite of the problems associated with dependence on amphetamines the authors still believe that they are invaluable in the management of mild to moderate depressive states and the neurasthenias. The harsh governmental restrictions placed upon the medical profession regarding the use of these drugs are questionable.

Cocaine

Cocaine is an alkaloid derived from the leaf of the shrub *Erythroxylon coca*, a plant indigenous to Bolivia and Peru, where its leaves have been chewed for centuries for their stimulating effects on the central nervous system. In this country the alkaloid extract is taken by ingestion, injection, or snuffing, and occasionally it is sprinkled on the genitals. The description of the high achieved with this is almost identical to that described by users of large doses of amphetamines. The most common aspects of the high, then, are the euphoria, the exhiliration, and the powerful rush of a sense of well-being and confidence. Also in common with the amphetamines, the user builds up a tolerance to the drug and may become physically dependent. It is estimated that those who become physically dependent may use as much as 500 mg. a day; the acute lethal dose is estimated to be in the range of 1 gm.

Acute and chronic toxic effects are similar to those of the amphetamines and are referable to stimulation of the central nervous system. The acutely toxic patient is excited, confused, restless, and very anxious and apprehensive. His pulse is rapid, his blood pressure is increased, and his respirations may become irregular. Usually his pupils are dilated. His temperature may be elevated. Death may result as a consequence of respiratory arrest. The treatment for the acute toxic physical effects involves limiting the further absorption of cocaine and the intravenous administration of a short-acting barbiturate. Chronic abuse of cocaine often leads to loss of weight and anemia, as the drug is anorectic. Perforation of the nasal septum is occasionally seen. Psychologically, there may develop a toxic psychosis with visual, auditory, and tactile hallucinations. And as with amphetamines, a paranoid delusional system may develop.

Barbiturates

Barbiturates are general depressants that have considerable effect on the activity of nerve, skeletal muscle, smooth muscle, and cardiac muscle and are also capable of depressing a wide range of biological functions.

The characteristics of barbiturate dependence are a psychological dependence owing to the user's subjective reactions of pleasure and release from tension and manifesting itself in a strong desire, even compulsion, to continue taking the drug, a tendency to increase the dosage to overcome the tolerance factor, and physical dependence when the presence of the drug is necessary for the maintenance of homeostasis. The last characteristic develops only when the drug is taken for over a period of one to two months or longer at doses above the recommended therapeutic level.

The barbiturates are legitimately manufactured in immense quantities and are readily available in numerous forms. For example, the long-acting barbiturate, phenobarbital, is an ingredient in at least 80 different proprietary drugs in combination with other barbiturates, bromides, tranquilizers, analgesics, antihistamines, vitamins, antibiotics, gastric antacids, and a number of other things. In 1954, it was estimated that at least 800,000 pounds of barbiturates were produced in the United States every year, enough to fill almost 6 billion capsules—about 30 capsules for every person in the country. Since 1962, production has increased to more than 1 million pounds a year, and by 1973 was sufficient to supply every person in the country with 50 doses. Because of these tremendous, legitimately manufactured quantities of barbiturates, there has been little pressure to establish illegal clandestine laboratories to produce the drug. Instead, the black market meets its need by diverting shipments of barbiturates from manufacturers to addresses in Mexico and then bringing them back across the border illegally. Additional supplies are obtained by robbing drug warehouses and doctors' offices.

The three major barbiturates common in the black market are secobarbital, pentobarbital, and a combination of secobarbital and amobarbital.

Patterns of Use

Clinical experience suggests that dependence generally occurs in the emotionally maladjusted person seeking relief from unbearable feelings of tension, anxiety, and inadequacy. Such people are frequently characterized as those who become dependent on other psychoactive agents, as passive-aggressive personalities or passive-dependent types. Almost without exception, persons with a dependence on barbiturates fall into one of three major patterns of use.

The first pattern, that of chronic intoxication, occurs for the most part in 30- to 50-year-old persons who obtain the drug from their physicians, rather than from an illegal source. Often the drug was initially prescribed in response to their complaints of difficulty in falling asleep or

nervousness. Their drug dependence may go unidentified by those around them for months or years or until their ability to work becomes impaired or such physical signs as slurred speech become apparent.

The second pattern of use is episodic intoxication, and users in this category are generally teenagers or young adults who ingest barbiturates with the same purpose for which they might consume alcohol, to produce a high or experience a sense of well-being. Factors such as the surroundings in which the abuser takes the drug (setting), the psychological makeup of the person, and, most important, his expectations of the effect (set) determine the end result. Like the so-called social drinker, these young people may become so accustomed to having episodically this sense of well-being engendered by the drug that barbiturates become a fairly constant aspect of their lives.

The third category is that of intravenous barbiturate use, and these users are mainly young adults who are intimately involved in the illegal drug culture and who can often be identified by the large abscesses covering accessible areas of their bodies. Their experiences with drugs have often been extensive, ranging from pill popping to speed and heroin. Barbiturates are injected for their rush effect, which is described as a pleasurable, warm, and drowsy feeling. Like speed freaks, these barb freaks are disliked by the rest of the subculture because of their irresponsibility and occasional tendency to be violent and disruptive.

In addition, some use barbiturates incidentally to their dependence on other drugs. Barbiturates are sometimes used by heroin addicts to boost the effects of weak heroin, and alcoholics are known to consider barbiturates a means of relieving the tremulousness of alcohol withdrawal. Some speed freaks inject secobarbital as a downer to help them avoid the paranoia and agitation usually experienced at the end of a trip.

Effects

All patterns of use present real dangers to the health of the user. It has been reported that barbiturates are the cause of death in 6 per cent of all suicides and cause more accidental deaths (18 per cent) than any other single drug. About 15,000 deaths in the United States are attributed annually to barbiturates. In New York City alone from 1957 to 1963, there were 8,469 cases of barbiturate poisoning, 1,165 of them fatalities. In the area of drugs, barbiturates rank second only to salicylates as a cause of accidental death in toddlers in the United States.

An average daily dose of 1.5 gm. of short-acting barbiturate is common, and some users have been reported to consume as much as 2.5 gm. daily over a period of months. Although marked tolerance develops to the sedating and intoxicating effects of the drug, the lethal dose is not much greater for the chronic abuser than it is for the neophyte. There is always the possibility of accidental death for the addict as he gradually increases his dosage. Once a user has developed tolerance at a specific dose level, he need raise the dosage by as little as 0.1 gm. to recapture intoxication. However, this continuing process leads the user to a point at which his doses are so massive that he may experience cardiovascular failure from the intense depressant effect of the drug. Barbiturate-induced depression of the central nervous system can range from mild sedation to deep coma, depending on the dose and route of administration, the degree of excitability of the central nervous system at the time the drug is being used, and the degree to which the user has already developed some tolerance to the drug.

The effects of mild barbiturate intoxication (both acute and chronic) resemble intoxication with alcohol. Symptoms include a general sluggishness, difficulty in thinking, poor memory, slowness of speech and comprehension, faulty judgment, narrowed range of attention, emotional lability, and exaggeration of basic personality traits. The sluggishness may wear off after a number of hours, but judgment may be defective, mood distorted, and motor skills impaired for many hours. Additional symptoms of barbiturate intoxication frequently include hostility, quarrelsomeness, and moroseness. Occasionally, paranoid ideas and suicidal tendencies surface. Neurological effects include nystagmus, diplopia, strabismus, ataxic gait, positive Romberg's sign, hypotonia, dysmetria, and decreased superficial reflexes. Diagnosis of barbiturate intoxication is based on the presence of at least some of these signs and symptoms, and this diagnosis may be confirmed by a number of laboratory tests; the most commonly used are paper chromatography and ultraviolet spectrophotometry.

Treatment

When a user's tolerance has grown to the extent that he is taking near-lethal doses, it is imperative that he withdraw or be withdrawn from the drug. The withdrawal syndrome can range from rather mild symptoms—such as anxiety, weakness, profuse sweating, and insomnia—to a severe reaction involving grand mal seizures, delirium, and cardiovascular collapse. A dosage of 0.6 mg. a day taken for at least 37 days may be necessary to produce signs of withdrawal. The greater the user's daily dose, the more severe are his withdrawal symptoms. Users with 400-mg.-a-day habits (pentobarbital or secobarbital) experience negligible symptoms, whereas those taking 800 mg. a day experience orthostatic hypotension, weakness, tremor, anxiety, and considerable discomfort, and about 75 per cent have convulsions. Users on even higher doses may experience apprehension, anorexia, confusion, delirium, hallucinations, psychoses, and convulsions. When seizures do occur, they are invariably of the clonic-tonic grand mal type, indistinguishable clinically from those of idiopathic grand mal epilepsy. The psychosis is clinically indistinguishable from that of alcoholic delirium tremens and is characterized by agitation, delusions, and hallucinations that are usually visual but may be auditory. Most of these symptoms appear within a day of the beginning of abstinence, but seizures generally do not occur until the second or third day, and psychosis, if it does develop, starts in the third to the eighth day. The various symptoms may last as long as 2 weeks.

To avoid seizures and sudden death, treatment of the patient during this period is very conservative. First, the magnitude of the user's daily habit must be determined. Family members and druggists should be consulted. The dose level must then be clinically verified. When a dose level has been attained in which the patient demonstrates a mild degree of intoxication and sedation, he should be stabilized on this dosage for 1 or 2 days. Then gradually this dose can be reduced, but by no more than 10 per cent a day. If, during this gradual withdrawal, the patient again begins to exhibit abstinence symptoms, the daily decrement should be halved. In the case of a patient who, when first seen, is comatose or grossly intoxicated, barbiturates are withheld until these symptoms have cleared.

After withdrawal is complete, the patient enters a crucial period in which he must overcome his desire to begin once again to take the drug. If a user is to remain drug-free, follow-up treatment, usually involving psychiatric help and the use of community resources, is vital. If this treatment is not forthcoming and successful, the patient will almost certainly return to barbiturates or a drug with similar hazards.

Methaqualone

Methaqualone is a nonbarbiturate sedative-hypnotic whose growth as a drug of abuse, particularly among young people, has accelerated rapidly over the last few years. These abusers, who enjoy the buzz they get from the drug, take large quantities, which they obtain through prescriptions from physicians and from illegitimate sources.

Methaqualone is a hypnotic. Among the undesirable effects reported are dryness of the mouth, headache, urticaria, dizziness, diarrhea, chills, tremors, hangover, paresthesia, menstrual disturbance, epistaxis, and depersonalization. Some users report the feeling that they will lose their minds. Chronic large doses have been reported to lead to epigastric distress, clumsiness, and forgetfulness. Methaqualone stimulates a considerable increase in the activity of the liver microsomal enzymes, more so than do the barbiturates. Furthermore, it is longer acting than amobarbital, secobarbital, and chloral hydrate. Like other drugs of dependence, methaqualone suppresses REM sleep, and REM rebound occurs upon its withdrawal. Tolerance to this drug may develop.

Like the barbiturates, to which it exhibits cross-tolerance, methaqualone is capable of producing a considerable degree of psychological dependence. A withdrawal syndrome has been observed in people using 600 to 3,000 mg. of methaqualone daily for prolonged periods of time. The syndrome consists of insomnia, headache, abdominal cramps, anorexia, nausea, irritability, and anxiety. In addition, hallucinations and nightmares have been reported and are thought to be related to use at the higher-dose levels. This withdrawal syndrome generally begins within 24 hours of cessation of drug use and persists for 2 to 3 days. It may be interrupted by giving the patient methaqualone, and this is the basis of treatment, which consists of tapering doses of the drug.

Overdose of methaqualone may result in restlessness, delirium, hypertonia, muscle spasms leading to convulsions, and death. Unlike the severe barbiturate toxic state, cardiovascular and respiratory depression are generally absent from the comparable methaqualone syndrome. Most fatal doses have involved a combination of methaqualone and alcohol. Treatment of overdosage involves supportive measures to maintain vital functions. In the case of recently ingested drug in a patient who is still conscious, gastric lavage is indicated.

Meprobamate

The acute toxic effects of large doses of meprobamate may include ataxia, somnolence, hypotensive reactions, shock, loss of consciousness, respiratory depression, and death. Somnolence is a common symptom of chronic toxicity. Tolerance does develop, and withdrawal symptoms occur in people who have chronically used large doses, usually more than several grams daily. When the drug is withdrawn abruptly, patients experience tremors, ataxia, headache, insomnia, and gastrointestinal-disturbances for several days; occasionally, convulsions occur with the cessation of the chronic use of very large doses (3 gm. or more daily). A syndrome resembling delirium tremens may occur within 36 to 48 hours. The symptoms include severe anxiety, tremors, muscle twitching, and hallucinations; grand mal seizures may develop.

Control of the convulsions is achieved with the intravenous administration of diphenyl-hydantoin sodium. The over-all treatment involves gradual withdrawal from the drug, but, because there is cross-tolerance with the barbiturates, a regime of short-acting barbiturate may be started and gradually withdrawn. Alternatively, the meprobamate can be reinstituted and gradually withdrawn over a period of about 10 days. Primarily because of the risk of convulsions, withdrawal,is perhaps best accomplished in a hospital setting.

Benzodiazepines

Like meprobamate, chlordiazepoxide and

diazepam are used for the symptomatic treatment of anxiety; in addition, they are commonly used as skeletal-muscle relaxants and in the treatment of alcoholism. The toxicity is relatively low; people who have ingested large amounts (more than 2 gm.) at one time in suicide attempts experienced drowsiness, lethargy, ataxia, and sometimes confusion and managed to depress their vital signs somewhat, but they have not succeeded in significantly harming themselves. However, chlordiazepoxide has been taken in doses that have caused comatose states. There is some question as to whether people can become psychologically dependent on the benzodiazepines since they apparently produce less euphoria, less of a high, than the other drugs mentioned here. But it is clear that those who take them over long periods of time, usually in large doses (several hundred milligrams or more daily), may experience a withdrawal syndrome when the drugs are withdrawn abruptly. The symptoms may include insomnia, anorexia, agitation, muscle twitching, sweating, and sometimes convulsions. The convulsions may not appear for several weeks after the withdrawal of these drugs, and this delayed reaction is thought to be due to the slowness with which the drugs are eliminated. Management of convulsions is similar to that described for meprobamate. The authors disagree with the severe governmental restrictions placed upon this class of drugs which are most useful in a variety of psychiatric disorders.

Glue and Other Volatile Solvents

Glue sniffing has received a lot of notoriety in recent years, possibly because it is a favorite psychoactive of the very young—from teenagers to children of 6 or 7 years. The glue is sniffed directly from tubes, from plastic bags, or from smears on pieces of cloth. At first, a few sniffs may lead to a jag, but, because tolerance develops over a period of weeks or months, chronic users may have to use up to seven tubes before achieving the desired effect of this central nervous system depressant. The intoxication is characterized by euphoria, excitement, a floating sensation, dizziness, slurred speech, and ataxia. Inebriation is accompanied by a breakdown of inhibitions, which is often reflected in a reckless abandon, and by a sense of greatly increased power and ability. The aggressiveness that accompanies alcoholic inebriation

is characteristic of that produced by glue sniffing, and, as in an alcohol drunk, amnesia for the acute intoxication may occur. Visual hallucinations sometimes occur. The duration of the intoxication is variable, anywhere from 15 minutes to several hours. Drowsiness usually accompanies small doses; stupor and even unconsciousness are occasionally sequelae of heavier use. Nausea and anorexia are acute symptoms, and weight loss may accompany chronic use.

Among the various psychoactive substances that are abused, the volatile solvents are among the most dangerous. There is no doubt that tolerance to these agents does occur, but it is not clear that there is a physical dependence with a withdrawal syndrome. There is no question, however, that young people may develop a severe psychological dependence on these substances. The habit is dangerous for two reasons. First, there is a risk of tissue damage—particularly to the bone marrow, brain, liver, and kidneys—resulting from high concentrations of toluene and other similar solvents, and the tissue damage may be irreversible; also, overdosage may lead to death from respiratory arrest. Second, young people intoxicated on these solvents appear to be more aggressive and impulsive, and at the same time they exhibit impaired judgment, a combination that can lead to dangerous and sometimes life-threatening behaviors and activities. Toluene appears to be the most widely used of the agents in this class, but xylene, benzene, lacquers, paint thinners, and lighter fluids have been used.

Hallucinogens

Among these drugs, d-lysergic acid diethylamide (LSD), peyote, mescaline, and psilocybin are the hallucinogens about which most is known. However, synthetic hallucinogens have recently been developed about which less is known. These newer drugs include 2,5-dimethoxy-4-methylamphetamine (DOM), sometimes called STP, N,N-dimethyltryptamine (DMT), the closely related substance N,N-diethyltryptamine (DET), dipropyltryptamine (DPT), phencyclidine hydrochloride (PCP), and 3,4-methylene-dioxyamphetamine (MDA). Some varieties of morning glory seeds contain lysergic acid amide-like alkaloids, derivatives that apparently have about one tenth the potency of LSD. A tea or brew may be prepared from the seeds, or they may simply be chewed. Other hallucinogens, such as Hawaiian wood-rose and nutmeg, are beginning to be experimented with, and there are reports of dried sea horses and small starfish being ingested to produce a new type of trip.

All these hallucinogens apparently act primarily on the central nervous system to produce some striking subjective effects. People who have taken these drugs often feel overwhelmed by auditory, visual, tactile, and other stimuli, which are perceived as especially brilliant and intense, and they may experience synesthesia, a unique alteration of perception wherein one sees sound and hears colors. Users may, on the one hand, experience a magnification of affective reactivity, with rapid change and much lability, and, on the other hand, achieve a state of relative calm and timelessness, which they often relate to a sense of eternity and which is frequently accompanied by a belief that during this state they have an exceptional capacity for being insightful and for integrating thinking and feeling.

These drugs seem to produce a whole range of contradictory effects, which appear to be experienced all at the same time but often in waves and with different constellations predominating at any particular time. Along with the underlying personality structure of the user, set and setting are important in determining the predominant kind of reaction a person has under the influence of the drug. Persons who are anxious, fearful, and rigid are more likely to experience a panic reaction than are persons who are more comfortable and open to the experience.

In the case of most of the hallucinogens, tolerance develops remarkably rapidly, so much so that, if they are used continually for 3 or 4 days, there is little psychedelic effect from the drugs. These drugs may have some slight capacity for psychological dependence, but they have none for physical dependence.

The risks involved in the use of hallucinogens are almost entirely mental and emotional in nature. Some users experience intense anxiety to the point of panic, paranoid reactions, and sometimes depression. Users sometimes become quite confused and have a frightening inability to separate fantasy from reality. Flashbacks—the recurrence after a drug-free period of an effect, usually of an anxiety-provoking nature,

that occurred during the drug experience—do occasionally occur. Prolonged psychotic reactions that seem to have been precipitated by the drug experience have been reported. Chromosome breakage was once thought to be a consequence of use, but considerable doubt has been raised by more recent studies.

The most important treatment approach to the person who is having a bad trip, one usually characterized by panic reaction, is talking down. This approach involves the giving of reassurance, comfort, and support to the patient, preferably by someone who is experienced in the use of hallucinogens.

Nicotine

Tobacco is the dried leaf of *Nicotiana tabacum*, and nicotine is the active principle in tobacco. The pure chemical compound was first isolated in 1828. The smoking, chewing, or snuffing of tobacco is a habit that afflicts more than 100 million Americans.

Nicotine has a markedly stimulating effect on the central nervous system. In large doses it produces tremors in humans and convulsions in animals. A wide range of cardiovascular responses has been attributed to nicotine. Among these responses are vasoconstriction, elevated blood pressure, and tachycardia. Acute nicotine poisoning has been reported in humans, with death occurring as a result of respiratory failure secondary to muscular paralysis from as little as 60 mg. Tolerance to nicotine develops when the compound is taken repeatedly, as in chronic cigarette smoking. The report of the Surgeon General, *Smoking and Health*, set forth the relationship of smoking to a variety of medical illnesses, including lung cancer, hypertension, bronchial asthma, bronchitis and other upper respiratory infections, cardiovascular disease, and chronic hypoxia.

Nicotine dependence is a well-defined syndrome, and a psychological and physiological withdrawal syndrome is associated with the abrupt cessation of smoking. This syndrome has been noted in both laboratory animals and humans. Studies have demonstrated that dogs and chimpanzees can become addicted to tobacco smoke. Although the incidence of smoking has been decreasing nationally, new smokers always seem to appear on the horizon, usually during adolescence. This attraction to smoking may be due to the adolescent's natural desire to experience the adult world. When the adolescent's parents smoke, the risk that the teenager will smoke is greater because of identification. In addition, advertising campaigns that encourage smoking, even though barred from television by governmental legislation, still appear in newspapers and magazines and appeal to the adolescent's need to maintain self-esteem to make his sexual role identification, and to quest for pleasure. Some advertising campaigns are particularly invidious in that they imply that to disregard hazardous warnings about cigarette smoking is a sign of independent thinking in the face of authoritarian caveat.

The cure of nicotinism is as difficult as the cure of other drug-dependent states. Self-help groups have been only partially successful. Hypnotic induction—in which the smoker is told that he will not want a cigarette and that, if he takes one, it will taste vile or produce nausea—has been attempted. Operant conditioning and other behavioral therapy approaches, particularly in group settings, are also used. Some people advocate gradual withdrawal and others favor a "cold-turkey" approach. In the latter approach, a minor tranquilizer may be useful in the early stages of abstinence. Regardless of method used, cessation of smoking is successful in only 40 per cent of all cases, and the relapse rate is high.

Studies of the personalities of those who smoke reveal conflicting pictures, ranging from the aggressive, hard-driving, ambitious personality to the more passive, oral-dependent personality. Nicotinism is not delimited by a particular psychiatric diagnosis, and it remains a prime public health problem.

REFERENCES

Ager, S. A. Luding-out, New Engl. J. Med., *287:* 51, 1972.

Beaubrun, M. H., and Knight, F. Pediatric assessment of 30 chronic users of cannabis and 30 matched controls. Am. J. Psychiatry, *130:* 309, 1973.

Connell, P. H. *Amphetamine Psychosis.* Chapman & Hall, London, 1958.

Gerald, M. C., and Schwirian, P. M. Nonmedical use of methaqualone. Arch. Gen. Psychiatry, *28:* 627, 1973.

Griffith, J. D., Cavanaugh, J. H., and Oates, J. A. Psychosis induced by the administration of *d*-amphetamine to human volunteers. In *Psychotomimetic Drugs,* D. H. Efron, editor, page 287. Raven Press, New York, 1970a.

Griffith, J. D., Cavanaugh, J. H., and Oates, J. A. Experimental psychosis induced by the administration of *d*-amphetamine. In *Amphetamines and Related Compounds: Proceedings of the Mario Negri Institute for Pharmacological Research, Milan, Italy,* E. Costa and S. Garattini, editors, page 897. Raven Press, New York, 1970b.

Grinspoon, L. *Marijuana Reconsidered.* Harvard University Press, Cambridge, Mass., 1971.

Hochman, J. S., and Brill, N. Q. Chronic marijuana use and psychosocial adaptation. Am. J. Psychiatry, *130:* 132, 1973.

Smoking and health. Report of the Advisory Committee to the Surgeon General of the Public Health Service. Public Health Service Publication No. 1103. U.S. Government Printing Office, Washington, D. C., 1964.

22.3.   ALCOHOLISM AND ALCOHOLIC PSYCHOSES

Introduction

An estimated 9 million Americans suffer from alcoholism. They are associated with an annual toll of 25,000 traffic fatalities, 15,000 homicides and suicides, and 20,000 deaths from alcohol-associated diseases. Alcoholism affects nearly 40 million spouses and children, and accounts for almost half of the five million arrests each year.

Definitions

In the second edition of the American Psychiatric Association's *Diagnostic and Statistical Manual of Mental Disorders.* (DSM-II), the A.P.A. encouraged the recording of the diagnosis of alcoholism separately, even when it begins as the symptomatic expression of another disorder. In such cases, the A.P.A. suggests that the diagnosis that most urgently requires treatment be listed first in the record. If there is no issue of disposition of treatment priority, the manual suggests the physician should list the more serious condition first. It also recommends that the physician underscore on the patient's record the disorder that he believes to be the underlying one.

The category of Alcoholic psychoses is a subclassification of Psychoses associated with organic brain syndromes and includes delirium tremens, Korsakoff's psychosis, other alcoholic hallucinosis, alcohol paranoid state, acute alcohol intoxication (not including simple drukenness, which is listed elsewhere as "Nonpsychotic OBS with alcohol"), alcoholic deterioration, pathological intoxication, and other [and unspecified] alcoholic psychosis.

Alcoholism itself is listed under Personality disorders and certain other nonpsychotic mental disorders. The category of alcoholism is for "patients whose alcohol intake is great enough to damage their physical health, or their personal or social functioning, or when it has become a prerequisite to normal functioning. DSM-II recognizes four types of alcoholism: 1. Episodic excessive drinking. "If alcoholism is present and the individual becomes intoxicated as frequently as four times a year, the condition should be classified here. 2. Habitual excessive drinking. "This diagnosis is given to persons who are alcoholic and who either become intoxicated more than 12 times a year or are recognizably under the influence of alcohol more than once a week, even though not intoxicated." 3. Alcohol addiction. This is defined as dependency; withdrawal symptoms are direct evidence: inability to go without drinking for a day is presumptive evidence, as is heavy drinking for 3 months or more. 4. Other [and unspecified] alcoholism. (See Table I.)

Here, alcoholism is defined as a chronic behavioral disorder manifested by an undue preoccupation with alcohol and its use to the detriment of physical and mental health, by loss of control when drinking is begun, and by a self-destructive attitude in dealing with personal relationships and life situations. Alcoholism results from a disturbance and deprivation in early life experiences and the associated related alterations in basic physicochemical responsiveness, from the identification by the alcoholic person with significant figures who deal with life problems through an unhealthy preoccupation with alcohol, and from a sociocultural milieu that causes ambivalence, conflict, and guilt in the use of alcohol.

Epidemiology and Social Consequences

The obvious deterioration of physical and social integrity of the skid-row habitué is well-known. (See Figure 1.) Much less apparent are the effects of alcoholism on persons in other socio-economic settings: the loss of income, the loss of potential and of productivity, the rupture of families, and the physical impairments. Courts, hospitals, clinics, agencies, industries, families, and individuals are constantly expending energies and resources on behalf of alcoholic persons.

Skid-row bums represent only 3 to 5 per cent of the estimated 9 million alcoholic persons in the United States. Most alcoholic people live with their families and are able to work and function, despite their problems. It has been estimated that up to 5 per cent of the country's work force are alcoholics and that almost another 5 per cent are serious abusers of alcohol.

Alcoholism costs the economy an estimated $15 billion each year. Of this sum, $10 billion comes from lost work time; $2 billion is spent for health and welfare services; and another $3 billion is attributed to property damage, medical expenses, and other overhead costs.

One third of each year's arrests are for public intoxication. If arrests for drunken driving, disorderly conduct, vagrancy, and other alcohol-related offenses are added in, the proportion rises to 40 to 49 per cent.

The ratio of male to female alcoholic persons is most commonly quoted as 5 ½ to 1. However, clinical observations suggest that more women are now seeking treatment and that this ratio is diminishing. The impression that there are far more male than female alcoholic persons could arise from the easier detection of the illness in men. Women may remain protected in their homes and for longer periods escape social or even family detection.

Physiological Effects of Alcohol

Alcohol lifted to the lips, from the initial sniff and sip, gets into the blood stream in very small amounts through the mucous membranes and lungs. Once ingested, alcohol is absorbed from the alimentary tract and carried by the blood to the brain and other organs. At what speed the alcohol enters the blood stream depends on many factors: the amount and type of food in the stomach, the type of beverage consumed and its alcohol concentration, the circumstances under which it is being drunk, and the drinker's constitutional state.

Mechanics of Absorption.

Foods in the stomach, especially mixed meals, slow alcohol absorption. Drinking water with alcohol increases absorption as does carbon dioxide; for that reason, champagnes and highballs are notorious for causing rapid and heightened effects.

The body has certain protective devices against being inundated by alcohol. For example, unlike other foodstuffs, alcohol can be absorbed into the blood stream directly from the stomach. If the concentration of alcohol

TABLE I

*Major Criteria for the Diagnosis of Alcoholism**

Criterion	Diagnostic Level	Criterion	Diagnostic Level
Track I: Physiological and Clinical		Fatty degeneration in absence of other known cause	2
A. Physiological dependency		Alcoholic hepatitis	1
1. Physiological dependence as manifested by evidence of a withdrawal syndrome when the intake of alcohol is interrupted or decreased without substitution of other sedation. It must be remembered that overuse of other sedative drugs can produce a similar withdrawal state, which should be differentiated from withdrawal from alcohol.		Laennec's cirrhosis	2
		Pancreatitis in the absence of cholelithiasis	2
		Chronic gastritis	3
		Hematological disorders:	
		Anemia: hypochromic, normocytic, macrocytic, hemolytic with stomatocytosis, low folic acid	3
a. Gross tremor (differentiated from other causes of tremor)	1	Clotting disorders: prothrombin elevation, thrombocytopenia	3
b. Hallucinosis (differentiated from schizophrenic hallucinations or other psychoses)	1	Wernicke-Korsakoff syndrome	2
		Alcoholic cerebellar degeneration	1
c. Withdrawal seizures (differentiated from epilepsy and other seizure disorders)	1	Cerebral degeneration in absence of Alzheimer's disease or arteriosclerosis	2
d. Delirium tremens (usually starts between the first and third day after withdrawal and minimally includes tremors, disorientation, and hallucinations)	1	Central pontine myelinolysis — diagnosis only / Marchiafava-Bignami's disease — possible post mortem	2 / 2
2. Evidence of tolerance to the effects of alcohol. (There may be a decrease in previously high levels of tolerance late in the course.) Although the degree of tolerance to alcohol in no way matches the degree of tolerance to other drugs, the behavioral effects of a given amount of alcohol vary greatly between alcoholic and nonalcoholic persons.		Peripheral neuropathy (see also beriberi)	2
		Toxic amblyopia	3
		Alcohol myopathy	2
		Alcohol cardiomyopathy	2
		Beriberi	3
		Pellagra	3
a. A blood alcohol level of more than 150 mg. without gross evidence of intoxication.	1	**Track II: Behavioral, Psychological, and Attitudinal**	
b. The consumption of ⅕ of a gallon of whiskey or an equivalent amount of wine or beer daily, for more than one day, by a 180-lb. individual.	1	All chronic conditions of psychological dependence occur in dynamic equilibrium with intrapsychic and interpersonal consequences. In alcoholism, similarly, there are varied effects on character and family. Like other chronic relapsing diseases, alcoholism produces vocational, social, and physical impairments. Therefore, the implications of these disruptions must be evaluated and related to the individual and his pattern of alcoholism. The following behavior patterns show psychological dependence on alcohol in alcoholism:	
3. Alcoholic blackout periods (differential diagnosis from purely psychological fugue states and psychomotor seizures).	2		
B. Clinical: major alcohol-associated illnesses Alcoholism can be assumed to exist if major alcohol-associated illnesses develop in a person who drinks regularly. In such individuals, evidence of physiological and psychological dependence should be searched for.		1. Drinking despite strong medical contraindication known to patient	1
		2. Drinking despite strong, identified, social contraindication (job loss for intoxication, marriage disruption because of drinking, arrest for intoxication, driving while intoxicated)	1
		3. Patient's subjective complaint of loss of control of alcohol consumption	2

* From Am. J. Psychiatry, *129:* 2, 1972.

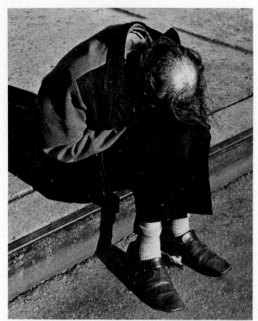

FIGURE 1. A "bowery bum" in New York City. (Courtesy of Dave Healey for Magnum Photos, Inc.)

becomes too high in the stomach, mucus is then secreted, and the pyloric valve closes. This action slows absorption and prevents the alcohol from passing into the small intestine, where no important restraints to absorption are available. Thus, a large amount of alcohol can remain unabsorbed for hours. Further, the pylorospasm often results in nausea and vomiting.

Once alcohol is absorbed into the blood stream, it is distributed to all the tissues of the body. Since it is uniformly dissolved in the water of the body, those tissues containing a high proportion of water receive a high concentration of alcohol. The intoxicating effects are greater when the blood alcohol is rising rapidly than when it is being destroyed or oxidized and falling. For this reason, the rate of absorption has a direct bearing on intoxicating responses.

Mechanics of Elimination

Immediately after absorption, destruction and elimination begin. The kidneys and lungs excrete about one tenth of the total alcohol ingested unchanged; the rest undergoes oxidation. The rate of oxidation of alcohol is independent of the body's energy requirements and fairly constant. The average person oxidizes three fourths of an ounce of whiskey an hour. If

his rate of sipping is equivalent, he does not accumulate alcohol in the body or become intoxicated.

Alcohol's oxidation provides heat and work energy. However, because excessive consumers receive so many calories as a consequence of their alcohol intake, they tend to neglect other sources of food and may ignore nutritional needs. The ultimate results are vitamin-deficiency diseases.

Effects on the Brain

Alcohol is a central nervous system depressant, similar to other anesthetics. At a level of 0.05 per cent of alcohol in the blood, thought, judgment, and restraint are loosened and sometimes disrupted. At a concentration of 0.10 per cent, voluntary motor actions usually become perceptibly clumsy. At 0.20 per cent, the function of the entire motor area of the brain is measurably depressed; the part of the brain that controls emotional behavior may also be affected. At 0.30 per cent, a person is commonly confused or may begin to be stuporous. At 0.40 or 0.50 per cent, he is in a coma. At higher levels, those primitive centers of the brain controlling breathing and heart rate are affected, and death ensues.

A moderate amount of alcohol, by releasing inhibitions, eases the way toward sexual activity, but too much has the effect noted by the porter in Macbeth: "it provokes the desire, but it takes away the performance." Similarly, people who have tied one on at a party note that they sleep only fitfully later that night. Several drinks before bedtime decrease the amount of REM sleep, with the anticipated aftereffects the next day.

Other Physiological Effects

Prolonged copious use of alcohol may produce withdrawal symptoms. Because alcohol affects the hypothalamus and the pituitary gland, chronic states of intoxication may result in disturbances of sexual function and mineral and water balance.

The liver is affected by alcohol and is the main site for its catabolism. A reversibly fatty infiltration of the liver is thought to occur with heavy consumption of alcohol. What relation, if any, this infiltration plays in the production of liver cirrhosis is not yet known. Acute intoxication can be associated with hypoglycemia that, when unrecognized, may have been responsible for some of the sudden deaths of intoxicated persons.

Chronic heavy drinking is associated with gastritis, achlorhydria, and gastric ulcers. Occasionally, maladies of the small intestine, pancreatitis, and pancreatic insufficiency are associated with alcoholism. Heavy alcohol intake may interfere with the normal processes of food digestion and absorption. As a result, the food that is consumed is inadequately digested. Alcohol abuse also appears to affect adversely the capacity of the intestine to absorb various nutrients, including vitamins and amino acids.

Muscle weakness is a side effect of alcoholism. And alcohol has been shown to affect the hearts of even nonalcoholic volunteers, increasing the resting cardiac output, heart rate, and myocardial oxygen consumption.

Alcohol and Other Drugs

The interaction between alcohol and other drugs may be dangerous, even fatal. Certain drugs, such as phenobarbital, are metabolized by the liver, as is alcohol, and their prolonged use may lead to acceleration of their metabolism and thus to increased tolerance, as is the case with alcohol. When the alcoholic person is sober, this accelerated metabolism makes him unusually tolerant to many other drugs, such as sedatives and tranquilizers; on the other hand, when he is drunk, these drugs are competing with the alcohol for the same detoxification mechanism, thus decreasing his tolerance. Tolerance is diminished with corresponding liver pathology.

The combined effects of alcohol and other drugs that depress the central nervous system are usually synergistic but may be additive. Drugs for inducing sleep, tranquilizers, sedatives, and drugs for pain relief, motion sickness, and head cold and allergy symptoms must be used with caution in alcoholic persons. Narcotics depress the sensory areas of the cerebral cortex, resulting in relief of pain, sedation, apathy, drowsiness, and sleep. High enough dosages can result in respiratory failure and death. Increasing dosages of such hypnotic-sedative drugs as chloral hydrate, paraldehyde, and bromides, like alcohol, produce a range of effects from tranquilization and sedation to motor and intellectual impairment to stupor,

coma, and death. They are synergistic with alcohol. Since tranquilizers can potentiate the effects of alcohol, patients should be instructed about the dangers of combining them and particularly about the increased dangers in driving or operating machinery.

Causes

Psychoanalytical Theories

Freud believed that alcoholism was the result of strong oral influences in childhood. Alcohol provides a mood alteration and a consequent redirection of thought processes, providing the impetus for regressive levels of thinking and for achieving gratification from thinking unrelated to logic. Alcohol provides an escape from reality.

Menninger advanced a self-destructive drive as the prime component of alcoholism. The child feels intense rage against his parents yet fears losing them. Later in life, alcohol becomes the means to achieve gratification and revenge: hostility experienced through antisocial behavior while under the influence of alcohol and the resultant punishment when sober to alleviate guilt. Therefore, Menninger sees alcoholism as a form of chronic suicide.

Adler attributed the cause of addiction to powerful feelings of inferiority related to a perpetual state of insecurity and a desire to escape responsibility. An alcoholic addiction may be heralded, according to Adler, by marked shyness, a preference for isolation, impatience, irritability, anxiety, depression, hypersensitivity, and sexual inadequacy. Adler incriminated overindulgence and excessive coddling, leading to an inability to face the frustrations of adulthood and the subsequent use of alcohol as a method of countering the demands of society.

Frustrated ambitions may play a role in the development of an alcoholic problem, according to McClelland. He suggests that the alcoholic may have an enhanced need for power but is inadequate to achieve his goals. He uses alcohol because it gives him a sense of release and of power and feelings of achievement.

Learning Theories

The learning theorists, in general, involve a drive setting responses into motion, responses that are also influenced by cues from other stimuli insufficient in strength to be drives.

Whenever a response is unrewarded by a reaction that lessens the drive, the response tends to disappear, letting others appear. In other words, the extinction of successive nonrewarded responses produces random behavior. When, however, a response is followed by a reward, the relation between stimulus and this response is strengthened. Consequently, in the presence of an identical drive and other cues, this response is more likely to occur. This strengthening of the cue-response connection is the essence of learning.

Dollard and Miller pointed out that alcohol results in a temporary reduction of fear and conflict. The attempt to adapt to fear and conflict through the release provided by alcohol, followed by the state of misery at its withdrawal, may produce the addictive cycle. Shoben feels that readily available release from anxiety arising from the first drinking experience is the method by which reinforcement principles operate in alcoholism.

Physiological Theories

Nutritional deficiencies have been incriminated as important links in the alcoholism chain. Williams postulates that, because of an inherited defect of metabolism, some people require unusual amounts of some of the essential vitamins. Since they do not get these amounts in their normal diets, they have a genetically caused nutritional deficiency. In those who drink alcohol, this deficiency results in an abnormal craving for liquor, and alcoholism results. But Popham, Wexburg, and Lester and Greenberg have criticized the findings of Williams.

Fenna and his associates wondered whether genetic factors account for the high alcoholism rates among American Indians and Eskimos. They found that the concentration of alcohol in the blood of Indians falls more slowly than it does in whites, suggesting that a genetic factor is at work. A similar inference was drawn by Wolff, who reported that alcohol in amounts that have little or no detectable effect on Caucasians consistently have a marked effect on Japanese, Taiwanese, and Koreans.

Sociological Theories

Horton believes that alcohol has the property of reducing anxiety and that its use is differentially determined, depending on the society's basic security and anxiety, as well as the availability of alcohol.

Bales relates social organization and cultural practice to alcoholism based on: "(1) The degree to which the culture operates to bring about acute needs for adjustment, or inner tensions, in its members. (2) The set of attitudes toward drinking which the culture produces in its members.... (3) The degree to which the culture provides suitable substitutive means of satisfaction."

Lemert distinguishes between primary deviance, which is conduct that may cause someone to be labeled by others as a deviant, and secondary deviance, which is behavior forced on him by being placed in a deviant role. The more advanced the secondary deviance, the more difficult it is for the person to return to society. Such behavior may result when there is too great a strain between perceived goals and the means available for attaining them. People may adapt to this conflict through conformity, ritualism, retreat, or rebellion; alcoholism may represent one of the latter two modes.

Alcoholic Psychoses

In many cases alcohol is merely the means by which severe, long-standing personality disturbances are brought to the surface.

Blackouts

The occurrence of blackouts is relatively frequent in the total alcoholic population and may be an early sign of alcoholism. Blackouts refer to a total amnesic state in which the patient has no recall of his activities or behavior when he has blacked out, although to the disinterested observer he is reasonably intact. Whether this phenomenon is a drug-induced amnesia attack or an acute dissociative response is unclear. The blackout may also sustain a system of psychological defense. The mean drunk may not recall the fight he picked; the normally prudish woman may not remember her drunken promiscuity and may not even recognize the stranger who wakens in her bed.

Pathological Intoxication

The onset of pathological intoxication is dramatic and sudden. Consciousness is impaired. The person is confused and disoriented and may suffer illusions, transitory delusions, and visual hallucinations. There is greatly increased activity, impulsive and aggressive, often to the point of destructiveness. Rage, anxiety, and depression are the emotional components, and attempts at suicide are frequent. This disorder may last for a few moments, a day, or more. It terminates in a prolonged period of sleep, with amnesia for the episode on awakening. Persons with hysterical or epileptoid temperaments are more prone than the general population to these outbursts; they have high levels of anxiety and tension, and alcohol may cause sufficient disorganization and loss of control to release aggressive impulses.

Delirium Tremens

Delirium tremens (D.T.'s) is an acute psychotic state, usually occurring after a prolonged, copious, and severe period of drinking. Delirium tremens is rarely seen in people under the age of 30 or in those who have not suffered serious alcoholism for 3 to 5 years. A lowering of the blood level alcohol may produce delirium tremens, as may acute injuries or infections in a drinking alcoholic person. The delirium is usually preceded by restlessness, irritability, anorexia, tremulousness, and disturbed sleep with terrifying dreams. Occasional illusions or hallucinations become more frequent. Confusion with disorientation for time and place is common, attention is fleeting, motor activity is marked, and sleep is impossible.

Physical examination reveals congestion of conjunctivae and face, with dilated pupils slow to react to light. A coarse tremor is almost always present and is increased by muscular tension. Tremulous tongue, lips, and face are often seen in fully developed cases. The pulse is rapid, irregular, and weak. Temperature is elevated, the skin moist, perspiration free, reflexes heightened, and speech indistinct. Epileptiform seizures may occur.

Delirium tremens is thought to be due to a disturbed metabolic state. Its course usually runs 3 to 10 days, with recovery preceded by prolonged sleep, clearer consciousness, and disappearance of hallucinations. Prognosis depends on the physical status of the patient and the presence or absence of concurrent disease. If the condition is left untreated, the mortality may be as high as 15 per cent.

The treatment of delirium tremens involves withdrawing alcohol and placing the patient in bed under excellent nursing conditions. Constant reassurance and the avoidance of physical restraints are advisable. Opiates should be avoided.

Chlordiazepoxide hydrochloride significantly alleviates agitation when no major psychiatric disease underlies the alcoholism. Reported side effects of chlordiazepoxide include syncope, drowsiness, ataxia, confusion, skin eruptions, idiopathic jaundice, menstrual irregularities, extrapyramidal symptoms and nausea. Alternatively, hydroxyzine may be used to eliminate agitation, anxiety, tension, confusion, and apprehension. It does not impair mental alertness, but drowsiness and dryness of the mouth may occur when high dosages are used.

Parenteral diazepam may be used to control recurrent seizures. Dosage should be individualized for maximum beneficial effect. Side effects most commonly reported are drowsiness, fatigue, and ataxia.

If the patient is in a state of dehydration, replacement of fluids and electrolytes is necessary. Nutritional needs must be carefully tended to with a high-calorie, high-carbohydrate diet supplemented by multivitamins.

Acute Alcoholic Hallucinosis

This condition represents a liberation of an underlying personality disorder as a consequence of alcoholic intake. Many observers see a close relation to schizophrenia. Patients who have suffered chronic alcoholic hallucinosis have, in time, become obviously schizophrenic.

Acute alcoholic hallucinosis usually follows a prolonged drinking bout. In contrast to the visual hallucinations and clouded consciousness of delirium tremens, in this reaction auditory hallucinations of a threatening nature appear in a clear sensorium. Ideas of reference and the acquisition of an elaborated delusional system are frequent, with the patient often responding to his ideas. Often the patient tries to involve the law in his defense or use other means of protection against the terrifying attacks. Although hallucinating, the patient is oriented to time and place, fits his hallucinations and delusions into his real environment, and, even after he recovers, can recall vividly the events, feelings, and ideas of the psychotic episode. The mood of the patient is apprehensive and fearful, frequently accompanied by anger or depression. Suicide attempts are common.

Treatment involves hospitalizing the patient, withdrawing alcohol, and providing medication to calm him. Adequate nutrition and vitamins should be supplied. Trifluoperazine, alone or in combination with chlorpromazine, is useful in treating thought disturbances and psychotic disorganization. The usual course runs 5 days to a month, but recurrences are common if alcohol is resorted to again.

Wernicke's Syndrome

Wernicke's syndrome is a rare, although once common, condition mainly seen in chronic alcoholic patients. It is due to vitamin and other nutritional deficiencies, especially thiamine deficiency. It begins with delirium and consists of ophthalmoplegia, memory loss, confabulation, apathy or apprehension, clouding of consciousness, ataxia, and, at times, coma. It results from neuronal and capillary lesions, particularly in the gray matter of the brain stem and structures near the third and fourth ventricles.

Alcoholic Paranoia

Patients who have been so diagnosed are those who in their premorbid period showed the same impairment of personality development and resultant psychopathological processes as seen in other paranoid psychoses. Alcohol use weakens repression; forbidden homosexual impulses may rise to the surface and are defended against by a paranoid delusional system.

The clinical picture is characterized by delusions of jealousy, associated with suspicion and distrust. Projection is intense. A paniclike state frequently occurs. The prognosis is not good, although the patient is more comfortable and less delusional when hospitalized. Return to the original environment results in a recurrence of symptoms in most cases.

Korsakoff's Syndrome

This syndrome may be preceded by an episode of delirium tremens. Korsakoff's syndrome consists of amnesia, confabulation or falsification of memory, disorientation as to time and place, and peripheral neuropathy. It is mainly the result of nutritional deficiency, especially of thiamine and niacin.

At first glance, the Korsakoff patient may appear clear, and the severity of his mental disturbance may not be apparent. Although he may be able to deal with immediate events, those requiring memory are beyond him. The memory loss is progressive, and he may respond to his amnesia by a lightness of attitude and confabulation. Disorientation as to time, misidentification of people, and a superficially jovial mood are common. The confabulation and mood are defenses against the patient's confronting himself with his defective functioning. The accompanying polyneuropathy is usually most marked in the lower limbs.

Many patients lose their symptoms after 6 to 8 weeks of treatment. In others, the syndrome is not completely reversible, improvement takes longer, and recovery of memory is not complete. Some patients always retain a certain degree of intellectual, emotional, and esthetic impairment. Neuropathy clears quickly and usually completely.

Treatment consists of the withdrawal of alcohol and the institution of a regimen of 20 to 50 mg. of thiamine hydrochloride daily for 1 week or more. A diet rich in all nutrients should be liberally provided. Rest for the symptoms of neuropathy is advisable.

Alcoholic Deterioration

In some patients who have suffered from a prolonged period of chronic alcoholism, one begins to see a gradual disintegration of personality structure, with emotional lability, loss of control, and evidence of dementia. The structural damage is probably due to brain damage from avitaminosis. The underlying pathological change is the result of a diffuse degeneration of nerve cells in the cerebral cortex. The symptoms are related to the underlying personality structure associated with the general findings of any dementia.

Personality Factors

No common personality disorder is predictive of alcoholism. There is no single personality configuration in alcoholism. Nor is there a predetermined course through which alcoholism sufferers pass. Little or nothing is known about the natural history of alcoholism or the rate of spontaneous remission. Nothing is known about the number of patients who reach a level of disturbance with alcohol and become stable or the incidence of patients who have a very malignant course.

Reactive Alcoholic Persons

These patients appear to have become preoccupied with alcohol only after being overwhelmed by some external stress. In many cases the temporary relief prevails, and avoidance of facing fears is prolonged. In other cases, the alcohol intensifies the depression, and the person, unaware of the causes of the deepened depression, consumes greater amounts of alcohol. With prolonged use of increasingly greater amounts of alcohol, physiological dependence on it may occur, and the person continues to drink heavily to prevent withdrawal symptoms.

Other reactive alcoholic persons may use alcohol to blur perceptions in the presence of an emotionally threatening milieu, such as a homosexual impulse. The most common reactive situation leading to a preoccupation with alcohol is that found in persons who need to break down psychological barriers—for example, the lawyer who must have a few drinks before he can address judge and jury.

In a reactive alcoholic person, premorbid adjustment has been reasonably satisfactory. The unhealthy encounter with alcohol has a determinable onset, it runs a course consistent with great tension release, and termination of the bout is related to a great effort of control by the person. The reactive alcoholic person may have one or more such periods of alcoholic distress.

Addictive Alcoholic Persons

The addictive alcoholic person shows gross disturbances in his prealcoholic personality, with marked evidence of inadequate and unsatisfactory interpersonal relations. Patients in this category have often been fascinated with alcohol from their first encounter; the onset of drinking bouts is undeterminate, without apparent reason, continuing until the person is physically unable to continue. Most striking in the total pattern of responses is the self-destructive component.

Interpersonal Relationships

The interpersonal relations of alcoholic persons tend to be rigid, stereotyped, and subjectively unrewarding. Discomforting feelings and responses are denied; aloofness, feelings of omnipotence, invulnerability, and a lack of dependence on others is common. An all-consuming hostility, associated with an inability to achieve satisfactory sexual adjustment, and depression are frequent. Most often, alcoholic persons do not get from the relationships they form just what they want, nor do they make others pleased, satisfied, or happy. These responses are related to disturbances and deprivation early in life.

Psychosexual Development

During early life, object loss may result in primitive excessive demands that cannot be satisfied and interpersonal relations that cannot succeed. At their failure, rejection is encountered, reawakening the feelings of the original loss and rejection. The intensity of these feelings is so great that an all-consuming hostility threatens the person, and he can deal with this hostility only by a self-destructive pattern, one facet of which is his preoccupation with alcohol.

At later stages of psychosexual development, a less intense disturbance and self-destructive pattern is possible. Only specific traumas reawaken feelings of deprivation and disturbance, with resulting self-limiting responses.

The gratification of sexual activity, the type of interpersonal relations, the intensity of hostility, and the pervasiveness of the self-destructive effort are similarly related to the level of development at which the impediment to psychological growth occurred. The earliest deprivation can be gratified only by oral satisfaction through incorporation and destruction of the love object, instituting the need to find another object.

The mechanism of denial is a patient's manner of dealing with life by denying feelings of isolation and inferiority, the absence of self-respect, and lack of sexual satisfaction, along with a dependence on alcohol and other external agents for security and care.

Depression is the prevailing mood in alcoholism. Object losses, isolation, anxieties, ungratified sexual impulses, unrealized goals, and thousands of feelings, real and fantasized, so plague the sufferer that relief must be sought. Hopelessness, sadness, and feelings of futility, failure, and worthlessness are sporadically or continuously present. Depression becomes so unbearable at times that only a bout with alcohol or a more direct suicidal attempt is the outlet.

Treatment

If the toxic state in acute alcoholic intoxication is not too profound, the patient may be treated with 10 to 25 mg. of chlordiazepoxide 4 times a day for 1 to 3 days without hospitalization. Whenever intoxication is severe enough to require hospitalization, minor tranquilizers such as chlordiazepoxide or hydroxyzine are initially useful.

If the patient is dehydrated, fluids fortified with vitamin B complex should be provided orally or parenterally. Thiamine hydrochloride in 200-mg. daily doses may be given intramuscularly or by mouth. When convulsions are expected or have occurred, diphenylhydantoin sodium in 1½ grains may be administered orally 3 times a day.

A cardinal rule of therapy is that the treatment program must be tailored to the needs and resources of the individual patient. A second cardinal rule of treatment is to remember the chronicity inherent in alcohol problems. Abstinence is not the only criterion for successful treatment. Family adjustment, occupational effectiveness, social adequacy, and intrapersonal contentment, along with posttreatment reduction of drinking behavior, may be equally effective indicators of improvement.

The most important treatment ingredient is the relationship of the patient with another person or group, whether it be clinic, therapy group, physician, psychiatrist, social worker, hospital, or Alcoholics Anonymous. The sooner the positive relationship takes place, the greater potential for a successful encounter. The therapist must often treat a marriage partner or members of a family, recognizing forces in the environment that operate in a negative therapeutic manner.

Substitution Therapies

Various substitution therapies—vitamins, hormones, carbohydrates, tranquilizers, and sedative drugs—have been used in alcoholism, but none appears to achieve a success rate above that seen with placebos, and all suggest that a compassionate, understanding human encounter must be an adjunct to treatment.

Aversion Therapy

This form of treatment uses emetine or apomorphine in an attempt to create a distaste for alcohol by developing a reflex association between alcohol and vomiting. Alcohol must be drunk shortly before the onset of the drug induces nausea and vomiting. Conditioning sessions, using the patient's favorite type of beverage, last for 30 to 60 minutes and are given on alternate days for a total of 4 to 6 treatments. Reinforcement to aversion by one or two reconditioning experiences is given any time a patient develops a desire to drink. At the end of 6 months, reconditioning experiences are administered.

There is a higher than average improvement rate among patients who have had a sustained relation with the therapist before or after treatment and who are in the high socio-economic groups. There is also an automatic selection factor in patients agreeing to undergo this treatment voluntarily.

Disulfiram Therapy

Five to 10 minutes after the ingestion of alcohol, the patient on disulfiram develops a sensation of heat in the face, along with intense lobster-red flushing of face, sclerae, upper limbs, and chest. The disulfiram reactor also suffers feelings of constriction in the neck, irritation of the trachea, spasms of coughing, and labored breathing. The most intense symptoms develop 30 minutes after the ingestion of alcohol. People who have consumed large amounts of alcohol become nauseated, and the flushing is replaced by pallor, owing to a considerable hypotension. Vomiting begins, and a feeling of uneasiness and apprehension develops, which most people find the most disagreeable symptom. The initial dose of disulfiram is 0.5 gm. once a day for 1 to 3 weeks. Because disulfiram is slowly metabolized, patients may be maintained on daily doses of 0.25 to 0.5 gm. and must be without alcohol for 4 days after the last dose. Most workers feel it is an adjunct to treatment and offers the greatest potential for delaying impulsive drinking episodes.

If a disulfiram-alcohol reaction occurs, the patient should be placed in shock position. Electrolytic balance may be maintained by dextrose and saline infusions. Plasma and oxygen should be provided when indicated. Antihistamine medication should be given either intramuscularly or intravenously. When disulfiram was first introduced, it was believed that patients should experience such a reaction. However, after some deaths from cardiac and respiratory failure, it was concluded that such reactions should be avoided. Now physicians simply describe what will happen if alcohol is drunk while the patient is taking disulfiram.

Psychological Treatment

Psychological therapies have been the most uniformly advocated in alcoholism, although there is no uniformity of opinion as to which type of psychological treatment is most effective. Group and individual psychotherapy, milieu therapy, family therapy, and casework have been used in alcoholism.

The initial contact with the alcoholic person is crucial to successful treatment. In the early encounter, therapists need to be active and supportive because patients with alcohol problems are depressed, anticipate rejection, and interpret the passive role of a therapist as rejecting. The therapist must also deal with alcohol as a defense. The pharmacological effect of alcohol acts as an emotional and intellectual barrier between patient and therapist, and therapeutic efforts are blunted. The removal of this barrier should be an early goal for effective progress.

Denial, a major mental mechanism in alcoholism, must be dealt with as soon and as often as it becomes recognizable. The therapist must be prepared to have the therapeutic bond tested again and again and cannot hide behind the screen of the patient's lack of motivation when relapses become threatening to the therapist and not a part of his understanding of the therapeutic process. Depressions can be countered by the active, supportive role of the therapist and at times by the addition of antidepressant medication.

In recent years, group therapy has become widely popular. It can help the alcoholic person see himself more honestly through the eyes of others who have been through the mill, view his relationship to others more clearly, and feel that he is an integral part of a social system. Psychodrama may also help to bring about self-realization.

Alcoholics Anonymous

Alcoholics Anonymous has been of great value in organizing self-help for alcoholic persons. It has assisted many thousands of troubled people, it has demonstrated that alcoholic persons can be helped, and it waged the fight and furnished the interest when others hid behind moralism and pessimism. It imparts comradeship, since all members suffer the same disturbance; it encourages introspection and confession; and it gratifies dependency needs through group identification and by caring for new intoxicated members. Switching from alcohol to Alcoholics Anonymous offers a less destructive social outlet for addictive needs. It is not the answer for everyone by any means; not all can accept its evangelistic tinge and its insistence that members confess to having hit bottom, and it has been of less value in the early detection of alcoholism. But it has done much for many and helped greatly to prod society into the realization that alcoholic people can be rehabilitated.

REFERENCES

Cahalan, D., Cisin, I. H., and Crossley, H. M. *American Drinking Practices: A National Survey of Drinking Behavior and Attitudes.* Rutgers Center of Alcohol Studies, New Brunswick, N. J., 1969.

Chafetz, M. E. New perspectives in the management of the alcoholic. In *Drugs and the Brain*, P. Black, editor, p. 341. Johns Hopkins University Press, Baltimore, 1969.

Dollard, J. A., and Miller, N. E. *Personality and Psychotherapy: An Analysis in Terms of Learning, Thinking, and Culture.* McGraw-Hill, New York, 1950.

Jellinek, E. M. *The Disease Concept of Alcoholism.* Hillhouse Press, New Haven, 1960.

National Council on Alcoholism. Criteria for the diagnosis of alcoholism. Am. J. Psychiatry, *129:* 127, 1972.

Noble, E. P., Parker, E., Alkana, R., Cohen, H., and Birch, H. Propranolol-ethanol interaction in man. Fed. Proc., *32:* 724, 1973.

Williams, R. J. *Nutrition and Alcoholism.* University of Oklahoma Press, Norman, 1951.

23

Normal and Abnormal Human Sexuality

23.1. INTRODUCTION TO SEXUALITY

Normal and Abnormal Sexuality

A decade ago psychiatrists were more certain than they are today about what constitutes healthy sexuality. At that time, the majority of psychiatrists seemingly believed, for example, that homosexuality is an illness. Currently, there is a sharp debate between two polarized groups—one still claiming that homosexuality is a disease, the other claiming that it should not even be regarded as deviation, since that word implies psychopathology, but simply as a sexual variation.

Theoretical considerations affect one's concept of normality. In the 1960's, the physiological research of Masters and Johnson made the issue of the vaginal versus the clitoral orgasm a debating point for dozens of workers in the field. Until then, except for a few debunkers, the vaginal transfer theory of Freud had led therapists to the mistaken notion that the woman who fails to transfer the seat of excitability from the clitoris to the vagina is immature. To be sure, the inability to have a coital orgasm does signify an inhibition, but the clitoral-labial mechanism has to work as a unit to produce orgasm, and the therapist needs to recognize the central importance of the clitoris in the orgastic process.

Freud argued that forepleasure or foreplay is infantile and that only the end pleasure (orgasm) is mature. Actually, orgasm occurs in early infancy. In Freud's view the mechanisms through which forepleasure is attained are an obstacle to the mature achievement of the sexual aim. Most sexologists now take the opposite view.

Current professionals are not nearly as worried about fixation points and compulsions as were Freud and the generation of psychoanalysts after him, provided the sexual activity is pleasurable and noninjurious to both partners. Hence, the range of normal sexual behavior has broadened enormously from the rather restricted one of Freud's time and place.

Normal functioning—that is, what society judges to be normal—has shifted from reproductive sex to relational sex and is now moving toward the sanctioning of recreational sex (physical pleasure accompanied by no more than affection). Men have always enjoyed all three levels; now women are discovering that they also have the capacity to enjoy sex at all three levels, including the initiation of recreational sex.

Today's concepts of normality are affected by new discoveries and new facts, new technological inventions and improvements, and shifting social patterns, belief systems, and attitudes—all of which affect people's thinking and feeling. Normality is a process—a dynamic, shifting, changing interplay among discovery, invention, dissemination of information, and behavioral and attitudinal changes.

Sexual System

Sexuality may be described in terms of a system analogous to the circulatory or respiratory system. The components of the sexual system are set forth in Table 1.

Biological Sex

The basic characteristics of the organism are the result of the interaction between the environment and the genetic code transmitted by the parents. The fetal environment may itself

TABLE I

Sexual System (Sexuality)

Biological sex—chromosomes, hormones, primary and secondary sex characteristics.

Sexual identity (sometimes called core gender identity)—sense of maleness and femaleness.

Gender identity—sense of masculinity and femininity.

Sexual role behavior, sex behavior—behavior motivated by desire for sexual pleasure, ultimately orgasm (physical sex); gender behavior—behavior with masculine and feminine connotations.

---

be highly significant in shaping sexual development and differentiation. A deficiency or excess of maternal hormones, viral infections, trauma, toxicity, nutritional deficiency, or maternal stress may affect the fetus adversely even before the environment at and after birth becomes effective. Ordinarily, the XX or XY chromosomal combination programs the undifferentiated gonad to become ovaries or testes. If testes, the gonad secrets androgen, which programs the fetus to become a male. The primordial fetus is female. Testicular secretions (or their absence) program the brain into patterns of organization, subsuming later sexual behavior. Abnormalities in biological sex may be minor or major. Major anatomical or physiological abnormalities create problems of intersexuality that may, if not corrected early in life, lead to conflicts in sexual or gender identity.

Sexual Identity

Sexual identity may be defined as the person's inner feeling of maleness or femaleness continued over time. The sense of one's maleness or femaleness is more or less reinforced by the ways in which people, notably parents, react. Of equal importance to the role of fetal androgens in organizing the brain for later masculine behavior (if androgen is present in sufficient amounts) or for female behavior (if androgen is insufficient) is the assignment of sex to the infant. Even in the presence of ambiguous biological characteristics, unambiguous sex rearing usually leads to a firm sexual and gender identity. A change in sex assignment is generally unwise after the child is older than 18 months.

Almost everyone goes through sexual develop-

ment differentiation without serious defects in sexual identity. The exceptions are some children with ambiguous sexual morphology who have ambiguous sex rearing and transsexuals who have the conviction that they belong to the opposite sex and reject their own body appearance and social status.

Gender Identity

With relatively rare exceptions, the development of sexuality leads to a secure sense of maleness or femaleness, which is generally complete by the age of three years. However, in American culture, doubts and conflicts about masculinity and femininity are ubiquitous. Serious disturbances lead to sex deviations.

Sexual Role Behavior

Sexual role behavior is divided into sex behavior and gender behavior. Sex behavior is based on a desire for sexual pleasure, ultimately for orgasm (physical sex); gender behavior is behavior with masculine and feminine connotations. The sexual response cycle and dysfunctions in performance come under the first category; sexual relatedness or relationships come under the second category. Gender role behavior was once handed down or assigned by tradition; today, roles are negotiable, and problems may become serious if negotiation is impossible to attain because of faulty communications.

REFERENCES

Freyhan, F. A. Scientific models for sexual behavior from the clinician's point of view. In *Contemporary Sexual Behavior: Critical Issues in the 1970"s*, J. Zubin and J. Money, editors, p. 259. Johns Hopkins University Press, Baltimore, 1973.

Gadpaille, W. J. Research into the physiology of maleness and femaleness. Arch. Gen. Psychiatry, *26:* 193, 1972.

Lief, H. I. Obstacles to the ideal and complete sex education of the medical student and physician. In *Contemporary Sexual Behavior: Critical Issues in the 1970's*, J. Zubin and J. Money, editors, p. 441. Johns Hopkins University Press, Baltimore, 1973.

MacLean, P. D. New findings on brain function and sociosexual behavior. In *Contemporary Sexual Behavior: Critical Issues in the 1970's*, J. Zubin and J. Money, editors, p. 53. Johns Hopkins University Press, Baltimore, 1973.

Masters, W. H., and Johnson, V. E. *Human Sexual Response*. Little, Brown, Boston, 1966.

Masters, W. H., and Johnson, V. E. *Human Sexual Inadequacy*. Little, Brown, Boston, 1970.

Money, J. and Ehrhardt, A.A. *Man and Woman, Boy and Girl*. Johns Hopkins University Press, Baltimore, 1972.

Sorensen, R. C. *Adolescent Sexuality in Contemporary America*. World, New York, 1973.

Stoller, R. J. Overview: The impact of new advances in sex

research on psychoanalytic theory. Am. J. Psychiatry, *130*: 241, 1973.

Zubin, J., and Money, J. editors. *Contemporary Sexual Behavior: Critical Issues in the 1970's.* Johns Hopkins University Press, Baltimore, 1973.

23.2   SEXUAL ANATOMY AND PHYSIOLOGY

Introduction

The sex of a human being is determined at the time of fertilization. Within the broad limits defined by normal variation, individual heredity, and environmental influence, the physiology, anatomy, and physical development of a person are, therefore, forecast at conception. To the extent that society dictates social and cultural roles according to sex, psychological development is also affected. Sexual physiology goes beyond reproduction, and hormonal changes affect libido, physical well-being, and behavior.

Embryology

Gonadal structures are recognizable in the embryo by the fourth week of development (see Figure 1). However, these structures do not assume male or female morphological characteristics until the seventh week of development. In addition to indifferent gonads, male and female fetuses have identical genital tubes. The development of the testes causes the female tubes, the Müllerian duct, to shrink away in the male fetus, and development of the ovary causes the disappearance of the male tubes, the Wolffian duct, in the female fetus.

Development of the Testes

Between the sixth and eighth weeks of development, the primitive sex cords in the male embryo proliferate and anastomose with one another in the medulla of the sex gland, forming the testis cords. While the testis cords are proliferating in the medulla of the sex gland, the cortex degenerates. The germ cells disappear from the cortex, and a dense layer of fibrous connective tissue, the tunica albuginea, separates the testis cords from the surface epithelium. This surface epithelium then disappears, leaving the tunica albuginea as the capsule of

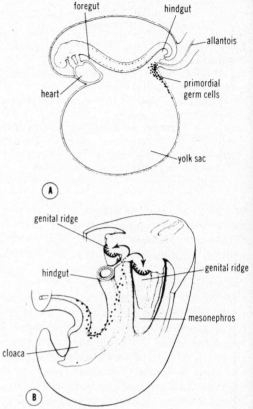

FIGURE 1. *A.* Schematic drawing of a 3-week-old embryo, showing the primordial germ cells in the wall of the yolk sac, close to the attachment of the allantois (after Witchi). *B.* Drawing to show the migration path of the primordial germ cells along the wall of the hindgut and the dorsal mesentery into the genital ridge. Note the position of the genital ridge and mesonephros. (Reproduced from J. Langman, *Medical Embryology,* ed. 2, Williams & Wilkins, Baltimore, 1972, by permission.)

the testes. During the fourth to eighth months of development, the interstitial cells of Leydig are formed from the mesenchyme between seminiferous tubules. The tubules themselves have formed from primitive germ cells and epithelial cells from the surface of the gland.

At this time the testes' initial attachment to the primitive kidney is reduced to a mesentery-like attachment called the gubernaculum testis, which extends from the caudal pole of the testes to the genital swelling of the fetus. In the second month of life, the fetus grows rapidly. The gubernaculum testis does not grow correspondingly, with the end result that the testes seem to descend. By the end of the third month, they lie near the inguinal region. At this time the prostate glands and scrotal sac form. The final descent through the inguinal ring into the scrotal swelling occurs in the seventh month of development.

Development of the Ovaries

The development of the ovaries involves primarily the development of the cortex of the gland. The sex cords of the medulla eventually disappear and are replaced by vascular stromata, which form the ovarian medulla. The surface epithelium of the gland thickens and proliferates, giving rise to cords that push into the gonad. These cords then split into clusters of cells that surround the primitive germ cells. The cord cells eventually develop into follicular cells; the germ cells develop into oogonia and then oocytes. At birth the follicles are very similar to the young follicles in the adult ovary.

Development of the External Genitalia

Until the seventh week, the external development of the genitalia appears the same in the male and female fetuses. In the presence of androgens, male development occurs; in the absence of androgens, female development occurs. These changes can occur under the influence of fetal testosterone or of exogenously administered androgens (see Figure 2).

Anatomy

Male

The external genitalia of the normal, adult male include the penis, scrotum, testes, epididymis, and parts of the vas deferens. The internal parts of the genital system include the vas deferens, seminal vesicles, ejaculatory ducts, and prostate.

The testis or male gonad is an oval gland measuring approximately 1½ inches by 1 inch by ¾ inch. There are two testes, each with an epididymis attached to its upper pole and posterior border. Each testis is surrounded by two coats—the tunica vaginalis and the tough, outer tunica albuginea—and is enclosed in the scrotal sac (see Figure 3).

The scrotum, the bag of skin and tissue in which the testes lie, hangs between the thighs. Externally, it is a single pouch. Internally, it is divided by subcutaneous tissue into right and left compartments, each containing a testis and epididymis. The left testis usually hangs lower than the right. The scrotal sac is responsive to temperature changes and responds with elevation to sexual stimulation.

Within the testes are the seminiferous tubules that produce the sperm cells. Between these tubules lie the cells of Leydig, which are involved in the production of testosterone. Testosterone is the male hormone responsible for development of masculine secondary sex characteristics. The seminiferous tubules join to form the straight tubules and then the rete testis at the apex of the gland. These, in turn, give rise to efferent ductules, which coil to form the head of the epididymis. They then empty into the duct of the epididymis (the head and tail). The tail of the organ continues as the vas

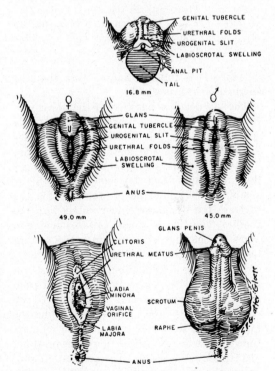

FIGURE 2. Differentiation of male and female external genitalia from indifferent primordia. Male differentiation occurs only in the presence of androgenic stimulation during the first 12 weeks of fetal life. (Redrawn from Van Wyk and Grumbach, 1968. Reproduced from J. R. Brobeck, editor, *Best & Taylor's Physiological Basis of Medical Practice*, ed. 9, Williams & Wilkins, Baltimore, 1973, by permission.)

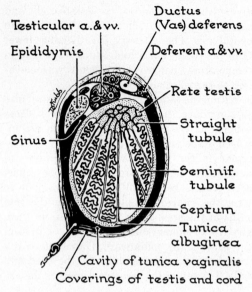

FIGURE 3. Right testis in transverse section. (Reproduced from R. L. Dickinson, *Atlas of Human Sex Anatomy*, ed. 2, Williams & Wilkins, Baltimore, 1949, by permission.)

deferens. It is through this network that the spermatozoa must travel.

The vas deferens passes over the pelvis into the lower abdomen and is here connected to the seminal vesicle. This vesicle secretes a substance believed to add motility to the sperm. The vas deferens, now called the ejaculatory duct, continues from its connection with the seminal vesicle into the prostate. Within the prostate the ejaculatory duct enters into the urethra. The duct is usually closed, opening to allow the passage of semen into the urethra under strong sexual stimulation (see Figure 4).

This passage of fluid into the urethra—sperm from the testicles and epididymis, fluid from the seminal vesicles, and fluid released by contraction of the prostate itself—provides the man with a sensation of impending climax. Indeed, once there is contraction of the prostate, ejaculation is inevitable. The ejaculate is propelled through the penis by urethral contractions. The ejaculate consists of about one teaspoon of fluid (2.5 cc.) and contains about 120 million sperm cells.

The urethra, through which the ejaculate travels, is 8 to 9 inches long, originating in the bladder, passing through the prostate (prostatic urethra), and following the ventral surface of

the penis to the glans (penile urethra) (see Figure 5).

The prostate is a gland weighing about 20 gm.; it surrounds the urethra and shares the bladder bed near the neck of the bladder. It can be palpated rectally. The gland is composed partially of smooth muscle cells and elastic tissue fibers. During sexual excitation this smooth muscle contracts, and prostatic secretions are emptied from the ductules of the gland into the urethra.

Cowper's glands, two pea-size structures located behind the membranous urethra, may provide a small amount of additional lubrication during sexual excitation.

The penis has been referred to by Freud as the executive organ of sexuality. The word "penis" has been traced from the Latin as meaning variously "tail" or "to hand," referring to the pendant position of the organ in its resting or flaccid state. The size of the penis varies within a range that is fairly constant—7 to 11 cm. in the flaccid state and 14 to 18cm. in the erect state. The flaccid dimension bears little relation to the erect dimension; the smaller penis erects to a proportionally greater size than does the

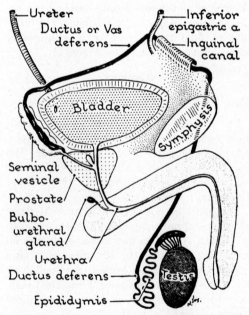

FIGURE 4. Diagram of the ductus (vas) deferens. (Reproduced from R. L. Dickinson, *Atlas of Human Sex Anatomy*, ed. 2, Williams & Wilkins, Baltimore, 1949, by permission.)

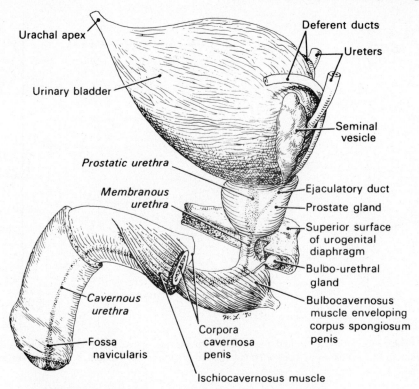

FIGURE 5. The male urethra and its relation to the urogenital organs. (Courtesy of R. F. Becker, Ph.D., Michigan State University.)

larger penis (see Figure 6).

The penis consists of the glans, shaft, and root and is composed primarily of erectile tissue. It comprises three parallel tubes: two corpora cavernosa, which lie side by side, and beneath them the single corpus spongiosum, which is traversed by the urethra. The anterior end of the corpus spongiosum fits over the corpora cavernosa and is called the glans. The foreskin covering the glans is known as the prepuce (see Figure 7).

All three fibrous tubes of the penis have innumerable spaces that can become engorged with blood, causing the penis to become erect. The three tubes extend backward, each corpus cavernosum attaching to an arm of the pubis and the corpus spongiosum extending into the urethral bulb. The muscles covering these backward extension (the bulbocavernosus and the ischiocavernosus) by their contractions, respectively, propel ejaculate through the urethra at the point of sexual climax and prevent blood from leaving the penis, so that erection can be maintained during sexual excitement.

Activation by the parasympathetic nervous system is involved in erection. The pelvic splanchnic nerves (S2, 3, and 4) stimulate the blood vessels of the area to dilate, causing the penis to become erect. The sympathetic nervous system in involved in ejaculation. Through its hypogastric plexus, the sympathetic nervous system innervates the urethral crest and the muscles of the epididymis, vas deferens, seminal vesicles, and prostate. Stimulation of this plexus causes ejaculation of seminal fluid from these glands and ducts into the urethra.

Female

The internal female genital system comprises the ovaries, fallopian tubes, uterus, and vagina. The external genitalia or vulva includes the mons pubis, major and minor lips, clitoris, glans, vestibule of the vagina, and vaginal orifice (see Figure 8).

The female gonads are the two ovaries, which lie on either side of the uterus. They are spherical glands, about 1 inch in diameter, and are supported by a fold of peritoneum called the

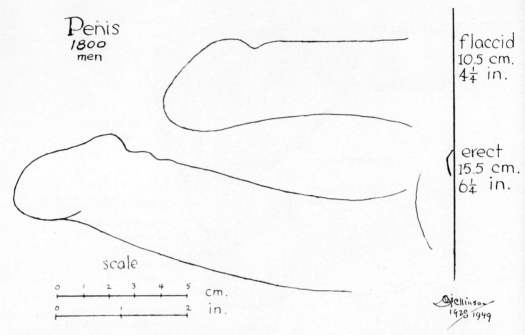

Penis
1800
men

flaccid
10.5 cm.
4¼ in.

erect
15.5 cm.
6¼ in.

scale

| 0 | 1 | 2 | 3 | 4 | 5 | cm. |

| 0 | | | 1 | | | 2 | in. |

Dickinson
1928 1949

FIGURE 6. The penis in the flaccid and erect states with average size as surveyed and drawn by Dickinson. (Reproduced from R. L. Dickinson, *Atlas of Human Sex Anatomy*, ed. 2, Williams & Wilkins, Baltimore, 1949, by permission.)

suspensory ligament. A newborn female has about 200,000 immature ova in each ovary. These ova decrease in number with age and disappear after menopause. Throughout her reproductive life, from puberty to menopause, a woman usually releases a total of 400 ova into the peritoneal cavity. Release of ova usually occurs once every lunar month. The ovaries also produce two hormones important to female sexual development, estrogen and progesterone (see Figure 9).

The ovum released by the ovary can be caught in the fingerlike processes of the fallopian tubes—either tube may service either ovary—and propelled through the tubes by occasional peristalsis and action of the hairlike processes in the tubes to the uterus. The tubes themselves are about 4½ inches long and curve from the ovaries to the uterus. Fertilization occurs in the tubes, and tubal secretion may be nourishing to the released ovum.

The uterus is a muscular, thick-walled, hollow organ about 3 inches in length, and shaped like an inverted pear. The uterus receives a uterine tube from above on each side and opens into the vagina below. When not harboring a fetus, the uterine cavity remains collapsed. It is held in place by two broad ligaments and two round ligaments. The endometrium, the internal mucous surface of the uterus, is composed of glands and stromata and goes through stages each month: (1) postmenstrual, (2) proliferative or nonsecretory, (3) secretory or progestational shedding of the upper two thirds of the endomedtium. It regenerates from the remaining basales, composed of stromata and stumps of glands (see Figure 10).

The vagina is usually in a collapsed state. It is about 3 inches long and extends from the cervix of the uterus above (see Figure 11) to the vestibule of the vagina or the vaginal opening below. In most virgins a membranous fold, the hymen, separates the vestibule and opening from the rest of the vaginal canal. The mucous membrane lining the vaginal walls rests in numerous transverse folds. This lining can stretch during the birth process. To accommodate the penis during sexual intercourse, the vagina expands in both length and width. In addition to its other functions, the vagina offers a passage for the release of menstrual fluid from the uterus. After menopause, the vagina loses much of its elasticity.

The blood supply to the internal genitalia

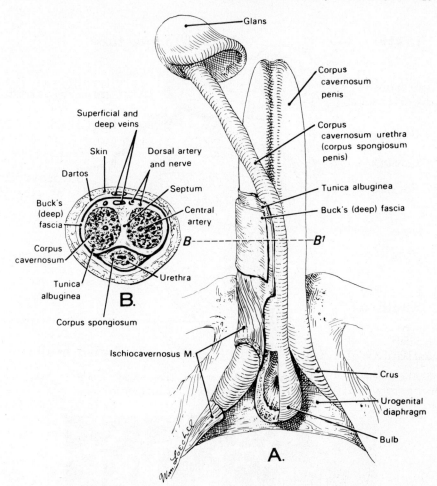

Glans

Corpus
cavernosum
penis

Corpus
cavernosum urethra
(corpus spongiosum
penis)

Tunica albuginea

Buck's (deep) fascia

Superficial and
deep veins

Skin

Dorsal artery
and nerve

Dartos

Septum

Buck's
(deep)
fascia

Central
artery

Corpus
cavernosum

Tunica
albuginea

Urethra

B.

Corpus spongiosum

Ischiocavernosus M.

Crus

Urogenital
diaphragm

Bulb

A.

FIGURE 7. *A.* Crural relationships and tunics of the penis. *B.* Cross-section taken through *A* at *B–B¹*. (Courtesy of R. F. Becker, Ph.D., Michigan State University.)

includes the ovarian artery, derived from the aorta, and the vaginal and uterine arteries, which arise from the internal iliac. Congestion of small vessels surrounding the vagina results in a transudate that lubricates the vaginal walls during sexual excitement.

The hypogastric plexus of the sympathetic nervous system supplies the uterus, tubes, and part of the vagina. The lower part of the vagina is supplied by the pudendal nerve. During sexual climax these nerves stimulate the genitalia to contract rapidly.

The most superficial aspect of the female external genitalia is the mons pubis (see Figure 12), a mound directly in front of the pubic bone. Hair growth occurs here at puberty. The pattern of hair growth in the mature woman varies but

follows roughly the shape of an inverted triangle.

The major lips are two broad cutaneous ridges that meet in the midline of the body and cover most of the other external genitals. They extend backward to the perineum.

Inside the major lips lie the minor lips, thinner folds devoid of fat that lie alongside the vaginal orifice and form the angle limiting the vestibule. Opening into the vestibule are the urethra, vagina, paraurethral glands, and vestibular gland. The minor lips are free posteriorly but join anteriorly to form the prepuce and frenulum of the clitoris.

Masters and Johnson have described the clitoris as the primary female sexual organ in that orgasm is dependent, physiologically, on

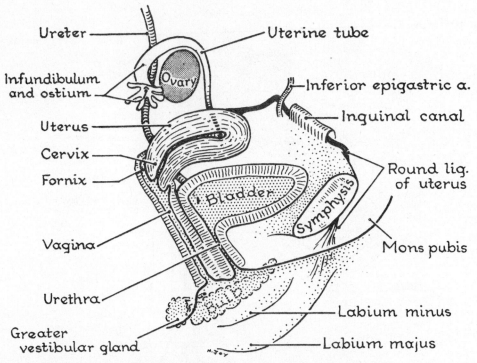

FIGURE 8. The female pelvis and perineum, median section. (Reproduced from R. L. Dickinson, *Atlas of Human Sex Anatomy*, ed. 2, Williams & Wilkins, Baltimore, 1949, by permission.)

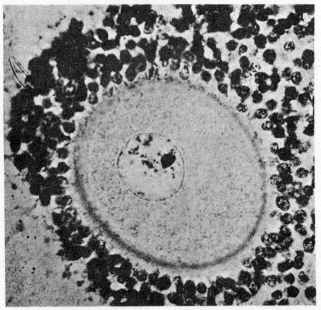

FIGURE 9. Human oocyte from a large graafian follicle (× 480). (Reproduced from Eastman and Hellman, *Williams' Obstetrics*, ed. 13, p. 60, Appleton-Century-Crofts, New York, 1966, by permission.)

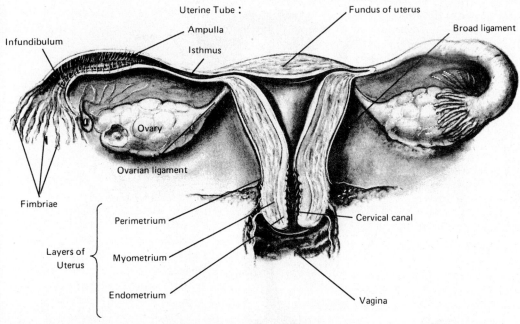

FIGURE 10. Internal female reproductive organs. (Reproduced from Dienhart, *Basic Human Anatomy and Physiology*, p. 215, W. B. Saunders, Philadelphia, 1967, by permission.)

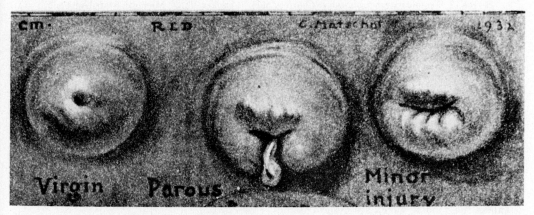

FIGURE 11. The cervix in the nulliparous and multiparous female. (Reproduced from R. L. Dickinson, *Atlas of Human Sex Anatomy*, ed. 2, Williams & Wilkins, Baltimore, 1949, by permission.)

adequate clitoral stimulation. It has a nerve net three times as large as that of the penis in proportion to its size. The clitoral prepuce is contiguous with the labia minora, and, during coitus there is no direct stimulation of the clitoris by the penis. Rather, traction exerted on the minor lips as a result of penile thrusting accounts for stimulation of the clitoris necessary for orgasm to occur.

The size of the clitoris varies considerably (see Figure 13) and is unrelated to the degree of sexual responsiveness of a particular woman.

Breasts are not specifically sexual organs but are important in sexual play and as erogenous areas. Breasts are much more fully developed in the human female than in the male. They function as suckling organs but respond in a definitive physiological pattern during intercourse as well. There is a wide variation in size, shape, and sensitivity of breasts in women. The breasts are attached to the chest muscles and are composed of glandular, fibrous and fatty

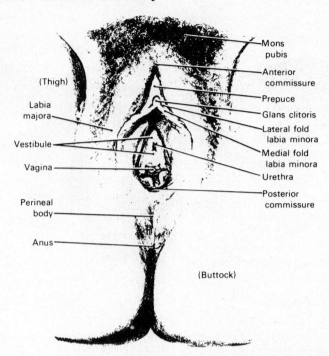

(Thigh)

Labia
majora

Vestibule

Vagina

Perineal
body

Anus

Mons
pubis

Anterior
commissure

Prepuce

Glans clitoris

Lateral fold
labia minora

Medial fold
labia minora

Urethra

Posterior
commissure

(Buttock)

FIGURE 12. Female external genitalia. (Courtesy of R. F. Becker, Ph.D., Michigan State University.)

tissue. The nipple and surrounding areola possess a darker pigmentation than the rest of the breast. This pigmentation increases with pregnancy and childbirth.

Physiology

Gonadal sex is chromosomally determined at the time of fertilization, and chromatic bodies (or lack of them) appear as indications of genetic sex in nonsexual body cells as well. These chromatin bodies are present only in the female (see Figure 14).

Unlike the gonads, which are under chromosomal influence, the fetal external genitalia are very susceptible to hormones, and exogenous hormonal administration may cause external genital development inconsistent with the fetal sex gland development. A female fetus, possessing an ovary, may develop external genitalia resembling that of a male if the pregnant mother received sufficient exogenous androgen.

In normal development, spermatogenesis and oogenesis begin embryonically and are continued and completed at puberty. Figure 15 summarizes the normal hormonal effect at the time of puberty.

The onset of menstruation after puberty marks the expulsion of the unfertilized egg from the ovary and the uterine bleeding that follows. At menarche, however, the female does not always release an egg and may not, at first, be fertile. The process of menstruation, involving ovulation and uterine changes, is intricately involved with hormonal changes (see Figures 16 to 19).

The hypothalamic-testicular interaction resulting in the release of sperm is also intimately connected with hormonal regulation (see Figure 20).

Fertilization

For fertilization, a mature ovum and a sperm must meet in the fallopian tube. The sperm is viable for about 36 hours and may be present in the tube before the egg arrives. Conception must occur within 48 hours of ovulation. Many sperm may enter the fallopian tubes, but only one can penetrate the capsule of the egg. Once this penetration has occurred, the egg becomes impenetrable to other sperm. The final maturation of the egg occurs after it has been fertilized. The egg divides and continues to divide into greater numbers of cells. The sperm determines the sex of the child. The egg always contains an X or female chromosome. If the sperm adds a male or Y chromosome, the embryo is a male. If

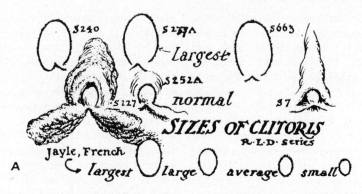

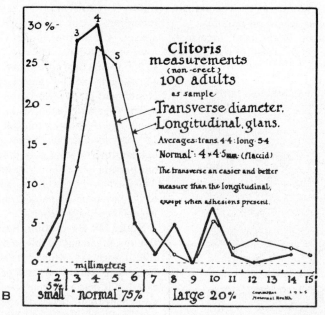

FIGURE 13. Size of clitoris. *A*. Anatomical drawings showing location and dimensions of clitoris (life size). *B*. Range of clitoral measurements in nonerect state. (Reproduced from R. L. Dickinson, *Atlas of Human Sex Anatomy*, ed. 2, Williams & Wilkins, Baltimore, 1949, by permission.)

the sperm adds another X chromosome, the embryo is a female. After about 3 days of division of the fertilized egg, at the 16-cell stage, the fertilized egg enters the uterine cavity.

Physiological Responses

In the normal man or woman, a sequence of physiological sexual responses exists that has been described by Masters and Johnson. These levels of sexual arousal consist of four discrete phases, each accompanied by unique physiological changes (see Tables I and II). These phases can be understood physiologically as increasing levels of vasocongestion and myotonia (tumescence) and the subsequent rapid release of this

vascular activity and muscle tone as a result of orgasm (detumescence).

Stage I: Excitement. This phase is brought on by psychological stimulation—fantasy, the presence of a love object—or physiological stimulation—stroking, kissing—or a combination of both. It is characterized by erection in the man and vaginal lubrication in the woman, both occurring within 10 seconds of effective stimulation. The nipples of both sexes become erect, although this erection is more common in the woman (see Figure 21). The clitoris becomes hard and turgid, and the labia majora and minora become thicker as a result of venous engorgement (see Figure 22). The excitement phase may last several minutes to several hours.

Stage II: Plateau. As stimulation continues, the testes increase in size 50 per cent and elevate. The vaginal barrel shows a characteristic constriction along the outer third, known as the orgasmic platform. The clitoris elevates and retracts behind the symphysis pubis and, as a result, is not easily accessible. Breast size in the woman increases 25 per cent. Continued engorgement of the penis and vagina produces specific color changes, most marked in the labia minora, which spread and become a deep purple-red color (see Figure 23). Voluntary contractions of large muscle groups occur. The plateau phase lasts 30 seconds to several minutes.

Stage III: Orgasm. In the man, orgasm is triggered by a subjective sense of ejaculatory inevitability, followed by the forceful emission of semen. In the woman, orgasm is characterized by 3 to 12 involuntary contractions of the vaginal orgasmic platform. Tetanic contractions of the uterus, flowing from the fundus downward to the cervix, also occur. Both sexes show involuntary contractions of the internal and external anal sphincter. The male orgasm is associated with four to five rhythmic spasms of the prostate, seminal vesicles, vas, and urethra. In both sexes the contractions of the various organs occur at intervals of 0.8 second. Other changes consist of further voluntary and involuntary movements of the large muscle groups, including facial grimacing and carpopedal spasm. Blood pressure rises 20 to 40 mm. (systolic and diastolic), and the heart rate rises to 120 to 160 beats a minute. Orgasm lasts 3 to 15 seconds and is associated with a slight clouding of consciousness.

The orgasmic potential in men is highest at about age 18 and in women at about age 35. The 18-year-old man may achieve as many as eight orgasms in a 24-hour period. In the man over 30, one orgasm in a 24-hour period is more common. The increased orgasmic potential in the woman of 35 has been explained on the basis of less psychological inhibition.

Stage IV: Resolution. Resolution consists of the disgorgement of blood from the genitalia (detumescence), which brings the body back to its resting state. If orgasm occurs, resolution is rapid; if it does not occur, resolution may take 2 to 6 hours and be associated with irritability and pain in the genitalia (see Figure 24). Successful resolution in both sexes is characterized by a subjective sense of well-being and a specific perspiratory reaction—a generalized excretion of sweat over the entire body, including the palms and soles.

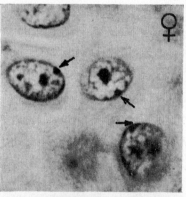
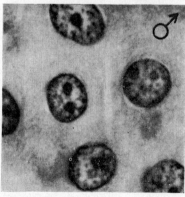

FIGURE 14. Nuclei of cells in the epidermal spinus layer of a genetic female (*top*) and a genetic male (*bottom*). The sex chromatin bodies are indicated by *arrows* in the female. (Redrawn from Grumbach and Barr, 1958. Reproduced from J. R. Brobeck, editor, *Best & Taylor's Physiological Basis of Medical Practice*, ed. 9, Williams & Wilkins, Baltimore, 1973, by permission.)

After orgasm, men have a refractory period that may last from several minutes to many hours; in this period they cannot be stimulated to further orgasm. The refractory period does not exist in women, who are capable of multiple and successive orgasms. Some women are capable of experiencing 20 to 30 orgasms by continued penile or manual stimulation, barring exhaustion. Psychosexual development, psychological development, and psychological attitude toward sexuality are directly involved with and affect the physiology of human sexual response (see Figure 25).

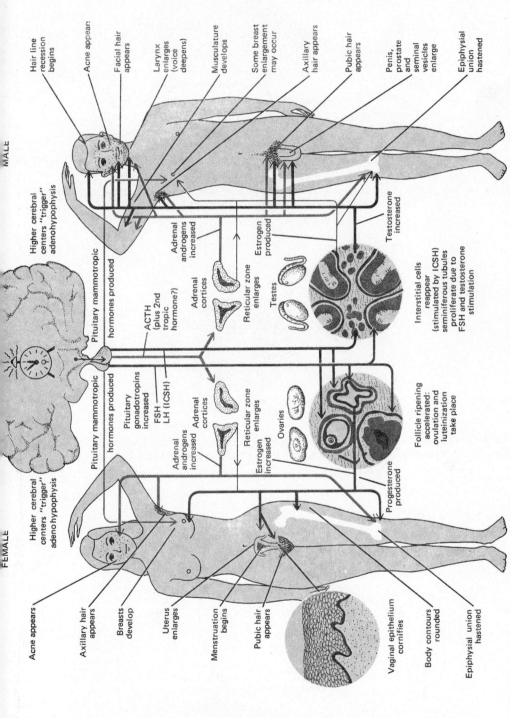

FEMALE

Acne appears

Axillary hair appears

Breasts develop

Uterus enlarges

Menstruation begins

Pubic hair appears

Vaginal epithelium cornifies

Body contours rounded

Epiphysial union hastened

Higher cerebral centers "trigger" adeno hypophysis

Pituitary mammotropic hormones produced

Pituitary gonadotropins increased
FSH
LH (ICSH)

ACTH (plus 2nd tropic hormone?)

Adrenal androgens increased

Adrenal cortices

Reticular zone enlarges

Estrogen increased

Ovaries

Follicle ripening accelerated: ovulation and luteinization take place

Progesterone produced

MALE

Hair line recession begins

Acne appears

Facial hair appears

Larynx enlarges (voice deepens)

Musculature develops

Some breast enlargement may occur

Axillary hair appears

Pubic hair appears

Penis, prostate and seminal vesicles enlarge

Epiphysial union hastened

Higher cerebral centers "trigger" adenohypophysis

Pituitary mammotropic hormones produced

Adrenal androgens increased

Adrenal cortices

Reticular zone enlarges

Estrogen produced

Testes

Testosterone increased

Interstitial cells reappear (stimulated by ICSH) seminiferous tubules proliferate due to FSH and testosterone stimulation

FIGURE 15. Effects of sex hormones on development puberty. (Copyright 1965 by CIBA Pharmaceutical Company, Division of CIBA-GEIGY Corporation. Reproduced with permission from the Ciba Collections of Medical Illustrations by Frank Netter, M. D. All rights reserved.)

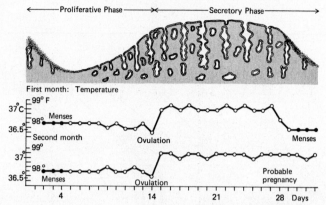

FIGURE 16. The phases of the menstrual cycle. (Reproduced from Benson, *Handbook of Obstetrics and Gynecology*, ed. 3, p. 26, Lange Medical Publications, Los Altos, Calif., 1968, by permission.)

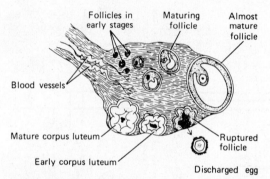

FIGURE 17. Composite view of ovum. (Reproduced from Crawley, Malfetti, Stewart, and Vas Dias, *Reproduction, Sex, and Preparation for Marriage*, p. 16, Prentice-Hall, Englewood Cliffs, N.J., 1964, by permission.)

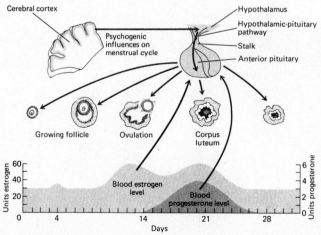

FIGURE 18. Ovulation during the menstrual cycle. (Reproduced from Benson, *Handbook of Obstetrics and Gynecology*, ed. 3, p. 26. Lange Medical Publications, Los Altos, Calif., 1968, by permission.)

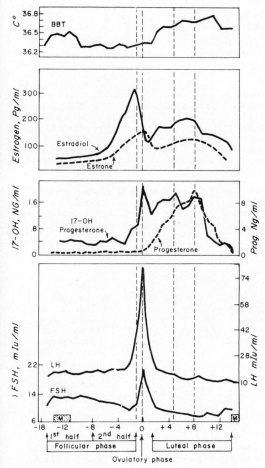

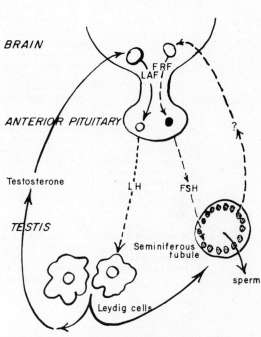

FIGURE 19. The hormonal events of the reproductive cycle are centered on the midcycle LH peak (day 0). Basal body temperatures (*BBT*) are shown on the *top line*. Plasma levels of luteinizing hormone (*LH*) and follicle-stimulating hormone (*FSH*) are shown on the *bottom two lines*. Gonadal steroid levels (estradiol, estrone, 17-hydroxyprogesterone, and progesterone) are shown in the *center*. Days of menstrual bleeding are indicated by *M*. (Redrawn from Ross et al., 1970, and Koreman et al., 1970. Reproduced from J. R. Brobeck, editor, *Best & Taylor's Physiological Basis of Medical Practice*, ed. 9, Williams & Wilkins, Baltimore, 1973, by permission.)

FIGURE 20. Testicular function in man. The hypothalamo-pituitary-Leydig cell axis is shown on the *left* with pituitary luteinizing hormone stimulating testosterone secretion. The hypothalamo-pituitary-tubular axis is shown on the *right* with follicle-stimulating hormone and testosterone stimulating spermatogenesis. A factor from the seminiferous tubules is believed to regulate the secretion of follicle-stimulating hormone. (Reproduced from J. R. Brobeck, editor, *Best & Taylor's Physiological Basis of Medical Practice*, ed. 9, Williams & Wilkins, Baltimore, 1973, by permission.)

TABLE I

*The Male Sexual Response Cycle**

	I. Excitement Phase (several minutes to hours)	II. Plateau Phase (30 sec. to 3 min.)	III. Orgasmic Phase (3–15 sec.)	IV. Resolution Phase (10–15 min.; if no orgasm, ½-1 day)
Skin	No change	Sexual flush: inconsistently appears; maculopapular rash originates on abdomen and spreads to anterior chest wall, face, and neck and can include shoulders and forearms	Well-developed flush	Flush disappears in reverse order of appearance; inconsistently appearing film of perspiration on soles of feet and palms of hands
Penis	Erection within 10–30 sec caused by vasocongestion of erectile bodies of corpus cavernosa of shaft. Loss of erection may occur with introduction of asexual stimulus, loud noise	Increase in size of glans and diameter of penile shaft; inconsistent deepening of coronal and glans coloration	Ejaculation: marked by 3 to 4 contractions at 0.8 sec. of vas, seminal vesicles, prostate, and urethra; followed by minor contractions with increasing intervals.	Erection: partial involution in 5–10 sec. with variable refractory period; full detumescence in 5–30 min.
Scrotum and testes	Tightening and lifting of scrotal sac and partial elevation of testes toward perineum	50 per cent increase in size of testes over unstimualted state due to vasocongestion and flattening of testes against perineum signaling impending ejaculation	No change	Decrease to base line size due to loss of vasocongestion. Testicular and scrotal descent within 5–30 min. after orgasm. Involution may take several hours if there is no orgasmic release
Cowper's glands	No change	2–3 drops of mucoid fluid that contain viable sperm	No change	No change
Other	Breasts: inconsistent nipple erection	Myotonia: semispastic contractions of facial, abdominal, and intercostal muscles. Tachycardia: up to 175 per min. Blood pressure: rise in systolic 20–80 mm.; in diastolic 10–40 mm. Respiration: increased	Loss of voluntary muscular control Rectum: rhythmical contractions of sphincter Up to 180 beats per min. 40–100 systolic; 20–50 diastolic Up to 40 respirations per min. Ejaculatory spurt: 12–20 inches at age 18 decreasing with age to seepage at 70	Return to base line state in 5–10 min.

* Table prepared by Virginia A. Sadock, M.D., after Masters and Johnson data.

TABLE II

*The Female Sexual Response Cycle**

	I. Excitement Phase (several minutes to hours)	II. Plateau Phase (30 sec. to 3 min.)	III. Orgasmic Phase (3–15 sec.)	IV. Resolution Phase (10–15 min.; if no orgasm, ½–1 day)
Skin	No change	Sexual flush inconstant except in fair skinned; pink mottling on abdomen, spreads to breasts, neck, face, often to arms, thighs, and buttocks—looks like measles rash	No change (flush at its peak)	Fine perspiration, mostly on flush areas; flush disappears in reverse order
Breasts	Nipple erection in two-thirds of subjects Venous congestion Areolar enlargement	Flush: mottling coalesces to form a red papillary rash Size: increase one fourth over normal, especially in breasts that have not nursed Areolae: enlarge; impinge on nipples so they seem to disappear	No change (venous tree pattern stands out sharply; breasts may become tremulous)	Return to normal in reverse order of appearance in ½ hour or more
Clitoris	Glans: half of subjects, no change visible, but with colposcope, enlargement always observed; half of subjects, glans diameter always increased 2-fold or more. Shaft: variable increase in diameter; elongation occurs in only 10 per cent of subjects	Retraction: shaft withdraws deep into swollen prepuce; just before orgasm, it is difficult to visualize; may relax and retract several times if phase II is unduly prolonged Intrapreputial movement with thrusting: movements synchronized with thrusting owing to traction on labia minora and prepuce	No change Shaft movements continue throughout if thrusting is maintained	Shaft returns to normal position in 5–10 sec.; full detumescence in 5–30 min. (if no orgasm, clitoris remains engorged for several hours)
Labia Majora	Nullipara: thin down; elevated; flatten against perineum Multipara: rapid congestion and edema; increases to 2–3 times normal size	Nullipara: totally disappear (may reswell if phase II unduly prolonged.) Multipara: become so enlarged and edematous, they hang like folds of a heavy curtain	No change	Nullipara: *increase* to normal size in 1–2 min. or less Multipara: *decrease* to normal size in 10–15 min.
Labia Minora	Color change: to bright pink in nullipara and red in multipara Size: increase 2–3 times over normal; prepuce often much more; proximal portion firms, adding up to ³⁄₄ inch to functional vaginal sidewalls	Color change: suddenly turn bright red in nullipara, burgundy red in multipara, signifies onset of phase II, orgasm will then always follow within 3 min. if stimulation is continued Size: enlarged labia gap widely to form a vestibular funnel into vaginal orifice	Firm proximal areas contract with contractions of lower third	Returns to pink blotchy color in 2 min. or less; total resolution of color and size in 5 min. (decoloration, clitoral return and detumescence of lower third all occur as rapidly as loss of the erection in men)
Bartholin's Glands	No change	A few drops of mucoid secretion form; aid in lubricating vestibule (insufficient to lubricate vagina)	No change	No change
Vagina	Vaginal transudate: appears 10–30 sec. after onset of arousal; drops of clear fluid coalesce to form a	Copious transudate continues to form; quantity of transudate generally increased only by prolonging	No change (transudate provides maximum degree of lubrication)	Some transudate collects on floor of the upper two thirds formed by its posterior wall (in supine po-

TABLE II—*Continued*

	I. Excitement Phase (several minutes to hours)	II. Plateau Phase (30 sec. to 3 min.)	III. Orgasmic Phase (3–15 sec.)	IV. Resolution Phase (10–15 min.; if no orgasm, ½-1 day)
	well-lubricated vaginal barrel (aids in buffering acidity of vagina to neutral pH required by sperm) Color change: mucosa turns patchy purple	preorgasm stimulation (increased flow occurs during premenstrual period) Color change: uniform dark purple mucosa		sition); ejaculate deposited in this area forming seminal pool
Upper two-thirds	Balloons: dilates convulsively as uterus moves up, pulling anterior vaginal wall with it; fornices lengthen; rugae flatten	Further ballooning creates diameter of 2½–3 inches; then wall relaxes in a slow, tensionless manner	No change: fully ballooned out and motionless	Cervical descent: descends to seminal pool in 3-4 min.
Lower third	Dilation of vaginal lumen to 1-1¼ inches occurs; congestion of walls proceeds gradually, increasing in rate as phase II approaches	Maximum distension reached rapidly; contracts lumen of lower third and upper labia to ½ or more its diameter in phase I; contraction around penis allows thrusting traction on clitoral shaft via labia and prepuce.	3–15 contractions of lower third and proximal labia minora at ¾-sec. intervals	Congestion disappears in seconds (if no orgasm, congestion persists for 20–30 min.)
Uterus	Ascent: moves into false pelvis late in phase I Cervix: passively elevated with uterus (no evidence of any cervical secretions during entire cycle)	Contractions: strong sustained contractions begin late in phase II; have same rhythm as contractions late in labor, lasting 2+ min. Cervix: slight swelling; patchy purple (inconstant; related to chronic cervicitis)	Contractions throughout orgasm; strongest with pregnancy and masturbation	Descent: slowly returns to normal Cervix: color and size return to normal in 4 min; patulous for 10 min.
Others	Fourchette: color changes throughout cycle as in labia minora	Perineal body: spasmodic tightening with involuntary elevation of perineum Hyperventilation and carpopedal spasms; both are usually present, the latter less frequently and only in female-supine position	Irregular spasms continue Rectum: rhythmical contractions inconstant; more apt to occur with masturbation than coitus External urethral sphincter: occasional contraction, no urine loss	All reactions cease abruptly or within a few seconds

* From *The Nature and Evolution of Female Sexuality*, by Mary Jane Sherfey, Copyright 1966, 1972 by Mary Jane Sherfey. Reprinted by permission of Random House, Inc.

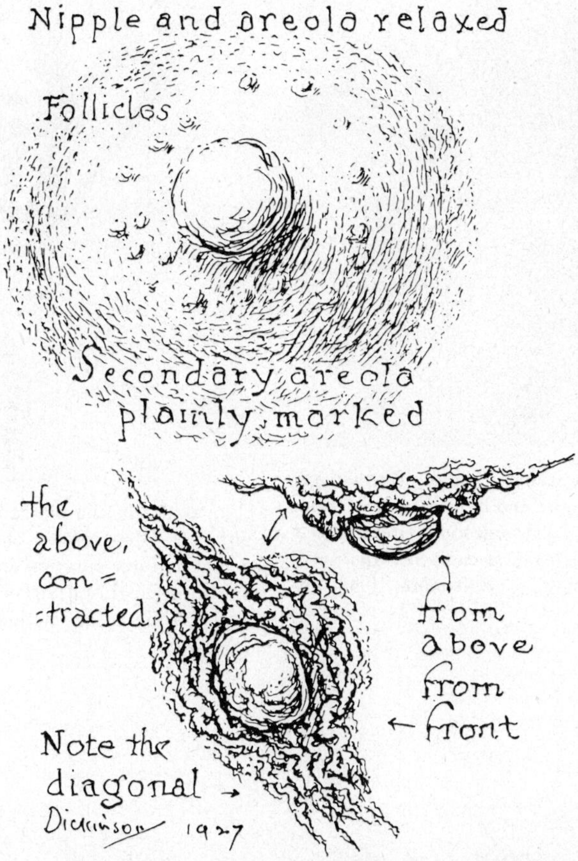

FIGURE 21. As sexual excitement increases, nipple erection and impingement of the areolar on the nipple is a finding in two thirds of women. (Reproduced from R. L. Dickinson, *Atlas of Human Sex Anatomy*, ed. 2, Williams & Wilkins, Baltimore, 1949, by permission.)

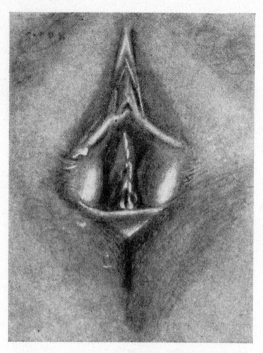

FIGURE 22. In the excitement phase of sexual responsivity, the labia majora and labia minora become thickened as a result of vasocongestion. (Reproduced from R. L. Dickinson, *Atlas of Human Sex Anatomy*, ed. 2, Williams & Wilkins, Baltimore, 1949, by permission.)

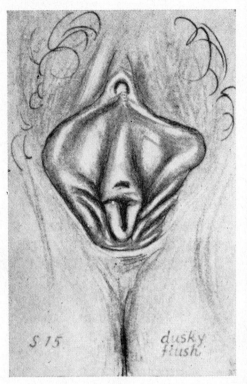

FIGURE 23. In the plateau phase of sexual responsivity, the labia minora elongate, spread, and thin out; the clitoris enlarges and elevates. (Reproduced from R. L. Dickinson, *Atlas of Human Sex Anatomy*, ed. 2, Williams & Wilkins, Baltimore, 1949, by permission.)

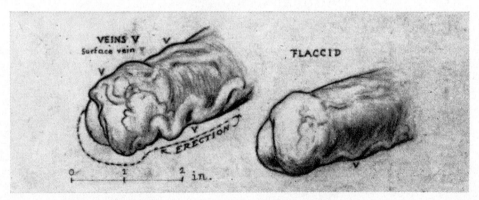

FIGURE 24. Venous engorgement without orgasm produces partial involution of the penis with associated pain (*left*). Complete involution occurs after orgasm, and the penis returns to its flaccid state (*right*). (Reproduced from R. L. Dickinson, *Atlas of Human Sex Anatomy*, ed. 2, Williams & Wilkins, Baltimore, 1949, by permission.)

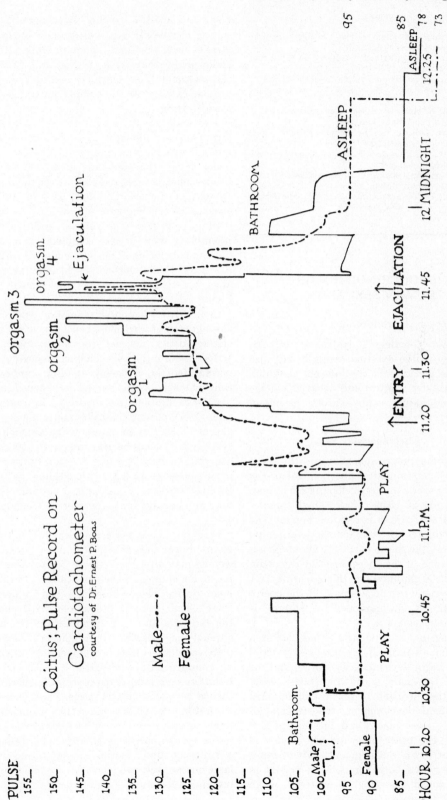

FIGURE 25. Coitus was performed with both partners monitored for pulse rate. Note the increased rate in both the man and the woman, the length of foreplay, the multiple orgasmic return of the woman, and the orgasm and resolution to the resting state with sleep. (Reproduced from R. L. Dickinson, *Atlas of Human Sex Anatomy*, ed. 2, Williams & Wilkins, Baltimore, 1949, by permission.)

REFERENCES

American Medical Association. *Human Sexuality*. American Medical Association, Chicago, 1972.
Basmajian, J. V. *Grant's Method of Anatomy*, ed. 8. Williams & Wilkins, Baltimore, 1971.
Brobeck, J. R. (editor). *Best & Taylor's Physiological Basis of Medical Practice*, ed. 9. Williams & Wilkins, Baltimore, 1973.
Dickinson, R. L. *Atlas of Human Sex Anatomy*, ed. 2. Williams & Wilkins, Baltimore, 1949.
Ellis, A., and Arbanel, A. *The Encyclopedia of Sexual Behavior*. Jason Aronson, New York, 1973.
Masters, W. H., and Johnson, V. E. *Human Sexual Response*. Little, Brown, Boston, 1966.
Masters, W. H., and Johnson, V. E. *Human Sexual Inadequacy*. Little, Brown, Boston, 1970.
Sherfey, M. J. *The Nature and Evolution of Female Sexuality*. Random House, New York, 1972.

23.3.   ENDOCRINOLOGY OF HUMAN SEXUALITY

Introduction

Maleness or femaleness involves not only the morphology of the external genitalia but also that of the gonads and the internal genitalia. Ultimate gender identity and behavior emerge from a combination of physical and psychosocial factors.

Chromosomal Sex

In the normal progression of events, the sex of a person is determined at the moment of the union of the sperm and egg cells. In each human cell, there are 22 pairs of autosomal chromosomes and one pair of sex chromosomes. The ovum contributes the X or female-determining chromosome; the sperm carries either an X or a Y chromosome. If the sperm meeting the ovum contains the X chromosome, the blueprint is set for the development of a female. If the sperm contains the Y chromosome, the embryo is destined to become a male.

According to Jost, maleness is imposed on a basically female fetus. The embryonal gonadal structures begin developing as ovaries, and the growth of the male gonad transpires consequent to the intrusion of the Y chromosome. Early in fetal development, the struggle for supremacy takes place, and one component suppresses the other, allowing the organs of one sex to begin development. When dominance fails, then both components persist in the same gonad, resulting in ovo-testis, or an

ovary and a testis develop independently, resulting in true hermaphroditism (see Figure 1). Here is seen the result of faulty chromosomal endowment—that is, both XX and XY sex chromosomal lines—gonadal inadequacy, ambiguous external genitalia, and confused gender identification.

The male gonad is believed to produce an organizing or inductor substance sometimes referred to as a fetal androgen, different from testosterone, that induces regresssion of the Mullerian structures and permits the full development of the Wolffian duct system. In the absence of this inductor substance, the basic femininity of the fetus persists, and a person resembling more or less completely a phenotypic female results. Thus, one endowed with an XY chromosomal pattern but lacking the organizer emerges as a phenotypic female (see Figure 2).

Some writers list chromosomal or genetic sex as diagnostic of sexuality when a person's sexual characteristics are not consonant. Barr described, within the cells of a buccal smear of the normal female, a deeply staining chromatin conglomerate located immediately beneath the nuclear membrane (see Figure 3). In a normal male or XY person, these chromatin masses are absent; however, in males with Klinefelter's syndrome (gynecomastia and testicular dysgenesis), an extra X is found; as a result, such a person posesses an XXY chromosomal pattern. Some of these males may appear normal; others may be eunuchoid; all are infertile (see Figure 4).

Fetal hormones, maternal hormones, or exogenous hormones administered to pregnant women may alter the external genital development, depending on the time in fetal development during which these hormonal influences come to bear. In congenital adrenal hyperplasia, the excessive androgens produced by the fetal adrenal may prevent the formation of a complete vagina, resulting in a urogenital sinus and an enlarged clitoris at birth; if the hormonal influence was mild or later in its appearance, then a normal vagina is formed, and only the clitoral enlargement is indicative of unnatural fetal hormonal influences (see Figure 5). So, too, a woman harboring an arrhenoblastoma or a virilizing tumor of the adrenal or receiving large doses of testosterone or androgenic progestational substances (norethindrone, ethister-

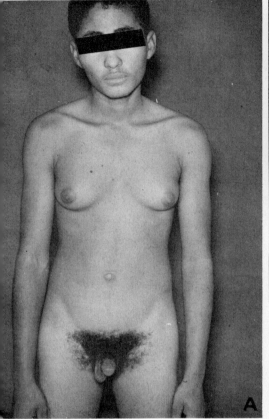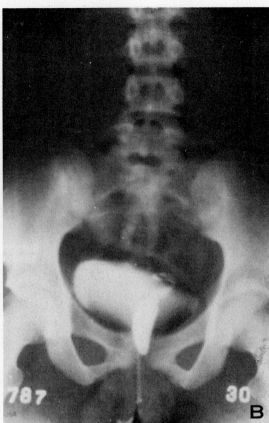

FIGURE 1. A true hermaphrodite. An abdominal ovary and a scrotal testis were found on biopsy of gonadal structures. Menses occurred each month from the urogenital sinus. *A*. Note gynecomastia. *B*. A cystogram and vaginal-uterosalpingogram revealed separate openings for the urethra and vaginal tract. The unicollis uterus and the Fallopian tube are outlined.

one) during pregnancy may give birth to an infant with anomalous external genitalia.

Maleness and Femaleness

Male Endocrinology

After the male gonad develops as the result of chromosomal endowment and fetal androgen, the testicular androgens permit the maturation of the external genitalia and masculine bodily habitus. Urinary 17-ketosteroid levels remain low in the male infant until the prepubertal age. at which time there are increments, reaching a peak at 18 to 20 years (see Figure 6) then tapering off to a fairly constant level. After the age of 50, plasma testosterone levels begin slowly to decline.

Pituitary interstitial cell-stimulating hormone stimulates the testes to produce androgens and estrogens. FSH (follicle-stimulating hormone), in the presence of testosterone, permits the maturation of the germ cells lying in between the sustentacular cells of the tubule to mature into spermatogonia. The Sertoli or sustentacular cells are thought by some to be capable of producing estrogen. Others postulate a specific kind of inhibitory property as a system for the control of hormonal secretion. Androgens affect other than sexual activities: nitrogen retention, skeletal growth, increase in muscle mass and somatic organ size (kidney, liver, spleen), salt and water retention, and fat metabolism. The Leydig cells of the testis release androgens during the first 6 months after birth and then become active again around the tenth to the thirteenth years of age with early manifestations of pubescence. At puberty, when the body is suffused with androgens in increasing amounts, sex drive and libido develop as a part of the total picture. Extensive

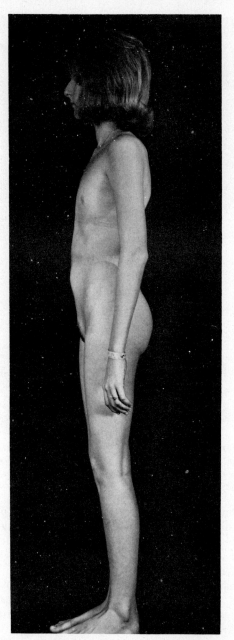

FIGURE 2. A phenotypic female with XY karyotype. The vaginal canal was normal without clitoral enlargement. At laparotomy, dysgenetic gonads and a uterus with Fallopian tubes were present. On cyclic estrogen-progestogen therapy, menses were induced at regular intervals, and good breast development resulted.

changes take place in the nervous system; in addition, there is growth of the secondary sex characteristics and maturation of the organs of reproduction.

The age of puberty varies widely within the normal range and may be conditioned by genetic background and by nutritional and environmental factors. Boys reach puberty (defined as the ability to ejaculate and produce spermatozoa) from 9 to 17 years, 15 being the average age. Other characteristics of the adult male also appear—activity of sweat and apocrine glands, growth of the larynx, and hair distribution. Muscular growth, with broadening of shoulders and generalized skeletal development, continues until 16 to 18 years for most.

Eunuchoid males whose condition is due to hypogonadotropic hypogonadism or primary testicular failure usually respond well to adequate androgen replacement therapy. The patient with secondary hypogonadism, caused by a pituitary chromophobe adenoma or other lesion disturbing the hypothalamic-pituitary axis, exhibits marked loss in sexual function; replacement hormonal therapy in such cases restores sexual capacity. When the pituitary or testes are removed, sexual potential usually fails; in an occasional man, the memory of past events may be sufficient to permit sexual arousal and function without androgens.

The adult male with sexual inadequacy may be said to have a psychogenic block if he has normal testicular function. Administration of the customary small dosages of androgens to such a patient most often proves futile unless the androgens are accompanied by psychotherapy to resolve some underlying emotional prob-

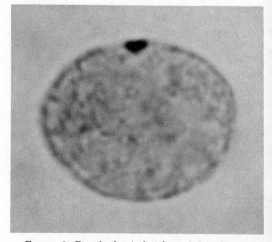

FIGURE 3. Barr body. A deeply staining chromatin mass just below the cellular membrane of the nucleus is found in more than 30 per cent of somatic cells in the normal female.

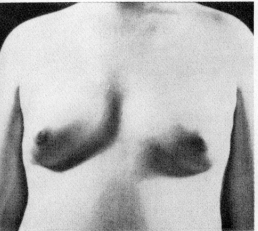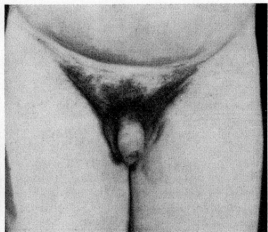

FIGURE 4. Gynecomastia in a male with Klinefelter's syndrome, with positive Barr bodies and an XXY karyotype. The testes are very small and show typical seminiferous tubule sclerosis.

lem or some severe psychogenic overlay. The man entering his fifties and later years frequently complains of loss of potency—loss of erectile ability, capacity for intromission, or ability to maintain an erection. Some men experience more or less complete loss of libido, personality changes, insomnia, loss of self-confidence, fatigue, and depression—symptoms thought by some to be components of the male climacteric. Testosterone, in sufficiently large amounts, may satisfactorily alleviate many of the complaints (see Tables I and II).

Men with uncontrollable sexual appetites (satyriasis) may be suffering from a compulsive neurosis. Excessive coitus in itself does not constitute satyriasis; the drive for sexual gratification must be so overpowering that it becomes the one dominant thought and purpose of the person's life. Genetic factors may be implicated. The finding of an XYY chromosomal pattern in markedly aggressive men with tendencies to commit sex crimes and murders adds another dimension to the problem. Therapy in the form of estrogens has been tried, but estrogens also stimulate nipple and breast development. However, ¼ to ½ tablet of an estrogen-progestogen contraceptive pill administered daily or every other day is effective in reducing the uncontrollable sex drive without much breast stimulation.

Female Endocrinology

Feminine body growth, development, and maturation of the organs of reproduction begin 1½ years earlier than in males, at about 13½ years of age. A second variation occurs in the woman's fifth decade, when sex hormone production comes to a virtual halt.

In the female, pubescence begins with the budding of the breasts, the appearance of sexual hair, and growth of the internal and external genitalia. The onset of puberty varies from 9 to 17 years of age. Menarche in the young girl frequently occurs without the release of an ovum during the early phase of this maturing process. Usually, several months to years elapse before optimal reproductive efficiency (monthly ovulation) is established.

The estrogens produced by maturing follicles stimulate the proliferation of the endometrium. This proliferation is made possible by the FSH and luteinizing hormone released from the pituitary. The Graafian follicle chosen for ovulation releases an ovum as a result of a marked surge of luteinizing hormone and a minor surge in FSH secretion. The ruptured follicle is rapidly converted into a corpus luteum, and the estrogen and progesterone produced by it arrest further proliferation and induce secretory changes of the endometrium, preparing it for nidation of the ovum. If fertilization does not take place, the corpus luteum regresses; the ovarian hormonal levels drop as a signal to the pituitary to begin a new cycle. When fertilization does occur, minute amounts of chorionic gonadotropin keep the corpus luteum viable to secrete the hormones requisite for maintenance and nutriment of the developing embryo while

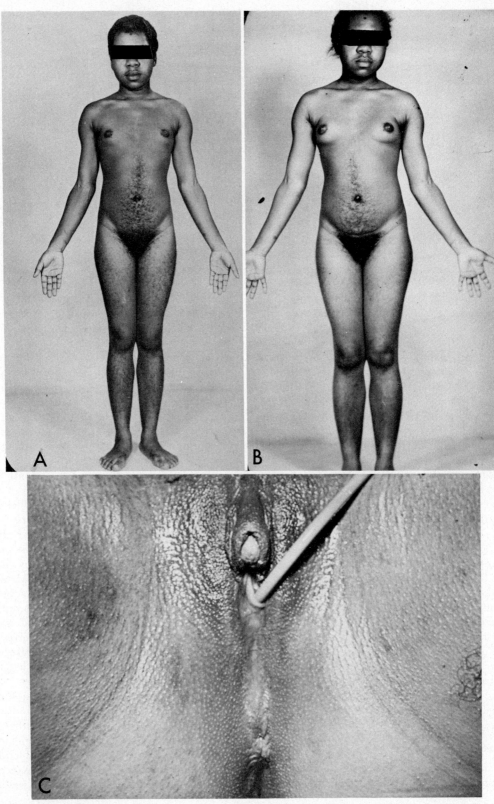

FIGURE 5. *A.* Female pseudohermaphroditism due to congenital adrenal hyperplasia. *B.* Note the breast development after 6 months of cortisone therapy; normal cyclic menses began within a few months. *C.* Note the enlarged clitoris and urogenital sinus.

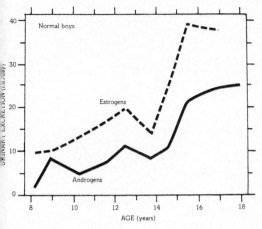

FIGURE 6. The excretion of sex hormones in boys (i.u., international units). (Data are from W. W. Greulich, et al. Somatic and endocrine studies of puperal and adolescent boys. Monogr. Soc. Res. Child Develop., 7: 26, 1942.)

minimizing uterine contractions. The corpus luteum continues to function for about 3 months; thereafter, the placenta assumes hormonal responsibility for gestation. At a time not precisely established, the fetal endocrinological system begins to function as dictated by fetal chromosomal inheritance.

Disorders due to inborn error in the enzymes needed for hormonal synthesis and utilization by the fetus may result in many endocrinopathies, such as congenital adrenal hyperplasia, resulting in pseudohermaphroditism in the female (see Table III) and macrogenitosomia precox in the male. Early treatment with glucocorticoids from childhood onward prevents the virilization of the afflicted girl by dampening excess androgen and pregnanetriol production by the adrenals. All the untoward effects of excess androgens can be thwarted or avoided, and normal feminine development, menstruation, and even conception may be expected.

Another example of an inborn enzymatic error interfering with proper progression of maleness is the insensitive androgen syndrome or the syndrome of feminizing testes. The estrogens but not the testosterone produced by the testes are effective in stimulating target tissues. The insensitivity to endogenous or even exogenous testosterone results from failure of the receptor sites to utilize this hormone. Such persons appear as well-breasted females, without pubic or axillary hair, acne, or oily skin, and

with a normal but blind vaginal canal (see Figure 7). The absence of a uterus and fallopian tubes indicates that the Y chromosome and the fetal androgens caused regression of the Mullerian duct structures. Such persons are feminine in outlook, sexual behavior, and response, despite the absence of menstruation and the presence of testes.

Women frequently have heightened sex interest at the time of ovulation; others have heightened sex interest during the week before menstruation. However, many women find sexual relations during the latter part of the luteal phase less than appealing. But the adult woman may have normal sex drives or suffer from frigidity or an overabundance of urges for sexual gratification—all independent of the phases of the menstrual cycle.

For many women, interest in sex wanes at the time of the menopause and thereafter. With the marked estrogen deficiency of the postmenopausal period, the vaginal mucosa thins and atrophies, and intercourse is frequently attended by dyspareunia. On the other hand, many women, freed from the fear of pregnancy, enjoy flight of fancy and fantasy, and sex drive may increase—in some, to nymphomaniacal proportions.

The ever-changing activity of the ovarian hormones of the woman finally comes to a halt in the fifth or sixth decade; sometimes the activity ceases abruptly with cessation of menses and sometimes with much troublesome menstrual irregularity, emotional changes, and depressive reactions that veer from slight to intense. Most endocrinologists agree that estrogen depletion is attended by severe vasomotor disturbances, psychosexual upheaval, and a raft of metabolic changes. It is considered good medical practice to correct the hormonal deficiency with estrogen replacement therapy. Many clinicians add a small amount of androgen to this regimen because it adds to well-being and rekindles waning sex drive.

Frigidity may be primary or secondary. Primary frigidity is regarded as psychogenic in origin and frequently necessitates the efforts of the endocrinologist, the psychiatrist, and a competent team of sex counselors. Secondary frigidity usually results from manifold causes and is far easier to manage. After a woman has had several pregnancies, she may become sexually inadequate. Her sexual response may be

TABLE I

Loss of Potentia and Personality Changes in a 50-Year-Old Man

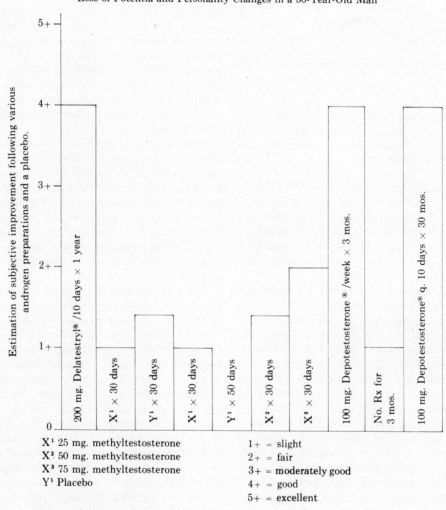

X¹ 25 mg. methyltestosterone
X² 50 mg. methyltestosterone
X³ 75 mg. methyltestosterone
Y¹ Placebo

1+ = slight
2+ = fair
3+ = moderately good
4+ = good
5+ = excellent

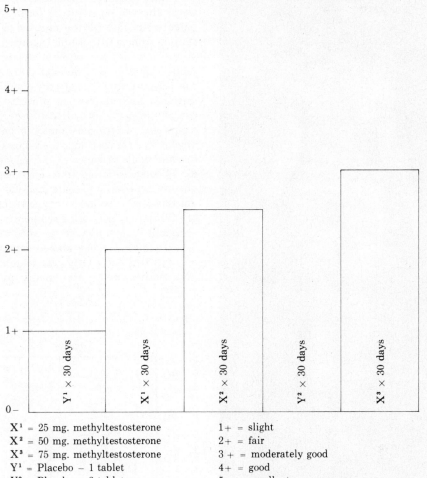

TABLE II

Loss of Potentia, Loss of Self-Confidence, and Asocial Behavior in a 60-Year-Old Man

X¹ = 25 mg. methyltestosterone   1+ = slight
X² = 50 mg. methyltestosterone   2+ = fair
X³ = 75 mg. methyltestosterone   3 + = moderately good
Y¹ = Placebo – 1 tablet   4+ = good
Y² = Placebo – 3 tablets   5+ = excellent

TABLE III

Personality Changes and Biochemical Data—Three Sisters with Congenital Adrenal Hyperplasia

Personality Disorder	Age (yrs)	Urinary Excretion (mg/24 hrs)		Response to Cortisone	Age at:			
		17-Keto steroids	Pregnane-triol		Menarche	Cessation of menses	Appearance of pubic hair	Onset of virilization
1. Nymphomania with homosexual tendencies*	34	35.9 18.6	24.5	Good	10	18	4	18
2. Religious fanatic	44	75.2	—	Good	11	15	?	15
3. Alcoholic†	51	43.0	23.5	Refused Rx	0	—	9	?

* During cortisone therapy, libido returned to normal, and homosexual tendencies disappeared.

† Surgery (abdominal) was performed at age 17. She had not menstruated before operation and did not menstruate afterward. (Possibly the operation was a panhysterectomy.)

Reproduced from R. B. Greenblatt and J. -J. Leng, Factors influencing sexual behavior, J. Am. Geriatrics, *20:* 49, 1972, with permission of the authors.

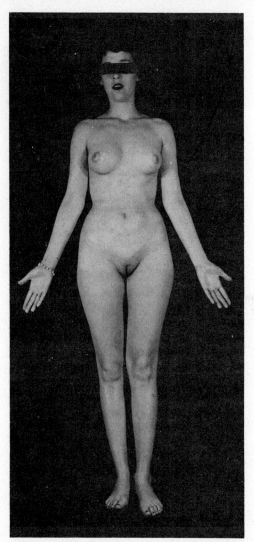

FIGURE 7. A phenotypic female with abdominal testes and an XY chromosomal karyotype. Note the excellent breast development and the absence of pubic hair. A normal blind vagina was present without clitoral enlargement.

revived readily in most instances. Testosterone administration restores the capacity for sexual gratification in almost all women who have once known libido. Estrogens alone are less effective but occasionally do as well as testosterone (see Table IV).

A third type of frigidity, amenable to gynecological therapy, may be a defensive mechanism because of dyspareunia due to endometriosis; bacterial, protozoal, or fungal vaginitis; atrophic (senile) vaginitis; or scarring of the

introitus. Correction of these conditions frequently overcomes the problem. Antibiotic and fungicidal agents cure the usual vaginal infections; the use of estrogens locally, orally, or parenterally restores the mucosa to a healthy state in women with senile vaginitis. Kraurosis vulvae, a moderately rare but advanced form of senile vaginitis, is complicated by atrophy of the perigenital skin, narrowing of the vaginal introitus, and unrelenting pruritus. The local use of ointments of hydrocortisone or its analogues and of estrogens, orally or parenterally, ameliorates the discomfort, assuages the pruritus, and tends to overcome the defensive frigidity. Women suffering from endometriosis frequently experience dyspareunia and avoid sexual relations. The use of progestational agents or testosterone may bring temporary relief.

Nymphomania may be regarded as a form of sexual gluttony. Some women cannot be sexually satisfied and continually search for sexual gratification. Some are unable to reach an

TABLE IV

Comparative Effects of Various Hormones on Libido in a 36-Year-Old Woman Who Complained of Frigidity

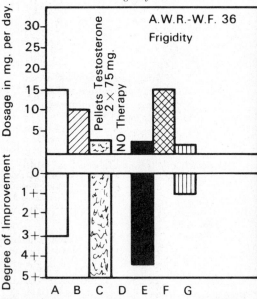

The responses (ranging from 1+ to 5+) are shown in the lower part of the graph. The sequence of hormone dosages is shown in the upper part of the graph. From left to right, (A) methyltestosterone, (B) placebo, (C) testosterone by implantation, (D) no therapy, (E) testosterone propionate subcutaneously, (F) progestogens, and (G) estrogens.

orgasm. Other women have multiple orgasms, but satiety escapes them. Progestational agents and tranquilizers, such as reserpine, may be used over a prolonged period of time to dampen their sexual ardor and to provide them with an opportunity to readjust to their new and decreased needs for sexual activity. Nymphomania is rarely the result of excess hormones; in most, the condition is of psychogenic origin, although women who harbor a virilizing tumor of the adrenal or ovaries may have excessive sexual drives.

REFERENCES

Dmowski, W. P., and Greenblatt, R. B. Abnormal sexual differentiation. Am. Fam. Physician, 3: 72, 1971.
Greenblatt, R. B. Clinical aspects of sexual abnormalities in man. Recent Prog. Horm. Res., 14: 335, 1958.
Greenblatt, R. B., Mortara, F., and Torpin, R. Sexual libido in the female. Am. J. Obstet. Gynecol., 44: 658, 1942.
Jost, A. Problems of fetal endocrinology: The gonadal and hypophyseal hormones. Recent Progr. Hormone Res., 13: 379, 1953.
Jost, A. "Maleness" is imposed upon a basically female fetus. Science Digest, 73: 4, 1973.
Masters, W. H., and Johnson, V. E. Human Sexual Response. Little, Brown, Boston, 1966.

23.4.   BRAIN MECHANISMS OF ELEMENTAL SEXUAL FUNCTIONS

Introduction

Specific brain structures are involved in such elemental sexual functions as penile erection and seminal discharge. In its evolution the human brain expands in hierarchic fashion along the lines of three basic patterns, which in Figure 1 are labeled reptilian, paleomammalian, and neomammalian. Because of the respective similarities in chemistry and anatomical organization of the three basic evolutionary formations, the comparative experimental approach can give important leads in regard to primal neural functions of the human brain.

Penile Erection

In all mammalian forms, the neomammalian formation consists of the most highly evolved form of cortex, called neocortex, and structures of the brain stem with which it is primarily connected. In the squirrel monkey, MacLean and co-workers explored all the medial, frontal,

and parietal neocortex. As illustrated in Figure 2, stimulation of the transitional region between medial frontal cortex and limbic cortex of the anterior cingulate gyrus evoked full erection. Stimulation within the medial part of the cerebral peduncles also elicited erection. Stimulation of the middle segment of the cerebral peduncle, which contains efferent fibers from that region, failed to induce erection.

In all existing mammals, most of the phylogenetically old cortex is contained in large convolution called the limbic system. This anatomically and functionally integrated system represents an inheritance from paleomammalian forms (see Figure 3). Evidence has accumulated that the limbic system derives information in terms of emotional feelings that guide behavior required for self-preservation and the preservation of the species.

Chemical or electrical stimulation of parts of the septal division in male cats has resulted in behavior suggestive of feline courtship and, in some instances, penile erection. The structures and pathways of the limbic system involved in penile erection are schematically shown in Figure 4. Stimulation of the lower part of the septum and the contiguous medial preoptic area elicited full erection. In a number of instances, stimulation within the dorsal psalterium or fimbria of the hippocampus resulted in recruitment of hippocampal potentials and penile erection.

In the third subdivision of the limbic system, positive loci for erection were found in the mammillary bodies, along the course of the mammillothalamic tract, in the anterior thalamus, and in the pregenual cingulate and subcallosal cortex which are known to receive projections from the anterior thalamic nuclei. The third subdivision articulates with the part of the medial dorsal nucleus that projects to the posterior part of the gyrus rectus. Stimulation at loci in either of these structures was highly effective in eliciting penile erection.

The hippocampus contains the so-called archicortex of the limbic lobe. Stimulation at positive points in the pregenual cingulate cortex and subcallosal region resulted in a build-up of high-voltage potentials in the hippocampus that coincided with the appearance of penile erection. Stimulation at positive sites in the septum and anterior thalamus commonly led to the development of self-sustained hippocampal

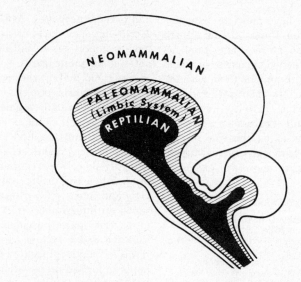

FIGURE 1. Diagram of the hierarchy of the three basic cerebrotypes that provide the anatomical and chemical blueprints for the evolution and growth of the human brain. (From P. D. MacLean, The brain in relation to empathy and medical eduction. J. Nerv. Ment. Dis., *144:* 374, 1967.)

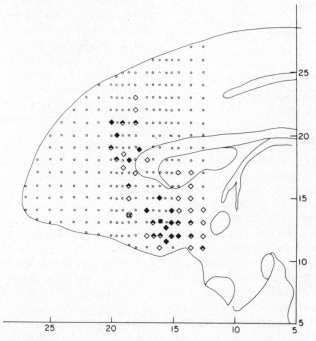

FIGURE 2. Diagram of medial frontal lobe of squirrel monkey, with *diamond* and *square* symbols indicating loci at which electrical stimulation resulted in penile erection. *Squares* give added information that stimulation was followed by hippocampal after-discharges. *White, half black,* and *solid black* symbols refer, respectively, to gradations of erection of 1+, 2 to 3+, and 4 to 5+. Rows of *small cirlces* overlie regions explored and found negative. Marginal scales, in millimeters, give distances forward and above zero axis of sterotaxic atlas. (From S. Dua and P. D. MacLean, Localization for penile erection in medial frontal lobe. Am. J. Physiol., *207:* 1425, 1964.)

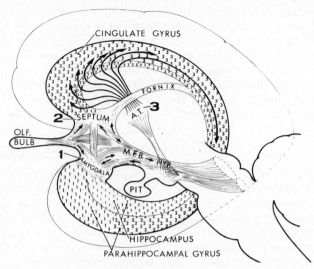

FIGURE 3. Diagram of three main corticosubcortical subdivisions of the limbic system discussed with respect to genital and oral functions. *HYP*, hypothalamus; *MFB*, medial forebrain bundle; *OLF*, olfactory; *PIT*, pituitary. (Based on P. D. MacLean, Contrasting functions of limbic and neocortical systems of the brain and their relevance to psychophysiological aspects of medicine. Am. J. Med., *25:* 611, 1958.)

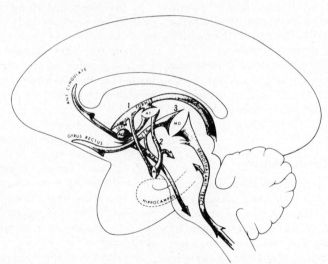

FIGURE 4. Anatomical diagram of cerebral circuits involved in elemental sexual functions. *AC*, anterior commissure; *AT*, anterior thalamic nuclei; *ITP*, inferior thalamic peduncle; *M*, mammillary bodies; *MD*, medial dorsal nucleus; *MFB*, medial forebrain bundle; *MT*, mammillothalamic tract; *SEPT*, septum. (From P. D. MacLean, New findings relevant to the evolution of psychosexual functions of the brain. J. Nerv. Ment. Dis., *135:* 289, 1962.)

afterdischarges associated with throbbing of the penis and an increase in the size of the erection. Afterward, spiking activity might appear in the hippocampus and persist for periods up to 10 minutes, during which time there was waxing and waning of penile erection. In view of the known hippocampal projections to the septum and anterior thalamus, these findings suggested that the hippocampus exerts a modulatory influence on genital tumescence. It seems likely that, in addition to its influence on genital function, the hippocampus also affects the regulation of the release of gonadotropin. In view of limbic system involvement in emotional behavior, these findings suggest neural mechanisms by which aspects of affective experience influence genital and gonadal function.

The major counterpart of the reptilian forebrain in mammals is represented by the corpus striatum (caudate and putamen) and globus pallidus. Stimulation at many points within the caudate, putamen, and globus pallidus elicited no genital responses.

Discharge

Seminal discharge, sometimes preceding erection, was elicited only when the electrodes lay along the course of the spinothalamic pathway and its ancient medial ramifications into the caudial intralaminar region of the thalamus. Characteristically, as the electrode approached one of these points, the monkey would begin to scratch in the region of the chest or abdomen and then, with the electrode at the critical locus, scratch the genitalia. However, emission containing motile sperm could occur independently of scratching. The thalamic structures involved in these manifestations lie in close relationship to the part of the midline thalamus involved in penile erection.

Robinson and Mishkin reported a single case of a macaque that ejaculated following self-stimulation through an electrode in the medial preoptic area. According to Herberg, stimulation in the posterior hypothalamus of rats may induce ejaculation.

Oral-Genital Behavior

Slow-frequency stimulation of the amygdala may elicit first either facial or alimentary responses—such as biting, chewing, and salivation—followed 30 or more seconds later by penile erection. Such a behavioral sequence may be due to recruitment of neural activity in the septum, mediodorsal nucleus, and hypothalamus, with which the amygdala is reciprocally connected. These observations give insight into mechanisms underlying erection seen in human infants and animals during feeding or attempts to feed. The close relationship between oral and genital functions seems attributable to the olfactory sense, which, dating far back in evolution, is involved in both feeding and mating.

In Figure 5 the shield and sword of Mars are used to indicate, respectively, the pathways from the amygdala and septum that are involved in oral and genital functions in a region involved in the expression of angry and defensive behavior. In the squirrel monkey, stimulation within a narrow compass of this region elicits penile erection, angry behavior, biting, and chewing. Since fighting is a preliminary to both feeding and mating, the same mechanisms for combat appear to be involved in each situation.

Social Communication

While defending its territory, the Uganda kob often develops penile erections. The same autonomic manifestation may be seen in the chimpanzee during its raucus display. The squirrel monkey provides an excellent example of multiple ways in which the genital organ may be used in social communication. The species variously uses a genital display in a show of aggression, courtship, and greeting. Ablation experiments show that the striatal complex plays a basic role in its performance.

In the communal situation, the displaying monkey vocalizes, spreads one thigh, and directs the fully erect penis toward the head or chest of the other animal. The display may involve grinding of the teeth, recalling that bruxism and penile erection have been observed in man during rapid eye movement sleep correlated with dreaming. If a new male is introduced into an established colony of squirrel monkeys, all the male monkeys approach it and display. If the stranger does not remain quiet, with its head bowed, it will be viciously attacked. Showing a remarkable parallel to reptiles and some lower forms, the male squirrel monkey displays to a female during courtship in the same manner as in an aggressive encounter with other males.

A variation of the display is also used as a form of greeting. One variety of squirrel monkey will display to its reflection in a mirror. After large bilateral lesions of the globus pallidus, monkeys no longer were inclined to display. Yet these animals were capable of defending themselves and even overpowering the dominant animal when introduced into an established colony of squirrel monkeys. Small bilateral lesions of pallidal projections in the ansa lenticularis may interfere with the somatic components of the display, whereas small lesions of the medial forebrain bundle affect the genital response.

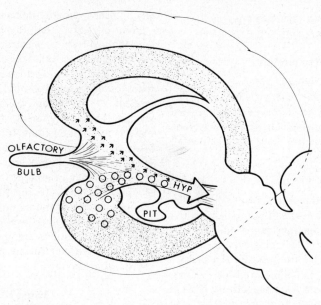

FIGURE 5. Diagram of medial view of squirrel monkey's brain illustrating convergence in hypothalamus of amygdala and septal pathways involved in oral (O) and genital (→) functions. *PIT*, pituitary; *HYP*, hypothalamus. (Adapted from P. D. MacLean, Man and his animal brains. Mod. Med., *32:* 95, 1964.)

Although squirrel monkeys in the wild are not territorial in the strict sense, they will defend their enclosure against the intrusion of strange animals. Sentinel monkeys in troops of baboons and green monkeys sit at lookout sites with their thighs spread and a display of partial erection while the troop feeds or naps.

Gajdusek has described a genital display in New Guinea tribes suggestive of the display in squirrel monkeys. I. Eibl-Eibesfeldt has presented cinematographic documentation of adolescent children in a primitive tribe elsewhere who display in a self-assertive manner.

The lemur, which represents a primitive primate with a well-developed septum, has a greeting display in which the male and female mutually lick the anogenital region. In contrast, the display of the squirrel monkey, which occupies an intermediate position on the phylogenetic scale of primates, involves primarily visual communication. The great development of the third subdivision of the limbic system in higher primates and man may reflect a shifting in emphasis from olfactory to visual factors in sociosexual behavior. It is of significance that, after large lesions of the medial dorsal nucleus, the squirrel monkey no longer shows an inclination to display.

REFERENCES

MacLean, P. D. Psychosomatic disease and the "visceral brain": Recent developments bearing on the Papez theory of emotion. Psychosom. Med., *11:* 338, 1949.

MacLean, P. D. Some psychiatric implications of physiological studies on frontotemporal portion of limbic system (visceral brain). Electroencephalogr. Clin. Neurophysiol., *4:* 407, 1952.

MacLean, P. D. Chemical and electrical stimulation of hippocampus in unrestrained animals. II. Behavioral findings. Am. Med. Assoc. Arch. Neurol. Psychiatry, *78:* 128, 1957.

MacLean, P. D. A chronically fixed stereotaxic device for intercerebral exploration with macro and micro electrodes. Electroencephalogr. Clin. Neurophysiol., *22:* 180, 1967.

MacLean, P. D. Effects of pallidal lesions on species-typical display behavior of squirrel monkey. Fed. Proc., *32:* 384, 1973.

MacLean, P. D. New findings on brain function and sociosexual behavior. In *Contemporary Sexual Behavior: Critical Issues in the 1970's,* J. Zubin and J. Money, editors. The Johns Hopkins University Press, Baltimore, 1973.

MacLean, P. D. A triune concept of the brain and behavior. Lecture I: Man's reptilian and limbic inheritance. Lecture II: Man's limbic brain and the psychoses. Lecture III: New trends in man's evolution. In *The Hincks Memorial Lectures,* T. Boag and D. Campbell, editors. University of Toronto Press, Toronto, 1973.

Poletti, C. E., Kinnard, M. A. and MacLean, P. D. Hippocampal influence on unit activity of hypothalamus, preoptic region, and basal forebrain in awake, sitting squirrel monkeys. J. Neurophysiol., *36:* 308, 1973.

Slotnick, B. M. Disturbance of maternal behavior in the cat following lesions of the cingulate cortex. Behavior, *24:* 204, 1967.

Stamm, J. S. The function of the median cerebral cortex in maternal behavior of rats. J. Comp. Physiol. Psychol., *48:* 347, 1955.

23.5.   STAGES OF SEXUAL DEVELOPMENT

Introduction

Sexual behavior is the end product of interacting systems that change over time. The interacting systems are biopsychosocial. Sexual development depends on constitutional factors, environmental influences, and the accidental, including the traumatic.

Freud

Libido was defined by Freud in 1905 as a quantitative force that measures the intensity of the sexual drives. This instinct represents the psychic counterpart of the biological (hormonal) sources and originates from within the person. It can, of course, be stimulated by outside forces. In "Three Essays on the Theory of Sexuality," Freud argued persuasively that the libido theory is applicable to children. They derive protoerotic pleasure in specific ways from given experiences or conditions. This infantile sexuality is qualitatively different from adult sexuality. The similarity is in the fact that the source of pain and pleasure, as well as the response to stimuli, gives rise to a specific set of responses.

The three essential characteristics of infantile sexuality are these: (1) At its origin, it attaches itself to one of the vital somatic functions. (2) It has as yet no sexual object; therefore, it is autoerotic. (3) The sexual aim is dominated sequentially by erotogenic zones. Because of these characteristics, a child goes through different stages in his psychosexual development—oral phase, anal phase, phallic phase, and genital phase.

During the genital stage of development, the Oedipus complex is initially resolved. With the passing of the Oedipus complex, the child has developed an independent, internalized, superego. The important defense of sublimation is beginning to develop. As the child goes through latency, sexual feelings, according to Freud, are held to a minimum. With the onset of puberty, the sexual drives re-emerge with considerable strength, threatening the relatively weak ego. The Oedipus complex re-emerges for the second and final time; the adolescent forever relinquishes the sexual attachment to the parent of the opposite sex and finds his sexual partner among peers, outside the home environment.

Freud stressed, that the bedrock of bisexuality is the biological substrate to which all later psychosexual and sociosexual developments are related. His theory does, therefore, leave much room for environmental influences on the development of the sexual potential in men and women. The development of neurotic conflicts results, to a large extent, from the libido's inability to obtain satisfaction along normal developmental lines. Freud strongly believed that sexual deviancy originates from a combination of three factors: (1) constitutional-biological, (2) accidental-environmental and (3) internal unconscious. In other words, sexual conflicts and neurotic conflicts are, at least in part, propelled by psychological mechanisms within the person himself.

Kinsey

The major influence on thinking about human sexuality after Freud was the work of Alfred Kinsey and his associates. The major contribution of Kinsey, beyond that of opening the way for nonclinical research, remains the broad imagery of sexual behavior within contemporary society, against which given theories can be examined.

Kinsey's data suggested the occurrence of prepubertal orgasm in a small number of girls and a smaller number of boys. A substantial proportion of people reported prepubertal sex play, making it something of a conventional aspect of development, but far fewer who reported sex play reported erotic arousal. For less than 10 per cent, preadolescent experience includes some sexual contact with adults. For most, this contact represented an isolated experience. Even when the child reacted negatively, the reaction was, for most, rather mild.

Past puberty, masturbation becomes a critical part of the experiences of males and something dramatically less than that for females. After adolescence, it declines in significance for men, although it remains a minor source of sexual outlet for a large number of men during the rest of the life cycle. Rates of activity are substantially lower for females than for males during adolescence. About one-half of all females who do masturbate to orgasm do so after having experienced orgasm in some form of sociosexual activity; for boys, masturbation is almost universally the introduction to orgasm. Frequencies of the activity among women tend to increase to middle age. Fantasy is more common among males than among females, but among those females who both masturbate and use fantasy, the context of fantasy tends to be more realistic than that among males. Females who engage in early masturbatory activity also tend to be generally more sexually active and report a higher rate of orgasm in subsequent marital intercourse.

Petting behavior—essentially the same behavior subsequently labeled foreplay—is most typically the mode of entry into sociosexual activity, but boys are more likely to engage in this behavior than are girls during midadolescence. The activity culminates in orgasm for about one-fifth of the boys (18 per cent) but for very few girls (3 per cent). By the early twenties the percentages even out, and orgasms occurs for about 30 per cent of both genders.

Kinsey established the normative nature of premarital activity for both genders. About one-half of all women reported premarital intercourse, with little difference across varied social levels. For men, it was an even more common event, with more marked social level differences. When educational backgrounds were considered, premarital coitus was reported by 98 per cent of the men with educational attainment of eighth grade or less, by 85 per cent of those with 9 to 12 years of school, and by 68 per cent of those with 13 years or more. More recent research has suggested a moderate increase in premarital intercourse rates for women, but the activity is still disproportionately confined to relationships marked by strong emotional involvement.

Orgasm almost always accompanied premarital intercourse for men, but only two-thirds of the women reporting premarital intercourse reported ever reaching orgasm. The difference, however, is not substantially different from a similar difference in reports of early marital coitus.

Frequencies of coital activity in marriage range from about 2.5 times a week for those couples in their twenties to 1.5 times a week for those in their forties to 0.5 times a week for those in their sixties. This decline tends to coincide with declining male interest in marital coitus, but it does not coincide with female

interest, which increases in association with greater orgasmic capacity.

Normal Sexual Development

Infancy (Birth to 18 Months)

In the first year of life, the major channel for libidinal satisfaction is through the mouth. The erotic attachments and pleasures achieved from self-stimulation and relationships with important others are forerunners of future development. If the normal curiosity of the young child is thwarted and his relationship with other persons is fragile, anxiety and uncertainty will develop in the child.

The autoerotic experiences of pleasure from touch and oral exploration are probably similar in boys and girls. Also, the internalized world of object representations develops along similar lines. Separation anxiety, primitive affects of satiation, and rage are not different.

Early Childhood (18 Months to 5 Years)

During the toilet-training period, the child first learns to associate the genitalia with privacy and cleanliness or dirt. The act of releasing the contents of the bowel and the bladder is a source of enjoyment for the child. He learns that he has control of these functions. The parent interferes with the sense of pleasure the child receives from the acts of evacuation by teaching him that his production are not beautiful and worthwhile but dirty and in need of control. Much of the fantasy life of the child at this stage is attached to his production. Nonsensitive child rearing can traumatize the child and give rise to future conflicts, which, on the emotional level, are tied to acts of giving and receiving.

Together with the developing sense of privacy, children experience a phallic exhibitionistic period. The pride in one's genitals and the wish to share this feeling with others is stressed. Sexually, the child discovers his genitalia and finds that they can bring him pleasure. The communication between the parents and the child concerning this exploratory sexual behavior is another milestone in the sexual development of the child. If parents are too strict and shame the child for his behavior or if they are too encouraging, the child associates negative feelings, such as guilt and shame, with something that gives him pleasure and is associated with the genitals. The fantasy life of the child is vivid and may give rise to unwarranted conclusions. For example, if a boy enjoys fondling his genitalia yet feels that he should not enjoy it, he may develop undue anxiety associated with his natural fears of losing something he cherishes (castration anxiety). If the parents verbalize threats in this area major neurotic problems concerning sexuality may develop in the child in later life.

For the girl, who does not develop as intense a castration anxiety as the boy, there does not seem to be as great a psychological need to give up the sought-for object, the parent of the opposite sex. Hence, her sexual development is not tied as intrinsically to castration anxiety as is the boy's. Her wish for a penis is modified, and she learns to want a child to compensate for what she perceives as a loss of a penis. It is unclear whether cultural factors can sway the psychological developments of the two sexes.

During the last two years of this stage, the child works through the beginning relationships with the parent of the opposite sex. In this relationship, the child lays the foundation for future healthy relationships with people of the opposite sex. The child has to realize that he cannot possess, emotionally or sexually, the parent of the opposite sex. This first love relationship has to be given up in favor of possible future gratifications.

Late Childhood (5 to 11 Years)

With the passing of the Oedipus complex, the period of latency is ushered in. Sex play, usually quite harmless, begins between boys and girls. The boys continue to be curious about sex; among girls, the curiosity is merely episodic. As the children grow older, parental concern regarding sexual matters increases.

The psychological task of the child and, in turn, the parental figure is to allow for a smooth transition from the home environment to the school. The child also slowly develops meaningful relationships with peers of the same sex with whom he or she shares interest, hobbies, activities, and, later on, fantasies relating to sexuality. These homosocial friendships solidify the sexual identity of the child.

Early Adolescence (12 to 15 Years)

Puberty develops slowly and, in its major aspects, can occur between 11 and 15 and still fall within the normal range, although earlier or later development need not imply pathology. The sociocultural referent represents a new set of age-graded expectations. Essential to these new role expectations are a granting of greater autonomy and a lessening of direct adult supervision; greater involvement in and importance of peer groups, largely same-sex in membership; and the social recognition of sexual interests and capacities.

For males, the major development, the capacity to ejaculate, is directly linked to the experiencing of sexual pleasure. Indeed, all but a few males experience orgasm within 2 years of puberty and this experience initiates a pattern of masturbation that occurs at fairly high levels of frequency during early, middle, and late adolescence. This pattern is particularly characteristic of middle-class males, who generally engage in limited direct sociosexual activity during this period. Lower-class and working-class males are substantially more likely to engage in heterosexual activity, including coital activity. However, this activity does little to reinforce heterosocial competence. A pattern of combined heterosexuality and homosociality continues to characterize patterns of sexual behavior during the rest of adolescence and much of adulthood. It is reinforced by and continues to reinforce the sexually segregated character of lower-class and working-class social life on many levels besides the sexual.

For females, the most direct expression of puberty, menses, is predominantly negative. Periodic flows heighten already existing ambivalences about their genitalia and serve as direct reminders of the potential reproductive consequence of coital activity. The most general pattern is to avoid genital involvement or exploration. Masturbation to orgasm is exceedingly rare during this period. Females resemble males in the basically homosocial nature of peer involvement, but the content of this homosocial interaction heavily reflects a commitment to anticipated heterosocial roles as girlfriends, wives, and mothers.

Much of the sexual behavior of adolescents—masturbation, necking, petting, and, especially, heterosexual intercourse—is performed with intense feelings of anxiety and guilt on the part of the adolescent. Optimally, adolescence brings with it the resolution of unconscious incestuous attachments to one's own parents. However, one often sees regression to earlier stages of development because of a variety of unresolved unconscious conflicts.

Late Adolescence (16 to 18 Years)

For both genders, heterosociality becomes fairly normative. The rating-and-dating system becomes an important—if not the central—aspect of adolescent society.

For males, particularly in the middle class, a commitment to masturbation persists with an increasing commitment to sociosexual activity. On all class levels, sociosexual activity is colored by homosocial attachments. Attempts at masculinity confirmation possibly serve ego more than libido. The effects of this homosocial component are more temporary for middle-class adolescents, where the general norms of social life are more heavily heterosocial, than among lower strata, where such behavior is more consistent with such general norms.

Most males, by this time, have engaged in heavy petting—genital involvement without coitus. A majority or near majority of lower-class and working-class males have experienced coitus, as have something less than that number of middle-class males. Initial coital acts tend to occur in relatively nonserious relationships. The relatively short duration of the relationship within which coitus occurs during this stage may reflect an inability to manage the emotional requirements of partners who are social and near-age peers.

For both males and females during late adolescence, the negotiation of this increased sexuality is rendered difficult by the conflicting pressures of parental attachment and peer attachment. This conflict remains somewhat simpler for the male than for the female.

Youth (18 to 23 Years)

The proximity of marriage makes this a period of maximum interpersonal and intrapsychic sexual self-consciousness. It is also the period when one's sexual status is a matter of public concern or when one's sexual status is part of one's public status. Premarital intercourse becomes virtually normative during this period, occurring for most men and a majority of women—the women extending greater degrees of physical intimacy in return for greater emotional commitment by the men.

Superficial problems of sexual competence—secondary impotence, premature ejaculation, and anxieties about penis size—commonly appear in otherwise normal men. Moreover, unresolved problems of relating the erotic to the sentimental and the prior training through masturbation and difficulties. As female partners become more emotionally secure in the relationships, their interest in and capacity to enjoy sexual activity increase, but the same emotional commitment creates an uncertain complexity of motivation for many men.

Early Adulthood (23 to 30 Years)

With formal engagement and marriage, sexual access is fully legitimated and regularized. For both sexes, sexual attractiveness and acceptance of the sexual facilitate an elaboration of sexual techniques, although this elaboration varies greatly across social class lines. As sexual access ceases to be problematic, more attention is focused on the activity itself.

The regularization of sexual access—with the addition of the density of interaction and the pressures of early pregnancy and child rearing—frequently creates a problem of declining eroticism for many men. For middle-class men, the complicated and lush eroticism cultivated by long periods of masturbation typically leads to a sense of erotic deprivation. For many such men, masturbation persists as a source of sexual outlet, allowing them to more fully tap their otherwise unexpressed and unconventional erotic imagery. Moreover, their training in and commitment to heterosociality and their commitments to careers often prevent the exploration of extramarital activity during these early years. However, working-class and lower-class men, although they are less trained in erotic imagery by earlier abandonment of masturbation for sociosexual activity, living in a less heterosocially oriented social world and being less committed to occupational success, experience a loss of homosocial masculinity confirmation by an abandonment of public sexual activity. For these men, both the pressures and the practice of extramarital sex appear fairly early in the marriage.

Middle Adulthood (31 to 46 Years)

This period, particularly for middle-class people, is a point of maximum involvement in careers, family, child rearing, and the social life of the surrounding community. Rates of marital intercourse decline, reflecting a decline of interest on the part of the husband. This declining rate of male interest in marital coitus frequently reflects an inability to connect marital sexual activity with (in the case of higher social strata) the elaborate sense of the erotic developed during adolescence or with (in the case of the lower strata) homosocial validation. For women, however, on all but the lowest social level, interest in marital competence increases. Typically, the woman's commitments to the sexual derive heavily from the sensual and from continuing confirmation of an emotional attachment. Marital intercourse rates during this period remain higher among higher social class groups.

For both genders, this is the period of rising extramarital activity, with well over one half of all men and about one-fourth of all women reporting at least one instance. The patterning of extramarital sexual activity continues to be expressive of earlier patterns of psychosexual development. For men, it predominantly has the capacity for detachment that in adolescence was directly related to the pursuit of sexual fantasies and the homosocial validation of masculinity. For women, it resembles a quest for circumstances that justify and confirm a romantic self-image, rather than a quest for lost orgasms.

Late Adulthood (46 to 60 Years)

As the biological drives decrease in intensity, the man takes longer to reach orgasm, and the pleasure associated with orgasm is no longer as powerful an event for him. In the woman, the decline in coital activity is not as marked; rather, she stabilizes at about the same level she was at previously. For both sexes, though, it is imperative to continue in sexual activity. Long sexual abstinence makes it harder for either sex to continue to function.

Menopause occurs sometime during this stage. The average age of menopause is 50. The biological changes may result in normal psychological problems for women, particularly those in the middle class. The fact that pregnancy can no longer occur often increases the woman's interest in sex, just at the time when the man's interest is often on the decline. The woman can no longer transfer her conflicts, feelings, and

gratifications onto her children, since they have left the home. Thus, husband and wife are compelled to resolve their problems directly.

Old Age (60 Years and Over)

Although sexual desire and ability have realistically decreased, sexual feelings are very much with people in this age range. Married couples in their seventies can have an active sexual life and enjoy it. Those who had sexual difficulties earlier often experience a re-emergence of the negative old feelings and problems.

REFERENCES

Borowitz, G. H. The capacity to masturbate alone in adolescence. In *Annals of Adolescent Psychiatry*. S. C. Feinstein and P. Giovacchini, editors. Basic Books, New York, 1973.
Freud, S. Three essays on the theory of sexuality. In *The Standard Edition of the Complete Psychological Works of Sigmund Freud*. vol. 7, p. 135. Hogarth Press, London, 1953.
Gagnon, J. H., and Simon, W. *Sexual Conduct: The Social Sources of Human Sexuality*. Aldine-Atherton, Chicago, 1973.
Kinsey, A. C., Pomeroy, W. B., and Martin, C. E., *Sexual Behavior in the Human Male*, W. B. Saunders, Philadelphia, 1948.
Kinsey, A. C., Pomeroy, W. B., Martin, C. E., and Gebhard, P. H. *Sexual Behavior in the Human Female*, W. B. Saunders, Philadelphia, 1953.
Masters, W. H., and Johnson, V. E. *Human Sexual Response*. Little, Brown, Boston, 1966.
Offer, D. *Psychological World of the Teen-ager: A Study of Normal Adolescent Boys*, Harper & Row, New York, 1973.
Stoller, R. J. *Sex and Gender: On the Development of Masculinity and Femininity*. Science House, New York, 1968.
Stoller, R. J. Overview: the impact of new advances in sex research on psychoanalytic theory. Am. J. Psychiatry, *130*: 241, 1973.

23.6.   GENDER IDENTITY

Development

Gender identity is a term used for one's sense of masculinity and femininity. It is the product of three kinds of forces: biological, biopsychic, and intrapsychic responses to the environment, especially the effects due to parents and to societal attitudes.

For mammals, the resting state of tissue is female, and male organs are produced only if an androgen pulse is added. Likewise, androgens at the critical period specific for each species are needed for the brain to be organized to maleness. Such organization then produces a reaction in lower animals typical of the males of that species—that is, masculine behavior. Natural experiments in human beings confirm the general rule that maleness and masculinity depend on fetal and paranatal androgens. In an ascending evolutionary scale, however, the general rule of behavior is that the organism is granted greater flexibility of response to a larger spread of environmental stimuli. This is also true for gender behavior.

Biopsychic forces originate in the environment and exert their influence throughout life outside awareness, conscious or unconscious; they are nonmental (nonpsychic). Environment here means not just stimuli coming from outside the organism but also those that come from within and that set up changes in the nervous system, more or less permanently instigating behavior. Those processes described so far are imprinting, classical conditioning, and visceral conditioning.

Enviornmental-intrapsychic forces are made up of the effects of shaping—reward and punishment that do not leave deposits of intrapsychic conflict—and the effects of trauma, frustration, conflict (at first with objects in the outside world and then with one part of oneself attempting to control another), and the efforts the person makes to resolve these conflicts in order to ensure gratification and tranquility.

The most notable description of the development of gender identity is Freud's. In brief, he believed that maleness and masculinity are the primary and more natural states and that both males and females consider femaleness and femininity to be less valuable. Both maleness and femaleness, however, are invaded by attributes of the other sex, and this innate bisexuality has its consequences for both normal and abnormal development.

According to Freud, the biologically normal infant boy is attached literally and figuratively to his mother. As his awareness of himself and the outside world grows, affection and erotic desire are focused exclusively on her. One zone followed by another becomes a source of his libidinal needs, giving rise to stages—oral, anal, urethral, phallic, and, finally, in the fortunate few, according to Freud, mature genitality. The last stage is defined by a full capacity for orgasmic and loving satisfaction with a person of the opposite sex.

However, the boy's father serves as a powerful rival whose threats, open or implied, are seen by the boy as directed at his maleness, invested in his genitals. Castration anxiety forces the boy to detour in his search for an ideal sex object. If the threats are not too great, the boy in time surmounts the danger and eventually finds other women as gratifying substitutes for his mother.

The little girl, on the other hand, has a more devious and uncertain gender development, Freud believed. First, her original love object is a person of the same sex. Then, too, she is supposed to possess an organ inferior for erotic pleasure. She wants a penis and fantasizes having one. The girl has to learn masochism and passivity.

The boy achieves masculinity on resolving the oedipal conflict: the desire for his mother versus the threat of castration from his father. The girl finds her femininity by entering into the oedipal conflict—that is, by turning to her father and risking her mother's wrath.

This development makes a bisexual solution possible. If the boy is too threatened, he may put on the disguise of femininity; in developing too great an attachment for his father, he may identify with his mother and offer himself, as if a female, to his father. If the little girl cannot renounce her desire for a penis and for mother, she is also forced to a bisexual solution.

However, for both male and female infants, the first months of life are spent in a state of symbiosis in which the child has not yet separated out himself or herself from the dimensions of the mother's body or psyche. This state of merging suggests that the earliest stages of infancy are experienced as if one were part of the mother. It may be that a protofemininity is the first stage in the development of both boys and girls.

In the most extreme form of femininity found in males, transsexualism, an excessively close, blissful symbiosis between the mother and her infant son is established from birth on and maintained for years. When the mother-infant son symbiosis is not relaxed, as it is in the boys who become masculine, no masculinity develops; rather, from the time one can first measure any sort of gender behavior, the boy is feminine.

The second clue to protofemininity is found in the ubiquitous fear in men of being unmanly. Once a male has developed a sense of masculinity, achieved in part in the struggle to separate from the symbiosis with his mother and to create for himself a distinct identity, an inner vigilance must be established.

The third clue comes from female transsexuals. Females whose symbiotic relationship with the mother is ruptured are in danger of masculinity. These little girls are encouraged by their fathers to be independent, tough, aggressive, and forceful. And, these girls become the most masculine of females.

Core gender identity is the sense of maleness or the sense of femaleness. It is the conviction, established in the first 2 or 3 years of life, that one belongs to the male or to the female sex. In the rare case of assignment to the wrong sex, core gender identity almost always follows that assignment, rather than the biological state. Core gender identity is created by biological factors, genital anatomy, sex assignment and rearing, imprinting, and classical, visceral, and operant conditioning.

There are conditions in which core gender identity formation is invaded from the start with elements of belief that one is not a member of the male or the female sex. In some intersexed people—those with hermaphroditic external genitals—the assignment of sex may be equivocal from the start. The transsexual, although clearly assigned to the proper anatomical sex, develops a belief that he or she is a member of the opposite sex, regardless of the information given by sex assignment, appearance and sensations of one's genitals, one's name, and one's parents' recognition of one's sex.

The two main factors in creating gender identity are the silent effects of learning and the more sharply experienced modifications resulting from frustration, trauma, conflict, and the attempts to resolve conflicts. Parents, siblings, and others outside the family may shape masculine and feminine behavior by complicated systems of reward and punishment, subtle and gross.

Disorders

The gender disorders can be divided into two groups, deviations (variants) and perversions (sexual neuroses). The deviations are made up of those aberrations of masculinity and femininity that are not the result of intrapsychic conflict; the perversious are the result of intrapsychic conflict.

Transsexualism

The most extreme form of gender reversal is transsexualism, the belief by an anatomically normal person that he or she is a member of the opposite sex. The gender reversal in both sexes is present as soon as any behavior that can be called masculinity or femininity begins. As gender identity develops, there are no episodes of behavior appropriate to one's sex; rather, the person continues unchanged from the femininity present since earliest childhood. Because of the sensed incongruity between sex and gender identity, the transsexual seeks sex-change procedures, surgical and hormonal techniques aimed at making the body appear and function like that of the opposite sex.

Male Transsexualism. At his birth, the male transsexual is clearly recognized as a male, and sex assignment is clear-cut. His mother establishes an extremely close and loving symbiosis with him. By the time he is a year or two of age, the first intimations of femininity appear; by rewarding the behavior, his mother permits it to flower, and it does.

As soon as the child can manage, he spontaneously begins putting on girls' clothes and, in all his play, takes girls' parts. He has no interest in masculine activities, and he joins girls in girls' games. By 3, 4, or 5 years of age, he has given himself a girl's name and is talking of becoming both a girl (an identity and a role) and a female (a biological state) when he grows up. He may even announce that he wishes his penis to be removed.

In school his femininity marks him for teasing by the other boys but not often by girls. Under the pressure of his peers, teachers, or neighbors—but not his parents—he may try to hide his femininity, but he does not succeed, and so he finds himself almost friendless. The ensuing state of sadness and loneliness leads to poor school performance, further isolation from other people, and a picture of a generalized neurosis. However, as soon as the transsexual is given permission by some authority in society, such as a physician, to embark on the task of passing into membership in the female sex, the anxiety, depression, and withdrawn behavior disappear.

The transsexual single-mindedly seeks out sex-change procedures and in time manages to arrange for estrogens to create breasts and otherwise feminize his body contours, electrolysis to remove the male hair distribution, and surgery to create female-appearing genitals by means of castration of the testes, amputation of the penis, and creation of an artificial vagina.

What factors cause male transsexualism? The boy's mother is a woman with a strong bisexual component in her personality. She chose a man, the transsexual-to-be's father, who was distant and passive; only occasionally do these men have an effeminate tinge. Almost invariably, only one son in the family is the transsexual. This boy is chosen because his mother finds him beautiful. Her desire for loving completeness with this son is profound. The two are all too close in the sharing of her femaleness. It is an endless continuation of the merging of their two bodies from earliest infancy.

The child's femininity begins to appear as soon as any gender is manifested; when it does so, the second part of the process of its creation is underway: the positive reinforcement of all behavior that the mother finds graceful, lovely, clean, tender—that is, what she should define as not masculine. To allow her son masculinity would arouse in her the envy that would ruin their love. The feminizing process is uninterrupted; she has ensured that in her choice of husband. He is not there to disturb the obviously intense symbiosis or to serve as a model for his son's masculinity, as other fathers do.

Although experts speculate that transsexualism must be the result of genetic, hormonal, or central nervous system factors, or a combination of these factors, no evidence has been found in human beings.

Although few cases have been reported, one can be cautiously optimistic that treating the very feminine boy may stop the progress of his developing femininity. In essence, the treatment is behavior modification. In addition to treating the boy, encouraging the pleasures of masculinity and discouraging femininity, the therapist must also treat the mother. Attempts to involve the fathers in treatment have so far failed. There is no report of an adolescent being treated by behavior modification alone and then developing masculinity and heterosexuality. So far, no treatment has been reported that will make the adult transsexual masculine.

Female Transsexualism. Female transsexuals are the most masculine of females. These anatomically normal females have been masculine since early childhood and have not had episodes in their lives when they expressed femininity. Like the males, they are exclusively homosexual if measured by the anatomy of their sex objects but heterosexual if measured by identity. They do not deny their anatomical sex but are unendingly preoccupied with the sense of really being men and with the desire to have their bodies changed to male. It is not yet possible to give her functioning testes or a penis. However, with testosterone, mastectomy, and panhysterectomy, the patient can pass as a man.

When a child, this girl refuses to be a girl. She gives herself a boy's name, dresses completely in boys' clothes, and is interested in and skillful in the same activities as are boys. As soon as she can, often in adolescence, she passes as a young man. Even before a sex change, the patient has found a partner with whom she lives for a long time, perhaps permanently. This partner is not an overt homosexual but is usually a woman who has not had homosexual relations, who has been married and had children, and who responds to the patient as if she were a man without a penis, not as if she were a homosexual.

Although the evidence is fragmentary, the following may account for female transsexualism. At the time this infant is born or in the early months of life, her mother is unavailable for mothering. The infant's father is either unwilling or unable to move in and by himself carry the burden of his wife's problem. The little girl is used for that; she is to be a comfort and a cure that the father will not provide. He encourages her in behavior he considers masculine, and so she spends much time with him successfully learning to be like his little boy. This process is furthered from the start by the girl's unlovely appearance. Had she been considered feminine, she would not have served as well for molding into masculinity.

As with male transsexualism, there is no reported evidence of biological factors in the etiology.

There are no cases reported in the literature of child, adolescent, or adult female transsexuals being successfully treated by any method that would make them feminine.

Fetishistic Cross-dressing (Transvestism)

Sexual excitement produced by garments of

the opposite sex is found exclusively in males. Although this deviation starts most often in adolescence, it has been seen in prepubertal boys and may even first manifest itself in adult men in their thirties or forties. There are two groups—those men who prefer a single type of garment, such as shoes, throughout their lives and those who, starting with a single garment, eventually prefer to dress completely as women and who, in addition to the penile gratification, also have the nonerotic pleasure of feeling themselves temporarily to be women with penises.

By whatever chance cicumstances the boy or man first puts on women's clothes, he is astonished to find himself intensely excited sexually. From the experience on, he recognizes this to be his greatest and sometimes only mode of sexual gratification. Because of the risks involved of being found in women's clothes, the activity is usually secretive. Many transvestites are married and work in professions requiring masculine interests and behavior; they dress, except when cross-dressed, in masculine clothes; and they have masculine interests and hobbies and engage in masculine sports. The greatest number cross-dress only intermittently. When doing so, they do not feel themselves to be females. Quite the opposite. Nothing could emphasize their maleness more than their intense, gratifying erection when dressed in women's clothes.

Many transvestites or their families report that the first episode of cross-dressing occurred when a female dressed the boy in girl's clothes in childhood, at which time he was not sexually excited. The cross-dressing was done to humiliate him; that is, it was done by a female attacking the boy's masculinity.

Evidence of a biological cause has not surfaced.

There are no reports of the treatment of a series of fetishistic cross-dressers who lost the perversion after psychotherapy or psychoanalysis. However, recent reports show that behavior modification techniques can be successful.

Cross-gender Homosexuality

Many male and female homosexuals have cross-gender qualities. Homosexuals like their own genitals and feel that these organs are appropriate. Sexually, they prefer people with the same genitals. Homosexuals are, in the vast majority, uninterested in sex change. Fetishistic excitement from clothes of the opposite sex is rare in homosexual males and unknown in transsexuals. Cross-dressing in homosexuals is not for the purpose of passing as a member of the opposite sex. In males, it derives from identification with women and hostility toward them; the undercurrent of mimicry reveals the disturbance in identifying with women that helps save the male homosexual from being transsexual. In butch female homosexuals, cross-dressing is used to increase the sense of masculinity, but it is not carried to such an extent that one would think the person is a male.

Psychoses and Borderline States

Although flagrant cross-gender behavior is not typical of psychoses and borderline states, it is occasionally seen. The gender disorder may be found with or without homosexuality and with or without fetishism; the main features, as in any psychosis, are the signs and symptoms of psychosis that always define the state.

A mild form of gender disorder typically found in paranoid males, psychotic or borderline, is accusations of homosexuality. On closer examination, these accusations are seen to be threats of transsexual disintegration; the hallucinations or delusions threaten the patient with losing attributes of the sex or gender he prizes. This finding is uncommon, however, in women; for them, the paranoid content is usually of heterosexual jeopardy and accusations.

Intersexuality

Today, the term "intersexuality" is used in discussing those with gross anatomical or physiological aspects of the opposite sex. These aspects may be found in the chromosomes (such as XXY and XO), external genitals (such as pseudohermaphroditism), internal sexual apparatuses (such as absent uterus and proximal vagina with concomitant masculinized external genitals in a female), gonads (such as ovotestes), and hormonal state and resultant secondary sex characteristics (such as androgen insensitivity syndrome).

Two distinct factors contribute to the development of gender identity in intersexed patients. The first is that sex assignment and parental influences during rearing account for the core gender identity in most patients. The second factor is that, when abnormal fetal hormonal-central nervous system development occurs, gender identity is bent in the direction predictable from animal studies—androgenization of the brain turns the child toward masculinity, and absence of androgenization tends the child toward femininity.

In Turner's syndrome, one sex chromosome is missing (XO), and so only a female chromosome is present to influence sex development. The result is absence or minimal development of the gonads; no significant sex hormone, male or female, is produced in fetal life or postnatally. The sexual tissues thus retain a female resting state. These girls are incomplete in their sexual anatomy and, lacking adequate estrogens, develop no secondary sex characteristics without treatment. They often suffer other stigmata, such as web neck. The infant is born with normal-appearing femal external genitals and so is unequivocally assigned to the female sex and thus reared. All these children develop as unremarkably feminine, heterosexually oriented girls, although later medical management is necessary to assist them with their infertility and absence of secondary sex characteristics.

In Klinefelter's syndrome, the patient (usually XXY) has a male habitus, under the influence of the Y chromosome, but this effect is weakened by the presence of the second X chromosome. Although he is born with a penis and testes, the testes are small and infertile, and the penis may also be small. In adolescence, some of these patients develop gynecomastia and other feminine-appearing contours. Sexual desire is usually weak. Sex assignment and rearing should lead to a clear sense of maleness, but these patients often have gender disturbances, ranging from a complete reversal, as in transsexualism, to homosexuality or an intermittent desire to put on women's clothes. There is a wide spread psychopathology in many of these patients, well beyond that of gender.

When adrenogenital syndrome occurs in females, excessive adrenal fetal androgens cause masculinization of the external genitals, ranging from mild clitoral enlargement to external genitals that look like a normal scrotal sac, testes, and a penis; hidden behind these external genitals are a vagina and a uterus. These patients are otherwise normally female. At birth, if the genitals look male, the child is assigned to the male sex and is so reared; the result is a clear sense of maleness and un-remarkable masculinity; but if the child is diagnosed as a female and so reared, a sense of femaleness and femininity results. If the parents are uncertain as to which sex their child belongs, a hermaphroditic identity results. However, fetal androgens organize the fetal brain in a masculine direction. Those children raised unequivocally as girls have a tomboy quality more intense than that found in a control series, but the girls nonetheless have a heterosexual orientation.

In a male pseudohermaphroditism, the genitals' appearance at birth, not the true biological maleness, determines the sex assignment, and the core gender identity is male, female, or hermaphroditic, depending on the family's conviction as to the child's sex.

Androgen insensitivity syndrome results from an inability of target tissues to respond to androgens. Unable to respond, the fetal tissues remain in their female resting state, and the brain is not organized to masculinity. The infant at birth appears an unremarkable female, although she has cryptorchid testes, which produce the testosterone to which the tissues do not respond, and minimal or absent internal sexual organs. Secondary sex characteristics as puberty are female because of the small but sufficient amounts of estrogens typically produced by the testes. These patients invariably sense themselves as females and are feminine.

These different disorders require different medical and psychiatric management. Attempts to change gender orientation should be based on careful investigation of the patient's present gender identity. The identity truth should prevail. In the newborn, in whom no gender identity has yet formed, the easier decision, hormonally and surgically, is to attempt reconstruction that results in female morphology.

REFERENCES

Barlow, D. H., Reynolds, E. J., and Agras, S. Gender identity change in a transsexual. Arch. Gen. Psychiatry, *28:* 569, 1973.

Freud, S. Three essays on the theory of sexuality. In *Standard Edition of the Complete Psychological Works of Sigmund Freud*, vol. 7, p. 135. Hogarth Press, London, 1953.

Green, R., and Money, J., editors. *Transsexualism and Sex Reassignment*. Johns Hopkins Press, Baltimore, 1969.

Jost, A. A new look at the mechanisms controlling sex differentiation in mammals. Johns Hopkins Med. J., *130:* 38, 1972.

Money, J., and Erhardt, A. A. *Man and Woman/Boy and Girl*. Johns Hopkins Press, Baltimore, 1972.

Money, J., Hampson, J. G., and Hampson, J. L. An examination of some basic sexual concepts: The evidence of human hermaphroditism. Bull. Johns Hopkins Hosp., *97:* 301, 1955.

Stoller, R. J. *Sex and Gender.* Science House, New York, 1968.

Stoller, R. J. The impact of new advances in sex research on psychoanalytic theory. Am. J. Psychiatry, *130:* 241, 1973.

Stoller, R. J., and Baker, H. J. Two male transsexuals in one family. Arch. Sex. Behav., *2:* 323, 1973.

23.7.   PREGNANCY AND SEXUAL BEHAVIOR

General Considerations

As a physical condition and at a purely biological level, the pregnant state confers on the pre-existing self of the woman new biogenetic ferment. Along with internal changes are the more obvious external changes in mammary and abdominal contour that progressively increase with advancing pregnancy (see Figure 1).

In the first trimester (see Figure 2), pregnancy is almost always accompanied by some degree of gastric distress, if not by nausea and vomiting. The ordinarily self-limiting nature of this probably hormonal phenomenon and its well known prevalence attenuate its disruptive impact on the sexual desires of the husband.

An aspect of pregnancy that may interfere with marital sexuality is the so-called introversion of pregnancy. This entity tends to be defensively perceived by the husband. In essence, it consists of self-absorbing, in-and-out preoccupations. These self-distant lapses are readily confused in the mind of the husband with communicative alienation, which he equates with loss of his wife's desire to sustain her intimacy with him both conversationally and sexually. The wife is, for the most part, unaware of her causative role in this couple-at-odds syndrome.

The volumetric effects of later pregnancy are attended by physical changes that, in many instances, constitute sexual impediments. The sheer abdominal bulk and height of the uterus and its contents near term often engender postural restlessness in futile search of comfort, along with exertional respiratory distress. These physical factors may form a distracting presence that places sexuality beyond enjoyable reach.

Intrauterine Fetal Death

Retention of the products of conception after loss of fetal life may occur at any time in pregnancy. In the absence of expulsive uterine activity, the patient, if in the early months of pregnancy, is ordinarily without subjective awareness of the fetal demise. The diagnosis is, at the outset, difficult to confirm. Later in pregnancy, after the uterus becomes abdominal and fetal movements and heart tones are discernible, the diagnosis is more easily made. Even then, however, the medical tendency is to wait for the spontaneous onset of labor, which usually occurs within a month.

The resultant periods of equivocal and watchful waiting are difficult and trying for the patient and her husband. Along with the feelings of loss is the frequently encountered conviction on the part of the wife that she must rid herself of this dead thing inside her and the companionate belief, on her part and on the part of the husband, that sexual relations under such circumstances are not only undesirable but insupportable to the point of ghoulishness.

Postorgasmic Contractions and Premature Labor

In some patients, particularly during the last trimester of pregnancy, orgasmic sexual activity may be followed by uterine contractions of a painfully prolonged order.

Ptyalism

This very distressing condition, characterized by round-the-clock salivation, is, in its severe form, disabling from almost every social aspect. Unlike the nausea of early pregnancy, it may persist until delivery. The copious secretion of saliva—some of which, particularly during sleep, is partially swallowed and regurgitated—frequently leads to nausea and vomiting. Sexual malaise is a frequent concomitant. This syndrome has been intransigent to a variety of therapeutic regimens. However, doxepin has been used with dramatic and sustained results.

Symphysial Separation

Relaxation of the supporting ligaments of the bony pelvis normally occurs preparatory to labor and in apparent response to the hormone relaxin. This relaxation is most frequently sub-

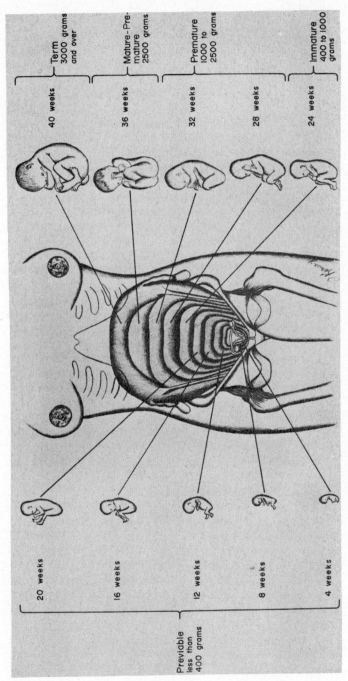

FIGURE 1. Uterofetal relationships as they develop during pregnancy.

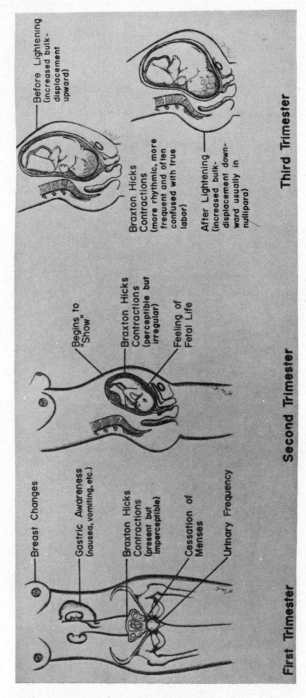

FIGURE 2. The symptoms most common to each trimester of pregnancy.

clinical and, when clinical, predominantly sacroiliac, but occasionally it is targeted to the connective elements that bind and immobilize the symphysis pubis. When this occurs in exaggerated form, the patient experiences severe pain on pelvic motion, which renders movement, locomotor or sexual, extremely uncomfortable. A tightly supportive hip binder provides some palliative relief, but such patients almost always sexually bench themselves for the duration of pregnancy in the almost certain knowledge that their pelvic disabilities will disappear after delivery (see Figure 3).

Pheochromocytoma

This adrenal tumor, when coexisting with pregnancy, can be deadly. It is frequently confused with toxemia, in which event death, as a result of hypertensive crisis, may result. Since the extreme hypertension associated with this tumor is paroxysmal and is usually detected at the time of crisis, anxiety, particularly of a recurrently severe nature, is a leading and all too frequently overlooked symptom.

Bleeding and Sexual Proscription

Bleeding may occur at any point in pregnancy, but it is most apt to occur in the first and third trimesters. Since bleeding early in pregnancy is frequently followed by spontaneous abortion, precautionary interdiction of sexual relations on a temporary basis is usually recommended. Bleeding in late pregnancy, because of its hemorrhagic potential—for example, placenta previa and abruption of the placenta—usually requires at least an evaluatory period of hospitalizations, as well as sexual proscription.

Proximate Considerations

The infertile couple may react to childlessness in highly individualized ways. The man, for example, in the course of a protracted medical work-up designed to overcome sterility, may dutifully conform to the masturbatory claims made upon him for repeated sperm analyses, to schedule sex, and to posthaste delivery of his wife to the doctor for postcoital cervical examination; and yet he may inwardly rebel at the medicated tenor of this prescriptive style of sexual life by becoming subject to premature ejaculation or to impotence or by seeking more spontaneous sexual pastures. The

wife, on the other hand, may become ritualistically involved in becoming pregnant. In the self-absorbing process, her capacity for erotic temperature is superseded by the temperature chart.

Habitual aborters, as a result of frustration and despair attending a succession of spontaneous abortions, frequently blame their husbands for their reproductive disabilities. They take the easy step to a self-curative extramarital pregnancy, which is almost always foredoomed to another abortive failure.

Some women—on the basis of what they consider to be hyperfertility, attested by a rapid succession of successful pregnancies—undergo tubal sterilization. Many of these women, particularly among the educationally and financially deprived, come to regard sexuality as the instrumentality that keeps them knocked up and barefooted. The sexual act becomes invested with more anticipatory dread than participatory pleasure. After tubal ligation and usually only after months of cautious appraisal, they frequently begin to experience their role as a sexual partner in a markedly enhanced way. But many notice no change in their sexual responsiveness, and some, particularly if sterilization was predicated on a medical complication aggravated by pregnancy, feel deprived and complain of decreased libido.

Contingent Considerations

The personalities of the wife and the husband, their desire for the pregnancy, financial circumstances, family size, material and nonmaterial aspirations, and unforeseen situations may impose on pregnancy sexually cordant or discordant patterns. Of essence, particularly in this age of contraceptive options, is desirability. When the pregnancy is mutually desired and there are no medical complications, sexuality is usually unaffected. Without desirability, in the minds of either or both of the partners, there frequently appears an element of recriminatory disaffection that, to some degree, is carried over into sexuality. When confronted with an unplanned pregnancy, the couple with marginal financial resources and with the education of their other children foremost in mind tend to blame themselves less than they blame each other. The immediate emotional tension of unacceptance is ordinarily followed by forced, grudging, and resigned acceptance. During the

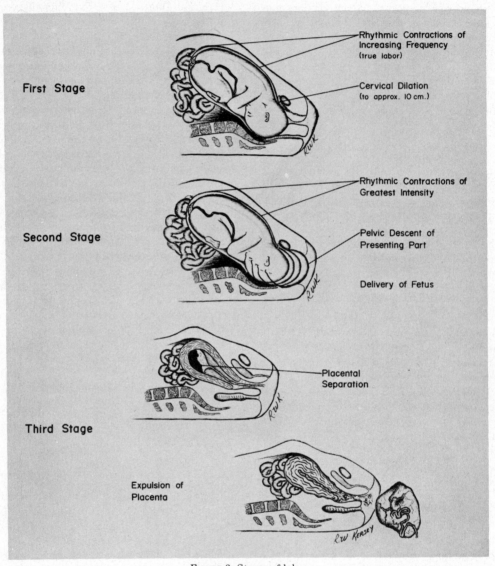

FIGURE 3. Stages of labor.

period of resolving accommodation to the reproductive fait accompli, there is often a disruption of the normally affiliative sexual relationship. The disruptiveness may take the form of pouting or punitive abstention. Or the husband may contentiously desensualize sex by dispensing with his usual amenities and foreplay. The wife may respond in kind.

The wife whose feminine security hinges on a bridelike figure becomes increasingly concerned over her disfigurement during pregnancy and more needful of husbandly reassurance, particularly sexual reassurance. Some such patients place the emotional lability of pregnancy, such as tearfulness at the slightest provocation, in the dominating service of their increasing sexual sensitivity and more or less extract sexual overtures from the husband; others, at subtle levels of awareness, regale the husband with an unaccustomed kind of sexual come-on that uniquely engages his arousal potential and that, in the absence of a motivated need specific to pregnancy, may be curiously inconspicuous in the nonpregnant state.

The lonely and dejected wife who feels that her unfaithful husband can be erotically recaptured and the gulf between her and her progressively more independent teenage children can be bridged by a familial event that in the past was always blessed usually compounds her difficulties when she preceives and attempts to resolve her problems in this way.

In a combined psychiatric-obstetric study of more than 500 women, each of whom had experienced at least three successive spontaneous abortions, it was found that about one third had undergone a criminal abortion before marriage. Unresolved guilt complexes associated with the criminal abortion represented a continuing unconscious conflict that, in somatic translation and after marriage, culminated in recurrently expiative spontaneous abortions. But most of these patients initially resisted insightful acceptance of any possible relatedness between the criminal abortion and their more current abortive difficulties. The most striking historical feature common to their preabortive backgrounds was the seductive and gamelike quality of the relationships between the patients and their fathers. The seductive interest was usually veiled until the patient entered into puberty, when it became operative at the level of sexual suspicion and punitive distrust. The

patient began to act the role that her father, in projection, had defined for her. Her cued sexual role was experienced as coming from within herself and had to be self-punitively undone.

Puerperal Considerations

The terminative climax of pregnancy, with the living birth of a healthy infant, ideally marks both a festive end and an auspicious beginning. Under these circumstances the climactic features, personified in the new addition to the family, clearly outweigh the anticlimactic features, the travail and tensions that may have occurred during pregnancy.

Although reaffirmative tendencies are usually dominant and ultimately prevail, they are frequently delayed by unaffirmative feelings experienced by the wife after her delivery. In minor form, the postpartal blues usually become manifest early in the postpartal period, perhaps in initial response to hormone withdrawal, and take the anticlimactic form of unredeemed let-down. Although usually of a self-limiting nature, these feelings of dejection may translate into feelings of doubt. Depression is not usually brought to the attention of the doctor. Instead, the wife toughs it out and only later, after it has been overcome, brings it to his attention. In the interim, however, there is an accompanying sexual detachment.

Much more infrequently, depressive reactions of a less concealable type develop. Along with the classic depressive hallmarks, including loss of libido, more contextual symptomatic features appear that typically interrelate maternal shortcomings with the newborn child. Phobic fears of hurting or dropping the baby while caring for it are almost invariable concerns and may be superseded by ruminative thoughts of willfully acting out such fears or by hallucinatory voices urging the mother in this direction. Functional psychoses of virtually every variety consonant with reproductive age may coexist with or follow pregnancy.

Conclusion

In the usual course of events, sexual behavior is only marginally affected by pregnancy. But its psychoendocrine effects, volumetric claims, and puerperal aftereffects exert, to some extent, a moderating influence on sexual activity.

In the unusual course of events, physical, hormonal, emotional, psychosocial, or situational determinants may disruptively modify sexual behavior to the extreme extent of elective or medical proscription.

REFERENCES

Asch, S. Mental and emotional problems. In *Medical Surgical, and Gynecologic Complications of Pregnancy*, J. Robinsky and A. Guttmacher, editors, p. 461. Williams & Wilkins, Baltimore, 1965.
Goodlin, R. C., Keller, D. W., and Raffin, M. Orgasm during late pregnancy: Possible deleterious effects. Obstet. Gynecol., *38:* 916, 1971.
Heitman, M. Pregnancy interwoven with people and problems. Med. Insight, *2:* 16, 1970.
Meares, R., Grimwade, J., Brickley, M., and Wood, C. Pregnancy and neuroticism. Med. J. Aust., *1:* 517, 1972.
Sawin, C. *The Hormones: Endocrine Physiology*. Little, Brown, Boston, 1969.
Shader, R., and DiMascio, A. *Psychotropic Drug Side-Effects*. Williams & Wilkins, Baltimore, 1970.

23.8.   SEX AND MEDICINE

23.8a.   SEX AND SURGICAL PROCEDURES IN MEN

Introduction

Surgical procedures can threaten potency, fertility, and excretory control. A procedure may affect the self-image of the patient and the reflected image imposed by the environment on the patient. Doubts, guilt, recrimination, and even hate may appear.

Sterilization

Castration

This operation can have profound depressing effects on a man of any age. Before puberty, the lack of testicular androgen can lead to exaggerated long-bone growth, eunuchoid facies, and small genitalia. Androgen replacement brings about salutary secondary sexual characteristics and allows normal potency. After puberty, castration does not reverse male characteristics, and such eunuchs are usually potent, since adrenal androgen output is adequate. With the implantation of testicular protheses, a sexual partner may be led to believe that the patient is intact.

The diseases requiring castration as therapy are malignancies that are fanned in the fire of testicular androgen. Even medical castration by the administration of estrogen carries the consequences of surgical castration.

Excessive androgen or gonadotrophin administration resulting in sterility (the male pill) is accompanied by increased sexual desire, satisfactory intercourse, and patient satisfaction. At the termination of such therapy, vasomotor episodes, mental depression, and feelings of muscular weakness and temporary loss of potency occur almost uniformly. All these symptoms disappear in about 2 months as normal testicular function returns. Patients with initially low sperm counts take longer to return to the pretreatment level of fertility.

Vasectomy

Because of the poor prognosis of reversibility (25 per cent), an in-depth interview with both partners is essential before a vasectomy. Patients who have difficulties with sexual function before vasectomy are likely (5 per cent) to have increasing difficulties postoperatively. A smaller number have alleviation of sexual dysfunction when that dysfunction was in any part due to fear of impregnation. Spontaneous reanastomosis is extremely rare but has been reported.

The psychological effect of knowing that the fertile years are ended can lead to depression.

Disorders of Ejaculation

Retrograde Ejaculation

Many operative procedures, such as prostatectomy, lead to retrograde ejaculation. Extensive dissections at the posterior bladder wall can lead to retrograde or absent ejaculation. The man with retrograde ejaculation complains of losing the urethral phase of orgasm but is usually reconciled to the idea of the infertility accompanying this condition by the life-threatening nature of the initial pathology.

Absent Ejaculation

In the course of aneurysm repair, back fusion, or sympathectomy for hypertension, the fourth lumbar sympathetic ganglion may be damaged, resulting in ejaculatory impotence. The impact on the patient is violent and intractable. The lesion is irreversible and leads to long-standing frustration and depression.

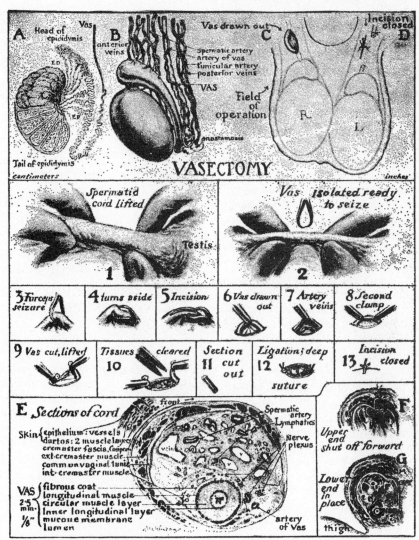

FIGURE 1. The technique and anatomy of vasectomy. (From R. L. Dickinson, *Atlas of Human Sex Anatomy*, ed. 2. Williams & Wilkins, Baltimore, 1949.)

Disorders of Potency Secondary to Surgical Procedures

Perineal prostatectomy or radical prostatectomy carries a high incidence of impotence and, in some cases, loss of urinary control. These complications are not well accepted by patients and reinforce the impression that they are falling into senescent decline. Depression is profound, and patients strive desperately for any procedure holding out any hope for repair.

The perineal plication operation carries a good chance of restoring potency for impotence of neural or vascular origin. Implantation of a silicone splint in the penis or fitting the patient with an external dildo is perferred only for poor-risk patients.

For carcinoma of the penis or urethra, amputation of the penis and dissection of associated nodes is usually the treatment of choice. The procedures are not well accepted by most men, and a marked change in attitude after the operations is the rule. Most men who have lost their penises involuntarily are anxious and acutely ashamed of their altered genital profile. Because of the loss of social face and masculinity, the incidence of suicide is high.

Quite the reverse is true when amputation

has been at the patient's own hands. The underlying guilt is relieved by the amputation, and the patient feels ennobled and inspired by his change.

The response to penile inversion in true transsexuals is extremely gratifying.

With an attack of priapism, which is usually due to underlying hematological disease, the untreated patient is left with a fibrotic, painful, and distorted penis. The most effective early treatment involves end-to-side shunt of the saphenous vein to the evacuated corpora cavernosa. This procedure results in impotence unless pressure is applied to the shunt. Some positions in intercourse apply such pressure, and manual pressure can be used to restore erection in all positions.

Ostomies

The attitude of patients to the permanent placement of an abdominal stoma is universally one of horror. The assault on human dignity and body image is severe.

Colostomy

The usual placement of the stoma in the left upper quadrant, the potential with constipating diets, and the option of daily irrigation to yield a dry colostomy make adjustment to this procedure the best of any stoma operations. However, if the rectum has been resected by the combined abdominoperineal approach, damage to the perineal nerves and the perivesical plexus is common, and disorders of potency occur.

Ileostomy

By presenting a continuously wet surface, the stoma makes normal sexual contact messy. The victims of these stomas are a remarkably well-adjusted group and are much reinforced by a self-help association that reviews and invents stratagems to deal with their new life pattern. On the other hand, the continuous care that this type of stoma demands changes many of these patients into emotional cripples, demanding and unable to give love.

Renal Transplant

The association of peripheral neuritis with uremia, even with dialysis therapy, may underlie the loss of potency that accompanies severe renal disease. This loss of potency may trigger the loss of libido that persists even after successful renal transplant.

REFERENCES

Goldfield, M. D., and Glick, I. D. Self-mutilation of the genitalia. Med. Asp. Hum. Sex., 7: 219, 1973.

Krock, N. Ileostomy catheter. Med. World News, 15: 38, 1974.

Levy, N. B. For dialysis patients, sex, too, is a washout. Med. World News, 14: 15, 1973.

Munnell, E. Total hysterectomy. Am. J. Ob. Gynecol., 54: 31, 1947.

Phoenix, C. H. Sexual behavior in Rhesus monkeys after vasectomy. Science, 179: 493, 1973.

Rodgers, D. A., Ziegler, F. J., Altrocchi, J., and Levy, N. A longitudinal study of the psycho-social effects of vasectomy. J. Marriage Fam., 27: 59, 1965.

Rodgers, D. A., Ziegler, F. J., and Levy, N. Prevailing cultural attitudes about vasectomy: A possible explanation of postoperative psychological response. Psychosom. Med., 29: 367, 1967.

23.8b. PSYCHOLOGICAL IMPACT OF SURGICAL PROCEDURES ON WOMEN

Introduction

Fantasies can stimulate emotional responses at the time of any surgery performed on women's genital organs, resulting in anxiety, guilt, or feelings of inadequacy, mutilation, and depression. With these attitudinal changes, the behavioral patterns of women after surgery on their reproductive tracts can be markedly changed.

Castrating and Sterilizing Procedures

Sterilization

Sterilization of a woman may produce either positive or negative emotional responses. Women who request sterilization have few negative emotional sequelae. Women for whom sterilization is recommended for such disorders as rheumatic heart disease and renal disease frequently respond with anxiety, guilt, depression, or psychosis. The degree of the negative responses seems to depend on the cultural attitude concerning reproduction. With changing attitudes and the movement of women into multiple roles, fewer negative responses are being noted in tubal sterilizations.

Most depressed patients have a combination of anger and guilt, and the anger is turned inward through the force of their guilt. In the case of sterilization, the anger stems from the surgeon's interference with their ability to reproduce and guilt from the fact that the physician may have been trying to improve their health. In addition, women develop concerns about changes in their bodies because of a lack of hormonal stimulation.

Bilateral Oophorectomy

When a bilateral oophorectomy is performed, fantasies may result in feelings of loss of femininity and loss of libido, depending on how the woman feels about the loss of her reproductive potential.

In addition, a woman may develop concerns about changes in her body because of a lack of hormone stimulation. Substitutional estrogen may, for the most part, prevent these changes.

Hysterectomy

After a hysterectomy, the response to the operation depends on the emotional maturity of the woman, on her cultural attitudes about the importance of reproduction, and on the preparation that her physicians gave her. Studies suggest that women who have had difficulty in forming a meaningful relationship in marriage and those with previous psychiatric histories are at greater risk than those women who do not fall into this category. Husbands of women who have undergone hysterectomies also show emotional difficulties.

In making a decision to perform a hysterectomy, the physician needs to evaluate the total patient and needs to give the patient an opportunity to express her fantasies, anxieties, and other emotional responses preoperatively. The physician should take care to correct any abnormal ideas if they exist. In addition, a hysterectomy should not be performed as a routine method of sterilization and should not be performed on women as an answer to symptoms related to emotional conflicts. The hysterectomy procedure should be limited to those women who have organic disease of the uterus and related structures.

Vaginal Procedures

Dilatation and Curettage

Dilatation and curettage is the most common operative procedure performed on the pelvic organs of women. Frequently, this operation is performed on women who have been infertile,

with pregnancy occurring after the diagnostic procedure, perhaps because it solves their guilt over sexuality and pregnancy. For other women this operation may represent a sadistic assault on their genitalia and internal organs. Most women feel that the operation either cleanses their reproductive organs or improves the function of these organs. Anger may result from disappointment when the operative procedure does not cure their symptoms, as in a woman with menometrorrhagia. It is, therefore, important for the physician to differentiate between the woman's fantasy and the reality of what the operative procedure will accomplish.

Abortion

In women who have spontaneous abortions in the first trimester, a dilatation and evacuation is frequently carried out. For these women the procedure may represent a cleansing procedure, relieving their guilt related to the negative feelings they may have had concerning their pregnancy. In women who have had abortions performed in the first trimester by suction curettage, few emotional sequelae are noted if they are well-adjusted emotionally. However, women who do not have good emotional adjustment may develop depression related to the guilt and anger they feel about the termination of the pregnancy. Women in whom abortion is brought about by saline instillation show a somewhat greater degree of depression because they frequently feel fetal movement before the termination of the pregnancy. This reaction is especially true in women who look on reproduction as a central part of femininity. However, even in this group of women, marked emotional depression is not a frequent occurrence.

Vaginal Plastic Procedures

Anterior and posterior colpoperineorrhaphy is usually followed by a positive emotional response. However, some women become depressed because their fantasies, such as the expectation that this operative procedure will enhance their sexuality, are not fulfilled.

Colpocleisis

A colpocleisis is frequently performed in older women who have a large cystocele, rectocele, or uterine prolapse. Frequently, this operative procedure results in a great deal of anger, feelings of inadequacy, and disappointment in women who wish to continue their sexual lives. The patient must be properly evaluated and prepared for the closing off of her vagina.

Creating an Artificial Vagina

A women who is born without a vagina or with just a pouch may have an artificial vagina developed for her. The expectations of the patient must be discussed, and she must be cooperative during the postoperative period for the artificial vagina to become a useful structure. When the operation is unsuccessful, the failure is usually caused by the patient's emotional reactions of fear and anxiety.

Obstetrical Operations

Many women feel that episiotomies are assults on their bodies. Some, therefore, respond with anger.

Sometimes a woman fantasizes that forceps are destructive to her and to her baby, and on occasion she feels that the necessity for forceps represents a failure on her part as a woman. These feelings and attitudes can result in depression during the postpartum period. Proper evaluation and communication with the patient can prevent many of these emotional responses.

A cesarean section can be associated with old fantasies related to birth through the umbilicus, resulting in anxiety and complicating the post-partum period. In addition, women on whom cesarean sections are performed may feel threatened by the fact that they could not have their babies normally.

Radical Pelvic Operations

Pelvic exenteration leaves the woman with a colostomy and an artificial urinary bladder. If the woman does not fully understand the postoperative effects, severe depression may occur. However, well-motivated women are able to continue leading useful lives after this type of surgery.

REFERENCES

Deutsch, H. *Psychology of Women*, vol. I. Grune & Stratton, New York, 1900.
Freud, S. *The Basic Writings of Sigmund Freud*, p. 907. Modern Library, New York, 1938.
Kistner, R. W. *Gynecology: Principles and Presentations*. ed. 2. Year Book Medical Publishers, Chicago, 1900.
Osofsky, H., and Osofsky, J. *The Abortion Experience*. Harper & Row, New York, 1973.
Richards, D. H. *Depressive Illness after Hysterectomy*. Physicians International Press, 1973.

23.8c.   SEX AND MEDICAL ILLNESS

Classification

Most sexual behavior problems are transient. If sexual behavior problems associated with terminal illness are excluded, sexual problems related to medical illness can be classified into four general groups: disinterest or lack of desire for sexual activity; physical incapacity or discomfort with sexual performance; fear of causing, precipitating, or aggravating a physical illness by sexual behavior; and use of medical illness as an excuse to avoid feared or undesired sexual experience.

Disinterest

Transient disinterest or lack of desire for sexual activity occurs in most persons whenever they become sufficiently preoccupied with the symptoms of their primary medical illnesses. The presenting symptoms are typically those of the primary medical illness, and the altered sexual behavior is a secondary complaint, if the patient notices it all. Complaints most commonly come from the patient's sexual partner. Therapy is typically directed toward the primary illness, and the sexual problem disappears or lessens as the primary medical illness improves.

Physical Incapacity

Acute Symptoms. Acute trauma to bones, muscle, skin, or internal organs frequently makes the patient's familiar sexual behaviors uncomfortable or embarrassing. When the duration of the medical illness is expected to be brief, treatment consists of reassurance and appropriate therapy for the primary medical illness. When the duration is predicted to be long but the prognosis is for eventual total recovery, additional understanding and reassurance are indicated. The patient frequently needs the physician's permission to experiment with new or modified patterns of sexual behavior. The physician can initiate this experimentation by low-key education about how similar sexual problems have been solved by other patients. However, unless the physician communicates to the patient the feeling that a discussion of sexual behavior problems is welcome, the patient is frequently too embarrassed to mention the fact that sexual problems exist. When the problem is handled early by the physician responsible for the medical illness, the patient should not need a referral to a sex therapist.

Crippling Sequelae. Other medical illnesses produce crippling and incapacitating sequelae that interfere with the patient's familiar sexual behaviors. The primary illness and its sequelae may be permanent and irreversible, but the sexual problems are usually transient or subject to acceptable adaptations. Some rehabilitation specialists enlist the assistance of former patients who have solved their own sexual problems. They serve as therapeutic assistants through reassuring rap sessions, frank, open, permissive discussions, and films of their own paraplegic sexual behaviors. Most paraplegic and quadraplegic patients are sexually adapted to an able-bodied partner.

Progressive crippling results in painful or awkward sexual behavior problems. Body-image changes can make the patient ashamed of being touched or seen. Therapy is directed at rehabilitation from the primary incapacitating illness, permission to experiment sexually, and education about the adaptive solutions used by other patients with comparable problems.

Fear

Fear that any sexual behavior may cause, precipitate, or aggravate a new or existing physical illness is common in patients recovering from life-threatening illnesses. The fear may last long after recovery and convalescence from the primary illness. Complaints may be expressed first by the patient's partner, rather than by the patient. The sexual partner may believe that requesting or demanding sex is likely to lead to homicide, and the patient may silently fear that allowing himself to become sexually aroused is risking suicide. One or both of the partners may become tense, guilty, and irritable and may seek permanent separation. The able-bodied spouse may seek extramarital sexual gratification. Whether this gratification is sought secretly or openly, guilt, resentment, hostility, and self-esteem problems complicate the sexual performance problems. Conscientious but extremely conservative medical management unwittingly aggravates the fear. At a very early stage of convalescence, the physician

managing the medical illness is obligated to explore what help the patient and the partner need in re-establishing the premorbid patterns of sexual behavior. When the problem becomes chronic, more specific psychiatric or sex therapy is likely to be needed.

When the medical problem has been abortion or a venereal disease, the punishment-guilt-abstention feelings frequently rob the patient of sexual gratification, precipitate performance difficulties, or bring about total cessation of all sexual behavior. Preventive reassurance and education can influence the long-term outcome.

Excuse

Human beings with problems about expressing sexual behaviors and feelings may welcome their physical illnesses as acceptable shields and justifications against having to perform sexually. However, physical illnesses or their sequelae can rarely be blamed for permanent sexual abstinence. The first step is separation of the two problems.

Management

The management of the patient with a physical medical illness plus a sexual hang-up problem is always difficult. An essential first step is for the physician to recognize and state that he knows the patient hurts and would like to be helped. He must be willing to protect the patient from the immediate demands of the sexual partner when the patient separates the medical illness and the sexual behavior problems. If the physician's competence is limited to the management of the medical illness, he must refer the patient for treatment of the sexual problem and maintain a cooperative liaison with the sex therapist. He must also be prepared for remissions of both the medical illness and the sexual behavior problems and remissions in the patient's recognition that medical illness is not causing the sexual incapacity.

REFERENCES

Belt, B. G. Some organic causes of impotence. Med. Asp. Hum. Sex., 7: 152, 1973.
Bennett, R. G. Gonorrheal proctitis. Med. Asp. Hum. Sex., 7: 188, 1973.
Birnbaum, M. D., and Eskin, B. A. Psychosexual aspects of endocrine disorders. Med. Asp. Hum. Sex., 7: 143, 1973.
Comarr, A. E. Sex among patients with spinal cord and/or cauda equina injuries. Med. Asp. Hum. Sex., 7: 222, 1973.
Dwyer, J. T. Psychosexual aspects of weight control and dieting behaviors in adolescents. Med. Asp. Hum. Sex., 7: 82, 1973.

Hastings, D. W. *Impotence and Frigidity*. Little, Brown, Boston, 1963.

Kolodny, R. Sexual dysfunction in diabetic females. Diabetes, *20:* 557, 1971.

Marbach, A. H. Sexual problems and gynecologic illness. Med. Asp. Hum. Sex., *4:* 48, 1970.

Parades, A. Marital sexual factors in alcoholism. Med. Asp. Hum. Sex. *7:* 98, 1973.

Rubin, D. Sex in patients with neck, back, and radicular pain syndromes. Med. Asp. Hum. Sex., *6:* 14, 1972.

Wershub, L. *Sexual Impotence in the Male*. Charles C Thomas, Springfield, Ill., 1959.

23.8d.   DRUGS AND SEXUAL BEHAVIOR

Introduction

Drug responses may be largely the result of the situation in which the drug is used. Some people find their sexual drive and activity increased by such depressant drugs as barbiturates. Others are completely inhibited by barbiturates. Lysergic acid diethylamide (LSD) impairs the sexual performance of some people; others have found it to be the wonder drug that finally brings full potency after years of humiliating failure.

Sufficient doses of heroin nearly always depress desire and ability to perform. However, with most drugs, there is no clear relation between drug ingestion and sexual behavior.

A person's current psychological status and his total personality makeup must be considered in evaluating the effects of drugs on his sexual behavior.

Sexual Effects of Drugs

Alcohol

Alcohol is an addicting and potentially dangerous drug, the most important drug of abuse in the United States today. Many persons who consider themselves social drinkers consume a quantity of alcohol sufficient to have depressive effects, particularly on sexual activity. Impotence in middle-aged men is often the result of excessive alcohol intake. In addition, one partner may be so repelled by the other's alcoholic behavior that he or she avoids sex.

Although it is well known that alcohol impairs sexual performance, it may foster the initiation of sexual activity by removing inhibitions and social restraints.

Marijuana

The sexual effects of marijuana are related to dosage and to expectations. There is no clear indication that it is an aphrodisiac; there is some evidence that it can contribute to impotence. Changes in sexual behavior are often the result of the letting go of controls and inhibitions. There is no evidence to indicate that marijuana contributes significantly to sexual promiscuity or immorality.

LSD and Related Drugs

There is no pharmacological evidence that LSD is sexually stimulating. Such drugs may increase or decrease sexual functioning, depending on individual expectations and conscious and unconscious forces.

Amphetamines

Amphetamines have inconsistent but dose-related effects. Sexual behavior may be bizarre, and violent sexual abuses have been reported. In stimulating the central nervous system, amphetamines reduce fatigue and increase alertness and mental clarity. Amphetamines such as methamphetamine produce a sense of thrill and excitement, but there is no evidence that the sexual drive or sexual performance is enhanced. High doses of some amphetamines can alter sensation.

Heroin

Confusion of sexual identity and of identity in general is one of the factors associated with the heroin addict. Heroin addicts show less interest in sex than do others their own age.

The typical addict, unable to deal with the conflicts and anxieties of normal life and of interpersonal relations, finds in heroin the ideal tranquilizer. Once addiction is well-established, heroin removes the desire and thus the anxieties associated with desire. The heroin addict wants to reduce sensory stimulation as much as possible. Sexual feelings may be absent, but sexual activity is often very much a part of an addict's daily life. Many female addicts must resort to prostitution to support their habits, and many male addicts act as pimps or homosexual prostitutes out of economic necessity.

Some observers have speculated that the addict's life-style imitates the rhythms of female sexual excitement and gratification—the procuring of the drug, the injection of it *into* the body, and the peak of excitement, followed by the postorgasmic stage of relaxation. These observers further suggest that the male addict has a confused sexual identity.

Amenorrhea, infertility, and lowered libido have been associated with heroin addiction and are believed to be a direct result of the physical action of the drug. The sexual impairment resulting from heroin use may be partly a psychological disturbance associated with the sedative and euphoric effects of the drug itself.

Cyclazocine

A sufficient amount of cyclazocine blocks the action of opiates, and an opiate addict, if given the antagonist, has withdrawal symptoms. Male addicts receiving cyclazocine during the initial phase, while the drug level is being built up, report markedly increased sexual interest and drive, more frequent erections, and the first wet dreams in years. The effect may be due to a release phenomenon. Opiate addicts have reduced sex drives. The cyclazocine may neutralize these effects and thus free the sex drive.

Methaqualone

Methaqualone may reduce inhibitions and thus facilitate the initiation of sexual activity. However, with larger doses and continued use, anaphrodisiac effects are reported. Difficulty in obtaining an erection and maintaining it and inhibition of ejaculation are described by men on significant doses of methaqualone. Women describe various depressions of sexual drive and difficulties in achieving orgasm.

Psychotropic Drugs

Antipsychotic Drugs. Phenothiazines, such as chlorpromazine and trifluperazine, may produce impotence as a result of their atropinelike effects. Thioridazine causes dry ejaculation.

Butyrophenones, such as haloperidol, act similarly to the phenothiazines in producing occasional episodes of impotence. In addition, libido may be decreased. Catalepsy, in which loss of muscle tone occurs with strong emotional states, may affect coitus adversely.

Antianxiety Agents. No specific side effects relate to the genitalia with these classes of drugs. Sexual functioning may improve as the anxiety, which may inhibit sexual expression, is reduced.

Antidepressants. The two major groups of antidepressants, tricyclics and monoamine oxidase inhibitors, have atropinelike side effects and may produce potency problems. But sexual performance improves as the depression lifts.

Miscellaneous Substances

In small doses, cocaine produces an intense euphoria that may enhance libido and increase erection time. With chronic use, restlessness, tremors, and a toxic psychosis occur. Tolerance, habituation, and a continued need for the drug eventually produce a complete loss of sexual interest.

Derived from the Spanish fly (*Cantharis vesicatoria*), cantharides have an intensely irritant action on mucous membranes. Large amounts of the drug are poisonous and cause vomiting, abdominal pain, renal damage, shock, and death.

Because of yohimbine's parasympathetic effect of increased vasodilation, it was believed to help induce erection. No evidence of effectiveness has been demonstrated.

Amyl nitrate, a strong peripheral vasodilator used in the treatment of angina pectoris, causes massive peripheral vasodilation and, when inhaled or popped at the moment of orgasm, is reported to enhance orgastic pleasure. This effect may be related to an altered state of consciousness.

Camphor is a mild respiratory and circulatory stimulant. Attempts have been made, without success, to find aphrodisiac effects.

Levodopa is an agent used for the relief of Parkinson's disease. In rare instances, increased libido has been observed in persons receiving the drug. The mechanism of action may be the result of the enhanced sense of well-being as the patient's tremor, dysphagia, and depression abate.

Pheromones are chemical substances produced by a member of a species that stimulates a response, usually sexual, in another of the same species. These chemicals may play a role in human sexuality, but human pheromones have yet to be demonstrated.

REFERENCES

Cushman, P. Sexual behavior in heroin addiction and methadone maintenance. N.Y. State J. Med., *27:* 1961, 1972.
Freedman, A. M. Drug addiction: An eclectic view. J. A. M. A., *197:* 878, 1966.
Halikas, J. A., Goodwin, P. H., and Guze, S. B. Marijuana

effects: A survey of regular users. J. A. M. A., *217:* 692, 1971.

Inaba, D. S., Gay, G. R., Newmeyer, S. A., and Whitehead, C. Methaqualone abuse. J. A. M. A., *224:* 1505, 1973.

Mathis, J. L. Sexual aspects of heroin addiction. Med. Asp. Hum. Sex., *4:* 98, 1970.

National Commission on Marijuana and Drug Abuse. *Drug Use in America: Problem in Perspective.* United States Government Printing Office. Washington, 1973.

Uhlenbuth, E. H., Rickels, K., and Fisher, S. Doctor's verbal attitude and clinical setting in the symptomatic response to pharmacotherapy. Psychopharmacologia, *9:* 392, 1966.

Ungerleider, J. T., and Fisher, D. D. LSD: Research and joy ride. Nation, May 16, 1966

23.8e.   PSYCHOLOGICAL ASPECTS OF CONTRACEPTION

Contraceptive Methods

Temporary or intermittent celibacy in the form of timed abstinence (the rhythm method) is used by a huge number of couples. Since normally only one egg is released a month and this egg has a life-span of only 12 to 24 hours, avoidance of intravaginal ejaculation during that time theorectically prevents conception. But difficulties in predicting the time of ovulation, uncertainties in ascertaining the duration of survival of previously introduced spermatozoa, and inconsistencies in the resolve to abstain render the method notoriously unreliable. (See Table I.)

The prevention of intravaginal insemination by withdrawal of the penis from the vagina before ejaculation is another contraceptive method that is theoretically efficient. But an uncommon alertness and a constancy of motivation are essential. In addition, the degree of emotional and physical control required of both partners by this method is not a universal attribute. Nor is the willingness to accept full sexual gratification by this coital technique universally acceptable.

The chemical methods of contraception include various spermicidal and sperm-immobilizing materials. These are constituted in the form of jellies, creams, foams, and suppositories and are inserted into the vagina precoitally or before ejaculation. For some people they increase the degree of coital lubrication to an objectionable level. Theoretically, their uncertain dispersal about and out of the vagina with coition renders them less than absolutely efficient. They do have a respectable order of effectiveness, but they must be used correctly and with consistency. The foams are the most efficient and are seemingly the least objectionable from the point of view of excess lubrication.

Obstructions to the flow of semen into the woman and to the upward motility of spermatozoa within the woman are also used to prevent the meeting of sperm and egg. The condom or penis-covering sheath (see Figure 1) effectively prevents the intravaginal deposition of semen. For some, its use is erotic. For others, it is disruptive and interferes with pleasure. As with all other coitally connected methods, it must be used for every intravaginal ejaculation.

The intravaginal diaphragm (see Figure 2) is the method most commonly used by women to prevent the upward progress of spermatozoa after the intravaginal deposition of semen. It is quite effective, especially when used with a spermicidal jelly or cream. However, its use requires a degree of intellect, an initial and possibly an intermittent fitting for appropriate size, and steadfast diligence in insertion for every ejaculatory encounter.

The method requiring the least diligence is the intrauterine device (IUD). Once it is correctly inserted by a physician or other skilled person, it may remain in place indefinitely, maintaining its effectiveness. The devices are manufactured in numerous forms and are most commonly composed of highly flexible, preformed plastic (see Figure 3). They have considerable efficiency and probably prevent pregnancy by interfering with zygote implantation. Each type of intrauterine device has its own rate of spontaneous expulsion, pregnancy failure, pelvic infection, uterine perforation, and requested removal because of excessive or abnormal uterine bleeding.

The dual oral contraceptive pill has absolute contraceptive efficiency. The combination and dosage of estrogen plus progestin present in dual oral contraceptive tablets consistently prevents ovulation when the tablets are taken daily for 3 of every 4 weeks. Neither 21 days of progestin alone (the minipill) nor 16 days of estrogen followed by 5 days of estrogen plus progestin (sequential oral contraceptives) have the absolute reliability of the dual contraceptive pill. The oral contraceptives available in the United States and their hormonal contents are listed in Table II. Many side effects have been ascribed to the use of these medications; all these side effects

Table I

Current Methods of Contraception

Type	Method of Action	Effectiveness*	Advantages	Disadvantages	Potential Complications
ˌythm	Timed abstinence	Low	No cost Always available No professional help required	Imposed coital timing (lack of spontaneity)	Essentially none
ˌthdrawal	Prevention of insemination	Low (but theoretically high)	No cost Always available No professional help required	Regular coital use required Requires considerable attention and control	Essentially none
ˌravaginal foams, creams, ˌellies, and suppositories	Spermicidal	Low	Inexpensive Generally available No professional help required	Regular coital use required Possible messiness Possible interference with enjoyment	Essentially none
ˌndom	Sperm barrier	Medium	Inexpensive Generally available No professional help required Decreased acquisition of coitally transmitted diseases	Regular coital use required Possible interference with enjoyment	Essentially none
ˌaphragm	Sperm barrier (plus spermicidal with jelly)	Medium	Inexpensive	Regular coital use required Possible interference with enjoyment Requires professional fitting Not anatomically adaptable to everyone	Essentially none
ˌrauterine device (IUD)	Unknown (possibly prevents zygote implantation)	Medium	Inexpensive Only single decision required Not coitally connected	Possible increase in bleeding and cramping Requires professional insertion	Uterine perforation, pelvic infection, spontaneous expulsion
ˌal (hormonal)	Prevention of ovulation (possible interference with sperm mobility)	High	Inexpensive Potential absolute efficiency Not coitally connected	Possible side effects Daily ingestion Requires professional prescription	Thromboembolism, neuro-ocular disturbances, hypertension

* Effectiveness is rated roughly as follows: low, more than 20 pregnancies per 100 woman-years of use; medium, 1 to 20 ˌegnancies per 100 woman-years of use; high, less than 1 pregnancy per 100 woman-years of use.

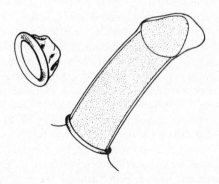

Figure 1. The condom, before and after being unrolled onto the erect penis.

are essentially minor, with the exception of thromboembolism, neuro-ocular disturbances, and protracted anovulation. Although the causative role of oral contraceptives has not been firmly established in these circumstances, the Food and Drug Administration has recommended that the pill not be given to women who have a history of thrombophlebitis or embolic phenomena, impaired liver function, breast cancer, estrogen-dependent tumors, or undiagnosed genital bleeding. The Food and Drug Administration has also recommended discontinuation of oral contraceptives in the event of migraine headaches, hypertension, modification of vision, or development of ocular abnormalities. The incidence of severe complications or death

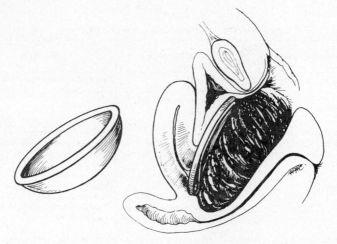

FIGURE 2. The intravaginal diaphragm and its position during coition.

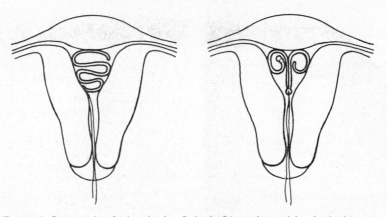

FIGURE 3. Intrauterine devices *in situ*. *Left*, the Lippes loop; *right*, the double coil.

associated with oral contraceptive ingestion is about one fifth to one tenth that associated with pregnancy.

With the exception of the intrauterine device, each of the methods requires sustained motivation. Error and inconsistency in use are far more commonly the cause of contraceptive failure than is failure of the method itself.

Contraceptive Use

Many religious groups have opposed pregnancy prevention. Varying degrees of guilt, emanate from conflict between deeprooted, childhood-imbued religious restrictions against contraception and the user's own modern, intellectualized belief in the inappropriateness of those restrictions. This guilt is magnified when both partners are subject to such conflicts but to different degrees.

The user of the rhythm method is characterized as somewhat rigid regarding her religious and social attitudes. Sexual drive is low, and body image is negative.

The user of the withdrawal method is characterized as having an excessive faith in luck, a denying attitude regarding fertility, and feelings of guilt if she is contraceptively prepared for coitus. Withdrawal deprives each partner of pleasure, but, inasmuch as pleasure and orgasm are not her goals, the method is punitively directed. Furthermore, if withdrawal fails and she becomes pregnant, it is obviously his fault, and her feelings about men are verified.

Women who enforce use of the condom are described as angry at men and distrustful. They figuratively reject men through the use of a barrier to exclude their dirty semen and to exclude any direct contact with the repugnant penis.

TABLE II

Oral Contraceptive Agents Currently Available in the United States

Trade Name (Pharmaceutical Company)	Estrogen	Progestin
Dual or Combined Oral Contraceptives		
Norinyl 1 + 50 (Syntex)	Mestranol 0.05 mg.	Norethindrone 1.0 mg.
Norinyl 1 + 80 (Syntex)	Mestranol 0.08 mg.	Norethindrone 1.0 mg.
Norinyl-2 (Syntex)	Mestranol 0.1 mg.	Norethindrone 2.0 mg.
Ortho-Novum 1/50 (Ortho)	Mestranol 0.05 mg.	Norethindrone 1.0 mg.
Ortho-Novum 1/80 (Ortho)	Mestranol 0.08 mg.	Norethindrone 1.0 mg.
Ortho-Novum-2 (Ortho)	Mestranol 0.1 mg.	Norethindrone 2.0 mg.
Ortho-Novum-10 (Ortho)	Mestranol 0.06 mg.	Norethindrone 10.0 mg.
Enovid-E (Searle)	Mestranol 0.1 mg.	Norethynodrel 2.5 mg.
Enovid-5 (Searle)	Mestranol 0.075 mg.	Norethynodrel 5.0 mg.
Ovulen (Searle)	Mestranol 0.1 mg.	Ethynodiol diacetate 1.0 mg.
Demulen (Searle)	Ethinyl estradiol 0.05 mg.	Ethynodiol diacetate 1.0 mg.
Ovral (Wyeth)	Ethinyl estradiol 0.05 mg.	Norgestrel 0.5 mg.
Norlestrin-1 mg. (Parke-Davis)	Ethinyl estradiol 0.05 mg.	Norethindrone acetate 1.0 mg.
Norlestrin-2.5 mg. (Parke-Davis)	Ethinyl estradiol 0.05 mg.	Norethindrone acetate 2.5 mg.
Loestrin 1/20 (Parke-Davis)	Ethinyl estradiol 0.02 mg.	Norethindrone acetate 1.0 mg.
Sequential Oral Contraceptives		
Norquen (Syntex)	Mestranol 0.08 mg.	Norethindrone 2.0 mg.
Ortho-Novum SQ (Ortho)	Mestranol 0.08 mg.	Norethindrone 2.0 mg.
Oracon (Mead Johnson)	Ethinyl estradiol 0.1 mg.	Dimethisterone 25 mg.
Minipill (Pure Progestin) Oral Contraceptives		
Nor-Q-D (Syntex)		Norethindrone 0.35 mg.
Micronor (Ortho)		Norethindrone 0.35 mg.
Ovrette (Wyeth)		Norethindrone 0.35 mg.

Women employing intravaginal foams and jellies are described as passive, motherhood-family directed, and highly satisfied with their femininity. Such women are joyfully dependent on men and see them as strong, supportive, protective and responsible. Highly effective contraceptive methods, especially if they exclude the mutual sharing of love and semen, conflict with her needs for passivity, for giving, and for motherhood.

The diaphragm user is considered independent, self-reliant, logical, career-oriented, and competitive with men. She likes to be in control of herself and her sexuality and of the men in the world about her.

The user of the intrauterine device is believed to be comfortable with her body, loving, masturbatory, and highly orgasmic. She is not anxious in passivity and does not feel threatened by events and situations beyond her control.

The woman who chooses oral contraceptives is described as modern, active, opportunistic, ambitious, accepting of the new role of women, acquisitive, and desirous of freedom. Passivity is threatening; although marriage may not be seen in that light, pregnancy and childbirth are. Personal control of a totally efficient contraceptive method relieves concerns of potential personal imprisonment in a sterotyped woman's role.

As superficially reasonable as these personality vignettes may seem, they are generalities. Even so, no contraceptive is ideal for all, and impressing one's own concepts of contraceptive use on another is inconsiderate and defeating.

Contraceptive Nonuse

Contraceptive nonusers may be characterized as immature, dependent, insecure, impulsive, and indecisive. They often have low self-esteem and little desire to control their lives or the world about them. They have a limited capacity to assume responsibility, to complete self-assumed tasks, to tolerate frustration, and to appreciate long-range goals.

This generality contains certain aspects of truth but describes only the most blatant and flagrant of contraceptive nonusers. Far more subtle personality characteristics and psychological factors control contraceptive disuse, misuse, or rejection in most people.

Denial

An unwillingness to acknowledge reality is one of the most common bases for contraceptive nonuse. It is especially operative during the early coital trials and experiences of high school and college students. It may simply be a denial that coitus will occur. It may be a denial that impregnation is possible, an assumption of invulnerability. Or the person may deny that contraception really works. Denial of personal responsibility for contraceptive use may also be present.

Opportunism (Desperation)

An exceptionally prevalent basis for contraceptive nonuse is simple opportunism, the availability of a coital opportunity and the unwillingness for whatever reason to put it off until a contraceptive can be obtained. The opportunity may be to initiate, cement, or protract a relationship, to gain status, to obtain infrequently available affection, to relieve peer group pressure or to be accepted.

In some circumstances, the opportunity and reward may merely be to please a partner. In most cases, however, the opportunity is that of obtaining immediate personal sensual pleasure. The psychological setting in nearly all such circumstances contains an aspect of desperation.

Sexual Identity Conflicts

Self-worth and self-esteem are frequently judged on the basis of virility, as demonstrated by impregnation, and femininity, as demonstrated by fecundity. If ego rewards in life are minimal and self-esteem can neither be built nor sustained through other efforts, the creative, productive accomplishment of pregnancy and reproduction may be compensatory and may be used as repetitively as required.

Contraceptive nonuse may also be seen in the insecure man who uses sexual activity to reinforce a marginal self-esteem. He may fear that the use of a contraceptive will diminish his partner's desire and responsiveness and thus reduce the availability of his sexual outlet. Conversely, he may anticipate that contraception will eliminate her fear of pregnancy and accentuate her lustful demands beyond his ability to fulfill.

Being rejected by a mate or partner may reinforce feelings of insecurity, low self-worth, and sexual inadequacy. Restitution may require proof of one's sexual ability or desirability through sexual activity. In some instances this may require that contraceptives not be used and that pregnancy be achieved as demonstrative proof of worth.

Certain childless women who sense their aging with despair, develop an engulfing, irresistable urge to demonstrate their feminity with motherhood.

Love

Risk-taking and self-sacrifice are readily accepted as demonstrations of one's love for another. This risk-taking extends to the willful risking of pregnancy. Occasionally, the rejection of contraception may arise from naive and idealistic adoration and an ethereal concept of the requirements of romantic devotion. In some minds a positive declaration for contraception destroys the illusion that coitus is a spontaneous, uncontrollable, and overwhelming consequence of love.

Guilt

To be sexually accessible at all times because of the use of noncoitally connected contraception can be distressing to some women. Accessibility is tantamount to prostitution and promiscuity, an open invitation to be used (or raped), rather than to be romantically seduced and loved. Additionally, many people have been raised to believe that sex was designed by God for making babies. Sex with contraception must be accepted as sex for lustful and sensual pleasure.

Shame (Embarrassment)

The presence or potentiality of feelings of shame or embarrassment is also counterproductive to the acquisition or use of a contraceptive. Embarrassment sufficient to preclude contraceptive use may arise from a necessity to admit ignorance to a partner, to a peer group, or to a physician. Embarrassment may also arise from the potentiality of discovery by parents, children, relatives, friends, or others that a contraceptive has been sought or is being used. This feeling is particularly prevalent among adolescents and those acting counter to their social or religious teachings.

Hostility

Resentment and hostility are frequently seen as motivating forces for contraceptive rejection. A hostile woman, by rejecting contraception, can also reject her partner, using the fear of potential pregnancy as her weapon. For the man, the hostile act may be to provoke fear, or it may be a revengeful enforcing of impregnation. For others, it may be a deliberate seeking of pregnancy to injure a parent, to rebel against a social group, to escape an undesirable environment, to punish a straying mate with guilt and additional responsibility, to retaliate against rejection.

In many instances, the rejection of contraception may be used as a statement to the partner that discontent exists and that noncontraceptive sequelae, celibacy or pregnancy, will result if the current resentment is not tended and 'resolved. Or it may possibly result from resentment against a shift in contraceptive responsibility.

Coital Gamesmanship

The male-female power struggle taken to bed may arise from a bilateral desire to control or manipulate or from a reactive expression of self-defense against a partner who would otherwise dominate to the point of obtaining total submissiveness and subservience. In this sense it is a struggle to maintain a desired degree of independence and self-identity.

The question may relate to who is going to control the frequency of coitus. Or the question may relate to who is going to be forced to accept the demeaning role of contraceptor and who is going to be forced to accept being the recipient of accusations of responsibility in the event of pregnancy.

Masochism

Hostility may be inwardly directed by persons having feeling of worthlessness and may manifest itself in self-deprecating and self-punishing behavior, such as, life-threatening self-abortion, necessitated or generated by deliberate contraceptive nonuse. Far milder forces may only require oneself to be used sexually. Or

pregnancy may be directly sought as a demeaning, degrading, socially reprehensible, imprisoning, figure-destroying subjugation.

Eroticism

A different approach to contraceptive nonuse is seen in persons who have a desire for self-indulgence, who have a rather insistent urge constantly to supersede previous pleasures. The erotic sensualization may be obtained by taking the risk of pregnancy through contraceptive nonuse. To risk is anxiety provoking, but to win is thrilling and ego satisfying in any endeavor, and the thrill is usually directly proportional to the degree of initial anxiety.

Entrapment

Pregnancy may be used to trap a partner into marriage or into a closer commitment to self or family. It may be used to prevent separation or divorce or to force a partner into providing previously limited emotional or financial support. It may even be undertaken to force the partner to confess socially that coitus has been occurring.

Nihilism

Feelings of apathy, hopelessness, and insurmountable poverty are not conducive to effortful and planned activity, including activity aimed at pregnancy prevention. Sufficiently grave emotional and intellectual nihilism may result in cessation of sexual activity, but this is uncommon except in the most severely depressed states. Sexual activity persists, and, although pregnancy itself is rarely sought, the dispatch of effort to prevent it is inconsistent with the nihilistic outlook over-all.

Affectional Poverty

Chronic or acute deprivation of love, companionship, and the feeling of being needed is frequently accompanied by conflicts regarding sexual identity. An unmet need to be needed and loved is commonly seen and socially anticipated in the unmarried. Indulgence in requested coitus after an ego-gratifying pursuit is a common method for temporary fulfillment of this need. A more emphatic and persistent need may be met by forgoing contraception, achieving pregnancy, and acquiring fulfillment through the acquisition of a needful and loving infant.

This, of course, may also occur within marriage whenever emotional and affectional gratification becomes unavailable for whatever reason.

The recent loss of a friend, parent, relative, partner, or even a deeply loved pet is a common finding in studies of women seeking abortion. For many, the loss of emotional support, love, or companionship may be temporarily mollified through coitus. And in these therapeutic encounters, contraception is often ignored or rejected.

Fear and Anxiety

Physically and emotionally directed fears of anxieties may cause certain persons to eschew specific types of contraception or contraception in general. There may be fears of manipulating, altering, or harming the body or of infection, cancer, uterine perforation, blood clots, or unknown diseases. The woman may fear a loss of personal control and the initiation of irrepressible sexual aggression or promiscuity if the threat of pregnancy is lifted. Or, conversely, there may be a fear of frigidity or loss of libido as a contraceptive side effect. The fear may relate to the potential of interference with future fertility. Or it may relate to the awesome responsibility one then has to control and to decide on one's reproductive fate.

Abortion Availability

Abortion availability becomes a rationally acceptable basis for using a less efficient but more acceptable means of contraception or for regular or occasional rejection of contraception. This is especially true for persons who have infrequent coitus, couples with apparent low fertility, or others in whom the potentiality for impregnation appears to be slight.

Becoming pregnant and having a child are often totally separate thoughts. Abortion can be salvaging and useful for the person who needs to demonstrate fecundity but for whom an infant would be anathema. Abortion offers the best of two worlds, satisfaction through achievement of pregnancy without a demanding requisite for protracted responsibility.

Iatrogenesis

Too frequently, the physician's attitude toward contraceptive use by others is colored by his own moral, religious, and social philosophy. The demeaning, opinionated, intimidating, and pronatalist attitude of some physicians; the ignorance, apathy, or inconsiderate unconcern of others; and the embarrassment, ambivalence, or punitiveness of still others are destructive of contraceptive enthusiasm and are substantial factors in patient's misuse or nonuse of contraception. Equally reprehensible is the much more common aspect of oversight.

REFERENCES

Calderone, M., editor. *Manual of Family Planning and Contraceptive Practice.* Williams & Wilkins, Baltimore, 1970.

23.8f.   ABORTION

Definition

Abortion is the expulsion of a previable fetus from the uterus before gestation is complete. The abortion may be spontaneous or artificially induced.

Spontaneous and Habitual Abortion

Spontaneous abortion may be defined as the expulsion of a previable fetus in the absence of external manipulation. Habitual abortion is characterized by three or more consecutive spontaneous abortions (see Table I).

The cause of spontaneous abortion is as yet unknown. Only a small percentage of fetuses from spontaneous abortions show fetal abnormalities. Factors known to affect spontaneous abortion have been summarized as follows: (1) Low hormone levels that seem to fluctuate with emotional stress. (2) The presence of microscopic degenerative changes in the chorionic villi of the majority of the abortions. (3) An incompetent cervix, which accounts for about 13 per cent of all spontaneous abortions. (4) Psychological factors.

There are a number of consistent findings in women suffering from habitual abortion. The mothers of these patients are often dominant, overpowering women who have difficulty in separating themselves from their children. The patients remain tied to their mothers from early infancy, never actually maturing as persons. The father of the patient may be absent,

TABLE I

Types of Abortion

Spontaneous abortion—the spontaneous expulsion of a previable fetus.

Habitual abortion—three or more consecutive spontaneous abortions.

Missed abortion—a state wherein a dead fetus is not expelled within 2 months.

Threatened abortion—more than one missed period with bleeding and cramps.

Incomplete abortion—continuous bleeding with the expulsion of chorionic tissue.

Therapeutic abortion—an induced abortion for medical indications. With the increasing sophistication of medical techniques, these indications have diminished markedly. Currently, the two main indications are psychiatric and the potential abnormality of the fetus.

Induced abortion—an abortion purposefully brought on by outside forces. The abortion may be criminal or medical. The technique used depends on the duration of the pregnancy; the principal techniques are dilation and curettage, suction curettage, saline injection into the amniotic sac at about the eighteenth week of gestation, and hysterotomy.

---

emotionally distant, or too involved and concerned with his daughter. As children, these patients are described as nice, quiet, and obedient. They are careful and constantly concerned about their physical health and well-being and often somatize their emotional problems. In adolescence, they never show much curiosity or even interest in the changes taking place within their own bodies.

The clinical picture of a woman having habitual abortions is usually presented in one of three ways. First, she is seen as a dependent, immature person who has terrible fears of her own growth and acceptance of herself as a woman. She usually marries a man who is protective. Childish and immature, she remains deeply attached to her mother. The second type of woman usually seems independent. She is career-oriented, and it is hard for her to accept womanhood, which she equates with dependence, weakness, and submission. The third type of woman is a rather hysterical and somewhat narcissistic person. Pregnancy represents an intolerable threat to her body image.

Induced Abortion

The most heated arguments concerning induced abortion cluster around three main issues. First, at what point does life begin? Second, has the individual woman the right to control her own body? Third, what are the psychological consequences?

The laws of Western civilization have been ambivalent concerning the issue of life and abortion.

In January 1973, in a decision concerning abortions, the U. S. Supreme Court rejected the idea that the fetus becomes a person on conception and is thus entitled to the due process and equal protection guaranteed by the Constitution.

Most women experience life with the onset of quickening.

Emotional Factors in Pregnancy

The first trimester is characterized by ambivalence, no matter how planned and desired the conception was. Dormant unconscious fears are reactivated; when reinforced by physiological processes, these fears give rise to symptoms. The patient also experiences new feelings, such as the need to mother and the wish to be mothered, to be taken care of. The outcome of this conflict is determined by the mental and emotional health of the woman and by her environmental support or its lack.

With the onset of quickening, in the twelfth to fourteenth week of gestation, the fetus becomes a reality. With the acceptance of this fact, the balance usually shifts to gratification of the need to mother. Refusal to accept the fetus as a psychological reality results in prolongation of the conflict, resulting in denial of pregnancy, psychosomatic ailments, or efforts at aborting the fetus.

In the second and third trimesters the fetus becomes a baby, an accepted reality, assuming a definite place in the psychic life of the woman. The subsequent development of feelings aroused by pregnancy has a maturing effect on the woman.

Motivations for Abortion

Initially, there may be an impulse to remove the disrupting factor and regain homeostasis. Social and moral considerations may contribute to feelings of shame and disgrace and concern over responsibility and the burden of financial support. Induced abortions are frequently sought to terminate pregnancy after rape, incest, sexual acting out, and "accidents." Married women who seek abortion because of too many children or for economic reasons seem to respond better than single women.

Psychiatric Considerations

Psychotic women are no better or worse after abortion. It is not possible to evaluate the problem of abortion-related suicide. Suicide in pregnant women is extremely rare. However, a pregnant woman who wanted an abortion desperately could get a criminal abortion or attempt to abort herself. Suicide statistics could change dramatically if these two avenues were totally cut off from her.

A pregnant patient who feels coerced by familial or social forces needs help to sort out her feelings and to cope more effectively with the problem. The patient has to cope with her personal feelings of guilt and deal with overt and covert attitudes of the personnel directly administering to her.

Psychiatric Sequelae

In evaluating the consequences of induced abortion, one must consider three aspects: (1) Immediate psychological effects of induced abortion. (2) Long-term psychological consequences of induced abortion. (3) Long-term psychological effects on unwanted children born to women denied induced abortion.

The immediate reaction to abortion is relief. The patient who has developed the least attachment to the fetus—that is, the woman who refers to the pregnancy as a "blood clot" or "tissue"—usually does best clinically. Pregnancy is experienced as a disrupting factor; its removal restores her to her previous homeostasis. The best time for termination of pregnancy is up to the fourteenth week of gestation. An exception is the medically sick woman who has to have a therapeutic abortion and experiences the loss of the fetus with reactive depression. Grief, mourning, and varying degrees of depression are necessary steps in the resolution of such a loss.

The most consistent postabortion psychiatric finding is guilt. The healthier patients are the least disturbed; they are better able to cope with guilt feelings.

What are the long-term effects of an abortion in shaping and changing the life pattern of the woman concerned? Psychoanalytic studies tes-

tify to the difficulty in assimilating the abortion experience. The psychiatrist should look beyond the immediate symptoms and acute decompensation.

And what of the unwanted child born after an abortion has been refused? If one has to single out one factor as most responsible for psychopathology, one can safely point to rejection. The effects of rejection, albeit before birth, can be crippling.

REFERENCES

Callahan, D. *Abortion: Law, Choice, and Morality*. Collier Books, London, 1970.
Ekblad, M. Induced abortion on psychiatric grounds: A follow-up study of 479 women. Acta Psychiatr. Neurol. Scand., *99:* 3, 1955.
Ewing, J. A., and Rouse, B. E. Therapeutic abortion and a prior psychiatric history. Am. J. Psychiatry, *130:* 1, 1973.
Floyd, M. K. *Abortion Bibliography for 1971*. Whitson, Troy, N.Y., 1973.
Group for the Advancement of Psychiatry. *The Right to Abortion: A Psychiatric View*. Charles Scribner's Sons, New York, 1970.
Mann, E. C. Habitual abortion. Am. J. Obstet. Gynecol., *77:* 706, 1959.
Minoro, M., editor. *Japan's Experience in Family Planning—Past and Present*. Family Planning Federation of Japan, Tokyo, 1967.
Rosen, H. *Abortion in America*. Beacon Press, Boston, 1954.

23.9.   SEXUAL BEHAVIOR AND MENTAL ILLNESS

Introduction

Until the last few years, the role of sexuality was considered to be of central importance in normal and abnormal personality development. Many psychiatrists still hold such views and believe that sexual functions are likely to be disturbed in mental disorders and that recovery from such illnesses may be retarded or endangered by patients' sexual activities. Others theorize that the struggle for mastery of the sex drive in adolescence must be won, or psychosis will result. Avoidance or postponement of the struggle may lead to characterological deficiencies, whereas neuroses may be derived from unresolved psychosexual conflicts.

However, many of these contentions must now be viewed in the light of evidence from recent human and animal research. Masserman has adopted the viewpoint that sexual dysfunctions are usually secondary considerations in human maladjustment, an opinion based on work with experimental neuroses in animals and on his own clinical experience. He concedes that behavior is mostly motivated by physiological needs but regards sexual desires as relatively unimportant because they are episodic, transient, and, viewed dispassionately, dispensable. In his framework, more important issues in the understanding of mental disturbances include the unique capacities and maturity of the patient, individual experience, and the range of adaptive behaviors. Patients with various kinds of mental illnesses have shown little or no evidence of sexual maladjustment. On the other hand, there is at least one clinical entity, hysteria, in which there are definite sexual components. Moreover, studies of patients with particular kinds of deviant sexual behavior often show an increased incidence of mental and emotional difficulties.

It is perhaps best at the present time to take the position that sexual function and dysfunction should be viewed as one facet of behavior that may or may not be affected by mental or physical disease.

Mental Retardation

The sexual development and physical growth of the mentally retarded person is often inversely proportional to the degree of mental subnormality. It is unusual for profoundly or severely retarded persons to engage in heterosexual relationships. Generally, they exhibit primitive sexual behaviors, such as individual or mutual masturbation. On the other hand, less retarded persons are capable of mature heterosexual relationships, including marriage.

Some of the sexual problems that have been reported in association with mental deficiency include sexual behavior that is appropriate for persons of younger chronological age, thus creating adjustment problems when the mentally deficient child attempts to function within normal groups. Other difficulties have to do with homosexual or heterosexual exploitation of dull or gullible persons. There are also parental conflicts about accepting the sexuality of their mentally retarded children.

Organic Brain Syndromes

Organic lesions of the brain may produce various kinds of sexual aberrations, depending on the extent and the area of the brain involved.

Characteristic of the Kluver-Bucy syndrome associated with bilateral lesions of the temporal lobes in both animals and humans is bizarre hypersexuality, which can probably be interpreted as release phenomena in the Jacksonian sense. More commonly, structural pathology of the central nervous system is associated with nonspecific changes in sexual behavior that may be understood in terms of dissolution, with a retreat toward lower or more primitive levels of behavioral organization. Commonly, such pathology is associated with a loss of social controls, with sexual behavior occurring at inappropriate times or circumstances, rather than hypersexuality or particular kinds of sexual deviations. Other considerations have to do with pre-existing personality characteristics. Further, the extent of intellectual and social deterioration in senile brain disease is directly proportional to the amount of neuropathological degeneration as measured by neurofibrillary tangles, ventricular size, senile plaques, and brain weight.

In other instances, patients with early organic disorders of the brain may present in depressed states, as in presenile dementia and in neurosyphilis. It may reasonably be assumed that sexual activity and interests are reduced in the presence of clinical depression.

Major Affective Disorders

Libido and potency may be reduced or abolished in endogenous depression, but sexual interests and desires are likely affected as a general consequence of the depressed state, rather than because of any specific physiological mechanism. Decreases in libido and impotence have been described in manic-depressive patients, but increased interest in sex is commonly associated with hypomanic episodes, with an increased incidence of promiscuity and illegitimate pregnancies. Sexual preoccupations and delusions are often found in patients during hypomanic and manic episodes. These delusions sometimes take the form of pseudocyesis. Another sexual problem that creates difficulties in the marital adjustment of manic-depressive patients is the common wish by the hypomanic patient for another pregnancy. This wish may arise in either male or female patients. This demand, coupled with impaired social and financial judgment and other typical features of the illness, frequently precipitates separation and divorce. However, follow-up studies have shown that the long-range prognosis in manic-depressive illness is relatively favorable, with a high percentage of patients achieving a good marital and social adjustment.

The depressive and paranoid psychoses are superimposed on a premorbid personality described as rigid, overconscientious, and restricted, with lifelong repression of sexual and aggressive drives. Obsessive-compulsive defenses predominate, and the illness may be viewed as a decompensation of this defensive system. Sexual adjustment is generally described as poor.

Studies of populations presenting with various complaints about sexual functioning show a relatively low incidence of psychotic illness in general and of affective disorders in particular.

Schizophrenia

Considerable pathology in sexual development and its expression might be expected in schizophrenia, which is postulated by some to have an unresolved pregential conflict at its core. Moreover, hormonal and metabolic alterations have been demonstrated in schizophrenic patients. Deviations in sexual functioning and responsiveness in schizophrenia would also be anticipated in the light of the lower rates of marriage and fertility among such patients and their tendency to avoid close relationships. Physical sexual intimacy may be accomplished quite easily by the schizophrenic patient, but such activity is detached from the partner and remains uncommitted, with frequent sick qualities, such as sadism and other hostile or perverted characteristics.

Neuroses

Psychoanalytic theory predicts that behavioral expression of sexuality will be inhibited or deviant in illnesses thought to result from unresolved conflicts arising during psychosexual phases of development. The available evidence does not support such a position. Nevertheless, many of the clinical discriptions of anxiety neurosis and the other kinds of neurotic disorders do mention sexual maladjustments.

A variety of psychological test instruments have been applied to studies of sexual behavior and its disturbances in relation to neurotic features. The majority of the studies show more neurotic features or, more usually, factor loadings suggesting more emotional difficulties in people who have problems with sexual adjustment than in those who do not. However, the explicit diagnostic criteria for neurosis are not usually considered. In fact, many such studies have made use of nonclinical populations, with neurosis defined in terms of cutting scores on various psychological test measures and personality inventories.

Personality Disorders

Hysterical Personality

The hysterical personality or hysteria is the only psychiatric diagnostic entity for which sexual dysfunctions have been specifically demonstrated. The most common difficulty among hysterical women is sexual indifference. Hysteria is characterized by conflicts between sexual motivation and behavior.

Antisocial Personality

Delinquent and antisocial behavior in childhood is highly predictive of both adult sociopathy and hysteria. Increased sexual activity and interest in sex was more typical of the girls than of the boys who became sociopathic adults. There is a high incidence of persons with antisocial personality disorders among populations of patients who are charged with sexual offenses. Endocrine studies have shown that hormones exert effects on both sexual and aggressive behavior and may be used therapeutically to modify both.

Passive-Aggressive Personality

Very little has been written about the sexual behavior of patients with a diagnosis of passive-aggressive personality disorder. The incidences of both marriage and divorce were higher in one cohort of passive-aggressives, with at least half having been divorced or remarried during the course of a 7- to 15-year follow-up study. One third of the subjects admitted to promiscuity —that is, multiple extramarital sexual relationships with more than one partner.

Emotionally Unstable Personality

Patients with emotionally unstable character disorders, particularly women, often experience sexual problems, with frequent promiscuous behavior.

Hypersexuality

Nymphomania and satyriasis signify excessive or pathological heterosexual interests and desires for coitus in women and in men, respectively. Although there is considerable descriptive literature, there have been few scientific studies. The medical descriptions of the subject mostly state that hypersexuality is associated with a lack of sexual gratification or release of tension and is accompanied by psychological difficulties.

REFERENCES

de la Cruz, F. F., and LaVeck, G. D. *Human Sexuality and the Mentally Retarded.* Brunner/Mazel, New York, 1973.
Epstein, A. W. The relationship of altered brain states to sexual psychopathology. In *Contemporary Sexual Behavior*, J. Zubin and J. Money, editors, p. 297. Johns Hopkins University Press, Baltimore, 1973.
Flor-Henry, P. Ictal and interictal psychiatric manifestations in epilepsy: Specific or nonspecific? Epilepsia, *13:* 773, 1972.
Hooshmand, H., Escobar, M. R., and Kopf, S. W. Neurosyphilis: A study of 241 patients. J. A. M. A., *219:* 726, 1972.
Jensen, G. D. Human sexual behavior in primate perspective In *Contemporary Sexual Behavior*, J. Zubin and J. Money, editors, p. 17. Johns Hopkins University Press, Baltimore, 1973.
Klein, D. F., Honigfeld, G., and Feldman, S. Prediction of drug effect in personality disorders. J. Nerv. Ment. Dis., *156:* 183, 1973.
Laschet, U. Antiandrogen in the treatment of sex offenders: Mode of action and therapeutic outcome. In *Contemporary Sexual Behavior*, J. Zubin and J. Money, editors, p. 311. Johns Hopkins University Press, Baltimore, 1973.
Luisada, P. V., and Pittard, B. A. The hysterical personality in males. In *Scientific Proceedings in Summary Form from the 126th Annual Meeting of the American Psychiatric Assoc.*, p. 313. American Psychiatric Association, Washington, 1973.
MacLean, P. D. Special award lecture: New findings on brain function and sociosexual behavior. In *Contemporary Sexual Behavior*, J. Zubin and J. Money, editors, p. 53. Johns Hopkins University Press, Baltimore, 1973.
Oppenheimer, H. *Clinical Psychiatry: Issues and Challenges.* Harper & Row, New York, 1971.
Robins, L. N. *Deviant Children Grown Up.* Williams & Wilkins, Baltimore, 1966.
Shiloh, A., editor. *Studies in Human Sexual Behavior: The American Scene.* Charles C Thomas, Springfield, Ill., 1970.
Smith, L. G., and Smith, J. R. Co-marital sex: The incorporation of extramarital sex into the marriage relationship. In *Contemporary Sexual Behavior*, J. Zubin and J. Money, editors, p. 391. Johns Hopkins University Press, Baltimore, 1973.
Tyrer, P. J. Relevance of bodily feelings in emotion. Lancet, *1:* 915, 1973.
Wahl, C. W. *Sexual Problems: Diagnosis and Treatment in Medical Practice.* Free Press (Macmillan), New York, 1967.
Zubin, J., and Money, J., editors. *Contemporary Sexual Behavior: Critical Issues in the 1970's.* Johns Hopkins University Press, Baltimore, 1973.

23.10. SEXUAL VARIANTS AND SEXUAL DISORDERS

23.10a. HOMOSEXUALITY AND SEXUAL ORIENTATION DISTURBANCES

Definition

Homosexuality was listed as a sexual deviation under the broad rubric of "Personality disorders and certain other nonpsychotic mental disorders" in the second edition of the American Psychiatric Association's *Diagnostic and Statistical Manual of Mental Disorders.* This classification reflected a more tolerant approach to this condition than existed in the previous edition's listing, which included sexual deviation under the category of "Sociopathic personality disturbance," or in earlier classifications, which places it in the group of psychopathic personalities with pathological sexuality. In April 1974, the American Psychiatric Association ruled that homosexuality would no longer be listed as a mental disorder. In its place it created a category of "Sexual orientation disturbance," described as follows:

"This category is for individuals whose sexual interests are directed primarily toward people of the same sex and who are either disturbed by, in conflict with, or wish to change their sexual orientation. This diagnostic category is distinguished from homosexuality, which by itself does not necessarily constitute a psychiatric disorder. Homosexuality per se is one form of sexual behavior and, like other forms of sexual behavior which are not by themselves psychiatric disorders, is not listed in this nomenclature of mental disorders."

Homosexuality can be defined in simple operational terms as any behavior involving sexual relations with a member of the same sex. Such a definition, however, fails to do justice to the wide variety of motivations that can underlie such behavior. Some persons enter into homosexual liaisons only because heterosexual objects are not available to them; others do so out of loneliness, boredom, rebelliousness, curiosity, or a neurotic need to please. Homosexual behavior also occurs among many adolescents and preadolescents as an expression of their intense sexual strivings in a society that forbids them the heterosexual explorations that they would prefer if they were free to choose.

The definition of homosexuality is further complicated by the fact that homosexual and heterosexual behaviors in human beings are not always discrete or clearly differentiated patterns. Rather, they are points on a continuum that ranges from exclusive heterosexuality to exclusive homosexuality, with various gradations of bisexual patterns in between.

In this discussion, the definition of homosexuality is restricted to persons with a strong preferential erotic attraction to members of their own sex.

Epidemiology

Homosexual activities of some kind probably occur in almost all societies, but the attitudes of different societies toward such practices vary widely. These variant societal attitudes toward homosexual behavior make the scientific study of its prevalence extremely difficult.

In American culture homosexuals can be encountered in all walks of life, at all socio-economic levels, among all racial and ethnic groups, and in both rural and urban areas. Their actual numbers are almost impossible to ascertain because many persons withhold this information from investigators. It is probable that actual incidence figures are higher than studies have reported.

The 1948 Kinsey study, based on interviews with more than 5,000 white American men, concluded that 37 per cent of the men in this society have had at least some overt homosexual experience to the point of orgasm between adolescence and old age. A more relevant statistic is the finding that 10 per cent of white men are more or less exclusively homosexual for at least 3 years between the ages of 16 and 55, and 4 per cent of them are exclusively homosexual throughout their lives. About 13 per cent of the sample revealed a potentiality for homosexual behavior, in that they reacted erotically to other males, despite the fact that they had had no overt homosexual contacts after the onset of adolescence.

Comparable studies of American women by the Kinsey group in 1953 revealed a lower incidence of homosexuality among them, as compared with men, although the figures were substantially higher for unmarried women than for married women. Between 2 and 6 per cent of the unmarried women in the sample but less than 1 per cent of the married women had been more or less exclusively homosexual in each of the years between 20 and 35 years of age. On the other hand, about 28 per cent of the women in the study reported some homosexual experiences or arousal in the course of their lives, 13 per cent of them to the point of orgasm.

Causes

Nineteenth century scientists leaned toward a genetic explanation of homosexuality or else regarded it as a stigma of some degenerative disease of the nervous system. With the advent of embryology, the ancient Greek conception of organic bisexuality was revived. Psychoanalytic explanations have combined this concept of bisexuality with a developmental theory based on psychosocial factors. Freud's view was that there is a normal psychic bisexuality, based on a biological bisexual predisposition in all human beings, and that all persons go through a homoerotic phase in childhood in the regular course of development. According to this view, if homosexuality develops in later life, it is the result of an arrest of normal development or else of regression as a result of castration anxiety mobilized by pathogenic family relationships. Even if development proceeds normally, certain vestiges of the homoerotic phase remain as permanent aspects of the personality. These latent homosexual tendencies are universal, Freud believed, and are reflected in sublimated patterns of affection for members of one's own sex or in certain passive tendencies in men and aggressive tendencies in women.

A more recent view rejects the theory of psychic bisexuality and argues that heterosexuality is the biological norm in all mammals, including humans, and that the development of homosexuality is always a pathological consequence of fears of heterosexual functioning that have been produced by unfavorable life experiences.

With the development of modern genetics and endocrinology, many efforts have been directed toward attempting to demonstrate either a genetic predisposition or a hormonal basis for homosexual behavior. The generally higher incidence of homosexual concordance in monozygotic as compared with dizygotic twins suggests that the possibility of a hidden genetic predisposition interacting with subsequent environmental experiences cannot be entirely ruled out. Chromosomal studies have thus far been unable to differentiate homosexuals from heterosexuals. And hormonal studies of homosexuals have failed to demonstrate any consistent difference between them and heterosexual controls. For the time being, therefore, the question of whether there may be innate genetic or endocrinological differences between obligatory homosexuals and heterosexuals must be regarded as unsettled.

The most prevalent theory concerning the cause of homosexuality attributes it to a pathogenic family background. The most significant factor in the genesis of homosexuality is a parental constellation of a detached, hostile father and a close-binding, seductive mother who dominates and minimizes her husband. Various other family patterns have been described—for example, distant or hostile mothers and overly close fathers, ambivalent relationships with an older brother, absent mothers, absent fathers, idealized fathers, and broken homes.

However, the fact that many heterosexual men have similar backgrounds and do not go on to become homosexual suggests that these familial patterns are not adequate in themselves as sole etiological explanations. The cause of homosexuality is not only multiply determined by psychodynamic, sociocultural, biological, and situational factors but also reflects the significance of subtle temporal, qualitative, and quantitative variables.

Clinical Features

Homosexuals may indulge in all the erotic practices that characterize heterosexual relations except for the limitations imposed by their same-sex anatomies. Kissing, tongue play, petting, mutual masturbation (either by hand or body friction), oral-genital relations, breast stimulation and kissing (by women), and anal intercourse (by men) are all common practices, although some persons show a preference for certain patterns and a distaste for others. The use of artificial phalluses (dildos) to simulate male-female intercourse is rare between homosexual women.

Most homosexuals do not fall into active or passive categories in their relations with one another. The majority vary their techniques, assuming the active and passive roles alter-

nately or taking different roles with different partners. Moreover, there is no reliable correlation between physical appearance, social mannerisms, and preferred sexual practices.

Male homosexuals are often quite promiscuous in their sexual behavior. If their avoidance of heterosexual involvement is related to fears of interpersonal commitment, intimacy, or responsibility, the same fears operate with regard to homosexual relationships. On the other hand, if heterosexual exchanges were as easily available as homosexual ones, is there any reason to doubt that heterosexual men would be just as promiscuous? In actual fact, there has been an enormous increase in heterosexual promiscuity in recent years, since the advent of the pill has made women less fearful of pregnancy and, consequently, less inhibited about undertaking sexual relations.

Gay bars, public baths, autos, and certain streets, parks, and public rest rooms are the locales where homosexuals meet one another, and, in some of them, liaisons frequently take place. Often, these liaisons are entirely anonymous. In some men, the drive for such contacts takes on a compulsive quality. Not all men who pursue these practices are obligatory homosexuals. The "heterosexual" group usually function as fellatees, rather than fellators, and apparently view their experiences not as homosexual encounters but, rather, as a quick, inexpensive, and impersonal way of achieving an orgasm. They are largely emotionally withdrawn men whose marriages have deteriorated and whose sex lives with their wives have become unsatisfactory.

Despite the relative ease with which homosexual contacts can be made, not all homosexuals pursue patterns of promiscuity. The more emotionally mature the person, the more likely is he or she to seek some kind of stable liaison with a genuine love object. Since such relationships have no legal bonds, many of them break up after a year or two. Such stable relationships are more frequent among female homosexuals than among male homosexuals.

Although most male homosexuals seem to be drawn to partners with attributes reflecting a high degree of masculinity—well-developed physiques and, particularly, large penises—there are wide variations of preference. Some are attracted by qualities of intellect or by cultural achievement, and some reach out for partners with obvious feminine characteristics, mannerisms, or dress. The popular assumption that homosexuals constitute a threat to young children is an unwarranted myth; the seeking out of children as sexual objects is much less common among homosexuals than among heterosexuals.

Psychopathology

There is no reason to assume that there is a specific psychodynamic structure to homosexuality any more than there is to heterosexuality. Nevertheless, it may well be that there is a higher incidence of neurotic personality distortion among homosexuals than among heterosexuals. In a culture like this, in which being homosexual is labeled as being queer and means being subjected to ridicule, humiliation, contempt, and rejection, it would be remarkable if most persons who found themselves growing up with such yearnings did not suffer from an impaired self-image, feelings of emotional insecurity, and various defensive personality consequences.

Female Homosexuality

American culture does not attach as much stigma to sexual intimacies between women as it does to those between men.

The female homosexual is not as likely as is her male counterpart to suffer from fears of disclosure, threats of blackmail, or feelings of insecurity and inadequacy. As a result, a greater proportion of female homosexuals maintain stable patterns of social adjustment than do male homosexuals, the degree of promiscuity among female homosexuals is much less than among male homosexuals, and there is a higher proportion of long-term relationships among female homosexuals.

Most studies agree that the incidence of homosexuality in women is only about half that for men. The achievement of a feminine identity is less difficult in this society than is the achievement of masculine identity; dependency patterns constitute an acceptable adaptation for women and are more easily achieved than are the patterns of self-reliance and vocational and paternal responsibility required of men. In the sexual act itself, it is much easier for a woman to stimulate competence than it is for a man. The degree of exclusive homosexuality in women is quite low. Most homosexual women have had some exposure to heterosexual relations. And women who have a fear of or aversion to heterosexuality have an option open to them that is evidently quite rare among men; 14 to 19 per cent of unmarried women and the 5 to 8 per cent of previously married women never have any sociosexual responses through all their adult years. The double sexual standard of this culture finds such asexuality acceptable in women but not in men.

The cause of female homosexuality is more obscure than that of male homosexuality. The evidence appears to be that their family backgrounds are as diverse as are those of male homosexuals. Some lesbians have had hostile, domineering mothers and detached, unassertive fathers, similar to those found in the families of male homosexuals. Others, however, had intense, seductive relationships with their fathers and had narcissistic, detached mothers. In others, the parental background does not appear particularly exceptional. In still others strong rivalry patterns with male siblings appear to have had a decisive influence, with resultant hostility to men and rejection of the female sex role. Others have grown up feeling that their parents would have preferred them to be boys. A common factor in most of their backgrounds is a strong antiheterosexual pattern in the home—stemming sometimes from the mother, sometimes from the father. As a result, relations with boys tend to be powerfully discouraged and laden with guilt and fear, but crushes on girls are either disregarded or covertly encouraged.

Significant numbers of women choose the homosexual route because—for reasons of unattractiveness, shyness, fears of rejection, or lack of available men—they feel closed off from the heterosexual relationships they might otherwise prefer.

Psychological Tests

No psychological tests pathognomonically differentiate homosexuals from heterosexuals in the absence of a clinical history. Homosexuality is not a single clinical entity, and there is no necessary correlation between a homosexual orientation and other aspects of a person's intrapsychic or interpersonal functioning.

Homosexuality and Mental Illness

This is one of the most disputed issues related to the subject of homosexuality. Should a homosexual orientation properly be regarded and classified as an illness requiring psychotherapeutic intervention whenever possible? Or is it merely a different way of life that falls within a normal psychobiological range but that happens to be regarded with disfavor in today's culture? Freud did not consider it an illness. However, many contemporary psychoanalysts do consider homosexuality as a form of psychopathology.

Psychiatric views in favor of considering homosexuality as a form of psychopathology generally rest on three major arguments: (1) that homosexuals are the product of disordered sexual development, (2) that they represent a deviation from the biological norm, and (3) that they are uniformly deeply disturbed, unhappy people.

When examined closely, the statement that homosexuality is the result of disordered sexual development really says nothing other than that the outcome of that development is not considered to be normal. Second, it is true that exclusive homosexuality is rarely seen in lower animals, except under extreme and unusual environmental conditions. By the same token, however, exclusive and obligatory heterosexuality is equally unusual. Third, the contention that all homosexuals are deeply disturbed and unhappy people, put forward primarily by psychoanalysts, is obviously based on therapeutic experience with homosexual patients and is as unwarranted as any similar generalization about heterosexuals would be if it were based only on work with disturbed or deeply troubled persons. Many homosexuals, both male and female, function responsibly and honorably, often in positions of the highest trust, and live emotionally stable, mature, and well-adjusted lives, psychodynamically indistinguishable from well-adjusted heterosexuals, except for their alternative sexual preferences.

Latent Homosexuality

The concept of latent homosexuality rests on Freud's theory of psychic bisexuality, a theory open to considerable doubt. It assumes that vestiges of an original homosexual phase of development remain in all persons and are manifested in sublimated form in tender feelings toward members of one's own sex and in certain psychic patterns considered to be identified with the opposite sex. Passive tendencies in men and aggressive tendencies in women fall into this category.

However, the assumption that certain psychological traits are innately masculine or feminine is questionable. Gender role patterns vary widely in different cultures and in different historical periods and are strongly influenced by the acculturation processes that the infant encounters in the first several years of life. Although, in the aggregate, males tend to be more aggressive and more physically active than females, the distributions of these traits in males and females constitute overlapping curves, with many perfectly normal female infants being constitutionally more aggressive and vigorous than many perfectly normal male infants.

Apart from its dubious theoretical basis, the concept of latent homosexuality carries with it some questionable clinical inferences. It is widely assumed, for example, that the syndrome of homosexual panic is due to life situations that have unduly stimulated the latent homosexuality of certain men to a point at which their egos become overwhelmed by the fear that these homosexual impulses may emerge. However, in a culture such as this one, where homosexuality is associated with weakness and effeminacy, many men who have doubts about their masculinity express these doubts in the form of fears that they may be homosexual or will be so considered by others.

Prevention and Treatment

If most homosexual patterns are acquired, rather than innate, the optimal time for preventive measures is in early childhood, prepubertally—before sexual object choice has begun to take clear form. Children who are failing to develop sex-appropriate gender role identifications or satisfactory peer relationships should be considered potentially vulnerable to homosexual development, and adequate family diagnosis and treatment should be undertaken as early as possible. The family as a whole should be regarded as the problem, not just the child. Emphasis in treatment should be placed on those aspects of the family dynamics that are interfering with the child's development of a positive identification with the same-sex parent, affectionate and unambivalent feelings toward the opposite parent, and good peer relationships. Important to explore are not only the patterns of mothering and fathering but also the antisexual bias that often exists in these families.

Once a homosexual predilection has clearly emerged, the question of whether treatment should be undertaken rests fundamentally on the person's motivation. Unless an adolescent wishes to change, not much can be accomplished, and it is more constructive to try to help the parents approach the issue of homosexuality with greater tolerance and understanding and, above all, not to reject their children on this account. At the same time, an effort should be made to help the homosexual youngsters accept themselves without shame or guilt and to cope with the social consequences of their variant sexual preference.

Homosexuals present themselves for treatment for a wide variety of reasons. Some come for help with problems analogous to those presented by heterosexuals—difficulties in attracting partners, break-up of important dyadic relationships, problems in self-realization, various neuroses, and depressive reactions. Most of these patients are not interested in changing their sexual orientation and should be treated as any corresponding heterosexual patient would be.

Other patients, however, are unhappy with their homosexual adaptation and would like to function heterosexually. These patients fall into the new diagnostic category of sexual orientation disturbance. If the psychotherapeutic process fails in the achievement of a heterosexual orientation, the effort should be directed toward enabling these patients to accept their homosexual identity without shame and to function as mature and responsible people within the context of that identity.

The myth that homosexuality is untreatable still has wide currency. True, the treatment of homosexuality is not easy. Part of the difficulty is the same as that found in any behavioral pattern in which the chief symptom carries with it a high potential for gratification. Counterbalancing this gratification, however, is the pressure of the social milieu, the impairment of self-image, and the unsatisfactory interpersonal adjustment that often accompany a homosexual way of life in this culture.

The reasons for seeking help have an important bearing on what can be expected from therapy. Those who undertake therapy for the specific purpose of altering their sexual patterns, all other things being equal, offer the best prognosis for achieving such change. Those who come unwillingly because of court orders growing out of legal violations tend to be least promising. A genuine shift in preferential sex object choice does take place in somewhere between 20 and 50 per cent of patients with homosexual behavior who seek psychotherapy with this end in mind. The single most important prerequisite to reversibility is a powerful motivation to achieve such a change. Given such motivation, other favorable prognostic indices are (1) youth—patients under 35 tend to do better, (2) previous heterosexual behavior or responsiveness, (3) recency of onset of homosexual activity, and (4) in men, aggressive personality patterns, as contrasted to strongly passive patterns and effeminate mannerisms, especially if they date back to childhood.

The treatment techniques used vary widely—from psychoanalysis to psychoanalytically oriented psychotherapies to group therapy to conditioning techniques using aversive and reinforcing stimuli. Despite differences in approach, all these methods share certain features in common. All require a high degree of motivation and cooperation from the patient. All tend to discourage homosexual behavior and encourage heterosexual behavior. The dynamic psychotherapies, in addition, place stress on other aspects of the patient's personality functioning, with special emphasis on increasing his self-esteem and his self-assertiveness.

However, all therapeutic approaches are of limited value in relation to the problem of homosexuality in its broadest aspects. The large majority of homosexuals do not seek to change their sexual patterns.

REFERENCES

Freud, S. Three essays on the theory of sexuality. In *Standard Edition of the Complete Psychological Works of Sigmund Freud*, J. Strachey, editor, vol. 7, pp. 135–243. Hogarth Press, London, 1953.

Kinsey, A. C., Pomeroy, W. B., and Martin, C. E., *Sexual Behavior in the Human Male*. W. B. Saunders, Philadelphia, 1948.

Kinsey, A. C., Pomeroy, W. B., Martin, C. E., and Gebhard, P. H. *Sexual Behavior in the Human Female*. W. B. Saunders, Philadelphia, 1953.

Marmor, J., editor. *Sexual Inversion. The Multiple Roots of Homosexuality.* Basic Books, New York, 1965.

Saghir, M. T., and Robins, E. *Male and Female Homosexuality.* Williams & Wilkins, Baltimore, 1973.

Tourney, G., and Hatfield, L. M. Androgen metabolism in schizophrenics, homosexuals, and normal controls. Biol. Psychiatry, 6: 23, 1973.

23.10b FRIGIDITY, DYSPAREUNIA, AND VAGINISMUS

Introduction

When emotional factors are thought to be playing a major role in their genesis, frigidity, dyspareunia, and vaginismus are classified as psychophysiologic genitourinary disorders in the American Psychiatric Association's *Diagnostic and Statistical Manual of Mental Disorders.* If the reasons for these dysfunctions are primarily anatomical or physiological, they should not be classified as mental disorders. Somatic and psychogenic factors can, however, coexist.

Frigidity

Frigidity or sexual anesthesia is a term applied to a wide range of inhibited sexual responses in women, from a complete lack of response to sexual stimulation to various inadequacies in orgasmic response, despite the fact that the woman finds sex otherwise pleasurable.

Masters and Johnson dispense with the value-laden term of frigidity and, instead, refer descriptively to orgasmic dysfunction. They consider primary orgasmic dysfunction as a condition in which a woman has never experienced an orgasm in masturbation, love play, or coitus. The term secondary or situational orgasmic dysfunction is used to refer to a condition in which the woman has experienced at least one previous orgasm, regardless of how or under what circumstances it was induced.

Incidence

A study of 1,000 married women found that only two of every five women experienced orgasms during intercourse, a figure roughly corroborated by other investigators. A Kinsey study revealed that about 36 per cent of the married women had never experienced orgasm from any source before marriage. Among married women, the percentage who had never experienced orgasm dropped to as low as 5 per cent, but a large proportion of these responded only occasionally. The Kinsey statistics indicate that there has been a gradual diminution in the incidence of orgasmic difficulties in women born in successive decades after 1900.

Causes

In the absence of detectable organic factors, it is fair to assume that the vast majority of orgasmic inadequacies in women are basically psychogenic. Girls growing up in societies dominated by a double sexual standard are generally subjected to considerably more sexual repression in the process of growing up than are boys. Because of this differential in early acculturation, a woman's ability to be sexually responsive is usually more dependent than is a man's on feelings of trust, security, tenderness, intimacy, and affection in the relation with her partner. Any life experiences that have rendered her less open to such feelings impair her capacity for orgasmic responsiveness. Traumatic sexual events may lead to the conviction that sex is an act of violent aggression. Orgasm may be unconsciously associated with loss of control or a state of dangerous vulnerability. Women with such backgrounds frequently present themselves with a history of never having had an orgasmic experience.

When, however, women have experienced orgasms but are unable to achieve them with a particular partner, the root of the difficulty can almost invariably be found in the nature of the relation with that partner. A frequent presenting factor is the partner's premature ejaculation, which does not allow the woman sufficient time to build up the erotic tension necessary for orgasmic release. Perhaps even more frequent is a disturbance in the nonsexual interpersonal relationship with the partner.

Orgasmic dysfunction can be a secondary consequence of any severe debilitating disease, general ill health, extreme fatigue, excessive indulgence in alcohol or other depressant drug, or depression. Hormonal factors are not usually involved in orgasmic inadequacy, nor is the administration of estrogen therapeutically effective.

Treatment

The therapeutic program initiated by Masters and Johnson has enabled these disorders to be treated with a high rate of success. The therapist must do more than improve the woman's insight to alter her behavior. He often needs to use specific measures designed to desensitize the patient's fears and guilt feelings and to enable the patient to confront the anxiety-provoking situation directly and in a new way. And in almost every instance of orgasmic dysfunction, the relation with the sexual partner must be taken into account. Frequently, the husband is equally inhibited about sexual matters; he may have potency or ejaculatory problems that accentuate the woman's orgasmic difficulties; or there may be significant interpersonal problems between them. The Masters and Johnson approach insists on treating the two sexual partners as a unit.

Masters and Johnson are also convinced that the treatment process should be conducted by a dual-sex team. They feel that a dual-sex team offers each partner a friend in court and prevents the development of transference reactions to a single therapist.

Dyspareunia and Vaginismus

These two disorders often coexist and have similar causative origins. Dyspareunia refers to painful intercourse. When present, it is usually but not always accompanied by vaginismus, an involuntary spasm of the pelvic musculature and lower third of the vagina. This spasm makes penile entry difficult, if not impossible.

Incidence

These disorders probably constitute only a small proportion of the total number of functional orgasmic disorders. Masters and Johnson indicate that, of 342 women with orgasmic dysfunction whom they treated, 29 also suffered from vaginismus.

Causes

When dyspareunia and vaginismus are psychogenic, the background factors are identical to those for frigidity. The pain in coition and the subsequent spasm are often the result of a failure in vaginal lubrication. Such failure is to be expected when there is a total inhibition of erotic reactivity as a consequence of intense guilt or fear underlying the sexual act. If these disorders have been manifest from the first attempt at coitus, one is dealing with psychodynamic factors identical to those in primary orgasmic dysfunction, although they are often more intense in these disorders. On the other hand, if these symptoms appear in a woman who was previously orgasmic in coitus, one must consider—once organic factors are excluded—the situational factors described for secondary orgasmic dysfunction. However, in the absence of any obvious traumatizing experience, such as a rape or a beating from a mate, there is a strong presumption that a somatic problem accounts for the painful coitus.

After a hysterectomy or other genital tract surgery, a transitory vaginismus may occur that is due not to any somatic factor but to the woman's anxiety that she may be hurt in coitus. Medical reassurance and a patient, gentle approach on the part of the sexual partner usually overcome this problem.

Treatment

In addition to the general principles involved in the therapy of the orgasmic disorders, the treatment of dyspareunia and vaginismus may require certain specific technical interventions, particularly the use of graduated vaginal dilators within the framework of the Masters and Johnson approach. If somatic factors are involved, they must be taken care of appropriately.

Orgasmic Dysfunction and Aging

There is no basis in fact for the myth that postmenopausal women are doomed to lose both the desire and the capacity for sexual pleasure. When this loss does occur, it is usually a consequence of the absence of sexual outlets, or else it represents a rationalized retreat from sexual participation on the part of a woman who has always been totally or relatively frigid.

Although the physiological reactions involved in the various phases of the sexual response cycle of the postmenopausal woman tend to be slowed or diminished in intensity in some respects, the capacity for orgasmic pleasure remains intact. The aging process does initiate a number of changes in the female genital apparatus as a result of the diminution in the production of the sex steriods. The most pertinent of these changes are the thinning of the vaginal mucosal lining and the gradual contracture of the vaginal barrel. In addition, the loss of fatty tissue in the area of the mons and the labia renders the clitoral glans and shaft more susceptible to irritation by manipulation and coitus. Sexual intercourse may become painful to the aging woman. Adequate sex-steroid replacement therapy retards these changes and prevents such secondary dyspareunia and vaginismus. However, if sexual intercourse continues regularly throughout the menopausal and postmenopausal years, this in itself, even without sex-steroid therapy, tends to retard the development of involutional changes in the vaginal mucosa and barrel.

REFERENCES

Benedek, T. The functions of the sexual apparatus and their disturbances. In *Psychosomatic Medicine*, F. Alexander, editor, p. 247. W. W. Norton, New York, 1950.
Freud, S. The psychology of women. In *New Introductory Lectures in Psychoanalysis*, p. 161, W. W. Norton, New York, 1933.
Marmor, J. Some considerations concerning orgasm in the female. Psychosom. Med., *16:* 240, 1954.
Masters, W. H., and Johnson, V. E. *Human Sexual Response.* Little, Brown, Boston, 1966.
Masters, W. H., and Johnson, V. E. *Human Sexual Inadequacy.* Little, Brown, Boston, 1970.
Salzman, L. Sexuality in psychoanalytic theory. In *Modern Psychoanalysis*, J. Marmor, editor, p. 135. Basic Books, New York, 1968.

23.10c. IMPOTENCE AND EJACULATORY DISTURBANCES

Impotence

Sexual impotence refers to the inability of a man to achieve a quality of erection sufficient to enable him to achieve coitus successfully. In primary impotence, the man has never been able to achieve a satisfactory coital erection. In secondary impotence, the man has been potent and has developed his impotence subsequently. The diagnosis of impotence should not be used to refer to an occasional erective failure caused by extreme fatigue, excessive alcohol, or some other transient unfavorable circumstance; such reactions are quite common in otherwise normal men. If, however, the erective failure becomes a frequently repeated pattern—Masters and Johnson suggest the arbitrary figure of failure in 25 per cent of coital attempts—a diagnosis of secondary impotence is warranted.

Incidence

Accurate figures concerning the incidence of primary and secondary impotence are difficult to come by, largely because to have such a problem is generally a source of shame and embarrassment in a society that places a high premium on masculine coital effectiveness. The Kinsey statistics reveal a gradual rise in the incidence of impotence with age, particularly after 45, with a more rapid increase after 55. By age 70, 27 per cent of the white men in the Kinsey study reported impotence; by age 75, 55 per cent; and by 80, 75 per cent.

Causes

Impotence can be caused by a broad spectrum of physical disorders and drugs, but such cases constitute only a small percentage of the total number of presenting potency problems.

Psychological Causes. Primary impotence is usually indicative of more serious intrapsychic disturbance than is impotence of secondary or situational origin. Men suffering from primary impotence often come from sexually repressed or religiously orthodox family backgrounds, where sex was either never discussed or treated as sinful, immoral, or ugly. They have often had abnormally close relations with seductive mothers. Any life experiences that make a man unusually fearful of intimacy and unable to love or feel loved, inordinately immature or inadequate, or deeply distrustful of, fearful of, or hostile to women may render him impotent. The cultural ambience, particularly in middle-class groups, often makes sexual intercourse a difficult process because it is surrounded by many taboos and societal restrictions.

Similar background factors can be found in patients with secondary impotence, although the effect of these factors has not been so severe as to preclude some capacity for subsequent potency. Situational factors play a major role in the causation of secondary impotence. Such factors include excessive indulgence in alcohol, a pre-existing pattern of premature ejaculation that leads to tension and unhappiness in the female partner, economic or work tensions, depressive reactions, marital discord, loss of attractiveness of the partner, and traumatic experiences that arouse feelings of hostility or rejection toward the partner or make the man feel particularly inadequate or guilty.

Somatic Causes. Any severe or debilitating illness can be a cause of impotence and is usually associated with loss of libido. In certain illnesses, such as cardiorespiratory disease, libido may be relatively intact, but the serious impairment of cardiac or pulmonary reserve may make sexual excitement and functioning difficult. In some cases of angina pectoris, the inhibiting factor may be the fear of triggering an attack of angina. Diabetes mellitus appears to be particularly capable of causing impotence, although the mechanism is obscure. Other metabolic conditions that may be associated with impotence are myxedema, thyrotoxicosis, pituitary disease, and Addison's disease.

The role of sex hormone deficiencies in disturbances of potency is not of major importance. Testicular castration before puberty usually leads to primary impotence, but post-pubertal castration need not. Large amounts of estrogen result in loss of libido and impotence in men, but testosterone has no significant effect on either libido or potency in normal men.

Any neurological disorder that destroys the function of the sacral cord or of the lower thoracolumbar sympathetic fibers can cause impotence. Hypothalamic lesions and temporal lobe lesions may also cause impotence, although temporal lobe lesions are sometimes associated with hypersexuality.

Local anatomical defects or diseases of the genital tract can create sexual dysfunction. Prostatectomy, particularly perineal prostatectomy, may result in impotence.

A wide variety of drugs can interfere with sexual potency. The most frequently implicated drug is alcohol, but all addictive drugs can produce secondary impotence and loss of libido. Most psychotropic drugs are capable, in large doses, of interfering with potency.

The correlation between the aging process and impotence is not inevitable. With age, almost all normal men experience a gradual lessening of libidinal urgency, and the frequency of the need for sexual discharge diminishes. However, the capacity for erection continues to an advanced age, even though the attainment of erection under sexual stimulation may take place more slowly than it did in the man's youth. Once erection is achieved, the aging man is generally able to maintain it for longer periods of time before experiencing ejaculatory urgency. The available evidence indicates that, with available opportunities for coitus, men can retain the capacity for satisfactory sexual intercourse well into their eighties.

One variety of secondary impotence develops when the man or his partner or both are unaware of the natural diminution in libidinal urgency that occurs in aging, and pressure develops—usually from the woman—for more frequent coital contacts than the man is motivated for. Or the man himself may develop an increasing concern over the fact that it is taking him longer to achieve erection than it used to. The result in such instances can be the development of performance anxiety in the man, with consequent secondary impotence.

Treatment

Contemporary treatment of impotence leans heavily on the contributions of Masters and Johnson, who treat the impotent man and his female partner together. Dynamic psychotherapy may be indicated as a prelude to or a concomitant of the Masters and Johnson approach, particularly in cases of primary impotence, in which underlying feelings of sexual guilt, anxiety, and emotional immaturity may be great. In cases of secondary impotence, attention must be given to the factors involved in the onset of the symptom, and these factors must be dealt with by appropriate psychotherapeutic techniques, including conjoint marital therapy where indicated. Masters and Johnson report a success rate, after a 5-year follow-up, of 60 per cent in cases of primary impotence and about 75 per cent in cases of secondary impotence. Others who use their approach report similar figures.

Ejaculatory Disturbances

Premature Ejaculation

Premature ejaculation is relative to the ability to satisfy a female partner, whose own time of response depends on her own psychodynamic patterns and on the degree of excitement to which the man has brought her during coital foreplay. Under some circumstances, 60 seconds of intravaginal penile movement is sufficient to bring both partners to a mutually gratifying climax; under other circumstances, 5 or 10 minutes or more of vigorous intravaginal penile activity leave the woman unsatisfied, and the man, as a result, feels inadequate. Therefore, premature ejaculation is defined as that condition in which a man, with any woman, achieves orgasm before or within seconds after vaginal intromission or in which a man, despite having a partner capable of achieving an orgasm without difficulty, is unable to delay his orgasm or ejaculation during intravaginal coitus for a sufficient length of time to satisfy her in at least half of their coital connections.

Incidence. Premature ejaculation is probably the commonest of all disturbances in male sexual function. In contemporary society, premature ejaculation has become a matter of increasing concern to both sexes, particularly among better educated people, and therapeutic help is being sought more frequently than in the past.

Causes. Difficulty in ejaculatory control tends to be closely associated with the existence of anxiety during the sexual act. The reaction of the female partner becomes an additional contributing factor. Idiosyncratic variations make certain persons more prone to its development than others and make for differences in its severity. The background factors in impotence should be looked for.

Treatment. Masters and Johnson approach premature ejaculation not as the man's problem alone but, rather, as a problem of an interacting sexual couple. Using their method—which involves desensitization of sexual guilt, removal of performance anxiety, and a practiced lowering of the threshold of penile excitability, all in a dyadic context—Masters and Johnson have reported almost 98 per cent success in the amelioration of premature ejaculation within a matter of weeks. Comparable rates of success have been reported by others who use this method or modifications of it. The lowering of the threshold of penile excitability is achieved by a squeeze technique that the female partner uses when the man begins to experience a sense of ejaculatory urgency.

Retarded or Inhibited Ejaculation

This disorder, the reverse of premature ejaculation, is sometimes called ejaculatory incompetence. It is a condition in which the man manifests difficulty or inability in achieving ejaculation during coitus. It can be designated as primary when it has always been present and as secondary when it develops after previous normal functioning.

Incidence. Retarded ejaculation is considerably less common than premature ejaculation. Masters and Johnson had 3.8 per cent in their series.

Causes. When retarded or inhibited ejaculation during coitus has always been present, the precursory factors are often similar to those for primary impotence. These factors include puritanical or orthodox religious backgrounds in which guilt and anxiety concerning sex have been strongly fostered. Fears of impregnating the partner, unconscious anxieties concerning the vagina as a contaminated organ, or anxious-hostile fantasies of the ejaculate as a contaminating substance that will defile the woman may be involved. Often, these men are rigidly compulsive personalities to whom orgasm means a terrifying loss of control, or their security systems are built around tightly holding on to everything they have.

Secondary ejaculatory incompetence of psychogenic origin is invarably the result of disturbances in the interpersonal relation between the man and his partner. The causative factors may include pressure from a wife who wants to become pregnant, a demand from an unmarried partner for marriage or some other form of commitment, a loss of sexual attraction to the partner, interpersonal friction, or a traumatic experience.

Ejaculatory difficulty may, however, be the result of organic factors, and these factors must always be ruled out. Neurological disorders interfering with the sympathetic innervation to the genitalia, such as lumber sympathectomy and syringomyelia, may cause ejaculatory incompetence. The condition has also been described in cases of parkinsonism. Drugs with antiadrenergic action have been reported as causing ejaculatory inhibition, as have various phenothiazine drugs.

Treatment. When the symptom of ejaculatory retardation or inhibition is a reflection of a deep-seated personality disorder, analytically oriented psychotherapy may be necessary. When the symptom is secondary to some situational problem, that problem must be dealt with by appropriate measures, including conjoint marital therapy where indicated. In addition, Masters and Johnson have found that a direct approach to the symptom itself, working with both partners, can often be effective. Masters and Johnson report 14 successes out of

17 cases of ejaculatory incompetence referred to them.

REFERENCES

Hastings, D. W. *Impotence and Frigidity*. Little, Brown, Boston, 1963.
Johnson, J. *Disorders of Sexual Potency in the Male*. Pergamon Press, Oxford, 1968.
Keen, H. Autonomic neuropathy in diabetes mellitus. Postgrad. Med. J., *35:* 272, 1959.
Masters, W. H., and Johnson, V. E. *Human Sexual Inadequacy*. Little, Brown, Boston, 1970.
Perloff, W. H. Hormones and homosexuality. In *Sexual Inversion: The Multiple Roots of Homosexuality*, J. Marmor, editor, p. 44, Basic Books, New York, 1965.
Semans, J. H. Premature ejaculation: A new approach. South. Med. J., *49:* 353, 1956.

23.10d. THE UNCONSUMMATED MARRIAGE

Introduction

The unconsummated marriage is not a rare complaint. Couples present with this problem after having been married several months or several years. Masters and Johnson have reported an unconsummated marriage of 17 years' duration.

The couple involved in an unconsummated marriage are typically uninformed and inhibited about sexuality. Their feelings of guilt, shame, or inadequacy are increased by their problem, and they are disturbed by a need to seek help and a need to conceal their difficulty.

Frequently, the couple do not seek help directly, but the woman may reveal the problem to her gynecologist on a visit ostensibly concerned with vague vaginal or somatic complaints. On examining her, the gynecologist may find an intact hymen. In some cases the wife may have undergone a hymenectomy. This surgical procedure is another stress, however, and often serves to increase the feelings of inadequacy in the couple. The wife may feel put upon, abused, or mutilated, and the husband's concern about his manliness is increased. The physician's questioning, if he is comfortable dealing with sexual problems, may be the first opening to frank discussion of the couple's distress.

Once presented, this complaint can often be successfully treated. The duration of the problem does not significantly affect the prognosis or outcome of the case.

Causes

Lack of sexual education, sexual prohibitions overly stressed by parents or society, neurotic problems of an oedipal nature, immaturity in both partners, overdependence on primary families, and problems in sexual identification—all contribute to nonconsummation of a marriage.

Clinical Features

In the unconsummated marriage, the husband frequently has a problem with impotence, and many wives present with vaginismus. It is often difficult to determine which problem arose first, as there has frequently been no premarital sexual experience for either partner. The woman may develop vaginismus after repeated sexual encounters with a dysfunctional man have caused her to feel rejected and frustrated; or the man may develop impotence owing to the same feelings after unsuccessful attempts at intercourse with a woman suffering from vaginismus. Occasionally, one partner is able to function outside of the marital situation, and, frequently, either partner would function better sexually with a less dysfunctional mate.

The man usually bears the burden of guilt for dysfunction, but the woman suffers equally, feeling that she is not sufficiently desirable or attractive to arouse her husband.

A frequent dynamic in the unconsummated marriage involves a husband who has been taught that there are two types of women—one for love and one for sex—and a wife has been brought up to expect the man to make all the advances. Their sexual life is paralyzed, as he is unable to move sexually toward his good woman, and she fears losing his love and her own self-respect if she is sexually aggressive with him. With little or no sexual play between them, they remain more attached to their primary families than to each other.

Another common pattern involves the couple for whom marriage is a power struggle and sex the major battlefield. The wife appears aggressive and controlling, and the husband appears passive and submissive. In bed, however, the husband withholds sex through impotence or premature ejaculation, and the wife is left feeling rejected and unfulfilled. She usually has her own sexual problems and is hesitant about self-stimulation or has difficulty in achieving climax. Both partners end up feeling inadequate and frustrated.

Treatment

The unconsummated marriage is best treated by seeing both members of the couple. Dual-sex therapy involving a male-female co-therapy team has been markedly effective. However, other forms of conjoint therapy, marital counseling, traditional psychotherapy on a one-to-one basis, and counseling from a sensitive family physician, gynecologist, or urologist are all helpful.

The couple need to receive factual sexual information from a sympathetic, accepting, but authoritative source. They need permission and encouragement to function sexually and to build confidence and pride in their own sexuality. Couples who come for treatment with this problem are usually highly motivated and respond quickly and positively to therapy.

The therapists represent for them authority or parental figures who for the first time recognize, accept, and encourage their sexuality. The therapists act as sex educators and provide positive models for sexual identification. In dual-sex therapy they take over the sexual lives of the couple by directing, through various prescribed sexual exercises, the patients' sexual play. In this way, the therapists suspend the couple's prohibitive and inhibiting superegos and introduce new and more permissive standards of appropriate sexual behavior.

The couple may be given specific instructions regarding their sexual behavior. Initially, intercourse may be prohibited and sexual contact limited to, first, general body caressing and, later, genital caressing. This initial limitation removes the pressure to perform from both partners. Before attempting intercourse, the couple learn to become physically comfortable with each other. At the same time, they receive factual information regarding anatomy and sexual physiology and are helped to restructure their attitudes toward sexuality.

When one or both partners present a serious maturational failure, when fear of the opposite sex is deeply ingrained or sexual identification is markedly distorted, or when there is little contact with reality or only a superficial commitment to the marriage, the couple present a poor prognosis.

Many women involved in unconsummated marriages have distorted concepts about their vaginas. There can be a fear of having no opening, fear of being too small or too soft, or a confusion of the vagina with the rectum, leading to feelings of being unclean. The man may share in these distortions of the vagina and, in addition, perceive it as dangerous to himself. Similarly, both partners may share distortions about the man's penis, perceiving it as a weapon, as too large, or as too small. However, many of these patients can be helped by simple education about genital anatomy and physiology, by suggestions for self-exploration, and by corrective information from a physician.

REFERENCES

Ellis, H. *Studies in the Psychology of Sex*. Random House, New York, 1942.
Friedman, L. J. *Virgin Wives: A Study of Unconsummated Marriages*. J. B. Lippincott, Philadelphia, 1962.
Hastings, D. W. *Impotence and Frigidity*. Little, Brown, Boston, 1963.
Masters, W. H., and Johnson, V. E. *Human Sexual Inadequacy*. Little, Brown, Boston, 1970.

23.10e. INCEST

Introduction

Incest comprises a group of clinical syndromes whose importance outweighs their infrequent occurrence. The incest theme is universal. The incest taboo is perhaps the most binding and ubiquitous moral constraint.

Definition

Most definitions of incest describe it as the occurrence of sexual relations between blood relatives. However, this definition does not include certain clinically incestuous situations. For example, sexual relations between stepfather and stepdaughter or among stepsiblings are usually considered incestuous, although no blood relationship exists. In psychiatry, incest denotes intimate physical contact accompanied by conscious sexual excitement between persons within the same socialization unit, other than husband and wife or the cultural equivalent, or between persons who are close blood relatives.

Epidemiology

Incest is universally prohibited but everywhere recognized and has been reported in almost all civilized societies. However, reliable estimates of its incidence and prevalence are not available. The vigor of the incest taboo and the shame and guilt associated with overt incest make full reporting impossible. Differential reporting according to social class further distorts the available data; incestuous behavior in families of lower socio-economic status and among persons with a history of social deviance is more likely to be detected and reported than is incest in prosperous, respectable families.

In Sweden, where every incest offender receives a mandatory pretrial psychiatric study, the yearly incidence has been estimated at 0.73 case per million population. Comparable figures from United States sources range from 1.1 to 1.9 cases per million. Estimates of incest offenses as a percentage of total sex offenses vary from 2.4 to 6.3 per cent.

The older participant in an incestuous relationship is much likelier to be male than female, reflecting, perhaps the relatively stronger taboo against mother-son incest and its symbolic equivalents than against father-daughter and sibling incest.

Causes

The incest taboo is determined by a variety of instigating and sustaining factors. In the oedipal situation, the child feels excluded from the passionate love between his parents, wishes to possess his mother, and regards his father as, in part, a hated rival. He perceives a jealousy and prohibitive demeanor in his father and responds to the perceived threat and to his own projected aggression with guilt and castration anxiety. The dreaded retaliation of his father revives anxieties from an earlier age, when his basic fear was of being abandoned.

Anthropologists have shown that the nature of the incest taboo is culturally determined. Sociologists have pointed out the role of the incest taboo in facilitating socialization and role learning, forcing members of a nuclear family to choose love objects outside their group.

Biological factors may have some role in determining the incest taboo. A human group practicing incest is selectively disadvantaged by the lesser fitness resulting from inbreeding vis-à-vis outbreeding human groups. Human groups that insist on outbreeding are favored and preserved by the process of survival of the fittest.

Incestuous acts are, at least to some degree, collusive. In father-daughter incest, for example, the father is aided and abetted in his liaison by conscious or unconscious seduction by his daughter and by his wife's collusion. The mother forces a heavy burden of responsibility onto her daughter by causing her to assume the role of wife and lover with her own father, thus absolving the mother of this unwanted role.

Lustig and co-workers proposed that incest is a transaction that protects and maintains a dysfunctional family structure. Five conditions of the dysfunctional family foster breakdown of the incest barrier: (1) emergence of the daughter as the central female figure of the household in place of the mother, (2) some degree of sexual incompatibility between the parents, with unrelieved sexual tension in the father, (3) unwillingness of the father to seek a partner outside the nuclear family because he needs to maintain the public façade of stable and competent patriarch, (4) shared fears of family disintegration and abandonment, making the family desperate for an alternative to disintegration, (5) covert sanction by the nonparticipant mother, who condones and colludes with the assumption by the daughter of a sexual role with her father.

Sociological factors associated with a breakdown of incest barriers are overcrowding, with physical proximity; alcoholism; geographic isolation such that extrafamilial social and emotional contacts are effectively impossible; in the case of father-daughter incest, prolonged absence of the father from the home and his subsequent return to find an aging wife and a young, attractive, and tempting daughter; and loss of the wife by divorce, separation, or death, leaving the father alone with an adolescent daughter. The contemporary pattern of small, mobile, vertical family units and the loss of the extended family may foster incestuous relationships. In cases of father-daughter incest, the father is generally in his late thirties or early forties, a period during which marital stress often develops.

Incest in the nuclear family may be related to an extension of neurotic endogamy. Desertion anxiety is often strikingly prominent in incestuous partners and their families.

Major mental illness is a factor in incestuous behavior, according to some studies. Intellectual deficiency and constitutional inferiority may play a part in some cases of clinical incest.

Psychodynamics

The psychodynamics of father-daughter incest has been described in detail by Kaufman. In his series, desertion anxiety is a pervasive theme. The father or stepfather deserted the children at some time through divorce, living away from home, alcoholism, or frank desertion. Similarly, the maternal grandfather had deserted the family. The maternal grandmother was consistently stern, demanding, cold, and hostile and reacted to desertion by her husband by singling out one daughter, on whom she lavished displaced feelings of hostility and resentment. These daughters, who became the mothers of the incestuous daughters, were hard, infantile, and dependent, and they married men who were similarly dependent and infantile.

The mother singles out one daughter, displacing hostility arising in her own unresolved oedipal conflict. She deserts her husband sexually and forces her daughter to assume the role of sexual partner for the husband. The mother feels guilty and denies the incestuous liaison, even in the face of obvious or very suggestive evidence.

Incest usually has its onset when the father and daughter feel abandoned because of the mother's giving birth to a new sibling, turning to the maternal grandmother, or developing some outside interest. The girl, lonely and fearful, then accepts her father's sexual advances as expressions of affection, acquiescing in the tacit encouragement she receives from her mother. The mother's denial freezes role relations and preserves them from change.

Paranoid traits and unconscious homosexual strivings are common in incestuous fathers. The paranoid component is related to strong unconscious hostility toward the paternal grandmother, subsequently transferred to the wife and the daughter. Incest is an expression of his unconscious hostility, fused with primitive genital impulses discharged toward the daughter. Some fathers appear to have had a disturbed relationship with their own harsh and authoritarian fathers, who were ambivalently hated but admired; passive homosexual longings promote a process whereby the father obtains a fantasied affection from his own father through an incestuous liaison with a daughter.

Clinical Features

Father-Daughter Incest

There is little consensus as to the severity of emotional disturbance among incestuous fathers. Incestuous fathers have made poor sexual adjustments. Wives of such men often describe their sexual relations as devoid of affection and state that their husbands appear to derive an exclusively physical satisfaction from intercourse. The inability of these men to achieve a stable heterosexual orientation is reflected in a variety of coping mechanisms: sexual withdrawal, hypersexuality, flagrant promiscuity, and virtual abstinence.

Incestuous fathers may suffer from some degree of guilt and depression during their incestuous activity, but most often they become remorseful and repentant after the incest has been disclosed. Such rationalization as parental duty, a necessity to teach the facts of life, and pacification of an angry daughter are used to try to cope with the massive guilt resulting from violation of the incest taboo. However, the guilt may arise not only from the incestuous behavior but also from the disgrace and embarrassment rendered to families.

Incestuous fathers seem to come from backgrounds of social deprivation in the form of parental conflict or broken homes, marginal economic circumstances or parental unemployment, poor education, and occupational instability. Apparently, the disposition toward incestuous behavior is not correlated with more general criminal tendencies.

The wives of incestuous fathers are often dependent and infantile, pathologically attached to their own mothers, and prone to panic in the face of responsibility. They promote the incestuous liaison by frustrating their husbands sexually or symbolically deserting them and by promoting a dysfunctional role allocation wherein the daughter is subtly encouraged to assume the role of sexual partner for the father. These mothers push their daughters prematurely into a mothering role. The wives do not usually report the incestuous activity. As a rule, they tolerate it with little protest or exercise massive denial. Conceivably, such wives identify with their daughters and gratify in fantasy their childhood incestuous wishes toward their own fathers. If they do report the incestuous liaison, their doing so is often precipitated by anger over some other matter. The wives are perhaps too guilty about their own collusion or too fond of their husbands to report the offense. Moreover, they are often extremely dependent on their husbands and seem prepared to pay a great price emotionally to remain with them.

Promiscuity among the wives of incestuous

fathers is common. Occasionally, promiscuity and elopement by the mother precedes and perhaps precipitates incestuous activity between father and daughter.

The daughters collude in the incestuous liaison and play an active and even initiating role in establishing the pattern. The girls may be frightened and lonely and welcome their fathers' advances as expression of parental love. The incestuous activity often continues until it is discovered, and the girls do not act as though they were injured.

Incestuous daughters often have a façade of pseudomaturity—they may be precocious in learning, reality-mastery, and motility, but object relations, feminine identification, and adolescent ego development are disturbed or impaired. The girls tend to develop character disorders, rather than neuroses or psychoses, and regression after the interruption of incest leads to promiscuity, antisocial behavior, frigidity, homosexuality, learning disabilities, and depression.

Like her mother, the incestuous daughter is unlikely to report the liaison at first or to protest about it. If she eventually does so, it is often precipitated by anger at her father for something else or by jealousy of his relationship with another woman. Oedipal guilt may play a role in reluctance to accuse the father. Some girls avoid guilt feelings through a denial of pleasure and by assuming a consistently passive role in the relationship.

Daughters who regret the incestuous behavior may seek forgiveness from their mothers, even though the mothers have not objected to their behavior or condemned them. The daughters' guilt may stem not only from violation of the incest taboo but also from hostile impulses toward the mothers.

Sibling Incest

The older participant tends to be male. The commonest pattern is of normal sexual play and exploration leading eventually to heterosexual intercourse but subsequent substitution of sibling partners with exogamous partners, with no psychological harm to either participant. Parents usually deny the incestuous behavior; the absence of strong sanctions or punishments minimizes feelings of guilt among the participants. Prepubertal sibling incest may be viewed as a normal variant of heterosexual development. Occasionally, sibling incest is associated with more serious psychopathology when the pattern is prolonged, rather than a transitional developmental phase.

Mother-Son Incest

Generally, the occurrence of mother-son incest bespeaks more severe psychopathology among the participants than does father-daughter incest (where personality disorder is common) and sibling incest (where the participants are sometimes almost normal). The psychodynamics of mother-son incest include the mother's profound dependency on her son, to whom she turns for emotional support and protection and eventually sexual gratification. The son is idealized, and the mother's youthful fantasy of a romantic lover is invested in her own son. The mother is angry with her husband and may even blame him for her incestuous behavior.

Other Forms of Incest

Grandfather-granddaughter incest is clinically and dynamically similar to father-daughter incest, with a tendency for the granddaughter to turn to promiscuity or show features of personality disorders after termination of the incestuous liaison.

Uncle-niece incest is similar to father-daughter incest—in fact, the incestuous object choices made by the uncle and the niece symbolically represent the daughter and the father, respectively.

Like mother-son incest, aunt-nephew incestuous relationships are uncommon and bespeak more severe emotional disorder among the participants than do other forms of incestuous activity.

In Western cultures, the clinical occurrence of homosexual incest is uncommon. Important dynamic determinants appear to be avoidance of feared but desired heterosexual incest, profound distortions of intrafamilial roles and boundaries, collusion by the opposite-sexed nonparticipant family members, and the maintenance of family secrets.

Course and Prognosis

In cases of father-daughter incest, the father usually begins the relationship with his oldest daughter, then proceeds to include one or more of her younger sisters. The activity may proceed for some time before discovery or disclosure; after that, recidivism is uncommon, and breakup of the family unit often occurs.

As a rule, if the adults harbor little anxiety or guilt about the relationship, the daughter will do the same. The incestuous daughter may be relatively free of guilt feelings until she is exposed to censure. Sometimes, however, the daughter's sense of guilt causes her to give up the relationship of her own accord; sometimes she gives up incestuous activity with the father only to turn to compulsive promiscuity with other men.

There is little agreement about the role of father-daughter incest as a cause of serious subsequent psychopathology. Among those girls who become involved in therapy, a façade of maturity, competence, and responsibility often masks a hostile-dependent way of relating to older women and a proneness to making impossible demands and acting out seriously when their demands are frustrated. However, incestuous relationships do not always have a traumatic effect.

Occurrence and especially disclosure of incest in a culture where that form of incest is strongly proscribed or carries institutionalized punishment is more damaging to the participants than if the cultural attitude were mild or indifferent. For father-daughter incest, the preadolescent daughter appears less harmed by the occurrence than is the older girl.

Treatment

The prevention and treatment of clinical incest are complicated by the multidetermined nature of its occurrence, by difficulty in ascertaining what weight to assign to each of the many contributing factors, and by the limited accessibility of many of these factors to therapy. Furthermore, is the occurrence of incest necessarily pathological? The need for and choice of treatment must be decided on the basis of the response of the participants to their alleged transgression and to personal factors that may be related to the incest.

Messer suggested some specific preventive measures. Legal adoption of stepchildren and, in reconstituted families, relinquishing of financial support provided by the absent parent may strengthen the family structure and thereby strengthen the incest taboo and diminish the likelihood of clinical incest. A couple may usefully reinvigorate and reconfirm their mutuality through second honeymoons, whereby exclusive possession in the children's absence is asserted. In reconstituted families, open discussion of the fact that remarriage involved no deliberate disloyalty to the deceased or departed spouse may help foster healthier relationships. Openly affectionate parents give their children firm models on which to develop healthy heterosexual role identification.

The terms "mother" and "father" buttress the incest taboo. However, parents should probably be encouraged to recognize the normality of the family romance.

When appropriate and warranted, intensive psychotherapy or psychoanalysis can be recommended. Other approaches to treatment include open and frank discussion of sex, emphasizing the normality of incestuous feelings and wishes but the inadvisability of acting on such wishes, substitution of alternative modes of symbolic expression in play or social interaction, and healthy affection from other adults in the environment. Where major emotional or psychiatric difficulties exist, institutionalization may be required.

Clinical incest may usefully be viewed as a symptom of family maladjustment, and family therapy aimed at healthier role allocation may be indicated. Interpretive work should focus on the pervasive use of denial as a defense, stressing not only the denial of the incestuous act but also the denial of the extensive dysfunctional role relationships within the family and the collusion of nonparticipating members.

Where the incestuous act occurs in association with acute psychiatric illness, effective treatment of the illness is likely to lead to a remission of symptoms. Once incestuous behavior is disclosed and discussed, it is not likely to reoccur.

REFERENCES

Freud, S. Totem and taboo. In *Standard Edition of the Complete Psychological Works of Sigmund Freud*, J. Strachey, editor, vol. 13. Hogarth Press, London, 1955.

Henderson, D. J. Incest: A synthesis of data. Can. Psychiatr. Assoc. J., *17:* 299, 1972.

Kaufman, I., Peck, A. L., and Tagiuri, C. K. The family constellation and overt incestuous relations between father and daughter. Am. J. Orthopsychiatry, *24:* 266, 1954.

Lukianowicz, N. Incest. Br. J. Psychiatry, *120:* 301, 1972.

Lustig, N., Dresser, J. W., Spellman, S. W., and Murray, T. B. Incest: A family group survival pattern. Arch. Gen. Psychiatry, *14:* 31, 1966.

Messer, A. A. The "Phaedra complex." Arch. Gen. Psychiatry, *21:* 213, 1969.

Weiner, I. B. On incest: A survey. Excerpta Criminol., *4:* 137, 1964.

23.10 f. OTHER SEXUAL DEVIATIONS

Introduction

The American Psychiatric Association's *Diagnostic and Statistical Manual of Mental Disorders* defines sexual deviations as follows: "This category is for individuals whose sexual interests are directed primarily toward objects other than people of the opposite sex; toward sexual acts not usually associated with coitus or toward coitus performed under bizarre circumstances as in necrophilia, pedophilia, sexual sadism, and fetishism. Even though many find their practices distasteful, they remain unable to substitute normal sexual behavior for them. This diagnosis is not appropriate for individuals who perform deviant sexual acts because normal sexual objects are not available to them."

In April 1974, the Association's official list of mental disorders was changed to include the terms "sexual orientation disturbance" for persons whose sexual interests are directed toward persons of the same sex and who are disturbed by or in conflict with that orientation or who wish to change. This diagnostic category is distinguished from homosexuality, which does not constitute a psychiatric disorder.

The A. P. A. list of deviations includes fetishism, pedophilia, transvestitism, exhibitionism, voyeurism, sadism, and masochism. Others that may be added are rape, lust murder, necrophilia, bestiality, and sodomy.

Deviant acts must be distinguished from deviancy. Much foreplay may be in the form of deviant acts, but if these acts serve only to stimulate for normal coitus, they are not considered part of a deviational pattern or performed by a sexual deviate.

Psychoanalytic theory indicates that sexual deviation is either a regression to or a fixation at an early level of psychosexual development, resulting in a repetitive pattern of sexual behavior that is not mature or genital in its application and expression. Psychoanalytic theory also states that castration anxiety is common to all sexual deviations. The sexual deviate uses sex as a vehicle for the expression of such feelings as hostility and anxiety.

Aggressive and Anonymous Deviations

A classification that is useful in understanding sexual deviations is that distinguishing anonymous sexual deviations from aggressive sexual deviations.

Aggressive deviants include those who commit rape, lust murder, sadomasochism, pedophilia, necrophilia, and sodomy. The aggression is directed toward another human being, alive or dead, using the vehicle of sexuality for the expression of the aggression and the hostility. The rapist may, with sufficient aggressive force, become a lust murderer, and those who commit lust murder may also practice necrophilia.

Sodomy is a general legal term, usually referring to unnatural sex acts and including almost anything that is not penovaginal intercourse. However, its common usage is for penile-anal or oral-genital contact. If anal intercourse in heterosexual relationships is found to be satisfying without penovaginal contact, it is considered an aggressive deviation.

Anonymous sexual deviations involve gradually decreasing contact with the object of sexual desire. In frottage the deviant touches in public places. The usual object of his touchings is the breast or buttocks of a woman in a crowded train or elevator. He wishes no further contact with her and appears to obtain gratification from this fleeting physical touch. Usually, the frotteur does not go beyond this form of touching and is not considered to be dangerous or likely to be involved in aggressive sexual deviations.

The exhibitionist exposes his genitals. The mode of operation is usually quite consistent and, in many cases, involves his automobile. Some expose themselves on buses and subways and others when walking down the street. There is often a hint of pedophilia. The exhibitionist is attempting to resolve particular problems within himself and is not considered dangerous nor will he graduate to more serious sexual deviations.

The voyeur or peeping tom is not interested in

making contact with the object of his sexual desires. His primary interest is to achieve orgasmic expression by viewing others involved in sexual relations or by viewing a woman in the nude in her home. He is usually apprehended for loitering and prowling; rarely does he become a more serious sexual deviant.

The obscene telephone caller achieves sexual gratification from calling young women on the phone and making obscene remarks that suggest that the woman on the other end will meet him for sexual relations. The obscene letter writer is further removed from the object of his sexual desire.

Still further away from the object of his sexual desire is the fetishist, who is interested in his sexual object only through a displacement to a part of her clothing—a shoe, a stocking, underwear, or a brassiere. Often, the fetishist is one who is able to achieve orgasm only through masturbation with the object of the fetish nearby.

These deviations are primarily, but not exclusively, male behaviors. Frequently, the exhibitionist masturbates as he is exposing himself, as does the voyeur as he is peeping. Occasionally, they return to their homes and fantasy the experience of either exposing or watching and then masturbate to the fantasy. These deviations are usually conducted alone.

Wife swapping, especially if conducted in public or if the sexual relations are viewed by the other spouses, may be seen as having sexual deviational qualities. Ménage à trois, in which two persons of the same sex and one of the opposite sex perform sexual acts on each other, reveals homosexual, voyeuristic and exhibitionistic tendencies. Group rape has homosexual qualities in that a number of men are inserting their genitals into the same receptacle and sharing a fairly intimate activity.

Rape

Rape is the penetration of the female by the male genital by means of force, fraud, or fear. Rape may be regarded as a fusion of aggressive and sexual impulses. Others see rape as a vehicle for the expression of hostility, especially toward women. Often, rape is not considered a sexual deviation unless it is aggravated or there is force attached. Some men are repeated rapists and have a compulsive urge to harm the

object of their sexual relations. This may be an expression of a need to expiate guilt and hostility toward the seductive mother.

Lust Murder

Lust murder or rape murder cases are rare and often occur in clusters or groups. Often, the victims are prostitutes or women the rapist finds to be immoral. In these cases, the rape comes first; the murder may be conducted at the time of the rape or shortly after it. Necrophilia, sexual intercourse with a corpse, is seen rarely but most frequently after a murder.

Sadomasochism

The sadist wishes to express harm or gain sexual satisfaction from harming another person. The masochist gains sexual gratification by experiencing pain before, during, or after a sexual act. Sometimes, the sexual pain is in lieu of sexual relationships. There are far fewer sadists than masochists. Often, sadists are prostitutes who get paid for acting sadistic. Masochists are most often men who enjoy being flagellated, bound, whipped, or insulted as a preliminary to sexual relationships. Many men prefer to undergo their masochistic experiences while dressed in women's clothes.

Sodomy

Sodomy refers to pederasty or anal intercourse between homosexuals. Sodomy is also used for abnormal acts with animals, which are now called bestiality or zoophilia.

Transvestism

The transvestite, usually a man, obtains sexual pleasure by wearing the clothing of the opposite sex and often by masturbating while so dressed. This deviation is related to castration anxiety; the man reassures himself that the woman has a penis because he is the embodiment of that conclusion. The transvestite is often homosexual; he may also reveal fetishistic and masochistic aspects.

The transvestite in adolescence may pose a danger to his own life. Occasionally, death results from strangulation when the adolescent boy dresses up in his mother's clothes and attempts to achieve orgasm by strangulation with one of her stockings. In many cases, the deviate goes too far and dies from strangulation shortly after orgasm.

Pedophilia

Pedophilia is a sexual desire for children. It may be homosexual or heterosexual. The greatest amount of pedophilic behavior is in families or among friends and neighbors. Often, it is a one-time activity in which a man who has been denied or deprived of adult female sexual gratification becomes intoxicated and turns to children.

The pedophile may feel impotent or unable to perform adequately with women. Unconscious feelings of hostility, resentment, and vindictiveness toward women may be expressed in the pedophilic behavior.

Exhibitionism

The exhibitionist compulsively exposes himself to others, often young women, in order to note their shocked response at the sight of his penis. The dynamics behind exhibitionism and pedophilia is often similar. There is a fear of castration and the need to reassure oneself that one is able to perform. Rarely does an exhibitionist succeed in enticing a woman to have relations with him by exposing his penis to her. In fact, if a woman were to show interest in the exhibitionist, the great majority would run the other way, preferring not to have to prove what they already fear, that they are sexually inadequate. Thus, they choose a victim who is unlikely to offer this type of confrontation.

Bestiality

The human being who engages in bestiality or zoophilia achieves sexual gratification by having intercourse with a living animal. In Kinsey's sampling, intercourse with animals was the least frequent form of human sexual behavior; it was most common in the preadolescent years and in rural areas. One-third of the males who lived in rural areas and were in the upper educational level had had sexual intercourse with an animal to the point of orgasm.

The animal symbolizes the phallus. Identification with a small animal gratifies the wish for tender, loving care that the helpless animal (child) requires; a large animal enables identification with the parental role in the child-parent relationship.

Hypersexuality

This condition in men (satyriasis) or women (nymphomania) is characterized by an excessive and constant preoccupation with the desire for coitus. It is usually associated with compulsive masturbation. It may result from organic dysfunction—such as temporal lobe disorders, cerebral syphilis, or excessive use of drugs, particularly marihuana, cocaine and testosterone. Psychological causes include the need to prove one's masculinity or femininity, the search for intimacy and love, and unresolved oedipal conflicts in which the person is searching unconsciously for the opposite-sex parent.

Excretory Perversions

Coprophilia

Sexual pleasure associated with the desire to defecate on a partner or to be defecated on or to eat feces (coprophagia) is associated with fixation at the anal stage of psychosexual development. Symbolically, the person attempts to deny castration fears by the equation feces = penis. A variant of the perversion is the compulsive utterance of obscene words (coprolalia), in which the person attempts to master sexual fears by magical incantations. Coprolalia is also associated with Gilles de la Tourette's disease, with accompanying spasmodic tics and echolalia.

Urolagnia

Sexual pleasure associated with the desire to urinate on a partner or to be urinated on is a form of urethral eroticism. It has been observed in persons who were overprotected by mothers with extreme ambitions for their children. Urethral eroticism may be associated with masturbatory techniques involving the insertion of foreign objects into the urethra for sexual stimulation in both men and women.

Treatment

The law may mandate psychiatric treatment for sexual offenders. Men are sometimes placed in group psychotherapy and are able to learn from each other about controlling or regulating their behavior. Usually, the sexual deviation is not cured by the treatment, but behavior is regulated so that the offender does not get into further difficulty with the law. Treatment for many of the deviations is quite difficult, especially if there is a fixation at an early level of psychosexual development. The person who has expressed his deviation under stress or under the influence of alcohol, leading to a temporary regression, is a much more successful candidate for treatment. More often than not, he learns what stresses bother him and how he has traditionally handled the stress by drinking, producing regressive sexual behavior.

REFERENCES

Freud, S. Three essays on the theory of sexuality. In *Standard Edition of the Complete Psychological Works of Sigmund Freud*, vol. 7, p. 123. Hogarth Press, London, 1953.
Mohr, J. W., Turner, R. E., and Jerry, M. D. *Pedophilia and Exhibitionism*. University of Toronto Press, Toronto, 1964.
Peters, J. J., and Sadoff, R. L. Clinical observations of child molesters. Med. Asp. Hum. Sex., *4:* 20, 1970.
Sadoff, R. L. Sexually deviated offenders. Temple Law Q., *40:* 205, 1967.
Slovenko, R. *Sexual Behavior and the Law*. Charles C. Thomas, Springfield, Ill., 1965.

23.11. TREATMENT OF SEXUAL DISORDERS

Introduction

Sexual counseling programs—patterned on the therapy at the Reproductive Biology Research Foundation in St. Louis, Missouri, offered by William Masters and Virginia Johnson—are springing up throughout the country. Most of these programs accept only married couples for treatment. Basic to the therapy is the concept of the marital-unit problem. Both partners are involved in a relationship in which there is sexual distress, and both, therefore, must participate in the therapy program.

Presenting complaints may include premature ejaculation, primary or secondary impotence, or ejaculatory incompetence in the man; lack of orgasmic response, dyspareunia, and vaginismus in the woman; and general sexual incompatibility resulting from lack of interest or desire in either the man or the woman. The presenting sexual problem often reflects other areas of disharmony or misunderstanding in the marriage. The marital relationship as a whole is treated, with emphasis on sexual functioning as a part of that relationship. Psychological and physiological aspects of sexual functioning are discussed, and an educative attitude is used.

Suggestions are made for specific sexual activity, and these suggestions are followed in the privacy of the couple's home.

The crux of the program is the roundtable session in which a male-and-female therapy team clarifies, discusses, and works through the problems with the couple. These four-way sessions require active participation on the part of the patients. The aim of the therapy is to establish or re-establish communication within the marital unit.

The therapy team approach is an essential part of the treatment plan. The woman of the patient couple is represented by the female therapist and the man by the male therapist. In this type of treatment, support, challenge, criticism, and encouragement are best accepted when offered by the therapist of the same sex. And a patient may really listen to his or her mate's words for the first time when they are restated or represented by the opposite-sex therapist.

Treatment is short-term and behaviorally oriented. The co-therapists attempt to reflect the situation as they see it, rather than interpret underlying dynamics. An undistorted picture of the relationship presented by a dual-sex team often corrects the myopic, narrow view held individually by each marriage partner.

Couples undergo thorough physical and psychological examinations before therapy proceeds. Initial histories are taken to determine suitability for this type of treatment. When there is evidence of major underlying psychopathology, further psychiatric evaluation is suggested, and participation in the program may be deferred until the patient seems more able to benefit from it. Concurrent psychotherapy with a psychiatrist while participating in these programs is frequently recommended.

Each patient is interviewed individually by both the male therapist and the female therapist before the roundtable sessions. A complete sexual history is obtained, and this history is later reflected back to the couple, with the aim of helping them understand their present problem. The individual sessions also enable the therapists to understand the lifestyle of the patients and enable them to make suggestions that fit into that lifestyle.

Specific exercises are prescribed for the couple to help them with their particular problem.

Most forms of sexual inadequacy involve lack of information, misinformation, and fear of performance. The couples are, therefore, specifically prohibited from any sexual play other than that prescribed by the therapists. Beginning exercises usually focus on heightening sensory awareness to touch, sight, sound, and smell. Initially, intercourse is interdicted, and couples learn to give and receive bodily pleasure without the pressure of performance. They are simultaneously learning how to communicate nonverbally in a mutually satisfactory way and learning that sexual foreplay is as important as intercourse and orgasm. Genital stimulation is eventually added to general body stimulation. The couple are instructed sequentially to try various positions for intercourse, without necessarily completing the union, and to use varieties of stimulating techniques before they are instructed to proceed with intercourse. The approaches vary with different presenting complaints, but the over-all goal is always to initiate an educational process, to diminish fears of performance felt by both sexes, and to facilitate communication.

Roundtable sessions follow each new exercise period, and problems and satisfactions, both sexual and in other areas of the couple's lives, are discussed. Specific instructions and the introduction of new exercises geared to the individual couple's progress are reviewed in each session. Gradually, the couple gain confidence and learn or relearn to communicate, verbally and sexually.

Specific instructions are given in the areas of verbal and nonverbal communication. Couples are urged to set aside prescribed periods each day just to talk to each other in order to overcome frequent patterns of withdrawal into silence or busy work. As far as possible, phone conversations, involvement with children, and television watching are banned during these periods of time. The couples are also taught techniques of communication that can help them keep in touch with their own feelings and express them to their partners. Each is encouraged to start as many sentences as possible with the word "I" and to question his or her mate directly, rather than to guess what the partner is thinking or feeling. The couples are also urged to use their angry feelings as a signal that they are severely threatened or hurt and to explore their anger within that framework. The

need to be vulnerable to one's mate if there is to be effective communication is stressed throughout the sessions.

Impotence

Sexual functioning in men is influenced by complex conscious and unconscious psychic factors, by such physiological factors as neurological and endocrine status and age, and by such sociocultural factors as income and education and the prevailing sexual mores and attitudes about women. These are all taken into account before dual-sex therapy. The patient is physically examined and questioned as to type and quantity of drug intake, and he undergoes laboratory tests, psychological tests, and a psychiatric interview.

After the initial history taking and examination, the couple and the dual-sex team proceed with the roundtable sessions. A good portion of these sessions deal with the extrasexual interaction of the couple to enable them to work through daily or long-standing hostilities, misunderstandings, and fears and to increase their communication. At the same time, they are given specific instructions in how to communicate physically. When impotence is the main complaint, intercourse is forbidden, and the couple begin with a series of nongenital caressing exercises. The couple's approach to and interaction during these exercises are often a microcosm of their usual way of relating. The man and the woman are alternately assigned the role of initiating a session of caressing, so that the responsibility for their sexual interaction is shared and does not rest with one partner. With emphasis removed not only from intercourse but from the genitalia, the couple relearn the more general pleasures of touching each other. The man, in particular, is relieved of the pressure to perform, and this relief is often enough to allow him to gain an erection quite easily. The couple next includes genital stimulation in their sessions of physical caressing, with each alternately guiding the partner's hand in the patterns of touch found most pleasing. At this stage, the patients may manipulate each other to orgasm when they so desire.

When the couple have had enough good sexual experiences without intercourse and can tolerate the idea of an unsuccessful coital experience, they are advised to try intercourse. The burden of the union is lightened for the man in that the woman is instructed to assume the superior position and encouraged to take charge of inserting the man's penis into her vagina. At this time, when the man has been achieving erections for several weeks and is able to sustain it through insertion and entry, the pathology of the woman may often emerge more clearly. She may balk at accepting equal responsibility for their sexual interactions or responsibility for her own sexuality. When the couple are quite at ease with insertion and entry, they are instructed to carry intercourse as far as they care to, including orgasm.

Setbacks are examined and learned from, and the couple are encouraged to take an optimistic attitude and to rely on sexual techniques not involving intercourse during difficult periods. The experience that sexual satisfaction can be achieved in other ways and the equal valuation of alternative methods by the therapists continue to relieve the man of performance pressure and the woman of her frustrations.

Unconsummated Marriage

Couples come with this complaint after suffering lack of consummation for periods varying from several months to several years. This is an unusually easy disorder to treat. The couple determined to remain together in spite of extreme sexual difficulties are highly motivated and make good material for this type of treatment. Typically, both husband and wife are misinformed or uninformed regarding all areas of sexuality and are very inexperienced. Sexual prohibitions absorbed from parents and society and lack of sexual education play large parts in the unconsummated marriage.

The couple are educated jointly about their sexual anatomy and physiology. They are then instructed in techniques of foreplay and genital stimulation. Initial prohibition of intercourse allays the usually present fear of penetration in the woman until she becomes more comfortable with her own sexuality. It also relieves performance pressure from the man. It is vital, early in therapy, to make clear that successful intercourse depends on both partners, as it is usually the husband in these cases who has assumed total responsibility for the couple's failure to function sexually. The wife is instructed early in treatment on the techniques of masturbation and is encouraged to enjoy her own sexuality. If she suffers from vaginismus, she is instructed in

the use of size-graded dilators. Fears of or desires for pregnancy in both partners are also discussed.

Usually, the immediate relief of pressure to have intercourse, a sound sexual education, contraceptive advice, dilators patiently used to alleviate vaginal constriction, and the presence of authority figures (in the form of the therapists) who encourage sexual interaction enable the couple to make rapid progress in treatment and to consummate their union.

The couple are advised to have intercourse first in the male superior position, as this position is generally most acceptable to both partners. The wife is, nonetheless, expected to help her husband during the process of intromission. Once successful intercourse has been experienced, the couple are able to repeat the experience with less and less anxiety. Follow-up sessions are held to help the couple through inevitable setbacks until they are secure enough to sustain an occasional unsuccessful attempt at coitus. At that point they are discharged.

Premature Ejaculation

In premature ejaculation the man arrives at orgasm and ejaculation before he wishes to do so. His dissatisfaction invariably relates to his having ejaculated and lost his erection before his sexual partner has reached orgasm.

The first step in treating this complaint is to re-establish a climate of comfort and acceptance for the couple's sexual interaction. By the time the couple come for treatment, the husband's sense of inadequacy and the wife's sense of frustration have usually led to a pattern of infrequent intercourse. The man is encouraged to masturbate, and a moratorium is placed on intercourse. The couple are re-educated to enjoy touch and body stimulation in general. When the anxiety of physical closeness has been diminished, they are instructed to proceed to genital stimulation and then intercourse and are simultaneously given specific techniques to deal with the premature ejaculation.

The man or the wife stimulates the erect penis until the premonitory sensations of impending orgasm and ejaculation are felt. The penile stimulation is stopped abruptly. Sexual excitement and possibly the erection subside over the course of the ensuing minutes. The stimulation is then started again and, as before, is stopped at the first sensation of impending orgasm. This technique appears to train the threshold of excitability to be more tolerant of the stimuli. This exercise is done two or three times a day for 20 to 30 minutes. After several days coitus is usually prolonged.

Reducing the tactile component involves reducing the amount or the intensity of vaginal friction or reducing the excitability of the receptor organs in the glans penis. Some find condoms to be a solution to their problem of premature ejaculation. The amount of vaginal friction may also be reduced by limiting the frequency of thrusts or the extent of penis travel within the vagina.

The female co-therapist must enlist the wife's cooperation in treating this complaint. With the knowledge that her own sexual needs will eventually be better met, with emphasis on the fact that the problem has been beyond the husband's conscious control, and with encouragement of manual stimulation and satisfaction of the wife by the husband, the wife is usually able to be a constructive part of the treatment program.

Vaginismus and Dyspareunia

Dyspareunia, painful or difficult sexual intercourse, and vaginismus, an involuntary spasm of the muscles surrounding the vagina that results in constriction of the vagina, are differentiated from frigidity, but the same underlying fear, hostility, and guilt lead to these consequences. Dyspareunia and vaginismus are less prevalent than frigidity and generally indicate the presence of more severe pathology.

In vaginismus, the involuntary muscle spasm that prevents penile penetration and renders coitus impossible may express the force with which the woman desires to prevent penile entrance into her body. Her perception of the male sexual organ as a dangerous weapon leads her to lose her capacity for sensation. Her concern with her inability to participate in sexual intercourse reinforces her distress and her fears that she is unfeminine or homosexual. Similarly, in dyspareunia the psychogenic fear of anticipated pain makes intercourse unbearable or unpleasant.

Ideally, the therapeutic plan includes education of both partners to increased awareness of sexual technique and relationship pitfalls and increased understanding of the part that each partner plays in the problem of the other. Social and internal pressures that characterize female development in society; ignorance of sexual techniques; moral, religious, and parental prohibitions; fear of dependency and of the expression of aggressive impulses; and excessive guilt and fear of coitus—all impinge on the freedom of the woman to develop her capacity for sexual pleasure.

A vital part of the treatment of vaginismus is the physical examination, with the husband present so that he is able to see the spasm of muscles resulting in constriction of the vagina. The involuntary nature of this spasm is explained to him by the therapist to lessen his feeling of rejection and to enable him to be supportive and encouraging of his wife throughout treatment. Intercourse is initially prohibited, relieving the wife of fears of penetration, pain, and her own sense of inadequacy and relieving the husband of his frustrations in literally coming up against a wall. The couple are then able to enjoy each other physically in a nongenital manner.

The wife is encouraged to take responsibility for her own problems and is taught to introduce dilators into her vagina in graduated sizes, beginning with a narrow size that could easily be accommodated by a virgin. Since she is performing these exercises herself, she is controlling the anxiety that may be caused by conscious or unconscious rape fantasies, by fear of hurting herself, and by her own vaginal manipulation, and she can stop the exercise at any time. The husband is thus relieved of the role of intruder or aggressor, and she is literally placed in touch with her own sexuality and encouraged to be conscious of it. Treatment usually proceeds rapidly, and intercourse is allowed only when the wife is comfortable with insertion of the largest size in the series of dilators. By that time she has also become more comfortable with her husband's penis through exercises in which she has manually stimulated him to orgasm.

With dyspareunia, thorough obstetrical examination is necessary to assure both the patient and the therapist that there is no physical cause for the woman's pain. The couple can then be informed that the dyspareunia is a result of lack of sufficient lubrication and excitement in the woman, involuntary muscle spasm—as in vaginismus—or sensation perceived as pain for psychological reasons.

With the initial prohibition of intercourse, the wife is relieved of her fears of penetration and anticipation of pain and is able to learn to relax and enjoy herself in sexual situations with her husband. The prohibition of intercourse may allow her to respond to other genital stimulation. This response enables the husband to learn what is most stimulating to her sexually and to restore the confidence he may have lost during their previous distressing sexual encounters.

Before the couple have intercourse, the husband is satisfied by the wife with either manual or oral manipulation of his genitals. In addition to fulfilling his needs, this manipulation enables the wife to be giving and active sexually and to become comfortable with her husband's genitalia.

She is encouraged to explore herself and to masturbate, and her husband also stimulates her manually before intercourse is attempted. At the first attempt at intercourse during treatment, a sterile lubricant may be prescribed to facilitate entry.

The female superior position is used during coitus because it accentuates the active role being cultivated in the woman and seems less threatening to women who approach intercourse with fear. In addition, the husband is free to play with the rest of her body in the ways that he has learned to please her. Only after the couple can achieve intromission easily and with pleasure do they proceed to movement and eventually to completion.

Nonorgasm

Frigidity or sexual anesthesia designates a variety of sexual disorders related to the inhibition of female sexual response, ranging from unsatisfactory orgasm but otherwise vigorous sexual response to complete lack of response to sexual stimulation.

Nonorgasm refers specifically to the inability to achieve orgasm by means of masturbation or coitus. The psychological factors associated with nonorgasm are variously ascribed to fear of impregnation, fear of rejection by the sexual partner, envy or hostility toward the man, guilt regarding the impropriety of the sex act, and fear of mutilation.

Unresponsiveness may be used as a weapon against the man. To the woman who feels inferior and, therefore, hostile toward the man, sexual nonparticipation may be a bid for independence. Frigidity may also be a defense against earlier unacceptable impulses, such as competitiveness with the mother and forbidden sexual fantasies. Orgasm may also be equated with loss of control and with aggressive, destructive, or violent behavior. Fear of these impulses contributes to sexual inhibition.

In dual-sex therapy, the nonorgasmic woman is educated about her sexual anatomy and physiology in conjunction with her partner. The man is instructed in the techniques of foreplay, particularly genital stimulation. In addition, the woman receives specific instructions in masturbatory techniques and may experience her first orgasm by this method.

She then shares with her husband what she has learned through self-stimulation. The couple proceed slowly from general body and genital stimulation to penile penetration, with the woman in the female superior position. This position allows her freedom of movement and facilitates a teasing technique, in which intercourse is interrupted by periods of rest and nongenital body contact. These enforced interruptions allow for progressive stimulation without the demand for a climax. The man is usually brought to orgasm manually or orally during these sessions. Only toward the end of treatment, when the woman has been able to achieve climax with manual stimulation are the couple instructed to complete intercourse.

Retarded Ejaculation

This disorder is characterized by the inability to achieve orgasm, even though the erection is satisfactory. At times, retarded ejaculation is selective. The man is able to achieve orgasm as a result of masturbation but not during coitus. There are usually severe conflicts present in these men, including deep-seated fears of women. In some, histories of incest with the mother are found. Hostility toward or fear of women and unconscious confusion of the wife with the mother are the dynamics most often encountered.

The couples are treated in an authoritarian, behavioral manner. Increased communication helps clear up projections and distorted percep-

TABLE I

*Success Rate Summary**

Complaint	Success Rate (%)
Male	
Premature ejaculation	97
Retarded ejaculation	72
Secondary impotence	69
Primary impotence	49
Female	
Masturbatory orgasmic dysfunction	91
Primary orgasmic dysʼunction	82
Coital orgasmic dysfunction	80

* After Masters and Johnson data.

tions of the opposite sex.

The support of the woman must be enlisted if therapy is to succeed. The way the woman plays into her husband's problem may emerge and be dealt with as treatment progresses. Physically, the couple move first to general caressing and then to genital caressing. The wife is guided by her husband to stimulate him satisfactorily. The couple stay with manual stimulation until the husband is thoroughly comfortable in coming to orgasm in front of his wife this way. The couple continue manual stimulation until the husband feels that he is approaching orgasm. Only then does he attempt penetration. Once he has been able to ejaculate in his partner's vagina, successive attempts become easier, with the man being able to enter the woman earlier in sexual play.

Results

Masters and Johnson report that about 80 per cent of persons treated for all types of sexual dysfunction have a successful outcome with the dual-sex therapy method. This figure has been replicated at other centers. There is variability in the success rate according to the particular disorder, as indicated in Table 1.

REFERENCES

Finkie, A. L., and Moyers, T. G. Sexual potency in aging males. J. Urol., *84:* 152, 1960.
Hastings, D. W. *Impotence and Frigidity.* Little, Brown, Boston, 1963.
Kinsey, A. C., Pomeroy, W. B., Martin, C. E., and Gebhard, P. *Sexual Behavior in the Human Male.* W. B. Saunders, Philadelphia, 1948.
Kinsey, A. C., Pomeroy, W. B., Martin C. E., and Gebhard, P. *Sexual Behavior in the Human Female.* W. B. Saunders, Philadelphia, 1953.
Masters, W. H., and Johnson, V. E. *Human Sexual Response.* Little, Brown, Boston, 1966.
Masters, W. H., and Johnson, V. E. *Human Sexual Inadequacy.* Little, Brown, Boston, 1970.

23.12. SEX AND THE LAW

Sex Offenders

As defined by the law, a sex offender is a person who commits a crime involving the expression of sexual urges. These offenses traditionally include rape, indecent assault, incest, assault with intent to commit sodomy, sodomy, assault with intent to ravish or rape, indecent exposure, child molestation, and homosexual assaults. A number of sexual deviations—including transvestitism, fetishism, and coprophilia—are not considered sex offenses.

The law has tended to group all persons committing crimes with sexual connotations into a class of criminals called "sex offenders" or "sexual psychopaths." Since 1938, a number of states have passed sexual psychopath statutes, which are aimed at the protection of society and the treatment of the offender. Most of these laws impose indeterminate sentences on the offender and provide for treatment or rehabilitation in a hospital or prison. But not all sex offenders are alike. A classification system has been suggested by Ellis and Brancale:

1. Normal sex offenders, who are not sexual deviates but who commit illegal sex acts.

2. Sex deviates who commit illegal sex acts but who are sufficiently stable and well-integrated to maintain their deviational patterns without usually getting into legal difficulty.

3. Sexually and psychiatrically deviated offenders who commit illegal sex acts and who are so emotionally disturbed and mentally impaired that they frequently come to legal attention.

4. Psychiatrically disordered but sexually nondeviated offenders who commit illicit sex acts because of their general disturbances and who are often apprehended.

The most recidivistic sex offense is exhibitionism, and that offense usually does not progress to more serious sexual crimes. The general recidivism rate of all sex offenses is low compared with other crimes.

Homosexuality

Homosexual behavior is illegal in all states except one, Illinois, where homosexual behavior between consenting adults has been decriminalized. Vice squads in police departments are active in rooting out homosexuals in the community. It is not true that there is greater violence in homosexual triangles than in heterosexual triangles. In the military, homosexual behavior is prohibited, ostensibly because of the fear of exposure and blackmail.

The danger of homosexual behavior exists in forced situations between adults and in adults' enticing children or adolescents to perform homosexual acts. Forced relationships and relationships with youngsters continue to be prohibited in all jurisdictions. The penalties for homosexual behavior appear to be excessively harsh, and the methods of arresting often seem underhanded.

Some homosexuals prefer to dress in women's clothes and may be harassed and accused of disturbing the peace or being nuisances.

Prostitution

Prostitution is defined as sexual activity for pay. It includes all forms of sexual encounter, homosexual and heterosexual. There are two principal types of heterosexual prostitutes:

1. Street prostitutes abound in large cities, where they accost men on the street. Many of these women are frequently arrested.

2. The private prostitute is contracted by a middleman or a pimp, who sets up private arrangements with women in their own apartments. Other prostitutes working privately make their own arrangements with repeat customers.

In many municipalities in this country, prostitution was allowed until recently. One municipality in Nevada openly supports prostitution and is proud of the medical attention it gives its tourist attractions. However, in most communities, prostitution is outlawed, and police vice squads round up prostitutes and get them off the streets. England attempted to regulate prostitution after the Wolfenden Report indicated that discreet prostitution was tolerable but that open lewdness on the street was not to be accepted. Criminal laws against prostitution are relatively ineffective.

Rape

Rape may be defined as sexual intercourse by use of force, fear, or fraud between persons of the same sex or the opposite sex. Homosexual rape occurs primarily in closed institutions, such as prisons and maximum-security hospitals. Homosexual rape is more frequent among men than among women and usually denotes a hostile, aggressive attitude, rather than a sexual one. The rapist often does not see himself as a homosexual but sees the victim as a passive homosexual.

Heterosexual rape is defined in the law as penetration of the penis beyond the introitus. Whether ejaculation occurs is irrelevant. By definition, a man who cannot have an erection is unable to commit rape. Oral sex is not rape; neither are other indecent touchings or assaults. In the law, rape is seen as a very serious offense. Some jurisdictions have a classification called aggravated rape, which includes rape by force with a deadly weapon or harm or assault in addition to rape.

Statutory rape refers to unlawful sexual intercourse between a male over the age of 16 and a female under the age of consent, which varies from 14 to 21, depending on the jurisdiction. This type of rape is not seen as a deviation, except when the age discrepancy is excessive, in which case the deviation is called pedophilia. In pedophilia the age discrepancy must be in excess of 10 years or the girl must be 12 or younger.

In rape prosecutions the victim has to be examined by a physician to prove that there has been penetration, evidence of semen at the time of her complaint, or evidence of bruises or other physical damage as a result of the assault. Often, the victim encounters negative attitudes by police and other examiners, who question whether she enjoyed it and test to see whether she succumbed to temptation or was actually forced into a sexual act.

Usually, the rapist is a one-timer who uses poor judgment or forces the issue under the influence of alcohol or drugs. At other times, he is a repetitive, aggressive person who has a pattern of uncontrollable reaction. Lust murderers, those who rape and then kill their victims are rare.

Castration

In some places in the world, sex offenders of serious aggressive tendencies are castrated to allow them to return to the community without danger to others. Many sex offenders would prefer to be castrated, rather than be locked up for the rest of their lives, as some laws have mandated. However, the American Civil Liberties Union and other civil rights groups have questioned whether it is appropriate for these men to have to make such a choice and whether their freedom to give informed consent to the procedure is abrogated by undue coercion by virtue of the indefinite or indeterminate sentence.

Sterilization

Sterilization procedures render a person incapable of reproduction. In a man the sterilization procedure is usually accomplished by vasectomy, a ligation of the vas deferens. For a woman the sterilization procedure is a tubal ligation, a ligation of her fallopian tubes.

Some states use legal formulae to determine whether a voluntary sterilization of a woman should be allowed. In one state, the formula is a multiplication of the woman's age by the number of her children; if that number is 100 or more, she may have the procedure. Sterilizing an unwed woman occasionally presents problems in the event that she marries and her husband wishes to have children. The husband-to-be must be informed that the woman is sterile. If he is not informed, he may file for annulment on the basis of fraud or concealment of essential information.

In the event of a failure of the sterilization procedure and a resultant pregnancy, there may be a lawsuit against the physician who performed the procedure unless he has carefully advised the couple that there is a minimal risk of becoming pregnant again. Voluntary sterilization produces relatively few legal ramifications.

Eugenic sterilization—the sterilization of men and women to prevent certain characteristics from being passed on to offspring—is usually designed for mentally retarded women. Schizophrenic women are also encouraged to have sterilization.

Many statutes have provided for sterilization of hereditary criminals, sex offenders, syphilitics, the mentally retarded, and epileptics. The American Civil Liberties Union and other human rights groups have been challenging the legality and ethical considerations of such sterilization procedures.

Bigamy

Bigamy is the condition of having two spouses; having more than two spouses is called polygamy. Bigamy has been outlawed in the United States.

In some cultures and some jurisdictions, common-law marriage is recognized without benefit of license or clergy. If two people of opposite sex present themselves as married, particularly if they raise a family, they may be assumed to have the same rights and liabilities as legally married people. In some areas, the cost of obtaining a divorce is prohibitive, and people may separate without obtaining a valid divorce certificate. The understanding is that they are divorced or separated and free to find other mates. Occasionally, a man marries another woman before he has achieved a valid divorce from his first wife and does not mention his previous marriage to anyone. Under the law, the second marriage is invalid if it is contested.

Another type of unintentional bigamy is the case of a man who falls into a fugue state from a neurotic dissociative reaction and leaves his home and family to seek a new life. He may be unaware that he has been previously married and may take a second wife and raise a family with her. If it is discovered that he has a first wife and children living, the second marriage is null and void. However, he may not be charged with deliberate bigamy, which is a misdemeanor, because it may be shown that his fugue state or dissociative reaction led to a loss of memory, for which he cannot be held consciously responsible.

Illegitimacy

The term "illegitimacy" refers to both parents and children. A mother is not usually referred to as an illegitimate mother because she bears the child and is the natural parent. However, the natural father who is not legally married to the mother of the child is called the illegitimate father. The child is referred to as an illegitimate child, born out of wedlock. Any child born to a married woman is considered the legitimate offspring of the woman's husband, whether or not it was medically possible for the husband to have fathered the child.

Until recently, the illegitimate child had no legal rights. He could not inherit from his father, nor could he take his father's name. The law, in its attempt to legitimize as many children as possible, has liberalized its formerly stringent views on illegitimate relationships.

Ordinarily, the mother of the child had the right and the option to keep the child or give him out for foster care. The illegitimate father was never consulted, nor did he have any rights in this regard. In a recent case, the Supreme Court of Illinois declared that the illegitimate father has special rights to his natural child and that the child has rights to his natural father.

Artificial Insemination

Artificial insemination is the injection of viable sperm into the vagina of a woman to induce a pregnancy. This is done by artificial means. The sperm may be from a donor or may be the woman's husband's sperm, condensed to make it more viable. In some cases, the donor's and the husband's sperm are mixed, so as to leave open the question of biological paternity.

The child born of artificial insemination has all the rights of a natural child and is legitimized. All records of the procedure—in most states a legal release is required of both husband and wife—are kept confidential. Artificial insemination is used almost exclusively with married women with the consent of their husbands. If a woman is impregnated by artificial means without the consent of her husband, a legal battle may ensue in which the husband may disown the child.

Abortion

Abortion is the termination of pregnancy, which can be spontaneous or induced. Induced abortions can be therapeutic or criminal. Until recently, all induced abortions that were not performed to save the life of the mother were considered illegal. In 1973 the United States Supreme Court held the following:

1. The decision to have an abortion during the first three months of pregnancy and the manner in which it is performed are dependent solely upon the medical judgment of the physician and may not be prohibited by the state.

2. Until viability—that is, between the twenty-fourth and the twenty-eight week of pregnancy—the state may regulate abortion procedures.

3. After the twenty-eight week the state may regulate or forbid abortion, unless medical judgment indicates to the contrary for the life or health of the mother.

REFERENCES

Ellis, A., and Brancale, R. *The Psychology of Sex Offenders.* Charles C. Thomas, Springfield, Ill., 1956.
Gagnon, J., and Simon, W., editors. *Sexual Deviance.* Harper & Row, New York, 1967.
Ploscowe, M. *Sex and the Law,* Ace Books, New York, 1962.
Sadoff, R. L. Sexually deviated offenders. Temple Law Q., *40:* 92, 1967.
Tappan, P. Some myths about the sex offender. Fed. Proc., *19:* 7, 1955.
Wolfenden Report. Lancer Books, New York, 1964.

24

Transient Situational Disturbances

24.1. ADJUSTMENT REACTION OF ADULT LIFE

Introduction

Psychiatrists do not know how many or what kinds of acute situational disturbances turn into chronic psychiatric or medical illnesses or contribute to other disabling but undiagnosed problems of living. They do know that chronic psychiatric illness and enduring life problems are difficult and costly to treat; a critical issue is the extent to which these problems would have been transient if treated earlier and more appropriately. Situational disturbances and adjustment reactions usually call for crisis intervention.

Primary crisis intervention occurs, for example, with persons given primary care by family physicians or in a general medical emergency department. They may receive crisis-oriented support during a bereavement or after the diagnosis of a serious physical illness has been made. Other life crises—such as loss of employment, severe marital disputes, and divorce—are mostly handled by the troubled persons themselves or with the assistance of friends, clergymen, the police, lawyers, family agencies, school counselors, and family physicians.

At a somewhat later point in crisis situations, after a patient has been identified, psychiatrists are more likely to be called in as consultants or therapists. Crisis intervention at this point is secondary prevention. The most common situation is attempted or threatened suicide. The diagnostic category of transient situational disturbances is a token acknowledgment of the existence of these problems.

Official Diagnostic Criteria

The second edition of the American Psychiatric Association's *Diagnostic and Statistical Manual of Mental Disorders* (DSM-II) specifies that the primary causative factor in transient situational disturbances is overwhelming environmental stress. Examples of overwhelming stress include an unwanted pregnancy and military combat. The subcategories of transient situational disturbances are called adjustment reactions, a term that implies that ordinary life events may be implicated. However, the criterion specifying that stress be overwhelming is thereby blurred if not contradicted.

DSM-II may cause confusion by specifying that the category of transient situational disorders be used only with persons "without any apparent underlying mental disorders." The question then arises: Why should the presence of a pre-existing or underlying disorder make the category of situational disturbance less useful? More importantly, the question of whether a precipitating event has occurred is valuable information, whether or not there is another disorder.

Although the DSM-II criterion of an acute onset seems clear enough, in practice this guideline often becomes difficult to apply. Problems of living accumulate, and situational disturbances are not necessarily acute in the sense of sudden onset; chronic situational reactions occur with chronic stress and are frequent in large segments of the population.

In DSM-II, no symptomatic criteria for situational disturbances are specified. DSM-II allows for disorders of "any severity (including those of psychotic proportions)." A symptomatic diagnosis can and probably always should accompany the diagnosis of situational disturbance.

DMS-II specifies that, if "the symptoms persist after the stress is removed, the diagnosis of another mental disorder is indicated." This recommendation, together with the qualifying term "transient," makes outcome, rather than prognosis, a diagnostic criterion. Most situational reactions are of brief duration. However, all follow-up studies of the bereaved, of disaster victims, and of concentration camp survivors show that a portion do have symptoms that are far from transient. It would be advantageous to retain the diagnosis of situational reaction and to examine the treatment of those situations and persons with disturbances that persist.

Diagnostic Usage

The Cumulative Psychiatric Case Register in Monroe County, New York, suggests that the DSM-II guideline that this diagnosis should not be used in the presence of an underlying mental disorder was often ignored. The rates for use of the diagnosis of adjustment reaction of adult life show striking differences by population subgroups divided by age, race, and sex (see Table I). By far the highest rate was for nonwhite women in the age range of 25 to 34—11.0 patients per 1,000 population in this demographic group. This rate contrasts with a low of 1.0 patients per 1,000 white men in the age group of 45 to 54. The diagnosis is used more commonly with women, both white and nonwhite, but somewhat more than twice as frequently in nonwhite women as in white women. However, the over-all rates for white men are essentially the same as for nonwhite men. The increase in stress for those in disadvantaged social groups is associated with a marked increase in diagnoses of situational disturbances, but the increase is similar to that found in disadvantaged social groups for all psychiatric diagnoses.

The predominant symptoms in 40 patients given the diagnosis of adjustment reaction of adult life in a 1971 Strong Memorial Hospital

TABLE I

Prevalence Rates* for Adjustment Reaction of Adult Life in Monroe County, New York, for 1971 by Sex and Race

	Men	Women
White	0.85 (2.20)	1.46 (4.28)
Nonwhite	0.88 (1.82)	3.41 (11.00)

* Rates are calculated per 1,000 population in each demographic group. The age range is 21 to 59. Figures for the age range of 25 to 34, which had the highest rates in each group, are given in parentheses.

series were strikingly depressive. During the episodes in which the diagnosis of adult adjustment reaction was given, 80 per cent of the patients had noteworthy depressive symptoms, with nine (22.5 per cent) of them making suicidal attempts. In 35 per cent of the patients, angry, hostile, destructive behavior, often including assaultive violence, characterized part of the symptomatic reaction, with this being the most salient feature in 10 per cent. Only 22.5 per cent of the patients had sufficiently severe anxiety or tension for this symptom to be reported in the case record. But 20 per cent of the patients had psychophysiologic disorders, such as anorexia, headaches, and asthmatic attacks. Another 25 per cent reported severe insomnia. As still another form of symptom manifestation, 22.5 per cent were reported to have a situation-related increase in problems with alcohol. And 10 per cent of the patients had begun or increased their use of illicit drugs during the situational episode.

By far the most frequent kind of precipitating problem for this series of patient was family or marital difficulties. These difficulties were described in the case records as major features of the problem in at least 75 per cent of the cases. Often, the family or marital upheaval involved the loss of a family relationship; 20 per cent of these patients were undergoing an acute grief reaction over the death of one or more family members, and another 37.5 per cent had suffered losses in the form of a recent divorce, a separation, or having their children taken away by a court. Thus, 57.5 per cent of the cases had incurred loss, separation, or death of a family member, which had helped precipitate the acute situational reaction. It is not surprising, then, that depressive symptoms were prominent.

In this series of 40 patients, 27 (67.5 per cent) were given the diagnosis of "adult adjustment reaction," despite having had previous psychiatric contacts. At least 15 had been seen previously with symptoms of depression, often associated with other situational difficulties. Six patients had had previous treatment for alcoholism, all reactivated in the present episode. Four had had problems with drug dependence; two were diagnosed as mentally retarded, one had congenital lues, and three carried diagnoses of chronic schizophrenia, borderline or residual. In addition, 20 (50 per cent) of the patients were described in the case records as having had long-standing personality disorders, previously undiagnosed and untreated.

Crisis Theory and Therapy

Caplan has described four phases in the crisis sequence: First, in the phase of impact, usually lasting from minutes to hours, the person tends to be in a state of dazed shock with emergency fight-flight responses and often considerable disorientation and distractibility. The second phase is typically associated with increasing turmoil, ambiguity, and uncertainty, with a flood of emotions, such as rage, guilt, anxiety, and depression. Previous modes of responding are temporarily either unavailable or ineffectual. In phase three, additional internal and external resources are mobilized. The environment is explored for new opportunities, and processes of reconstructing a new world of activities and relationships are underway, sometimes with certain goals relinquished as unobtainable. The fourth phase involves long-term reconstruction and re-equilibrium, with an outcome that may go in either of two directions. On the one hand, there may be growth and an improved level of functioning; on the other hand, psychological, somatic, or interpersonal disorders may become more or less chronic.

Langsley and Kaplan found that the hospitalization of patients who had been scheduled for admission could be avoided indefinitely by a team approach to families at the point of intake. The patient with the presenting symptoms was seen and treated as part of a disordered or disrupted family system.

Conceptually, crisis theory needs to give greater attention to disequilibrium of social systems. Concepts of transactional interplay between persons and groups in which sequences unfold with the continual, active participation of everyone concerned need to replace the simplistic notion of one-way causal effects manifest in the continuing dichotomy between endogenous and reactive disorders.

Crises of parenthood and changes in middle life may have clear transitional qualities—for example, when an occupational career goal becomes unattainable or ambitions for one's children must be abandoned. In such circumstances, it is appropriate for the therapist to consider whether symptoms are primarily evidence of enduring mental disorder or are adaptive signals indicating a need and readiness for change. Therapy can then be oriented to facilitating and supporting change through the transition if such readiness exists.

Conclusion

The concept of crisis includes developmental transitions having the potential either for pathology or for improved health and altered interpersonal relationships. The adequate understanding of crises requires attention to multilevel transactions, including the biological functioning and the psychodynamics of the person, but also explicit assessment of the social context, especially the family as a small social system.

REFERENCES

Bartolucci, G., and Drayer, C. An overview of crisis intervention in the emergency rooms of general hospitals. Am. J. Psychiatry, *130:* 953, 1973.
Beck, J. C., and Worthen, K. Precipitation stress, crisis theory and hospitalization in schizophrenia and depression. Arch. Gen. Psychiatry, *26:* 123, 1972.
Caplan, G. *Principles of Preventive Psychiatry.* Basic Books, New York, 1964.
Langsley, D., and Kaplan, D. *The Treatment of Families in Crisis.* Grune & Stratton, New York, 1968.
Lindemann, E. Symptomatology and management of acute grief. Am. J. Psychiatry, *101:* 141, 1944.
McPartland, T., and Richart, R. Social and clinical outcomes of physical treatment. Arch. Gen. Psychiatry, *14:* 179, 1966.
Tyhurst, J. The role of transition states—including disasters —in mental illness. In *Symposium on Preventive and Social Psychiatry*, p. 149. U. S. Government Printing Office, Washington, 1957.

24.2.   TRAUMATIC WAR NEUROSIS

Introduction

The term "war neurosis" encompasses a wide variety of abnormal reactions that occur in military personnel in wartime. There has been considerable reluctance to apply diagnoses of neurosis or psychosis to these cases of transient reactions to unusual, severe, or overwhelming military stress. There is a clear-cut relationship between the severity of stress—the real danger of the combat situation—and the chance of emotional breakdown. This premise led to the dictum that every person has his breaking point, that there are limits to the amount of stress each person can tolerate.

Causes

Gillespie noted, for England, that the heaviest air raids of World War II seemed to affect the mental health of the civilian population in a negligible way. In fact, he observed that evacuated children were greater psychiatric problems than were children under the air raids.

In Germany, Bonhoeffer and others felt that war neuroses were caused by secondary psychological mechanisms, such as the wish to escape from danger and eventually to receive compensation. It was the general experience in the German Army that symptoms more often appeared after the danger was over; rarely did they appear during combat. The Germans reported that the majority of cases were depressive reactions, with apathy and psychosomatic complaints. These conditions were treated by limited rest, away from the hospital. In general, it was assumed that a strong preventive factor was provided against war neurosis by the unsympathetic attitude shown by men in the front line toward one who showed "weakness" and "nervous failure."

In France it was theorized that suffering in a group is easier to bear than is individual suffering. If one becomes symptomatic, others undergoing the same ordeal tend to show little sympathy; there is, then, no gain from such symptoms. Restated, one may propose that, in states of emergency, the group becomes more important than the individual, perhaps as a primitive survival mechanism, and external pressure strengthens rather than weakens resistance against the expression of neurotic symptoms.

The Battlefield Milieu

One of the most striking impressions on soldiers entering combat for the first time is the silence, the apparent absence of human beings, and the lack of movement of any kind that usually exists in the no-man's land between them and the enemy except during periods of attack by either side. Inactivity, together with the natural fear of the unseen enemy, helps to lay the groundwork for the feeling of anxiety that is common to all soldiers. In actual battle the soldier crouches down and conceals himself, Indian fashion. One antidote for relief of the anxiety caused by inactivity is the tactical use of the General Patton technique of continuous, unremitting attack to expedite the termination of the particular battle action. The value of isolated examples of courage in battle is well-documented.

Reactions to Battle

Before entering the combat situation, the normal soldier experiences anticipatory uneasiness, varying in intensity according to his previous experience or lack of it. The average untested soldier enters combat with an intellectual appreciation of the dangers he will face, but the situation has little emotional immediacy. Succeeding experiences in battle cause him to feel greater apprehension.

Immediately after relief from combat, the most striking reaction is overwhelming physical fatigue, combined with apathy and subnormal reactiveness to stimuli. As a variant, there may be irritability or, occasionally, moderate euphoria and psychomotor overaction, with laughing and pressure of speech. Some soldiers pace about restlessly; others sit and stare blankly. Eventually, the tension under which the soldier has operated and which continues to assert itself may make an outlet seem essential. Thus arise the common reactive alcoholic, sexual, and social excesses of soldiers after combat.

Normal combat fear may be understood in three manifest components: (1) fear of death, pain, injury, or mutilation; (2) fear of gross incapacitation by fear reactions, with resulting inability to guard one's self or discharge duties adequately; and (3) fear of exhibiting fear and of thus losing caste with the combat group. Panic, the pathological counterpart of normal fear, involves temporary major disorganization of thinking and control by fear. Consciousness is usually clouded. The soldier's actions are usually wholly unadaptive and often compromise his safety. The most common expression of true panic in the battlefield is the panic run, in which, usually during a shelling, the soldier deserts cover and dashes about impulsively, exposing himself to flying shell fragments or other gunfire.

Muscular tension normally increases under combat stress. From this elevated base line it is exaggerated momentarily by the impact of more acute combat stresses. Tension headaches of moderate degree are the results in some normal soldiers of increased muscle tension.

"Freezing," a soldier's term denoting temporary immobilization while subjected to heightened combat stress, is a normal reaction if it is extremely transitory. It is abnormal if it is more than transitory, if it is inappropriately induced, or if it prevents the soldier from accomplishing movements necessary to his own safety or that of others.

Shaking and tremor accompany the increased muscle tension. They occur in normal soldiers subjected to close shelling or bombing, particularly after they have been sensitized to combat stimuli, and disappear rather rapidly after cessation of the stimulus. These transient reactions are most likely to develop when the soldier is forced to remain passive and take it—for example, while taking cover during a shelling. The reactions should not be evaluated as symptoms of pathological reaction to battle. The abnormal shaking response is grosser and more incapacitating and tends to last for hours after the immediate combat stimulus has ceased.

Excessive perspiration is a common psychosomatic response to combat stress. Some soldiers experience anorexia or nausea. Vague abdominal distress and mild diarrhea are frequent. Urinary frequency is one of the most common normal responses to combat stress. It is often accompanied by urgency and nocturia.

Tachycardia is a frequent battle response. Breathlessness, a sense of thoracic oppression, and sensations of faintness and giddiness may occur in moments of extreme stress.

When generalized muscular weakness and lassitude, caused by extreme physical fatigue, are added to the symptoms already described, a transitory picture resembling neurocirculatory asthenia may develop.

Subjective sensations of fear are almost invariably present among personnel in battle. In susceptible persons or under special circumstances of severe stress, combat tension may overwhelm personality integration and produce a psychiatric casualty. Combat anxiety is clearly perceived by the combatant as a fear of mutilation or loss of life. It may be defended against by denial mechanisms.

Casualties

The wounded exhibit little external evidence of a recent psychic trauma, particularly when severe pain is relieved. Their apparent absence of anxiety is in marked contrast to the visible tension of psychiatric casualties and of soldiers evacuated for mild nonbattle injuries or illness. Yet, the wounded casualty has suffered an equal, if not greater, emotional stress.

The relative freedom from tension displayed by battle casualties can be explained by their status of definite removal from further danger for honorable reasons. In contrast, evacuation from combat for slight injuries, subjective complaints, or emotional breakdown may result in only temporary relief. Even more important is the inner turmoil due to self-directed condemnation for apparent failure to withstand battle stress. Such a conflict is not present in the wounded, whose combat injuries are positive proof to themselves and others of their courage.

Stressful combat experiences, including injury, demonstrate that an aggressive attitude toward danger can easily result in catastrophe. Consequently, confidence in one's ability to conquer external problems may become seriously impaired. As a result, there may be regression to a more helpless form of adaptation. Persons of passive or insecure personality are most vulnerable to the mental component of injury.

Advances in surgery and allied specialties have steadily increased the number and types of wounded who are rapidly restored to full function. This success in the organic sphere of therapy only intensifies the psychological problems of convalescence, for patients become acutely aware that recovery is equated with return to combat, and its tensions and fears. The previously hidden psychic trauma from battle becomes more and more manifest as physical improvement slowly but surely removes the protective safeguards of disability. At this time, wound scars and operative sites may become painful and injured extremities remain tender, with limited motion, and new symptoms are added, such as headache, giddiness, and gastrointestinal complaints. Overt anxiety may come to the surface in the form of insomnia, battle dreams, excess sweating and tremor, irritability, outburst of rage, and excessive alcoholism.

However, intrapsychic influences exert strong pressure toward return to combat duty. The most potent of these mechanisms is group identification. The injured casualty is still psychologically bound to members of his squad, platoon, and company. Prolonged hospitalization reduces the power of group identification.

Related to group motivation is the self-critical component of the personality. Conscience impels conformity with the moral and ethical demands of society. It presses the soldier toward duty, despite fear and tension.

Fresh casualties are preoccupied with uncomfortable bodily sensations produced by the injury or surgical procedures. Only days or weeks later, when there is a decrease of discomfort, does the patient come to a realization of permanent dysfunction and its potential adverse effect on future living. At this time, clinical signs of depression may appear, owing to a feeling of irreparable loss, comparable to the mourning that follows the death of a loved one. The problem of adjustment becomes a conflict between continuing a dependent, sponsored existence and attempting the difficult pathway toward adult goals. At this stage, patients require strong support and encouragement, with realistic demonstrations that practical objectives are possible.

One study of traumatic war neuroses observed that cases of war neuroses were still coming into the Veterans Administration hospital 5 years after World War II ended. The clinical picture was one of intense anxiety, recurrent battle dreams, startle reactions to loud noises, tension, depression, guilt, and a tendency to sudden, explosive, aggressive reactions. Secondary symptoms were the tendency to avoid people, a fear of exposure to criticism, difficulty in making decisions, and various types of sleep disturbances.

Another report, a 15-year follow-up on cases of traumatic war neurosis, stressed that the combat syndrome persists as a chronic state of overvigilance. Needing to avoid noisy and overstimulating situations, worn out by nightmares and sleep difficulties, these veterans are often more disabled than is generally recognized.

Treatment

In most cases, early treatment includes some combination of evaluation, crisis intervention, brief psychotherapy, inpatient treatment, outpatient psychopharmacological treatment, and medical consultation to assist in clarifying the somatization reactions.

REFERENCES

Brill, N. Q., and Beebe, G. W. *A Followup Study of War Neurosis.* United States Government Printing Office, Washington, 1955.

Glass, A. J. Principles of combat psychiatry. Milit. Med., *117:* 27, 1955.

Kalinowsky, L. B. Problems of war neuroses in the light of experience in other countries. Am. J. Psychiatry, *107:* 340, 1950.

Mayfield, D. G., and Fowler, D. R. Combat plus twenty years: The effect of previous combat experience on psychiatric patients. Milit. Med., *134:* 1348, 1969.

Ranson, S. W. The normal battle reaction: Its relation to the pathological battle reaction. Bull. U. S. Army Med. Dept. (Suppl.), 3, 1949.

25

Psychophysiologic Disorders

25.1. HISTORY OF PSYCHOPHYSIOLOGIC MEDICINE

Mind-Body Problem

Prehistory

In prehistoric times, the storehouse of reliable cause and effect relationships was small. Spirit was the prime force, the unseen power that controlled events as sure-handedly and with as much determination as a dream overtakes one. Pain or weakness was attributed to the force of an evil spirit or will. It could be the will of an enemy or rival, the spirit of a violated place, the world-controlling spirits threatening out of whimsy, or the spirits of the dead, angry at not receiving appropriate libations.

Bad things existed outside of the individual person and entered the body to attack. Even death was not an indwelling potential but a visitor who could suddenly be seen standing nearby during the moments before the stiffening of the body. Disease in its more serious forms was the result of a body's being possessed by an ill-intentioned spirit. Holes were bored in the skulls of sick persons to let the evil out. Whatever the approach of the healer, he always gave his patient a renewed will to health by the power of suggestion. Thus did primitive people emphasize a holistic concept, rather than a dichotomized psyche and soma. (see Table I).

Egyptians

Egypt's embalmers were a separate caste of the hereditary priesthood; when they cut into the bodies of the dead to draw out, wash, and wrap the organs in linen, they were sure to leave the heart intact, for here rested the soul, the person's intelligence and emotions, his personal self. Like earlier people, the Egyptians imagined death and disease to come into the body from the outside: the gods, spirits—especially those of the dead—and the evil wishes of humans.

Thoth, Isis, her son Horus, and the vizier Imhotep (circa 2800 B.C.), who was eventually deified as a healing god because of his medical knowledge, were all called upon for aid in exorcising bad spirits. But Egypt's three classes of famous physicians, magicians, and priests of Sekhment did not rely on the gods. They compiled medical observations to aid themselves and their descendents in diagnosis and treatment. Treatments suggested included oral rites, manual rites, and specific drug dosages. The choice might be rational and effective, irrational and effective, or magical and ineffective.

Babylonians and Assyrians

The medical texts of the conglomeric Sumerian-Babylonian-Assyrian civilization (circa 2500 to 500 B.C.) are similar to the contemporary but more famous texts of Egypt. However, these texts are heavily weighted toward magic, and no existing text is totally rational.

The ultimate source of disease might be the gods who had sent pain as punishment for ritual or moral error, the neglected and angered dead, the hand of a ghost escaped from an unburied body, an ill wind, sorcery purchased by the pocketbook of a malevolent person, or the patient himself if he had committed a ritual or moral sin. Accordingly, a person in pain was disgraced and urged to look into his soul and examine his sins until the charms of the priest should free him from sickness. Disease was thought of as having a cause within the patient, rather than coming on him from the outside.

TABLE I

History of Psychosomatic Medicine

Date	Historical Period	Psychosomatic Orientation
10,000 B.C.	Primitive society	Disease is caused by spiritual powers and must be fought by spiritual means; the evil spirit that enters and affects the total being must be liberated through exorcism, trepanation, etc.
2500–500 B.C.	Babylonian-Assyrian civilization	Medicine is dominated by religion, and suggestion is the major tool of treatment. Sigerist: "Mesopotamian medicine was psychosomatic in all its aspects."
400 B.C.	Greek civilization	Socrates: "As it is not proper to cure the eyes without the head, nor the head without the body, so neither is it proper to cure the body without the soul." Hippocrates: "In order to cure the human body, it is necessary to have a knowledge of the whole of things."
100 B.C.–400 A.D.	Late Greek-Early Roman civilization	Galen's humoral theory postulates that disease is caused by disturbances in the fluids of the body. Medicine adopts a holistic approach to disease.
500–1500	Middle Ages	Mysticism and religion dominate medicine. Sinning is the cause of mental and somatic illness.
1500–1700	Renaissance	Renewed interest in the natural sciences and their application to medicine; advances in anatomy (Vesalius), autopsy (Morgagni), microscopy (Leeuwenhoek). Psychic influences on soma are rejected as unscientific; the study of the mind is relegated to religion and philosophy.
1800–1900	19th century	Modern laboratory-based medicine of Pasteur and Virchow. Virchow: "Disease has its origin in disease of the cell." Psychosomatic approach discarded, since all disease must be associated with structural cell change. The disease is treated, not the patient.
1900–present	20th century	Freud's early psychoanalytic formulations emphasize the role of psychic determinism in somatic conversion reactions (Dora case). These early concepts are limited to major hysterical conversions; subsequently, Alexander differentiates conversion reactions from psychosomatic disorders.

Jews

For the Hebrews, disease was predominantly the punishment suffered for the sin of having disobeyed God or His laws. Healers in the form of doctors were scorned. For group sin there was the group punishment of pestilence or plague. Sabbath rest, abstaining from carnivorous animals, isolating lepers, and burying excrement in camp were some of the laws enforced by the priesthood.

Like the Egyptians, the Jews considered the heart to be the seat of intelligence and will. They believed the will and the body to be interacting and bound together.

Jesus, too, saw the body and the spirit as a whole. He does not appear to have thought of disease as a punishment for disobedience to law but more as an imbalance within the patient, an imbalance correctable by a psychic act of faith.

Greeks

Like the rest of the ancient world, the Greeks were impressed by Egypt's medicine. As in Egypt, the priest-physicians of Greece passed on to their sons observations on wounds and diseases. They did so through the centuries at medical schools. Eventually, this priesthood lost its requirement that the status be inherited.

The deities brought disease and healing; spirit and body were an interralated unity. The priest-physician might talk to the patient and make suggestions; if surgery was required, it might be done on a drugged sleeper by a priest wearing the robes of the god; or perhaps no interview took place, and the arrival of the god occurred only within dreams. By isolation, the patient was brought in touch with his emotions, with his private spirit world, and perhaps reunified himself toward health. His dreams were interpreted by a priest-physician, who pointed out elements of the dreams that could be used for motivation.

Disease, wrote Hippocrates (460–355 B.C.), originated within the body and was due not to spirits but to an imbalance in fluid matter. This imbalance could be related to or even caused by a similar imbalance in the patient's external environment. Physical or fluid imbalance could be caused by emotional upset, too. Hippocrates reported that fear produced sweat and that shame brought on palpitations of the heart.

The search for the location of the mind occupied the Greeks in a discussion of the organ housing that faculty and became temporarily complicated but ultimately clarified by a tendancy to separate the functions of mind into various subdivisions, such as life force, reason, consciousness, and the emotions. Hippocrates considered the brain to be the center of the senses and of reason, but he agreed with others that a certain life force called pneuma was more basic. Since pneuma controlled the brain, it was the ultimate source of intelligence and feeling.

Plato (427–347 B.C.) imagined an ideal world; each palpable bird and each tangible tree he saw was but a copy of the ideal bird and the ideal tree in a perfect pre-existing mental world. Plato saw spirit as superior to matter. As an idealist, he went against the tendency of the preceding generations to dignify and study matter, developed into the theories of Democritus, the atomist (born 460 B.C.).

Asclepiades (1st century B.C.) founded a medical theory stemming from atomism. In his system, the soul had no location but was the convergence of all perception; disturbances of the passions could cause mental disease, whereas too much constriction or relaxation in the vacuum or space between the gyrating atoms of the body caused physical disease.

In *Timaeus* Plato remarked that trouble in the soul could bring trouble to the body. Aristotle (384–322 B.C.) observed that the emotions of anger, fear, courage, and joy affect the body; and Aretaeus (1st century A.D.) pinpointed a disturbance of the emotions as one of the six major causes of paralysis.

Middle-Ages

The European tribesmen who occupied Rome brought with them a slighter tradition of medical observations. Objective observation was run to ground by the return of belief in spiritual powers, demons, witches, and sin. All these agents were accused of having produced disease, and healing again became a spiritual issue. The evil was within and without; a sick person might consult a priest or the relics of a saint and promise to give up his own sin or lack of faith or evil impulses in exchange for health.

Renaissance

After 1,000 years of religious dominance, interest in natural causes and cures of disease returned. During the Renaissance the study of the material world was renewed, but the material eventually became the dominant and virtually only credited field. This dominance was reflected in the study of human health, which was divided into the fluorishing investigation of the body's structures and an atrophying study of the emotions.

René Descartes (1596–1650) dismissed every assumption and came quickly into himself, to his mind and its self-awareness, not to his senses. Both spirit and matter are real, although spirit precedes matter. Cartesian dualism gave matter more importance than Platonic idealism had but less importance than the atomists had given it.

The telescope and the microscope brought more of the unseen external world into the domain of the seen and known. Renewed interest in mathematics, chemistry, and physics produced a similar widening of objective knowledge, and new information from these fields was applied to medicine in biochemistry and bacteriology. Knowledge regarding the soma multiplied, and the psyche was pushed out of the field of scientific study. Its sector called mind was discussed only by philosophers, its sector called soul was discussed by the theologians, and its sector of the emotions was ignored. Indeed, psychic influence on the soma was rejected as unscientific; it eventually became common to treat the disease and not the patient.

19th and 20th Centuries

In the 19th century, the mind-body schism spread to its furthest division. The 20th century witnesses a new attempt to view mind-body holistically. It was Freud (1856–1939) who brought psyche and soma back together, using memory as the laboratory of the psyche. He demonstrated the importance of the emotions in producing both mental disturbances and somatic disorders. With transference and countertransference, Freud pulled the doctor-patient relationship out of the religious framework of hope and faith and into an intellectually understandable dynamism.

Representatives from both fields of study, psyche and soma, have agreed for more than 100 years that, in a small body of disorders, emotional and somatic activities overlap. These disorders were first called psychosomatic disorders by Heinroth in 1818, when he used the term in regard to insomnia. The disorders other than insomnia that were classed as psychosomatic grew to include conversion hysteria (later excluded because it operates through the central nervous system, rather than through the autonomic nervous system), ulcerative colitis, peptic ulcer, migraine, bronchial asthma, and rheumatoid arthritis.

The American Psychiatric Association's second edition of *Diagnostic and Statistical Manual of Mental Disorders*, defines psychophysiologic disorders as follows: "This group of disorders is characterized by physical symptoms that are caused by emotional factors and involve a single organ system, usually under autonomic nervous system innervation. The physiological changes involved are those that normally accompany certain emotional states, but in these disorders the changes are more intense and sustained. The individual may not be consciously aware of his emotional state."

Treatment of psychophysiologic disorders by psychological methods has not produced good enough results to encourage psychological treatment alone. Indeed, investigators have raised the question of the validity of the concept of psychophysiologic medicine.

Emotions and Cell Tissue

Using Freud's insight, a number of workers in the early decades of the 20th century tried to expand the understanding of the interrelationship of psyche and soma. Two trends developed, one suggesting that specific emotions lead to specific cell and tissue damage, and the second holding that generalized anxiety creates the preconditions for a number of not necessarily predetermined diseases.

Franz Alexander believed that, if a specific stimulus or stress occurred, it expressed itself in the specific response of a predetermined organ. He applied the fight-flight alert of the body against stress to the problem. Alexander saw conflict as a stress and suggested that, when conflict presents itself to a person, he may suppress this stress and produce, through the voluntary nervous system, a reaction such as the conversion reaction described by Freud. On the other hand, after suppressing stress, he may, through the autonomic system, keep his sympathetic responses alert for heightened aggression or flight or his parasympathetic responses alerted for heightened vegetative activity. Prolonged alertness and tension can produce physiological disorders and eventual pathology of the organs of the viscera.

A number of investigators have developed the pathway concept of constellations into theories involving the whole personality. The competitive, restless, time-haunted, and coronary-bound type A person has certain physiological characteristics: high plasma triglyceride, high cholesterol level, hyperinsulinemic response to glucose challenge, and high levels of noradrenaline present in urine. Some investigators have suggested correlations between cancer proneness and personalities who repress and deny emotional stress, seldom project for defense, and only slowly recover from depression after loss; they hypothesize that depression may be somatized as neoplasm.

There are, it appears, four general types of reaction to stress; the normal, in which alert is followed by an action of defense; the neurotic, in which the alert or anxiety is so great that the defense becomes ineffective; the psychotic, in which the alarm may be misperceived or even ignored; and the psychophysiologic, in which defense by the psyche fails, and the alert is translated into somatic systems, causing changes in body tissue.

In recent reports on the disorders classified as psychophysiologic, there is a tendency to isolate what becomes of the stress produced by conflict. The conflicts are often seen as unresolved holdovers from the pregenital period; dependence versus independence and resultant tensions leading to ulcer; riddance versus retention and resultant tensions leading to intentinal disorders; expression or suppression of anxiety or rage and resulting tensions leading to cardiovascular problems and vascular headache.

A genetic predisposition to physiologic exaggeration of normal functioning is related to the excessive pepsinogen production of the potential ulcer patient. A genetic enzyme deficiency is projected. A congenitally high sensitivity to parasympathetic stimulation is noted in cases of irritable colon. To conflict as a source of stress have been added the crises of human chronology—such as puberty, parenthood, and aging—and those of situation, such as success and failure or loss of key persons.

REFERENCES

Alexander, F. *Psychosomatic Medicine: Its Principles and Application.* W. W. Norton, New York, 1950.

Freud, S. Fragment of an analysis of a case of hysteria. In *Standard Edition of the Complete Works of Sigmund Freud.* Hogarth Press, London, 1953.

Freud, S. On narcissism: An introduction. In *Standard Edition of the Complete Works of Sigmund Freud*, vol. 14, p. 73. Hogarth Press, London, 1957.

Reeves, J. W. *Body and Mind in Western Thought.* Penguin Books, Baltimore, 1958.

Sigerist, H. E. *A. History of Medicine*, vols. 1 and 2. Oxford University Press, New York, 1951 and 1961.

Zilboorg. G., and Henry, G. W. *A History of Medical Psychology*, W. W. Norton, New York, 1941.

25.2.   CURRENT THEORETICAL CONCEPTS IN PSYCHOPHYSIOLOGIC MEDICINE

Social Sphere

The focus of a number of studies has been on social environmental factors and the correlation of these factors with indices of physiologic dysfunction or illness in various populations. This ecological approach began with broad surveys attempting to establish over-all indices of illness in different socio-economic groups. Many studies have focused on diseases of poverty. Their conclusions are clear—that the poor suffer selectively from a wide number of disorders. The intermediate links remain obscure, including such probable factors as heightened exposure to noxious environmental agents, decreased access to or ability to utilize medical care, and chronic culturally fostered adverse emotional stimulation.

A somewhat more specific group of studies has suggested that a wide variety of illnesses may be preceded by general disruption or life change. A more precise approach has been to take a naturally occurring event with presumed psychological impact, such as the closing of a factory, and to document in some detail the physiologic changes and symptomatic episodes associated with it. An intrinsically appealing concept is that social stability or lack thereof is reflected in intrapersonal organization or disorganization. The immediate implications for medical management concern the nature of the social milieu and its effect on medical and surgical care in the hospital itself.

The general conclusion seems warranted that disruption of the interpersonal environment may result in adverse biophysiologic effects through a variety of channels, although these effects have not yet been clearly elucidated.

The concept of stress has led to somewhat more sharply focused investigations of milieu effects. Unfortunately, the word "stress" is used in a variety of ways. At times, it designates a kind of stimulus to coping methods of the fight-flight variety. These methods are relatively homogeneous, but one must distinguish among chronic anxiety, mobilization of active strivings, and increased likelihood of aggressive responses, any or all of which may, if sustained, be pathogenic. At other times, the word "stress" is used as a touchstone for all sorts of psychological stimuli. Indeed, stressful experiences appear to have highly variable effects. Patterns of stress are multiple, as are the chains of reaction set off within coping organisms. A large number of environmental stimuli lead to sustained mobilization of adaptive agonistic systems, which can result in dysfunction, particularly of the sympathoadrenal system, and eventually in illness.

Another form of adversive environmental stimulation is separation and loss. Reactions to separation and loss provide a powerful set of stimuli leading to dysfunction and illness in animals and human beings.

Biological Sphere

Studies of neurophysiologic and neuroendocrine regulation have done much to establish the bodily pathways and control systems that serve as potential avenues for communication between brain and periphery. The sympathetic nervous system and its cardiovascular effects were prototypic of the body's rapid adaptations. Studies revealed subtle complexities. Specific affect patterns showed their own variations, and different persons had specific combinations of response patterns. Learned influences may enter in a variety of ways.

More sustained reactions are mediated by endocrine systems. Studies have shown the responsivity of the adrenal cortex to psychological states of sustained anxiety, anger, and acute depression. These responses are characteristic in normal persons threatened by loss of a loved relative, in patients suffering from acute depression, and in patients in acute schizophrenic turmoil. Human studies have been extended by animal work that has indicated the intricate relationship between the limbic system and diphasic anabolic and catabolic endocrine responses.

The peripheral autonomic nervous system has been shown to be highly complicated and specialized. Catecholamines and other transmitter substances appear to be of key importance not only in the peripheral autonomic nervous system but also in the brain and hence in states involving profound disturbance of central functioning, such as depression. Studies are beginning to reveal interactions between catecholamines and other messenger substances, such as prostaglandins and cyclic adenosine monophosphate. Avenues of communication exist between neuroendocrine processes and the immune system, which itself constitutes a vast, buffered system, remembering and recognizing foreign substances and continuously being mobilized or demobilized by interaction with the material environment.

Psychological Sphere

Distorted Adaptive Response

A number of investigators have suggested that psychosomatic disorder represents some exaggeration of habitual responses that have become maladaptive. A competitive, hard driving, time-dominated, urgent mode of habitual functioning is characteristic of patients with coronary artery disease. Engel suggested that, in contrast to the flight-fight reaction mobilizing the organism for activity, there is a response characterized by inactivity and demobilization, which he called conservation-withdrawal. He noted a chronological relationship between the onset of a number of disease states and the antecedent occurrence of depression, despair, or giving up. Such psychological reactions, together with closely related physiologic concomitants, may lead to some failure of key adaptive responses, leaving the sufferer vulnerable to a variety of noxious influences. Such a chain of events could serve as a partial, nonspecific precipitating cause in many diseases.

Specific Habitual Emotional Response Patterns

The most classical formulation of emotional specificity was developed by Franz Alexander. Using the available physiology of his day, he developed an ingenious set of hypotheses, characterizing seven classical psychosomatic disorders; essential hypertension, bronchial asthma, neurodermatitis, peptic ulcer, ulcerative colitis, rheumatoid arthritis, and thyrotoxicosis. He saw all these disorders as embodying a psychophysiologic expression of chronic dammed-up emotions—for example, in ulcer the chronic desire to take in and be fed, opposed by shame and guilt; in hypertension, the chronic partial emergence of aggressive tendencies never efficiently repressed.

Conversion

Alexander's hypotheses were framed in terms of quasiautomatic manifestations of the physiologic components of emotional life. For example, he saw asthma as largely determined by dammed-up urges to cry out to a mother. An alternative view stressed the symbolic elements, the conflict over expression and concealment, and a compromise formation in partial, distorted expression. This view categorized many of the psychosomatic disorders listed above as primitive forms of a conversion disorder.

Engel has distinguished between true conversion symptoms—triggered by percepts, persisting as memory traces, and involving functions in some way under the purview of conscious experience—and what he calls complications of conversion—physiologic processes that result from the conversion disorder. The hysteric may be not so much the victim of automatic stereotyped patterns triggered by environmental stimuli as locked into a pattern of using certain methods to achieve foreordained ends. Some of these ends may be partly conscious, as in the case of secondary gain; most of them are remote from awareness, based on powerful primitive fantasies and associated emotions.

Mind and Body

Problems of mind and body or brain and consciousness can be clarified by philosophic rigor and attention to levels of discourse. They are highlighted by the Western European conception of science as dealing with a "real" mechanical world, thus relegating psychological states to some subjective ineffable realm. Scientists have still not been able to trace the routes whereby a social stimulus leads to an elevation in blood pressure.

Four concepts that have been explored in recent years contribute, each in an incomplete fashion, to the understanding of emotion and psychophysiologic disease. These are the principle of multifactorial causes, the principle of genetic variability and somatopsychic disorder, contributions from the knowledge of learning in the widest sense, and the role of symbolic systems.

REFERENCES

Alexander, F., French, T. M., and Pollock, G., editors. *Psychosomatic Specificity: Experimental Study and Results*, vol. 1. University of Chicago Press, Chicago, 1968.

Engel, G. L. Personal theories of disease as determinants of patient-physician relationship. Psychosom. Med., *35:* 184, 1973.

Fabrega, H., and Manning, P. K. An integrated theory of disease: Ladino-Mestizo views of disease in the Chiappas highlands. Psychosom. Med., *35:* 223, 1973.

Harburg, E. Socio-ecological stress, suppressed hostility, skin color, and black-white male blood pressure: Detroit. Psychosom. Med., *35:* 276, 1973.

Kaj Jerne, N. The immune system. Sci. Am., *229:* 52, 1973.

Knapp, P. H. Revolution, relevance, and psychosomatic medicine: Where the light is not. Psychosom. Med., *33:* 363, 1971.

Luborsky, L., Docherty, J. P., and Penick, S. Onset conditions for psychosomatic symptoms: A comparative review of immediate observations with retrospective research. Psychosom. Med., *35:* 187, 1973.

Mason, J. W., Brady, J. U., Polish, E., Bauer, J. S., Robinson, J., and Dodson, E. Concurrent measurements of 17-hydroxy-corticosteroid and pepsinogen levels during prolonged emotional stress in the monkey. Psychosom. Med., *21:* 432, 1959.

Mendelson, M., Hirsch, S., and Webber, C. S. A critical examination of some recent theoretical models in psychosomatic medicine. Psychosom. Med., *18:* 363, 1956.

Regestein, Q. R., Pegram, G. V., Cook, B., and Bradley, D. Alpha rhythm percentage during four- and 12-hour feedback periods. Psychosom. Med., *35:* 215, 1973.

Schildkraut, J. J., and Kety, S. S. Biogenic amines and emotion. Science, *156:* 21, 1967.

Shapiro, A. P., Gottschalk, L., Knapp, P. H., Reiser, M., and Sapira, J. D., editors. *Psychosomatic Classics: Selected Papers from "Psychosomatic Medicine."* Karger, Basel, 1971.

25.3.   PSYCHOPHYSIOLOGIC GASTROINTESTINAL DISORDERS
I. PEPTIC ULCER

Definition

The term "peptic ulcer" is used to refer to both gastric ulcer and duodenal ulcer. Both require the presence of acid gastric juice, but duodenal ulcer is characterized by chronic hypersecretion of acid and pepsin, whereas this chronic hypersecretion is not the case for gastric ulcers, except for those occurring in the immediate prepyloric region.

Somatopsychic-Psychosomatic Concept

The primary factor in the genesis of the disorder is a somatic process that not only is responsible for the nature of the final organic state but also is capable of contributing directly or indirectly to the development of specific psychological characteristics. With duodenal ulcer, this process involves the influence of feeding activity and gastric hypersecretion on psychic development. The consequent psychological features define in more or less specific ways the circumstances that prove to be psychologically stressful for the person and hence identify the psychodynamic conditions under which the organic process may become activated. The somatic factor must be present and exerting an influence from early in life, placing it in the category of a genic, congenital, or early-acquired defect. Once initiated, the disorder is characteristically chronic or recurring. (See Figure 1.)

Psychological Processes and Gastric Function

In the course of mounting hunger and then nursing, the infant periodically achieves relief of tension in the mother's arms, laying the basis for the ultimate association in the nervous system of an intrinsic drive (hunger) and its relief through an environmental influence (mother). This is a reciprocal process, the mother being required to recognize and respond appropriately to the infant's cues indicating hunger and the infant being required to fit into

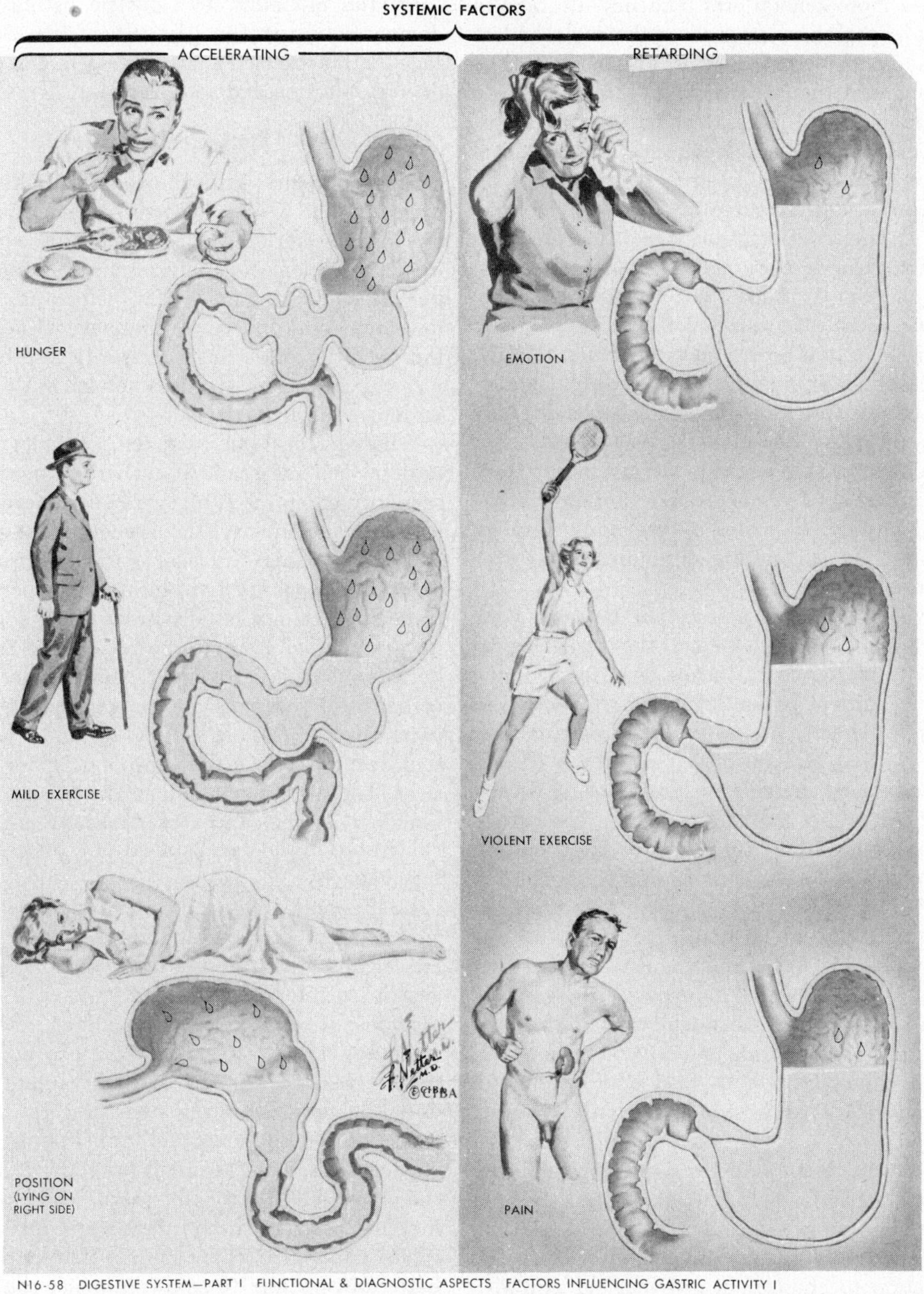

N16-58 DIGESTIVE SYSTEM—PART I FUNCTIONAL & DIAGNOSTIC ASPECTS FACTORS INFLUENCING GASTRIC ACTIVITY I

FIGURE 1. Systemic factors influencing gastric activity. (© Copyright CIBA Pharmaceutical Company, Division of CIBA-GEIGY Corporation. Reproduced, with permission, from THE CIBA COLLECTION OF MEDICAL ILLUSTRATIONS by Frank H. Netter, M.D. All rights reserved.)

the mother's particular patterns of nursing. If successful, the process is a source of mutual gratification; if unsuccessful, it becomes a source of tension and frustration for both infant and mother.

For the infant, this experience is associated

with a more general oral tendency—to take in what is perceived as good or desirable and to refuse or spit out what is felt as bad. The feeding experiences of infancy also provide a nidus around which may cluster a whole complex of associations related to such fundamental human needs as the need to be taken care of, supported, and nurtured.

With the eruption of teeth and the transition from sucking to chewing comes another contribution of a body activity to psychic development—the expression of aggression and hostility in oral terms, such as biting, tearing, and even consuming cannibalistically. Characteristically, the thwarting of oral needs, literally or figuratively, may elicit aggressive impulses to take by force that which is not given or to force the others to give, expressed literally by the child and symbolically by the adult through grabbing, tearing, biting, or holding firmly with the teeth.

Evidence for an association between such psychodynamic trends and the physiological activity of the stomach has been forthcoming from studies of patients with gastric fistula. In infancy, when the relationship between mother and child is still intimately linked to the repeated cycles of relief of hunger being associated with the mothering figure, one would expect behavioral expressions of affection and aggression to be accompanied by an increase in gastric secretion. These, indeed, were the findings in a 15- to 18-month-old infant with a gastric fistula. Active relating patterns, whether affectionate or hostile, induced gastric secretory behavior, such as one might expect when the stomach was preparing to receive food; however, in the absence of both food and meaningful human relationship, stomach activity virtually ceased.

With the infant's further psychological development, particularly the acquisition of language and more sophisticated ways of relating, one might expect this relationship with gastric secretion to change. In a 4-year-old girl with gastric fistula, gastric secretion of acid and pepsin remained at a low basal level as long as she was relating comfortably and happily. On the other hand, when the 4-year-old had to make an effort to relate, gastric secretion rose, as it did when she was angry or anxious. Secretion was low when she became detached or withdrawn.

Studies of adults with gastric fistulas also demonstrate a rise in gastric secretion during rage, both expressed and suppressed, and a fall during dejection and withdrawal.

Pathogenesis

Most patients with duodenal ulcers have large and chronically hypersecreting stomachs, but hypersecretion alone is not sufficient for ulcer formation. Not only may hypersecretion be present for many years before an ulcer develops—and, indeed, it may never develop—but secretion does not necessarily rise before ulcer development and does not fall with healing unless gastritis develops.

Whether the large stomach, with its large parietal cell mass and its generally increased secretory potential, is a genetically determined anatomical characteristic or whether the stomach hypertrophies in response to some primary central nervous system influences operating from birth cannot be answered. Some support for genetic factors comes from twin and family data. Thus, there is a significantly higher concordance of ulcer disease among monozygotic twins than among dizygotic twins and a highly significant excess of ulcers among close relatives. On the other hand, an increased functional demand, for whatever reason, may also contribute to the development of a hypersecretory capacity.

Infants may differ in the activity characteristics of their feeding apparatuses, and it is conceivable that those with the more active gastric secretory potential also have a more vigorous drive to nurse. The infant with the more active gastric secretory pattern may behave more of the time like a hungry infant than does the normosecreting or hyposecreting infant. Further, mothers differ in their ability and capacity to satisfy the infant's oral drive. When the mother's ability to gratify oral needs matches or exceeds the infant's oral drive, the infant has a good chance of satisfaction and a better opportunity to gain confidence that oral tensions will not become intolerable or remain unrelieved. On the other hand, when the ability of the mother to satisfy the oral needs is lower than the infant's oral drive, the infant will be repetitively or chronically exposed to periods of oral tension and will have difficulty gaining confidence that the environment can be depended on to fulfill these needs. Such tensions projected over the entire developmental span of the child may be expected to exert a significant influence on his ultimate psychic structure as an adult.

Oral character traits and conflicts around dependence and independence, although expressed in many different ways, are prominent characteristics of duodenal ulcer patients. But not all persons with such psychological characteristics develop ulcers or are ulcer-prone. Whether a duodenal ulcer develops later in life depends on the secretory capacity of the stomach, the greatest potential for ulcer formation being among those who are hypersecretors and were orally frustrated in infancy.

Ulcer formation depends on current psychosocial factors and the degree to which they are psychologically stressful for the particular person. The psychosocial situations specifically stressful for each person make up the precipitating circumstances determining the time at which an ulcer ultimately forms in the ulcer-prone person.

Psychological Characteristics

The basic psychodynamic trends in the hypersecretor-duodenal ulcer group cluster around strong needs to be taken care of, to lean on others, to be fed, to be nurtured, and to have close body contact of a succoring type. Many developmental factors determine how such a central organizing psychodynamic tendency is eventually expressed.

In the seudoindependent patient, underlying dependent needs may be largely or completely denied and an opposite façade presented. These patients appear to be highly independent, self-reliant, aggressive, controlling, and overactive. The interpersonal relationships of these patients are controlling, rather than warm.

In the passive-dependent patient, the underlying dependent needs are overtly expressed and to a considerable degree are conscious. These persons are outwardly compliant, passive, ingratiating, and eager to perform for others; yet they are also clinging and dependent and may even be demanding in a passive-aggressive way. They tend to get into social and interpersonal relationships in which they can depend on a nurturing figure or a paternal, supportive social organization.

In acting out patients, the dependent needs are taken care of by blatant acting out and by insistent demanding. Irresponsible, with little investment in achievement, they may drift from job to job and are often unemployed. Addiction to tobacco, alcohol, and drugs is common. In their relationships they are parasitic and without consideration of others.

Among many patients these tendencies are much more subtly manifest or defended against.

Pathogenic Psychological Stress

Effective frustration of ongoing dependent needs is the common denominator of the psychological stresses leading to activation of a duodenal ulcer. Precipitating events are characterized by their capacity to mobilize fears of loss of love or security through intensification or frustration of persistent infantile, passive-dependent wishes, usually with feelings of helplessness and anger.

The pseudoindependent person is likely to develop ulcer symptoms when his own efforts no longer succeed in forcing others to provide or when external circumstances beyond his control become frustrating. The passive-dependent person may develop ulcer symptoms when the person or organization on whom or which he is dependent refuses or fails to satisfy his needs. The acting out or demanding person may get symptoms when he is forcibly restrained from acting out, as when he is jailed or when supplies are simply not forthcoming.

In most cases the sequence of events in response to such a psychological stress is for the patient (1) to intensify the psychological and social devices that he characteristically uses to assure gratification of needs, (2) when these devices fail, to experience increasing anger, which usually must be suppressed or denied if it threatens still further the sources of supply, (3) to turn on the self or internalize the aggressive impulse, and the development of corresponding feelings of guilt, and (4) when he no longer feels able to cope, to give up, with feelings of helplessness in some patients, hopelessness in others. Once the symptoms begin, this sequence may be terminated or reversed by the altered expectation from the self and the changed behavior of the environment toward the patient. The exact point in this sequence when ulcer activity begins has not yet been clearly delineated.

Treatment

Anything that assures gratification of the patient's dependent needs without undermining his pride and self-respect should have a salutary effect in reversing the conditions that led to ulcer activation. The physician must know, for example, to what extent and under what circumstances the pseudoindependent patient will permit himself to be controlled by the physician. The clinician must know who in the family or among friends is acceptable to and capable of supporting the patient. He must recognize that, for the pseudoindependent patient, respite may be achieved not by rest or inactivity but by permission to engage in some other activity, to escape temporarily from burdens of responsibility. He must know that the passive-dependent patient may need a much longer period of babying and indulgence but also that a few of these patients are insatiable in their needs to be taken care of. He must recognize that the excessively passive-dependent patient may respond to surgery by prolonged invalidism, even though the ulcer heals, and that the guilt-ridden patient may have intractable pain long after the ulcer is healed.

No form of psychotherapy can be expected to eliminate the underlying somatic determinants—that is, the lifelong chronic hypersecretion and the as yet unidentified factors determining the vulnerability of the duodenal mucosa. On the other hand, psychotherapy, including psychoanalysis, may improve the capability of some patients to manage their lives, to deal with unconscious conflicts, and to gratify needs in personally and socially acceptable ways. However, nothing can be expected to protect a patient from the vicissitudes of life, and it is possible that even the best adjusted hypersecretor may, under sufficient provocation, develop a duodenal ulcer.

REFERENCES

Engel, G. L. Psychogenic pain and the pain-prone patient. Am. J. Med., 26: 899, 1959.

Kapp, F., Rosenbaum, M., and Romano, J. Psychological factors in men with peptic ulcers. Am. J. Psychiatry, 103: 700, 1947.

Kezur, E., Kapp, F., and Rosenbarum, M. Psychological factors in women with peptic ulcer. Am. J. Psychiatry, 108: 368, 1951.

Mirsky, I. A. Physiologic, psychologic, and social determinants in the etiology of duodenal ulcer. Am. J. Digest. Dist., 3: 285, 1958.

Weisman, A. D. A study of the psychodynamics of duodenal ulcer exacerbations. Psychosom. Med., 18: 2, 1956.

Wolf, S., and Wolff, H. G. Human Gastric Function. Oxford University Press, New York, 1947.

25.4 PSYCHOPHYSIOLOGIC GASTROINTESTINAL DISORDERS II. INTESTINAL DISORDERS

Introduction

Some bowel-function disorders are purely psychogenic in origin, some are psychophysiologic phenomena, and some are symptoms of organic bowel disorders. The organic bowel disorders are called somatopsy chic-psychosomatic because of the role of organic factors in the primary predisposition and of psychological factors in the course.

Psychophysiologic and Psychogenic Disorders

The eliminative function of the bowel determines its involvement in psychophysiologic patterns of riddance and retention. The conflict between physiological function and the social and interpersonal demands for bowel control and cleanliness determines the role of the bowel in psychogenic disorders.

Evacuation of the bowel during fear presumably represents a primitive reaction to acute stress. During acute anxiety there may be periodic peristaltic rushes, sometimes with cramps and diarrhea. On rare occasions, diarrhea may accompany acute feelings of sadness, discouragement, and depression. More commonly, these affects are associated with constipation.

Conversion Reactions and Anal Drive

The rich symbolism associated with feces and defecation and the erotogenicity of the anus, plus the fact that its function is learned and partially under voluntary control, predispose the rectum and anus to conversion and anal drive patterns. These patterns include constipation, frequent bowel movements, rectal spasm, sphincter spasm, rectal sensations, and pruritus ani. The repressed fantasies and the corresponding conversion manifestations include ideas of rectal pregnancy (severe constipation, abdominal distension, followed by a huge evacuation), anal intercourse and homosexual wishes (sphincter spasm, rectal spasm, pruritus ani, constipation, rectal sensations), and aggression expressed in soiling terms (constipation, frequent evacuations, pain in the rectum).

Patients manifesting such conversion symptoms are likely to have a predisposition to conversion, and many have the personality features of hysteria. A few, especially men with such rectal symptoms, may be latently paranoid.

In some persons constipation and diarrhea are expressive of psychological trends deeply embedded in the matrix of the personality. Among these conflicting personality trends, control versus lack of control, generosity versus miserliness, stubbornness versus compliancy, order versus disorder, and cleanliness versus sloppiness may increasingly be equated with the corresponding bowel behavior and be so expressed. Thus, such a person may become constipated or have diarrhea when called on to give or perform more than he feels capable of, when in a messy place, when angry, or when he feels deprived.

Disorders of Elimination Secondary to Psychopathological States

Some inappropriate or bizarre patterns of elimination differ from conversion reactions in that they represent complex disturbances in the behavior associated with elimination, rather than representing the use of a body part or function in a symbolic or a defensive manner.

Addiction to Laxatives, Enemas, and High Colonic Irrigation. Psychological inquiry often demonstrates, as the basis for excessive purging, morbid psychological concepts of something bad or destructive within the body—actually displacements of bad or disturbing thoughts or fantasies. Assocrdingly, the patient sees the contents of the bowel as bad or dangerous. These strange notions are not restricted to the functions of the gastrointestinal system but extend to many other spheres as well. Some patients are obviously schizophrenic, and most reveal at least an inclination toward the persecutory delusional attitude of the paranoid.

Encopresis and Psychogenic Megacolon. Encopresis begins either as a failure to achieve proper toileting or as a loss of previously achieved bowel control and only infrequently extends into adulthood. It takes the form either of the promiscuous and causal expulsion of feces whenever the impulse so moves or of prolonged retention of stool, with leakage of feces or periodic huge movements. The prolonged retention may be associated with enormous distention of the colon, sometimes designated as

psychogenic megacolon. Giant megacolon or megasigmoid is thought to reflect a failure to respond to defecation stimuli.

Bowel Manifestations with Psychosis. Extreme constipation may develop during psychotic depression, and incontinence may develop during acute and chronic brain syndromes and schizophrenia. Persistent and bizarre anal and rectal sensations, sometimes frankly delusional or persecutory in character, are occasionally the presenting complaint of a paranoid patient.

Somatopsychic-Psychosomatic Disorders

Ulcerative Colitis

Ulcerative colitis is a chronic or remitting disorder involving primarily the mucosa and submucosa of the large bowel. A significant familial occurrence suggests a genetic determinant. Various factors, including psychic insult, are seen as capable of triggering the breakdown of defenses in immunologically primed patients to produce the overt disease.

The manifest disease may develop at any age, including neonatally, and, once initiated, may be marked by remissions and relapses or by a chronic, unremitting course. A clear-cut chronological relationship exists between psychological stress and onset or exacerbation on the one hand and between psychological support and remission on the other hand.

Psychological Characteristics. Many ulcerative colitis patients are described as neat, orderly, punctual, conscientious, indecisive, obstinate, and conforming. Often noted are a guarding of affectivity, overintellectualization, rigid attitudes toward morality and standards of behavior, meticulousness of speech, avoidance of dirty language, a defective sense of humor, obsessive worrying, and timidity. Some patients are petulant, querulous, demanding, and provocative, but well-directed aggressive action and clear-cut expressions of anger are uncommon. Many are characterized by an extreme sensitivity, with an almost uncanny perception of hostile or rejecting attitudes on the part of others. Patients feel inferiority, an acute sense of obligation, and a need to experience some sense of security. By and large, they avoid chances and do not deal daringly with their environment.

The patient appears to have a dependent

relation with one or two key persons, usually a parent or parent figure; on the other hand, he reveals a limited capacity to establish warm, genuine friendships with others. The quality of expectation from the key figure is magical, imperious, and omnipotent.

In general, the mothers of such patients are described as controlling and dominating. They are either cold, unhappy, pleasureless, gloomy women with no great zest or enjoyment in life or hard-driving, businesslike, perfectionistic women who are active and concerned with many outside interests but often dissatisfied with their own or others' accomplishments, especially their children's. The woman patient is inclined to portray her father as a gentle, kind, passive, usually ineffective man to whom she is quite attached. The male patient describes his father either as brutal, punitive, threatening, coarse, and very masculine or, less often, as passive and weak and unable to stand up to the mother.

Ulcerative colitis patients display low interest and participation in sexual activity. Frigidity and degrees of impotence are common. Many acknowledge a preference for being fondled or cuddled. In marital relationships the spouse commonly fulfills the role of the succoring, sustaining mother or takes a role subordinate to the patient's mother.

Precipitating Psychological Stress. Psychologically stressful events are likely to fall into three categories: (1) real, fantasied, or threatened interruption of a key relation, (2) demands by others for performance that the patient feels incapable of fulfilling, and (3) overwhelming threat from or disapproval by a parental figure. As a rule, hostility and rage toward the disappointing figure are repressed. Common to all these circumstances is an acute or gradually developing feeling on the part of the patient that he has become helpless to cope with what is happening. The disease becomes active in the course of giving up psychologically and is marked by the affect of helplessness.

Treatment. The first step in the treatment of an acutely ill ulcerative colitis patient is to establish a relationship. This step is best achieved through the sensitive quality of the physician's first inquiry and his prompt attention to relief of discomfort. Thereafter, constant awareness of the patient's needs and of his characteristic ways of functioning is of the utmost importance in enabling the patient to

use the relationship with his physician as a means of re-establishing his psychological equilibrium and health. The patient readily endows his physician with the omniscient and omnipotent qualities of the key object.

Awareness of the kind of relationship that exists with other members of the family, especially with the mother or the spouse, prepares the physician for the kinds of difficulties that may arise. Usually, the important other figure is experiencing a considerable amount of guilt concerning the patient's illness and may have a strong need to reassert her control over both herself and the patient. The physician must not take a retaliative or a punitive attitude toward the other members of the family. On the other hand, to the patient he must appear stronger than the dominant family member.

There is no evidence at present that psychotherapy, no matter how intensive, can eliminate the biological defect underlying colitis. Therefore, an expectation of complete cure is unjustified. Remission and complete healing are common, but psychotherapy cannot ensure against a recurrence in the face of sufficient stress. The major contribution that psychotherapy can make is to modify the basic psychological structure and capacity to relate, so as to render the patient less vulnerable to situations in which the disease had become manifest in the past.

Insight therapy is useful with the relatively more active, independent patients. Patients who are strongly symbiotic or transitional are helped more by support, catharsis, and suggestion than by interpretation.

Granulomatous (Regional) Enteritis and Colitis (Crohn's Disease)

The available data indicate many similarities between these patients and those with ulcerative colitis. Indeed, the diseases may occur in the same family, suggesting a common genetic factor. The psychological resemblance is greatest in respect to the prominence of obsessive-compulsiveness, the patterns of relating, and the vulnerability to object loss and the subsequent development of giving up as the setting in which onset or relapse of active disease occurs.

Celiac Sprue

Celiac disease of childhood and many instances of idiopathic steatorrhea of adulthood probably represent the same disorder. In both conditions identical and, to a large extent, reversible damage to the small intestinal mucosa is produced by low molecular weight, glutamine-rich polypeptides isolated from the breakdown products of gluten, the water-insoluble protein moiety of wheat. Evidence for a genetic determinant has been brought forth.

The underlying mucosal defect and the presence of gluten in the diet may both be necessary but not sufficient for the development of the malabsorption syndrome. Some researchers have suggested that psychological stress may be a contributing factor. Among children, a disturbance in the mother-child relation, including changes in patterns of handling and feeding, appears to be associated with exacerbations; remissions have been brought about by improving the mother-child relation, even without removing gluten from the diet. Among adults, the onset or recurrences are noted in settings in which real or threatened loss of support eventuates in psychological giving up, with feelings of sadness, despair, and helplessness.

Irritable Bowel Syndrome

This is the classic functional bowel disorder, characterized by alternating diarrhea and constipation, abdominal cramps, flatulence, and, at times, increased mucus in the stools. Patients with spastic colon have lower abdominal pain and cramps as the main symptom and, in addition, have constipation that alternates with diarrhea or with periods of normal bowel movements. Patients with functional diarrhea have little or no abdominal pain, their chief symptom being constant or intermittent diarrhea. There may be as yet unidentified organic factors influencing the bowel response to psychological stress.

Patients with spastic colon are said to be rigid, obsessional, and compulsive persons; those with functional diarrhea show more diffuse free-floating or phobic anxiety. Many tend to be orderly, methodical, conscientious, precise, preoccupied with cleanliness, tidiness, regularity, punctuality, and schedules. Such patients place a high premium on intellectual control and performance and are restrained in their expression of emotions. They are hypersensitive and easily hurt, to the point at times of paranoid suspiciousness. Important in the underlying psychodynamics are conflicts about giving and receiving and the control of aggression. Distrustful and fearful of rejection, espe-

cially if aggressive or sexual impulses are displayed, they tend to hold on to what they possess and not to give. Feelings of depression are common, and there is a relatively high incidence of significant clinical depression.

REFERENCES

Engel, G. L. Studies of ulcerative colitis. II. The nature of the somatic processes and the adequacy of psychosomatic hypotheses. Am. J. Med., *16:* 416, 1954.

Engel, G. L. Studies of ulcerative colitis. III. The nature of the psychologic processes. Am. J. Med., *19:* 231, 1955.

Karush, A., Daniels, G. E., O'Connor, F. G., and Stern, L. O. The response to psychotherapy in chronic ulcerative colitis. I. Pretreatment factors. Psychosom. Med., *30:* 255, 1968.

Karush, A., Daniels, G. E., O'Connor, F. G., and Stern, L. O. The response to psychotherapy in chronic ulcerative colitis. II. Factors arising from the therapeutic situation. Psychosom. Med., *31:* 201, 1969.

McKegney, F. P., Gordon, R. O., and Levine, S. M. A psychosomatic comparison of patients with ulcerative colitis and Crohn's disease. Psychosom. Med., *32:* 153, 1970.

Whybrow, P. C., Kane, F. J., and Lipton, M. A. Regional ileitis and psychiatric disorder. Psychosom. Med., *30:* 209, 1968.

25.5.   OBESITY

Definition

Obesity is a condition characterized by excessive accumulations of fat in the body. By convention, obesity is said to be present when body weight exceeds by 20 per cent the standard weight listed in the usual height-weight tables.

Epidemiology

Social factors in the United States exert a powerful influence on the prevalence of obesity. The most striking influence is that of socio-economic status. One study found obesity six times more common among women of low status than among those of high status (see Figure 1). A similar, although weaker, relationship was found among men. Social mobility, ethnic factors, and generation in the United States also influence the prevalence of obesity.

Age is the second major influence on obesity. There is a threefold increase between ages 20 and 50. At age 50, prevalence falls sharply, presumably because of the very high mortality of the obese from cardiovascular disease in the older age groups. Women show a higher prevalence of obesity than men, particularly past age 50.

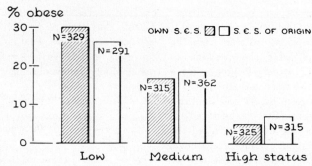

FIGURE 1. Decreasing prevalence of obesity with increasing socioeconomic status (S. E. S.) among women in a large American city. Socio-economic status of origin is almost as strongly linked to obesity as is the person's own socio-economic status. (P. B. Goldblatt, M. E. Moore, and A. J. Stunkard, Social factors in obesity. J. A. M. A., *192:* 1039, 1965)

Causes

One accumulates fat by eating more calories than are expended as energy. But we understand only imperfectly the regulation of body weight. (See Figure 2.)

The fat stores of an average nonobese man constitute 15 per cent of his body weight —enough to provide for all his caloric needs for nearly a month. During a year, he consumes approximately one million calories; his body fat stores remain unchanged during this time because he expends an equal number of calories. An error of no more than 10 per cent in either intake or output would lead to a 30-pound change in body weight within this year.

What normally activates the apparatus regulating body weight? One stops eating at the end of a meal because he has replenished some nutrient that had been depleted. And he becomes hungry again when the nutrient, which had been restored by the meal, is once again depleted. It seems reasonable that some metabolic signal, derived from food that has been absorbed, is carried by the blood to the brain. There, this signal activates receptor cells, probably in the hypothalamus, to produce satiety. Hunger is the consequence of the decreasing strength of this same metabolic signal, secondary to the depletion of the critical nutrient.

But single-factor theories of obesity encounter two specific problems. First, how can a mechanism of short-term, meal-to-meal control of food intake account for the remarkable stability of body weight over long periods of time and in the face of often marked short-term fluctuations? Second, how can a single-factor theory or indeed, any physiological theory account for the function of satiety? For satiety occurs so soon after the beginning of a meal that only a small proportion of the total caloric content of the meal can have been absorbed.

If humoral factors do not terminate eating, what does? A full stomach may be a better answer than one would have thought even a few years ago.

People learn, as do other animals, to change their food intake and meal size in response to changes in energy expenditure and in the nutritive value of their food. Oral and gastric factors may serve as conditioned stimuli; humoral factors absorbed from the gastrointestinal tract may serve as the latter, unconditioned stimuli. Impaired alimentary learning may be involved in the eating disorders found in obesity. An impairment of satiety appears to play a major role in these disorders.

The precision of regulation of body weight, even among obese organisms, suggests that the causes of obesity are to be sought in the determinants of the set point of the regulation. Besides social and emotional determinants, there are genetic, developmental, physical activity, and brain-damage determinants.

Genetic Determinants

The existence of numerous forms of inherited obesity in animals and the ease with which adiposity can be produced by selective breeding make it clear that genetic factors can play a determining role in obesity. These factors must also be presumed to be important in human obesity. Evidence of the heritability of somatotypes is stronger than that of obesity, and obesity occurs with much greater frequency in

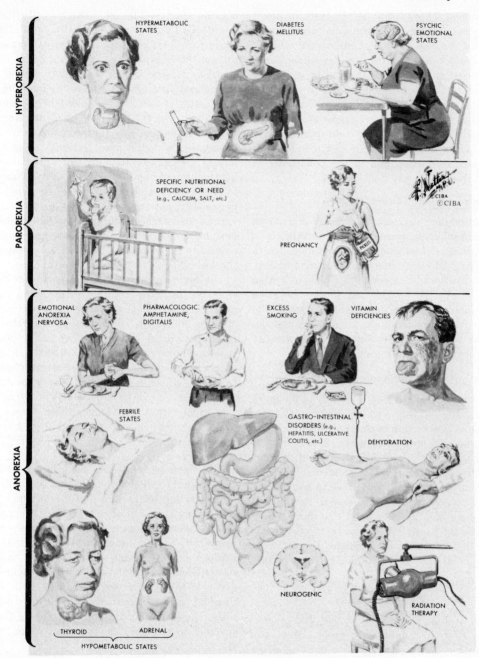

FIGURE 2. Disturbances of hunger and appetite. © Copyright 1959 CIBA Pharmaceutical Company, Division of CIBA-GEIGY Corporation. Reproduced, with permission, from THE CIBA COLLECTION OF MEDICAL ILLUSTRATIONS by Frank H. Netter, M.D. All rights reserved.)

some physical types than in others. Obese adolescent girls, for example, show extremely low ratings for ectomorphy; the presence of even a moderate degree of ectomorphy appears to protect against obesity.

Developmental Determinants

Early in life, adipose tissue grows by both increases in cell number and increases in cell size. Once the number of adipocytes has been established, it does not seem to be susceptible to change. Obesity that began early in life is characterized by adipose tissue with an increased number and size of adipocytes. Obesity that began in adult life, on the other hand, results solely from an increase in the size of the adipocytes. In both instances, weight reduction produces a decrease in cell size. The greater number of such cells—perhaps as much as fivefold—in juvenile-onset obese persons may be a factor in their widely recognized difficulty in weight reduction and in the persistence of their obesity.

Physical Activity Determinants

The marked decrease in physical activity in affluent societies seems to be the major factor in the recent rise of obesity as a public health problem. Physical inactivity restricts energy expenditure and may contribute to an increased food intake. Although food intake increases with increasing energy expenditure over a wide range of energy demands, intake does not decrease proportionately when physical activity falls below a certain minimum level.

Brain-damage Determinants

Brain damage can lead to obesity, although it is probably a very rare cause of obesity in humans. Destruction of the ventromedial hypothalamus can produce obesity. There is growing evidence that the central nervous system, particularly the lateral and ventromedial hypothalamic areas, adjusts food intake in response to changing energy requirements so as to maintain fat stores at a baseline level determined by a specific set point. There is no reason to assume that the nervous system defends the same set point in all persons of the same height and body build.

Clinical Features

Many obese persons report that they overeat when they are emotionally upset, often soon thereafter. But many nonobese persons report similar experiences, and it is difficult to ascertain the specificity for obesity of such short-term contingencies. Reports linking emotional factors and obesity over the long range seem more specific. It is common for obese persons to lose large amounts of weight when they fall in love and to gain weight when they lose a loved one.

The habitual eating patterns of many obese persons seem similar in many ways to those found in different forms of experimental obesity. Impaired satiety is a particularly important problem. Obese persons seem inordinately susceptible to food cues in their environment, to the palatability of foods, and to the inability to stop eating if food is available. Obese persons are usually susceptible to all kinds of external stimuli to eating, but they remain relatively unresponsive to the usual internal signals of hunger. Some are often unable to distinguish between hunger and other kinds of dysphoria.

The view that obese persons have a specific personality pattern is no longer held. Of the various emotional disturbances to which obese persons are subject, only two are specifically related to their obesity. The first is overeating; the second is a disturbance in body image.

The night-eating syndrome seems to be precipitated by stressful life circumstances and, once present, tends to recur daily until the stress is alleviated. The binge-eating syndrome is characterized by the sudden, compulsive ingestion of very large amounts of food in a very short time, usually with great subsequent agitation and self-condemnation. It, too, appears to represent a reaction to stress. But, in contrast to the night-eating syndrome, these bouts of overeating are not periodic, and they are far more often linked to specific precipitating circumstances.

The obese person whose body image is disturbed characteristically feels that his body is grotesque and loathesome and that others view it with hostility and contempt. This feeling is closely associated with self-consciousness and impaired social functioning. Emotionally healthy obese persons have no body image disturbances, and only a minority of neurotic obese persons have such disturbances. The disorder is confined to those who have been obese since childhood; and, even among these juvenile onset obese, less than half suffer from it.

Course and Prognosis

The prognosis for weight reduction is poor, and the course of obesity tends toward inexorable progression. There is a threefold increase in the prevalence of obesity with advancing age, and both individual humans and animals show increasing amounts of body fat with increasing age. The prognosis is particularly poor for persons who become obese in childhood. Juvenile-onset obesity tends to be more severe, more resistant to treatment, and more likely to be associated with emotional disturbance.

Treatment

The basis of weight reduction is simple—establish a caloric deficit by bringing intake below output. The simplest way to reduce caloric intake is by means of a low-calorie diet. The best long-term effects are achieved with a balanced diet that contains readily available foods. For most people, the most satisfactory reducing diet consists of their usual foods in amounts determined with the aid of tables of food values available in standard works. Such a diet gives the best chance of long-term maintenance of the weight loss achieved by dieting. But it is the most difficult kind of diet to follow during the period of weight reduction.

Many obese persons find it easier to use a novel or even bizarre diet. Whatever effectiveness these diets may have results, in large part, from their monotony. When the dieter stops the diet and returns to his usual fare, the incentives to overeat are multiplied.

Effective pharmacological treatment of obesity is largely confined to the amphetamines. These agents suppress appetite; when used in conjunction with diet in a carefully planned treatment program, they have some limited usefulness. In the face of today's widespread drug abuse, however, the mild and transient value of amphetamines in the treatment of obesity is probably outweighed by the danger posed by their abuse.

Thyroid or thyroid analogues are indicated for the occasional obese person with hypothryroidism and probably not otherwise. Bulk producers may help control the constipation that follows decreased food intake, but their effectiveness in weight reduction is doubtful.

Increased physical activity is frequently recommended as a part of weight-reduction regimens, but its usefulness has probably been underestimated. Since caloric expenditure in most forms of physical activity is directly proportional to body weight, obese persons expend more calories with the same amount of activity than do those of normal weight. Furthermore, increased physical activity may actually cause a decrease in the food intake of sedentary persons.

This combination of increased caloric expenditure and probably decreased food intake makes an increase in physical activity a highly desirable feature of any weight-reduction program.

Surgical treatment of severe obesity has been attempted by means of an intestinal bypass that short-circuits most of the absorptive surface of the intestine. But a jejunoileal shunt is fraught with danger and should be considered an investigative procedure.

Group therapy extends the number of obese patients the physician can treat and probably also increases the effectiveness of treatment. Group methods are being applied by TOPS (Take Off Pounds Sensibly), a self-help group, and Weight Watchers, a commercial organization.

As many as half of the patients routinely treated for obesity by family physicians may develop mild anxiety and depression. In addition, a high incidence of emotional disturbance has been reported among obese persons undergoing long-term, in-hospital treatment by fasting or severe caloric restriction. Obese persons with extensive psychopathology, those with a history of emotional disturbance during dieting, and those in the midst of a life crisis should attempt weight reduction, if at all, cautiously and under careful supervision.

There is no evidence that uncovering the unconscious causes of overeating can alter the symptom choice of persons who overeat in response to stress. Years after successful psychotherapy and successful weight reduction, persons who overeat under stress continue to do so. Furthermore, many obese persons seem particularly vulnerable to the overdependency on the therapist and the inordinate regression that may occur during the uncovering psychotherapies.

Two conditions may constitute specific indications for psychodynamic psychotherapy: disturbances in body image and the binge-eating syndrome. Both have been successfully treated, with enduring weight losses. Neither condition has been influenced by other forms of treatment, including weight reduction. Psychotherapy of patients with these conditions frequently requires years to ensure enduring results.

The most important new development in the treatment of obesity has been the introduction of behavior modification. However, its greater effectiveness is in contrast to ineffective traditional methods of treatment and by no means implies a solution to the problem of obesity.

REFERENCES

Bruch, H. *Eating Disorders: Obesity and Anorexia Nervosa and the Person Within.* Basic Books, New York, 1973.

LeMagnen, J. Advances in studies on the physiological control and regulation of food intake. Prog. Physiol. Psychol., *4:* 203, 1971.

Mayer, J. *Overweight: Causes, Cost, and Control.* Prentice-Hall, Englewood Cliffs, N. J., 1968.

Schachter, S. Some extraordinary facts about obese humans and rats. Am. Psychol., *26:* 129, 1971.

Stuart, R. B., and Davis, B. *Slim Chance in a Fat World: Behavioral Control of Obesity.* Research Press, Champaign, Ill., 1971.

Stunkard, A. J. New therapies for the eating disorders: Behavior modification of obesity and anorexia nervosa. Arch. Gen. Psychiatry, *26:* 391, 1972.

25.6   ANOREXIA NERVOSA

Introduction

Persons with psychogenic malnutrition are a heterogenous population. There is a group of adolescents, many overweight, who become desperately concerned about their weight, feel self-conscious and ugly, and then diet excessively to escape obesity. Most then become phobic about food, dread a return to obesity, and continue in a state of semistarvation lest they lose control again and become fat. Another group seem to develop the syndrome as a result of hysterical or somatic disturbances. Gastralgias, dysphagias, abdominal distress, and other somatic problems lead to a diminution in eating to avoid the distress. Some patients are obsessional. They spend their waking hours ruminating about food and weight, sometimes fluctuating between starvation and bulimia, often using semistarvation as a form of self-punishment or a means of purification for presumed sins. Finally, there are those few sexually naive adolescent girls who fear a fantasized pregnancy. They starve themselves to prevent the development of an abdominal protrusion that will reveal their imagined plight.

Epidemiology

Anorexia nervosa is an uncommon disorder in its severe forms. Mild disturbances are probably not rare. The annual incidence in the general population has been reported as 0.24 to 1.3 per 100,000. The sex ratio reflects a remarkable preponderance of females. A disproportionate number belong to the upper and middle social classes, which may reflect the worth attributed to leanness by these groups.

Causes and Psychodynamics

For some of these patients, antecedent circumstances focused attention on eating and adiposity. In some cases, one or both parents had a special preoccupation with food, eating, or obesity. Some parents were obese, food faddists, or unduly concerned with calories. In many cases, food early became a familial concern and a basis for conflict and strife. Some had many aversions to food; others were overweight. Some were temperamental eaters or developed gastrointestinal ailments. Many appear to have been good quiet children who were obedient and helpful, as well as excellent students. As adolescents, many were shy, timid, neat and controlled but frequently uninformed and fearful about sexual matters. Naivete, constrictuion, and a lack of personal initiative are common.

The precipitating events, anteceding the loss of weight, include such traumatic experiences as separations from critical people, puberty, sexual experiences, and failures. Some of these patients were initially overweight, but their obesity led to self-consciousness, discontent, and social isolation. A common instigator of a diet is the ridicule of friends or family. Some lose their appetites, but many struggle to restrain their eating lest they revert to their former obese plight.

A prominent feature in some cases is the attribution of symbolic meaning to food and obesity. Eating comes to signify evil and self-indulgence. Like ascetics, these patients select semistarvation to attain a sense of control over their sordid body, its impulses and carnal desires. Mastery over a masturbatory, homosexual, or heterosexual conflict may be achieved by this tactic. For others, semistarvation serves as a form of self-punishment and purification, often to expiate guilt. Some perceive cachexia as a form of inconspicuousness or anonymity. It is associated with a return to childhood, infantile dependency, and repudiation of responsibility, feminine contours, and sexuality.

In many cases, the dieting and malnutrition

are conspicuous, powerful behaviors that provoke family and friends. They become ways to gain attention, express anger or combat one's family.

A few patients starve themselves to inanition and die. Most do not seem aware of auorexia nervosa's lethal potential.

Clinical Features

The average patient with anorexia nervosa is a female who weighed 122 pounds before her illness and lost 44 pounds to a weight of 78 pounds. The age of onset is usually in the late teens and early 20's. Most patients with anorexia nervosa are females.

Eating patterns vary widely. Some patients go on diets and lose their appetites; others never had big appetites. Others retain their appetites but curb them because of the fear of somatic distress or apprehension about obesity. In a few patients hatred for food reinforces the diet. Internal signals of hunger and satiety that guide most people are misinterpreted or lost. Eating habits become disorganized, and peculiar food preferences and cravings emerge. Some patients hide or dispose of their food to avoid nourishment. Others induce vomiting. Others concentrate on the distal end of their gastrointestinal tract by resorting to cathartics and enemas to rid the body of calories.

Menstrual changes are usually found. Amenorrhea is a frequent but not invariable finding.

The remarkable energy and activity of these patients has been repeatedly cited. Some, perhaps one fourth of them, exhibit this trait. Most patients lose weight slowly, so that adaptation to malnutrition has time to occur.

Constipation is another common finding. The usual explanation has been the diet of small bulk that these patients consume. Many take laxatives to relieve the constipation, but others use purgatives chronically and addictively to rid their bodies of the offending nutriments.

There are also reports of compulsive stealing of food or other articles. A few patients narcissistically spend time before mirrors, admiring their emaciated form. Some react to their personal ambivalence about food by showing an inordinate interest in recipes and cooking.

From 3 to 15 per cent of patients die of malnutrition or intercurrent infection. Perhaps 3 per cent eventually commit suicide.

Severely cachetic patients present hypotension, slow pulse, hypothermia, cyanosis of the extremities, peculiar pigmentation and hyperkeratosis of the skin, increase of lanugo hair over the body, atrophy of the breast, and reduction in axillary and pubic hair. Leukopenia, lymphocytosis, and anemia may appear. Hypoglycemia, hypercholesterolemia, hypoproteinemia, and hypercarotemia have all been observed. All are probably a consequence of the malnutrition and abnormal diet. Those patients who persistently induce vomiting develop hypokalemia as a complication. (See Figure 1.)

Differential Diagnosis

The diagnosis is usually not difficult, particularly when there is a history of a fear of obesity, the onset of a diet, unwillingness to eat, self-induced vomiting, food binges, and amenorrhea in a late adolescent female. The clinican may occasionally be deceived when there are gastrointestinal symptoms and other somatic complaints. A routine examination may uncover no organic pathology and a premature psychiatric diagnosis may be made. The weight loss may be due to esophageal, gastric, duodenal, or pancreatic pathology or granulomatous disease of the small bowel. Anorexia nervosa is also found in children, middle-aged women, and men. A great loss of weight in these groups is not always due to chronic disease, neoplasm, or occult infection.

Treatment

There is at this time no specific therapy that is generally accredited or experimentally confirmed. One must first decide whether the malnutrition is life-threatening. When a patient approaches a weight of 65 pounds or loses 50 per cent of ideal weight, the physician should not delay. If the patient does not begin to eat voluntarily, forced feeding by gastric intubation should be started.

About two thirds of these patients emerge as improved or recovered; one third remain unchanged or die. Some patients fully recover; others recover only to relapse. Some swing from malnutrition to obesity; others remain cachectic for many years. A few die from inanition or intercurrent infection.

At present, the indicated therapies are eclec-

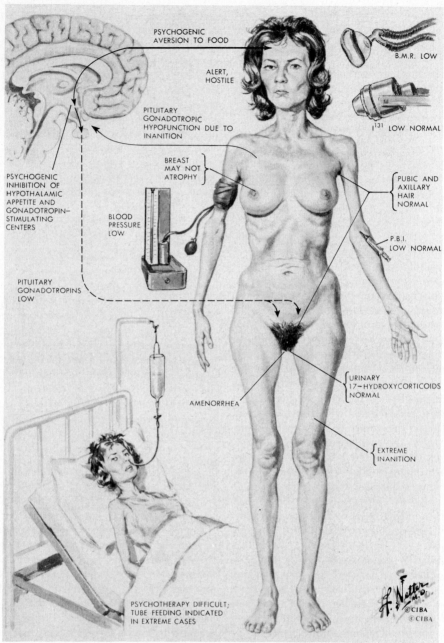

PSYCHOGENIC
AVERSION TO FOOD

B.M.R. LOW

ALERT,
HOSTILE

I¹³¹ LOW NORMAL

PITUITARY
GONADOTROPIC
HYPOFUNCTION DUE TO
INANITION

BREAST
MAY NOT
ATROPHY

PSYCHOGENIC
INHIBITION OF
HYPOTHALAMIC
APPETITE AND
GONADOTROPIN–
STIMULATING
CENTERS

PUBIC AND
AXILLARY
HAIR
NORMAL

BLOOD
PRESSURE
LOW

P.B.I.
LOW NORMAL

PITUITARY
GONADOTROPINS
LOW

URINARY
17–HYDROXYCORTICOIDS
NORMAL

AMENORRHEA

EXTREME
INANITION

PSYCHOTHERAPY DIFFICULT;
TUBE FEEDING INDICATED
IN EXTREME CASES

N61·62 VOLUME 4—ENDOCRINE SYSTEM PITUITARY GLAND ANOREXIA NERVOSADR. EZRIN

FIGURE 1. Anorexia nervosa. (© Copyright 1959 CIBA Pharmaceutical Company, Division of CIBA-GEIGY Corporation. Reproduced, with permission, from THE CIBA COLLECTION OF MEDICAL ILLUSTRATIONS by Frank H. Netter, M.D. All rights reserved.)

tic. Tranquilizers and antidepressant drugs may be used to reduce anxiety or treat depression. A wide range of other treatments may be applied, ranging from supportive strategies through hypnosis and insightful tactics.

REFERENCES

Bliss, E. L., and Branch, C. H. H. *Anorexia Nervosa.* Harper & Row, New York, 1960.
Crisp, A. H. Clinical and therapeutic aspects of anorexia nervosa: A study of 30 cases. J. Psychosom. Res., *9:* 67, 1965.
Dally, P. *Anorexia Nervosa.* Grune & Stratton, New York,

1969.

Nemiah, J. C. Anorexia nervosa. Medicine, *29:* 225, 1950.

Russell, G. F. M. Metabolic, endocrine and psychiatric aspects of anorexia nervosa. In *The Scientific Basis of Medicine Annual Reviews*, p. 236. Athlone Press, London, 1969.

Theander, S. Anorexia nervosa. Acta Psychiatr. Scan., *214* (Suppl.): 29, 1970.

25.7   PSYCHOPHYSIOLOGIC CARDIOVASCULAR DISORDERS

Introduction

Changes in the functioning of the cardiovascular system are commonly associated with emotional arousal. Fear, anxiety, anger, elation, and excitement are all accompanied by changes in the rate, rhythm, output, and stroke volume of the heart, changes in arterial blood pressure, and changes in other indices of cardiovascular function. These affective and physiological responses may be evoked by stimuli emanating from the environment, particularly those subjectively interpreted as signifying threat, loss, or gain. Information inputs derived from the body and spontaneously arising thoughts and images may have similar effects, depending on their subjective meaning. Further, perception of changed cardiac action or of chest pain, regardless of its origin, may give rise to fearful appraisal and thus intensify the affective arousal and associated cardiovascular symptoms.

Life situations and events that make heavy adaptive demands on the person are often viewed as potential codeterminants of cardiovascular pathology. Once such a pathology is present, intense affective arousal may lead to cardiac decompensation and other potentially lethal effects. On the other hand, the occurrence of a myocardial infarction or the development of hypertension or angina may have a meaning for the patient that results in the development of anxiety or depression or both. Pyschological responses may not only aggravate cardiovascular dysfunction and symptoms but also lead to maladaptive coping strategies.

Coronary Heart Disease

The alarming rise in the incidence of CHD is attributed to changing ways of life, to sociocultural and economic factors. There is no evidence that any constellation of psychological factors can by itself cause CHD. But many psychological variables have been postulated to predispose to CHD. The most impressive empirical evidence supports a hypothesis that a behavior pattern, designated type A, distinguishes coronary-prone persons. This pattern is an overt life style characterized by extreme competitiveness, drive for success, impatience, restlessness, hyperalertness, and a subjective sense of time urgency and pressure of commitments and responsibilities. People lacking these behavioral characteristics have been designated as type B. Men with a type A behavior pattern tend to have elevated plasma triglyceride and cholesterol values, hyperinsulinemic response to a glucose challenge, and increased diurnal secretion of noradrenaline. Type A men have increased prevalence and incidence of CHD and of myocardial infarction and angina pectoris. Since the chance of recurrent and fatal myocardial infarction is associated with type A behavior, it appears that this behavior pattern increases the probability of developing manifest CHD and influences its severity.

Psychodynamically oriented workers claim that an obsessive-compulsive neurotic personality style underlies the type A behavior pattern. Differences have been found between patients with angina pectoris and those who suffered a myocardial infarction. The angina patients tend to be more hypochondriacal, anxious, and overtly emotionally unstable. The myocardial infarction patients are more outwardly controlled and successful in repressing and denying anxiety, anger, and depression.

Other psychosocial variables postulated to predispose to CHD include status incongruity, job dissatisfaction, work overload, and prolonged psychological stress. In this country, the incidence and prevalence of CHD appear to be greater in the blue-collar group than in the managerial one.

Certain personality attributes predispose a person to react and act in a manner described as type A behavior pattern. Such behavior, however, depends for its full expression on living in a social environment that provides opportunities and rewards for competitive striving. Affluent societies are characterized by a value system and socio-economic conditions that allow extreme forms of type A behavior to flourish.

Further, the ubiquity in such societies of such living habits as cigarette smoking, excessive consumption of a diet rich in saturated fats and calories, and physical inactivity adds a set of factors that, in conjunction with restless striving, predispose to CHD. In addition, frequent exposure to information inputs that are excessive, novel, attractive, discrepant, or threatening characterizes living in technological societies and results in frequent affective and autonomic arousal, which is accompanied by the increased secretion of catecholamines. The catecholamines increase the oxygen requirements of the myocardium, release free fatty acids from body fat deposits, increase the heart rate, and contribute to the elevation of blood pressure. These sympatho-adrenal concomitants of emotional arousal may contribute directly and indirectly to atherogenesis and CHD.

Myocardial Infarction and Angina

Psychological Precipitants

Myocardial infarction, angina pectoris, and cardiac arrhythmias may follow in the wake of subjectively stressful life changes or situations. What constitutes psychological stress is determined by the person's particular vulnerabilities, his appraisal of the event, and the consequent intensity of his emotional arousal. Some life changes, however, are likely to be deleterious for many persons. Bereavement is one of them. Losses of valued relationships, prestige, and job have been implicated antecedents of myocardial infarction. Losses usually evoke grief, depression, a sense of emotional drain or exhaustion, helplessness, and hopelessness. There is some evidence that any event that elicits one or more of these emotional responses in a person already suffering from CHD may trigger a myocardial infarction.

Patients with angina pectoris show a tendency to anxiety, compulsiveness, somatic concerns in response to stress, and a lower pain threshold long before their illness. Anger, anxiety, elation, excitement—states sharing heightened autonomic arousal—are able to trigger and exacerbate anginal attacks. Anxiety evoked by anginal pain and its threatening meaning increase the frequency and severity of the attacks. Nocturnal anginal attacks can be precipiated by frightening dreams.

Psychological Responses

The most important immediate responses to myocardial infarction are fear and minimization of danger. Intense fear may contribute to the onset of lethal arrhythmias. Minimization or denial interferes with the decision process to seek immediate medical help. The resulting delay in initiating treatment may be fatal.

More than 50 per cent of patients hospitalized for treatment of ischemic heart disease show moderate or severe depressive symptoms or anxiety. The more severe the disease, the more chronic the depression. The most disturbed patients tend to be those who were tense and upset before hospitalization. On discharge from the hospital after a myocardial infarction or severe angina pectoris, the crucial task is to avoid patient disability unwarranted by the actual cardiac impairment. About one of every six cardiac patients fails to return to work because of psychological reasons.

Several types of response to and coping with manifest CHD may be distinguished: (1) realistic acceptance of the damage and judicious attempts at full attainable rehabilitation, (2) excessive dependence and related perpetuation of the sick role, (3) minimization of the significance of the disease and attempts to live as if it did not exist, (4) the use of the heart disease to manipulate and control others by playing on their sympathy and feelings of guilt.

These responses and coping strategies are influenced by personality, family, and medical factors. Persons who habitually deny or minimize the threatening significance of events tend to do so after a myocardial infarction. Such patients tend to disregard medical advice on restrictions of physcial activity and smoking. Persons who fear dependence, passivity, and enforced inactivity are also liable to fail to comply with medical management and rehabilitation advice. In contrast, persons characterized by trait anxiety and habitual overconcern about bodily integrity tend to respond to the heart attack with an overt anxiety neurosis and hypochondriasis. Patients complaining of left chest pain after an infarction have high neuroticism scores and are frequently disabled out of proportion to their cardiac impairment. They refuse to resume their vocational, recreational, and sexual activities. Those disabled by a psychiatric disorder may respond to adequate information, reassurance, the use of minor tranquilizers or antidepressants, and, in some cases, interpretative psychotherapy dealing with the underlying conflicts and guilt feelings. Patients who derive primary or secondary gains from the illness may respond to group therapy and to help in finding more adaptive coping strategies.

The behavior of the patient's spouse may augment his anxiety, dependence, and invalidism or, on the contrary, impel him to undertake efforts inimical to his health. The wives of patients with myocardial infarction often develop anxiety, depression, and somatic symptoms. They tend to blame themselves for the husband's illness. Some develop chest pains and palpitations. Anxiety in the spouse is liable to increase that in the patient and either enhance his dependence and disability or lead to a premature return to work and sexual activity, minimization of symptoms, and a general attitude of forced independence and vigor. Interviews with and emotional support for the spouse should be part of the rehabilitation of a cardiac patient. Marital couple psychotherapy may be helpful in selected cases. Counseling about sexual activity for the patients should be a rule. Postinfarction patients may return to sexual activity at the same time they are able to perform ordinary activities without symptoms, cardiac arrhythmias, or electrocardiogram changes.

The behavior of the doctor also influences the patient's attitude. Inadequate, vague, or frightening statements may increase the patient's apprehension or noncompliance. Treating the symptoms of anxiety and depression as if they were manifestations of cardiac pathology tends to prolong the patient's disability.

The incidence of adverse psychological reactions to a stay in an intensive care unit varies in different studies. It is distinctly lower in coronary care units than in the intensive care units receiving patients after open-heart surgery. A coronary care unit has little adverse effect on the patient's psychological state. Some patients become anxious or depressed on transfer to a general ward and require special emotional support and reassurance from the staff to overcome their separation anxiety. Anxiety may be present in 80 per cent of the coronary care unit patients, but it is rarely extreme and is related to a threatening illness, rather than to the physical setting of the unit.

Cardiac surgery, especially open-heart surgery, is followed by psychiatric complications more often than are other major operations. The incidence of psychiatric disorders after open-heart surgery is at least twice as high as after closed-heart surgery. It ranges from 25 to 50 per cent. Four psychiatric syndromes have been reported to follow open-heart surgery: delirium, which is the most common complication; hallucinosis; paranoid psychosis; and a mixed affective syndrome, psychotic or neurotic, with varying degrees of depression, anxiety, elation, or apathy. Psotcardiotomy delirium may be reduced by the careful selection of patients, preoperative psychological preparation, shortened bypass time, avoidance of hypotension, and the provision of optimal sensory input, sleep, and supportive nursing care in the intensive care unit. Treatment of severe postcardiotomy peridol and, at times, electroshock treatments.

Essential Hypertension

Psychosocial Predisposing Factors

A wide range of environmental stimuli engendering fear, anger, and frustration may bring about an elevation of arterial blood pressure. (See Figure 1.) Hypertensive patients tend to respond with higher and more prolonged blood pressure rises than do normotensives. Anger tends to be associated with an increase in diastolic pressure. Experimental subjects exposed to an anger-arousing task and allowed to aggress against the provocateur displayed a fall of their raised distolic pressure as long as they experienced little guilt about their aggression. Acute elevations tend to subside over a period of a few weeks to a few months. The reduction of blood pressure in hypertensive patients may occur in the setting of a good doctor-patient relationship, in psychotherapy, or during hospitalization. These findings, however, do not prove the causative role of psychological factors in essential hypertension.

Certain occupations appear to be associated with an increased frequency of essential hypertension. Cobb and Rose found high prevalence and incidence rates of hypertension in air traffic controllers, especially those working at high traffic-density centers. Suppressed hostility when arbitrarily attacked and feeling guilt about the display of hostility are both related to

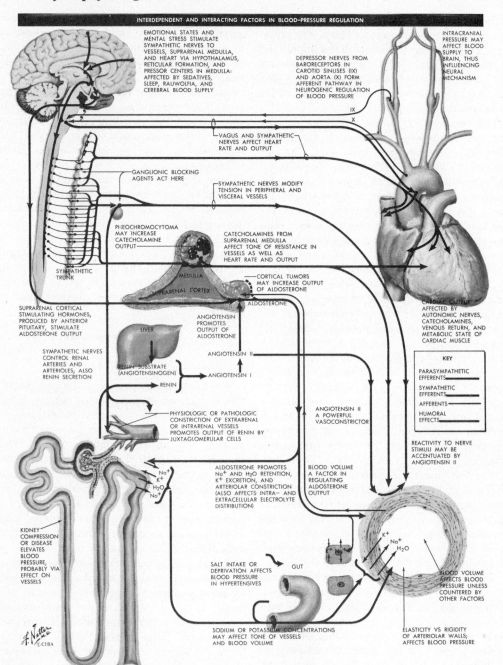

INTERDEPENDENT AND INTERACTING FACTORS IN BLOOD-PRESSURE REGULATION

EMOTIONAL STATES AND MENTAL STRESS STIMULATE SYMPATHETIC NERVES TO VESSELS, SUPRARENAL MEDULLA, AND HEART VIA HYPOTHALAMUS, RETICULAR FORMATION, AND PRESSOR CENTERS IN MEDULLA: AFFECTED BY SEDATIVES, SLEEP, RAUWOLFIA, AND CEREBRAL BLOOD SUPPLY

DEPRESSOR NERVES FROM BARORECEPTORS IN CAROTID SINUSES (IX) AND AORTA (X) FORM AFFERENT PATHWAY IN NEUROGENIC REGULATION OF BLOOD PRESSURE

INTRACRANIAL PRESSURE MAY AFFECT BLOOD SUPPLY TO BRAIN, THUS INFLUENCING NEURAL MECHANISM

VAGUS AND SYMPATHETIC NERVES AFFECT HEART RATE AND OUTPUT

GANGLIONIC BLOCKING AGENTS ACT HERE

SYMPATHETIC NERVES MODIFY TENSION IN PERIPHERAL AND VISCERAL VESSELS

PHEOCHROMOCYTOMA MAY INCREASE CATECHOLAMINE OUTPUT

CATECHOLAMINES FROM SUPRARENAL MEDULLA AFFECT TONE OF RESISTANCE IN VESSELS AS WELL AS HEART RATE AND OUTPUT

SYMPATHETIC TRUNK

MEDULLA

SUPRARENAL CORTEX

CORTICAL TUMORS MAY INCREASE OUTPUT OF ALDOSTERONE

ALDOSTERONE

SUPRARENAL CORTICAL STIMULATING HORMONES, PRODUCED BY ANTERIOR PITUITARY, STIMULATE ALDOSTERONE OUTPUT

ANGIOTENSIN PROMOTES OUTPUT OF ALDOSTERONE

CARDIAC OUTPUT AFFECTED BY AUTONOMIC NERVES, CATECHOLAMINES, VENOUS RETURN, AND METABOLIC STATE OF CARDIAC MUSCLE

SYMPATHETIC NERVES CONTROL RENAL ARTERIES AND ARTERIOLES; ALSO RENIN SECRETION

LIVER

RENIN SUBSTRATE (ANGIOTENSINOGEN)

RENIN

ANGIOTENSIN II

ANGIOTENSIN I

PHYSIOLOGIC OR PATHOLOGIC CONSTRICTION OF EXTRARENAL OR INTRARENAL VESSELS PROMOTES OUTPUT OF RENIN BY JUXTAGLOMERULAR CELLS

ANGIOTENSIN II A POWERFUL VASOCONSTRICTOR

KEY

PARASYMPATHETIC EFFERENTS

SYMPATHETIC EFFERENTS

AFFERENTS

HUMORAL EFFECTS

REACTIVITY TO NERVE STIMULI MAY BE ACCENTUATED BY ANGIOTENSIN II

Na+
K+
H2O
Na+

ALDOSTERONE PROMOTES Na+ AND H2O RETENTION, K+ EXCRETION, AND ARTERIOLAR CONSTRICTION (ALSO AFFECTS INTRA– AND EXTRACELLULAR ELECTROLYTE DISTRIBUTION)

BLOOD VOLUME A FACTOR IN REGULATING ALDOSTERONE OUTPUT

K+
Na+
H2O

KIDNEY COMPRESSION OR DISEASE ELEVATES BLOOD PRESSURE, PROBABLY VIA EFFECT ON VESSELS

SALT INTAKE OR DEPRIVATION AFFECTS BLOOD PRESSURE IN HYPERTENSIVES

GUT

BLOOD VOLUME AFFECTS BLOOD PRESSURE UNLESS COUNTERED BY OTHER FACTORS

SODIUM OR POTASSIUM CONCENTRATIONS MAY AFFECT TONE OF VESSELS AND BLOOD VOLUME

ELASTICITY VS RIGIDITY OF ARTERIOLAR WALLS; AFFECTS BLOOD PRESSURE

FIGURE 1. Interdependent and interacting factors in blood-pressure regulation. (© Copyright CIBA Pharmaceutical Company, Division of CIBA-GEIGY Corporation. Reproduced, with permission, from THE CIBA COLLECTION OF MEDICAL ILLUSTRATIONS by Frank H. Netter, M.D. All rights reserved.)

higher blood pressure levels.

It appears that genetic or early learning factors predispose a person to respond to subjectively stressful life events and situations with

increases in blood pressure. In the labile or borderline stage of hypertension, extending over months or many years, episodes of raised blood pressure are intermittent. They are readily provoked by emotional and autonomic arousal in response to personally significant environmental stimuli evoking a defensive attitude of vigilance, uncertainty, preparedness for fight or flight, and concomitant affective states, conscious or not.

Management

(1) Early detection. Blood pressure determination should be conducted in every health care facility, including psychiatric facilities. (2) Early and consistent treatment of detected cases with hypotensive drugs. (3) Support of the patient's motivation for continued treatment, coupled with allaying his fears related to the diagnosis. (4) Psychotherapy aimed at helping the patient identify life situations and events that repeatedly arouse his resentment or anxiety. (5) Psychotropic drugs as an adjunct to other therapies, especially during periods of excessive emotional arousal and related increase in vasomotor lability.(6) Biofeedback techniques.

Cardiac Arrhythmias

Psychological Factors

Psychological factors can predispose to and precipitate disturbances of cardiac rate and rhythm, regardless of whether heart disease is present. Emotional influences are particularly prominent in the commonest arrhythmias, those most likely to occur in the absence of heart disease—sinus tachycardia, paroxysmal atrial tachycardia, and atrial and ventricular ectopic beats.

Clinical studies have shown a relationship between psychological variables and paroxysmal supraventricular arrhythmias—atrial and AV junctional tachycardia and atrial fibrillation. Half of the subjects had structural heart disease. The patients tended to be hostile but afraid to express anger, compulsive, and chronically anxious. Many showed sustained sinus tachycardia, palpitations, and poor exercise tolerance. Paroxysmal arrhythmias often occurred in a setting of heightened anxiety, hostility, guilt feeling, or depression provoked by interpersonal conflicts and other subjectively distressing life events. At such periods, the patients were more susceptible to physical precipitants of arrhythmias, such as exercise, abrupt postural changes, and sneezing. Some

developed an arrhythmia in response to sudden fright or an outburst of anger or during a frightening dream. Since most people with similar personality characteristics who are subjected to similar stresses do not develop ectopic tachyarrhythmias, the persons who do must have an organic predisposition to disordered heart rhythm.

Repetitive, sustained paroxysmal tachycardia may occur in the absence of organic heart disease. It usually starts in adolescence or young adulthood and shows an association with neurosis and emotional stress. Supraventricular tachycardia is only occasionally fatal, but, if organic heart disease develops in such a patient, the prognosis may become grave.

Lethal cardiac arrhythmia is a possible cause of sudden death in response to overwhelming emotional arousal or giving up. During REM sleep, ectopic ventricular beats and other ectopic rhythms may be associated with outbursts of sympathetic activity and elevation and variability of heart rate and systolic blood pressure.

Management

Psychotherapy is indicated in patients who suffer frequent, prolonged, or severe arrhythmias clearly related to interpersonal and intrapsychic conflicts and associated emotions. The relief of anxiety, indecision, and guilt and improved coping with hostility are the usual goals. Fear of cardiac disease and of sudden death is often aroused by awareness of even a benign arrhythmia, and the psychodynamic meaning of the fear may have to be explored. Benzodiazepines are useful in reducing anxiety without producing autonomic side effects. Patients have been successfully trained to voluntarily decrease ectopic ventricular beats and to slow and speed heart rate.

Congestive Heart Failure

Psychological Factors

Patients with compensated heart disease may develop heart failure in response to psychological factors acting directly or indirectly. Direct effects include intense affective arousal, such as anxiety or anger, and feelings of grief, depression, and hopelessness. Indirect effects result from the patient's illness behavior, which may take the form of excessive physical activity, failure to take medication, or failure to follow dietary restrictions. Psychological precipitation has been reported in 50 to 75 per cent of patients. The commonest events are violent interpersonal conflicts and actual or threatened loss of an important relationship.

Anxiety and anger are commonly associated with increased heart rate and blood pressure, decreased cardiac filling time, and increased venous pressure.

Management

Inquiry into the patient's emotional state and social situation before the development of unexpected heart failure or when the heart fails to respond to medical treatment should be routine. The detection of deviant illness behavior and its psychosocial basis is needed. Noncompliance with the medical regimen may be an expression of rejection or eager acceptance of the sick role; of depression and suicidal tendencies; of the denial of illness; or of resentment toward a close person or doctor. Sometimes the patient was never adequately informed about his illness and his need for treatment.

Psychotherapy, usually of a supporting and information-giving type, is best provided by the physician responsible for the patient's continuous medical care. Psychotropic drugs—especially those with prominent cardiovascular side effects, such as phenothiazines and tricyclic antidepressants—should be used cautiously.

Organic Brain Syndromes

Organic brain syndromes may result from diseases of the heart and circulation. The most important pathophysiologic factor is generalized hypoxia and focal or widespread cerebral ischemia. The generalized hypoxia results in cerebral hypoxia as part of circulatory failure; the cerebral ischemia is due to mechanical obstruction of cerebral circulation by local vasospasm, embolism, or thrombosis. Delirium may be caused by drugs used for cardiac disorders. Drugs such as diuretics may give rise to delirium indirectly by causing hyponatremia and hypotension.

Neuroses

A patient with heart disease or essential hypertension may develop reactive anxiety neurosis related to the meaning of the illness and its symptoms to him. Anxiety is often accompa-nied by sinus tachycardia, ectopic rhythms, and elevated systolic blood pressure, which increase the burden on the diseased heart and predispose to paroxysmal tachyarrhythmias, congestive heart failure, acute pulmonary edema, angina pectoris, and myocardial infarction. Acute anxiety attacks may precipitate any of these complications in a patient with ischemic or other heart disease. Hyperventilation, which often accompanies acute anxiety attacks, may imitate coronary insufficiency or thrombosis and, on occasion, accompany and mask it. Conversion symptoms, mostly chest pain, may follow infarction and lead to psychogenic invalidism. Depressive neurosis is common. Patients told that they have elevated blood pressure often develop neurotic symptoms, such as insomnia, headache, fatigue, weakness, and dizziness.

A different problem is presented by neurotic and, occasionally, psychotic patients who complain of symptoms suggestive of heart disease but without any evidence of it. Some patients fear heart disease without having any suggestive somatic complaints. The fear may range from anxious concern through severe phobia or hypochondriasis to a delusional conviction.

The management of neurocirculatory asthenia is often difficult, and the results are poor. Psychotherapy aimed at uncovering psychodynamic factors—usually conflicts relating to hostility, dependence, guilt, and death anxiety—may be effective in some cases. The more primary and secondary gains the patient derives from his symptoms, the poorer the outlook. Minor tranquilizers and β-adrenergic blocking agents may help symptomatically. Physical training programs aimed at increasing the patient's effort tolerance may be helpful, especially if the programs are combined with group psychotherapy.

REFERENCES

Blanchard, E. B., and Young, L. D. Self-control of cardiac functioning: A promise as yet unfulfilled. Psychol. Bull., 79: 145, 1973.

Cay, E. L., Vetter, N., Philip, A., and Dugard, P. Return to work after a heart attack. J. Psychosom. Res., 17: 231, 1973.

Cobb, S., and Rose, R. M. Hypertension, peptic ulcer, and diabetes in air traffic controllers. J. A. M. A. 224: 489, 1973.

Friedman, M. Pathogenesis of Coronary Artery Disease. McGraw-Hill, New York, 1969.

Harburg, E., Erfurt, J. C., Hauenstein, L. S., Chape, C., Schull, W. J., and Schork, M. A. Socio-ecological stress, suppressed hostility, skin color, and black-white male blood pressure: Detroit. Psychosom. Med., 35: 276, 1973.

Hinkle, L. E., Coronary heart disease and sudden death in

actively empolyed American men. Bull. N. Y. Acad. Med. *35:* 276, 1973.

Kavanagh, T., and Shepard, R. J. The immediate antecedents of myocardial infarction in active men. Can. Med. Assoc. J., *109:* 19, 1973.

Lane, F. M. Mental mechanisms and the pain of angina pectoris. Am. Heart J., *85:* 563, 1973.

Lipowski, Z. J. Affluence, information inputs and health. Soc. Sci. Med., *7:* 517, 1973.

Mayou, R. The patient with angina: Symptoms and disability. Postgrad. Med. J., *49:* 250, 1973.

Morrelli, H. F. Propranolol. Ann. Intern. Med., *78:* 913, 1973.

Perlman, L. V., Ferguson, S., Bergum, K., Isenberg, E. L., and Hammarsten, J. F. Precipitation of congestive heart failure: Social and emotional factors. Ann. Intern. Med., *75:* 1, 1971.

Rathe, R. H., Tuffi, C. F., Suchor, R. J., and Arthur, R. J. Group therapy in the outpatient management of post-myocardial infarction patients. Psychiatry Med., *4:* 77, 1973.

Rosenblatt, G., Hartmann, E., and Zwilling, G. R. Cardiac irritability during sleep and dreaming. J. Psychosom. Res., *17:* 129, 1973.

Saunders, B. A., and Jenkins, L. C. Cardiac arrhythmias of central nervous system origin: Possible mechanism and suppression. Can. Anaesth. Soc. J., *20:* 617, 1973.

Skelton, M., and Dominian, J. Psychological stress in wives of patients with myocardial infarction. Br. Med. J., *2:* 101, 1973.

Stamler, J. Epidemiology of coronary heart disease. Med. Clin. North Am., *57:* 5, 1973.

Thulesius, O., Hansson, R., and Lisi E. Cardiospecific beta-adrenergic blockade in the treatment of nervous heart symptoms. Curr. Ther. Res. *15:* 805, 1973.

25.8. PSYCHOPHYSIOLOGIC RESPIRATORY DISORDERS

Introduction

The respiratory system is closely related to a variety of behavioral activities that have considerable emotional meaning. Crying, sucking, smelling and the expulsion of irritants by means of coughing and sneezing are all associated with respiration from the earliest moments of life. The respiratory system is involved in the earliest significant relationships that a person has with other people and provides one of the earliest means of expressing emotional reactions and needs.

Recently, Dudley and his coworkers have shown that the hypnotic suggestion of situations inducing anxiety or anger results in an increase in ventilation and oxygen consumption. In contrast, the suggestion of depression or deep relaxation produces a decrease in alveolar ventilation and oxygen consumption and elevates carbon dioxide concentration. They suggest that a primary factor in determining a person's respiratory response to adverse life situations is his psychological orientation. They report that subjects oriented to action after a short term adverse life situation developed hyperventilation and that nonaction-oriented subjects responded with hypoventilation.

Hyperventilation

One of the most common complaints of anxious patients is difficulty in breathing. Patients often demonstrate this difficulty by deep sighs or state that they cannot get enough air. The hyperventilation syndrome is characterized by diverse symptoms, such as fainting, light-headedness, feelings of unreality, numbness or tingling sensations, palpitations, chest pain, dyspnea, and headaches. Occasionally, the syndrome is accompanied by feelings of impending death.

In the differential diagnosis it is important to consider other causes, such as febrile illnesses, high external temperature, hypoparathyroidism, brain tumor, and encephalitis. Most frequently, however, the syndrome may be mistaken for cardiovascular disease or asthma.

Replication of the symptoms by requested hyperventilation has considerable explanatory and reassuring value. Patients may be given specific instructions aimed at controlling the symptoms by modifying their breathing. Psychotherapy is often effective in the treatment of the underlying anxiety. Psychopharmacological medication may also be used in selected cases.

Dyspnea

One of the frequent symptoms associated with cardiac or respiratory illnesses is shortness of breath or dyspnea. Dyspnea has been associated with both the hyperventilation and the hyperpnea accompanying anger and anxiety and with the reduction in ventilation associated with depression. Patients tend to overrate or underrate breathlessness, depending on their psychological attitude.

Asthma

The major psychophysiologic respiratory disorder is bronchial asthma. The primary pulmonary change in asthmatic breathing is bronchiolar obstruction, resulting from a combination of bronchospasms, bronchial edema, and mucous plugs. The obstructive processes produce the signs and symptoms.

Causes

A specific etiological determinant has not been isolated. It appears that a variety of factors are involved in the development of asthma and in the precipitation of asthmatic attacks.

Emotions may modify the immunologic or allergic mechanisms responsible for some cases of asthma. Emotional phenomena may also be related to the development of asthma by means of central nervous system control of bronchiolar function. A combination of both of these processes in varying proportions occurs in most cases.

A number of studies have suggested a relationship between asthma and a cyclothymic or hysterical personality. Investigations have shown that there is a wide variation in personality disturbances among asthmatic patients and that there is no single personality type.

A number of specific conflicts have been reported as leading to bronchial asthma. Much of the emphasis on the psychological genesis of asthma has been concerned with the view that the significant psychodynamic process in asthma is the unconscious fear of loss of the mother or mother figure. Sexual temptations, competitive feelings, narcissistic desires, and hostile impulses may precede asthmatic attacks. Behavior of fantasies with such themes become sources of emotional tension to the asthmatic because they stimulate fears of retaliatory withdrawal or estrangement from a parental figure.

The dependency observed in asthmatics may be secondary to the disease process. The asthmatic attack itself could give rise to an acute need to cling to a mother figure and may, therefore, tend to reinforce the helpless dependency seen in these patients.

Stimuli regularly associated with the presence of an allergic substance may precipitate an attack in a susceptible person.

Treatment

Many factors are involved in the development and precipitation of asthma. Therefore, the joint efforts of internist and psychiatrist are important in handling the medical and psychological aspects of the illness. A wide range of psychiatric treatment modalities have been used, including individual psychotherapy, group therapy, hypnosis, and psychopharmacological agents. Behavior modification techniques have also been used.

REFERENCES

Freeman, E. H., Feingold, B. F., Schlesinger, K., and Gorman, F. J. Psychological variables in allergic disorders: a review. Psychosomat. Med., *26:* 543, 1964.

Knapp, P. H., Mushatt, C., Nemetz, S. J., Constantine, H., and Friedman, S. The context of reported asthma during psychoanalysis. Psychosomat. Med., *32:* 167, 1970.

Luparello, T., Lyons, H. A. Bleecker, E. R., and McFadden, E. R. Influences of suggestion on airway reactivity in asthmatic subjects. Psychosomat. Med., *30:* 819, 1968.

McFadden, E. R., Luparello, T., Lyons, H. A., and Bleecker, E. The mechanism of action of suggestion in the induction of acute asthma attacks. Psychosomat. Med., *31:* 312, 1969.

Schiavi, R. C., Stein, M., and Sethi, B. Respiratory variables in response to a pain-fear stimulus and in experimental asthma. Psychosomat. Med., *23:* 485, 1961.

Stein, M., Schiavi, R. C., and Luparello, T. J. The hypothalamus and immune process. Ann. N. Y. Acad. Sci., *164:* 464, 1969.

25.9.   PSYCHOPHYSIOLOGIC ENDOCRINE DISORDERS

Physiologic Mechanisms

The hypothalamus directly influences endocrine funtion. It exerts its influence both by secreting hormones that affect the anterior pituitary and by regulating the sympathetic and parasympathetic neurons that terminate in endocrine glands. The hormonal influences of the hypothalamus, pituitary, and target endocrine glands on one another are characterized by three kinds of feedback—long, short, and ultrashort. Long feedback systems are those in which hormones produced by the target endocrine gland inhibit or activate hypothalamic or pituitary function. The effects of steroid hormones on other brain regions may also be included here. Short feedback systems are those in which hormones synthesized by the anterior pituitary influence the hypothalamus. Ultrashort feedback systems are those in which the hypothalamic releasing factors directly influence their own rate of production and release (see Figure 1).

Endocrine Function and Emotional States

No pattern of endocrine functioning has been shown to be characteristic of particular emo-

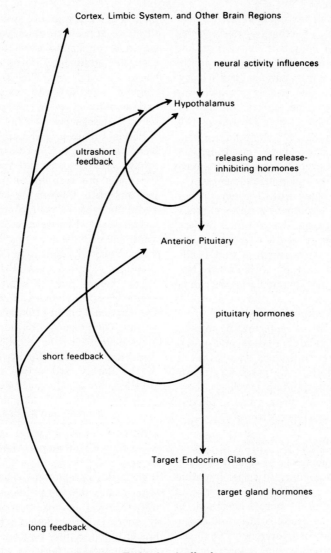

Cortex, Limbic System, and Other Brain Regions

neural activity influences

Hypothalamus

ultrashort
feedback

releasing and release-
inhibiting hormones

Anterior Pituitary

pituitary hormones

short feedback

Target Endocrine Glands

target gland hormones

long feedback

FIGURE 1. Endocrine feedback systems.

tions. However, adrenal medullary and adrenal cortical secretion rates are moderately increased in states of anxiety and diffuse emotional arousal.

In acute schizophrenic episodes adrenocortical activity is increased in proportion to the degree of emotional turmoil (psychotic turmoil, ego disintegration), and 24-hour corticosteroid production may be 2 to 3 times normal. In chronic schizophrenia the secretion and metabolism of cortisol, aldosterone, and estrogens are normal.

In psychotic depression the increase in adrenal cortical activity seems proportional to the degree of diffuse emotional arousal or anxiety present. A decreased sensitivity to endogenous insulin and a decreased growth hormone response to hypoglycemia have also been reported.

Hypopituitarism

The symptoms of hypopituitarism result from the lack of pituitary tropic hormone stimulation of target endocrine glands, especially the adrenals and thyroid. Hypopituitarism is caused by postpartum necrosis of the anterior pituitary (Sheehan's syndrome) and by cranial injuries, infections, and tumors, such as chromophobe adenoma and craniopharyngioma. Early symptoms are fatigability, lethargy, marked cold intolerance, loss of body hair, impotence, and loss of libido. Patients may die early in the course of the disease from adrenal insufficiency. In later stages of the disease, patients are usually deeply depressed and exhibit apathy, inactivity, and mental torpor. They frequently have delusions and signs of mild chronic organic brain syndrome, particularly impairment of memory for recent events. Some patients have periods of irritability and quarrelsomeness. Delirium, stupor, or coma with hypotension and hypothermia may accompany a physical crisis.

If panhypopituitarism, due to tumor or cyst, occurs in childhood, it results in dwarfism and the psychological consequences of that condition. Replacement therapy with growth hormone and adrenal and thyroid hormones can be of great help to growth if the diagnosis is reached before the epiphyses close.

Treatment consists of replacing the missing target endocrine gland hormones and giving attention to tumors or infections, should they be present. The prognosis for the psychiatric symptoms is good. Long-standing psychosis, however, may be resistant to treatment. Lack of drive may persist in some patients.

Cushing's Syndrome

Cushing's syndrome may be caused by adrenal hyperplasia (secondary to either hypothalamic dysfunction or ACTH-secreting tumors of the pituitary or other tissues), adenoma, or carcinoma or by the administration of exogenous ACTH or glucocorticosteroids. The physical signs and symptoms include truncal obesity, abdominal striae, moon facies, hirsutism, amenorrhea, hypertension, glycosuria, osteoporosis, and weakness. Psychological disturbances are present in more than 50 per cent of patients in many series. The syndrome is more common in women than in men and occurs most often in the third or fourth decade.

Psychological difficulties are among the presenting signs and symptoms in 40 to 50 per cent of patients. Impotence and loss of libido are common. Brief episodes of disturbed behavior characterized by excitement, acute anxiety, emotional lability, or apathy are seen.

Patients often experience increased appetite, sleeplessness, and hypersensitivity to environmental and emotional stimuli. Psychiatric disturbance appears to be only one-third to one-fourth as common in association with ACTH or cortisone administration as with endogenous Cushing's syndrome. Euphoria is much more common in patients given exogenous hormones, and anxious or retarded depression predominates in endogenous Cushing's syndrome.

Patients frequently complain of memory defects, and nonpsychotic organic brain syndromes with confusion and disorientation occur. Psychoses are seen in 15 to 25 per cent of patients with Cushing's syndrome. Paranoia and hallucinations are common.

Treatment of endogenous cases of Cushing's syndrome includes surgery and pituitary irradiation. Phenothiazines may decrease the hypothalamic secretion of ACTH-releasing factor. Psychotherapy may be helpful in helping patients adjust to changes in appearance and to the emotional lability that accompany the syndrome. The prognosis for patients with psychiatric disturbances is excellent. In psychosis associated with ACTH or cortisone, a reduction of the dosage and active treatment of the psychosis are usually successful.

Addison's Disease

Adrenal insufficiency, Addison's disease, may result from disturbed hypothalmic, pituitary, or adrenal functioning. It is much less common than Cushing's syndrome. The signs and symptoms usually develop insidiously and are slowly progressive. They include weakness, fatigability, anorexia, weight loss, nausea and vomiting, loss of libido, diffuse pigmentation of the skin, and hypotension. Patients with advanced disease almost always have psychological symptoms. Depressive mood, irritability, psychomotor retardation, and apathy are common. Most patients have some degree of mild organic brain syndrome, with a prominent memory defect. Hallucinations, delusions, and frank psychosis are rare but may resemble paranoid or catatonic states or manic-depressive psychosis. Addisonian crisis is accompanied by acute organic brain syndrome.

The mental symptoms usually respond to cortisone treatment. The presence of hypotension in the Addisonian patient should make clinicians cautious in using antidepressants and phenothiazines.

Hyperthyroidism

Hyperthyroidism is a relatively common disorder that occurs most frequently in the third and fourth decade and more frequently in women than in men. The clinical picture, except for the exophthalmos, results from the actions of excessive amounts of thyroid hormones. The physical signs and symptoms include staring, protruding eyes; goiter; warm, moist skin; weight loss and weakness despite normal or increased appetite; menstrual disorders; fine tremor; restlessness; heat intolerance; and, in older patients, signs and symptoms of cardiac failure. Mild to moderate emotional and cognitive disturbances are present in almost all cases. (See Figure 2.)

There is a growing evidence that thyroid hyperfunction in hyperthyroidism results largely from a serum 7 S globulin, long-acting thyroid stimulator, rather than from pituitary TSH. It has been hypothesized that stress may increase the secretion of TSH and vasoconstrictor substances, which, acting together, damage the thyroid and expose thyroid cell wall components to the body's immune system. The immune system is hypothesized to respond by producing long-acting thyoid stimulator.

Hyperthyroid patients are almost always anxious, tense, hyperexcitable, irritable, and emotionally labile. Frequently, they exhibit a fluctuating depressive mood without psychomotor retardation. A less common but clinically important variety of hyperthyroidism, termed apathetic thyrotoxicosis, more often affects middle-aged and elderly patients and seems to occur in patients whose disease has been undiagnosed for long periods of time. These patients are lethargic, listless, depressed, and mentally slow. Severe muscle wasting, weight loss, and congestive heart failure are usual, but the classical tremor, eye signs, and moist, hot skin of thyrotoxicosis are usually absent. The patients can lapse rapidly into semistupor or coma and die.

No psychotic picture is typical of hyperthyroidism. Patients have presented clinical pictures resembling schizophrenia, manic-depressive psychosis, paranoid state, and involutional melancholia. Antithyroid durgs can produce an acute brain syndrome.

It is frequently important to differentiate hyperthyroidism from anxiety neurosis. The signs in order of their diagnostic specificity for hyperthyroidism are cardiac arrhythmia, hyperkinetic movements, pulse rate of more than 90 a minute, palpable thyroid, bruit over thyroid, lid retraction, hot hands, lid lag, and fine finger tremor. The discriminating symptoms in order are excessive sensitivity to heat and preference for cold, increased appetite, weight loss, excessive sweating, palpitations, tiredness, and dyspnea on effort.

Hyperthyroidism is treated with antithyroid drugs, radioactive iodine, or surgery, depending on such factors as the severity of the illness, the patient's age, and his medical condition. Psychotherapy may help the patient adjust to the symptoms of his disease while they are being treated and may be helpful in preparing him for surgical operation. To the degree that stress appears to be related to the onset and course of a patient's hyperthyroidism, psychotherapy may help him manage stress more adaptively.

Psychotropic drugs must be used with some caution. Chlorpromazine may increase tachycardia. Tricyclic antidepressants may induce cardiac arrythmias. Benzodiazepines may cause false normal results of ^{131}I uptake and resin-triiodthyronine uptake studies in patients who are clinically hyperthyroid. They may be useful, however, in managing anxiety. Phenothiazines apparently do not significantly alter the PBI or ^{131}I uptake.

Hypothyroidism

Hypothyroidism occurs most often after the administration of radioactive iodine to control hyperthyroidism or after a subtotal thyroidectomy for hyperthyroidism, Hashimoto's thyroiditis, or multinodular goiter. Idiopathic hypothyroidism is probably usually the result of Hashimoto's thyroiditis but may also occur in hypopituitarism, pituitary failure to produce TSH, and severe iodine deficiency in areas of endemic goiter. Mental changes are always present. In infants, hypothyroidism leads to cretinism. The infant is sluggish, somnolent, and a poor feeder. In 3 to 6 months the full-blown picture is seen, including protruding tongue, unbilical hernia, poor muscle tone, wide-set eyes, and low forehead. Untreated, the infant shows dwarfed stature, evidence of retarded bone age, delayed eruption of teeth, and severe mental retardation. Cretinism is usually

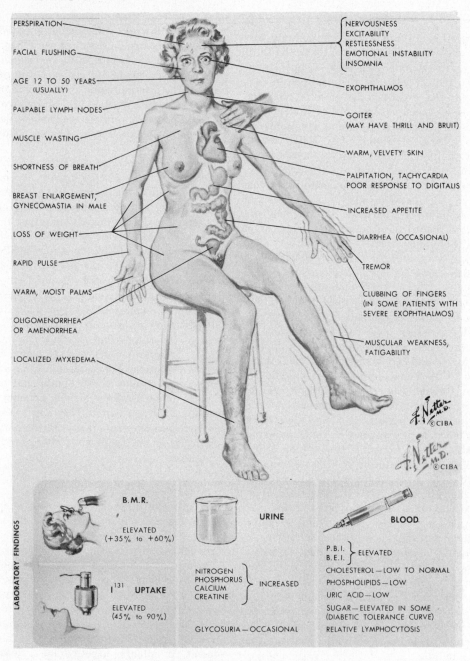

PERSPIRATION

FACIAL FLUSHING

AGE 12 TO 50 YEARS
(USUALLY)

PALPABLE LYMPH NODES

MUSCLE WASTING

SHORTNESS OF BREATH

BREAST ENLARGEMENT,
GYNECOMASTIA IN MALE

LOSS OF WEIGHT

RAPID PULSE

WARM, MOIST PALMS

OLIGOMENORRHEA
OR AMENORRHEA

LOCALIZED MYXEDEMA

NERVOUSNESS
EXCITABILITY
RESTLESSNESS
EMOTIONAL INSTABILITY
INSOMNIA

EXOPHTHALMOS

GOITER
(MAY HAVE THRILL AND BRUIT)

WARM, VELVETY SKIN

PALPITATION, TACHYCARDIA
POOR RESPONSE TO DIGITALIS

INCREASED APPETITE

DIARRHEA (OCCASIONAL)

TREMOR

CLUBBING OF FINGERS
(IN SOME PATIENTS WITH
SEVERE EXOPHTHALMOS)

MUSCULAR WEAKNESS,
FATIGABILITY

LABORATORY FINDINGS

B.M.R.
ELEVATED
(+35% to +60%)

I^{131} **UPTAKE**
ELEVATED
(45% to 90%)

URINE

NITROGEN
PHOSPHORUS
CALCIUM   } INCREASED
CREATINE

GLYCOSURIA—OCCASIONAL

BLOOD

P.B.I.
B.E.I.   } ELEVATED

CHOLESTEROL—LOW TO NORMAL
PHOSPHOLIPIDS—LOW
URIC ACID—LOW
SUGAR—ELEVATED IN SOME
(DIABETIC TOLERANCE CURVE)
RELATIVE LYMPHOCYTOSIS

N27-61 ENDOCRINE SYSTEM—Vol 4 THYROID GLAND GRAVES' DISEASE—CLINICAL MANIFESTATIONS DR. RAWSON

FIGURE 2. Diffuse hyperthyroidism (Graves' disease): medical manifestations (© Copyright 1959 CIBA Pharmaceutical Company, Division of CIBA-GEIGY Corporation. Reproduced, with permission, from THE CIBA COLLECTION OF MEDICAL ILLUSTRATIONS by Frank H. Netter, M.D. All rights reserved.)

due to maternal iodine deficiency but may also be seen in congenital thyroid aplasia and congenital metabolic defects in thyroid hormone formation.

A hypothyroid patient often has a dull expression, puffy eyelids, loss of the outer third of the eyebrows, swollen tongue, hoarse voice, and rough, dry skin. Constipation, cold intolerance, and prolonged menstrual bleeding are common. Anemia, rhinorrhea, deafness, arthralgia, and

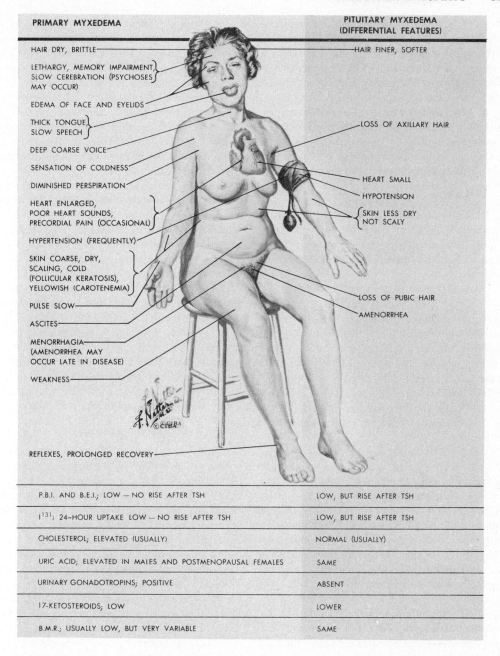

PRIMARY MYXEDEMA	PITUITARY MYXEDEMA (DIFFERENTIAL FEATURES)

HAIR DRY, BRITTLE

LETHARGY, MEMORY IMPAIRMENT, SLOW CEREBRATION (PSYCHOSES MAY OCCUR)

EDEMA OF FACE AND EYELIDS

THICK TONGUE, SLOW SPEECH

DEEP COARSE VOICE

SENSATION OF COLDNESS

DIMINISHED PERSPIRATION

HEART ENLARGED, POOR HEART SOUNDS, PRECORDIAL PAIN (OCCASIONAL)

HYPERTENSION (FREQUENTLY)

SKIN COARSE, DRY, SCALING, COLD (FOLLICULAR KERATOSIS), YELLOWISH (CAROTENEMIA)

PULSE SLOW

ASCITES

MENORRHAGIA (AMENORRHEA MAY OCCUR LATE IN DISEASE)

WEAKNESS

REFLEXES, PROLONGED RECOVERY

HAIR FINER, SOFTER

LOSS OF AXILLARY HAIR

HEART SMALL

HYPOTENSION

SKIN LESS DRY NOT SCALY

LOSS OF PUBIC HAIR

AMENORRHEA

Primary Myxedema	Pituitary Myxedema
P.B.I. AND B.E.I.; LOW — NO RISE AFTER TSH	LOW, BUT RISE AFTER TSH
I¹³¹; 24-HOUR UPTAKE LOW — NO RISE AFTER TSH	LOW, BUT RISE AFTER TSH
CHOLESTEROL; ELEVATED (USUALLY)	NORMAL (USUALLY)
URIC ACID; ELEVATED IN MALES AND POSTMENOPAUSAL FEMALES	SAME
URINARY GONADOTROPINS; POSITIVE	ABSENT
17-KETOSTEROIDS; LOW	LOWER
B.M.R.; USUALLY LOW, BUT VERY VARIABLE	SAME

N67-60   VOLUME 4 — ENDOCRINE SYSTEM   ADULT MYXEDEMA — SYMPTOMS AND SIGNS DR. RAWSON

FIGURE 3. Adult myxedema: clinical manifestations and etiology. (© Copyright 1959 CIBA Pharmaceutical Company, Division of CIBA-GEIGY Corporation. Reproduced, with permission, from THE CIBA COLLECTION OF MEDICAL ILLUSTRATIONS by Frank H. Netter, M.D. All rights reserved.)

muscle weakness are also seen. (See Figure 3.) The mental signs and symptoms include psychomotor retardation, decreased initiative, slowness in comprehension, drowsiness, and impairment of recent memory. If psychosis (myxedema madness) develops, it usually takes the form of an organic brain syndrome, with clouding of consciousness, which may progress to delirium, stupor, or coma.

In cretinism, thyroid replacement should be begun as early as possible. Thyroid hormone is essential for normal brain development in the last few prenatal months and first few postnatal months.

Thyroxin replacement therapy should be gradual to avoid physiological and psychological disturbances. For example, if the metabolic rate is increased too rapidly, cardiac failure can occur. Moreover, thyroid replacement can precipitate or temporarily worsen a psychosis in a hypothyroid patient. A precipitated psychosis clears over a period of weeks, during which thyroid replacement treatment should be continued. Phenothiazines should be used cautiously in hypothyroid patients.

Although residual impairment of intellectual functions may occur in patients with long-standing disease, the prognosis for the reversal of most mental symptoms in most patients is good.

Diabetes Mellitus

Diabetes mellitus consists of both metabolic and vascular disturbances. The metabolic disturbances, due to a relative or absolute lack of insulin, include an inappropriately elevated blood glucose level and changes in lipid and protein metabolism. The vascular disturbances include a microangiopathy, particularly affecting the eye and the kidneys, and accelerated atherosclerosis.

Emotional distress can exacerbate diabetes, either directly through physiological changes or indirectly by leading the patient to neglect the proper management of his disease. Stress interviews can produce ketosis in diabetic patients and a similar metabolic shift in normal persons, particularly when the interviews threaten dependency needs or cause the interviewees to feel deprived of affection and emotional support. Conflicts with significant persons, actual or threatened loss of these persons, and chronic situations engendering feelings of loneliness, rejection, and resentment may exacerbate patients' diabetes and produce a relative increase in insulin requirements. Young patients with labile diabetes are more subject to this stress than are older patients with mild diabetes.

The classic symptoms of polydipsia, polyuria, and polyphagia in association with weight loss raise the suspicion of diabetes. Children or adolescents, however, may experience episodes of unconsciousness associated with ketoacidosis as an early symptom of diabetes. Adults with maturity-onset diabetes may complain of a number of symptoms that can easily be ascribed to psychological causes—moderate weight loss or gain, blurred vision, fatigue, impotence, faints, paresthesias, and loss of sensation.

The medical management of diabetes depends on the severity of the disease. Attention to diet, to attaining and maintaining ideal body weight, and to preventing or delaying the complications of diabetes are central concerns. Oral hypoglycemic agents or insulin may be required in severe cases. Parents may overprotect children with diabetes. Diet or insulin often become an issue for rebellion in adolescents. The need to attend to diet and the complications of diabetes may provoke maladaptive responses in adults.

Diabetic patients who become psychotic or depressed can be treated with psychotropic drugs. Phenothiazines can induce hyperglycemia in some previously well-regulated diabetic patients but, by bringing a psychosis under control, permit better management of the diabetes. Both tricyclic and monamine oxidase inhibitor antidepressants may lower blood glucose levels in diabetic patients but can be used if the clinician is aware of this possibility.

Hypoglycemia

Almost all cases of hypoglycemia (blood glucose level less than 50 mg. per ml.) have an organic cause. However, some evidence suggests that essential reactive hypoglycemia (functional hypoglycemia), a milder syndrome that occurs in relation to meals, may be induced or exacerbated in part by stress.

The most common cause of hypoglycemia is exogenous insulin overdose in diabetic patients. Hypoglycemia may also be caused by pancreatic and other tumors; pancreatitis; liver, adrenal, thyroid, or pituitary insufficiency; malnutrition; malabsorption syndromes; gastrectomy; alcoholism; hereditary disorders of carbohydrate metabolism; and the prediabetic state. Stress may play a role in the onset and course of this syndrome. These patients are frequently described as emotionally labile. Hypoglycemia can be induced by conditioning, and patients with essential reactive hypoglycemia and psychic tension states may be cured of both by psychotherapy.

Hypoglycemia frequently presents with mental symptoms, including episodes of anxiety, fugue, uncharacteristic behavior (irritability, anger, indecency, or violence), confusion, apathy, psychomotor agitation or retardation, depression, delusions, hallucinations, convulsions, and coma. Repeated episodes of hypoglycemia may damage the brain, producing personality changes or clinical pictures of presenile or senile dementia. Acute episodes of hypoglycemia usually begin with tremor, light-headedness, perspiration, anxiety, irritability, hunger, nausea, pallor, and increased pulse rate and blood pressure. Because mental symptoms are frequent in hypoglycemia, it is easy to misdiagnose.

Spontaneous remissions are common in essential reactive hypoglycemia. A diet low in carbohydrates and high in protein and fats is often beneficial, but this benefit may be a placebo effect. Psychotherapy has been reported to be curative in one study. Monoamine oxidase inhibitors of both the hydrazine and the nonhydrazine classes lower blood glucose levels in some normal and diabetic persons and, therefore, probably should not be used in patients with essential reactive hypoglycemia.

The treatment of hypoglycemia due to other causes should be directed at the underlying cause and is frequently quite beneficial. Only 25 per cent of pancreatic adenomas are malignant.

Puberty

Puberty is a time not only of sexual changes but also of a general growth spurt. There are substantial increments in height and weight, changes in facial contours, fat distribution, pelvic proportions, and muscular development. All these changes are under hormonal control.

The age of onset of puberty is likely to have psychological consequences, and these consequences tend to be sex-differentiated. For boys, early maturation tends to elicit greater prestige, but this is not generally true for girls. Most girls who accept the menarche and do not find it highly stressful show the following characteristics: (1) They do not experience the menarche in an information vacuum. Information is obtained in advance from mothers, friends, and physicians. (2) They perceive menstruation as a necessary, if inconvenient, step toward desired roles as women and mothers. (3) The experi-

ence of menstrual cramps localizes and makes understandable a diffuse set of preceding internal changes. (4) Once the menstrual cycle becomes regular, the uncertainty associated with irregular bleeding is reduced, and anxiety is diminished.

Much of the unpredictable moodiness, hostility, depressions, and other signs of distress in adolescence may be related to the major changes in sex hormone levels that are characteristic of pubertal development.

Menstrual Cycle Distress

About a third of young women in the general population are bothered to some extent by premenstrual cramps, backaches, headaches, irritability, mood swings, tension, or depression; about 10 per cent experience these symptoms in sufficient severity to interfere with their everyday activities. The four days before menstruation and the days of menstrual bleeding are marked by a definite increase in the proportion of women who commit suicide, engage in acts of violence, and encounter other serious difficulties.

Estrogen and progesterone have effects on brain function and behavior. Estrogens, for example, lower seizure thresholds, and progesterone raises such thresholds. Large doses of progesterone produce general anesthesia, and moderate doses produce sedation. The rise and fall of progesterone during the menstrual cycle may produce a mild sedation, followed by withdrawal phenomena of the sort associated with sedative drugs. Some women during the premenstrual phase report impaired concentration and show alterations in time judgments and visual perception.

The changes in progesterone concentrations are accompanied by changes in the secretion of other hormones. Changes in aldosterone, for example, may be important in a subgroup of patients who experience premenstrual bloating and edema.

The 20 per cent of women who regularly experience moderate to severe cyclic changes in moods and symptoms may benefit from a careful charting of their experiences over several successive months. In this way, they can be helped to prepare themselves psychologically for days of emotional instability associated with changes in hormonal condition.

If the pattern and type of distress are known, appropriate medication can be prescribed for a specific phase of the menstrual cycle. Antianxiety medication may be useful for a woman who has severe and recurrent bouts of anxiety in the premenstrual phase. For a patient who becomes deeply troubled by distortions of her body image, secondary to premenstrual water retention, a diuretic may be advisable. For a patient with severe dysmenorrhea, an effective analgesic may be useful.

Amenorrhea

Primary amenorrhea is the delay of menarche beyond the age of 18. Secondary amenorrhea is the absence of menstruation after normal cycles have been well-established. Amenorrhea of variable lengths is normally associated with the immediate postmenarchal and the menopausal periods and with the puerperium. Both primary and secondary amenorrhea may result from a large number of organic conditions that affect the vagina, uterus, ovaries, and hypothalamic-pituitary axis. Some progestational drugs may induce long-lasting amenorrhea. However, psychogenic amenorrhea is the most frequent single cause of amenorrhea in young women.

Cases are reported in which amenorrhea began immediately after an acute psychic trauma, and normal cycles returned when the psychic stress was alleviated. Reported traumatic events have included rape, being jilted, discovery of a husband's infidelity, sudden death of a loved one, illegal abortion, and giving birth to a malformed child. Women with chronic psychiatric disturbances appear to have a high incidence of menstrual dysfunction. And amenorrhea becomes more prevalent in times of social distress, such as war. Some patients with secondary amenorrhea are psychosexually immature, rejecting the female role and not focusing on or comfortable about intercourse.

Psychogenic amenorrhea also occurs in anorexia nervosa, in which it may be an early sign, and as part of the syndrome of pseudocyesis. Psychologically, pseudocyesis may represent the fulfillment of a wish for the satisfactions and other personal meanings of being pregnant or a denial of symptoms that the patient associates with uterine or cervical cancer.

No pattern of reproductive hormone excretion in the urine is characteristic of psychogenic amenorrhea. The most common pattern is one of low urinary levels of both gonadotropins and estrogen, suggesting hypothalamic-pituitary dysfunction.

Treatment of psychogenic amenorrhea varies with the cause. In anorexia nervosa, the amenorrhea disappears as the underlying disorder and poor nutrition are remedied. Phenothiazines can cause amenorrhea, particularly if given in high doses. In pseudocyesis, several simple treatment approaches have been successful, including telling the patient that she is not pregnant, re-education, hypnosis, and suggestion. More formal psychotherapy can be directed at underlying conflicts. Alleviating the stress associated with psychologically traumatic events should restore normal menstrual function in most cases in which specific psychological trauma is important.

Infertility

A couple is commonly defined as infertile when pregnancy has not occurred after a year of sexual activity without contraception. Infertility is frequently psychogenic, resulting from psychologically based impotence or frigidity, premature ejaculation, too frequent or too infrequent ejaculation, and aberrant sexual behaviors. Psychophysiologic endocrine reactions are only rarely cited as possible etiological pathways in cases of infertility, and the clinical evidence for their role is entirely anecdotal. In women, disordered hypothalamic-pituitary functioning could lead to infertility by causing anovulation, an inhospitably viscous cervical mucus, or improper preparation of the uterus for implantation—changes that have all been observed in patients with psychogenic amenorrhea. In men, disordered hypothalamic-pituitary functioning could produce oligospermia or poor motility and morphology of sperm.

Postpartum Distress

Women in their reproductive years have a fourfold to fivefold increase of risk of mental illness, especially psychosis, during their first 3 months postpartum. Besides the severe postpartum psychiatric reactions, about two thirds of normal women develop a brief period of increased emotional lability in the first 10 days postpartum; this lability is termed the postpartum blues. Although many women complain of minor disturbances during pregnancy, most evidence indicates that women are at low risk for severe psychological distress at this time. There is a drastic increase of risk associated with delivery.

Throughout pregnancy, there are gradual increases in the secretion of many hormones—chorionic gonadotropin, estrogens, progesterone, adrenocortical steroids, androgens, and thyroid hormone. Concentrations of most of these hormones decrease precipitously within 3 days postpartum. An abrupt withdrawal of these hormones may foster syndromes similar to those following the withdrawal of psychoactive drugs. The changes in a particular hormone are more drastic for some women than for others. Genetic and nutritional factors may influence the rate and extent of endocrine changes.

Despite its gratifications, the postpartum period is not without its stresses. For example, the father's reaction to the advent of an infant has an important bearing on the mother's ability to cope with the new demands of the situation. Moreover the mother is likely, especially at the end of her first pregnancy, to experience changes in body image and other aspects of her self-concept that are highly pertinent to self-esteem and relations with significant other people. Her sense of adequacy as a mother and the extent of her motivational conflict over her mothering role seem to be important factors in postpartum psychiatric illness.

In respect to postpartum blues, the physician can be helpful through anticipatory guidance in prenatal care. The patient can be prepared for a period of emotional lability after delivery. For mothers who are unusually upset, mild tranquilizers are often helpful. If the patient has difficulty in sleeping, chloral hydrate may be indicated.

In respect to severe postpartum psychiatric reactions, an awareness of predisposing factors may be useful to the physician. If the woman has a history of repeated and severe psychiatric reactions after previous pregnancies, therapeutic abortion deserves serious consideration. In less severe situations, psychotherapy during pregnancy may help the patient work out relevant problems, such as conflicts with her mother. Specific preparation for the tasks of infant care and her mothering role may be useful. A careful prenatal history may be helpful in clarifying recurrent depressive or manic-depres-

sive episodes. Close medical guidance is needed. When there is no history of a previous psychiatric disorder but there is an intense motivational conflict regarding the prospect of motherhood, psychotherapy is in order. Current conflicts with the woman's mother and her husband deserve close scrutiny, as they can undermine a woman's capacity to cope with the new situation that delivery brings.

Prenatal and postpartum classes can be useful in dealing with such problems. If well-conducted, they can provide models of effectiveness, interpersonal support, and increased understanding of shared problems. Physicians responsible for routine postnatal care are well advised to see their patients about 2 weeks after delivery, rather than wait for the customary 6 weeks postpartum follow-up. If unusual distress, such as prolonged crying spells, has lasted beyond the tenth day postpartum and is accompanied by such symptoms as severe insomnia, confusion, and feelings of hostility toward the baby, early referral to a psychiatrist is in order. Early detection and treatment of postpartum psychiatric disorders offer significant prospects for improvement.

Menopausal Distress

Cessation of the menses takes place gradually in most women over a 2- to 5-year period. Symptoms of the normal menopause, such as hot flashes and increased irritability, probably have some relation to changes in ovarian hormones and gonadotropins, but the relation between endocrine changes and the severe involutional psychiatric disorders remains obscure.

The menopause usually takes place between ages 45 and 49. With advancing age, the decline of ovarian secretory activity occurs gradually over several years. Ovulation and menstruation become irregular. Menses cease when the amount of estrogen secreted is too little to stimulate uterine endometrial growth. In due course, estrogen levels become so low that they fail to inhibit the pituitary, and large quantities of pituitary gonadotropins are secreted. These high, sustained levels of gonadotropins may have adverse effects in some women. But it is not clear that they cause hot flashes.

There is a tendency toward decline in sexual activity around the age of 60. This decline is often related to the husband's diminishing sexual interest at about that age. Many menopausal women experience a loss of sexual interest, but this loss can be reversed by estrogen replacement therapy. The decrease in sexual interest may be due to regressive changes in the female genitalia induced by estrogen deficiency, predisposing to discomfort in sexual intercourse. Estrogens may also be helpful in the treatment of hot flashes and associated anxiety and irritability, sometimes relieving depression as well. The clinician should be aware of the possible carcinogenic effects of long term estrogen replacement therapy.

A few coping strategies are avoidance tendencies, involving psychological processes through which people minimize awareness of threatening implications of their life circumstances; patterns of behavior that have the functional effect of reassuring oneself about the persistence of youthfulness; seeking of information about the menopause itself, about new bases for self-esteem, and about changes in interpersonal relations; the making of new friendships or the deepening of existing ones; the initiation or deepening of occupational and recreational activities; a search for substitute children, both within and beyond the family; exploring new ways of relating to one's children; seeking out new satisfactions in the role of grandparent; intensifying religious commitment; self-appraisal, especially in placing greater value on personal qualities of experience, judgment, and maturity.

REFERENCES

Frankenhaeuser, M. Experimental approaches to the study of human behavior as related to neuroendocrine functions. In *Society, Stress, and Disease*, L. Levi, editor, vol. 1, p. 22. Oxford University Press, London, 1971.

Froberg, J., Karlsson, C. G., Levi, L., and Lidberg, L. Physiological and biochemical stress reactions induced by psychosocial stimuli. In *Society, Stress, and Disease*, L. Levi, editor, vol. 1, p. 280. Oxford University Press, London, 1971.

Gibbons, J. L. Steroid metabolism in schizophrenia, depression, and mania. In *Biochemistry, Schizophrenia, and Affective Illnesses*, H. F. Himwich, editor, p. 308. Williams & Wilkins, Baltimore, 1970.

Globus, G. Consciousness and brain. I. The identity thesis. Arch. Gen. Psychiatry, *29:* 153, 1973.

Hamburg, B. A., and Hamburg, D. A. Stressful transitions of adolescence: Endocrine and psychosocial aspects. In *Society, Stress, and Disease*, L. Levi, editor. Oxford University Press, London, 1974.

Melges, F. T., and Hamburg, D. A. Psychological distress during the menstrual, postpartum, and menopausal periods. In *Views on Human Sexuality*, F. Beach, editor, p. 235. McGraw-Hill, New York, 1974.

Sachar, E. J. Endocrine factors in psychopathological states. In *Biological Psychiatry*, J. Mendels, editor, p. 175. Wiley, New York, 1973.

Sachar, E. J., Halpern, F., Rosenfeld, R. S., Gallagher, T. F., and Hellman, L. Plasma and urinary testosterone levels in depressed men. Arch. Gen. Psychiatry, *28:* 15, 1973.

Sachar, E. J., Hellman, L., Roffwarg, H. P., Halpern, F. S., Fukushima, D. K., and Gallagher, T. F. Disrupted 24-hour patterns of cortisol secretion in psychotic depression. Arch. Gen. Psychiatry, *28:* 19, 1973.

25.10. PSYCHOPHYSIOLOGIC ALLERGIC AND SKIN DISORDERS

Skin Disorders

The skin serves as a mirror of emotional states. Because of its rich endowment with sense receptors for pain, touch, and temperature, the skin becomes the matrix for the body ego. The sexual function of the skin and the significance to normal development of its successively libidinized erogenous zone were hypothesized by Freud.

Abnormal Cutaneous Sensations

Generalized Pruritus. Itch, tickle, and pain are all conveyed by the same afferent fibers and are differentiated only by the frequency of impulse. The neurohumoral basis of naturally occurring pruritus is still unclear.

Anxious and tense persons or normally well-adjusted persons at times of anxiety and tension may be more conscious than usual of itching sensations from a lesion. Guilt, anger, boredom, irritation, and sexual arousal may all predispose the person to itching and subsequent scratching, which evidently derives from reflexive movements that serve to clear the skin of irritants. In humans it may be both painful and highly pleasurable and may thus serve both self-punitive and autoerotic purposes. Scratch-induced, self-inflicted neurotic excoriations are encountered frequently by dermatologists. In some cases they may be successfully treated by direct confrontation and supportive psychotherapy. Sexualized aggressive feelings originally aimed at key figures during the first years of life may induce the conflicts that are displaced onto the self in scratching episodes, frequently during sleep.

Localized Pruritus. *Pruritus Ani.* The investigation of this disorder commonly yields a history of local irritation—threadworms, irritant discharge, fungal infection—or general systematic factors, such as nutritive deficiencies or drug intoxications. However, after running a conventional course, it often fails to respond to therapeutic measures and acquires a life of its own, apparently perpetuated by scratching and superimposed inflammation.

Personality deviations often precede this condition, and emotional disturbances often precipitate and maintain it. Some workers feel that many character traits of these patients are based on compliance with or opposition to parental dictates regarding bowel training. Fixation at or regression to this anal stage of development leads to conflicts that frequently involve sadistic impulses, which may be dealt with by a variety of defenses: reaction formation manifesting as gentleness and subservience toward authority, projection with suspiciousness and ideas of reference, and turning on the self, of which the scratching is a vivid manifestation.

A pleasurable component of the anal activity is usually obliterated by an unconscious sense of guilt, which changes the pleasurable rubbing into self-punitive scratching. In both men and women, defective heterosexual relationships are common.

Pruritus vulvae. Both itching and scratching may have a painful and pleasurable quality. In some patients, pleasure derived from rubbing and scratching is quite conscious, but more often the pleasurable element is repressed. Most patients give a long history of sexual frustration, which was frequently intensified at the time of the onset of pruritus. For many of these patients, a powerful father fixation and a severe code of morality interfered with adult sexual expression and in some cases led to pronounced masochistic trends. At times of intense frustration, these patients regress to a masturbatory level of psychosexual development, but, because of their intense guilt, self-punitive feelings also become intense. Thus, the pruritus vulvae strikes a balance between pleasure and pain.

Abnormal Cutaneous Manifestations

Hyperhidrosis. States of fear, rage, and tension can induce an increase of sweat secretion. Emotional sweating appears primarily on the palms, soles, and axillae; thermal sweating is most evident on the forehead, neck, trunk, and dorsum of hand and forearm. Excessive sweating (hyperhidrosis) may, under conditions of prolonged emotional stress, lead to secondary skin changes and may thereby underlie a number of other dermatological conditions that are not primarily related to emotions. Hyperhidrosis may be viewed as an anxiety phenomenon mediated by the autonomic nervous system.

Rosacea. This condition is more common in women than in men and usually occurs in the thirties and forties. It features an increased vascularity, with papule formation on the blush area of the face and upper chest. Sufferers from rosacea display a heightened responsiveness not only to heat but also to hot drinks, spiced food, hurried meals, and a variety of emotions.

Some workers feel that these patients present specific personality features, the most outstanding characteristics of which are their abnormally high level of self-esteem, anxious dependence on the good opinion of others, compulsive desire to please, and constant fear of attracting attention. Underlying these personality features are unreasonably strong feelings of inferiority, guilt, and shame. Rosacea is usually preceded by life situations that led to the production or activation of shame. Rosacea appears to represent a state of permanent blush.

Urticaria. In a study of 35 urticaria suffers, two-thirds stated spontaneously that, as children, they had been deprived of their mother's love. In the majority of cases, this belief seemed to be ill-founded. As children, some openly expressed their resentment; others suppressed or repressed the aggressive response and turned to its opposite—exemplary, compliant behavior—to secure affection.

These two behavioral patterns were carried forward into adult life. Roughly half the patients displayed an ingratiating and excessively compliant attitude toward their environment, an attitude that was further intensified by criticism or disapproval. The other group demanded what they regarded as their due, complained bitterly if it was not forthcoming, and presented a vindictive and bellicose appearance. Patients of both groups showed an inability to tolerate the denial of love and reacted with anger to such a situation. The aroused anger found token expression in urticarial eruptions.

Other authors relate urticaria attacks specifically to anxiety.

Atopic Dermatitis. Atopic dermatitis is usually accompanied by itching that often appears disproportionate in severity to the visible lesions. This condition is found in both a childhood and an adult form, both frequently appearing in the same person, with an intervening period of several years. The literature abounds with references to the appearance of atopic dermatitis after an emotional disturbance. The recurring theme that seems to pervade all the varieties of precipitating events is that of loss of love.

Patients studied by Wittkower and Edgell felt that they had not had their fair share of affection as children and tended to maintain in adult life an inordinate childlike dependence on a parent, in most cases the mother. For some, a need for affection, attention, and support found its expression in a submissive, docile, or even overtly helpless attitude. In others, the same need was concealed behind self-assertive, ambitious, or even provocative behavior. For many, the lack of self-confidence impaired their social and occupational progress. Many remained single or married partners who appeared to serve as parent substitutes.

Psoriasis. The primary cause of psoriasis is not known, but aggravating factors include systemic infection, an excess or deficiency of sunlight, damp or cold, and emotional stress. The nature of the emotional event that proves significantly stressful is related to the particular personality difficulty. If a person is emotionally maladjusted for reasons unrelated to the psoriasis, the emotional maladjustment may take charge of the psoriasis and may determine its onset and further relapses.

Alopecia Areata. This disorder has frequently been described as a condition in which the emotional factor plays an important role. Characteristic features are symbiotic loss at an early age, subsequent management of the loss with other symptoms present, and a precipitating event, such as a real or threatened abandonment or the birth of a sibling, leading to the collapse of the management system, precipitating extensive hair loss.

Acne Vulgaris. No claim is made that psychological factors alone explain the development of acne. Rather, both physiologic processes and emotional disturbances of puberty are relevant to its common onset at this period. A retardation of emotional and psychosexual de-

velopment is related to its onset and persistence beyond the normal span of puberty.

Autoerythrocyte Sensitization

This condition of a chronic purpuric state is characterized by episodes of painful spontaneous bruising of a particular sort: a sudden pain, usually of some severity, draws the patient's attention to some part of the skin surface; thereupon, a lump appears, which soon becomes erythematous, and soon thereafter shows a characteristic ecchymotic change. This last phase lasts a week or longer. The pain is frequently disabling. The patient otherwise experiences normal bruising susceptibility.

The factor of suggestion plays a role. In several cases investigators produced characteristic lesions by direct suggestion under hypnosis. Subsequently, they demonstrated convincingly that highly consistent personality findings (hysterical and masochistic) are uniformly present. Moreover, a clear time relationship to a psychological stress was present in a great many cases.

Distribution of Lesions

Repeatedly, cases are cited in which the bodily area affected appears to be related to a current and presumably related conflict. A young woman in conflict over sexual intimacy with eruptions in the breast and girdle area is cited, and a number of cases of wedding-ring dermatitis are related to an extramarital affair.

Women with psychosomatic and organic conditions, as well as men with psychosomatic conditions whose lesions produced a visible disfigurement, have been found to be more disturbed than those with similar conditions that were concealed. The secondary effects on the psyche of the social handicap of a disfiguring disease must be considered in any study that proposes purely causative ties from anxiety or neuroticism to cutaneous disorders.

Psychodynamics

Certain emotional states may correlate highly with various forms of skin disorder: aggression with generalized pruritus, sexual frustration with genital and anal pruritus, anxiety with hyperhidrosis, shame with rosacea, anger with urticaria, and the longing for love with atopic dermatitis. None of these mood states is disease-specific; all are found not only in normals and neurotics but also in other psychosomatic disorders. None of the disorders described is believed to be psychogenic. All are multicausal and determined by a combination of factors.

Allergic Disorders

Constitutional Factors

Both urticaria and atopic dermatitis are frequently connected with exposure to substances, generally proteins, that act as allergens. Commonly, particularly in the case of atopic dermatitis, the victim gives a history of past or present allergies involving different systems. A strong family history of allergic responsiveness is often elicited.

Psychological Factors

In allergic disorders, there is a strong correlation with emotionally disturbing events that, according to some observers, tend to be somewhat illness-specific and specific in the emotional reaction they induce. An allergic skin reaction can be altered by suggestion or an experience that activates significant emotions.

Certain features of personality structure and psychodynamics are common to patients with different allergic disorders. The most outstanding is a strong longing for love, a longing of the infantile dependent kind that arises from a sense of deprivation of maternal love in childhood and leads to a passive-dependent relationship with the mother and to a fear of estrangement from her and a fear of being left alone. Situations that precipitate allergic attacks are those that reactivate these fears. A wide spectrum of defense mechanisms may be used to deal with these fears, and a wide variety of personalities are found who, on the surface, appear to have little in common.

For certain persons, psychosis and allergic disorder represent alternative modes of expression of unconscious conflict. Allergic patients and psychiatric patients have in common an oversensitivity to stimuli that are innocuous to others; and in both instances, the oversensitivity, if not inborn, can be traced back to previous sensitizing experiences. More important, certain psychological features are so commonly found in allergic patients that it is hard to believe that this combination is due merely to chance. More likely, the personality features described are concomitant with an allergic

diathesis, and the nature of the response to stressful life situations is determined by the allergic predisposition of the patients concerned.

Treatment

The therapeutic approach may be from the allergic angle, provided evidence of an existing allergy can be elicited, or from the psychological angle, provided evidence of emotional maladjustment can be elicited. Each of these measures may have a beneficial desensitizing effect, but the removal of a distressing symptom does not resolve emotional conflicts. Psychological disorders arising from them may be more distressing than the psychosomatic disorder was.

It appears advisable to offer psychotherapy to those allergic patients in whom the onset and exacerbations of their disorders are clearly related to emotional factors. In recent years, group psychotherapy has been increasingly used in allergic diseases. Psychotherapy directed at intrafamily relationships has proved to be quite successful.

The tranquilizers and antidepressants are most effective in the relief of the somatic effects of psychosomatic allergic disorders when the disorder of affect or behavior is most conspicuous. Results have been least gratifying in those cases in which psychopathology appears negligible.

A demonstrable cutaneous allergy cannot be produced by hypnotic suggestions, but demonstrable cutaneous allergic response can be reduced by hypnotic suggestion.

A number of behavioral therapy approaches appear to be gaining increased application in the treatment of skin disorders. And autogenic training is increasingly used in the treatment of psychosomatic conditions.

REFERENCES

Engel, G. L. *Psychological Development in Health and Disease.* W. B. Saunders, Philadelphia, 1962.
Hirt, M. L., editor. *Psychological and Allergic Aspects of Asthma.* Charles C Thomas, Springfield, Ill., 1965.
Lester, E. P., Wittkower, E. D., Katz, F., and Azima, H. Phrenotropic drugs in psychosomatic disorders (skin). Am. J. Psychiatry, *119:* 136, 1962.
Wittkower, E. D. Studies of the personality of patients suffering from urticaria. Psychosom. Med., *15:* 116, 1953.
Wittkower, E. D., and Edgell, P. G. Eczema: A psychosomatic study. Arch. Derm. Syph., *63:* 207, 1951.
Wittkower, E. D., and Engels, W. D. Psyche and allergy. In *Psychological and Allergic Aspects of Asthma,* M. Hirt, editor, p. 143. Charles C Thomas, Springfield, Ill., 1965.

25.11. RHEUMATOID ARTHRITIS

Introduction

Rheumatoid arthritis is a systemic disorder whose cause or causes are still unknown. Although the prime symptoms and the inflammatory changes are characteristically found in articular and associated structures, there are also a number of extra-articular signs and symptoms.

Causes and Pathogenesis

There may be a genetic predisposition toward immunologic abnormalities that may be a necessary substrate for the disease. If there is a genetic substrate, it could lead to manifest disease through environmental factors. Some of these environmental factors may be psychological in nature.

Immunologic Factors

It seems reasonably certain that immune mechanisms are important. Present theories suggest that an as yet unidentified antigen stimulates antibody production by the plasma cells in the synovium. The resulting antigen-antibody complexes somehow lead to the alteration of the antibody, so that it is no longer regarded as self by the body. This alienated antibody stimulates the production of rheumatoid factor, leading to phagocytosis and release of lysosomes, which results in tissue damage and inflammation. The rheumatoid factor is believed to play a role in perpetuating disease activity by virtue of the immunologic reactions that take place with immunoglobulin G (IgG), but it is not thought to initiate rheumatoid arthritis.

Possible Psychophysiologic Mechanisms

Among the factors involved in the regulation of connective tissue synthesis in general and collagen in particular are growth hormone, thyroxin, androgens, estrogens, and the adrenal corticosteroids—all of which vary with emotional stimulation. Corticosteroids, in particular, interfere with the immune mechanisms and with the production of collagens.

Further, the synovium is surrounded by a dense network of capillary vessels adjacent to the joint cavity and is well supplied with lymphatics and nerve fibers. These nerves are widely distributed in the ligaments and joint capsules as well and come from several spinal segments carrying autonomic fibers and sensory fibers. Thus, the possible mechanisms underlying a psychosomatic cause and pathogenesis should certainly include the hormonal and autonomic nervous system pathways.

Loss of the sensory fibers, resulting from either peripheral nervous system disease or central nervous system disease, can lead to joint pathology, neuropathic arthropathy. The joint deformities that develop in rheumatoid arthritis are thought to have their origin in muscle spasm, with flexor contraction and extensor spasm, similar to that occurring in injury.

Life Events

A number of investigators have demonstrated that changes in the psychological and social milieu are important as antecedents of a variety of illnesses. The central hypothesis is that life changes of major importance evoke psychological responses that are frequently associated with psychophysiologic reactions. These bodily function alterations may lead to dysfunction and disease. An additional hypothesis suggests that the stress of these life events makes people more vulnerable and susceptible to disease.

Psychoimmunologic Relationships

Some authors have suggested that stress predisposes patients to the so-called autoimmune disorders by leading to alterations in immunologic reactivity. There appears to be some relationship between elevated proteins and high life-change events. However, because many patients with rheumatoid arthritis do not have elevated immunoglobulin levels, other factors must be involved in the pathogenesis of this illness.

Body Boundaries

Patients whose symptoms involve the exterior of the body, such as rheumatoid arthritics, tend to perceive firm body boundaries, as shown by barrier scores derived from the Rorschach test. On the other hand, patients whose symptoms involve the interior of the body, such as peptic ulcer patients, perceive their body boundaries as indefinite and reveal higher penetration responses on Rorschach examination.

Arthritic children have been described by their mothers as much more active than the average child before the onset of the illness. This finding is similar to the description of arthritic adults, who are described as being quite competitive and vigorous athletes before the onset of their arthritic symptoms. Arthritic children scored higher on tests measuring perceptual motor skills than on problems involving purely verbal material. They also scored higher than asthmatic children on Rorschach scales measuring body-image barriers.

Outer control has been positively related to barrier scores and inner control negatively related to penetration scores. A combination of high barrier and low penetration appeared to be associated with good psychological control.

Psychosocial Findings

In our study, women with rheumatoid arthritis tended to come from homes in which there were high discrepancies between the social status indicators of the mother and the father. They tended to recall their mothers as being arbitrary, severe, unreasonable, and controlling. Further, their reaction to their mothers was a high degree of covert anger but very little actual overt aggression and resistance. Nevertheless, rheumatoid arthritic women chose them as role models as often as did women without rheumatoid arthritis. Recollections of the father and reactions to the father showed no differences between the arthritics and the nonarthritic subjects. In their current personality functioning, rheumatoid arthritic women showed a continuation of conflicts over the expression of aggressive impulses. They revealed a high level of anger but wished to control it, and their guilt about expressing it was found to be as strong as for women without rheumatoid arthritis. On a variety of measures of poor mental health, rheumatoid arthritic women reported a greater number of symptoms. Their marriages were characterized by high discrepancies between their own and their husband's status variables; they showed high status stress and they tended to be married to men whose own status variables were incongruent. Rheumatoid arthritic women and their husbands expressed a great deal of anger and aggression toward one another. Husbands of rheumatoid arthritic women were also found to be more likely to have peptic ulcers than was the general population.

Like the women, the men with rheumatoid arthritis reported more symptoms of poor mental health, but, in contrast to the women, the men were found to be low on anger and aggression. Since their wives were equally low on this factor, the marriages of the rheumatoid arthritic men and healthy women were low on marital hostility.

Other investigators have concluded that certain traits not found in the criminal or mentally ill make a person more vulnerable to trigger mechanisms that precipitate the onset of rheumatoid arthritis. They identified these traits as those characterizing the law-abiding good citizens who live by the golden rule, are overly conscientious, have a high degree of social consciousness, are unduly sensitive to criticism, and have an exaggerated sense of responsibility to social and moral obligations.

Personality Characteristics

A number of investigators have employed the Minnesota Multiphasic Personality Inventory (MMPI) in an attempt to characterize personality traits among rheumatoid arthritics. A number of investigators are in agreement that, compared with various control groups, rheumatoid arthritics tend to be, in Moos' words, "self-sacrificing, masochistic, conforming, self-conscious, shy, inhibited, perfectionistic and interested in sports and games. They also tend to overreact to their illness." There is however, much disagreement in the literature about other issues, such as the expression of anger, separation, traumata, and the amount of impulsivity and defiance shown. Although emotional stress may initiate or aggravate muscular pain, there is no final proof of the relationship of psychophysiologic factors to rheumatoid arthritis. This question remains unanswered for the time being, most of the studies being merely provocative, rather than definitive. Work with the Maudsley Personality Inventory (MPI) on patients with early or chronic rheumatoid arthritis found that people with rheumatoid arthritis do differ significantly in personality from normal people and from neurotic people but that the differences are more extensive in the chronic arthritics. The differences may develop as the result of the arthritis.

Clinical Features

In some cases, the illness begins suddenly with high fever, extensive polyarticular inflammation, and the rapid development of severe deformities. Most usually, however, the onset is slower, with minimal to moderate discomfort and only the gradual development of minimal deformities.

Frequently, the disease begins with systemic symptoms, such as fatigue, weight loss due to anorexia, and occasional fever. Later, fleeting or long-lasting pain develops in joints and the muscles near them. Early-morning joint stiffness is a particularly frequent complaint. The most commonly attacked joints are the hands, feet, and knees in a symmetrical manner. Once attached, a joint tends to remain involved for long periods of time, other joints gradually being added to the progressive disability. Tenosynovitis is quite common. A variety of joint deformities occur, owing to the joint disease itself, to shortening of tendons, or to the muscle imbalance associated with splinting or myositis. Ulnar deviation of the fingers is frequently noted.

When the disease is active, lymph nodes may be enlarged to such an extent as to suggest a primary lymphatic disease.

Although clinical heart disease is unusual, postmortem examinations of patients with rheumatoid arthritis frequently reveal granulomatous and fibrous heart lesions.

Prognosis

Of the patients who have the symptoms of the illness for less than a year, about 75 per cent improve, and as many as 20 per cent have a complete remission. Factors related to a poor prognosis in respect to joint function include disease that persists longer than a year in a patient below the age of 30, disease that is sustained, the presence of subcutaneous nodules, and high titers of rheumatoid factor. However, even in these cases, up to 70 per cent of the patients remain capable of full employment.

Treatment

Because of the possibility of early remission and the uncertainty of the future course of events, most physicians avoid strenuous medications in the case of a patient with early rheumatoid arthritis. Since there is no definite evidence that the natural progress of the illness is altered by any of the therapies available,

conservative management offers a prognosis at least no worse than that of the more heroic measures.

Immediate management goals are relief of pain and reduction of the inflammatory process. Long-range goals include prevention and correction of deformities, maintenance of function, and prevention or treatment of other health problems that arise. Because of the comprehensive nature of the management, interpretation to and education of the patient and his family are important. Motivation for following the proposed regimen must be maintained. The physician and the other health professionals involved in the care of the patient must keep close watch for the development of depression, apathy, and a helpless, hopeless outlook.

The value of a carefully designed program of rest and exercise has been well-documented. Such a program helps prevent muscular atrophy, maintains the mobility of the affected joint, and decreases the psychological distress associated with immobility.

Heat and cold applications are also effective in relieving the pain and stiffness that result from spasm of the muscles. When joints are actively inflamed, splints are effective in helping to release muscle spasms and pain.

Since one of the most important goals is to maintain active functioning, the use of adaptive equipment in helping the patient to cope may become important. Physiotherapy, physical therapy, and occupational therapy are essential in the comprehensive management of cases of rheumatoid arthritis. Further, a skilled social worker or psychiatric nurse may be of help in assessing the emotional status and life situation of the patient and in maintaining motivation and adequate defenses. Psychiatrists often work as regular members of the rheumatology team. On occasion, frank depression or other psychiatric disturbance may develop, and psychiatric consultation or intervention is important.

Aspirin is most frequently prescribed for the relief of pain and for its anti-inflammatory action. When the disease is active, this medication should be taken on a regular daily basis. Because of the possibility of mucosal irritation, aspirin should be taken with food or with an antacid. Other side effects of aspirin include loss of auditory acuity or tinnitus.

A bland sleeping medication and relaxing

tranquilizers may be helpful when used judiciously. However, potentially addicting drugs should be given with great care because of the chronicity of the illness. Pills should not replace an ongoing attempt to help the patient understand himself and his conflicts and the necessity of making appropriate adaptations to his situation.

If conservative measures do not control the progress of the disease, most authorities consider gold salts to have a definite place in the management of rheumatoid arthritis. Toxic reactions of varying severity occur in about 50 per cent of cases.

Because of the waxing and waning nature of the illness, the efficacy of a given medication is extremely difficult to assess.

The physician should be alert to the kinds of life stresses that may influence exacerbations. Life events of particular significance, such as separation or loss of loved objects, are particularly important. Psychotherapy can be valuable in the management of certain patients with rheumatoid arthritis. One valuable aspect of psychotherapy is its provision of a structured, predictable, and dependable interpersonal relationship. Hypnosis may be useful in cases of rheumatoid arthritis as an aid in muscle relaxation and the control of pain.

The ravages of a chronic, deforming, painful illness such as rheumatoid arthritis cannot help but involve the entire organism. One's body image and the concept of self and what one can do are sharply altered. In some patients, this alteration may lead to cataclysmic distress, with breakdown of defenses and ego disorganization. At the very least, the associated decreased motivation for self-help may have a devastating effect in the management of the patient.

REFERENCES

Bourestom, N. C., and Howard, M. T. Personality characteristics of three disability groups. Arch. Phys. Med., *46:* 626, 1965.

Cobb, S., Schull, W. J., Harburg, E., and Kasl, S. The intrafamilial transmission of rheumatoid arthritis: Summary of findings. J. Chronic Dis., *22:* 295, 1969.

Heisel, J. S. Life changes as etiologic factors in juvenile rheumatoid arthritis. J. Psychosom. Res., *16:* 411, 1972.

Hendrie, H. C., Paraskevas, F., Baragar, F. D., and Adamson, J. D. Stress, immunoglobulin levels, and early polyarthritis. J. Psychosom. Res., *15:* 337, 1971.

Moldofsky, H., and Chester, W. J. Pain and mood patterns in patients with rheumatoid arthritis. Psychosom. Med., *32:* 309, 1970.

Moos, R. H. Personality factors associated with rheumatoid arthritis: A review. J. Chronic Dis., *17:* 41, 1964.

Rodnan, G. P., editor. Primer on the rheumatic diseases. J. A. M. A., *224:* 663, 1973.

Shafii, M. Psychotherapeutic treatment for rheumatoid arthritis. Arch. Gen. Psychiatry, *29:* 85, 1973.

25.12. PSYCHOGENIC PAIN

Introduction

In its simplest form, pain is a somatopsychic phenomenon, a signal of actual or potential danger to body tissues and to the person, and, as such, it is an important adaptive mechanism. Under some circumstances, pain can become nagging and persistent and impair the sufferer's ability to work, to think, to sleep; it can even destroy his will to live.

For a person to experience pain, consciousness, attention, and self-concern are necessary. Intense stimulation of other senses, such as loud noises, may reduce or abolish pain. Activities that narrow attention, such as those practiced by yogis, seem to cancel pain.

In infancy and childhood, pain is perceived when impulses from the surface and internal organs of the body are initiated by noxious stimuli. As the personality develops, pain sensations become associated with feelings, ideas, and actions related to life experiences. Memories of painful experiences in childhood may be recalled later, fantasied, or even hallucinated. As the human mind develops the capacity to form symbols by associating sensations with feelings and ideas, pain becomes invested with increasingly complex meanings. Specific painful experiences in childhood are influential in how a person perceives and experiences pain in later life.

During childhood, pain is frequently associated with punishment. This association may be exaggerated in children who are made to submit to painful forms of punishment to an excessive degree. As adults, they may suffer pain as a neurotic symbol to evade feeling guilty for some impulse or action by reviving a pain from their past and experiencing it as if it were in the present.

Some children receive love and attention only when they are suffering from a painful injury or disease. Later in life, they may exaggerate a current minor ache or hallucinate a past pain in an attempt to regain the sympathy and concern they received when they suffered as children.

For other persons, pleasure and pain are inextricably intertwined. The equation, set up in childhood, that pain and suffering accompany forbidden pleasures and unacceptable impulses allows them to express both sides of the conflict.

Clinical Features

Psychogenic pain may be a secondary symptom of a psychophysiologic disorder, or it may be a neurotic conversion symptom. In both situations, an underlying conflict, outside the patient's awareness, is active and involves clashes between dependent, hostile, or sexual impulses and opposing intrapsychic inhibitions, ideals, or cultural mores.

Pain as a symptom in psychophysiologic disorders results from the stimulation of peripheral end organs, triggered by the emotionally induced physiologic dysfunction. Sometimes, as with pain of a peptic ulcer, the discomfort originates with organic damage, which is the end result of chronic gastrointestinal dysfunction secondary to psychic conflict.

A neurotic conversion pain originates in the mind but is experienced as if it were in the body. It derives from psychic representation (memories) of bodily functions that are used to represent unconscious conflicts in a symbolic manner. The patient is aware neither of the conflict nor of the mechanism used to express it.

A conversion pain develops when the patient is unable to resolve a current frustrating life situation. It permits the expression of the forbidden wish in a form not recognizable by the patient, and at the same time it imposes suffering for such a wish. It also removes the patient from the disturbing life situation and provides a different way of relating—that is, the sick role, which is sanctioned by society. The patient for whom such a pain is serving well feels little or no anxiety or depression and is indifferent to the pain.

Conversion pain may be based on pains reported to the patient by someone with whom he has or had an intense ambivalent relationship. Such a pain is an identification with the other person with whom the patient is or has been in a conflict that he will not allow himself

to recognize. And conversion pain may be a punishment wished on someone else.

Frequently, conversion pain is associated with localized tenderness, changes in autonomic function, motor weakness, and hyperalgesia.

To make a positive diagnosis of conversion pain, the psychiatrist must have evidence that the pain was precipitated by a current conflict that is being solved symbolically through the symptom.

Masochism

In the masochistic lifestyle, the patient suffers pain as a neurotic form of adaptation. Masochistic persons have learned to enjoy suffering in order to assuage guilt that would otherwise be experienced for unacceptable impulses, fantasies, or actions. By combining forbidden gratification with self-inflicted pain, they avoid guilt. The pain itself is not originally a source of gratification; it is the price the patient pays in order to avoid feeling guilty. The unacceptable impulses are often sexual ones, often cruel ones, and frequently a combination. Masochists seek out situations that will be painful or make the most of an organically induced pain. Yet they are unaware of their mechanisms and think that they suffer from bad luck or mistreatment.

Pain Proneness

In this partially successful type of masochism, persons use pain to avoid or alleviate guilt. Such persons also have episodes of depression and difficulty in controlling aggression. They tend to be accident-prone and often have difficulty in handling success. They struggle with intense aggressive impulses, which they attempt to control by being loners and by suffering from various chronic intractable pain syndromes, often connected with injuries at work.

Phantom Limb Pain

Although temporary phantom sensations of the distal portion of a severed limb are experienced normally, the sensations gradually disappear as the patient learns to accept the loss of part of himself and to modify his body image accordingly. People whose phantom sensations become chronic, painful, and disabling are expressing their inability to accept the loss and are turning on themselves the resentment and hate connected with their misfortune.

Painful Posttraumatic States

These are overlapping syndromes in which a trivial injury leads to chronic pain, often associated with a nonhealing wound and depressive symptoms and frequently complicated by litigation involving accidents.

Differential Diagnosis

Pain associated with psychophysiologic disorders results when coping mechanisms, including conversion, are ineffective or fail. Failure to cope with problems is experienced by these patients in terms of anxiety, fear, and feelings of helplessness; the activation of their biological systems leads to physiologic changes, such as tachycardia, sweating, vasoconstriction, and hyperperistalsis.

Conversion symptoms are common among persons with hysterical character structures. These patients are apt to be histrionic in describing their pain and vague in describing the circumstances surrounding its development. This pain does not correspond to anatomical or physiological reality. Such patients demand attention, admiration, and support from the people they are involved with, including their physicians. Women of this type are often seductive in their manner and, at the same time, find sex distasteful. A past history of previous conversion symptoms, phobias, and repeated surgical operations for abdominal pain of obscure origin is common.

Psychogenic pain is sometimes a symptom in neurotic and psychotic depressive reactions. A masked depression may be manifested by a conversion pain—for example, a toothache or other mouth pain in a patient with an intense conflict over biting impulses.

Complaints of pain play a large role in hypochondriacal syndromes. Such pains are widespread, vaguely and bizarrely described, and linked with feelings of anxiety and depression, often with hints of paranoid thinking.

The malingerer who complains of pain is usually evasive, in contrast to the patient with conversion pain, who relates well to the physician. Malingering occurs in persons who have an obvious gain to be achieved by being sick.

The differentiation of psychogenic pain from neurogenic pain, that due to damage to the peripheral or central nervous system, is made on the basis of a history of injury to the nervous system and the burning, persistent, disagreeable, and diffuse quality of neurogenic pain.

Management

The doctor should learn about his patient's life adjustments before the development of the painful syndrome and about the psychological and social setting in which the pain was first experienced. To gather this information, the physician should use an interview style that elicits psychological and interpersonal data concurrently with the bodily complaints.

Insight psychotherapy is indicated for patients who are willing and able to deal with their emotional problems. However, patients who are unable or unwilling to face their problems are likely to become depressed or to develop another complaint or a behavioral symptom when confronted with their intrapsychic conflict. The physician can best treat these patients by helping them to learn to live with their pain.

Analgesic drugs probably owe their effect in eliminating psychogenic pain to their role as placebos. For patients in whom pain represents a depressive equivalent, antidepressant drugs and, if the drugs are ineffectual, electroshock therapy are of value. The phenothiazines are effective in relieving pain that represents a somatic delusion.

Behavioral modification therapy trains the patient to give up his pain habit and to learn healthier patterns of adjustment. Hypnotherapy is of value in some cases for the short-term relief it offers, but it rarely gives the patient lasting relief. When patients are relieved of psychogenic pain, persuasion, suggestion, and a positive doctor-patient relationship are the essential ingredients.

Neurosurgical procedures are resorted to in patients with chronic psychogenic pain when other measures fail. Incisions, excisions, and electrical stimulations at all levels are often followed by pain relief, but the relief is usually short-lived.

Whatever medical, surgical, or psychological measures the physician uses in the management of psychogenic pain, it is imperative that he understand and deal with his patient as a person and, insofar as possible, deal with the forces that drove him to his dismal choice of pain.

REFERENCES

Aring, C. D. Nature and significance of chronic pain. Med. Clin. North Am., *42:* 1467, 1958.

Casey, K. L. Pain: A current view of neural mechanisms. Am. Scientists, *61:* 194, 1973.

Engel, G. L. Primary atypical facial neuralgia: An hysterical conversion symptom. Psychosom. Med., *13:* 375, 1951.

Engel, G. L. Conversion symptoms. In *Signs and Symptoms.* C. M. MacBryde and R. S. Blacklow, editors, ed. 5. p. 650. Lippincott, Philadelphia, 1970.

Engel, G. L. Pain. In *Signs and Symptoms.* C. J. MacBryde and R. S. Blacklow, editors. ed. 5, p. 44. Lippincott, Philadelphia, 1970.

Fabrega, H., and Manning, P. K. An integrated theory of disease: Ladino-Mestigo views of disease in the Chiapas highlands. Psychosom. Med., *35:* 223, 1973.

Ramzy, O., and Wallerstein, R. S. Pain, fear, and anxiety: A study in their interrelationships. In *Psychoanalytic Study of the Child,* R. S. Eisler, A. Freud, H. Hartmann, and M. Kris, editors, vol. 13, p. 147. International Universities Press, New York, 1958.

Sternbach, R. A. *Pain: A Psychophysiological Analysis.* Academic Press, New York, 1968

25.13. ACCIDENT PRONENESS

Introduction

Accidents are the leading cause of death in the age range of 3 to 36 and even in later years are surpassed only by heart disease, cancer, and stroke. Certain people tend to have many more accidents in the course of their work than do others.

The unplanned and unanticipated nature of an accident, together with the actual physical injury or property loss involved, lends an air of shock, and at times feelings of guilt and responsibility may be aroused. To the extent that the general public believes there is no cause for an accident, individual responsibility and guilt can be dissipated and the occurrence ascribed to pure chance. Causes can sometimes be determined and possibly corrected. However, causes are often multiple and require a many-faceted approach to the problem. Many studies have attempted to determine the nature of the personality involved in accident proneness.

Accidents Involving Adults

Personality Type

A survey of the literature on the personality types of people involved in accidents gives a general impression that people who are subject to repeated accidents seem to be oriented toward action as a specific way of dealing with conflicts and anxiety and of restoring mental equilibrium. Regardless of the personality type, intrapsychic and interpersonal difficulties are partly resolved by the accident.

Motivation

There has been a tendency to emphasize unconscious conflicts involving aggressive drives and a defensive sense of guilt seeking either expression or expiation. An unconscious wish to escape or avoid something is often apparent. This desire to escape may be related to external situations in which an accident provides a convenient way of avoiding a possibly humiliating experience.

Psychophysiologic Considerations

A physical condition such as fatigue may lead to distraction or an inability to respond quickly enough to avoid an accident. More important is the role of such toxic factors as barbiturates, antihistamines, marijuana, and particularly alcohol. The increased lethargy experienced by women as a result of menstruation and the premenstrum may lead to a reduction in judgment and a slower reaction time and, therefore, more accidents.

Accidents Involving Children

Many minor injuries of childhood are considered within normal limits and to be expected in view of the greater motor activity associated with childhood and the relative lack of neuromuscular control. However, some children seem to be accident-prone.

Accident proneness may be related to the development of the function of self-preservation and to the existence of certain age-specific conflicts occurring in infancy, childhood, and adolescence. These conflicts occur specifically around 2 to 2½ years of age, about 4 to 6, and at the onset of puberty, ranging from 13 to 15. These children tend to express mental conflicts in bodily terms. The occurrence of accidents at certain age periods suggests that accident proneness is not necessarily an inherent character trait but is, rather, a mode of resolution of intrapsychic or external conflicts that may arise from time to time in the course of development and in adult life.

Critique

Statistical studies indicate that over a long period of time the number of accidents in a given industrial situation remains constant but that the membership of the group having the accidents changes. This finding suggests that accidents result from both environmental and personal factors, with different emphasis possible at various times.

Early studies leading to the concept of accident proneness failed to take into account the degree of exposure to dangerous situations. Obviously, a person who drives 100,000 miles a year is more exposed to the possibility of automobile accidents than is someone who drives 1,000 miles a year.

Many persons with a so-called accident-prone personality have few accidents. And it is possible that accident-prone persons have a greater incidence of perceptual distortions than do other people. The concept of personality type may be too vague or too superficial to deal with the type of intrapsychic or interpersonal conflicts that lead to repeated accidents.

Diagnosis

The diagnosis of accident proneness is based on a history of repeated accidents. A detailed personality study most likely indicates a tendency to action and to bodily expression of mental conflicts with a less marked tendency to introspection. Still deeper study might show the existence of problems in interpersonal situations or the existence of unresolved intrapsychic conflicts centering about expressions of hostility and a sense of guilt. This finding may appear in the form of a defensive denial of a sense of guilt and a need for expiation mediated through a fantasy of invulnerability and disbelief in the possibility of injury.

Treatment

The treatment of accident proneness is based, first of all, on identification of the existence of the syndrome and the correction of any environmental factors that may play a part. Work habits, driving habits, sleep patterns, and drug-taking habits may have to be altered.

The correction of the underlying personality problems depends on the ability of the patient to enter into a psychotherapeutic relationship with a therapist and to alter his life situation.

Correction may involve treating a depressive state, dealing with an unconscious sense of guilt based on fantasized misdeeds, dealing with masochistic tendencies expressed through accident proneness, or helping someone to recognize how a particular event or life situation—marriage, for example—has contributed to the accident-prone condition. If depression is the underlying condition, treatment with antidepressant medication may be effective.

Individual therapists report varying degrees of success in dealing with the syndrome of accident proneness, but their reports tend to regard the problem only as part of the total deviant pattern, and the improvement of this specific syndrome is related to the general success of psychotherapy.

REFERENCES

Conger, J., Gaskill, H., Glad, D., Hassell, L., Rainey, R., and Sawrcz, W. Psychological and psychophysiological factors in motor vehicle accidents. J. A. M. A., *169:* 1581, 1959.

Dunbar, F. *Psychosomatic Diagnosis.* Paul B. Hoeber, New York, 1943.

Finch, J., and Smith, J. *Psychiatric and Legal Aspects of Automobile Fatalities.* Charles C Thomas, Springfield, Ill., 1970.

Frankl, L. Self preservation and the development of accident proneness in children and adolescents. Psychoanal. Study Child, *18:* 464, 1963.

Menninger, K. A. Purposive accident as an expression of self-destructive tendencies. Int. J. Psychoanal., *17:* 6, 1952.

Statistical Bulletin. Metropolitan Life Insurance Company, New York, 1973.

Tabachnick, N., editor. *Accident or Suicide?* Charles C Thomas, Springfield, Ill., 1973.

Tabachnick, N., Litman, R., Osman, M., Jones, W., Cohn, J., Kasper, A., and Moffat, J. Comparative psychiatric study of accidental suicidal death. Arch. Gen. Psychiatry, *14:* 60, 1966.

25.14. HEADACHES

Introduction

The complaint of headache may be divided into two broad diagnostic categories. One category comprises the migraine and tension headaches. These headaches have characteristic features that enable a diagnosis to be made from the history. The second category comprises headaches associated with intracranial lesions, systemic diseases, and local diseases of the eyes and nasopharynx. In these cases, diagnosis is primarily by physical examination and laboratory findings.

A headache may arise from stimulation of pain-sensitive tissue outside and adjacent to the skull or as a result of the stimulation of intracranial structures. Headache may also occur by conversion reaction in hysteria and in hypochondriacal and delusional states.

Psychological Factors

No one specific personality type describes all headache or migraine patients. Personality disorders manifested by recurring maladaptive behavior include passive-aggressive, obsessive-compulsive, and hysterical types, which usually co-exist with neurotic conflicts. Although in one study of headache patients, anxiety was found to be the predominate symptom, other neuroses also occurred.

The migraine personality has been described as rigid, pent-up, perfectionistic, overconscientious, ambitious, and obsessional in nature. Many migraine patients do have these characteristics, but so do many headache-free persons.

Observations by psychoanalysts suggest that hostile impulses are the chief source of neurotic conflict in patients with migraine and other types of headache. The headache typically develops when the patient reaches the limit of his capacity to tolerate his suppressed or repressed anger. A given patient's headaches may be partly caused by suppressed rage and partly by hysteria. Positive or negative identification with a family figure and introjection of that figure also play a role when symptoms arise from the patient's desire to gain attention or affection. In some patients, a headache may reflect a need to remain dependent.

The mechanism of psychological factors occurs (1) directly, by precipitating changes in specific physiologic functions, such as cranial vascular changes, sustained muscle contractions, and increased or decreased activity of various glands, (2) indirectly, by conversion of an emotional conflict into a physical dysfunction, and (3) in delusional or hypochondriacal states. These psychological mechanisms simulate a number of organic processes that must be ruled out before a definitive diagnosis can be established.

Vascular Headache of the Migraine Type

The cause of migraine is unknown. In an attack of migraine, there first occurs a preheadache phase, in which cortical ischemia, associated with a secondary process of spreading cortical depression, accounts for the focal and other neurological symptoms observed during an attack. Secondly, there occurs a headache phase of arterial vasodilatation of the extracranial or scalp arteries; this vasodilatation is accompanied by a sterile inflammation of the arterial walls.

Clinical Manifestations

Recurrent head pain—typically unilateral and accompanied by anorexia and, less frequently, nausea and vomiting—is the most common characteristic. Motion sickness and cyclical vomiting are typical in children. Women are apparently more often affected than men. In common migraine, the prodromal period is not sharply defined but is generally marked by mood, gastrointestinal, or fluid-balance disturbances preceding the headache phase by hours or days. The location of the pain may be bilateral; the duration is variable. This is the most frequent type of migraine. In classic migraine, the prodromal period is sharply defined by contralateral neurological manifestations that are usually visual but may be sensory or motor. The headache is characteristically unilateral, pulsatile, and shorter in duration than the hours to days of the common migraine.

Management

The total patient, rather than just the symptom, must be treated. The therapeutic program should include relaxation, a reasonable amount of physical exercise, adequate rest, a well-rounded diet, and the treatment of any associated medical disorders. Supportive therapy also includes the removal or reduction of precipitating or provoking factors, such as exposure to glare or flickering lights, the missing of meals, overloaded environmental demands, offending allergens, fatigue, the ingestion of foods containing tyramine or monosodium glutamate, and, whenever possible, such drugs as vasodilators. Since emotional factors appear to be a frequent precipitant of a migraine attack, the treatment of psychological problems is paramount.

The most effective agent for treatment of an attack of migraine is ergotamine tartrate which can be given orally, subligually, as a rectal suppository, or parenterally. The recommended oral or rectal dose is 2 mg. at the onset of headache, followed by 2 mg. within the hour but not more than 6 mg. for any single attack. Administration of the first 2 mg. early in the course of an attack is of paramount importance. Ergotamine restores the dilated vessels to a nonpainful, constricted state and reduces the pain threshold to normal. Caffeine and ergotamine in combination can reduce the amount of ergotamine needed to provide relief. Daily use of ergotamine tartrate may result in dependency, with withdrawal manifestations if the drug is stopped. Most such patients have an underlying depression, and their use of ergotamine is not primarily related to relief from the headache. Gradual withdrawal of the drug and appropriate psychotherapeutic management of the underlying depression are necessary.

Methysergide maleate has proved to be an effective prophylactic agent. Methysergide simulates the action of serotonin and, by occupying the same receptor sites on blood vessels, may act as competitive antagonist.

Minor and major tranquilizers and the barbiturates may be of temporary benefit in migraine prophylaxis by providing a reduction of anxiety and an improvement in the patient's ability to handle stress.

The treatment of choice for migraine with underlying depression is an antidepressant agent such as the dibenzazepine derivative imipramine hydrochloride or amitriptyline hydrochloride. The use of antidepressant drugs for a migraine patient with depressed mood is not sound therapy in most instances.

Muscle-Contraction Headache

Also termed tension, psychogenic, nervous, and rheumatic headache, the muscle-contraction headache is a common type of nonpulsatile headache; it may be transitory or intermittent or may persist for hours, days, or weeks. Patients with migraine frequently have muscle-contraction headaches between their attacks of migraine.

Long-sustained contraction of the skeletal muscles of the scalp, shoulders, neck, and face in patients suffering from anxiety, environmental and situation tension, and depressed states results in the headache. Concurrent vascular and local chemical changes within skeletal muscles are factors in the production of pain.

Clinical Features

There are no prodromal signs. The majority of patients locate their discomfort in the occipital and nuchal areas, usually bilaterally. The pain is described as a steady ache, pressure, tightness, or bandlike pain. Tautness of the muscles of the neck, scalp, and face may be found on examination. There may be localized painful nodules or areas, and occasionally neck movement is limited.

Treatment

Psychotherapy is the basic tool in management of muscle-contraction headaches associated with emotional tension and life stress. The patient who is depressed benefits from the use of antidepressants. Muscle relaxants with a tranquilizing action, analgesics, and sedatives play a useful but limited role in treatment. Correction of faulty posture, massage, hot packs, manipulation, manual stretching of the nuchal and occipital muscles, and the induction of anesthesia in local areas of tenderness are helpful temporary measures.

Nonmigrainous Vascular Headache

Electrolyte imbalance, vasodilatation, and altered intracranial dynamics resulting from cerebral edema or dehydration are related factors in a nonmigrainous type of vascular headache. Systemic conditions may also cause such headaches.

The ingestion of foods containing tyramine or monosodium glutamate may precipitate a headache. The abrupt withdrawal of a usually high intake of caffeine is a common cause of headache. Drugs and other chemical agents that may provoke headache include nitrates and nitrites, nitroglycerine, hydralazine hydrochloride, reserpine, corticosteroids, antipyrine and its congeners, and such hypoglycemic agents as insulin and the sulfonylureas. Some of the monoamine oxidase inhibitors may produce headache. Cranial artery vasodilation is the underlying mechanism.

Intracranial (Traction) Headache

Intracranial Tumors

The headache of an intracranial mass is usually of moderate intensity and intermittent in its early phase. When the head pain is unilateral, it is usually on the same side of the head as the tumor, but, in the presence of increased intracranial pressure, the pain becomes generalized.

Intracranial Vascular Headache

Sudden or insidious headache is the most frequent initial symptom in brain abscess. Vascular malformations, especially angiomas (most often in the parieto-occipital region), may lead to sudden, severe headaches, usually on the ipsilateral side and often confined to the area over the malformation. Aneurysm of the internal carotid or posterior communicating artery may cause recurring headaches resulting from irritation of the dura. Headache occurs in 90 per cent of subdural hematomas. Headache has been reported as occurring in 32 per cent of patients after a lumbar puncture. Basilar and carotid artery insufficiency may cause intermittent headache accompanied by sensory and motor disturbances.

Headache Resulting from Overt Cranial Inflammation

The headache resulting from intracranial inflammation (meningitis and encephalitis) is generally gradual in onset over hours or days, thus differing from the headache resulting from subarachnoid hemorrhage. The symptoms are determined by the location of the inflammatory process, the degree of inflammation, and the type of structure involved. Temporal arteritis (cranial) is primarily a disease of older persons; it is characterized by headache, constitutional symptoms, and ocular complications.

Sinusal, Dental and Other Cranial Neck Structures

Acute sinusitis is usually associated with severe headache of a dull, aching quality. Movement and change of position of the head intensify the pain.

Congestion and edema of the nasal and paranasal mucous membranes result in pain and nasal discomfort, usually occurring as a reaction to stress.

Optic neuritis, an ocular condition commonly associated with pain in the eye and frontal headache, may be accompanied by sudden visual loss and pain on movement of the eye. Extremely severe pain deep in the eye, around the orbit, or in the brow is symptomatic of glaucoma.

Headache may result from noxious stimulation of structures of the neck, joints, ligaments, muscles, or cervical roots. Headache may also be associated with disease of or injury to the cervical spine.

Posttraumatic Headache

There is no direct correlation between the severity of injury and the development of posttraumatic headache, which may simulate almost any type of chronic recurring headache. The headache may begin when the patient regains consciousness or when he begins to walk. In most cases, the frequency and severity of the headache diminish with the passage of time, although there is considerable variation from patient to patient.

Headache is a common symptom after a head injury, and it may persist for months or years. It is most frequently associated with dizziness, insomnia, fears and anxieties, irritability, fatigue, and inability to concentrate. Such factors as domestic or financial difficulties, a hazardous occupation, and the desire to obtain compensation, financial or otherwise, tend to produce and prolong the symptoms once they have developed. The severity and duration of the posttraumatic syndrome depend on the circumstances of the injury and the patient's psychological status before the injury.

REFERENCES

Friedman, A. P. Pharmacological approach to the treatment of headache. Dis. Nerv. Syst., *22:* 36, 1961.
Friedman, A. P., and Elkind, A. H. Appraisal of methysergide in the treatment of vascular headaches of the migraine type. J. A. M. A., *184:* 125, 1963.
Friedman, A. P. Classification of headache. J. A. M. A., *179:* 717, 1962.
Friedman, A. P., Harter, D. H., and Merritt, H. H. Ophthalmoplegic migraine, Arch. Neurol., *7:* 320, 1962.
Friedman, A. P., Rowan, A. J., Wood, E. H., and Frazier, S. H. Observations on vascular headache of the migraine type. In *Background to Migraine*, J. N. Cumings, editor, vol. 5. Heinemann, London, 1973.
Wolff, H. G., Kunkle, E. C., Lund, D. W., and Maher, P. J. Studies on headache: Induced mechanical stress in the analysis of headache mechanisms. Trans. Am. Neurol. Assoc., *72:* 93, 1947.

25.15.   TREATMENT OF PSYCHOPHYSIOLOGIC DISORDERS

Introduction

Psychomedical treatment emphasizes the interrelation of mind and body in the genesis of symptom and disorder. From a multicausal point of view, every disease can be considered psychophysiologic, since every disorder is affected in some fashion by emotional factors.

Hostility, depression, and anxiety are at the root of most psychophysiologic disorders. However, the presenting complaint is usually physical.

Types of Patients

Psychophysiologic Illness Group

These patients suffer from such classic psychophysiologic disorders as peptic ulcer and ulcerative colitis. In these disease processes one cannot posit a strictly psychogenic explanation. Both somatic and emotional factors must be assumed to be causing the illness. The patients are best approached by a combination of psychiatric and medical means.

Psychiatric Group

Patients in this group suffer from physical disturbances caused by psychological illness. Their somatic disabilities may be real or unreal. When real, the disability involves the voluntary nervous system and is termed a hysterical neurosis of the conversion type. Among the unreal disabilities are hypochondriasis and delusional preoccupation with physical functioning, which is often seen in schizophrenics. Patients in this group suffer primarily from a psychological disturbance that requires psychiatric treatment, but auxiliary medical therapy may be necessary.

Reactive Group

These patients have organic disorders, but they also suffer from an associated psychological disturbance. For example, a patient with heart disease may develop a reactive anxiety regarding his life-threatening condition. This anxiety in turn may produce physical manifestations that complicate the somatic situation. On the other hand, a patient with a preexisting emotional disturbance may develop an apparently independent organic condition; for example, a patient with a phobia may develop a tumor. Not only can the psychological status of such a patient deteriorate rapidly if not properly managed, but the organic condition may be worsened if the emotional problems are not resolved. A patient's own physician may be successful in treating a reactive psychological state if he is supportive and encouraging, offering continuous reassurance and showing concern for the patient's welfare.

Combined Treatment Approach

The combined treatment approach, in which the psychiatrist handles the psychiatric aspects of the case and the internist or other specialist treats the somatic aspects, requires the closest collaboration between the two physicians. Such disorders as bronchial asthma, in which psychosocial processes play a distinct role in the development and course, may respond well to the combined treatment approach. Although the asthmatic attacks themselves may be treated successfully by the physician, psychiatric treatment can be useful in the short run by helping to alleviate the anxiety associated with the attacks and in the long run by helping to uncover the cause of the interdependency involved in the disorder.

In the acute phase of a somatic illness, such as an acute attack of ulcerative colitis, medical therapy is the primary form of treatment; psychotherapy, with its more long-range goals, consists at this stage of reassurance and support. As the pendulum of disease activity shifts and the illness progresses to a more chronic state, psychotherapy assumes the primary role and medical therapy the less active position. The symptoms themselves must be treated by the internist, but the psychiatrist can help the patient focus on his feelings about the symptoms and gain understanding of the unconscious processes involved.

If during an initial attack of a psychophysiologic disorder the patient responds to active medical therapy in association with the superficial support, ventilation, reassurance, and environmental manipulation provided by the internist, additional psychotherapy by a psychiatrist is not required. Psychosomatic illness that does not respond to medical treatment or that is in a chronic phase should receive psychophysiological evaluation by a psychiatrist and combined therapy as indicated.

Treatment should aim at a more mature general life adjustment, increased capacity for physical and occupational activity, amelioration of the progression of the disease, reversal of the pathology, avoidance of complications of the basic disease process, decreased use of secondary gain associated with the illness, and increased capacity to adjust to the presence of the disease.

Psychiatric Aspects

When the psychophysiologic patient first becomes ill, he is usually convinced that the illness is purely organic in origin. He rejects psychotherapy as treatment for his sickness. The very idea of emotional illness may be repugnant because of personal prejudices concerning psychiatry.

In the initial phase, physical treatment and psychotherapeutic procedures must be combined subtly. A good arrangement in this early stage is treatment by a psychologically oriented physician, one who is sensitive to unconscious and transference phenomena and who is working with a psychotherapist.

Psychotherapy must often proceed more slowly and cautiously than with other psychiatric patients. Postive transference should be developed gradually. The psychiatrist must be supportive and reassuring during the acute phase of the illness. As the disorder enters a chronic stage, the psychiatrist may make exploratory interpretations, but a strong patient-physician relationship is essential for any such exploration. During therapy a great deal of hostility appears—first in the form of overt ventilation and then in the framework of the transference. Free and appropriate expression of the patient's hostility is to be encouraged.

The therapist must pay particular attention to current problems in the patient's immediate life situation and deal with his reaction to the therapist and to treatment. There should be increased emphasis on evaluation of the patient's characterological difficulties and on his habitual reactions, particularly his reactions to himself and his environment. The psychiatrist should also analyze the patient's anxieties and how he copes with stress situations, such as asking for complete care, always having to be right, refraining from self-assertion, and suppressing all forbidden impulses. Most orthodox Freudian analysts feel that deep unconscious material in these patients must be handled with care and has limited application in the treatment of acute psychophysiologic illness.

The patient is often involved in a repetitious pattern involving stress in his interpersonal relations. Since he is usually unaware of this pattern, it is helpful to show him that the pattern is not accidental but is determined by factors of which he is unaware, and it is essential to show him how he may change this disturbing pattern and act in a new and healthier manner.

Psychophysiologic patients tend to drive toward psychologically regressed mental and physical behavior. Usually their regression is to a traumatic or highly conflictual period. By re-enacting certain specific attitudes of childhood or infancy, they are attempting to master the anxiety and illness first manifested during those earlier stages. They are bound closely to and dependent on home and family. Their interaction with the environment is significant and even more apparent than in many neurotic patients.

In the treatment of psychophysiologic disorders, the key concept is flexibility in technique. Because of the patient's poor motivitation and because of their poor physical condition, frequent changes in the psychotherapeutic approach may be necessary.

In many patients the motivation for entering treatment is so poor that they drop out of therapy for minor reasons. The patient's neurotic needs are often well served by his illness.

The psychotherapist must be careful not to overburden the ego by too rapid uncovering of repressed impulses. When anxiety is allowed to develop too suddenly—as a result, say, of too active an interpretation of a psychological defense—there may be severe exacerbation of physical symptoms.

During a course of psychotherapy, patients with psychophysiologic disorders may require medical or surgical treatment for their organic disorders. The psychiatrist should cooperate closely with surgeons or medical personnel and should maintain contact with the patient during this emergency. Such interest offers valuable emotional support in a time of crisis. If the patient requires a major surgical procedure, psychological preparation for the operative procedure is important. After the operation, psychotherapy should be continued.

Psychophysiologic patients often require special privileges and attention not usually given to the average patient.

A psychiatrist working with a patient suffering from a psychophysiologic disorder should acquaint himself with the medical aspects of the patient's illness and the medication the patient is receiving. And the internist should be aware of the psychiatric problems involved. To facilitate their understanding of each other's role, the two physicians should hold an occasional conference.

Medical Aspects

The internist's treatment of psychophysiologic disorders should follow the established rules for their medical management. Generally, the internist should spend as much time as possible with the patient and listen patiently to his many complaints. He must be reassuring and supportive. Before he performs a physically manipulative procedure—particularly if it is painful, such as a sigmoidoscopy—he should explain to the patient just what will happen. The explanation allays the the patient's anxiety, makes him more cooperative, and facilitates the examination.

Because these patients are frequently regressed and infantile, they tend to look to drugs and medication for magical results and cure. Injudicious administration of drugs may result in addiction. This danger is particularly significant because psychophysiologic illnesses are characteristically chronic and drawn out, and the drugs administered are essentially palliative. On occasion, it is useful to allow limited quantities of hypnotics or tranquilizers because of the immediate relaxation afforded.

The dosage and pharmacologic action of drugs are sometimes unpredictable, particularly when the patient is receiving psychotherapy. For example, psychotherapy may dramatically alter the insulin requirements of diabetics. A patient suffering from diabetes who does not accept his illness and who has self-destructive impulses of which he is unaware may purposely not control his diet and, as a result, end up in a hyperglycemic coma. In the case of cardiac patients, some refuse to curtail their physical activity after a myocardial infarction because of a reluctance to admit weakness or because of a fear that they will somehow be considered less manly. Others use their illness as a welcome punishment for guilt or as a way of avoiding responsibility. Therapy in such cases must strive to help the patient minimize his fears and focus on self-care and the re-establishment of a healthy body image.

REFERENCES

Alexander, F. *Psychosomatic Medicine.* Norton, New York, 1950.

Bernard, V. Discussion of failures in psychosomatic case treatments. Am. Psychopathol. Assoc. *37:* 118, 1948.

Gilbert, M. M. Reactive depression as a model psychosomatic disease. Psychosomatics, *11:* 426, 1970.

Miller. L. The mind and the body. Int. J. Psychiatry. *7:* 518, 1967.

Winnicott, D. W. Psychosomatic illness in its positive and negative aspects. Int. J. Psychoanal., *47:* 510, 1966.

Wolff, H. H. The psychodynamic approach to psychosomatic disorders: Contributions and limitations of psychoanalysis. Br. J. Med. Psychol., *41:* 343, 1968.

26

Unusual Psychiatric Disorders and Atypical Psychoses

Introduction

The following classification of unusual psychiatric syndromes is proposed: (1) Situation-specific syndromes, or behavioral manifestations that arise from certain specific environmental conditions that are essential factors in the pathogenesis of the syndrome. (2) Idiopathic syndromes, in which there is only a postulated constitutional predisposition to the syndrome and certain hypothesized psychodynamic factors. Under the heading idiopathic, a further distinction between autonomous and associated phenomena can be made, depending on whether the observed syndrome presents itself as an isolated phenomenon or as a particular modification of another mental disorder. (3) Culture-bound syndromes, or psychiatric syndromes that are restricted to specific cultural settings. (4) Atypical psychoses, or psychotic syndromes that seem to belong to a well-known diagnostic entity but that show certain symptomatic features that cannot be reconciled with the generally accepted typical characteristics of this diagnostic category.

Situation-Specific Syndromes

Ganser's Syndrome

In this psychiatric disorder the patient gives an utterly incorrect and often ridiculous reply to a question, although it is clear that he has understood its sense. These patients often appear to be disoriented in time and place, but their general behavior gives the distinct impression that they are alert. They are not confused in the usual sense. They give the impression of selecting purposely—although unconsciously— the wrong, approximate answer.

Auditory and visual hallucinations, hysterical analgesia, true spatial and temporal disorientation, circumscribed amnesia, and lack of insight are often symptoms associated with the Ganser state. Thus, this syndrome frequently bears the marks of a psychosis.

The premorbid personality of the patient is often characterized by hysterical features. This condition has never been observed in persons of superior intelligence.

The central phenomenon is the patient's unconscious attempt to mimic the disorganized behavior and thinking of a psychotic patient according to his naive and personal mental image of madness. The patient's secondary gain seems to lie in the fact that he escapes a threatening or frustrating reality by conveying the impression that he is insane. In almost every case the patient is in a confining situation, such as prison. Ganser's syndrome may occur as an isolated dissociative state or may be temporarily superimposed on other functional or organic mental diseases.

Ganser's syndrome is usually short-lived, and the patient recovers within a few days or weeks. Psychotherapy, tranquilizers, and possibly intravenous injections of amobarbital are usually effective in speeding the patient's recovery.

Folie à Deux (Double Insanity)

Folie à deux is characterized by the occurrence of psychotic symptoms, including delusions, shared by two or more persons living in close and intimate association. Psychotic symptoms—most frequently, delusions—are transmitted from a sick person to a healthy one, who often elaborates on these induced delusions. Lasègue and Falret, who published the first paper on *folie à deux*, summarized their observations in nine conclusions, many of which are still valid and may be summarized as follows:

Under ordinary circumstances, psychotic symptoms are not contagious from a psychotic to a healthy person or to another psychotic person.

Such contagion of psychotic symptoms can only occur in an exceptional combination of conditions.

These conditions are: (1) One person is the dominant one. He or she is usually more intelligent than the other and gradually imposes his or her delusions on the more passive and originally healthy partner. (2) The two persons have lived a very close-knit existence in the same environment for a long period of time, relatively isolated from the outside world. (3) The shared delusion is usually kept within the limits of possibility and may be based on past events or certain common expectations.

The observations and conditions relating to this disease are similar in character wherever they are found.

This type of psychosis is found more frequently among women than among men.

Heredity may be the predisposing cause, particularly when the two persons come from the same family.

The main therapeutic indication is to separate the two patients, in which case the passive one may recover, once he is cut off from his source of delusions.

The nondominant patient is usually not as deeply affected as the dominant patient.

In some cases the pressure of the psychotic person may be extended to a third person or even to more persons in the environment. However, it is usually sufficient to isolate only the actively psychotic person from his sphere of influence.

The mechanism of identification probably plays a key role. The recipient or passive partner has much in common with the dominant partner because of many shared life experiences, common needs and hopes, and a deep emotional rapport with and concern for the partner. He is faced with the choice of either losing the only person to whom he has been—

and perhaps ever will be—very close or joining this person in his pathological world in order to avoid the loss.

In a number of cases the passive partner loses his delusions and regains his reality testing after he has been separated for some weeks or months from the actively psychotic partner. The dominant partner has to be treated like any other patient suffering from a functional psychosis—that is, with pharmacotherapy or electroconvulsive treatment. The passive partner may require physical treatment to speed his recovery, or he may recover spontaneously over a period of time. He almost certainly requires psychotherapy to help him work through the loss of the other person and accept the fact that the other one is—and he himself has been—mentally ill.

Idiopathic Syndromes

Gilles de la Tourette's Disease

The symptoms begin in childhood, usually in children between the ages of 2 and 12 years. The patients exhibit an expanding repertoire of motor tics that involve not only spasmodic grimacing but also violent steryotyped tics—hopping, skipping, jumping, grinding of the teeth, and other sudden compulsive motor outbursts that, nevertheless, may involve a certain amount of coordination. A compulsive coprolalia in which, the patients are compelled to utter swear words or obscenities, is sometimes accompanied by compulsive coughing, spitting, blowing, or barking sounds. There may also be echolalia, consisting of the repetition of words or short phrases immediately after the patient has heard them.

Males outnumber females in a ratio of 4 or 3 to 1, and the parents seem to show paranoid and dominant traits in a higher than expected proportion.

Organic pathology of the central nervous system has always been suspected of playing a role in the development of the unusually gross physical symptoms these patients display. However, soft neurological signs of central nervous system abnormalities and nonspecific electroencephalographic findings are observed in only about half the patients. A genetic cause is not probable, since there are few familial cases reported. The syndrome may be precipitated by physical or mental stress. The patient's symptoms may be understood as a desparate attempt to draw attention to himself and also as the automatized, inhibited rage reaction of a rejected child.

Until recently, no reliable, effective treatment of the condition was known. The outcome was almost always poor. Eventually, many patients had to be institutionalized or live as recluses. One of the major tranquilizers, haloperidol, a butyrophenone derivative, seems to offer the most effective treatment.

Autoscopic Phenomena

These autonomous phenomena are, as a rule, not symptomatic of any particular mental disorder. They consist of hallucinatory experiences in which the person's own body is perceived as appearing in a mirror. This specter is usually colorless and transparent, but it is seen clearly, appears suddenly and without warning, and imitates the person's movements. The appearance usually lasts only a few seconds, and in most cases these phantoms are seen at dusk. In addition, there may be hallucinatory perceptions in the auditory and other modalities. The person usually retains a certain detached insight into the unreality of the experience and reacts with bewilderment and sadness.

The cause of the autoscopic phenomenon, like the cause of other complex hallucinations, is not known. One theory holds that the phenomenon reflects an irritation of areas in the temporoparietal lobes; another holds that it represents the projection of specially elaborated memory traces. Occasionally, the phenomenon is symptomatic of schizophrenia or depression. Many authors believe some normal persons with well-developed imagination, a visualizer type of personality structure, and narcissistic character traits may occasionally see their doubles under conditions of emotional stress.

There is rarely any need for special treatment of this condition, which in most cases is neither incapacitating nor progressive. In certain instances, treatment of the accompanying neurological, neurotic, or psychotic condition may be indicated.

Capgras' Syndrome

The characteristic feature of this condition is the patient's delusional conviction that certain persons in his environment are not their real selves but, instead, are doubles who assume the role of the persons they impersonate and behave like them. This syndrome occurs more frequently in women than in men. No cases are known in which the condition did not occur as a manifestation of another psychosis, usually schizophrenia.

The uncoupling of normally fused components of perception and recognition may have a neurophysiologic cause that so far remains unknown. It may, on the other hand, be determined psychodynamically. The patient may reject the person involved and attribute bad features to him, but he cannot allow himself to become conscious of this rejection because of guilt feelings and ambivalent attitudes. What he really feels about the person with whom he is confronted is displaced to the double, who is an impostor and, therefore, may be safely and righteously rejected.

The outcome depends on therapeutic success with the psychosis of which it is only an aspect. It often responds to electroconvulsive treatment and pharmacotherapy, at least temporarily.

Cotard's Syndrome (Délire de Négation)

Patients complain of having lost not only their possessions, status, and strength but also their heart, blood, and intestines. The world beyond them may also be reduced to nothingness. Trees, houses, and other people do not really exist any more. Time stops, and, as a result, the patient has become immortal.

The syndrome is seen most frequently in patients suffering from agitated depression, but occasionally it occurs in acute schizophrenic breakdowns and in certain brain syndromes, particularly of the senile and presenile type. The syndrome usually lasts only a few days or weeks, and it responds to any treatment that influences the basic disorder of which it is a part. Chronic forms of the syndrome are today almost exclusively associated with senile psychoses.

Munchausen Syndrome

Patients wander from hospital to hospital, where they manage to be admitted because of the dramatic stories they tell about being dangerously ill. They usually have a history of multiple surgery, and they often succeed in fabricating signs and symptoms of serious pathology—hemorrhages, emesis, fever, seizures, and dermatologic lesions. Once admitted to a hospital, these patients are usually troublesome and hostile, may become threatening or physically aggressive toward the staff, and commonly sign out against advice. When they are seen by psychiatrists, female patients are usually diagnosed as hysterical and male patients as psychopaths.

These patients perform willful acts to evoke their symptoms, but the acts are unconsciously determined and must involve considerable masochistic needs. Deprivation in childhood and disturbed relationships with aloof or sadistic parents may provide the background for the persistent need to receive attention for traumatic illness in a hospital setting.

The patients are, as a rule, poorly motivated to accept and follow through with psychiatric treatment. Prolonged psychotherapy by therapists who are not easily discouraged by repeated setbacks is the treatment of choice for the basic syndrome.

Culture-Bound Syndromes

Amok

The amok syndrome consists of a sudden, unprovoked outburst of wild rage that causes the affected person to run madly about, armed with a knife, firearm, or grenade, and to attack and maim or kill indiscriminately any men and animals in his way before he is overpowered or is killed himself. This savage homicidal attack is generally preceded by a period of preoccupation, brooding, and mild depression. After the attack, the person feels exhausted, has complete amnesia for it, and often commits suicide.

The condition used to be almost exclusively associated with the people of Malaya, where it occurred only among men, but it has also been reported occasionally in African and other cultures in the tropics. It has been theorized that a culture that imposes heavy restrictions on adolescents and adulthood but allows children free rein to express their aggression may be especially prone to psychopathologic reactions of the amok type. The belief in magical possession by demons and evil spirits may be another cultural factor that has contributed to the development of the amok syndrome. Loss of face and shame has been proposed as a determining factor for amok behavior.

The only immediate treatment consists of overpowering the amok patient and getting complete physical control over him. The attack is usually over within a few hours. Afterward, the patient may require treatment for the toxic confusional state or the chronic psychotic condition that was the underlying cause.

Koro

This is an acute anxiety reaction characterized by the patient's desperate fear that his penis is shrinking and may disappear into his abdomen, in which case he will die. The Koro syndrome occurs almost exclusively among the people of the Malay archipelago and among the South Chinese (Cantonese). Corresponding female cases have been described, the affected woman complaining of shrinkage of her vulval labia and breast.

Koro is a psychogenic disorder resulting from the interaction of cultural, social, and psychodynamic factors in especially predisposed personalities. Culturally elaborated fears about nocturnal emission, masturbation, and sexual overindulgence seem to give rise to the condition. The patient's insight into his own condition is usually quite impaired.

Patients have been treated with psychotherapy, tranquilizing drugs, and, in a few cases, modified insulin and electroplexy. The prognosis is related to the premorbid personality adjustment and the associated pathology.

Latah

This syndrome has been observed mostly among the Malaysian people, and it occurs clinically in two forms. One is the startle reaction, in which a sudden stimulus provokes the suspension of all normal activity and triggers a set of unusual and inappropriate motor and verbal manifestations, over which the affected person has no voluntary control. The other type of latah is a mimetic or echo reaction, in which a sudden stimulus compels the affected person to imitate any action or words to which he is exposed. He remains aware of the situation and may verbally protest against any unacceptable action he is forced to carry out, such as disrobing in public. Latah may become a chronic disease that leads to permanent automatic obedience and echo reactions, forcing the affected person into hiding and inducing marked personality deterioration.

The disorder is found in women of all Malaysian races, especially the Javanese, but it is also observed in a smaller proportion of men in

Malaysia. Conditions similar to and often identical with latah have also been reported among Africans, aboriginal Siberians, Laplanders, and North Americans.

Latah may be an intense fright reaction involving disorganization of the ego and obliteration of the ego boundaries. A sudden fright may provoke inhibition of proper perceptual-motor integration and may, through loosening of the ego boundaries, render the patient powerless to resist any stimuli coming from the environment. As a result, the patient's behavior is determined by echolalia and echopraxis. The coprolalia that is sometimes observed may be a symbolic defensive act.

There is usually no personality disturbance outside of the attacks, intelligent people are more frequently affected than are mentally defectives, and it may be difficult to get a person out of the state if he is of the neurotic or hysterical type. The traditional belief of the Malayan people in possession states, their children's games of producing trance states, and the frankness and absence of disguise for sexual imagery may contribute significantly to the specificity of the latah reaction among the Malayan people.

Treatment should consist of psychotherapy and pharmacotherapeutic tranquilization. When the latah reaction is associated with a chronic mental disorder, pharmacotherapy and electroplexy are indicated.

Piblokto

Occurring among the Eskimos and sometimes referred to as Arctic hysteria, this condition is characterized by attacks lasting from 1 to 2 hours, during which the patient, who is usually a woman, begins to scream and to tear off and destroy her clothing. While imitating the cry of some animal or bird, she may then throw herself on the snow or run wildly about on the ice. After the attack, she appears quite normal and usually has amnesia for it. Piblokto is almost certainly a hysterical state of dissociation.

Wihtigo

Wihtigo or windigo psychosis is a psychiatric illness confined to the Cree, Ojibway, and Salteaux Indians of North America. They believe that they may be transformed into a wihtigo, a giant monster that eats human flesh.

During times of starvation, a man may develop the delusion that he has been transformed into a wihtigo, and he may actually feel and express a craving for human flesh. Symptoms concerning the alimentary tract—such as loss of appetite and nausea from trivial causes—may sometimes cause the patient to become greatly excited for fear of being transformed into a wihtigo.

Voodoo and Other Possession States

The voodoo cult that is practiced in African societies and among native West Indians is particularly widespread in Haiti. At a typical Voodoo ceremony, dozens of people, after 2 or 3 hours of dancing to the wild rhythms of the drums and under the incantations of the voodoo priest (houngan), fall into hysterical trance states, during which they exhibit convulsions, excitement, the arc en cercle, and short-lasting twilight states. The people of these cultures believe in the possibility of being involuntarily possessed by evil spirits. Because of this belief, chronic hysterical and psychosomatic symptoms may be induced, and appropriate treatment for such conditions and for major psychoses due to other causes may be delayed.

Atypical Psychoses

Atypical Cycloid Psychoses

The cycloid psychoses, which are characterized by phasic recurrences, have been subdivided into three forms: motility psychoses, confusional psychoses, and anxiety-blissfulness psychoses.

The motility psychosis in its hyperkinetic form may resemble a manic or catatonic excitement. It may be distinguished from a manic state by the presence of many abrupt gestures and expressive movements, which seem to be the result of autonomous mechanisms and are apparently not responses to environmental stimuli or expressions of the patient's mood. These disorders may be differentiated from catatonic excitement by the absence of stereotyped and bizarre movements. The akinetic form motility psychosis seems to be identical with a typical catatonic stupor. These states are separated from typical schizophrenia mainly on the basis of their rapid and favorable course, which does not lead to any personality deterioration.

The excited confusional psychosis can be distinguished from some confused manic states by the greater lability of the patient's emotional state, which may be characterized by prevailing anxiety, rather than euphoria. These patients are not as distractible as manic patients are, they often misidentify persons in their environment, and the incoherence of their speech seems to be independent of a flight of ideas.

The inhibited confusional psychosis shares with the catatonic stupor and the akinetic motility psychosis the symptoms of mutism and greatly decreased motor behavior, but it differs from these states by the preservation of better self-care and greater spontaneity and by the absence of negativism.

The anxiety phase of the anxiety-blissfulness psychosis may resemble agitated depression, but it may also be characterized by so much anxious inhibition that the patient can hardly move. Periodic states of overwhelming anxiety and paranoid ideas of reference are characteristic of this condition, but self-accusations, hypochondriacal preoccupations, and other depressive symptoms, as well as hallucinations, may accompany it. The blissfulness phase manifests itself most frequently in expansive behavior and grandiose ideas, which are concerned less with self-aggrandizement than with the mission of making others happy and of saving the world. In women the dominant emotion is usually one of passive ecstasy, often the result of fantastic religious delusions.

Periodic recurrences are most frequent in the motility psychoses; they are less frequent in the anxiety-blissfulness psychoses and are still rarer in the confusional psychoses. Complete recovery of the patient is the rule in all these conditions.

Atypical Schizophrenias

Patients suffering from affect-laden paraphrenia express manifold delusions, which may be well-systematized. The strong and sustained affect that pervades them is pathological, although it may be an appropriate reaction to the content of the delusions, and it may be expressed as irritability, anxiety, or ecstasy.

Periodic catatonia, which differs from typical schizophrenic catatonia by the periodicity of its excited or stuporous phases, may sometimes resemble an akinetic or hyperkinetic motility psychosis, but it usually presents distinctive symptoms of stereotypy, bizarreness, grimacing, and a mixture of akinetic and hyperkinetic manifestations.

Schizophasia is characterized by a profound thought disturbance that results in a disorder of concept formation and abstract thinking and expresses itself in marked incoherence of speech. Such patients may at times resemble excited confusional psychotics; at other times they may resemble excited catatonics.

The prognosis is, in general, much poorer for the atypical schizophrenias than for the cycloid psychoses, and it is most guarded for the schizophasic patients, who often remain chronically ill or may recover with a permanent personality defect.

REFERENCES

De la Tourette, G. Etude sur une affection nerveuse caractérisée par l'incoordination motrice accompagnée d'écholalie et de coprolalie. Arch. Neurol. (Paris), *9:* 158, 1885.

Dow, T. W., and Silver, D. A drug-induced koro syndrome, J. Florida Med. Assoc., *60:* 32, 1973.

Enoch, M. D., Trethowan, W. H., and Barker, J. C. *Some Uncommon Psychiatric Syndromes.* Wright, Bristol. 1967.

Fish, F. A guide to the Leonhard classification of chronic schizophrenia. Psychiatr. Q. *38:* 438, 1964.

Friel, P. B. Familial incidence of Gilles de la Tourette's disease, with observation on aetiology and treatment. Br. J. Psychiatry, *122:* 655, 1973.

Klempel, K. False recognition on the pattern of the "Capgras syndrome" and related phenomena. Psychiatr. Clin., *6:* 17, 1973.

Lucas, A. R., and Rodin, E. A. Electroencephalogram in Gilles de la Tourette's disease. Dis. Nerv. Syst., *43:* 85, 1973.

Murphy, H. B. M. History and the evolution of syndromes: The striking case of latah and amok. In *Psychopathology: Contributions from the Social, Behavioral, and Biological Sciences,* M. Hammer, K. Salzinger, and S. Sutton, editors, p. 33. Wiley, New York, 1973.

Sanders, D. G. Familial occurrence of Gilles de la Tourette syndrome: Report of the syndrome occurring in a father and son. Arch. Gen. Psychiatry, *28:* 326, 1973.

Shapiro, A. K., Shapiro, E. and Wayne, H. Birth, developmental, and family histories and demographic information in Tourette's syndrome. J. Nerv. Ment. Dis., *155* 335, 1973.

Shapiro, A. K., Shapiro, E., and Wayne, H. Treatment of Tourette's syndrome. Arch. Gen. Psychiatry, *28:* 92, 1973.

Sirois, F. Les épidémies d'hystérie: Revue de la litérature: Réflexions sur le problème de la contagion psychopathologique. Union Med. Can., *102:* 1906, 1973.

Spiro, H. R. Chronic factitious illness: Munchausen's syndrome. Arch. Gen. Psychiatry, *18:* 569, 1968.

Tsoi, W. F. The Ganser Syndrome in Singapore: A report on ten cases. Br. J. Psychiatry, *122:* 604, 1973.

27

Psychiatry and Other Specialties

27.1 PSYCHIATRY AND MEDICINE

Patient's Emotional Reactions to Illness

When a person develops a symptom and realizes that this feeling is a deviation from his expectation of normal or his feeling of well-being, he concedes that he is no longer as self-sufficient as before, and he may feel threatened, depressed, anxious, or fearful. Since the patient-physician relationship is one that involves dependency of the patient on the physician, dependent needs or conflicts usually color the relationship.

Dependency Problems

Those who crave dependency and develop an overly dependent relationship with helping professionals either were overprotected as children and conditioned not to want to leave a protected environment or did not have their dependency needs satisfied and are still seeking what they never got in childhood. Both types tend to be hypochondriacal, to prolong convalescence, and to be prone to drug dependency. Concerned attention from relatives, physicians, or others may prolong the illness and the dependency ties.

Persons who were overprotected as children often grew up as only children or were selected by their parents for special attention. Since the patient's dependency needs are often insatiable, his persistent complaints or demands for help are eventually met by the physician's frustration and anger. By caring for the patient, by listening, by setting realistic limits, and by not giving direct advice in any area other than that related to health, the internist can meet the patient's dependency needs without getting involved in a hostile antitherapeutic conflict.

In patients whose dependency needs were never quite satisfied during their developmental years, overt signs of rejection may often be detected in the history. Sometimes the concerned physician seems omnipotent and the long-lost source of kindly attention.

The management of the superdependent patient by the internist is often difficult. Recognition of the problem may alleviate the anxiety of those caring for the patient. It is helpful to minimize secondary gain. With hospitalized patients, a flexible discharge policy may be needed, and sometimes setting limits of inpatient stay may be necessary. In the outpatient setting, the frequency of appointments may be decreased. The consultation time may be shortened. And it often helps for the physician to be more than normally talkative during the interview, since dependency is fostered by silence. It is imperative that the physician not prescribe excessive medications. Drugs to a dependent patient are usually felt as caring, loving, giving gestures that further cement the dependency.

Those who are afraid of dependency are often basically dependent but fearful of losing control of their destiny; by the mechanism of reaction formation, they have developed an independent façade. Often, they were frightened by feelings of helplessness when they were children. They fear illness because it makes them feel helpless again.

Some persons who are afraid of a dependent state are ashamed of helplessness. In childhood, such persons were usually pushed prematurely into independent activity by their parents.

Anxiety

During the initial medical interview, anxiety is usually present. Some patients manifest overt anxiety, most often detected by the moist palm at the time of the handshake. Restlessness and difficulty in speaking are sometimes seen early in the interview. Other patients may become garrulous. Often the circumstantial, verbal patient is manifesting a clinging, dependent relationship with the physician.

Some view the physician as a benevolent, paternalistic protector, others with hostility or suspicion, and still others with an apprehensive fear of the unknown. Some female patients may relate to their male physicians as they have related to all other men, through an expression of their sexuality.

Denial

Denial may be manifest in some patients who minimize their symptoms. The tendency may be a way of averting anxiety, or it may represent a character trait in people with hysterical personality disorders. Denial is usually betrayed by the obvious disparity between the patient's condition and how he reports it. Many patients smilingly insist that all is well or that a symptom does not exist.

Many patients are unaware of the degree to which they are distorting the facts. Some patients deliberately distort or consciously deny information about which they are ashamed or afraid. Eventually, time and the persistence of the illness make denial untenable in most cases. Depression, with or without regression, may occur as a sequel to denial.

Regression

Illness—especially if it requires bed rest, hospitalization, and nursing care—normally promotes a degree of regression. This regression is an emotional and physical retreat from adult standards of independence and self-determination to a more infantile level of weakness, passivity, and dependence on others. This state is the culturally accepted sick role, which in an acute illness is tolerated and often fostered by physicians. The regressed patient is submissive, trusting, and cooperative, with child-like obedience. Problems arise when such a patient regresses excessively and becomes unable or unwilling to cooperate. For him, regression and dependency represent a tempting retreat from the overwhelming or unsatisfying task of recovery. The illness may seem incurable to the patient, and a hopeless depression may ensue. Occasionally, the demands of family, job, or social life encourage prolonged illness.

The management of the regressed patient usually requires a tolerant but gently insistent push program by the physician, nurses, and other personnel in contact with him. A hovering, caring, and often guilty spouse tends to foster regression either by solicitude or by angrily rejecting the patient. Counseling with appropriate family members can help overcome the withdrawal and reluctance of a regressed patient.

Hostility

Other difficult patients are demanding, obtuse, hypochondriacal, and often litigious. Many are overtly paranoid, but usually they are emotionally troubled people who are seeking attention in the only way they believe possible. They may be emotionally cold and disliked by their associates and relatives, completely unable to receive affection from anyone without experiencing emotional discomfort or fear. Feelings of estrangement and loneliness may cause them to decide unconsciously that negative attention is better than none. Some chronically guilt-ridden patients cannot tolerate a warm, close, pleasant contact with a physician or being made well. These patients unconsciously resist every step toward successful treatment.

Sometimes, the uncooperative patient is an overly dependent person who is childishly expressing jealously and resentment that he cannot have the physician all to himself and completely under his control. On the other hand, the overly polite patient may be fighting unconscious hostility.

The peripatetic patient always seems dissatisfied and may go to great extremes in his doctor shopping. Some of these patients are threatened by any close relationship and can handle closeness only by self-imposed rejection. Many are emotionally immature and unable to tolerate the threat of illness and eventual death. Many have hysterical personality disorders, and some manifest specific conversion reactions. These patients are quite suggestible and usually identify with an older father-figure physician, who, they feel, possesses magical powers. Initially, they may take a flight into health. The improvement is usually short-lived.

Physician's Emotional Attitudes

Many of the problems that confront an internist are vague, nonspecific, and unclassifiable. The internist's ability to feel comfortable with such patients may indicate how secure he is in his professional role or how well he understands the psychodynamics of his patients. Unfortunately, some physicians do not gain insight and continue to experience frustration.

The basic reasons students enter the field of medicine are usually intellectual, manifest, and unconscious. One unconscious reason may be curiosity, a voyeuristic need to know about or to see other people, perhaps to reassure the physician that he is normal. Some people enter medicine as a counterphobic reaction to the fear of death. Some dependent persons enter medicine with a strong reaction formation to their dependency needs. They satisfy their needs by helping others but deny their needs and often express their independence through aggressiveness, solo practice, and resistance to third-party intervention in the patient-physician relationship. Sometimes they encourage patients to rely on them excessively. Some students enter medicine because of unconscious parental fostering or because they identify with a secure father figure, who is perceived as an older wise physician.

Many physicians feel uncomfortable and anxious when involved with a critically ill patient. Their anxiety may be manifested by psychomotor restlessness, impatience, and irritability with the hospital staff. On occasion, they blame the patient. This projection of blame is especially common in physicians who deal with drug-dependent or alcohol-dependent patients.

The insecure but hard-driving, overly ambitious physician may try to prove himself through his work. It is common for such a physician to be flamboyant, to pursue a challenging diagnosis diligently, and to put down those who question his motives. He may institute dramatic therapeutic procedures that do more for his own morale than for his patient's welfare. Frequently, a young internist orders an elaborate array of laboratory tests in order not to miss a diagnosis. On the other hand, some physicians who have experienced a financially impoverished background project their own parsimony into the medical setting and avoid ordering valid diagnostic tests and adequate medications. A more frequent problem is the physician who prescribes an excessive number of drugs because he cannot explain a symptom

complex and cannot tolerate his patient's demands for more help. Often, the patient is asking for more of the physician's time, rather than for more drugs. This situation often results in an impasse between the continued demands of the patient and the reluctance of the physician to be further controlled by the patient. When the physician senses that he is in a servile role with the patient, he may rebel, resist, or refer.

Some internists respond to the hypochondriacal patient as though the patient were weak-willed or were not trying hard enough. Such an attitude can be destructive to the development of a trusting relationship.

The physician must have a compassionate, tolerant understanding of the patient, even though he personally may not agree with the life style of the patient. Likewise, the physician must understand the uncooperative patient who is seemingly attempting to scuttle the therapeutic regime. The lack of cooperation may reflect a depression or a displacement of anger by the patient.

Patient-Physician Encounters

Compensation Problems

The physician often rejects a patient with a medical-legal problem because of possible involvement in court or deposition proceedings. Such testimony is time-consuming and emotionally unrewarding. Also, the physician often finds incapacity beyond the level expected from the objective findings and may conclude that there are elements of hypochondriasis, hysteria, or malingering. He may react with disdain and subtly reject the patient at a time when support and compassion are most needed.

After an injury in an automobile or industrial accident, an early posttraumatic syndrome is manifest by a psychophysiologic response to the fear of annihilation. This reaction may last from a few minutes to several months and has a variety of symptoms associated with it, such as fearfulness, startle reaction, repetitive dreams or nightmares, palpitations, headache, dizziness, insomnia, irritability, anxiety, and fatigue. In patients with a tenuous emotional equilibrium, the acute symptoms may persist or may be replaced by other more chronic neurotic symptoms. These neuroses are nonspecific and generally begin 3 to 6 months after the accident. The reaction usually arises along the lines of previous personality patterns, whereas the traumatic syndrome manifests symptoms uniformly seen in everyone, regardless of the previous personality pattern.

Secondary gain associated with a traumatic neurosis is often misunderstood. Dependent longings to be cared for, masochistic needs to experience pain and misery, and hostile desires for revenge against an employer, insurance company, or spouse—all on an unconscious level—are psychologically more important than fantasied financial remuneration. However, the possibility of monetary compensation often influences the course of the neurosis. Secondary gain of any type may prolong the symptoms. Physicians may unconsciously foster secondary gain by failing to look at the emotional issues involved and by using excessive symptomatic therapy. Loss of time from work, disruption of a tenuous family equilibrium, and disappointments may contribute to the neurotic pattern.

The physician must remain objective. Psychotherapy should be supportive. Generalizations and false reassurance may be as harmful as overtreatment, but a better understanding of the patient and his problem and giving him the opportunity to express his feelings put the physician in the best position to develop a healthy patient-physician relationship.

Diabetes Mellitus

Provoked unexpressed hostility seems capable of causing significant physiologic changes in diabetics. Stressful life situations that adversely affect the course of diabetes usually involve significant persons in the patient's life. Circumstances that provoke feelings of frustrations, loneliness, or dejection are frequently accompanied by glycosuria and increased insulin requirements.

When the patient learns he has diabetes, a reactive depression is almost inevitable. Many patients are shocked and have an incredulous attitude. Sometimes the initial effective shock is compounded by a physician who instills a fear of complications, and a hypochondriacal overconcern develops. If a patient has developed the rigid defense of an obsessive-compulsive personality, he can usually accept the restrictions that diabetes usually requires, but some patients overemphasize control and become so inflexible that their entire lives are rigidly governed by their disease. The aggressive person may become hostile, resistive, and sometimes paranoid. The passive person may become acquiescing and regressed.

Most patients adjust to diabetes. Endogenous depression occasionally occurs, but the incidence is probably not higher than in the general population. Nevertheless, the adequate management of diabetes requires an understanding of personality traits and the life situation of the individual patient.

Alcoholism

Most alcoholics minimize the quantity of alcohol they consume and often deny obvious physical, family, or job problems. Physicians are often hostile in their approach with alcoholics, and many physicians feel that direct confrontation and an aggressive approach to therapy are more effective than logic or insight. Treatment is often difficult and fraught with frustration because the patient's motivation is poor. It is important that the internist develop a rapport with the patient, so that some degree of trust will develop.

Long-term supportive follow-up seems helpful in maintaining a state of sobriety. Most alcoholics have intense dependency needs.

Intensive Care Units

The initial emotional responses of a patient in an intensive care unit are usually fear and overt anxiety. Depression occurs later, usually on the third or fourth day. Various behavioral problems also develop later, after the initial fear and anxiety abate. Psychotic reactions occur commonly in neurosurgical and postcardiac surgery intensive care units but are rarely seen in medical intensive care units.

Psychiatric treatment includes the proper use of tranquilizers and nighttime sedation, careful and detailed explanations of the significance of myocardial infarction and the attending psychological stresses, environmental manipulation, bolstering of optimism, and confrontation of inappropriate behavior. It is also important for all unit personnel to maintain open communication. Group psychotherapeutic approaches can be helpful, and the involvement of spouses is beneficial.

Chronic Illness

With the realization that his illness is chronic, the patient is in greatest need of emotional support. There is often a period of depression, which may result in a helpless regression, with melancholy and self-pity; or denial of the depression may occur, with a pseudogaity.

Frequently, patients feel angry about their plight. This anger may be projected to various aspects of the care or to the patient's family. Abused relatives and medical personnel are initially dismayed, later defensive, and finally retaliatory. Early recognition of such problems, counseling of nurses and the family, and helping the patient verbalize and abreact his anger can channel hostility and aggressiveness into more constructive efforts or rehabilitation.

Chronically ill patients often crave constant expressions of their physician's commitment to their comfort and continued survival. This commitment is often in the form of medication. The dependent and insecure patient may easily become drug dependent. The patient who trusts and respects his physician is likely to get good effects from his medication. The distrustful and angry patient has a higher incidence of adverse reactions and inadequate results. The physician may prescribe unnecessary drugs because of his insecurity in dealing with a chronically ill or incurable patient. A rejecting physician may prescribe large quantities of drugs, with infrequent recheck examinations, in a not too disguised wish that the patient would go away.

When used with care and understanding, drugs furnish a mutually acceptable reason for regular visits, periodic re-evaluations, and repeated reinforcements of the physician's concern for his patient's welfare. Regular reviews of medication and maintenance of a good patient-physician relationship minimize the problem of overmedication and drug dependency.

Some patients with chronic illness require hospitalization and may become dependent on the care they receive in the hospital. Discharge from the hospital may result in a separation anxiety. A common reaction is for a relapse to occur a day or so before the planned hospital discharge. Some patients may become depressed and withdrawn; they may develop insomnia or become increasingly dependent on nursing care. In such instances, it is important that the patient discuss his fear and anxiety about leaving the protected hospital environment. Also, close family members must learn to accept the patient's feelings of irritation and anger, which are usually related to the frustrations of a changed life pattern associated with a chronic illness but which may be displaced to the spouse, children, or other close associates.

Malignancy

The inevitability of death poses the question of disclosure of the diagnosis and prognosis to the patient. Most people have sufficient ego strength to be able to tolerate reality. Whether to tell a patient he has a malignancy must be an individual decision. This decision may depend on the patient's emotional assets.

For the patient who is told he has cancer, there is initially shock, fear, and depression. This period is short-lived and is followed by denial and mourning; there may be frenzied planning and meaningless activity. Finally, there is an acceptance of altered goals in life, with a realistic adjustment to the illness and cooperation with the attending physicians.

What is said and done to a patient is far less important than the manner in which it is said and done. The patient can sense the physician's anxiety, unrealistic promises, or uninvolvement. Ideally, the physician should portray warmth, understanding, and compassion while allowing the patient to ventilate his feelings. Many fears may be allayed by open discussion.

Renal Disease

Unlike patients with terminal malignancies, patients with renal disease always have hope of complete cure and rehabilitation with a successful kidney transplant. When a transplanted kidney is rejected, the patient must be dependent on hemodialysis. Hemodialysis units have produced a plethora of unique problems. There is the agonizing decision as to whether to include a patient in an already overcrowed hemodialysis program. Patients who receive hemodialysis are totally dependent on the dialysis machine and the unit staff for their continued survival. The mortality rate among patients on dialysis varies from 5 to 20 per cent a year. Suicide is one of the more frequent causes of death.

Death

The fear of death is universal. If the patient has felt insecure, if he has been exposed to the loss of significant figures in his life, or if he is guilt-ridden, he may be unable to accept the inevitability of death. The support of loved ones, and the physician is imperative as death approaches.

Often, the detached concern that is taught in medical school becomes either aloofness or over-involvement. The feeling of helplessness or impotence at the time of death is widespread. The physician may be trapped by valiant efforts to prolong life and then be unable to stop the machines without feelings of guilt. A realistic view of the patient's status, discussions with relatives, and consultations with colleagues help put this problem into perspective.

Psychiatric Consultation

Hospital Consultation

Consultations requested about patients who are already hospitalized on a medical service are influenced by such factors as the patient's knowledge of the need for psychiatric evaluation and help, his current emotional status, and his behavior. Some factors are related to the physician's tolerance of or insight into his patient's emotional problems and his awareness of his own need for help in further evaluation and treatment of the patient.

Probably the most frequent reason for psychiatric consultation is a request for diagnostic help. Many patients are admitted to the hospital on a medical service for diagnostic evaluation of symptoms that prove to be solely or primarily the result of psychophysiologic disorders or somatization reactions. Patients with depression often enter the hospital on medical services for evaluation of their somatic symptoms.

All medical problems have emotional components with regard to how the patient feels about and reacts to his illness. But many medical problems may present as though they were primarily psychiatric illnesses. A thorough medical evaluation and mental status examination should always be done with a patient whose condition is unclear. Table I lists some medical problems that may masquerade as psychiatric syndromes.

If the problem is of sufficient magnitude to require inpatient psychiatric care, a transfer to a psychiatric unit may be advised. More often, the consultant outlines a therapeutic program for the internist to institute and conduct. Or the psychiatrist may recommend that the patient be dismissed from the hospital, with outpatient psychiatric follow-up therapy.

Behavioral problems are often the reason for the psychiatric consultations. These problems may include suicidal behavior, overt hostility, regression, the breaking of hospital rules, and general deviation from the role expected of a hospitalized patient. The internist may be perplexed or threatened by his patient's behavior. Some physicians equate tearfulness with depression; others are intolerant of emotional problems and request psychiatric help at the first sign of emotional instability. Some internists are eager to discuss the psychodynamics of their patients in detail, often to confirm their own formulations. Other physicians merely want hard facts; these physicians may be quite impatient with a consultant who is vague or unable to be helpful in the way the referring physician wants help.

Many hospital psychiatric consultations are requested on an emergency basis because of suicidal or homicidal ideation, acute excitement due to delirium or psychosis, and adverse reactions to psychopharmacologic agents.

Sometimes an acutely ill patient insists on leaving the hospital against medical advice. Some patients who do this have angrily complained that they are not receiving adequate medical care. They provoke active staff hostility, which causes their complaints to be real and reinforces their justification for leaving the hospital. They often find flaws in the hospital procedures that justify a complaint. The consultant must work directly with the patient, employing face-saving measures that allow the patient to stay in the hospital and maintain his dignity. The psychiatrist must also interpret the patient's behavior to the medical and nursing staff so that they can deal with it as an illness and overcome their ambivalence about the resistive patient. Sometimes patients want to leave the hospital against advice because they are frightened or deny the seriousness of their illness. They may be unable to submit to the dependent status of a patient. In such

TABLE I

Medical Problems That May Present as Psychiatric Symptoms

	Sex and Age Prevalence	Common Medical Symptoms	Psychiatric Symptoms and Complaints	Impaired Performance and Behavior	Diagnostic Problems
Hyperthyroidism (thyrotoxicosis)	Females 3:1, 30 to 50	Tremor, sweating, loss of weight and strength	Anxiety if rapid onset; depression if slow onset	Occasional hyperactive or grandiose behavior	Long lead time; a rapid onset resembles anxiety attack
Hypothyroidism (myxedema)	Females 5:1, 30 to 50	Puffy face, dry skin, cold intolerance	Anxiety with irritability, thought disorder, somatic delusions, hallucinations	Myxedema madness; delusional, paranoid, belligerent behavior	Madness may mimic schizophrenia; mental status is clear, even during most disturbed behavior
Hyperparathyroidism	Females 3:1, 40 to 60	Weakness, anorexia, fractures, calculi, peptic ulcers	Either state may cause anxiety-hyperactivity and irritability or depression—apathy and withdrawal	Either state may proceed to a toxic psychosis: confusion, disorientation, clouded sensorium, etc.	Anorexia and fatigue of slow-growing adenoma resemble involutional depression
Hypoparathyroidism	Females, 40 to 60	Hyperreflexia, spasms, tetany			None; rare condition except for surgery
Hyperadrenalism (Cushing's disease)	Both sexes, adults	Weight gain, fat alteration, easy fatigability	Varied; depression, anxiety, thought disorder with somatic delusions	Rarely produces aberrant behavior	Bizarre somatic delusions caused by bodily change resemble schizophrenia
Adrenal cortical insufficiency (Addison's disease)	Both sexes, adults	Weight loss, hypotension, skin pigmentation	Depression—negativism, apathy; thought disorder—suspiciousness	Toxic psychosis with confusion and agitation	Long lead time; weight loss, apathy, despondency resemble involutional depression
Porphyria—acute intermittent type	Females, 20 to 40	Abdominal crises, paresthesias, weakness	Anxiety—sudden onset, severe; mood swings	Extremes of excitement or withdrawal; emotional or angry outbursts	Patients often have truly neurotic life styles; crises resemble conversion reactions or anxiety attacks
Pernicious anemia (Addisonian anemia)	Females, 40 to 60	Weight loss, weakness, glossitis, extremity neuritis	Depression—feelings of guilt and worthlessness	Eventual brain damage, with confusion and memory loss	Long lead time—sometimes many months; easily mistaken for involutional depression; normal early blood studies may give false reassurance
Hepatolenticular degeneration (Wilson's disease)	Males 2:1, adolescence	Liver and extrapyramidal symptoms, Kayser-Fleischer rings	Mood swings—sudden and changeable; anger—explosive	Eventual brain damage, with memory and I.Q. loss; combativeness	In late teens, may resemble adolescent storm, incorrigibility, or schizophrenia

Hypoglycemia (islet cell adenoma)	Both sexes, adults	Tremor, sweating, hunger, fatigue, dizziness	Anxiety—fear and dread; depression with fatigue	Agitation, confusion; eventual brain damage	Can mimic anxiety attack or acute alcoholism; bizarre behavior may draw attention away from somatic symptoms
Intracranial tumors	Both sexes, adults	None early; headache, vomiting, papilledema later	Varied; depression, anxiety, personality changes	Loss of memory, judgment, self-criticism; clouding of consciousness	Tumor location may not determine early symptoms
Pancreatic carcinoma	Males 3:1, 50 to 70	Weight loss, abdominal pain, weakness, jaundice	Depression, sense of imminent doom but without severe guilt	Loss of drive and motivation	Long lead time; exact age and symptoms of involutional depression
Pheochromocytoma	Both sexes, adults	Headache, sweating during elevated blood pressure	Anxiety, panic, fear, apprehension, trembling	Inability to function during an attack	Classic symptoms of anxiety attack, intermittently normal blood pressures may discourage further studies
Multiple sclerosis	Females, 20 to 40	Motor and sensory losses, scanning speech, nystagmus	Varied; personality changes, mood swings, depression; bland euphoria uncommon	Inappropriate behavior due to personality changes	Long lead time; early neurological symptoms mimic hysteria or conversion reactions
Systemic lupus erythematosus	Females 8:1, 20 to 40	Multiple symptoms of cardiovascular, genitourinary, gastrointestinal, other systems	Varied; thought disorder, depression, confusion	Toxic psychosis unrelated to steroid treatment	Long lead time, perhaps many years, psychiatric picture variable over time; thought disorder resembles schizophrenia

instances it may be necessary to confront the patient's excessive denial in a firm yet understanding manner. Discussion of the problem with the medical staff and continued follow-up and often supportive, brief psychotherapy may be indicated.

Outpatient Consultation

If the psychiatrist is in solo practice, the patient usually sees him in his office at an appointed time. The psychiatrist then communicates the results of his evaluation to the referring physician by letter. In group practices, the psychiatric consultant usually interviews the patient in the internist's office after discussing the reasons for the consultation with the internist and reviewing the patient's history and laboratory test results. After the interview, the consultant then makes a notation in the patient's record and discusses his evaluation with the internist responsible for the patient's care.

Psychiatric consultants are frequently asked to evaluate the medical-legal aspects of a patient's problems. In such situations it is important to develop all aspects of the patient's problem and keep complete records for testimony that may be required later. Opinions about the influence of emotional issues on the patient's symptoms, pre-existing psychopathology, the degree of incapacity, and the possibility of malingering are difficult but necessary assessments. The psychiatric consultant may also be asked to evaluate the competence of patients to negotiate wills or contracts or to take marriage vows.

REFERENCES

Emotional stresses of patient-physician encounters, J. A. M. A., *223*: 1037, 1973.
Lief, H. I., Leif, V. F., and Lief, N. R. *The Psychological Basis of Medical Practice.* Harper & Row, New York, 1963.
Morgan, W. L., and Engel, G. L. *The Clinical Approach to the Patient.* Saunders, Philadelphia, 1969.
Saul, L. J. *Emotional Maturity.* Lippincott, Philadelphia, 1971.
Schwab, J. J. *Handbood of Psychiatric Consultation.* Appleton-Century-Crofts, New York, 1968.
Solomon, P., and Patch, V. D. *Handbook of Psychiatry.* Lange, Los Altos, Calif., 1969.

27.2.   THANATOLOGY

Introduction

Thanatology may be defined as the study of the physical and psychosocial contexts of death.

Attitudes about death and its meaning can be reduced to four main ideas: death as an illusion and extension of life, death as an inevitable and inexorable fact of life, death as an explanation and expiation of life, and death as exigency and defeat of life. All theories about death are beliefs about life. It is simply futile, a chance for retribution and reward, a stark symbol of finitude, or a way station to another existence. The existential and operational viewpoints declare: (1) Death is not the same as dying. (2) Death is not the opposite of life. (3) One can live out a full span of years but may not. (4) Regardless of the length of life, one meets and copes with many small deaths. (5) One reaches out and relinquishes, accepts, and forsakes, using different lifestyles and deathstyles.

There are only a few ways to perish: accident, intention, illness, allotment, and decrepitude. Simply to be alive is to be at risk.

Death-Related Situations and Syndromes

Two major concepts help to understand how people face extinction. These are: my death versus your death and partial death versus total death. Impersonal death is the demise of someone who means little or nothing. Interpersonal death occurs when someone dies about whom one cares, yet one is exempted to a degree (partial death). One can be sad but also feel guilty, relieved, and even secretly pleased. Interpersonal death matters in proportion to the disruption that such deaths make in one's own life. Interpersonal death is the most significant situation. It means one's own extinction as an autonomous, self-aware person. However, one does not need to die in order to undergo and experience intrapersonal death. Key transitions during development symbolize these changes. One can die by degrees, in which restitution and replacement cannot keep pace with loss and disability, or all at once.

Fatal Illness and Timely Death

Just as a good patient is expected to conform to hospital rules and to a schedule of recovery, a dying patient is implicitly expected to follow an anticipated course. Awareness of incipient death often leads to premature and preliminary bereavement, but the patient may not die on time. When this happens, the survivors, including members of the professional staff, are often found to be disappointed, frustrated, and even openly angry.

Stages of dying have been classified as denial, anger, bargaining, depression, and acceptance. However, many patients show other responses: humor, self-pity, compassion, love, apathy, apprehension, and so forth.

Although dividing fatal illness into stages is sometimes a mere abstraction, time, space, and reality do change during the course. One can recognize different coping styles and psychosocial issues in the intervals between the initial diagnosis and death itself. Stage I, prediagnostic and diagnostic, is the interval from the onset of symptoms to the definitive diagnosis. Stage II, established disease, extends from the time of diagnosis and early treatment until relief and remission cease. The purpose of treatment may be curative or palliative during established disease. Stage III, decline and deterioration, starts at the time when there is nothing left to do and the patient becomes more disabled but not necessarily preterminal or terminal. During stage III, families ask, physicians answer, but patients rarely ask how much longer. The salient psychosocial problems of patients during stage I are those of postponement and denial. In stage II the major areas of concern are those of work, family, religion, economics, self-esteem, physical incapacity, and emotional vulnerability. As stage III appears, patients must call on others for what they have heretofore done for themselves. Patients take more medication, have fewer interests, need more assistance, have less autonomy, show more regression, and have fewer options. Simultaneously, the hospital staff and family are faced with their shortcomings and futility, bereavement, and intimation of their own mortality.

Untimely Death

Some deaths take place suddenly and without warning. There are three kinds of untimely deaths: premature death, unexpected death, and calamitous death.

Terminality

Dying and death are closely related, but they are not the same. It would be much less ambiguous to call dying "terminality." From the physical standpoint, dying is the near absence of healthy organ functions, and death is their total cessation.

In death-related situations, people tend to draw away from each other. Revulsion about sickness, noxious smells and sights, bitterness and regrets, futility and resentment conspire with natural fears about death and dying to separate one person from another. The major exception is found in common calamities—such as floods, shipwrecks, and wartime disasters—when one becomes the equal of everyone else, and all cling together for mutual protection.

Fear of death is universal. To know what any person fears in death, one needs to know what he has suffered and endured during life, as well as what has given him most fulfillment and what he dreads losing. Because to most people death is life with a negative sign, fear of death may be defined as how one systematizes his sufferings, actual and anticipated.

Fear of dying occurs often in the course of life, without necessarily being related to actual death. It consists of an existential anxiety about one's being, presence, and consciousness. One feels utterly helpless, slipping away into anonymity and unreality. This sense of imminent disaster rarely happens to dying patients, even those who have experienced acute anxiety during healthier days.

Three general forms of anxiety occur during terminality, largely unaccompanied by autonomic signs of fear. These syndromes are alienation, annihilation, and endangerment. Alienation is characterized by a sense of loneliness, isolation, abandonment, and derealization of the surrounding world. Annihilation is anxiety about becoming nothing at all. Endangerment combines a feeling of imminent danger with resentment and anger about being so frail, mortal, and destructible. Endangerment is to destructiveness what anxiety is to specific fears; endangered people look for someone to blame, just as anxious people find objects and situations to fear.

Acceptance and Denial of Death

Awareness of dying is a result of the equilibrium between acceptance and denial. Neither exists without the other, but they exist in varying proportions. Both are social strategies that enable patients to accommodate and to reduce apprehensions. The balance between acceptance and denial can be analyzed by establishing three orders of denial and acceptance. The first and most conspicuous is denial of the facts about illness, including the diagnosis. This is direct repudiation of immediate experience.

The second form is denial of the implications or inferences to be drawn from the illness and its signs. The third is denial of death itself, the unimaginable cessation.

Hope and despair are reciprocally related, but it is erroneous to believe that hope is contingent on major denial. Hope does not depend on belief in an incorrect diagnosis, extended survival, or cure. Indeed, vain hope can be a cause of despair. Authentic hope stems from unwavering self-esteem, not faith in something that will never come. Despair does not necessarily result from acceptance; more often, despair without an outlet in open communication leads to anger, frustration, and more vigorous denial.

Life-Threatening Behavior

Not every instance of life-threatening behavior starts with a wish to die, to kill, or to be killed. However, innate fears of death frequently evoke an antithetical inability or unwillingness to recognize danger. Risky behavior is not necessarily equivalent to life-threatening behavior.

The most common types of life-threatening behavior that a psychiatrist is apt to encounter and that carry a risk of serious physical danger are self-injury and intoxication; rash, regretted, incautious, or bizarre acts; significant ommissions; significant excesses; and countertherapeutic behavior.

Suicide is a prototype of life-threatening behavior. There are no specific causes of sucide but many predisposing factors. Suicide attempters usually talk about problems of retribution and revenge, release from suffering, insoluble differences and dissonances with significant key others, loss of self-esteem, and either excessively controlled impulses or overwhelming destructiveness. In addition, patients may feel utterly hopeless and helpless about doing anything corrective for themselves or others.

Bereavement

Bereavement is like dying itself, except that it refers to the process by which a person suffers, sustains, and then recovers from the wound inflicted by the loss of someone essential to his reality. Like any other wound, it may be short and trivial or very serious, life-threatening, and prolonged. During the bereavement process, healing can be impaired, delayed, and exaggerated, with many secondary complications, including that of chronic invalidism.

Whenever someone cared about is very ill, is operated on, or even recovers from a serious disease, one tends to be anxious and to undergo anticipatory grief. It is an important phase because preparation is self-knowledge, and opportunity for early acceptance of the departure of part of one's own reality.

The initial response to death is usually one of intense anxiety, followed quickly by denial. In the immediate shock, a survivor may go numb, shut down, close off, seem to become indifferent or dazed. Then numbness is typically followed by either copious weeping or unnatural control. Both extremes represent craving and searching for the one who is lost.

After the acute mourning subsides, depression and grief follow—dejection, disorganization, depletion, sleeplessness. Dreams that resurrect the dead are later phenomena: in the immediate period of bereavement, they are less common than semihallucinatory feelings that the dead still survive in some way.

In American society, bereaved people frequently suffer from loneliness and isolation in the months after the death because there are few rituals of support available. Consequently, many survivors find a resurgence of anxiety, dejection, and despair from 4 to 6 months after the death. In self-healing efforts, they may rush to divest themselves of attachments to their previous reality—selling possessions, moving away, shunning friends, trying to change their personality in some drastic fashion. Anger, depression, and guilt may reappear; bitterness leads to withdrawal, and this cycle perpetuates itself into a syndrome of feeling deadened and yet insisting that all is well.

Sooner or later, bereavement comes to an end, although memories continue. The mourner finds it more and more difficult to visualize the deceased and becomes restless, searching for new outlets and things to do. Normal bereavement duration is decided by personal and cultural expectations, which may range from a few days of decorous depression to many months of intense emotional impoverishment. Bereavement ceases when a person becomes operational again, active and responsive to work, recreation, and emotional life.

It is appropriate to diagnose abnormal bereavement only under the following conditions:

(1) arrest of the process, in which afflicted patients show typical symptoms for long periods without evidence of relief, recovery, or restitution, (2) exaggeration of symptoms during the course, (3) deviant behavior that violates conventional expectations or jeopardizes physical health and safety.

Psychiatric Management of Terminality

Not every preterminal or terminal patient requires psychiatric intervention. But many patients can be helped, directly and indirectly, by psychiatric contributions. Psychiatrists can participate in the following ways: consultation with the staff about the psychosocial diagnosis and management of patients and families; regular sessions with nurses and social workers who are exposed to the frustrations and conflicts of terminality and lethality; psychotherapeutic interviews with patients; assessment of patients who endanger themselves through life-threatening behavior; teaching medical students about death, dying, bereavement, and life-threatening behavior; promulgation of psychosocial management principles to other professionals who care for terminal and preterminal patients; closer contact with colleagues who are directly charged with the primary responsibility of diagnosis, treatment, and everyday care; self-instruction in contemporary medical and surgical knowledge, problems, and procedures; introduction of the psychological autopsy; and constant search for death-related situations and psychodynamic analysis of clinical problems related to self-inimical behavior.

Three principal aims and objectives should guide the psychiatric management of terminality; safe conduct, dignified dying, and appropriate death. Safe conduct is the alleviation of secondary suffering due to the personal crisis of dying. Dignified dying means that one continues to regard a dying patient as a responsible person, capable of clear perceptions, honest relationships, and purposeful behavior, consistent with the inroads of physical decline and disability. Dignity, in contrast to demoralization, also means to look on a patient as even more than he is, was, or might be. An appropriate death can be defined as a death one might choose, were there a choice.

Certain recommendations can be made to promote the three principal aims and objectives. First, sit down, listen, and allot time for direct conversation on a person-to-person basis. Cliches, brisk reassurance, lugubrious commiseration, and overly professional ploys and poses are transparent clues that the therapist is uneasy and is looking for the exit. The most important element in psychiatric management is the capacity to be there. Even silence, a touch, a gesture, or a small gift can be eloquent.

To tell or not to tell the patient that he is dying is seldom a crucial question. Most patients already know at least the tenor of the situation, even though members of the family may not realize it.

Appropriate interventions include adequate relief of pain and suffering; informed consent about the diagnosis, treatment, and course; preservation of self-esteem and autonomy; open and candid communication with significant key others; and courage to accept what cannot be changed.

Special Topics and Problems

Death and Children

Discussing death with an inquiring child requires simplicity, candor, and none of the fairy tales that frighten more often than clarify. Adults are cautioned not to invent answers when they know none. It is important that the explainer show minimal anxiety. People who are deeply grieved should be brief, and the task of informing should be delegated to someone not intimately involved in the bereavement. Children can and do grieve, and crying should not be the cause of reproach.

Experts seem to agree that children should be permitted to attend funerals and to realize the finality of death in the company of trustworthy adults. If, however, there is a strong possibility that otherwise controlled adults will break down and be a disturbing influence, discretion is desirable. In any event, the adult may take the child to the cemetery later to show the peace, serenity, and repose that a well-tended memorial evokes. A child who is not permitted to mourn and is discouraged from believing in death may undergo alienation anxiety.

Children have a fairly clear idea of death at an early age, but their concepts evolve from thoughts of death as a temporary state to a notion that death happens only to old people. Later on, death is accepted as irreversible.

Longevity and Old Age

Fear of death seems more acute among young adults and middle-age people than among the very old. Thanatology's task with the very aged is neither to prolong nor to shorten life but to emphasize significant and competent survival on the best terms possible—economic, social, physical, residential, and emotional. Suicide rates go up with age, isolation, lack of significant social role, disabling illness, and alcoholism.

Euthanasia, Organ Transplantation, and Informed Consent

Euthanasia means "good death". Candidates for euthanasia and organ transplants are both victims of incurable illnesses, and they face death in the near future. In addition, their incapacity is so severe that the quality of their lives is almost negligible. To carry out either of these procedures, one must obtain informed consent from everyone concerned.

There are, of course, differences: Organ transplantation seeks to relieve suffering and to extend life. Euthanasia also seeks to relieve suffering, but it seeks to shorten the course of dying in situations where extended living is unlikely.

Arguments against euthanasia are many, but lack of informed consent or no consent whatsoever is perhaps the most significant. Similar arguments could be mustered about overly enthusiastic organ transplantations by surgeons with consummate skill but impervious narcissism. Medicine needs operational criteria for its life-and-death decisions. People generally want to be in charge of their own fate, including their dying, or at least to have the options of informed collaboration.

REFERENCES

Feifel, H. *The Meaning of Death.* McGraw-Hill, New York, 1959.
Feifel, H., Freilich, J., and Hermann, L. Death fear in dying heart and cancer patients. J. Psychosom. Res., *17:* 161, 1973.
Fulton, R., editor. *Death and Identity.* John Wiley, New York, 1965.
Gruman, G. J. An historical introduction to ideas about voluntary euthanasia: With a bibliographic survey and guide for interdisciplinary studies. Omega, *4:* 87, 1973.
Hanlan, A. More notes of a dying professor. Penn. Gazette, *71:* 29, 1973.
Kastenbaum, R., and Aisenberg, R. *The Psychology of Death.* Springer, New York, 1972.
Kubler-Ross, E. *On Death and Dying.* Macmillan, London, 1969.
Resnik, H., and Hathorne, B., editors. *Suicide Prevention in the Seventies.* National Institute of Mental Health, Rockville, Md., 1973.
Shneidman, E. S. *Deaths of Man.* Quadrangle/New York Times, New York, 1973.
Weisman, A. D. *On Dying and Denying: A Psychiatric Study of Terminality.* Behavioral Publications, New York, 1972.

27.3. PSYCHIATRY AND SURGERY

General Psychodynamic Principles

In both a realistic and symbolic sense, surgery represents a threat to bodily integrity and at times to life itself. A minor surgical procedure may appear major to the patient. Memories of past operations or other traumatic assaults are revived and become attached to the present intervention. In addition, the underlying symbolic meaning of the involved organ system, the use of anesthesia, and the surgeon-patient relationship can determine the post-operative outcome.

Loss of consciousness is equated with death. Organ loss or loss of body parts becomes associated with castration anxiety, infantile fears of punishment, and whatever cathexes are attached to the organ.

Motivations for multiple surgical procedures include the use of operations to avoid other conflicts in one's life, a transference phenomenon to the surgeon as a strong and unyielding father figure, infantile and unfulfilled wishes to have a child, and the erotized wish for punishment—that is, for castration. The desire for an operation may also be a form of partial suicide.

Regression with the reactivation of past conflicts is a common reaction of the surgical patient. The protected environment of the hospital, the dependency on care-giving personnel, and the incapacity brought about by a physical illness encourage regression in that they place the patient in a position of passivity reminiscent of infantile and childhood experiences. In such a position it becomes difficult for the patient to delay gratification or tolerate frustration, and his behavior thus becomes demanding and aggressive.

In the preoperative period patients' reactions may vary from utter and supreme calm to panic and overt psychosis. Patients with moderate anxiety or anticipatory fear are less likely to develop emotional disturbances during or after the stress of an operation than are patients with excessive or low anxiety; patients with high levels of anticipatory fear are more likely to display intense fear of body damage postoperatively, and patients with low preoperative anxiety are more likely to display reactions of anger and resentment. Excessive preoperative anxiety, denial, and unrealistic surgical expectations are accurate prognosticators of postoperative psychiatric complications.

Postoperative complications include exacerbations of previous neurotic symptoms, delayed convalescence, disruptive ward behavior, and psychosis. The psychotic disturbances precipitated by the multiple stresses of surgical intervention consist mainly of affective disorders, schizophreniclike psychoses, and delirious states. Postoperative delirium occurs most frequently in elderly patients.

Cardiovascular Operations

The patient facing a heart operation mobilizes various defense mechanisms to cope with the severe stresses associated with the procedure. The patient experiences these stresses as threats to his life on both a realistic and a symbolic level. The emergency defenses are immobilization, hysterical amnesia or depersonalization, belligerence, excitement, and desperate denial.

The lowest death rate (5.5 per cent) has been found in patients with the best motivation and the least anxiety, the highest mortality (47 per cent) occurred in patients with an ambivalence weighted against surgery. The group with the lowest mortality also had the fewest psychiatric complications. Those with the highest percentage of adverse psychological reactions exhibited preoperative panic.

Postoperative psychosis is the major psychiatric complication of cardiac operations. The incidence after closed-heart procedures is reported at about 15 per cent. Open-heart procedures have increased post-operative psychosis to an average of 50 per cent. Multiple variables are associated with the psychoses, and there appears to be more than one form of psychosis. The two broadest categories are those of delirium or an organic brain syndrome and a schizophreniclike psychosis.

Preventive measures have included suggestions for improving intensive care units so that they are less foreboding and foreign to the patient. Adequate preoperative psychological preparation and establishing a relationship with the patient that continues postoperatively have also been effective.

Genitourinary Operations

Pelvic Operations

In preoperative evaluations and postoperative follow-ups in 40 women 12 to 18 months after pelvic operations, Lindemaan reported typical signs and symptoms of depression in 13 patients. An agitated depression began 3 to 4 weeks after the operation and lasted more than 3 months. In addition, the frequency of postoperative complications was higher in these patients than in women having cholecystectomies. The uterus is regarded by many women as an important symbol of femininity.

Renal Transplantation

The living related donor, usually a parent or sibling, faces several potential conflicts. He is asked to give up a functioning organ to save another's life and to risk an operation himself and the possibility that in the future his life may be in jeopardy if his remaining kidney becomes diseased or injured. These risks can stir underlying psychological conflicts between donor and recipient. Postoperative depression in the donor is common.

The recipient of a renal homograft is relieved of the rigors of chronic dialysis and yet exposes himself to other problems, such as the pervasive fear of organ rejection and the side effects of immunosuppressive and steroid medication. Psychosis after the transplantation procedure is rare. Generally, over-all psychological adaptation is superior to that of the patient maintained by chronic dialysis alone, although suicidal behavior may ensue if the homograft fails and dialysis again becomes necessary. Ambivalent and hostilely dependent relationships can develop between recipient and donor. Additional conflicts may center around the manner in which the patient emotionally incorporates his new kidney into his body image if the donor is of the opposite sex. Recipients of cadaveric donors may experience guilt if they cannot resolve conflicts over their living having been dependent upon the death of another.

Gastrointestinal Operations

Vagotomy and Gastrectomy

Patients with little gratification from their illness and with minimal secondary gain tend to have a better prognosis than patients emotionally invested in their illness and treatment. Some patients show a significant increase in other psychosomatic and neurotic symptoms, such as, hypertension, migraine headaches, asthma, and psychocutaneous disorders.

Colectomy, Ileostomy, and Colostomy

In 41 patients with total colectomies and permanent ileostomies for ulcerative colitis, all but one were found to be in good general health and preferred their present situation to living with chronic ulcerative colitis. They reported no evidence of psychosis or the establishment of a new psychosomatic target organ after the operation. However, 46 per cent described subjective states of discomfort and uneasiness with the ileostomy, such as concern over sexual functioning, fear of contamination by fecal material, and other feelings of embarrassment. Most believed that acceptance by key figures in their lives was essential.

In a comparable examination of 36 patients with permanent colostomies after abdominoperineal resection for carcinoma of the large bowel, depression, shame, and helpless anger in the postoperative phase were common. In the first year, regaining bowel control through successful colostomy training was associated with obsessional defenses. Patients unsuccessful in reestablishing bowel habits became fearful, isolated, and unable to handle the responsibilities of everyday life.

Musculoskeletal Operations

Lower-extremity amputation has greater significance in the aged patient for whom amputation symbolizes the encroachment of death and a form of defeat. A pervasive postoperative depression is characterized by feelings of hopelessness and by preoccupation with impending death.

Rhinoplasty

Psychiatric illness, distortions in body image, sexual identity conflicts, and thwarted interpersonal relations have been noted in patients overconcerned with the nose. The operation, rather than being seen as psychologically hazardous, initiates a chain reaction in the patient's social relationships, enhancing emotional security and growth. Thus, rhinoplasty is viewed as facilitating psychotherapy and as a positive measure in improving a distorted body image.

Mastectomy

The breast is the emotional symbol of a woman's pride in her sexuality and her motherliness. Postmastectomy depression is viewed as a form of mourning over the loss of the breast and is common in women who have invested excessive feeling in their breasts. The trauma of the operation is seen as greater in women in the childbearing age range than in older women. Concern over death becomes more in postclimacteric patients.

Conclusion

The surgeon-patient relationship as a therapeutic agent is a powerful force shaping the patient's postoperative destiny. Through the development of mutual trust, the fostering of hope, and an empathetic approach toward the patient's plight, the surgeon encourages postoperative adaptive mechanisms that strengthen the patient's ability to withstand the regressive pulls of the postoperative phase and thereby aid in his recovery.

An operation should be performed only for surgical reasons and not for psychological reasons. If the surgeon or the patient has unrealistic expectations for the procedure, psychiatric complications are likely. There is evidence that a collaborative effort between surgeon and psychiatrist is helpful in the preparation and evaluation of patients for open-heart operations, removal of cataracts, and rhinoplastics. Postoperatively, the continuation of a preoperatively established relationship can diminish or prevent severe psychiatric complications, such as postcardiotomy delirium.

REFERENCES

Abram, H. S., and Gill, B. F. Predictions of postoperative psychiatric complications. New Engl. J. Med., 265: 1123, 1961.

Deutsch, H. Some psychoanalytic observations in surgery. Psychosom. Med., 4: 105, 1942.

Hackett, T. P., and Weisman, A. D. Psychiatric management

of operative syndromes. II. Psychodynamic factors in formulation and management. Psychosom. Med., *22:* 356, 1960.

Lindemann, E. Observations on psychiatric sequelae to surgical operations in women. Am. J. Psychiatry, *124:* 132, 1941.

Menninger, K. A. Polysurgery and polysurgical addiction. Psychoanal. Q., *3:* 173, 1934.

Weisman, A. D., and Hackett, T. P. Psychosis after eye surgery; establishment of specific doctor-patient relationship in prevention and treatment of "black-patch" delirium. New Eng. J. Med., *258:* 1284, 1958.

28

Psychiatric Emergencies

28.1. SUICIDE

Introduction

Suicide is defined as the human act of self-inflicted, self-intentioned cessation, and it embraces a multitude of conscious motivational states. However, every case of overt self-destruction involves the pressure of phenomenologically felt unbearable anguish. In this sense, suicide is better understood as an escape from, rather than a going toward. Therapy by the psychiatrist should consist essentially of reducing the terror of the external and internal pressures and of increasing the avenues for both psychological and real escape.

In addition to the intrapsychic and interpersonal elements of suicidal crisis, there may be biological and physiological components related, for example, to drug intake or to the menstrual cycle. A familial history of suicide can cloud the life of a person and become a factor in his own penchant toward suicide.

Statistics

The reported suicide rate for the United States is between 10 and 12 per 100,000. The number of suicides in the United States every year is given at about 22,000, but many experts believe the actual number to be at least twice as high. Suicide is ranked among the first five causes of death for white males aged 10 to 55; it is the second ranked cause of death for white males aged 15 to 19.

More men than women commit suicide (about 3 to 1), and more women than men attempt suicide (again about 3 to 1). In the 1970's, there is some evidence that the ratio for committed suicide seems to be changing, moving toward, but not yet achieving, an equal proportion between the sexes.

Evaluation of Suicidal Patients

Lethality, Perturbation, and Inimicality

Perturbation or subjective distress refers to how upset (disturbed, agitated, sane-insane, discomposed) the patient is. Lethality refers to the probability of that patient's committing suicide—not simply hurting or injuring or harming himself but dying by his own hand.

One can be highly perturbed and not necessarily be suicidal; the converse is also true. It is elevated lethality, not heightened perturbation, that kills a patient. The treatment of the highly suicidal person needs to focus on reducing or mollifying the lethality and on reducing the perturbation only as it exacerbates the lethality. The prodromal clues to suicide seem to be contained best in the word "change"—changes in the patient's interests, lifestyle, ties to life, habits, sexual patterns, attitudes toward life, eating patterns, and so on.

Inimicality refers to the person's general lifestyle—the extent to which he is his own worst enemy. Inimical behaviors can include self-defeating patterns involving alcohol, drugs, maiming, and neglecting one's medical regimen in diseases like diabetes and may even include telling the boss off or not studying for board exams.

Psychological Characteristics

Suicide has been related to many emotions; hostility, despair, shame, guilt, dependency, hopelessness, and ennui. If there is one general psychological state commonly assumed to be associated with suicide, it is a state of intolerable emotion or unbearable or unrepeatable despair.

The treatment of the highly lethal person ought to take into account three psychological features that characterize the suicidal state—brief duration, ambivalence, and dyadic event.

The acute suicidal crisis or period of high and dangerous lethality is an interval of relatively short duration—to be counted, typically, in hours or days, not usually in terms of months or years. A person is at a peak of self-destructiveness for a brief time and then is helped, cools off, or is dead.

The prototypical psychological picture of a person on the brink of suicide is that of one who wants to and does not want to. He makes plans for self-destruction and, at the same time, entertains fantasies of rescue and intervention.

As a therapeutic tactic, the therapist should address himself to the life side of the patient's ambivalent inner struggle. The psychodynamic heart of the suicidal act is ambivalence; the characteristic suicidal sound is the cry for help; the prototypical suicidal act is to cut one's throat and plead for help and fantasy rescue and intervention—all at the same time.

Most suicidal events are dyadic events—that is, two-person events. Although the suicidal drama takes place within the person's head, most suicidal tensions are between two people keenly known to each other; spouse and spouse, parent and child, or lover and lover. Some modes of death are more stigmatizing to the survivors than are other modes of death, and generally speaking, suicide imposes the greatest stigma of all on its survivors.

Intentionality

All deaths can be thought of as intentioned, subintentioned, or unintentioned. An intentioned death is any death in which the decedent plays a direct, conscious role in effecting his own demise. An unintentioned death is any death in which the decedent plays no effective role in effecting his own demise, in which death results entirely from independent physical trauma from without or from nonpsychologically laden biological failure from within. Subintentioned deaths are deaths in which the decedent plays some partial, covert, or unconscious role in hastening his own demise through poor judgment, imprudence, excessive risk taking, abuse of alcohol, misuse of drugs, neglect of self, self-destructive style of life, disregard of prescribed lifesaving medical regimen, and so on—in which the person fosters, facilitates, exacerbates, or hastens the process of his dying.

Myths of Suicide

Even among professional persons, there exist a number of misconceptions and myths about suicidal phenomena. Here briefly, is a list of some of the more outstanding misconceptions on this topic:

Fable: People who talk about suicide do not commit suicide. *Fact:* Of any ten persons who kill themselves, eight have given definite warnings of their suicidal intentions.

Fable: Suicide happens without warning. *Fact:* Studies reveal that the suicidal person gives many clues and warnings regarding his suicidal intentions.

Fable: Suicidal people are fully intent on dying. *Fact:* Most suicidal people are undecided about living or dying, and they gamble with death, leaving it to others to save them. Almost no one commits suicide without letting others know how he is feeling.

Fable: Once a person is suicidal, he is suicidal forever. *Fact:* Persons who wish to kill themselves are suicidal only for a limited period of time.

Fable: Improvement after a suicidal crisis means that the suicidal risk is over. *Fact:* Most suicides occur about 3 months after the beginning of improvement, when the person has the energy to put his morbid thoughts and feelings into effect.

Fable: Suicide strikes much more often among the rich, or, conversely, it occurs almost exclusively among the poor. *Fact:* Suicide is neither the rich man's disease nor the poor man's curse. Suicide is represented proportionately among all levels of society.

Fable: Suicide is inherited or runs in the family. *Fact:* It is an individual pattern.

Fable: All suicidal persons are mentally ill, and suicide is always the act of a psychotic person. *Fact:* Studies of hundreds of genuine suicide notes indicate that, although the suicidal person is extremely unhappy and always perturbed, he is not necessarily mentally ill.

Attempted Suicide

Although one has to attempt suicide in order to commit it, attempting suicide does not always have death as its objective. Often, the goal of attempted suicide is to change one's life or to change the significant others around one, rather than to end life. On the other hand, death is sometimes intended and only fortuitously avoided. After that, one's life is forever somewhat different. It is useful to think of two sets of overlapping populations: (1) those who attempt suicide, few of whom go on to commit it, and (2) those who commit suicide, many of whom have previously attempted it. The ratio between suicide attempts and actual suicides is about 8 to 1—1 suicide for every 8 attempts. Suicide attempts have many meanings and, whatever their level of lethality, should be taken seriously.

Partial Death and Substitutes for Suicide

Sometimes, the lifestyle of a person seems to truncate and demean his life so that he is as good as dead. Alcoholism, drug addiction, mismanagement of physical disease, and masochistic behavior can often be seen in this light. Menninger writes of (1) chronic suicide, including asceticism, martyrdom, neurotic invalidism, alcohol addiction, antisocial behavior, and psychosis, (2) focal suicide, focused on a limited part of the body, including self-mutilations, malingering, multiple surgery, purposive accidents, impotence, and frigidity, and (3) organic suicide, focusing on the phychological factors in organic disease, especially the self-punishing, aggressive, and erotic components.

Management

Some special therapeutic stratagems or orientations with a highly lethal patient include:

A continuous, preferably daily, monitoring of the patient's lethality rating.

An active outreach, dealing with some of the reality problems, patient's giving direction without exhortation, actively taking the side of life. It relates to befriending and caring.

Use of community resources, including employment, Veterans Administration (when applicable), social agencies, and psychiatric social work assistance.

Consultation with a peer. The items to be discussed might include the therapist's treatment of the case; his own feelings of frustration, helplessness, or even anger; his countertransference reactions generally; and the advisability of hospitalization for the patient.

Hospitalization.

Transference. The therapist can be active, show his personal concern, increase the frequency of the sessions, invoke the magic of the unique therapist-patient relationship, be less of a *tabula rasa*, and give transfusions of realistic hope and succor.

The involvement of significant others. It is not suggested that the significant other be seen as often as the patient is seen, but other people in the suicidal patient's life should be directly involved and, a least, their roles as hinderers or helpers in the treatment process assessed.

Careful modification of the usual canons of confidentiality. The therapist should not ally himself with death. Statements given during the therapy session relating to the patient's overt suicidal or homicidal plans cannot be treated as a secret between two collusive partners.

Limitation of one's own practice to a very few highly lethal patients. Such patients demand a great deal of investment of psychic energy, and one must beware of spreading oneself too thin in one's professional life.

Prodromal Clues to Suicide

Almost everyone who seriously intends suicide gives some clues to his imminent action. Sometimes there are broad hints, sometimes only subtle changes in behavior. But the suicide decision is usually not impulsive.

Fully three-fourths of all those who commit suicide see a physician 4 months, at most, before they kill themselves. They are always disturbed, and often they are depressed. They feel hopeless about the direction of their lives and helpless to do anything about it. Usually, their attitude reflects itself in various verbal or behavioral clues. Most obvious are the statements of those who threaten, "I'm going to kill myself." They usually mean it, at least unconsciously. All verbal suicidal indications should be taken with some seriousness. A suicide attempt, no matter how feeble or unlikely to succeed, is the starkest testimony of the suicidal state. Four of five persons who kill themselves have attempted to do so at least once previously.

Once a person has finally decided to kill himself, he begins to act differently. He may withdraw. He may drastically reduce eating or refrain from conversation or ignore normal sexual drives. He may either sleep more soundly or suffer from insomnia. He may have a will drawn up or act as if he were going on a long and distant trip. In the final days of his life, he frequently gives away what, for him, have been highly valued material possessions.

Occasionally, the situation itself may be the final straw and is the crucial indicator of imminent suicide. People already suffering from suffocating depressions often kill themselves on learning—or believing erroneously—that they have a malignant tumor.

There are also life-course clues to suicide—indices that seem by the age of 29 to be related to suicide at the age of 55. These factors, related to intelligent Caucasian males, include a number of subtle features: (1) early evidence of instability, including dishonesty, (2) early rejection by the father, (3) multiple marriages, (4) alcoholism, (5) an unstable occupational history, (6) ups and downs in income, (7) a crippling physical disability, especially one involving dyspnea, (8) disappointment in the use of one's potential—that is, a disparity between aspiration and accomplishment, (9) any talk or hint of self-destruction, and (10) a competitive or self-absorbed spouse.

Patient Suicides

The most common suicidal crisis in psychiatry occurs when a psychiatrist is faced by a self-destructive patient. But another kind of crisis arises when a patient in therapy with a psychiatrist commits suicide. Psychotherapists seem to react to the suicide of a patient much as do other human beings. Their first reactions are often those of pain and defense. They also experience fears concerning blame, responsibility, and inadequacy.

The psychological mechanisms seen in therapists are essentially those found in other survivor-victims, such as relatives: denial and repression, including, on occasion, denial of the obvious nature of the death, forgetting of details, and omissions and distortions of the facts. The therapeutic effects of supportive consultation with colleagues and of review of the case with peers, to examine what might have been done or what could have been overlooked, seem to be of great psychological benefit.

Postvention and the Survivor-Victim

A person's death is not just an ending; it is also a beginning for the survivors. In suicide, the largest public health problem is the alleviation of the effects of stress in the survivor-victims of suicidal deaths. This is the process called postvention—those appropriate and helpful acts that come after the event. Its purpose is to help survivors live longer, more productively, and with less stress than is likely otherwise.

Survivor-victims of suicides are invaded by an unhealthy complex of disturbing emotions; shame, guilt, hatred, and perplexity. They are obsessed with thoughts about the death, seeking reasons, finding targets, and often punishing themselves. There is marked increase in dependency needs, with regressive behavior and traumatic loss of feelings of identity, and, over-all, a kind of affective anesthesia, an unhealthy docility, a cowed and subdued reaction.

Postventive efforts are not limited to this initial stage of shock but are more often directed to the longer haul, the day-to-day living with the sense of mourning during the year or more after the first shock of loss. Postvention shares many of the characteristics of psychotherapy: talk, opportunity for ventilation, abreaction, interpretation, reassurance, direction, and even gentle confrontation. It provides an arena for the expression of hidden emotions, especially such negative affective states as anger, shame, and guilt. It puts a measure of stability into the grieving person's life and, at the least, provides an interpersonal relationship with the therapist.

A few tentative conclusions about postventive work can be drawn:

1. In working with survivor-victims of dire deaths, the therapist should begin as soon as possible after the tragedy—within the first 72 hours, if possible.

2. Remarkably little resistance is met from survivor-victims; most are willing—some are passively eager—to talk to a professional person.

3. The role of negative emotions toward the deceased—irritation, anger, envy, and guilt—needs to be explored but not necessarily at the very beginning.

4. The professional plays the important role of reality tester. He is not so much the echo of conscience as the quiet voice of reason.

5. Medical evaluation is crucial. One should be alert for a possible decline in physical health and in over-all mental well-being.

Three final points: Postvention can be viewed as prevention for the next decade or for the next generation. Postvention can be practiced by psychiatrists, nurses, lawyers, social workers, physicians, psychologists, good neighbors, and friends—thanatologists all. A comprehensive program of mental health concern on the part of a benign and enlightened community should include all three elements of care: prevention, intervention, and postvention.

REFERENCES

Alvarez, A. *The Savage God: A Study of Suicide.* Random House, New York, 1972.
Dublin, L. I. *Suicide: A Sociological and Statistical Study.* Ronald Press, New York, 1963.
Durkheim, E. *Suicide.* Free Press of Glencoe (Macmillan), New York, 1951.
Kelly, W. A. Suicide and psychiatric education. Am. J. Psychiatry, *130:* 463, 1973.
Kiev, A. Cluster analysis profiles of suicide attempters. Am. J. Psychiatry, *133:* 2, 1976.
Shneidman, E. S. Perturbation and lethality as precursors of suicide in a gifted group. Life-Threatening Behavior, *1:* 23, 1971.
Shneidman, E. S., Farberow, N. L., and Litman, R. E. *The Psychology of Suicide.* Science House, New York, 1970.
Stoller, R. J. *Splitting: A Case of Female Masculinity.* Quadrangle Books, New York, 1973.

28.2. OTHER PSYCHIATRIC EMERGENCIES

Introduction

A psychiatric emergency is a disturbance in thoughts, feelings, or actions for which immediate treatment is deemed necessary. The physician may respond with condemnatory attitudes toward a patient whose psychiatric emergency has been precipitated by alcohol or drug abuse. Chronic mental illness may have led to social deterioration and lack of personal cleanliness. Many acutely disturbed patients are irritable, demanding, hostile, and provocative. For all these reasons, the physician may respond to the patient with negative feelings. The physician must subject himself constantly to self-criticism and self-appraisal and must alert himself to feelings and attitudes that may adversely affect his relationship with the patient and thus impair his clinical judgment.

Psychological Emergencies

Depression

Suicidal depression is the single most important category in emergency psychiatry. One must be alert to the danger signs—a relatively abrupt onset in a previously competent person, early-morning insomnia and agitation, a loss of all appetites and interests, feelings of hopeless despair, inability to express one's thoughts or feelings, and progressive social withdrawal. The appearance of delusions, such as having committed an unpardonable sin, is a particularly ominous sign, calling for emergency inpatient care under constant nursing supervision and probably calling for electroconvulsive therapy.

Violence

Outwardly directed destructive behavior is relatively rare in mental illness. Violent patients are usually frightened of their own hostile impulses and desperately seek help to prevent loss of control.

The violent patient is often engaged in a desperate and panic-stricken struggle to prevent his imagined total annihilation, either through the destruction of his physical self or, even more frightening at times, through the destruction of his self-esteem. The psychiatrist must express his respect for the violent patient and by direct verbal reassurances inform him of his positive commitment to the patient's welfare and the fact that no harm will be inflicted on him. However, the psychotic violent patient is relatively inaccessible and uncontrollable.

Violent psychotic patients are sometimes placed in mechanical restraints. This procedure creates a vicious cycle by intensifying the patient's psychotic terror and, if prolonged, can cause hyperthermia. In some instances of catatonic excitement, it can cause death.

Transient situational disturbances in all age groups may result in tantrumlike outbursts of rage. These outbursts are seen particularly in marital quarrels. Wounded self-esteem is a big issue. Therefore, patronizing or contemptuous attitudes must be avoided and an effort made to communicate an attitude of respect and an authentic peacemaking concern. In this category of nonpsychotic violent behavior, there is the best opportunity for psychological resolution through crisis intervention. A show of force—that is, the mere display of a sufficient number of helping hands—with appropriate comments of reassurance, usually suffices to bring this type of patient under control.

In evaluating the possibilities of recurrent episodes of violence, one should inquire concerning a history of previous acts of violence by the patient, of violent parental behavior during the patient's developmental years, of a childhood history of fire setting and cruelty to animals; the possession of weapons; and drug dependency states involving, most of all, alcohol but including the barbiturates, amphetamines, and LSD.

These patients share in common a low frustration tolerance, and they react violently when crossed. Although violence is usually directed against family members, it may be expressed indiscriminately during periods of acute stress. Such people often come to the emergency room voluntarily, asking for help because of impending loss of control. One should not add to their frustrations by red tape and prolonged waiting in the emergency room.

Fugue States

A patient is occasionally brought to an emergency room with an expression of bewilderment on his face. In spite of negative findings on physical and laboratory examinations, the patient describes a total amnesia for the events of the preceding several hours or days. Often, the patient claims to have forgotten all data of personal identification. These patients are usually suffering from a hysterical dissociative reaction or fugue state.

Such patients should be hospitalized and the life circumstances preceding the fugue state carefully scrutinized. The patient has usually taken a twofold flight from an unbearable life situation—a physical flight so that he is usually some distance from his appropriate habitat and a psychological flight into the dissociative state. The traumatic situation often involves a personal interaction filled with rage and threats to self-esteem and fraught with the danger of loss of impulse control.

The most important aspect of treatment is to assist the patient in relation to the overwhelming environmental trauma from which he has taken flight. If discharged to an unchanged home situation, another fugue state will probably supervene, in the course of which the patient may commit murder and suicide.

Related to the fugue state is hysterical psychosis, psychotic reaction of acute and dramatic onset, temporally related to a profoundly upsetting event or circumstance. Clinical manifestations include delusions, hallucinations, depersonalization, and grossly unusual behavior. The acute episode seldom lasts more than a week or two, and on recovery there is practically no residue.

The essential diagnostic feature of hysterical psychosis is the pressure of an overwhelming environmental trauma. Treatment consists of a brief separation from the traumatic environment and the provision of appropriate supportive social and psychological assistance.

Homosexual Panic

This transient situational disturbance of adult life is characterized by delusions and hallucinations that accuse the patient, in derisive and contemptuous terms, of a variety of homosexual practices. The panic typically occurs in patients with schizoid personality disorders who have successfully protected themselves in the past from physical intimacy. Breakdown occurs in settings of enforced intimacy, such as a college dormitory or a military barracks. There may be a history of alcohol or drug use preceding the acute episode.

Treatment first involves rescuing the patient from the traumatic situation by hospitalization. With male patients, female staff members, preferably those cast in a matronly model, should be used as therapeutic allies. If this simple maneuver does not result in symptomatic relief, chlorpromazine should be administered orally in 100-mg. doses repeated every 1 to 4 hours until remission has occurred. Such patients usually resume their prepsychotic level of adaptation.

Other Panic Reactions

Panic reactions without psychotic content can occur as part of agoraphobia, episodes of acute anxiety occurring in crowded public settings. These episodes may present clinically as a fear of an impending fatal heart attack. Typically, there is a history of anxiety and depression during the preceding months, based on an increasingly stressful life circumstance.

Treatment of the acute episode is by simple reassurance and the use of a mild sedative such as chlordiazepoxide or diazepam. A long-term treatment program should be instituted to prevent the development of a chronic incapacitating phobic reaction.

Neurosis

Acute anxiety symptoms may appear after a near escape from death in combat, an accident, or a natural catastrophe. Usually, the patient retains self-control during the actual period of danger, although a panic reaction can occur, characterized by terror and ineffective efforts at flight. Such panic-stricken patients are extraordinarily suggestible and easily hypnotizable, so that reassurance and firm instructions concerning appropriate behavior are usually followed with childlike obedience. Typically, gross neurotic symptoms appear only after evacuation to safety has occurred. At such times, one may observe coarse tremors and a variety of symptoms of conversion hysteria involving sensory and motor abnormalities. Treatment should encourage an immediate return to previous responsibilities in the danger area. One should avoid prolonged diagnostic and therapeutic inpatient procedures, which encourage regression and chronic invalidism.

Mania

Manic excitement occurs in the manic phase of manic-depressive psychosis. In a pathologically elated state, the patient may impoverish himself with extravagent expenditures, engage in inappropriate sexual involvements, and commit traffic violations because of reckless driving. Commonly, the frantic family consults the psychiatrist without the patient. In communicating with the patient, the family should be encouraged to adopt an attitude of nonpunitive sobriety and firm insistence on the need for a physician's help. Every manic patient teeters on the brink of depression. It is usually possible to quiet the patient down long enough for him to accept medications and hospitalization, if necessary. If the manic pressure is considerable, chlorpromazine should be administered intramuscularly and repeated until the symptoms are under control.

Paranoid Schizophrenia

Paranoid schizophrenics occasionally display psychotic excitement in which they barricade themselves against imagined enemies or declare themselves the principal figure in some grandiose plot. It is usually possible to establish contact with a rational ego core and to talk the patient down to the point where he will accept the need for medication and hospitalization. Depending on the degree of excitement, it may be necesssry to administer chlorpromazine.

Catatonic Schizophrenia

The patient with catatonic stupor usually displays automatic obedience and accepts inpatient care without resistance. Unless there is some physical contraindication, ECT in an inpatient setting is the procedure of choice for interrupting an attack of catatonic stupor. The patient should not be discharged until the environmental precipitating factors are corrected.

Catatonic excitement may be more difficult to manage as a psychiatric emergency. Hospital admission is the necessary first step. Shock therapy is the safest, swiftest, and most dependable way of interrupting the condition. Discharge should be delayed until the traumatic environment has been improved.

Anorexia Nervosa

Anorexia nervosa is an obsessional preoccupation with the desire to be thin. It usually occurs in females. The compulsive avoidance of food may reduce the patient to such an extreme degree of inanition that death by starvation occurs. For this reason, hospitalization usually becomes necessary.

These patients have a curious intolerance for inactivity and physical confinement. In the hospital, a regimen of rewards, consisting of opportunities for increased physical activity after weight gain, and punishment, consisting of confinement to quarters on weight loss, can usually achieve an upward drift to acceptable weight levels.

These patients usually have a deep-seated yearning to remain tiny and to retain a practically intrauterine state of passive dependency on parental figures. These difficult psychotherapeutic issues must be taken up when the starvation emergency has been treated.

Acute Psychosomatic Issues

In intensive care units, coronary care units, and surgical recovery rooms, symptoms of severe anxiety may appear on the first or second days of confinement, inability to cooperate in a treatment procedure may appear during the next two days, and reactions of depression may appear thereafter. Toxic metabolic problems and impaired cerebral circulation add an organic factor that may precipitate a reaction of psychotic delirium.

Postoperative reactions of delirium are best controlled with chlorpromazine. Organic delirium tends to be at its worst at night. Premature cessation of medication or night nursing can result in psychotic panic reactions, with flight through windows, leading to crippling and death. Letting a trusted relative sit by the bedside is a particularly helpful nursing procedure. On recovery from an organic psychosis, the patient has a usually transient reaction of depression, requiring supportive psychotherapy.

Patients who press for elective surgery as a device to escape from unbearable life situations may be detected at times with careful preoperative psychiatric evaluation.

One of the complications of accident surgery is a postoperative flareup of dependency needs.

Patients who are to undergo mutilating surgery—such as amputation, mastectomy, or colostomy—should be psychologically prepared.

Rhinoplasty is occasionally followed by a psychotic reaction. Adolescents in the midst of an identity crisis may react to an excellent cosmetic result with ambivalence and psychotic decompensation. Treatment of these cases requires hospitalization, antipsychotic medications, and psychotherapy that focuses on sexual questions and other issues involved in the identity crisis.

Reserpine is particularly liable to precipitate an acute depressive reaction in a patient undergoing treatment for hypertension.

Insomnia

Insomnia may occur as a relatively benign symptom in relation to a period of unusual personal stress. It may mark the onset of a more severe depressive reaction, in which case it is associated with early-morning agitation and other signs and symptoms of depression. There may be a fear of falling asleep, because of frightening dreams, as part of a traumatic neurosis after a battle, accident, or other personal catastrophe. Insomnia may be part of a hysterical neurotic sleep disorder.

A helpful remedy to produce a night's sleep is a combination of amitriptyline and diazepam at bedtime. Flurazpam (Dalmane) has been especially successful in the treatment of insomnia at a dose of 30 mg. upon retiring. Only nonfatal quantities of medication should be prescribed at any one time, and these should be entrusted to a reliable relative to prevent the accumulation of a potentially fatal cache of medication.

When insomnia is due to psychotic excitement, manic or catatonic, and there is physical exhaustion or it is due to an agitated depression with suicidal trends, electroshock therapy is the most dependable way of restoring the sleep cycle.

Headache

In the absence of positive physical findings and in the presence of positive signs and symptoms of depression, headache may be treated as an element in the depressive syndrome, with appropriate caution concerning the dangers of drug dependency or suicide by overdose.

Dysmenorrhea

When dysmenorrhea is associated with premenstrual depression and hostility, marital disharmony, sexual difficulty, a variety of medical and gynecological complaints, and suicidal attempts in the past, suicidal precautions are indicated.

Hyperventilation

Anxious patients may pant in terror. After a few seconds of overbreathing, a state of alkalosis sets in, owing to excess carbon dioxide output. A reduction in consciousness occurs, with giddiness, faintness, and blurring of vision. Treatment consists of reassuring explanations and instructions to relax and to breathe into a paper bag held over the mouth and nose. The accumulation of carbon dioxide thus produced reverses the hyperventilation syndrome. Follow-up treatment of the basic emotional disorder should focus on the life circumstances that precipitated the attack.

Dying

Most clinicians do not tell the patient he is dying. It is enough to be honest and to acknowledge that the situation is serious. It is important to listen to the patient and to take one's lead from him. Most patients want to be told about the possible outcome of the illness; they just prefer not to be told that their case is hopeless.

Organic Emergencies

Alcoholism

The chronic alcoholic usually has chronic liver, brain, and heart diseases. He has nutritional deficiencies, is prone to infection, and is even more prone to certain malignancies. The odor of alcohol may disguise behavioral abnormalities due to schizophrenia, hypoglycemia, or subarachnoid hemorrhage. The analgesic effect of alcohol may obscure the presence of broken bones and other serious injuries. One should be alert to the problem of mixed addiction.

When the possibility of a major physical disease requiring inpatient care has been eliminated, the treatment of the acute alcoholic is aimed at making him ambulatory as swiftly as possible.

The severity of the withdrawal syndrome depends on the chronicity and severity of the preceding alcoholic state. When there is doubt, the patient should be hospitalized. Chlordiazepoxide is administered by mouth and repeated in 1 to 6 hours, depending on the patient's condition. When the patient has been stable for 24 to 36 hours, the medication should be gradually discontinued by reducing the dosage over a 2-day period. If overt psychosis appears as alcoholic hallucinosis or delirium tremens, diazepam may be given intramuscularly until the patient has improved enough to cooperate for oral medications.

Drug Abuse

Drug abuse tends to occur in epidemics, contagion is a basic factor, and newly involved cases are more contagious than are chronic cases. The overdosed heroin patient is pale and cyanotic. He has pinpoint pupils and is areflexic. He may not be breathing at all, or he may take three or four shallow gasping breaths a minute. His tongue should be pulled forward and out of the way, the angles of his jaws should be strongly pushed forward and his mouth wiped free of blood and mucus, and then he should be given a few mouth-to-mouth respirations until his color improves. An oropharyngeal airway should be inserted, and the physician should continue breathing for him via mouth-to-mouth resuscitation.

A needle should be placed in a vein, blood drawn for a study of drug levels, and the patient given intravenous naloxone hydrochloride. Naloxone is a narcotic antagonist that reverses the opiate effects, including respiratory depression, within 2 minutes of the injection. If the desired degree of counteraction and respiratory improvement is not obtained, this dose may be repeated after 2 or 3 minutes.

If the overdose is due to methadone, breathing should be monitored for 24 hours. It may be necessary to provide naloxone in the form of a continuous intravenous drip overnight.

In sedative overdose, whoever finds the patient should make him vomit by giving ipecac syrup. However, a patient who is only partially responsive should not be provoked to vomit. In a hospital setting, vomiting can be induced by apomorphine if the patient is fully alert and cooperative.

When the patient reaches the hospital, the most imperative step is to establish and maintain a good airway. Central nervous system stimulants should not be used. If arterial hypotension occurs, the treatment of choice is the administration of whole blood, 5 per cent albumin, or normal saline to expand the blood volume.

Once cardiorespiratory functioning is assured, the next step is to get the offending agent out of the patient by gastric lavage with saline and activated charcoal. However, gastric lavage should not be attempted in a patient with depressed and sinking consciousness until he has been intubated. Otherwise, aspiration pneumonitis may occur and lead to a fatal outcome. After the patient's stomach is washed with 500 ml. of saline and charcoal, lavage with normal saline should be continued until the return is clear. This procedure is followed by the instillation and withdrawal of castor oil. Forced diuresis is initiated with intravenous urea. (See Figure 1.)

With hallucinogens, psychotic reactions are associated with perceptual distortions and hallucinations. Panic may occur, with impulsive flight and suicide. Occasionally, there may be impulsive acts of violence.

These patients should be provided with special nursing care and supportive psychotherapy. They tend to maintain human contact and can often be talked down from the psychotic flight.

With amphetamines and cocaine, patients

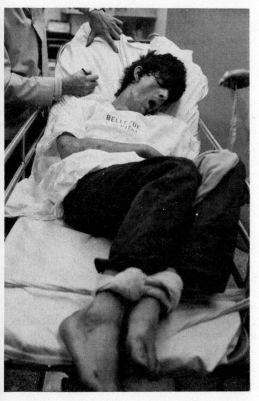

FIGURE 1. Bellevue Hospital emergency ward: a drug addict brought in after having taken an overdose. (Courtesy of Leonard Freed for Magnum Photos, Inc.)

are often paranoid, subject to tactile hallucinations, irritable, and capable of violent aggressive behavior. Chlorpromazine is the medication of choice for symptom control and for stabilization of cardiovascular and autonomic irregularities.

Hypertensive Crisis

This type of emergency can occur in a patient treated for depression with a monoamine oxidase (MAO) inhibitor if he has eaten food with a high tyramine content or if he has taken sympathomimetic drugs, particularly by injection. The hypertensive crisis is characterized by a severe occipital headache that may radiate frontally, palpitation, neck stiffness and soreness, nausea, vomiting, sweating, photophobia, constricting chest pain, and dilated pupils. Intracranial bleeding, sometimes fatal, has been reported.

The MAO inhibitor should be discontinued at once and therapy instituted to reduce blood pressure. Phentolamine should be carried by the patient and taken by mouth if a severe headache occurs after a dietary infraction. If the crisis is severe and the patient is brought to a hospital emergency room, he should receive phentolamine.

Postseizure Excitement

After an electroconvulsive treatment, some patients, particularly men, awaken with terror, become dangerously assaultive, and try to escape. They attack anyone who tries to control them. The episode may be associated with piercing, blood-curdling screams.

If the patient is permitted to sleep quietly after the treatment for as long as he wants and is permitted to awaken spontaneously, the likelihood of postseizure excitement is reduced. In a patient known to be subject to this pattern of postseizure behavior, a needle may be placed in his vein before full awakening and a small quantity of a barbiturate injected very slowly as he starts to stir, in order to prolong the postseizure sleep period.

Delirium

This psychotic reaction, characterized by disorientation and frightening delusions, can occur in any acute, organically caused disorganization of brain functioning. Chlorpromazine may be repeated every hour or two as necessary. Delirium tends to be worse at night, so careful nursing and adequate medication should be continued, even after daytime improvement has been achieved.

Heatstroke

Patients with a history of head injury, alcoholism, or phenothiazine medication are prone to respond adversely to excessive exposure to hot weather, particularly if this exposure involves physical exertion and direct exposure to the sun. The patient may become mute, stuporous, or delirious. Diagnosis depends on the history, the presence of a hot dry skin, and an elevated pulse and body temperature. Treatment consists of removal of the patient to a cool place, cold-water sponges to reduce body temperature, and saline.

Emergencies in Child Psychiatry

The emergency is usually the last stage in a long history of psychopathology, family disorganization, and physical and emotional exhaustion. The emergency becomes manifest when the significant adults can no longer provide ego support and control.

Accidental Poisoning

The child's stomach should be emptied as quickly as possible. Vomiting is best induced if one or two glasses of water or milk are given beforehand. Warm saline and mustard water are not effective. Syrup of ipecac can be given in doses of 10 to 15 ml. and repeated in 15 to 30 minutes if emesis does not occur. The subcutaneous injection of apomorphine is most dependable. Never provoke vomiting or attempt gastric lavage in a patient only partially responsive until he has been intubated.

Emesis should not be induced after the ingestion of corrosives, strychnine, or petroleum products or if a state of coma exists.

If vomiting cannot be induced and if emptying of the stomach is not contraindicated, the parents or physician should institute gastric lavage at once. The safest lavage fluid is isotonic or one-half isotonic saline solution. Lavage should be repeated 10 to 12 times or until the returns are clear. Lavage may be completed with an activated charcoal suspension.

It is important to maintain the child under continued observation to guard against the effects of delayed intestinal absorption of toxic substances or the continuing toxic effects of opitates that have been temporarily reversed by naloxone. The child should not be discharged until an appointment has been made for the child and his parents for psychodiagnostic studies and a family-centered treatment program.

Battered-Child Syndrome

Perhaps the most important aspect of this problem is its episodic character. There is a premonitory phase, during which the parent of the child is struggling actively with fear of loss of self-control. The child may show evidence of poor nutrition and hygiene and of general failure to thrive.

In all suspicious cases, even when the injury is not serious, the child should be hospitalized. It is important to avoid accusations or premature confrontations, so as not to cause defensive parental reactions. The parents should be interviewed separately. One should look for a history of violence in their childhood backgrounds. Emotional deprivation in the parents' childhoods may be a cause of low self-esteem, social isolation, and a lack of mothering skills.

The maltreated child is usually different from his siblings in some way to make him more vunerable to abuse. Precocious and hyperactive children, prematures, adopted children, and stepchildren are all abuse-prone. In terms of the current crisis, one should inquire for the presence of a major setback in the child's family situation. The child battering may take place in a dissociative state for which the guilty parent is amnesic. Recent changes in the child are also important. A febrile condition causing fretfulness may provoke an already teetering parent to lose control.

It is essential to set up a long-term program of help for the parents. They should have opportunities for regular absences from their children, making use of day care centers and similar facilities. There should be provision for emergency short-term hospital admissions for the endangered child. If the family cannot be rehabilitated, suitable foster home placement should be arranged.

Adoption

Adopted children have an increased incidence of mental disorders. These disorders tend to become manifest primarily during adolescence. The identity crisis that erupts normally at this time is typically associated with rebellion and parental rejection. Adopted children may run away from home at this time in search of their natural parents. There may be intense daydreaming, with romantic fantasies concerning one's natural origins. If the adoptive parents are middle-class, there may be sexual acting out with partners from lower social strata. Overt psychotic reactions may occur.

The adoptive parents need support in relation to their feelings of bewilderment, disappointment, and guilt. The patient needs help in understanding his rejection of the adoptive parents as a normal adolscent quest for identity.

Hyperkinesis

Minimal brain dysfunction in the hyperkinetic child is probably the single most common disorder seen by child psychiatrists. It is characterized by overactivity, distractibility, impulsivity, and excitability.

Hyperactivity is a nonspecific symptom and not a total personality disorder. It occurs more or less normally in the infant and young preschool child and frequently appears with fatigue in normal children. It is considered a sign of developmental immaturity only when it persists after age 7 or when it is excessive. The hyperkinetic child may become a psychiatric emergency if the significant adults can no longer tolerate his behavior.

The treatment of choice in virtually all cases depends, first, on the use of proper medications; second, on counseling and guidance for the family; and, third, on psychotherapy for the child. Many of these children improve around puberty. There is need for ongoing assistance to overcome social handicaps and to treat chronic depression and severely impaired self-esteem.

Bereavement

Many children seen in emergency psychiatric consulation give a history of the loss of a parent, sibling, or other close relative through illness, hospitalization, or death within weeks of the onset of symptoms. The symptoms include suicidal behavior, acute phobias, hysterical conversion, hypochondriasis with panic-stricken reactions to minor injuries, fear of death and dying, regression in toilet training, fire setting, cruelty to pets, and even psychotic reactions. In teenagers, there may be drug abuse, delinquency, sexual promiscuity, and out-of-wedlock pregnancy.

The disturbance in the child is almost always an expression of a disturbance in the family. The child may feel that a grief-stricken parent has withdrawn his love. Coming on top of guilt based on oedipal or sibling rivalry, this experience may be emotionally crushing to the bereaved child.

The parents should encourage the child to discuss the death with them. If they cannot do so, some other responsible adult should do it for them. The child should be given the opportunity to suffer the loss but not be overwhelmed by it.

The child's main problems relate to the loss of a significant adult, which suddenly highlights his own vulnerability to abandonment and the fact that ne himself is vulnerable to death.

Many children play at death and dying as a way of coping with this complex life experience.

Fatal Illness

A psychiatric emergency can arise in relation to the parents of a dying child. The child is often bewildered. He usually suffers much guilt in relation to his illness and is apt to misinterpret his parents' frantic behavior as evidence of withdrawal of their love.

School Phobia

Without apparent reason, a child may suddenly refuse to go to school. When pressured, he panics unless permitted to stay home. This is a serious psychiatric emergency because of a vicious circle that quickly sets in—the longer the child stays out of school, the more severe are his social and educational impairments and the more difficult is the problem of treatment.

Lassers and associates have proposed an eight-step program to cope with acute school phobia. A careful physical examination is the first step. Psychiatric examination is the next step. Finding a therapeutic ally is the next step; this ally can be a teacher, a clergyman, the family doctor, or a family friend. The interpretive interview is a single, family-centered session with the therapist to explain to the family the danger of prolonged absence from school and to insist on hospitalization in a psychiatric unit with classroom facilities as the alternative to immediate resumption of schooling. Planning the details of a return to school involves setting an exact date in a face-to-face meeting between family and school authorities. Continuing support for the child, the family, and the school authorities must be maintained by means of phone calls and office, home, and school visits. Follow-up refers to the need for a continuing open-ended availability of the therapist after regular schooling has been resumed. Psychotherapy for the child and his family should be offered.

Fire Setting

Fire setting is commonly associated with enuresis and hyperkinetic behavior and is most likely an expression of anxiety and depression. Treatment requires a careful diagnostic evaluation and a family-centered treatment program. The use of amphetamines, tricyclic antidepressants, and other appropriate medications is often of considerable value.

Anorexia Nervosa

It is usually helpful to set a limit, with the understanding that, if the child's weight drops below the agreed-on level, hospitalization is obligatory.

Sexual Assault

Sexual assault in childhood can be divided into two categories—those involving an adult's act of exhibitionism or indecent exposure and those involving physical contact and rape. The exhibitionism is much more common and involves both boys and girls. Treatment should be directed at diminishing the reactions of panic and outrage on the part of the parents and at exploring the family pathology that may have contributed to the child's vulnerability. The adult exhibitionist who does not establish physical contact with the child is suffering from a relatively benign disorder that may be safely treated in an outpatient setting.

The child who has been physically molested has suffered a much more serious trauma, particularly if rape has occurred. In most rape cases, the perpetrator is a family member or family friend. Subsequent promiscuity as an adolescent and prostitution as an adult seem to represent, in part, efforts to overcome the trauma of the early sexual assault, feelings of self-hatred, disillusionment, and contempt for men.

Physical treatment of the rape victim is directed at repair of the injuries, prevention of venereal disease, and prevention of pregnancy. The gynecologist should be experienced in examining children, so as not to further traumatize the child.

From the psychological point of view, a family-centered treatment approach is crucial. If at all possible, hospitalization should be avoided. The treatment plan aims to permit free ventilation of the child's thoughts and feelings. The usual pattern of suppressing all discussion has the effect of intensifying the child's guilt and sets the stage for long-range chronic psychopathology. If the family pathology is severe, foster home placement may be indicated.

Newborn Abstinence Syndrome

In heroin addiction in newborn infants, the newborn may appear normal, but, somewhere between 6 and 48 hours after birth, the abstinence syndrome begins. The infant develops a high pitched, ear-piercing cry that is continuous and far louder than a normal cry. In its mildest form, the infant displays hypertonic muscles with an exaggerated Moro reflex and tremulousness. In more severe forms there are, in addition, sweating, salivating, yawning, sneezing and loose stools. In the most severe reaction there may also occur vomiting, diarrhea, and convulsions.

Treatment consists of chlorpromazine. The signs of autonomic dysfunction can be relieved by small doses of paregoric.

Women receiving barbiturates in the last trimester of pregnancy may give birth to barbiturate-addicted babies. The abstinence symptoms do not start until 4 to 7 days after birth. The cry is loud, shrill, and continuous. These infants eat voraciously but often gag and vomit, so that pyloric stenosis may be suspected. There is irritability and fitful sleep.

Treatment consists of protecting these babies from extraneous stimuli and the liberal use of a pacifier and, if necessary, sedatives—chlorpromazine, phenobarbital, diazepam. Treatment must be continued for 2 to 6 months before the baby becomes normal. In all cases, the first sign of progress is the infant's ability to sleep for longer periods, up to several hours during the night.

Psychiatric Complications of Encounter Groups

Quasitherapeutic groups are characterized by a lack of any screening procedures for admission to the group; a certain amount of coercion to participate in the group; a failure to obtain informed consent from persons entering the group; a failure to delineate clearly the rules and goals of the group, so that a passive, frightened person may feel unable to disengage himself from the group; a lack of available mental health professional consultation; a lack of follow-up concerning the subsequent clinical course of a group member; and, most important, a lack of proper training of the leaders.

With this spectrum of deficiencies as a background, it becomes understandable why there are increasing reports in the literature of acute psychotic episodes, suicidal acting out, homosexual panic, depression, sexual and aggressive acting out, and ill-advised upheavals in personal life, including the breakup of families and divorce.

If these complications occur in settings away from home, it is advisable to have the patient return home at once—if possible, accompanied by his parents or responsible relatives. Treatment of the individual case depends on the results of a careful diagnostic study.

REFERENCES

Babigian, H. M., and Odoroff, C. L. The mortality experience of a population with physiatric illness. Am. J. Psychiatry, *126:* 470, 1969.

Barton, W. *The Psychiatric Emergency.* American Psychiatric Association and National Association of Mental Health, Washington, D.C., 1966.

Blachly, P. H., Naloxone for diagnosis in methadone programs. J. A. M. A., *224:* 334, 1973.

Bogdonoff, M. D. Counter transference as a source of error in medical care. In *Frontiers in General Hospital Psychiatry.* L. Linn, editor, pp. 301–307. International Universities Press, New York, 1961.

Kalinowsky, L. B., and Hippius, M. *Pharmacologic Convulsive and Cther Somatic Treatments in Psychiatry.* Grune & Stratton, New York, 1969.

Kubler-Ross, E. *On Death and Dying.* Macmillan, New York, 1969.

Lassers, E., Nordan, R., and Bladholm, S. Steps in the return to school of children with school problems. Am. J. Psychiatry. *130:* 265, 1973.

Linn, L. Emergency room psychiatry: A gateway to community medicine. Mt. Sinai J. Med., *38:* 110, 1971.

Waldron, V. D., Klimt, C. R., and Seibel, J. E. Methadone overdose treated with naloxone infusion. J. A. M. A., *225:* 53, 1973.

29

Psychotherapies

29.1. PSYCHOANALYSIS AND PSYCHOANALYTIC PSYCHOTHERAPY

Introduction

The problems that bring people to psychiatrists for treatment are of two kinds: those that seem to have their origins largely in the remote past of the patient's life and those that seem to arise largely from current stresses, both internal and external. However, current external stresses may occur in combination with older problems. And some patients who have old but still active and unsolved problems may arrange their lives in such a way that they appear to be victims of current external situations.

When a patient's problems seem to come mainly from the past, however much they appear to be current problems, psychoanalysis may well be the treatment of choice. The conditions of the analytical situation are designed to evoke regressive feelings and fantasies, bringing them to the surface in an atmosphere in which they can be carefully studied. In contrast, evocation of regressive phenomena may be neither necessary nor desirable if the problems are predominantly current ones. In that event, some form of psychoanalytic psychotherapy—a therapy in which there is considerably less emphasis on the study of the archaic patterns of responses to the treatment situation—may well be the treatment of choice.

Psychoanalysis and psychoanalytic psychotherapy both apply psychoanalytic understandings of human behavior; both attempt to modify behavior by such psychological methods as confrontation, clarification, and interpretation; both require introspection by the patient and empathic understanding by the therapist; both require consistent attention to the countertransference. But psychoanalysis attempts to rely solely on interpretation as its technical modality, and it concentrates on the events of the analytical relationship, tending to treat the relationship as a closed system when a transference neurosis has been established. Psychoanalytic psychotherapy, on the other hand, often minimizes the events of the relationship of the patient and therapist except when they clamorously obstruct the treatment process and may use supportive measures, advice, environmental manipulation, and other maneuvers in addition to interpretation.

Psychoanalysis

The Psychoanalytic Situation

The externals of the psychoanalytic situation, the setting, are little changed from Freud's day. The patient lies on a couch or sofa, and the analyst usually sits behind him, remaining for the most part outside the patient's field of vision and intruding as little as possible into the patient's thought processes. Sessions are usually four or more times a week. Most analyses last at least 2 years, and analyses of more than 5 years are common. The patient is guided in his behavior by the fundamental rule, and the analyst endeavors to maintain an evenly suspended attention. For the most part, the analyst's activity is limited to timely interpretation of his patient's associations. Although the analyst tries not to impose his own personality and system of values on his patient, he nevertheless must enter into some reality negotiations with his patient. There are schedules and fees to be arranged; and weekends, vacations, and illnesses may interrupt the course of treatment.

Realistic aspects of the analyst's personality become apparent to the patient in many ways, and it is neither possible nor desirable for the analyst to maintain a blank screen. Thus, a real relationship underlies the analytical setting, and the handling of the real relationship may make the difference between success and failure in the treatment endeavor.

The reclining position of the patient on the couch, with the analyst seated nearby, attending to every word, reproduces symbolically an ancient parent-child situation, the nuances of which vary from patient to patient. Preoedipal anxieties derived from the early mother-child dyad may be revived early in the analysis. The patient's difficulties in trusting the analyst, whom he does not see, to maintain that trust in the absence of immediate gratification and feedback, and to maintain an appreciation of the separateness of the patient from the analyst may occupy the center of the stage during the opening phases of analysis. The capacity of the patient to call on these ego functions throughout the analysis is indispensable for ultimate success, and an estimate of this capacity is one of the important considerations in the assessment of analyzability.

The couch also introduces an element of sensory deprivation, since visual stimuli are limited, and tends to promote regression. In the analytical situation, however, regression must remain controlled and in the service of the treatment. Almost any verbal input from the analyst tends to counteract regression by its sensory impact.

Fundamental Rule

The patient agrees to be completely candid with his analyst and to reveal things about himself that he does not even know that he knows. There is a clear emphasis on the value of recognition and verbalization of psychic contents—of ideas, impulses, conflicts, and emotions. And action based on impulse without adequate prior consideration is to be avoided. The supine and relatively immobile attitude of the patient on the couch favors verbalization instead of action. Properly observed, the fundamental rule leads to the patient's use of the technique of free association.

Free Association

The associations are directed by three kinds of unconscious forces: pathogenic conflicts of the neurosis, the wish to get well, and the wish to please the analyst. The interplay among these factors becomes very complex and at times threatens the progress of the analysis, as when some impulse that is unacceptable to the patient and that is a part of his neurosis comes into conflict with his wish to please the analyst, who, he assumes, also finds the impulse unacceptable.

Rule of Abstinence

The patient must be prepared to endure delay of gratification of instinctual wishes so that he can talk about them in the treatment. It is only through the optimal frustration of the patient's wishes in the framework of the analysis that the analytical process is propelled forward, that the patient becomes conscious of his psychic tensions, instead of reducing them in unproductive gratification or keeping them in repression. The key phrase is "optimal frustration," with the implication that there is also an "optimal gratification," since few patients could tolerate for long a totally sterile, nongiving analytical environment. But the analyst's temptation to play the role of the indulgent parent and to give beyond the requirements of the analytical process must be strongly resisted if the work of the analysis is to proceed.

Analytical Process

The process of clinical psychoanalysis is slow and tedious. Although the goal of analysis remains the undoing of repression and the recovering of lost memories, the gradual integration of previously repressed material into the total structure of the personality is the chief requirement of analytical work. The work of analysis is much concerned with preparing the patient to deal with the material uncovered. Patient and analyst seldom follow a straight path to insight.

Transference. One criterion by which psychoanalysis can be differentiated in principle from other forms of psychotherapy, including psychoanalytic psychotherapy, is the management of transference. In general psychiatry, the term "transference" has come to be used as a loose designation for all aspects of the patient's feelings and behavior toward the physician. When it is used in this encompassing sense, it may be more appropriate to refer to transference as a relationship. In contrast, transference in psychoanalysis is conceived of as an endopsychic phenomenon that occurs entirely within the mind.

The analyst must conduct himself in such a fashion that he does not interfere with the development of the transference processes that indicate to him the nature of the pathology. This is best done by maintaining a nonjudgmental, even somewhat cold or remote, stance toward the patient. But the analyst should not be so remote that he is, in fact, cruel to his patient. The reliving or repetition in the transference always involves elements of both past and present.

Therapeutic Alliance. In recent years, analysts have given increasing attention to those aspects of the patient's relationship with them that do not involve displacement of a childhood wish onto the current figure of the analyst. Classical transferences in that sense always involve some degree of regression, repression, and repetition. Various writers have delineated two additional categories of object relationships within the analytical situation: the therapeutic alliance and the real relationship with the analyst.

In therapeutic analysis, basic trust must predominate if analytical work is to proceed. The patient's capacity to maintain a satisfactory working object relationshp with the analyst is challenged when he enters the analytical situation. A period of trial analysis may show that his sense of basic trust is not stable enough to tolerate analysis and that some other form of therapy must be attempted. In the most favorable cases, there may be almost no disturbance of the therapeutic alliance.

Real Relationship. This term includes that part of the analytical relationship between two adults entering into a joint venture and the necessity for them to conduct themselves realistically around such matters as fees, illnesses, interruptions—in short, all the reality arrangements necessary to conduct the analysis. The real relationship between analyst and patient also includes the patient's realistic perceptions of his analyst. A patient may accurately perceive objectionable character traits in his analyst that make in impossible for the analysis to continue. He may also perceive the analyst's countertransference reactions quite astutely. The patient's perceptions of his analyst may be sidetracked by unrealistic transference considerations, but eventually they should be brought into the field of the analysis.

Transference Neurosis. The central event in a classical therapeutic analysis is the establishment of the transference neurosis and its ultimate resolution by interpretation. The transference neurosis announces its existence with an increase in the patient's concern and preoccupation with his analysis, which becomes temporarily the most important concern of his life. The transference neurosis is a somewhat variable but more or less sustained set of transferences, focused on the analyst, in which the patient repeats much of the crucial material from his past. The crucial issue is whether the patient is beginning to develop his power of self-observation in the analysis.

In the repetitions manifested in the transference neurosis, the analyst can observe firsthand many of the important conflicts and conflict solutions of a patient's childhood, conflicts that had undergone repression long since but that had not been otherwise resolved. In the analytical situation, however, under the conditions of the therapeutic alliance, the patient's besieged ego finds a new and strong ally in the analyst.

Resistance. Since the undoing of pathological repression is the hub of analytical work, the analyst, by insisting on a recognition of unwanted impulses, may seem to his patient to be siding with those impulses in repression, instead of with his reasonable ego. Sooner or later the patient feels impelled to repeat old ego or superego defenses against threatening impulses, but now these defenses are also directed against the analyst, who appears to stand for such impulses. In the simplest situation, an infantile sexual or aggressive impulse that is now directed toward the analyst becomes the occasion for a variety of equally infantile guilt feelings. At times, the hope of finally gratifying ungratifiable infantile strivings overrides all other concerns, including analytical progress. In either event, motives have arisen for resisting the progress of the analysis. The analysis of resistance is at the heart of the analytical work.

Some clinical manifestations of resistance are an absence of affect, lateness, missed hours, forgetting to pay the bill, obvious avoidance of some topics, a preoccupation with trivia, and the use of cliches and technical terms. Any persistent stereotyped bit of behavior is a clue to the operation of resistance.

Working Through. The analyst generally proceeds from the surface down, which means that resistances are raised to awareness in advance of the drive derivatives against which they are defending. First, the defensive maneuvers must be isolated from the judging part of the patient's ego. Next, the patient may come to see that he has a part to play in his behavior, that he is actively bringing about some condition he had previously passively experienced as happening to him. The analyst's next task is to demonstrate to the patient that the defense has a purpose and that the purpose is to evade something. Furthermore, the patient learns that what is evaded and how it is evaded are both historically determined. In this way, the patient is gradually led to sort out past from present, the confusion of which is the essence of neurosis.

This sequence of interpretation leads to the integration by the ego of some previously warded-off drive derivative. Once having been made conscious, with appropriate affect, the drive derivative becomes permanently available to the patient's ego instead of remaining split off from it. However, the patient soon comes up with another resistance and the process begins all over again. The process of confronting the patient's ego again and again with the same material is called working through.

Narcissistic Transferences. Some patients are analyzable but do not develop typical transference neuroses in the classical sense. Often, these patients are fairly well-adjusted and well-functioning people whose personality disturbance prevents them from achieving a full measure of satisfaction in life. The central pathology involves the relationship between the self and the archaic narcissistic objects. These archaic narcissistic objects are the grandiose self and the idealized parent imago, the reactivations of which constitute a threat to the patient's sense of integrity of the self.

If the analyst does not interfere with the spontaneous unfolding of the transference, one of those archaic narcissistic states may make its reappearance, instead of the expected oedipal transference neurosis. Much of the work of analysis of these patients is concerned with discovering the current stimuli that set off regressive responses in them. Often, these stimuli are subtle slights, perhaps hardly noticeable to an observer.

Termination of Treatment. The termination phase begins when the patient has finally relived much of the primary infantile situation and has begun to resolve infantile conflicts in various ways. Old conflicts are successfully reworked, with different, more adaptive results. The goals of the analysis have been reached if the patient becomes free enough to develop in his own way. An important task of the termination phase is the dissolution of those positive but illogical bonds that at first served to propel the analysis forward.

Interpretive Process

The intervention of the analyst in the neurotic conflicts of his patient is virtually limited to the process of interpretation, making intelligible and meaningful to the patient those psychological events he has not hitherto understood.

Relation to Transference. The analyst in psychoanalysis directs the patient's attention primarily to the events within the analysis itself and to intrapsychic events. The transference constitutes the principal frame of reference for interpretation. Great attention is paid to material that provides access to the deeper layers of the ego and to the id. This attention includes the interpretation of dreams and the analysis of fantasies and parapraxes, particularly when they seem to involve the analysis and the analyst.

Dream Interpretation. A dream is a sort of commentary on the events of the preceding day that arises from the deeper—that is, unconscious—layers of the ego. The unconscious portions of the ego also include memory traces from the more distant past. The study of current distortions, as they are revealed by the mechanisms involved in the formation of the dream, provides valuable clues to the specific nature of those aspects of the past being relived by the patient in his relationship with the analyst.

Current Conflicts in Historical Perspective. Ideally, a complete psychoanalytic interpretation incudes meaningful statements of current conflicts and of the historical factors that influence them. Such an interpretation contains formulations of both sides of current and past conflicts, the defensive maneuvers used to lessen the impact of the conflicts, and the reasons why the conflicts are currently active. However, complete interpretations of this kind are seldom made to the patient in the course of an analysis; when they are, they are most often used as a summarization of a long period of analytical work. Most of the comments made to the patient are more limited in scope and deal with matters of immediate concern.

Timing. Proper timing often boils down to the analyst's tact and his empathic understanding of his patient. The analyst may interpret something just before the patient sees it anyway, interpret material charged with feeling, or interpret at the level of the focal conflict.

Dynamics of Cure

Although the process of analysis depends on the effects of suggestion at some stages, these effects must, in the long run, be removed. Otherwise, the cure may depend on the continued influence of the analyst.

The process of cure in analysis involves the undoing of repression safely and effectively, and both the repressing forces and the repressed strivings must be accounted for. If the cure is to be a lasting one, the patient's superego must undergo a permanent modification. Changes in superego functioning are a logical result of changes in ego functioning; conditions for the adult are no longer what they were for the child. The ego of the adult has less to fear from the repressed impulses themselves; his ego is finally in a position either to accept these impulses or to renounce them.

Frequently, toward the end of an analysis, a patient recalls some positive memories about the parent figure he has consistently maligned. In erecting defensive processes to repress the memory of some of the experiences of childhood, the ego may shrink away not only from negative memories but also from positive memories. Analysis may have as one of its effects the emancipation from repression of certain non-traumatic memories, as well as traumatic ones. Such a process may be significant in the development of greater strengths in ego functioning.

The impulses themselves undergo change. Once freed from repression, their infantile forms, characterized by the primary process, undergo modification. Analysis offers the possibility of reduction in the intensity of the components of the conflicts and the possibility of finding more acceptable ways of handling impulses of unreduced intensity. Instead of the new solution being largely a more acceptable method of channeling unmodified infantile strivings, the primary-process quality of the drives themselves is lessened, and they take on a more reality-adaptive form. The goal of analysis with respect to the drives is to transfer them from the area of transference to the area of progressive neutralization.

Indications

The primary indication for psychoanalysis is the finding that, in all probability, the patient has had long-standing conflicts that continue into the present in an active but unconscious form and that produce signs or symptoms or character problems sufficient to justify extensive treatment. The analytic patient has a conflict within the structure of his own personality. That conflict is inaccessible to consciousness, and the frustrated drives that are part of the conflict repetitively press for discharge or expression.

Ideal Patient Population. Psychoanalysis was considered by Freud to be the ideal treatment for the hysterias and the compulsion neuroses. Analysis has also been considered the best treatment for certain perversions. The psychoanalytic treatment of personality disorders has become commonplace. The individual patterns within the diagnostic group must be considered carefully from all metapsychological points of view. For example, a hysteric suffering from a monosymptomatic conversion may be defending himself against an underlying psychosis that could be seriously aggravated by analysis. Also, a severe obsessive-compulsive neurotic may be paranoid.

Patient's Motivation. Of the essence in assessing analyzability is the estimate of the patient's ability to form an analytical pact and to maintain a commitment to a progressively deepening analytical process that attempts to bring about internal change through increasing self-awareness. The ego of a patient in analysis must be such that he can tolerate the frustrations of his impulses without responding with some serious form of acting out or by shifting from one pathological pattern to another. Most psychotic patients are excluded from traditional psychoanalysis because of the difficulty they have in forming the affective and realistic bonds that are essential parts of the transference neurosis. Most patients with addictions are regarded as unsuitable because their egos are unable to tolerate the frustration of primitive impulses.

Contraindications

The various contraindications to the use of psychoanalysis seem generally valid. (1) There may be an apparent absence of a moderately reasonable and cooperative ego. Adults over 40, for example, are often believed to lack sufficient flexibility for major personality changes. However, if there are good opportunities for libidinal and narcissistic satisfactions, analysis of patients over 40 may have a favorable outcome. (2) The neurosis may be so minor that the expenditure of time, effort, and money in a full-scale analysis cannot be justified. (3) A neurosis may have elements of such pressing urgency that there is not enough time to wait for the establishment of a transference neurosis. (4) A patient's life situation may be unmodifiable, on realistic grounds, so that a successful analysis only results in greater difficulties for him. (5) The analysis of friends and relatives by the same analyst is contraindicated because the many previous points of relationship can seriously cloud the patient's understanding of his current transference responses. A short period of trial analysis may be the only way to decide whether a patient is analyzable and whether he should be analyzed by a specific analyst.

Psychoanalytic Psychotherapy

Basis for Therapeutic Intervention

The diagnostic process on which the psychiatrist bases his therapeutic intervention in his patient's life must include a comprehensive formulation of the essential issues in the patient's life. It should consist of a general statement of the dynamics and genetics of the individual patient, based on adequate study of the somatic, intrapsychic, interpersonal, and cultural aspects of his life.

The basic conflicts of a persistent neurosis are, in general, primarily intrapsychic, an opposition between segments of functions of the personality. The conflict usually rages over some force or drive, biological or psychological, that is unacceptable to other segments of the personality—that is, to other intrapsychic forces. Or, in another type of conflict, two unconscious strivings of a mutually contradictory nature may be seeking simultaneous expression.

Interpersonal factors may be deeply involved. A patient may be seriously at odds with those in his environment in a variety of ways. At times, the conflict with others is actually the manifestation of an intrapsychic conflict on an interpersonal stage.

Conflict may be due primarily to the environment. In some patients, dynamic patterns have been so seriously distorted in the process of development that ego functions that ordinarily play a role in a fairly successful adaptation to the environment remain relatively undeveloped or otherwise distorted.

A reliable diagnostic evaluation requires an assessment of those aspects of the patient's functioning that are free from conflict, as well as an assessment of the areas of conflict. Many people manage to function successfully for the most part, despite limited neurotic symptoms or character traits, until they are subjected to severe environmental stress. They may then discover that their ego lacks sufficient flexibility and resourcefulness to master the stressful situation to which they are suddenly exposed.

Definition

Psychoanalytic psychotherapy is psychotherapy based on valid psychiatric diagnosis and on psychoanalytic formulations. The diagnostic work-up should give the therapist an understanding of the patient's major conflicts and permit an evaluation of his areas of ego strength and weakness. Psychoanalytic psychotherapy also takes into consideration the available information about a patient's historical development, especially his relationship with the crucial figures of his childhood.

Unlike analysis, which has as its ultimate concern the uncovering and subsequent working through of infantile conflicts as they arise in the transference neurosis, psychoanalytic psychotherapy takes as its focus current conflicts and current dynamic patterns. Unlike psychoanalysis, which has as its technique the use of free association and the analysis of the transference neurosis, psychoanalytic psychotherapy uses interviewing and discussion techniques that use free association much less frequently. And, unlike analysis, the work on transference in psychoanalytic psychotherapy is usually limited to a discussion of the patient's moderately superficial transference reactions toward the psychiatrist and others.

Guidelines

The psychiatrist may throw his weight behind one or more components of the patient's conflict or try to foster a new and more effective solution. The psychiatrist may work intentionally toward strengthening the defensive forces of the ego or superego to lessen the strivings that are seeking expression and that are stimulating conflict and anxiety. Or, by a leading question based on incisive understanding, he may bring out into the open for discussion some pathological material that has been conscious or preconscious. There may be a limited attempt to arrive at insight into conscious and preconscious dynamic patterns, but almost never into deep unconscious patterns. Or a patient may have lost his bearings temporarily as the result of some difficult emotional problems. With a moderate amount of direction, support, and clarification of the issues by the psychiatrist, the patient may be able to make his own way again without much difficulty.

Flexibility. Psychoanalytic psychotherapy does not exclude such measures as the use of psychotropic drugs. In fact, the use of such medication is indicated for specific kinds of patients. Nor does it exclude the use of electroshock therapy or other legitimate somatic methods.

Flexibility of technique and adaptability to the patient's needs can be emphasized in psychoanalytic psychotherapy, whereas the analysis of genetic sources is emphasized in psychoanalysis. Psychoanalytic psychotherapy can range from a single supportive interview centering on a current but pressing problem to many years of treatment with one or two interviews a week. In contrast to psychoanalysis, psychoanalytic psychotherapy can be used to treat a major portion of the disorders listed in the field of psychopathology.

Treatment Techniques. One point of difference from classical analysis is that psychoanalytic psychotherapy does not involve the use of the couch. The stimulation of temporary regressive patterns of feeling and thinking, a necessary development in psychoanalysis, is much less appropriate in psychoanalytic psychotherapy, with its greater focus on more current dynamic patterns. The fact that the therapist is in the patient's line of vision in psychoanalytic psychotherapy may make him seem a more real person and less a composite of projected fantasies. Furthermore, since psychoanalytic psychotherapy has a strong focus on the current dynamic patterns causing the patient difficulty in his extratherapeutic life, transference responses to the therapist are not inclined to become as intense as in an analysis.

In analysis, everything possible is done to promote the controlled regression of the transference neurosis in order to bring to the surface those specific dynamic patterns from the past that are producing the neurosis. In most psychotherapy an effort is made to avoid inducing any more regression that the patient brings with him into the treatment.

Transferences. Transference attitudes and responses to the therapist may arise from time to time and can be used productively. Spontaneous transferences in the therapeutic situation may give valuable clues about the patient's behavior in extratherapeutic situations and at times about his childhood. They may inform the therapist about what probably is in focus for the patient at any given time, within or outside of the treatment relationship.

The central focus of psychoanalysis is the analysis of transferences to the analyst. The central focus of psychoanalytic psychotherapy is the analysis of the patient's problems with other persons and within himself. The analysis of the trasferences to the therapist is often a peripheral matter. If during the course of therapy, it becomes necessary to interpret some transference strivings toward the therapist, an interpretation away from the therapist can be of great value. By placing the emphasis away from the patient-therapist axis, the therapist can lessen the possibility of the development of an unmanageable or unrecognized transference neurosis.

Types

Insight Therapy. A stringent, critical, but affectionate self-scrutiny, as well as an outwardly directed scrutiny, can lead to the growth of a person and his creative potential. A new perception may occur in the preconscious while listening to an interpretation, but the interpretation does not result in the undoing of a bit of repression. This limited effect leads to intellectual insight. In another instance, however, the timing and accuracy of the interpretation may lead to the release of affect, the production of important new material, a sudden surprised feeling of recognition often called an "Ah-ha! experience." This leads to emotional insight based on an affective experience blended with cognitive factors. Emotional insight is often much more productive than intellectual insight.

The emphasis by the psychiatrist in such therapy is on the value to the patient of gaining a number of new insights into the current dynamics of his feelings, his responses, and his behavior, primarily in his current relation with other persons. To a lesser extent, the emphasis is on the value of developing some insight into his responses to the therapist and into his responses in childhood.

Insight psychotherapy is the treatment of choice for a patient who has fairly adequate ego strength to bring to bear on his problems but who for one or another reason should not or cannot have an analysis.

The effectiveness of insight psychotherapy does not depend solely on the insights developed or used. The patient's therapeutic response is based on other factors as well—for example, on the ventilation of his feelings in a nonjudgmental but limit-setting atmosphere and on his identification with the therapist.

A therapeutic relationship does not require an indiscriminate acceptance of all that the patient says and does. The therapist stands for long-term as well as short-term values, for the reality principle as well as the pleasure principle. At times, the therapist must intervene on the side of a relatively weak ego by giving unmistakable evidence of his expectation that the patient will try seriously for a better level of adjustment or by setting realistic limits to the patient's maladaptive behavior. In doing this, the therapist sincerely tries to be guided by his dynamic assessment of the situation and not by his own countertransference responses.

Inevitably, the attitudes of the therapist and his responses to the patient and his ideas and impulses are different from those of important figures in the patient's childhood. At times the therapist discusses the differences between their attitudes and his own. The patient may come to see that he had generalized his parents' attitudes as being universal and had generalized his own responses to his parents' attitudes so that they became automatic responses to all parental or older figures. At times, the techniques of insight therapy and corrective emotional experience can focus on the effect of pathogenic fantasies about the figures of childhood.

Intellectual insight may be sufficient to tide the patient over until the equilibrium with his environment is more favorable. He may learn through the educational influence of his therapist how to avoid some of the problems he has

been creating or encountering, without ever knowing about their roots.

Insight psychotherapy is frequently complicated by spontaneous strong transferences to the therapist that threaten at times to disrupt the treatment. The therapist should discuss transference chiefly when transference reactions seem to block the patient from continuing his open discussion of his experiences, his feelings, and his problems. In addition, transference manifestations can occasionally be pointed out, discussed, or dealt with in some other ways, even when they are not blocking the progress of the psychotherapeutic interviews, although the therapist rarely attempt to induce a transference neurosis. He can deal effectively with the significance of the transference as it throws light on the patient's contemporary life and problems, with only limited reference to his childhood.

Supportive Therapy. This therapy offers support by an authority figure during a period of illness, turmoil, or temporary decompensation. It has the goal of restoring or strengthening the defenses and integrative capacities that have been impaired. It provides a period of acceptance and dependence for a patient who is acutely in need of help in dealing with his guilt, his shame, or his anxiety and in meeting the frustrations or the external pressures that have been too great for him to handle.

Supportive psychotherapy uses such techniques as a warm, friendly, strong leadership; a gratification of dependency needs if that can be done without evoking undue shame; support in the development of legitimate independence; help in the development of hobbies and of pleasurable but nondestructive sublimations; adequate rest and diversion; the removal of excessive external strain if that is a productive step; hospitalization when it is indicated; medication that may alleviate symptoms and often does more; and guidance and advice in current issues. It uses those techniques that may make the patient feel more secure, accepted, protected, encouraged, or safe or less anxious and less alone.

A danger in supportive psychotherapy is the possibility of fostering too great a regression and too strong a dependency. From the beginning, the psychiatrist must plan to work persistently and with good timing toward weaning the patient to a resumption of a greater inde-

TABLE I

Psychoanalysis and Psychoanalytic Psychotherapy

	Psychoanalysis	Insight Therapy	Relationship Therapy	Supportive Therapy
Basic theory Goals	Psychoanalytic psychology Reorganization of character structure, with diminution of pathological defenses, integration or ultimate rejection of warded-off strivings and ideation. Understanding rather than symptom relief the objective, but symptom relief usually results. Correction of developmental lags in otherwise relatively mature personalities	Psychoanalytic psychology Resolution of selected conflicts and limited removal of pathological defenses. Understanding the primary goal, usually with secondary relief of symptoms	Psychoanalytic psychology Growth of the relatively immature personality through catalytic relationship with the therapist offset the neurotogenic effects of prior significant relationships	Psychoanalytic psychology Restoration of prior equilibrium, reduction of anxiety and fear in new situations help in tolerating unalterable situations
Activity of patient and therapist	Freely hovering attention by the analyst, free association by the patient. Interpretation of transference and resistance. Suggestion ultimately interpreted	Freely hovering attention by the therapist but with more focusing than in analysis. Less emphasis on free association, more on discussion by the patient. Suggestion usually eventually interpreted	Therapist participates as a real person around current issues, becomes a helpful parental figure	Expressive techniques generally avoided, except for some cathartic effects. Therapist actively intervenes, advises, fosters discussion, selects focus
Interpretive emphasis	Focus on resistance and transference to the analyst	Greater emphasis on interpersonal events, less on transferences to the analyst than in analysis, but transference interpretation often effective. Transferences to persons other than the therapist often effectively interpreted	Discussion and clarification of interpersonal events. Transference may or may not be interpreted	Interpretations of transferences to therapist generally avoided unless significantly interfering with the therapeutic relationship. Strong focus on external events
Transference	Transference neurosis fostered on foundation of the therapeutic alliance and the real relationship	Transference neurosis discouraged, therapeutic alliance fostered	Transference neurosis discouraged. Real relationship and therapeutic alliance emphasized	Transference neurosis discouraged. Therapeutic alliance may be firm or weak
Confidentiality	Absolute	Absolute	Usually absolute but may be abrogated in some situations	Usually absolute but may be abrogated in some situations
Regression	Fostered in the form of the transference neurosis	Generally discouraged except as necessary to gain access to fantasy material and other derivatives of the unconscious	Regression generally discouraged	Generally discouraged but may occasionally be fostered for its own sake
Adjuncts	Couch	Couch rarely used. Psychotropic drugs used occasionally	Couch contraindicated. Group methods, family therapy, or family contacts on a planned basis. Other therapists and agencies may be involved	Couch usually contraindicated. Psychotropic drugs, occupational therapy hospitalization (including day hospitalization). Family contact on planned basis. Other therapists and agencies may be involved
Frequency and duration	4–5 times weekly, 2–5+ years. Sessions usually about 50 minutes	1–3 times weekly. Few sessions to several years. Sessions usually from ½ to 1 hour	1 or 2 times weekly. 1 month to several years. Sessions usually ½ to 1 hour	Daily sessions to once every few months. One session to a lifelong process. Sessions may be brief, ranging from a few minutes to an hour
Prerequisites	Relatively mature personality, favorable life situation, motivation for long undertaking, capacity to tolerate frustration, capacity for stable therapeutic alliance, psychological mindedness	Relatively mature personality. Capacity for therapeutic alliance, some capacity to tolerate frustration. Adequate motivation and some degree of psychological mindedness	Capacity for therapeutic alliance. Personality capable of growth. Reality situation not too unfavorable	Personality organization may range from psychotic to mature. At least some capacity to form a therapeutic alliance

pendence. But some patients require supportive measures indefinitely, often with the goal of maintaining a marginal adjustment outside a hospital.

The verbalization of unexpressed strong emotions may bring considerable relief. The goal of such talking out is not necessarily or primarily that of gaining insight into the unconscious dynamic patterns that may be intensifying current responses. Rather, the reduction of inner tension and anxiety may result from the expression of emotion and its subsequent discussion and may lead to greater insight and objectivity in evaluating a current problem.

Relationship Therapy. This treatment method not only aims at a restoration of the *status quo ante* but to some extent also aims at a change in personality patterns and at a decrease in vulnerability to external pressures. Relationship therapy can be described as a fairly prolonged period of contact between a patient and a therapist in which the therapist can maintain, without too much conscious effort, a productive psychotherapeutic approach. The patient responds in various ways, and there develops an interplay of feeling, of communication, and of new experience. Certain therapeutic experiences occur for the patient, such as acceptance as worthwhile or potentially so, absence of condemnation or rejection because of defensive distortion, identification with some of the more successful achievements and adjustments of the therapist as they may fit his own needs, and spontaneous corrective emotional experiences as a result of the therapist's not responding in the neurotic fashion expected by the patient. The cornerstone of the relationship is that the therapist's fairly consistent attitudes toward the patient are like a composite of those attitudes of a good, deeply helpful father or mother or of a good, deeply helpful older brother or sister.

The psychiatrist is not so much treating the patient as rearing him or providing a setting in which the patient can rear himself, can grow and develop. For this reason, relationship therapy is often recommended for patients who are in some sort of developmental turmoil, such as the transition from adolescence to adulthood, at whatever chronological age the change may occur.

Relationship therapy provides the therapist with frequent opportunities to behave in a fashion different from the destructive or unproductive portions of the behavior of the patient's parents. At times, such experiences seem to neutralize or to reverse some of the effects of the parents' mistakes. If the patient had overly authoritarian parents, the therapist's friendly, flexible, nonjudgmental, nonauthoritarian, but at times firm and limit-setting attitude provides the patient with opportunities to adjust to, be led by, and identify with a new type of parent figure.

Relationship therapy is suitable for a variety of psychogenic illnesses. It may be useful when a patient is very resistive to expressive psychotherapy or is considered too ill for such a procedure. It may be chosen when the diagnostic assessment indicates that a gradual maturing process based on the elaboration of new foci for identification can be regarded as the most promising path toward modification.

Brief Psychotherapy. Brief psychotherapy is characterized by a limited number of interviews, usually 10 to 15, agreed upon in advance with the patient. Brief psychotherapy concentrates on current problems, only rarely touches on transference issues unless they are negative, and seldom deals with character problems; dependence and regression are discouraged. The therapist takes a more active role in determining the focus of the interviews than is the rule in open-ended therapies.

It is the treatment of choice for a great many patients, especially those in an acute crisis who are not interested in reorganizing their character structures. Patients who are somewhat psychologically minded are likely to benefit the most from brief therapy, since the format requires that the patient be able to look at himself realistically, have a strong ego, be in a favorable reality situation, and be able to work well with the therapist.

Techniques used in brief psychotherapy are derived from psychoanalytic concepts and methods, but there is greater latitude to deal with spouses and relatives, the use of psychopharmacologic agents, and other matters. The therapist usually selectively ignores the genetic origins of his patient's problems in brief treatment.

Focal Psychotherapy. Focal psychotherapy is a form of brief, insight-oriented treatment. In focal psychotherapy the therapist chooses a focus in the first two or three sessions, instead of allowing a focus to crystallize gradually over the first 10 or 20 sessions, as in the more open-ended forms of psychotherapy. The focus should be such that it can be presented as a meaningful and acceptable interpretation near the end of the therapy. Material that does not contribute to an understanding of the focus is selectively ignored.

Environmental Manipulation. At times, the removal of a patient from a stressful environment or the effecting of some change in the environment so that it is less stressful holds the greatest hope for successful treatment. Common instances of this treatment adjunct range from direct contact with the patient's family through the recommendation of a vacation for an overworked patient to foster home placement for a child.

Activity Therapies. Activity therapies depend for their effect not on the verbalization of psychic contents but on the reduction of intense and perhaps unacceptable or conflict-filled strivings through active expression of derivative and related drives. In this group of therapies are the occupational, recreational, industrial, dance, and music therapies. The activity therapies are often used in hospitals.

A basic assumption is that some activities are more therapeutic than others in specific problems. For example, it is often observed that depressed hospitalized patients seem to benefit from monotonous tasks they can regard as demeaning, thereby giving some expression to their wish to suffer in a harmless and even constructive way, refocusing some of their aggression away from themselves onto their environment.

The process and not the product of the process is of greatest importance. It is more important that a patient *do* leatherwork or *make* a finger painting than that the purse or the picture be of good quality, although that may also be important to the patient. There is a growing tendency to use occupational therapy for the fostering of better interpersonal relationships among the patients and with the therapists.

Competitive games may give acceptable expression to hostile urges. And a dance therapy, in the form of expressive physical movement, may drain off intense drives. But of greater importance is the almost inevitable psychologi-

cal contact with other human beings that helps to reverse regression.

Bibliotherapy. Some patients, by virtue of their work or profession, are required to read technical materials about mental health. The reading of technical material may well become a locus of resistance in these patients. The therapist or analyst usually cannot forbid the reading of technical books and articles; he must deal interpretively with the resistance that the reading serves. For one thing, any article or book about psychiatry is a generalizing statement about a class of people; its uncritical application to the individual reader is, at best, a risky proposition.

But for some patients, the use of literature for therapeutic purposes, bibliotherapy, does seem to have a limited usefulness. Some persons whose conflicts are not severe may derive comfort and support from the Bible. Others may gain some limited, though genuine, insight into their own dynamics by reading some books on mental health. A good marriage manual may be therapeutic for the emotional problems of a marriage. In some psychiatric hospitals, patient groups have been formed for the study of great books; but the socialization may be more beneficial than the insights obtained from the books.

Dynamics of Cure

The emphasis in psychoanalytic psychotherapy is more on current dynamic trends than on genetics and more on the understanding of contemporary relations and dynamics than on the understanding of the transference. Unlike psychoanalysis, psychotherapy tends to discourage regression and dependence except when the need for support is great. The greater flexibility in the choice of techniques open to the therapist may help compensate for a less reliable therapeutic alliance.

Therapy may become a way of life for the patient, a possible manifestation of uncontrolled or uncontrollable regression. Some patients whose egos are such that they are unable to stand alone may need permanent supportive treatment. But, most often, terminable therapy seems to result from a subtle interplay of silent transference and countertransference factors, with the therapist finding unconscious gratification in fulfilling some parental roles for his patient, who finds the re-enactment of childhood or the apparent fulfillment of ungratified childhood wishes seductive.

If intense transference responses appear without adequate preparation, a sort of wild analysis or wild psychotherapy may result. Usually, the patient then breaks off treatment, convinced either that his therapist has problems more severe than his own or that psychotherapy is not for him.

Some inexact interpretations can be a comfort to the patient to the extent that they permit him to rationalize his own problems, to lessen his anxiety by making a displacement away from prime causes. In this event, a new intellectual idea has been substituted for a possible true insight.

REFERENCES

Dewald, P. *Psychotherapy: A Dynamic Approach*, ed. 2. Basic Books, New York, 1970.
Fenichel, O. *Problems of Psychoanalytic Technique*. Psychoanalytic Quarterly, Albany, 1941.
Fromm-Reichmann, F. *Principles of Intensive Psychotherapy*. University of Chicago Press, Chicago, 1950.
Greenson, R. R. *The Technique and Practice of Psychoanalysis*. International Universities Press, New York, 1967.
Kohut, H. *The Analysis of the Self*. International Universities Press, New York, 1971.
Levine, M. *Psychotherapy in Medical Practice*. Macmillan, New York, 1942.

29.2. BEHAVIOR THERAPY

Introduction

The origins of behavior therapy or behavior modification can be traced to the animal learning laboratories of Bekhterev and Pavlov in the Soviet Union and Thorndike in the United States. The principles of learning that evolved from these early researchers continue to be modified and elaborated in contemporary laboratories of experimental behavioral science.

Nature of Behavior Therapy

Behavior therapy is the systematic application of principles of learning to the analysis and treatment of behavior disorders.

Strictly speaking, behavior refers to the organism's skeletal muscle activity—in man, both what he does and what he says (verbal behavior). To understand most clinical problems, one must also take into account what the patient thinks and feels. These private events cannot be directly observed but must be inferred from observable events—what the patient says, his facial expression, physiological measures.

Behavior therapy is a particular way of approaching clinical problems and of collecting and analyzing clinical data. The first step is to conduct a behavioral analysis. This analysis consists of describing in as objective, explicit, and quantitative terms as possible the maladaptive responses that constitute the patient's disorder—that is, the behaviors that cause him distress or that limit his satisfactions and effectiveness in familial, social, vocational, and other important life areas. The behavioral analysis generates a series of clinical hypotheses about the variables that are controlling and maintaining the patient's problematic behaviors.

The next step is to use this behavioral analysis to design a tentative treatment program. Such a program consists largely of testing out the clinical hypotheses by manipulating the behavioral and environmental variables thought to be functionally related to the patient's adjustment problems. The patient's responses to the therapeutic intervention provide additional data and allow further development and refinement of the behavioral analysis.

In behavior therapy, emphasis is placed on what is directly observable and measurable—the behavior of the patient and its relationship to environmental events. By using both the methods and the results of experimental behavioral science, this approach strives to develop the clinical discipline of psychiatry in the natural science tradition.

Systematic Desensitization

A person can overcome unadaptive anxiety that is elicited by a class of situations or objects by approaching the feared situations gradually and in a psychophysiologic state that inhibits anxiety. The therapist uses deep muscular relaxation to induce a psychophysiologic state that counterconditions anxiety responses. Rather than use actual situations or objects that elicit fear, the patient and the therapist prepare a graded list or hierarchy of anxiety-provoking scenes associated with the patient's fears. The learned relaxation state and the anxiety-provoking scenes are then systematically paired in the treatment.

A variety of procedures can be used to induce profound muscular relaxation. Most are based on a method called progressive relaxation. It consists of having the patient tense and then relax major muscle groups of the body in a fixed and systematic order, usually beginning at the top of the body and working down. Some clinicians use hypnosis with selected patients to facilitate relaxation. Tape-recorded procedures offer the advantage of allowing the patient to practice relaxation on his own.

In hierarchy construction the clinician determines all the antecedent (stimulus) conditions that elicit inappropriate anxiety in the patient. These conditions are grouped into themes. For each theme, a list or hierarchy of 10 to 12 scenes is then developed and arranged in order of increasing anxiety.

The deconditioning of the anxiety attached to each theme is then accomplished by having the patient vividly imagine each hierarchy scene while in a deeply relaxed state. This is done systematically, beginning with the least anxiety—provoking scene and proceeding through the list at a rate determined by the patient's responses. In general, the patient should experience only minimal anxiety with a given scene before proceeding to the next scene. Several repetitions of each scene may be required before the anxiety reaches the minimal level. The expectation is that, when the patient can vividly imagine the highest or most anxiety-provoking scene with equanimity, he will experience little anxiety in the corresponding real-life situation. However, the process of carry-over is facilitated by having the patient enter, between treatment sessions, actual anxiety-provoking situations that he has overcome in therapy.

The therapist should respond to the patient's reports of entering situations on his fear hierarchy with enthusiastic approval. Such approval usually constitutes a powerful reinforcer for the patient to continue to confront his fears and thus facilitates progress. However, the patient should not be urged to enter high-anxiety situations prematurely. A heroic effort by the patient to do so may result in his fleeing the situation in an intensely fearful state, thereby reinforcing his phobic-avoidance behavior and losing some of the progress he has made.

Indications

Systematic desensitization is applicable when one can identify the stimulus antecedents that elicit anxiety, which, in turn, mediates unadaptive or disruptive behavior. Often, obsessive-compulsive behaviors are mediated by the anxiety elicited by specific objects or situations. Desensitization has been used effectively with some stutterers by deconditioning the anxiety associated with a range of speaking situations. Certain sexual problems are amenable to desensitization therapy. A number of psychophysiologic disorders have been treated by desensitization, using a hierarchy of stimuli that elicit anxiety-related physiologic reactions. These reactions include such diverse disorders as bronchial asthma and dysmenorrhea.

Limitations

Systematic desensitization alone may not be sufficient to alleviate anxiety-mediated symptoms in some clinical situations. The behavioral analysis may reveal that multiple environmental variables are maintaining the patient's disordered state. The behavior of stuttering is so overlearned and habitual in some severe adult cases, for example, that reducing situational anxiety may not be sufficient to remove the speech problem. Often, retraining of speech habits is also required. Other examples are provided by many patients with severe, chronic phobias.

Procedural Variations

Numerous variations on the standard procedure have been described. Two are mentioned here because of their theoretical and practical importance: in vivo desensitization and the adjunctive use of drugs.

In vivo desensitization, also called reinforced practice, entails the use of actual, rather than merely imaginal, objects and situations in helping the patient overcome irrational, unadaptive fears. The object may be brought to the patient—as in the treatment of a phobia of cats, spiders, or other small, portable objects—or the patient may be brought to the feared situation, as in treating acrophobia. Typically, the therapist accompanies the patient along the steps of the hierarchy—increasing heights for the acrophobic patient—and relies on the emotional state induced by the psychotherapeutic relationship to countercondition anxiety. This procedure has the advantage of obviating the problem of carry-over, since the actual fear-eliciting situation is approached. A limitation is that practical problems are sometimes posed with particular classes of phobic situations, such as fear of social criticism. However, the consensus is that in vivo desensitization is more reliable and more rapid-acting than desensitization with imaginal scenes.

Various drugs have been used in an effort to hasten desensitization. The widest experience is with the ultrarapid-acting barbiturate sodium methohexital (Brevital), which is given intravenously in subanesthetic doses. Usually, up to 60 mg. of the drug are given in divided doses in any session. If certain procedural details are carefully followed, almost all patients find the procedure pleasant, with few detracting side effects. The advantages of Brevital-aided desensitization are that preliminary training in relaxation can be shortened, almost all patients are able to become adequately relaxed, and the treatment itself appears to proceed more rapidly.

Positive Reinforcement and Extinction

The core notion in positive reinforcement and extinction is that behavior is determined in part by its consequences. If a behavioral response is followed by a generally rewarding event (for example, food, avoidance of pain, or praise), it tends to be strengthened and to occur more

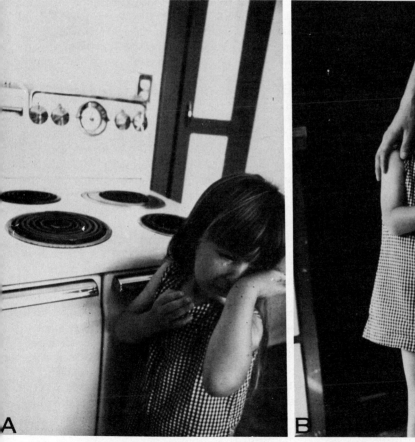
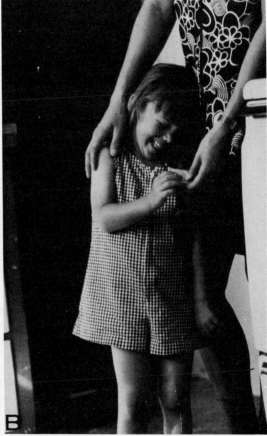

FIGURE 1. Touching a hot burner (A) is an example of punishment—that is, response-contingent aversive stimulation. Running to mother (B) is rewarded by mother's comforting, succoring behavior (positive reinforcement). Courtesy of Bill McDonald, CRM Books, *Psychology Today: An Introduction.*

frequently under the same environmental circumstances. If a response is followed by an aversive stimulus (punishment) or by no stimulus at all (extinction), it tends to be weakened and occur less frequently under the same environmental circumstances.

Token Economy

The power of operant-reinforcement procedures in the treatment of psychotic patients in a ward setting was first systematically demonstrated by Ayllon and Axrin. They were impressed by the number of eating problems on a ward for chronic psychotic patients. After a period of detailed observation, they hypothesized that most of the eating problems exhibited by the patients were being inadvertently reinforced by the medical and nursing staff and by other patients. Frequently, on this understaffed ward, the problem patient's main social contact with the nursing staff occurred at mealtimes, when coaxing, help with utensils, and other forms of rewarding social attention occurred as a consequence of his apparent inability to attend to his own needs. To foster more adaptive behavior, Ayllon and Azrin changed the contingencies of reinforcement. Eating problems of all kinds were simply ignored, and any patient who failed to enter the dining room within a designated period of time simply did not eat. Within a few days, the problem patients were eating all meals virtually unaided.

Freed from the time-consuming task of helping the patients maintain their state of nutrition, the nursing staff now increased their social interactions with each patient in the form of interest, attention, and praise, contingent on prosocial and self-help behaviors. With this use of positive reinforcement and the extinction of putative eating problems and other inappropriate behaviors, much of the socially disruptive, disorganized, and regressive behavior of the patients disappeared.

Ayllon and Azrin then introduced tokens as a convenient medium for the delivery or withdrawal of positive reinforcement. In their token economy, a patient received a set number of tokens for self-help behaviors, such as adequate grooming, rising at an appropriate hour, and making his bed. He could earn additional tokens for adaptive, prosocial behaviors, such as adequately performing meaningful tasks off and on the ward. The patient could spend tokens for meeting his ordinary needs (food, decorating his room) and for additional goods, pleasures, and privileges (cigarettes, watching television, a trip off the hospital grounds). The patient was fined tokens according to a prescribed schedule for dyssocial behaviors, such as being obstreperous, destructive of property, or physically assaultive.

This arrangement provided a convenient means of insuring that each patient's specific behaviors had specific consequences—an arrangement close to the complex network of contingencies that operate in the world outside the hospital ward. A therapist can also design treatment strategies for individual patients for the removal of unadaptive, deviant behavior or to remedy specific behavior deficits.

Applications to Neurotic Behaviors

The treatment of specific neurotic and habit disturbances entails five steps—selecting and specifying the target behavior, measuring the target behavior, choosing an adequate reinforcer, setting up a contingency, and monitoring progress.

The choice of behavior to be modified must follow from a complete behavioral analysis of the clinical problem. Measuring the target behavior is crucial, since evidence that the intervention is being effective comes from measurable changes in this dependent variable. The therapist and patient must then search the environment for an available reinforcer that will be sufficiently powerful to shape and maintain new behavior. One general procedure for doing this is to determine what the patient now does a lot of. Such high-frequency behavior tends to be reinforcing. The patient, with the aid of the therapist, sets up an arrangement in which access to the reinforcer is contingent on first emitting the weak target behavior. In general, a reinforcer is maximally effective if it immediately follows the behavior to be strengthened. Shaping may also be necessary. Another principle involves the schedule of reinforcement. An intermittent schedule of reinforcement has the advantage of generating behavior that is more resistant to extinction; the new behavior gradually becomes less immediately dependent on the specific reinforcement. The patient keeps records of his progress, so he and the therapist can ascertain whether or not the procedures are working.

Contingency Contracting

Contingency or behavioral contracting illustrates two recent emphases in behavior therapy; working more in the patient's natural environment and identifying the locus of clinical problems in the interactions among sets of persons, such as spouses and other family members, rather than in a single individual.

Some frequently recurring characteristics of unsatisfying and disturbed marriages make contingency contracting an especially suitable mode of intervention. Often each partner has no clear idea of what the other wants or expects from the relationship, and negotiating behavioral contracts tends to make these expectations more explicit. Also, the interaction in disturbed marriages often entails each trying to get his needs met largely by the exchange of punishment and negative reinforcement rather than positive reinforcement.

To apply contingency contracting, the therapist helps the couple identify and specify the behaviors they most want from each other and helps them negotiate a contract for their exchange. To avoid ambiguity and misunderstanding, the therapist usually has the couple write out the various contingencies.

Contingency contracting is often quite effective in improving marital relationships by beginning the process of unscrambling the many punitive and ineffective ways in which the couple have come to deal with each other. In addition to the benefit derived from removing specific aversive control measures (nagging, withdrawal of affection, reticence), another benefit may result from the mutual experience of negotiating contracts. Negotiation entails trying to understand the partner's wants and needs, expressing one's own wants and needs, and often finding that the other is willing and able to carry out an agreement to change the behavior. Changes in expressed feelings and attitudes tend to follow these behavioral alterations.

Metronome-Conditioned Speech Retraining

This behavioral procedure illustrates the development of behavioral prostheses—mechanical or electronic devices worn or carried by the patient in his natural environment to facilitate the learning of more adaptive behavioral patterns. The procedure and prosthesis described here are for the treatment of severe and chronic stuttering in adolescents and adults. Often, stuttering in these patients is so practiced and overlearned that other procedures used alone, such as the rearrangement of reinforcement contingencies or the deconditioning of speech-related anxiety, are not sufficient to bring about substantial improvement.

Most stutterers show an immediate and striking increase in fluency if they pace their speech to the rhythmic beats of an auditory metronome. The patient wears a miniaturized electronic metronome, which resembles a hearing aid, behind his ear (see Figure 2). This metronome enables the patient to carry his prosthetic device and hence his treatment into the natural environment. It is equipped with a rate control (30 to 150 beats a minute).

In the first treatment session, the therapist finds the conditions under which the patient can be highly fluent with the aid of a desk metronome, like the ones used in piano practice. If the patient is clearly fluent at 40 syllables a minute, the therapist gradually in-

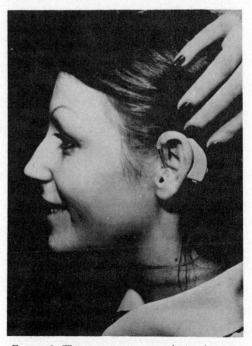

FIGURE 2. The pacemaster, an electronic metronome, as worn by a stutterer. This instrument is made by Associated Auditory Instruments, Inc., 6795 Market Street, Upper Darby, Pennsylvania 19082.

creases the metronome to 50, 60, and eventually 90 or 100 beats a minute. Also, the patient begins to pace more than one syllable to each beat. He practices daily at home at the current rate between his weekly sessions with the therapist. At the same time, the patient gradually makes the speaking situations in which he practices fluency more complex and potentially more anxiety-provoking. Thus, he may speak alone during home practice for the first week but have a roommate, parent, or friend present during the second week. Once easy fluency is possible with one other person present, he may ask a third person to be present and so forth. Most well-motivated patients are speaking fluently in the normal range (100 to 160 words a minute) in low-stress situations after 3 to 5 weeks of treatment.

At this point, the patient begins to use the miniaturized metronome, which allows him to extend his fluency practice into the more and more complex situations he encounters in his daily life. He proceeds hierarchically from low-stress situations, where the probability of stuttering is small, to higher-stress situations, where the probability of stuttering was previously great. The experience of fluency, with its attendant increased confidence and sense of mastery at each step, set the stage for success at the next step.

If the patient experiences unanticipated difficulty speaking fluently in a given situation, he may decrease the rate of the metronome and thereby reduce the rate of his own speech. Other things being equal, this slower rate of speech allows him to regain fluency.

When the patient is highly fluent in most speaking situations that arise in his daily life, he begins to discontinue the use of the metronome. He stops using it in the easiest situation first, then in the next most easy, and so on, until he no longer uses the prosthesis. This stage may require many months.

REFERENCES

Bandura, A. *Principles of Behavior Modification.* Holt, Rinehart and Winston, New York, 1969.
Brady, J. P. Metronome-conditioned speech retraining for stuttering. Behav. Ther., *2:* 129, 1971.
Brady, J. P. Systematic desensitization. In *Behavior Modification: Principles and Clinical Applications.* W. S. Agras, editor. Little, Brown, Boston, 1972.
Brady, J. P. Behavior therapy: Fad or psychotherapy of the future? In *Advances in Behavior Therapy, 1970,* R. D. Rubin, J. D. Henderson, D. K. Pumroy, and J. P. Brady, editors. Academic Press, New York, 1973.
Brady, J. P., and Brady, C. N. Behavior therapy of stuttering. Folia Phoniatr. (Basel), *24:* 355, 1972.
Brady, J. P., and Rieger, W. Behavioral treatment of anorexia nervosa. In *Proceedings of the International Symposium on Behavior Modification* (Minneapolis, Minn., Oct. 4–6, 1972). Appleton-Century-Crofts, New York, 1974.
Liberman, R. P. Behavioral modification of schizophrenia: A review. Schizophrenia Bull., *6:* 37, 1972.
Lovaas, O. I., Koegel, R., Simmons, J. Q., and Long, J. S. Some generalization and follow-up measures on autistic children in behavior therapy. J. Appl. Behav. Anal., *6:* 131, 1973.
Wolpe, J. *The Practice of Behavior Therapy,* Pergamon Press, New York, 1969.
Yates, A. J. *Behavior Therapy.* John Wiley, New York, 1970.

29.3. CLIENT-CENTERED PSYCHOTHERAPY

Introduction

The central hypothesis of the client-centered approach is that the potential of any person tends to be released in a relationship in which one person (usually thought of as the helping person) is experiencing and communicating his own realness, his caring, and a deeply sensitive, nonjudgmental understanding. This approach is unique in being oriented to the process of the relationship, rather than to the symptoms or their cure; in drawing its hypotheses from the raw data of therapeutic and other relationships, making special use of recorded and filmed interviews; and in its determination to test all its hypotheses through appropriate research. The term "client" rather than "patient", indicates that this is not a manipulative or medically prescriptive model.

Characteristics

The characteristics that distinguish this point of view from other forms of psychotherapy include: (1) the developing hypothesis that certain attitudes in the therapist constitute the necessary and sufficient conditions of therapeutic effectiveness, (2) the developing concept of the therapist's function as that of being immediately present and accessible to his client and relying on his moment-to-moment experiencing in the relationship with the client, (3) continuing focus on the phenomenal world of the client, (4) a developing theory that the therapeutic process is marked by a change in the client's manner of experiencing, with increasing ability to live more fully in the immediate moment, (5) continued stress on the self-actualizing quality of the human organism as the motivational force in therapy, (6) a concern with the process of personality change, rather than the structure of personality, (7) emphasis on the need for continued research to gain essential learnings regarding psychotherapy, (8) the hypothesis that the same principles of psychotherapy apply to all persons whether they are categorized as psychotic, neurotic, or normal, (9) a view of psychotherapy as one specialized example of all constructive interpersonal relationships, with the consequent generalized applicability of all knowledge gained from the field of psychotherapy, (10) a determination to build all theoretical formulations out of the soil of experience, rather than twisting experience to fit a preformed theory, and (11) a concern with the philosophical issues that derive from the practice of psychotherapy.

Therapeutic Relationship

Therapeutic success is dependent not primarily on the technical training or skills of the therapist but on the presence of certain attitudes in the therapist. When they are effectively communicated to and perceived by the client, these attitudes are the crucial determinants of therapeutic progress and constructive changes in personality. Three attitudes or conditions appear to be most important for the success of therapy: (1) the therapist's genuineness or congruence, (2) the therapist's complete acceptance of or unconditional positive regard for his client, and (3) a sensitive and accurately empathic understanding of the client by the therapist.

Therapeutic Process

When the conditions for therapy are present, a process of therapeutic change is set in motion. This process can be viewed from the outside as a sequence of phenomena. It can also be viewed from the inside, from the client's perceptions.

In a broad sense, the process may be described as the client's reciprocation of the therapist's attitudes. As he finds someone listening to him with consistent acceptance while he expresses his thoughts and feelings, the client, little by little, becomes increasingly able to listen to communications from within himself; he becomes able to realize that he *is* angry or that he *is* frightened or that he *is* experiencing feelings of love. Gradually, he becomes able to listen to feelings within himself that previously seemed so bizarre, so terrible, or so disorganizing that they had been shut off completely from awareness. As he reveals these hidden and "awful" aspects of himself, he finds that the therapist's regard for him remains unshaken. Slowly, he moves toward adopting this same attitude toward himself, toward accepting himself as he is, and thus prepares to move forward in the process of becoming. As the client is able to listen to more of himself, he moves toward greater congruence, toward expressing all of himself more openly. He is, at last, free to change and grow in the directions that are natural to the maturing human organism.

In client-centered therapy, there is a continuum of process that can be divided into seven stages. The client enters therapy at some point on this continuum and changes in ways that move him toward the endpoint of the scale. Essentially, the scale is from a rigid fixity of attitudes and constructs and perceptions to a changingness and flow in all these respects. It moves from remoteness from experiencing to immediacy of experiencing. It is a shift in the quality of life from stasis to process, from structure to fluidity.

Stage 1

The person is rigidly structured in the constructs he forms about himself and his world. He is so remote from the immediate experiencing going on within himself that he is unaware of it. There is no awareness of any desire to change or grow. No problems are recognized. Feelings and personal meanings are neither recognized nor owned. The person in this state lives in a sure world of fixed constructs, all external to himself. He communicates only about externals. He is unlikely to come voluntarily for therapy, and, if he is sent for help, the hope of progress is dim, unless he is in a situation such as play therapy or group therapy, in which, without taking any verbal initiative, he can gradually relax and experience the reality of a therapeutic climate.

Stage 2

The person is able to express himself on nonself topics and about problems which are perceived as external. Feelings are sometimes described as unowned or as past objects. Personal constructs are rigid, thought of as facts.

Stage 3

If a client at stage 2 experiences himself as being fully received as he is, a loosening begins to take place. There is freer expression about self as an object. Even self-related experiences are described as objects. There is now much expression about feelings and personal meanings that are not now present. Experiencing is also described in the past or as remote from the self. Constructs are, however, beginning to be recognized as such, not as facts.

Stage 4

Feelings are described as objects in the present. Occasionally, feelings are even expressed in the present, breaking through against the client's wishes. There is a fear that feelings may be experienced in the immediate present. Experiencing is less remote and may occasionally occur with little postponement. There is a loosening of the way experience is construed and a beginning questioning of the validity of such structures. There is a beginning sense of self-responsibility for problems. Close relationships are still seen as dangerous, but occasionally the client risks relating himself to some extent on a feeling basis.

Much of therapy—probably in any type of therapy—exists at about the stage 4 level. The client is exploring, he is beginning to sense himself as a feeling, experiencing creature; he is frightened and disorganized by elements he dimly senses or occasionally blurts out.

Stage 5

The client feels safe in the therapeutic relationship and less frightened of the discoveries in himself. Feelings are now expressed freely as existing in the present. The personal meanings or feelings that have been denied to awareness are close to being fully experienced—sometimes with fear, distrust, or amazement. The client has a desire not only to own his self-feelings, but to be the "real me." There is an increasing recognition of and facing of the disparities between the self as it has been built up and the actual experiencing. The client is far more fluid than in stages 1 and 2. He is much closer to his organic, visceral being, which is always in process. He is far more aware of himself and

beginning to sense that the self he exhibits or wears can be checked for accuracy against the organic flow going on within him.

Stage 6

The sixth stage is distinctive and often dramatic. Perhaps its most compelling element is the full and accepted experiencing, in the immediate present, of feelings previously denied to awareness. Often, the client is hit by this experiencing, and physiological concomitants, such as sighs and tears and muscular relaxation, are frequent. There is no longer any particular awareness of self as an object. The self *is* the experiencing, the ongoing process, changing from moment to moment. The constructs by which the client has been living as though they were solid guides dissolve in this immediacy of experiencing and are seen for what they are—namely, construings that have taken place in him. Consequently, the person sometimes feels shaky or cut loose from his foundations.

Stage 7

This stage is a trend or goal, rather than something fully achieved. It is a description of the fully functioning person. Here, the person is no longer fearful of experiencing feelings with immediacy and richness of detail. This occurs not only in therapy but in outside relationships as well. This welling up of experiencing in the moment constitutes a referent by which the person is able to know who he is, what he wants, and what his attitudes are—both positive and negative attitudes. He is acceptant toward himself, has a trust in his own organismic process, which is wiser than his mind alone. Each experience determines its own meaning and is not interpreted in terms of a past structure. His self is the subjective awareness of what he is experiencing.

Theory of Therapy

Basic Concepts

Actualizing Tendency. It is hypothesized that man, like every other living organism, plant or animal, has an inherent tendency to develop all his capacities in ways that serve to maintain or enhance the organism. This tendency, when free to operate, moves the person toward what is termed growth, maturity, and life enrichment. Innumerable environmental circumstances can prevent the human organism from moving in actualizing directions. The elements that surround him—physical and psychological—can mean that the actualizing tendency is stunted or stopped altogether; that it may be able to exert itself only in warped or bizarre or abnormal manifestations; that it may turn in socially destructive, rather than constructive, ways.

Self. The infant becomes aware of experiences that he discriminates as being "me." Slowly, a self-concept is formed. It may be thought of as an organized, consistent, conceptual Gestalt composed of the perceptions of the "me" or "I" and the perceptions of the relationships of this "I" to the outside world and to others. It includes the values attached to these perceptions. It is a fluid, changing Gestalt, but, at any given moment, it is an entity. It is available to awareness but not necessarily in awareness. It is a constant referent for the person who acts in terms of it.

Experiencing. Experiencing is the process that includes all that is going on within the envelope of the organism that is available to awareness. When it is close to awareness, it is a dimly felt meaning but also a referent. When an experience has been denied to awareness because it is inconsistent with the self concept, it may, in therapy, come into awareness with a rush. This is the phenomenon of being hit by a feeling. It can be termed experiencing a felt meaning *fully* in the immediate moment.

Incongruence. Incongruence is the discrepancy that can come to exist between the experiencing of the organism and the concept of self. It is most clearly evident in therapy when it disappears. Thus, the person may be—in awareness—a self with no hostile feelings toward another (spouse, mother, whatever). But as he comes in touch with his experiencing organism, he discovers that he is full of rage. In this moment, his concept of himself is significantly altered.

When there is a high degree of incongruence, the actualizing tendency comes to have a confused or bifurcated role. On the one hand, the selfconcept becomes supported by this tendency as the person struggles to enhance the picture he has of himself. At the same time, the organism is striving to meet its needs, which may be at odds with the conscious desires of the person. This conflict is clearly evident in therapy.

Conditions for Therapy

For therapeutic change to occur, it appears necessary for these conditions to exist:

1. The client is experiencing at least a vague incongruence, which causes him to be anxious.

2. The therapist is congruent (genuine or real) in the relationship—his picture of himself and the way he communicates matching his immediate experiencing.

3. The therapist is experiencing a prizing or caring or acceptant attitude toward the client.

4. The therapist is experiencing an accurately sensitive understanding of the client's internal frame of reference, the world of internal and external reality as perceived by the client.

5. The client perceives, to some minimal degree, the realness, the caring, and the understanding of the therapist. His perception is based only in part on the therapist's words, often more deeply on other cues.

Process of Therapy

When these conditions exist and continue, a process is set in motion:

1. The client is increasingly free in expressing his feelings and personal meanings through both verbal and motor channels.

2. His expression has increasingly to do with self, rather than nonself.

3. He is able more accurately to differentiate his feelings and perceptions and their objects, whether others or self. His experiencing is more accurately symbolized in awareness.

4. He begins to deal more and more with the incongruence between what he is immediately experiencing and the concept he has of himself.

5. He comes to experience *fully*, in awareness, some of these descrepancies. He lives feelings and meanings that have previously been denied to awareness.

6. His picture of himself keeps changing and reorganizing to assimilate these previously denied experiences.

7. He recognizes that the structures by which he has guided his life are products of his own construings, not real structures.

8. His concept of self becomes both more congruent with his immediate experiencings and also more fluid and changing. Increasing congruence between self and experiencing is

synonymous with improved psychological adjustment.

9. Because he is more congruent and thus experiencing fewer internal threats, he can relate more freely and openly to the therapist and to others.

10. He increasingly regards himself as the locus of evaluation, the source of the valuing process.

Changes in Personality and Behavior

The conditions of therapy and the process of therapy bring about certain changes:

1. Being more congruent, with less to defend, the client is more open to his experience, takes in more data more accurately.

2. He is consequently more effective in meeting and coping with life's problems and in handling relationships.

3. Tension of all kinds is reduced—the anxiety level, the physiological and psychological tensions.

4. With the locus of choice in himself, he becomes more confident and self-directing.

5. His values are determined by an organismic valuing process that discriminates between the satisfying, enhancing experience and that which is unsatisfactory. He regards his experiencing as positive, constructive, and a useful guide.

6. His behavior is more within his own control, is more mature, and is better related to others.

Applications

In client-centered therapy, the therapeutic relationship has always been conceived of as a special instance of interpersonal relationships in general. Change and growth in therapy have also been seen as a special instance of growth and development in any human being. Perhaps it is because of these two points of view that client-centered theories and methods have been used in a wide variety of settings that bear no resemblance to the formal therapy situation.

The Intensive Group

Whether a number of persons come to a group because they are experiencing serious problems, as in group therapy, or come together to enrich and enchance their personal development, as in the encounter group, a client-centered approach

has been found to be directly applicable. The responsible person is more accurately described as a facilitator, rather than a leader, because he sees his function as that of releasing the potentialities for self-understanding and behavioral change in the group members, rather than manipulating, interpreting, or persuading. A process is set in motion that bears definite resemblances to the course of psychotherapy.

Education

The basic concepts, theory, and even the methods of the client-centered approach have clear relevance to schools. Just as one-to-one therapy creates a climate for learning about oneself, so the educator can create a climate in which both cognitive and affective learning can go forward at the student's own pace in a classroom.

In two school systems, large-scale change efforts have been based on the client-centered approach, with generally favorable results in promoting self-directed change but not without turbulence and divisiveness in the organizational structures. Often, the encounter group plays a part in bringing about the initial attitudinal change on the part of educators.

Other Applications

The client-centered approach has had a wide and positive reception by a large number of professional groups other than therapist, including school and vocational counselors, marriage counselors, business executives, clergymen of many faiths, and workers in community development. It has been used effectively in widely different cultural settings—France, Belgium, Italy, and Japan, for example. It has been used in situations of sharp racial tension between whites and blacks, whites and chicanos. It has brought striking changes in groups of Jesuit leaders, as well as other religious thinkers. It has been used with a group representative of the deep tensions in Northern Ireland.

REFERENCES

Hart, J. T., and Tomlinson, T. M., editors. *New Directions in Client-Centered Therapy*. Houghton Mifflin, Boston, 1970.

Meador, B. D. Client-centered therapy. In *Current Psychotherapies*. R. Corsini, editor. F. E. Peacock, Itasca, Ill., 1973.

Rogers, C. R. *Client-Centered Therapy*. Houghton Mifflin, Boston, 1951.

Rogers, C. R. Persons or science: A philosophical question. Am. Psychol., *10:* 267, 1955.

Rogers, C. R. The necessary and sufficient conditions of therapeutic personality change. J. Consult. Psychol., *21:* 95, 1957.

Rogers, C. R. A theory of therapy, personality, and interpersonal relationships as developed in the client-centered framework. In *Psychology: A Study of Science*, S. Koch, editor. *Vol. 3, Formulations of the Person and the Social Context*, p. 184. McGraw-Hill, New York, 1959.

Rogers, C. R. *On Becoming A Person.* Houghton Mifflin, Boston, 1961.

Rogers, C. R. My philosophy of interpersonal relationships and how it grew. J. Human. Psychol., *13*, 3, 1973.

29.4. HYPNOSIS: AN ADJUNCT TO PSYCHOTHERAPY

Introduction

Everything done in psychotherapy with hypnosis can also be done without hypnosis. The advantage of hypnosis is that it accelerates the impact of psychotherapeutic intervention.

The word "hypnosis" (from the Greek word *hypnos*, meaning sleep) can be misleading because it is not a form of sleep; rather, it is a complex process of heightened or aroused concentration. Although peripheral awareness is reduced in sleep and hypnosis alike, focal awareness, which is almost obliterated in sleep, is at optimal capacity in hypnosis.

Characteristics

Hypnosis can be described as an altered state of intense and sensitive interpersonal relatedness between hypnotist and patient, characterized by the patient's nonrational submission and relative abandonment of executive control to a more or less regressed, dissociated state.

Capacity for Hypnosis

The patient must have a latent capacity for aroused concentration that can be tapped and then structured by the hypnotist-therapist. The hypnotist can provide an appropriate occasion for the subject to activate his own capacity for the trance experience. This capacity or lack of it is not necessarily identified by the patient's conscious evaluation of his hypnotizability.

To determine the efficacy and possible extent of the use of hypnosis in therapy, the clinician should make some test of the patient's hypnotizability. Subjects who are deeply hypnotizable seem to have an impressive capacity

to roll their eyes upward. The degree of eye roll as studied by Herbert Spiegel roughly correlates with hypnotizability (see Figure 1).

Trance Induction

The phenomenon of trance induction is a three-stage operation. The patient's perception of the aura is an anticipatory phase. If the reputation of the hypnotist, his appearance, or his presentation is such that it coincides with the patient's transference predisposition or expectancy, the necessary rapport is comparatively easy to establish. The patient becomes more receptive to the physician's signals to enter the trance and is able to accept more fully the directions given to him during the trance state.

During psychophysiologic enhancement, the hypnotist indicates, in advance, the probable and, therefore, the predictable psychophysiologic phenomena that will occur. The hypnotist also implies that these phenomena are due to his signals. In addition, the patient's suspense accentuates the psychophysiologic effect.

During the third phase of trance induction, the patient more or less abandons his executive controls and shows nonrational submission to a dissociated state. The hypnotist has the broad power to structure the nature of the patient's nonrational plunge into submission; however, he cannot determine either the moment or the manner of the patient's submission.

The induction technique is almost inconsequential in the production of the trance. Creating an atmosphere of appropriate security and relaxation is important. But these elements are secondary compared with the expectation of both the patient and the doctor and the relationship between them. The patient is encouraged to make himself comfortable and to concentrate. The therapist may then ask him to gaze at a dot on a card, a spot on the ceiling, or a pencil point; to roll his eyes up, as if he were trying to look at his eyebrows; to concentrate on holding one hand in a raised position; to sway back and forth from a standing position until he falls back into a chair placed behind him; or to perform any one of an almost limitless number of procedures that involve concentration. In brief, the therapist chooses a technique with

UP-GAZE   ROLL

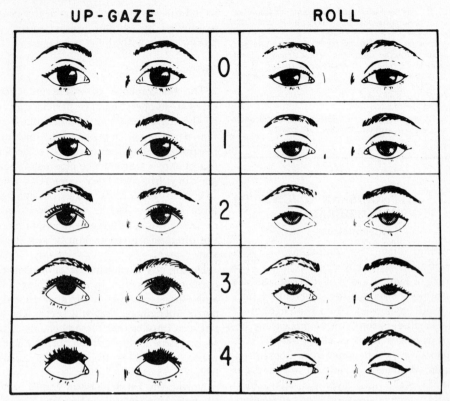

FIGURE 1. Hypnotizability, as measured by up-gaze and eye roll.

which he feels comfortable and confident and that the patient finds acceptable and sometimes even expects.

Phenomenology

The objective and subjective phenomena that occur vary widely, depending on the expectations of the subject and the hypnotist. In Western culture the trance state generally exists at one of three levels. The light trance is most readily identified by motor alterations, such as hyperkinesis and retardation. The middle range is usually distinguished by these changes, plus such sensory alterations as paresthesia, analgesia, anesthesia, partial amnesia, and posthypnotic compliance with simple signals. The deep, somnambulistic level is characterized by the additional features of posthypnotic compliance, even with bizarre signals; visual, auditory, and tactile hallucinations; time distortion; age regression; hypermnesia or selective amnesia; profound anesthesia; and the ability to maintain the trance state with the eyes open.

While hypnotized, a patient may be told that, when the hypnotist lights a cigarette after the trance, the patient will ask for one, puff at it once or twice, and then put it out. It can be predicted with confidence that after the trance the patient will do precisely this. It is also predictable that (1) he will have an amnesia, more or less, to the general context of the instruction, technically called the signal, (2) he will comply with the instruction compulsively, and (3) he will rationalize his act of snuffing out the cigarette by saying, "This cigarette is stale," or "I must be catching a cold," or something along these lines.

Psychotherapeutic Application

Hypnosis enables the psychiatrist to focus the patient's intense concentration on certain areas. The desired information can be reached more directly through hypnosis than when the psychiatrist must depend on the patient's free association, with its mass of resistances, irrelevant information, and conscious censure. An atmosphere of receptivity enhances the patient's capacity for exploration and change.

Prerequisites for Therapeutic Effectiveness

If the therapist believes that the dissociation and concentration obtained in hypnosis can facilitate treatment, he must assume certain responsibilities: He must identify the capacity of the patient for the trance experience. He must provide the optimal conditions necessary for the trance, including patient-doctor rapport, security, and physical comfort. He must structure the trance in accordance with his therapeutic goals. And he must educate the patient to respond at a given signal in the service of the treatment program.

As in all psychotherapeutic encounters, the effectiveness of hypnosis depends on the patient's well-being, which is determined by the restoration of the patient's previous level of self-esteem, the alleviation of stress in his environment, the patient's reformulation of the symbolism of his symptom into a less extreme form, although the basic language remains the same, and the provision of a clinical atmosphere of flux that allows the patient to reorder his own evaluation of the complex balance between the possible secondary gains derived from invalidism and the loss of his self-respect as a result of that invalidism.

Basic Strategies

The use of hypnosis to facilitate psychotherapy involves two basic strategies. The first strategy is to enhance the patient's control; the second is to uncover the material the patient has repressed.

Control Enhancement. Control enhancement is usually focused on symptom alteration or attitude alteration. These are essentially suppressive and containment operations, designed to increase the patient's control so that he can learn more effective ways of achieving the defined goals of his therapy.

Symptom alteration is direct guidance that diverts the patient's attention from his symptoms and reminds him that more resourceful and effective means are available for his use in coping with problems of adaptation. For example, an embarrassing exposed head tic may be converted to a hidden toe tic.

Attitude alteration presents the patient with an alternative attitude toward a chronic, recurrent disability or a pending problem-posing event. By invoking the power of compulsive compliance with the posthypnotic signal, it influences the patient to abandon old perspectives and adopt new ones in the service of more effective adaptation. For example, compulsive cigarette smoking can be stopped when the patient concentrates on his need to respect his body and to protect it from poison.

Uncovering Repressed Material. Uncovering what is repressed may be accomplished by simple abreaction or by more complex exploration of past events.

The release of repressed material can sometimes be provoked by design. Frequently, however, such material bursts through without an evocative signal from the therapist when the appropriate therapeutic atmosphere has been established. The sanctioned abandonment of the patient's executive control to the therapist may be sufficient to permit the release of highly charged affect. Often, just the opportunity for release provided by the treatment setting and the subsequent reconstitution of self-esteem are all that are needed for clinical success. For example, the battle casualty can re-enact the traumatic event, recall forgotten details, give vent to his fears and guilt, and discover that he can still live with honor.

Exploratory uncovering is the most subtle form of hypnotic intervention in psychotherapy. It makes use of hypermnesia and permits a piecemeal collection of presumably isolated data from the past. A remembered episode of being choked may reawaken old attitudes toward an older brother. When the connections and trends become apparent, an insight is permitted that frees the patient sufficiently to change toward health.

Precautions and Contraindications

Usually, the suspicious or paranoid patient avoids or resists efforts at hypnosis. Occasionally, however, such a patient may go into the trance state, only to have the experience evoke latent fears and suspicions that present a potential threat to the physical safety of the therapist. As a safeguard against this type of reaction, the hypnotist should pace the hypnotic intervention in accordance with the interests and desires of the patient, and he should never use coercive ploys. The patient needs the freedom to stop whenever he feels threatened by the interaction.

The sensitive, fragile patient who has already suffered many painful failures may have unrealistic expectations regarding the rewards to be derived from hypnosis. The probable failure may be so traumatic that the risk of disappointment is not clinically justifiable. However, with time and clarification, the patient's high expectations and the impact of disappointment may be attenuated and the experiment may be attempted with reasonable safety.

Generally, a hypnotized subject cannot be coerced into performing an action that violates his values and beliefs. However, during the time period necessary to discover the disparity between the patient's compulsion to comply with the therapist's signal and his resistance to it, he may feel confused and unable to exercise his best judgment. During this transient period, the patient may commit an act that is somewhat disparate with his usual conduct. Therefore, the therapist must assume a degree of responsibility for the patient. An explosive abreaction may require psychological restitutive measures. Therapist-induced explorations into amnesic realms of the past must be conducted in a disciplined manner within a designed treatment program.

When a therapist commits an error in a nonhypnotic setting, the patient who has ready access to his own faculties can critically judge and cope with the error to some extent. However, this capacity for critical appraisal is not readily available to the patient in a trance state, so correction of the error either is delayed or may not be made at all. The existence of such a possibility lends support to the contention that, as a general rule, intensive short-term insight therapy should be practiced only by experienced psychotherapists. Similarly, the risk of error emphasizes the needs to limit the general use of hypnosis to symptom and attitude alteration and to reserve the uncovering techniques for those clinicians who have been trained in the psychodynamics of intervention.

REFERENCES

Brenman, M., and Gill, M. M. *Hypnotherapy*. International Universities Press, New York. 1947.
Erikson, M. H. Hypnosis in medicine. Med. Clin. North Am., 28: 639, 1944.
Gill, M. M., and Brenman, M. *Hypnosis and Related States*. International Universities Press, New York, 1959.
Haley, J. *Strategies of Psychotherapy*. Grune & Stratton, New York. 1963.
Katz, R. L., Kao, C. K., Spiegel, H., and Katz, G. J. *Advances in Neurology*, vol. 4. Raven Press, New York, 1974.
Spiegel, H. An eye-roll test for hypnotizability. Am. J. Clin. Hypn., *18:* 26, 1972.
Spiegel, H. *A Manual for Hypnotic Induction Profile*. Soni Medica, New York, 1973.
Spiegel, H., and Shainess, N. Operational spectrum of psychotherapeutic process. Arch. Gen. Psychiatry, *9:* 477, 1963.

29.5   GROUP PSYCHOTHERAPY

Introduction

Group psychotherapy is a form of treatment in which carefully selected emotionally ill persons are placed into a group, guided by a trained therapist, for the purpose of helping one another effect personality change. By means of a variety of technical maneuvers and theoretical constructs, the leader uses the group members' interactions to bring about this change.

It is important to differentiate the new groups—encounter groups, T-groups, and sensitivity training groups—from traditional group psychotherapy. Only the psychotherapy group should be composed of members who are suffering from a variety of mental disorders.

A distinction should also be made between group psychotherapy and group management methods, which do not emphasize the salient features of the therapy group—careful screening and selection of patients, special organization of the group, limited size, skilled and specific leadership, and well-defined therapeutic goals.

Classifications

The types of group therapy can be compared and classified along a number of parameters: the population of which the group is composed, the particular group processes and mechanisms emphasized, leadership styles, theoretical frame-works, types of interaction, and specific goals to be achieved. At the present time there are such a great variety of approaches to the group method of treatment that none can be considered superior to the others. Most clinicians work within a psychoanalytically oriented frame of reference—Freudian or neo-Freudian. Recently, the transactional approach developed by Berne—in which greater emphasis is placed on the current interactions between members, the here and now approach—has become popular, as has the application of behavior therapy. And a group-centered psychotherapy, in which the therapist is nondirective and noninterpretive, has been introduced by Rogers. In Table I only the major group psychotherapeutic methods are outlined.

Role of the Therapist

Regardless of the makeup of the group, the group psychotherapist stands as the single most important group member. This position sometimes leads to patients' overreacting to his behavior or to their endowing him with magical abilities that he cannot live up to. The group leader must be knowledgeable about the causes and diagnosis of mental illness and in the varieties of treatment modalities available—not just the group method. Only then can he determine who can best benefit from group therapy.

In psychoanalytically oriented group psychotherpy the therapist traditionally plays a relatively passive role, acting as an all-accepting neutral screen onto which patients can project their thoughts and feelings. However, some workers advocate that the therapist involve himself actively and demonstrate his caring attitude by open interpretation and intervention when necessary.

Although there are differences in opinion regarding how active or passive a role the therapist should play, it is generally agreed that his role is primarily facilitative. Group members themselves should be the primary source of cure and change.

The therapist must exercise great skill and delicacy in helping the group to function productively without allowing himself to control the interaction. By promoting self-reliance, encouraging members to overcome resistance, and using social reinforcement, he can help patients gain in self-esteem and function effectively within the group. His direction of the group, although rarely obvious, is nonetheless firm.

Directive Role

The business of the therapy group is interaction, and one of the therapist's main functions is to see that this interaction takes place. He must help members focus on how they are dealing with one another and must explore possible reasons for lack of interpersonal contact between particular group members. As director, the therapist must also steer discussion away from irrelevant material and must help patients explore the connections between their past, present, and future.

Stimulative Role

The therapist must function as a catalyst for group interaction. When the group activity becomes nonproductive, he should stimulate discussion and be able to get the group moving again. Bringing up previously discussed issues, asking pertinent questions, and retracing earlier discussions are just a few of the ways for the leader to accomplish this.

Extensional Role

Sometimes group activity becomes bogged down on a particular point. The therapist elaborates on or adds to the theme at hand so as to open up the group to new psychological awareness.

Interpretive Role

When a particular patient is ready to accept certain insights, the therapist makes appropriate interpretations that help the patient change his maladaptive behavior. Timing is critical, since interpretation offered when the patient is not psychologically ready can often do more harm than good. Although group members are encouraged to offer interpretations to one another, the therapist may have to intervene with questions and explanations. The therapist may have to offer interpretations many times and in many different ways before the patient comes to understand his own faulty reactions.

Selection of Patients

Group psychotherapy cannot be applied as a blanket form of psychiatric treatment for all types of emotional disorders. Even if an accurate determination is made regarding a particular patient's suitability for group therapy, the success or failure of treatment may depend on the group into which he is placed. Whether or not a therapy-fostering group atmosphere is achieved often depends on the types of patients

TABLE I

Comparison of Different Types of Group Psychotherapy

Parameters	Supportive Group Therapy	Analytically Oriented Group Therapy	Psychoanalysis of Groups	Transactional Group Therapy	Behavioral Group Therapy
Frequency	Once a week	1 to 3 times a week	1 to 5 times a week	1 to 3 times a week	1 to 3 times a week
Duration	Up to 6 months	1 to 3 years	1 to 3 years	1 to 3 years	Up to 6 months
Primary indications	Psychotic and neurotic disorders, transient situational reactions	Neurotic disorders, borderline state	Neurotic disorders	Neurotic and psychotic disorders	Phobias, passivity, sexual problems
Individual screening interview	Usually	Always	Always	Usually	Usually
Communication content	Primarily environmental factors	Present and past life situations, intragroup and extragroup relationships	Primary past life experiences, intragroup relationships	Primary intragroup relationships; rarely, past history; here and now stressed	Specific symptoms without focus on causality
Transference	Positive transference encouraged to promote improved functioning	Positive and negative transference evoked and analyzed	Transference neurosis evoked and analyzed	Positive relationships fostered, negative feelings analyzed	Positive relationships fostered, no examination of transference
Dreams	Not analyzed	Analyzed frequently	Always analyzed and encouraged	Analyzed rarely	Not used
Dependency	Intragroup dependency encouraged; members rely on leader to great extent	Intragroup dependency encouraged, dependency on leader variable	Intragroup dependency encouraged, dependency on leader variable	Intragroup dependency encouraged, dependency on leader not encouraged	Intragroup dependency not encouraged; reliance on leader is high
Therapist activity	Strengthen existing defenses, active, give advice	Challenge defenses, active, give advice or personal response	Challenge defenses, passive, give no advice or personal response	Challenge defenses, active, give personal response rather than advice	Create new defenses, active and directive
Interpretation	No interpretation of unconscious conflict	Interpretation of unconscious conflict	Interpretation of unconscious conflict extensive	Interpretation of current behavioral patterns in the here and now	Not used
Major group processes	Universalization, reality testing	Cohesion, transference, reality testing	Transference, ventilation, catharsis, reality testing	Abreaction, reality testing	Cohesion, reinforcement, conditioning
Socialization outside group	Encouraged	Generally discouraged	Discouraged	Variable	Discouraged
Goals	Better adaptation to environment	Moderate reconstruction of personality dynamics	Extensive reconstruction of personality dynamics	Alteration of behavior through mechanism of conscious control	Relief of specific psychiatric symptom

n the group and on the therapist's style of leadership and theoretical orientation.

To determine a patient's suitability for group psychotherapy, the therapist needs a great deal of data that can be gathered only in individual sessions. In the screening interview, the psychiatrist should take a careful psychiatric history and give a mental status examination, so that he has certain dynamic, behavioral, and diagnostic factors in hand.

Dynamic Factors

Authority Anxiety. Those patients whose primary problem centers on their relationship to authority and who are extremely anxious in the presence of authority figures often do better in the group setting than in the dyadic setting. They gain support from the peer group and are thus aided in dealing with the therapist more realistically. Able to identify with others in the group who may have less difficulty in this area, they are eventually better able to perceive the therapist as less punitive or authoritarian than they had believed him to be. Adolescents generally manifest authority anxiety, and for this reason many workers see group psychotherapy as the treatment of choice for this age group.

Peer Anxiety. The patient who has destructive relationships with his peer group or who has been extremely isolated from peer group contact generally reacts negatively or with increased anxiety when placed in the group setting. For those patients whose nuclear problem is rooted in the sibling relationship, the group can provide the corrective emotional experience necessary for cure; but the psychiatrist must determine the patient's ability to tolerate the degree of discomfort that will be produced.

For the child who was raised without siblings, the group may produce anxiety because his central position is jeopardized—perhaps for the first time. Within the group these patients demand to have their narcissistic needs gratified by the therapist. But the group setting demands that sharing occur.

The central position that some only children cherish may be anathema to others who were deprived of peer interaction within the family unit. This reaction is especially common if the parents were harsh and punitive and the overwhelmed child longed for allies from whom he could derive support.

Behavioral Factors

Defense mechanisms are mental processes that a person uses to protect himself from consciously experiencing anxiety; they enable him to cope with a variety of internal and external stresses.

Projection. One of the positive indications for group psychotherapy is the finding that a patient uses the defense mechanism of projection, in which he attributes to others impulses that he finds unacceptable in himself. In the group setting, the other group members constantly confront such a patient with his distortions. Such group processes force introspective analysis to occur, and the projective mechanism is thereby eroded.

Repression, Denial, and Suppression. These defenses are characterized by the elimination from consciousness of all thoughts, feelings, memories, strivings, impulses, and other mental experiences that constitute a threat to one's self-image and the image he wishes others to have of him or her. Repression is similar to denial except that in denial it is external reality, rather than internal reality, that is transformed so as not to be painful. Suppression—not to be confused with repression, which occurs outside of the person's awareness—is a conscious attempt to withhold painful material.

Repression, denial, and suppression are particularly well-suited for examination in group psychotherapy. When one member recalls an event, other members recall repressed material. But should the repressed material enter consciousness before it can be assimilated effectively, the patient may be overwhelmed with intolerable anxiety. Suppression—the conscious witholding of information about oneself because of fear, anxiety, guilt, shame, or embarassment—is one of the mental processes attended to by the well-functioning psychotherapy group. In the group, a patient may reveal his most hidden secret only to realize that others harbor a similar thought, feeling, or life even. When denial is the major mental mechanism employed the group is not only able to correct the distortion but is capable of helping the patient examine a variety of ways in which he can cope with the situation more effectively.

Transference Reactions. One of the characteristics of all in-depth psychotherapies, particularly those that are psychoanalytically oriented, is a close examination of distortions in the feelings of the patient toward the therapist. Such transference examination rests on the premise that the patient reacts to the therapist in the same way that he reacted to significant figures in his past life, and, as this reaction is analyzed, emotional growth and development occur. But sometimes the transference is so intense that it cannot be analyzed in the one-to-one relationship.

Patients who are likely to develop a psychotic transferential reaction to the therapist are best placed in a group in addition to or in place of individual therapy. If the transference is negative, the patient has the opportunity to observe his or her co-patients' distinctly different reactions to the therapist. If the transference is positive, the group setting provides the opportunity for certain elements of the transference to be diluted.

Diagnostic Factors

The diagnosis of the patient's disorder is important in determining the best therapeutic approach and in evaluating his motivation for treatment, his capacity for change, and the strengths and weaknesses of his personality structure. Group psychotherapy has been conducted with patients in practically every diagnostic category. (See Table II for a comparison of group therapy with neurotics and psychotics.)

The diagnostic process routinely includes an extensive examination of the patient's chief complaint, a detailed evaluation of his past developmental history, and a review of his levels of functioning in various life areas—vocational, familial, social, marital, sexual. The mental status examination provides clues to the psychopathological processes at work currently, in the past, and under stress. It also helps predict the patient's characteristic response to stress. Diagnosis includes a variety of postulates about the psychodynamics and defense mechanisms involved, the causes of the patient's emotional disorder, and the desired goals to be achieved. In addition, no patient should be placed in psychotherapy for an emotional disorder without a physical examination to rule out the presence of an organic disease that may account for some if not all of the patient's symptoms.

Schizophrenia. The group experience can provide the schizophrenic patient with a thera-

peutic atmosphere that supports reality orientation and encourages him to relate to others so as to combat his feelings of fear and distrust. The group setting is geared to be socially supportive, and outside group contact has been advocated by some workers because, for many schizophrenic patients, the group provides their only socialization experience in an otherwise bleak and dreary existence.

Affective Disorders. Patients in this category have the least successful outcome in group psychotherapy. When depression is the major symptom and suicide represents a real risk, hospitalization is preferable to outpatient treatment of any kind. Placing the severely depressed patient, who requires a high degree of emotional support and nurturance, in a group as the first therapeutic intervention may aggravate his symptoms, since he is unable to receive sufficient nurturance from the leader. No severely depressed, suicidal patient should be placed in a new group on an outpatient basis without first having established a strong positive relationship with the therapist.

Manic patients are extremely difficult to manage in the group setting. They tend to display excessive elation, talkativeness, and irritability, traits that often antagonize both the group members and the leader, and they are given to accelerated speech and motor activity, which the group is often unable to control.

Paranoid States. Paranoid patients usually resist most forms of psychotherapy. When there is a risk that the patient will incorporate the group into his paranoid delusion, it is unlikely that effective reality testing will be possible. But when the patient is still capable of being influenced by the consensual validation of the group, group therapy may be quite effective and, in fact, superior to the one-to-one therapeutic situation. The paranoid's use of projection lends itself to accurate and effective interpretation by the group.

Neuroses. Most group psychotherapy approaches have been attempted with neurotics, and every category of neurosis has been treated with success. Psychoanalytically oriented group psychotherapy has been used with the majority of neurotic conditions, but recently phobic disorders have been treated with increasing success by means of behavioral group therapy. Generally, a depressed patient who does not require

TABLE II

Differences in Group Psychotherapy with Neurotics and with Psychotics*

Comparison Parameters	Neuroses	Psychoses
Indications	All neurotic diagnostic categories can be included; special care is needed with depressive neurosis and suicidal ideation.	Latent schizophrenia is most amenable to treatment, but all schizophrenias can be included; poor results are obtained with psychotic depressions, mania, and paranoia.
Composition	Patients are generally treated in groups that are homogeneous for neurotic traits, although one or two mild psychotics can be included.	Patients are treated in groups homogeneous for psychotic states.
Reality testing	Reality testing by the group as a whole is excellent; irrational attitudes are not prominent and are easily corrected when they do appear.	Reality testing by the group as a whole may be poor; delusions and hallucinations not subject to reality testing may appear.
Leadership	Less activity by the leader is necessary for effective group functioning; generally, less hostility toward the leader is expressed.	The leader is generally more active and directive; potential and actual hostility toward the leader is greater because of schizophrenic ambivalence.
Socialization	The group is little or no substitute for social experience and offers less direct gratification of emotional needs; outside social contact is usually discouraged.	The group may provide the only real social experience for the majority of patients; it offers more direct gratification of emotional needs; outside social contact may be encouraged.
Dependency	Members show little exclusive dependency on the leader, many peer transactions, great tendency toward autonomous functioning.	Members show great dependence on the leader; peer transactions need to be encouraged; autonomous functioning by the group as a whole is difficult to achieve.
Cohesiveness	Cohesiveness is generally high; members value the group and are more susceptible to group pressure than to therapist approval.	Cohesiveness is difficult to achieve; members may resent participation and devalue the group; they are more susceptible to therapist approval than to group pressure.
Standards	Group standards, such as confidentiality, are easily adhered to.	Group standards require repeated confirmation by the leader; they are not adhered to consistently.
Communication	Communication level is high, with members sharing experiences; mutual identifications among the members are easily made; patients do not feel completely alone.	Communication is inhibited, with little sharing of experiences; mutual identifications are not prevalent; patients tend to feel alone.
Associations	Associations of members may be centered on a single theme or group event.	Associations of members may have autistic qualities, not influenced by a group event or possessing a common theme.
Acting out	Group is more prone to sexual acting out than to aggressive acting out; expression of affect needs to be encouraged.	Group is more prone to aggressive acting out than to sexual acting out; expression of affect may have to be curbed.
Interpretation	Unconscious conflicts are accessible and can be interpreted accurately; dream interpretation of latent content is prevalent.	Accurate interpretations of unconscious conflicts may be suppressed by the leader; dream interpretation receives little emphasis.
Insight	Patients are able to accept and examine group behavior as a manifestation of intrapsychic conflict and are able to see connection to original family group.	Patients tend to project intrapsychic conflict and do not accept group behavior as related; they deny that behavior is a manifestation of original family group experiences.
Problem patients	Group monopolist is not common and is easily managed by patients; suicidal ideation is not prevalent; group tends to deal with crises effectively.	Monopolist is common and is poorly managed by members; suicidal ideation is common; members usually withdraw in crisis, and leader must exert control.
Goals	Goal is to achieve complete reconstruction of the dynamics of personality organization for the majority of patients.	Goal is to relieve specific psychiatric symptoms and to improve functioning in one or more areas for the majority of patients.

* Adapted from Max Day and Elvin Semrad in *Comprehensive Group Psychotherapy*, H. I. Kaplan and B. J. Sadock, editors. Williams & Wilkins, Baltimore, 1971.

hospitalization will do best in a group after he has established a warm, supportive relationship with the therapist.

Personality Disorders. Group psychotherapy is ideal for these patients because, when they display their characteristic behavioral patterns in the group, the members reflect back to the patient the effects of these patterns on his interpersonal relationships. These vigorous confrontations force the patient to examine his behavior. However, certain modifications in technique or frank contraindications to group treatment exist in the following subgroups.

Explosive Personality (Aggressive Personality). Patients who have explosive outbursts of physical or verbal aggressiveness often cannot control themselves and may represent a physical risk to the other group members, for whom the therapist is responsible. If there is a real danger that a patient will act out his aggressive impulses, he should not be included in a therapy group.

Schizoid Personality. Patients with schizoid personality are generally shy and oversensitive and avoid close or competitive relationships with others. There is a risk that more verbal, healthier patients will overshadow the schizoid member. Patients with schizoid personality require a supportive group milieu.

Passive-Aggressive Personality. In the passive pattern, the patient is unable to assert himself and assumes a role of chronic submissiveness and compliance. But beneath the unassuming facade may be a great deal of hostility and resentment. The group setting exposes the passivity to analysis by allowing the patient to become consciously aware of what he may have denied and rationalized previously. Group members confront him whenever he behaves too passively, and he is thus encouraged to become more outgoing and to react more spontaneously with a true expression of feelings.

In the aggressive pattern, the patient expresses angry feelings covertly by being stubborn, obstructionistic, or intentionally inefficient. The group usually reacts hostilely to these disguised expressions of anger, thus communicating to the patient the effects of his passive-aggressive behavior on others, but the group members also try to be of help, rather than overtly rejecting the patient, as usually happens outside the group.

Antisocial Personality. Antisocial persons are irresponsible and incapable of significant loyalty to individuals or groups. Unable to learn from experience, they are resistant to all forms of psychotherapy and may be particularly unsuited for group psychotherpay, since they do not constructively assimilate the interpretations made by other group members or by the therapist. Because of their inability to adhere to group standards of any sort, they are unable to maintain the confidentiality of the group, and for this reason, they may have to be excluded from group treatment.

Adolescent Disorders. The adolescent characteristically shows fluidity of behavior in his attempts to consolidate his identity. In addition, he often has a fear of authority. The group setting allows the adolescent to explore attitudes toward authority more effectively than does the one-to-one situation because in the group he has the support of his peers.

Other Disorders. Sexual orientation disturbances, transvestitism, voyeurism, alcoholism, drug dependence, psychosomatic illnesses, and such special symptoms as speech disturbance, deafness, and mental retardation are suitable for the group method of treatment. Patients suffering from any of these disorders may be placed in homogeneous groups, composed of patients with similar problems, or may be integrated into heterogeneous groups.

Structural Organization

Size

Group therapy has been successful with as few as 3 members and as many as 15, but most therapists consider 8 to 10 members optimal. With fewer members there may be too little interaction, unless they are especially verbal. With a larger group the interaction may be too great for the members or the therapist to follow.

At times the composition of the group may determine its size. If, for example, a group contains an extremely verbal, aggressive, dominating member, it may be necessary to increase the size to provide counterforces to offset the monopolist. A group composed primarily of withdrawn, schizoid members may require additional members to heighten the level of interaction.

Frequency of Sessions

Most group psychotherapists conduct group sessions once weekly. When alternate sessions are used, the group meets twice a week, once with the therapist and once without him.

At times it may be necessary to increase the frequency of sessions during a particular period and for specific reasons. A member of the group may be undergoing a life stress of such magnitude that he requires more frequent meetings of the group to provide him with support. Or the group as a whole may be in crisis—a member may have died, for example—and extra meetings are needed for the crisis to be worked through.

Length of Sessions

In general, group sessions last from 1 to 2 hours, with the average length being 1½ hours. The time limit set, however, should be constant. This limit allows the group to become aware of patterns that may be of significance—such as a particular member's always bringing up a topic meaningful to him just before the end of a session. For patients who have difficulty controlling impulses, the fixed length of the session serves as a model for the setting of limits. And the time limit can be reassuring for those patients who fear a loss of control.

In 1963 Bach and Stoller introduced the concept of time-extended therapy, in which the group meets continuously for 12 to 72 hours. The participants are pushed to a heightened level of emotional interaction by virtue of their enforced proximity for an extended period of time. Enforced interactional proximity and sleep deprivation produce a breakdown in certain ego defenses, release affective processes, and promote a less guarded type of communication. However, in time-extended groups—marathons, as they have come to be called—careful selection procedures are necessary to determine the capacity of the participants to deal with the increased affective tone of these groups and their ability to maintain cognitive thinking, which normally disintegrates when one is deprived of sleep.

Homogeneous Versus Heterogeneous Groups

Most therapists support the view that the group should be as heterogeneous as possible to ensure maximal interaction. Thus, the group should be composed of members from different categories of illness and with varied behavioral patterns; from all races, social levels, and educational backgrounds; and of various ages and both sexes.

Diagnostic Factors

Some borderline schizophrenic patients can be placed in groups with neurotic patients. The schizophrenic, who is more vulnerable to the evocation of unconscious processes, can provide the neurotic with the necessary stimulation to break through repressive barriers, which are more intact in neurotics. Conversely, the neurotic can provide a high degree of reality testing and support for those ego defenses that have become weakened in the schizophrenic.

Although it is not advisable to place the schizophrenic who suffers from delusions or hallucinations in a group made up of neurotics, such schizophrenic patients can be treated in group therapy. Delusional and hallucinating patients can help one another within the group setting. The delusional patient can provide effective reality testing for the hallucinating patient and vice versa. And patients with different delusions can challenge one another.

Dynamic Organization

If the oedipal conflict is used as a basis of organization, a patient who is competitive with his father can be placed in a group with a patient who competes with his son and a patient who was subject to an overprotective or seductive mother can be placed in a group with such a close-binding mother. Each patient should be the mirror image of another.

Behavioral Patterns

The patient whose lifestyle is marked by isolation, withdrawal, and a fear of close relationships should be exposed to a member whose lifestyle is marked by an extrovertive or pathologically outgoing personality organization. The patient who is helpless, indecisive, and overly dependent should be matched with one who is impulsive, quick to make decisions, and overly independent. Similarly, a patient dealing with the problems of leaving his parents' home can benefit from contact with one who is contemplating or who has successfully negotiated such a move. Patients who have experienced divorce or marriage can help others who are anxious about such life decisions.

Sexual Patterns

The group setting provides a unique opportunity for the patients and the therapist to learn whether a sexual problem is the result of faulty education or psychological problems or a combination of both. Group members who openly share accounts of their sexual activities are reassuring. Furthermore, the sharing of experience has an educational effect. The group should cover the broad range of sexual behavior as much as possible.

Men and women should be placed in the same group, so that attitudes toward sex can be examined more effectively. Even though there may be initial inhibitions to a frank and open discussion of sexual matters in the mixed group, such an exchange will eventually take place, and the anxieties attached to the interchange will be fruitfully examined. The mixed group also allows for a variety of familial surrogates—mother, father, brother, sister—and patients can more quickly gain insight into the way past relationships motivate present behavior toward the opposite sex.

In certain situations, such as homosexuality, the group may be organized unisexually. The homosexual's anxiety about discussing and examining the genesis and dynamics of his situation may be overwhelming if the other members of the group do not have a similar problem. The therapeutic goal—whether conversion to heterosexuality or better adaptation to homosexuality—also plays a part in determining whether to place the homosexual in a mixed group. In general, most heterosexually oriented groups are tolerant of deviant sexual behavior but tend to pressure the homosexual patient to change his orientation.

Socio-Economic Factors

Patients from different socio-economic levels can be integrated into the same group with salutary effects. If, for example, a patient who has achieved financial success but who is anxious about not having earned a college degree is placed in a group with a patient who is anxious about his limited financial means but who does have a college degree, one can predict the potential value of their interaction.

Racial, religious, and ethnic variations in group composition can also be used effectively. When this is done, it is desirable to include more than one member from any given background; two members with similar backgrounds provide mutual support and identification and

so enable each to tolerate the minority position. Early on, the therapist should make a statement to the effect that one of the group standards is to respect the differences between members.

Of particular relevance today is group work with the poor conducted by a middle-class therapist. Poor patients may feel the therapist cannot understand their situation, and sometimes this is so. The mutual support and understanding among group members help to close this cultural gap and aid the therapist in making distinctions.

Age

Patients between 20 and 50 can be effectively integrated into the same group. Age differences aid in the development of parent-child and brother-sister models.

In organizing the adult group, the therapist should be careful not to have only one member representative of the extreme age group. It is likely, for example, that a woman of 50 in a group of adults between 20 and 25 would be subject to a variety of transferential mother surrogate reactions on the part of the younger members. This situation may be intolerable and antitherapeutic if all the younger patients had mothers whom they despised.

Both the child and the adolescent are best treated in groups composed of patients in their own age group. Some adolescent patients are capable of assimilating the material of the adult group, regardless of content, but they should not be deprived of a constructive peer experience that they might otherwise not have. In addition, adolescents often have severe authority problems, which would increase their anxiety level in an adult group. With peers they are better able to express feelings toward the authority figure represented by the therapist and to find support from their co-patients.

Mechanisms

Developmental Phases

There have been a number of interpretations of the sequential development of a therapy group. One system differentiates three stages: (1) inclusion—the members' striving to be accepted and loved by the leader, (2) power—the members' attempting to gain autonomy from the leader, and (3) affection—the members' looking to one another for aid and both giving and receiving help.

Not every member is in the same developmental phase at the same time. For example, the patient whose major problem is oriented about his relationship to authority may immediately begin competing with the leader rather than seeking his approval. And the extremely dependent patient may be unwilling to leave the inclusion phase as others move on to more autonomous functioning.

Group Formation

Members may behave differently within the group from the way they behave individually outside the group. Each patient approaches the group initially in a way unique to him. But a process inherent in group formation requires that the patient suspend his previous ways of coping. In entering the group, he allows his executive ego functions—reality testing, adaptation to and mastery of the environment, and perception—to be taken over to some degree by the collective assessment provided by the total membership, including the leader. To do this, the patient must have developed a sense of basic trust and must feel that he is able to rely on the group as a whole.

Group Processes

Reality Testing. Reality testing—that is, objectively evaluating the world and being aware of oneself and others as they really are—is no easy task. The group setting serves as a reality-testing forum as each member verbalizes his thoughts and feelings toward the others and as these verbalizations are examined by the leader and the membership. When one member's perception of another is distorted, others in the group are able to bring their own observations to bear on the misperception. As a result, a constant assessment of reality takes place.

Transference. Freud originally defined transference as the unconscious attachment to others of feelings and attitudes toward important persons in the patient's early life, but it has become more loosely constructed to include feelings toward others of which the patient is consciously aware. The feelings evoked between members of the group and between members and the therapist are transferential when they are irrational and not consonant with reality.

Stimulation of Transference. As patients observe one another's interactions, feelings that may have been repressed or suppressed can emerge. In general, negative feelings are expressed sooner in the group setting than in the one-to-one situation. A group patient may be reassured as he observes the therapist's nonpunitive reaction to another patient's anger and so be willing to express similar feelings of which he may not have been aware.

Multiple Transference. A variety of group members may stand for the people significant in a particular patient's past or current life situation. He may see one co-patient as wife, another as mother, and others as father, sibling, and employer. The patient can then work through actual or fantasized conflicts with the surrogate figures to a successful resolution. Role-playing techniques make use of this concept extensively.

Collective Transference. A member's pathologically personifying the group into a single transferential figure, generally his mother or father, is a phenomenon unique to group therapy. Or he may see the therapist as one figure and the group as a whole as another. The collective transference may be either positive or negative in feeling tone. The therapist should be aware of this common reaction and, when it occurs, encourage the patient to respond to members as individuals and to differentiate them, one from the other, in order to work through this distortion.

Transference Neurosis. When a patient's transferential attachment to the therapist or to another patient becomes excessively strong, a transference neurosis is said to exist. Feelings toward the leader are diluted and lessened in intensity because of the presence of other members, who draw off many of the emotions that might otherwise be directed toward him. A co-patient may more nearly resemble the important figure in the patient's past life and so become a major transferential object.

Identification. In the group setting, various models are available, and a passive patient may identify with certain qualities of a more outgoing member, a process that may occur consciously by simple imitation or unconsciously, outside of awareness.

The sense of alienation is lost as patients develop feelings toward one another and toward the group as a whole. The group provides a sense of security, and a feeling of belonging develops. Members are tolerant of one another and attempt to understand varieties of behavior, regardless of how deviant they may be. This mechanism, acceptance, is therapeutic in that members realize there is an appropriate place for differences of opinion.

Universalization. In the group the patient recognizes that he is not alone in having an emotional problem and that others may be struggling with the same or similar problems. This process of universalization is one of the most important in group psychotherapy.

The mechanism of universality and its derivatives—support, altruism, advice giving, reassurance—are processes that continue throughout the life of the group. But premature, ill-timed, capricious advice that is based on distorted perceptions of the patient's situation or that he is unable to follow because it exceeds his capacities may be hazardous. Ideally, the patient should be able to formulate his own course of action, aided by different points of view.

Cohesion. Group members feel a sense of belonging. They value the group, which engenders loyalty and friendliness among them. They are willing to work together and to take responsibility for one another in achieving their common goals. They are also willing to endure a certain degree of frustration to maintain the group's integrity. A cohesive psychotherapy group is a group in which members are accepting and supportive and have meaningful relationships with one another. Cohesion is the single most important factor in group therapy.

At times, a group may become too cohesive. The participants may find such security with one another and find that their group activities give them such marked relief from anxiety that they lose the therapeutic goal of more independent functioning for each member.

Group Pressure. Every group member is susceptible to group pressures to alter his behavior, thinking, or feeling; how susceptible he is depends on how attracted he is to the other members of the group and how much he values his group membership. Whether the effects of group pressure are beneficial or harmful rests largely with the therapist's management of this

mechanism, a derivative of group cohesion.

Much of the effectiveness of the behavioral approach to group psychotherapy rests on the observation that a patient is motivated by the reinforcement of member and therapist approval to embark on a new behavioral pattern. Similar reinforcements, including environmental approval, motivate him to maintain that new pattern of behavior.

Intellectualization. This process implies a cognitive awareness of oneself, others, and the various life experiences that account for current functioning. Feedback, in which each member confronts the others with his immediate responses to events as they occur, serves as a learning device. Each member is helped thereby to evaluate his own defense mechanisms and ways of coping. Confrontation groups rely on this feedback mechanism extensively. Interpretation, a derivative of intellectualization, also provides the patient with a cognitive framework within which he can understand himself better, whether that interpretation comes from the therapist or other group members.

Intellectualization does not necessarily lead to change; experiential factors must be added if effective learning is to take place.

Ventilation and Catharsis. Ventilation is the open expression of one's innermost thoughts and secrets. Catharsis is the evocation of feeling tones and affects that may be attached to the ventilated thought or secret. Ventilation allows for the amelioration of guilt feelings and anxiety through confession and provides the group with important information about the patient's thoughts, fantasies, and problems. It also stimulates associations in other members.

Each group develops its own mix of ventilatory and cathartic processes, the mix depending on the composition of the group, the style of leadership, and the theoretical framework. A group composed primarily of members with poor impulse control is generally characterized by a heightened emotional tone. Conversely, a group composed primarily of obsessive-compulsive personalities tends to be restricted emotionally. For the impulsive group a leadership style that encourages catharsis may be antitherapeutic, but for the impulsive group it may be quite therapeutic.

Abreaction. Abreaction is the reliving of past events and the emotions associated with them;

it is a more heightened process than catharsis, in that the discharge of affect is greater. Moreover, it is associated with increased insight, since the patient is able to recognize the link between current irrational attitudes and previous emotional states. Abreaction also brings about an awareness, often for the first time, of degrees of emotion previously blocked from consciousness. It is often a highly therapeutic experience, even though it may produce an unavoidable sense of distress in all concerned as the process unfolds.

Techniques geared to release strong emotion must be well-timed and used only when the patient is well-integrated into a group capable of providing as much support as is necessary to allow the patient to pass through the abreacted experience. When the experience is not well-timed, psychological decompensation may occur.

Motor abreaction is the experiencing of an unconscious impulse through physical activity. Motor activity among patients in a group may heighten psychological awareness. For example, two members between whom the therapist has postulated unconscious competitive feelings can be made to experience these emotions by having them hand wrestle.

A vast array of techniques are available to aid in achieving motor abreaction. Falling backward into the arms of another member to elicit feelings related to trust, pounding a pillow to release unconscious aggressive impulses, and hand wrestling are only a few. The encounter movement has had a marked impact on traditional group therapy in the development of techniques for the release of repressed and suppressed emotions and for a heightened awareness of feeling tones. But, to be most effective, motor abreaction must be coupled with other processes, especially intellectualization and its derivatives, cognitive awareness, interpretation, and rationality.

Therapeutic Considerations

Most of the processes used in group therapy result, directly or indirectly, from a number of technical maneuvers available to the therapist working within a specific theoretical framework. The therapist must determine which group mechanism ought to be activated and then choose the technique to be used.

Dream Analysis

The techniques of dream interpretation used in individual therapy can be applied to the group setting with only minor changes. The associations come not only from the dreamer but from the other members as well. In addition, the other members can also give directions. The dream serves as a communication by the dreamer of material he might not otherwise be able to ventilate. Accordingly, it can be used to integrate an otherwise fearful member into the group.

Dream analysis is used primarily in groups that operate within a psychoanalytic framework. But other therapy approaches also use the dream. In Gestalt therapy the dream may be acted out, with different members taking different roles. The dreamer may himself take different parts while the other group members observe and comment. Other approaches, such as transactional and behavioral therapy, rarely use dream analysis.

Free Association

The process of free association occurs within the group as one member's thought or feeling is followed by another member's thought or feeling, which may or may not be logically related. The therapist does not direct the group but encourages spontaneity and a free-floating discussion. His task is to find a common theme in the various productions elicited, reflect these back to the group, and examine the way the theme applies to each member by eliciting further associations.

Go-Round

In this technique the therapist asks each member of the group to respond in turn to a specific thought, feeling, behavioral pattern, topic, or theme introduced by a patient or by the therapist himself. Since each member must participate and no one is allowed to withdraw, this technique can be especially valuable for the schizoid member, who might not otherwise contribute, and for the passive member, who might be too intimidated to do so. It also helps control the monopolist, who might otherwise dominate a session.

Co-Therapy

Ideally, in co-therapy each therapist becomes actively involved, so that neither is in a position of greater authority or dominance. Co-therapists of different sexes can stimulate the replication of parental surrogates in the group; if the two interact harmoniously, they can serve as a corrective emotional experience for the members. Even if the co-therapists are of the same sex, one often tends to be confrontative and interpretative and is seen as masculine, and the other tends to be evocative of feelings and is seen as feminine. Styles of leadership and the personality characteristics of the co-therapists, regardless of their gender, also elicit transferential reactions.

Co-therapists are able to observe more interactions than a single therapist can. They are also able to pick up blind spots in one another; therefore, their countertransference feelings are less apt to interfere with effective therapy. The co-therapy relationship should be amiable, but the two therapists need not hold to the same theoretic framework.

New Member

A new member may be welcomed and quickly integrated into a group, or he may be the object of overt or covert hostility, irrespective of his personality pattern. If the group welcomes him, the therapist need only examine the process of integration and its significance. If the other members are covertly hostile to the new member, ignoring him or discussing old themes or group events that he knows nothing about, the therapist must point out these hostile maneuvers and examine their significance. If the hostility is overt, the therapist's responsibility is to protect the new member from attack and to explore the causes of the hostility.

Acting Out

A patient may attempt to avoid tension through activity, usually sexual or aggressive. The action gratifies an impulse, and the patient feels relief. But the relief is temporary, providing no lasting solution to the conflicts that contribute to the patient's inability to delay gratification and tolerate frustration. Two people in a group may be sexually attracted to each other and may gratify the impulse by having extragroup activity, which may include sexual intercourse. But if this happens, motivating factors behind their attraction may be inaccessible for examination.

Most group therapists prohibit sexual or aggressive contact between patients. When such contact does occur, the therapist attempts to analyze its significance retrospectively. The atmosphere of the group should be such that sexual attractions and aggressive feelings can be ventilated openly, thereby providing the therapist and the members with the opportunity to make proper and timely interpretations.

Alternate Sessions

Alternate sessions are held without the therapist but are specifically organized by him, and all members are expected to attend. The time and place for the alternate sessions may be left up to the group. A variation of the alternate session is the aftersession, which differs only in that it takes place immediately after the session at which the therapist is present. The alternate session is generally held a few days after the regular session.

These procedures give the patients more time to get to know one another and to clarify and stimulate their interaction. The members become aware of variations in their behavior related to the presence or absence of the therapist. Their dependency on the therapist is lessened as reliance on one another is fostered. The alternate session also allows the members to compare feelings toward the therapist and to correct whatever distorted views they may have about him. The alternate session may be protective by enabling the group to recognize aberrant behavior on the part of the therapist.

Electronic Recordings

Both audio tape and video tape have been used extensively in group psychotherapy. Tapes can be stored and played back at a later date, allowing group members to observe change over a period of time. Patients may see themselves first hand on a television monitor while they interact, with dramatic effect on their insight into their own and one another's behavior.

Termination

The discharge of a patient from group therapy implies that goals have been achieved. Ideally, there should be consensual validation by the patient involved, the therapist, and the other members. The greater the divergence from such concensus, the greater is the likelihood that termination is premature.

Although discharge is the goal sought by all

the members, it is an event that may cause turmoil and upheaval. Some members become competitive with the departing member. Others are not able to tolerate the loss involved and may feel rejected and abandoned. Some react as if the discharged member had died, and they experience grief. For some members leaving the group, the vehicle that enabled them to achieve their goals and a healthier adaptation, there is also a sense of loss, and a complex array of emotions may be stimulated. Because of these complexities, the therapist should allow sufficient time, generally 2 to 3 months (8 to 12 sessions), for these various reactions to be explored, examined, and analyzed.

REFERENCES

Cartwright, D., and Zander, A. Group cohesiveness. In *Group Dynamics and Research and Theory.* D. Cartwright and A. Zander, editors, Harper & Row, New York, 1960.
Gottschalk, L. A., and Pattison, E. M. Psychiatric perspectives on T-groups and the laboratory movement. Am. J. Psychiatry, *126:* 823, 1969.
Kaplan, H. I., and Sadock, B. J., editors. *Comprehensive Group Psychotherapy.* Williams & Wilkins, Baltimore, 1971.
Moreno, J. L. *Who Shall Survive?* Beacon House, New York, 1953.
Sadock, B. J., and Kaplan, H. I. Long-term intensive group psychotherapy a part of residency training. Am. J. Psychiatry, *126:* 1138, 1970.
Stoller, F. H. Accelerated interaction. Int. J. Group Psychother., *18:* 244, 1968.
Whitehorn, J. C., and Betz, B. J. Further studies of the doctor as a crucial variable in the outcome of treatment with schizophrenic patients. Am. J. Psychiatry, *117:* 215, 1966.

29.6. COMBINED INDIVIDUAL AND GROUP PSYCHOTHERAPY

Introduction

In combined individual and group psychotherapy, the patient is seen individually by the therapist and also takes part in group sessions on a regular basis. The therapist for the group and individual sessions is usually the same. The patient sees the therapist on an individual basis anywhere from one to five times a week; group sessions are usually held once a week and may vary in length from 1 to 2 hours.

Combined therapy is a particular treatment modality. It is not a system by which individual therapy is augmented by an occasional group session, nor does it mean that a participant in group therapy meets alone with the therapist from time to time. Rather, it is an ongoing plan in which the group experience interacts meaningfully with the individual sessions, and there is reciprocal feedback that helps to form an integrated therapeutic experience.

Rationale

The human personality develops not only from genetically based constitutional determinants but also from the interaction of the child with a number of other persons—mother, father, teachers, friends, and siblings. The quality of these experiences determines the presence or absence of psychopathology. Although the one-to-one doctor-patient relationship allows for a deep examination of the transference reaction, it may not provide the corrective emotional experiences necessary for therapeutic change. The addition of the group situation provides the patient with a variety of persons toward whom transferential reactions can develop. In the microcosm of the group, the patient can relive and work through familial and other important influences in his life.

Formation of the Group

Heterogeneous groups tend to function more successfully than homogeneous ones, although an atmosphere of compatibility is necessary for interaction to take place. It is desirable for the group to contain both men and women, in equal numbers if possible, as well as a variety of ages and personality problems. Married couples should usually not be treated in the same group, although they may both be patients of the same therapist and may participate in separate groups.

Transference

Theoretically, the doctor-patient relationship and the distortions attached to it constitute the transference neurosis, and analysis of this state is the basis of all psychoanalytically oriented therapies. In combined therapy, the transference becomes more complicated because it is directed to the other patients as well as to the therapist. At times, the feelings the patient has toward the therapist may remain unconscious and be displaced onto a fellow group member. The opposite may also occur, with the patient able to express feelings only toward the therapist when realistically they ought to be directed toward a group member.

Whereas the group provides multiple transference models and thus elicits a wider range of reactions, individual therapy allows for a closer handling of transference and for more control of the situation. Transference should be worked out in the dyadic setting before the patient begins group psychotherapy, and each patient should be well aware of the nature of his transference.

Dyadic Setting

Much of the work in the dyadic setting consists of examining, in greater depth than is possible in the group, the thoughts and feelings the patient has toward his fellow group members. Most therapists hold these communications to be confidential, but they encourage the patient to be as open in the group as they are in the dyadic setting. In addition, individual sessions permit the emergence and examination of the transference neurosis, as in classical analysis. The one-to-one, doctor-patient relationship also allows for the easy introduction of a patient into a group for the first time. The presence of the known therapist is reassuring as the patient learns to deal with a group of strangers. The one-to-one setting permits the patient who is sensitive about certain subjects to discuss them in a more private setting. The dyadic relationship also gives the therapist an in-depth understanding of the patient. Whereas the group experience focuses on here-and-now responses, individual therapy is able to delve into the origins, meaning, and implications of these responses.

Group Setting

The group setting superimposes on the dyadic setting all the processes at work in therapy groups, such as support, imparting of information, ventilation, interaction, and reality testing. The patients in combined therapy have the unique distinction of all sharing the same therapist for individual sessions. Because group therapy, unlike individual therapy, is more like a real-life situation, the insights and emotional reactions that occur in the group take on new significance.

Therapeutic Process

There is a constant interplay between the group setting and the dyadic setting. In a general way, however, the group session focuses on the various defenses used by the patient, whereas the individual session examines the underlying psychic conflict against which the defense was erected in the first place. As the group processes erode a particular defense mechanism, the individual session may serve as a stabilizing force and prevent the patient's anxiety from reaching intolerable levels. Dream analysis, revelation of certain personal data, and deep interpretation are best suited to the individual sessions. Group members sometimes help one another out of personal crises, and, in many groups, members are available to one another for practical assistance in a variety of circumstances.

Resistance

In the group, patients see one another improve, they place pressure on one another to open themselves up for psychic exploration, and they confront each other with interpretations of resistant behavior. At one time or another, nearly all patients display resistant behavior in either group or individual therapy, manifested by stubborness, silence, unexcused absences, irrelevant filibusters, and the like.

Since resistance impedes therapeutic progress, it is important that it be analyzed. Group pressure is usually more effective than therapist pressure in breaking down resistance, but it is not without dangers. Too sudden or ill-timed breakthroughs can sometimes have disastrous effects. It is up to the therapist to guard against assaults that may strip away defenses at the wrong time or in the wrong way.

Insight

Just as resistance, which prevents insight, is lessened in combined psychotherapy, insight is frequently facilitated by the combined method. Insight is attained as the patient undergoes changes in both conceptualization and behavior. Formulated concepts can be explored in individual therapy, and experience can be formalized into concepts through the vehicle of group therapy. The group gives the patient opportunities to test and reinforce insights gained in individual therapy.

Interpretation

Interpretation may come from other group members as well as from the therapist. One of the tasks of the therapist is to evaluate the interpretations that are made by the members and place these interpretations in proper perspective. Although interpretation in group therapy is most effective when it comes from the group, the therapist must validate accurate interpretations and point out the inaccuracy of inaccurate ones.

Techniques

A variety of techniques, based on different theoretical frameworks, have been used with the combined therapy format. Such workers as Bieber, Stein, and Fried increase the frequency of the individual sessions to encourage the emergence of the transference neurosis. In the behavioral model, individual sessions are regularly scheduled but tend to be less frequent. Depending on the therapist's orientation, the patient may use the couch or a chair during the individual sessions.

Structured Interaction

Structured interactional group therapy developed by Harold I. Kaplan and Benjamin J. Sadock is based on strong leadership and a structured framework in which spontaneous interaction can take place. Since the therapist takes an active leadership role and is responsible for therapeutic maneuvers that control group interrelationships and interaction, it is imperative that he have sufficient knowledge of each individual patient's needs and emotional status. This kind of data can only be accumulated in the one-to-one setting. The dyadic setting also provides the therapist with a personal relationship with each individual patient, thus softening the image of authoritarianism that can result from his efforts to structure the activity of the group.

Confidentiality

Both group and individual psychotherapy are based on a cornerstone of trust, and confidentiality is one block in this structure. The patient must be assured that information he reveals or behavior he displays will not be discussed outside the therapeutic setting and that all material will be treated as strictly confidential.

REFERENCES

Bieber, T. B. Combined individual and group therapy. In *Comprehensive Group Psychotherapy*, H. I. Kaplan and B. J. Sadock, editors, p. 153. Williams & Wilkins, Baltimore, 1971.

Durkin, H. Relationship of transference to acting out. Am. J. Orthopsychiatry, *25:* 644, 1955.
Hulse, W. C. Transference, catharsis, insight, and reality-testing during concomitant individual and group psychotherapy. Int. J. Group Psychother., *5:* 45, 1955.
Kaplan, H. I., and Sadock, B. J., editors. *Comprehensive Group Psychotherapy*. Williams & Wilkins, Baltimore, 1971.
Kaplan, H. I., and Sadock, B. J. Structured interaction: A new technique in group psychotherapy. Am. J. Psychother., *31:* 418, 1971.
Stein, A. The nature of transference in combined therapy. Int. J. Group Psychother., *14:* 413, 1964.

29.7.   FAMILY THERAPY

Introduction

Definition

Family therapy is not a treatment method but a clinical orientation that includes many different therapeutic approaches. Having developed independently in different parts of the United States, each school of family therapy has different operations. Some family therapists continued with an individual orientation and theory of change and merely added more people in the interview room. Others made a radical shift and instituted entirely new procedures and new theories of change. What distinguishes the family approach from that of other therapy is the basic premise that the unit with the problem is not the single individual but two or more people. It is not that there is a patient with something wrong who is put under stress by other people, but that symptomatic behavior is a contract between two or more people. How to change such contracts is the focus of the many different family therapy approaches.

Approaches

Some forms of family therapy are spontaneous and unplanned with the therapist using interpretations and uncovering techniques. Other forms are carefully planned and the outcome is documented. Some therapists require that the whole family always come to each interview, while others are quite willing to interview individuals or sections of families. This reflects the fact that some family therapists are method oriented and others are problem oriented in the sense that they change their approach depending on the problem. In some approaches, the therapist is central and works hard in negotiating among family members, whereas in others the therapist focuses the family members on each other and may even spend most of the time out of the room behind a one-way mirror watching the family work by itself. Family therapy can range from being a happening to an occasion of planned directives. The focus can be on expressing emotions or on changing family structure.

Some family therapists work largely with the marriage as the fundamental dyad in the family or at least the nuclear family; others emphasize the importance of bringing in the network of extended kin and even friends and neighbors on the supposition that everyone in the system is involved. In multiple family therapy, a number of families are seen together in a large group. Of course, many family therapists change their approach over time as they find new ways of working. For example, Bowen shifted from hospitalizing the whole family to largely seeing individual family members to seeing couples or families in groups.

Family therapy sessions may range from the 45-minute hour to marathon sessions of many hours a day, as in Multiple Impact Family Therapy, which is geared to families who cannot attend regular sessions because of long distance travel problems. As family therapy has developed in Canada, in Latin America, and Europe, the number of different approaches tends to multiply.

Indications and Contraindications

When all therapy is considered from a family orientation, one cannot say that family therapy is indicated in one case and individual therapy in another. From the family point of view, individual therapy is, in fact, one way of intervening in a family. To interview a child alone and not see the parents is a way of doing therapy with a family, even if the therapist thinks he is engaged in individual therapy. To hospitalize an adolescent, whether the parents are interviewed or not, is a clinical intervention into a family. Therefore, the question is not when is family therapy indicated but when is it appropriate to interview one person and when to interview several people. For example, if a married couple is in crisis and violent, the first interview might better be individual until the groundwork is laid for seeing the family members together.

Family Theory

There is no comprehensive, coherent theory of family therapy; as with psychodynamic theory, more emphasis is placed on a theory of pathology than a theory of therapy. What characterizes a family orientation is the fact that the choice of who is to be the focus of diagnosis and therapy is made arbitrarily. An individual, a dyad, or a triad can be chosen. For example, the same problem can be regarded in the following ways:

1. Individual. A 10-year-old boy will not go outside the house alone, claiming to be afraid of dogs. From the individual point of view, he has a dog phobia. Inside him is a fear of dogs.

2. Dyad. If one notices the boy's mother is constantly with him because of this problem and that she has no interest in life except him and his fears, one can say that the unit with the problem is the dyad of mother-child. The fear of dogs helps to maintain an overinvolved relationship between mother and child.

3. Triad. If one observes the sequence between mother, father, and child, it becomes apparent that mother and father avoid each other except in relation to the son's problem. When mother and father have too much conflict, they make peace by consoling each other about the boy's fears. In the triadic view, the boy helps to hold the marriage together by having this problem.

Although these are ostensibly descriptions of the same problem, obviously the therapeutic intervention will be quite different in each case —helping a boy to get over his introjected fear of dogs, changing a mother-child relationship, or changing a triangulated child-parent relationship involve different interventions.

Terminology

The dyad is the smallest unit in family theory, and so most problem descriptions are of that unit or larger ones. To formulate a scientific description of these units is difficult, since there is no language for relationships and all terminology is based on individual characteristics. One can use the work "symptom" to mean the way one person responds to another, but the word carries a connotation of individual psychopathology. To speak of a depression, a phobia, a compulsion, or a psychotic episode as adaptive behavior involving several people leads to confusion; as originally developed, those terms were not meant to describe more than one person. Thus, traditional psychiatric diagnostic categories are not appropriate to family therapy. Equally inappropriate is the traditional intake procedure in which an individual is interviewed, given psychological tests, and classified. The appropriate intake procedure is to bring together all the people involved in the situation.

Natural Groups

By the term "family," many family therapists mean unit of several people but not necessarily blood relatives. Family therapy actually concerns itself with natural groups any relationship with a history and a future. A man can manifest symptoms in relation to his work if the people there are highly significant to him and he has long term patterns of behavior established with them. A child's disturbance may relate to the family or to school or to a conflict between home and school. The more disturbed the child, the more there is a replication of conflictual relationships in different settings. For example, a patient's psychotic episode on a hospital ward can be a response to a covert conflict between his therapist and ward administrator, as was pointed out as long ago as 1954. However, if the situation is examined more fully, it usually becomes clear that he is in a similar situation in a variety of contexts. At the same time he is responding to a covert conflict between his parents, he is also caught in a conflict between parents and hospital staff. When it was discovered that symptoms have a function in relation to other people, the total interpersonal context became part of the diagnosis of a psychiatric problem.

Theoretical Models

Because most family therapists were originally concerned with individuals, it was natural that theories about changing individuals would be adapted and expanded by the family therapy theoreticians. Just as therapists made interpretations to individuals to bring their unconscious ideas into awareness, they did so with whole families gathered together. In the early days, therapists would interpret the transference and help the family members to understand their unconscious dynamics. This approach changed when therapists shifted to

making interpretations to family members about how they were dealing with each other. Wives might be helped to understand, for example, that they were provoking their husbands, and if a wife objected to this interpretation she could be offered an interpretation about her resistance and transference involvement. Therapists also carried from individual therapy into family therapy the idea that if an individual expressed his feelings he would change. Therefore, early family therapists tried to encourage the expression of affect.

As family therapists gained more experience, they began to do therapy on the basis of new premises, ones that had not existed previously in individual therapy. One theoretical approach was based on the communication theory ideas that were developing as whole families were observed. In this approach, the therapist emphasized specificity and clarity of communication as a cause of therapeutic change because of the increased harmony and togetherness brought about. Another set of theories about change developed around the idea of differentiating people from one another. As it was recognized how intimately involved family members could be, therapy focused on shifting the family members toward more independence and autonomy. The goal was not to bring about family togetherness but disengagement.

Systems Theory and Structural Theory

As family therapy moved further from individual theory, the theoretical model that emerged as most characteristic of family therapy was one based on cybernetics. The concept of a system of repeating sequences limited by governors was proposed in the 1940's and began to influence the social sciences. It appeared in psychiatry with the recognition that change in one person could affect, sometimes adversely, another person in the family. From that point on, families began to be described as made up of people responding to one another in repeating ways so that the system was stable, as in any governed system. For example, if the father exceeds the limits of behavior within the system, the mother reacts, and if the mother introduces new behavior, the father reacts. Should the mother and father behave in ways that exceed the limits of the system, the child will react. Stability is maintained because the participants respond in "error activated" ways to any deviation from the habitual behavior within the system. When that habitual behavior includes psychiatric symptoms expressed by one or more family members, then the symptoms cannot change unless the behavior of the various family members change. Family therapy became a way of changing sequences of behavior among intimates in ongoing, ruled governed systems.

Although the cybernetic, or systems, model became the most popular one with family therapists, other theoretical dimensions are also important. One is the concept of family structure. All learning animals organize in hierarchies based on power and status. Family structure can be described in terms of hierarchy, and most family theorists argue that pathology expressed by an individual occurs when there is a confusion in a hierarchy or a violation of rules innate in hierarchical organizations. For example, if a mother sides consistently with child against father, she is breaching generation lines and so violating the rules of hierarchical structures. Similarily, if a grandmother consistently forms a coalition with a child against the child's mother, the levels of hierarchy in the organization are in confusion and the individuals will experience distress. These structural principles apply to other natural groups besides families. If a ward doctor consistently sides with a mental hospital patient against a psychiatric resident, a hierarchical confusion occurs and odd behavior will result.

This point of view does not assume that it is pathological for a mother occasionally to save a child from father's wrath. Coalitions form and change in any flexible system. It is the consistent, repeating, cross-generational coalitions that lead to distress, particularly when they are secret. The ward doctor who is constantly siding covertly with a patient against a resident is expressing a pathological situation, but this does not mean that it is pathological occasionally to protect a patient from a resident.

It is in relation to repetitive sequences that systems theory and structural theory come together. In a dynamic system, structure appears with the repetition of sequences. When one observes a person repeatedly telling another what to do and the other doing it, one concludes that there is a hierarchical structure with two people of different status. A hierarchical structure is shaped by the behavior of the people involved, and, insofar as the behavior is repetitive and redundant, it is an error-activated, governed system. If one person deviates from the repeating behavior, the other reacts against that deviation.

Pathological behavior appears when the repeating sequences simultaneously define two opposite hierarchies, or when the hierarchy is unstable because the behavior indicates one shape at one time and another at other times, as when parents sometimes take charge and at other times accept their child as an authority over them.

The following is an example of the repeating behavior in an abnormal system:

A mother and her 11-year-old boy are in an overinvolved relationship of mutual exasperation. The mother insists that the boy be more independent while simultaneously condemning him if he becomes so. The father is peripheral to the family, holding down two jobs and seldom at home. In the typical family sequence, the mother becomes overtaxed in dealing with her son, and in exasperation asks her husband for assistance and support. Her behavior defines the hierarchy as two parents dealing jointly together as authorities in relation to the child. The husband steps in to deal with the son, usually demanding from the son more independent behavior and less fear and dependence on his mother. When this occurs, the mother reacts and condemns that father for not understanding the son, shifting to a coalition with the son against the father. The father withdraws to the periphery. The mother has redefined the hierarchy as one in which she and her son have special status and the father is not to interfere. Later, in exasperation with the son, the mother will ask for support from the father. She defines them as two parents in charge of the child. The father begins to deal with the son or advise his wife how to deal with him, and the mother reacts against the father, indicating that he is not to interfere. Once again, the husband withdraws to the periphery. This sequence repeats itself endlessly and the hierarchy is undefined and confused. The homeostatic process prevents a clarification of the hierarchy or a resolution of symptomatic behavior.

Family Development

Besides a theory of systems and of hierarchical structure, there is a third dimension of family theory. A recent concern has been with the stages of family development over time. It is obvious that families change over the years as part of a natural process. As children mature and parents and grandparents age, coalition structures shift and the hierarchy changes. In the family life cycle, there is a major reversal of the hierarchical structure. Children shift from being taken care of by their parents to being peers of parents to taking care of parents in their old age. Some spontaneous change in families may be related to this developmental process over time; sometimes, therapy is given credit for a change that is a product of a natural process.

In summary, a comprehensive family theory, if developed, would have to include the homeostatic behavior of intimates, the nature of hierarchical structure, and developmental changes in the life cycle of natural groups. Family research has found a complication that makes the task of creating theory more difficult. Just as it was discovered that an individual behaves differently in different contexts, it has become apparent that families change in different contexts of observation. Family members can respond to each other in one way in a research setting and in another way in a therapy setting. To accumulate evidence in support of a hypothesis can be a problem when the data fluctuate with the circumstances under which they are gathered.

Theory of Therapeutic Change

Family theory, particularly homeostatic theory, has provided a model for explaining how a system remains unchanged. The clinical problem lies in providing a theory of how to bring change about. Granting that one needs a theory of how to stabilize a change when it is obtained in therapy, it is also necessary to theorize about how to start a change happening.

Two Major Approaches

In recent years, family therapy ideas have led to a concern with how to produce systematic changes in governed systems. Two major approaches characterize many diverse family therapies. In one approach, the therapist introduces a small change in the system and begins to amplify it. As this deviation from usual behavior is amplified, the entire system must go through a reorganization to adapt to the deviation. Thus, the system is changed. The other approach is just the opposite. A therapist forces a change in the family by introducing a crisis. To adapt to this new extreme situation, the family must reorganize.

For example, in a structure in which a grandmother joins in a coalition against the mother, the grandmother takes care of the grandchild while the mother withdraws. At a certain point, the grandmother insists that the mother take responsibility for the child. As the mother does so, the grandmother intrudes and insists that the mother does not know how to take care of the child or is irresponsible, and she takes over. The mother withdraws while the grandmother takes care of the grandchild. At another point, the grandmother insists that the mother take care of the child, and the sequence begins again. The hierarchy is confused because the grandmother is crossing generation lines and joining with a child against its mother. The goal of the therapy is to put the mother in charge of her child and the grandmother in an advisory capacity, dealing with the grandchild through the mother.

In this kind of situation, the goal can be achieved by a step-by-step process. The therapist can encourage the mother to take care of the child in one small area and restrain the grandmother from interfering in that area. As this change is accepted, it can be enlarged by having the mother deal with the child effectively in another small area while the grandmother is restrained. The therapist introduces a small deviation and then amplifies it, forcing the system to reorganize to adapt to the deviation.

In the crisis approach, the therapist might insist that for a period of 2 weeks the grandmother have full care of the grandchild while the mother does as she pleases. If the child misbehaves, the grandmother must deal with it. After 2 weeks of this burden, the therapist shifts to the opposite extreme. He insists that for the next 2 weeks the mother is to have full responsibility for the child. If the child misbehaves, the mother must deal with it. At the end of the second 2 weeks, the therapist has the family adopt an organization whereby the mother is primarily in charge and the grandmother is her adviser. (Often, the grandmother accepts this arrangement, since she is threatened with having full charge of the child if she does not.) To adapt to the crisis of an extreme change, the organization has had to shift.

Certain premises follow from conceiving of the problem of therapy as one of changing a governed, stable system. One premise is that change can most easily be accomplished if the family situation is unstable, which is often the case when a person with a problem first enters treatment. If the therapist intervenes actively at the beginning with a crisis approach, he takes advantage of the instability that led to the call for help. This approach is not feasible if the psychiatrist is functioning as an agent of social control and is stabilizing problem people for the community. If he uses drugs and custody to quiet a problem person or situation, or if he does extensive diagnosis, the problem sequence becomes stabilized and after that it is difficult to change.

The family systems view leads logically to the idea that therapy should be active and directive, but it also leads to a change in past ideas about therapeutic change. Since the problem is defined as changing the behavior of more than one person, focusing on insight and self-understanding, expressing affect, or exploring fantasies or the past is not relevant to therapy. Therapeutic change is defined as a shift in the interaction of intimates, including the interaction with the therapist. The therapist should not interview a person alone to help him understand his fantasies, but he can interview him alone to change the way he is dealing with an intimate.

Stages of Therapy

In the systems approach, whereby individual change is brought about by changing the system, therapy must proceed through stages. One cannot go directly from the problem situation to the structure that is the goal. For example, stages of therapy can be applied to the problem of an overinvolved mother and child, and peripheral father, with the boy expressing a symptom of a fear of dogs. In the first stage of the therapy, the therapist insists that the father deal with the child in relation to a dog while the mother withdraws from the scene. As father and child become more involved, the mother will become upset at being left out and will attempt to re-engage herself. If she is blocked off from dealing with the child, she will deal with the father, complaining about his neglect of her and lack of appreciation of her problems. The therapy then enters the next stage, in which the emphasis is on the married couple. The child is moved out to dealing with peers rather than parents. The hierarchy has been stabilized in a structure in which parents are together in relation to child. If the marriage issues are resolved and the marriage is stabilized, the therapist can leave the system with the problem solved.

Therapist Coalitions

In the systems approach, a crucial problem for a therapist is the way he becomes part of the coalition patterns in families. A fundamental rule in family therapy is that one should not *consistently* side with any one member or part of a family against any other. If this happens, therapy has a poor outcome. To be helplessly caught in coalitions is a therapeutic misfortune. For example, when a therapist involuntarily and without plan attempts to rescue a child from his parents, he has formed a coalition with the child against the parents. Often, he is duplicating a family situation whereby someone of higher status, such as a grandmother, attempts to rescue the child from the parents. Thus, he is not introducing change but stabilizing an abnormal structural pattern. Similarly, to side consistently with a wife against a husband or with parents against in-laws can lead to a poor outcome.

As one observes therapists at work, it becomes evident how difficult it is for a therapist not to join one faction of a family against another as he becomes personally involved. For example, if the therapist is young he tends to side with adolescents against parents. There is a generational pull that he can hardly resist. If the therapist is older and having problems with his own children, he may side with parents against their problem child. These coalitions are formed even if the therapist is not interviewing the whole family. The therapist who hospitalizes and medicates an adolescent is aligning himself with the family faction that presents the child as the problem even if he has never met the family.

A further premise of the systems view is that the therapeutic milieu can replicate the problem situations of patients. For example, a child can become disturbed if the mother and grandmother are in a struggle in which they use the child in their conflict. Yet, a "child" can also be disturbed if a psychiatric resident and his supervisor are in a struggle in which they use the patient in their conflict. Should the supervisor attempt to rescue the patient from a resident he considers incompetent or too emotionally involved, and the resident attempt to save the patient from the supervisor, who is too in-human, a typical family pattern is being repro-duced that consistently leads to symptoms.

From a systems view, the interaction of a psychiatric staff becomes as important as the interaction of family members. If a resident is assigned a patient for intensive individual therapy while a social worker sees the parents, each professional can respond with conflictual territorial struggles that replicate the behavior in a problem family. Unlike other therapeutic modalities, the family view requires a contextual view of the problem in that everyone involved must be considered as part of the problem situation.

REFERENCES

Glick, I., and Haley, J. *Family Therapy Research: An Annotated Bibliography.* Grune & Stratton, New York, 1971.
Haley, J. *Uncommon Therapy.* W. W. Norton, New York, 1973.
Jackson, D. D. The question of family homeostasis. Psychia-try *31* (Suppl.): 79, 1957.
Minuchin, S., and Montalvo, B. Techniques for working with disorganized low socioeconomic families. Am. J. Orthopsy-chiatry, *37:* 880, 1967.
Pittman, F. S., Langsley, D. G., Flomenhaft, K., DeYoung, C. D., and Machotka, I. Therapy techniques of the family treatment unit. In *Changing Families*, J. Haley, editor. Grune & Stratton, New York, 1971.
Speck, R. V., and Attneave, C. *Retribalization and Healing.* Pantheon Books, New York, 1973.

29.8.   MARITAL THERAPY

Introduction

Marital therapy is designed to modify psy-chologically the interaction of two married peo-ple who are in conflict with one another along one or a variety of parameters—social, emotion-al, sexual, economic. Marital therapy is a form of psychotherapy in that a trained person estab-lishes a professional contract with the patient-couple and, through definite types of communi-cation, attempts to alleviate the disturbance, reverse or change maladaptive patterns of be-havior, and encourage personality growth and development.

Marriage counseling may be considered more limited in scope than marital therapy in that only a particular conflict related to the immedi-ate concerns of the family is discussed. Or marriage counseling may be primarily task-ori-ented, geared to solving a specific problem, such as child rearing. In marriage therapy, there is a greater emphasis on restructuring the interac-tion between the couple, including, at times, an exploration of the psychodynamics of each of the partners. Both therapy and counseling place emphasis on helping the marital partners to cope more effectively with their problems. Most important is the definition of appropriate and realistic goals, which may involve extensive reconstruction of the union, problem-solving approaches, or a combination of both.

Types of Therapy

Individual Therapy

Marital partners may be seen by different therapists, who may not necessarily com-municate with one another. Indeed, they may not even know one another. Treatment in these situations is individually oriented, with the goal being to strengthen the adaptive capacities of each partner. At times, only one of the partners is in treatment; in such cases a visit by the spouse who is not in treatment with the thera-pist may be of value. The visiting partner may provide the therapist with data about the pa-tient that may otherwise be overlooked; overt or covert anxiety in the visiting partner as a result of change in the patient can be identified and dealt with; irrational beliefs about treat-ment events can be corrected; and attempts by the partner to consciously or unconsciously sabotage the treatment of the patient can be examined.

Individual Marital Therapy

This form of treatment involves each of the marriage partners in therapy. When the same therapist conducts the treatment, it is called *concurrent* therapy; when one therapist sees one of the partners and a different therapist the other, it is called *collaborative* therapy.

Conjoint Therapy

Conjoint therapy is the treatment of partners in joint sessions conducted by either one or two therapists; it is the most common treatment method used in marital therapy. Co-therapy with therapists of both sexes working with a couple prevents a particular patient from feeling ganged up on when confronted by two members of the opposite sex.

Four-Way Session

In this approach each partner is seen by a different therapist, with regular joint sessions in which all four participate. A variation of the four-way session is the round-table interview, developed by Masters and Johnson for the rapid treatment of sexually dysfunctional couples. Two patients and two opposite-sex therapists meet regularly.

Group Psychotherapy

Therapy for married couples placed in a group, usually three to four couples and one or two therapists, allows for a variety of group dynamics to exert their effects on the married units involved. The couples identify with one another and recognize that others have similar problems; each gains support and empathy from fellow group members of the same or opposite sex; they explore sexual attitudes and have the opportunity to gain new information from their peer group; each receives specific feedback about his or her behavior, either negative or positive, that may have more meaning and be better assimilated coming from a more neutral nonspouse member.

When only one partner is in a therapy group, the other spouse may visit the group on occasion, so as to allow the members to test reality more effectively. At times, a group may be so organized that only one married couple is part of the larger group.

Combined Therapy

Combined therapy refers to any or all of the above described techniques used concurrently or in combination. Thus, a particular patient-couple may begin treatment with one or both partners in individual psychotherapy, continue to conjoint therapy with his or her partner, and terminate therapy after a course of treatment in a married couples group. The rationale for combined therapy is that no single approach to marital problems has been demonstrated as superior to another. Familiarity with a variety of approaches allows the therapist a degree of flexibility that will provide maximum benefit for the couple in distress.

Indications

Regardless of the specific therapeutic technique used, certain guidelines for starting marital therapy are agreed on: when methods of individual therapy have failed to resolve the marital difficulties or would be likely to fail because of insufficient motivation, when the onset of distress in one or both partners clearly relates to marital events, and when marital therapy is requested by a couple in conflict and unable to resolve it.

Problems in communication between partners are a prime indication for marital therapy. In such instances, one spouse may be intimidated by the other, may react with anxiety when attempting to tell the other about thoughts or feelings, or may project onto the other unconscious expectations. The therapy is geared to enable each of the partners to see the other realistically.

Conflicts in one or several areas, such as the partners' sexual life, are indications for treatment. Similarly, difficulty in establishing satisfactory roles in the social, economic, parental, or emotional area is an indication for help. The clinician should evaluate all aspects of the marital relationship before attempting to treat only one problem, which may be a symptom of a more pervasive marital disorder.

Contraindications

Contraindications for marital therapy include patients with severe forms of psychosis, particularly those with paranoid elements and patients in whom the homeostatic mechanism of the marriage is a protection against psychosis; one or both of the partners really wants to get a divorce; one spouse refuses to participate because of anxiety or fear.

Models of Therapy

Psychoanalytic Model

Marital therapy based on psychoanalytic principles assumes that conscious and unconscious feelings exist between the spouses and that these feelings are based on the past familial experiences of each. The therapist sees marital conflict emerging from unfulfilled infantile expectations that one or both partners hope the other will gratify. In therapy, these strivings are interpreted, as are the various transferences made by the partners toward the therapist.

Behavioral Model

In therapy based on learning theory, particularly operant conditioning, the therapist shapes the behavior of each of the spouses in such a way that destructive patterns are replaced by constructive patterns. As behavior changes, a reciprocal reward system is established between the partners and between the partners and the therapist, who, by his approval or disapproval, reinforces healthy interaction.

Client-Centered Model

This approach, based on the work of Carl Rogers, helps the couple clarify their own thinking and feelings. The therapist follows the lead of the patients and does not introduce material based on a preconceived scheme, other than the basic assumption that the client possesses the ability to improve.

Transactional Model

In therapy based on the theories of Eric Berne, the therapist examines the transactions between the spouses as they occur in the here-and-now. A determination is made about whether the patient is acting as parent, child, or adult—different ego states assumed at various times. The therapist provides the couple with active feedback about their interactions as they occur.

Systems Theory Model

Derived from general systems theory, this model sees the marital unit as a system in equilibrium. Disequilibrium is equivalent to discomfort and produces stress, which is felt by the partners. The role of the therapist is to monitor the emotional forces from moment to moment as they unfold through the interactions of the couple. Therapy is geared to modify whatever tension states exist.

Eclectic Model

This model requires that the therapist be able to take the best of a variety of schools and apply them where applicable. Accordingly, the therapist may be a participant-observer at one mo-

ment—active, forthright, open—and a passive observer of the couple's interaction the next. If a psychoanalytic interpretation is called for, it is made. If, on the other hand, a didactic presentation of sexual technique or child-rearing practices is required, that is given.

Goals

Ackerman has defined the aims of marital therapy as follows: "The goals of therapy for marital disorders are to alleviate emotional distress and disability and to promote the levels of well-being of both together and of each partner as an individual. In a general way, the therapist moves toward these goals by strengthening the shared resources for problem-solving; encouraging the substitution of more adequate controls and defenses for pathogenic ones; enhancing immunity against the disintegrative effects of emotional upset; enhancing the complementarity of the relationship; and promoting the growth of the relationship and of each partner as an individual."

Included in the therapeutic task is the notion that each partner in the marriage must take responsibility in attempting to understand the psychodynamic makeup of his or her personality. Accountability for the effects of behavior on one's own life, the life of the spouse, and the lives of others in the environment is emphasized. This emphasis often results in a deeper understanding of the problems that created marital discord and in a working through of individual psychopathology.

Marital therapy does not ensure the maintenance of any marriage. In certain instances it may show the partners that they are in a nonviable union that should be dissolved.

REFERENCES

Ackerman, N. W. *The Psychodynamics of Family Life.* Basic Books, New York, 1958.
Ackerman, N. W. *Treating the Troubled Family*, p. 114. Basic Books, New York, 1966.
Bowen, M. Family therapy and family group therapy. In *Comprehensive Group Psychotherapy*, H. I. Kaplan and B. J. Sadock, editors, p. 384. Williams & Wilkins, Baltimore, 1971.
Lidz, T. *The Person.* Basic Books, p. 411. New York, 1968.
Papanek, H. Group psychotherapy with married couples. In *Comprehensive Group Psychotherapy*, H. I. Kaplan and B. J. Sadock, editors, p. 691. Williams & Wilkins, Baltimore, 1971.

29.9.   PSYCHODRAMA

Introduction

Psychodrama is primarily a form of group psychotherapy that involves a structured, directed, and dramatized acting out of the patient's personal and emotional problems and his immediate group interaction problems. Originally promulgated by Moreno (Figure 1), it has been modified by him and by others, using different psychological (Jungian, Pavlovian, hypnotic) and psychoanalytic (Freudian) theories.

Psychodrama is based on the underlying principle that dramatic psychotherapy permits greater depth and breadth of awareness than is obtainable through merely verbal means. It includes such procedures as catharsis, abreaction, free association in acting, and encounters between persons. Interpretations may be used but are not often needed. The goal is not only insight but spontaneity, total perception of unhealthy responses, a more accurate perception of reality, involvement with other persons, and learning through experiencing.

Elements of Psychodrama

The Group. The group—the audience and the participants—must be moved toward acting out through a warm-up, which may take one of three forms: (1) the cluster warm-up, in which different discussion groups merge into a single predominant one; (2) the association warm-up, in which a chain of ideas leads to a final theme; and (3) the directed warm-up, in which an already familiar topic is introduced for portrayal.

The Protagonist (Figure 2). The acting subject, the patient, must be motivated by some need, such as relief from anxiety or frustration in a real-life situation. Resistances to participation may be due to private fears, social or ethnic conflicts, or symbolic problems.

The Director. The director or therapist leads the production in accordance with clues provided by the patient, instructing all the performers as to their roles. His own role varies with the dramatic situation; he must constantly change his role to bring out and correct the patient's maladaptive patterns. The relationship between the patient and therapist is not only transferential but also telic: The patient has a direct, primary, intuitive feeling about the immediate behavior of the therapist.

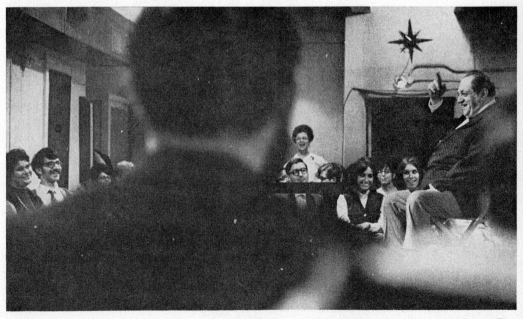

FIGURE 1. Illustration of psychodrama session conducted by J. L. Moreno, at right. (Courtesy of George Zimbel.)

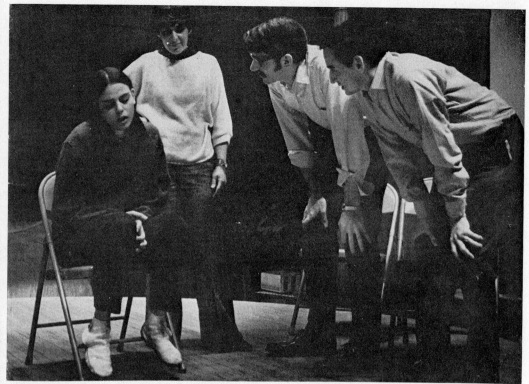

FIGURE 2. The protagonist on the chair is in a mood of depression. Multiple doubles, standing, represent various aspects of her personality. The double establishes identity with the protagonist by moving, acting, and behaving like her. (Courtesy of George Zimbel.)

Auxiliary Egos. Auxiliary egos are other persons in the group who act out the roles assigned to them by the director in order to intensify the impact or clarify the meaning of the therapeutic situation. These persons represent the patient's perceptions of the significant people in his environment.

Techniques

The drama may focus on a special area of functioning such as a delusion or hallucination, or on a dream, a family or community situation (Figure 2), a symbolic role, an unconscious attitude, or an imagined future situation. Techniques to advance therapeutic progress, productivity, and creativity include the soliloquy (a recital of overt and hidden thoughts and feelings), role reversal (the exchange by the patient of his role for the role of a significant person), the double (an auxiliary ego acting like the patient), the multiple double (several egos acting as the patient did on different occasions), and the mirror technique (an ego imitating the patient and speaking for him when he cannot

act for himself). Other modifying techniques include the use of hypnosis, barbiturates, alcohol, or stimulants to modify the acting behavior in various ways.

REFERENCES

Enneis, J. M. The hypnodramatic technique. *Int. J. Group Psychother.* *3:* 11, 1950.
Moreno, J. L. *Psychodrama.* Beacon House, New York, 1945.
Moreno, J. L. Philosophy of the third psychiatric revolution, with special emphasis on group psychotherapy and psychodrama. *Progr. Psychother.* *1:* 24, 1956.
Moreno, J. L. Psychodrama. In *Comprehensive Group Psychotherapy,* H. I. Kaplan and B. J. Sadock, editors. Williams & Wilkins, Baltimore, 1971.
Yablonsky, L., and Enneis, J. M. Psychodrama theory and practice. *Progr. Psychother.* *1:* 149, 1956.

29.10.   RECENT METHODS OF PSYCHOTHERAPY

Introduction

Techniques of psychotherapy are not designed on the drawing board, nor do they originate in the philosopher's armchair; they are typically the creation of clinicians concerned with practical problems. The goal of psychotherapy—mental health—is relative to the culture, and it embodies rules of conduct, moral values, and cultural norms to a significant extent.

There has been a profound disenchantment with the traditional model of individual, intensive, long-term psychoanalytic psychotherapy that evolved from the teachings of Freud and his successors. Criticisms have been leveled at its inordinate length, cost, questionable effectiveness, relative unavailability to the less affluent members of society, and alleged general obsolescence. This disillusionment refers to the psychoanalytic model of a human as an instinct-ridden being who must be socialized, molded, and adapted to prevailing social conditions in order to mature. The model is similarly criticized for its idealization of reason and rationality as the guiding forces in a person's search for salvation in a civilized society; its preoccupation with the past at the expense of experiences in the here-and-now; its advocacy of individuality, liberalism, achievement, productivity, acceptance of existential loneliness, the finiteness of human existence, and pragmatic acquiecence in the social status quo.

A major counter trend discernible in several of the newer systems of psychotherapy is their thoroughgoing anti-intellectualism and their large-scale abandonment of traditional social values. Their emphasis rests on experience in the here-and-now, the supremacy of experience for the sake of experience regardless of its long-range consequences, the group as a vehicle and goal of relatedness, and the wholesale rejection of reason and contemplation as viable forces in solving human problems. Although this trend is most clearly exemplified by encounter groups and the so-called humanistic forms of psychotherapy, it is also embodied in some of the approaches described here (for example, primal therapy and Gestalt therapy), and it is undoubtedly a part of their current popularity and appeal.

Almost all the founders of the therapies examined here have either implied or flatly stated that ours is a sick society that inevitably produces neurotic or psychotic persons. Janov (primal therapy), Perls (Gestalt therapy), and Berne (transactional analysis) paint the picture of the inherently healthy child tormented and twisted into bizarre molds of conduct and thought by powerful cultural influences and social figures, usually parents. Janov suggests that therapy should be a process of returning to the moment this burden was accepted, denouncing it, rejecting it, and abandoning the imposed sense of responsibility to others. Perls exhorts man to labor against the influences of a society that makes him deaf to his own needs and slave to its unnatural demands. Berne invokes the pitiful scene of the child striving for order in a threatening world, adopting legends and fantasies as reality, and struggling to protect his private myth from chaos. Assuming that the human being is innately healthy and strong, these authors suggest that the unnatural order of his social existence stymies his healthy growth and grinds him into the miserable dust of mental illness. Repeatedly, it is a twisted sense of moral responsibility to others that is proclaimed the villain of the drama.

At odds with this view are Glasser and Frankl, who argue that a failing sense of moral responsibility to others is the chief cause of current distress. Reflecting the influence of his practice with juvenile delinquents, Glasser makes this the explicit theme of his therapy. However, Glasser's failure to examine the meaning of responsibility in any modern context has deprived the notion of substance. It remains for Frankl to examine consciously the philosophical and psychological import of a person's sense of responsibility to something other than himself. However, Frankl's excursion into existentialism gives his system a philosophical, if not mystical, air that is suspect in a profession dominated by logical positivist doctrine. Nonetheless, Frankl vividly demonstrates the fact that the contemporary therapist must be prepared to examine his own culture and come to grips with those features of it that uniquely contribute to the distress he confronts in his patients each day.

Frank distinguishes the following common, nonspecific factors in the psychotherapeutic influence: (1) an intense, emotionally charged, confiding relationship with a helping person, (2) a rationale or myth that includes an explanation of the cause of the patient's distress and that indirectly strengthens the patient's confidence in the therapist, (3) provision of new information concerning the nature and sources of the patient's problems and possible alternative ways of dealing with them, (4) strengthening the patient's expectations of help through the personal qualities of the therapist, (5) provision of success experiences, that further heighten the patient's hope and enhance his sense of mastery and interpersonal competence, and (6) facilitation of emotional arousal.

At one extreme, the common ingredients may account for the most substantial part of change, with specific techniques—such as role playing, interpretations, abreaction, and primal screaming—playing only an insignificant role. At the other extreme, specific techniques may greatly overshadow effects attributable to the nonspecific features of the patient-therapist relationship.

Primal Therapy

Primal therapy is the creation of the psychologist Arthur Janov. He relates that he stumbled onto the basic technique of primal therapy when he asked a patient in group therapy to repeatedly cry out "Mommy" and "Daddy." As the patient did so, he became increasingly emotional and his body began to twitch and be shaken by minor convulsions; he than gave out a jolting scream of agony. Afterward, he claimed he had regained his ability to feel. Proceeding to use the technique with other patients, Janov found that it consistently led to a piercing scream that was followed by insights. Janov applied variations of the technique to more and more patients and generated a theory to explain the phenomenon.

Theory

Primal theory asserts that neurosis is the result of failure to satisfy basic infantile needs. If the environment does not allow direct gratification of these basic needs, the person substitutes symbolic—that is, neurotic—means of gratification. A critical juncture is reached when the child realizes that his needs for love and acceptance will never be adequately met. Although this experience may derive from an event that is minor in itself, it is the most shattering, destructive experience in the neurotic's life and the bedrock of his disorder. This crucial event, referred to as the major primal scene, triggers the complete repression of the real self with its basic needs and the emergence of an unreal self, presumably acceptable to others, which becomes the neurotic's facade.

The infant's instinctive defense against life-threatening pain is the separation of feeling from consciousness, a separation that Janov calls the split. According to him, each denial of basic needs results in cumulative pain, the sum of all pains experienced forming the primal pool. Separated from consciousness, the repressed pain manifests itself in physiological tension, the major characteristic of neurosis. In therapy, efforts are made to reverse the neurotic process by forcing the patient to re-experience and integrate the repressed primal pain.

Technique

The patient undergoes a physical examination; he then provides the therapist with a written life history and other information relevant to his problems. If he is selected for therapy, he must comply with an elaborate set of instructions (for example, isolation in a hotel room for 48 hours before the initial appointment) aimed at softening up his defenses. Therapy thus begins with the patient in a state of heightened frustration, which is designed to facilitate violent overthrow of his defenses, seen as the major task of therapy.

Primal therapy itself consists of 3 weeks of intensive individual therapy, each session lasting until the patient is exhausted and calls for a halt. The setting is a quiet, darkened room, in which the patient lies on a couch in a spreadeagle position to enhance feelings of defenselessness. The therapist tries to identify such salient defense mechanisms as intellectualizing and instructs the patient not to use them. When the patient expresses a strong feeling, the therapist orders him to give in to it, to let it overtake him. Early childhood experiences and feelings are emphasized, and the patient is encouraged to re-enact specific scenes. Resulting pre-primals are eventually followed by overwhelming pain and the reinstatement of forgotten memories (the full primal). The primal is a totally engulfing experience, in which the patient may assume the fetal position and use baby talk.

At the end of the period of intensive individual therapy, the patient enters group therapy on an outpatient basis for 8 months. Patients, without apparent awareness of their surroundings, engage in their respective primal experiences. At the end of a group session, the patients describe their feelings during the primals and explore how these feelings lead to neurotic behavior.

Most patients are reported to be well at the end of about 8 months. Primals become more infrequent, and pain is experienced directly, without help or instruction. Neurotic patterns are said to end, and old habits no longer have appeal. The patient is said to become a real person, seemingly more content with himself and less dominated by unconscious needs.

Comment

Primal therapy is clearly an outgrowth of traditional psychodynamic therapy. It seeks to uproot basic traumas by direct and frontal attack on the patient's defenses. The weight of the therapeutic effort is borne by abreaction and catharsis.

Although Janov is undoubtedly operating with powerful psychological mechanisms, his assertions flatly contradict and deny clinical observations made by legions of clinicians. His approach represents a gross oversimplification.

The evidence of therapeutic results rest predominantly on testimonials from former patients. The controlled studies cited by Janov are based on highly questionable assumptions and inadequate experimental designs.

Transactional Analysis

Transactional analysis evolved from the work of Eric Berne, a Canadian-born psychiatrist with psychoanalytic training. Revolting against the alleged complexity and elitism of professional psychotherapy, Berne undertook to establish therapeutic procedures that, presented in layman's terms, would be simple to understand and apply.

Theory

Berne postulated that the human personality is composed of three ego states—Parent, Adult, and Child—which are coherent organizations of intellect and emotion. The Parent ego state consists of introjected parental values and admonitions; the Adult ego state evaluates the demands of the environment objectively, although it can be influenced by the other two ego states; the Child ego state is the spontaneous, childlike component of the personality. Any given behavior reflects the ego state in control of the personality. Criticism and orthodoxy are associated with the Parent; unemotional calcu-

lation of the reward potentials of possible behaviors is associated with the Adult; and irrational fear, inferiority, and joy are associated with the Child.

The influence of these ego states is witnessed in the communicative exchanges between people called transactions. Since transactions take place between individual ego states, there is always the potential for complementary transactions (the ego state addressed replies) or crossed transactions (an ego state other than the one addressed replies). When complementary transactions take place, communication may continue indefinitely, but it abruptly halts after crossed transactions. Transactions may occur simultaneously on overt and covert levels; an ostensible Adult-to-Adult transaction may hide a more important Child-to-Child transaction. Intrinsic to the nature of transactions is the inclusion of rewards or payoffs for their use; whatever the form of a transaction, each party receives a payoff of some sort. Games are transactions that include covert and overt exchanges and afford the players well-defined payoffs.

Currently, increasing emphasis is placed on analysis of lifescript, a preconscious organization of one's entire life, laid down in childhood, that dictates how a person will feel about himself and interact with others. The lifescript reflects one of four possible introjected self-judgments: (1) I'm O.K. and you're (that is, others are) O.K., (2) I'm not O.K., but you are, (3) you're not O.K., but I am, or (4) neither of us is O.K. Such feelings, which reflect parental evaluation of the infant, are said to form the basis of how the child will experience his life.

Technique

Most commonly, indoctrination in the principles of transactional analysis theory is the first step in the treatment of neurotic disorders. During initial interviews, the therapist listens carefully for verbal cues to the patient's lifescript and points out the role of the ego states in the patient's interactions with the therapist and with others. After a potent level of rapport has been attained, the therapist may attempt to explicate the entire lifescript for the patient and instruct him in constructing another that is more reality-oriented and more suitable to the patient's needs. At all points, the therapist resists becoming involved in the games that typify the neurotic's frustrating interactions with others, while pointing out to the patient that such games are not only self-defeating but unnecessary. No attempt is made to destroy the different ego states—indeed, this is considered impossible—or to castigate their function; however, the therapist does attempt to protect the patient from the authoritarian demands of the Parent or the impulsive actions of the Child, while attempting to maximize the influence of the Adult. The patient may also become involved in group therapy sessions in which the therapist intervenes at certain points to map out the nature of the transactions among the patients, pointing out how they reflect neurotic lifescript patterns or the emergence of more productive modes of interaction.

Comment

Although Berne has inveighed against elitism and vague jargon in psychotherapy, the everyday words and phrases used in transactional analysis have meanings no less esoteric than those associated with terms used in other therapies. The therapist's active involvement with the patient is hardly unique; and, despite pleas for egalitarianism, the patient is still confronted by the therapist, still told what is wrong with him and what to do about it.

Although Berne had a gift for startling insights into the nuances of social exchanges, the theoretical underpinnings of his approach are weak. A human being is more than a social manipulator; emotional well-being is more than introjected feelings of self-worth. If the patient is destined to follow his lifescript, how can he almost arbitrarily drop it and choose another one?

As is true of most forms of psychotherapy, evidence for the efficacy of transactional analysis techniques rests primarily on case histories, which raise more questions than they answer. For example, to what extent does the adoption of a new lifescript simply reflect the influence of the patient's trust in the therapist? What are the personality characteristics considered prerequisite for therapeutic change? If humans are so addicted to games, what evidence is there that therapy itself is not simply a game? By this reasoning, transactional analysis therapy may be no more than a process of learning powerful strategies of social manipulation and subtle ways to use them.

There are compelling parallels between transactional analysis theory and psychoanalytic theory (the ego states, for example). The perpetuation of characteristic modes of interactions with others, in which Berne finds evidence for the lifescript, can be explained just as easily in terms of reinforcement theories. Finally, it is not evident that transactional analysis achieves unique results with a broad spectrum of the patient population. On the contrary, it requires patients who are mildly disturbed, well-integrated, and socially aware.

Gestalt Therapy

The evolution of Gestalt therapy is closely associated with the work of F. S. Perls (See Figure 1.), a European émigré trained in the psychoanalytic tradition. Although acknowledging its influence, Perls largely rejected the tenets of psychoanalysis and founded his own school of therapy, borrowing the name "Gestalt" from Gestalt psychology, an influential school of thought in academic psychology whose exponents advocated holistic analysis of psychological phenomena, asserting that the whole, rather than being determined by its parts, determines the meaning of the parts.

Theory

Gestalt theory proposes that the natural course of biological and psychological development of the organism entails a full awareness of physical sensations and psychological needs. Such awareness is said to trigger inherent tendencies of the organism to organize its behavior in a manner leading to the fulfillment of needs and the appropriate expression of affect—for example, hunger leads to eating, anger to aggression. When a need is satisfactorily met or an emotion satisfactorily expressed, it is essentially destroyed, allowing other needs and sensations to dominate the field of awareness. This process leads to proper biological and psychological adjustment to the environment, but any interference with it damages the holistic nature of organismic functioning and may threaten the healthy survival of the organism.

Repression is considered the most common form of interference with the process of adjusting to the environment. An inevitable by-product of civilized existence, repression is said to effect a split in the personality, resulting in neurotic anxiety. Because repression mech-

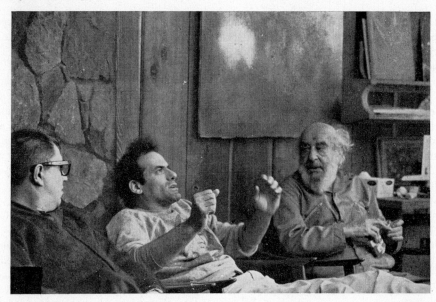

FIGURE 1. Fritz Perls, at right, conducting a group session in which feeling tones are emphasized. (Courtesy of Michel Alexander.)

anisms are typically immune from overthrow by intellectual means, the therapeutic effort must stress sensorimotor awareness and the physical expression or acting out of repressed desires.

Technique

The therapist takes an active role in the encounter, seeking to find perceptual blocks that blind the patient to his real feelings and forcing him to attend to psychological and physical stimuli in his environment that he had previously blocked out. Concentrated effort is focused on actual behaviors executed during therapy.

Group work may be either an adjunct or a substitute for individual therapy. Emphasis rests on actions in the present and on direct expression of needs and feelings. The therapist takes an active role, insisting that the exchanges among group members faithfully reflect their true feelings about each other. The patient may be prevented from slipping into stereotyped social roles that allow him to remain unaware of his feelings by role reversal, such as having a shy patient boast of his accomplishments, or by having him participate with others in an elaborate stage production representing a rehearsal of how he will act in particular social situations.

Comment

Gestalt therapy makes significant use of psychoanalytic teachings while seeking to overcome the heavy emphasis on verbal expression in the secrecy of the analytical chamber. The insistence that the direct experiencing of emotion in the present forms the bedrock of all therapeutic change is well-taken, although hardly original. Many Gestalt techniques, although quite ingenious and therapeutically valuable, have a gimmicky quality. There is an absence of clearly formulated therapeutic goals, with the result that Gestalt therapy does not appear to be an orderly process.

No significant efforts have been made to assess the therapeutic outcomes of Gestalt therapy, and most therapists who work within the Gestalt tradition have shown little inclination to subject the method to objective study.

Reality Therapy

Reality therapy is associated with the work of the American psychiatrist William Glasser. His objections to conventional therapy are: (1) Conventional categories of mental illness and efforts to treat patients in accordance with them are useless. (2) Probing the past for insights into present behavior is futile. (3) Reliving the past in the context of the transference has scant therapeutic value. (4) Insight and understanding of unconscious conflicts do not lead to behavior change. (5) Conventional psychiatry actively avoids the problem of morality. (6) Conventional therapy fails to teach the patient better behavior, resting its hopes on insight and understanding that, in some vague way, are expected to result in behavior change.

Glasser's basic premise is that all persons in need of psychotherapeutic help deny reality and are unable to fulfill their essential needs. Basic needs relevant to psychiatry are the need to love and be loved and to be worthwhile to others and oneself. Responsibility, another key concept of reality therapy, is defined as the ability to fulfill one's needs and to do so in a way that does not deprive others of the ability to fulfill their needs.

Essentially, responsibility is taught through love and discipline. In significant respects, the psychotherapist is not different from the parent or teacher who is responsible, tough, human, and sensitive and who cares, sets an example, demonstrates, and instructs. Glasser stresses the importance of therapeutic involvement, a major task that may take a long time. Once involvement has occurred, the therapist mediates the crucial lesson that the patient is responsible for his behavior. The patient begins to assume this responsibility when he becomes convinced that he is involved with a responsible therapist. A growing sense of self-worth is concomitant with the patient's efforts to become responsible for his behavior. The goal of therapy is not happiness but the acceptance of reality and the willingness to struggle with it in a responsible way.

Reality therapy has deep roots in religious teachings over the centuries, and it echoes the precepts of moral therapy popular in the nineteenth century. One of the most articulate spokesmen for this position is O. H. Mowrer, who, like Glasser, became deeply disenchanted with the teachings of psychoanalysis—in particular, its ethical neutrality. The task of therapy is to exhort the patient to recognize the evil of his ways, to conform to prevailing moral standards, and to go and sin no more.

Neurotic and psychotic patients do suffer from guilt, avoid facing reality, and have abdicated responsibility for important personal decisions and the conduct of their lives. However, they frequently do so for a variety of reasons, including the fact that their efforts toward independence, mastery, and interpersonal competence have frequently been discouraged and thwarted by significant persons in their early lives. Glasser's statement that "People do not act irresponsibly because they are 'ill'; they are 'ill' because they act irresponsibly," denies the history of dynamic psychology of almost 100 years and constitutes a throwback to a primitive view of human conduct and its mainsprings.

Glasser's emphasis on the therapist's genuine involvement, the need for autonomy and independence on the patient's part, and specific behaviors is forward-looking and cognate with contemporary developments in psychotherapy. Another positive contribution is his willingness to focus serious therapeutic effort on such patients as adolescent delinquents, who have traditionally been considered rather unpromising candidates for psychotherapy.

Rational-Emotive Psychotherapy

This form of psychotherapy, developed by the psychologist Albert Ellis, grew out of the originator's practice as a psychoanalyst. In significant respects, it reflects Ellis' dissatisfaction with the slowness, tedium, and indirectness of traditional psychoanalytic practices. Rational-emotive therapy seeks to confront neurotic conflicts in a straightforward and direct manner, thus undermining and uprooting their irrational and illogical bases. By short-circuiting the slow process of working through, rational-emotive therapy mounts a frontal attack on core conflicts, rather than permitting them to emerge slowly and haltingly. The therapist's stance is that of an unquestioned expert and authority who is in charge of the change process at all times. Emotional disturbances, according to Ellis, are the end product of irrational or illogical thinking. The patient continually indoctrinates himself with phrases and sentences that become his thoughts and emotions, thus governing his behavior. The task of therapy is to make these phrases and sentences explicit, to confront the patient with their irrationality, and thereby to force him to abandon them. This objective is accomplished by the therapist's active and direct interventions. The patient must learn to oppose actively the irrational ideas that continue to beset him and to combat them on his own. Therapy, therefore, is merely the beginning, albeit an auspicious one, of a battle the patient must wage throughout life.

Rational-emotive therapy appears to be most suitable for patients who are not severely disturbed, who have a fairly high level of intelligence, and who have sufficient inner strength to take active steps in directing their destiny. Shyness, nonassertiveness in social situations, phobic avoidance reactions, marital problems, and fears surrounding sexual situations are prime conditions.

In assigning prominence to the erosion of illogical beliefs and attitudes through the power of reason, Ellis underestimates the therapist's directiveness, which is focused on persuading, indoctrinating, and encouraging the patient in ways the therapist deems appropriate and desirable.

Logotherapy

Developed by Victor E. Frankl, a Viennese psychiatrist whose early training was in the psychoanalytic tradition, logotherapy reflects the influence of existential philosophers. According to Frankl, today's psychotherapist is increasingly confronted with patients whose basic source of discomfort and unhappiness is traceable to their inability to find meaning in their lives. Frankl describes this situation as an existential vacuum, a significant symptom of which is boredom. People often become acutely aware of the lack of content of their lives, which they seek to combat by a frantic search for pleasure through superficial sexual encounters and other means. Frankl castigates dynamic psychology and psychoanalysis for failing to recognize and respond to the patient's existential problems.

The ultimate task of psychotherapy, as Frankl sees it, is to come to grips with the patient's existential frustration and to aid him in his search for meaning. He must become conscious and responsible, and he must discover and develop the meaning of his own idiosyncratic existence. In accordance with existential teachings, he must realize himself by recognizing his human destiny, including the inevitability of suffering and death. Psychotherapy must always be concerned with the total person,

never with isolated symptoms or maladaptations. Logotherapy is not meant to replace psychotherapy in the traditional sense; instead, it is described as a supplement stressing the spiritual dimension of human existence.

As therapy progresses, the patient learns that the goal of human aspirations is not pleasure, happiness, or enjoyment—a lesson the therapist conveys through patience, reasoning, and demonstration; rather, it is the infusion of life with meaning, a task the patient must undertake himself and for which he must assume responsibility. As the patient succeeds in ceasing to blame the past and as he takes charge of his own destiny, he achieves freedom and self-realization. Love, the intimate community of oneself with another, and creative work are seen as supreme values. Above all, the patient must become responsible and active.

Frankl's approach is implemented by two specific techniques, paradoxical intention and dereflection. Frankl argues that, if the neurotic deliberately attempts to bring about the events he fears, he will come to recognize the unrealistic nature of his anxiety as the feared consequences fail to eventuate. Dereflection refers to the process of changing the center of attention from oneself to some external goal.

Although weak in technique, logotherapy has added a dimension to traditional psychotherapy—the emphasis on spiritual nature and the meaning of human existence. Logotherapy has forcefully called attention to philosophical problems and the question of meaning that are undeniably a part of all psychotherapeutic work. Its range of applicability is restricted to persons with reasonable intelligence who are not severely impaired in their day-to-day functioning and whose general outlook on life includes a reflective bent that makes them receptive to searching self-examination.

Direct Analysis

This method of psychotherapy, designed primarily to treat acutely ill schizophrenic patients, was developed by the psychiatrist John N. Rosen. Based on fundamental psychoanalytic principles, direct analysis is primarily a total-push approach intended to combat the patient's terror in acute schizophrenic episodes. To accomplish this end, Rosen directly interprets the symbolic meanings of the patient's unconscious conflicts as they manifest themselves in his current illness. Commensurate with the patient's desperate state, Rosen will stay with the patient for many hours, rapidly build rapport, and push through to the core conflict as it emerges from the patient's verbalizations, gestures, and symptomatic acts.

Rosen typically treats his patients outside the hospital setting, usually in the context of a therapeutic community of former patients and assistants, often graduate students and others with whom Rosen has developed close and trusting interpersonal relationships.

Rosen has been criticized for an undue emphasis on the acute phase of the patient's illness and neglect of the long-term characterological aspects of the treatment program. Efforts to assess the therapeutic effectiveness of direct analysis have produced equivocal results. Nevertheless, Rosen deserves credit for adapting psychoanalytic insights to specific exigencies.

Short-Term Psychotherapy

In recent years, the mental health professions have shown considerable interest in time-limited forms of psychotherapy and crisis intervention. Exemplifying this trend is the form of brief psychotherapy developed by Peter Sifneos, an American psychiatrist who has pioneered in developing a focused, problem-solving approach to brief psychotherapy. His approach is based on psychoanalytic principles. He distinguished two forms of brief psychotherapy, anxiety-provoking and anxiety-suppressive. The former came to occupy the focus of his attention. It is a goal-oriented form of psychotherapy that typically lasts from 2 months to 1 year, with an average of 4 months.

Patient Selection

Patient selection is crucial in Sifneos' brief psychotherapy. The patient must be of above-average intelligence, as demonstrated by work or educational achievement; he must have had at least one meaningful relationship with another person during his lifetime; he must be flexible, capable of expressing some affect, and able to interact with the therapist; he must have a specific chief complaint; he must be motivated to work hard during his treatment and have fairly realistic expectations of what

can be achieved. Motivation for psychotherapy is perhaps the single most important prerequisite.

Technique

The patient typically meets with the therapist in weekly face-to-face interviews. The therapist, relying on the patient's motivation and positive attitude, encourages the rapid development of rapport and a productive working alliance that serves as a major therapeutic tool. With focus resting on circumscribed emotional conflicts underlying the patient's symptoms, character traits such as masochism, excessive passivity, and dependence are deliberately bypassed. Relying and capitalizing on the patient's personality assets and adaptive resources, the therapist fosters active problem solving in the areas previously identified as targets for therapy. To this end, confrontation and anxiety-provoking questions are used to mobilize the patient's emotions and to enable him to become aware of his feelings. As the patient learns to master his conflict, he gains strength, competence, and increasing self-reliance. This process is undergirded by the quality of the therapeutic relationship, which also promotes a growing identification with the therapist. Therapy terminates when the patient has mastered the circumscribed problem.

Results

In several studies, Sifneos has used questionnaires, follow-up interviews, and a controlled design to assess treatment outcomes. Although the samples were relatively small and the designs were lacking in rigor, the results are clearly encouraging. Symptom changes were less impressive than other gains derived from therapy. Becoming aware of salient aspects of one's emotional difficulties and being able to talk about them was clearly a factor in the patient's sense of achievement, competence, and mastery. Sifneos regards the patient's growing identification with the therapist as another salient factor in this process. He also recognizes that the patient's initial determination to change clearly played a part.

Comment

Sifneos' short-term psychotherapy exemplifies an important contemporary trend that will undoubtedly gain increasing momentum in the next decade. Brief psychotherapy based on psychoanalytic principles effectively draws on the patient's inner resources and uses to therapeutic advantage those forces within the patient and the therapeutic relationship on which change ultimately hinges in all forms of psychotherapy. Among its major virtues are a realistic appraisal of what is therapeutically possible in a given instance, a clear formulation of therapeutic goals that are sharply kept in focus throughout the course of treatment, and a careful selection of candidates that renders this therapeutic approach feasible.

EST

EST stands for Erhard Seminars Training developed by Werner Erhard from California. It consists of attempts to change behavior by using certain consciousness altering techniques such as the evoking of strong emotional states and abreaction in groups. It uses a combination of encounter, zen, positive thinking, gestalt, Taoism and other approaches which contribute to an eclectic amalgam that is of questionable value regarding long-term beneficial effects.

REFERENCES

Bergin, A. E., and Strupp, H. H. *Changing Frontiers in the Science of Psychotherapy.* Aldine-Atherton, Chicago, 1972.

Brown, P., editor. *Radical Psychology.* Harper & Row, New York, 1973.

Frank, J. Therapeutic factors in psychotherapy. Am. J. Psychother., *25:* 350, 1971.

Patterson, C. H. *Theories of Counseling and Psychotherapy.* Harper & Row, New York, 1973.

Shapiro, A. D., Placebo effects in medicine, psychotherapy, and psychoanalysis. In *Handbook of Psychotherapy and Behavior Change,* A. E. Bergin and S. L. Garfield, editors. John Wiley, New York, 1971.

30

Organic Therapies

30.1. ANTIPSYCHOTIC DRUGS (MAJOR TRANQUILIZERS)

Introduction

Antipsychotic drugs are known also as the *major* tranquilizers, as represented by chlorpromazine. Although chlorpromazine does not usually produce a permanent cure in schizophrenia, it does benefit greatly many patients in a way no treatment ever did before. Previously, many mental hospitals had been primarily custodial in character. The fact that clinically significant therapeutic effects could be produced by a drug created an atmosphere that emphasized positive treatment and led to the vigorous application of milieu therapy, psychotherapy, group therapy, and occupational therapy. Some patients were helped so much that they were able to remain out of the hospital and function in the community. Other patients were discharged to nursing homes or halfway houses. For those remaining in the mental hospital, the hospital became a more humane place. The changes have resulted in a massive reduction in the number of hospitalized schizophrenic patients, a finding all the more remarkable because, up to the introduction of the new drugs, there had been a steady increase in the hospitalized mental patient census (see Figure 1).

Classification

The major classes of antipsychotic drugs are as follows: phenothiazines, butyrophenones, thioxanthenes, dibenzoxapines, dihydroindolones, and rauwolfia alkaloids (see Tables I and II). Unlike many drugs commonly used in psychiatry these agents have little or no abuse potential and are thus not classified as controlled substances. Table III outlines the characteristics of drugs at each Drug Enforcement Administration control level.

Efficacy

Chlorpromazine and the other antipsychotic drugs have now been studied in hundreds of double-blind studies, the results of which are summarized in Table IV. The vast majority of these studies indicate that antipsychotics are superior to placebos in the treatment of acute and chronic schizophrenic patients. In some of the smaller studies, the dosage was too low to show an effect, but, when adequate doses were administered, chlorpromazine was quite consistently proved to be superior to a placebo (see Table V). The phenothiazines both prevent the emergence of new psychotic symptoms and suppress pre-existing symptoms of schizophrenia.

For the average patient, most of the therapeutic gain occurs in the first 6 weeks of phenothiazine therapy, although further treatment gains are made during the subsequent 12 or 18 weeks. Phenothiazine therapy brings about a cognitive restoration, with a decrease in psychotic thinking, projection, suspiciousness, perplexity, and ideas of reference and a normalization of psychomotor behavior in both retarded and hyperactive patients. There is a reduction of both fundamental symptoms of schizophrenia—such as thought disorder, blunted affect, indifference, withdrawal, retardation, psychotic behavior, and mannerisms—and accessory symptoms—such as hallucinations, paranoid identification, hostility, belligerence, resistiveness, and uncooperativeness.

Comparative Effects

With the exception of promazine, all the phenothiazine drugs are clearly superior to a placebo. Comparisons against chlorpromazine

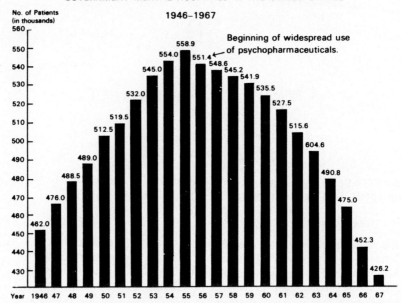

NUMBER OF RESIDENT PATIENTS IN STATE AND LOCAL
GOVERNMENT MENTAL HOSPITALS IN THE UNITED STATES

FIGURE 1. Population of public mental hospitals in the United States, 1946–1967. Note the progressive decline in the number of patients beginning in 1956, corresponding to the widespread introduction of the phenothiazines followed shortly thereafter by other psychoactive agents. Based on data from United States Public Health Service.

in control trials found promazine clearly inferior to chlorpromazine. All the other antipsychotic agents were equal to chlorpromazine in therapeutic efficacy. Some control trials did not include chlorpromazine as a comparison group but did include thioridazine or trifluoperazine. The other antipsychotic compounds are equal in therapeutic efficacy to thioridazine and trifluoperazine, these two drugs being equal to chlorpromazine in therapeutic efficacy. Thus, there is considerable evidence from many controlled studies that the antipsychotic compounds, with the exception of promazine, are equal to chlorpromazine in therapeutic efficacy. The differences are primarily in side effects. Some may produce more sedation than others. However, all the antipsychotic compounds increase psychomotor activity in the retarded patient to make him more normally active and reduce psychomotor activity in the agitated patient, making him more normally active.

It is unwise to change antipsychotic drugs every few days. One should try to find the optimal dose of a single drug and give the drug a reasonable time to exert its behavioral effect.

However, at some point—often after days in a severely disturbed acute patient and after weeks in a less dramatically impaired patient—a trial with a different antipsychotic agent is warranted, since patients who fail to respond to one phenothiazine occasionally show a good response to another.

Dosage

Different patients may respond to widely different doses, so there is no set dose for any given antipsychotic agent.

There is a wide therapeutic range between effective dose and toxic overdose with the antipsychotic agents. In research studies, patients have been treated with safety with 10 to 100 times the therapeutic dose.

The level at which antipsychotic drug therapy is instituted and the manner of its use vary widely from one psychiatric setting to another. Generally, crisis-oriented, overcrowded, acute public facilities start drug therapy in the emergency room, use intramuscular medication freely in turbulent or severely withdrawn patients, and raise dosage rapidly over 2 or 3 days to a high level—perhaps, 1,000 mg. of chlor-promazine—reducing dosage only after the patient is clearly much less aroused and agitated and is beginning to look quiet and even sleepy. In better-staffed, more selective, private acute facilities, a more thoughtful drug-free evaluation period of days or even weeks may precede a rather gradual initiation of drug therapy, with levels of 300 mg. a day of chlorpromazine being much more common than levels of 1,000 mg. No reasonable evidence indicates which procedure leads to a better long-term remission. Sometimes side effects limit the dosage level attainable and may require shifting to another drug.

The most common side effects, sedation and extrapyramidal symptoms, do not usually make a shift to another drug necessary. Sedation can be handled by dose reduction or by giving most of the drug at bedtime. Neurological side effects present a quandary. One can block them with an antiparkinsonian agent or reduce the dose or both. There is no clear evidence favoring either strategy. The therapeutic decision should probably rest on the patient's level of improvement. If the patient is much better, decrease the dose. If the patient is still very psychotic, add an antiparkinsonian drug and raise the antipsychotic drug dose if clinically necessary.

Most clinicians gradually reduce the dosage of the antipsychotic drug once the patient appears maximally improved and raise the dose again if symptoms recur. A prophylactic modest elevation of dosage is sometimes used when the patient is about to undergo a special stress, such as returning home or starting a new job.

The antipsychotic effects of phenothiazines are of relatively long duration, on the order of days not hours, but their sedative effects generally last only a few hours. The common medical habit of administering medication three times a day may make the patient oversedated when he should be working or learning. The same total dose given at bedtime may well promote better sleep and leave the patient calm but not sedated during the day.

The cost of these drugs is not a function of dose. A 25-mg. chlorpromazine tablet costs almost as much as a 100-mg. tablet. Therefore, giving the largest available indicated dosage form once a day saves considerable money over time and, in hospitals, substantially reduces nursing time and costs. For patients in aftercare, a bedtime or evening dose may be harder for the patient to forget and easier for the family to monitor than a three-times-a-day regimen. Spansules or other delayed release oral forms of some phenothiazines are available for prescription use, but there is no evidence that these more expensive formulations have any advantage over standard tablet preparations.

Blood Levels

Different patients manifest widely different blood levels with comparable doses. Some patients receiving a moderate dose of chlorpromazine are found to have an extremely high blood level and to be excessively sedated. When the dose is reduced, the patient improves remarkably. This patient may have a deficit in metabolism and may have built up a psychotoxically high level of blood chlorpromazine. In contrast, some patients have extremely low blood levels, even on high doses. These patients may metabolize chlorpromazine so rapidly that, even on high doses, adequate amounts of chlorpromazine do not reach the brain.

High-Dosage Treatment

A number of patients do not benefit significantly from any antipsychotic drug medication. The question arises whether they would have experienced a remission in their disease had they been treated with higher than normal doses.

The NIMH performed two collaborative studies to test this question. In one study, chronically hospitalized patients received a high dose of chlorpromazine (2,000 mg. a day); in the other study, similar patients received trifluoperazine (70 mg.). The controls were patients receiving normal doses or a placebo. In young, acute patients the high-dose treatment resulted in somewhat more improvement than was seen at normal doses. The high-dose treatment did not benefit older, chronic, burned out schizophrenics.

Treatment-resistant patients deserve a trial on moderately high-dose treatment. Perhaps in selective cases megadose treatment is indicated on an experimental basis. Because of the larger clinical literature on megadose fluphenazine therapy, this drug is recommended for high-dose use.

TABLE I

Phenothiazine Antipsychotic Agents (Major Tranquilizers)

| Class | Name | | Manufacturer | Structure | Adult Dose Range | | Adult Single Dose Range |
	Generic	Trade			(mg./day)		(mg)
					Acute	Maintenance	
Aliphatic	Chlorpromazine	Thorazine	Smith, Kline & French		25–2,000 Oral 25–2,400 IM	200–1,000 Oral	10–400 Oral 10–400 IM
	Triflupromazine	Vesprin	Squibb		100–200 Oral 25–150 IM	50–150 Oral	10–50 Oral 10–50 IM
	Promazine	Sparine	Wyeth		25–1,000 Oral 25–1,000 IM	200–600 Oral	10–400 Oral 10–100 IM
Piperazine	Prochlorperazine	Compazine	Smith, Kline & French		15–150 Oral 30–100 IM	15–75 Oral	5–25 Oral 10–20 IM
	Perphenazine	Trilafon	Schering		16–64 Oral 10–20 IM	8–16 Oral	2–16 Oral 5 IM
	Trifluoperazine	Stelazine	Smith, Kline & French		10–40 Oral 1–6 IM	5–15 Oral	1–10 Oral 1–2 IM

Class	Generic	Brand	Manufacturer	Structure	Dose 1	Dose 2	Dose 3
Piperazine	Fluphenazine	Prolixin, Permitil	Squibb, Schering		20–60 Oral, 5–20 IM (HCl)	5–20 Oral, 25–50 IM (Decanoate or enanthate, weekly or biweekly)	
	Acetophenazine	Tindal	Schering		40–120 Oral	20–40 Oral	20–40
	Butaperazine	Repoise	Robins		15–100 Oral	5–50 Oral	5–30
	Carphenazine	Proketazine	Wyeth		100–200	50–150	12.5–50
Piperidine	Thioridazine	Mellaril	Sandoz		300–800 Oral	100–300 Oral	50–300
	Mesoridazine	Serentil	Boehringer		50–400 Oral, 25–200 IM	25–200 Oral	10–100 Oral, 25 IM
	Piperacetazine	Quide	Dow		40–60 Oral	20–50 Oral	10–60

Table I.—continued

| | Available Preparation | | | | | | | | | Equivalence* |
| | Oral | | | | | Injection | | | Suppository | |
	Tablet (mg.)	Capsule (mg.)	Syrup	Elixir	Concentrate	Ampul	Vial	Syringe	(mg.)	(mg.)
Chlorpromazine	10, 25, 50, 100, 200	Sustained release: 30, 75, 150, 200, 300	10 mg./ml.		30 mg./ml. 100 mg./ml.	25 mg./ml. 50 mg./ml.	25 mg./ml.		25, 100	100
Triflupromazine	10, 25, 50		50 mg./5 ml.					10 mg./ml.		25
Promazine	10, 25, 50, 100, 200		10 mg./5 ml.		30 mg./ml. 100 mg./ml.	25 mg./ml.	10 mg./ml.			100
Prochlorperazine	5, 10, 25	Sustained release: 10, 15, 30, 75	5 mg./5 ml.		10 mg./ml.	5 mg./ml.	5 mg./ml.		2.5, 5, 25	15
Perphenazine	2, 4, 8, 16				3.2 mg./ml.	5 mg./ml.	5 mg./ml.			10
Trifluoperazine	1, 2, 5, 10				10 mg./ml.					5
Fluphenazine	0.25; 1, 2, 5, 10; sustained release: 1			0.5 mg./ml.	5 mg./ml.		2 mg./ml. HCl (decanoate or enanthate) 25 mg./ml. (decanoate or enanthate)			2
Acetophenazine	20									20
Butaperazine	5, 10, 20									10
Carphenazine	12.5, 25, 50				30 mg./ml.					25
Thioridazine	10, 15, 25, 50, 100, 150, 200				100 mg./ml.					100
Mesoridazine	10, 25, 50, 100				25 mg./ml.	25 mg./ml.				100
Piperacetazine	10, 25									10

* Dose required to achieve therapeutic efficacy of 100 mg. chlorpromazine.

TABLE I.—*Continued*

	Side Effects
Dry mouth and throat	Sedation
Blurred vision	Insomnia
Cutaneous flushing	Bizarre dreams
Constipation	Impaired psychomotor activity
Urinary retention	Somnambulism
Paralytic ileus	Confusion
Mental confusion	Paradoxical aggravation of psychotic symptoms
Miosis	Hyperpyrexia
Mydriasis	Skin eruptions (urticarial, maculopapular, petechial, or edematous)
Postural hypotension	Contact dermatitis
Broadened, flattened, or clove T waves and increased Q-R intervals on electrocardiogram	Photosensitivity reaction
	Blue-gray metallic discoloration of the skin over areas exposed to sunlight
Parkinsonian syndrome	Deposits in the anterior lens and posterior cornea (visible only by slit-lens examination)
Masklike face	Retinitis pigmentosa
Tremor at rest	Abnormal glucose-tolerance curve
Rigidity	Breast engorgement and lactation in female patients
Shuffling gait	Weight gain
Motor retardation	Delayed ejaculation
Drooling	Orgasm without ejaculation
Dyskinesias	Loss of erectile ability
Bizarre movements of tongue, face, and neck	Agranulocytosis
Buccofacial movements	Eosinophilia
Salivation	Leukopenia
Torticollis	Hemolytic anemia
Oculogyric crisis	Thrombocytic purpura
Opisthotonos	Pancytopenia
Akathisia	Jaundice
Lowered seizure threshold	
Convulsive seizures	

TABLE II

Nonphenothiazine Antipsychotic Agents (Major Tranquilizers)

| Class | Name | | Manufacturer | Structure | Adult Dose Range (mg./day) | | Adult single Dose Range |
	Generic	Trade			Acute	Maintenance	*mg.*
Butyrophenones	Haloperidol	Haldol	McNeil		1–15 Oral 2–15 IM	1–15	0.5–5 Oral 2–5 IM
Thioxanthenes	Chlorprothixene	Taractan	Roche		75–600 Oral 75–200 IM	75	25–150 Oral 25–50 IM
	Thiothixene	Navane	Roerig		6–60 Oral 8–30 IM	6–60	2–20 Oral 4–5 IM
Dibenzoxapines	Loxapine	Loxitane	Lederle		20–100	20–100	10–60
Dihydroindolones	Molindone	Moban	Endo		15–225	15–225	5–75

TABLE II.—*continued*

Rauwolfia alkaloid	Reserpine*
	Serpasial, Rau-sed, Sandril, Raurine, Reserpoid, Vio-serpine
	Ciba, Squibb, Lilly, Westerfield, Upjchn, Rowell

Dosages: 0.1–5; 2.5–10.0 IM (following a small initial dose to test patient responsiveness); 0.1–5; 1; 0.1–5 Oral

| Class | Available Preparations | | | | | | Drug Enforcement Administration Control Level | Side Effects |
| | Oral | | | Concentrate | Injection | | | |
	Tablet	Capsule	Elixir		Ampul	Vial		
	mg.	*mg.*						
Haloperidol	0.5, 1, 2, 5, 10			2 mg./ml.	5 mg./ml.		0	Same as for phenothiazine antipsychotic agents
Chlorprothixene	10, 25, 50, 100	1, 2, 5, 10, 20		20 mg./ml.	12.5 mg./ml.		0	
Thiothixene				5 mg./ml.		2 mg./ml.	0	
Loxapine		10, 25, 50						
Molindone	5, 10, 25							
Reserpine	0.1, 0.25, 1, 2, 5	0.25, 0.5	0.05 mg./ml.		2.5 mg./ml.	2.5 g./ml.	0	Reserpine is associated with many of the same side effects as the phenothiazine antipsychotic agents. However, in addition it frequently produces depression. Approximately 6 per cent of all patients on reserpine require hospitalization or electroconvulsive therapy for depression caused by the drug.

* Rarely prescribed for psychosis.

TABLE III

Characteristics of Drugs at Each Drug Enforcement Administration (D.E.A.) Control Level

D.E.A. Control Level (Schedule)	Characteristics of Drugs at Each Control Level	Examples of Drugs at Each Control Level
I	High abuse potential No accepted use in medical treatment in the United States at the present time and therefore not for prescription use	LSD, heroin, marihuana, peyote, mescaline, psilocybin, tetrahydrocannabinols, nicocodeine, nicomorphine, and others
II	High abuse potential Severe physical dependence liability Severe psychological dependence liability	Amphetamines, opium, morphine, codeine, hydromorphine, phenmetrazine, cocaine, methaqualone, amobarbital, secobarbital pentobarbital, methylphenidate, and others
III	Abuse potential less than levels I and II Moderate or low physical dependence liability High psychological dependence liability	Glutethimide, methyprylon, phencyclidine, nalorphine, sulfonmethane, benzphetamine, phendimetrazine, clortermine, mazindol, chlorphentermine, compounds containing codeine, morphine, opium, hydrocodone, dihydrocodeine, and others
IV	Low abuse potential Limited physical dependence liability Limited psychological dependence liability	Barbital, phenobarbital, the benzodiazepines, chloral hydrate, ethchlorvynol, ethinamate, meprobamate, paraldehyde, and others
V	Lowest abuse potential of all controlled substances	Narcotic preparations containing limited amounts of non-narcotic active medicinal ingredients

Maintenance Treatment

After the patient is substantially improved with pharmacotherapy, the question arises as to how long he should be kept on maintenance antipsychotic drug treatment. Properly controlled double-blind studies in 24 countries have shown that significantly more patients relapse on placebo than on continued pharmacotherapy. Maintenance phenothiazines are necessary to prevent relapse in most schizophrenic patients. Phenothiazines, although they do not in any sense cure patients, do alter the course of their disease in a quantitative way, certainly lessening the period of hospitalization and increasing the quality and amount of normal behavior outside the hospital.

The number of relapses within a given time period may vary with the sickness of the population studied—that is, sick patients have more relapses than those less seriously ill. About 50 per cent of a moderately ill population will relapse within 6 months after their drugs are discontinued. These data can be used to argue both for and against discontinuing phenothiazines. Since 50 per cent do not relapse, half the patients continuing medication must be taking a drug they do not need. On the other hand, 50 per cent do relapse, and a relapse can often have a serious impact on a patient and his family.

The decision to continue on the drug for a long time should be arrived at clinically for each individual patient and should be based on a knowledge of his illness and his life situation. It seems reasonable to continue most patients on phenothiazines for 6 months to 1 year after a psychotic episode; however, over longer periods, treatment should be individualized. A history of relapse after discontinuation of phenothiazines is an indication for a longer period of maintenance. Psychotherapeutic and social interventions during the recovery phase and in posthospital care are important in prompting improved social adjustment and may help prevent relapse.

Drug Holidays

Since there is some risk of long-term toxicity with the antipsychotic drugs, it is reasonable to

TABLE IV

TABLE IV

Drug-Placebo Comparisons in Controlled Studies of Schizophrenia

Drug		Number of Studies in Which Drug Was	
Generic name	Trade name	More effective than placebo	Equal to placebo
Chlorpromazine	Thorazine	54	11
Reserpine	Serpasil	20	9
Triflupromazine	Vesprin	9	1
Perphenazine	Trilafon	5	0
Prochlorperazine	Compazine	7	2
Trifluoperazine	Stelazine	16	2
Fluphenazine	Prolixin	15	0
Butaperazine	Repoise	4	0
Thioridazine	Mellaril	7	0
Mesoridazine	Serentil	3	0
Mepazine	Pacatal	2	3
Carphenazine	Proketazine	2	0
Promazine	Sparine	3	4
Phenobarbital	Luminal	0	3
Chlorprothixene	Taractan	4	0
Thiothixene	Navane	2	0

TABLE V

Chlorpromazine-Placebo Comparisons at Different Dose Levels

Dose (mg. a day)	Number of Studies in Which Chlorpromazine Was		
	More effective than a placebo	Slightly more effective than a placebo	Equal to a placebo
300 or less	11	6	9
301–400	4	3	1
401–500	4	0	1
501–800	14	0	0
800 or more	12	0	0
Totals (all doses)	45	9	11

kinetics of intramuscular versus oral absorption, distribution, and metabolism of the drugs. In any case, the depot intramuscular medication should be considered for patients who do not have optimal responses to oral medication or who are suspected of failing to take the medication, as evidenced by frequent relapses.

Combined Therapy

Antipsychotic Drugs and Somatic Therapies

Phenothiazines and the other antipsychotic drugs have largely replaced insulin coma and electroconvulsive therapy (ECT) in the treatment of the schizophrenic patient. Studies show that ECT is no more effective than the phenothiazines. Some clinicians are of the opinion that ECT is helpful in the treatment of selected schizophrenics when given concurrently with phenothiazine therapy.

Drug Combinations

It has not been demonstrated experimentally that combining one phenothiazine with another phenothiazine results in a treatment superior to comparable amounts of a single phenothiazine. In a large collaborative Veterans Administration study it was found that the addition of imipramine or a monoamine oxidase inhibitor to chlorpromazine did not benefit chronic schizophrenics more than did chlorpromazine alone. Combining tricyclic antidepressants with phenothiazines suggests that this mixture may

look for ways of maintaining a remission by use of minimal amounts of antipsychotic drugs. Drug holidays, one way to reduce dosages, have been studied, chiefly by Veterans Administration in chronic inpatients. For the large majority of chronic patients, 2- or 3-day-a-week drug holidays do not result in a significant deleterious effect. Of course, this should not be interpreted to mean that an intermittent schedule should be used indiscriminately.

A number of long acting antipsychotic agents are under study, and two are currently available in the United States for general use. These intramuscular depot forms, fluphenazine enanthate and fluphenazine decanoate, provide a useful treatment approach for patients who do not take their oral medication. On the basis of available evidence from double blind studies, the depot fluphenazine is as effective as oral fluphenazine. In open trials, there have been clinical reports of patients who were particularly benefited by the depot medication, presumably because they had failed to take oral medication but also possibly because of the benefit some patients, both depressed patients and patients with catatoniclike symptoms, but the results are not uniform, and differences are small, sometimes negligible.

When working with a combination, one is often well advised to prescribe both medicines individually until the optimal ratio is arrived at. Clinical experience indicates that the judicious use of combinations can be helpful to some patients, although indiscriminate polypharmacy is not to be encouraged because controlled studies fail to indicate that there are marked advantages in combinations. Table VI lists some commonly used drug combinations compounded by the manufacturer in a single preparation.

Drugs and Psychological and Social Treatments

A study conducted at the Massachusetts Mental Health Center by Greenblatt and co-workers compared four variations in drug and social therapies. Intensive social therapy—consisting of a variety of psychotherapies, social work, occupational therapies, psychodrama, total-push therapies, and so on—was administered at the center. The minimal social therapy was administered to chronic state hospital patients. Two groups were transferred to the center and received intensive social therapy, one group with drugs and the other without drugs. The two groups remaining at the state hospital received minimal social therapy, one group with drugs and one group without drugs. In terms of symptomatic improvement, the patients who received drugs in both milieux did show greater improvement, although there was a slight nonsignificant trend for greater symptomatic improvement in the drug-plus-intensive-social-therapy group (33 per cent) than in the drug-plus-minimal-social therapy group (23 per cent). Both these improvement rates were significantly higher than that observed in the nondrug groups in the state hospital milieu (10 per cent) or at the Massachusetts Mental Health Center (0 per cent). Those patients who were able to leave the hospital because of symptomatic improvement were those who had both drug therapy and the social therapies (see Table VII). If anything, the intensive social therapies without drugs militated against improvement. This group of patients, when placed on drugs again after having been off them for 6 months, never did catch up with the group that

was continuously treated with drugs plus social therapies.

In no sense do social therapies substitute for phenothiazines. The social therapies did not have the antipsychotic activity of the drugs. Conversely, phenothiazine therapies may be beneficial in reducing the patient's psychotic symptoms, but they do not necessarily help him get a job, adjust to his family situation, or give him the motivation and judgment to stay out of the hospital. There is good reason to believe that in older, chronic patients the value of drug therapy declines, and social therapies are of relatively greater importance. It is in chronic patients generally that behavior modification programs without drugs have been most effective.

Clinical Use

In manic, destructive, socially disruptive, or violent patients, the rapid control of symptoms is of paramount importance, not only for short-term safety but also because the patient has to live with the knowledge of any destructive act he performed while severely disturbed. Rapid control can prevent such potentially destructive or embarrassing actions. Rapid control of the symptoms of a patient in catatonic excitement can be lifesaving.

For quick and maximal antipsychotic action, it is often advisable to give large doses of parenteral medication—for example, 50 to 100 mg. of chlorpromazine intramuscularly three or four times a day or equivalent doses of another antipsychotic drug, such as haloperidol, perphenazine, or fluphenazine. In some patients chlorpromazine may be preferred because of its sedative properties. In many cases, the patients may be alarmed at being oversedated, and less sedative drugs—such as trifluoperazine perphenazine, fluphenazine, or haloperidol—may be indicated. Intramuscular chlorpromazine should be given deeply into the buttocks, and the injection site should be rotated, since this drug is irritating. Oral medication should be administered at the same time, so that after a few intramuscular doses one can switch gradually to high oral doses at a level of 1.0 to 1.5 gm. of chlorpromazine a day or equivalent amounts of any other antipsychotic. During the period of the change to oral medication, the patient should be observed closely for worsening, so that

Preparation	Manufacturer	Ingredients and Amount of Each Ingredient	Recommended Dosage*	Indications	D.E.A.† Control Level
		mg.			
Triavil Etrafon	Merck, Sharp & Dohme Schering	Perphenazine and Amitriptyline Tablet—2:25, 4:25, 2:10, 4:10	Initial Therapy Tablet of 2:25 or 4:25 t.i.d. or q.i.d. Maintenance Therapy Tablet of 2:25 or 4:25 b.i.d. or q.i.d.	Depression and associated anxiety	0
Deprol	Wallace	Meprobamate and Benactyzine Tablet—400:1	Initial Therapy One tablet t.i.d. or q.i.d. Maintenance Therapy Initial dosage may be increased to six tablets a day then gradually reduced to the lowest levels that provide relief	Depression and associated anxiety	IV
Milpath Pathibamate	Wallace Lederle	Meprobamate and tridihexethyl chloride Tablet—400:25, 200:25	Tablet of 400:25 t.i.d. at mealtimes and two tablets at bedtime	Peptic ulcer and irritable bowel syndrome	0
Tuinal	Lilly	Secobarbital and Amobarbital Capsule—25:25, 50:50, 100:100	50 to 200 mg. at bedtime or 1 hour preoperatively	Insomnia Preoperative sedation	II
Dexamyl‡	Smith, Kline & French	Dextroamphetamine and Amobarbital Tablet—5:32 Sustained release capsule—15:97, 10:65 Elixir—5:32/5 ml.	Should be administered at the lowest effective dosage Capsule—one capsule in the morning Tablets and Elixir—one tablet (or one teaspoonful of the Elixir) b.i.d. or t.i.d. 30 to 60 minutes before meals	Exogenous obesity	II
Eskatrol‡	Smith, Kline & French	Dextroamphetamine and Prochlorperazine Sustained release capsule—15:7.5	1 capsule in the morning	Exogenous obesity	II
Biphetamine‡	Pennwalt	Amphetamine and Dextroamphetamine Capsule—3.75: 3.75, 6.25: 6.25, 10:10	Should be administered at the lowest effective dosage, one capsule daily, 10 to 14 hours before retiring	Exogenous obesity	II
Librax	Roche	Chlordiazepoxide and clinidium bromide Capsule—5:2.5	One or two capsules t.i.d. or q.i.d. before meals and at bedtime	Peptic ulcer, gastritis, duodentitis, irritable bowel syndrome, spastic colitis and mild ulcerative colitis	0

* t.i.d., q.i.d., and b.i.d.
† Drug Enforcement Administration.
‡ The United States Food and Drug Administration does not recommend the use of amphetamine or its derivatives for depression. However, the authors have found these medications of use in selected cases of depression and neurasthenia when used judiciously.

one can act quickly by increasing the oral dose or by reinstituting a few more intramuscular injections.

After the initial psychotic behavior is controlled, one lowers the dose and then makes adjustments to arrive at an optimal dose for cognitive restoration. When high doses are required, the sedative effects of chlorpromazine limit its usefulness, and an agent with fewer sedating and autonomic effects without local irritation at the site of injection is preferable. High doses of the more potent antipsychotics possess considerable sedative properties. There is little need to use nonantipsychotic sedatives in addition.

Side Effects

Many of the psychotropic drugs share common pharmacologic modes of action that produce categories of related side effects. For example, most of the antipsychotic and antidepressant medications alter biogenic amines and block cholinergic receptors, both centrally and peripherally, and can produce a family of autonomic side effects, such as blurred vision, dry mouth, constipation, and urinary retention. In addition, all the antipsychotic compounds produce extrapyramidal side effects.

Autonomic Side Effects

The autonomic side effects are due to the anticholinergic and antiadrenergic properties of the antipsychotic drugs. Autonomic side effects that can occur include dry mouth and throat, blurred vision, cutaneous flushing, constipation, urinary retention, paralytic ileus, mental confusion, miosis, mydriasis, and postural hypotension. Patients develop tolerance to the dry mouth and to the other autonomic side effects, so that these are most troublesome early in treatment. Postural hypotension can usually be managed by having the patient lie down with his feet higher than his head. With cardiac patients, a predrug electrocardiogram for baseline purposes is indicated.

Extrapyramidal Effects

The most dramatic of the common side effects produced by the antipsychotic drugs, and pharmacologically a theoretically important group of side effects shown by all the antipsychotic agents, are the extrapyramidal reactions.

TABLE VII

Drug Therapy versus Social Therapies in Chronic Schizophrenia: Results of Four Treatment Regimes (Data from Greenblatt et al., 1965)

	Intensive Social Therapies	Minimal Social Therapies
	%	%
Patients showing high improvement at 6 months		
Drug therapy	33	23
No drug therapy	0	10
Patients discharged after 6 to 9 months		
Drug therapy	27	9
No drug therapy for 6 months	7	5
Patients showing high improvement after 36 months		
Drug therapy	35	19
No drug therapy for 6 months	26	6

This family of side effects is typically classified into three arbitrary categories: parkinsonian syndrome, dyskinesias, and akathisia. The parkinsonian syndrome consists of a masklike face, tremor at rest, rigidity, shuffling gait, and motor retardation. The dyskinesias consist of a broad range of bizarre movements of the tongue, face, and neck, including buccofacial movements with salivation, torticollis, oculogyric crisis, and opisthotonus. Akathisia is a motor restlessness in which the patient manifests a great urge to move about and has considerable difficulty in sitting still.

If one diagnoses these manifestations as an increase in psychosis, the treatment is to increase the dose of the antipsychotic medication. However, if one diagnoses them as extrapyramidal effects, the treatment is to decrease the dose of the antipsychotic medication or to add an antiparkinsonian drug. Particularly helpful in making a correct diagnosis is a therapeutic trial of antiparkinsonian agents.

Among the phenothiazines, thioridazine produces the fewest extrapyramidal effects; haloperidol, thiothixene, butaperazine, trifluoperazine, and fluphenazine produce the most extrapyramidal effects. Chlorpromazine, chlorprothixene, and acetophenazine occupy an intermediate position.

Antiparkinsonian agents are of use in drug-induced extrapyramidal effects (see Table VIII). Roughly speaking, one can prescribe 5 mg. of procyclidine or an equivalent amount of other antiparkinsonian medication for every 400 mg. of chlorpromazine or its equivalent. Procyclidine is a short-acting drug; therefore, three-times-day administration is used initially, although later one can use one dose at bedtime or a twice-a-day schedule for convenience. It is not necessary to increase the dose about 15 mg. a day. The minimal dose of any antiparkinsonian drug should be used, and dose adjustment is often required.

Antiparkinsoniam medication should be given with caution in the presence of benign prostatic hypertrophy or narrow-angle glaucoma, so as to avoid augmenting the atropine-like properties of phenothiazines with antiparkinsonian drugs.

An extrapyramidal syndrome that is said to emerge relatively late during the course of treatment with antipsychotic compounds, particularly when these drugs have been used in high doses over years, has been called tardive dyskinesia or terminal extrapyramidal insufficiency. It occurs late in the course of treatment (sometimes appearing after the drug has been discontinued), may persist for years, is relatively treatment-resistant, and is absent during sleep. Tardive dyskinesia is characterized by grimacing, by buccofacial-mandibular or buccolingual movements—including sucking, smacking movements of the lips, lateral or fly-catching movements of the tongue, and lateral jaw movements—choreiform-like jerky movements of the arms, athetoid movements of the upper extremeties or fingers and ankles and toes, and tonic contractions of the neck and back. The symptoms may occur or become intensified a few days to weeks after the drug has been stopped or reduced, although they may also appear during drug therapy. The reappearance or intensification with reduction of dosage or cessation of drug treatment may be an unmasking of the symptom, since the phenothiazine-induced rigidity can damp the dystonic movements. Hence, paradoxically, the symptom may be suppressed by putting the patient on large doses of phenothiazines or butyrophenones. The symptoms may persist for long periods of time in some patients, and in

others they may disappear within weeks or months after cessation of treatment. They are not particularly helped by antiparkinsonian medication; indeed, this treatment may occasionally aggravate them. Reserpinelike drugs may produce a beneficial effect on this side effect. Deanol (Deaner) has also been reported to be of use.

Other Central Nervous System Effects

Most of the antipsychotic compounds lower the threshold of seizures in animals. Seizures rarely occur in human beings treated with high doses of antipsychotic compounds. The question therefore arises whether phenothiazines are contraindicated in patients with seizure disorders and psychosis. In the absence of controlled data, one is left with the clinical opinion that patients with epilepsy generally show an improvement in both their behavioral disorder and their seizure disorder with antipsychotic drug treatment. When seizures do occur, they generally occur with high doses of the drug and consist of a single isolated seizure. They often do not recur, even on the same dose, and one can often treat the patient with a slightly lower dose without any seizures. On occasion, one can add an anticonvulsant, such as diphenylhydantoin (Dilantin), to the treatment regime and continue antipsychotic drugs with no seizures even at higher doses.

On occasion, the antipsychotic agents produce sedation, particularly in the first few days of treatment. Patients rapidly develop tolerance to the sedative properties. Of the phenothiazines, chlorpromazine and thioridazine produce more sedation than fluplenazine, haloperidol, thiothixene, and trifluoperazine. The drowsiness can be controlled by reducing the dosage by switching to a less sedating phenothiazine, or by giving the whole daily phenothiazine dose at bedtime.

The term "behavioral toxicity" has been applied to adverse behavioral change produced by any psychotropic drug. It is often difficult to evaluate such a change in seriously ill schizophrenic patients, since it would be necessary to separate non-drug-related worsening of the schizophrenic state from drug-induced toxicity. Such symptoms as insomnia, bizarre dreams, impaired psychomotor activity, aggravation of schizophrenic symptoms, toxic confusional

Table VIII
Antiparkinsonian Agents

Class	Generic	Trade	Manufacturer	Structure	Adult Dose Range (mg./day)	Adult Single Dose Range (mg.)	Tablet	Capsule	Concentrate	Elixir	Ampul	Vial	Syringe
Piperidines	Biperiden	Akineton	Knoll		2–6	2	2				5 mg./ml.		
	Procyclidine	Kemadrin	Burroughs Wellcome		2–20	2–5	2, 5						
	Trihexyphenidyl	Artane Tremin Antitrem Pipanol	Lederle Schering Roerig Winthrop		1–15	1–3	2, 5	Sustained release: 5	2 mg./5ml.				
Ethanolamine Antihistamines	Diphenhydramine	Benadryl	Parke, Davis		10–400	10–50	25, 50			12.5 mg./5 ml.	50 mg./ml.	10 mg./ml. 50 mg./ml.	50 mg./ml.
	Orphenadrine	Disipal	Riker		50–150	50	50						

TABLE VIII—*continued*

| Tropines | Benztropine | Cogentin | Merck, Sharpe & Dohme | 1-8 | 1-4 | 0.5, 1, 2 | 1 mg./ml. |

Side Effects

Drowsiness
Confusion
Nervousness
Restlessness
Nausea
Vomiting
Diarrhea
Blurred vision
Diplopia

Difficulty in urination
Constipation
Nasal stuffiness
Vertigo
Palpitation
Headache
Insomnia
Tightness of the chest and wheezing
Thickening of bronchial secretions

Dryness of mouth, nose, and throat
Urticaria
Drug rash
Photosensitivity
Hemolytic anemia
Hypotension
Epigastric distress
Anaphylactic shock
Tingling, heaviness, and weakness of hands

states, and somnambulism do occur in patients under treatment with psychotropic drugs. Akathasia or a worsening of psychosis can be reversed in minutes by intramuscular antiparkinson agents. Some of these effects may be dose-related and can be lessened by an alteration in the dose, the addition or deletion of drugs, or the use of a different type of antipsychotic agent. Some of the confusional states may be related to the anticholinergic properties of the drugs. In addition, patients differ in their rate of metabolism of a specific drug, and slow metabolizers may build up psychotoxic levels of the drug or its metabolites.

Allergic Reactions

The jaundice induced by chlorpromazine used to be one of the more striking side effects of the drug. Recently, for some unexplained reason, the incidence of chlorpromazine jaundice has dropped considerably; the incidence now is probably in the range of one out of every 1,000 patients treated. The jaundice most often occurs 1 to 5 weeks after initiation of phenothiazine therapy. It is generally preceded, for 1 to 7 days, by a flulike syndrome of malaise, abdominal pain, fever, nausea, vomiting, and diarrhea. Clinical factors that may point to a diagnosis of a phenothiazine-induced jaundice are the temporal association of the jaundice with the beginning of the phenothiazine therapy, the lack of an enlarged or tender liver, and chemical evidence of choleostasis. The jaundice generally disappears within several weeks. Most cases of chlorpromazine jaundice are benign, and complete return to normal liver function occurs.

Jaundice has also been reported with promazine, thioridazine, and prochlorperazine and very rarely with fluphenazine and triflupromazine. There is no convincing evidence that haloperidol can produce a chlorpromazine-type jaundice. The majority of cases of phenothiazine-induced jaundice reported in the medical literature have occurred with chlorpromazine.

Agranulocytosis

Agranulocytosis is probably the most serious side effect observed with phenothiazines, but fortunately it is quite rare. It generally occurs in the first 6 to 8 weeks of phenothiazine treatment, its onset being abrupt and consisting of the sudden appearance of sore throat, ulcerations, and fever. When it occurs, the mortality rate is generally high—often 30 per cent or more. Phenothiazine medication should be immediately discontinued, and the patient should be transferred to a medical facility for reverse isolation procedure. Energetic treatment of the infection is indicated, although prophylactic antibiotic therapy may not be indicated because of the danger of propagation of drug-resistant organisms. It is said that the adrenal corticosteroids do not hasten recovery. Cross-sensitivity to other phenothiazines may occur, but hard data are lacking. The incidence of agranulocytosis is probably about one out of 500,000 patients, but no accurate data exist. Very rarely it has been reported to occur with promazine, prochlorperazine, and thioridazine, although it may occur with almost any phenothiazine.

Phenothiazine-induced agranulocytosis usually occurs in older female patients with other complicating systematic diseases and is considerably rarer in young, healthy patients.

Skin and Eye Effects

A variety of skin eruptions—including urticarial, maculopapular, petechial, and edematous eruptions—have been associated with phenothiazine treatment. These eruptions occur early in treatment, generally in the first few weeks. A contact dermatitis can also occur in personnel who handle chlorpromazine.

A photosensitivity reaction of the phototoxic type that resembles severe sunburn can occur in patients on chlorpromazine. Treatment consists of avoidance of sunlight.

One long-term side effect consists of blue-gray metallic discoloration of the skin over areas exposed to sunlight. Histological examination of skin biopsies reveals pigmentary granules similar to but not histochemically identical with melanin.

In addition, eye changes have been noticed after long-term high-dose chlorpromazine treatment. These changes have been described as whitish brown, granular deposits concentrated in the anterior lens and posterior cornea, visible only by slit-lens examination. They progress to opaque white and yellow-brown granules, often stellate in shape. Occasionally, the conjunctiva is discolored by a brown pigment. These lens changes are quite different from those of senile cataracts and are in no way related to them.

Statistically, these opacities occur more frequently in patients with skin discoloration. Retinal damage is not seen in these patients, and vision is almost never impaired. The occurrence and severity of these opacities is related to the duration and total dose of chlorpromazine, the majority of patients who show these deposits having ingested 1 to 3 kg. of phenothiazine throughout the therapeutic course. Hospitals differ in their reported prevalence of these skin and eye effects, estimates varying from less than 1 per cent to more than 30 per cent.

Sunlight plays a role in both the skin and eye effects, and part of the difference between hospitals may relate to the differential exposure of patients to the sun. It has been thought that this condition can be treated by removing the patient from the sun.

Thioridazine has a much more dangerous effect on the eye than chlorpromazine does. In doses over 800 mg. a day, retinitis pigmentosa occurs, which can cause substantial visual impairment or even blindness. This condition is said not to remit when the drug is stopped. Doses of thioridazine over 800 mg. a day are, therefore, to be strenuously avoided.

Endocrine Effects and Impotence

The effect of antipsychotic drugs in producing breast engorgment and lactation in female patients is well known, although incidence figures are lacking. If every patient were checked for lactation by manual pressure on the breast, an incidence of 20 to 40 per cent might be found. Subjective complaints of overt lactation are quite rare, less than 5 per cent, and are often adequately handled by dose reduction or by shifting the patient to another drug. Drug-related gynecomastia in male patients has been described.

Clinical studies show small and inconsistant effects of these drugs in other sex hormones and adrenocortical, thyroid, and pituitary hormones. The marked weight gain sometimes associated with phenothiazine treatment has not been explained on any endocrine basis.

Sexual impotence, beginning with delayed ejaculation but progressing to orgasm without ejaculation and ultimately to loss of erectile ability, can probably occur with other antipsychotic agents, but is most frequently reported to occur with thioridazine, perhaps because this drug has more autonomic and fewer extrapyramidal side effects than do higher-potency antipsychotic agents.

Side Effects in the Elderly

Elderly psychotic patients tolerate and require lower dosages of antipsychotic drugs than do younger adult schizophrenics. A dose of 10 or 25 mg. of thioridazine or 0.25 mg. of haloperidol is a safe dose in elderly patients, and clinically effective dosages are usually 100 mg. or less of the former or 1 mg. of the latter a day. Hypotension or ataxia, with resulting high risk of hip fracture, can result if such patients are placed rapidly on high-dose drug levels. Also, the higher prevalence of tardive dyskinesia in elderly patients makes one cautious. Nevertheless, these drugs can be very effective in psychotic geriatric patients. Where clear hyperarousal exists at doses of the sort suggested above, careful gradual raising of the dose until symptomatic relief is obtained is clearly indicated.

Implications for Theory

The most likely common denominator of the antipsychotic drugs is their effect on central neurotransmitter systems. Basically, the information carried by nerves is passed down the neuron by an action potential. However, this information is transmitted from nerve to nerve by a means of a chemical messenger, a neurotransmitter substance. In the peripheral nervous system, norepinephrine (NEP) and acetylcholine are the transmitter substances. In the central nervous system there may be a wide variety of transmitters—such as acetylcholine, NEP, serotonin, and dopamine. Figure 2 presents a schematic outline of a noradrenergic neuron. The neurotransmitter substance is synthesized within the nerve. In the case of norepinephrine, this synthesis is from tyrosine. The substance (NEP, for example) is stored in a storage vesicle. When the action potential comes down, the nerve part of the neurotransmitter substance is released; this stimulates a receptor site on the next nerve effectively to transmit the information from nerve to nerve. In the case of norepinephrine, the transmission is terminated by the membrane pump's actively accumulating the norepinephrine in the presynaptic neuron. The most likely place for the common denominator of the antipsychotic drugs to act is on this system.

All the antipsychotic drugs cause parkinsonian side effects. Since Parkinson's disease has been shown to be a dopamine deficiency disease, one would assume that the parkinsonian side effects caused by the antipsychotic drugs are through the dopaminergic mechanism. In addition, all the antipsychotic drugs block central dopamine receptors. It is reasonable, therefore, to form the hypothesis that the common denominator underlying all the drugs that benefit schizophrenia is their ability to block central dopamine receptors. All antipsy-

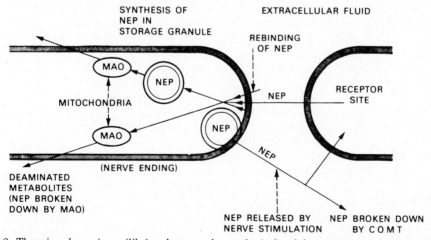

FIGURE 2. There is a dynamic equilibrium between the synthesis, breakdown, storage, release, and rebinding of norepinephrine (*NEP*) in the nerve ending. *MAO*, monoamine oxidase; *COMT*, catechol-*O*-methyltransferase.

chotic drugs do block central dopamine receptors and compensatorily increase dopamine synthesis. Chlorpromazine has a molecular configuration similar to that of dopamine. This similarity may account for chlorpromazine's ability to block dopaminergic receptors. Deviation from the structural characteristics of chlorpromazine—as in promazine hydrochloride, promethazine hydrochloride, and imipramine hydrochloride—results in loss of antipsychotic activity.

If the antipsychotic drugs do benefit schizophrenia through a dopaminergic mechanism by blocking the receptor site, one might assume that, of one could reduce the amount of dopamine in the brain by giving an inhibitor of dopamine synthesis, one could potentiate the action of the antipsychotic drugs. Indeed, if one blocks dopamine synthesis with α-methyl-p-tyrosine, one can reduce the amount of antipsychotic agents necessary for a beneficial effect in schizophrenia. This observation that α-methyl-p-tyrosine reduces the antipsychotic dose of the neuroleptics is evidence that they produce their antipsychotic action by means of an interaction with a catecholamine. Thus, there are several lines of evidence that the antipsychotic drugs may benefit schizophrenia by blocking the receptors for the catecholamine or interfering with catecholamine storage, the former being potentiated by catecholamine synthesis inhibitors.

If decreasing dopaminergic activity benefits schizophrenia, then could schizophrenia be worsened or produced by increasing dopaminergic activation? The psychomotor stimulants, such as amphetamine and methylphenidate, are potent releasers of dopamine. Large doses of amphetamine can cause a paranoid schizophrenic episode. This has been shown experimentally in normal volunteers.

The activation of psychotic symptoms by methylphenidate allows for certain inferences concerning the cause of schizophrenia. This phenomenon is consistent with the hypothesis that methylphenidate intensifies psychotic symptoms by affecting central dopamine activity.

If brain monoamine oxidase is decreased in a schizophrenic brain, it is tempting to speculate that the methylphenidate-induced psychosis activation is related to the monoamine oxidase deficit, particularly in that central catecholamines released by methylphenidate could be expected to be released in active form, since they would not be effectively metabolized intraneuronally. Methylphenidate releases preferentially from the monoamine stores, a finding that is consistent with the greater potency of methylphenidate, relative to amphetamine, in worsening psychosis.

A substantial body of evidence indicates that stereotyped behavior is controlled by a balance between the dopaminergic and cholinergic systems. When physostigmine was administered prior to methylphenidate, it prevented the psychosis from worsening. This effect indicates that the worsening of the psychosis produced by methylphenidate and presumably mediated by dopamine is controlled by a dopaminergic-cholinergic balance, as is stereotyped behavior. Is the underlying psychosis also controlled by an endogenous dopaminergic factor that is balanced by the cholinergic system? The observation that physostigmine does not reduce psychosis suggests that the underlying psychotic process is not as easily amenable to the effects of altering cholinergic tone as is the worsening of the psychosis produced by methylphenidate. There is evidence that schizophrenic patients have low amounts of the enzyme monoamine oxidase in their platelets. Furthermore, identical twins have similar platelet monoamine oxidase, in contrast to dizygotic twins. Since there is a hereditary predisposition for schizophrenia, this suggests that perhaps the mechanism by which schizophrenia is inherited is by a genetically determined deficit in the amount of monoamine oxidase in the brain.

Whether the dopamine theory of schizophrenia turns out to have any validity or not, some understanding of the basic pharmacologic mechanisms involved in neurotransmitters in the central nervous system will be important both to the understanding of mental illness and to the understanding of side effects.

REFERENCES

Davis, J. M. Overview: maintenance therapy in psychiatry: schizophrenia. Am. J. Psychiatry *132:* 1237, 1975.

Davis, J. M. Recent developments in the drug treatment of schizophrenia. Am. J. Psychiatry, *133:* 208, 1976.

Engelhardt, D. M., Rosen, B., Freedman, N., and Margolis, R. Phenothiazines in prevention of psychiatric hospitalization. IV. Delay or prevention of hospitalization: A reevaluation. Arch. Gen. Psychiatry, *16:* 98, 1967.

Gardos, G., and Cole, J. O. Maintenance anti-psychotic

therapy. Am. J. Psychiatry, *133:* 32, 1976.

Greenblatt, M., Solomon, M. H., Evans, A. S., and Brooks, G. W., editors. *Drug and Social Therapy in Chronic Schizophrenia.* Charles C Thomas, Springfield, Ill., 1965.

Hogarty, G. E., and Goldberg, S. E. Drugs and sociotherapy in the aftercare of schizophrenic patients. Arch. Gen. Psychiatry, *28:* 54, 1973.

Hollister, L. E. Complications from psychotherapeutic drugs. Clin. Pharmacol. Ther., *5:* 322, 1964.

Janowsky, D. S., El-Yousef, M. K., Davis, J. M., and Sekerke, H. J. Provocation of schizophrenic symptoms by intravenous administration of methylphenidate. Arch. Gen Psychiatry, *28:* 185, 1973.

Lehmann, H. E. Drug treatment of schizophrenia. In *Psychopharmacology.* Little, Brown, Boston, 1965.

Miller, E. Deanol: a solution for tardive dyskinesia. N. Engl. J. Med., *291:* 796, 1974.

Prien, R. F., Levine, J., and Cole, J. O. High-dose trifluoperazine therapy in chronic schizophrenia. Am. J. Psychiatry, *126:* 53, 1969.

30.2   ANTIDEPRESSANT DRUGS

Introduction

In the late 1950's two classes of drugs were discovered that proved effective in the therapy of depression—the imipramine-type drugs (tricyclic antidepressants) and the monoamine oxidase (MAO) inhibitors. These discoveries added a new dimension to depressive illness therapy, which had previously consisted primarily of electroconvulsive therapy, sedatives, narcotics, psychomotor stimulants, and psychotherapy. Although the tricyclic and MAO inhibitor drugs have been widely used since their initial discovery, there are still problems with their use. The available drugs of each class are listed in Table I, along with their approximate effective dose ranges.

The antidepressant drugs do not markedly influence the normal organism in a baseline state but, rather, correct an abnormal condition. Table II summarizes the results of many well-controlled studies of the antidepressants.

Tricyclic Drugs

The tricyclic antidepressants—imipramine, amitriptyline, desipramine, nortriptyline, protriptyline—are structurally similar to the phenothiazines, the sulfur atom in the phenothiazine molecule having been replaced by a dimethyl bridge. These drugs all appear to be active antidepressants. Other drugs of this class that are slightly different in structure—such as chlorimipramine, ketoimipramine, trimipramine, and opipramol—also appear to have considerable antidepressant activity. The tricyclic antidepressants are readily absorbed from the gastrointestinal tract. In human beings, imipramine and amitriptyline are partially metabolized to their respective desmethyl derivatives. Amitriptyline is reported to be more sedating than imipramine, and protriptyline is less so.

Clinical Effects

In normal persons, imipramine and amitriptyline produce slight sedation. However, in severely depressed psychotic patients, they produce a striking improvement in behavior and a marked lessening of depression, generally within 3 to 10 days after the onset of treatment. Patients who do not respond after receiving an adequate dose of these drugs for a 3-week period probably will not respond at all. Furthermore, the degree of response in the first 3 weeks of treatment predicts the ultimate therapeutic response; 70 per cent of the depressed patients are substantially benefited by tricyclic antidepressants, in contrast to 40 per cent who are helped by a placebo in the same time period.

Dosage

Many psychiatrists favor dose levels of 150 to 250 mg. of imipramine or amitriptyline a day—a level that should be gradually obtained over a period of several days. Other investigators think that the ideal therapeutic dose lies between 75 and 350 mg. a day, although, with many patients, increasing the dose above 250 mg. does not produce greater improvement. Protriptyline and nortriptyline are more potent on a milligram-per-milligram basis than the other tricyclic antidepressants, and smaller daily doses of these drugs are required for effective therapy.

Although the tricyclic drug may have an effect within 3 days of the onset of treatment, it may take as long as 3 weeks before there is any evidence of improvement.

Imipramine

Table II lists the number of double-blind studies in which imipramine was shown to be

TABLE I

Tricyclic and Monoamine Oxidase Inhibitor Antidepressant Agents[a]

Class	Name (Generic)	Name (Trade)	Manufacturer	Structure	Dose Range — Initial Week (mg./day)	Dose Range — After Second Week[b] (mg./day)	Adult Single Dose Range[b] (mg.)	Oral — Tablet (mg.)	Oral — Capsule (mg.)	Oral — Concentrate	Injection — Ampul	Injection — Vial	D.E.A.[c] Control Level
Tricyclic	Imipramine	Presamine Tofranil SK-Pramine	USV Geigy Smith, Kline & French	$CH_2-CH_2-CH_2-N(CH_3)_2$ (dibenzazepine)	50–100	75–300	10–200	10, 25, 50	75, 100 125, 150		25 mg./2 ml. in 2 ml. 12.5 mg./ml.		0
	Desipramine	Norpramin Pertofrane	Merrel-National USV	$CH_2-CH_2-CH_2-N(CH_3)H$ (dibenzazepine)	50–150	75–200	25–150	25, 50	25, 50				0
	Amitriptyline	Elavil Endep	Merck, Sharp & Dohme Roche	$H_3C-CH_2-CH_2-N(CH_3)_2$ (dibenzocycloheptene)	50–150	40–300	10–200	10, 25, 50 75, 100				10 mg./ml.	0
	Nortriptyline	Aventyl	Lilly	$H_3C-CH_2-CH_2-N(CH_3)H$ (dibenzocycloheptene)	25–50	50–100	10–100		10, 25	2 mg./ml.			0
	Protriptyline	Vivactil	Merck, Sharp & Dohme	$CH_2-CH_2-CH_2-N(CH_3)H$ (dibenzocycloheptene)	10–30	10–60	5–30	5, 10					0
	Doxepin[d]	Sinequan Adapin	Pfizer Pennwalt	$CH-CH_2-CH_2-N(CH_3)_2$ (dibenzoxepine)	50–100	75–200	10–100	10, 25, 50 100		10 mg./ml.			0

TABLE I—*Continued*

Monoamine Oxidase Inhibitor	Isocarbox-azid	Marplan	Roche	$CH_2-NH-NH-C-C-CH=C-CH_3$ (with O and N, O ring)	10-30	10-60	10-30	10	0
	Phenelzine	Nardil	Warner-Chilcott	$CH_2-CH_2-N-NH_2$ (H)	30-45	45-75	15-45	15	0
	Tranylcy-promine	Parnate	Smith, Kline & French	$C-C-NH_2$ (H, H, CH$_3$ cyclopropane)	20-30	20-40	10-40	10	0

Side Effects

Dry mouth	Aggravation of narrow-angle glaucoma
Palpitations	(not chronic simple glaucoma)
Tachycardia	Urinary retention (caution in benign
Heart block	prostatic hypertrophy)
Myocardial infarction	Paralytic ileus
Loss of accommodation	Peculiar taste
Orthostatic hypotension	Skin rash
Fainting	Galactorrhea
Dizziness	Gynecomastia (in males)
Nausea	Bone marrow depression
Vomiting	
Constipation	
Sedation	
Agitation	
Hallucinations and delusions	
(in latent psychotics)	
Diarrhea	
Black tongue	
Edema	

[a] Monoamine oxidase inhibitors withdrawn from market: Iproniazid (Marsilid), Pheniprazine (Catron), Etryptamine (Monase), and Nialamide (Niamid).
[b] When satisfactory improvement is attained, dosage should be reduced to the lowest level that will maintain symptomatic relief.
[c] D.E.A., Drug Enforcement Administration.
[d] The manufacturers of doxepin claim that it is useful as an antianxiety agent.

TABLE II

Summary of Controlled Double-Blind Evaluations of Antidepressant Drugs*

Drug		Number of Studies in Which the Effect of Treatment Was				
Generic name	Trade name	Greater than placebo	Equal to placebo	Greater than imipramine	Equal to imipramine	Less than imipramine
Tricyclic drugs						
Imipramine	Tofranil	26	12			
Amitriptyline	Elavil	9	2	2	5	0
Desipramine	Norpramine, Pertofran	3	2	0	6	1
Nortriptyline	Aventyl	4	0	0	0	0
Protriptyline	Vivactyl	2	0	0	2	0
Opipramol	Insidon	4	0	0	0	0
Trimipramine	Surmontil	1	0	2	0	0
MAO inhibitors						
Tranylcypromine	Parnate	2	1	0	3	0
Iproniazid	Marsilid	4	3	0	1	1
Isocarboxazid	Marplan	2	4	0	2	2
Nialamide	Niamid	0	3	0	0	1
Pheniprazine	Catron	1	1	0	1	1
Phenelzine	Nardil	4	3	0	4	3
Pargyline	Eutonyl	2	0	0	0	0
Etryptamine	Monase	1	0	0	0	0
Other treatments						
Electroshock therapy		7	1	4	3	0
Chlorpromazine	Thorazine	3	0	0	3	0
Thioridazine	Mellaril	0	0	0	1	0
Chlorprothixene	Taractan	0	0	0	1	0

* The figures include controlled studies only. A drug was not considered better than another drug unless a statistically significant difference existed between the two drugs in their relative effectiveness. Nortriptylene = amitriptyline in three studies.

more effective than a placebo, as opposed to the number of studies in which imipramine was equal to a placebo in therapeutic effectiveness. Most of the studies demonstrated the therapeutic effectiveness of imipramine. Those studies that failed to show a clear-cut drug effect sometimes suffered from such methodological inadequacies as inadequate dosage, inappropriate rating scales, and small patient populations that included elderly patients, schizo-affective patients, and patients with compensation neuroses.

Only a few recent studies make any real claim to have identified a group of patients for whom imipramine has proved to be particularly effective. In general, attempts to identify drug-susceptible populations, as opposed to those populations whose response is negligible, have not been sufficiently exhaustive. Nor have the studies been cross-validated.

Amitriptyline

Most studies that have compared amitriptyline with imipramine have found the drugs to be about equally effective (see Table II). No studies have shown amitriptyline to be less effective than imipramine. Several double-blind studies show amitriptyline to be superior to imipramine. However, this finding may be a dosage artifact; when these drugs are compared on a milligram-per-milligram basis, amitriptyline may be slightly more potent. The effective dose for amitriptyline is 150 to 250 mg. a day.

Desipramine and Nortriptyline

The desmethyl derivatives of imipramine and amitriptyline, desipramine and nortriptyline, are similar in many pharmacologic parameters to their parent compounds but appear to be more stimulating and may aggravate anxiety and tension. Based on drug-placebo and drug-imipramine comparisons, these drugs are approximately comparable to imipramine in efficacy. Desipramine was less effective than imipramine in one study but equally effective in six studies. Desipramine showed no superiority over a placebo in a study of depressed Veterans Administration patients, a group who might be expected to have schizo-affective psychoses and compensation neuroses with depression. Nortriptyline has appeared to be an effective antidepressant in controlled studies.

Other Tricyclic Antidepressants

Recently, several new tricyclic antidepressants have been synthesized. Trimipramine was found to be at least as effective as imipramine in several studies. Protriptyline is an imipramine-type drug that has been shown to be roughly equivalent to imipramine in outpatient populations, although it seems to be more potent on a milligram-per-kilogram basis. It has not been well studied on inpatients with severe depression. Opipromol has been shown to be more effective than a placebo. Doxepin is a new psychotherapeutic agent that has been suggested to have properties in common with both imipramine and diazepam, an antianxiety agent. Doxepin has been found to be effective in both depression and anxiety states.

Clinical Use

The tricyclic drugs are the most effective class of antidepressants. They have the least risk of side effects and are probably the drugs of choice for most depressed patients. First, the patient's psychiatric and medical status is assessed. If the patient is extremely depressed or suicidal, the physician may move rapidly to a high dosage. If the patient has pre-existing cardiovascular disease, a more cautious approach—low initial dosage, less rapid increase—is used. Under ordinary circumstances one starts with a modest dose, such as 25 mg. of imipramine or amitriptyline three times a day; if the dosage is well tolerated, one moves to 50 mg. three times a day within several days. After 1 week, the dose is adjusted up to 200 mg. a day or, in some patients, up to 250 mg. a day. The systematic recording of postural hypotension with lying and standing blood pressures and the monitoring of therapeutic results and side effects can be helpful in dosage

adjustments. Once the patient is stabilized on a safe and clinically effective dose, medication can gradually be switched, so that the patient takes the entire daily dose at bedtime. This dosage proves as satisfactory as three times a day dosing; in addition, it is easier for the patient to remember, and it produces peak side effects when the patient is asleep. Dosage is reduced by about 50 per cent for maintenance treatment; here again, the entire dose can be given at bedtime. Because of the sedative effects of amitriptyline, adequate sleep is frequently induced without the necessity of giving a sleeping medication.

After patients have responded to tricyclic drugs and have been discharged from the hospital, the next therapeutic decision that faces the clinician is when to discontinue the antidepressant drugs. Continued treatment with tricyclic drugs or lithium is indicated for some patients for at least a year or so. In patients with a history of frequent recurrent depressive episodes, more prolonged maintenance therapy is indicated. Lithium is indicated in bipolar patients, since it has a prophylactic action in preventing both mania and depression.

Blood Levels

At least 70 per cent of depressed patients are helped by antidepressant drugs. Undoubtedly, some of the patients who are not helped are suffering from a form of depression unresponsive to this class of drugs. However, others may not respond for clinical, pharmacologic reasons. As the tricyclic drugs are administered, blood levels build up until they reach a fairly constant level, in about 1 week, and remain that way for the next several weeks. There is a wide individual difference in levels between different patients. Some patients may metabolize the drug very rapidly, fail to build up the blood level adequately, and hence have low brain levels. Other patients may have a defect in metabolism; therefore, high plasma levels and high brain levels may accumulate, and the patients may fail to improve clinically because they are receiving toxic doses. The clinician should make an effort to find the best tricyclic dose for a given patient.

Side Effects

All the tricyclic drugs produce side effects that are roughly similar, although there are slight quantitative differences—for example, amitriptyline is said to be more sedating and protriptyline less sedating than imipramine. All the tricyclic antidepressants can cause the typical autonomic effects expected as a result of their anticholinergic pharmacological properties, such as dry mouth, palpitations, tachycardia, loss of accommodation, postural hypotension, fainting, dizziness, vomiting, constipation, edema, and aggravation of narrow-angle glaucoma. In rare instances, urinary retention and paralytic ileus have also been observed and can lead to serious or even fatal complications, particularly if the tricyclic drug has been combined with other drugs having similar anticholinergic effects—for example, a phenothiazine plus an antiparkinsonian drug. Other rare side effects include galactorrhea and profuse sweating. In general, dry mouth is the most noteworthy of the autonomic side effects, and patients should be warned that it may occur. Postural hypotension is not usually a problem, but when it is troublesome, some authors advise the use of fluorohydrocortisone (0.025 to 0.05 mg. twice a day). The autonomic side effects are, on the whole, very mild and tend to become even less troublesome after the first few weeks of treatment; in any event, they can be controlled by adjusting the dosage of the drug.

The imipramine-type antidepressants, particularly amitriptyline, have also been reported to have a potentiating effect when taken in combination with ethyl alcohol.

Two important properties of the tricyclic antidepressants are (1) their ability to inhibit the reuptake of released norepinephrine, thus potentiating noradrenergic function (norepinephrine remains at the receptor site for a longer period of time because its action is not terminated by the reuptake pump), and (2) anticholinergic blockage, an atropinelike action. Both properties may play roles in producing many of the autonomic side effects.

Skin reactions are noted early in therapy and often subside with reduced dosage. Jaundice, which occurs early, of the cholestatic type, similar to that attributed to chlorpromazine. Agranulocytosis is a very rare complication of these drugs. Rare cases of leukocytosis, leukopenia, and eosinophilia have been observed.

When administered in the usual therapeutic doses, the tricyclic drugs may cause flattened T-waves, prolonged QT intervals, and depressed S-T segments in the electrocardiogram. Cardiovascular incidents have occurred in patients with pre-existing heart disease. However, it is sometimes difficult to separate a side effect causally related to a drug from a cardiovascular incident precipitated by other factors but, by chance, coincident with drug therapy. In predisposed patients, tricyclic drugs should be started in low doses, with gradual dose increment and careful monitoring of cardiac function.

Tricyclic drugs may cause a persistent, fine, rapid tremor, particularly in the upper extremities but also in the tongue. Twitching, convulsions, dysarthria, paresthesia, peroneal palsies, and ataxia may occur in rare instances. Disturbance of motor function is rare but is more likely to occur in elderly patients. Insomnia has also been noted in elderly patients on occasion, but it is transitory and responds well to nightly sedation. From time to time, both amitriptyline and imipramine may cause episodes of schizophrenic excitement, confusion, or mania. Such episodes usually occur in patients with a predisposition to schizophrenia, chronic brain syndrome, or bipolar manic-depressive disease, rather than neuroses, which suggests that a pre-existing substratum of disease must be present for the drug to exert its psychotomimetic properties. Such symptoms usually subside 1 to 2 days after withdrawal of the drug, and they can be controlled by administration of the phenothiazine derivatives. Mild withdrawal reactions have been observed on abrupt termination of imipramine after 2 months of treatment with 300 mg. daily; the reactions consist of nausea, vomiting, and malaise. Since a gradual reduction in dosage is usually carried out in preference to abrupt withdrawal, these reactions should not pose a clinical problem. The central anticholinergic syndrome can occur and is best treated by discontinuing the tricyclic drug.

Overdosage

An overdose of an imipramine-type antidepressant produces a clinical picture characterized by temporary agitation, delirium, convulsions, hyperreflexive tendons, bowel and bladder paralysis, disturbance of temperature regulation, and mydriasis; the patient then progresses to coma, with shock and respiratory depression. Disturbances of cardiac rhythm—such as tachycardia, arterial fibrillation, ventricular flutters, and atrioventricular or intraventricular block—can also occur. Coma is generally not protracted more than 24 hours. All the above signs and symptoms may be present to a greater or lesser degree or even absent, depending on the amount of drug ingested. The lethal dose of these drugs has been estimated as being from 10 to 30 times the daily dose level.

Treatment of tricyclic overdoses should include gastric aspiration and lavage with activated charcoal, the use of intramuscular anticonvulsants such as paraldehyde or diazepam, coma care, and support of respiration.

Although tricyclic coma is generally of short duration, it can result in death from cardiac arrhythmia, and management of cardiac function is critical. If the patient survives this period, recovery without sequelae is probable, and vigorous resuscitative measures, cardioversion, continuous electrocardiogram monitoring, and chemotherapy to prevent and manage arrhythmias should be applied in an intensive-care unit. Arrhythmias may be mediated in part by the tricyclic's anticholinergic properties and in part by a direct myocardial depression. Physostigmine (0.25 to 4 mg. intravenously or intramuscularly) is useful to prevent or reverse anticholinergic tachycardia. It also relieves central psychotoxity of the tricyclic-induced central anticholinergic syndrome. Administration of bicarbonate is also helpful to prevent arrhythmias, and propranolol is useful to treat them. Late cardiac difficulties can occur even several days after the patient has regained consciousness; thus patients should be under medical supervision for this time period.

Care should be taken so the suicidal depressed patient does not have access to excessive numbers of antidepressant tablets, since several grams—20 to 40 of the 50-mg. tablets—can be fatal.

Monoamine Oxidase Inhibitors

Iproniazid was the first widely prescribed monoamine oxidase inhibitor. The discovery that this drug could produce rare but troublesome liver toxicity then led to the synthesis of the other hydrazine MAO inhibitors—isocarboxazid, nialamide, and phenelzine—and the nonhydrazine MAO inhibitors—tranylcypromine and pargyline. Table I lists the available MAO inhibitors and gives approximate dose ranges.

Results of Treatment

Table II lists the number of controlled studies showing the efficacy of these drugs versus that of a placebo. Comparisons with imipramine are also presented, since imipramine constitutes the best-studied and most widely used alternate chemotherapy for depressed patients. The therapeutic effect of tranylcypromine is greater than that of a placebo. There is evidence, in well-controlled studies, that iproniazid, phenelzine, and pargyline are also therapeutically effective. Pargyline is marketed only as an antihypertensive, however. Tranylcypromine and iproniazid appear to be most effective; nialamide and isocarboxazid are least effective; and phenelzine occupies a position somewhere in the middle. Roughly speaking, reported toxicity parallels clinical effectiveness.

As a class, the MAO inhibitors seem less effective than the tricyclic antidepressants. Some patients who do not respond to tricyclics may respond to MAO inhibitors, so that a trial on MAO inhibitors for tricyclic nonresponders can be useful. But, since tricyclic drugs are more effective, they are the drugs of choice in most depressions.

Improvement with MAO inhibitors often occurs 4 to 8 weeks after initiation of therapy, its onset frequently being quite dramatic.

Side Effects

Severe hepatic necrosis, which occurred very rarely but with a high fatality rate (about 25 per cent), was reported initially with iproniazid, which led to its withdrawal from general prescription use. Hepatocellular damage has also been very rarely reported in patients treated with other hydrazine MAO inhibitor antidepressants—phenelzine, nialamide, and isocarboxazid—although it is believed that the reactions occur less frequently with these MAO inhibitors than with iproniazid.

The MAO inhibitors cause autonomic side effects, such as dry mouth, dizziness, orthostatic hypotension, epigastric distress, constipation, delayed micturition, delayed ejaculation, and impotence. A side effect of special importance that may result from the use of the MAO inhibitors, particularly tranylcypromine, is the hypertensive crisis, which is occasionally accompanied by intracranial bleeding. Severe occipital headache, stiff neck, sweating, nausea and vomiting, and sharply elevated blood pressure are common prodromal symptoms. The possibility of such side effects can be reduced by careful attention to diet and by avoidance of pressor drugs and related substances. Patients should be appropriately warned. Should these side effects occur, they can be treated by the administration of α-blockers such as phentolamine. Chlorpromazine can also be used.

The combination of an MAO inhibitor with an imipramine-type drug can lead to a syndrome characterized by restlessness, dizziness, tremulousness, muscle twitching, sweating, convulsions, hyperpyrexia (104° to 109°F.), and sometimes death. These reactions can also occur when an MAO inhibitor is replaced by an imipramine-type drug or meperidine in high doses or given intramuscularly. Consequently, a washout period of 7 days is recommended to allow the MAO enzyme to regain activity before such a substitution is made.

The MAO inhibitors potentiate a great variety of drugs, including sympathomimetic amines (such as ephedrine), opiates (meperidine), barbiturates, methyldopa, ganglionic blocking agents, procaine, anesthetic agents, chloral hydrate, and aspirin.

MAO inhibitors can convert a retarded depression into an agitated or anxious one and can occasionally cause hypomania or an acute schizophrenic psychosis. MAO inhibitors can also produce an acute confusional reaction, with disorientation, mental clouding, and illusions. The MAO inhibitors have been associated with altered erotic desires, edema, and muscle tremor. And they can cause dizziness, generalized weakness, slurred speech, increased muscle tone, hyperreflexia, and clonus. An occasional peripheral neuropathy can also occur.

Overdosage

Intoxication caused by MAO inhibitors is, in general, characterized by agitation that progresses to coma with hyperthermia, an increase in respiratory rate, tachycardia, dilated pupils, and hyperactive deep-tendon reflexes. Involuntary movements may be present, particularly in the face and jaw.

Toxicity occurs 1 to 6 hours after ingestion of the drugs.

Acidification of the urine markedly hastens the excretion of tranylcypromine, phenelzine, and amphetamine, and dialysis has been used with success in tranylcypromine poisoning. Chlorpromazine, presumably because of its adrenergic blocking action, is a useful drug in the treatment of poisoning with MAO inhibitors. In cases of hypertensive crises, α-adrenergic blocking agents such as phentolamine may be helpful.

Psychomotor Stimulants

Amphetamine, dextroamphetamine, methamphetamine, methylphenidate, and deanol are classified as psychomotor stimulants (see Table III).

Methylphenidate may be of value in treating patients with mild depression and psychiatric outpatients. There is no evidence that the drug has a beneficial effect on moderate to severe depression.

Amphetamine is of value in mild to moderate depression, but there is less evidence of its effectiveness in severe depression. The amphetamine-type drugs can cause jitteriness, palpitation, psychoses, and other toxic effects and therefore should be used judiciously. Psychic dependence can occur with dextroamphetamine. High doses of amphetamine can produce a florid psychosis that usually resembles paranoid schizophrenia.

There is excellent evidence that amphetamines and methylphenidate are effective in the reduction and control of hyperkinetic behavior in children. These stimulants are also effective in postponing the deterioration to psychomotor performances that often accompanies fatigue.

Phenothiazines

Phenothiazine derivatives have proved to be effective antidepressants. Studies have shown that chorpromazine and imipramine are equally effective, both being superior to a placebo in the treatment of agitated depression. The Veterans Administration (VA) has done a series of closely controlled studies using multivariate analysis. Because the VA population is relatively homogeneous and is studied with identical or similar rating scales, it is possible to combine results from different VA hospital studies, as shown in Table IV. There appears to be some therapeutic efficacy both for phenothiazines and for tricyclic antidepressants. Thioridazine and perphenazine proved to be effective antidepressants in anxious depression.

TABLE III
Psychomotor Stimulants[a]

Name		Manufacturer	Structure	Adult Dose Range (mg./day)	Adult Single Dose Range[b] (mg.[b])	Available Preparations			D.E.A.[c] Control Level
Generic	Trade					Tablet (mg.)	Capsule	Elixir	
Amphetamine	Benzedrine	Smith, Kline & French	phenyl–CH₂–CH(CH₃)–NH₂	5–30	5–10	5, 10			II
Dextroamphetamine	Dexedrine	Smith, Kline & French	phenyl–CH₂CHCH₃–NH₂	5–30	5–10	5	Sustained release: 5, 10, 15	1 mg./ml.	II
Methamphetamine	Desoxyn Fetamin	Abbott Mission	phenyl–CH₂–CH–CH₃, NH–CH₃	5–15	2.5–5	2.5, 5; sustained release: 5, 10, 15			II
Methylphenidate	Ritalin	Ciba	[structure: phenyl–CH(piperidyl)–COOCH₃]	20–60	5–20	5, 10, 20			II
Deanol	Deaner	Riker	HO–CH₂–CH₂–N(CH₃)₂ · CH₃C₆H₄–CONH–C₆H₄–COOH	75–300	75–300	25, 100			0

Side Effects: High abuse potential, Tachycardia, Hypertension, Cardiac arrhythmia, Angina, Overstimulation, Insomnia, Headache, Nervousness and increased tension, Dizziness, Skin rash, Dry mouth and may produce or aggravate psychosis in large doses.

[a] The United States Food and Drug Administration does not recommend the use of amphetamine or its derivatives for depression. However, the authors have found these medications of use in selected cases of depression and neurasthenia when used judiciously.

[b] Except for sustained release preparations which are equivalent to the effective adult daily dose (mg./day).

[c] D.E.A., Drug Enforcement Administration

TABLE IV

*Results of Drug Treatment: Response of Veterans Administration Patients Classified by Overall-Hollister Subtypes**

Drug Treatment	Change Score			
	Overall-Hollister Subtype			Entire Population
	Anxious	Hostile	Retarded	
Study 1				
Imipramine	38	38	66	43
Thioridazine	64	51	32	56
Study 2				
Amitriptyline	50	52	72	54
Amitriptyline-perphenazine	66	74	36	64
Study 3				
Tranylcypromine	47	72	15	44
Dextroamphetamine	65	39	38	50
Study 4				
Dextroamphetamine-amobarbital				34
Placebo				43
Isocarboxazid				27
Imipramine				57
Study 5				
Placebo				45
Desipramine				23
Atropine				39
Imipramine				45
Amitriptyline				54
Study 6				
Amitriptyline	53†	38†	120†	75
Perphenazine	93†	64†	−4†	35
Amitriptyline-perphenazine	84†	77†	62†	65

*Change measured by IMPS manifest depression score both for subtypes and for the population as a whole (except where noted).

†Mean change scores on IMPS total pathology were used, since manifest depression data were not available.

Phobic-Anxiety Syndrome

A syndrome characterized by panic attacks often occurs when the patient is in some sense separated from significant others—traveling alone in subways, tunnels, bridges, out in the streets. The patient then begins to show anticipatory anxiety and dread of situations that may get him in the situation of which he is phobic. The patients typically have been fearful, dependent children with a great deal of separation anxiety. Imipramine dramatically stops the panic attacks, and minor traquilizers are sometimes useful to overcome the anticipatory anxiety and help the patient go back into the situation in which he experienced the panic attack so that he can demonstrate to himself that he no longer gets the panic attack. Imipramine seems to be specific for the panic attack, as opposed to the anticipatory anxiety. The childhood version of the syndrome (school phobia) is also helped by imipramine.

Anxiety-Depression Syndrome

A common disorder of outpatients is the mixed anxiety-depression syndrome (nonpsychotic). Doxepin (see Table V), a tricyclic drug having antidepressive and antianxiety properties, has been shown to be superior to a placebo and equal to diazepam (Valium) and to chlordiazepoxide (Librium) in efficacy. In one study, doxepin was slightly superior to diazepam, possibly because many patients with depression were included in the sample studied and possibly because a relatively low dose of diazepam was used. Conventional tricyclic antidepressants have also been used to treat this syndrome, and doxepin is approximately as effective as they are. Doxepin is approximately equal to amitriptyline-perphenazine in treating anxious-depressed patients.

TABLE V

Therapeutic Effects of Doxepin in Anxiety-Depression Syndrome and in Depression: Comparison of Doxepin with Standard Drug

Syndrome and Standard Drug	Doxepin		
	Superior	Equal	Inferior
Anxiety-Depression			
Placebo	6	0	0
Chlordiazepoxide	0	11	0
Diazepam	1	7	0
Amitriptyline	1	1	0
Amitriptyline-perphenazine	1	4	1
Thioridazine	0	1	0
Depression			
Placebo	2	0	0
Imipramine	0	3	0
Amitriptyline	0	8	0
Amitriptyline-perphenazine	0	1	0

For mixed outpatient anxiety-depression, typical doses of doxepin consist of 100 to 300 mg. a day. Doses for anxiety are slightly lower.

The perphenazine-amitriptyline combination seems to show particular promise with the hostile type of depression. In several studies based on outpatient populations with anxiety and depression, the amitriptyline-perphenazine combination proved superior to chlordiazepoxide and a placebo. However, the British General Practitioner Research Group, in its study of drug combinations, did not find this combination to be superior to perphenazine alone.

It is also a common clinical observation that many patients treated with imipramine are often helped by the addition of a phenothiazine derivative at the point in their recovery when they begin to get high.

In the absence of studies that clearly predict which drug to use for which patients, it seems reasonable to use antipsychotic drugs with or without amitriptyline in treating anxiety and depression when this syndrome is seen in patients with signs of schizophrenia, endogenous depression, psychotic depression, or manic-depressive illness. When the anxiety-depression syndrome shades into outpatient nonpsychotic anxiety, doxepin seems to be as effective as the above classes of drugs.

Choice of Treatment

In Table II the efficacy of imipramine in the treatment of depression is compared with ECT and other antidepressant medications. In four of the seven studies comparing imipramine with electroshock therapy, ECT proved more effective; in the remaining three studies, ECT was equally effective. However, ECT acts faster than imipramine, a factor of importance in the treatment of the acutely suicidal patient. Since ECT produces temporary memory loss, postshock confusion, and perhaps subtle but permanent central nervous system changes, some psychiatrists prefer not to use it as a routine measure. With ECT, maintenance therapy with imipramine is necessary to prevent recurrence of depression after remission. The recurrence rate of depression after ECT is high (18 to 46 per cent after 6 months). Yet, of the depressed patients who do not respond to imipramine, amitriptyline, or phenelzine, about 50 per cent respond to ECT.

Phenelzine has been shown to be inferior to ECT in four studies. Isocarboxazid has also been found less effective than ECT. However, a tranylcypromine and trifluoperazine combination has been reported to result in rapid antidepressant effect, and there is some evidence that this combination can be uniquely effective in a small proportion of patients.

It has been suggested that a patient with a relative who responded well to either an imipramine-type drug or an MAO inhibitor will respond better to that type of drug than to another. And it has been suggested that cases of hysteria with secondary depression respond best to MAO inhibitors. However, studies that identify a specific type of patient as responding differentially to a drug should be regarded as only tentative until they have been cross-validated.

Imipramine-type (tricyclic) drugs are probably slightly more effective and slightly safer than MAO inhibitors. Phenothiazine derivatives or MAO inhibitors may also be of value in selected cases.

In general, the antidepressants are quite safe; although potentially dangerous side effects do occur, they are rare. Since they do occur, however, and since these drugs are quite potent, they should be prescribed only when there are definite indications that such treatment is necessary. Under normal circumstances. there is no medical need for weekly routine laboratory tests when an antidepressant is used, but appropriate investigations should be made before administration of the drug when there is evidence of physical disease.

Effective psychotherapy may greatly enhance the patient's response to antidepressant drugs and prevent recurrence. Moreover, depression in patients with underlying neuroses or personality disorders may respond dramatically to psychotherapy and not respond at all to existing drugs.

Many untreated serious depressions often run for 6 months or more before remission occurs. About 15 per cent of patients with recurrent depressive disease eventually commit suicide. Acute depression can be very painful, and chronic depression leads to much disability and unhappiness. Most cases of true depressive disease are readily treatable and should be vigorously and quickly treated.

Implications for Theory

The fact that the tricyclic antidepressants, the MAO inhibitors, ECT, the antipsychotic agents, and lithium benefit affective disorders may provide clues as to the causes of these diseases. The most likely common pharmacologic pathways on which all these agents may interact are the neurotransmitters. Norepinephrine (NE) and dopamine (DA) have been shown to be some of the transmitters involved with the reward centers. In a common-sense manner, elation and sadness relate to reward or no reward. Specifically, if drive in some sense energizes behavior—turns up the gain, as it were, in mania—the gain could be set too high and in depression set too low. Serotonin (5-hydroxytryptamine (5-HT)) may be involved in punishments. Acetylcholine (ACh) antagonizes NE's effect on the reward center in the sense that the noradrenergic reward center may have a cholinergic input that acts in such a direction as to inhibit or tone down the reward or pleasure component.

Reserpine lowers brain levels of serotonin and catecholamines and often causes depression. The MAO inhibitors increase brain levels of amines by inhibiting their degradation, but the tricyclic antidepressants may make more norepinephrine or serotonin available at the receptor site through inhibition of reuptake. Both of these latter classes of drugs are beneficial in depression. Electroconvulsive therapy increases norepinephrine synthesis and utilization and also relieves depression. Lithium may act by increasing the net reuptake or accumulation of norepinephrine or serotonin, thereby suppressing mania.

Monoamine Oxidase Inhibitors

The monoamine oxidase (MAO) inhibitors probably act by the irreversible inhibition of the enzyme monoamine oxidase, which intracellularly deaminates DA, NE, and 5-HT. This leads to the accumulation of higher levels of these amines in the brains of many species, which may result in more transmitter substances being available for use. The evidence that these drugs act by the inhibition of monoamine oxidase rather than by other mechanisms is based primarily on the fact that there are many MAO inhibitors, differing in chemical properties and structure yet sharing the properties of inhibiting monoamine oxidase and relieving depression. Evidence that therapeutic doses of MAO inhibitors do alter MAO and increase brain amines (5-HT, NE, DA) in human beings is provided by autopsy studies. The elevation of 5-HT occurs several weeks after the onset of treatment with MAO inhibitors, the time at which the antidepressant effect occurs.

Tricyclic Antidepressants

The potentiation by imipramine and similar drugs of the action of NE in a variety of systems has been explained by the observation that imipramine blocks the uptake of NE into the nerve ending, thereby leaving newly released NE at the receptor site of a longer time. A similar mechanism exists for the neuronal uptake of serotonin. Tricyclic drugs do increase the urinary excretion of O-methylated amines and decrease the excretion of vanillylmandelic acid. Platelets, structurally and functionally, have many similarities to nerve endings and may, in fact, provide an accessible model of the nerve ending. Imipramine decreases uptake of 5-HT into platelets drawn from patients under treatment with the tricyclic drug, in comparison with platelets drawn from controlled drug-free patients.

Reserpine-Induced Depression

A significant percentage of hypertensive patients treated with high doses of reserpine develop depressions similar to endogenous depressive reactions. Hypertensive patients treated with reserpine show significantly more depressive reactions than do similar patients treated with other antihypertensive drugs. In addition, the incidence of reserpine-induced depression is dose-related, with most cases occuring in patients receiving 0.75 mg. of reserpine a day or more. Generally, the onset of depression occurs between 1 and 7 months after the initiation of reserpine therapy. The depression usually subsides when the patient is taken off reserpine and recurs when reserpine therapy is resumed.

Reserpine depletes the brain of serotonin and norepinephrine. A variety of evidence suggests that reserpine disrupts the process by which the intracellular vesicles store norepinephrine. Norepinephrine is released into the cell sap, where it is destroyed by mitochondrial oxidase; hence, most of the transmitter is inactivated intracellularly, without exerting any physiologic effect.

Electroconvulsive Therapy

Animal studies indicate that after ECT there is an increase in the synthesis and utilization of NE. Other studies have yielded disparate results, however, so there is no present consensus on the mechanism by which ECT benefits depression.

Lithium

Schildkraut and associates found that lithium administered to animals before the injection of intracisternal NE decreased the levels of labeled normethanephrine and increased the levels of tritiated, deaminated catecholamine metabolites in the brain. Lithium pretreatment has increased the net uptake of NE and 5-HT into brain; 5-HT uptake in platelets is enhanced in the patient who is receiving lithium. Futhermore, lithium decreases the pressor response to intravenous infusion of NE, an effect consistent with increased uptake or decreased receptor sensitivity or both. The effects are small, and there is no consensus on how lithium affects neurotransmitters.

Amphetamine

Acute administration of amphetamine causes elation in humans and hyperactivity in animals, an effect that, in animal studies, has been shown to depend on the presence of catecholamines in the brain. Fawcett and his collaborators have noted that a behavioral response of elation to a 3-day trial of amphetamine predicts which depressed patients will respond to tricyclic drugs. In large doses, it depletes the brain of NE, and prolonged use of this drug is sometimes followed by depression.

Indirect Measurement of Brain Amines

Since it has been postulated that depression is associated with low brain NE levels and since it has been suggested that significant quantities of brain catecholamines are metabolized to 3-methoxy-4-hydroxphenylglycol (MHPG), the amount of MHPG excreted in the urine may reflect the metabolism of NE in brain. It was found that the urinary levels of MHPG were significantly lower in a group of seriously depressed patients than in controls. The signifi-

cance of these results depend on the demonstration that MHPG levels in urine do reflect NE metabolism in brain. Furthermore, increased excretion of MHPG has been found in mania. Studies indicate that some depressed patients may have a modest decrease of brain serotonin.

Other Evidence

The β-blocking drug propranolol can be associated with depression when given in high doses in those patients who developed reserpine depression when reserpine was previously used to treat their hypertension. Thyroid hormones can shorten the lag period in female depressives treated with tricyclics, and thyroid interacts with catecholamines in complex ways. Depression is associated with excess secretion of cortisol and other endocrine abnormalities. The central control of these neuroendocrine systems involves neural circuits that may use norepinephrine, dopamine, and serotonin as their neurotransmitter substances.

Cholinergic Involvement

Preliminary data provide evidence that increasing central acetylcholine levels with the cholinesterase inhibitor physostigmine antagonizes manic symptoms, decreases the intensity of the manic syndrome, and causes an anergic syndrome, consisting in part of lethargy, drained feelings, slowed thoughts, and motor retardation. In a number of cases, physostigmine appears to cause symptoms characteristic of a depressive mood. A rebound worsening of mania has been reported several hours after physostigmine treatment. The cholinesterase inhibitors appear to decrease mania and increase depression and psychomotor retardation in manic-depressive patients and excited schizo-affective patients. Since mania has previously been thought to be due to a depletion of norepinephrine, these data raised the possibility that a given affective state may represent a balance between adrenergic and cholinergic factors. Mania could be considered to represent a relative predominance of adrenergic activity. Depression could represent a relative cholinergic prodominance.

The central effects of the monoamine depleter reserpine, the depressant effects of which have been used to support the monoamine hypothesis of depression, are remarkably similar to those of the cholinesterase inhibitors. Overlapping symptoms include apathy, lassitude, sloweddown thinking, psychomotor retardation, lack of interest, fatigue, lethargy, nightmares, and depression. Indeed, reserpine has been reported to have central cholinergic properties. Thus, reserpine-induced depression could be due to a combination of monoamine depletion and cholinergic activation, shifting adrenergic-cholinergic balance to a cholinergic predominance. Likewise, tricyclic-antidepressant-induced manic reactions and antidepressant effects could be due to a combination of decreased central cholinergic activity associated with increased adrenergic activity, shifting adrenergic-cholinergic balance toward an adrenergic predominance.

Critique

A number of lines of circumstantial evidence implicate neurotransmitters in depression, but the evidence is indirect. The antidepressants are clinically neither specific nor highly effective. Depression may not be a single diagnostic entity. Evidence related to the MAO inhibitors, tricyclic drugs, reserpine, and lithium fails to implicate clearly either NE, 5-HT, DA, or ACh. The reduced levels of 5-HT or 5-HIAA in brain and cerebrospinal fluid in depression implicate serotonin. The observation that propanolol can cause depression implicates NE. It may be inappropriate to designate a preferred amine, since most of the evidence is not definitive; both amines could be involved.

Hyperactivity Syndrome

Psychomotor stimulants, such as amphetamine and methylphenidate, often produce dramatic improvement in the performance of hyperkinetic children. It can be postulated that the basic neurophysiologic disorder of hyperkinesia of childhood is a disorder of inhibitory mechanisms in the central nervous system, such that irrelevant stimuli are not filtered out, and the child is at the mercy of his environment. Psychomotor stimulants seem to improve areas of cognitive function that are impaired in these children.

Rather than give these drugs indiscriminately, one should give the drug as a therapeutic trial. After assessing the child's behavior both at home and at school, the clinician can start with a relatively small dose, such as 5 mg. of D-amphetamine or 10 mg. of methylphenidate, given in the morning, and increase the dose every 2 to 3 days to a maximum of 30 mg. of D-amphetamine or 60 mg. of methylphenidate, taken morning and noon. About two thirds to three fourths of all hyperactive children show a marked to moderate improvement. It is often advisable not to continue the drug for unusually lengthy periods of time but to interrupt treatment on occasion to determine whether the child continues to need treatment.

In general, side effects of psychomotor stimulants are minimal. Occasionally, insomnia and anorexia occur, but these side effects can be controlled by giving the medication with meals, by altering the dosage, or by giving the medication only in the morning.

REFERENCES

Asberg, M., Cronoholm, B., Sjoquist, F., and Tuck, D. Relationship between plasma levels and therapeutic effect of nortriptyline. Br. Med. J., 3: 331, 1971.
Bunney, W. E., Jr., and Davis, J. M. Norepinephrine in depressive reactions. Arch. Gen. Psychiatry, 13: 483, 1965.
Fawcett, J., Maas, J. W., and Dekirmenjian, H. Depression and MHPG excretion response to dextroamphetamine and tricyclic antidepressants. Arch. Gen. Psychiatry, 26: 246, 1972.
Klerman, G. L., and Cole. J. O. Clinical Pharmacology of imipramine and related antidepressant compounds. Pharmacol. Rev., 17: 101, 1965.
Kragh-Sorenson, P., Asberg, M., and Eggert Hensen, C. Plasma nortriptyline levels in endogenous depression. Lancet, 1: 113, 1973.
Mindham, R. H. S., Howland, C., and Shepherd, M. Continuation therapy with tricyclic antidepressants in depressive illness. Lancet, 2: 854, 1972.
Schildkraut, J. J. The catecholamine hypothesis of affective disorders: A review of supporting evidence. Am. J. Psychiatry, 122: 509, 1965.

30.3.   MINOR TRANQUILIZERS, ANTI-ANXIETY AGENTS, SEDATIVES, AND HYPNOTICS

Minor Tranquilizers

These minor tranquilizers share the sedative, hypnotic, central muscle relaxant, anticonvulsant, central nervous sustem depressant, and habituating potential of the barbiturates. There are many workers who feel that minor tranquilizers should be classified as sedatives in view of their similar effect.

Antianxiety Drugs vs. Anti-Psychotic Drugs

Antianxiety drugs are indicated in neuroses. They act as sedatives, are hypnotic, produce somnolence, relax muscles, produce ataxia, and have anticonvulsant effects. They are also habituating, tolerance develops, and they produce withdrawal symptoms upon cessation of the drug. Suicide attempts with antianxiety drugs are often successful because of their depressive effect on medullary centers.

Anti-psychotic drugs are indicated in psychoses. They do not produce somnolence or have hypnotic effects. Increased muscle spasticity and extrapyramidal symptoms are common. The convulsive threshold is lowered and convulsions may result. These drugs are not habituating, tolerance does not develop, and they do not have a serious suicide abuse potential.

Clinical Considerations

The antianxiety drugs are used to reduce anxiety in neurotic patients and to treat delirium tremens and epilepsy. Treatment with the antianxiety drug is simpler than with the anti-psychotic drug. There is little reason to prefer one drug over another for oral therapy, which is the usual mode of administration. Since tolerance to the antianxiety effects of these compounds develops rapidly, they are useful only for relatively short periods of continuous treatment, such as 3 or 4 weeks. If unusual circumstances require a longer administration, intermittent drug-free periods may restore effectiveness.

The minor tranquilizers resemble the sedative-hypnotic drugs more closely than they do the antipsychotic drugs. Physicians have been using meprobamate in the treatment of anxiety and related symptoms for more than 15 years. Newer therapeutic agents—such as chlordiazepoxide (Librium), diazepam (Valium), oxazepam (Serax), tybamate (Solacen), and clorazepate (Tranxene)—have come into increasing use in the intervening years. These drugs have all been called minor tranquilizers and have been alleged to be superior to the barbiturates as antianxiety agents. All these drugs, at appropriate dosages, reduce anxiety and can produce drowsiness (sedation) and sleep (hypnosis).

Meprobamate and Tybamate

Derivatives of meprobamate include tybamate, another antianxiety agent, and carisoprodol (Soma, Rela), which has selective properties as a skeletal muscle relaxant but negligible antianxiety effects.

Table I compares meprobamate and tybamate with a placebo. Meprobamate is significantly more effective than a placebo in some of the double-blind studies, and tybamate is significantly more effective than a placebo in most of the double-blind studies that have made this comparison. Most of the studies found meprobamate to be equal to the barbiturates in efficacy, and in some studies there was a trend for meprobamate to be superior.

The usual dosage of meprobamate is 400 mg. three or four times a day. The usual dosage of tybamate is two 250-mg. capsules three or four times a day (see Table II). Tybamate appears to be particularly effective in the somatically oriented hypochondriacal patient.

About half the patients on meprobamate develop drowsiness as a side effect. It is, there-

TABLE I
Summary of Controlled, Double-Blind Evaluations of the Minor Tranquilizing Drugs*

Drug		Number of Studies in Which Drug Was					
Generic name	Trade name	Better than placebo		Better than barbiturates		Better than meprobamate	
		Yes	No	Yes	No	Yes	No
Barbiturates		13	6				
Meprobamate	Miltown, Equanil	18	9	3	7		
Chlordiazepoxide	Librium	27	1	3	4	2	3
Diazepam	Valium	16	2	4	1	1	1
Oxazepam	Serax	8	1				
Tybamate	Solacen, Tybatran	15	1			2	1

* Figures include controlled, double-blind studies only. A drug was not considered better than another drug unless a statistically significant difference existed between the two drugs in their relative effectiveness.

Name		Manu-facturer	Structure	Adult Dose Range	Adult Single Dose Range	
Generic	Trade				Sedative*	Hypnotic‡
				mg./day		mg.
Meprobamate	Equanil Miltown	Wyeth Wallace	$H_2N-\overset{O}{\underset{}{C}}-OCH_2-\overset{C_3H_7}{\underset{CH_3}{C}}-CH_2O-\overset{O}{\underset{}{C}}-NH_2$	400–1,600	200–400	
Tybamate	Tybatran	Robins	$H_2NCOOCH_2(CH_3)C(C_3H_7)$ $CH_2OCONH(CH_2)_3CH_3$	250–2000	250–500	
Ethinamate	Valmid	Dista		500–1000		500–1000
Glutethimide	Doriden	USV		125–500	125–250	500
Methyprylon	Noludar	Roche		50–400	50–100	200–400
Ethchlorvynol	Placidyl	Abbott	$HC\equiv C-\overset{OH}{\underset{C_2H_5}{C}}-CH=CHCl$	500–750		500–750
Methaqualone	Quaalude Sopor	Rorer Arnar-Stone		75–300	75	150–300
Diphenhydra-mine	Benadryl	Parke, Davis		10–400	50	
Hydroxyzine	Vistaril Atarax	Pfizer Roerig		25–400	25–100	
Chloral hydrate	Noctec Kessodrate Felsules Aquachloral	Squibb McKesson Fellows Webcon	$CCl_3CH(OH)$	250–100	250	500–2000
Promethazine	Phenergan	Wyeth		12.5–150	12.5–50	12.5–50
Paraldehyde	Paral	Fellows		4–10 ml.		4–10 ml.

* Sedative dose is that amount given at one time sufficient to reduce anxiety without inducing sleep.
‡ Hypnotic dose is that amount given at one time sufficient to induce sleep.
§ D.E.A., Drug Enforcement Administration.

tives, Hypnotics and Antianxiety Agents

Available Preparations									Addictive		D.E.A.§ Control Level
Oral					Injection				Psychological Dependence	Physiological Dependence	
Tablet	Capsule	Syrup	Elixir	Ampul	Ampul	Vial	Syringe	Suppository			
mg.	*mg.*						*mg.*				
200, 400, 600	400								+	+	IV
	125, 250 350								–	–	0
	500								+	+	IV
125, 250 500	500								+	+	III
50, 200	300								+	+	III
	100, 200, 500, 750								+	+	IV
150–300									+	+	II
	25, 50		12.5 mg./ 5 ml.		50 mg./ml.	10 mg./ml. 50 mg./ml.	50 mg./ ml.		–	–	0
10, 25, 50, 100	25, 50, 10	2 mg./ml. 5 mg./ml.				25 mg./ml. 50 mg./ml.	25 mg./ ml. 50 mg./ ml.		–	–	0
	250, 500	100 mg./ml.						325 650 975 1,300	+	+	IV
12.5, 25, 50		1.25 mg./ ml. 5 mg./ml.			25 mg./ml. 50 mg./ml.			25 50	–	–	0
	1000 (1000 mg. = 1 ml.)		30 ml.	2 ml. 5 ml. 10 ml.					+	+	IV

Side Effects: Impaired judgment and performance, Drowsiness, Lethargy, Residual sedation ("hangover"), Skin eruptions, Nausea, Vomiting, Paradoxical restlessness or excitement, Exacerbation of symptoms of organic brain syndrome, Ataxia, Atropine psychosis with hypnotic doses of diphenhydramine or hydroxysine, Unpredictable clinical course after glutethimide overdose, High addictive potential and low margin of safety in suicide attempts with glutethimide, and With promethazine, a phenothiazine without antipsychotic activity, side effects of the phenothiazine class may be observed.

TABLE III
Benzodiazepines

Name		Manu-facturer	Structure	Adult Dose Range	Adult Single Dose Range	Available Preparations					Addictive		D.E.A. Control Level
Generic	Trade					Oral		Injection					
				mg/day	*mg.*	Tablet	Capsule	Ampul	Vial	Syringe	Psycho-logical Depen-dence	Physio-logical Depen-dence	
					mg.								
Chlordiazep-oxide	Librium Libritabs	Roche Roche		15–100	5–25	5, 10, 25	5, 10, 25	5 mg. dry filled with 2 ml. diluent			+	+	IV
Diazepam	Valium	Roche		6–40	2–10	2, 5, 10		5 mg./ml.	5 mg./ml.	5 mg./ml.	+	+	IV
Oxazepam	Serax	Wyeth		30–120	10–30	5					+	+	IV
Clorazepate	Tranxene	Abbott		11.75–60	3.75–60	22.5	3.75, 7.5, 15				+	+	IV

Flurazepam	Dalmane	Roche	CH₂CH₂N(C₂H₅)₂ structure	15–30	15–30	15, 30	?	?	IV
Clonazepam	Clonopin	Roche	structure	1.5–20	0.5–7	0., 1, 2	+	+	IV

*Unlike the other benzodiazepines available for clinical use, clonazepam is not indicated for use as a sedative or hypnotic. It is classified as an antiepileptic agent, use ful alone or as an adjunct in the treatment of the Lennox-Gastaut syndrome (petit mal variant), akinetic and myoclonic seizures. Clonopin may also be useful in patients with absence seizures (petit mal) who have failed to respond to succinimides.

Side Effects: Paradoxical excitement, Hypnagogic hallucination, Phlebitis, Fatigue, Drowsiness, Somnolence, Muscle weakness, Nystagmus Ataxia, Dysarthria, Impaired reaction time, motor coordination, and intellectual function: and Central nervous system depression.

fore, wise to start with a small dose and build up to a therapeutic dose within 3 or 4 days. The sedative effect of meprobamate is potentiated by alcohol and other central nervous system depressants.

Large doses of meprobamate may be addicting. Sudden withdrawal after high doses of meprobamate may cause anxiety, restlessness, weakness, convulsions, and delirium. This condition is best treated by slow withdrawal in a supervised setting.

Benzodiazepine Derivatives

The first of the benzodiazepine derivatives was chlordiazepoxide. Five additional derivatives of this class are now available in the United States: diazepam, oxazepam, clorazepate, flurazepam, and clonazepam (see table III). Table I shows comparisons of chlordiazepoxide, diazepam, and oxazepam with a placebo, meprobamate, and barbiturates. All three of the benzodiazepine drugs are better than a placebo in almost all the studies that have been done. About three fourths of the double-blind studies find the benzodiazepines to be more effective than the barbiturates.

Clorazepate (Tranxene) is decarboxylated in the stomach into its principal metabolite, nordiazepam. Diazepam itself is demethylated in the liver to nordiazepam. The nordiazepam is metabolized in the liver to oxazepam (Serax), which is then conjugated and excreted as an inactive metabolite. There is excellent evidence that clorazepate is an effective antianxiety agent. It has been shown in double-blind studies to be at least as effective as diazepam and definitely superior to a placebo.

Typical daily dose schedules for the benzodiazepine minor tranquilizers are: chlordiazepoxide, 10 to 25 mg. three or four times a day; diazepam, 2 to 10 mg. three or four times a day; oxazepam, 15 to 30 mg. three times a day; and clorazepate, 3.75 to 15 mg. four times a day. The drug effect usually manifests itself in a few days.

The benzodiazepines, like other antianxiety agents, cause sedation. Because of this effect, it is wise to start with a small dose and build up to the full therapeutic dose in 3 or 4 days.

When given by mouth, the drugs are effective in reducing chronic anxiety, but they can also overcome acute anxiety when given intravenously. For example, 10 mg. of diazepam intravenously infused over 10 minutes reduces symptoms of anxiety. The maximal effects are seen 20 to 30 minutes after the end of administration of the drug.

The most striking pharmacologic action of the benzodiazepines in laboratory animals has long been their ability to disinhibit behavior suppressed by fear of punishment without seriously interfering with appetitive behavior. Benzodiazepines may well be given mainly at bedtime, so that the sedative side effects will be dissipated during the night and the antianxiety effect will persist during the next day.

Diphenylhydantoin

This effective, relatively nonsedative anticonvulsant drug has been claimed to be effective in the treatment of a range of neurotic and behavioral symptoms. The drug is relatively benign in low doses (200 mg. a day) and may uniquely benefit occasional outpatients who fail to respond to other drugs. However, diphenylhydantoin toxicity is frequently seen in epileptics on higher dosages; they may manifest ataxia and confusion. Diphenylhydantoin toxicity is more common in patients with low serum albumin due to decreased protein binding. It may also come on 2 or 3 weeks after phenobarbital is discontinued in patients who had been receiving both drugs when phenobarbital-induced enzyme induction disappears.

Propranolol and Related Drugs

Anxiety is characterized by palpitations rapid heart beat, tremor, tingling, cold sweats, chest constriction, and twitching. Physiologically, many of these symptoms can be caused by epinephrine secreted during stress. This point raises the question of whether one of the components in anxiety is the perception of these internal epinephrine-induced physiological events or even a hyperawareness of normal adrenergic functioning.

Many of these peripheral autonomic events can be blocked by β-adrenergic blocking agents, such as propranolol (Inderal). The hypothesis here is that the β-adrenergic agent may block the autonomic signals of anxiety and, thus, may benefit anxiety through a peripheral mechanism. Propranolol, given either intravenously or orally in β-receptor-blocking doses, produces improvements in patients with anxiety, particularly improvements in the somatic manifestations of anxiety.

The use of β blockers for anxiety is still in the investigational stage and is mentioned here for its theoretical relevance. When such drugs become available for general use with a psychiatric indication, one must be mindful of the side effects and contraindications of the β-blocking drugs, such as asthma and cardiac conditions in which a slowing of the heart would be harmful.

Antihistamines and Over-the-Counter Sedatives

Patent medicines marketed for the treatment of nervousness usually contain a sedative antihistamine, such as methapyriline, and a little scopolamine. There is the remote possibility that the advertising of these patent remedies potentiates either their real efficacy or their placebo effect to the point where people who buy them in drug stores actually are helped. Antihistamines have antianxiety and sedative side effects in some adults, and one such drug, diphenhydramine, is used as a sedative in children. Hydroxyzine, usually used as an antianxiety agent, also belongs in this class.

Methaqualone

This modest nonbarbiturate sedative and hypnotic came into prominence as a favored drug among drug abusers in the early 1970's. It is alleged to produce a more intense peak experience than do barbiturates.

Hydergine

Hydergine has been used for several years as an agent for treating mental problems in the aging, presumably because of its vasodilating action. It apparently alleviates anxiety, agitation, and irritability. This improvement is slow in onset; in placebo-controlled studies, significant differences become more and more obvious over a 3-month period but may be minimal or absent after only 1 month.

Alcohol

Alcohol is clearly usable as a sedative and mild antianxiety agent. It is usually self-prescribed and has been evaluated as a therapy only in institutionalized patients.

Effectiveness

A large body of data, summarized in Table I, supports the superiority of the benzodiazepines, chlordiazepoxide, diazepam, and oxazepam, over both a placebo and barbiturates as treatments for anxious outpatients. Tybamate also has a reasonably impressive box score; meprobamate looks somewhat less consistently superior to other treatments.

Patients with anxiety accompanying acute or chronic schizophrenia or depression or severe personality disorder usually do not do well on either an antianxiety drug or a placebo. Patients with anxiety symptoms of less than 6 months' duration and with little prior experience with drug therapy do remarkably well on a placebo, showing 85 per cent improvement, but they show only 80 per cent improvement on chlordiazepoxide. For more chronic patients with several previous trials on drug therapy, the drug-improvement rate stays at 80 per cent, but the placebo rate drops to 20 per cent.

The nature of the improvement produced by minor tranquilizers may go beyond a simple antianxiety effect. More instances of positive life events and fewer instances of negative life events have been reported by outpatients receiving chlordiazepoxide, as compared with a placebo control group. This result may be due to a perceptual alteration, producing a tendency for the patients to see events in a positive light. Alternatively, chlordiazepoxide may provide relief of incapacitating psychiatric symptoms and a secondary increase in vigor, thus allowing the patient to deal with life situations in a more constructive manner. Or the drug may have a mild disinhibiting action, similar to that seen socially after modest doses of alcohol.

Outpatient neurotics constitute an extremely heterogeneous group, and the most important aspect of drug therapy is the identification of which patient will do well on which drug. Some patients have episodic, irregular attacks of acute, severe anxiety and may be free of obvious psychiatric symptoms between attacks. These attacks can be aborted by the intravenous administration of barbiturates or diazepam. Some patients prefer to carry a few tablets of a barbiturate or diazepam with them so that they can take one if they should have an attack, and they find this method preferable to the three-times-a-day administration of drugs.

Other patients who have attacks of apparent anxiety, characterized by panic attack of severe and pervasive fright of overwhelming proportions, also have an incapacitating secondary set of phobias, chiefly fears of being alone or fears of going outside or on the subway without company, occasioned by their anticipation that they may have a panic attack and be helpless. These panic attacks do not respond to either phenothiazines or minor tranquilizers but have been shown to respond to antidepressant drugs, such as imipramine.

Diagnosis becomes important in deciding which drug to give to which patient in an outpatient situation, since it is mandatory to treat incipient schizophrenics with antipsychotics, and some patients with depression may do better on one or another of the various antidepressants than on a minor tranquilizer. Although barbiturates may be adequate for acute anxiety attacks, there is a definite therapeutic benefit from some of the minor tranquilizers in chronic anxiety. The clinician must try a patient on what seems to be the drug most likely to help him and, if this fails, try him on another drug of a different class.

In general, the chlordiazepoxide (Librium, Valium, Serax) family of drugs is probably the best for the majority of anxious outpatients, but many other drugs may be indicated for specific symptoms (see Tables II and III).

Sedatives and Hypnotics

Barbiturates, meprobamate, and the benzodiazepine-type drugs are extensively used as sleeping medications. Controlled studies indicate that all have significant hypnotic properties. At the doses commonly used, barbiturates and nonbarbiturate sedatives are comparable in hypnotic properties to flurazepam, which is slightly more potent than diazepam, meprobamate, chlordiazepoxide, and oxazepam. The chief advantage of flurazepam is that is is alleged to have less liability for death in overdose situations and less liability for abuse. This relative freedom from toxicity is an important advantage of all the benzodiazepine drugs. Sedatives should be used with caution in patients with liver, cardiac, and kidney diseases and diabetes, hyperthyroidism, and congestive heart failure. The nonbarbiturate sedatives, such as glutethimide, have the same side-effect liabilities for abuse and overdose as do the barbiturates. They are extremely lethal in overdose. The nonbarbiturate sedatives have considerable liability for barbiturate-type abuse and cause the same withdrawal syndrome as do barbiturates.

Barbiturates

The first barbiturate to be used in medicine was barbital (Veronal), introduced in 1903. It was followed by phenobarbital (Luminal), amobarbital (Amytal), pentobarbital (Nembutal), secobarbital (Seconal), thiopental (Pentothal), and hexobarbital (Evipal). In all, about 2,500 barbiturates have been synthesized, and 50 barbiturates have been used clinically.

Patients who have difficulty in falling asleep but then sleep soundly can be given short-acting barbiturates. Patients who wake up frequently throughout the night may require a medium-acting barbiturate. Long-acting barbiturates are useful as sedatives in chronic anxiety but are relatively poor hypnotics. Commonly used barbiturates are noted in Table IV.

Medium-acting barbiturates are effective in chronic anxiety and can produce a dramatic antianxiety effect in an acute anxiety attack. Sometimes a patient derives a sense of control over episodes of acute anxiety from the knowledge that he has a few barbiturate tablets in his pocket and can control an anxiety attack if it develops.

In general, the barbiturates are probably a bit more effective than a placebo as antianxiety agents and a bit less effective than the benzodiazepines. They are frequently used to commit successful suicide. However, they are inexpensive in their generic forms and may be used for anxious patients who must pay for their own medications if suidal risk appears remote.

In large doses, the barbiturates produce a depression of the central nervous system; the respiratory center is particularly vulnerable, and respiratory depression is common from barbiturate overdose. This effect may constitute a particular danger in patients with severe pulmonary insufficiency. Barbiturates have no analgesic action of their own. Because of this lack, the barbiturates do not cause sleep when insomnia is due to pain; instead, they can produce restlessness and confusion.

Phenobarbital is said to be an excellent anticonvulsant and a potent inducer of hepatic enzymes. It is known to speed the body's metabolism of dicoumarin in this manner, thereby lowering prothrombin time if the patient's dicoumarin dose is not adjusted upward concomitantly.

Nonbarbiturate Hypnotics

Drugs like glutethimide are chemically not at all like barbiturates but are either pharmacologically as bad as the barbiturates or, in the case of glutethimide in particular, are worse. It is hard to find a special indication for any of these drugs at the present time. Barbiturates are slightly cheaper, and benzodiazepines are safer and as effective.

Chloral hydrate is the oldest hypnotic, having been introduced into medicine in 1869. It is a relatively short-acting drug that is useful in initial insomnia, but it has less value as a daytime sedative. Chloral hydrate is an effective hypnotic. It is widely assumed to be a safe, mild hypnotic. It is rapidly changed in the body to trichloroethanol, which is also an effective hypnotic. Chloral hydrate's lethal dose is about 5 to 10 times its hypnotic dose of 1 to 2 gm.

Paraldehyde is another traditional hypnotic, first introduced into medicine in 1882. Paraldehyde, 5 cc intramuscularly or 5 to 10 cc. by mouth, is an old-fashioned treatment for both alcoholic withdrawal symptoms and psychiatric conditions with severely disturbed behavior. Paraldehyde is mostly metabolized, but its excretion by the lungs limits its usefulness because of its offensive taste and ubiquitous odor.

Glutethimide (Doriden) has been widely used as a hypnotic and a daytime sedative. It should be prescribed with the same vigilance that is exercised in the prescription of barbiturates. Glutethimide is dependency-producing and can be lethal in overdose. In glutethimide poisoning the patient is more likely to go into shock than is the case with barbiturates, and his level of consciousness may vary up and down erratically. Convulsions sometimes occur. The drug's anticholinergic properties cause pupillary dilatation and may cause patients in glutethimide coma to be misdiagnosed as being in atropine coma.

Methyprylon (Noludar) is similar in structure to glutethimide, and, like glutethimide, it is used as both a hypnotic and a daytime sedative. It is addicting and can be lethal in large doses.

TABLE IV
Barbiturates

Name			Side-Chain Substitutions				Adult Dose Range	Adult Single Dose Range		Common Therapeutic Uses				D.E.A. Control Level
Generic	Trade	Manu-facturer	R₁	R₂	N₃	C₂	*mg./day*	Seda-tive *mg.*	Hyp-notic	Seda-tive	Hyp-notic	Anti-Con-vulsive	Gen-eral Anes-thetic	
Long-acting (duration of action, more than 8 hours)														
Phenobarbital	Luminal	Winthrop	Ethyl	1-Methylbutyl	H	O	15–600	15–30	100–200	+	+	+	–	IV
Butabarbital	Gemonil	Abbott	Ethyl	Ethyl	CH₃	O	– –	30–60	–	–	–	+	–	III
Pentobarbital	Mebaral	Winthrop	Ethyl	Ethyl	CH₃	O	32–600	32–100	–	+	–	+	–	IV
Intermediate-acting (duration of action, 5 to 8 hours)														
Amobarbital	Amytal	Lilly	Ethyl	Isopentyl	H	O	15–480	15–120	100–200	+	+	+	+	II
Butabarbital	Butisol	McNeil	Ethyl	*sec*-Butyl	H	O	15–120	15–30	50–100	+	+	–	–	III
Pentobarbital	Nembutal	Abbott	Ethyl	1-Methylbutyl	H	O	30–200	30–40	100–200	+	+	+	+	II
Short-acting (duration of action, 1 to 5 hours)														
Secobarbital	Seconal	Lilly	Allyl	1-Methylbutyl	H	O	100–300	–	100–200	–	+	+	+	II
Talbutal	Lotusate	Winthrop	Allyl	*sec*-Butyl	H	O	120	–	100–120	+	+	–	+	III
Ultra-short acting (duration of action, less than 1 hour)														
Methohexital	Brevital	Lilly	Allyl	1-Methyl-2-Pentynyl	CH₃	O	–	–	–	–	–	–	+	IV
Thiamylal	Surital	Parke, Davis	Allyl	2-Pentynyl	H	S	–	–	–	–	–	–	+	III
Thiopental	Pentothal	Abbott	Ethyl		H	S	–	–	–	–	–	–	+	III

Side Effects: Residual sedation, Vertigo, Headache, Hebetude, Nausea, Vomiting, Emesis, Skin rash, Excitement, Hypersensitivity reactions, Confusion, Depression, Gastric distress, Megaloblastic anemia, Respiratory depression, including apnea, Circulatory depression, Psychological dependence, and Withdrawal symptoms.

Flurazepam (Dalmane) is a benzodiazepine hypnotic agent that has real advantages over the other hypnotics. It produces adequate hypnosis, approximately equal in effectiveness to barbiturates and nonbarbiturate sedatives. It does not alter liver microsomal enzymes insofar as is known, so it is easier to use in cardiac patients. There is no evidence that it is dangerous in suicide attempts, and generalizing from the relative safety of the other benzodiazepines, one can expect it to be a much safer drug in regard to liability to overdose toxicity.

Untoward Drug Effects

Behavioral Toxicity

Behavioral toxicity is impairment produced by drugs on various aspects of behavior, such as motor behavior and thinking. Most psychotropic drugs, when given in large doses, produce some behavioral impairment in normal volunteers. However, when antipsychotic or antidepressant drugs are used effectively to treat schizophrenia or depression, respectively, there is often an improvement in cognitive functions. Presumably, the improvement in the mental disease results in an improvement in performance in the behavioral task that more than compensates for whatever behavioral toxicity the drug may have.

The sedative drugs and the minor tranquilizers produce a slight impairment on many behavioral tasks. They may improve performance on certain tasks in certain situations, but they fail to alter performance in other behavioral tasks. For example, 30 mg. of chlordiazepoxide or 5 mg. of diazepam reduce the peak velocity of saccadic eye movements by about 10 per cent. Behavioral toxicity is typically dose-dependent. Since tolerance may develop to minor tranquilizer or sedative drug-induced sedation, it is highly desirable to do chronic as well as acute studies of behavioral toxicity. In the clinical situation the anxious patient may do better in cognitive functions in his work and social life because the antianxiety effects of the drug free him from his disruptive influence, which more than counteracts the behavioral toxicity produced by the drug. The behavioral toxicity of the minor tranquilizers is slight and barely measurable at normal doses, but its occurrence should be balanced against the therapeutic benefit in a given case. The sedative effects of different sedative agents can have an additive effect. When chlordiazepoxide, diazepam, sedative agents, or phenothiazines are administered in normal doses along with alcohol, significant behavior impairment is noted.

Drug-Drug Interaction

With large numbers of patients taking multiple drugs, the potentialities for drug-drug interactions are considerable. Drug interactions can be classified as to whether they involve interaction between drugs on absorption, interactions in the mechanisms by which the drugs get to the receptor site (binding to plasma proteins, either displacement or increased binding; drug distribution; or drug transport and release to and from tissue), interactions between drugs on receptor sites, or interactions between drugs during their metabolism or excretion—stimulation of metabolism (induction) or inhibition of metabolism, increased or decreased urinary excretion.

The classical example of drug-drug interaction is the induction of liver microsomal enzymes by barbiturates, which then speed up the metabolism of anticoagulants. When a patient, who has been taking a barbiturate sleeping pill daily, returns home from the hospital and stops taking his barbiturates, the induced enzymes regress, and the patient metabolizes the anticoagulants more slowly. Blood levels of the anticoagulants increase, and the patient begins to bleed.

The nonbarbiturate sedative glutethimide is said to stimulate the liver drug-metabolizing microsomal enzymes and thus antagonizes the therapeutic actions of the oral anticoagulants. There is also preliminary evidence that ethchlorvynol antagonizes the therapeutic actions of these anticoagulants. Present evidence indicates that the benzodiazepines do not potentiate anticoagulants.

Side Effects

The side effects of the minor tranquilizers are usually of minor importance and generally constitute no more than an inconvenience to the patient. The most common side effect is drowsiness, and patients should be advised not to drive or operate machinery until they can accurately gauge their own reactions to the drug.

When used as hypnotics, the drugs do produce a slight cognitive impairment that is still present the next morning.

In general, the barbiturates produce more sedation than do the minor tranquilizers. At the doses used in controlled studies, barbiturates produced about as much sedation as the minor tranquilizers and were less effective in reducing anxiety; therefore, the empirical evidence suggests that at doses producing equal amounts of sedation the minor tranquilizers have more antianxiety action than do the barbiturates.

Paradoxical excitement can occur with all the drugs, but it probably occurs more frequently with the barbiturates. This adverse effect has been particularly noted in hyperkinetic children and in elderly or organically impaired adult patients.

Diazepam use has been observed to be associated with an increase in suicidal ideation in a small proportion of the patients treated in a placebo-controlled study. This finding may account in part for diazepam's failure to be superior to a placebo in two recent multiunit studies of depression.

With meprobamate, urticarial or erythematous rashes, anaphylactoid reactions, other allergic reactions, and angioneurotic edema occur infrequently; even more rarely, cases of dermatitis, blood dyscrasias, gastrointestinal upsets, and extraocular muscular paralysis have been reported. With chlordiazepoxide and diazepam, the major side effects are drowsiness, dizziness, and ataxia.

In general, the side effects of the minor tranquilizers do not constitute contraindications for their use. The side effects can usually be controlled by dosage reduction or by stopping the medication. Many of the minor complaints may be not pharmacologic side effects but somatic complaints that the patient would experience with a placebo as well. The fact that the minor tranquilizers are relatively safe is an advantage over the antipsychotics and antidepressants, which produce side effects with greater frequency and of somewhat greater severity.

Suicide Potential

The possibility of suicide with most of the minor tranquilizers is minimal. Only rarely have successful suicides been reported with meprobamate at high doses. There is controversy about suicides with benzodiazepines. With meprobamate. 20 to 40 gm. of the drug—50 to 100 of the 400-mg. tablets—are required to commit suicide. Meprobamate overdose can be effectively treated by forced diuresis.

Physical Dependence and Tolerance

Of the drugs discussed in this section, the barbiturates, chlordiazepoxide, diazepam, and meprobamate have been clearly shown to produce physical dependence of the barbiturate type in human studies. Glutethimide and methaqualone clearly have the same property, documented by clear cases of patients experiencing the usual withdrawal syndrome. It must be assumed that the other nonbarbiturate hypnotics and the other benzodiazepines share this undesirable pharmacological property. Alcohol certainly has shown this property for centuries, as evidenced by delirium tremens and rum fits. The sedative antihistamines lack this potential, as do phenothiazines and tricyclic antidepressants.

The only hypnosedative antianxiety drug that is clear of physical dependence liability is tybamate; this drug is clean because of its very short half-life in the body.

On the basis of limited available information, a dose of 3,200 mg. of meprobamate a day for 40 days or of 300 mg. of chlordiazepoxide daily for a month can cause clear physical dependence.

Since it takes a relatively high constant blood level of a sedative drug to induce physical dependence of any serious sort—for example, 600 mg. or more of a medium-acting or short-acting barbiturate a day—one or two sleeping pills a night will not produce marked dependence. On the other hand, data from sleep laboratories suggest that tolerance develops after a few nights to the sleep-increasing and electroencephalographic effects of hypnotics when they are given nightly. On this evidence, long-term use of hypnotics may have little usefulness in insomniacs other than as a friendly nightly placebo.

Cross-tolerance exists among all these drugs, so one can be used to suppress early withdrawal symptoms caused by physical dependence on another. Although pentobarbital has long been used as a standard detoxification agent, it seems more logical to use a longer-acting drug, such as diazepam, a practice already in vogue in some facilities for the detoxification of alcoholics.

REFERENCES

Davis, J. M., Bartlett, E., and Termini, B. A. Overdosage of psychotropic drugs. Dis. Nerv. Syst., *29:* 157, 246, 1968.

Hollister, L. E., Motzenboker, F. P., and Degan, R. O. Withdrawal reactions from chlordiazepoxide (Librium). Psychopharmacologia, 2: 63, 1961.

Klein, D. F. Delineation of two drug-responsive anxiety syndromes. Psychopharmacologia, *5:* 397, 1964.

Klein, D. F., and Davis, J. M. *Diagnosis and Treatment of Psychiatric Disorders.* Williams & Wilkins, Baltimore, 1969.

Klein, D. F., Honigfeld, G., and Feldman, S. Prediction of drug effect in personality disorders. J. Nerv. Ment. Dis., *156:* 183, 1973.

Lader, M. H., and Wing, L. Physiological measures, sedative drugs, and morbid anxiety. *Maudsley Monograph No. 14,* p. 1. Oxford University Press, London, 1966.

Lipman, R. S., Covi, L. Derogatis, L. R., Rickels, K., and Uhlenhuth, E. H. Medication, anxiety reduction, and patient report of significant life situation events. Dis. Nerv. Syst., *32:* 240, 1971.

Robinson, D. S., and Amidon, E. L. Interaction of benzodiazepines with warfarin in man. In *The Benzodiazepines.* S. Garattini, E. Mussini, and L. O. Randall, editors. p. 641, Raven Press, New York, 1973.

Stein, L. S., Wise, C. D., and Berger, B. D. Antianxiety action of benzodiazepines: Decrease in activity of serotonin neurons in the punishment system. In *The Benzodiazepines.* S. Garattini, E. Mussini, and L. O. Randall, editors, p. 299, Raven Press, New York, 1973.

30.4.   NARCOTHERAPY

Use in Psychotherapy

The use of an intravenous injection of a drug that may facilitate the uncovering of emotionally laden material in psychotherapy is known as narcotherapy. It consists of two aspects: the abreactive or cathartic aspect and the narcosynthesis or narcoanalytic aspect. The former refers to the uncovering, reliving, or otherwise experiencing of an emotionally traumatic event; the latter refers to the psychotherapeutic working through of this material and the integration of the resultant insights into the total personality.

Just as catharsis in psychotherapy or hypnosis may not be sufficient for full, long-lasting improvement, catharsis in narcoanalysis is not sufficient by itself. The rationale pursued relates to the ability of barbiturate-type drugs to produce a mild euphoria and weakened inhibitory mechanisms, allowing the easier uncovering of traumatic events, and to the ability of the psychomotor stimulants to produce a euphoria and an increase in talkativeness and social interactions, which may also facilitate the breaking through of anxiety-laden material into consciousness. Both facilitate exploration and catharsis.

Psychomotor stimulants are used at present for this purpose, although they are not routine treatment. For example, 25 to 40 mg. of methylphenidate can be slowly injected intravenously to produce a psychostimulant-induced narcotherapy session. Another technique is the use of a 5 per cent solution of Pentothal Sodium (thiopental sodium), given at a rate of about 2 cc. a minute; the rate and the total dose can be varied and should be adjusted to the clinical state achieved. The total dose may vary between 0.25 and 0.5 gm., although occasionally some patients need up to 1.0 gm. A combination of sedatives and psychostimulants can also be used.

Narcotherapy relates to psychotherapy in many ways as hypnosis related to hypnotherapy. Many of the dangers that apply to hypnosis also apply to narcotherapy. However, like hypnosis, narcotherapy may be useful in special situations. Mute psychotic patients can sometimes be induced to give useful historical material under Amytal (amobarbital) or Pentothal Sodium.

Intravenous barbiturates have been used and can still be used to produce rapid hypnosis in disturbed correlative patients. The phenothiazines take longer to act, given intramuscularly, but are much more helpful in the long run. The barbiturates should only be used in those rare major emergencies when instantaneous behavior control is vital. In all usage of intravenous barbiturates, the state of the patient's larynx requires consideration.

Other Uses

Pentothal Sodium can be useful to distinguish organic conditions from functional conditions, essentially as a provocative test for organic brain disease. Neurological symptoms that are normally present in mild degree can become markedly worse after the administration of intravenous barbiturates, and symptoms such as confabulation, denial of illness, and disorientation may appear in blatant form after

Pentothal when they were present in mild form in the baseline state. Patients with significant organic brain disease may have markedly less tolerance for barbiturate sedation than do normal patients. One must beware of giving a toxic dose to the patient, since small doses may result in serious sedation or mild coma.

These agents are also useful to distinguish catatonic stupor from retarded depression. The depressed patient becomes sleepy; the catatonic patient sometimes experiences a temporary clearing of the catatonia, with a rational, lucid interval. Patients who do not eat owing to catatonia can eat during the lucid interval. Diazepam may prove a slightly safer and slightly more convenient intravenous sedative agent than Pentothal for such purposes.

What a patient says under the influence of these agents may be no more true than what he says under the influence of alcohol. These agents are not truth serums.

REFERENCES

Freed, H. The use of Ritalin intravenously as a diagnostic adjuvant in psychiatry. Am. J. Psychiatry, *114:* 944, 1958.
Guile, L. A. Intravenous methyl phenidate: A pilot study. Med. J. Aust., *2:* 93, 1963.
Hope, J. M., Callaway, E., and Sands, S. L. Intravenous Pervitin and the psychopathology of schizophrenia. Dis. Nerv. Syst., *12:* 67, 1951.
Horsley, J. S. Narcoanalysis. J. Ment. Sci., *82:* 416, 1936.
Pennes, H. H. Clinical reactions of schizophrenics to Sodium Amytal. Pervitin hydrochloride, mescalin sulfate and D-lysergic acid diethylamide. J. Nerv. Ment. Dis., *119:* 95, 1954.
Witton, K. Directive psychotherapy with parenteral Ritalin in advanced schizophrenia. Dis. Nerv. Syst., *21:* 1, 1960.

30.5. CONVULSIVE THERAPIES

Pharmacological Convulsive Treatment

Convulsive therapies were introduced by von Meduna on the basis of two different observations: First, patients suddenly lose their symptoms when they have a spontaneous convulsion. Second, epilepsy and schizophrenia hardly ever occur in the same patient. Von Meduna induced actual convulsions in schizophrenic patients, first with camphor in oil and later with a soluble synthetic camphor preparation, pentylenetetrazol (Metrazol), which could be injected intravenously as a 10 per cent solution. In the majority of cases it produced a convulsion

within 30 seconds with a dose of 5 to 10 cc. injected rapidly.

Several pharmacological convulsive agents were used after the introduction of Metrazol. The only one still being used is the inhalation of hexafluorodiethyl ether, known under the trade name of Indoklon. It is applied as an inhalant by means of a mask and a vaporizer loaded with gauze saturated with the liquid. Since it has an anesthetizing phase, the patient first loses consciousness, then has some myoclonic movements, and finally develops a tonic-clonic convulsion. Today Indoklon is used with barbiturate anesthesia and muscle relaxation.

Indoklon inhalation therapy has the same indications and the same effectiveness as electric convulsive therapy (ECT). Some clinicians find Indoklon more effective in resistent types of schizophrenia. The side effect of confusion is the same in Indoklon treatment, thus contradicting the notion that the electric current in ECT is responsible for the confusion. One disadvantage of Indoklon is that nausea is more frequent than with ECT and must be counteracted by an intravenous injection of 5 mg. of Compazine (prochlorperazine).

Electric Convulsive Treatment

In 1938 Cerletti and Bini replaced pharmacological convulsive therapy with electrically induced convulsions. Bini built a simple apparatus using alternating current. Most machines are still based on his original model. Some workers use unidirectional current and claim that it produces less confusion. No convincing evidence has ever been given to prove that the memory impairment is actually reduced with modified currents.

The only true innovation in the application of ECT is the use of unilateral stimulation. The unquestionable advantage of this method, if applied to the nondominant hemisphere of the brain, is that it avoids confusion and memory impairment. So far, unilateral ECT has not replaced bilateral ECT.

In the standard technique, electrodes are applied to both temples. Skin resistance must be decreased by a salt water solution or electrojelly similar to the one used in electrocardiography. The amount of current applied by the originators of the method was 70 to 130 volts for 0.1 to 0.5 second.

The present technique used by the majority of workers is modified by the use of muscle-relaxant drugs. Such muscle relaxation is needed to prevent fractures during the convulsion. A concentrated aqueous extract of curare was later replaced by various synthesized curarelike preparations. Because fatalities occurred, probably as the result of some central effect of the curare, it was replaced by succinylcholine. Since succinylcholine suppresses the patient's respiration, he is first anesthetized with a short-acting intravenous barbiturate injection, such as a 0.2 per cent solution of methohexital (Brevital) in a 5 per cent dextrose solution and a 0.2 per cent solution of succinylcholine chloride, also dissolved in 0.2 per cent dextrose. The drip method is preferable for the introduction of the barbiturate, as well as for the succinylcholine.

Cardiovascular and pulmonary complications can occur in ECT modified by anesthesia and muscle-relaxant drugs. Premedication with barbiturates in patients with cardiac complications should be avoided.

The manifestations of electrically induced convulsions resemble those of a spontaneous convulsion with certain differences. If the amount of current given is not sufficient, the nonanesthetized patient will only lose consciousness (petit mal response). If somewhat more current is given, the patient may have a delayed convulsion—that is, he will lose consciousness and, after only a few seconds, will go slowly into the tonic phase, followed by the clonic phase. If still more current is used, he will have an immediate convulsion in which the tonic phase starts at the moment of the stimulation.

The tonic phase lasts for about 10 seconds, and the clonic phase lasts 30 to 40 seconds. In modified convulsions with muscle-relaxant drugs, it is sometimes difficult to see any movements. However, a slight plantar flexion of the feet can be noticed as evidence of the tonic phase; after about 10 seconds some toe or other movements should indicate the clonic phase. A nonmotor manifestation of a convulsion is the appearance of gooseflesh.

The amount of current necessary for a convulsion changes among different people. Male patients usually have a lower threshold than female patients, and young people have a lower one than old persons. Barbiturates may raise the threshold considerably. No patient fails to convulse if an adequate amount of current or repeated electric stimulation is given.

After the convulsive movements have stopped, the patient remains in a state of apnea, which may be prolonged if muscle-relaxant drugs are used. Oxygen is given until the patient resumes breathing.

Medication should be withheld on the morning of the treatment; psychotropic drugs with hypotensive effects are to be particularly avoided. The patient should be treated in the morning without breakfast or in the afternoon after having a light breakfast of coffee and toast and no other food for at least 4 hours before treatment. His bladder must be voided. Dentures are usually removed, although in patients with partial dentures it is safer to leave them in because irregularly spaced teeth may break during the contraction of the jaw. Mouth gags of various types are used to protect the teeth and the tongue. Even when muscle-relaxant drugs are used, the jaw muscles may contract quite strongly because of their direct stimulation by the electrodes.

The patient regains consciousness after a few minutes but remains in a clouded state for 15 to 30 minutes. It is advisable to keep him in the treatment area for at least an hour. Headache is a frequent complaint. Nausea can be prevented with 100 mg. of Dramamine (dimenhydrinate), given intramuscularly, or 5 mg. of Compazine, given intramuscularly or intravenously. Succinylcholine causes an unexplained pain in jaw and neck muscles after the first treatment but not after subsequent ones. Confusion is also present.

Changes during ECT

Arrhythmias are frequent, and a brief asystole is usually observed during the tonic phase of the convulsion. Hematological and serological changes are contradictory in the reports available.

The most frequent endocrinological observation is an increase in weight, which may be due to an effect on diencephalic centers. Menstrual changes in the form of amenorrhea for 1 or 2 months occur frequently.

Neurovegetative changes were the basis for the prognostic Funkenstein test. Patients have a good prognosis for ECT if they have more than a 50 mm. Hg rise in systolic blood pressure after an intravenous injection of 0.5 mg. of epinephrine and a fall of blood pressure after 10 mm. of Mecholyl (methacholine), given intramuscularly, with failure to return to their normal blood pressure within 25 minutes. The same is true for those who respond to Mecholyl with chills.

Psychopathological Changes. Psychopathological changes consist primarily of amnesia for the whole treatment procedure and, after several treatments, memory impairment, which may last for one or several weeks after termination of treatment. No lasting loss or impairment of memory occurs.

Some patients, on waking up from the treatment, misinterpret their surroundings and react with an excitement state. They should receive an intravenous injection of 2 to 3 cc. of Valium (diazepam) or a barbiturate drip for 20 minutes after the convulsion. In rare cases the psychopathological changes during a course of ECT may be complicated by various types of organic reactions, such as hallucinatory symptoms different from those for which the patient is being treated.

Patients also show such emotional changes as euphoria and complete affective dullness. The intensity of the reaction depends on the number and the spacing of the treatments.

A vexing psychopathological phenomenon is the fear the patient has of the treatment before the first treatment. He is relieved of this fear after the first treatment, when he realizes that he did not have any discomfort during the treatment. However, after several treatments another type of fear sets in and does not leave the patient until he has finished the series. He remains aware of the fear, although he cannot give a reason for it, and it recurs when he has to undergo treatment again, even after years have passed. This fear seems to be a result of the unpleasant experience of waking up after the treatment and not knowing who he is or where he is.

Neurological Changes. Neurological observations are essentially identical to those seen in any generalized convulsion. No reflexes can be elicited during and shortly after the convulsion. After a period of flaccidity, pyramidal signs may appear. The pupils do not react for a while, and then they may oscillate between rigidity and reflex activity. Constriction of the retinal vessels has been observed in delayed reactions before the onset of the convulsion, as is seen in epileptics, and is followed by vasodilation of the retinal vessels. Postconvulsive motor phenomena may consist of various involuntary movements and automatisms, which should not be mistaken for a second convulsion. Aphasia, agnosia, and other disturbances of cortical function can also be observed temporarily.

Electroencephalographic findings essentially repeat those seen in spontaneous convulsions. After each convulsion there is a slow-wave pattern that returns to normal after 5 to 30 minutes. After several treatments the abnormal pattern remains, and various electroencephalographic changes indicate the cerebral dysfunction during a series of electrically or pharmacologically induced convulsions. After the treatments have been discontinued, the electroencephalogram may remain abnormal for several days or weeks. After 2 or 3 months, the electroencephalogram returns to normal in all cases.

Complications

With the exception of fractures in unmodified ECT, complications are extremely rare. Most physical ailments do not represent a contraindication to ECT. The same is true for such physiological conditions as pregnancy. ECT is not dangerous to mother or child, nor does it accelerate the termination of pregnancy. Age is no contraindication to ECT; both young children and very old persons can be treated.

Before the introduction of muscle-relaxant drugs, the most frequent complications in convulsive therapy were fractures. The most frequent ones were those occurring in the dorsal spine between the fourth and eighth dorsal vertebrae. They consisted of varying degrees of compression in these vertebrae. No neurological complications were ever observed in connection with these fractures. Another type of fracture was that of the long bones, which occurred in the head of the humerus and the head of the femur. They were rare, although clinically much more serious than those of the spine. As with all fractures in convulsive therapy, they are explained by the muscular contraction.

Fatalities have been extremely rare, even before the introduction of anesthesia techniques in convulsion therapy. Some statistics found a death rate of up to 0.1 per cent but they probably included cases in which death occurred during a course of ECT but was unrelated to the treatment. If death occurs as the result of cardiac arrest or myocardial infarction, a contributing effect of the barbiturate anesthesia cannot be ruled out. In hypertensives, both the barbiturate anesthesia and the convulsion have a hypotensive effect. Coronary occlusion has been observed 30 minutes or 1 hour after treatment.

Contraindications

Brain tumors are the only definite contraindication. Although all other neurological conditions can be treated without any damage, it appears that the sudden increase of intracerebral pressure during a convulsion represents great danger to patients with brain tumors.

There is a danger that the muscle relaxant succinylcholine will increase intraocular pressure. In patients with glaucoma, eserine drops should be given before ECT.

Indications and Results

Convulsive therapy was introduced as a treatment for schizophrenia. Only 4 years after its introduction, it became noticeable that the best results were obtained in depressions. This type of therapy is useful in many conditions. Since the introduction of drug therapy, the indications for ECT have become more restricted.

Depression. Both retarded and agitated depressions clear up after three or four convulsive treatments. It is then advisable to give two or three more treatments at increasing intervals to stabilize the result.

Most depressions respond to ECT. This is as true for manic-depressive patients, who change from a manic to a depressive state (bipolar depressions), as it is for those who have only recurrent depressions (unipolar depressions). Involutional melancholia not complicated by schizophrenic features also responds to a short course of six to eight ECT sessions. This is equally true for depressions of old age, as long as they are not caused by arteriosclerotic or senile brain changes.

In neurotic or reactive depressions the results are less reliable. However, many of these patients respond well, especially those who have true depressive episodes. The atypical depressions, which last longer and are mixed with neurotic and often schizoid features, respond less well.

The danger of suicide is a definite indication for immediate ECT. Time is another important consideration in favor of ECT. Patients unable to continue in their work frequently risk the loss of their job if the slow-acting drugs are not effective and later have to be followed with ECT. In hospitalized patients the expense of several weeks' stay for an often unsuccessful antidepressant medication may suggest an immediate course of ECT.

Convulsive therapy does not prevent subsequent depressive episodes. The shortening of a depressive phase by convulsive therapy may even shorten the intervals between episodes. In such cases antidepressant medication can be given. A monthly preventive ECT has been shown to be another effective means to forestall future episodes. Today such monthly ECT has been replaced in bipolar depressions by prophylactic medication with lithium.

Mania. Lithium is the treatment of choice in manic patients. However, if these patients are severely disturbed, ECT can be given until the more slowly acting lithium is effective.

Schizophrenia. ECT has never been very successful in chronic cases of schizophrenia, and it has been replaced to a large extent by the neuroleptic drugs. In acute schizophrenia the preference of the therapist is often what determines whether he administers medication first or starts immediately with ECT.

When it is successful, ECT removes acute schizophrenic symptoms with three or four treatments. It is necessary, however, to continue treatment up to 10 and possibly up to 20 treatments because in schizophrenia, in contrast to depression, termination after the removal of all symptoms almost invariably leads to a relapse within less than a week's time.

Two prognostic factors are decisive in any group of schizophrenics treated with convulsive therapy. The acute onset of illness is the most favorable prognostic factor. Duration of illness of less than a year is the other favorable factor.

Of the various subtypes of schizophrenia, catatonic excitement responds best. In catatonic excitement with severe agitation and frequent febrile temperatures, two or three ECT treatments given within 24 hours often have a lifesaving effect. Catatonic stupors respond well temporarily, usually after two or three treatments, but the long-term results are often disappointing. Acute paranoid schizophrenia in young patients also responds well to ECT. Paranoiacs in the middle-age group respond symptomatically but relapse easily, even after a long series of treatments. Simple and hebephrenic schizophrenics have the poorest results.

In chronic schizophrenia, pharmacotherapy has replaced ECT to a large extent, but there are still some indications for ECT. A patient with catatonic stupor may tend to become more withdrawn every few weeks and, like most withdrawn schizophrenics, not respond to drugs. Patients with short flare-ups of their symptoms may respond quickly to a few ECT treatments. Patients unwilling to take drugs regularly represent another group in whom maintenance ECT may be indicated.

Neurosis. Neurotics do not represent a promising indication for ECT. The only exceptions are neurotics with depressive symptoms and those in whom acute anxiety or panic states can be removed with one or two ECT treatments in a purely symptomatic way. Neurotics are apt to react to the side effects of ECT, such as memory impairment and physical complaints, in an exaggerated manner and sometimes with gross hysterical manifestations. Therefore, indications for ECT in neurotic patients are rare.

Other Disorders. Psychiatric patients with organic cerebral conditions, epileptics, and mentally retarded patients may have psychotic episodes that respond well to a few ECT treatments. In particular, arteriosclerotic or senile psychoses may show symptoms that can be removed with a minimal number of treatments if such patients stop eating or become severely agitated and do not tolerate or respond to neuroleptic medication. Acute organic reactions such as toxic infectious psychoses also respond well, but pharmacotherapy is usually adequate except in severe excitement.

REFERENCES

Abrams, R. Recent clinical studies of ECT. Semin. Psychiatry, *4:* 3, 1972.

Abrams, R., and Taylor, M. A. Anterior bifrontal ECT: A clinical trail. Br. J. Psychiatry, *122:* 587, 1973.

Cerletti, U., and Bini, L. L'Elettroshock. Arch. Gen. Neurol. Psichiatr. Psicoanal., *19:* 266, 1938.

Cronholm, B., and Ottosson, J. O. The experience of memory function after electroconvulsive therapy. Br. J. Psychiatry, *109:* 251, 1963.

Impastato, D. J. The safer administration of succinylcholine without barbiturates: A new technic. Am. J. Psychiatry, *113:* 461, 1956.

Kalinowsky, L. B., and Hippius, H. *Pharmacological, Convulsive and Other Somatic Treatments in Psychiatry.* Grune & Stratton, New York, 1969.

Krantz, J. C., Jr., Truitt, E. B., Spears, L., and Ling, A. S. C. New pharmacoconvulsive agent. Science, *126:* 353, 1957.

Lebensohn, Z. M. In defense of electroshock therapy. Med. Ann. D. C., *42:* 6, 1973.

Stromgren, L. S. Unilateral versus bilateral electroconvulsive therapy. Acta Psychiatr. Scand. [Suppl.], 240, 1973.

30.6. INSULIN COMA TREATMENT

Technique

The original technique consisted of injecting increasing amounts of insulin until hypoglycemic coma occurred. Because of the possibility of an allergic reaction and, more important, hypersensitivity to insulin in individual patients, treatment is usually started with 10 or 15 units. This amount is increased each day by 5 or 10 units. A coma is usually obtained with 100 or 200 units.

Manifestations

About an hour after the injection of insulin, the patient shows the first signs of hypoglycemia—perspiration and feelings of tiredness and somnolence. During the second hour, the patient's sensorium becomes clouded, and he falls asleep. Some patients become restless, toss around, and yell. Others are disoriented or have hallucinations. Speech becomes dysarthric. Aphasia and apraxia may be noticed. The motor phenomena during the second hour consist of automatic movements, forced grasping, myoclonic twitchings, and various dystonic manifestations.

Convulsions are frequent, during the second hour of hypoglycemia. Patients who are inclined to have convulsions often receive anticonvulsant medication before the insulin injection. Convulsions during the later hours of hypoglycemia are considered a danger sign and require immediate termination of hypoglycemia.

During the third hour, the patient can go into a true coma. The coma stage is reached when the patient is unable to respond to stimuli. Spasms similar to those of decerebrate rigidity may occur, the pupils do not react to light, and the deepest stage is characterized by a change of the pupils from dilation to miosis, absence of the corneal reflex, and disappearance of tendon reflexes. At first, the patient is usually left in coma not longer than 15 minutes; in subsequent treatments the coma can be slowly prolonged up to an hour.

Termination

Termination is facilitated by the hormone glucagon, which can be used in doses of 0.33 to 1 mg. intravenously or intramuscularly. Awakening usually begins after 10 or 20 minutes. If the patient does not react by then, the dose is repeated. Small amounts are usually sufficient to awake the patient so that he is able to drink a sugar solution or other carbohydrate preparation. Laqueur also found adrenalin and thiamine to be effective in many patients for termination of hypoglycemic coma.

An aftershock may appear several hours after termination of treatment. The patient may perspire or feel tired and lie down for a nap. He should be watched carefully because such patients may be in a second hypoglycemic coma. Patients should have some sugar with them and be told to eat some at the first sign of uneasiness. They should be warned against sleeping in the afternoon of treatment days and should be engaged in group activities so that they can be watched. If a second coma develops, the usual measures of termination must be undertaken.

Number of Comas

The number of comas is uaually determined by the response of the patient in his psychiatric symptoms. Improvement in insulin treatment occurs more slowly than in convulsive therapy; therefore, treatment should be continued to the point of maximal improvement. Forty to 60 comas are considered a minimum. After the patient has reached his optimal improvement, a few more comas should be given.

Complications and Contraindications

Changes in pulse rate are normal manifestations in hypoglycemia. Complications can be due to acute cardiac insufficiency in patients who have an unrecognized cardiac illness or to sudden vasomotor collapses.

The most important and most frequent complications is the protracted coma, which is actually an encephalopathy. The patient remains in coma after the hypoglycemia is eliminated by means of glucagon or repeated intravenous glucose administration and even after abnormally high blood-sugar levels are obtained.

The most important treatment for this emergency is prevention. Techniques that anesthesiologists use with patients in deep states of unconsciousness should be applied, particularly adequate oxygenation and all measures to maintain cardiovascular activity.

Fatalities in insulin coma treatment were originally reported as 0.5 per cent of patients treated. Modern techniques have considerably reduced or even eliminated fatalities.

An activation of the psychosis may occur, but probably more frequent are short-lasting organic reactions that may follow protracted comas. Permanent organic brain damage is extremely rare.

Neuropathological changes due to hypoglycemia are usually reversible, but there are a few irreversible cell changes and areas of rarefaction.

There are more contraindications in insulin coma treatment than in convulsive therapy. Any patient with cardiovascular pathology should be excluded from insulin coma treatment. Patients over 50 years of age and those with renal, respiratory, and other general medical diseases are rarely accepted. Diabetes is not necessarily considered a contraindication. Insulin should be avoided during pregnancy.

Indications and Results

Schizophrenia is the main indication for this method but it is rarely used today.

Modified Insulin Therapy

Modified insulin therapy has been used in various conditions, including schizophrenia. It consists of the usual induction of hypoglycemic states but avoids coma. Such mild hypoglycemias have a sedative effect and improve the patient's appetite, weight, and general physical condition. It is usually combined with other somatic treatments.

REFERENCES

Horwitz, W. A., and Kalinowsky, L. B. Combined insulin coma and electric convulsive therapy in schizophrenia. Am. J. Psychiatry, *104:* 682, 1948.

Kalinowsky, L. B., and Hippius, H. *Pharmacological Convulsive and Other Somatic Treatments in Psychiatry.* Grune & Stratton, New York, 1969.

Laqueur, H. P., and La Burt, H. A. Coma therapy with multiple insulin doses. J. Neuropsychiatry, *1:* 135, 1960.

Laqueur, H. P., and La Burt, H. A. Experience with low-zinc insulin with semilente insulin with glucagon and adrenalin-thiamine in insulin coma treatment. J. Neuropsychiatry, *2:* 86, 1960.

Sakel, M. *The Pharmacological Shock Treatment of Schizophrenia. Nervous and Mental Disease Monograph Series,* No. 62. Nervous and Mental Diseases Publishing Company, New York, 1938.

Sargant, W., Slater, E., and Kelly, D. *An Introduction to Physical Methods of Treatment in Psychiatry.* Churchill Livingstone, Edinburgh, 1972.

30.7. PSYCHOSURGERY

History

In 1936, Moniz in Portugal, together with Lima, reported on frontal lobe surgery as an approach to the treatment of certain psychoses, particularly schizophrenia. Much later, it was noted that a Swiss psychiatrist, Burckhardt, in the 1880's had operated on the cerebral cortex to treat disturbed mental patients, but this had soon been forgotten. Moniz based his work on certain clinical observations and on experimental work by Fulton and Jacobsen. The removal of frontal lobes in monkeys changed the aggressive behavior of these animals without interfering with their intellectual functioning. Moniz and Lima, therefore, injected alcohol into the white matter of the frontal lobe and later used a blunt instrument to separate frontal lobe tissues. In the United States, this work was pioneered by Freeman and Watts; it was also used extensively by many British workers. Various operations in different parts of the brain were subsequently introduced, and in recent years stereotaxic procedures have been devised in the field of psychosurgery. The appearance of neuroleptic drugs made surgery in the majority of chronic schizophrenics obsolete. However, other indications had been demonstrated, and, in well selected cases, this therapeutic approach continues to be an important tool in the treatment of otherwise intractable cases of emotional illness (Kalinowsky and Hippius, 1969).

Technical Procedures

Bilateral prefrontal lobotomy, also called leukotomy, was performed by Moniz and Lima by means of several spherical cuts in the white matter in both hemispheres. The more widely used standard lobotomy by Freeman and Watts was a bilateral blind operation. They cut the white matter in a plane anterior to the anterior horns of the lateral ventricles. Others used an open procedure under direct vision. Later on, partial frontal lobe destructions, such as rostral frontal lobotomy, were used. Then it was realized that the more important areas for the removal of undesirable psychiatric symptoms are the lower orbital parts of the frontal lobes, and operations in this area replaced the standard bilateral lobotomy.

Bimedial lobotomies leaving intact the lateral part of the frontal lobe were used extensively by Greenblatt and Solomon. Grantham used coagulation in an inferior medial bifrontal lobotomy.

The trend toward smaller operations grew out of the observation of personality changes that were a disturbing aftereffect, although intellectual impairment was negligible in even the larger operations. One of the smaller methods was the transorbital lobotomy, in which the cuts were performed with a leukotome introduced through the vault of the orbit.

Cortical undercutting was introduced by Scoville, who experimented with undercutting in various parts of the frontal lobe and got his best results with undercutting of the orbital surface. A more restricted orbitoventromedial undercutting was used by Hirose in Japan. These operations left the cortex intact, but topectomies, devised by Pool, removed cortical tissue in Brodmann's areas 9, 10, and 46.

Stereotaxic operations in various locations are the latest development in this field. They were first practiced by Spiegel and Wycis in thalamotomy, with destructions of the dorsal medial nucleus of the thalamus. Today, in England more than in other countries, stereotaxic operations are used in many parts of the limbic system. Anterior cingulectomies and stereotaxic lesions in these areas avoid larger destruction of brain tissue and also guarantee a more exact localization of the lesion. Extensive use of sterotaxic tractotomies has been made by Knight, who, in a large number of orbital undercuttings, realized that it was the posterior part of the incision in the substantia innominata that led to the best therapeutic effects. He introduced seeds of radioactive yttrium Y-90 into this area. Multiple stereotaxic lesions in different areas in the limbic system, depending on the patient's psychopathology, are recommended by Kelly and others.

The deepest part of the brain operated on is the posteromedial part of the hypothalamus near the third ventricle. When this area, designated the ergotropic triangle, is stimulated, a strong sympathetic discharge is elicited; its electrocauterization produces a marked calming effect.

Linstrom uses ultrasonic waves to produce local necrosis in the prefrontal white matter to avoid extensive anatomical destruction, a method that he calls prefrontal sonic treatment.

The postoperative course is usually uneventful as far as surgical complications are concerned. With closed operations, vessels may become injured. Open operations, performed with an osteoplastic flap, have no serious surgical complications.

Anatomical and Psychopathological Considerations

Meyer demonstrated that localization of the cut and outcome have little relationship, and that only the number of fibers cut made a difference. This finding was the main reason that partial frontal lobotomies were recommended. Later developments, such as the introduction of stereotaxic operations in the limbic system, did not essentially change the therapeutic results, although they did reduce the side effects.

Psychopathologically, the common feature of all psychosurgical interventions is the diminished reaction to unpleasant sensations. The larger operations also led to personality changes. Psychosurgery does not remove certain psychiatric target symptoms but, rather, the emotional response of the patient to such symptoms. A severe obsessive-compulsive patient is able to overcome his phobias or compulsive urges because their emotional impact is reduced. At the same time, such a patient may show side effects that are explained by his reduced concern over his relationship with family and co-workers. The smaller operations that follwed the standard lobotomy and particularly the minimal lesions of stereotaxic operations have practically eliminated the undesirable side effects.

The immediate psychopathological changes hardly differ from those after other brain operations. These changes are transitory and have manifold characteristics of an acute brain syndrome with Korsakofflike symptoms and emotional blunting, often followed by euphoria. Loss of initiative can be extreme. The duration of these symptoms is unpredictable, but they may last several weeks. They are usually absent after the smaller stereotaxic operations.

Indications

Psychosurgery is not specific for any individual mental illness. Before the era of pharmacotherapy, psychosurgery was widely used to reduce disturbed behavior in schizophrenic patients. Such conditions as schizophrenia, obsessive-compulsive neuroses, and chronic depressions unresponsive to the usual antidepressive treatments, represent the largest number of patients in whom psychosurgery has been used and for which it may be indicated.

The use of psychosurgery is objectionable to many psychiatrists as well as to the general public, who object to the irreversible damage to the brain for whatever reason.

REFERENCES

Brown, M. H., and Lighthill, J. A. Selective anterior cingulotomy: A psychosurgical evaluation. J. Neurosurg., 29: 613, 1968.
Freeman, W. Transorbital lobotomy. Am. J. Psychiatry, 105: 734, 1949.
Greenblatt, M., and Solomon, H. C. Frontal Lobes and Schizophrenia. Springer, New York, 1953.
Kalinowsky, L. B., and Hippius, H. Pharmacological, Convulsive, and Other Somatic Treatments in Psychiatry. Grune & Stratton, New York, 1969.
Kelly, D., Richardson, A., and Mitchell-Heggs, N. Technique and assessment of limbic leucotomy. In Surgical Approaches in Psychiatry, L. V. Laitinen and K. E. Livingston, editors, p. 201. Medical and Technical Publishing, Lancaster, 1973.
Thorpe, F. T. An evaluation of prefrontal leucotomy in the affective disorders of old age. A follow-up study. J. Ment. Sci., 104: 403, 1958.

30.8.   LITHIUM THERAPY

Introduction

Lithium therapy is remarkable in combating episodes of mania and hypomania. Moreover, the therapeutic effects of this drug are apparently unrelated to the patient's age, sex, or duration of illness.

In contrast to other psychoactive drugs, lithium retains its physical integrity in the body. After several days of intake, its concentration in blood and tissues enters into dynamic equilibrium. This property makes it possible for the physician to monitor the amount of active agent present by determining its concentration in the blood.

Manic-Depressive Illness

Among the outstanding symptoms of mania are elated mood, grandiosity, and hyperactivity. Although the manic person may feel wonderful, his normal judgments about the real world around him and his own capabilities may be distorted and exaggerated. He is, in turn, irritable, argumentative, expansive, distractible, and volatile, and his good mood is apt to turn readily into rage when he is frustrated.

Mania is most often one phase of the bipolar manic-depressive illness. It may either precede or follow a period of normal mood or a depressed phase.

Hypomania is the term used to describe manic behavior of lesser intenstiy. However, the hypomanic can be even more of a danger to himself than is the manic, since his disturbance is less evident to the observer.

The response and future progress of the manic-depressive treated with lithium is good to excellent, in contrast to the schizophrenic, who responds poorly to lithium treatment.

Treatment

Patients on lithium carbonate must be maintained under close clinical supervision. Contraindications for its use include renal conditions, decompensated heart disease, and central nervous system pathology.

During an acute manic phase, the ability to tolerate lithium may be increased, but this tolerance decreases sharply as soon as the manic symptoms subside. Furthermore, since toxicity of lithium has been shown to be potentiated when sodium intake is restricted, it is essential for the patient to maintain a normal diet, including salt and adequate fluid intake.

Dosage

Patients in acute mania can tolerate and often need high doses of lithium to achieve a therapeutic effect. However, the dosage must be rapidly reduced to maintenance levels when the acute attack has subsided and evaluation of the patient's psychiatric status, along with frequent lithium blood levels the first 10 days, must be continued to avoid excessive serum concentration and toxic reactions.

For the patient in a moderately severe manic state, the initial daily dosage of lithium carbonate ranges from 1,500 mg. to 2,100 mg. for a 70-kg. patient. After 5 to 10 days of lithium treatment, when the mania usually abates, daily dosage must be reduced to 900 to 1,200 mg. The precise amount required by the individual patient is determined by continuous periodic observation of the clinical state, achievement of a blood lithium level of 0.8 to 1.5 mEq/liter, and avoidance of side effects.

Side Effects and Complications

In some patients with serum levels of lithium over 1.5 mEq/liter and occasionally in patients with lower serum levels, there may be a number of side effects, including hand tremor, abdominal cramps, nausea, vomiting, diarrhea, thirst and polyuria, fatigue or sleepiness, and weight gain, perhaps 5 to 10 pounds in several weeks.

These symptoms often occur during the first 2 to 4 weeks of lithium stabilization, but they disappear either spontaneously or with a lowering of the dosage. A slight tremor may persist, but it is of no particular significance.

In some instances, goiter may be another side effect of lithium treatment. Lithium may act as a secondary contributing factor in precipitating thyroid disease in some patients, particularly in those with existing thyroid dysfunction or goiter.

Skin rash and allergic reactions have not been proved to be due to lithium, and they usually disappear with time.

If lithium is given in excessive amounts or if the renal mechanisms fail to eliminate it properly, the serum lithium rises above 2.0 mEq/liter, and signs and symptoms of lithium poisoning or intoxication ensue. Early symptoms of poisoning are sluggishness, lethargy, tremor or muscle twitchings, ataxia, slurred speech, loss of appetite, and vomiting or diarrhea. Within days, the patient lapses into a state of semiconsciousness and coma, with hyperactive deep reflexes, muscle tremors, and fasciculations. There may be epileptiform seizures and severe electrolyte changes and consequent cardiac impairment, which may result in death.

A diagnosis of lithium poisoning is determined by the clinical condition of the patient and by a serum lithium value that exceeds 2.0 to 3.0 mEq/liter. Treatment consists of stopping the drug at once and applying the supportive measures usually used with patients in coma. Maintenance of normal fluid and electrolyte balance is of particular importance. Use of special agents that induce a diuresis of lithium, including mannitol and aminophylline, along with alkalinization of the urine, is reported to help in reversing the toxicity. Correction of extracellular fluid and electrolyte depletion must be instituted. In some cases, potassium and sodium salts are indicated, but these require the careful analysis of extracellular and intracellular electrolyte shifts. Daily electrolytes, body weight, hematocrit, and lithium levels must be determined serially during the acute stages of lithium poisoning. In addition, antiepileptic medications should be instituted because of the high incidence of seizure phenemena.

Bipolar II patients can be defined as those who have had previous attacks of mild hypomania and depression but in whom only the depressed phases have been severe enough to require admission to the hospital or medical management in the office or home. Indeed, in many of those mild bipolar II patients, the hypomanic phases have positively augmented the patient's personal, business, or creative life. Lithium in maintenance dosage not only counteracts manic episodes of psychotic intensity but also balances these bipolar II hypomanic and depressive mood swings. These patients often prefer to settle for their highs and lows rather than a middle-of-the-road mood achieved on lithium.

In addition some patients are reluctant to accept lithium therapy as a lifetime need. The mere idea suggests permanent commitment to a drug and periodic blood tests, similar to the enslavement of diabetics.

Evaluation of Therapy

Patients suffering from episodes of mania or hypomania have shown remarkable improvement within 5 to 10 days after starting lithium carbonate therapy. Apparently, lithium affects the underlying manic process without sedating the patient, whereas chlorpromazine and haloperidol control the manic behavior by sedation without basically affecting the underlying biochemical defect.

The therapeutic value of lithium in the treatment of unipolar or bipolar depression has to date not been established. Lithium has been established as an effective prophylactic agent for future episodes of mania. There is much controversy about the effectiveness of lithium in the treatment of various types of depression. The authors agree with the U.S. Food and Drug Administration (F.D.A.) position that it should be used in those manic-depressive patients with a history of mania. The dosage for prophylactic maintenance lithium must be adjusted to the individual patient, but, in general, 900 to 1,200 mg. a day for a 150-pound person is most adequate, provided the serum levels are maintained between 0.8 and 1.5 mEq/liter.

Patients on lithium maintenance therapy should be advised to discontinue the drug if they expeience side effects or if they become febrile or are exposed to profound sodium loss. There should be continued monthly monitoring of blood lithium levels, along with repeated reminders to the patient not to go on crash diets or submit to diuretics.

REFERENCES

Coppen, A., Noguera, R., Bailey, J., Burns, B. H., Swani, M. S., Hare, E. H., Gardner, R., and Maggs, R. Prophylactic lithium in affective disorders. Lancet, 2: 275, 1971.

Fieve, R. R., and Mendlewicz, J. Lithium prophylaxis of bipolar manic-depressive illness (abstract). Psychopharmacologia, 26 (Suppl.): 93, 1972.

Fieve, R. R., Mendlewicz, J., and Fleiss, J. L. Dominant X-linked transmission in manic-depressive illness: Linkage studies with the Xga blood group. Proceedings of the VIII International Congress of the CINP-Copenhagen, 1972. Avicenum Czechoslovak Medical Press, Prague, 1973.

Fieve, R. R., Mendlewicz, J., and Fleiss, J. L. Manic-depressive illness: Linkage with the Xg blood group. Am. J. Psychiatry, 130: 1355, 1973.

Geyer, H., and Gershon, S. Exploration of the antidepressant potential of lithium. Psychopharmacologia, 28: 107, 1973.

Mendlewicz, J., Fieve, R. R., Rainer, J. D., and Fleiss, J. L. Manic-depressive illness: A comparative study of patients with and without a family history. Br. J. Psychiatry, 120: 523, 1972.

Prien, R. F., Caffey, E. M., and Klett, C. J. Prophylactic efficacy of lithium carbonate in manic-depressive illness. Arch. Gen. Psychiatry, 28: 337, 1973.

Prien, R. F., Klett, J., and Caffey, E. M. A comparison of lithium carbonate and imipramine in the prevention of affective episodes in recurrent affective illness. Prepublication Report No. 94. Central Neuropsychiatric Research Laboratory, April 1973.

Stallone, F., Shelley, E., Mendlewicz, J., and Fieve, R. R. The use of lithium in affective disorders. III. A double-blind study of prophylaxis in bipolar illness. Am. J. Psychiatry, *130:* 22, 1973.

Zubin, J. Cross-national study of diagnosis of the mental disorders: Methodology and planning. Am. J. Psychiatry, *125* (Suppl.): 12, 1969.

30.9 MISCELLANEOUS ORGANIC THERAPIES

Niacin Therapy

Large doses of niacin (vitamin B³, nicotinic acid) were first used by Hoffer to treat patients with schizophrenia. The rational for this method derives from the notion of faulty transmethylation as a biochemical precursor of schizophrenia; large doses of the methyl acceptor niacin should absorb the putative excess methyl groups in the brain of schizophrenic patients and therby correct the imbalance.

Despite the demonstrated lack of therapeutic effect in schizophrenia, niacin therapy is widely touted by self-styled orthomolecular psychiatrists with a proselytizing fervor. The niacin regimen is frequently combined with high-dose ascorbic acid, special diets, and, fortunately, neuroleptic drugs and convulsive therapy. In *The Eden Express* by medical student Mark Vonnegut, a remarkable personal account of schizophrenia is described. His therapeutic encounters with megavitamin therapy, antipsychotic drugs and ECT are vividly presented.

Electrosleep Therapy

This treatment method originated in the Soviet Union, where it is used extensively for a variety of neurotic, psychotic, and psychophysiologic conditions. The term "electrosleep" is a misnomer, since sleep does not usually occur during the treatment session.

The treatment consists of the passage of a low milliamperage (0.4 to 2.0 mA) pulsed unidirectional current through electrodes placed over the orbits and mastoid processes,producing a slight tingling sensation without sleep. Treatments are given daily for 30 to 60 minutes, for a total of 5 to 10 sessions. No unwanted secondary effects are reported.

In a double-blind clinical comparison of genuine and sham electrosleep in anxious or depressed neurotic outpatients, Rosenthal found the active treatment more effective in relieving anxiety, insomnia, and depression. However, patients with psychotic depression were made worse by electrosleep.

Polarization Therapy

A technique similar to electrosleep was introduced by Lipold and Redfearn. They used smaller currents (0.25 to 0.5 mA) passed through electrodes applied over the orbits and one leg. With their method, the patient experiences no sensation of current flow, and the authors found the treatment superior to a placebo in a controlled trial in depressed patients. Because of the placement of the electrodes and the very small currents used, the suspicion arises that the treatment exerts no direct physiologic effects on the brain.

Nonconvulsive Electrical Stimulation Therapy

Treatment techniques very, but patients are generally anesthetized and given bitemporal stimulation at 60 to 100 mA, which is gradually lowered to 0.5 mA and discontinued over 3 to 15 minutes as the patient regains consciousness. The therapeutic value of the marked emotional release or abreaction that frequently follows cessation of the current is stressed, especially for neurotic patients and those with traumatic neuroses.

Two controlled studies have demonstrated that nonconvulsive electrical stimulation is therapeutically inferior to ECT. Psychiatrists using the nonconvulsive method, however assert that it is effective for those patients who have not done well with ECT or for whom ECT is not indicated—patients with anxiety neurosis, phobic neurosis, depressive neurosis, and personality disorders. Their illness is subject to spontaneous fluctuation, and their symptoms may respond readily, if transiently, to suggestion, persuasion, hypnosis, and other nonspecific approaches.

Diphenylhydantoin (Phenytoin) Therapy

The anticonvulsant diphenylhydantoin (Dilantin) or DPH achieved widespread publicity in the late 1960's, when a prominent businessman reported in the lay press that his long-standing neurotic symptoms were relieved by a course of treatment with this drug. A number of controlled studies of DPH were performed without showing any therapeutic action in the neurotic and psychotic patients treated. The potential side effects of DPH include agranulocytosis, toxic psychosis, and gingival hypertrophy, so this medication should probably be reserved for the treatment of patients with demonstrated or suspected seizure disorders, which is the only U.S. Food and Drug Administration (F.D.A.) approved use. Interesting investigational uses of phenytoin are in the treatment of cardia arrhythmias, antisocial behavior disorders, and trigeminal neuralgia.

Continuous Sleep Therapy

This somatic treatment method was introduced by Kläsi in 1922 for the treatment of psychotic patients. He used injections of a barbiturate mixture to keep patients in a state of continuous narcosis for about 10 days, with brief daily dose reductions to permit the patient to take nourishment and use the bathroom. Complications were frequent, with seizures and delirious states commonly observed at treatment termination, and there was a substantial mortality rate.

Today chlorpromazine (Thorazine) is given in daily doses of 400 to 1,600 mg. in combination with various adjuvant hypnotics to keep the patient asleep for about 20 hours daily. Reports of over-all results of 70 per cent recovered or much improved for patients with chronic anxiety states (the rates are much lower in schizophrenia and obsessional neurosis) are difficult to interpret in light of the fact that almost all patients received concomitant ECT and antidepressant drug therapy. Also, it is not possible to separate the putative effects of narcosis from the well-known therapeutic effects of chlorpromazine.

Four out of 500 patients died during treatment (two from aspirated vomitus), for a mortality rate of 0.8 per cent, about 100 times that for ECT alone. Since no controlled studies of continuous narcosis are available, there is no satisfactory way to assess the possible therapeutic effects of this method.

Acetylcholine Treatment

In 1937 Fiamberti recommended acetylcholine as a less drastic method of shock therapy. Its intravenous injection causes cardiac arrest for 30 to 50 seconds and unconsciousness of short duration. Injections of up to 600 mg. were used on schizophrenics. Lopez Ibor used smaller amounts of up to 200 mg. in anxiety neuroses. In the treatment of neuroses, only slight respiratory difficulty, coughing, and slow pulse were noticed, and repeated intravenous injections were considered valuable. This treatment is rarely used today.

Atropine and Scopolamine Therapy

Toxic doses of atropine sulfate, injected intramuscularly, were recommended by Forrer in 1951. Various vegetative symptoms, restlessness, and delirious states can be observed, followed by a coma with spontaneous awakening. The treatment was given primarily in neuroses, but it also seemed to be effective in various excitement states. Hyperthermia was the most dreaded complication.

Goldner has recommended scopolamine sleep treatment. After a period of 4 to 6 hours of coma, the patient wakes up in a confused state, showing various organic reactions, including visual hallucinations. The doses of scopolamine range from 5 to 30 mg. initially and are increased to a maximum of 100 mg. Schizophrenics and other patients have been treated, partly in combination with psychotropic drugs. This treatment is still used in some parts of the world, particularly Poland, but is rarely used in the United States.

Carbon Dioxide Therapy

Inhalation of carbon dioxide for the treatment of neurotic patients was introduced by Meduna, the orginator of convulsive therapy. The method consists of administering 20 to 100 inhalations of a 30 per cent carbon dioxide-70 per cent oxygen mixture, producing unconsciousness followed by muscular rigidity and spastic flexion of the extremities. From 20 to 150 treatments are given, and the uncontrolled clinical trials published have reported the usual beneficial effects in patients with anxiety and personality disorders, with poor effects in obsessional or hypochondriacal neurotics. The few controlled trials undertaken with carbon dioxide therapy fail to show any clinical effects in neurotic patients. In view of the recent reports of fatal outcome in opiate addicts receiving this treatment, it can no longer be considered innocuous.

REFERENCES

Aaron, H. Phenytoin. Med. Lett. *18:* 5, 1976.
Hoffer, A., and Osmond, H. Treatment of schizophrenia with nicotinic acid. Acta Psychiatr. Scand., *40:* 171, 1964.
Lippold, O. C. F., and Redfearn, J. W. T. Mental changes resulting from the passage of small direct currents through the human brain. Br. J. Psychaitry, *110:* 768, 1964.
Rosenthal, S. H. Electrosleep: A double-blind clinical study. Biol. Psychiatry, *4:* 179, 1972.
Walter, C. J. S., Mitchell-Heggs, N., and Sargant, W. Modified narcosis, ECT, and antidepressant drugs. Br. J. Psychiatry, *120:* 651, 1972.

31

Milieu Therapy

31.1. THE HOSPITAL AS A THERAPEUTIC COMMUNITY

Introduction

Professionals and institutions dealing with mental illness intend that all psychiatric hospital experiences should be therapeutic for the patient involved. However, many anti-therapeutic interactions among the staff and patients occur in all institutions, and many aspects of the institution and its environment may be neither therapeutic nor a therapeutic community.

The therapeutic community is based on the premise that a psychiatric ward or hospital is a social system. As such, it is influenced by the persons who are its members, both patients and staff; they are influenced, in turn, by the surroundings in which they find themselves. Thus, the therapeutic community approach attempts to make maximum use of the social system and its constituents, the personnel and the hospital community, to modify the patient's behavior so that he may manage his life and his personal relationships in a more constructive fashion.

The principles and the practices under which the therapeutic community operates include:

Communication is open and direct between the staff and the patients.

Patients are encouraged to participate actively in their own treatment.

The governing system offers frequent opportunities to participate in administrative and therapeutic decision making by both the patients and the staff.

Although the staff is in the position of final authority, much of the operation of the unit is in the hands of the patients.

Often, there are systems of patient government that have some features of a democratic society.

The unit and the hospital remain in close contact with the outside community, and there is frequent communication and interrelationship between them.

Usually, the unit has an open door, and patients have freedom within the hospital and its grounds.

The emphasis on physician authority is reduced. Rather than an authoritarian-submission model or a guidance-cooperation model between physician and patient, the predominant model of interrelating is a mutual collaborative one.

The therapeutic community attempts to avoid the social isolation and the dehumanization of the large institution, the withdrawal of the patient from meaningful interpersonal relationships and extensive psychological regression, the physician being regarded as a powerful and all-knowing authority, and the separation of the patient from his family, his community, and his usual responsibilities.

Administrative Organization and Leadership

If the leadership of the community provides opportunities for open communication, for participation in the decision-making processes, for increased esteem, for status and monetary rewards for excellence in performance, for satisfying and humane working conditions, and for appropriate and rewarding human personal relationships, then the entire organization is likely to deal with its peers and its subordinates in a similar fashion. If the leadership is authoritarian, is organized according to a narrow hierarchy, inhibits communication, and interferes with the participation of the staff and the patients in decision making about the day-to-day functioning of the unit or of the hospital, then very often morale is low among the patients and the staff, and therapy is impeded. The 24-hour-a-day formal therapy program and informal therapy experiences are shaped by these factors.

Staff

The staff determine the details of the operation of particular units. The staff include all personnel—professional, technical, nonprofessional, and support personnel. Frequently, the staff leadership of a unit or the team leader in a particular functional unit is the key person for that organizational or functional unit. He sets the emotional tone for that aspect of the system.

There have been some differences of opinion as to how these interactions and outcomes are best accomplished. One group advocates natural and spontaneous responses, and these responses become the subject of retrospective evaluations by the staff and the patients. An attempt is made to use these interactions as a learning experience in daily living for the patients and the staff. In this kind of approach, the patient's attitudes and behavior, including both adaptive and maladaptive behaviors and transferences, evoke in the staff certain spontaneous reactions. The staff must retain a generally therapeutic and humane response and must avoid excessive responses. When more understanding is acquired about the patient's behavior, the staff may begin to react to this behavior by interpreting the responses usually evoked, by clarifying the nature of the interaction, or by interpreting what the patient is doing and why.

Another approach to the question of how the staff respond to patient behavior is the prescribed attitude. In this approach, the team's leadership or the team leader forms a diagnostic understanding of the patient's behavior and prescribes an attitudinal approach to the patient based on this understanding. The staff of such a unit may create milieu homogeneity, which can be thought of as a corrective emotional experience. Examples of such attitudes include kind firmness, permissiveness, and limit setting.

Both approaches are used in most therapeutic communities. The trend, however, has been away from the more formal attitude prescrip-

tion and the creation of a planned environment. Instead, the spontaneous natural approach has been used more widely in recent years. One exception has been the therapeutic approach in units oriented to behavior modification. There, the milieu is structured and planned, based on behavioral principles, understanding, and therapeutic interventions.

The therapeutic community approach also suggests that the staff foster the development of multidisciplinary therapeutic teams, with a good deal of role sharing and role overlap. Another characteristic is the frequent and open sharing in verbal and written form of observations about patient and staff behaviors on the unit.

Patients

Instead of adopting the usual sick role—which emphasizes being cared for, being dependent, being passive, and being acted on—the patient is encouraged to be active, independent, and a collaborator and participant in his treatment to the degree that such activity and behavior are possible.

Patients, along with the staff, become members of a community that governs and administers many aspects of the unit or hospital in which they find themselves. Day-to-day matters concerning group living and the management of the hospital are important aspects of the matters that patient-staff groups decide. The governance possibilities may extend into such matters as over-all unit policy, individual or group privileges and restrictions, and therapeutic objectives and decisions.

The patient takes increasing responsibility for his current life situations. He participates in living in a community where his contacts with others become therapeutic and rehabilitative encounters from which he learns about himself and how he expresses adaptive and maladaptive features of his personality. He becomes a therapeutic person for other patients in that he is responsible for their ward behavior and adaption as well as his own. He tends to be more active in his own day-to-day living needs, and he is responsible for his person and his behavior.

His participation should reduce regression and shorten his hospital stay, thereby encouraging the patient to resume his ordinary out-of-hospital roles earlier than usual and to separate from the hospital as quickly as possible. The community offers a stable and consistent milieu in which interpersonal transactions are visible. The behavior of the participants may be reflected to the persons involved relatively accurately and, thereby, be subject to clarification, analysis, and understanding.

Ecology of the Hospital

The location of the hospital in a rural or urban area, its size, its architecture, the materials used in its construction, the distribution and use of space, the number of beds, the number of patients, the furnishings, the use of color and materials in its decor, the attitudes about the use of the facility—all help determine the therapeutic atmosphere of a hospital.

Ideally, the therapeutic institution is small or medium-sized. It is located near the population it serves. It is attractive in architecture and decor, with adequate space and furnishings. There are appropriate spaces for living, sleeping, activity, and work. Most units are open, and there is considerable communication and movement between the inside and the outside. Patients have many of their personal belongings and their own clothes available to them. Small groups of patients and staff may come together in social, therapy, or work groupings of 4 to 15 people. Also, there is space for large group meeings. The patients and the staff need time alone on occasions, and there are provisions for that need.

Optimism and hope gradually accrue and replace discouragement and despair. This change is often reflected in the outcome of treatment—shorter hospital stays and quicker resumption of usual life roles. Often, part-time hospital programs are begun. Rehabilitation in the community is encouraged and enhanced.

Treatment Potential

The implicit and explicit communications by professional and nonprofessional employees and by the other patients establish a series of expectations that may become self-fulfilling prophecies. Hope becomes an important positive attitude and is frequently followed by positive outcomes.

The ward, the therapy team and the other personnel, the patients, and the hospital begin a process with the recently admitted patient in which he or she is socialized into patient roles. These persons, the setting, the use of space, the decor, and many other facets of living transmit messages about how things are done and what it takes to become a success as a patient. There are both overt and covert messages, so that the manifest content of the communication may be quite different from the latent content. Small and large group meetings, informal communication, and other interactions should, under optimum conditions, clarify the preferred responses and assist the patient in his adaptation, resolving his own confusion and any ambiguity he may feel.

Theoretical Basis

The orientations of those who operate therapeutic communities are usually psychodynamic, psychoanalytic, or behavioral.

In the psychodynamic, psychoanalytic framework, hypotheses about the therapeutic effects of the therapeutic community center on the interface between ego functions and environment. The environment may alter or shape certain psychodynamic balances that are intrapsychic. Some of these structures or functions are the adaptive functions of the ego, ego defenses, the self systems, and object representations. The inputs from the environment of the hospital ward are intended to provide predictability, certainty, and continuity of experience for the patient, thereby reducing anxiety, guilt, and shame. The corrective experience of an environment that is reality-oriented and humane promotes the reduction of painful tensions and the associated structural and economic imbalances. If successful, the therapeutic community promotes more appropriate and more realistic interpersonal relations. It enhances self-esteem and reduces feelings of wrongdoing or sinfulness.

The therapeutic community offers opportunities to influence and shape behavior through systems of rewards and punishment, both overt and covert. Such interventions may be thought of as theoretical and therapeutic extensions of behavioral therapy. Therapeutic decisions about privileges, constraints, and discharge may be viewed by the staff and the patients as rewards or punishments. As such, they may influence behavior in desired therapeutic outcomes, or they may become antitherapeutic if applied in an arbitrary or authoritarian fashion. Thus, almost every therapeutic community uses some therapeutic elements of psychoanalytic understanding and some elements of behavioral understanding.

REFERENCES

Caudill, W. *The Psychiatric Hospital as a Small Society.* Harvard University Press, Cambridge, 1958.
Cumming, J., and Cumming, E. *Ego and Milieu.* Atherton Press, New York, 1962.
Greenblatt, M., Levinson, D. J., and Williams, R. H. *The Patient and the Mental Hospital.* Free Press of Glencoe (Macmillan), New York, 1957.
Jones, M. *The Therapeutic community.* Basic Books, New York, 1953.
Rapoport, R. N. *Community as Doctor.* Charles C Thomas, Springfield, Ill., 1960.
Stanton, A. H., and Schwartz, M. S. *The Mental Hospital.* Basic Books, New York, 1954.

31.2.   PARTIAL HOSPITALIZATION

Introduction

Partial hospitalization may include day hospitalization, night hospitalization, and evening or weekend hospital care. Day hospitalization is a structured psychiatric treatment program that patients attend 5 days a week, excluding weekends, from 9:00 A.M. to 5:00 P.M. Ordinarily, patients eat breakfast and dinner at home and have lunch at the day hospital. In night hospitalization, patients usually work or go to school and return to the hospital for dinner. They then participate in evening activities and sleep in the hospital. In evening and weekend hospital care, patients function in jobs or school and return to the hospital for evening or weekend treatment programs.

Day Hospitals

Functions

A day hospital may be an alternative to inpatient care, a transition from inpatient care to full-time life in the community, or an alternative to outpatient care. Day hospitals have also been used for crisis intervention and for specific types of patients, such as alcoholics, drug addicts, those with character disorders, children, adolescents, and the elderly.

Structure

The term "day hospital" is reserved for a unit in which every form of treatment provided in a psychiatric hospital is available. A day center, on the other hand, is independent of a hospital and provides social and occupational services with little or no medical supervision. Such centers are more suitable for patients who require supportive care alone and for those who need a long-term social rehabilitation program to upgrade their vocational and social skills.

Characteristics

A typical day program is located in an urban area. It is usually affiliated with a large hospital or community mental health center. The number of patients ranges between 20 and 40 at any one time. The age of the patients is between 18 and 65 years. There are usually more women patients than men. The usual criteria for admission are: (1) The patient must be able to spend nights and weekends at home. (2) The family must be willing for the patient to remain at home, and the home environment must not be so grossly pathogenic that it would be destructive for the patient to remain. (3) The patient or the family must be able to provide transportation, or transportation must be provided by the service. (4) The patient cannot be suicidal, homicidal, assaultive, or grossly out of contact and disorganized. (5) The patient cannot be primarily alcoholic or drug-addicted. (6) The patient should not have a severe organic brain syndrome or be severely mentally retarded. (7) The patient must be ambulatory—that is, he must not be medically ill or have a severe physical handicap.

The largest diagnostic category is schizophrenia. Day hospital hours are 9 A.M. to 5 P.M. Monday through Friday. The average length of stay is 2 to 3 months. The staff includes at least one part-time or full-time psychiatrist, with the majority of the staff members being psychiatric nurses, social workers, and mental health workers. Occupational therapists are desirable as long as they emphasize preparation for job rehabilitation, including prevocational therapy, as opposed to an emphasis on leisure-time activities.

The location may vary: (1) Day patients may be treated on the inpatient service along with inpatients. (2) The day hospital may be located in the same hospital but in different quarters from the inpatient service. (3) It may be located in a separate building within the local community, preferably not far from the hospital. Easy access should be provided for those day patients who need an occasional overnight stay on the inpatient service.

Advantages

Day care is preferable to inpatient and outpatient care for many patients. Most patients have low self-esteem. Putting a patient away in a psychiatric hospital usually lowers his self-esteem further and attaches a stigma to him. Day hospitalization should cause less lowering of self-esteem. The expectation of healthier functioning in a day hospital probably leads to less regression than occurs on an inpatient service. Patients can maintain some social and vocational roles because they are home evenings and weekends. There is no separation from family and friends, and, although the family may have pathological aspects, it often offers a great deal of emotional support for patients. It is not necessary for patients to adapt to a total institution with a deviant culture. Many psychiatric patients have severe problems managing their dependent and passive needs. Once such a patient is hospitalized and subjected to a regressive environment, the likelihood increases that he will regress in the face of a subsequent life stress.

The family as a social system is not permitted to extrude the patient as the sick member and has less opportunity to close ranks. Instead, it is confronted with the necessity of integrating him into the family system.

The staff, especially the nursing staff, can lead a more regular life, working 5 days a week with no evening or weekend shifts. The cost should be less because only one meal a day is served, space is not needed for beds, and only one shift of staff is required. Day patients may experience less sexual frustration because there is no prolonged period of sexual abstinence. And the community learns to adopt more realistic attitudes toward the mentally ill and to recognize that they are not all dangerous and to be feared.

Disadvantages

When the family is in crisis and at the breaking point, it may be impossible to deal with the situation effectively unless the patient is removed to an inpatient service, thus relieving the strain. Separating the patient from his family enables him to achieve not only symptom remission but also psychological growth because he is no longer subjected to the pathological interaction with family members that tends to perpetuate and exacerbate psychopathology.

Some patients are unable to control unacceptable impulses, such as aggression and self-destruction, and may need the protection afforded by inpatient care.

While the patient is in the hospital, the staff can observe his behavior and manage it in a therapeutic manner. Many staff members are more comfortable with the availability of 24-hour observation and control for patients.

The external controls offered by the hospital allow psychotherapy to deal with threatening material that may potentially lead to ego disorganization of the patient.

Patients may have harmful effects on other family members, especially children, if they are home during psychotic episodes.

It is easier for day patients than for inpatients to drop out of the program.

Regression can occur in a day hospital as well as on an inpatient service, and some patients may prefer to remain dependent in a protected environment indefinitely.

There is often a problem with transportation, especially in rural areas where patients must travel great distances from home to the day hospital.

Many patients do not have families or friends to live with.

Day care costs more than outpatient care, and attending a day program interferes with employment or school. Many insurance policies cover inpatient care but not day care.

Night Hospitalization

Many inpatient services use night hospital status for previously full-time inpatients as a means of easing the transition from hospital to community life. This status allows patients to gradually become less dependent on the hospital while beginning to function in jobs, housekeeping, or student roles or while seeking employment or housing. Return to the hospital in the evening can offer support until the patient feels secure enough for full discharge. Ordinarily, this process should not take more than a few weeks. If a longer period of supervised living is indicated, other more economical and less regressive arrangements, such as half-way houses, should be used. Of course, many patients may return directly to their homes and jobs without the need for night hospital status.

Supervised Residences

Supervised residence programs are not forms of partial hospitalization, but they are needed to enable day programs to treat many patients without families. Many community mental health centers operate halfway houses that have a limited stay of about 6 months for patients in transition from the hospital. The expectation for these patients is that they will be able to manage their own living arrangements after making an adjustment to community life. In addition, many programs obtain apartments in the local community that are supervised by a mental health team, which may consist of a social worker or nurse and a mental health worker. Patients living in the supervised apartments can remain indefinitely if they are not able to move on to their own independent living. Apartment living with four or five patients in an apartment house seems to most closely approximate family living in a community. The use of hostels or lodges has been of value for some patients, but in some senses there are mini-institutions within the community. Foster homes may be helpful, but the screening of such homes is of vital importance

Evening and Weekend Programs

The indications for evening and weekend programs are not yet clearly defined, nor are there many such programs in existence. Per-haps the reason is that persons who can function adequately in vocational and social roles during the weekdays ordinarily should not be in need of such extensive therapeutic programs.

Since many patients, especially those from the lower classes, are not able to leave their jobs during the work day for therapeutic sessions, a comprehensive community mental health cen-ter should offer a variety of evening therapeutic activities, such as group and individual therapy and social clubs.

Conclusion

Although the concept of partial hospitaliza-tion has been widely accepted in principle, programs based on this concept are generally underutilized. A major cause has been the lack of clear-cut criteria for the selection of suitable patients for such programs.

The results of controlled research studies and of clinical experience appear to warrant the following conclusion: The day hospital not only is a feasible alternative to inpatient care but is generally preferable to it except for the most seriously disturbed acutely psychotic patients, who require full-time hospitalization. The day hospital is useful in reducing the length of inpatient hospitalization and in facilitating the patients' re-entry into the community. It is helpful in upgrading the social and vocational skills of some chronic schizophrenic patients, and for others it is a necessary support to make it possible for them to be maintained in the community. Outpatient therapy is preferable to day hospitalization for the great majority of neurotic patients.

REFERENCES

Belyaeva, T. V., and Kabanov, M. M. Partial hospitalization in a psychiatric clinic. Sov. Neurol. Psychiatry, 5: 71, 1972–73.
Bennett, D. H. The day-hospital. Bibl. Psychiatr. Neurol. (Basel), 142: 4, 1969.
Epps, R. L., and Hanes, J. D. Day Care of Psychiatric Patients. Charles C Thomas, Springfield, Ill., 1964.
Glasscote, R. M., Kraft, A. M., Glassman, S. M., and Jepson, W. W. Partial Hospitalization for the Mentally Ill: A Study of Programs and Problems. Joint Information Service and National Association for Mental Health, Washington, 1969.
Herz, M. I., Endicott, J., Spitzer, R. L., and Mesnikoff, A. Day versus inpatient hospitalization: A controlled study. Am. J. Psychiatry, 127: 107, 1971.
Koltun, L. V. Possibilities of stabilizing remissions in schi-zophrenics transferred from a psychiatric hospital to a day hospital. Sov. Neurol. Psychiatry, 5: 109, 1972–73.
Kramer, B. M. Day Hospital. Grune & Stratton, New York, 1962.
Zwerling, I., and Wilder, J. F. An evaluation of the applica-bility of the day hospital in treatment of acutely disturbed patients. Isr. Ann. Psychiatry, 2: 162, 1964.

31.3.   OCCUPATIONAL THERAPY AND OTHER THERAPEUTIC ACTIVITIES

Introduction

For the mentally ill, the emptiness of institu-tional life can oppress the mind even more than the fetters of the past oppressed the body. With time on their hands, many patients accept work gladly. But many patients elect not to work, to go for walks, to play games, or to attend religious services. In an attempt to involve this larger group of patients who are incapable of participating on their own initiative in the hospital's industries and social programs, therapists developed the field of occupational therapy.

Occupational therapy is a method of treating the sick or impaired by means of purposeful occupation. Its goals are to arouse interest, courage, and confidence; to exercise mind and body in healthy activity; to overcome disability; and to re-establish the capacity for industrial usefulness and social fulfillment.

It is important to fit the occupational therapy assignment to the needs of the individual patient. The treatment should be prescribed and administered with medical advice and correlated with other forms of treatment.

Although some patients do best alone, group activities are usually preferred to facilitate the development of social skills and to enable patients to benefit from the example and encouragement of fellow patients. Occupational therapy is used to improve the quality of the patient's relations.

This frame of reference requires that the work-centered focus of occupational therapy be broadened to encompass play. With the advent of more effective treatment methods, there came a demand for still another service for the recovering patient who was emerging from years of psychiatric invalidism and who lacked the elementary life skills for shopping, cooking, cleaning, personal hygiene, posture, gait, social deportment, job hunting, and dating. Thus these three activities areas relating to work, play, and personal life skills are usually combined in a single program under the auspices of a single department of therapeutic activities, whose goal is to prepare the patient for life outside the hospital.

Work as Activities Therapy

Every psychiatric history should include a detailed work history. The need to work exists in chronic psychotic patients more frequently than is ordinarily realized. Patients manifest pride and satisfaction in their ability to make a contribution to the welfare of the hospital. In one study, they struck up friendships, went to work together, chatted and ate together; mute patients became communicative; all became more tidy personally and in their behavior on the wards; they used their leisure time constructively and socially, rather than in autistic reveries, as previously. In some instances, patients have been hired as hospital employees.

Vocational rehabilitation usually comprises five interrelated services, all of which are aimed at establishing and maintaining the client or patient in a job—vocational counseling, vocational training, restoration services, job finding and placement services, and personal counseling.

Some hospitals permit patients to go off the grounds to work in the community by day and return to the hospital in the evening. Some states maintain sheltered workshops for the mentally handicapped. There, vocational training and further psychiatric treatment may take place on an outpatient basis. In some instances, a sheltered workshop is a permanent solution for the patient's needs.

Dance Therapy

Dance therapy is the planned use of dance to aid in the physical and psychic integration of the patient. Dance therapy is an outgrowth of modern dance. The essence of modern dance is self-expression—freedom of form, deliberate avoidance of a set vocabulary of steps, and the willingness to borrow from the other dance forms, such as ballet, folk, and social dance. Eclecticism is a keynote of dance therapy.

The prime goals in dance therapy are heightened body awareness, expression of affect, fostering communication and interaction, reduction of idiosyncratic behavior, and re-establishing a sense of self through movement. Rhythmic body action is the road to these goals. The therapist must assure his patient that judgments as to correctness of movement or aesthetic results are irrelevant. Neither is prior dance training required for a participant in a dance therapy session.

The patient's psychic state is revealed through his movement patterns. And it is the patient's specific movement repertory that the therapist seeks to recognize, analyze, and treat. Verbal imagery and music are used to further motor responsiveness. In group dance therapy, the participants usually work in a circle to promote a sense of unity and empathy. The therapist functions as a member of the group, the empathic catalyst, the cohesive force in the over-all structure.

REFERENCES

American Occupational Therapy Association. Occupational therapy: Its definition and functions. Am. J. Occup. Ther., *26:* 204, 1972.

Fairweather, G. W., Sanders, D. H., Cressler, D. L., and Maynard, H. *Community Life for the Mentally Ill.* Aldine Publishing Company, Chicago, 1969.

Fleischl, M. F., and Wolf, A. Techniques of social rehabilitation. In *Current Psychiatric Therapies,* J. Masserman, ed., vol. 7. Grune & Stratton, New York, 1967.

Glasscote, R. M., Cumming, E., Rutman, I., Sussex, J. N., and Glassman, S. M. *Rehabilitating the Mentally Ill in the Community.* Joint Information Service of the American Psychiatric Association and National Association for Mental Health, Washington, 1971.

Jones, M. *The Therapeutic Community: A New Treatment Method in Psychiatry.* Basic Books, New York, 1953.

Linn, L., Weinroth, L. A., and Shamah, R. *Occupational Therapy in Dynamic Psychiatry.* American Psychiatric Association, Washington, 1962.

Reich, R., and Siegel, L. The chronically mentally ill shuffle to oblivion. Psychiatr. Ann., *3:* 35, 1973.

32

Evaluation of Psychiatric Treatment

32.1. EVALUATION OF PSYCHIATRIC TREATMENT

Criteria of Improvement

Success in achieving the goals of certain forms of psychotherapy, such as helping the patient to achieve a more integrated personality or greater self-realization, can never be determined objectively. However, the goals of many forms of treatment are more circumscribed, and the extent to which they have been achieved in a given patient can be specified.

Over-All versus Specific Measures

Psychiatric improvement is seldom unitary. A patient's subjective symptoms and his interpersonal behavior may vary independently, or there may even be an inverse relationship between the two. A patient's headaches may occur less frequently when he begins to express his anger openly. Or he may recover from one symptom only to substitute another. Furthermore, different forms of treatment focus on different aspects of personality functioning. The behavior therapies, for example, concentrate on the amelioration of specific behavior disorders, whereas the insight therapies try to correct certain distorted perceptions of self and others.

However, an estimate of the patient's over-all improvement cannot be dispensed with. Such an estimate permits the rater to assign appropriate weights, on an intuitive basis, to improvement in particular facets of the patient's behavior. The over-all rating "much improved," for example, may be based on the disappearance of headaches in one patient, on a second patient's improved relationship with his wife, and on some combination of both factors in a third.

Face Validity versus Construct Validity

All criteria of improvement ultimately reflect implicit value judgments of the patient, the people important to him, and the therapist. Some of these values are so widely shared that any measure of improvement based on them receives universal acceptance; they are said to have face validity. These criteria include subjective comfort, the capacity to establish mutually rewarding relationships with other persons, the ability to do one's job adequately and to derive some satisfaction from working, and the possession of certain social skills.

But treatment techniques require improvement measures derived from the specific theoretical constructs on which the treatment method is based. Such measures may be said to have construct validity.

Because such measures are closely bound to the theories from which they derive, they do not permit comparison of therapies based on different views. Moreover, all measures with construct validity are justified by the fact that they are closely related to measures with face validity. There is little point in trying to increase a patient's insight or self-congruence if this change is not reflected in an improvement in subjective comfort and personal functioning.

Issues of Baseline and Improvement Interval

The ideal criterion for the evaluation of the effectiveness of treatment is a comparison of the patient's status at the end of therapy with his normal or potentially best state. The only practical alternative for such a baseline is the patient's state at the moment he seeks treatment, since only then can he be observed directly. Most patients, however, come for help when environmental stress and internal vulnerability have reduced their well-being to an abnormally low state. These patients are more distressed and incapacitated when they come to psychotherapy than they were a few months before or will be a few months later, regardless of the effects of psychotherapy. In many instances, the patient's acute symptoms would disappear without therapy.

The choice of the proper time interval for evaluating improvement presents related problems. The medical tradition of a 5-year follow-up fosters the conception of long-term improvement as the ultimate test of therapeutic efficacy. Before the advent of the phenothiazines, no form of psychiatric treatment produced a higher 5-year improvement rate than any other form, and the 5-year improvement rate for persons who had received any kind of psychiatric treatment was no higher than the rate for those who had received no specific treatment at all. Typically, a treated group of neurotics improves more rapidly than the control group and maintains its improvement, but the controls catch up eventually. But even if psychiatric treatment did no more than speed up the improvement that would occur in any case, it would be worthwhile.

Criteria of Outcome

There are three major classes of criteria by which to evaluate outcomes of treatment: the patient's subjective state, his behavior, and his state of physiological tension. The patient is the sole source of information as to how he feels, and he can also report on his behavior as he perceives it. However, his reports need to be supplemented by direct observations. In the therapy situation, these can be made by the therapist or by trained observers not directly involved in therapy.

Self-Reports

Only the patient knows how troubled he was when he applied for treatment and whether or not treatment has brought relief. However, unstructured self-reports, solicited by the therapist, are subject to error. The patient may lack the insight and sensitivity required for good self-observation. Even a good self-observer may allow his self-reports to be colored by his fears, disappointments, hopes, and clues that implicitly suggest to the patient what is expected of him. All forms of psychotherapy contain the implicit expectation that the patient adopt the therapist's view of mental illness and treatment. Various ways of structuring reports represent partial solutions to these problems.

Symptom Checklists. An obvious way of determining the results of treatment is to have the patient report at intervals how he feels by checking the symptoms he is experiencing and their degree of severity. Such scales can be analyzed to yield mean distress scores and scores based on categories of symptoms. In neurotics, for example, the degree of over-all distress seems to be determined primarily by the severity of symptoms related to anxiety and depression. Mean distress scores are too labile to distinguish the relative effectiveness of different types of treatment, but subscales may be useful.

Analysis of Target Complaints. These are the complaints the patient cites as his reasons for seeking treatment. They are considerably more stable than mean distress scores over a short time span and permit comparison of different forms of treatment. The analysis of target complaints has proved particularly useful in the evaluation of drug therapies.

However, the patient's target complaints may change as therapy progresses. As he develops confidence in his therapist, the patient may reveal problems he had concealed at the outset, and the insight he gains in the course of treatment may lead him to reformulate his initial complaints. Also, the comparison of one patient's complaints with another's presents problems.

Q-Sort. In the Q-sort the patient arranges a large number of cards—on each of which is written a complaint, personality attribute, or attitude—in accordance with how applicable they are to him personally. Those that are most applicable are placed at one end of a scale, those least applicable at the other, and the remainder in between. Statistical analysis follows.

Semantic Differential. This test consists of a series of nine-point, bipolar scales, such as sharp-dull, clean-dirty, hot-cold, good-bad. The patient is asked to rate certain concepts on each of these dimensions. Concepts are chosen that are relevant to the patient's problems and the goals of therapy, such as "myself," "my mother's influence on me," and "my sexual feelings." By means of appropriate statistical analysis, each concept can be located in a three-dimensional meaning space, whose axes are good-bad, strong-weak, and active-passive, as well as along other dimensions appropriate to particular groups of patients. It is then possible to determine in quantitative terms how the meanings of the concepts are affected by therapy.

Minnesota Multiphasic Personality Inventory. This test yields a general overview, including those symptoms and personality attitudes that may be resistant to treatment. The significance of the individual patient's answers emerges only by their statistical comparison with norms based on large patient populations.

Ratings of Behavior

Patients' self-reports require supplementation and validation by observations of their behavior, especially outside of therapy, to determine the extent to which changes observed in the treatment situation have generalized to the rest of their lives. Obtaining this information for hospitalized patients is relatively simple because they can be continuously observed. Typically, this procedure involves the observation and rating of the patient's behavior at regular time intervals around the clock and a subsequent check of the reliability of these observations by a comparison of the ratings made by various members of the treatment staff.

With regard to outpatients, information about behavior outside therapy must be based on home visits or relatives' reports, which are subject to distortions. These distortions in relatives' reports can be reduced by the use of structured scales and especially by interviews that try to elicit from the informants specific information in support of their judgments.

Outpatient group therapies offer an intermediate vantage point, since presumably the therapy group resembles many situations of everyday life more closely than the individual interview. However, one must determine the extent to which behavior observed in therapy groups carries over into other situations.

Objective Indices of Emotional States

Some objective indices of emotional states measure lexical and nonlexical aspects of speech, and others a variety of autonomic measures, such as heart rate, skin resistance, and skin temperature. Biochemical correlates of emotional states, such as the rise of free fatty acids with anxiety and the close correlation of increased urinary levels of 17-hydroxycorticosteroids with clinical estimates of severity of depression, can also be measured.

REFERENCES

Bergin, A. E. The evaluation of therapeutic outcomes. In *Handbook of Psychotherapy and Behavior Change: An Empirical Analysis*. A. E. Bergin and S. L. Garfield, editors, p. 217. John Wiley, New York, 1971.

Derogatis, L. R., Lipman, R. S., Rickels, K., Uhlenhuth, E. H., and Covi, L. The symptom distress checklist (HSCL): A measure of primary symptom dimensions. In *Psychological Measurement: Modern Problems in Pharmacopsychiatry*, P. Pichot, editor. S. Karger. Basel, 1974.

Lang, P. J. The application of psychophysiological methods to the study of psychotherapy and behavior modification. In *Handbook of Psychotherapy and Behavior Change: An Empirical Analysis*, A. E. Bergin and S. L. Garfield, editors, p. 75. John Wiley, New York, 1971.

Meltzoff, J., and Kornreich, M. *Research in Psychotherapy*. Atherton Press, New York, 1970.

Orne, M. T. Demand characteristics and the concept of quasi-controls. In *Artifacts in Behavioral Research*, R. Rosenthal and R. L. Rosnow, editors, p. 143. Academic Press, New York, 1969.

Paul, G. L. *Insight vs. Desensitization in Psychotherapy: An Experiment in Anxiety Reduction*. Stanford University Press, Palo Alto, Calif., 1966.

Strupp, H. H., and Bergin, A. E. Some empirical and conceptual bases for coordinated research in psychotherapy: A critical review of issues, trends, and evidence. Int. J. Psychiatry, 7: 18, 1969.

32.2.   PSYCHIATRIC RATING SCALES

Introduction

Evaluating response to psychiatric treatment differs from evaluating response to treatment in other fields of medicine because no readily available or clearly useful physiologic measures reflect changes in the severity of the patient's psychiatric condition. Except for a few limited indices—such as discharge from the hospital, readmission, and return to work—the evaluation of severity requires judgments made by the patient himself, someone who knows him, or a trained professional observer. Unless these judgments are made in a standardized manner that lends itself to statistical analysis, it is impossible to compare different therapies and different patients or to compare and integrate the judgments of more than one observer. An approach to solving this problem was the development of rating scales—techniques for recording judgments of a dimension, trait, or behavior along a continuum.

Definitions

The term "scale" is commonly used in three different ways. At the broadest level, it denotes an entire procedure or instrument that yields one or more quantitative indices. An example is the Inpatient Multidimensional Psychiatric Scale. At the next level, scale refers to a score based on some computed value that used data from two or more judgments. For example, the scales of the Minnesota Multiphasic Personality Inventory (MMPI) are based on ratings of many different true-false judgments. At the narrowest level, scale refers to a single judgment of some trait or dimension, sometimes referred to as an item. For example, the scale of suicidal thoughts or impulses, one of the 75 individual scales of the Inpatient Multidimensional Psychiatric Scale, calls for a single judgment on a 9-point scale. The number of discriminations called for in a single rating scale varies from 2, such as present-absent, to as many as the scale designer believes feasible. The actual judgment may call for selecting a number, an adjective, a brief description, or a point along a line that reflects distance from two defined end points.

The term "rating scale," as applied to an entire procedure or instrument, is often limited to instruments that call for judgments made by someone other than the subject himself. In this section, however, the term includes any procedure that yields a quantitative index of a subject's condition, whether dependent on self-rating or on ratings made by others.

Selecting and Developing Rating Scales

Coverage

The coverage of the rating scale should be appropriate to the type of patients being studied and the treatment being evaluated. A measure of long-term personality traits is hardly relevant as a criterion measure of improvement in a study of the short-term effects of an antidepressant agent on acutely depressed inpatients. Failure to include relevant dimensions in a study comparing two treatments may falsely lead to the conclusion that there are no differences in outcome when, in fact, there are. On the other hand, the inclusion of a large number

TABLE I

Critical Areas for the Evaluation of Treatment for Five Types of Mental Disorder

Type of Condition	Critical Areas
Acute schizophrenia	Reality-testing impairment Thought disorder Sensorium Behavioral disorganization Suicide and violence
Chronic schizophrenia in the community	Social adjustment (role-functioning, interpersonal relations, self-care)
Major affective disorder	Reality testing Behavioral disorganization Mood and subjective distress Vegetative signs and symptoms Social adjustment
Outpatient neurotic condition	Subjective distress Social adjustment Personality traits (if long-term psychotherapy) Ego functions and patterns of defense (if psychoanalytic therapy)
Addiction	Addiction pattern Social adjustment Subjective distress

of variables for which there is no reason to expect differential change complicates the final interpretation of the results of the data analysis.

Table I lists certain critical areas for the evaluation of treatment for five different types of mental disorders. The list is by no means exhaustive but merely indicates those areas likely to be the focus of treatment evaluation.

Any patient characteristic that can be explicitly defined can be measured by a rating scale.

Manifest Psychopathology. Most psychiatric rating scales evaluate the kinds of manifest psychopathology that have been traditionally included in a mental status examination, such as disturbed mood, impairment of reality testing, psychomotor disturbance, and orientation and memory disturbance. Some rating scales that focus on manifest psychopathology are all-purpose scales that cover a broad range of dimensions. Others are limited to particular dimensions, such as depression or anxiety, or to the use with particular subgroups of patients, such as schizophrenics or those with affective illnesses

Social Adjustment. There is fair agreement on what constitutes adequate functioning in the occupational and marital aspects of social adjustment but much less agreement on what constitutes impairment in the use of leisure time, relationships with the extended family, and participation in community affairs. Social adjustment includes performance level, satisfaction, and discrepancy between what is expected by the community or the family and the actual level of performance. The rating scales that focus on social adjustment vary with regard to which of these aspects of social adjustment they cover. Measures of social adjustment usually have items that refer to behavior that can be expected to occur only when the subject is living in the community.

Personality. Most personality scales are self-report measures completed by the patient himself. They are rarely used in evaluating psychiatric treatment because personality refers to stable traits and there is little expectation that it will change with the most commonly used forms of psychiatric treatment.

Psychoanalytic Concepts. Only a few rating scales use psychoanalytic concepts, such as ego strength, ego balance, ego functions, and patterning of defenses. The high level of inference required for making judgments of these variables tends to lower interjudge reliability.

Over-All Severity of Illness. A rating scale measuring over-all severity of illness attempts to allow the clinician to use all aspects of the patient's symptoms and functioning to arrive at a single summary judgment. Table II presents an example of a rating scale for measuring over-all severity of illness, the Global Assessment Scale. Some of the standard rating scales of psychopathology have included a few items reflecting positive functioning, such as being cooperative, being cheerful, having a sense of humor, and being responsible. More complete coverage of good or superior functioning is available in the rating scales that tap social adjustment and in those that are global assessments of over-all severity of illness.

Change. Evaluating change requires an initial evaluation, a subsequent evaluation, and some type of statistical manipulation. It is also possible to evaluate change by having the rater rate his perception of change itself at a follow-up evaluation. Or the patient, rather than the clinician, may make improvement ratings on self-selected target complaints.

Time Period Covered

Whatever coverage is selected as appropriate must be limited to a specific time period. This period can vary from the moment at which the patient is being evaluated to his entire lifetime. The decision regarding the time period is obviously related to the specific dimensions being covered. For example, personality traits usually refer to characteristic or long-standing patterns of behavior. Mood can be evaluated on a short-term or a long-term basis. When rating scales are used for diagnostic purposes, rather than for measuring change, a long time period is often used so that the entire current illness can be evaluated.

Collecting the Data

Self-Report Questionnaire. The major advantage of having the patient himself make ratings of his condition is that it saves professional time and expense. In addition, for evaluation of subjective distress in patients who are not very disturbed, self-report measures are more sensitive than evaluations made by professionals based on a clinical interview. On the other hand, if the patient is too disturbed to complete the task, cannot read or understand the intent of the questions, or is motivated in some way to falsify his responses, the self-report procedures are not very useful. Certain important dimensions of psychopathology—such as reality testing, thought disorder, sensorial disturbance, inappropriate behavior or affect, and some aspects of interpersonal relations—cannot be adequately evaluated with self-report measures.

Questionnaire Completed by Informant. Having an informant fill out a questionnaire about the patient also results in a saving of professional time and expense and provides an opportunity to get information about the patient's functioning that does not depend on observations of him in an artificial or limited setting. Informants' ratings of patients' behavior are sensitive measures of differential treatment response.

However, many patients have no informants available, particularly in urban settings, or the informants are unwilling or unable to give useful information. They may give the best information for those aspects of behavior that

TABLE II

Global Assessment Scale (GAS)

Robert L. Spitzer, M.D., Miriam Gibbon, M.S.W., Jean Endicott, Ph.D.

Rate the subject's lowest level of functioning in the last week by selecting the lowest range which describes his functioning on a hypothetical continuum of mental health-illness. For example, a subject whose "behavior is considerably influenced by delusions" (range 21 to 30) should be given a rating in that range even though he has "major impairment in several areas" (range 31 to 40). Use intermediary levels when appropriate (e.g., 35, 58, 63). Rate actual functioning independent of whether subject is receiving and may be helped by medication or some other form of treatment.

Name of Patient_____ID No._____Consec. No._____Code No._____

Admission Date_____Date of Rating_____Rater_____Rating_____

100–91   No symptoms, superior functioning in a wide range of activities, life's problems never seem to get out of hand, is sought out by others because of his warmth and integrity.

90–81   Transient symptoms may occur, but good functioning in all areas, interested and involved in a wide range of activities, socially effective, generally satisfied with life, "everyday" worries that only occasionally get out of hand.

80–71   Minimal symptoms may be present but no more than slight impairment in functioning, varying degrees of "everyday" worries and problems that sometimes get out of hand.

70–61   Some mild symptoms (e.g., depressive mood and mild insomnia) *or* some difficulty in several areas of functioning, but generally functioning pretty well, has some meaningful interpersonal relationships and most untrained people would not consider him "sick."

60–51   Moderate symptoms or generally functioning with some difficulty (e.g., few friends and flat affect, depressed mood and pathological self-doubt, euphoric mood and pressure of speech, moderately severe antisocial behavior).

50–41   Any serious symptomatology or impairment in functioning that most clinicians would think obviously requires treatment or attention (e.g., suicidal preoccupation or gesture, severe obsessional rituals, frequent anxiety attacks, serious antisocial behavior, compulsive drinking).

40–31   Major impairment in several areas, such as work, family relations, judgment, thinking, or mood (e.g., depressed woman avoids friends, neglects family, unable to do housework), *or* some impairment in reality testing or communication (e.g., speech is at times obscure, illogical or irrelevant), *or* single serious suicide attempt.

30–21   Unable to function in almost all areas (e.g., stays in bed all day(*or* behavior is considerably influenced by either delusions or hallucinations *or* serious impairment in communication (e.g., sometimes incoherent or unresponsive) or judgment (e.g., acts grossly inappropriately).

20–11   Needs some supervision to prevent hurting self or others or to maintain minimal personal hygiene (e.g., repeated suicide attempts, frequently violent, manic excitement, smears feces) *or* gross impairment in communication (e.g., largely incoherent or mute).

10–1   Needs constant supervision for several days to prevent hurting self or others, or makes no attempt to maintain minimal personal hygiene.

are directly observable or that affect other members of the family.

Naturalistic Observations. Most rating scales that rely on observations by professionals in a naturalistic setting are designed for use in an institutional setting, such as a psychiatric ward. Such ward observation scales are among the most sensitive measures. Most of the focus of such scales is an overt behavior that is of high frequency when significant and that is relatively easy to rate. Naturalistic observations are most appropriate for severely disturbed adults and children who manifest overt behavioral disturbance, such as temper tantrums, hyperactivity, or shyness. Many studies using naturalistic observation techniques call for the frequency with which certain target behaviors occur during a specified time period. However, it is expensive to obtain adequate time samples to make valid judgments of the patient's behavior, and the presence of an observer may influence the frequency of the behavior being studied.

Interview of Informant. A professional may interview an informant and record his judgments of the material provided. In this method, questions that the informant has difficulty in understanding can be rephrased or otherwise clarified. Further, more complex judgments can be made by the professional rater than can be made by an informant. In addition, the professional can make a judgment about the quality of the information.

Interview of Patient. The most commonly used method for obtaining data for rating scales used in studies evaluating treatment is the direct interview of a patient by a professional. The clinical interview combines elements of both self-report and naturalistic observation. In addition, the clinical interview enables the rater to obtain information with which to make judgments about clinical phenomena. The interviewer can interact with the patient in such a manner as to increase the patient's ability and willingness to provide valid information.

One of the main limitations of the clinical interview as a data-gathering technique is the variability among interviewers in the topics they cover and in the manner in which they phrase their questions. In addition, an interviewer often varies his interviewing procedure on subsequent occasions and with different patients. In terms of interrater agreement, ratings based on structured interviews have been found to be highly reliable, with coefficients generally higher than those based on unstructured clinical interviews.

Level of Judgments

The rater can be required to make judgments at different levels of complexity. At the simplest level, the rater can be required merely to record the presence of a small unit of clearly defined behavior, such as "Patient cries" or "Says he has felt anxious or tense." An example of an item requiring more complex judgment is, "Indicates that he cannot trust other people or

that he is unduly suspicious of their intent." Still more complex judgment is needed for items that require the rater to take into account the context in which a behavior occurs—for example, "Unable to work because of his psychopathology" or "Has delusions." The highest level of clinical judgment is generally required for ratings of psychoanalytic concepts.

Because simple judgments are generally more reliable, concepts should be defined at the lowest level of inference possible without lowering the validity of the item as a measure of the dimension under consideration. However complex the item to be judged, it should be clearly defined so that the rater knows what behavior is included.

Recording

Many rating scales contain dichotomous (true-false or present-absent) items. However, most phenomena included in psychiatric rating scales are obviously continuous and can only arbitrarily be dichotomized as present or absent. Therefore, each item should preferably allow the rater to choose from many levels of severity. Most rating scales contain items that have four to nine levels of severity. Usually, the same number of scale points is used for all items in the instrument.

A small number of scales, usually measures of personality traits or self-concept, call for ipsative ratings, in which the reference is the patient himself. The rater does not consider how the patient compares on the trait with other patients.

For the vast majority of scales, the task of the rater is to select an adjective or a number that corresponds to an adjective that indicates the magnitude of severity of a trait for a given patient relative to the full range of the trait in a hypothetical population of people. The adjectives used for scale points are the same kind of descriptive terms that clinicians commonly use when describing clinical phenomena: slight, mild, moderate, severe, and extreme. Such terms usually describe severity by taking into account both intensity and duration. Other scales may call for judgments of frequency: rarely, occasionally, fairly often, very often. In an effort to increase reliability and validity, some scale developers provide definitions or examples for each of the scale points. Table III

TABLE III

Two Common Item Formats Used in Rating Scales

A. Undefined scale points (from Brief Psychiatric Rating Scale, Overall and Gorham)

Suspiciousness—belief (delusional or otherwise) that others have now, or have had in the past, malicious or discriminatory intent toward the patient. On the basis of verbal report, rate only those suspicions which are currently held, whether they concern past or present circumstances.

Not present   Very mild   Mild   Moderate   Moderately severe   Severe   Extremely severe

B. Defined scale points (from Schedule for Affective Disorders and Schizophrenia, Spitzer and Endicott)

From slight distrustfulness through suspiciousness and delusions of persecution. Does not include feelings or beliefs which are completely justified by the situation.	0 No information
	1 Not at all or fully warranted by the situation
	2 Slight feelings of distrustfulness which may be realistically based and are of doubtful clinical significance
What kinds of trouble do you have with people?	
(Do you feel you have to be on guard with people?)	3 Suspiciousness definitely not warranted by the situation, but only occasional and of mild intensity, e.g., often feels taken advantage of
(Has anybody been against you or been giving you a hard time?)	4 Often suspicious or distrustful, but clearly without delusional conviction, or transient ideas of reference that he recognizes as his imagination
(Are people too critical of you?)	5 Pervasive suspiciousness or paranoid feelings of borderline delusional intensity, e.g., not sure if a plot exists against him
(Have you felt that people were talking about you behind your back, or taking special notice of you, or laughing at you?)	6 Clearcut paranoid delusions, pathological ideas of reference, or hallucinations of persecution
	7 As above, but preoccupied with delusions or hallucinations, or behavior greatly influenced by them
(Have you felt distrustful of others or afraid that you would be taken advantage of?)	

presents examples of scales with both undefined and defined levels of severity.

Administration

Short self-report scales and rating scales completed after routine clinical evaluations usually require no more than 10 to 15 minutes to complete. However, the clinical evaluation on which the rating scales are based usually lasts at least 20 minutes. On the other hand, rating scales using structured interview schedules that assess both current and historical information may take 2 hours or more to complete. Generally, patients who are very disturbed or who exhibit a wide range of psychopathology take more time to evaluate than do patients who are not very disturbed or whose psychopathology is limited to a circumscribed area.

Training

No training is required for self-report instruments other than some familiarity on the part of the person who explains to the patient the procedure he is to follow. But all rating scales require some experience with patients who exhibit the behaviors being rated, as well as specific training with the instrument.

Purely observational techniques require less professional training than procedures that require the rater to interact with the patient, as in conducting a clinical interview. Structured interviews enable raters to conduct a clinical evaluation even when they have had little formal training in interviewing or have had little prior contact with disturbed patients. However, unless a considerable amount of on-the-job training is done, the raters often do not know when and how to probe for additional information or how to clarify ambiguous responses. On the other hand, prior experience and formal professional training are no guarantees that the rater will make accurate judgments.

Summarizing the Data

Summarizing the data into a limited number of indices is desirable. The reliability of individual items is generally lower than that of a score based on a number of items, and decreasing the number of variables being evaluated decreases the likelihood of finding statistically significant relationships by chance alone. On the other hand, it is generally not good practice to reduce all the data from a rating scale into a single score unless there are data showing that the scale is truly unidimensional. Most rating scales measure several dimensions that are usually sufficiently uncorrelated with each other to contraindicate their being combined into a single index.

Three procedures are commonly used for deriving dimensional scoring systems for rating scale data. The procedure that has been most widely used in recent years is factor analysis. Another procedure for summarizing the data into a smaller number of variables is to group the items together on the basis of a clinical concept. A less commonly used technique is to develop a scoring system based on the responses of groups of subjects known to differ in some particular way.

When scoring systems for a particular instrument tap a number of different dimensions, the investigator is usually interested in comparing scores across different dimensions for the same subject or in comparing the subject's scores with scores from some reference group. For such purposes the raw scores are usually useless because there is no standard against which they can be compared to determine their relative severity. Therefore, raw scores are usually converted into standard scores, whereby each subject's score is an expression of how far it deviates from the mean score of the reference group. The most common standard score is the T-score, which sets the mean of the reference group at 50 and the standard deviation at 10. Most rating scales of psychopathology use, as a reference group, psychiatric inpatients because they show more variability on all traits than do outpatients and nonpatients, thus maximizing the ability to make fine discriminations.

Less commonly used methods for summarizing the data in a rating scale are procedures that classify subjects into various diagnostic categories. This is done by using one of several mathematical models or by using a logical decision-tree approach. Some of these procedures classify the patient according to the standard American Psychiatric Association nomenclature, whereas others classify the patient into one of several syndromal categories that overlap with or are subsets of standard diagnostic categories.

Often, an instrument has several scoring systems, such as a multidimensional system based on factor analysis and a typological system. In addition, the factor analytically based system may provide for scores at different levels of summarization. The investigator has to decide which level of summarization is appropriate for the needs of his particular study, since summarizing too broadly or not broadly enough is likely to obscure important differences among subjects.

Data Processing

Some of the short rating scales are easily hand-scored and do not require any elaborate statistical procedures. Others require procedures that usually involve specially written computer programs.

Reliability

A basic property of any measuring instrument is its reliability—that is, the consistency with which subjects are discriminated one from another. In the case of rating scales using clinicians as observers, reliability is expressed by the agreement between two or more observers who evaluate the same series of patients (interjudge reliability). In the case of self-report measures, it may be expressed by agreement between scores computed from two halves of the instrument (split-half reliability). Consistency or reliability can also be determined by comparing the results of an evaluation at one time with the results obtained on a later occasion (test-retest reliability). However, test-retest reliability is a measure of reliability only to the extent that the subject's true condition can be assumed to have been stable across the interval between evaluations. Therefore, this form of reliability is usually limited to studying characteristics not expected to change markedly with time.

Sometimes the internal consistency of an instrument—that is, the extent to which items in a scale co-vary—is referred to as yet another form of reliability. An internal consistency index gives an estimate of the correlation of the scale score with the score that would be obtained with a comparable set of items from the same behavioral domain. Internal consistency of a scale is high when subjects tend to be rated in the same manner on the component items. Ideally, high internal consistency indicates that the scale items are tapping different aspects of the same behavioral domain. A scale with high internal consistency may or may not be reliable in the interjudge sense of discriminating among subjects.

A common misunderstanding is the confusion between interjudge reliability and agreement among raters. Whereas it is possible to speak of agreement among raters on ratings for a single patient, one cannot speak of reliability because the essence of reliability is shared discrimination between subjects. When there is only one subject, there is no discrimination; hence, reliability is indeterminate. Similarly, in the unlikely event that two clinicians agree that 100 per cent of a sample of patients have the same rated amount of improvement in response to a given treatment, agreement would be perfect, but reliability would again be indeterminate.

Low interjudge reliability of a rating scale on a series of subjects may be due to inaccuracy in the actual ratings or a lack of variability in the sample studied. Inaccuracy in the actual ratings may be the result of problems in the instrument, such as poor item definitions, or of problems in the ratings, such as lack of training, carelessness, and poor judgment. Lack of variability in the sample may be caused by homogeneity of the sample, such as the rarity of hallucinations in normals or the ubiquity of worrying among hospitalized depressed patients. Reliability may be spuriously high because raters share the same biases or misconceptions or because, as a result of working together, they have developed shared methods for making ratings that are not actually a function of the rating scale being used.

Another source of spuriously high reliability is the inclusion of samples of subjects that increase subject variability far beyond what would be expected in the samples on which the instrument would actually be used. An example would be to include both normals and acutely disturbed schizophrenics in a reliability study for an instrument whose primary use would be to discriminate among outpatients.

Strictly speaking, therefore, reliability is not a property of a rating scale per se but, rather, of the rating scale applied to a particular sample by particular raters in a particular setting. A rating scale or any of its component scales, that is reliable when applied to a heterogeneous population may be found to be unreliable when applied to a sample that demonstrates no variability on the dimension tapped by the scale. Similarly, a rating scale that is reliable when used by well-trained raters may be found to be unreliable when used by poorly trained raters. Ideally, therefore, the reliability of an instrument should be determined on samples and with rates and under conditions as similar as possible to the actual conditions of a study.

It is impossible to give precise guidelines as to what are acceptable levels of reliability. Generally, however, one would be hesitant to use a rating scale in which reported intraclass reliabilities are consistently below 0.70. Well-trained raters can obtain reliability coefficients above 0.80 with many rating scales of psychopathology.

Validity

Validity is the extent to which an instrument is useful for a specific purpose. An instrument may be generally valid for one purpose but invalid for another.

Content Validity. Content validity refers to the extent to which the items in a scale sample the universe of behaviors of interest. As applied to an arithmetic test, this kind of validity is determined by examining whether the types of arithmetic problems included in the test items are representative of the types of arithmetic problems that the testees are expected to be able to solve.

Concurrent Validity. Concurrent validity refers to the relationship between the test results and some external criterion measure evaluated at roughly the same time. As applied to rating scales, this type of validity often involves demonstrating that groups of patients, differing from each other in some known characteristic external to the rating scale evaluation, are discriminated from each other by the rating scale.

TABLE IV

Some Rating Scales for the Evaluation of Psychiatric Treatment

Method and Rating Scale	Authors	Coverage
I. Self-report questionnaires		
Beck Depression Inventory	Beck, Ward, Mendelson, Mock	Depressive symptoms
Sixteen Personality Factor Questionnaire	Cattell	Personality traits
Personality and Social Network Adjustment Scale	Clark	Social adjustment
Symptom Distress Check List (SCL-90)*	Derogatis, Lipman, Covi	Symptoms
Personal Adjustment and Role Skills (PARS III)†	Ellsworth	Social adjustment
Eysenck Personality Inventory	Eysenck	Personality traits and symptoms
Minnesota Multiphasic Personality Inventory (MMPI)†	Hathaway, McKinley	Symptoms, attitudes, and personality traits
Katz Adjustment Scale-Subject Form (KAS-S)*· †	Katz	Social adjustment and symptoms
Fear Survey Schedule	Lang, Lazovik	Fearsome situations
Profile of Mood States (POMS)	McNair	Symptoms
Zung Self-Rating Depression Scales (SRS)	Zung	Depressive symptoms
II. Informant as data source		
Katz Adjustment Scale-Relative Form (KAS-R)*· †	Katz	Social adjustment and symptoms
Family Evaluation Form (FEF)‡	Spitzer, Gibbon, Endicott	Patient and family psychopathology and effect of patient on family
III. Naturalistic observation		
Manic-State Rating Scale	Beigel	Manic symptoms
Ward Behavior Inventory*	Burdock, Hardesty, Hakerem, Zubin, Beck	Observable evidence of psychopathology
Nursing Patient Behavior Index	Glueck, Rosenberg	Observable psychopathology
Systematic Nursing Observations of Psychopathology*	Hargreaves	Observable psychopathology
Nurses' Observation Scale for Inpatient Evaluation (Nosie-30)	Honigfeld	Observable psychopathology
Psychotic Inpatient Profile*	Lorr, Vestre	Observable psychopathology
Timed Behavioral Checklist for Performance Anxiety	Paul	Behavioral manifestations of anxiety
IV. Interview or other assessment of subject		
Ego Function Scales	Bellak, Hurvich, Gediman	Ego functions
MACC Behavioral Adjustment Scale (Form II)	Ellsworth	Observable evidence of psychopathology
Minnesota-Hartford Personality Assay*	Glueck, Meehl, Schofield, Clyde,	Personality traits and psychopathology
Structured and Scaled Interview to Assess Maladjustment (SIAM)‡	Gurland, Yorkston, Stone, Frank	Social adjustment
Hamilton Anxiety Scale	Hamilton	Anxious symptoms
Hamilton Rating Scale for Depression*	Hamilton	Depressive symptoms
Discharge Readiness Inventory	Hogarty, Prien, Derogatis, Bonato, Oliver	Ward behavior and potential for community adjustment
Social Dysfunction Rating Scale (SDRS)	Linn	Social adjustment
Inpatient Multidimensional Psychiatric Scale (IMPS*)	Lorr, McNair, Klett, Lasky	Psychopathology
Health—Sickness Rating Scale (HSRS)	Luborsky	Global mental health
Brief Psychiatric Rating Scale (BPRS)*	Overall, Gorham	Psychopathology
Phillips Prognostic Scale	Phillips	Premorbid adjustment and some clinical features
Social Disability Scale	Ruesch	Physical impairment and social disability
Mental Status Schedule (MSS)*	Spitzer, Burdock, Hardesty	Psychopathology
Problem Appraisal Scales (PAS)*	Spitzer, Endicott	Psychopathology and social adjustment
Mental Status Examination Record (MSER)*	Spitzer, Endicott	Psychopathology

* Scale reviewed in S. B. Lyerly, *Handbook of Psychiatric Rating Scales,* 1973.
† Selected as one of a core battery of instruments for the evaluation of psychotherapy by a National Institute of Mental Health working conference on psychotherapy outcome measures.
‡ Contains an interview schedule.

TABLE IV—(continued)

Method and Rating Scale	Authors	Coverage
Current and Past Psychopathology Scales (CAPPS)*·†	Spitzer, Endicott	Psychopathology and social adjustment, current and past
Schedule for Affective Disorders and Schizophrenia (SADS)‡	Spitzer, Endicott	Psychopathology and social adjustment, current and past
Psychiatric Status Schedule (PSS)*·†·‡	Spitzer, Endicott, Cohen	Psychopathology and social adjustment
Psychiatric Evaluation Form (PEF)*·‡	Spitzer, Endicott, Cohen, Mesnikoff	Psychopathology and social adjustment
Global Assessment Scale (GAS)	Spitzer, Gibbon, Endicott	Global mental health
Vaillant Prognostic Scale	Vaillant	Premorbid adjustment and some clinical features
Social Adjustment Scale (SAS)‡	Weissman, Paykel	Social adjustment
Present State Examination‡	Wing	Psychopathology
Wittenborn Psychiatric Rating Scales*	Wittenborn	Observable evidence of psychopathology

The ability of an instrument to evaluate change (necessary for evaluating therapy) is a form of concurrent validity, since the notion of change involves a difference in clinical condition at two or more points in time. One can obtain premeasures and postmeasures of patient status and correlate them with other measures of change that are external to the rating scale. One can compare the amount of improvement shown by an experimental group that receives an active treatment with a control group that receives a placebo or no treatment; differences in favor of the experimental group are evidence of the instrument's validity to measure change. One can contrast the scores for a single group of patients on admission, when one expects the disturbance to be at its height, with an evaluation performed at a later follow-up period, when patients usually show less disturbance, regardless of the treatment they receive.

Predictive Validity. Predictive validity refers to the ability of the instrument to predict some criterion measure external to the scale at a later time. The only distinction between predictive validity and concurrent validity is in the time period when the criterion measure is obtained.

Construct Validity. Construct validity involves demonstrating that certain explanatory constructs—such as anxiety, thought disorder, dependence, behavioral, and diagnostic types —account for some portion of the variability of the ratings. To do this, one must make predictions as to what empirical data are likely to be obtained if the explanatory constructs are validly reflected in the test. For example, a rating scale of anxiety is said to have construct validity if, in a variety of situations involving the expectation of possible physical harm or loss of self-esteem, the rating scale yields higher scores than in situations not so characterized.

As applied to the use of rating scales in evaluating treatment, construct validity deals with the question, "In what way have the patients really changed?" Only by examining all the other kinds of validity information can construct validity be determined.

Conclusion

In evaluating psychiatric treatment, one can seldom rely on a single criterion of improvement. Therefore, in evaluating psychiatric treatment, one must usually use several rating scales that employ different methods of collecting the information and that tap different behavioral domains (see Table IV).

REFERENCES

Bellak, L., Hurvich, M., and Gediman, H. K. *Ego Functions in Schizophrenics, Neurotics, and Normals.* Wiley, New York, 1973.

Buros, O. K., editor. *Personality Tests and Reviews.* Gryphon Press, Highland Park, N. J., 1970.

Derogatis, L. R., Lipman, R. S., and Covi, L. SCL-90: An outpatient psychiatric rating scale—preliminary report. Psychopharmacol. Bull., 9: 13, 1973.

Goldberg, L. R. Objective diagnostic tests and measures. Ann. Rev. Psychol. 25: 102, 1974.

Lyerly, S. B. *Handbook of Psychiatric Rating Scales,* ed. 2. National Institute of Mental Health, Bethesda, Md., 1973.

McGlashan, T., editor. *The Documentation of Clinical Psychotropic Drug Trials.* National Institute of Mental Health, Rockville, Md., 1973.

McNair, D. M. *Self-Evaluation of Antidepressants*. Report prepared for American College of Neuropsychopharmacology, Subcommittee of the Task Office on Antidepressants, 1973.

Spitzer, R. L., and Cohen, J. Common errors in quantitative psychiatric research. Int. J. Psychiatry, *6:* 109, 1968.

Spitzer, R. L., and Endicott, J. Computer diagnosis in an automated record keeping system: A study of clinical acceptability. In *Progress in Psychiatric Information Systems: Computer Applications*. J. L. Crawford, D. W. Morgan, and D. T. Giantinco, editors, p. 103. Ballinger Books, Cambridge, 1973.

Spitzer, R. L., and Endicott, J. *Schedule for Affective Disorders and Schizophrenia*. New York State Department of Mental Hygiene, New York, 1973.

Spitzer, R. L., Gibbon, M., and Endicott, J. *Global Assessment Scale*. New York State Department of Mental Hygiene, New York, 1973.

Waskow, I. G., and Parloff, M. B. *Psychotherapy Change Measures: Report on the Clinical Research Branch—NIMH Outcome Measures Project*. National Institute of Mental Health, Rockville, Md., 1974.

Wittenborn, J. R. Reliability, validity, and objectivity of symptom-rating scales. J. Nerv. Ment. Dis., *154:* 79, 1972.

33

Child Psychiatry: Introduction

33.1. HISTORY OF CHILD PSYCHIATRY

Introduction

The origins of a new health service are the obvious and expressed needs of a segment of the population. However, American child psychiatry did not arise from adult psychiatry and the American Psychiatric Association nor from child psychiatry as a distinct profession developed through close association with and nurturance from the professions of social work, psychology, and the social sciences. Also, the child guidance movement was a distinctly American contribution to culture.

Origins of a New Health Service

The recognized pioneer of foremost importance in this field was William Healy, and the place of origin was Chicago in 1909. However, one has to refer to the work of Lightner Witmer in 1905 in Philadelphia. Witmer established a child mental health project or clinic in Philadelphia that was active for a few years and that, in its organizational structure and functions, had some of the features inherent in the child guidance centers or clinics that had their direct lines of origins in the work of Healy.

Healy, who was first in general practice and later an instructor in gynecology, became interested in child health—physical, emotional, and intellectual—through Ethel S. Dummer and her friends, who were concerned with the inadequate care and disposition of delinquent, abandoned, and traumatized children appearing before the judges of the Cook County courts. One of the basic needs in this setting was a more accurate evaluation or diagnosis of the children, some of whom suffered from many serious physical and mental disorders.

After neurological training in Europe and a survey of pertinent children's services in the United States, Healy and his associates established the Institute for Juvenile Research in 1909. The primary functions of the institute as an administratively nonaffiliated adjunct of the court were those of evaluation and diagnosis.

The Institute for Juvenile Research established a unique model for child mental health care, involving not only the physician but also psychologists (mental testers) and volunteer home visitors, the harbingers of trained psychiatric social workers. Professionals and nonprofessionals interested in child care came to the institute to study and observe the methods used there and returned home to start similar institutes in their own communities.

Healy went to Boston in 1917 as the director of the Judge Baker Foundation, later the Judge Baker Guidance Center. It was independent of the Boston Juvenile Court but worked, in the early years, with children referred to the court. In the 1920's and early 1930's, its functions were essentially the same as those carried out in Chicago—namely, evaluation and diagnosis. But Healy also used the consultation method with outside social and health agencies. One or more of Boston's child-serving agencies continued the treatment of the child, with continuing follow-up consultation from the Judge Baker Guidance Center.

In the late 1920's and early 1930's there was a marked change and expansion in the types of behavioral problems accepted for evaluation and treatment by the child guidance centers. The professional personnel of the centers who first dealt with the delinquent child became more and more convinced that the delinquent child was basically an unhappy child or an emotionally disturbed child and that this unhappiness and disturbed condition existed long before the first incidences of antisocial behavior. Therefore, the child showing such prodromal signs should be treated at the center before he became delinquent, with a view to prevention of the delinquent activity. When this concept became widely accepted throughout the centers, nondelinquent children were accepted as patients.

By the middle of the 1950's, few reasonably large cities had not established a child guidance center, and even many small cities had such centers. This growth in child guidance centers and mental health centers for children led to the citation of the obvious need for clarified and adequate standards for the clinical operations of the centers and the need for the adequate academic education and clinical training in child development and child psychopathology of those mental health professionals and paraprofessionals who were offering child mental health care.

Emergence of a New Medical Specialty

American Orthopsychiatric Association

The American Orthopsychiatric Association was established in 1924. The leaders in its establishment were Lawson G. Lowrey, David M. Levy, Karl Menninger, William Healy, and Augusta F. Bronner. The association had at its inception and up to fairly recent times a primary interest in child mental health care. Although the leaders in the early years were, in the main, child psychiatrists, the association membership included psychologists and social workers.

National Committee for Mental Hygiene

From its beginning in the early years of this century, the National Committee for Mental Hygiene was concerned with the promotion of better health care for the mentally disturbed and particularly with the prevention of mental health problems through the early detection and care of children exhibiting the prodromal signs of emotional difficulties. It exerted influence and pressure to help communities establish child guidance centers and offered professional consultation and advice in their planning stages.

Commonwealth Fund

In 1922, the Commonwealth Fund adopted as its project of major concern the betterment of mental health care for adults and children. The fund created fellowships for the training of possible future leaders in this country and abroad. This fellowship program was continued into the 1940's, until the establishment of the National Institute of Mental Health by the Federal government in 1946. The Commonwealth Fund also contributed to the training of child mental health personnel through its establishment and funding of the Child Psychiatric Institute in New York in the 1930's.

American Association of Psychiatric Clinics for Children

The AAPCC was the first voluntary, standard-setting organization for child guidance clinics and their personnel. The AAPCC was founded in 1945. Membership was by clinics, not by persons, and clinics were admitted to membership if they voluntarily agreed to meet and maintain certain standards of excellence in clinic operations. As clinics met these standards, they were, after a review by the committee on membership, approved and admitted. Through review feedback to the clinic directors and their boards of trustees, scores of clinics throughout the country that were hitherto unapproved raised their standards to meet the membership requirements.

In addition, training committees in each of the disciplines of child psychiatry, clinical psychology, and social work were appointed, and each committee worked out the optimal and the minimal training standards that had to be met by a clinic that wished approval as an AAPCC-approved training center.

Through the review work of the training committees, glaring deficiencies in the training of child psychiatrists became apparent. The content of the training programs, the methods of training, and the length of the training period varied from clinic to clinic. There were no fixed training requirements, and there was no official, approving, or accrediting body for this profession. The disciplines of social work and psychology, in contrast, did have national approving and accrediting organizations.

In 1947, the Committee on Training in Child

Psychiatry of the AAPCC established its first approved standards for training. The standards stipulated a minimum of 1 year's training, individual supervision of the trainee, an adequate number of cases seen in diagnosis and treatment, a diversification in age and clinical problem of the trainee's case load, adequate case recording, and readings in the field.

National Institute of Mental Health

Through the National Institute of Mental Health, government funds for faculty salaries and stipends for trainees in all the mental health disciplines became available. Although the NIMH was not itself a standard-setting body, it did insist on excellent training programs in those institutions it funded. Although it never required the child guidance or child psychiatry centers to be approved AAPCC clinics, almost all the clinics receiving training funds did meet the standards of that association.

American Academy of Child Psychiatry

The American Academy of Child Psychiatry was established in 1953, with George E. Gardner as its president. The status of fellow was open only to those who were accredited by the American Board of Psychiatry and Neurology and who had practiced child psychiatry for at least 5 years. However, it became increasingly apparent in the 1960's that the 200 fellows were not representative of the estimated 1,000 men and women in America who were in the active practice of child psychiatry. The membership requirements were changed, and various new classifications were added.

Subspecialty Accreditation

In 1957, the American Board of Psychiatry and Neurology recognized child psychiatry as a subspecialty of psychiatry and established a subspecialty board to proceed with the enactment of policies and standards relative to accreditation and the creation of an examination committee. Hundreds of child psychiatrists have been accredited since that date.

REFERENCES

Curran, F. *The American Association of Psychiatric Clinics for Children—History, Purpose, and Organization.* American Association of Psychiatric Clinics for Children, New York, 1957.
Gardner, G. E. American child psychiatric clinics. Ann. Am. Acad. Pol. Soc. Sci., *286:* 26, 1953.
Gardner, G. E. William Healy, 1869–1963. J. Am. Acad. Child Psychiatry, *11:*1, 1972.
Kanner, L. *Child Psychiatry*, ed. 3. Charles C Thomas, Springfield, Ill., 1971.
Lowrey, L. G., and Sloane, V., editors. *Orthopsychiatry, 1923–1948.* American Orthopsychiatric Association, New York, 1948.

33.2. NORMAL CHILD DEVELOPMENT

Introduction

It is appropriate to distinguish among *growth*, increase in the number and size of cells; *experience*, summation of all previous internal and external stimulation; and *maturation*, altered function resulting from interaction between growth and experience. Maturation, according to the viewpoint adopted here, is not linear but discontinuous. Stages of development follow an age sequence, but stages and ages are not equivalent terms. The sequence of stages is not automatic but depends on both central nervous system growth and life experience; chronological change can proceed while psychological maturation lags. There is some evidence that particularly favorable environmental stimulation can accelerate progression from one stage to another, and there is clear evidence that unfavorable environments can markedly delay some aspects of development. Table I describes the commonly accepted landmarks of behavioral development.

There appear to be lower limits of age for the appearance of each stage, limits determined by central nervous system maturation; thus, no amount of verbal stimulation will lead to speech within the first half year of life. On the other hand, verbal stimulation during this period does play an important role in preparing the ground for the later acquisition of language. What is not known is whether there are upper time bounds for the acquisition of a given cognitive stage—that is, are there critical periods for the development of certain abilities, such that, if the appropriate stimulus conditions are not provided within a given interval. the ability will never appear?

TABLE I*

Landmarks of Normal Behavioral Development

Age	Motor Behavior	Adaptive Behavior	Language	Personal and Social Behavior
Under 4 weeks	Makes alternating crawling movements Moves head laterally when placed in prone position	Responds to sound of rattle and bell Regards moving objects momentarily	Small, throaty, undifferentiated noises	Quits when picked up Impassive face
4 weeks	Tonic neck flex positions predominate Hands fisted Head sags but can hold head erect for a few seconds	Follows moving objects to the midline Shows no interest and drops objects immediately	Beginning vocalization such as cooing, gurgling, and grunting	Regards face and diminishes activity Responds to speech
16 weeks	Symmetrical postures predominate Holds head balanced Head lifted 90 degrees when prone on forearm	Follows a slowly moving object well Arms activate on sight of dangling object	Laughs aloud Sustained cooing and gurgling	Spontaneous social smile Aware of strange situations
28 weeks	Sits steadily, leaning forward on hands Bounces actively when placed in standing position	One-hand approach and grasp of toy Bangs and shakes rattle Transfers toys	Vocalizes "m-m-m" when crying Makes vowel sounds such as "ah"	Takes feet to mouth Pats mirror image
40 weeks	Sits alone with good coordination Creeps Pulls self to standing position	Matches two objects at midline Attempts to imitate scribble	Says "da-da" or equivalent Responds to name or nickname	Responds to social play such as "pat-a-cake" and "peek-a-boo" Feeds self cracker and holds own bottle
52 weeks	Walks with one hand held Stands alone briefly		Uses expressive jargon Gives a toy on request	Cooperates in dressing
15 months	Toddles Creeps up stairs		Says three to five words meaningfully Pats pictures in book Shows shoes on request	Points or vocalizes wants Throws objects in play or refusal
18 months	Walks, seldom falls Hurls ball Walks up stairs with one hand held	Builds a tower of three or four cubes Scribbles spontaneously and imitates a writing stroke	Says 10 words, including own name Identifies one common object on picture card Names ball and carries out two directions—for example, "put on table" and "give to mother"	Feeds self in part, spills Pulls toy on string Carries or hugs a special toy, such as a doll
2 years	Runs well, no falling Kicks large ball Goes up and down stairs alone	Builds a tower of six or seven cubes Aligns cubes, imitating train Imitates vertical and circular strokes	Uses three-word sentences Carries out four simple directions	Puts on simple garment Domestic mimicry Refers to self by name
3 years	Rides tricycle Jumps from bottom steps Alternates feet going up stairs	Builds tower of nine or 10 cubes Imitates a three-cube bridge Copies a circle and a cross	Gives sex and full name Uses plurals Describes what is happening in a picture book	Puts on shoes Unbuttons buttons Feeds self well Understands taking turns

* Table by S. Chesso, M.D.

TABLE I (*continued*)

Age	Motor Behavior	Adaptive Behavior	Language	Personal and Social Behavior
4 years	Walks down stairs, one step per tread Stands on one foot for 4 to 8 seconds	Copies a cross Repeats four digits Counts three objects with correct pointing	Names colors, at least one correctly Understands five prepositional directives: "on," "under," "in," "in back of," or "in front of," and "beside"	Washes and dries own face Plays cooperatively with other children
5 years	Skips using feet alternately Usually has complete sphincter control	Copies a square Draws a recognizable man with a head, body, limbs Counts 10 objects accurately	Names the primary colors Names coins: pennies, nickels, dimes Asks meanings of words	Dresses and undresses Prints a few letters Plays competitive exercise games

Prenatal Factors

Significant experiential factors influence intrauterine development. Movements of the limbs *in utero* are important in maintaining joint mobility. The administration of androgenic hormones in the effort to prevent miscarriage affects sex differentiation in the fetus. Maternal stress, through the production of adrenal hormones, may influence the behavioral characteristics of the newborn. Complications of pregnancy and parturition are precursors of prenatal and paranatal injury to the central nervous system of the infant.

Infant Stage

The survival systems—breathing, sucking, swallowing, and circulatory and temperature homeostasis—are relatively functional at birth. But sensory systems are only incompletely developed; sensory impulses register at thalamic levels with no evidence of specific cortical responses. Further differentiation of neurophysiological functions depends on stimulatory reinforcement.

Stimulus Deprivation

In children with strabismus severe enough that images fall on nonequivalent parts of the two retinas, the image from one eye is suppressed; if left uncorrected to the age of 6 years, there is an irreversible loss of sight in the suppressed eye, amblyopia exanopsia.

Simple passive visual experience is not enough for the acquisition of visual-motor coordination. The development of visual placing responses and the ability to discriminate moving objects from stationary objects are functions of active exercise. The development of intersensory integration is an active, not an automatic, process. The organism begins with its initial given capacities, and these capacities are differentiated and interrelated by exercise so that higher order capabilities emerge.

In the terminology of Piaget, two fundamental processes are at work: assimilation and accommodation. Assimilation is the process of using and incorporating stimulus aliments in the environment, just as the organism uses foods. In assimilation, the organism takes in the new in terms of the familiar and acts in the present as it has in the past. In the process of accommodation, the organism is modified by the demands—that is, the novelties—of the environment. Accommodation leads to a reorganization of the programs of the organism as it struggles to cope more effectively with the mismatch between its available action patterns and the new requirements of its current environment.

Development of the Social Bond

As sensory development progresses, there is for all social organisms a parallel task of fashioning a tie between the newborn and its species. In recent years, much attention has been focused on the concepts of ethology. Ethologists have demonstrated, primarily in birds but also in ungulates, that there is a critical period shortly after birth in which the newborn becomes imprinted on a moving, sound-producing object that from then on serves to elicit following behavior, just as the mother does in the natural situation. Birds imprinted on artificial objects become isolates from the flock and may be unable to mate. For all the undoubted importance of imprinting in certain species, imprinting has not been demonstrated in man or in other primates.

The effects of total social isolation in subhuman species are of great interest in studying the socialization process. Puppies isolated in individual cages for 6 months exhibit a peculiar syndrome characterized by overactivity, distractibility, inadequate response to pain, whirling fits, inferiority to pet-reared and colony-reared dogs in problem solving and in food competition, and inability to be effectively socialized thereafter. Monkeys reared as isolates, even when offered surrogate mothers (objects for clinging), are subsequently unable to adjust to a colony existence and have extraordinary difficulty in learning to mate. When impregnated, isolate-reared females fail to mother their young. The behavioral peculiarities of these isolates were initially attributed to the lack of mothering in infancy, but Harlow's more recent studies have demonstrated that an opportunity for peer interaction between two non-mothered infant monkeys apparently suffices for the development of social behavior.

Harlow traced five affectional systems in the development of the monkey: infant-mother, peer, heterosexual, maternal, and paternal. The infant-mother affectional system is modulated by body contact, clinging, nursing, rocking, warmth, and visual stimulation. It passes through four stages: reflex, attachment, security, and separation. The peer system exhibits successive stages of presocial exploration, interactive play, aggressive play, and developing social status. Heterosexual differentiation includes the passivity pattern and pelvic thrusts of the female; the threat pattern, pelvic thrusts, and clasps of the male; grooming behavior; and full adult sexual behavior. The maternal affectional system develops through stages of attachment and protection, ambivalence, and separation and rejection. The paternal system includes such behaviors as retrieval, protection, and punishment.

Social Deprivation Syndromes

Pediatricians have long known and repeatedly recorded the severe developmental retardation that accompanies maternal rejection and neglect. Infants in institutions characterized by low staff-to-infant ratios and frequent turnover of personnel, even when physical care and freedom from infection are adequate, display marked developmental retardation. The same infants, if placed in adequate foster or adoptive care, undergo a marked acceleration in development. In 1952, on the basis of an extensive review of the literature, Bowlby concluded that early separation had persistent and irreversible effects on personality and intelligence. His stress on the irreversibility of the damage was unfortunate; the early studies confounded the effects of separation and institutionalization with the poor care provided the children once they were removed from the initially depriving situation. The consequences of deprivation vary with the severity and duration of the depriving experience, the age of the child at which the deprivation occurs, and the adequacy of restitutive measures.

Temperamental Differences

But what of the normal newborn in his own family? Is he a smooth slate on which characteristics are engraved with greater or lesser ease? There are strong suggestions of congenital differences. Researchers have demonstrated wide individual differences among infants in autonomic reactivity, differences that persist over the newborn period but whose long-range consequences are not yet known. Other researchers were able to identify nine behavioral dimensions on which reliable ratings can be obtained: activity-passivity, regularity-irregularity, intensity, approach-withdrawal, adaptive-nonadaptive, high-low threshold of response to stimulation, positive-negative mood, high-low selectivity, and high-low distractibility. The ratings on individual children showed substantial correlations between 3 months and 2 years but much lower correlation at 5 years. The researchers were able to discern a relationship between the initial characteristics of the infant, the mode of parental management, and the subsequent appearance of symptoms.

Clinicians are coming to the view that the infant is an important actor in the family drama, one who in part determines its course. The behavior of the infant serves to control the behavior of his mother, just as her behavior modulates his. The calm, smiling, predictable, good infant is a powerful reward for tender maternal care. The jittery, irregular, irritable infant tries a mother's patience; if her capacities for giving are marginal, his traits may cause her to turn away from him and thus complicate his already inadequate beginnings.

Cognitive Development.

At birth, all infants have a repertoire of reflex behaviors—breathing, crying, defecating, head turning toward the stimulated cheek, mouthing of a nipple touching the lips, sucking, and swallowing. Studies have indicated that both vision and hearing are more highly developed in the newborn than they had been thought to be. By 1 to 2 weeks of age, the infant smiles; this response is endogenously determined, as evident by smiling in blind infants. By 2 to 4 weeks of age, visual fixation and visual following are evident. By 4 to 8 weeks, social smiling is elicited by the face or the voice of the caretaker. By 16 to 18 weeks, vocalization or babbling has appeared in the child in a language-rich environment. The persistence and the further evolution of this vocalization depend on rewarding consequences from the human environment. By 18 to 20 weeks, selective social smiling is apparent to familiar faces. This smile has been shaped by the response of adults and is a powerful mechanism for controlling the adults. By 6 to 8 months, the child sits; by 9 to 12 months, he stands; and between 12 and 15 months, he usually walks and speaks his first words.

In contrast to the normative approach taken by Gesell, who views development as the unfolding of a genetically determined sequence, is Piaget's epigenetic theory of intelligence. To Piaget, intelligence is but a special instance of biological adaptation within the context of life, which he views as a continuous creative interaction between the organism and its environment. The outer manifestation of this interaction is coping behavior; the inward reflection is the functional organization of the mental apparatus. Adaptive coping continuously reorganizes the structures of the mind.

Piaget divides the development of intelligence into three major periods: sensorimotor, birth to 2 years; concrete operations, 2 to 12 years; and formal operations, 12 years through adult life. The sensorimotor period is one in which the congenital sensorimotor schemata or reflexes are generalized, related to one another,

and differentiated to become the elementary operations of intelligence. The period of concrete operations is divided into a preconceptual phase, from 2 to 4 years of age, during which symbols are constructed; the intuitive phase of acquiring concepts of space, causality, and time, from 4 to 7; and the phase of concrete operations, in which thought becomes decentered from perception and action—that is, the increasing autonomy of central processes permits the activities of classifying, ordering, and numbering. In the period of formal operations, the logical structures of abstract thought are mastered.

A review of the first few stages of the sensorimotor period may serve to convey Piaget's method of analysis. In its first stage, from birth to 2 months, the exercise of the ready-made reflexes leads to a transition from passive release by stimulation to active groping. Reflex sucking is accompanied by search and discrimination; vision moves from the pupillary reflex response to light to following and active search; prehension moves from the grasp reflex to separate finger movements. The exercise of a function brings inherent satisfaction or what Buhler called function pleasure. This notion of function pleasure is to be distinguished from the widely held concept that the satisfaction of a physiological need is the governing principle of behavior. The varying circumstances of stimulation during this period promote accommodation of the organism to the necessities of the external world; that is, the infant shapes his response to the particularities of the stimulating object—be it finger, nipple, or spoon—and, in so doing, changes himself.

The next stage, primary circular reactions, from 2 to 5 months, is one of reciprocal coordination between the hand and the sucking movements of the mouth, between the hearing and the seeing of a visible and audible object, between the seeing and the grasping of a visible and palpable object. New objects elicit greater interest than overly familiar ones. Recent studies have demonstrated that infants view complex patterns for longer periods than they view simple patterns. As the infant's hands come into his visual field by chance, he stares at them and then begins to move them as he watches them. Something looked at becomes something to grasp, and something grasped becomes something to suck. However, at this stage reality remains subjective—that is, there is no further search for an object that disappears from the visual field. The child has no general space but only a buccal, a kinesthetic, a visual, an auditory space.

The third stage, secondary circular reactions, from 5 to 9 months, is one in which the coordinations of the second stage become dissociated and regrouped in new ways and acquire the independence of learning sets. The rudiments of intentionality appear as the child begins to anticipate the consequences of his own acts. The infant no longer merely uses adventitious circumstances but begins to bring definite actions to bear on these circumstances. Ends, the outcomes sought, are differentiated from the means, his own actions. The infant dandled on his father's knee begins to bounce up and down when the knee stops, as if this were intended to cause the knee to bounce him. Recognition is manifested by outlined or abbreviated acts. Thus, the infant who had enjoyed the movements of a toy brought about by the shaking of his legs briefly shakes his legs when he sees the toy again. It is at this stage that the elementary construction of reality is undertaken. Objects begin to acquire permanence. Before this point, the rest of the world exists for the infant only insofar as it impinges on his sensations or is subject to his actions. Once removed from his immediate presence, objects have no further meaning for him. But now, if an object is dropped in front of him, he looks down to the ground to search for it; that is, he behaves for the first time as though the object had a reality outside of him, although true object permanence is not attained until well into the second year of life. Another important acquisition in this stage is the beginning of imitation.

The remaining stages of the sensorimotor period—coordination of the secondary schemata, the tertiary circular reactions, and the invention of new means through mental combination—cannot here be described, nor can the periods of concrete operations and formal operations. They do, however, repay careful study in Flavell's synthesis of Piaget's many volumes or, better yet, in the originals. Piaget has emphasized throughout the role of intervening experience on the maturation of cognitive functions. It is the richness, complexity, and diversity of stimulation in a favorable environment that result in the accommodation of mental structures to the nuances of reality and in the elaboration of the highest mental functions. Although Piaget's studies have until recently been limited to normal children of favorable circumstances, the framework he has developed is a useful one in cross-cultural and cross-class comparisons. Currently, there are active efforts to develop intelligence tests based on the Piagetan scheme of the epigenetic development of intelligence.

Emotional Development

Parallel to the stages of cognitive development are the stages of emotional development. Despite the conventional practice of separating them, they are clearly interdependent. Indeed, it is the caretaking person who provides the major stimulus to both aspects of mental growth. The human infant is totally dependent on adult caretakers for sheer survival. It is in relation to regular and hence predictable events of caretaking that an affectional tie between infant and caretaker develops; the infant's behavioral repertoire expands as his acts have consequences in the form of social responses from the caretakers.

The Freudian formulation that the tie to the mother develops solely or principally by extension from the nursing act is a far too restricted view. Touch, smell, sight, sound, warmth, kinesthetic stimulation, and the infant's own behavior enter into the complex of care. As perceptual and cognitive maturation occurs, the infant is able to relate these initially disconnected and separate experiences to the person who provides them and is able to distinguish her from other persons in the environment.

The severity of the effects resulting from deprivation of mothering care attests to the central role of mothering—and fathering—in the normal developmental process. However, Erikson's concept that sense of trust—confident expectation that needs will be met—is elaborated primarily from need satisfaction in the first year of life is one-sided and incomplete. The basis for trust in others begins to emerge from good care in infancy, but trust is in no sense a final acquisition of this first year; it must be continuously reinforced during childhood and adolescence if it is to become a prevailing trait. A more accurate formulation would be that the nucleus of trust is established in infancy but that the issue is far from settled. A comparison of the stage theories of Piaget, Freud, and Erikson is presented in Figure 1.

Toddler Stage

Physical and Intellectual Development

The second year of life is marked by acceleration of motor and intellectual development. The ability to walk confers on the toddler a degree of control over his own actions that allows him to determine when to approach and when to withdraw. The acquisition of speech profoundly extends his horizons. Typically, the child learns to say "no" before he learns to say "yes". The negativism of the toddler is a vital stage in individuation.

The second and third years of life are a period of increasing social demands on the child. Toilet training serves as a paradigm of the general training practices of the family—that is, the mother who is overly severe in this area is likely to be punitive and restrictive in others as well. The child's ability to accommodate himself to social demands by the acquisition of self-control can lead to pride in self and zestful striving for a new accomplishment; if he surrenders to parental coercion with shame at his physiological functions and doubt as to his own worth, he emerges inhibited, fearful, and stereotyped; if

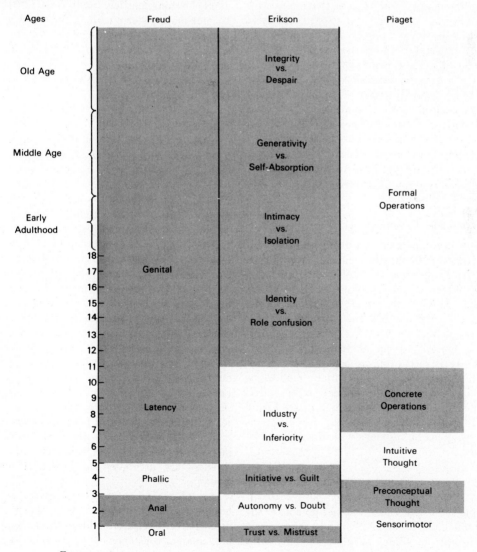

FIGURE 1. A comparison of the stage theories of Freud, Erikson, and Piaget.

he rebels, he may remain stubborn and oppositional.

Parallel to the changing tasks for the child are
changing tasks for his parents. Whereas in
infancy the major responsibility for parents is to
meet the infant's needs in a sensitive and giving
fashion, without so anticipating and so fulfilling
his needs that he never experiences tension, the
parental task at the toddler stage requires
firmness about the boundaries of acceptable
behavior and encouragement of the progressive
emancipation of the child. The child must be
allowed to do for himself insofar as he is able,
but he must be protected and assisted when the
challenges are beyond him.

In the fourth year of life, there is further
augmentation of the youngster's capacities,
which still run well behind his aspirations; he
often undertakes things he cannot complete
successfully. He becomes capable of anticipation as a basis for accepting the postponement
of immediate gratification. There is a flowering
of imagination, as revealed in controlled fantasy
and play, a central psychological activity for
this period. The trial roles assumed in dramatic
play allow the child to try out the adult identities he will one day have to understand and
assume. It is during this era that sexual identity
is firmly established.

Psychosexual Development

The forerunners of sexual differentiation are
evident from birth, when parents dress infants
differently and treat them differently because of
the differential expectations evoked by sex
typing. Through imitation, reward, and coercion, the child assumes the behaviors that his
culture defines for his sexual role. He exhibits
active curiosity about anatomical sex. If this
curiosity is recognized as healthy and is met
with honest and age-appropriate replies, he
acquires a sense of the wonder of life and is
comfortable about his own role in it (see Figure
2). If the subject is taboo and his questions
are rebuffed, he responds with shame and discomfort.

At this stage he is likely to struggle for the
exclusive affection and attention of his parents.
This struggle includes rivalry both with his
siblings and with one or another parent for the
star role in the family. Although he is beginning
to be able to share, he gives up only with

difficulty. If the demands for exclusive possession are not effectively resolved, the result is
likely to be jealous competitiveness in relations
with peers and lovers. The fantasies aroused by
the struggle lead to fear of retaliation and
displacement of fear onto external objects. In an
equitable, loving family, the child elaborates a
moral system of ethical rights freely contracted.
Conscience based on terror, with fear of retaliation for unchecked cupidity, leads to ritualized
and rigid moralism.

School Period

When the child enters kindergarten and elementary school, the formal demands for academic learning, particularly in Western society,
become major determinants of further personality development. So crucial is this task of
developing competence that success or failure in
it molds the child's image of himself as a
capable and adequate person or as an inferior
and feckless one.

Intelligence Measurement

Although the child's intelligence as measured
by I.Q. tests is the single variable that correlates
most highly with academic success, the coefficient of correlation between I.Q. and grades
does not exceed 0.6 to 0.7, thus accounting for
no more than a third to a half of the variance.
Equally salient are motivation, work habits,
creativity, and other traits for which there are
no quantitative measures. The disadvantageous
circumstances associated with urban slum life
depress motivation, measured I.Q., and academic accomplishment. From a third to a half
of children from urban slums are more than 2
years retarded in reading by the sixth grade,
and the gap is even greater by the ninth grade.
These are the youngsters who are likely to drop
out of school and to join the mass of chronically
unemployable adults because of lack of salable
skills. Unfortunately, by a process of circular
reasoning, the poor school performance is commonly explained by the low I.Q., and the
inferior academic accomplishments of slum
dwellers are attributed to biological inadequacy.

One of the most pernicious myths is the
notion of constancy of the I.Q. Although I.Q.
measures on groups of children show remarkable apparent constancy over a period of several

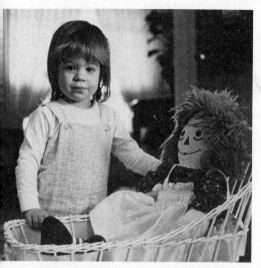

FIGURE 2. The child learns culturally appropriate behavior by identification with the same sex parent. (Courtesy of Nancy Barrett.)

years, the scores for individual children within the group, even of middle-class children, show wide variations. Children who at 5 display the traits associated with achievement motivation—independence, competitiveness, self-initiation—are among those likely to show I.Q. gains, whereas those low on these measures are characterized by declining I.Q. figures.

There is no innate intelligence. Intelligent is as intelligent does, for it is *behavior* that is measured. Intelligent behavior emerges from the interaction between the characteristics of the child and the demands and opportunities of his environment.

Aggressive Behavior

In the normal child, aggression can be effectively understood in terms of the motives—defense, mastery, curiosity—for which aggressiveness is a suitable mediator. Its greater frequency in the abnormal child can be correlated with defects in the organism, as in the case of brain injury, or with distortions in his environment, as in the case of faulty identification models. Moreover, the frequency of the display of aggressive behavior is a function of the culture in which the child is reared. Aggressive fantasy materials—movies, crime comics, and so on—rather than affording catharsis for instinctual aggressiveness, generate the very

tensions they profess to release. It is not the ubiquity of aggression that needs to be accounted for; it is its remarkably wide variation from culture to culture, from time to time in a given culture, and from person to person in a given culture at a given time.

A central issue is the meaning to be ascribed to the term "aggression." If a child is observed taking apart a watch, this behavior can be described as aggressive. In a given instance, it may be—if, for example, the watch belongs to the child's father, and the father has just punished him. On the other hand, if the watch is an old one in his stock of toys, his motive may be curiosity about its mechanism—a belief more readily accepted if his delight as he is able to reassemble it in working order is observed. If he strikes another child, this can be an act of aggression, if the victim is the baby sister his parents have just embraced. Or it may be defensive if the victim has made a threatening gesture or has tried to seize a favorite toy.

Humans are by nature neither aggressive nor peaceful but, rather, are fashioned into one or the other as the result of a complex interaction between a widely modifiable set of biological givens and the shaping influences of the biological environment, the cultural envelope, and individual experience.

The ubiquity of violence in Western society guarantees that children are surfeited with opportunities to learn violent behavior. The child sees that violence pays off; he is provided with adult models of violent behavior with whom to identify (television pales beside real life); violence as an appropriate response to intergroup conflict is sanctioned by national leaders. When violence is sanctioned, it increases predictably.

Adolescence

Adolescence is a period of variable onset and duration, marking the end of childhood and setting the foundation for maturity. Biologically, its onset is signaled by the final acceleration of growth and the beginnings of secondary sexual development, and its termination is marked by epiphyseal fusion and the completion of sexual differentiation. Psychologically, it is marked by an acceleration of cognitive growth and personality formation and is succeeded by the stage of parenthood and the acquisition of an adult work role. Socially, it is a period of intensified preparation for the assumption of an adult role, and its termination is signaled when the person is accorded full adult prerogatives, the timing and nature of which vary widely from society to society. Development at the biological, psychological, and social levels of integration is marked by significant interaction between levels, with events at any one level being able to impede or accelerate development at each of the others.

Biological Factors

Biological factors set wide limits for the onset, termination, and achievements of adolescence. Onset in normal children may occur as early as age 7 or 8 or as late as 17 or 18; termination may be as early as 15 or 16 or as late as 24 or 25. The timing is a function of internal factors, such as sex and inheritance, and of external factors, such as nutrition and medical care.

Social Factors

Adolescence as a social phenomenon, although restricted by biological limits, is a function of cultural norms. The more sophisticated a society is in its technology, the more prolonged is the period of adolescence, since the complexity of the preparation required for adult roles depends on the demands the society sets. In the United States the long period of study required for specialized occupational roles delays the age of self-support, the opportunity for marriage, and the age of creative contribution to society—all attributes of the adult role.

In many cultures the onset of adolescence is clearly signaled by puberty rites, usually in the form of tests of strength and courage. In technologically advanced societies, there is no such clear sign of the end of childhood; moreover, the requirements for adulthood are less sharply defined; the adolescent must undergo a more prolonged and, at times, confused struggle to attain adult status.

Psychological Factors

At a psychological level, the most striking attainment during adolescence is the capacity for abstract conceptualization, which lays the foundations of scientific contribution and of creativity. The adolescent's capacity for abstract thought accounts for his increasing concern with national and international problems and with the basic meanings and values of human existence. This idealism of adolescents is shaped by the cultural envelopes that surround them; but its very existence leads to questioning, to examination of basic premises, and to dissatisfaction with the imperfections of the world as it is. Fostering and strengthening this suprapersonal psychological trait in adolescence leads to the creation of adults who enhance the society that bred them. Denial of opportunity for its positive expression warps development and leads to a generation of self-preoccupied adults.

A related theme of adolescence is the search for a sense of personal identity. No longer a child and not yet an adult, the adolescent engages busily in determining who he is and what he is to become. He examines his parents from a more critical perspective and leans more to peer groups for his sense of belonging. If his relations with his parents have been soundly constructed and if they meet his doubts and criticisms with sympathetic understanding, this temporary unsettling of his prior role leads to a resynthesis of his relations with them on a firm and lasting basis, one marked by reciprocal respect and by personal independence without abandonment of filial loyalty. If the prior parent-child relationship has been one of excessive dependence or excessive hostility, adolescent turmoil may be prolonged and lead either to failure of emancipation or to rejection of family ties and a lasting sense of isolation.

A third major psychological issue is the further evolution of psychosexual role. The development of adult sexual characteristics and the experience of a bewildering array of new physical sensations challenge the psychosexual structures of childhood. The role of hormones is limited to priming the organism for biological maturation and to influencing but not determining the level of libido; the direction, nature, and adequacy of sexual performance are controlled by psychosocial factors.

The ambivalence of Western society toward sexuality—manifested by the conflicts between official attitudes and private behaviors and the pervasive emphasis on sex side by side with sanctions against its expression—contributes to the difficulty, so common in adolescence, of attaining the basis for a sense of competence, freedom, and pleasure as a sexually functioning adult. Adolescents are entitled to full and unambiguous information about the physiology of sex *and* its ethical significance as an intimate relationship between human beings. Ignorance of sex and impoverishment of human relationships account for sexual misadventures. A sense of inadequacy in sexuality not only impairs sexual function but also leads to disabilities in other adult roles.

The search for identity is markedly influenced by peer groups. If these are constructive social groups that provide creative outlets for adolescent energy, the result is a sense of meaningful membership in the community and identification with its goals. But if the peer group is a delinquent gang, with values antagonistic to the larger society, the result is likely to be antisocial personality organization.

The family is an important agent in transmitting the behavior patterns and values expected of the adolescent by society. Distortions in family structure, whether idiosyncratic or socially induced, inevitably have profound effects on individual development. The social consequences of economic disadvantage erode family structure.

The sensitivity of the adolescent to the good opinion of his peers and the dependence of his sense of identity on the attainment of competence in an adult role render him psychologically vulnerable to variations in physiological development, such as precocious or delayed growth, acne, obesity, enlarged mammary glands in boys, and inadequate or overabundant breast development in girls. These deviations from expected patterns of maturation, although they may be without medical significance, can lead to major psychological harm. The adolescent with limited intellectual or physical capacity can develop a persisting and even unchangeable feeling of inferiority if he is forced to compete in situations in which he repeatedly experiences failure.

The characteristic fluidity of psychological structure in adolescence results in the common display of transient symptoms, many of which resemble the psychopathological syndromes of adulthood. Incorrect diagnostic formulations may lead to social consequences that freeze into permanence an otherwise readily correctable deviation in the normal growth pattern. Schizophrenia and manic-depressive psychosis appear at significant rates for the first time in adolescence. However, they remain relatively uncommon disorders and must be discriminated from panic states in a youngster confronted by overwhelming internal and external stimulation.

The psychological basis for a sense of individual worth as an adult rests on the acquisition of competence in a work role during adolescence. A sense of competence is acquired by experiencing success in a socially important task. The sustained motivation necessary for mastering a difficult work role is possible only when there is a real likelihood of fulfilling that role in adult life and of having it respected by others.

After Adolescence

Development continues as long as life continues. As social roles change, as intellectual and physical capacities first advance and later recede, new challenges demand new adaptations. Sensory input helps maintain reality testing and perceptual organization. Social input is necessary for the maintenance of personality organization. Constancies of personality over a lifetime result from the constant reinforcement of personality traits by the social environment in which the person moves. Changes in the social field can lead to profound alterations in personal function.

REFERENCES

Birch, H. G., and Gussow, J. D. *Disadvantaged Children.* Harcourt, Brace & World, New York, 1970.

Eisenberg, L. Student unrest: Sources and consequences. Science, *167:* 1688, 1970.

Eisenberg, L. The human nature of human nature. Science, *176:* 123, 1972.

Flavell, J. H. *The Developmental Psychology of Jean Piaget.* D. Van Nostrand, New York, 1963.

Hamburg, D. A., and Brodie, H. K. H. Psychological research on human aggressiveness. Impact (UNESCO), *23:* 181, 1973.

Jensen, B. Human reciprocity. Am. J. Orthopsychiatry, *43:* 447, 1973.

Lehrman, D. S. The reproductive behavior of ring doves. Sci. Am., *211:* 48, 1964.

Raisman, G., and Field, P. M. Sexual dimorphism in the neurophil of the preoptic area of the rat and its dependence on neonatal androgen. Brain Res., *54:* 1, 1973.

34

Child Psychiatry: Assessment

34.1. PSYCHIATRIC EXAMINATION

Introduction

The psychiatric examination of a child constitutes a set of inquiries into and observations of his behavior, personality, and social relationships. The examination provides the data for an initial evaluation of the presenting clinical problem—its nature and circumstances, who are involved and concerned and their nature, the presumptive causes and determinants of the problem, and the possible avenues of correction and relief. In addition to the mental status that it seeks to elucidate, the examination aims to reveal constitutional givens and pertinent physical findings that may be observed or inferred and to reveal the significant environmental influences interacting with the growing child in the past and in the present.

Role of Parents

Interviews with the parents augment the history and provide information about the child that he may not know or that he may be unable or unwilling to reveal. Parents can provide facts about themselves, the family, and the child's social environment that cannot be obtained from the child. In addition, interviews with parents enable the psychiatrist to make an objective assessment of their psychological and emotional states, their attitudes, relationships, child-rearing practices, and reactions to the child. In most cases, parental attitudes and behavior are no less a part of the problem than the feelings and thoughts of the child himself. Usually, a complicated interplay of parental attitudes, the child's temperament, and fate

best explains his condition. An effective interview with the parents provides serial clues to the origins of the problem and the process of its development. The interview also suggests what further data should be sought from the examination of the child, from outside the family, from psychological tests, and from physical and other special examinations.

Interview Techniques

Parents can be spontaneous and candid if they perceive that their thoughts and feelings are accepted and respected. The interviewer should be alert, sensitive, and responsive to signs of tension that occlude sincere, honest communication.

Tension may also stem from the unfamiliarity of the examining situation. A simple description of the examining procedure and a brief explanation of its purposes are helpful. Often, these purposes become self-evident in the early course of a tactful and expert interview if it has achieved the desired, mutually informative quality of a conversation among a group of people with a common interest.

Other sources of tension may be the memory of prior frustrating experiences in relation to the problem, the circumstances of the referral, the expectation of criticism, feelings of injustice, or fears of the consequences of the examination. Such matters must be aired and worked out.

Because emotionally conflicted material is painful, it is unlikely to be revealed spontaneously as long as the flow of the interview is left entirely up to the parents. Flagrant omissions of obviously relevant topics, repetitious and verbose speech, gratuitously provocative statements, prolonged silences, and extreme passivity—all represent the suppression of disturbing thoughts bearing on the problem or the interview or both. The clinician may elect, by sympathizing with the parents' discomfort about the suppressed material, to bring the material into the discussion. Or he may feel that it is too sensitive and should be stored away until an appropriate occasion for its use arises.

The examiner should express in his own behavior the same good faith he desires from his informants. He should be aware that his own experiences in growing up may unwittingly affect his judgment of parental attitudes and behavior. He should keep in mind that parents of normal children cannot be differentiated, on the basis of consciously stated attitudes, from parents of maladjusted children and that no regular relationship has been demonstrated between specific parental attitudes and adjustment. It is the total constellation of a parent-child interaction that affects the child's development. Also, evidence is accumulating that parent-child interaction has to be assessed not only for parental influences on the child but also for the influence of the child's characteristics on the parents.

Interview Data

The interview must provide the developmental history and its ecology, the emotional climate and the obstetrical facts of the pregnancy and delivery, constitutional and temperamental characteristics, and the medical history. Further, it provides the data on the family and social environment, milestones and stresses in this environment, and their conjunction with the crucial milestones of the developing child. It must provide impressions of the personality and the mental status of each important person in the child's life. A family history, including the personal histories of the parents, the family relationships, the marital history and present marital relationship, a school history, and prior efforts to resolve the current or preceding psychiatric problems of the family should be obtained.

Such a complex potpourri can hardly be expected to be achieved solely by a systematic inquiry into facts, no matter how thorough and extensive. Conversely, the necessary facts will not be obtained by an unstructured, nondirective, evocative, psychodynamically oriented approach alone. The orderly accumulation and organization of significant facts need not pre-clude spontaneity, compassionate attention to suffering, and education about the purposes of the procedure.

Family group interviews may be helpful in clarifying areas of disagreement on salient points of the presenting problem. Separate interviews with each of the parents may facilitate any or many of the goals of the examination. Under special circumstances of broken homes, neglect, physical or mental illness, or institutionalization, adults other than the child's parents are of primary importance to the examination and the assessment.

Simmons suggests the following outline for interviewing parents:

1. Child's history
   a. Parents' main concerns about the child (chief complaint or presenting problem)
   b. Course of symptoms and current adjustment
   c. Past developmental, medical, social, and psychological history, including peer and school adjustments
   d. Child's relationships with siblings and each parent
2. Parents' marital history
3. Parents' personal history
   a. Parents' primary family, past and present
   b. School and vocational adjustment
   c. Social and avocational interests and activities
   d. Review of any specific medical or psychological problems suffered by either parent
4. Other family problems (other children, previous marriages, in-laws, neighbors, and so on)
5. Parents' opinions about possible causes and a review of their feelings about various treatments that may be proposed

Chess offers a practical and useful history guide (see Table I).

Examination

Physical Examination

To carry out an effective psychiatric examination of a child, the clinician has to have a good working knowledge of normal child development.

When possible, the pediatrician or family doctor—one with whom the child psychiatrist has easy, effective communication and rap-

TABLE I

History Guide

Date:

Referral:

Name: Sex: Date of birth:

Address:

Father's name: Mother's name:

Occupation: Occupation:

Sibs: Sex: Age: Grade:

Informants:

Presenting problems:

BIRTH AND INFANCY:

Parents' ages when child was born:

Planned baby: Problems of conception?

History of pregnancy, labor, and delivery:

Birth weight and neonatal history:

Feeding history:

Daily care of the baby given by:

DEVELOPMENTAL MILESTONES (AGES OF):

Sitting: Standing: Walking:

First word: First phrase or sentence:

Toilet training: Time of initiation, mode of proce-
                   dure:

TEMPERAMENT IN INFANCY:

TEMPERAMENT AT LATER STAGES:

HEALTH:

Operations:

Childhood diseases:

Other illnesses:

Accidents:

SCHOOL HISTORY:

Nursery:

Kindergarten:

First grade:

Present:

INTERPERSONAL RELATIONSHIPS:

ADDITIONAL FACTORS OF IMPORTANCE:

FURTHER DEVELOPMENT OF BEHAVIOR
  PROBLEMS:

IMPRESSION OF PARENTS:

---

port—should be responsible for the general medical care of the patient. Usually, the patient's medical status has been determined and is available to the examiner. The child psychiatrist must decide whether further studies are indicated. This decision may be of importance if the referring physician has been provoked unwittingly by the behavior of the child or the parents into overemphasizing emotional factors to the relative neglect of somatic disorders. However, a routine physical examination merely to rule out organic disease is not indicated.

Adequate medical studies involve much more than the detection or elimination of organic disease; they are crucial—along with studies of the patient's perception, cognitive status, and motor coordination—in determining the relative importance of genetic or acquired deficits and derangements in the development of psychiatric problems.

Careful observation of the child in his activities, with special emphasis on neurophysiological patterns, is more significant diagnostically than a formal neurological examination, which may reveal no discernible derangement. The history should have brought to light any event suggesting the possibility of brain damage. Early or late physical maturation may be a factor contributing to stress. The question of drug use for existing psychological disturbances or physical illness should not be neglected.

If physical studies are indicated, the examiner should help parents prepare the child and should himself help the child to understand the basis for them. It is often wise to postpone a physical examination until after at least one interview with the parents and after having a chance to discuss the procedure with the child.

Psychological Examination

Psychological testing need not be routine. However, it is a valuable aid in revealing inner states otherwise obscured by defenses or by inhibitions in communication. When time for the assessment is limited, tests may indicate limitations of ego functions. Testing is particularly indicated when there are questions involving learning difficulties, mental retardation, the possibility of brain damage, or the possibility of a severe disturbance of thinking.

Interview and Direct Observation

Before he examines the child, the child psychiatrist ordinarily has had ample briefing on the problem and on what the child is like to have formed a tentative working hypothesis. Even so, he should be prepared for occasional surprises.

It is the clinician's task to provide an emotional setting within which he and the child may interact so that the child can express directly or by implication what he is concerned about and what kind of a person he is. The examiner tries to facilitate the child's relationship to him, at the same time leaving leeway for the patient to bear only what stress he is ready and able to bear. The child's behavior in the interview is observed, appraised, and evaluated in the light of the history and the social milieu. The manner of the interview depends on the child's age. An adolescent may seek help himself and be the principal informant, especially if he is attempting to be independent of his parents.

Advice to parents on how to inform the child and prepare him for the interview ought to be given whenever necessary. The child's age, the nature and the severity of his problem, and his relationship with his parents greatly affect this advice. It is helpful if the appointment is related to a problem the child would like to overcome. Parents should explain that they have sought the psychiatrist's advice on how best to help the child and themselves.

Maximum advantage should be taken of the opportunity provided to observe the child's behavior in the waiting room and his ability to separate from his parents. A child with severe separation problems may have to be examined with a parent in the room. The results of an examination carried out under such circumstances are never fully satisfactory when there is not enough time to enable the child to tolerate being alone with the examiner. It is better to proceed as with a family group interview than to try to ignore the presence of the parent. Severe separation anxiety should be addressed sympathetically as an aspect of the problem for which help is sought and not as an obstacle to proper examination.

The child should not be expected to sit quietly in a chair throughout the interview. Aside from being inconsistent with the nature of childhood, it constricts the range of behavioral observations. A conversational approach should be attempted with all children who are old enough. Along with the presumptive task of the moment, the examiner should remember such niceties as pointing out the bathroom, explaining the unfamiliar setting, referring to the consequences of the disruption of the child's regular routine, and so forth.

Whether in play or in conversation, the child should be allowed and encouraged to take the initiative. It is important, especially at the outset, for the child to perceive the psychiatrist as a responsive human being. It is virtually useless to push diagnostic questions at a child who is unready or unable to lower his guard.

In the first interview and as long as the stresses dominate the atmosphere, it is a good rule to limit one's efforts to change behavior to the interview itself and to refrain from interpretations or suggestions that refer to the child's problem in his outside or real life.

Limit Setting. If the examiner succeeds in making the examination reasonable to the child—that is, no more threatening than the patient can tolerate—the child will be able to recognize, acknowledge, and communicate within limits of behavior that facilitate the investigative goals. Limits tend to take care of themselves when the examiner is involved in the child's spontaneous play or conversation as a sensitive participant and an auxiliary ego, compensating for such deficits as may reside in the child's own regulatory apparatus by virtue of his immaturity or pathology. Limits are important to avoid mobilizing excessive anxiety and guilt feelings. At the outset, therefore, direct but compassionate restraint of destructive or regressive behavior may be unavoidable.

Confidentiality. Some degree of mistrust and communication breakdown is inherent in psychopathology. Any child who needs to be examined has to be assumed to have secrets he is afraid to have his parents know. The psychiatrist needs to make the child feel that the danger of trusting other adults does not exist with him. A long step forward can be taken, even in the initial interview, if the examiner undertakes to inform the child what communications with his parents are indicated. Absolute confidentiality is unrealistic with young children, but a relationship of reasonable trust can be achieved without it.

Play. Children express themselves in action when words fail them. Comprehension of the action language of children expressed in play and other motor activity is the goal of the diagnostic examination. The psychiatrist has to note its content, form, and associated affect. Through play, the child attempts to regulate the stimuli affecting him. The play of a child with personality problems is directed toward these problems and contains both expressive and defensive reflections.

The examining room should be open enough

to allow for the physical activity required to reduce tension but not so large as to attenuate a reasonably intimate contact between the examiner and the patient. Toys and materials should be available to suit children of different ages, sexes, and interests. The room should be furnished and arranged so that toys and materials inappropriate for a particular child can be removed from view. Too great a choice may be overstimulating or distracting; too little may fail to accommodate important fantasies or concerns.

Mental Status. With an admixture of reassurance, sympathy, acceptance, listening, careful observation, tactful suggestions, and questions appropriate to the age, temperament, and prior emotional set of the patient, the examiner should be able, in one or more sessions, to learn how his patient's mind is functioning. The mental functions thus revealed constitute the mental status of the child. The psychopathology of the child is included within his mental status, but it is by no means identical to it. If the examiner attributes symptomatic significance to everything a child says and does, he not only risks confusion but may fail to appreciate healthy elements in the personality of his patient, their roles in his over-all adaptation, and the nature and function of his defenses.

From the child's appearance, his relationship to the examiner, his physical activity, and his facial expressions; from the interests, relationships, moods, thoughts, and fantasies that he reveals in spontaneous play and speech; from his responses to suggestions and questions, his defensiveness, and what he avoids—from all this, a behavioral profile of the child is gleaned. This profile includes signs in (1) the sensorimotor, (2) the perceptual, (3) the affective, (4) the intellectual-cognitive, (5) the interpersonal, (6) the ideational, and (7) the social spheres. These signs are the indicators of the mental status.

Diagnosis and Assessment

Diagnosis, which is a classificatory concept, is not synonymous with assessment, which has broader, more individualized, and more clinically useful connotations.

A number of classifications have been advanced, most notably by the American Psychi-

atric Association and the Group for the Advancement of Psychiatry. Descriptive classification is difficult in child psychiatry because the patient, whether disturbed or not, is in a growing, developing, constantly and rapidly changing state.

Mental functions are normally fluid. In pathological states, multiple causation is the rule. Different factors may cause similar symptom pictures; various behaviors may be the result of similar or even identical agencies. The direct relation of organic disturbances to specific symptoms is often uncertain. The problem of determining a primary cause has little meaning for the clinician in child psychiatry. At the same time, his understanding of the relation of mental function derangement to the clinical problem is essential to the planning of treatment.

In general, the younger the child, the more severe the effect of psychological traumata, and the greater the duration of the trauma, the more severe is the effect. Yet genetic constitutional, and social variables affect the reliability of this generalization.

The examiner can derive a clinical assessment from his various data by integrating them into a genetic dynamic formulation based on the accumulated body of theory and facts about disordered personality development during childhood. This formulation complements the diagnosis and individualizes it in behalf of a treatment plan by pointing out where change is required to ameliorate distress and to reduce pathogenicity.

The assessment must be understood by the parents and, to the extent appropriate to his development, by the child himself. The examiner should be able to communicate his opinion of what is wrong in such a way that his recommendations for intervention make sense.

REFERENCES

Chess, S. *An Introduction to Child Psychiatry*. ed. 2. Grune & Stratton, New York, 1969.
Goodman, J. D., and Sours, J. A. *The Child Mental Status Examination*. Basic Books, New York, 1967.
Group for the Advancement of Psychiatry. *The Diagnostic Process in Child Psychiatry*. Report No. 38. Group for the Advancement of Psychiatry, New York, 1957.
McDonald, M. The psychiatric evaluation of children. J. Child Psychiatry, 4: 569, 1965.
Simmons, J. E. *The Examination of Children*. Lea and Febiger, Philadelphia, 1969.

34.2. PSYCHOLOGICAL TESTING

Test Evaluation

Reliability

Test reliability refers essentially to the consistency of scores obtained by the same person. The principal procedures for computing test reliability include retest, parallel form, split-half, and Kuder-Richardson techniques. Retest reliability is the correlation between scores on the identical test administered at different times. When different forms of a test are administered on the two occasions, the correlation between them represents parallel-form reliability. Differences attributable to item sampling only are measured by split-half reliability. The usual way to compute split-half reliability is to find each person's score on the odd-numbered items and on the even-numbered items. Like split-half reliability, Kuder-Richardson reliability is derived from a single test session. Ultimately based on interitem consistency, it is also influenced by homogeneity of test content. In a test consisting of 50 vocabulary and 50 arithmetic items, the Kuder-Richardson reliability is lower than in a test composed of 100 items of either type alone.

Most tests provide such highly standardized procedures for administration and scoring as to leave little room for examiner variance, particularly in group tests designed for mass administration and machine scoring. But in most infant and preschool tests and in other individual instruments for clinical testing, there is more opportunity for the examiner's judgment to operate. Certain types of tests, such as projective personality tests, present special problems of scorer reliability. Whenever qualitative judgment is required in scoring, a sample of papers should be independently rescored by another examiner and the degree of agreement determined (see Table I).

Reliability is directly related to test length. An abbreviated form of a test can be expected to show some loss in reliability. Similarly, subtests or parts of a test have lower reliability than the complete test. Also, single-trial reliability coefficients found by odd-even or Kuder-Richardson techniques are inapplicable to speeded tests.

The standard error of measurement indicates the range of fluctuation to be expected in a person's score at a specified confidence level. Similarly, it permits an estimate of the score interval within which the examinee's true score, free from error variance, is likely to fall.

Validity

The most important property of a test is undoubtedly its validity. The concept of validity concerns the relationships of a test to other data about the person. An analysis of such relationships makes it possible to state what the test measures and how well it does so.

Content validity concerns primarily the adequacy with which the test items sample the content area to be measured. An achievement test, for example, may be checked against relevant course syllabi, textbooks, and the judgment of subject matter specialists.

In criterion-related validity, test scores are correlated or otherwise compared with an outside criterion. A test of emotional instability may be validated by administering it to persons known to have exhibited neurotic behavior as well as to a normal control group.

Construct validity is concerned primarily with an experimental verification of hypotheses regarding the psychological traits or theoretical constructs that account for performance on the test. If, a test is designed to detect anxiety, it could be administrered to children before and after an anxiety-provoking experience.

Norms

A raw score on any psychological test is meaningless until interpreted by comparison with the scores obtained by other persons. In the process of standardizing a test, one administers it to a large, representative sample of the population for which it is designed. The scores obtained by this group provide the test norms. A person's position in relation to the norms may be expressed in ratio I.Q.s, percentile ranks, and standard scores.

The traditional intelligence quotient, or ratio I.Q., is found by dividing a child's mental age by his chronological age. Theoretically, mental age represents the age of normal children whose test performance the child equals. If a 10-year-old does as well on a test as the average

12-year-old, his mental age is 12. Dividing this child's mental age (M.A. = 12) by his chronological age (C.A. = 10) and multiplying by 100 to avoid decimals yields an I.Q. of 120.

The percentile rank indicates the percentage of cases in the normative sample falling at or below the subject's score. Although percentile ranks correctly indicate the relative position of

TABLE I

Psychological Tests

Title	Major Category*	Author(s)	Publisher	Date(s)	Age or Grade Range	MMY†
Bayley Scales of Infant Development	C & P	N. Bayley	Psychological Corporation, New York	1969	2 mos.–2½ yrs.	7, 402
California Psychological Inventory (CPI)	P	H. G. Gough	Consulting Psychologists Press, Palo Alto, Calif.	1956–1969	13 yrs. and over	7, 49
Children's Apperception Test (CAT)	P	L. Bellak and S. Bellak	C. P. S. Co., Larchmont, N. Y.	1949–1965	3–10 yrs.	6, 206; P 419
Children's Personality Questionnaire	P	R. B. Porter and R. B. Cattell	Institute for Personality and Ability Testing, Champaign, Ill.	1959–1968	8–12 yrs.	6, 122; P 38
Columbia Mental Maturity Scale	C	B. B. Burgomeister and L. H. Blum	Harcourt, Brace Jovanovich, New York	1954–1972	3½–10 yrs.	X (6, 517)
Differential Aptitude Tests (DAT)	C	G. K. Bennett, H. G. Seashore, and A. G. Wesman	Psychological Corporation, New York	1947–1973	Grades 8–12	X (7, 673)
Early School Personality Questionnaire	P	R. W. Coan and R. B. Cattell	Institute for Personality and Ability Testing, Champaign, Ill.	1966–1970	6–8 yrs.	7, 171
Holtzman Inkblot Technique	P	W. H. Holtzman	Psychological Corporation, New York	1958–1966	5 yrs. and over	7, 169
Jr-Sr. High School Personality Questionnaire	P	R. B. Cattell, R. W. Coan, and H. Beloff	Bobbs-Merrill, Indianapolis	1953–1969	12–18 yrs.	7, 97
McCarthy Scales of Children's Abilities	C	D. McCarthy	Psychological Corporation, New York	1972	2½–8½ yrs.	X
Metropolitan Readiness Tests	C	G. H. Hildreth, N. L. Griffiths, and M. E. McGauvran	Harcourt, Brace Jovanovich, New York	1933–1969	Kindergarten and grade 1	7, 757
Rorschach	P	H. Rorschach	Hans Huber (U. S. distributor: Grune & Stratton, New York)	1921–1966	Ames *et al.,* norms, 2–16 yrs.	7, 175
Rosenzweig Picture-Frustration Study: Form for Children (P-F)	P	S. Rosenzweig	S. Rosenzweig, St. Louis, Mo.	1948–1960	4–13 yrs.	6, 238; P 471
Rotter Incomplete Sentences Blank (RISB)	P	J. B. Rotter	Psychological Corporation, New York	1950	Grades 9–12, 13–16 and adult	4, 130; P 472
Sequential Tests of Educational Progress (STEP)	C	Cooperative Test Division, Educational Testing Service	Educational Testing Service, Princeton, N. J.	1956–1969	Grades 4–14, in 4 levels	X (6, 25)
Stanford Achievement Test	C	R. Madden, E. F. Gardner, H. C. Rudman, B. Karlsen, and J. C. Merwin	Harcourt, Brace Jovanovich, New York	1923–1973	Grades 1½–9½ in 6 levels (also batteries K–1 and H. S.)	(7, 25)
Stanford-Binet Intelligence Scale	C	L. M. Terman and M. A. Merrill	Houghton Mifflin, Boston	1916–1973	2 yrs. and over	(7, 425)
STS Junior Inventory	P	H. H. Remmers and R. H. Bauernfeind	Scholastic Testing Service, Bensenville, Ill.	1957–1968	Grades 4–8	P 232A

* Test designed to measure primarily cognitive (C) or personality (P) traits.

† Volume and entry number in *Mental Measurements Yearbook* where latest information and critical reviews of the test can be located, including references to earlier reviews. Letter P preceding reference number indicates that latest information is in *Personality Tests and Reviews* (Buros, 1970); X signifies test is too recent for inclusion in MMY; citation in parentheses following X refers to review of earlier edition of test.

Table I—(*continued*)

Title	Major Cate-gory*	Author(s)	Publisher	(Date(s))	Age or Grade Range	MMY†
STS Youth Inventory	P	H. H. Remmers and B. Shimberg	Scholastic Testing Service, Bensenville, Ill.	1956–1971	Grades 7–12	P 233
Thematic Appercep-tion Test (TAT)	P	H. A. Murray	Harvard University Press, Cambridge, Mass.	1935–1943	4 yrs. and over	7, 181
Torrance Tests of Creative Thinking	C	E. P. Torrance	Personnel Press, Prince-ton, N. J.	1966	Kindergarten to adult	7, 448
Washington Univer-sity Sentence Com-pletion Test (WUSCT)	P	J. Loevinger, R. Wessler, and C. Redmore	Jossey-Bass, San Fran-cisco	1962–1970	12 yrs. and over	7, 182
Wechsler Intelligence Scale for Children Revised (WISC-R)	C	D. Wechsler	Psychological Corporation, New York	1949–1974	6-0 to 16-11 yrs.	7, 431
Wechsler Preschool and Primary Scale of Intelligence (WPPSI)	C	D. Wechsler	Psychological Corporation, New York	1967	4–6½ yrs.	7, 434

different persons, they do not accurately reflect differences in the amount of a trait.

The most precise measure is provided by standard scores and their various derivatives. In all such scores, the person's distance from the mean is expressed in standard deviation units (σ). If the normative sample has a mean of 38 and a standard deviation of 4, a raw score of 34 would correspond to a standard score of -1.00.

In addition to norm-referenced tests, an alternative interpretive model known as criterion-referenced testing is attracting increasing interest. Criterion-referenced scores use as their frame of reference a clearly defined content domain, rather than a specified population of persons. An examinee's raw score on a test, for example, may be interpreted in terms of the specific kinds of arithmetic operations he has mastered.

Test Administration

Standardized Procedure

The need for uniformity applies to such obvious factors as time limits and wording of directions and to more subtle conditions, such as the rate at which the examiner speaks, where he places emphasis, when he pauses in his presentation, his facial expression while pronouncing key words that may reveal the correct answer, and the position of materials to be used by the subject.

Any unusual condition of the subject—such as illness, fatigue, or excessive worry—may affect test scores adversely. Even the nature of the subject's activities immediately preceding a test must be taken into account.

Emotional and Motivational Factors

Among the emotional and motivational conditions found to affect test performance are praise, reproof, ridicule, knowledge of results, presence of observers, competition and rivalry, and various conditions evoking feelings of frustration, failure, and discouragement. With preschool children, experience with adults outside the immediate family is likely to affect performance on individually administered intelligence tests. There is evidence that children vary widely and consistently in their susceptibility to anxiety while taking tests and that high degrees of anxiety have a deleterious effect on test performance.

Movtivational factors may be especially influential in the test performance of preschool children, emotionally maladjusted children, ethnic minorities, and members of lower socioeconomic classes. Juvenile delinquents may approach tests with unfavorable attitudes, such as suspiciousness, insecurity, fear, or cynical indifference. Because of early failure and frustration experienced in school work, some children may have developed feelings of hostility and inferiority toward any academic task, which most intelligence tests resemble.

Rapport

The establishment of rapport is a process for arousing interest and eliciting cooperation from the subject so that the objectives of the test will be most fully attained. In tests of preschool children, special factors to be considered include shyness with strangers, distractibility, and negativism. A friendly, cheerful, and relaxed manner on the part of the examiner helps to reassure the child. The shy, timid child may need more time to become familiar with his surroundings before testing is begun. Test sessions should be brief and the tasks should be varied and intrinsically interesting to the child. The testing should be presented as a game and the child's curiosity aroused before each new task if introduced.

In tests of children in the primary grades, the game appeal is still the most effective way of arousing interest in the test. The older school child, on the other hand, can usually be motivated by an appeal to his competitive spirit and his desire to do well on all kinds of tests. However, every test presents an implied threat to the person's prestige. Some reasssurance is needed at the outset. The examiner should explain, for example, that no one is expected to finish or get all items right.

Examiner and Situational Variables

Test performance, particularly on individually administered intelligence tests and on projective tests, is significantly affected by examiner and situational variables. Such extraneous variables are more likely to operate with unstructured and ambiguous stimuli and with difficult and unfamiliar tasks than with clearly defined and well-learned functions. In general, children are more susceptible to examiner and situational influences than are adults.

Among the significant examiner variables are age, sex, professional and social status, appearance, and such behavioral characteristics as self-confidence, aggressiveness, responsiveness, and social warmth. Situational variables are illustrated by the place where the test is given (school, clinic, hospital, prison, psychology laboratory), the expectations and attitudes established by the way the forthcoming test is presented to the subject, and the nature of specific instructions.

Practice, Coaching, and Test Sophistication

Scores on intelligence tests can be appreciably improved by practice and coaching. The effects differ widely with the nature of the test and with the age, ability, and previous experience of the subjects. General test sophistication must also be considered in interpreting test performance. The child who has had extensive test-taking experience usually scores higher than the one who is taking his first test.

Intelligence Tests

Testing the School Child

Intelligence tests measure primarily those abilities essential for academic achievement. They are often more accurately described as tests of scholastic aptitude.

Typically, intelligence tests provide a global score purporting to indicate the person's general intellectual level. In actual practice, however, intelligence tests are overweighted with certain functions, usually verbal aptitudes, and may completely omit others.

In America, the most notable adaptation of the original Binet-Simon scale is the Stanford-Binet. Extending from the 2-year level to three superior-adult levels of increasing difficulty, the test yields a mental age and a deviation I.Q. Objects, pictures, and drawings are used largely at the younger ages (see Figure 1); printed verbal and numerical materials occur increasingly at the older age levels. Oral questions and answers are common throughout the scale.

Another individual test commonly used in the clinical examination of children is the Wechsler Intelligence Scale for Children Revised (WISC-R). This scale provides separate verbal and performance I.Q.'s based on different sets of tests, as well as a full-scale I.Q.

Both the Stanford-Binet and the WISC-R are individual tests, which must be administered to each subject singly and which require a highly trained examiner. Group tests are designed for rapid mass testing. They enable a single examiner to test a large group during one session and are relatively easy to administer and score. They are useful when a crude index of intellectual level suffices or when facilities for more intensive testing are unavailable.

An example of a nonlanguage test is the Columbia Mental Maturity Scale. Originally developed for use with cerebral palsied children, this scale uses a set of cards, each containing from three to five large drawings. The child identifies the drawing that does not belong with

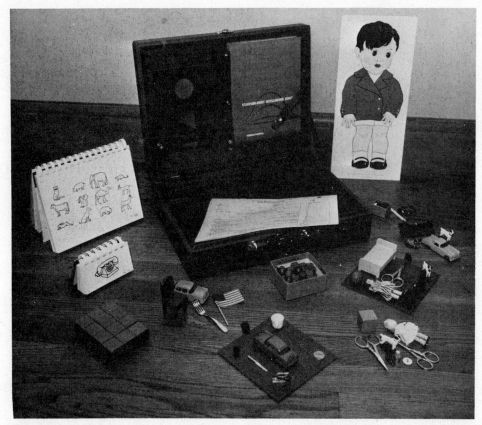

FIGURE 1. Test materials used in administering the Stanford-Binet. (Courtesy of the Houghton Mifflin Co.)

the others, indicating his choice by pointing or nodding.

Preschool and Infant Testing

Tests applicable before school entrance are subdivided into infant tests, designed for the first 18 months of life, and preschool tests, covering the ages of 18 to 60 months. The infant must be tested while lying down or supported on someone's lap. Speech is of little or no use in giving test instructions, although the child's own speech development provides relevant data. Many of the tests at this level are actually controlled observations of sensorimotor development. At the preschool level, the child can walk, sit at a table, use his hands in manipulating test objects, and communicate by language. The child is also much more responsive to the examiner as a person.

In the Gesell Developmental Schedules, data are obtained through direct observation of the infant's responses to standard toys and other stimulus objects, supplemented by information provided by the mother. The Bayley Scales of Infant Development (see Figure 2), covering the period from 2 months to 2½ years, include a mental scale, a motor scale, and an infant behavior record. Both the mental and motor scales yield a developmental index, expressed as a standard score within the child's own age level. The infant behavior record is a rating scale designed to assess various aspects of social and emotional behavior.

At the preschool level, the McCarthy Scales of Children's Abilities, suitable for children from 2½ to 8½ years of age, yield separate standard scores in verbal, perceptual-performance, quantitative, memory, and motor scales as well as a general cognitive index. The Wechsler Preschool and Primary Scale of Intelligence (WPPSI) is designed for ages 4 to 6½. In both content and form, it follows closely the

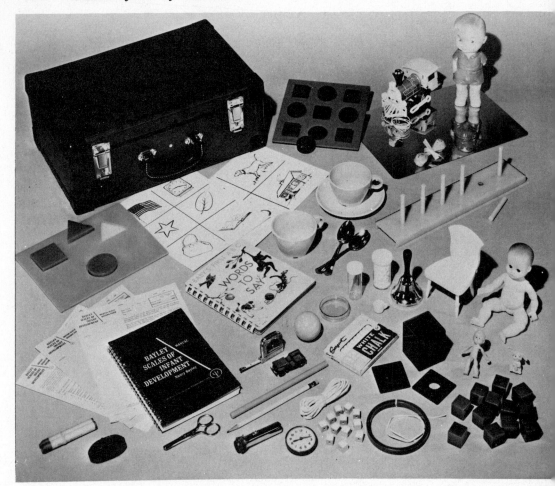

FIGURE 2. Test objects used with the Bayley Scales of Infant Development. (Courtesy of The Psychological Corporation.)

pattern of the earlier Wechsler scales, yielding verbal, performance, and full-scale deviation I.Q.'s.

Long-Term Prediction

Theoretically, if a child maintains the same status relative to his age norm, his I.Q. remains the same at all ages. The I.Q. has, in fact, proved to be fairly constant for most children. But scores on infant tests are virtually useless in predicting intellectual level in late childhood. Infant tests find their chief usefulness in the early detection of severe retardation resulting from organic causes.

Even in later childhood the I.Q. cannot be regarded as rigidly fixed. A major reason for the usual stability of the I.Q. is that most children remain in the same type of environment throughout their development. Another reason is that their previous experiences determine their level of attainment in prerequisite intellectual skills needed for subsequent learning. An early deficiency becomes cumulative unless corrected by special remedial programs.

Large shifts in I.Q. are usually associated with the cultural milieu and emotional climate of the home. Children in disadvantaged environments tend to lose with age and those in superior environments tend to gain. Changes in I.Q. are also related to certain personality characteristics of the child, such as emotional independence and achievement motivation.

Aptitude Tests

Since most intelligence tests concentrate on the more abstract verbal and numerical abilities, a need was felt for tests measuring the more concrete and practical intellectual skills. Mechanical aptitudes were among the first for which special tests were developed. Tests of clerical aptitude, measuring chiefly perceptual speed and accuracy, and tests of musical and artistic aptitudes followed.

Multiple aptitude batteries provide a profile of scores on separate tests. The Differential Aptitude Tests (DAT) yield scores in eight abilities: verbal reasoning, numerical ability, abstract reasoning, clerical speed and accuracy, mechanical reasoning, space relations, spelling, and language usage. Multiple aptitude batteries are most useful in the testing of older children and adolescents. One of their chief applications has been in educational and vocational counseling.

Education Tests

Readiness Tests

Educational readiness tests are designed to assess the child's specific qualifications for schoolwork. Essentially, readiness refers to the development of prerequisite skills and knowledge that enable the learner to profit maximally from a certain kind of instruction.

Special emphasis is placed on those abilities found to be most important in learning to read; some attention is also given to the prerequisites of numerical thinking and to the sensorimotor control required in learning to write. Among the specific functions covered are visual and auditory discrimination, motor control, verbal comprehension, vocabulary, quantitative concepts, and general information. A well known example is the Metropolitan Readiness Tests.

Tests of Special Educational Disabilities

Reading tests are customarily classified as survey and diagnostic tests. Survey tests indicate the general level of the child's achievement in reading. They usually provide a single score, although some differentiate between speed of reading and comprehension. These tests serve largely to screen children in need of remedial instruction. Diagnostic tests are designed to analyze the child's performance and to identify specific sources of difficulty. All such tests yield more than one score, and some include detailed checklists of specific types of errors. The examiner also needs information about possible emotional difficulties and a complete case history.

Educational Achievement Batteries

Achievement tests aim to measure the effects of a course of study. Some are comprehensive achievement batteries, designed to assess the pupil's over-all progress in schoolwork; others test for mastery of specific subjects or courses. Some achievement tests measure the attainment of relatively broad educational goals cutting across subject matter specialties.

An outstanding example of comprehensive achievement batteries is the Sequential Tests of Educational Progress (STEP). These tests are available at several levels, extending from the fourth grade of elementary school to the sophomore year of college. At each level, there are seven multiple-choice tests: English expression, reading, mechanics of writing, mathematics computation, mathematics basic concepts, science, and social studies. Major emphasis is placed on the application of learned skills to the solution of new problems.

Somewhat more emphasis on factual content and specific educational skills is to be found in the Stanford Achievement Test (SAT). Extending from the first through the ninth grade, with additional batteries for kindergarten-first grade and high school levels, the SAT provides a somewhat different set of subtests at different grade levels. A typical set includes 11 subtests, covering such functions as reading, comprehension, listening comprehension, vocabulary, spelling, social science, science, and mathematics. Certain subtests are also separately available for testing within a specified area.

Creativity Tests

The growing recognition that creative talent is not synonymous with academic intelligence, as measured by traditional intelligence tests, has been accompanied by vigorous efforts to develop specialized tests of creativity. Guilford and his associates have produced a variety of new types of tests. The tests involve principally various aspects of fluency, flexibility, and originality. The Torrance Tests of Creative Thinking have much in common with the Guilford tests. One test from the Torrance series is product improvement, in which the child suggests ways of changing a toy so it would be more fun to play with.

Personality Tests

In comparison with tests of ability, personality tests are much less satisfactory with regard to such technical properties as norms, reliability, and validity. Any information obtained from personality tests should be verified and supplemented from other sources, such as interviews with the child and his associates, direct observations of behavior in natural situations, and case history material.

Self-Report Inventories

Self-report inventories consist of a series of questions that the examinee answers about himself concerning emotional problems, persistent worries, and other behavior. Some inventories designed for children and adolescents are basically checklists of personal problems. The questions pertain directly to the information the examiner wishes to elicit about the child's feelings and actions. The responses are taken at face value as an indication of the behavior to which they refer. A clear example of this approach is the STS Youth Inventory, for grades 7 to 12. The 167 items constituting the current edition are grouped into five categories: my school, after high school, about myself, getting along with others, and things in general.

Another approach to the development of personality inventories is through empirical criterion keying. The procedure involves the selection of items and assignment of scoring weights by reference to some external criterion, such as psychiatric diagnosis, ratings by associates, educational and occupational data, or other independent information about persons in the standardization sample. In such inventories, items are used not as a means of eliciting specific information but as verbal stimuli whose correlates. The outstanding example of criterion keying is the Minnesota Multiphasic Personality Inventory (MMPI).

Projective Techinques

The chief characteristic of projective techniques is that the subject is assigned an unstructured task that permits an almost unlimited variety of possible responses. The test stimuli are typically vague and equivocal, and the instructions are brief and general. These techniques are based on the hypothesis that the way the subject perceives and interprets the test materials or structures the situation reflects basic characteristics of his personality. The test stimuli serve as a screen on which the subject projects his own ideas.

One of the most widely used projective techniques is the Rorschach, in which the subject is shown a set of bilaterally symmetrical inkblots and asked to tell what he sees or what the blot represents. Ames and her co-workers at the Gesell Institute of Child Development have published two sets of Rorschach norms, one for children between the ages of 2 and 10 years and the other for adolescents between the ages of 10 and 16 years.

The Holtzman Inkblot Technique, modeled after the Rorschach, was designed to eliminate the major technical deficiencies of the earlier instrument. It provides two parallel series of 45 cards each and requires only one response to a card, thereby holding response productivity constant for each examinee and avoiding some of the pitfalls of traditional Rorschach scoring. Scores are obtained for 22 response variables, including most of the Rorschach form variables and such additional variables as anxiety, hostility, and pathognomic verbalization.

The Thematic Apperception Test (TAT) presents more highly structured stimuli and requires more complex and meaningfully organized verbal responses. The TAT materials consist of a set of cards containing vague pictures in black and white. The examinee makes up a story to fit each picture, telling what led up to the event portrayed, describing what is happening at the moment and what the characters are feeling and thinking, and giving the outcome. Responses are interpreted largely through content analysis.

The Children's Appreception Test (CAT) is an adaptation of the TAT specially developed for children between the ages of 3 and 10 years. The CAT cards substitute animals for people on the assumption that young children project more readily to pictures of animals than to pictures of humans. The animals are portrayed in typically human situations and are designed to evoke fantasies relating to problems of feeding and other oral activity, sibling rivalry, parent-child relations, aggression, toilet training, and other childhood experiences. Contrary to the stated assumption, research with children from the first grade up has revealed either no difference or more often, greater productivity of clinically significant material with human than with animal pictures. As a result, a human modification of the CAT was prepared (CAT-H) for use with older children, especially those with a mental age above 10.

Another type of picture test is illustrated by the Rosenzweig Picture-Frustration Study (P-F). This test presents a series of cartoons in which one person frustrates another (see Figure 3). In the blank space provided, the child writes what the frustrated person would reply. Responses are classified with reference to type and direction of aggression. Types of aggression include obstacle-dominance, emphasizing the frustrating object; ego-defense, focusing attention on the protection of the frustrated person; and need-persistence, concentrating on the constructive solution of the frustrating problem.

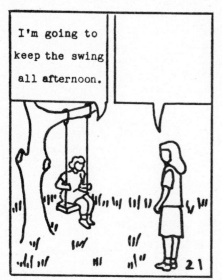

FIGURE 3. Sample item from Rosenzweig Picture-Frustration Study, Form for Children. (Reproduced by permission of Saul Rosenzweig.)

Direction of aggression is scored as extrapunitive, turned outward toward the environment; intropunitive, turned inward on the subject; and impunitive, turned off in an attempt to gloss over or evade the situation.

Certain projective instruments are wholly verbal, using only words in both stimulus materials and responses. Common examples include word association and sentence completion. In the typical sentence completion test, the opening words or sentence stems are formulated to elicit responses relevant to the personality trait or behavior domain to be assessed. The Rotter Incomplete Sentences Blank (RISB) consists of 40 sentence stems. The Washington University Sentence Completion Test (WUSCT) classifies the responses with reference to a seven-stage scale of ego development.

Drawings, toy tests, and other play techniques represent another application of projective methods. Special attention has centered on drawings of the human figure. Play and dramatic objects—such as puppets, dolls, toys, and miniatures—have also been used in projective examinations. The objects are usually selected because of their associative value, often including dolls representing adults and children, bathroom and kitchen fixtures, and other household furnishings. Play with such articles is expected to reveal the child's attitudes toward his family, sibling rivalries, fears, aggressions, and conflicts.

When evaluated as standardized tests, most projective techniques have fared quite poorly. In their present state of development, these techniques should be regarded not as tests but as aids to the clinical interviewer.

Cultural Differentials in Test Performance

In the measurement of both abilities and personality traits, tests yield significant mean differences between children reared in different cultures or subcultures, such as different socioeconomic levels, urban and rural environments, and minority groups. Several attempts have been made to develop culture-free or culture-fair tests. The earliest culture-free tests were designed on the premise that hereditary intellectual potential could be measured independently of the impact of cultural experiences. However, hereditary and environmental factors operate jointly at all stages in the development of the organism, and their effects are inextricably intertwined in the resulting behavior. The present objective is to construct tests that presuppose only experiences common to different cultures. Available culture-fair tests eliminate one or more parameters along which specific cultures differ, such as language, reading, speed, or culturally loaded content.

No existing test is universally applicable or equally fair to all cultures. Although less restricted than other tests, culture-fair tests are never completely unrestricted in their cultural reference. Any test tends to favor persons from the culture in which it was developed.

Culture fairness in testing depends on the elimination of relevant cultural parameters. A nonlanguage test may reduce the cultural handicap for children from one culture but increase it for children from another culture. Available culture-fair tests, moreover, differ among themselves in the extent to which they measure different abilities. When spatial content is substituted for verbal content, for example, the nature of the abilities sampled by the test may thereby be altered drastically. Although an I.Q. on one such test may be largely a measure of abstract reasoning, on another it may depend chiefly on spatial and perceptual abilities.

In psychometric terms, test bias refers specifically to overprediction or underprediction of criterion measures. If a test consistently underpredicts criterion performance for a particular group, it shows unfair discrimination or bias against the group.

The most important consideration in testing culturally dissimilar groups pertains to the interpretation of test scores. An inferior score on an arithmetic test could result from low test-taking motivation, poor reading ability, or an inadequate knowledge of arithmetic, among other reasons. Test scores should be used to facilitate an understanding of persons, not to label or classify them into rigid categories.

REFERENCES

American Psychological Association. *Standards for Educational & Psychological Tests*. ed. 3. American Psychological Association, Washington, 1974.

Anastasi, A. *Psychological Testing*, ed 4. Macmillan, New York, 1975.

Buros, O. K., editor. *The Seventh Mental Measurements Yearbook*. Gryphon Press, Highland Park, N. J., 1972.

Buros, O. K., editor. *Tests in Print*, ed. 2. Gryphon Press, Highland Park, N. J., 1973.

Cronbach, L. J. *Essentials of Psychological Testing*, ed. 3. Harper & Row, New York, 1970.

Goldman, L. *Using Tests in Counseling*, ed. 2. Appleton-Century-Crofts, New York, 1971.

Sattler, J. M., and Theye, F. Procedural, situational, and interpersonal variables in individual intelligence testing. Psychol. Bull., *68*: 347, 1967.

35

Child Psychiatry: Adjustment Reactions (Transient Situational Disturbances)

35.1.   ADJUSTMENT REACTIONS OF INFANCY AND CHILDHOOD

Introduction

In childhood behavioral disorders, direct cause-and-effect relationships are rare. The majority of behavioral deviancies of children fall into many inconsistent and inconstant patterns. Infants and children are constantly growing and changing physically, psychologically, socially, and in all their interactions with the world. What is normal behavior at one age becomes abnormal at another.

Diagnosis of deviant behavioral patterns is chancy at best. Some 30 systems have been developed over the past 40 years. Just as unsatisfactory as the other systems is the second edition of the American Psychiatric Association's *Diagnostic and Statistical Manual of Mental Disorders* (DSM-II). The most common diagnosis of children seen in psychiatric clinics in the United States is listed in this system under transient situational disturbances as "adjustment reactions of infancy and childhood."

Definition

Adjustment reactions, according to DSM-II, are relatively transient disorders that occur in emotionally normal persons. The reactions are acute symptoms of emotional strain and are the result of overwhelming environmental stress. If the patient is lucky enough to have good adaptive capacities, his symptoms usually recede as the stress diminishes. The stress may last from weeks to months or, rarely, years. The time

required for the reduction of stress varies enormously. If the symptoms persist, despite removal of the stress, the diagnosis of adjustment reaction becomes inappropriate, and another mental disorder is indicated. Since transient disorders can occur at any time of life, DSM-II lists adjustment reactions of infancy, childhood, adolescence, adult life, and late life. As defined, adjustment reactions are very little more than lists of symptoms.

Epidemiology

Arriving at an accurate estimate of the incidence of adjustment reactions of infancy and childhood is impossible. These disorders are transient and relatively unimportant in the long run of the child's life. No one can go through the stresses of infancy and childhood without sustaining strain that manifests itself in symptoms that can be characterized as temporary maladjustment. Seen this way, adjustment reactions are ubiquitous and inevitable. By the time a child psychiatrist is called in, the adjustment reaction is usually no longer a transient syndrome but signifies a more serious emotional disorder of greater fixity and poorer prognosis.

Causes

The behavioral abnormalities labeled adjustment reaction are too diverse and heterogeneous to provide specific etiological hypotheses. One must focus on each individual case to understand its cause. Despite the heterogeneity of the term, which covers everything from excessive crying in infancy to recurrent displays of ill temper and minor stealing at age 10, there are certain general principles of etiology.

Family Interaction Model

Every adjustment reaction, whether in infancy or childhood, involves a disturbance of interaction between the child and his environment, particularly the significant adults. More often than not, the child's disturbed behavior serves as a loudspeaker for a larger family disturbance. It may also serve as a tension-releasing device in the family system of emotional checks and balances, as in the case of scapegoating.

The child's disturbed reaction has multiple determinants. On the child's part, they are concerned with his age, physical health, genetic inheritance, temperament, stage of development, maturation, drives, modes of coping with anxiety (defenses), and previous experience with stress. On the environmental side, the determinants are concerned with the adequacy of the physical and psychosocial environment and the specific stresses to which the child must adapt. These stresses include family pathology, parental health, unemployment, and poor housing. The form, content, and duration of the abnormal reaction depend on the relationship between the child characteristics and the environmental characteristics at the time.

Behavior Theory Model

The behavior theorist suggests that the syndrome results from parental or other familial positive reinforcement of deviant behavior. If that maladaptive behavior is maintained by its consequences, eliminating or changing these consequences should modify the behavior.

Child Development Model

Conflict results from the frustrations of libidinal cathexis. Transient disorders are inevitable, being the result of interferences with the normal progression of the child's libidinal development and with the growth of his ego and superego. These interferences are seen primarily in terms of the mother's failure to provide caretaking and nurturance consonant with her child's needs. From this point of view, the developmental conflicts underlying adjustment reactions are phase specific and are related to the child's level of development. The conflicts arise when environmental demands are inappropriate to or incongruent with the level of development of the child.

Feedback Model

The closed system consisting of mother and child is defined by the rudimentary ego structure and intense psychobiological dependency of the infant and by the mediation of his universe through the mother. Infant behavioral disorders can be of two kinds—psychotoxic or the wrong kind of mother-child relationship and emotional deficiency related to maternal deprivation or an insufficient amount of mother-child relations.

Psychotoxic disturbances of infancy and childhood, are disturbances of the delicately balanced give-and-take between the mother and the child, in which the right response at the right time is required of each. This is a form of a behavioral feedback system between infant and mother. Disruption stimulates the child beyond his emotional and cognitive abilities and produces psychological overloading.

Developmental Lag Model

Together with the effects of physical illness and handicaps, the major attributes of the child that influence the interaction with his environment are those involving developmental disturbances and temperament. The organic neurological syndromes are a major cause of developmental disturbances in behavior. Developmental lags, on the other hand, are unrelated to organic lesions or defects and are nonpermanent. Once these lags have occurred, the child tends to catch up with time, so that his functioning at a later date is unremarkable. These lags or delays in development may appear in any of the child's psychological functions. Since mental retardation is a major cause of developmental lags, one must clarify whether or not the behavioral deviation is due to organic causes or is a transient defect in a child of normal intellectual abilities.

Language lags are common examples of transient developmental defects. They can be used as the paradigm for delays in other functions—motor skills, perceptual organization, and coordination. Whether or not a specific language disability produces secondary behavioral disturbances in an otherwise normal child depends on the severity of the disability, his previously learned modes of coping with stress (defenses), his temperament, and the kind of support and handling that he receives from his parents. If the child has poor sending power owing to his lag in language development, he has had little chance to develop adequate basic trust and self-esteem. His parents have become excessively anxious about his inability to communicate and have pressured him to the point that his use of language has become fraught with their anxiety and his. Finally, he is hyperactive and irritable and becomes disorganized when placed under stress. These factors combine into a whole that is more than the sum of its parts. Each factor exacerbates the others until a full-blown adjustment reaction appears, characterized by temper tantrums, alternation between hostile approach and withdrawal, crying spells, and long periods of silence.

Temperamental Quality Model

The effect of the child's temperamental qualities have been studied extensively, and 10 temperamental attributes have been identified —activity level, rhythmicity, approach or withdrawal, adaptability, intensity of reaction, threshold of responsiveness, quality of mood, distractibility, attention span, and persistence of attention. Certain temperamental clusters are associated with stressful parent-child interactions and the probability of behavior problems. Conversely, other temperamental clusters are associated with benign interactions and the absence of behavior pathology. A child who is highly reactive and slow to adapt, has intense moods, and withdraws from new situations is more likely to develop maladjustive reactions of negativism and detachment than the child whose adaptation rate and temperamental qualities are more suited to the stresses of changing environments.

Clinical Features

Since the diagnosis of adjustment reaction includes any transient disorder of behavior occurring in an otherwise normal child, the presenting symptoms are enormously varied. The specific behavioral constellation is determined by the chronological and maturational level of the child, his physical and psychological needs, his developmental phase, and the interaction of these factors with the physical, psychological, and social environmental variables.

Diagnosis

It is important to determine whether the deviant behavior of a child is symptomatic of a transient adaptive disorder or of a more serious disturbance. An adequate differential diagnosis depends on a detailed history, physical and psychiatric examinations of the child, direct observation of family life, and, when indicated, a school visit and specialized laboratory and psychological testing.

Treatment

The treatment of any psychiatric disorder should rest on an adequate understanding of its cause, its psychopathology, and the biological, psychological, and social factors that cause the disorder to persist. In adjustment reaction of infancy and childhood, the diagnosis does not automatically bring to mind a specific form of therapy. However, there are communalities of causal factors within the multitude of syndromes labeled adjustment reaction. One must consider the various goals to be achieved and the treatment modalities that would be appropriate.

Attenuation of Pathological Feedback

This can be accomplished in several ways— medication, behavior modification, and psychotherapy. Each method is capable of resolving the disturbed parent-child interaction. In the long run, the preference of the therapist and the attitudes of the family toward treatment may be the determining factors as to which of these treatment methods is the most successful. All have been used with considerable effectiveness.

Multiple Intervention

Since the child's disturbance has multiple origins, a single approach is unlikely to be as effective as a combined approach. Home visits, school consultations, and an insistence on the father's participation add up to greater effectiveness than does, say, drug therapy alone. A flexibility of approach is also necessary.

Family Intervention

Treatment of the child alone is not as effective as therapy of the entire family. Parents, siblings, and often, extended kin should be appropriately involved in the treatment process. The interactive effect of their participation is more than simply additive. The prognosis is much more guarded for the child whose family resists being involved in treatment.

REFERENCES

Bell, N. W., and Vogel, E. F., editors. *A Modern Introduction to the Family.* Free Press, Glencoe, Ill., 1960.
Bloch, D. A. The clinical home visit. Semin. Psychiatry, *5:* 132, 1973.
Bloch, D. A., and LaPerriere, K. Techniques of family therapy. Semin. Psychiatry, 5: 121, 1973.
Coddington, R. D. Significance of life events as etiologic factors in the diseases of children. J. Psychosom. Res., *16:* 7, 205, 1972.
Erikson, E. H. *Childhood and Society,* ed. 2, revised, pp. 255–258. W. W. Norton, New York, 1963.
Franklin, P. and Prosby, P. A standard initial interview. Semin. Psychiatry, 5: 149, 1973.
Lapouse, R. The epidemiology of behavior disorders in children. Am. J. Dis. Child. *111:* 594, 1966.
Ross, A. O. Behavior therapy. In *Manual of Child Psychopathology.* B. B. Wolman, editor, p. 900. McGraw-Hill, New York, 1972.
Stone, L. J., and Church, J. *Childhood and Adolescence,* ed. 3. Random House, New York, 1973.
Thomas, A., Chess, S., and Birch, H. *Temperament and Behavior Disorder in Children.* New York University Press, New York, 1963.

35.2.   ADJUSTMENT REACTION OF ADOLESCENCE

Definition

Adjustment reaction of adolescence includes the severe adolescent turmoil involved in the emotional vicissitudes of dealing with the tensions of the adolescent stage of growth and development. Symptoms are generally individual rather than multiple, mild rather than severe, and episodic rather than chronic. Common symptoms are:

1. Affective: anxiety, depression, hypomania, hypochondriasis, psychosomatic complaints, phobic anxiety, acting out.

2. Characterological: schizoid trends, immaturity, aggressivity, passivity, obsessive-compulsive behavior, character defenses (intellectualization, asceticism, detachment, perfectionism, oversensitivity).

3. Cognitive: school failures, diffusion of time perspective.

4. Psychosocial: conflict with family and community, negative identity.

Efforts to clarify diagnostic considerations in adolescence are difficult because of the rapid developmental, psychosomatic, and psychosocial changes that characterize this period of life.

Epidemiology

Adolescence is characterized by considerable physical, emotional, and social change, which results in pattern alterations condensed into a short time span. However, the difficulties in clarifying the diagnosis of adjustment reactions of adolescence make an epidemiological study uncertain, particularly since many workers believe normal adolescence is characterized by severe discomfort and turmoil. A conservative estimate is that 10 to 15 per cent of the adolescent population at some point in their development manifest an adjustment reaction requiring either a diagnostic evaluation or treatment.

Causes

During adolescence, aggressive and libidinal motivations must be dealt with, and the important tasks of modification of unconscious concepts of parents, assumption of moral standards, sexual role identification, and selection of an educational or career choice must be accomplished before the potential adult can achieve a characterological synthesis. This synthesis results from the correct establishment of identifications and reformation of the ego-ideal, leading to consolidation of the superego.

The demand for the loosening of ego structures presses from both emotional and physiological sources. During adolescence the ego has the opportunity of revising solutions of the oedipal conflict selected during latency development. This second chance is carried out by the dissolving or liquefaction of some ego structures, during which regressive features are certain to appear. Anna Freud describes a defensive regression to the ego state of primary identification, a response to intolerable anxiety produced by potentially close and threatening object relations. Geleerd views the adolescent as dealing with the intense demands of object relationships, heightened physiological processes resulting in continuous states of alertness and vigilance, and an increased sensitivity to stimuli. The adolescent uses the mechanism of partial regression to the undifferentiated phase of object relationships as an essential step in eventually furthering ego development. She regards this partial ego regression as a normal phenomenon and explains that the ego needs to withdraw various object cathexes in order to prepare itself for adult object relationships. During this process, the ego may show a spurt in development accompanied by increased growth and mastery of intellectual pursuits and a general widening of interest in human endeavors.

Ego Identity

Erikson uses the term "ego identity" to denote the results of certain gains the person has achieved by the end of adolescence. These derivatives of preadult experiences eventually connote a persistent sameness within oneself (self-sameness) and a persistent sharing of some kind of essential character with others. Intermediary periods known as latency and adolescence are more or less sanctioned psychosocial moratoria, during which a lasting pattern of inner identity is scheduled for relative completion.

The steps by which the ego grows follow a psychosocial schedule that includes: (1) the mechanisms of introjection and projection, which depend on a satisfactory mutuality between the mother and the child, (2) childhood identifications, which depend on satisfactory and trustworthy family experiences, and (3) identity formation, which arises from the repudiation of childhood identifications and the assumption of new configurations with both internal and societal recognitions.

The clinical picture of acute identity diffusion is recognized in young people who are unable to use the social or intrapsychic moratoria provided. The transitory regression is manifested by being unable to make decisions, a sense of isolation and inner emptiness, an inability to achieve relationships and sexual intimacy, a distorted time perspective resulting in a sense of great urgency and a loss of consideration for time as a dimension of living, an acute inability to work, and at times the choosing of a negative identity, a hostile parody of the usual roles in one's family or community.

Turmoil

Anna Freud refers to the difficulty of drawing the line between normality and pathology. She views adolescence as an interruption of peaceful growth that resembles a variety of emotional upsets. Adolescent reactions approximate symptom formation and merge, almost imperceptibly, into borderline states of almost all mental illnesses.

Among the defenses against infantile object ties, displacement of attachment anxiety to the parents may occur rapidly, leading to passionate longings for relationships. Intense substitute attachments may be made to other adults, leader types, friends, or heterosexual and homosexual relationships.

Another defense is reversal of affect: love is turned into hate, dependence into revolt, and respect and admiration into contempt and derision. If hostility and aggression are turned against the self, intense depression, masochism, and suicidal wishes and gestures may develop.

The other major category of defense is against the impulses themselves. The ascetic adolescent fights all his impulses and may extend the defense to fulfillment of the physiological needs—depriving himself of food, sleep, body comforts, and ordinary pleasures. The uncompromising adolescent uses intellectualism to attempt to control his impulses and to prevent any communication between his mind and his body.

Offer sees adolescent turmoil as only one route for passing through adolescence, and he contracts this disturbed group with those adolescents whose development is continuous and undisturbed. The antecedent of this nonturmoil path is believed to be a nonstressful childhood with maximal developmental opportunities.

Nagera describes special environmental conditions that affect adolescents and may lead to overwhelming of ego defenses—parental or familial developmental interferences, social development interferences, peer group pressures, and collective traumatic neuroses.

Clinical Features

The adolescent may display behavior that indicates some change in his capacity to cope with stress. Aggression that once was comfortably handled is now expressed more intensively toward family members, school and community authorities, and friends. On the other hand, the teenager may become passive and withdrawn.

Preadolescence (9 to 13 Years)

The frequently described mutual antagonism between preadolescent boys and girls is actually the expression of a mutual striving to strengthen sexual identity. An increase in libidinal and aggressive drive is characteristic.

Blos notes that boys and girls show significant differences in their regressive capacities during latency, boys using regression to the pregenital levels more frequently. The peer pressure to socialize, increasingly abstract educational demands, and increasing responsibilities in the family can create stress reactions in both boys and girls, resulting in psychopathology.

An increase in aggression as a means of dealing with environmental stress is a common and troublesome symptom. Increased fighting among boys and picking on girls may reach serious proportions. Girls, too, may manifest increased aggression and engage in fights with siblings, friends and parents. Affective expressions of regression are common in preadolescence. Depressive states can be precipitated by school failures, rejection by peers or groups, and disappointments in self-esteem systems involving sports, material acquisitions, and other disappointments. Bipolar affective expressions may also appear at this age.

Early Adolescence (12 to 16 Years)

The early adolescent differs from the preadolescent in the emergence of a definite genital drive organization. The adolescent displays a richer, increasingly varied emotional life and adandons the regressive positions of preadolescence. During the early adolescent phase there is an increase in the intensity of friendships with the same sex and a decrease in sustained interests and creativity. The main tasks to be accomplished involve the dissolution of intense ties to parents, siblings, and parental surrogates as the primary source of love and the shifting of these needs to friends, groups, and ideologies.

Common symptoms complexes derived from partial regression emphasize oscillating patterns of behavior. Extreme behavioral patterns may manifest themselves in fixation points, with a remarkable increase in anxiety and depression.

Affective reactions may be intense, with considerable moodiness, depression, and hypomanic behavior. Dealing with any type of loss becomes difficult, and these adolescents suffer from acute depressions that, however, respond well to relief from stress. Suicidal preoccupa-tions and gestures are common and obviously contain a poignant plea for help.

Acting out behavior and delinquent acts are common during this period. Adolescent rebellion may become exaggerated, resulting in running away, isolation, and alienation.

Middle Adolescence (14 to 18 Years)

Middle adolescence is characterized by attempts at mastery of the basic aspects of object relationships and the achievement of a growing feeling of comfort with heterosexual objects. Defensive and adaptive mechanisms are subject to intense stress as the adolescent is faced with the task of establishing dyadic relationships without the inner readiness for such activities.

Partial regressions during this phase may affect narcissistic defenses and result in unstable defense operations. Object hunger results in constantly changing superficial attachments, partial identifications with religious or social archetypes, and intense crushes on peers and adults.

Mild to severe feelings of depersonalization may occur and are usually precipitated by external stresses that demand that the adolescent behave autonomously and master demands of reality. School events may create an ego stress that calls forth an adjustment reaction evoking severe anxiety.

Overintense concern with the state of the world and politics may also precipitate an adjustment reaction, as the adolescent shifts his object cathexis from the family to an imperfect society.

Homosexual episodes may occur as an attempt to deal with overwhelming feelings of object hunger and may also constitute an adjustment reaction. In girls, anxiety related to questions of feminine identification, in which there is a slavish dependency on the mother, may result in a few experimental homosexual experiences. In boys, the fear of inadequacy in heterosexual relationships, coupled with incomplete identification with the father and continued dependence on the mother, may lead to similar episodes.

Acting out episodes involving short periods of leaving home and aggressive outbursts against parents, teachers, or other adults and other impulsive acts are attempts to avoid the partial regression required to work through to adolescent progressions. These acts may communicate a plea for help.

Late Adolescence (17 to 21 Years)

During this phase, previously resisted identifications with parental attitudes become acceptable, and it is now possible to make realistic career choices, become interested in household tasks, and assume moral, political, and ethical positions that may vary from but generally resemble those of parents.

Prolongation of this late stage of adolescence prevents resolution and delays the choice of permanent love objects, career selection, and social commitments. The termination of adolescence may act as a trauma on the developing ego with the demand finally to separate and individuate from infantile objects and to mourn the loss of the maternal symbiosis. The late adolescent reacts with the classical stages of mourning: denial, depression, separation-individuation, rage at the lost object, and reconstitution. Prolonged mourning with phasic fixations is clearly related to neurotic or other pathological diagnoses associated with unresolved residual fixations; the adjustment reaction, at times delayed, is characterized by resolution.

Differential Diagnosis

An adjustment reaction can simulate a psychiatric illness, but it can also color and intensify the clinical picture and serve as the precipitating stress in a subclinical process. Adolescent turmoil and psychiatric illness can both be present and influence one another. However, the symptoms in patients with adjustment reaction are primarily anxiety and depression; the more serious psychiatric symptoms of schizophrenia, neuroses, and personality disorders gradually become clearer with further study of symptoms, functioning of the patient, and family relationships.

The adolescent patient should be seen individually as well as within the family context in order to clarify his functioning capacities. Many times, an adolescent who relates well individually reveals a substantially different picture when seen within the family constellation.

Only one-third of hospitalized adolescents diagnosed eventually as schizophrenic present no diagnostic difficulty. Two-thirds of the schizophrenics may initially present clinical pictures of severe adjustment reactions of psychotic proportions or severe personality disorders. Further study demonstrates the underlying pathological process, although a clear differentiation between severe characterological disorders and schizophrenia may be difficult.

Personality disorders manifest lifelong patterns of behavior demonstrating developmental defect and fixation. A careful past history is necessary to reveal the true nature of the disturbances.

Anxiety, depression, phobias, conversion symptoms, and other symptoms experienced as subjective distress are common features of neuroses. Patients tend to be cooperative and to give frank, reliable histories. Many manifest personality traits that seem uninfluenced by adolescent adjustment reactions. The onset of the neurotic process can be traced to early trauma, losses, and conflicts, resulting in failure of early developmental resolutions.

Adolescent adjustment reactions seen in a clinic are characterized mainly by rapid regression, with evident ability to recover and master the conflict.

Treatment

Mild adjustment reactions usually respond well to reassurance or short-term psychotherapy. Support given to parents, patients, and concerned teachers and other adults that these reactions are in the service of ego mastery usually provides enough of a moratorium for eventual integration and synthesis to occur.

More severe adjustment reactions require careful diagnostic evaluation and psychotherapeutic interventions. Individual psychotherapy and psychoanalysis are effective in the treatment of adjustment reactions, but the therapist must be alert and flexible and must maintain objectivity and tolerance for the rapidly shifting ego states.

Collaborative or simultaneous therapy with the parents is of crucial importance. Parents should be brought into the treatment situation at the onset; at times they are crucial in making environmental adjustments or in breaking up intense interfamilial resistances to orderly growth.

A therapeutic approach to adolescents' adjustment reactions may be effectively achieved through group and family therapy.

REFERENCES

Blos, P. *On adolescence.* Free Press (Macmillan), New York, 1962.
Erickson, E. H. The problems of ego identity. J. Am. Physchoanal. Assoc., *4:* 56, 1956.
Feinstein, S. C., and Wolpert, E. A. Juvenile manic-depressive illness. J. Am. Acad. Child Psychiatry, *12:* 123, 1973.
Freud, A. Adolescence. Psychoanal. Study Child, *13:* 255, 1958.
Geleerd, E. R. Some aspects of ego vicissitudes in adolescence. J. Am. Psychoanal. Assoc., *9:* 394, 1961.
Grinker, R. R., and Holzman, P. S. Schizophrenic pathology in young adults. Arch. Gen. Psychiatry, *28:* 168, 1973.
Masterson, J. F. *The Psychiatric Dilemma of Adolescence.* Little, Brown, Boston, 1967.
Nagera, A. Adolescence: Some diagnostic, prognostic, and developmental considerations. In *Adolescent Psychiatry,* S. C. Feinstein and P. L. Giovacchini, editors, vol. 2, p. 44. Basic Books, New York, 1973.
Offer, D. *The Psychological World of the Teen-ager.* Basic Books, New York, 1969.
Stierlin, H., Levi, L. D., and Savard, R. J. Centrifugal versus centripetal separation in adolescence. In *Adolescent Psychiatry.* S. C. Feinstein and P. L. Giovacchini, editors, vol. 2, p. 211. Basic Books, New York, 1973.

35.3. CHILDREN'S REACTIONS TO ILLNESS, HOSPITALIZATION, AND SURGERY

Physical, Psychological, and Social Factors

Stressful stimuli of a physical, psychological, or social nature may bring about a derangement of the child's adaptive equilibrium and the appearance of illness or a disease state. Parental patterns of handling the ill child may be significantly altered because of anxiety or guilt, causing further changes in the behavior of the child or occasioning rivalrous or other responses in siblings. In seriously disturbed families, the child who falls ill may be made a scapegoat for family tensions, may be treated unrealistically as a chronic invalid, or may be handled in other ways that reflect the unconscious tendency of the parents or other family members to respond to his illness in terms of their own needs, rather than his. Families from different socioeconomic and ethnic backgrounds may respond quite differently to the illness of a child and may react positively or negatively to the need for dependence on medical personnel or other helping agencies.

With serious burns, spinal cord injuries, and respiratory polio, the impact phase involves initial realistic fears, followed by marked regression, sweeping denial, and the use of primitive fantasy. The recoil phase includes a lessening of regression and the appearance of mourning for the loss of the self, which may lead to depression, warded off for a time by eating disturbances or hostile, demanding behavior. The restitution phase permits beginning adaptation to and attempts at mastery of the situation, during which individual patterns related to premorbid personality trends emerge.

Psychological and social factors may act as predisposing and precipitating forces. Active children with inadequate parental supervision or with conflicts over acceptance of parental controls may be involved in frequent accidents. Maternal deprivation may lead to failure to thrive or delayed development or both. Parental problems in impulse control may produce the battered-child syndrome or drug intoxication of the child from repeated use of sedatives. And stressful stimuli such as competitive pressures or the loss or threat of loss of a parental figure seem to be involved in the precipitation of various illnesses.

Reactions of parents to serious or disabling illnesses tend to parallel the phasic responses in children. Initial realistic fear is often followed by (1) a phase of denial disbelief, persisting for weeks or months, (2) fear and frustration as well as depression, guilt, and self-recrimination, with intensified marital strife occurring in some families as the parent attempts to deal with such feelings by blaming each other, the physician, or others, and (3) rational inquiry and planning, involving the need to live with some uncertainty.

Whether a child's illness or injury produces a deleterious effect on his adaptation or the family equilibrium depends on the developmental level of the child, the child's previous adaptive capacity, the prior nature of the parent-child relationship, the existing family equilibrium, the nature of the illness or injury, and the meaning of the illness to the child and his family.

Acute Illness or Injury

Direct Effects

Malaise, discomfort, or pain may produce listlessness, prostration, disturbances in sleep and appetite, and irritability in children, much as in adults. However, restlessness is more common in children.

Reactive Effects

Regression. In infants and young children, regression may take the form of the reappearance of thumb sucking; return to the bottle; more demanding, clinging, negativistic, or aggressive behavior; and the temporary giving up of recently learned patterns, such as speech, walking, and bowel or bladder control. In older children, regression occasions the reappearance of more immature social patterns, including greater dependence on the parents, particularly the mother; demanding or aggressive behavior; limitations in the capacity to share with siblings or others; and difficulties in concentration and learning.

Depression. Depression may arise partly from the direct effects of the illness, as in infectious mononucleosis or infectious hepatitis, and partly from discouragement or restriction of activity and separation from the parents resulting from hospitalization. Eating and sleeping disturbances are frequent in young children as depressive equivalents, as are changes in motoric behavior from hypoactive to hyperactive. Wide mood swings often appear in older children and adolescents.

Misinterpretation. Preschool children ordinarily view pain or discomfort arising from illness or accident as punishment for real or imaginary transgression. Early school-age children show fears of bodily mutilation related to treatment procedures.

Physiological Concomitants of Anxiety. Tachycardia, palpitation, hyperventilation, diarrhea, or other signs and symptoms may be exhibited. Such physiological changes, ordinarily reversible, may compound the effects of the predominantly physical illness.

Conversion Reactions. These disturbances affect the voluntarily innervated striated musculature and the somatosensory apparatus. Transient mild to moderate symptoms are frequently encountered during convalescence from a predominantly physical illness. Such an illness may temporarily block a child's intense developmental need to achieve scholastically, athletically, or socially. Or the illness may precipitate conflict between a regressive wish to continue to be cared for by the mother and guilt over such wishes as the result of the pressure to return to the competitive arena.

Dissociative Reactions. Dissociative reactions, such as amnesia and pseudodelirious states, may compound or be compounded by an actual delirium, which is often of a subclinical nature.

Perceptual Motor Lags. Lags in perceptual motor functions after a systemic illness may persist for several weeks or months without apparent damage to the central nervous system. Such children may exhibit learning difficulties after returning to school.

Chronic Illness or Handicap

Many of the considerations mentioned for acute illnesses and injuries are applicable to chronic illness and handicapping injury. Those variables relating to the child's previous adaptive capacity and the parent-child-family balance appear to be of more importance than the nature of the specific disease or handicap.

Effects on Personality

The personality pictures seen in children with various diseases or handicaps appear to fall along a continuum, ranging from overdependent, overanxious, and passive or withdrawn patterns—with strong secondary gains from illness—to overindependent, aggressive modes of behavior—with strong associated tendencies to deny illness.

Parental reactions also fall along a continuum, ranging from overanxiety, overprotectiveness, and overindulgence to problems in acceptance of the child's disability. Little correlation appears to exist between extremes of unhealthy parental and family response and specific types of personality distortion on the part of the child.

Effects on Body Image

Size, strength, and attractiveness play some role in the child's confidence and social adjustment, but only in severe cases or in individual family situations do these factors appear to be of the utmost importance. In adolescents, who need acceptance by the peer group, reactions to a damaged body image may interfere with rehabilitative procedures.

Effects of Treatment

A small group of children may show paradoxical responses, with psychological decompensation, conversion, and other symptomatic reactions. In an unhealthy family situation in which the child with a chronic disease or handicap has taken on a central role as an invalid, the child's precipitation into health may upset the tenuous balance of adapative forces, making it difficult for the child to return quickly to a healthy role within the family.

Hospitalization

Short-Term Hospitalization

Infants in the first half-year of life exhibit **temporary, global responses, arising** from different methods of feeding and handling. Infants in the latter part of the first year experience stranger anxiety and separation anxiety, often with some regression and depression.

Children under 4 years of age are most vulnerable to separation from the mother. This separation is often misinterpreted as punishment or desertion, resulting in feelings of helplessness or fears of attack related to the child's limited capacities for reality testing. The phasic sequence of protest, despair, and detachment is frequently seen after a few days of hospitalization, even in well-adjusted children.

For the child from 4 years through the early school-age period, the psychological meaning of the illness and its treatment appears to have **greater potential effects than the actual separa**tion from his parents. Fears of bodily mutilation and the tendency to misinterpret painful treatment procedures as punishment often invoke anxiety, regression, and the other manifestations mentioned earlier; boys ordinarily exhibit more aggressive responses than girls do.

Older school-age children may show mild regression and anxiety over the functioning of certain organs. Fears of genital inadequacy, muscular weakness, and loss of body control or mastery contribute to feelings of anxiety and inferiority. In adolescents, many of the same trends are seen in more muted fashion. There are also struggles to establish a sense of identity and independence, and these struggles sometimes interfere with the teenager's cooperation in treatment programs.

Parental reactions show some similarity to the pattern seen during acute illness. Denial and disbelief are less marked with less serious illness.

Posthospitalization

Posthospitalization reactions may occur even in children who have been able to maintain control throughout the hospital experience. Regressive tendencies, outbursts of anxiety, and fears of doctors or needles may appear in children after the return home. Most children are able to adapt successfully to the experience of hospitalization, showing self-limited reactions that ordinarily subside after several weeks to several months.

Long-Term Hospitalization

Long-term hospitalization may lead to serious emotional deprivations. In large institutions, especially, children exhibit chronic depression and detachment, often leading to shallow social relationships, distorted time concepts, limited capacities for learning, lowered resistance to disease, and rebellious or antisocial behavior.

Surgery

Special problems may arise in regard to operations with necessarily mutilating effects, such as amputation. If a young child misinterprets the procedure as punishment or a hostile act, he may become aggressive in fantasied self-defense; fear, withdrawal, or other types of behavior may result. Strenuous denial may lead to difficulties with prosthetic devices. In older children and adolescents, an unconscious need to suffer may produce recurrent pain.

Anesthesia may evoke fears of loss of self-control. Older children may have fantasies about what may be done under narcosis. Preschool children are often stimulated, rather than sedated, by certain barbiturates. Marked anxiety over operative procedures may significantly raise the sedation or anesthetic threshold.

Treatment and Prevention

Treatment and prevention of unhealthy psychological reactions to illness or injury begin with the diagnostic and are involved in the interpretation of diagnostic findings and treatment recommendations to the parents. Anxious confused parents need careful explanations and opportunities to ask repeated questions and to air their misconceptions. The physician must avoid critical, judgmental attitudes toward the parents, and he should minimize their guilt and self-recrimination.

Acute Illness and Hospitalization

The physician should carefully explain each procedure to the child in advance, using terms and concepts appropriate to his developmental level. Ideally, the parents should be prepared in order to prepare the child. For the preschool child, his mother's overnight stay in the hospital with him is the most valuable preventive and supportive measure. For the older child, daily visiting is important, whatever his illness.

Special recreational programs in the hospital, permitting the child to play out his anxieties before and after treatment procedures, have real value. Also valuable is schooling even for the briefly hospitalized child.

Children should be cared for at home whenever possible. When hospitalization is indicated, the parents' concerns and needs, as well as the child's should be kept in mind. Most parents can make vital contributions to the hospital program through their participation. The handling of crucial phases in convalescence should be worked out co-operatively with parents. Explanations of regressive or other post-hospitalization behavior should be given in advance so that they will see this behavior as a characteristic of childhood and not as a personal failure.

Chronic Illness or Handicap

The use of a supportive psychotherapeutic relationship with child and parents underlies all other therapeutic steps. The physician should call on the skills of other members of the rehabilitation team. Group discussions among parents of children with particular kinds of disabilities are also helpful.

With a very young or seriously disturbed child, special arrangements to have the mother in the child's room when he undergoes preoperative sedation and to have her there when he awakens can afford continuity for the child. Opportunities to ask questions after as well as before such procedures can help children work through their misconceptions and anxieties.

Terminal Illness

The child's concept of death is not fully developed until he is about 10 years old. Therefore, children can deny fears of death but show other, more immediate fears of pain or treatment. Even in adolescents, fears of death are often expressed in terms of fear of pain or of need for someone to be with them to help them in difficult moments. The important thing is for the child and his parents to have someone to whom they can express their feelings, rather than to maintain an unrealistic silence. Psychiatric consultation may be helpful in understanding such situations and in working out a plan for supportive help.

REFERENCES

Heisel, J. S., Ream, S., Raitz, R., Rappaport, M., and Coddington, R. The significance of life events as contributing factors in the disease of children. J. Pediatr., *83:* 119, 1973.

Korsch, B. M., Gozzi, E. K., and Francis, V. Gaps in doctor-patient communication. I. Doctor-patient interaction and patient satisfaction. Pediatrics, *42:* 855, 1968.

Nagera, H. Children's reaction to the death of important objects: A developmental approach. Psychoanal. Study Child, *25:* 360, 1970.

Oremland, E. K., and Oremland, J. D., editors. *The Effects of Hospitalization on Children.* Charles C Thomas, Springfield, Ill., 1973.

Oremland, E. K., and Oremland, J. D. The immediate and prolonged psychological implications of transplants in children. In *The Effects of Hospitalization on Children,* E. K. Oremland and J. D. Oremland, editors, p. 166. Charles C Thomas, Springfield, Ill., 1973.

Plank, E. M. *Working with Children in Hospitals,* ed. 2. Case Western Reserve University Press, Cleveland, 1971.

Prugh, D. G. Toward an understanding of psychosomatic concepts in relation to illness in children. In *Modern Perspectives in Child Development,* A. I. Solnit and S. A. Provence, editors, p. 246. International Universities Press, New York, 1963.

Robertson, J. *Young Children in Hospitals,* ed. 2. Tavistock Publications, London, 1970.

36

Child Psychiatry: Special Symptoms

36.1. SPEECH, READING, AND LEARNING DISTURBANCES

Introduction

The broad category of *Special Symptoms* is for the occasional patient whose psychopathology is manifested by discrete, specific symptoms. It is discussed in the area of child psychiatry only because these symptoms are most often found in this age group. The reader should note that the specific symptoms outlined here can occur in adults as separate entities not elsewhere classified. Most often, however, such a discrete symptom in the adult is usually part of a more generalized psychopathological disorder.

In every case of a language, reading, or learning dysfunction, a variety of interrelated factors is operating. The child has constitutional strengths and weaknesses, and linguistic endowment apparently varies in different persons. The child makes adjustments to his constitutional or acquired deficit, and the defenses that he develops determine much of his functioning. The emotional climate in which he makes this adjustment modifies his response to his original difficulty.

Disorders

Aphasia. Aphasia is defined as the loss of the ability to transmit ideas of language in any of its forms—reading, writing, speaking—or failure in the appreciation of the written, printed, or spoken word. In acquired aphasia, both decoding and encoding processes are disordered. Acquired aphasia in children is rare. If it occurs in association with infectious processes, it usually results in only a temporary lowering of functional competence.

Congenital aphasia is the failure to develop language as a result of demonstrable central nervous system impairment. However, not all children who are unable to comprehend or to use symbols at relatively advanced ages have a verifiable history of brain injury or show positive neurological signs.

Some children show severe difficulties in language reception and expression and a markedly positive family history of language disability. Orton felt that this syndrome belongs in the category of developmental language and learning disturbances. Since investigation of the linguistic dysfunction does not permit deductions with regard to cause, a descriptive term such as "communicative disorders of early childhood" may be preferable to "aphasia," which has etiological connotations.

Early severe communicative difficulties are characterized by inattention to auditory stimuli and inability to assign symbolic significance to input events. Children with such difficulties hear, but they do not necessarily apprehend.

The degree of expressive impairment varies. Speech, if it is present at all, mirrors the diffuse reception. Echolalic responses or jargon may be substituted for meaningful communication.

Children with these disorders frequently show pervasive deviations in nonlinguistic motor and behavioral areas. And the absence of serviceable language tools tends to interfere with developing ego functions of mastery, impulse control, and the ability to postpone gratification. The fact that these children are unable to discharge tension by way of words often results in severe emotional problems. The intensity of psychological disturbance depends not only on the degree of impairment but also on the ability of the environment to tolerate and support this kind of child.

Eventually, with the help of appropriate

therapy, a number of such children do learn to use words, although paucity of verbal output, primitive sentence construction, and learning disabilities usually follow in the wake of severe retardation in the acquisition of language.

Dyslalia. Dyslalia is defined most simply as a disorder in talking. Between the ages of 4 and 7, dyslalic children have difficulty in making themselves understood. Their severe articulatory difficulties, their tendency to omission, substitution, and distortion of sounds, and their telescoping of words all tend to obscure more subtle receptive language deficits: short auditory memory span, diffuse auditory discrimination, and trouble with the sequential ordering of incoming information. Dyslalic children usually understand the language of others, but they may be unable to interpret the small, grammatical words that represent spatial, causal, and temporal relationships.

The dyslalic child's infantile sound substitutions and primitive sentence construction may suggest regressive modes of functioning. Some children for instance, find it hard to give up lisping. Secondary emotional problems tend to arise as the result of difficulties with expression and communication.

As dyslalic children mature, their speech usually improves, but articulatory immaturities and subtle residual problems with formulation and organization of language can be observed at later ages.

Cluttering. Cluttering, like dyslalia, is one of the constitutionally determined linguistic disturbances, and severe difficulties with the organization of language often persist into adulthood. Cluttered speech is characterized by excessive rate, fluctuations in rhythm, monotony, frequent repetitions of syllables and sounds, articulatory instability, and a tendency to reverse the order of sounds and words. On the receptive side, one finds disorders of auditory attention, deficient auditory discrimination, and diminished psychoacoustical ability.

Reading and Spelling Disabilities. These difficulties may occur as the result of organic brain disease: however, severe reading and spelling disorders frequently occur in families and are thus assumed to be genetically determined.

Reading disability is known as *dyslexia* and affects 12 per cent of all school children. Boys are affected four times more frequently than are girls. These children often have above average intelligence, vocabulary, and social development and are usually, though not always, left-handed. Characteristically, there is confusion of one consonant for another and a reversal of syllables or words (mirror-writing) so that they are unable to recognize a word. Some of these children may be able to correct the disability by learning to read via a phonic method, not commonly taught in school. Dyslexic children show visuomotor and preceptuamotor weaknesses on testing. Their reading disability may become a learning disability as they are unable to acquire knowledge through reading. The defect may be lifelong and lead to depression, low self-esteem, and a sense of futility. As adults, they may write poorly and tend to be inarticulate. In school it is important to distinguish dyslexia and poor school performance from scholastic difficulties that result from neurotic problems leading to underachievement. Children in the latter group are more articulate, verbal, and competent with abstractions. The dyslexic child requires specific training in remedial reading; the neurotic child requires psychotherapy.

Children with severe reading and spelling disabilities show a fluid, diffuse mode of perceptuomotor organization. Their responses in most areas of functioning reflect a maturational lag. Bright and highly motivated children whose self-image has not been damaged as a result of early failure may compensate spontaneously for their early perceptual fluidity and may eventually do well in reading. In more severe cases, intensive and long term remedial reading therapy is indicated (Figure 1). With such help, the large majority become adequate readers. In extreme cases the goal can be only functional reading.

In cases of severe spelling disabilities, remedial help is a necessity; however, it is usually of limited effectiveness. Although the children may remember the way that a word looks when it is printed in bold black letters on a white card, they are likely to lose the configuration when required to reproduce the same word in context.

Severe spelling disorders are often complicated by writing disabilities. These children's jerky, dysrhythmic handwriting mirrors their dysrhythmic speech. Their compositions reflect their cluttered, disorganized verbal output.

Stuttering. Stuttering is usually first noted between the ages of 2 and 4, when the child

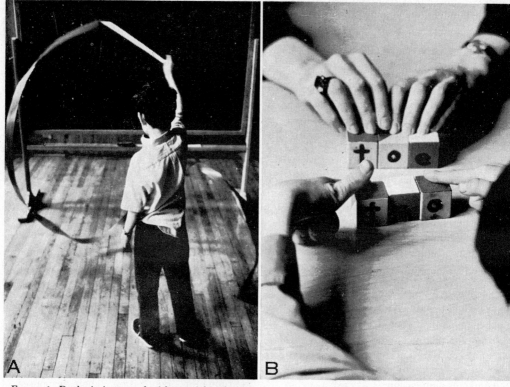

FIGURE 1. Dyslexia is treated with special techniques that reinforce different senses in addition to sight. In *A*, the child whirls ribbon to get the feeling or writing "3." In *B*, the child tries to arrange his blocks like the teacher's. (Courtesy of Joe Baker, *Medical World News*.)

begins to struggle with complex grammatical forms. At that age his neurophysiological maturation may lag far behind his emotional and intellectual need to express relatively complex content. At the same time, he has to renounce early instinctual gratifications, aggressive impulses are discouraged, a new sibling often threatens his place in the family, and his ties to his mother are being loosened. Primary stuttering, with its easy, effortless repetition of syllables, sounds, and words, disappears as the child's neurophysiological maturation enables him to cope with a heavy linguistic load. In older children, stuttering with its severe blocking, tension, and avoidance rituals becomes part of the ego's defensive system; it is rarely amenable to treatment by speech therapy alone and has to be regarded as a psychiatric disorder with psychotherapy indicated.

Differential Diagnosis

Severely limited speech output, fluid perceptual experiences, defects in body image, and overwhelming anxiety are characteristic both of schizophrenic children and of children who are suffering from early and severe communicative disorders. In schizophrenic children, however, fluidity is pervasive and involves the total personality organization, including the establishment of ego boundaries; in children with severe language deficits, the instability is confined to the perceptuomotor realm.

Psychotic Language

The verbal output of psychotic children is bizarre and idiosyncratic. They often show a total absence of communicative intent, which is a reflection of their failure to establish stable object relationships. Their echolalic speech has a mechanical, birdlike quality; sentence melody and pitch are usually inappropriate. Children with severe communicative disorders may echo words for purposes of clarification; pitch and inflection are usually normal.

In schizophrenics, words are no longer referents but instead become the things themselves, and as such they acquire magic properties. As in dreams, words may be distorted or telescoped; a whole train of thought may be condensed into a single word. Language in psychotic children often expresses primary processes.

REFERENCES

Bender, L. Psychiatric aspects. In *The Concept of Congenital Aphasia from the Standpoint of Dynamic Differential Diagnosis*, S. F. Brown, editor, p. 15. American Speech and Hearing Association, New York, 1958.
de Hirsch, K. Two categories of learning difficulties in adolescents. *Amer. J. Orthopsychiat. 33:* 87, 1963.
de Hirsch, K. The concept of plasticity and language disabilities. *Speech Path. Ther. 8:* 12, 1965.
de Hirsch, K., Jansky, J., and Langford, W. *Predicting Reading Failure.* Harper & Row, New York, 1966.
Gardner, G. E. Aggression and violence—the enemies of precision learning in children. *Amer. J. Psychiat. 128:* 445, 1971.
Johnson, W. *Stuttering in Children and Adults.* University of Minnesota Press, Minneapolis, 1955.
Laffal, J. *Pathological and Normal Language.* Atherton Press, New York, 1965.
Weiss, D. *Cluttering.* Prentice-Hall, Englewood Cliffs, N.J., 1964.
Werner, H., and Kaplan, B. *Symbol Formation.* John Wiley, New York, 1963.
Whitehurst, G. J. Discrimination learning in children as a function of reinforcement condition, task complexity, and chronological age. *J. Exp. Child Psychol. 7:* 314, 1969.

36.2. ENURESIS AND ENCOPRESIS

Enuresis

Enuresis is manifested as a repetitive, inappropriate, involuntary passage of urine. It can be defined as bed wetting or clothes wetting in persons over the age of 3 who fail to inhibit the reflex to pass urine when the impulse is felt during waking hours and those who do not rouse from sleep of their own accord when the process occurs during sleep.

Epidemiology

Enuresis is found in all countries, among rich and poor in both sexes. It afflicts those in normal and subnormal ranges of intelligence. No race is exempt.

Boys are twice as likely as girls to be enuretic. About 88 per cent of children are dry by age 4½; by age 7½ only 7 per cent are enuretic; between 7½ and 18 the percentage of enuretics drops to about 2 per cent. In highly selected military populations, such as volunteers to the United States Navy, the incidence varies between 0.5 and 3 per cent.

Those patients who are enuretic only at night are much less likely to have any associated or causative organic pathology. Since 80 per cent of enuretics are only nocturnal in their habit, this means that organicity must be sought more vigorously in 1 of 5 cases; 15 per cent of sufferers are both nocturnal and diurnal enuretics; 5 per cent are diurnal enuretics only.

Enuresis seems to be more common in the winter, and it occurs in cold rooms more than in better-heated quarters. Enuretics may form a disproportionately large number of delinquents.

In those who persist with enuresis into adolescence, compared with controls, there is a greater frequency in combination with passive-aggressive or passive-dependent reactions, past history of sleepwalking, family history of sleepwalking, inferior dentition, chronic genitourinary tract complaints, and family history of enuresis.

Causes

There is a growing corpus of opinion that maturational or developmental factors are more critical in causation than are psychodynamic considerations. The psychological position assumes that the presence of the symptom of enuresis is evidence of both a disturbed family and a maladjusted child. The developmental position cites the relationship between occurrence of a family history of enuresis and the symptom of enuresis. It is contended that genetic influences determine whether one is retarded in developing bladder control and whether one is psysiologically capable of being trained to have bladder control. Most enuretic patients remit spontaneously. When one looks at numbers of enuretics, they seem to have no problems other than the symptom of enuresis.

MacKeith presents data to the effect that a sensitive learning period in the third year of life is crucial to effective handling of the bladder. Anxiety in year 3 is correlated with persistent enuresis. Illness, one root of such anxiety, is more frequent at age 3 in enuretics than in nonenuretics. Maturation delay or developmental abnormalities are alleged to be involved in many instances of reported bladder function abnormality in enuretics. The correction of the abnormality may not cure bed wetting.

Many psychodynamic speculations are

deemed to be of causative significance. The enuresis is viewed as a desire for regression, a bid for attention, an active plea for help, a stated resentment to parents, a masturbatory equivalent, a clinging to infancy, and an expression of anger and resentment. Still other theories suggest that the enuretic is upset over sibling rivalry or feelings that he is an unwanted child or that he may be castrated. Enuresis is thought, too, to demonstrate an unwillingness to grow up and a need to deny strength.

Pathophysiology

Genitourinary tract investigation of enuretics reveals that they have small functional bladder capacity. Studies of adolescent enuretics reveal minimal but frequent organic abnormalities in the genitourinary tract.

Bed wetters are heavy sleepers. Bed wetting seldom occurs during rapid eye movement sleep, the stage in which the sleeper is relatively wakeful.

Bladder filling during sleep is most crucial in enuresis. Compared with controls, the enuretic has an increased frequency and magnitude of bladder contractions, which are prominent just before micturition. At the time of urine passage, the electroencephalogram shows an arousal, associated with mental confusion, autonomic behavior, poor reactivity to external stimuli, and retrograde amnesia, which lasts longer in enuretics than in nonenuretics.

During the flurry of autonomic activity associated with enuresis (tachypnea, tachycardia, compensatory bradycardia, penile erection, bladder contractions), the enuretic child's dreams are often of a hostile and aggressive nature. On the nights that adult enuretics wet, the content of their dreams involves dependency.

Clinical Features

There are two general categories of enuretics: the primary, persistent enuretic and the secondary, transient, or neurotic enuretic. Four-fifths of all enuretics are primary, which means that a period of sustained dryness has never developed. The secondary enuresis appears after a person has stopped wetting. A neurotic conflict, such as the birth of a sibling, or a transient emotional stress, such as making an adjustment to military service, may precipitate enuresis.

Here the enuresis is a regressive phenomenon. At least one of every 1,000 enuretics has an associated encopresis (involuntary passage of feces).

Studies of adolescent enuretics reveal that the teenager has grown up in a household in which there was conflict and bickering. The parents have had many child-rearing problems and seem to have encouraged acting out yet have discouraged the child in his efforts toward maturity. The parents may be permissive and unperturbed by enuresis. Since the enuretic uses his symptoms to express aggression and hostility and to get attention, enuresis may be a manifestation and a reflection of psychopathology in a family.

On the journey to dryness, the patient suffers relapses. These relapses occur in enuretics who are becoming dry spontaneously as well as in those who are being treated. Lapses that occur at night are often associated with fatigue or emotional turmoil. Lapses that occur during the day are often associated with excitement or excessively hard play.

Course and Prognosis

The overwhelming bulk of enuretics desist from the habit whether or not treatment is instituted. Although most children are dry by age 10, any child who is enuretic should be treated early, since it is impossible to distinguish the child who will continue to suffer enuresis into adolescence and adulthood.

Diagnosis

Enuresis produces no characteristic findings on direct examination of the mental status.

Bed wetting may be the presenting symptom in children with obstructive uropathy. These disorders include bladder outlet abnormalities at the neck and urethral anomalies, strictures, and stenoses. Or the obstruction may be due to neuromuscular abnormalities, with resultant megacystitis or neurogenic bladder. Urinary infections are commonly associated with enuresis. Dribbling by day usually suggests urethral obstruction or malfunction. Bouts of unexplained fever in enuretic children should demand a careful search for genitourinary illness.

Another possibility to be ruled out is epilepsy. The doctor must be certain that the nightly passage of urine is not part of a seizure pattern that is present but has not yet appeared during the child's waking hours.

Many enuretics are sleepwalkers, and they attempt to urinate during somnambulism. Therefore, sleepwalking must be differentiated from both enuresis and epilepsy.

In young children the sudden development of enuresis is a common presentation of diabetes mellitus.

Spinal tumors have a low incidence in childhood, but the loss of sphincter control in a child with progressive weakness, clumsiness, pain, and gait disturbance should alert the doctor to this possibility.

Other diagnoses to be considered when a child presents with enuresis include diabetes insipidus, spina bifida, lumbosacral myelodysplasia, sickle-cell anemia, foreign body, calculus, paraphimosis, vaginitis, mental retardation, and the presence of intestinal parasites.

In adolescents who develop enuresis after a period of dryness, the most likely cause is a transient emotional stress. However, when there is a long history of genitourinary complaints, the doctor must decide whether organic pathology is present.

Treatment

No treatment method is so successful as to win universal endorsement. After any underlying organic problem has been located and treated, the selection of the appropriate method depends on the individual circumstances. Usually, the doctor elects a combination of methods.

Placebos. In the literature marvelous successes are reported by using placebos. Since treatment of any sort depends largely on the ability of the therapist to promote a climate of mutual trust, confidence, and respect, the use of placebo methods runs the great risk of destroying such a relationship should the hoax be discovered.

Conditioning devices. The most effective way of banishing the symptom of bed wetting is to use a conditioning device that awakens the patient by an alarm bell or a buzzer as soon as a drop of urine contacts a wire pad on which he is sleeping. The conditioning process quickly leads to cessation of bed wetting, since the patient learns to awaken and void before the stimulus of the bell or buzzer. Although no substitute

symptoms develop after conditioning, adjunctive psychotherapy is often helpful to correct serious family psychopathology when conditioning devices are used.

Psychotherapy. Critical to the management of any case of enuresis is psychotherapy. The doctor must be supportive and must be capable of promoting and sustaining feelings of confidence and hope in the patient.

The largest barrier to successful psychotherapy is the wish by the patient (often with the psychological encouragement of his parents or spouse) that he contine the symptom. The therapist, by indicating explicitly and implicitly that he has confidence that the patient can cease his habit, may be the factor causing the patient to wish to correct his problem. The therapist must get the parents, too, to indicate genuinely to the patient that they wish him to stop bed wetting.

Drugs. If the physician believes there is a need for increased bladder retention, he chooses an anticholinergic, such as tincture of belladonna, five to 10 drops 3 times a day, or ephedrine sulphate capsules, 25 mg. at the hour of sleep.

Should the doctor elect to combat the deep sleep of the enuretic, he uses a sympathomimetic, such as dextroamphetamine sulfate tablets (Dexedrine), 5 mg. a day.

A decision that a child needs to be calmed down and rested results in the use of a sedative, such as phenobarbital tablets (Luminal), 15 mg. at the hour of sleep. Some doctors believe that rest can be facilitated by use of a relaxant, such as diphenhydramine hydrochloride (Benadryl), 50 mg. at the hour of sleep.

When the physician believes a daytime diuresis would be beneficial, caffeine, 2 or 3 gr. twice a day, is recommended. If the therapist thinks that a drug should be used to stop urine output at night, he may elect to use an antidiuretic, such as pitressin tartrate in oil, 0.2 ml. intramuscularly at 8 P.M.

By far the most studied drug in the past decade has been imipramine hydrochloride tablets (Tofranil). The usual dosage for 6 to 12 years olds is 25 mg., although some children may require as much as 75 mg.

A number of side effects can result from the use of tricyclic antidepressants. These side effects can be handled by reduction or elimination of the drug. Among the common side effects are dysuria, retention, and loss of appetite. On especially high doses, erythematous maculo-papular rashes may occur.

At the present time, antidepressants are the drugs of choice in the treatment of enuresis. Often, drug therapy is most efficacious when used in conjunction with other management methods.

Bladder Training. Enuretics have small functional bladder capacities. In bladder training the patient is asked to quantify his ability to drink measured volumes of fluid and to withhold urination for as long as possible. The desired result is that the patient becomes able to withhold increasingly larger volumes of fluid over greater periods of time. At night the patient's heightened threshold for retention eliminates the problem of bed wetting.

Sleep Interruption. Parents sometimes wake up the child to have him void during the night. Favorable responses may be due to the focused concern by the parents and the child as well as to positive behavioral reinforcement.

Hypnosis. Success with hypnosis may be related to the special quality of the treatment dyad in the hypnotherapeutic process.

Encopresis

Encopresis is a symptom marked by fecal soiling past the time that bowel control is physiologically possible and after toilet training should have been accomplished, between the ages of 2 and 3 years. It is defined as the repeated, involuntary passage of stool into clothing without the presence of any organic cause to explain the symptom.

Epidemiology

Encopresis is found much more frequently in boys than in girls. The ratio is about 5:1. The malady is found in relatively few persons. Of 1,000 consecutive cases referred from pediatricians to a child guidance clinic, only 15, or 1.5 per cent, were encopretic. Cases of encopresis are found throughout Western civilization. There seem to be no social or class barriers to encopresis. About one-fourth of encopretics have an associated constipation, which results in an overflow encopresis. Most cases of encopresis are not associated with voluminous fecal impaction.

Causes

Since the definition of encopresis excludes any known organicity, the origin of the disorder is related to psychodynamic and developmental factors. Most investigators believe that the mother-child interaction is crucial. Many neurodevelopmental learning and behavior problems are found in encopretics.

Clinical Features

Encopresis is characterized by passage of stool at inappropriate times and places, seemingly on an involuntary basis. Such children may be enuretic as well as encopretic. The stool passage accidents usually form no pattern as to their frequency, location, volume, or association with life events.

Course and Prognosis

The child who fails to attain bowel control may soon suffer from hostile behavior by one or more family members. As he associates outside the home, he finds himself liable to ridicule by his peers and alienation from his teachers. Many encopretics have had, from early life, excessive focus on their gastrointestinal functioning. They have had enemata, suppositories, and an incredible array of bowel-training techniques.

A rash of mechanical problems may result in organic defects in the lower gastrointestinal tract as the condition continues. The sufferer may require treatment for fissures, rectal prolapse, rectal excoriations, or impaction.

The natural history of the disorder seems to be self-limited.

Diagnosis

Encopresis provides no pathognomonic features in the psychiatric examination, including the direct examination of the mental status.

A chief problem in differential diagnosis is to be certain that the child is not suffering from Hirchsprung's disease (true aganglionic megacolon). A barium enema and fluoroscopy may be required to be certain of the diagnosis. Sometimes, a rectal examination or proctoscopy can be performed to see whether there is a large bolus of stool plus a dilated bowel just past the spincter.

Treatment

All who treat encopretics emphasize the importance of banishing punitive methods and the need to reassure the parents that the odious action is not willful. The family climate must be made warmer for the encopretic. Some mothers do not need psychotherapy but need to learn how to do a happier bowel training. Other children or their mothers or both need intensive psychotherapy aimed at protecting the child from his mother's too rigorous ministrations.

There is little evidence that drugs are useful in the treatment of encopresis. Imipramine (Tolfranil), 50 mg. at bedtime, has been used with encopretics who have no significant constipation. After a trial of a few weeks, the patient must be taken off the drug to see whether a relapse occurs.

Hypnosis has also been used in the treatment of encopresis. The difficulties in enduring true hypnosis in children plus the need to be conversant with the contraindications makes this treatment mode little recommended for general use.

The best results for symptom elimination seem to come from the use of reinforcers that reward the child for continence after the therapist has taken pains to include the family and the child in the treatment plan. With symptom reduction or elimination, the therapist can proceed with any necessary psychotherapy.

REFERENCES

Anthony, E. J. An experimental approach to the psychopathology of childhood; Encopresis, Br. J. Med Psychol., *30:* 146, 1957.
Henoch, E. H. How Henoch treated children with encopresis. Pediatrics, *46:* 802, 1970.
Hoag, J., Norriss, N., Himeno, E., and Jacobs, J. The encopretic child and his family. J. Am. Acad. Child Psychiatry, *1 :* 242, 1971.
MacKeith, R. C. A frequent factor in origins of primary nocturnal enuresis: Anxiety in the third year of life. Dev. Med. Child. Neurol., *10:* 465, 1968.
Muellner, S. R. Primary enuresis in children: New concepts of therapy. Med. Sci., *13:* 707, 1963.
Werry, J. S., and Cohrssen, J. Enuresis: An etiologic and theraputic study. J. Pediatr., *67:* 423, 1965.

36.3.   OTHER SPECIAL SYMPTOMS

Introduction

Nail biting, thumb sucking, and finger sucking are common symptoms. Generally, they are thought to be of only mild importance. However, thumb sucking and finger sucking may do considerable damage to dentition.

Epidemiology

Nail biting may begin as early as 1 year of age. From that point on, it shows a steadily increased incidence until about age 12. At age 17 to 18 in a select population of recruits, as many as one of four persists in the habit. By age 37, one of 12 persons continues to bite his nails.

Finger sucking is still present in about 31 per cent of children around 12 years old. This habit is more common in girls than in boys. There seems to be some coincidence of finger sucking and nail biting.

No co-variability can be found between nail biting and thumb sucking. Epidemiological research on thumb sucking is difficult because it is seldom the cause of a presenting or chief complaint.

Cause

Nail biting has been believed to be caused by psychological efforts at suicide or as an equivalent for masturbation. Or the nail biting is thought to be caused by intense or competitive impulses toward a parent. If such impulses were actualized, the child would destroy his source of dependency gratification. To resolve this conflict, the child bites his nails, thus denying his hostility, injuring himself, and demonstrating his punishment. He is able to express aggression but spare the object of his aggression.

Finger sucking and thumb sucking are thought to be the result of regression to oral satisfactions when the person is placed under the duress of tension or fatigue.

Pathology

Nail biting, thumb sucking, and finger sucking are considered socially offensive. In a few cases, nail biting may be so severe as to cause physical discomfort. In severe cases there may be psychological damage to the child's image of himself.

Clinical Features

Nail biting is an active process; finger sucking and thumb sucking are more passive.

Although nail biting is an oral-aggressive, tension-reducing impulse that is most likely to occur when the patient is bored or anxious, the habit is often present in persons in whom there is no obvious emotional disturbance.

Finger sucking and thumb sucking are present in nearly all babies in the first year of life. Such sucking should cause no concern. By age 2 to 5, children may resort to finger sucking when under emotional stress. The persistence of this habit may be associated with general immaturity.

Treatment

With young children who do not bite their nails severely, treatment techniques relying on suggestibility and self-reliance have been successful. The doctor should help the family reduce tension on the child. The child may participate in the treatment by means of pla-cebo tasks, such as taking the responsibility of soaking his nails daily in olive oil.

In patients with obvious emotional illness, the therapist must attend to the urgent and pressing life stresses. Behavior therapy is becoming widespread as a treatment for this symptom, particularly in young adults.

REFERENCES

Baalack, I. B., and Frisk, A. K. Fingersucking in children. Acta Odontol. Scand. *29:* 499, 1971.

Ballinger, B. R. The prevalence of nailbiting in normal and abnormal populations. Br. J. Psychiatry, *117:* 445, 1970.

Bucher, B. D. A pocket portable shock device with application to nailbiting. Behav. Res. Ther. *6:* 389, 1968.

Gale, E. N., and Ayer, W. A. Thumbsucking revisited. Am. J. Orthod., *55:* 167, 1969.

Klein, E. T. Thumbsucking habit: Meaningful or empty? Am. J. Orthod., *59:* 283, 1971.

Noyes, A. P., and Kolb, L. C. *Modern Clinical Psychiatry*, ed. 6. W. B. Saunders, Philadelphia, 1963.

37

Child Psychiatry: Behavior Disorders

37.1. BEHAVIOR DISORDERS

Introduction

The American Psychiatric Association's *Diagnostic and Statistical Manual of Mental Disorders* (DSM-II) defines behavior disorders of childhood and adolescence as follows: "This major category is reserved for disorders occurring in childhood and adolescence that are more stable, internalized, and resistant to treatment than transient situational disturbances but less so than psychoses, neuroses, and personality disorders. This intermediate stability is attributed to the greater fluidity of all behavior at this age. Characteristic manifestations include such symptoms as overactivity, inattentiveness, shyness, feelings of rejection, over-aggressiveness, timidity, and delinquency."

Epidemiology

The behavior disorders are among the most common conditions requiring psychiatric attention during latency and early adolescence. General population surveys suggest that 5 to 15 per cent of all children show some manifestations of disordered behavior.

Causes

With the exception of the hyperkinetic reaction, the behavior disorders are clearly related to faulty parental attitudes or child-rearing practices. Although temperamental factors within the child and accidental occurrences, such as illness in the youngster or parent, may play significant roles in the development of some behavior disorders, most problems appear to be related to relatively specific patterns of family malfunction that are chronic and that extend over much of the child's early development.

Types of Behavior Disorder

Hyperkinetic Reaction

DSM-II has this to say about hyperkinetic reaction: "This disorder is characterized by overactivity, restlessness, distractibility, and short attention span, especially in younger children; the behavior usually diminishes in adolescence."

"If this behavior is caused by organic brain damage, it should be diagnosed under the appropriate non-psychotic organic brain syndrome."

Although hyperkinesis caused by demonstrable organic brain damage is excluded from this category, there is considerable evidence that more subtle dysfunction of the central nervous system is a basic cause in a large number of cases. The current state of knowledge suggests that central nervous system maturational factors interact with environmental stresses in varying degrees to produce hyperactive behavior and the accompanying symptoms. It may be that those youngsters who are dealing primarily with a stressful environment respond poorly to stimulant medication and that those whose difficulty is largely maturational are benefited by such treatment.

The hyperkinesis is most marked in the young child and tends to disappear with age. In some children, however, motor hyperactivity is replaced by antisocial behavior or overt mental illness. Some cases of intermittent hyperactivity in children may represent juvenile forms of manic-depressive illness.

The diagnosis of hyperkinetic reaction is

made on the basis of parental reports of excessive activity, distractibility, restlessness, and short attention span, especially when these observations are confirmed by school reports and direct observation of the child.

Organic causes include damage to the central nervous system during pregnancy or delivery, neonatal anoxia, kernicterus, infectious illnesses of the central nervous system and their sequelae, chronic exposure to central nervous system toxins (especially lead), degenerative diseases of the central nervous system, and destructive brain lesions, including tumors.

Treatment of the hyperkinetic reaction is directed toward parental counseling and education, environmental manipulation, and, usually, medication for the child. Supportive and educative individual psychotherapy is indicated for the child in some cases.

Parental counseling emphasizes education regarding the nature of the disorder and management techniques. A calm, consistent, and repetitious restatement of reasonable expectations and rules often allows constructive channeling of the high activity level.

For school-age youngsters, consultation with school administrators and teachers is often necessary. Most educators are aware of the problem and the special educational techniques tailored to the needs and limitations of the hyperactive child. In severe cases, special placement may be necessary to avoid educational failure and the repeated clashes with peers and authority that may gradually establish a pattern of defeat, hostility, and secondary emotional problems.

Effective medications include dextroamphetamine, methylphenidate, chlorpromazine and other phenothiazines, and, most recently, imipramine.

The amphetamines were the first drugs successfully used in the pharmacotherapy of the hyperkinetic reaction. Multiple reports have substantiated beneficial and even dramatic results in 30 per cent to 75 per cent of treated hyperkinetic youngsters. Most clinicians have come to prefer dextroamphetamine to other amphetamines. Addiction does not seem to be a problem in youngsters who receive amphetamines for hyperactivity. Rather than producing euphoria, the amphetamines may produce depression in some successfully treated hyperactive youngsters.

Methylphenidate (Ritalin) appears to be roughly comparable to dextroamphetamine in effectiveness. It has the same adverse side effects of nervousness, insomnia, and anorexia as dextroamphetamine and also has a higher reported rate of hypersensitivity reactions. Methylphenidate has not been cleared for use in children under the age of 6 years. Toxic psychoses have been reported with methylphenidate administration.

Chlorpromazine (Thorazine) appears to benefit some hyperkinetic youngsters who do not respond to the cerebral stimulants. The phenothiazines are also effective in youngsters who are positive responders to stimulant medication. Serious systemic side effects have been reported with chlorpromazine, including jaundice and blood dyscrasias. Excessive drowsiness is a frequent complaint, especially early in treatment.

All these drugs are basically symptomatic and palliative. They are used to control target symptoms that make the youngster impossible to educate and socialize. They will not be of major benefit in improving the child's overall future adjustment unless this greater approachability is used to re-educate the child and his parents. Drug therapy should be accompanied by parental counseling, special education, and, if needed, psychotherapy, to establish a new adaptational pattern in the child.

Withdrawing Reaction

DSM-II says: "This disorder is characterized by seclusiveness, detachment, sensitivity, shyness, timidity, and general inability to form close interpersonal relationships. This diagnosis should be reserved for those who cannot be classified as having schizophrenia and whose tendencies toward withdrawal have not yet stabilized enough to justify the diagnosis of schizoid personality."

Temporary withdrawal from social interaction is a common defensive and adaptive technique in children, especially during periods of unusual stress. Withdrawal may also be noted as a significant element in reactions of grief or depression in children and adolescents. These transient reactions should be diagnosed under the heading of the transient situational disturbances (see Figure 1).

The withdrawing reaction as a behavior disorder is especially common in the 5- to 7-year age

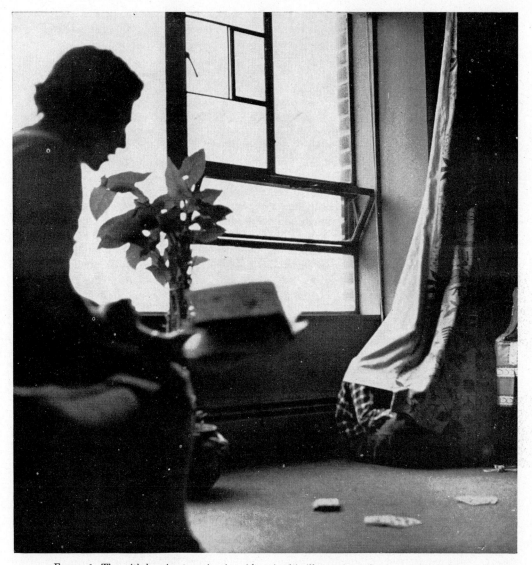

FIGURE 1. The withdrawing reaction is evident in this illustration. (Courtesy of Paul Berg.)

range and is frequently related to enrollment in preschool, kindergarten, or the first grade. Withdrawing reaction may be precipitated or exacerbated later in the development by similar stresses, such as moving to a new city, loss of important adults, or circumstances that publicly embarrass the youngster.

The child who is slow to adapt, has a low activity level, initial withdrawal responses to new stimuli, low intensity of reactions, and a relatively high frequency of negative mood responses has an inherent tendency to withdraw, especially in unfamiliar surroundings. These youngsters require an unusual degree of pa-

rental encouragement, patience, flexibility, and persistence if they are to be successfully socialized and gradually assimilated into a reasonable range of activities and environments. If the parents and other adults are either overprotective or excessively harsh and impatient, the child's difficulty in meeting new situations can become a generalized withdrawal from the world.

Another type of child may develop problems because his adaptability allows parents to impose idiosyncratic styles of behavior during early childhood that later conflict with extrafamilial expectations and lead to rejection in school or on the playground. Withdrawal then appears as a defensive tactic to avoid criticism, teasing, and other painful encounters with the larger world. Covert anger at the parents may lead to withdrawal at home as well.

Other children whose temperamental make up seems closer to average may develop the withdrawing reaction in response to family psychopathology or other factors that prevent predictable, confortable, and pleasant interpersonal encounters in early childhood.

Statistical studies of youngsters with withdrawing reaction show an unusually high incidence of maternal mental or physical illness. The mother herself is often a product of a home where alcoholism, chronic illness, or disability existed in one or both parents. The withdrawn child's father is often uninterested or tends to minimize the youngster's difficulties.

The withdrawing reaction appears to follow naturally from unpleasant or unpredictable experiences with early dependency and social interaction or from a conflict between parental values and those of the wider world. In the first case, the child emerges from the home with little reason to expect that interpersonal experiences will be pleasant or rewarding. In the second instance, the child learns patterns of behavior that are regarded as strange or unacceptable outside the family.

In either case, these youngsters present clinically as shy, uncommunicative children who seem unwilling or unable to open up to the examiner. Evidence of difficulty in separating from the mother may be observed. A slow approach that respects the child's caution may succeed over a period of time in thawing this reserve, but some youngsters remain suspicious, silent, and isolated for long periods of time. The mother's cooperation and even her presence in the interview situation may be necessary, especially with the younger child.

Some withdrawing youngsters drift into schizoid or schizophrenic adjustments, but many appear to overcome their shyness and develop normally in adulthood.

In the young child, parental counseling may be preferable to direct treatment of the youngster. In cases in which severe maternal psychopathology or a physical handicap interferes with the mother-child relationship, it may be necessary to provide substitute mothering experiences in the form of supportive psychotherapy or placement outside of the home.

Many youngsters respond rapidly to supportive psychotherapy that offers consistent warmth. The therapist should be available over a relatively extended period of time, since abrupt termination of the relationship may confirm the child's fear that caring for others is more painful than rewarding. Often group psychotherapy is a valuable way to assist the patient to generalize his trust in the therapist to other youngsters.

In older youngsters, especially adolescents in whom prolonged isolation has led to extensive dependence on compensatory grandiose daydreams, treatment is often more difficult and prolonged. Extreme patience is required to gain access to this fantasy world. Once the child shares his fantastic dreams with the therapist, there follows a prolonged delicate balancing between necessary challenges of the unrealistic ideas and the tact required to maintain the relationship. Group psychotherapy may be a valuable adjunct, especially in the later stages of treatment.

Every effort should be made to coordinate the treatment approach, so that the child encounters similar expectations, rewards, and limits in the treatment relationship, at home, and at school. Important adults in the child's life should be warned of the possibility of a transitional period, during which the child may become excessively aggressive.

Some authors have reported the use of antidepressants and cerebral stimulants to encourage greater activity. Such artificial activation is rarely beneficial except in those youngsters in whom depression is the primary cause of withdrawal.

Overanxious Reaction

DSM-II says: "This disorder is characterized by chronic anxiety, excessive and unrealistic fears, sleeplessness, nightmares, and exaggerated autonomic responses. The patient tends to be immature, self-conscious, grossly lacking in self-confidence, conforming, inhibited, dutiful, approval-seeking, and apprehensive in new situations and unfamiliar surroundings. It is to be distinguished from neuroses."

The basic pathology can be attributed to the youngster's premature effort to control his spontaneity and impulse expression in order to obtain the approval of achievement-oriented and constrictive parents, who themselves are often neurotic and anxious. The presenting symptoms include school avoidance, phobic concerns, sleep and eating disturbances, and diffuse fearfulness.

The traditional techniques of dynamically oriented psychotherapy are ideal for these youngsters. The exploratory, permissive, and accepting atmosphere of the individual play therapy session or psychiatric interview is ideally suited to the emergence of spontaneity and impulse expressions, which permits the child to correct his previously distorted idea of acceptable ranges of behavior and to raise his self-esteem. It is often necessary to provide collaborative counseling for the overly restrictive parents to make sure that they do not undo the beneficial freedom of expression the youngster is permitted in his own therapy.

Group therapy with the youngster or his parents may be useful at some stages of treatment to provide new peer models of greater emotional flexibility, open expression of affection, and true intimacy. In families in which the child's anxiety pattern seems to represent an identification with anxiety in the parent, to represent a necessary psychological underpinning to a neurotic family homeostasis, or to be the result of a scapegoated position in the family, conjoint family therapy may be the treatment of choice. Although the minor tranquilizing agents may be required for brief periods, they should not be used to suppress anxiety while basic family psychopathology is ignored.

The long-range prognosis for the overly anxious child appears to be reasonably good, at least for adequate adjustment to the requirements of adult social living. Effective treatment, especially if it alters noxious family patterns, may be of great benefit in preventing hidden neurotic suffering.

Runaway Reaction

DSM-II says: "Individuals with this disorder characteristically escape from threatening situations by running away from home for a day or more without permission. Typically they are immature and timid, and feel rejected at home, inadequate, and friendless. They often steal furtively (see Figure 2).

To be diagnosed as a youngster with runaway reaction, the child should show a repetitive pattern of flight from home and should also show other behavioral patterns that fit the constellation of symptoms described below.

The runaway reaction group contrast with the unsocialized aggressive reaction group in that the runaways respond to their frustration and anger with flight, rather than fight. The runaway reaction children are likely to be less physically robust than the openly aggressive unsocialized youngsters. They are also significantly less likely to have siblings than are socialized delinquents. This family constellation not only deprives the runaway of the opportunity for socialization experiences with peers, which might partially compensate for parental deficiencies, but provides little training in the successful expression of direct aggression. The result is that the youngster with runaway reaction feels weak, abandoned, mistreated, worthless, helpless, and hopeless. His anger leads to devious efforts at revenge, often clearly aimed at his harsh, rejecting parents. Very often he steals money from the home to finance a runaway.

The youngster with runaway reaction is basically a loner. He may associate with a delinquent gang, but he remains a fringe member, since he lacks both the courage and the loyalty to gain full acceptance in a cohesive and daring

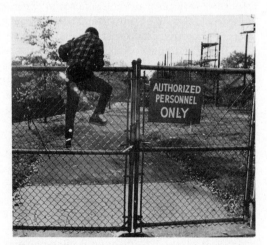

FIGURE 2. Running away. (Courtesy of Bob Adelman for Magnum Photos, Inc.)

group. The inability to assert himself and his hunger for acceptance frequently leads to passive homosexual experiences. Many youngsters with runaway reaction seem involved in an eternal search for a strong protector.

The runaway's description of conditions in his home is often bleak. Objective evaluation usually confirms his unpleasant account of cruelty, flagrant inconsistency, neglect, and profound emotional coldness in the family. The most common immediate cause of the runaway episode is fear of punishment or criticism at the hands of the parents or parent substitutes. Almost as frequently, the youngster runs away to revenge himself against the parents for some injustice. Once established, the runaway pattern may become so routinized that it is virtually unrelated to external circumstances.

Youngsters with runaway reaction are extremely difficult to treat, and their long-term prognosis is poor. Since the basic cause of the runaway reaction is rejection in the home, alteration of the home atmosphere is essential. Parental counseling, provision of needed family assistance in financial and other practical matters, and sometimes family therapy are indicated forms of therapeutic intervention. It may also be necessary to assist the runaway in achieving success in other areas of life. Most runaways are chronic school failures and detest traditional classroom learning. They often require special educational help to experience academic success. Active efforts to provide the youngster with pleasant and safe social experiences may also be an important part of treatment. Supportive group therapy, organized social clubs, and supervised recreational experiences may help.

If the home situation cannot be improved, it is usually necessary to remove the runaway to a more constructive environment. It should be anticipated that the youngster will repeat his pattern of running away through the early stages of the treatment program. An extended period of gradual resocialization, interrupted by many episodes of immature and impulsive behavior, should be anticipated.

Unsocialized Aggressive Reaction

DSM-II says: "This disorder is characterized by overt or covert hostile disobedience, quarrelsomeness, physical and verbal aggressiveness, vengefulness, and destructiveness. Temper tantrums, solitary stealing, lying, and hostile teasing of other children. are common. These patients usually have no consistent parental acceptance and discipline. This diagnosis should be distinguished from antisocial personality, runaway reaction of childhood, and group delinquent reaction of childhood."

The unsocialized aggressive child is very likely to be a boy with well-developed musculature who has experienced severe parental rejection, often alternating with unrealistic overprotection, especially shielding against the consequences of unacceptable behavior. His lack of socialization is revealed not only in his excessive aggressiveness but in a lack of sexual inhibition that is frequently expressed aggressively and openly. Punishment almost invariably increases his maladaptative expression of rage and frustration, rather than ameliorating the problem.

In evaluation interviews, the unsocialized aggressive child is typically hostile, provocative, and uncooperative. He rarely volunteers information regarding his personal difficulties and, even if confronted with them, may deny their occurrence. If he is cornered, he may blandly justify his behavior, go into a suspicious rage regarding the source of the examiner's information, or bolt from the room.

His hostility is not limited to adult authority figures but is expressed with equal venom toward his agemates and younger children. He often bullies those who are smaller and weaker than himself. Boasting and lying with little interest in the response of the listener reveal his profoundly narcissistic orientation.

The family situation often reveals severe marital disharmony. Because of a tendency toward family instability, there is often a stepparent or stepparents in the picture. Many unsocialized aggressive youngsters are only children who were unplanned and unwanted.

The child's aggressive behavior rarely seems directed toward any definable goal and provides him with little pleasure, success. or sustained advantage with his peers or authority figures. He has an inner core of self-hatred, depression, and helplessness. camouflaged with bravado, boastfulness, and grandiose self-presentations. Most anger is directed outward. Even when the unsocialized aggressive child feels sad or anxious. he blames others for his plight.

The age at which treatment is begun is an important determining factor in success, not only because of the tendency of this behavioral pattern to become increasingly internalized and fixed in the face of the counterhostility that these youngsters engender in others but also because of the greater practical ease with which overt aggressiveness can be managed in the younger child.

Involvement of the family is essential. Unless the parents can come to feel some acceptance and warmth for the youngster and provide consistent guidelines for acceptable behavior, there is small likelihood that the most intensive work with the child can be helpful. Conjoint marital therapy and family therapy with these families is extremely demanding. The therapist often feels overwhelmed by the intensity of the hostile interactions in the family group and frustrated by the parental inability to reach and persist in firm decisions regarding child management. Firmness and impartiality are essential but difficult to maintain in the atmosphere of mutual recrimination and contradictory accounts of family interactions.

It is often necessary to separate the child from his home situation. Even outside the home, the youngster can be expected to continue his aggressiveness, testing of limits, and provocation. Foster parents or treatment facility staff members require considerable support in order to tolerate prolonged periods in which their best efforts to be kind and fair are met with misbehavior, denial of personal responsibility, quibbling over rules, and paranoid accusations of unfairness and hostile intent.

Medications, especially the phenothiazines, may be of temporary value in some unsocialized aggressive children. They cannot substitute for the consistent and affectionate socializing experiences the child needs for the development of internal controls and new adaptational skills.

Behavior Modification

Since the symptoms of the behavior disorders are primarily reactions to faulty parental training and represent learned behavior, various techniques of behavior modification play an important role in their treatment. A prominent example is the use of token economies. In some cases, their effect on behavior patterns appears to be temporary unless the schedules of rein-

forcement are continued for long periods. Most successful treatment programs use a combination of behavior modification techniques, family therapy, relationship psychotherapy, and peer pressure.

REFERENCES

Feinstein, S. C., and Wolport, E. A. Juvenile manic depressive illness: Clinical and theoretical considerations. J. Acad. Child Psychiatry, *12:* 123, 1973.

Greenberg, L. M., Deem, M. A., and McMahon, S. Effects of dextroamphetamine, chlorpromazine, and hydroxyzine on behavior and performance in hyperkinetic children. Am. J. Psychiatry, *129:* 532, 1972.

Jenkins, R. L. The varieties of childrens's behavioral problems and family dynamics. Am. J. Psychiatry, *124:* 1440, 1968.

Jenkins, R. L. Classification of behavior problems of children. Am. J. Psychiatry, *125:* 1032, 1969.

Jenkins, R. L. *Behavior Disorders of Childhood and Adolescence.* Charles C Thomas, Springfield, Ill., 1973.

Jenkins, R. L., and Hewitt, L. Types of personality structure encountered in child guidance clinics. Am. J. Orthopsychiatry, *14:* 84, 1944.

Stierlin, H. A family perspective on adolescent runaways. Arch. Gen. Psychiatry, *29:* 56, 1973.

Thomas, A., Chess, S., and Birch, H. G. *Temperament and Behavior Disorders in Children,* New York University Press, New York, 1968.

37.2 GROUP DELINQUENT REACTION

Introduction

The second edition of the American Psychiatric Association's *Diagnostic and Statistical Manual of Mental Disorders* (DSM-II) says: "Individuals with this disorder have acquired the values, behavior, and skills of a delinquent peer group or gang to whom they are loyal and with whom they characteristically steal, skip school, and stay out late at night. The condition is more common in boys than girls. When group delinquency occurs with girls it usually involves sexual delinquency, although shoplifting is also common."

Epidemiology

No comprehensive data on the incidence of group delinquent reaction exists. Research suggests that the incidence varies both geographically and historically. The condition appears to be more common under any conditions that impair community and family stability. Such conditions include generalized social chaos as in natural disaster or war, neighborhoods undergoing rapid change, situations of cultural dissonance between the family and the larger society, and communities in which values are at variance with the norms of the larger society.

Causes

Sociological theories of group delinquency view the problem as an essentially normal reaction to socio-economic conditions. But many youngsters become neither delinquent nor emotionally ill in communities where juvenile crime is rampant (see Figure 1).

The youngster who fits the diagnostic category of group delinquent reaction might best be described as incompletely socialized. Early family experiences, especially with the mother, have been satisfactory, but later training is inadequate, usually because of paternal indifference or abuse in the father-child relationship. The father may be inept because of illness, absence, or alcoholism. The family is often poorly adapted to the social mores of the dominant society and often lacks status in the social hierarchy.

The delinquent gang takes over the adolescent or late childhood socialization of the child. The youngster brings to the peer gang a capacity for warmth, loyalty, courage, and commitment, even though these positive feelings may be directed toward some gang members who do not deserve it and cannot reciprocate. His delinquent acts arise not from hostility or vengence but from a desire for material gain, excitement, and peer acceptance.

Group delinquent reaction is currently considered an adaptive response to a variety of forces, including predisposing factors in the child, his family situation, and external social conditions. The youngster with group delinquent reaction is involved in unacceptable behavior because of the overriding importance of his delinquent peer group in his life. He does not show the incapacity for normal human relatedness of the antisocial personality.

Clinical Features

There is a history of adequate or even excessive conformity that ended when the youngster became a member of the delinquent peer group, usually in preadolescence or early adolescence. There may have been marginal or poor school performance, mild behavior problems, neurotic symptoms, or shyness.

Some degree of family pathology is usually evident. Patterns of paternal discipline may vary from harshness and excessive strictness to inconsistency or relative absence of supervision and control. The mother has often protected the child from consequences of early mild misbehaviors but does not appear to actively encourage delinquency. There is usually evidence of a relatively warm relationship between the mother and child, especially in infancy and early childhood. Some degree of marital disharmony may be present, and there is typically an absence of genuine family cohesion and comfortable interdependence. The group delinquent is likely to be from a large family living under poor economic circumstances.

The youngster himself is rarely guilty of criminal or antisocial acts alone. His misdeeds commonly occur in the company of his peer group. The parents often recognize the role of the peer group in the youngster's difficulties and complain of his wish to spend all his time with his friends.

Stealing and other minor delinquencies are the rule, rather than violent crimes against persons or severely destructive acts of vandalism. Stealing in the home is relatively rare.

The important constant is the influence of the group on the youngster's behavior and his extreme dependency on maintaining membership in the gang. Often multiple causative factors render the youth vulnerable to the gang's influence. These may operate in the middle- and upper-class settings, where socio-

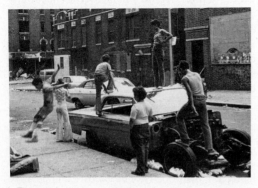

FIGURE 1. A gang in Bronx, New York, a manifestation of group delinquent reaction. (Courtesy of Sepp Seitz for Magnum Photos, Inc.)

logical factors are less evident, as well as in disadvantaged areas.

Course and Prognosis

The long-term prognosis for the youngster with group delinquent reaction appears to be relatively favorable in comparison with the youngster with unsocialized aggressive reaction or antisocial personality. Many group delinquent youngsters are not totally committed to a delinquent pattern and give it up. This change may occur in response to fortuitous positive occurrences, such as academic or athletic successes and romantic attachments, or in response to the influence of interested adults. Many other youngsters seem to be dissuaded from the pattern through the unpleasantness of arrest and appearance in a juvenile court. Such occurrences may also awaken the family to their responsibilities. It is difficult to determine the impact of therapy on the course of the illness.

Diagnosis

Group delinquent reaction is a descriptive diagnosis based on the finding of repetitive minor delinquencies occurring in a group matrix within which the youngster is capable of attachment, social interaction, and loyalty. Dynamic understanding of the factors predisposing the youngster to group delinquency depends on an evaluation of sociological and psychological forces impinging on the child, family, and neighborhood.

A youngster exhibiting group delinquent reaction shows a relative absence of the hostile, belligerent callousness and lack of empathy characteristic of the antisocial delinquent. Although rationalization and self-justification occur, there is less deliberate distortion and denial than is usually encountered in interviews with the more narcissistic antisocial delinquent. A capacity for trust and openness may be apparent if the examiner can demonstrate fairness and a desire to help.

Evidence of neurotic conflict may be apparent, expecially in the form of depressive tendencies. These self-doubts are not as malignant as those seen in the unsocialized delinquent and are not usually accompanied by grandiosity. A history of anxiety episodes is common.

The youngster with group delinquent reaction frequently complains of neglect, lack of love and understanding, or ineptitude, rather than accusing his parents of cruelty, strictness, and excessive punishment. There is often an insistence that his fellow delinquents understand and care for him in a way that his parents and other adults never have. Social immaturity is often evident in the youngster's difficulty in facing strangers and in his naive conviction that even the most self-centered of his delinquent friends has a deep affection for him.

Affective responses are often more genuine, spontaneous, varied, and appropriate than those of the antisocial delinquent, but they may show varying degrees of sentimentality, immaturity, crudeness, and lack of refinement in comparison with normal children of the same age.

The developmental history is often relatively normal during early childhood. Although marital discord and family difficulties may be apparent, there is usually evidence of adequate maternal care, at least during infancy. Overt rejection and hositility are not as apparent as in the history of the antisocial personality. Maternal hostility toward the child, if present, tends to be recent in origin and clearly related to the child's misbehavior and the real problems it has caused. The father is usually more remiss in his parental duties than the mother.

The psychiatric interview with the youngster and his parents may reveal the existence of living conditions and community organization patterns that make membership in a delinquent gang unusually attractive.

Neither the antisocial personality nor the child with unsocialized aggressive reaction has the group delinquent's capacity for commitment and loyalty to other persons and the group. The family of the youngster with group delinquent reaction may have been neglectful, but the family of the youngsters with unsocialized aggressive reaction or antisocial personality has often been actively aggressive and cruel.

Treatment

One element of the preventive approach to delinquency is the variety of general welfare programs that have been mounted to ameliorate the sociological conditions that seem to produce a high incidence of delinquent behavior. It is difficult to evaluate the impact of programs aimed at raising the standard of living, correcting early cognitive deficiencies of disadvantaged children, and providing appropriate supervised recreational facilities as an alternative to gang membership. Delinquency continues in spite of such programs, but their proponents can argue with justification that efforts have been inadequate and may have prevented the delinquency statistics from being worse than they are.

Another preventive approach has provided workers who enter the neighborhoods of the delinquent gangs and try to influence the entire gang. Systematic comparison of neighborhoods where such techniques are used with others where they are not applied may be methodologically impossible.

Individual outpatient psychotherapy appears to be ineffective. There is some evidence that reality therapy may be most effective in a group setting, either in self-help groups or in professionally directed groups. These groups use a core of reformed delinquents who understand the rationalizations, denials, and self-justifications of the gang member and vigorously confront the youngster with the realities of his predicament and the inevitibility of eventual negative consequences to him if he persists in delinquency.

In residential living institutions, the delinquent is approached with great tolerance, a minimum of control, and much warmth and personal attention.

In spite of an impressive body of evidence that even dedicated delinquents can be successfully treated, many programs fail, and even the effort to provide this kind of care is unusual. Such programs require not only an enormous expenditure of money and manpower but also unusually dedicated workers with extraordinary patientce, flexibility, and personal stability.

The consensus seems to favor various forms of group therapy for the youngster with group delinquent reaction. Group-oriented approaches capitalize on the gang member's natural proclivity to turn to peers for direction and emotional support. The crucial task is to convert the group orientation toward more conventional values. This may require separation from the previous peer group and transplantation to an entirely new environment. Other approaches—such as individual psychotherapy, family therapy, and more traditional residential treatment programs—may succeed in individual cases, although it is difficult to overcome the influence of a well-knit delinquent group.

A high percentage of these youngsters improve spontaneously as they become interested in heterosexual relationships, assume family responsibilities, and secure employment. Since their basic capacity for human relatedness is intact, they often discover their own passage out of delinquency.

Any approach that alters the attitudes of the entire group or that separates the youngster from the delinquent peer group and offers him contact with strong adult male leaders and less delinquently oriented peers is quite likely to improve the group delinquent's behavior.

REFERENCES

Adams, S. The P.I.C.O. project. In *The Sociology of Crime and Delinquency.* N. A. B. Jonston, editor, pp 213-224. Wiley, New York, 1962.

American Psychiatric Association. *Diagnostic and Statistical Manual of Mental Disorders* (DSM-II), ed. 2. American Psychiatric Association, Washington, 1968.

Argyle, M. *A New Approach to the Classification of Delinquents with Implications for Treatment.* California Board of Corrections, Monograph No. 2, 1961.

Jenkins, R. L. *Behavior Disorders of Childhood and Adolescence.* Charles C Thomas, Springfield, Ill., 1973.

Jenkins, R. L., and Glickman, S. Patterns of personality organization among delinquents. Nerv. Child, 6: 329, 1947.

Loughmiller, C., *Wilderness Road.* The Hogg Foundation, University of Texas, Austin, 1965.

38

Child Psychiatry: Other
Psychiatric Disorders

38.1.   NEUROSES

Introduction

In a brilliant series of logically linked clinical and theoretical inquiries, Freud gradually demonstrated the scientific validity of the poetic truth that the child is father to the man. He found that adult neurotic patients almost invariably gave a history of having undergone a similar type of disturbance at some time during childhood. Freud called this disturbance the Oedipus complex and looked on it as crucial in the development of both childhood and adult neuroses.

Causes

The normal development conflict is at first largely external, stemming from incompatibilities between the child's needs and the external demands of the environment. Gradually, the external demand is internalized, and the balance shifts from the need to gratify pleasurable impulses to the need to comply with the new internal representatives of the external order. When the conflict is unresolved, two forms of neurotic disturbance tend to occur. The first is circumscribed and restricted to the phase of the conflict. The second and more common form is a diffuse neurotic disturbance that presents itself as a polymorphous mixture of two or more neuroses. There is often gross familial pathology, with a plethora of constitutional dispositions. The defense mechanisms used tend to be various and primitive. As a result of the multiple fixation points, a sequence of different neurotic reactions appears during the course of development (see Table I).

Neurosis in childhood is said to occur as a result of unconscious conflicts over the handling of sexual and aggressive impulses that, although repressed, remain active and unresolved. These conflicts derive from the relation of the child to significant family members and belong almost exclusively to the preschool years. During early childhood, such conflicts may be expressed in various symptomatic reactions, but in older children they become internalized and relatively encapsulated and tend to be chronic. Mild reactions may resolve spontaneously as the child reworks the conflicts at a later stage of development and a higher level of maturation. The response to treatment is generally good.

Reactive disorders, developmental deviations, crises within healthy development, and certain predominantly physical disorders have a symptomatic resemblance to the neurotic picture. These conditions may act as precursors in the development of a full neurosis. In certain instances, the precipitating situational stress may be so overwhelming and unexpected to the child that it produces a traumatic neurosis. In certain cases, symptom formation may not occur. Instead, the personality structure of the child may be affected by neurotic conflicts, altering the patterns of reaction to internal demands and adaptations to the environment, and these patterns may assume the character of personality traits that cause little or no conscious anxiety. When these personality traits become fully crystallized, they coalesce to form a personality disorder.

TABLE I

*Classical Psychoneurotic Reactions of Childhood**

	Conversion Reaction (Dora)	Phobic Reaction (Hans)	Obsessive-Compulsive Reaction (Rat Man)	Mixed Neurotic Reaction (Wolf Man)
Family history	Striking family history of psychiatric and physical illness.	Both parents treated for neurotic conflict but not severe.	No family history of mental illness.	Striking family history of psychiatric and physical illness.
Symptoms	Enuresis and masturbation, 6–8 yr. Onset of neurosis at 8. Migraine, nervous cough, and hoarseness at 12. Aphonia at 16. "Appendicitis" at 16. Convulsions at 16. Facial neuralgia at 19. Change of personality at 8 from "wild creature" to quiet child.	Compulsive questions at 3–3½ yr. in regard to sex difference. Jealous reaction to sibling birth at 3½. Overt castration threat. Overt masturbation at 3½. Overeating and constipation at 4–5. Phobic reaction at 4–5. Attack of flu at 5 worsens phobia. Tonsillectomy at 5 worsens phobia.	Naughty period at 3–4 yr. Marked timidity after beating by father at 4. Recognizing people by their smells as a child (*Renifleur*). Precocious ego development. Onset of obsessive ideas at 6–7.	Tractable and quiet up to 3¼ yr. "Naughty" period at 3¼–4 yr. Phobias at 4–5 with nightmares. Obsessional reaction at 6–7 (pious ceremonials). Disappearance of neuroses at 8.
Causes	Seduction by older man. Father's illness. Father's affair.	Seductive care by mother. Sibling birth at 3½.	Seduction by governess at 4. Death of sibling at 4. Beating by father at 4.	Seduction by older sister at 3¼. Mother's illness. Conflict between maid and governess.

* Adapted from S. Freud, Collected Papers, Vol. 3. Hogarth Press, London, 1959.

Role of Anxiety

Freud came to regard anxiety as playing a primary role in the development of all types of disordered behavior, the elements of which could be regarded basically as techniques for reducing or avoiding anxiety. The anxiety may remain undefended, without an object, and may be experienced both psychologically and physically, as in the typical anxiety reaction; or it may be displaced onto some symbolic object or situation, as in the phobic reaction. It may be converted into various somatic symptoms, as in conversion reactions; or it may overwhelm the person and cause aimless activity or freezing, as in dissociative reactions. It may be transposed by means of various repetitions, rituals, and reactions, as in the obsessive-compulsive reactions; or it may allay itself by self-deprecation, as in the depressive reaction.

Role of Depression

Both anxiety and depression are appropriate reactions under normal conditions of danger and desertion, but both can become abnormal when they occur in inappropriate circumstances, when they persist for an undue length of time, or when the child is unable to make a developmentally appropriate adaptation to them.

Regression is often the mechanism of choice in depression. The other defenses mobilized against the danger of its emergence include obsessive-compulsive reactions (which magically compensate for loss of self-esteem), reversal of affect (characterized by excitement and clowning), identification with idealized objects, acting out (in the form of delinquency), and the development of psychosomatic states. All these defenses are means of averting the passive experience of helplessness in the face of frustration or disappointment.

Anxiety Reaction

Anxiety is a form of fear reaction that is different from normal object fear in the following ways: (1) It is diffuse or free-floating and not restricted to definite situations or objects. (2) It is not accompanied by any degree of insight into its immediate cause. (3) It tends to be experienced in terms of its physical manifestations, but these are not recognized as such by the person concerned. (4) It is prompted by anticipation of future threats, against which current avoidance responses would not be effective. (5) It is not controlled by any specific psychological defense mechanisms, as are the other neurotic reactions.

The American Psychiatric Association's second edition of *Diagnostic and Statistical Manual of Mental Disorders* DSM-II) defines anxiety as "the chief characteristic of the neuroses. It may be felt and expressed directly, or it may be controlled unconsciously and automatically by conversion, displacement and various other psychological mechanisms." Anxiety neurosis is characterized by anxious overconcern and is frequently associated with somatic symptoms.

Epidemiology

Anxiety and fear, varying in degree and nature, are encountered in all young children. Anxiety neurosis has been referred to not only as *the* neurosis of childhood but also as the form of neurosis most commonly reactivated in adult life.

Anxiety-prone persons have been estimated to make up between 5 and 10 per cent of the general population. These figures include the small percentage of vulnerable children who respond to the challenge of ordinary experience—such as sibling birth, illness, and hospitalization—with anxiety and regression, rather than with growth and maturation.

Causes

The majority of anxious children start as early as the first month of life to show behavior patterns that later develop into frank expressions of anxiety. The children show stress sensitivity from the very beginning, overreacting to both internal and external stimuli. They are easily startled and react poorly to change.

Infantile reactions considered indicative of anxiety—apathy, motor excitement, sleeplessness, refusal to eat, and autonomic disturbances—have been related to gross rejection and neglect on the part of the mother. Prenatal maternal anxieties, translated into muscular tensions involving the birth canal, may increase the frequency of abnormal birth conditions, which enhance the disposition to anxiety in the child. The predisposition is evident in the amplification of the universal anxieties—separation anxiety, stranger anxiety, and nocturnal anxiety—normally associated with the early anaclitic relationships.

At the later stages of development, the anxiety is generated from three different sources. Contagious anxiety is communicated to the child by any neurotically fearful adult with whom he is in close contact. Traumatic anxiety results from some unexpected fright that overwhelms the child's defenses. Conflict anxiety arises out of the intrapsychic sphere and is the most important source of neurotic anxiety.

Clinical Description

The principal psychological symptom is a diffuse and vague feeling of apprehension, as if something terrible were going to happen. The anxiety attacks sometimes begin after some manifest trauma which externalizes an accumulation of latent anxieties.

In addition, the child is generally irritable, worried about his health, and prone to episodes of acute anxiety. During acute attacks, physical symptoms may come to the fore and dominate the clinical picture. These symptoms may include disturbances of the heart's action, disturbances of respiration, gastrointestinal disturbances, and attacks of giddiness, trembling, sweating, and paresthesias. Urinary urgency and frequency are also usually present.

Nocturnal and Diurnal Anxiety Attacks. These attacks are characterized by acute terror or panic, with cataleptic features, profuse sweating, disorientation, and visual hallucinations. A waking terror may be brought about by visual illusions elaborated in the dark; a half-waking terror is often triggered by hypnagogic or hypnopompic hallucinations occurring during the twilight phase between sleeping and waking; a sleeping terror is brought about during light to moderate sleep, when anxiety dreams have their greatest incidence; a sleep-waking terror (the classical night terror) occurs when the predisposed child is roused from deep sleep into half-wakefulness; a day terror is similar to the night terror in its clinical picture and may alternate with it (see Figure 1).

The anxiety attacks in these cases are associated with such factors as interparental aggression, mental illness in the family, sleeping in the parental bedroom, undue parental pressures, traumatic experiences, and phobic, anxious mothers.

Chronic Anxiety Reaction. In certain immature children, there is a permanent attitude of apprehensiveness and an overreaction to almost every unexpected environmental stimulus. This combination causes the child to reverberate for long periods after a disturbing experience and produces a clinical picture of a timid, undecided, withdrawing child who has always been afraid of everything and who has been overwhelmed in turn by separation anxieties, stranger reactions, animal fears, dread of going to school, and general social anxiety. Night-

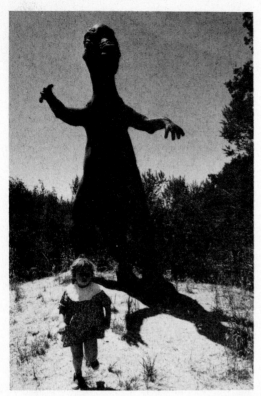

FIGURE 1. This surrealistic photograph symbolically represents a childhood nightmare reported by a patient in psychoanalysis. (Courtesy of Arthur Tress for Magnum Photos, Inc.)

mares are frequent, enuresis is common, and anxious preoccupation with bodily functioning is almost the rule. The child tends to be delicate and finicky about food to the constant concern of his equally nervous mother.

Hypochondriacal Reaction. A chronic hypochondriacal attitude in the child is made up of current complaints of vague ill health and anxious anticipation of future illness. A variety of factors in the child, the family, and the caring physician may contribute to the genesis of hypochondriasis. Factors in the child include identification with ill parents and siblings and the adoption of familial somatization techniques for dealing with stress: self-mothering in the absence of parental figures; attention seeking aimed at obtaining a greater acceptance and approval within the family; a flight into sickness to avoid threatening situations or pressures; reactivation of the sickness role, which once obtained for the child a suspension from regular routine and the loving solicitude of the parents; a compensation for social and educational failures linked to a lowering of self-esteem; a need to ward off indefinite, formless anxiety by the adoption of a definite form of sickness that might be cured; the effect of naive, infantile theories of disease that logically systematize bodily discomforts; and, above all, atonement for guilt feelings in relation to hostile and sexual impulses and acts.

The parents, particularly the mother, may be grossly hypochondriacal and may treat the child as a somatic extension of themselves. Their oversolicitude and protectiveness may thinly veil strong feelings of rejection, but, more frequently, the dislike and hostility are relatively unmasked. If there is much family history of disease, the anxious anticipation of the parents may fill the child with foreboding about his inheritance. Some mothers are at their best in the sickroom and enjoy the acts of ministration. The child's sickness then becomes an essential part in the relation with the mother, and he literally becomes her patient.

Prognosis

The prognosis is related to the stress sensitivity and the predisposition to anxiety accompanying it. When the development of anxiety has been late, the constitutional factors slight or absent, the birth history uneventful, and the first 2 or 3 years relatively peaceful, the anxiety reaction can be treated as a developmental neurotic conflict, with relatively favorable prognosis. On the other hand, when chronic insecurity dates from infancy and one or both parents are chronically anxious themselves, frequent relapses may occur throughout development, even though the prognosis for the current attack is good.

Management

A careful physical examination may be reassuring to some anxious and hypochondriacal children, but the dangers of iatrogenesis must be kept in mind if new complaints and new anxieties are to be avoided. Psychotherapy with the child should be coupled with guidance for the parents and, if necessary, psychiatric treatment when anxious concerns have reached neurotic proportions. The parents particularly need help when the repressed hostility of the anxious child comes to the surface with psychotherapy and is carried back into the home. With hypochondriacal children, medication must be cut down gradually and carefully, since the child has come to rely on its magical efficacy. When anxiety is acute and disruptive and sleep is much disturbed, the tranquilizing group of drugs may tide the child over a rough period before psychotherapy is able to control his anxieties.

Phobic Reaction

In this disorder, the child displaces the content of his original conflict onto an object or situation in the external environment that has some symbolic significance for him. Among the feared external objects or situations frequently chosen by children are animals, school, dirt, disease, high places, elevators, and dying. DSM-II notes that the apprehensiveness may be experienced as faintness, fatigue, palpitations, perspiration, nausea, tremor, and even panic.

Epidemiology

It is difficult to assess the incidence of phobic reactions because they are so often confused in clinics with the presence of fears. Fears occur regularly during the development of a normal child, and certain types of fears are characteristic of certain stages of development. The reaction of the child to a simple fear often seems to be disproportionate, persisting for long periods of time, and many simple fears of the preschool child may represent phobias. If this theory is true, phobic reactions are probably much commoner than would be supposed from an examination of clinical records. In guidance clinics, the phobic reaction is seen most frequently between the ages of 4 and 7 years and is seen equally in boys and girls.

Causes

In the immediate premorbid history of the phobic child, one frequently encounters a period of objectless anxiety, marked by restlessness, irritability, and naughtiness. Then comes an incident, and almost immediately there is a restructuring of internal forces, leading to a diminution of general anxiety and to the formation of a phobia. The choice of phobia may have some relation to a frightening, infantile experience, but, more often than not, the connection

between the phobia and the primary fear has been lost. The relation between the inner conflict and the specific content of the phobia is also obscure and complex.

Clinical Description

Constitutional and hereditary factors are generally insignificant. The children are physically well, cheerful, amiable, and active-minded, with a suggestion of emotional and social precocity.

Animal Phobia. Animal fears and anxiety dreams about animals are frequent between the ages of 3 and 5, and frightening experiences with animal pets are not unusual in this age group. Animals seem much freer in their sexual and aggressive behavior and much less hampered by social restrictions. Animals can, therefore, serve admirably for the projection of unacceptable feelings.

School phobia. This crucial psychopathology has been attributed to an anxiety over separation from the mother and to a concomitant anxiety on the part of the mother with regard to separation from her child; the two partners are dependent on, demanding of, and dominating each other in turn.

The school phobias that begin early are different clinical entities from those beginning at puberty or in early adolescence. The latter group tend to comprise severe character disorders and borderline psychoses, and there is often an associated family pathology of some severity, particularly depression in the mother. The external types of precipitating factors—disapproving teachers, poor grades, bullying, or shaming incidents in which the child loses face—may carry a more favorable prognosis than those connected with home and family, such as illness in the child, illness or death in the family, an accident involving the parents, or the development of mental illness in some crucial figure, such as the mother. The child may also show psychophysiologic reactions, such as abdominal pain, diarrhea, vomiting, and headache.

Death Phobia. This phobia might be referred to as 8-year anxiety, since it tends to occur at about that age. The child becomes preoccupied with ideas of death and dying. The main presenting fear is that the mother will die. At about 8 years, death, for many children, becomes irreversible, and death wishes, both conscious and unconscious, take on a new emotional coloring. The child becomes aware of a peculiar kind of helplessness in the face of the inevitability of death, with the additional feeling that no one can help, since everyone else is in the same predicament. An experience of death sometimes precipitates the crisis or brings it out at an earlier age, but it soon becomes clear that the emotional conflicts have been growing uninterruptedly since preschool days and that the fear of death is frequently a fear of punishment and retaliation.

Prognosis

Freud referred to the phobic neurosis of childhood as the model for all repressive disturbances. In the adult neurotic patient one frequently finds a residue of the childhood phobic reaction. The symptom is transient, but one cannot say the same for the neurotic substratum.

Management

The child's phobia, especially school phobia, may create serious problems for the family as a whole. In most of the phobias, other than the late school phobias, the prognosis for symptomatic cure is reasonably good within a short period of time, and the parents can be prevailed on to resist forceful and punitive measures during the period of therapy. In school phobia, the parents form an integral part of the treatment program. The current practice is to return the child as rapidly as possible to the school environment. In death phobia, a tranquilizing agent may relieve the panic that besets the child before sleep in the acute stage, since sleep may be associated with separation and death. With some acute phobias of recent onset and a clear-cut precipitating trauma, Levy's release therapy may be highly effective, especially if it is followed up by more traditional psychotherapy. Wolpe's method of systematic desensitization has been used in the treatment of child phobic patients, with good reported success.

Conversion Reaction

Freud introduced the concept of conversion as a mechanism for transforming anxiety into a dysfunction of bodily structures or organs supplied by the voluntary portion of the central nervous system, involving the striated musculature and the somatosensory apparatus. The symptoms serve to lessen conscious anxiety and to symbolize the underlying mental conflict. Since they also meet the immediate needs of the patients, they serve as a source of secondary gain. DSM-II differentiates conversion types of hysterical neurosis from psychophysiologic disorders (mediated by the autonomic system), from malingering (which is done consciously), and from neurological disorders (which cause anatomically circumscribed symptoms).

Epidemiology

About three to five cases of hysterical contractures, aphonias, and amblyopias can be expected in the outpatient department of a children's hospital every year. Conversion reactions occur predominantly in adolescent girls, but there is no appreciable sex difference during childhood. The incidence before school age is negligible, although cases have been reported in children as young as 1 to 3 years of age. It is now more frequent in working-class children and adults than in upper-class patients.

Causes

The choice of the afflicted region is determined by the unconscious sexual fantasies and the corresponding erotogeneity of the area, the point of least resistance, the situation in which the decisive repression occurred, and the ability of the organ to symbolize the unconscious drive.

Clinical Description

All the physical symptoms in the conversion reaction can be produced by volition or by emotion, although the patient may be able to maintain these symptoms for only a short time. The motor symptoms include paralyses, tics, and tremors; the sensory symptoms include anesthesias, paresthesias, and hyperesthesias (the distribution is not according to anatomical lines, varies at different examinations, and is susceptible to suggestion); and the visceral symptoms include anorexia, vomiting, bulimia, hiccups, respiratory tics, and abdominal complaints. Ocular hysteria occurs in children about as frequently as in adults, with peak frequencies in the 9- to 10-year and the 13- to 14-year groups and in a sex ratio of three girls to one boy. Hysterical contractures have been reported as frequent in the 10- to 15-year age group, with a female predominance of five to one. Precipitating factors include minor trauma or orthopedic procedures. Psychological factors include disturbed parents and parental relations, rigid authoritarian attitudes toward the child, and early feeding and behavior difficulties in the child. A period of severe emotional stress coincides with the onset of the symptoms.

Tic Syndrome. The tic syndrome can be roughly differentiated into two groups. In the first of these, the tic represents a conversion symptom in a genital syndrome; in these cases, tics are usually single and simply patterned. There is often a history of psychological trauma at the onset, and the psychopathology evoked has an oedipal configuration, with associated castration anxiety. The child often occupies a special position in the family, such as being the only boy, and his parents, especially his mother, are inclined to pressure and restrict him. From early life, he has shown a tendency to hyperactivity, and the parents have had difficulty in keeping him quiet and still. The prognosis with psychotherapy is favorable, and some of the mild varieties may clear up spontaneously within weeks or months.

The second type of tic disturbance has a mixed clinical picture and is generally associated with a neurotic character disorder, sometimes close to a borderline psychotic state. Anal sadism, exhibitionism, and voyeurism are prominent, and the symptoms may include coprolalia.

Hysterical Paresis. This type of conversion response is common at puberty and is sometimes brought about by a strongly worded suggestion from a parental figure, indicating possible loss of function or disability. In girls, there is often a marked ambivalent attitude toward boys, alternatively rejecting and inviting. The girl is usually highly contemptuous and disparaging of boys, and her crude and rough demeanor overlies a masculine identification. She is also outspokenly envious of boys and may list their many unfair advantages. The precipitating factors are often menarche, which serves as a reality confirmation of her no-longer-deniable femininity, and exposure to some violent sexual incident that may weaken the defense of masculine identification and necessitate the conversion of the emerging anxiety. In boys, the background is usually one of a passive, feminine character configuration, with submission to parental expectation. The conversion symptom is usually precipitated by a mobilization of anxiety in reference to guilt and punishment associated with pubertal masturbation and an excessively harsh superego structure, leading to a marked inhibition of any form of aggression.

Prognosis

The purer the conversion reaction and the freer the personality from character disorder, the better is the prognosis. The absence of gross pathology in the parents is also more conducive to a favorable outcome.

Management

Many different treatment procedures have been tried successfully with hysteria; most of these procedures incorporate some mode of suggestion. They aim at removing the symptoms, but they leave the underlying conflict unresolved. The use of hypnosis with children, especially with girls at puberty or approaching puberty, has iatrogenic dangers. Insight therapy is aimed at uncovering the neurotic conflict that has led to the conversion and at helping the child to reconvert. Environmental manipulation is sometimes more successful with hysterical children than with hysterical adults.

Dissociative Reaction

Neurotic anxieties belonging to this category may bring about a temporary disorganization of the personality that culminates in such aimless behavior as fugue states, catalepsy, amnesia, twilight states, narcolepsy, and pseudodelirious and stuporous states. Self-representation may be disturbed.

Epidemiology

Fugue states have been described in girls around the age of 8 and again at puberty. Somnambulism is rarely found below the age of 8, and it increases in frequency toward the end of childhood. The incidence appears to be higher in children from low socioeconomic areas.

Causes

There is sometimes a dissociative tendency in the family. The predisposition to gross reactions of the dissociative kind includes heavy constitutional factors, disturbed family relations, and unfavorable environments. Mental or physical illness in the family can act as a powerful model for abnormal behavior in a hypersuggestible, predisposed child.

Clinical Description

Children with a tendency to dissociation seem fairly well adjusted in their normal states, although somewhat shy and subdued. More than with the other hysterias of childhood, the dissociative type tends to be monosymptomatic, massive, and acute.

Somnambulism. This reaction can be defined as a fugue state that begins during sleep and is usually of shorter duration than a fugue. The movements of the somnabulist seem to be in response to the manifest or latent content of the dream, and the meaning may be an escape from the temptation of the bed or a movement toward a particular goal that represents gratification or reassurance. It becomes increasingly common after the age of 8, reaching a peak frequency around middle adolescence. In the majority of cases there is often a combination of approach and avoidance. At the point of greatest ambivalence, the patient may wake up. Compared with children who suffer from night terrors and nightmares, the sleepwalker appears to be less intelligent, less imaginative, and less prone to conscious anxiety but more suggestible. The patient tends to express himself more frequently through activity than in words, and dreaming is somewhat sparse and poorly recalled.

Twilight States. The typical early childhood is usually described as easy and uneventful, with a close relationship with both parents. A sibling is born when the child is about 3 or 4 years of age; soon after, the older child undergoes some traumatic sexual experience with an older person; the child at first keeps the experience secret but has guilt feelings. At about the fifth or sixth year, the child begins to show an exaggerated affection toward her mother and alienates herself from her father. The child appears to become increasingly disturbed; about her eighth year, she begins to suffer from twilight states, in which she both re-enacts her sexual seduction and shows marked hostility to the mother. As soon as the attack subsides, she once again reverses her behavior and clings affectionately to her mother, pleading for protection. Afterward, she shows complete amnesia for the whole event.

Prognosis

The dissociative state often disappears spontaneously in the course of a few months, to be replaced by some other symptom. One occasionally sees alternations of fugue states, somnambulism, and twilight states. The prognosis is less favorable for reactions beginning in childhood and reactions associated with personality disorders or with dissociative tendencies within the family.

Management

Psychotherapy should be aimed at the underlying conflict situation, rather than at the symptom itself. Hypnosis or amobarbital (Amytal) abreaction is often successful in relieving the acute symptoms.

Obsessive-Compulsive Reaction

The anxiety aroused by unconscious conflict is counteracted by the occurrence of thoughts (obsessions), acts or impulses to act (compulsions), or mixtures of both, which are all isolated from the original, unacceptable impulse. The external behavior often represents the opposite of the unconscious wish. Counting and touching ceremonials and recurrent thoughts appear frequently, resulting in marked anxiety if they are interfered with. DSM-II makes the point that anxiety appears when the patient becomes concerned at being unable to control his rituals himself.

Epidemiology

About 20 per cent of all cases of obsessional neurosis begin before the age of 15, and 50 to 60 per cent begin earlier than age 20. Of the childhood cases, about half have an acute onset. There is a slight preponderance of females, and females are more inclined to have an acute onset. The condition tends to occur in the upper brackets of social class, intelligence, and education. About 10 per cent of parents of obsessional children also suffer from obsessional illness, and between 40 and 60 per cent show obsessional traits. From 4 to 15 per cent of the parents may be psychotic.

Causes

According to psychoanalytic theory, the reaction is a defense against aggressive and sexual impulses, particularly in relation to the Oedipus complex. The initial defense is by regression to the anal-sadistic level, but the impulses at this level are also intolerable and must be warded off by reaction formation, isolation, and undoing.

The child-rearing of obsessional parents is rigidly scheduled. The child learns early that strict adherence to what he is taught is right and that to do otherwise is wrong. The child's world is inevitably clean, neat, and orderly, and the child develops just-so attitudes.

Clinical Description

Children who develop obsessional neurosis in late childhood or adolescence have often exhibited a variety of symtoms, including phobias, hypersensitivity, anxiety, inhibitions, obsessiveness, and shyness. Introversion is common. Clinicians describe the obsessional personality as cautious, deliberate, persistent, conscientious, dependable, dogged, austere, and perfectionistic. Psychoanalysts, elaborating on the original anal-erotic triad of Freud—orderliness, frugality, and obstinacy—emphasize the patient's stubbornness, egocentricity, and inflexibility and portray him as tyrannical, power-loving, dictatorial, hypercritical, vindictive, avaricious, parsimonious, irritable, malcontented, and hypochondriacal. The positive and negative pictures seem to depend on the degree of adjustment shown by the obsessional person. If the child is doing well in school, his ambitious and intellectual parents are inclined to treat his obsessional traits with respect.

The child begins his obsessional illness with the emergence of unacceptable thoughts—sometimes blasphemous, sometimes sexual, and sometimes aggressive. Unlike the adult obsessional, the child usually cannot keep his thoughts or ruminations to himself and may force his parents to participate in his rituals, answer his repetitious questions, and cater to his obsessional wants. The mother's compulsions may not fit those of the child, and she tends to become increasingly impatient with his insistence and may attempt to turn him aside from his demands, first by reason and argument and finally by punishment, so that child and mother are soon locked in an interminable sadomasochistic battle. Invariably, anxiety and depression supervene, together with vague psychosomatic symptoms.

Prognosis

Unfavorable factors are obsessional symptoms in early childhood, a premorbid obsessional personality, obsessional acts, and a severe clinical picture on first admission. Sometimes the obsessional symptoms subside spontaneously, but the background of anxiety, sensitivity, and inhibition may remain, with the result that the child continues to be nervous. Sometimes, the child begins to hide or camouflage his symptomatic acts. The prognosis, with treatment, of childhood obsessional states is fairly good, especially after prolonged intensive psychotherapy. About 30 to 40 per cent of the patients become completely symptom-free, with another 40 to 50 per cent improved or much improved. About 10 to 15 per cent of the patients apparently do not improve.

Management

Therapy takes place in a series of stages. In stage one, the child is relieved to talk about his peculiar symptoms without being mocked, criticized, or punished. He can also express his anger at the repercussions that his illness brings about in his home environment. In stage two, the child attempts to use the therapist in the same way he uses his mother, as a participant in his ceremonials; when the therapist balks at assuming this role, a stormy situation ensues. In stage three, which is often heralded by freer dream material, the child's defenses appear less inflexible. The stage that follows is characterized by messiness and aggression, and the child seems for a while to wallow in his regressions. As this stage abates, frank oedipal wishes and thoughts begin to emerge, and from then on the treatment resembles that of other neurotic children.

Depressive Reaction

Neurotic depressive disorders involve internalized conflicts in relation to deeply ambivalent feelings and are not commonly seen in their fully developed adult form in children, although depressive equivalents may take the place of the depression, varying in their composition with the child's stage of development. The conflict anxiety is said to be mitigated by self-deprecation and the sagging of mood. In older children, a loss of self-esteem, associated with feelings of guilt and ambivalence toward loved persons, has been reported. Psychomotor retardation and agitation are occasionally present but are much less marked than in adults.

The depressive reaction in children is characterized by sadness, helplessness, loneliness, homesickness, and inadequacy. The depressed child experiences a feeling of pain over real or supposed deprivation and may resign himself in a helpless, impotent way to the painful situation or react with aggression against the source of pain. The depressive response is always associated with undischarged aggression, and fear of superego sanctions leads to repression or displacement of the aggression onto the self.

DSM-II differentiates neurotic depression on two counts: as an excessive reaction to internal conflict and as a reaction to some identifiable event, such as the loss of a cherished person or thing.

Epidemiology

One is faced with an almost hopeless task in attempting to ascertain its prevalence. The few studies in the literature are merely descriptive of a small number of cases.

Causes

The depressive reaction has a close relation to aggressive feelings directed toward the loved parent of the same sex, thereby generating a conflict of ambivalence. Even the resolution of that conflict and the preservation of the rival involves some degree of loss in the renunciation of the basic desires. Some children who are predisposed to depression react to the dilemma with depressive feelings, the castration anxiety in such cases remaining relatively mild.

Clinical Description

The depressive picture in children between 8 and 11 years includes weeping bouts, some flatness of affect, fears of death for self or parents, irritability, somatic complaints, loss of appetite and energy, varying degrees of difficulty in school adjustment, and vacillation between clinging to and unreasonable hostility

toward their parents. Self-deprecation is often marked. The child may look sad and depressed, talk in a low and weak voice, turn his head to the wall, cry frequently, and constantly iterate his loneliness. The precipitating factors are usually specific events, such as accidents and physical illnesses, but not the real loss of either parent.

Instead of depression, a child may present with depressive equivalents, which can include eating and sleeping disturbances, antisocial behavior, accident proneness, running away from home, boredom and restlessness, fatigue, difficulty in concentration, and sexual acting out. These depressive equivalents also represent modes of defense adopted to ward off feelings of depression, isolation, loneliness, and emptiness.

The wish to die may stimulate suicidal ruminations, suicidal attempts, and actual suicide. Suicide is said to be rare under the age of 10; only three children in the United States were reported in this group in 1958. The number of suicides varies between 35 and 60 each year in the age group 10 to 14 years and between 250 and 300 each year in the age group of 15 to 19 years. Girls outnumber boys in attempting suicide three to one, and boys outnumber girls in successful suicides three to one; the ratio of attempted to successful suicide is about 100 to 1. The suicidal method most in favor was the use of drugs—aspirin, barbiturates, and tranquilizers. Some attempts at suicide seem to be manifestations of risk-taking behavior.

The core factor in the formation of a suicidal personality in childhood is thought to be a loss of love, real and fantasied. The part played by depression may be relatively small. In the adolescent, identity crisis may play the role that depression plays in the adult.

Prognosis

Symptomatic treatment is usually effective but offers no safeguard against the occurrence of similar reactions in the future, unless the underlying neurotic conflict is resolved and some measure of insight furnished to the child.

Management

As with the other neurotic conditions, intensive psychotherapy is the treatment of choice for the depressive reaction. Antidepressive drugs, such as amitriptyline (Elavil), may be indicated when the phenomenological picture is similar to the depressions of adult life, with marked loss of self-esteem, withdrawal from social interaction, depressive affect, self-accusation, and self-deprecation. In cases of attempted suicide in children, it is better to hospitalize the patient for a period after the attempt. Tranquilizers and antidepressants can be used as adjuncts, but the therapeutic aim should be insight, rather than reassurance.

REFERENCES

Anthony, E. J. An experimental approach to the psychopathology of childhood—Encopresis. Br. J. Med. Psychol., *30:* 146, 1957.
Anthony, E. J. An experimental approach to the psychopathology of childhood—Sleep disturbances. Br. J. Med. Psychol., *32:* 19, 1959.
Freud, S. *Collected Papers*, vol. 3. Hogarth Press, London, 1959.
Hartmann, H. Problems of infantile neurosis: A discussion. Psychoanal. Study Child, *9:* 16, 1954.
Kanner, L. *Child Psychiatry*, ed. 3. Charles C Thomas, Springfield, Ill., 1957.
Sandler, J., and Joffe, W. G. Notes on childhood depression. Int. J. Psychoanal., *46:* 88, 1965.

38.2. PSYCHOPHYSIOLOGIC DISORDERS

Introduction

Psychophysiologic disorders in children are a rather heterogeneous group of conditions in which the symptoms are due to a chronic and exaggerated state of the normal physiological expression of emotion, with feeling repressed. Such long-continued visceral states may eventually lead to structural changes.

Anorexia Nervosa

Anorexia nervosa is a serious and sometimes life-endangering condition characterized by a self-imposed, severe dietary limitation that leads to extreme loss of weight, serious malnutrition, malaise, and other associated symptoms.

Although it is most common in young adults, anorexia nervosa can occur at puberty or even before. The most typical history is that of the slightly obese youngster who decides to go on a self-imposed and often severe diet. The child and his parents are often pleased with the resulting weight loss until it becomes excessive, at which point efforts to encourage the child into a more reasonable intake are found to be futile. The child becomes increasingly malnourished and gaunt but clings to the idea that he is improving his health. He may continue with exercises, again of a self-imposed nature. Restlessness is common. Body reserves are generally used up. Blood sugar drops, and the youngster may suffer a circulatory collapse.

The premorbid personality of the youngster with anorexia nervosa is usually constricted, compulsive, and rigid. Hypersensitivity is a common characteristic, and some of these children have schizoid traits. The mechanism of denial is prominent.

It has been postulated that the psychodynamics of the anorexic child involves the entanglement of sexual and aggressive instincts with the concept of food intake. These basically immature youngsters fear growing up. Eating becomes a destructive oral-aggressive act, and it also has sexual connotations. In attempting to ward off dangerous instinctual impulses, the child also wards off eating.

Most of these youngsters have probably been overprotected by one or both parents. As with most other psychosomatic disorders, the child has had a close and markedly ambivalent tie to one parent. The disorder tends to occur somewhat more commonly in girls than in boys. By the time the disorder is well-advanced, one parent, if not both, has usually become overconcerned and oversolicitous and may spend long hours bribing, threatening, and otherwise attempting to get the child to eat.

Anorexia nervosa is a nonclassic psychophysiologic disorder in which it is difficult to postulate the existence of a biological factor. Most of the symptoms can be explained on the basis of severe psychological difficulties. Once the child begins to eat again, all the physical problems disappear. However, there is apt to be a swing back to obesity, which probably does include a biological factor.

The parents must be convinced that there is a large psychological contribution. All parental efforts toward enticing or threatening the child into eating must be discontinued, and the child must be convinced that his dietary intake is totally up to him.

The child must be helped to understand not

only that his dieting is excessive and harmful to himself but also that it is based on his unwillingness to grow up. His nutritional intake must be detached from his aggressive and sexual struggles while these other problems are dealt with.

If it becomes necessary to feed the patient intravenously or by nasal tube, the child must be helped to understand that he himself has caused the situation and that the measures undertaken are not provoked by the physicians' hostility but are practical requirements. When the child divorces his eating from his other difficulties, his physical status begins to improve, and his emotional problems can be worked on in a more leisurely and classical fashion.

Obesity

Obesity in youngsters begins to be diagnosed as a recognized and clearly identified syndrome during the grade school years. The obesity is apt to interfere with the child's participation in normal childhood activities, particularly athletics. Taunts from other children further isolate the obese child, who turns increasingly to eating and less to ordinary physical activities. Sensitivity about obesity tends to become enhanced at puberty. At this time, many of these youngsters begin to take dieting more seriously. Also, families tend to pay less attention to obesity during prepuberty than at adolescence. Statistically, obesity in children is more prevalent when the parents are obese.

Some children become overweight because of purely endocrine difficulties, but such cases are relatively rare. Most obese youngsters may have developed this condition as a result of perpetuated and exaggerated oral needs. The orally oriented child has great needs and demands much from his environment. Rarely is anyone able to meet such excessive needs for love and attention, and so the child tries to assuage them by an increase in caloric intake. Many obese children come from families in which food is overvalued. Mothers who themselves are oral in nature tend to feed the infant whenever he is uncomfortable, regardless of the reason for his discomfort. The young child builds a pathway from need to eating. He often has little if any motivation to diet because there are no other routes through which he can meet his oral needs.

There may be genetic, constitutional, biological, and psychological factors contributing to the overeating that results in obesity. Certain children, although obese, are not particularly maladjusted, and their obesity can be kept under control without great difficulty.

Proper management of the obese child involves a thorough study of the family and of the child himself. If the family tends toward overweight and the youngster's obesity is not excessive, few if any therapeutic measures may be necessary. If, on the other hand, the youngster reveals the psychological characteristics typical of many obese children—immaturity, hypersensitivity, and insatiability—more stringent therapeutic measures may be necessary.

Some physicians, especially pediatricians and child psychiatrists, have found group therapy for obese adolescents to be effective. However, it is not a good approach until a youngster develops more desire to become attractive than he had during the latency years.

Bronchial Asthma

Bronchial asthma is characterized by recurrent episodes of a wheezing type of dyspnea with labored and prolonged expiration. The symptoms are primarily due to a narrowing of the smaller bronchi and bronchioles. Although the condition may occur at almost any time in life, it often originates during childhood.

The recurrent attacks of wheezing dyspnea may come on as a result of exposure to a particular allergen, during a period of emotional stress, or without apparent reason and may last from a few minutes to several days. The labored breathing may be mild or reach the point where the child needs the assistance of an artificial respirator.

An attack of bronchial asthma is physically uncomfortable and produces anxiety in the child and the parents. Children with bronchial asthma frequently reveal overt emotional difficulties. Some physicians attribute them to the asthma itself, but others feel that they are a contributing cause. Probably both factors are involved.

As a result of repeated asthmatic attacks and the additional limitations imposed by medical management, many of these youngsters lead relatively secluded, quiet lives. They often have other psychosomatic difficulties, such as eczema and other skin problems.

Asthmatic children can be broadly divided

into two groups. One group show a number of neurotic symptoms and relatively few strong allergic reactions. They respond well to treatment in special residential centers for asthmatic children. The other group show fewer neurotic symptoms and less improvement when separated from parents and treated in a residential center.

A complete physical and psychiatric evaluation often gives important clues to the biological and psychological factors involved. Some youngsters do not respond well to psychiatric measures and present a lesser amount of psychopathology; immunologic and autoimmunologic factors appear to be predominant in these children. In other youngsters, the neurotic features are more prominent, and environmental manipulation and psychiatric treatment are more effective. There are, of course, children with combinations of both; for them, total team management is essential. In some children, separation from the family psychopathology leads to marked improvement in the asthma, even without medication or other therapeutic measures. The children most apt to benefit by this environmental manipulation are those with more neurotic features and fewer allergic problems.

Treatment of the child's parents is essential when the youngster's emotional difficulties are predominant, and some therapeutic assistance to parents is usually necessary even when the child's asthma is primarily of an allergic nature. Secondary gain accruing to the child from his asthmatic attacks should be minimized. Physical activities should be encouraged whenever they are not contraindicated by the asthma itself.

Functional Constipation

Functional constipation is a chronic condition primarily due to emotional problems in which the bowel is evacuated only at long intervals and with difficulty.

The typical history of a child with functional constipation reveals that his difficulty began early, usually during his first year. The child did not have a daily bowel movement as the parents wished, so they used manipulations to produce a daily movement. Slowly, the child became increasingly recalcitrant about evacuation, and the parents became increasingly concerned. By the time a youngster has reached school age with this condition, he is often quite constipated. The parents have often instituted a regimen of suppositories, enemas, or mineral oil. The evacuations the child does produce may be large and painful.

The majority of cases of chronic constipation in children result from emotional problems, rather than neurological problems. Once the child begins to resist parent demands and withhold feces, an atonic colon that performs poorly tends to develop. Such atonicity is further enhanced by parental use of laxatives, enemas, and suppositories.

Children with functional constipation have literally chosen to resist parental demands by not giving the very thing the parent seems most anxious to receive—a bowel movement every day. The personality of one or the other parent may be predominantly anal in nature, leading the parent to focus on the child's bowel habits in a demanding and forceful way. The children may present predominantly anal characteristics, being obstinate, ambivalent, and generally passive-aggressive.

Treatment is primarily directed to the parents, first to help them see how preoccupied they are with the child's bowel function and to understand their behavior as causative. They usually need considerable support and encouragment to reduce their intervention. Although the child usually reduces or gives up his symptom with the removal of the parental pressure, the characterologic traits may require psychotherapy. In the beginning of treatment, it may be useful to prescribe regular doses of mineral oil or some other stool-softening agent to prevent painful defecation.

Ulcerative Colitis

Ulcerative colitis is a serious chronic condition characterized by recurrent episodes of severe, bloody diarrhea. It is accompanied by anorexia, weight loss, and anemia. There are characteristic changes in the mucosa of the lower bowel and occasionally in the terminal ileum. An individual attack may last from a few weeks to a few months, after which the symptoms may abate but rarely disappear entirely. Further attacks tend to occur when the child is under emotional tension.

It has been suggested that children with ulcerative colitis can be divided into two relatively distinct personality types. By far the most common are those with obsessional personalities. Their pseudomature adjustment is interrupted by brief episodes of infantile dependent behavior. When the child develops an attack of ulcerative colitis, he characteristically becomes whiney, depressed, and demanding. A smaller number of children with ulcerative colitis are querulous, demanding, and manipulative. Their symptoms are somewhat less dramatic but more constant.

The parents of children with ulcerative colitis present more than the average amount of psychopathology, but there does not appear to be any single type of family dynamics characteristic of this disorder.

The peripheral circulating blood of the patient with ulcerative colitis contains some as yet unidentified substance that is toxic to colon cells. Two basic questions remain unanswered. What is the specific antigen in the blood and its exact location? What is the original triggering device that sets off the attack of colitis? One can presume, but as yet not prove, that emotional tension is the original triggering device. It is also presumed, but as yet not proved, that, once the process begins, the reduction in emotional tension does not necessarily lead to a remission in the disease.

Management usually involves some dietary restrictions, particularly during an exacerbation of the disease. Iron may be prescribed to combat the anemia. A considerable number of these children eventually come to surgery, where a one-stage or two-stage colectomy is performed. The most successful management of children with ulcerative colitis is based on a team approach involving a child psychiatrist, surgeon, pediatrician, and social worker. The child and his parents are seen by all members of the team, and a joint decision is reached on the basis of the findings of each team member. Psychotherapy for the child and case work for the parents are helpful.

Juvenile Diabetes Mellitus

Juvenile diabetes mellitus is a chronic condition that involves faulty carbohydrate metabolism as a result of difficulties in pancreatic function. It persists throughout life.

Emotional problems play a role in the juvenile diabetic. There is the likelihood that emotional trauma is a triggering mechanism to the onset of the diabetes. The general assumption is that there is a physiological predisposition and that in some fashion emotional unrest brings on the disorder. Some studies have shown that a high percentage of these children come from emotionally disordered families.

The parents need a reasonably full education concerning diabetes. They should be allowed the opportunity to ask questions and receive honest answers. The parents may have to assume the majority of the responsibility for insulin dosage and diet. As soon as the youngster is sufficiently capable, he should take over increasing responsibility for these matters. He also should be given an explanation of diabetes commensurate with his age. Whenever psychiatric difficulties are uncovered, they should be dealt with as adequately as possible.

REFERENCES

Bruch, H. Psychiatric aspects of obesity in children. Am. J. Psychiatry, *99:* 752, 1943.
Chess, S., Thomas, A., and Birch. H. *Your Child Is a Person*. Viking Press, New York, 1965.
Finch, S. M., and Hess, J. Ulcerative colitis in children. Am. J. Psychiatry, *118:* 819, 1962.
Frank, I., and Powell, M. *Psychosomatic Ailments in Childhood and Adolescence*. Charles C Thomas, Springfield, Ill., 1967.
Solnit, A., and Province, S., editors. *Modern Perspectives in Child Development*. International Universities Press, New York, 1963.
Weiss, E., and English, O. S. *Psychosomatic Medicine*, ed. 3. W. B. Saunders, Philadelphia, 1957.

38.3.   ANTISOCIAL PERSONALITY

Introduction

Modern concepts of juvenile delinquency suggest that children who are called delinquent are ill primarily in terms of society, in their inability to conform to the social milieu. Laws tend to reflect current morality, and children are caught up in intense personal conflicts in this rapidly shifting and changing culture.

Two types of sociopathic patterns can be described: (1) antisocial personality, characteristic of children and adolescents who are always in trouble, who seem not to profit from experience or punishment, and who have no loyalties to persons other than themselves; (2) dyssocial behavior, characteristic of children and adolescents who have been brought up in amoral or immoral families or institutions and who have identified with strong loyalties to a criminal element. Antisocial personality is listed in the standard nomenclature of the American Psychiatric Association under personality disorders and certain other nonpsychotic disorders, and dyssocial behavior is listed under conditions without manifest psychiatric disorder and nonspecific conditions.

The diagnosis of antisocial personality, "is reserved for individuals who are basically unsocialized and whose behavior pattern brings them repeatedly into conflict with society. They are incapable of significant loyalty to individuals, groups, or social values. They are grossly selfish, callous, irresponsible, impulsive, and unable to feel guilt or to learn from experience and punishment. Frustration tolerance is low. They tend to blame others or offer plausible rationalizations for their behavior. A mere history of repeated legal or social offenses is not sufficient to justify this diagnosis."

The diagnosis of dyssocial behavior "is for individuals who are not classifiable as antisocial personalities, but who are predatory and follow more or less criminal pursuits, such as racketeers, dishonest gamblers, prostitutes, and dope peddlers."

These types of personality disorders emerge out of a complex set of interactions among the genetic, constitutional, psychological, and social environmental factors. False learning, inadequate learning, or overlearning from one or both parents plays a special role in shaping the final behavioral pattern.

Epidemiology

The incidence of antisocial personality and dyssocial behavior varies from about 2 per cent to about 7 per cent of the childhood population. In boys, the major offenses are truancy, stealing, fire setting, vandalism, and cruelty to animals and human beings; in girls, the major offenses are stealing, shoplifting, and sexual promiscuity. The incidence of antisocial personality is higher in boys and in low-income, minority, and culturally deprived groups; it rises with the industrialization and urbanization of a population.

Causes

Any illness or defect that contributes to misperception of the external environment or the inability to identify with healthy personalities or the inability to inhibit hyperaggressive or hyperlibidinal behavior may contribute to the delinquent behavior pattern. This pattern may be influenced by mental retardation, epilepsy, brain damage, hyperkinesis, compulsion neurosis, childhood psychosis, and affect deprivation.

Current ideas about the psychopathology in delinquent behavior usually contain these four elements: (1) The child feels significant emotional deprivation and strongly resents it. (2) The child cannot establish his own range of skills because his parent have not set limits for him. (3) The parents, especially the mother, are very often overstimulating and inconsistent in their attitudes toward the child. (4) The child's behavior usually represents a vicarious source of pleasure and gratification for a parent and is often an expression of the parent's unconscious hostility toward the child, as the behavior is either overtly or covertly self-destructive to the child.

Clinical Features

In the absence of confusion due to toxic or organic factors, the child is usually superficially tense when he is brought to a psychiatrist by a parent, court worker, or social worker. He is often sullen, defiant, and flippant; he answers questions briefly and in a matter-of-fact tone, uses denial extensively, and tends to minimize the reasons for the referral. The child is usually reluctant to discuss inner emotional experiences, feelings, daydreams, jokes, favorite books, or television programs. He frequently projects personal difficulties onto a parent, sibling, or peer and almost always minimizes his involvement in any meaningful personal relationship. Guilt feelings are frequently not present or are glossed over quickly without much evidence of personal discomfort.

Those who are antisocial tend to be abrupt, cantankerous, impulsive, and easily frustrated. As the interviews progress, transient rage reactions often develop, and the explosive quality of their affective state is quite evident.

The dyssocial type of patient is usually shyer and more reticent in the interviews. Comments are rarely spontaneous, and answers to questions are usually clipped and abrupt. Inevitably, the issue of trust is brought up by the patient, and efforts are made to extract promises about confidential matters. It is apparently difficulty for these children to share dreams, daydreams, early memories, and favorite humorous stories.

Differential Diagnosis

Differential diagnosis requires a thorough and careful evaluation of the biological, psychological, and social factors that may contribute to the development of maladaptive behavior. A detailed and accurate history, physical and neurological examinations, and psychological and various laboratory tests are required to evaluate brain damage, mental retardation, and similar causes of the behavior. Direct observation of the child in an interview and skilled evaluation of the parents and perhaps of the parents and child together may give valuable clues to the possibility of a conscience defect, affect deprivation, major and significant loss of a loved person, or a connection between the parents' behavior and the child's antisocial symptoms.

Prognosis

The prognosis in treating antisocial personality and dyssocial behavior is poor to fair. The prognosis is much better if the behavior pattern emerges for the first time after the child starts school, if it is recognized promptly, if proper and adequate intervention occurs, and if both the child and his parents are motivated to explore the underlying sources of the behavior.

Management

Treatment involves a thorough diagnostic study and a definition of the extent and nature of the clinical problem. In most instances, it is necessary to work with the child and with the parents in a collaborative team approach.

Individual therapy usually has some special features that vary considerably from most other child psychotherapy. The presence of early childhood defects or distortions makes it necessary for the therapist to present himself consistently as a warm, understanding person. There should be a strong reality orientation in the collaborative process, with specific emphasis on requiring parents to set consistent and realistic limits on the child's behavior. There should be recognition of the high probability that the parents may not want to give up their vicarious and usually unconscious pleasure in the child's behavior.

Residential Treatment

In many instances, it is necessary to treat the delinquent in some type of residential institution to break the ties with the stimulative and destructive parent or to compensate in part for the absent or unavailable parental figure. The residential group attempt to focus on a child with weak and inadequate personality resources and to provide him with some nurture to compensate for his feeling of being unloved earlier in life.

Psychotherapy

Therapeutic work with delinquents, especially adolescents, requires much activity by the therapist. He should keep the patient talking, keep him active, keep him reality-oriented as much as possible, try to establish enough of a relationship so that the child can inhibit his tendency to act out impulses and can develop, instead, feelings of guilt, shame, and remorse—that is, the more classical neurotic personal feelings. The therapist should not encourage the emergence of instinctual behavior. The therapist should recognize the child's fear of loss of control over his own impulses. And the therapist should recognize the child's inevitable wish for consistent limit setting.

Drugs

The possibility of using antidepressants in conjunction with specific brief abreactive psychotherapies, phenothiazine drugs in the management of childhood psychoses, and mild tranquilizers and stimulants to aid in the management of hyperkinetic and impulse-ridden children seems promising.

REFERENCES

Aichhorn, A. *Wayward Youth.* Viking, New York, 1935.
Cloward, R. A., and Ohlin, L. E. *Delinquency and Opportunity: A Theory of Delinquent Gangs.* Free Press of Glencoe (Macmillan), New York, 1960.
Conger, J. J. A world they never knew: The family and social change. Daedalus, *100:* 1105, 1971.
Drucker, P. Rise of the knowledge worker. In *Britannica Book of the Year, 1973,* p. 15. The University of Chicago Press, Chicago, 1973.
Harris, T. G. Era of conscious action. In *Britannica Book of the Year, 1973,* p. 6. The University of Chicago Press, Chicago, 1973.
Johnson, A. M., and Szurek, S. A. The genesis of antisocial acting out in children and adults. Psychoanal. Q., *21:* 323, 1952.
Redl, F., and Wineman, D. *Controls from Within.* Free Press of Glencoe (Macmillan), New York, 1952.
Woolf, M. The child's moral development. In *Searchlights on Delinquency,* K. R. Eissler, editor, p. 263. International Universities Press, New York, 1949.

38.4. OTHER PERSONALITY DISORDERS

Concept of Personality

Personality or character is determined in large measure by the interaction between the instincts and the environment. A person's habitual patterns of behavior, the nature and design of which are unconsciously determined, are the outward manifestation of his inner interests and, in particular, his instinctual impulses.

Personality formation is a process of progressive integration. The organization of primitive faculties and impulses in the infant is chaotic. Later, as the child learns to adapt needs to external conditions, these impulses and the faculties that permitted their expression and fulfillment are organized to form specific patterns of behavior. Because these patterns assure gratification of the child's basic needs, he is—at least theoretically—no longer completely dependent on the crucial adults in his environment. However, the child's personality structure reflects his responses to the conscious and unconscious components of his parents' personalities and his perception of their conscious and unconscious attitudes toward him.

According to psychoanalytic theory, the ego seeks to regulate instinctual expression to conform with the demands of the external world. In the early stages of development, the parents function as auxiliary egos and assist in the control of the instincts. Subsequently, parental dictates with regard to instinctual discharge are internalized to form the child's superego or conscience. The superego imposes further controls on instinctual expression, insofar as violations of internalized parental values give rise to guilt feelings. The nature of the child's instinctual expressions and his capacity to delay discharge determine personality structure.

In adolescence there is a quantitative increase of instinctual pressure. The results are an abrupt withdrawal of cathexis from the parents. Narcissism occurs when self-inflation takes the form of arrogance, rebellion, defiance of rules, and flouting of authority. The sex drive, emancipation from parental authority, the aggressive drive to achieve and dominate, and the search for identity are the outstanding challenges that confront an adolescent, and these challenges are conditioned by previously established relationships and reactions. A previously well-knit personality is loosened under the impact of the profound biological changes and drives clamoring for satisfaction and of the prohibitions opposing the expression of such drives. Modes of behavior, previously satisfactory, are often not adequate to cope with the changes, and the resulting behavior may frighten teachers, parents, and doctors. Yet, the adolescent's behavior may be quite normal.

Assessment of Psychopathology

It is difficult to draw a line of demarcation between mental health and mental illness in childhood and adolescence. During the early years of life, the relative strengths of the id and the ego are in a constant state of flux; adaptive and defensive mechanisms, normal and pathogenic processes, frequently merge. The transition from one developmental level to the next may constitute a potential psychological hazard, for at this point major or minor stress is most likely to produce arrest in development, malfunction, fixation, or regression.

Symptoms manifested in childhood and adolescence do not necessarily carry the same significance they do in adult life, when typical symptom complexes lead to specific diagnoses. The presenting symptoms of immature persons are too unstable to provide reliable criteria for purposes of assessment. Instead, the assessment of child psychopathology hinges on one crucial variable—the child's capacity to move forward in progressive stages until maturation has been achieved, his personality is sufficiently integrated, and he has adapted successfully to the social community. Emotional upsets become significant when they exert an adverse effect on the child's over-all development.

Indications of possible psychopathology in childhood and adolescence cannot be properly evaluated if they are viewed in isolation or according to preconceived, rigid standards and criteria. They must be considered in relation to the person's total functioning and in terms of their potential effect on his development.

Personality Disorders

Personality disorders represent relatively fixed pathological trends in personality development and functioning that have become a way of life. According to the American Psychiatric Association's second edition of *Diagnostic and Statistical Manual of Mental Disorders* (DSM-II), "this group of disorders is characterized by deeply ingrained maladaptive patterns of behavior that are perceptibly different in quality from psychotic and neurotic symptoms. Generally, these are life-long patterns, often recognizable by the time of adolescence or earlier."

Personality disturbances are deep-seated disturbances; as such, their inherent structure can rarely be altered by therapy. However, prolonged therapy may lead to an improvement in functioning.

Children and adolescents with personality disorders solve their conflicts simply by changing their personalities. This change does not cause subjective feelings of discomfort unless they are confronted with the harsh realities of life, at which time they are forced to realize that their adaptive capacities are inadequate.

Clinical syndromes in childhood and adolescence are shaped by age and developmental status, level of personality organization, and the nature and quality of the child's interaction with his environment.

Paranoid Personality

Many of the elements described below in connection with the schizoid personality are present in this syndrome, coupled with an exquisite sensitivity in interpersonal relations. Suspiciousness, mistrust, envy, jealousy, and stubbornness are characteristic. Most marked is the tendency toward projection, a mechanism of defense by which one's own internal inadequacies and immaturities are attributed to others. The child's sensitivity may be due to an unusual constitutional sensitivity of the ego, enhanced by a sense of insecurity and inadequacy and by the turbulent, suspicious, distrustful attitudes of disturbed parents.

The goal of treatment is to strengthen the child's confidence, sense of security, and safety; to help him to develop appropriate reality-testing; and to ameliorate family pathology. The mechanism of projection is always dealt with directly and focused on clearly with adolescents.

Cyclothymic Personality

Adult cyclothymic personalities, according to DSM-II, are characterized by "recurring and alternating periods of depression and elation." These mood swings "are not readily attributable to external circumstances." This diagnosis is almost never applied to a child and infrequently to an adolescent. Mood changes in a child are influenced by parental attitudes, the family milieu, and peer relationships. Mood swings are part of adolescent change.

Children who are subjected to the chronic disapproval of their parents may be predisposed to the development of a cyclothymic personality. At first glance, they appear mature, happy, and active, but they are extremely sensitive, react with tears or depression when they are punished, and reveal marked mood variations, alternating between happiness and sadness, with minimal stimuli. However, not all children with these characteristics develop this disorder, nor do all adolescents.

The basic pathology stems from a conflict between a severe, punitive superego and powerful primitive unconscious impulses. Early childhood traumata, such as desertion, precipitate hostility, which is turned inward and is manifested clinically as depression.

Treatment is intensive and should involve the parents.

Schizoid Personality

Isolation is the most prominent symptom of the persons in this group (see Figure 1). They are further characterized by an inability to form close relationships with others, an inability to express normal feelings of aggression, and, in general, a tendency to withdraw emotionally from the environment. These children and adolescents are quiet, shy, obedient, sensitive, and retiring. Frequently, they become more withdrawn and introverted at puberty, and sometimes they become eccentric. Children with schizoid personalities show a marked infantilism, so that even their attempts to meet the ordinary problems of childhood evoke feelings of frustration, which give rise to poorly handled hostility. Fantasy becomes a common refuge. Most of these children grow up to be isolated adolescents and adults; some develop psychotic episodes.

The histories of these patients point up their life-long isolation from parents, siblings, and others; there is a strong possibility that this pattern is constitutionally determined. However, almost without exception the parents of such children are themselves without close

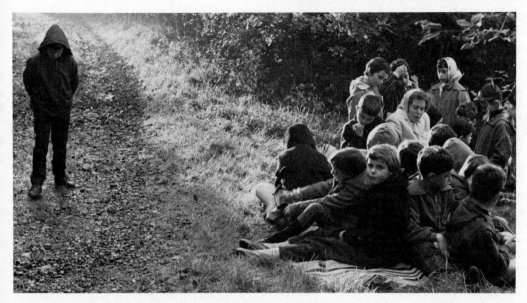

FIGURE 1. In this illustration a youngster appears isolated from the group. If rejection or alienation by peers occurs during preadolescence, future adjustment may be damaged. This is particularly noteworthy in the schizoid personality. (Courtesy of Leonard Freed for Magnum Photos, Inc.)

relationships, despite a facade of sociability. These parents also manifest a marked ambivalence toward their child; they attach great importance to his physical care but are incapable of providing him with emotional warmth or acceptance.

With therapy, such children and adolescents may develop some warmth and social facade, but they return to their solitary activities with relief. The more severe cases may develop psychoses in adolescence under the stress of phase-specific tasks.

Explosive Personality

This behavior is characterized by gross outbursts of rage expressed verbally or physically. The child may be repentant after a particular outburst, but recurrences are invariable. These patients are excitable, aggressive, and overresponsive to environmental pressures. According to DSM-II, "it is the intensity of the outbursts and the individual's inability to control them which distinguishes this group." Frustration, irritability, temper tantrums, destructive behavior, and a fierce resentment provoke him to strike out at the environment.

Treatment aims are twofold. One is to help the patient to develop healthier modes of expression and adequate gratifications. The other

is to work with the family to relieve the parents' pathological attitudes toward the child.

Obsessive-Compulsive Personality

Excessive rigidity and conformity, overconscientiousness, and inhibition of emotional expression are marked in these children and adolescents. They show an obsessive concern with adherence to standards of conscience or conformity, and they may have an inordinate capacity for work, without the usual capacity for relaxation.

Such children and adolescents are fixated at the anal stage of libidinal development. The resulting immaturities are countered by a punitive superego. The parents of such children are compulsive, driving, perfectionistic persons with very high standards who serve as models, and their rearing of the child is guaranteed to produce an obsessive-compulsive person.

Treatment seeks to develop a more balanced intrapsychic relationship among instinctual expressions, coping mechanisms, and the dictates of the superego. The parents' attitudes must also be altered.

Hysterical Personality

These behavior patterns are characterized by excitability, emotional instability, overreactivity, and self-dramatization, which is always attention-seeking and often seductive. These patients are also immature, self-centered, often vain, and usually dependent on others. Symptom formation of a conversion or dissociative nature may occur with stress and is more frequent in adolescence. Cultural influences play a role in encouraging conversion symptoms.

No matter what immaturities are present, the rigid superego finds them unacceptable, and thus the ego must create defenses to keep the impulses unconscious. Often, the environment invites the gratification of these mature impulses. The symptom symbolically solves the conflict; the real problem remains unsolved.

The intrapsychic conflicts must be worked out, and the family must be involved in any therapeutic program where possible.

Asthenic Personality

This diagnosis is rarely made in children or adolescents. In adults it is characterized by easy fatigability, low energy level, lack of enthusiasm, marked incapacity for enjoyment, and oversensitivity to physical and emotional stress, according to DSM-II. Constitutional factors may predispose the patient to this disorder. If the syndrome is identified, the patient should not be pushed to perform beyond his abilities, and the environment should be supporting and nonstressful. Usually, asthenia is a defense against murderous rage, suicidal ideation, and punitive behavior directed toward the family.

Passive-Aggressive Personality

Passive-Dependent Type. Dependence on one's parents is normal during childhood. This diagnosis is applied to those whose dependency needs exceed normal limits. Such a child or adolescent appears helpless and indecisive, clings to others, and is obviously neither autonomous nor independent to the degree considered healthy for his age or stage of development. Typically, he is overprotected by parents who often have mixed reactions about him, encourage a helpless and clinging attitude, and inhibit his development of independence because of their own guilt feelings. Treatment is designed to facilitate the healthy maturation of the child or adolescent and to correct unhealthy parental attitudes.

Passive-Aggressive Type. This clinical picture occurs most frequently in children and adolescents. Passive obstructionism, inefficiency, procrastination, stubbornness, and pouting are hallmarks. This behavior is an expression of resentment, invoked by excessive parental demands. If any overt expression of hostility is deemed unacceptable by the parent, the child may develop more subtle rebellious behavior. A classic reaction to such parental behavior is the child who dawdles endlessly over meals. The goal of treatment is to help the child or adolescent express his resentments and hostilities openly and in more acceptable ways. At the same time, his parents are made aware of their suppressive. critical attitudes and are helped to correct them.

Inadequate Personality

According to DSM-II, this behavior pattern is characterized by ineffectual responses to emotional, social, intellectual, and physical demands. Physical examination shows the patient to be within normal limits. The patient manifests inadaptability, ineptitude, poor judgment, social instability, and a lack of physical and emotional stamina. The plasticity of the child and the workability of the adolescent and their families can make this diagnostic category less gloomy and foreboding. Such a label is difficult to support, is questionable, and is rarely made.

REFERENCES

Chess, S., and Thomas, A., editors. *Annual Progress in Child Psychiatry and Child Development*. Brunner/Mazel, New York, 1972.
Feinstein, S. C., Giovacchini, P., and Miller, A. A. *Adolescent Psychiatry*, vol. 1. Basic Books, New York, 1971.
Group for the Advancement of Psychiatry. *Basic Concepts in Child Psychiatry*. Group for the Advancement of Psychiatry, New York, 1957.
Group for the Advancement of Psychiatry. *Normal Adolescence*. Group for the Advancement of Psychiatry, New York, 1968.
Teicher, J. D. Normal psychological changes in adolescence. *Calif. Med. 85:* 171, 1956.
Teicher, J. D. Psychotherapy of adolescents. *Calif. Med. 90:* 29, 1959.

38.5.   DRUG DEPENDENCE AND ALCOHOLISM

Definition

The second edition of the American Psychiatric Association's *Diagnostic and Statistical*

Manual of Mental Disorders (DSM-II) states that the category of drug dependence applies to patients who are addicted to or dependent on drugs other than alcohol, tobacco, or ordinary caffeine-containing beverages. The diagnosis requires evidence of habitual use or a clear sense of need for the drug. Withdrawal symptoms are not the only evidence of dependence; although always present when opium derivatives are withdrawn, they may be entirely absent when cocaine or marijuana is withdrawn. The category of alcoholism, according to DSM-II, is for patients whose alcohol intake is great enough to damage their physical health or their personal or social functioning or when it has become a prerequisite to normal functioning.

Drug dependence resides in the psychological structure and functioning of the person, rather than in the pharmacological effect of the drug. Drug dependence is a mode of adaptation, a behavior reflection of psychological stress, an attempt to master intrapsychic imbalance. The three areas of ego functioning to focus on are the ego and awareness of affects, especially anxiety and depression; object- and self-representation; and modification of consciousness.

Substances

Opioids

Heroin, meperidine, and other opioids are the drugs of choice for most American addicts. Some patients suffer only mild withdrawal symptoms when they are deprived of heroin, indicating that they have been using very diluted heroin. In such cases they may be addicted not only to the drug but to the needle and to the ritual of shooting up.

Marijuana

Marijuana cigarettes are prepared from the flowering tops of the hemp plant, cannabis. Like alcohol, marijuana relaxes inhibitions. Unlike opiates, marijuana is not associated with physical dependence, and persons who use it do not develop increasing tolerance necessitating larger and larger doses.

Amphetamines

Truck drivers who must remain awake for long stretches, students cramming for examinations, and writers faced with deadlines have long known the power of amphetamines to induce wakefulness. Amphetamines can be addictive and extremely dangerous. When amphetamines are used in large doses and then suddenly withdrawn, serious consequences may result. Also, large doses may produce psychotic reactions.

Barbiturates

Barbiturates are the most lethal of all drugs when alcohol is excluded. Withdrawal from a confirmed dependence requires careful procedures to avoid lethal results and often fatal convulsive reactions. Adolescents using barbiturates usually use other drugs, and the drugs are symbolic of their personality disturbances.

Proprietary Drugs

Cough medicines that contain codeine or alcohol can provide an easy path to addiction. Among hospitalized adolescent addicts, tremendous quantities of such drugs have been taken either before or with heroin.

Hallucinogenic Drugs

Mind-expanding drugs alter sensory perception and produce hallucinations. Such substances as lysergic acid diethylamide (LSD-25), mescaline or peyote, and psilocybin may precipitate psychosis, have serious side effects, or lead to addiction to other drugs.

Glue

The glue used in making model airplanes is both a stimulant and an intoxicant, and sniffing it can have serious toxic effects. The underlying depression of the young child is marked.

Gasoline

Gasoline is used as an intoxicant, particularly when money is not available for drugs or other costly substances.

Alcohol

Although alcoholism is generally considered an adult disorder that develops over a period of many years, the use of alcohol by adolescents and young people is very common and is increasing. Wine and beer are readily available, and they are cheaper than barbiturates and often used with barbiturates. Actual alcoholism is seen increasingly in young people. Treatment is both medical and psychiatric.

Epidemiology

Data about the incidence and prevalence of addiction and about the distribution of narcotics addicts in the United States are limited. However, an increasing number of high school and college students are arrested for possession, use, or sale of drugs of all varieties. The changes in patterns of drug use, the increasing involvement of young people from all socio-economic classes, and the movement of drug dependence downward into ever-younger groups of children suggest the widening dimensions of the problem.

Treatment

Most deaths associated with addiction are from overdoses of narcotics. Furthermore, addicts of all ages are particularly susceptible to infectious diseases—including malaria, tetanus, syphilis, bacterial and mycotic endocarditis, and infectious hepatitis—that can result from using shared, unsterile needles for injecting heroin.

Most treatment programs for addicts have been failures. Maintenance is being seen as a possibility for adults, but it is difficult to accept maintenance on drugs as a satisfactory aim in the case of children and adolescents.

To treat addiction successfully, one must study the society in which it flourishes. If necessary, schools and recreational institutions must be altered so that they provide positive growth experiences. At the same time, realistically oriented medical and psychiatric care must be provided for those youngsters who have succumbed to drug use.

The addict's ambivalence and fear of aggressive wishes usually make dyadic situations unbearable, but clinic or group therapy is useful. The patient becomes aware of painful affective feelings and finds that they are self-limiting and nondestructive. Supportive explanations and didactic instruction help the youth discover his ego disturbances and deal with his feelings. The therapist must interpret and deal with impulses acted out.

REFERENCES

California Conference of Local Mental Health Directors. *Position Paper on Substance Abuse, Alcoholism and Other Drug Abuse.* San Diego, 1972.
Freedman, A. M., and Wilson, E. A. Childhood and adolescent addictive disorders. Pediatrics, *34:* 283, 425, 1964.
Glasscote, R. *The Treatment of Drug Abuse.* American Psychiatric Association, Washington, D.C., 1973.
Group for the Advancement of Psychiatry. *Drug Misuse: A Psychiatric View of a Group for the Advancement of Psychiatry: Modern Dilemma.* New York, 1971.
Krystal, H., and Raskin, A. A. *Drug Dependence.* Wayne State University Press. Detroit, 1970.
Shick, J. F. E. The use of amphetamine in the Haight-Ashbury sub-culture. J. Psychedelic Drugs, 1973.
Wikler, A. Drug addiction. In *Practice of Medicine,* F. Tice, editor, p. 627. Prior, Hagerstown, Md., 1953.

38.6.   SEXUAL DEVIATIONS

Introduction

Sexual deviation is a label that should rarely be used in childhood. Fixed disorders in adolescence may warrant a diagnostic term, but it should be used only when the condition is regarded as the major personality disturbance, with such a degree of chronicity and pervasiveness in personality functioning as to dominate the adolescent's orientation toward social life. Some transiently homosexual behavior is known to be characteristic of many healthy boys and girls in the late preadolescent and early adolescent years. The label of sexual deviation applied to a child is associated with more immature emotional development than when applied to an adult.

The fact that many sexual activities, such as masturbation, are practically universal in society does not mean that they are necessarily normal. How a child achieves genital sexual satisfaction usually depends on his period of sexual development. In normal development, he passes through periods of early masturbation, homosexual attachment to peers, and sexual strivings that lead toward intercourse with a mature partner of the opposite sex. However, normal development does not always proceed smoothly. There may be departures from the normal sexual patterns at any point during childhood.

Masturbation

Children begin masturbating when they are very young: 1- and 2-year-olds play with their genitalia and obtain satisfaction from doing so. Some children continue to masturbate more actively than others, in which cases the activity is almost always stimulated, consciously or unconsciously, by the parents. Small gangs, usually of boys, sometimes use masturbation as an acting-out behavior. Oral copulation and other kinds of sexual deviation are frequently associated with it. Adolescent masturbation is characterized by an end point of satisfaction and is thus a more overtly sexual activity. Childhood masturbation is normal and is regarded as pathological only when it is excessive or when it is a source of anxiety for the child. Children who masturbate excessively usually suffer from guilt, as a result of cultural values imparted to them by their parents. Some young children become excessively involved with masturbation and seem to have a compulsion to carry it on. These children usually masturbate because of anxiety. Such children are nearly always involved with other sexual activities at the same time.

Masturbation is accompanied by fantasies. The content of the masturbation fantasies during the latter part of the anal-sadistic period and during the phallic and latency periods and adolescence is erotic or aggressive or both. The erotic fantasies are sensual in nature, and the love object is the parent of the opposite sex if the fantasy is heterosexual and the parent of the same sex if homosexual. The fantasies also have a sadistic or masochistic and an active or passive coloring. The aggressive fantasies are hostile and destructive in nature and have as the object one or the other parent.

The fantasies produce great mental torture and severe feelings of fear, guilt, and horror. The suffering becomes more than the child can tolerate. He tries to get rid of it by altering his behavior. Since he has the fantasies while masturbating, he comes to regard the masturbation as the cause of the fantasies, although actually they are coincidental. Therefore, he becomes frightened of his desire to masturbate and tries hard to stop it. At the same time he tries to deny the fantasies either by repressing them or by thinking of other things. That is why there is partial or complete cessation of masturbation during the latency period. During adolescence the sexual desires and, therefore, the desire to masturbate increase because of the physiologic changes of puberty. This increase reactivates the unconscious fantasies, which attempt to break through the repression and become conscious again. This attempt of the

repressed fantasies to become conscious is the cause of the adolescent's worry about the effects of masturbation on him. He is unconsciously afraid that the old horrifying repressed fantasies will return to torment him or will come true. His turmoil is only increased by threats, warnings, or punishments by parents.

Sexual Orientation Disturbance

It is normal for the child to engage in nongenital relationships with peers of his own sex. As he begins adolescence, the youngster develops relationships with children of both sexes. Homosexuality can then be regarded as part of the older child's confusion about his sexual identity. Whenever children are placed together in institutions, such as schools and residential homes, there is a stirring up of homosexual activity.

Some children seem to have confused gender identification and demonstrate at a young age that they are uncomfortable with the opposite sex. Typical is the boy who is overly attached to his mother and dresses and behaves in a feminine manner.

Certain preconditions in the family unit contribute to the development of homosexuality. Often stressed is the combination of a weak or absent father and a dominating, harsh mother. Boys in such households are unable to form an appropriate identification with the anatomical, psychological, and social roles of the man. Their attitudes toward women are distorted by sado-masochistic impulses, and toward men they develop passive and submissive homosexual attitudes. In girls, the same fear of and aggression toward the mother may be observed. The girl harbors a secret wish to be loved exclusively by the father and interprets his indifference as rejection because of her phallic deficiency. During adolescence she may turn away from men entirely and seek the company, admiration, or love of other females.

In early adolescence the avoidance of girls is a homosexual defense that may carry over into the late teens. Usually, there are homosexual fantasies of mutual masturbation and fellatio, a seductive mother, and a passive, retiring father. The occurrence of homosexual behavior or the fear of being a homosexual is often related to anxiety over not attaining the masculine ideal. A perception of marked deviance from the masculine ideal is one antecedent of the feeling that one has homosexual wishes and facilitates the probability of engaging in homosexual behavior.

Exhibitionism

The little child examines and displays his genitals with pride. In the adult, various activities such as exhibiting, looking, and stroking are preludes to the sexual act. Where exhibiting becomes an end in itself, it is a perversion. Such behavior always serves as a reassurance against castration. The purpose is not to seduce; seeing a nude female body destroys sexual desire. Exhibitionists enjoy the terror and fear engendered in the spectator. They confess to impotence with girls and have scorn and hatred for them. Often shy, they fear close relationships but seek admiration and reassurance about genital development in their display of it. Usually, there is a history of self-examination before the mirror.

Transvestitism

In transvestitism the child may be said to be deprived of normal gender identity. This development phenomenon may or may not be related to homosexuality. The child who practices transvestitism is usually involved in a pathological relationship with the parent of the opposite sex. Transvestitism is transitory but undetected in most adolescents. The boy really wishes to see the female figure—garbed in bra, swim suit, corset—but with the reassurance that his penis is there.

Abnormal Relations

Adults sometimes use children for their own sexual pleasure and encourage youngsters to indulge in sexual activity with animals and objects. Children who are brought to a psychiatrist because of excessive sexual activity have often suffered from adult sexual exploitation, including rape. Consummated incest is most common between fathers and daughters, but a *forme fruste* occurs frequently between mothers and sons. Because they are exposed to such intense sexual stimulation, these children have a compulsive need to relieve their own sexual tension.

Fetishism

As the child gradually separates from the parent he may want to cling to an object—a blanket, toy, or similar item—that for him represents the parent. This is an entirely normal development and can be considered a deviation only when the object becomes the primary choice of sexual satisfaction, a situation that can only develop much later. It is normal and common for adolescents to use an object to enhance sexual satisfaction.

Prostitution

Parents tend to push heterosexuality and sexual experiences too early. When standards are low at home, girls often engage in sexual relations quite early. When there has been considerable sexual seduction of the girl by the father or another man, the sexual drive is often intensified in adolescence. When coldness and rejection exist in the family and there is an aura of self-depreciation, girls often seek warmth and acceptance in physical contact, even though it may be destructive. When girls become involved in excessive sexual activity early in adolescence, it is almost always brought on by their having been exploited and sexually stimulated by adults. The deviant behavior leads to an increase in neurotic tension, which can only be relieved by excessive sexual activity. Classically, these adolescents present a bland, hysterical personality pattern.

Other Deviations

Other sexual devations are rarely seen in children and adolescents. Pedophilia, molesting a child sexually, is occasionally seen in adolescents. Sadism and masochism do occur, but they are clinical curiosities.

Treatment and Prognosis

Treatment consists mainly of understanding what the symptom means to the patient, understanding the compulsion and its repetitious activity, and relieving the patient's tension and redirecting his growth into healthy channels by attempting to make the compulsive process less satisfying to him.

The prognosis in these cases depends to a great extent on how early the child receives treatment and on how well the therapist is able to understand the family pattern and to view the symptoms as part of the child's total life experience. Management should involve a combination of psychiatric and legal approaches.

Older children are less responsive than young

children to treatment. When sexual deviation is present in the young child, he can be treated along with the entire family, thus exposing intrafamily tensions and abnormal relationships to therapeutic intervention. Workers have reported success with behavior modification therapy. Adolescents who are not engaging in homosexual activity but are using homosexual defenses seem to respond well to dynamically oriented treatment.

REFERENCES

Freud, S. Three essays on the theory of sexuality. In *Standard Edition of the Complete Psychological Works of Sigmund Freud*, vol. 7, p. 135. Hogarth Press, London, 1953.
Sperling, M. A study of deviate sexual behavior in children. In *Dynamic Psychopathology in Childhood*, L. Jessner and E. Pavenstedt, editors, p. 221, Grune & Stratton, New York, 1959.
Taylor, G. R. *Sex in History*. Thames & Hudson, London, 1962. *Wolfenden Report*. Stein & Day, New York, 1963.
Work, H. H. Sociopathic personality disorders. II. Sexual deviations. In *Comprehensive Textbook of Psychiatry*. A. M. Freedman and Harold I. Kaplan, editors, p. 1426. Williams & Wilkins, Baltimore, 1967.

38.7.   FUNCTIONAL PSYCHOSES

Introduction

Functional psychoses in childhood refer to syndromes for which the applicability of psychological forms of treatment is suggested. Special consideration is given to educational and environmental methods of prevention, psychotherapy, group psychotherapy, behavior therapy, milieu treatment, hospitalizations, or any or all of them combined. Minimum stress is placed on the use of medical or surgical treatment modalities. In this context, functional disorders in the area of childhood psychosis refer to those serious disturbances in psychological functioning that are reversible.

Phenomenology

The early forms of childhood psychosis, of faulty development, are established as infantile autism or autistic psychosis and as symbiotic syndromes, childhood schizophrenia, and the adolescent schizophrenic syndrome. All these extreme forms of difficulty have milder forms that are usually referred to as childhood or adolescent borderline conditions. Certain forms of autism, if untreated or unyielding to treat-

ment in the early stages, may later develop into schizophrenic conditions of childhood. For each of these major pictures of childhood psychosis, it is possible to predict from early forms a disease process that moves along developmental lines to severe pathology.

The autistic child is without a system of communication or communion, is out of reach within his own world, and is usually without verbal speech. This inability to engage the surrounding world results in the inability to develop the necessary internal world, together with its differentiation of functions, without which the child is limited in moving beyond the art of defense toward the art of encounter. The autistic personality remains empty, without further development of functions or of self, and thus maintains a pathological identity through individualism without the world.

In childhood schizophrenia are found conditions such as the break with reality; severely impaired reality testing; thought disorders of a primary nature; language systems in which there is often no clear separation among thought, act, and impulse; constant returns to fusion states; and temporary, complete autistic withdrawals. These childhood and adolescent disorders frequently resemble adult conditions except that in most cases the states of mental disorganization fluctuate and, therefore, are frequently seen as borderline conditions.

From a very early age, these children suffer from extreme sensitivity; they quickly regress under stress and are extremely vulnerable to separation, mild forms of rejection, and parental malfunctioning. Vulnerability of this kind has to do with inner constellations. This connection suggests that the psychological treatment forms used must accord with the specific personality structures available to the vulnerable child.

Many psychotic disorders in latency and in adolescence can be related to earlier difficulties, a fact indicating that disease processes seem to develop their own epigenetic scheme. But, frequently, latency children and young people during puberty and adolescence suffer sudden breakdowns or psychotic and schizophrenic illnesses that do not fall into these categories, even though early vulnerability can usually be detected.

Psychotic conditions of adolescence are much nearer those of adulthood. These conditions include problems of hysterical psychosis, schizophrenia, paranoid states, catatonic states, severe psychoticlike psychopathology, psychotic acting out, and the many borderline conditions of childhood and adolescence.

In schizophreniclike conditions of childhood, particularly the latency period, one of the characteristic ways of managing human relations is to maintain distance between self and object. The therapist must overcome the distance. The reduction in distance can be used as a way to establish the degree of increased mental health.

Certain conditions of hysterical psychosis—that is, exaggerations of hysterical symptoms—and of symbiotic conditions of childhood psychosis offer the reverse gauge. The measure of improvement lies in widening the distance and helping the children maintain increasing separation. But the attempt to maintain distance may fall apart and bring about states of fusion. Such children seem to fluctuate between total autistic withdrawal and total fusion. The problem is maintaining appropriate distance between self and object, between inner and outer, between thought and impulse, between the past, present, and future.

Diagnosis

The psychiatrist usually gathers clinical impressions about the child in play-therapy sessions or interviews. The social worker is involved with the parents, prepares the social history, participates in establishing a workable relationship with the parents, and collects data about the upbringing of the child. The psychological tester uses the standard situation to get a test picture. The neurologist looks for gross neurological signs to establish whether or not the problem is one of a functional psychosis. The speech pathologist contributes an assessment of the availability of or dysfunctioning in speech and of the degree of communication possible. All these data have to be reconciled with each other.

The diagnostic procedures require an understanding not only of the child but also of the parents. The total social situation must be assessed to ascertain whether the parents are able to maintain the treatment and make use of the professional resources to help create the facilitating environment.

Diagnosis, therefore, must go beyond the mere classification, the mere abstract treatability of the child. It must concern itself with the total social configuration, the family unity, the available resources, the technical skill available in the community, the dedication possible by the staff, the training conditions, and the research atmosphere.

Prognosis is not implicit in the picture of the illness but, rather, remains an infinite issue because of the complexity of the total social situation. One of the powerful aspects of diagnostic processes with psychotic children deals with the fact that they are seen after many other attempts at finding help have been made.

Therapy

Individual Psychotherapy

A classical analytical treatment allows for the development of a stable therapeutic situation, the development of transference neurosis, the analysis of the transference and the resistances, the solution of conflicts, and the dissolution of the transference neurosis, that repetition of the infantile neurosis. In the case of the psychotic child, there is no layer after layer of defense organization or adaptive capacity. Instead, behind the thin facade of logical, reality-oriented communications of the verbal representations can be found the primary process, the logic of the dream, the psychotic thought disorder.

The therapist's task must include the development of techniques by means of which a system of communication can be discovered and developed, a system that avoids the extremes of distance and closeness. The therapist must develop modes of interpretation that lead neither to loss of contact nor to fusion and that can be tolerated by the patient. Metaphorical language can be the link to the patient's unconscious material and, simultaneously, the patient's safety valve, by means of which optimum distance can be created and preserved.

In the case of autistic children, the problem of making nonthreatening and helpful contact is particularly difficult. The autistic, nonspeaking position, seemingly without contact, is a sort of defiance. The negativism of the autistic child is his way of insisting that he does not want to believe in communication, in committal—only in communion. He sees communion without language as the guarantee to maintain the object, albeit only an anaclitic object. His positive world is the symbiotic world, in which there is no clear separation between self and nonself, where there has not yet been the discovery of the other self, the object.

The therapist's task is to find methods by means of which he can guarantee that language is a system of communication between mother and child, a guarantee of their bond, and that communion without language is merely the bondage of the autistic or symbiotic child's dependency. The therapist's function is to help the child experience language as the warrant of growing autonomy, achievable without having to lose the mother. The therapeutic stance is to convince the child that there will be an emotional atmosphere that allows separation leading to individuation, rather than annihilation.

Only certain selected cases can be treated in office practice; therefore, psychotherapy in itself is not often the dominant treatment method of choice. Whether or not it is depends on the degree of the psychotic illness and on the ability of the family to support such treatment. Frequently, psychotherapy has to be a part of a total psychiatric armamentarium.

Group Psychotherapy

The treatment techniques—focusing on the variables of biological defects in the child, the pathology of the mother, the tenacious mother-child symbiosis, the psychologically absent father, and the total dynamics of the family interaction—afford the therapeutic leverage to alter the psychosis and the network of pathological reactions enmeshing all the family members. This treatment modality does not speak of cure but of sufficient improvement to return the child to more normal group experiences. In clinical situations in which group therapy and individual therapy are united, more effective modes of therapeutic interaction may occur.

Behavior Therapy and Behavior Modification

Behavior modification uses such operant conditioning techniques as positive reinforcement, such as reward through food or praise, and negative reinforcement, such as pain and punishment. These methods can be used to reinforce acceptable behavior, such as using words or giving up mutism or bizarre and unacceptable behavior.

If behavior modification and similar therapies, such as speech therapy, are used alone, it is found that improvement lasts only as long as these techniques are applied. When the techniques are stopped, the gains are soon extinguished, and the schizophrenic core is revealed as not having been touched.

Work with Parents

Psychotic conditions in childhood usually carry a strong component of pathology concerning the child's tie with the mother or parent surrogate. It is, therefore, necessary to develop special modes of technical help for the parent. With very young children, it is frequently useful to see the mother and the small child at the same time. The therapist then literally teaches the mother to respond appropriately to the child and to pick up cues. As the nonpathological link between mother and child, he is able to break the pathological pattern between them.

The main problem is helping the mother to separate from the child and to give up the symbiotic arrangement and its pathological consequences for both. In some cases, mere counseling and case work, focused on social planning, suffices. In other cases, family psychotherapy has to be initiated. In still other cases, individual psychotherapy with the parents is indicated.

The work with parents is directed first at the treatment of the child, but it is also concerned with the parents' adequate functioning. The psychiatric task with the parents is to free them from all possible burdens, to help them to allow separation, to work through their mourning in having to give up the illusion of possible recovery of the child, and to enable them to accept whatever improvement is possible or whatever further planning, such as permanent institutionalization, is necessary. The early fiction of the omnipotentiality of the child has to be given up and replaced by painful reality.

Work with the parents never allows smooth continuity. The same emergencies that the child creates are created by the parents, so that maintenance of the treatment situation is constantly endangered. A part of the parents' transference paradigm in regard to the worker is their fluctuation between the naive expectation that the worker is the omnipotent miracle worker and the equally dangerous fantasy that the worker has nothing to offer, does not help at all, and is a destroyer of hopes. This attitude of the parents seems to create a counterreaction in the therapeutic team—the fluctuation between despair and hope that accompanies the challenge of treating the psychotic child.

Milieu Treatment, Residential Centers, Hospitalization

Psychotic children, particularly when they are very young, are usually treated as long as possible at home, occasionally in boarding homes. Hospitalization is often considered merely a temporary measure for acute situations, since it is assumed that the home is the best place for the child. Hospitalization is considered in terms of added trauma as an undesirable intervention and is postponed as long as possible—feared by parents and treating physicians alike. Acute psychotic conditions may require no more than temporary therapeutic residential arrangements, but there are many borderline conditions.

The range of illness sometimes indicates that outpatient or office treatment alone is not the treatment of choice. Most authors look at the hospital as a positive milieu or a facilitating environment and discuss methods of arranging the milieu to help restore functioning.

Most treatment centers bring the children to a point at which separation from the hospital program is indicated. Interim steps are encouraged, such as day treatment centers, special schools, boarding and foster homes, and partial return to the family home.

REFERENCES

Bender, L. Childhood schizophrenia: A review. J. Hillside Hosp., *16:* 10, 1967.
Bettelheim, B. *The Empty Fortress.* Free Press of Glencoe (Macmillan), New York, 1967.
Bettelheim, B. *A Home for the Heart.* Alfred A. Knopf, New York, 1974.
Bowlby, J. *Attachment and Loss: Separation, Anxiety and Anger,* vol. 2. Basic Books, New York, 1973.
Brunstetter, R. W. Milieu treatment for psychotic children. In *Clinical Studies in Childhood Psychoses,* p. 174. Brunner/Mazel, New York, 1973.
Ekstein, R. *Children of Time and Space, of Action and Impulse.* Appleton-Century-Crofts, New York, 1966.
Ekstein, R., and Caruth, E. From the infinite to the infinitesimal: The play space of the schizophrenic child. Reiss-Davis Clin. Bull., *10:* 89, 1973.
Ekstein, R., and Cooper, B. The dividing of the working alliance in the parallel casework and therapy process of a schizophrenic young man. Reiss-Davis Clin. Bull., *10:* 79, 1973.
Kanner, L. Early infantile autism. J. Pediatr., *25:* 211, 1944.
Mahler, M. S. *On Human Symbiosis and the Vicissitudes of Individuation. Vol. 1: Infantile Psychosis.* International Universities Press, New York, 1968.
Ornitz, E. M. Childhood autism: A review of the clinical and experimental literature. Calif. Med., *118:* 21, 1973.
Spitz, R. A. *The First Year of Life: A Psychoanalytic Study of Normal and Deviant Development of Object Relations.* International Universities Press, New York, 1965.
Szurek, S. A., and Berlin, I. N. *Clinical Studies in Childhood Psychoses.* Brunner/Mazel, New York, 1973.

38.8.   ORGANIC BRAIN SYNDROMES

Introduction

Clinical symptoms referable to the neural system can occur with or without demonstrable structural or biochemical alterations in the neurons, their processes, or the supporting and surrounding cells. The clinical distinction between a functional and an organic brain syndrome is not always easy or clear cut. The second edition of the American Psychiatric Association's *Diagnostic and Statistical Manual of Mental Disorders* (DSM-II) defines organic brain syndromes as "disorders caused by or associated with impairment of brain tissue function."

Clinical Manifestations

The clinical manifestations of this group of disorders are the following:

Impairment of orientation to time, place, and person.

Impairment of remote and recent memory. Confabulation may result as a secondary phenomenon.

Decreased attention, brought out by testing digit span. Confusion may be present as a secondary effect.

Impaired ability to manipulate acquired knowledge, brought out by testing calculation and ability to interpret proverbs.

Impairment of judgment and insight.

Impairment of speech and praxis.

Impaired ability in construction (figure drawing).

Lability and shallowness of affect.

If, in addition, alternation of cranial nerve functions or focal signs are found in the motor or sensory system examination, the distinction becomes easier.

Focal or paroxysmal changes in an electroencephalogram (EEG), alteration of spinal fluid formula, or changes from normal in radiological and isotope studies confirm the organic nature of the clinical syndrome in most instances.

Psychiatric Examination

The psychiatric evaluation in such conditions differs in no way from the examination used in other conditions. The history can be particularly useful in indicating an absence of precursors of stress, conflict, and inhibition likely to lead to psychodynamically based problems. The way the child plays, speaks, and behaves may suggest organically based dysfunctions, and distortions of language, thinking, and visual-motor performance may become apparent. The way the child relates to the interviewer and fluctations in this relationship may also be significant.

Psychological Testing

Many test signs are suggestive of cerebral involvement of some kind. Small suggests the use of a basic test battery consisting of the age-appropriate form of the Wechsler Intelligence Scale; the Bender Visual-Motor Gestalt Test; lateralization tests; motor-test of lateralization; and projective tests, including the Rorschach, Thematic Apperception, and Human Figure Drawings.

Outcome

The manifestations of organic brain disease in childhood vary, depending on the nature of the cause, the particular time in the neurological maturation of the child at which the causative factor begins to operate, and the duration of time in which it does so. The severity of the insult and the general status of the child are also decisive factors. Parental management and interaction modify the outcome.

Causes

The popular concept of brain damage implies traumatic insult to the brain. It is more appropriate to consider three general categories. The first is maldevelopment, a structural deviation from the normal due to a variety of possible causes other than trauma. The second reflects actual damage to central nervous system structures being formed or already formed, due to such factors as trauma, infection, hemorrhage, and hypoxia. The third is malfunction without known structural change—for instance, the results of insufficient or excessive stimulation at significant points in development or the results of distortion in the child-parent interaction.

There seem to be critical periods for the development of various functions. If there is interference at one of these times, it may be difficult for the function ever to be developed adequately. In addition, early interference may have a profound and ever-increasing effect, since subsequent phases of development are distorted by what has previously gone awry.

However, an early insult may be overcome in several ways. One way is by compensatory overdevelopment of other functions. Or an uninjured area may to some extent take over the role of the injured area. Or, in later phases of development, what was deficient earlier may no longer be critical in terms of total functioning.

Prenatal causes of central nervous system dysfunction are metabolic, genetic, infectious, toxic, and psychogenic factors. Perinatal causes are prematurity, postmaturity, prolonged or rapid labor, abnormalities of presentation, induction of labor, accidents of labor, effects of medication, immunologic incompatibility, and normal mechanics of labor. Postnatal (to 5 years of age) causes are infections, injuries, medications, poisons, toxins, metabolic or vascular disturbances, psychogenic-environmental factors, neoplasms, and convulsive disorders.

Syndromes of Cerebral Dysfunction

Syndromes of cerebral dysfunction are possible results of aberrations of central nervous system function. The symptom picture in a given child is the final result of the organically based tendency toward a deviation of function and the way the child adapts to and compensates for this tendency. The adaptation and compensation are a composite of the child's ego strength and coping mechanisms and the state of the child-parent equilibrium (see Table I).

Hyperkinetic Reaction of Childhood

The DSM-II definition of hyperkinetic reaction of childhood reads: "This disorder is characterized by overactivity, restlessness, distracti-

TABLE I

Syndromes of Cerebral Dysfunction

Area	Clinical Manifestations
Neuromotor	Cerebral palsy
Neurosensory	Central blindness, deafness, anesthesia
Consciousness	Epilepsy
Intellectual	Some forms or components of mental retardation
Communication	Dysphasias, aphasias, more subtle language disabilities
Perception, association, retention, abstraction, expression	Specific learning disabilities
Object relations; reality testing	Some forms or components of psychoses of childhood
Motility, impulse, attention	Hyperkinetic impulse disorder

bility, and short attention span, especially in young children; the behavior usually diminishes in adolescence." DSM-II lists this disorder under the category behavior disorders of childhood and adolescence and states: "If this behavior is caused by organic brain damge, it should be diagnosed under the appropriate nonpsychotic organic brain syndrome." In the section of nonpsychotic organic brain syndromes, it is noted: "In children mild brain damage often manifests itself by hyperactivity, short attention span, easy distractibility, and impulsiveness. Sometimes the child is withdrawn, listless, perseverative, and unresponsive. In exceptional cases there may be great difficulty in initiating action."

Prevalence. Data regarding prevalence of this disorder vary from 4 per cent to 20 per cent. The figure quoted in most studies is 10 per cent of school population. Prevalence among boys compared with girls varies from three to one to nine to one. Among psychiatric clinic referrals, 50 per cent of school-age children are found to have this disorder.

Causes. Gross structural disease of the brain, such as trauma and encephalitis, can lead to hyperkinesis as a sequel. Children suffering from lead encephalopathy have also been shown to be impulsive and to have short attention spans. A genetic basis seems to be present in some instances. Social and emotional deprivation during development also seems to predispose to such behavior. The behavior manifested by these children seems to be the final common pathway for the expression of diverse pathologies.

Mechanism. The underlying mechanism for the development of this hyperkinetic picture is not known. A neuroanatomical basis has not been established.

Clinical Features. Hyperkinetic impulse disorder is particularly common in first-born boys. The new mother is apt to be tense and fearful of inadequacy as a woman. A newborn who is already afflicted with hyperkinetic impulse disorder may be unduly sensitive to stimuli and may respond in an undifferentiated, massive, aversive manner. When the mother picks up the infant and he stiffens, arches his back, spits, squalls, and thrashes in wild protest, to the frantic mother this behavior may represent the awful confirmation of her secret dread—that she has been rejected by the baby as inadequate. Her subsequent attempts to force the baby to conform only stimulate further negative reactions in the baby and may lay the groundwork for an ambivalent but predominatly negative relationship (see Figure 1).

It is common for the infant to be active in the crib, have a rapid developmental schedule, sleep little, and cry much past the traditional first 3 months of colic. The infant often gets out of the crib on his own very early. Once out of the crib and able to get about, the infant is apt to do so relentlessly, getting into everything and generally fingering, breaking, or disintegrating objects. As time goes on, his sphere of activity widens.

The toddler phase is replaced by a gallop. The activity may be relatively continuous and not turned off in appropriate situations, such as school and church. The child is unable, without great and conscious effort, to inhibit his response to any stimulus that comes along. In addition, the child seems incapable of attending to more than one stimulus at a time. He is a short sampler, incapable of attending to any stimulus for more than 10 seconds. Irritability may be set off by relatively minor stimuli.

Not all the phenomena are always seen together; there may be just one or two of these characteristics. If so, distractibility is often the only one. Further, each item of behavior can

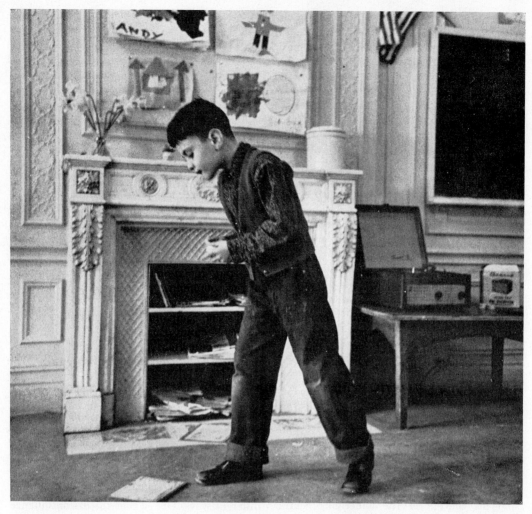

FIGURE 1. A hyperactive child. (Courtesy of Paul Berg.)

also be induced by difficulties in the emotional sphere, as in the child who is hyperactive and irritable as a result of inner tension and anxiety. But these behavioral phenomena may have their origin in altered central nervous system functions as well as in emotional disturbance.

The impaired functions are ego functions, and their poor performance may both create and worsen difficulties in a circular manner. Because of them, the child performs poorly and unacceptably, resulting in criticism and other pressures. The impaired ego may also make it harder for the child to tolerate and adapt to the feelings evoked in him by these pressures. Such children are prone to develop almost any kind of psychiatric disability in response to those spe-

cial problems, to the normal needs for adjustment required in the process of psychological-sexual-social maturation, and to the needs that may be imposed by psychological difficulties within the parents.

Diagnosis. A history suggests the diagnosis. The most striking finding is hyperactivity, but it may not always be manifested during a limited office interview. The neurological examination may be negative or show a variety of soft neurological signs. Perceptual-motor impairment, coordination deficits, disorders of attention, impulsivity, specific learning difficulties, disorders of speech and hearing, strabismus with central facial weakness, and mixed dominance are common.

The value of electroencephalograms in diagnosis remains a disputed issue. Most reports suggest that 50 to 60 per cent of hyperkinetic children show varying kinds of abnormalities, in contrast with 10 to 15 per cent of normal children in the same age group. A main reason for obtaining an EEG is to recognize the child who has frequent bilaterally synchronous discharges resulting in short *absence* spells and who reacts with hyperactivity in school out of sheer frustration.

Psychological testing may also be of value. Children showing only the behavioral aspects of hyperactivity tend not to show classical organic signs but on projective testing manifest their characteristic behavior in having a flow of associations, contaminations, and inability to delay. In those who show visual-perceptual difficulties, problems with spatial organization, and other phenomena suggesting cortical and diencephalic involvement, the classical test signs become more common.

Psychiatric examination, in addition to clarifying the particular defense mechanisms and conflicts, may suggest the presence of a basic, pervading, organically based anxiety.

Prognosis. Continuing learning difficulties and a tendency to sociopathic behavior may persist into adult life, despite the general diminution and final disappearance of motor hyperactivity in adolescence.

Treatment. The first requisite is that the physician communicate to both parent and child his concept of the underlying central nervous system aspect and the rationale for treatment. He can state with confidence that the hyperkinetic behavior most often is outgrown—treated or untreated—when the child is between 12 and 20 years of age. Nonetheless, it is important that the hyperkinetic picture be treated without waiting for its eventual disappearance. The mode of treatment is pharmacological, but there is some disagreement as to which medications are most efficacious.

There has been extensive experience with the central nervous system stimulants; amphetamine sulfate, dextroamphetamine sulfate, and methylphenidate hydrochloride. The customary recommended starting dose of dextroamphetamine is 5 mg. for children over 6 years of age and 2.5 mg. for children between 3 and 5 years of age. Clinical experience has suggested a beginning dosage and successive increments half that size. Daily dosage may be doubled at weekly increments if there is no response. Some older children may need as much as 40 mg. for optimal response. As to amphetamine sulfate, the customarily recommended dosage is to begin with 2.5 mg. daily for children between 3 and 5 years of age, increasing by the same amount weekly. For children 6 years of age or older, the recommended dosage is to begin with 10 mg. once to twice daily, increasing by 10 mg. weekly. Experience has suggested a more cautious approach, beginning with 5 mg. once daily and increasing by the same amount. If bothersome adverse reactions appear, such as insomnia or anorexia, the dosage should be reduced. The manufacturers do not recommend the use of this drug in children under 3 years of age. Methylphenidate may be given similarly, starting with 10 mg. daily for children above 6 years of age and 5 mg. for those between 3 and 5 years.

Common side effects of stimulants include anorexia, abdominal pain, insomnia, and headache. A common complaint is that the child has become quiet and very sensitive, crying at the slightest provocation. In most cases, a single dose after breakfast is efficacious, but it may be necessary to add another dose later during the day or to use long-acting forms. The dose should be reviewed at 6-month intervals.

With time, the need for the medication vanishes, and this point may be recognized in two different ways. One is that the discontinuance of the medication does not bring on the return of hyperkinetic symptoms. The other is that, instead of reducing overactivity, the usual effects of amphetamine—that is, overstimulation—begin to appear.

Various phenothiazines have been suggested as helpful when there is anxiety. Thioridazine hydrochloride is particularly useful for children more than 2 years of age. For children aged 2 to 12 years the recommended dosage is 0.5 mg. to a maximum of 3.0 mg. per kg. per day. The use of phenobarbital should be avoided in these children, since it frequently worsens behavior.

Although these medications may control the organically based hyperkinetic aspects, they do nothing directly for the emotionally based aspects.

The over-all treatment plan should include counseling the parents and the child and finding suitable programs that can meet the child's special needs. Appropriate educational planning is of special importance. Psychotherapy is sometimes needed.

Environmental manipulation should include decreasing external stimulation, decreasing alternatives, and encouraging patterns of behavior. These children often do better in a closed, structured classroom setting. Involvements in group activities should not be stopped, but providing more structure can help.

Specific Learning Disability

Special learning disability is frequently associated with hyperkinetic impulse disorder, but each may occur alone. Specific learning disability refers to an impairment of the ability to learn scholastically up to a level appropriate to the child's intellectual endowment as a result of inefficiencies in information processing. The disability is due to some disorder of cerebral dysfunction, rather than being emotionally, intellectually, or socially determined. There are many possible reasons for impairment of learning ability. Abnormal cerebral function may in itself be a significant cause in 5 to 10 per cent of school children.

Organic Brain Syndromes

Viral Encephalitis

Encephalitis caused by a virus is fairly common in childhood and may present initially as a sudden alteration in behavior. Arthropod-borne viruses and the herpes simplex virus are common pathogens. Delirium, confusion, and lethargy leading to stupor with seizures are the common manifestations in the acute phase. Hyperactive behavior with or without intellectual retardation is a common sequela. Focal neurological deficits noted in the acute phase may or may not persist. Herpes simplex virus accounts for 10 per cent of all reported cases of viral encephalitis in the United States today. Behavioral and speech abnormalities always precede focal motor signs. Herpes encephalitis has been treated with antiviral agents (5-Iodoxyuridine) with some success. Lasting neurological and intellectual handicap after encephalitis or meningitis is most likely when the infection takes place during the first 2 years of life.

Subacute sclerosing panencephalitis is a chronic form of encephalitis resulting from infection with the measles virus. The disease begins several years after a clinical episode of measles and starts with a subtle deterioration of intellect and personality. Extrapyramidal signs appear later. Myoclonic seizures are characteristic of the terminal stages. Often a hemorrhagic maculopathy is present.

Postinfectious Encephalomyelitis

An abrupt monophasic illness, with involvement of the central nervous system at multiple sites simultaneously, sometimes follows a variety of common viral infections of childhood. Smallpox, measles, mumps, rubella, and some nonspecific respiratory infections produce a disseminated encephalomyelitis. Alteration of sensorium, meningeal signs, seizures, and focal neurological signs are common. Most cases undergo complete spontaneous recovery.

Other viruses

Other forms of slow virus central nervous system infections in childhood are due to the rubella virus and the cytomegalo virus. Both viruses occur as congenital infections, and the virus continues to be present in the affected child for long periods of time. Failure to thrive, seizures, and irritability are common manifestations in infancy. Microcephaly and intellectual retardation are common sequelae. Autistic behavior is disproportionately common in rubella embryopathy and in association with toxoplasmosis and syphilis.

Encephalitis Lethargica

Von Economo's disease produces a clinical picture of lethargy and confused delirious behavior, with hallucinations in the acute phase. In the chronic phase, uninhibited, aggressive, and destructive behavior; emotional lability; sexual preoccupation; and selfish, suspicious behavior are common. A parkinsonian syndrome with oculogyric crises is a common sequela. Instances of this particular form of encephalitis have not been recorded in the past three decades.

Bacterial Infections

In most forms of purulent meningitides in childhood, some degree of cerebral parenchymal involvement occurs and is clinically manifested by seizures or other focal phenomena. Cerebral abscess due to contiguous spread or occurring as a metastatic infection also shows similar clinical features. These features are more likely to result in neurological and intellectual defects than in significant psychiatric residuals.

Congenital Syphilis

The now rarely seen juvenile general paresis may result in progressive mental deterioration. There may be apathy, forgetfulness, irritability, restlessness, night terrors, temper tantrums, and impulsive behavior, often antisocial. Less often than in adults, children may display euphoria, expansiveness, delusions, and hallucinations.

Epilepsy

Common to all the diverse manifestations of epilepsy is some alteration in the state of consciousness and some impairment of complete control of actions. Regardless of the type of seizure, there is often a distortion of the body image and self-concept. A child may view himself as crazy, impotent, or out of control and may respond by aggressiveness, withdrawal, inability to learn, counterphobic mechanisms, and a vast variety of behaviors that either act out or deny his distorted view of himself.

Grand Mal Seizures. In the most common form of epilepsy, grand mal, the patient may suddenly regain consciousness to find himself bruised, soiled, and wet, with bitten tongue, surrounded by a ring of curious and horrified on-lookers. This experience is enough to make him think that there must be something horribly wrong with him. Very often, parents react, consciously or unconsciously, to the presence of grand mal seizures as a curse and affliction, a punishment for them, retribution for some misdeed in act or thought.

One of the most common reactions is overprotection. A variant of this reaction is to set no limits for the child or to require performances from the child unlike those the parents require from their other children. Both modes of overprotection confirm the child's view of himself as someone different and interfere with the process of socialization and internalization of controls.

Petit Mal Seizures. The child with petit mal, who has sudden lapses of consciousness, may find it inexplicable and distressing that he seems to have missed something the teacher was saying or that he is suddenly behind the others in what they are reading. A child with akinetic or myoclonic seizures may be disturbed over the fact that, while drying the dishes, he suddenly drops or hurls a dish—not just once but many times.

Seizures with Behavioral Alterations. Temporal lobe or psychomotor seizures may be characterized by automatisms and aggressive outbursts, ranging from verbal expressions of rage to actual destruction or assault. The types of psychic phenomena that may be encountered in temporal lobe epilepsy include hallucinations, perceptual illusions, change of emotional tone, disorders of thought or language, and automatisms.

There have also been accounts of behavioral disorders in children who show a temporal or occipital spike focus without any overt evidence of seizures. These children may show oscillations in behavior, difficulty in relating to others, withdrawal or hostile aggressive attacks, enuresis or nightmares, or poor school work and paroxysmal headaches.

Contrasted with this picutre are prolonged episodes of behavioral disturbance that seem similar to temporal lobe epilepsy but that, on the EEG, show only generalized and not temporal lobe abnormalities. These episodes last as long as 72 hours, with confusion, hostility, negativism, and withdrawal, with or without automatisms but with apparent retention of consciousness.

Intracranial Neoplasms

Increased intracranial pressure, secondary to a neoplasm located anywhere intracranially, can produce behavioral changes. Most reviews suggest that there is nothing specific about a child's reaction to an intracranial tumor. Regressive tendencies, emotional instability, irritability, anxiety, withdrawal, and learning difficulties seem to reflect the fact that cerebral functioning is impaired. This impairment interferes with the child's ability to deal with emotional stresses already present and now intensified.

Degenerative Diseases

Most of the degenerative diseases occurring in childhood present a regression in behavior. A loss of previously acquired mental and motor skills is common. Degenerative diseases involving the basal ganglia can often simulate functional disorders in the beginning.

Brain Trauma

In the acute phase, the patient may be delirious, confused, and stuporous to comatose. But the sequelae are of more concern. The child may display marked irritability, restlessness, difficulty in concentration, ready fatigability, emotional instability, headaches, vertigo, sensitivity to change in position and to lights, noise, and confusion. Some degree of amnesia is characteristically present, and there may be some degree of impairment of intellectual functioning. Withdrawal, aggressiveness, and enuresis are common. So are sleep disturbance and the persistent recurrence of anxiety dreams in which the real or fantasied circumstances of the accident are recapitulated.

Because of the characteristics of childish and primary process thinking the child reacts to the traumatic accident as punishment and retaliation for his unacceptable wishes and thoughts. The situation is often worsened by implicit parental prohibitions against some catharsis and working-through of the traumatic event and the child's feelings. Psychotherapy for the child and counseling for the parents are often indicated.

A complication of head injury, subdural hematoma is more apt to result in neurological and intellectual deficit than in any significant psychiatric picture.

Endocrine Disorders

Personality disturbances consisting of anxiety, irritability, and emotional instability are common in thyrotoxicosis. A hypothyroid state is manifest as apathy and lack of interest in life. Behavioral abnormalities secondary to episodes of hypoglycemia are common in poorly regulated juvenile diabetes. Idiopathic hypoglycemia can often masquerade as a behavior disorder, with or without a seizure disorder.

Chromosomal Disorders

An increased incidence of XXY syndrome (Klinefelter's syndrome) has been noted in prisons and penal institutions. A definitive correlation has been suggested among aggressive antisocial behavior, tall stature, and the XXY genotype. A review of the literature indicates that children with Down's syndrome exhibit less antisocial behavior then do other children.

Metabolic Disorders

A variety of inherited errors in the metabolism of amino acids, carbohydrates, or fat result in intellectual retardation and seizures. Behavioral disturbances are present in most of these children. Phenylketonuric children may have dull and expressionless faces, be negativistic and apprehensive, and have speech disturbances. Others display striking psychoticlike behavior, manifested by withdrawal from reality, failure to relate to people, echolalia, and stereotyped, catatoniclike posturing. There may be loosening of associations, rambling, and bizarre and disconnected primary process thinking. The psychiatric disturbance in phenylketonuria may be at least partly attributable to the stress imposed on the child and his family by the rigorous feeding regimen given as treatment. Autistic behavior is alleged to be disproportionately common in phenylketonuria and has been reported in association with galactosemia. Self-mutilation has been found as a characteristic abnormality in a syndrome (Lesch-Nyhan) with mental retardation, choreoathetosis, and hyperuricemia due to an inherited deficiency in the enzyme hypoxanthine guanine ribosyltransferase. Porphyria is uncommon in childhood but can produce a confusional state during an acute episode.

Malnutrition from birth has been consistently shown to affect brain weight and intellectual growth. Accompanying behavioral disturbances include apathy and irritability. Thiamine deficiency, as in beri beri, and niacin deficiency in pellagra also lead to organic mental syndromes.

Mucopolysaccharidosis often results in storage of the mucopolysaccharides within neurons, resulting in organic deficits, such as retardation and seizures. Closely related sphingolipidoses result in lipid storage within the brain. The late onset, slowly progressive form, Spielmeyer-Vogt, can often present as a personality disorder in the initial stages. It has frequently been confused with childhood schizophrenia.

Toxins and Drugs

Acute lead encephalopathy presents irritability, coma, and convulsions. Mortality is high unless chelating and supportive treatment are immediately given. Most cases in the United States are associated with the ingestion of lead-bearing paint. Clinical lead poisoning produces anemia and often renal abnormalities, but its most important effects occur in the central nervous system. Widespread encephalopathy with perivascular cuffing and edema occurs in the acute stage.

Barbiturates may result in clouded sensorium, impaired judgment, and mental deterioration.

Amphetamines—along with barbiturates, marijuana, alcohol, and such agents as lysergic acid diethylamide (LSD)— are being used by adolescents for alterations of mood, alertness, energy, and states of consciousness, which are their acute effects. Depression and psychotic states have been described with continued use.

While sniffing gasoline, children may have hallucinations, auditory and visual, then become drowsy and lose consciousness. In the chronic phase, there are predominantly signs of neurological disability. The acute phase of glue sniffing is characterized by euphoria, excitement, exhilaration, and altered body sensations. There may be neurological phenomena, such as ataxia, diplopia, tinnitus, drowsiness, stupor, and unconsciousness. In the subacute phase, there may be irritability, inattentiveness, and episodes of drowsiness and unconsciousness. There have been no reports of chronic brain syndrome.

Medication given for therapeutic purposes may induce hallucinations.

REFERENCES

Arnold, L. E., Kirilcuk, V., Corson, S. A., and Corson, E. O'L. Levoamphetamine and dextroamphetamine: Differential effect on aggression and hyperkinesis in children and dogs. Am. J. Psychiatry, *130:* 165, 1973.

Laufer, M. W. Long-term management and some follow-up findings on the use of drugs with minimal cerebral syndromes. J. Learn Disabil., *4:* 518, 1971.

Laufer, M. W. Psychiatric diagnosis and treatment of children with minimal brain dysfunction. Ann. N. Y. Acad. Sci., *205:* 303, 1973.

Laufer, M. W., Denhoff, E., and Solomons, G. Hyperkinetic impulse disorder in children's behavior problems. Psychosom. Med., *19:* 38, 1957.

Randt, C. T., and Derby, B. M. Behavioral and brain correlations in early life: Nutritional deprivation. Arch. Neurol., *28:* 167, 1973.

Reitan, R. M., and Boll, T. J. Neuropsychological correlates of minimal brain dysfunction. Ann. N. Y. Acad. Sci., *205:* 65, 1973.

Satterfield, J. H. EEG issues in children with minimal brain dysfunction. In *Minimal Cerebral Dysfunction in Children*, S. Walzer and P. Wolff, editors, p. 35. Grune & Stratton, New York, 1973.

Shaffer. D. Psychiatric aspects of brain injury in childhood: A review. Dev. Med. Child Neurol., *15:* 11, 1973.

Small, L. *Neuropsychodiagnosis in Psychotherapy.* Brunner/Mazel, New York, 1973.

Walzer, S., and Wolff, P. H. Minimal Cerebral Dysfunction in children. *Seminars in Psychiatry*, M. Greenblatt and E. Hartmann, editors, vol 5. Grune & Stratton, New York, 1971.

Wender, P. H. *Minimal Brain Dysfunction in Children.* Wiley Interscience, New York, 1971.

Werry, J. S. Organic functions in childhood psychopathology. In *Psychopathological Disorders of Childhood*, H. C. Quay and J. S. Werry, editors, p. 83. Wiley, New York, 1972.

39

Child Psychiatry: Psychiatric Treatment

39.1. INDIVIDUAL PSYCHOTHERAPY

Theoretical Assumptions

Psychoanalytic Theory

Psychoanalytic theory conceives of exploratory psychotherapy working, with patients of all ages, by reversing the the evolution of psychopathological processes. The younger the child, the more intertwined are the genetic and dynamic forces.

Pathological processes begin with experiences that have proved to be particularly significant to the patient and have affected him adversely. The reason for this effect may reside in the nature of the experiences or of their intensity or both. Unconscious elements are subject to a pathological misuse of adaptive and defensive mechanisms. The result is the development of distressing symptoms, character attitudes, or patterns of behavior that constitute the emotional disturbance.

Increasingly, the psychoanalytic view of emotional disturbances in children has assumed a developmental orientation, stressing maladaptive defenses against unconscious conflicts between those impulses that are characteristic of a specific developmental phase and the influence of the environment, which may be experienced indirectly through the child's internalized representation of the environment. The result is difficulty in achieving or resolving developmental tasks and in achieving the capacities specific to ensuing phases of development.

Expressive and exploratory psychotherapy endeavors to reverse this evolution of emotional disturbance through a re-enactment and desensitization of the traumatic events by free expression of thoughts and feelings in an interview-play situation. The therapist helps his patient understand the warded-off feelings, fears, and wishes that have beset him.

At the center of resistances to treatment are the psychic functions that facilitate forgetting and repetition and that lead the patient to re-experience certain feelings out of context, without recalling their relevancy. In the therapeutic setting, the therapist becomes the object of these re-experienced thoughts, feelings, and reactions, known as transferences. The therapist attempts to use these transferred reactions to discover the genesis of the patient's problems and to formulate interpretations that will help the patient understand his enigmatic stance. The goal of these interpretations is to enable the patient to increase conscious control over heretofore automatic mental processes. The end result is a rearrangement of his personality structure and an enhanced ability to realize his potential.

Suppressive-supportive-educative psychotherapy works in an opposite fashion, aiming to facilitate repression. Capitalizing on the patient's desire to please him, the therapist encourages the patient to substitute new adaptive and defensive mechansims. In this type of therapy, the therapist uses interpretations minimally; instead, he emphasizes suggestion, persuasion, exhortation, operant or classical reinforcement, counseling, education, direction, advice, abreaction, environmental manipulation, intellectual review, gratification of the patient's current dependent needs, and similar techniques.

Learning-Behavioral Theories

Since disturbed behavior is acquired, its evolution and treatment can be understood within the framework of established theories of learning, such as Hull's reinforcement theory, Pavlov's conditioned reflex theories, and Skinner's operant conditioning theory. Systematic behavioral techniques are designed to eliminate symptoms and encourage positive behaviors in a wide range of childhood psychopathology.

Developmental Theories

Underlying child psychotherapy are a variety of interrelated psycho-socio-biological developmental sequences, including age-appropriate behavior, psychosexual development, and Piaget's sequence of intellectual evolution. Children react to hunger, other frustrations, injury, illness, separation, and death in ways representative of their stages of development.

Such information must be supplemented by personal knowledge and observation of children, with the resultant view of the child as a fluid, maturing, and developing organism who is not complete. The child's personality must be viewed in the perspective of his past, present, and future; the focus must be on questions of regression-progression and transience-permanence, rather than on static assessments.

Play serves a number of important purposes for children, such as facilitating the mastery of many of children's developmental crises through playful transformation into activity of what was passively experienced. Play is simultaneously a medium of communication, a vehicle for expression, and a means of sublimation.

Types of Psychotherapy

Psychotherapy can be classified in several ways. A common frame of reference for classification is the global aim and mode of the treatment—that is, supportive-suppressive-directive or expressive-exploratory-ventilative. It is possible also to describe psychotherapy in terms of its depth, duration, and intensity. Focusing on the therapist's approach, one can classify psychotherapy as being abreactive, interpretive, suggestive, persuasive, or educative. Eponyms such as Freudian, Kleinian, Rankian, and Rogerian refer to preferred theoretical concepts.

Among the common bases for classification of child therapy is identification of the factor presumed to be helpful for the young patient. Before the ascendency of psychoanalysis, the most prominent were suggestion, persuasive

exhortation, and reassurance. In the infancy of psychoanalysis, symptomatic relief tended to be attributed to the fact that the patient had rediscovered a lost memory. Shortly thereafter, the release of dammed-up emotions was highlighted. With further development of psychoanalytic thinking, the emphasis shifted to modification of superego standards, identification with the therapist, development of increased emotional discipline in the working-through process, development of insight, and expansion of ego functioning.

There has been a waxing and waning of prominence accorded conditioning factors such as motivating needs, stimulating cues, and the reinforcement of reward and punishment. Similarly, improvement has been perceived as developing from a deconditioning process that may involve systematic desensitization or a manipulation of the therapeutic relationship so as to provide a corrective emotional experience.

Many of these factors overlap, and efforts to attribute therapeutic progress with all patients to a single factor are unconvincing. None of these factors appears to be specific for any particular developmental stage, but the relationship itself and corrective emotional experiences, generally exert a greater influence with children than with adults.

Remedial, educational, and patterning psychotherapy endeavor to teach new attitudes and patterns of behavior to children who persist in using immature and inefficient patterns, which are often presumed to be the result of a maturational lag.

Supportive psychotherapy can help a well-adjusted youngster cope with the emotional turmoil engendered by a crisis. It is also used with disturbed youngsters whose ego functioning might be seriously disrupted by expressive-exploratory therapy.

Release therapy facilitates the abreaction of pent-up emotions. It is indicated primarily for preschool-aged children who are suffering from a distorted emotional reaction to an isolated trauma.

Psychotherapy with children is often psychoanalytically oriented; it endeavors through the vehicle of self-understanding to enable the child to develop his potential further. This goal is achieved by liberating for more constructive use the psychic energy presumed to be expended in defending against fantasied dangers. With awareness facilitated, the patient can evaluate the usefulness of his defensive maneuvers and relinquish the unnecessary ones that constitute the symptoms of his emotional disturbance.

This form of therapy is to be distinguished from child psychoanalysis, a more intensive and less common treatment, in which the unconscious elements are interpreted systematically in an orderly direction from outside in, resulting in the sequence of affect-defense-impulse. Under these circumstances, the therapist anticipates unconscious resistances and allows transference manifestations to mature to a full transference neurosis, through which neurotic conflicts are resolved.

In all psychotherapy, the child should derive support from the consistently understanding and accepting relationship with the therapist, while varying degrees of remedial educational guidance and emotional release are inevitably present.

Differences between Children and Adults

Children show a relative absence of some elements that contribute to successful treatment. A child, for example, typically does not seek help. As a consequence, one of the first tasks for the therapist is stimulation of the child's motivation for treatment. It is also common for children to begin therapy involuntarily and without the benefit of true parental support. Whereas adult patients frequently perceive advantages in getting well, children may envision therapeutic change as conforming to a disagreeable reality and may see the therapist as the parents' punitive agent.

Children tend to externalize internal conflicts, finding it difficult to conceive of problem resolution except by altering an obstructing environment.

The tendency of children to re-enact their previous feelings in new situations facilitates the early appearance of spontaneous and global transference reactions that may prove troublesome. Concurrently, the eagerness that children have for new experiences, coupled with their natural developmental fluidity, tends to limit the intensity and therapeutic usefulness of subsequent transference developments.

Children have a limited capacity for self-observation, with the notable exception of some obsessive children. These obsessive children, however, usually isolate the vital emotional components.

Typically motor-minded children may demand a degree of physical stamina that is not of consequence in therapy with adults. The age appropriateness of such primitive mechansims as denial, projection, and isolation hinders the process of working through, which relies on a patient's synthesizing and integrative capacities, both of which are immature in children. Also, environmental pressures on the therapist are generally greater in work with children than in work with adults.

However, children have the advantage of active maturational and developmental forces.

Therapeutic Techniques

Playroom

Therapists tend to change their preferences in equipment as they accumulate experience and develop confidence in their ability. Some inexperienced therapists seem to derive a sense of security from having a large variety of playthings available. However, these toys can be so absorbing that they help the child resist therapy.

Although individual considerations should be decisive, the following equipment can constitute a well-balanced playroom or play area: multigenerational families of flexible but sturdy dolls of various races, a policeman doll, a doctor doll, soldier dolls, a dollhouse and furnishings, toy animals, puppets, paper, crayons, paint, blunt-edged scissors, clay or something comparable, guns, rubber knives, rubber hammers, other tools, building blocks, cars, trucks, airplanes, and eating utensils. These toys should enable children to communicate through play. Mechanical toys tend to break, which may contribute to children's guilt feelings and to clutter.

A special drawer or box should be available to each child in which to store items the child brings to the therapy session or to store projects, such as drawings and stories, for future retrieval.

Initial Approach

A variety of approaches are derived from the therapist's perception of the child's needs and his individual style. The range extends from those in which the therapist endeavors to direct the child's thought content and activity—as in release therapy, some behavior therapy, and certain educational patterning techniques—to those exploratory methods in which the therapist endeavors to follow the child's lead. Even though the child determines the focus, it remains the therapist's responsibility to structure the situation.

The clinician's initial stance should be an empathic one.

Forcefully separating a struggling young child from his parent to accompany the therapist does not further future efforts at understanding. Rather than entering into a power struggle, the therapist is well-advised to have the parent accompany the terrified child to the therapy room and remain until the anxiety is diminished.

The therapist may communicate to the child that he does not intend to get angry or to be pleased in response to what the child says or does but that he will try to understand him. Such an expressive climate should not neglect geographical and behavioral limits. There is no therapeutic or developmental advantage in allowing a child to run wild, invading others' privacy. Setting limits establishes a setting and structure in which the child can be assessed, understood, and helped.

Children whose disagreeable behavior has typically evoked a negative reaction from everyone in the past may be threatened by the neutral, apparently unconcerned, even friendly therapist. At the other extreme, an inhibited, neurotic child who is the product of a rigid home and a highly organized school may experience mounting anxiety in response to the apparent absence of structure in the psychotherapeutic situation. From his superego-oriented view of the world, the constricted child feels that the therapeutic situation invites forbidden instinctual expression. The therapist's verbalization of his understanding of the child's apprehensions about the neutral therapeutic approach can help clear the air.

An explicit statement of a contractual nature, asserting that the child's play and fantasies will be considered a communication about himself and his problems, is in order. Although the child may not fully appreciate the significance of this assertion, it minimizes the prospect of some future therapeutic intervention derived from play being perceived by the child as an intrusive attack.

Although most children do not respond well to being greeted at the outset by a statement of their problem, it is rarely empathic to allow an entire initial session to pass without any mention of the presenting problem.

The closer the child is to adolescence, the greater the possibility that the therapist's offer of help will be perceived as an infantilizing demand for dependency.

Communication

Some children participate in play activities immediately and verbalize spontaneously without assistance from the therapist, but others appear to require considerable help. Responsive to the child's apparent needs, the therapist either assumes a relatively passive, observing role or a more active, intervening one.

Children generally are not as verbal as adults. The child's facies, gestures, posture, and motility and the content, form, and configuration of his play and art may say more than his words. Silent children in psychotherapy are common. A therapist's stance of countersilence is rarely fruitful because most children are capable of outlasting a therapist's silence. It is the therapist's task to assess the extent to which the child's silence represents defensive functioning, attack, contemplative reflection, or the quietude of comfortable love.

What appears to be a particularly rich therapeutic session may be followed by unprecedented silent resistance, expressive of the child's feeling guilty or experiencing a loyalty conflict between the therapist and his parents. Generally, the therapist's reassuring interpretation alleviates the child's concern.

Varying connotations are attached to the same words and phrases by people of different ages. A striking example is the word "why," probably the most common word in psychotherapy with adults. Children, however, often react to the question "Why?" as if it were an accusation.

Therapeutic Interventions

Therapeutic interventions with children encompass a range comparable to those used with adults in psychotherapy, but there are vital differences in the ways these interventions are used with children and adults. To encourage verbal and nonverbal associations, the child therapist needs to be specific in focusing his questions on what the child is just about ready to express. The best clues come from what the child has already communicated. In essence, the therapist asks the child to elaborate on what he has already said or done. It is important that the therapist avoid sounding as though he is quizzing the child and invading his privacy. The more the therapist can imply curiosity, not unlike that of another interested youngster, the greater the likelihood of fruitful response. This apparent naiveté should be tempered with an awareness of the risk of asking questions that may seem devious to the child, such as those to which the therapist obviously knows the answer.

Certain interventions vital in therapy with children are generally superfluous if not insulting to most adults. For example, to tell an angry adult that he is angry would be a confrontation that could readily prove offensive. However, telling a child that he is angry may be a necessary interpretation of affect, inasmuch as everyone may know about the child's anger except the child himself.

With children, it may be unwise to undo the projection into play that is characteristic of child therapy. When a child with adequate reality testing causes two dolls to fight, the therapist's running commentary might be limited to a description of the dolls' affect, without attributing the anger to the child. Under these circumstances, this displacement is viewed as an age-appropriate, adaptive mechanism, rather than as a pathological defensive maneuver. If the therapist told the child that he had the dolls fight because of his own anger, the child's resistance and defensiveness might be increased to the extent that he would stop the activity, thereby interrupting the communication. With children whose ego functioning is so defective that they confuse play and reality, the therapist may have to devote his efforts to educating the child about the distinction between play and reality before it is judicious to deal with the content of the play.

As a general rule, therapeutic interventions begin at the surface before proceeding deeper.

Attention is generally directed first to superficial behavior and affects, followed by defenses and other resistances, before dealing with conflict and impulse.

Nurturing and maintaining a therapeutic alliance may entail some education of the child regarding the process of therapy. Another educational intervention may entail assigning labels to affects that have not been part of the youngster's past experience.

Parental Involvement

Psychotherapy with children is characterized by the need for parental involvement. This involvement does not necessarily reflect parental culpability for the youngster's emotional difficulties, but it is a reality of the child's dependent state.

With preschool-aged children, the entire therapeutic effort may be directed toward the parents, without any direct treatment of the child. At the other extreme, children can be seen in psychotherapy without any parental involvement beyond the payment of fees and perhaps the transportation of the child to the therapeutic sessions. Most therapists agree that relatively few neurotic children who have reached the oedipal phase of development can sustain therapy by themselves. Even in the cases of those who can, the majority of practitioners maintain an informative alliance with the parents to obtain additional information about the child.

Probably the most frequent arrangement is parent guidance (focused on the child or on the parent-child interaction or on both) or therapy for the parents' own needs concurrent with the child's therapy. The parents may be seen by the child's therapist or by someone else. In family therapy, all or selected members of the family are treated simultaneously as a family group.

Confidentiality

There are advantages to creating an atmosphere in which the child can feel that his words and actions do not bind him to a commitment but are too important to be communicated to a third party without his permission. However, it can be risky to promise a child that the therapist will not tell the parents what transpires in therapeutic sessions, since the bulk of what children do and say in psychotherapy is common knowledge to the parents and the child could manipulate the situation so as to produce circumstantial evidence that the therapist has betrayed his confidence. Accordingly, if confidentiality requires specific discussion during treatment, the therapist may not want to go beyond indicating that he is not in the business of telling parents what goes on in therapy, as his role is to understand children and to help them. It is important also to enlist the parents' cooperation in respecting the privacy of the child's therapeutic sessions.

Routinely reporting to children the essence of all communications with third parties regarding the child underscores the therapist's reliability and his respect for the child's autonomy.

Indications for Psychotherapy

Psychotherapy is indicated for children with emotional disorders that impede maturational and developmental forces or induce reactions in the environment that are considered pathogenic. Ordinarily, such disharmonies are dealt with by the child with his parents' assistance, but, when these efforts are persistently inadequate, psychotherapeutic intervention may be indicated. Psychotherapy should be limited to those instances in which there are positive indicators pointing to its potential usefulness.

Contraindications

Psychotherapy is contraindicated if the emotional disturbance is judged to be an intractable one that will not respond to treatment. However, certain patients may elicit a reaction from one therapist that is a contraindication for psychotherapy with that therapist but not necessarily with another therapist.

Another contraindication is evidence that the therapeutic process will interfere with reparative forces. The forces mobilized as a consequence of psychotherapy may have dire social or somatic effects. For example, psychotherapy may upset a precarious family equilibrium, so as to cause more difficulty than the original problem posed.

Choice of Technique

For most neurotic children, a form of interpretive psychotherapy aimed at uncovering intrapsychic conflicts is indicated. But, if the youngster's ego functioning, particularly in the area of reality testing, is borderline, such an approach may precipitate psychosis.

If hyperactivity seems to represent a means of avoiding depression or of expressing anxiety resulting from an intrapsychic conflict over aggression, one would be inclined to approach that child with interpretive psychotherapy, exposing the child's conflicts over aggression to rational scrutiny. On the other hand, if the hyperactivity is presumed to result from minimal brain dysfunction, the therapist's primary task is to supply externally the controls that are lacking internally. To do so may require regulation of the child's life, isolating him from distressing stimuli, and similar supportive-suppressive measures.

Symptomatic treatment may be harmful at times. Consider the youngster with the symptom of reading retardation secondary to underlying emotional factors. The child may take his failure to respond to tutoring as further evidence of his stupidity and hopelessness. Furthermore, such a symptomatic approach may unwittingly repeat a pertinent trauma for the child.

Psychoanalytically derived individual psychotherapy seems to be most effective with youngsters who have internal, self-sustaining, neurotic conflicts that have not originated earlier than the phallic stage of development and have resulted in circumscribed, ego-alien symptoms. Such expressive-exploratory-interpretive therapy is generally less helpful for those children whose disturbance has not caused them much immediate discomfort. Frequently, these disturbances are a consequence of conflicts derived from prephallic phases, in which the resulting disturbance tends to permeate the child's entire character structure. Psychoanalytically oriented therapy is least effective when the therapist cannot establish a therapeutic alliance with the child, as in cases in which there has been an arrest in ego development, resulting in a diminished capacity for abstract thinking and object relationships. When the capacity for establishing and maintaining object relationship is severely limited, the treatment may need to be based on a foundation of need satisfaction. In such instances, it may be advantageous for the therapist to be the person who cares for the child, as is possible in residential treatment.

Time-limited, focused therapy is particularly effective in helping children deal with situational crises, particularly those that entail separation or loss. But deeply entrenched, rigid defensive operations can render brief therapy useless, and primitive, brittle defenses, such as massive denial of parental divorce, may signal that brief, focused therapy will engender additional primitive defenses or leave the child vulnerable to major ego disruption.

Termination

Terminating psychotherapy inevitably has its painful aspects, whether the termination is positively determined by the happy accomplishment of goals or whether it represents a sad acknowledgement of failure to achieve the desired results. If therapy is not going to be effective, one typically tries to make the termination as supportive as possible, with suggestions of alternate strategies to cope with the problem. With successful termination, it is generally best to agree to a termination date sometime in the future, thereby permitting anticipatory psychotherapeutic work about separation feelings. A child's expressed eagerness to end therapy should never be accepted as an indication that there is no accompanying anxiety about separation

Results

Investigators have amassed data suggesting favorable results in 65 to 80 per cent of the cases surveyed. But one is left with the question as to what would have happened to these children had they not been exposed to psychotherapy.

REFERENCES

Anthony, E. J. Communicating therapeutically with children. J. Am. Acad. Child Psychiatry, *3:* 106, 1964.
Freud, A. *Normality and Pathology in Childhood.* International Universities Press, New York, 1965.
Group for the Advancment of Psychiatry. *From Diagnosis to Treatment: An Approach to Treatment Planning for the Emotionally Disturbed Child.* Group for the Advancement of Psychiatry, New York, 1973.
Kessler, J. W. *Psychopathology of Childhood.* Prentice-Hall, Englewood Cliffs, N. J., 1966.
Lippman, H. S. *Treatment of the Child in Emotional Conflict.* McGraw-Hill, New York, 1956.
Proskauer, S. Focused time-limited psychotherapy with children. J. Am. Acad. Child Psychiatry, *10:* 619, 1971.
Strupp, H. H. *Psychotherapy: Clinical, Research, and Theoretical Issues.* Jason Aronson, New York, 1973.

39.2. GROUP THERAPY

Basic Principles

Despite different theoretical backgrounds of therapists, certain assumptions pervade their work. These assumptions include the unconscious, some constructs of the mind (such as ego), psychic determinism (uneasily coexisting with many theoreticians' philosophical allegiance to free will), and infantile sexuality.

Activity—such as artwork, play, dancing, gestures, and interactions—is based on the inner fantasies of the child that seek expression and resolution in development, family transactions, and other aspects of growth-promoting adaptation. The child exerts power plays and will in the constant search for gratification of his needs within his time-space complex. His behavioral patterns reveal to the perceptive therapist implied content, the meaning of which is inferred within the therapist's primary theoretical orientation.

The role of peer relationships for latency-age children underpins the use of group therapy for certain disorders of that age child.

Data for living, especially when interpreted in transmission by parents and other care-taking persons, strongly influence behavioral patterns of all age groups of children and adolescents. Rapid, oscillating, changing inputs often seem to overwhelm the child, not permitting adequate associative and dwelling time for purposive decision making. Part of the therapeutic responsbility in group psychotherapy of children and adolescents consists of sifting with the patients and helping them sort out faddish messages.

Children learn to operate in varying systems, constantly calling for rearrangements of equilibria. Therapy offers settings and techniques to glimpse the role of the child's family as a message center and processor. With this focus not on individual psychopathology but on systems of negotiation, the group leader and the group itself confront this structured segment of their lives primarily in the here-and-now of that group session.

Age and developmental considerations have dominated the group therapies used for children. In the general schemata of group therapy, several classifications are available (see Figure

1). One such grouping bases itself on psychoanalytic approaches: (1) psychodrama, which is based on techniques for the symbolic expression of conflicts, (2) nondirective therapy, in which structure and the active interference of the therapist are kept to a minimum, (3) psychoanalytic therapy, which relies on psychoanalytic concepts and seeks to impart these concepts to the patients to some degree, and (4) transactional analysis, another educative type of therapy that imparts to the child some understanding of his actions and that encourages him to apply this knowledge. Therapists differ in their reliance on verbalization and conceptualization in therapy as opposed to symbolic expression of conflicts, in the degree to which group interaction is spontaneous or structured, in their views of the role of the therapist, and in their understanding of how group therapy actually works.

However, these approaches do not well describe the techniques developed over the years for children. Characteristics of developmental stages influenced the growth of group psychotherapy techniques more than perhaps any other factor. Investigators tended to group children by age and the nature of the presenting difficulties. They also assumed that the verbalization of children could not be used extensively much before puberty or adolescence, so that play and activity dominated their approaches.

Preschool and Early School-Age Groups

Work with the preschool group is usually structured by the therapist through the use of a particular technique, such as puppets or artwork, or it is couched in terms of a permissive play atmosphere. In therapy with puppets, the children project their fantasies onto the puppets, as in ordinary play. The main value lies in the cathexis afforded the child, especially if he shows difficulty in expressing his feelings. The group aids the child less by interaction with other members than by action with puppets.

A provocative approach to early school-age children emphasizes model reinforcement in group therapy in a school setting. The therapists assume that the children retain their behavioral repertoires.

In play group therapy, the emphasis rests on the interactional qualities of the children with one another and with the therapist in a permis-

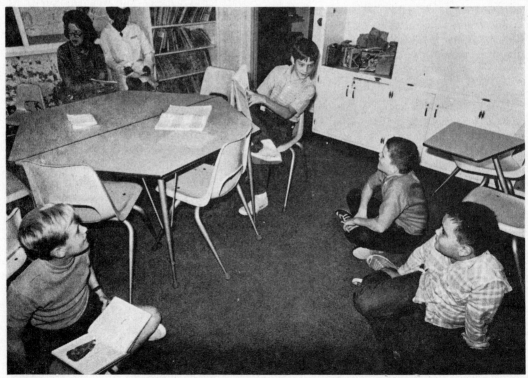

Figure 1. Interactional group therapy with latency age children conducted by cotherapists. (Courtesy of Irvin Kraft, M.D.)

sive playroom setting. The therapist allows the children to produce fantasies verbally and in play but uses active restraint when the children undergo excessive tension. The toys are the traditional ones used in individual play therapy, such as water, Plasticine, a doll's house, and toy guns. The children use the toys to act out aggressive impulses and to relive their home difficulties.

The mechanism of identification affords the child major opportunities for therapeutic gain as he identifies himself with the other group members and with the therapist. Since the individual child constitutes the focus of the treatment, little attention is given to the group as an entity in itself. As in ordinary play relationships of children, attachments to peers and toys and the formations of subgroups shift for each child.

The children show social hunger, the need to be like their peers and to be accepted by them. Usually, the therapist excludes children who have never realized a primary relationship, as with their mothers, since individual psychotherapy could better help those children. Ginott also rejects children with murderous attitudes toward siblings, sociopathic children, those with perverse sexual experiences, habitual thieves, and extremely aggressive children. Usually, the children selected include those with phobic reactions, effeminate boys, shy and withdrawn children, and children with primary behavior disorders.

Latency-Age Groups

Activity-interview group psychotherapy combines elements of activity, play, and interview group therapies. It differs from activity group therapy in that the therapist actively interprets to the children their actions and verbalizations as they involve themselves with the usual materials used in play therapy and activity therapy.

The children can be more disturbed than in activity group therapy, since dreams and other dynamically laden verbalizations undergo group discussion. The children verbalize in a problem-oriented manner, with the awareness that problems brought them together and that the group aims to change them.

Composition of the Group

In some clinic and private practice situations in which an activity therapy setting may not be

feasible, the emphasis can be shifted to an interview type, with little toy play and no use made of tools or arts and crafts. The children can be of both sexes, and their selection depends more on the over-all structure of the group than on the individual patient's characteristics. The optimum size of the group is six children. If the group contains several withdrawn and taciturn members, it behooves the leader not to include another withdrawn child.

The patients not usually taken into these groups include the incorrigible or psychopathic child, the homicidal child, and the overtly sexually deviant child. The severely threatened, ritualistic, socially peculiar children who cannot establish effective communication at any useful level with the group members fail to do well in these groups.

Intellectual ability should be well distributed, for too many retardates in the group impede interaction and tend to enhance motoric patterns of all the group members. Children with physical deformities, tics, protruding teeth, or behavior based on maturational brain dysfunction find the group situation helpful (see Figure 2). Vehement interactions or taunts about their disabilities produce in time a group response of support as the members perceive the victim's sensitivities and feelings.

Since the sex ratio inherent in child psychiatric work with latency children runs 3 to 1 of boys to girls, finding enough girls becomes a problem. If possible, equal numbers of each sex should be sought. The girls act as a modulating influence and diminish extremes of behavior.

Psychodynamics

During exposures to the groups, the child demonstrates his customary and usual adaptational patterns. If, for example, he has used his haplessness to elicit dependency fostering and psychological feeding responses from adults and peers, the neutrality and passivity of the therapist impede these patterns and create enough frustration to initiate different behavior in time. Similarly, the provocative, extremely aggressive child finds no rejection or punishment for his behavioral distortions. In time, he begins to react differently toward the therapist and his fellow group members.

Milieu therapy is a related technique in that it involves structured activities and projects, but it sees itself as constituting a therapeutic

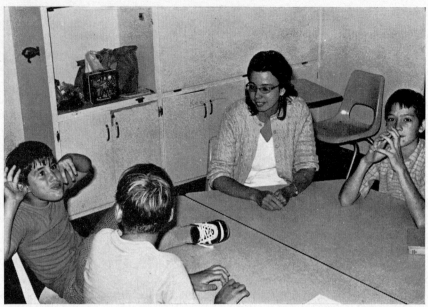

FIGURE 2. Group therapy with a hyperkinetic youngster. (Courtesy of Irvin Kraft, M.D.)

home or milieu, and the primary emphasis is on the associative element, rather than the activities involved. The central technique is the formation of a club by the children themselves.

Functions

The latency age grouping centers on the child's attuning himself to peers, teachers, leaders, community groups, ideals, and sublimated interests. Conscience formation, deriving from the resolution of oedipal strivings, involves both behavioral and cognitive vectors.

The function of group psychotherapy in this age-band is to aid the organizations of drives into socially acceptable behavior modes. The child gains in coping patterns and in understanding certain levels of psychological material. He gains experiential insight as he seeks his place in the group by modifying his behavior. Beyond certain fundamental rules established by the therapist, children set their own group behavioral standards openly and explicitly, as well as the usual covert ones that any group constructs automatically.

Rules

The therapist usually states that none of the children's verbalizations will be censured and that he will not permit behavior destructive to persons or the building. The therapist also reserves the right to notify parents if a serious

matter significantly affecting health emerges. Also, he notifies the children of telephone and other contacts their parents make with him about them.

Pubertal Groups

Pubertal children are often grouped monosexually. Their problems resemble those of late latency children, but they are also beginning to feel the impact and pressures of early adolescence. Since children of this age experience difficulties in conceptualizing, pubertal therapy groups tend to use play, drawing, psychodrama, and other nonverbal modes of expression. The therapist's role is active and directive.

Activity group psychotherapy has been the recommended type of group therapy for preadolescent children. The children, in groups of not more than eight, freely act out in a setting especially designed and planned for its physical and milieu characteristics. Games, structures activities, and projects must be planned and carried out. For children with neurotic-type difficulties, equipment is minimal in order to reduce the potential for frustration and failure, the goal being maximal elicitation of fantasies and expression of feelings about others. Anxiety, however, is allowed to develop, and the therapist works to help the group members cope with it. In the ego-impaired group, the sessions are highly structured, and anxiety is reduced to a minimum, although the structure is progressively loosened as their frustration tolerance rises. In the neurotic-type groups, limit setting is maintained only to protect personal safety and to prevent property damage, whereas in the ego-impairment group, all destructive behavior is actively discouraged.

When boys reach the preadolescent age range, especially in residential treatment, aggressive feelings drive and perplex them to impulsive actions. Group therapy, especially when combined with other techniques, affords opportunities for positive interpersonal transactions that diminish their basic mistrust, enhance low self-esteem, and affect their dependency-independency conflicts.

Activity groups provide an emotionally corrective experience by using a highly permissive setting to encourage freedom of expression of pent-up feelings along with regression. Interview-activity and other variants along the spectrum of therapeutic techniques also provide effective opportunities for experiential insight. Consistency, warmth, flexibility, and empathic qualities of the therapist, coupled with adequate knowledge of personality theory and therapeutic techniques, provide the ingredients for good group therapy in this and other age bands.

Parent Groups

Parent groups are a valuable aid to the group therapy of the children themselves. The parent of a child in therapy often has difficulty in understanding the nature of his child's ailment, in discerning the line of demarcation between normal and pathological behavior, in relating to the medical establishment, and in coping with feelings of guilt. A parents' group helps members formulate guidelines for action. In discussion groups mothers of disadvantaged children acquire new understanding of their children and change their attitudes, which improves the behavior of the children.

Adolescent Groups

Peer group affiliation and identification offer a basic opportunity for working on self-esteem, devices to enhance ego strength, personal consistency, and a feeling of environmental mastery. When the adolescent has failed to obtain these structural members, he can, through group psychotherapy, retrieve his lost opportunity in a helpful psychosocial therapeutic context and head on more directedly to adulthood.

Techniques of group therapy with adolescents vary widely, usually correlating well with the therapist's background and present outlook. Ackerman places both genders, ranging in age from 15 to 23, in the same group and suggested that the group functioned to "provide a social testing ground for the perceptions of self and relations to others." He emphasized the importance of nonverbal behavioral patterns as material for the group.

Group therapy deals more with conscious and preconscious levels than does an intensive, deeply introspective approach. Clarification, mutual support, facilitation of catharsis, reality testing, superego relaxation, and group integration are ego-supportive techniques.

Composition of the Group

The group format is that of an open-ended, interview-interaction, activity organization. The preferred number of adolescents is 8 to 10, but often circumstances require screening perhaps 30 or more to produce a group of 15. Of these, about 6 form a core group with constant attendance and effort, another 3 or 4 constitute an intermediate group who attend more than they miss, and the remainder make up a peripheral group who attend occasionally. Some therapists suggest separation of patients in early adolescence (ages 13 and 14) from older patients, since boys of 13 and 14 find 17-year-old girls difficult to deal with in these groups. Certain behavioral patterns—such as overt homosexuality, a flagrant sociopathic history, drug addiction, and psychosis—contraindicate inclusion in these groups.

Aims and Techniques

Interview mixed-group psychotherapy offers opportunity for the adolescent to relearn peer-relating techniques in a protective and supportive situation. Diminution of anxiety over sexual feelings and consolidation of sexual identification occur. The adolescent participates in group interaction in time and feels the pull of group cohesiveness. He also goes through relationship, catharsis, insight, reality testing, and sublimation as he reacts to the group's pace and its changes. The mechanism of identification affords the adolescent major opportunities for therapeutic gain as he identifies himself with other groups members and the therapist. The individual adolescent constitutes the focus of treatment, but he and the therapist are continually involved with the group as a sounding board and testing ground.

The therapist must be active, ego-supportive, and in control of the group situation at all times. He interprets cautiously to avoid the patient's misconstruing interpretation as personal criticism. Interpretations also focus on reality, rather than on symbolisms. They are couched in simple, direct references to basic feelings and to unconscious intent of behavior when it lies quite close to awareness.

Brief group responses to significant experiences narrated by a patient fulfill his needs, for he can return to the subject later if necessary. The group often prefers short discussions, since anxiety is too high to dwell at length on a topic.

The encounter group uses psychodrama, role play, and other active forms of interaction. The raw material offers opportunities from which insight develops. The group becomes the vehicle for heightened emotional interaction between therapist and patient and between patient and patient. The groups is expected to experience and share the feelings of a member, rather than merely attending to them, in order to increase group interaction. A key concept is free role experimentation, which facilitates the resolution of the adolescent ego identity crisis by allowing the adolescent to experiment with a wide variety of feelings, thoughts, and behaviors in a group setting.

Transactional analysis emphasizes treatment with specific goals defined in terms of observable changes in behavior and in attitudes. The concepts of transactional analysis provide a common vocabulary and frame of reference that are readily intelligible to adolescents and preadolescents for group discussions and analysis. Behavior is changed primarily by increasing the group members' understanding of themselves and of each other. Transactional analysis uses role play, Gestalts, psychodrama, and other group therapy techniques that involve verbalization and analysis. It also uses verbal contracting, in which the patient defines specific goals to work toward and the length of time in which he expects to achieve them.

Behavioral contracting schedules the exchange of positive reinforcements between two or more persons. A good contract specifies five requirements: (1) the privileges each party expects for fulfilling his responsibilities, (2) the responsibilities essential to securing each privilege, (3) a system of sanctions for failure to meet responsibilities, (4) a bonus clause, and (5) a feedback system to keep track of reinforcements given and received.

Modeling and peer reinforcement recognize the group itself as an active therapeutic factor in addition to being something acted on by the therapist, a trend also visible in transactional analysis and encounter therapy.

Therapy for Delinquent Adolescents

Delinquent adolescents differ in their dyssocial patterns from those who, in an adjustment reaction of adolescence or a transitional neurotic acting-out incident, violate the legal, moral, and social values of the community. The adolescent with a delinquent character disorder is persistently truant, runs away, or engages in other activities that usually mean removal to an institution.

In a study of group psychotherapy with male delinquents in an institution, group psychotherapy improved intellectual and school functions and psychological tests indicated some enhancement of emotional maturity. Another study indicated sequential steps in the responses, the first being episodes of testing and the second a series of acceptance operations.

The character distortions to be dealt with use aggression predominantly to reduce the internalized anxiety. The delinquents show a weak ego structure and a defective superego. As the therapist continues to model early life experiences for the adolescent—but without the inconsistencies of feelings, exploitations. and dishonesties—he becomes an ego-ideal for an embryonic superego.

With other therapists, the goal is real autonomy for the patient, not adjustment to the institution. They adhere to a leader role of permissiveness and support contrary to the over-all patterns of the institution.

Role of the Therapist

The traditionally passive role of the therapist has come under attack. Encounter therapy, for instance, incorporates several active techniques, such as environmental intervention, to stimulate positive, meaningful, and concerned encounters between the therapist and his group, to foster a positive transference to the therapist, and to motivate group members to attend sessions. Transactional analysis provides an active, intervening role for the group therapist, and the very nature of contractural techniques assures that he will state his expectations and premises in a manner proscribed by psychoanalytic theory.

Another aspect of the therapist's task is specificity of intervention. Therapists upholding the value of specific, highly directed intervention maintain that it is not enough for them to project a benevolent, supportive, and permissive presence. Specific intervention on the part of the therapist necessarily involves the projection of his values and expectations on the group.

The use of parapsychiatric personnel reflects another change in the role of the therapist.

Evaluation

Group psychotherapy helps children feel unconditionally accepted by the therapist and the group members. Failures are seen as part of each child's development. Complexes of feeling and ideation gain expression. Feelings of guilt, anxiety, inferiority, and insecurity find relief. Affection and aggression are evidenced without retaliation and danger.

REFERENCES

Barcai, A., Umbarger, C., Pierce, T., and Chamberlain, P. A comparison of three group approaches to underachieving children. Am. J. Orthopsychiatry, 43: 133, 1973.
Duffy, J. H., and Kraft, I. A. Beginning and middle phase characteristics of group psychotherapy and early adolescent boys and girls. Pschoanal. Groups, 2: 23, 1966–1967.
Gibson, R. E. The ambassador and the system (electronic and otherwise). Johns Hopkins Magazine, 24: 2, 1973.
Kraft, I. A., and Delaney, W. Movement communication with children in a psychoeducation program at a day hospital. J. Am. Dance Therapy Assoc., 1: 6, 1968.
Kraft, I. A., and Vick, J. Flexibility and variability of group psychotherapy with adolescent children. In Group Therapy 1973: An Overview, E. Schwartz and L. Wolberg, editors. Intercontinental Medical, New York, 1973.
Melville, K. Changing the family game. Science, 13: 17, 1973.
Rachman, A. W. Encounter techniques in analytic group psychotherapy with adolescents. Int. J. Group Psychother., 21: 319, 1971.
Rose, S. D. Treating Children in Groups, Jossey-Bass, London, 1972.
Sands, R. M., Blank, R., Brandt, B., Golub, S., Joelson, R., Klappersack, B., Levin, E., and Rothenburg, E. Breaking the bonds of tradition: reassessment of group treatment of latency children in a community mental health center. Am. J. Orthopsychiatry, 43: 212, 1973.
Vick, J., and Kraft, I. A. Creative activities. In Group Therapy for the Adolescent, N. S. Brandes, editor, p. 127. Jason Aronson, New York, 1973.

39.3. ORGANIC THERAPIES

Introduction

Physician attitudes limit the effectiveness of drug treatment because of the tendency to promote use in too large or too small amounts and because the attitude of the physician has a profound impact on the patient and family. The most experienced practitioners and researchers in child psychopharmacology typically report dosage values considerably in excess of the recommended dosages on the package insert on a milligram-per-kilogram basis.

Except for hospitalized children, the majority of illnesses for which pharmacotherapy is indicated are treated within a family context, where the parents and siblings are aware of and participate in the treatment. Drug abuse in an older sibling or parental doubts based on misapprehensions gained from sensational newspaper articles can defeat a sound treatment plan. It is incumbent on the physician to explain the rationale for the treatment and deal with misapprehensions by factual but sensitive handling of the family's concerns. In addition, all psychiatric complaints in children require psychological methods of management. Drugs do not cure, educate, or unlearn the basic causes of the disorder but only alleviate the most prominent symptoms. For children with the most severe pathology—such as organically retarded, hyperactive, or psychotic children—drugs can frequently make the difference between institutionalization and managing the child at home when parental support is adequate and appropriate therapeutic support can be given to the entire family.

Most children accept medication without a fuss if they are convinced it will help them and if the adult role models are accepting and supportive. Some children, however, feel embarrassed and regard the illness and the medication as something shameful. The child's fear may be augmented by peers who link his

TABLE I

Currently Available Phenothiazines: Status and Dosage for Children

Class	Generic	Trade	Manufacturer	Status* (PDR-1976)	Dosage (PDR-1976)	D.E.A.† Control Level	Remarks
Aliphatic	Chlorpromazine	Thorazine	Smith Kline & French	1	*Oral:* ¼ mg./lb. body weight q. 4–6 hr. prn for outpatients. *Rectal:* ½ mg./lb. body weight gm. 6–8 hr. prn for outpatients. *IM:* ¼ mg./lb. body weight q. 6–8 hr. prn for outpatients. With hospitalized patients higher doses may be used.	0	
	Triflupromazine	Vesprin	Squibb	1	*Oral:* 2 mg./kg. (1 mg./lb.) up to a maximum total daily dose of 150 mg. in divided doses. *IM:* 0.2 to 0.25 mg./kg. (⅒ to ⅛ mg./lb. up to a maximum total daily dose of 10 mg.)	0	Should not be administered to children under 2½ years of age and not recommended for IV use in children
Piperazine	Promazine	Sparine	Wyeth	0	Not listed	0	
	Prochlorperazine	Compazine	Smith Kline & French	1	*Oral* or *Rectal:* For children 2 to 12 years, starting dosage is 2.5 mg. b.i.d. or t.i.d., with maximum first day total dosage of 10 mg. For ages 2 to 5, total daily dosage usually does not exceed 20 mg. For ages 6–12, total daily dosage usually does not exceed 25 mg. *IM:* For ages under 12 calculate each dose on the basis of 0.06 mg./lb. body weight.	0	Not recommended for children under 20 lbs. in weight or 2 years of age. Children seem more prone to develop extrapyramidal reactions, even on moderate doses.
	Perphenazine	Trilafon	Schering	2	*Oral:* 2 to 4 mg. t.i.d. for neurotic anxiety and tension states. 4 to 8 mg. t.i.d. for moderately disturbed nonhospitalized psychotic patients. 8 to 16 mg. b.i.d. to q.i.d. for hospitalized psychiatric patients. Avoid dosages in excess of 64 mg. daily. *IM:* Children over 12 may receive the lowest limit of adult dosage.	0	Pediatric dose not yet established.

	Generic	Trade Name	Manufacturer	*	Dosage	†	
	Trifluoperazine	Stelazine	Smith Kline & French	1	*Oral:* Start with 1 mg. once a day or b.i.d. Daily dosage in excess of 15 mg. is rarely needed. *IM:* 1 mg. once a day or b.i.d.	0	These dosages are for children, ages 6 to 12 who are hospitalized or under close supervision.
	Fluphenazine HCl	Prolixin	Squibb	0	Safety and efficacy in children have not been established.	0	
		Permitil	Schering				
	Fluphenazine Decanoate	Prolixin	Squibb	2	Dosage for children over 12 not listed	0	
	Fluphenazine Enanthane	Prolixin	Squibb	2	Dosage for children over 12 not listed	0	
	Acetophenazine	Tindal	Schering	2	Dosage for children over 12 not listed	0	Not recommended for the pediatric age group
	Butaperazine	Repoise	Robins	2	Dosage for children over 12 not listed	0	
	Carphenazine	Proketazine	Wyeth	0	Not listed	0	
Piperidine	Thioridazine	Mellaril	Sandoz	1	For children 2 to 12 years, the dosage ranges from 0.5 mg./kg. to a maximum of 3.0 mg./kg. per day. For children with moderate disorders 10 mg. b.i.d. or t.i.d. is the usual starting dosage. For hospitalized, severely disturbed or psychotic children, 25 mg. b.i.d. or t.i.d. is the usual starting dosage.	0	Not intended for children under 2 years of age
	Mesoridazine	Serentil	Boehringer Ingelheim	2	Dosage for children over 12 not listed	0	
	Piperacetazine	Quide	Dow	2	Dosage for children over 12 not listed	0	

* 0 = No reference to children under 12; 1 = Recommended for children under 12; 2 = Not recommended for children under 12. PDR, *Physicians' Desk Reference*, Charles E. Baker, Jr., 1976.
† D.E.A., Drug Enforcement Administration.

deviant behavior with the fact that he is taking medication. The child has to be made to understand that medication does not absolve him from the responsibility to try, to exert control, and to obey authorities.

Guidelines for the proper dose range for different conditions have not been well-established for children. The time of day at which medication is given and the number of doses each day have to take into account the routines of the child during the day, especially his educational and peer considerations. There is also, apparently, a much wider range of dosage idiosyncrasy among children than among adults, so each patient must be carefully titrated, starting at the lowest recommended dose and proceeding to the amount that gives satisfactory benefit with the fewest side effects. Deleterious effects on cognitive function or peer relationships and beneficial educational changes can be ascertained only by careful inquiry and follow-up in the child's school.

Major Tranquilizers

Phenothiazines are recommended for only the most severely disturbed children. In general, the more potent piperazine drugs are used with the more severely impaired schizophrenic, autistic, and organically damaged children, particularly those who become sedated with chlorpromazine and require the presumed stimulating effects of these drugs to counteract apathy, withdrawal, retarded speech, and inadequate social interaction. However, controlled studies do not document the supposed stimulating effect in the severely withdrawn and apathetic child.

Such medications should be used only after an attempt at environmental or psychotherapeutic management has been made. Behavior modification provides an alternative method for all but the most agitated and uncontrolled children, and those techniques should be tried before pharmacotherapy is maintained over long periods of time.

Treatment should start with the lowest recommended dosage and be increased gradually over a period of weeks. A trial of 2 to 4 weeks is generally required as a minimum to establish efficacy and to adjust dosage. Retarded schizophrenic children may tolerate much larger doses of trifluoperazine or fluphenazine than do less

impaired, older children; retarded schizophrenics may show improvement in motor skills, social responsiveness, and language as a result of this drug regimen. The adult dose, adjusted strictly for body weight, may be 2 to 5 times too high for such a child, and a high incidence of dystonic effects has been reported. Small doses of the piperazines may cause irritability, agitation, or dyskinesia. Table I shows recommended phenothiazine usage with children.

The most common side-effect is lassitude and drowsiness, but this effect disappears after a few days in many children. Extrapyramidal symptoms may range from mild tremors to severe parkinsonism. The most disturbing side-effect is the syndrome of dyskinesia, including torticollis, aphonia, and dysphagia. Table II presents the side-effects found in an investigation of children with childhood psychosis in five single-blind trials.

Occasional reports of blood dyscrasias in children being treated with phenothiazines suggest that weekly blood counts are advisable during the first few months of therapy, inasmuch as this symptom occurs relatively early in treatment.

Minor Tranquilizers

Table III presents the recommended dosages for the most commonly used agents of this class. The minor tranquilizers have been extensively used in outpatient children with a variety of symptoms, including school phobias, night terrors, anxiety attacks, enuresis, encopresis, insomnia, muscular tension, tics, hypochondria, sexual precociousness, and depression. However, there is a marked discrepancy in the rates of success found in controlled and uncontrolled reports. The controlled trials almost always show equivocal or minor benefits, and the effect on cognitive function has not been adequately investigated.

The beneficial use of the minor tranquilizers in children who exhibit muscular tension, mild spasticity, or athetosis has been reported in a number of controlled and partially controlled trials. The effects are somewhat equivocal but are more convincing than findings with anxiety states, for which they are more commonly used. It has also been reported that chlordiazepoxide may disinhibit some impulsive and anxious children, making them paradoxically more aggressive.

TABLE II

Phenothiazine Side-Effects Data in Five Single-Blind Studies*: Distribution of Complaints by Symptom Areas (Percentage of Total Complaints in Parentheses)

	Chlorpro-mazine	Thioridazine	Triflupro-mazine	Prochlor-perazine	Fluphen-azine
Number of trials	12	24	14	7	28
Number of trials with positive treatment emergent symptoms	7	17	9	3	19
Total complaints	14	132	51	13	98
Adverse behavior effects	5 (36)	16 (12)	10 (20)	3 (23)	19 (19)
Lethargy, listlessness	2 (14)	4 (3)	2 (4)	1 (8)	8 (8)
Increased appetite	0	46 (35)	8 (16)	1 (8)	14 (14)
Weight gain	1 (7)	7 (5)	3 (6)	1 (8)	10 (10)
Gastrointestinal symptoms	0	0	0	3 (23)	0
Anorexia	0	1 (1)	0	2 (15)	4 (4)
Extrapyramidal symptoms	6 (43)	7 (5)	28 (55)†	1 (8)	33 (34)
Genitourinary symptoms	0	47 (36)	0	1 (8)	10 (10)
Photosensitivity	0	4 (3)	0	0	0

* D. M. Englehardt, P. Polizos, and R. A. Margolis. The drug treatment of childhood psychosis. In *Drugs, Development, and Cerebral Function*, W. L. Smith, editor, p. 230, Charles C Thomas, Springfield, Ill., 1972.

† This figure is an underestimate, since 6 of the 14 children received procyclidine HCl (Kemadrin) prophylactically and exhibited no extrapyramidal symptoms.

Antidepressants

These drugs, although not recommended for use with children under age 12, appear to have some value in the symptomatic control of persistent nocturnal enuresis, school phobia, and hyperkinetic impulse disorders. The drugs provide a useful alternative when other treatments have failed. A number of clinical trials suggest definite value for some depressed adolescents when they are carefully diagnosed to eliminate those depressions due to temporary stress, identity crisis, and other temporary adjustment reactions.

Central Nervous System Stimulants

These drugs have generally been used most successfully with the less severe behavior disorders, particularly minimal brain dysfunction and the hyperkinetic impulse syndrome. Their action is immediate and often dramatic in producing a calm, more integrated behavior pattern. Controlled trials have shown positive benefits on cognitive and perceptual functions, motor behavior, learning, and school achievement.

Children who do not have severe psychopathology but who do have attentional deficits, with or without hyperactivity, show significant benefit from these agents. Children with learning disorders without hyperactivity have shown significant gains in attention and achievement in short-term trials.

Early clinical reports that the stimulants relieve anxiety and inhibitions in neurotic children have not generally been confirmed in controlled trials, and measures of anxiety have generally been unaffected by treatment. However, clinical experience indicates that some inhibited and apathetic children without serious psychopathology show improvement.

The stimulants have not been found useful in schizophrenic and autistic children and may, in fact, exacerbate psychotic thought processes and behavior. Children with obsessional traits may become more withdrawn and preoccupied, and even children with apparently classical hyperkinetic impulse disorders sometimes become tearful and depressed.

The most common side-effects are insomnia and anorexia. These effects tend to diminish in most children over a 4-week period, and adjustment of dosage with respect to time of day and amount is frequently necessary.

Table IV presents the recommended dosages for the stimulants. Most experience shows that these agents are effective in a majority of cases within the dosage ranges given, but some chil-

TABLE III

Minor Tranquilizer Usage with Children

Brand Name	Generic Name	Manufacturer	Status* (PDR-1976)	Dosage (PDR-1976)	DEA† Control Level	Remarks
Benzodiazepines						
Librium	Chlordiazepoxide	Roche	1	5 mg., 2–4 times daily (may be increased in some children to 10 mg. 2 or 3 times daily)	IV	Not recommended for children under age 6
Valium	Diazepam	Roche	1	1–2.5 mg., 3 or 4 times daily initially; increase gradually as needed and tolerated	IV	Not for use in children under 6 months
Serax	Oxazepam	Wyeth	1	Absolute dosage for children 6–12 years of age is not established	IV	Not indicated in children under age 6
Tranxene	Clorazepate	Abbott	2		IV	Not recommended for patients under age 18
Substituted propanediols						
Miltown	Meprobamate	Wallace	1	100–200 mg. 2 or 3 times daily	IV	Not recommended for children under age 6
Tybatran	Tybamate	Robins	1	For children 6–12 years of age 20–35 mg./kg. body weight in 3 or 4 equally divided doses	0	Not recommended for children under age 6
Diphenylmethane derivatives						
Atarax Vistaril	Hydroxyzine	Roerig Pfizer	1	Under 6 years: 50 mg. daily in divided doses. Over 6 years: 50–100 mg. daily in divided doses	0	
Benadryl	Diphenhydramine	Parke, Davis	1	5 mg./kg./24 hrs., daily dose not to exceed 300 mg.; given in 3–4 divided doses a day	0	

* 0 = No reference to children under 12; 1 = Recommended for children under 12; 2 = Not recommended for children under 12. PDR, *Physicians' Desk Reference*, Charles E. Baker, Jr., 1976.
† DEA, Drug Enforcement Administration.

TABLE IV

Stimulant Drug Use with Children

Brand Name	Generic Name	Manufacturer	Dosage (1976 PDR)*	Remarks	DEA† Control Level
Benzedrine	Amphetamine sulfate	Smith Kline & French	Children 3–5 years of age: start with 2.5 mg. daily; dosage may be raised in increments of 2.5 mg. at weekly intervals until optimal response is obtained. Children 6 years of age and older: start with 5 mg. once or twice daily; daily dosage may be raised in increments of 5 mg. at weekly intervals until optimal response is obtained. Daily dosage may range from 5 mg. to 40 mg., although rarely some older children may require more than 40 mg. a day for optimal response.	Not recommended for use in children under 3 years of age	II
Dexedrine	Dextroamphetamine sulfate	Smith Kline & French	Children 3–5 years of age: start with 2.5 mg. daily; dosage may be raised in increments of 2.5 mg. at weekly intervals. Children 6 years of age and older: start with 5 mg. once or twice daily; daily dosage may be raised in increments of 5 mg. at weekly intervals. Daily dosage may range from 5 mg. to 40 mg., although rarely some older children may require more than 40 mg. a day for optimal response.	Not recommended for use in children under 3 years of age	II
Ritalin	Methylphenidate hydrochloride	Ciba	Start with small doses (such as 5 mg. before breakfast and lunch) with gradual increments of 5–10 mg. weekly. Daily dosage above 60 mg. is not recommended. If improvement is not observed after appropriate dosage adjustment over a 1-month period, the drug should be discontinued.	Not recommended for use in children under 6 years of age	II
Cylert	Pemoline	Abbott	Start with 37.5 mg. a day. This daily dosage should be gradually increased at weekly intervals in increments of 18.75 mg. until the desired clinical response is obtained. The mean daily effective dose ranges from 56.25 to 75 mg. a day. The maximum daily recommended dose is 112.5 mg.		IV
Deaner	Deanol acetamidobenzoate	Riker	Start with 300 mg. in the morning. After 3 weeks, if satisfactory improvement has occurred, most children may be maintained on 100 mg. daily doses. The maximum maintenance dose should not exceed 300 mg. daily.	Not recommended for use in children under 6 years of age	0

* PDR, *Physicians' Desk Reference*, Charles E. Baker, Jr., 1976.

† DEA, Drug Enforcement Administration.

dren tolerate and require somewhat higher levels. Careful diagnosis, follow-up, and continued monitoring of progress must be maintained, and frequent drug holidays must be implemented so that treatment is discontinued when no longer indicated.

Other Somatic Therapies

Insulin shock therapy, electroconvulsive therapy, and lobotomy are no longer considered justifiable or of value in children. Recently use of megavitamin therapy for a variety of psychiatric conditions in children has not been shown to have any definite value.

REFERENCES

Arnold, L. E., Huestis, R. D., Smeltzer, D. J., Scheib, J., Wemmer, D., and Colner, G. Levoamphetamine vs dextroamphetamine in minimal brain dysfunction. Arch. Gen. Psychiat., 33: 292, 1976.
Conners, C. K. Symposium: Behavior modification by drugs. II. Psychological effects of stimulant drugs in children with minimal brain dysfunction. Pediatrics, 49: 702, 1972.
Conners, C. K. Symposium: Behavior modification by drugs. minimal brain dysfunction. Ann. N. N. Acad. Sci., 205: 283, 1973.
Eisenberg, L., and Conners, C. K. Psychopharmacology in childhood. In Behavioral Science in Pediatric Medicine, N. Talbot, J. Kagan, and L. Eisenberg, editors, pp. 397–423. Saunders, Philadelphia, 1971.
Engelhardt, D. M., Polizos, P., and Margolis, R. A. The drug treatment of childhood psychosis, In Drugs, Development, and Cerebral Function, W. L. Smith, editor, pp. 224–234. Charles C Thomas, Springfield, Ill., 1972.
Laufer, M. W. Psychiatric diagnosis and treatment of children with minimal brain dysfunction. Ann. N. Y. Acad. Sci., 205: 303, 1973.
Lipman, R. S. Pharmacotherapy of children. Psychopharmacol. Bull., 7: 14, 1971.
Millichap, J. G. Drugs in management of minimal brain dysfunction. Ann. N. Y. Acad. Sci., 205: 321, 1973.
Satterfield, J. H., Lesser, , L. I., Saul, R. E., and Cantwell, D. P. EEG aspects in the diagnosis and treatment of minimal brain dysfunction. Ann. N. Y. Acad. Sci., 205: 274, 1973.
Snyder, S. H., and Meyerhoff, J. L. How amphetamine acts in minimal brain dysfunction. Ann. N. Y. Acad. Sci., 205: 310, 1973.
Solomons, G. Drug therapy: Initiation and follow-up. Ann. N. Y. Acad. Sci., 205: 335, 1973.
Wender, P. H. Minimal Brain Dysfunction, in Children. Wiley-Interscience, New York, 1971.

39.4.   RESIDENTIAL TREATMENT

Introduction

It has been estimated that there are 450,000 seriously distrubed children in need of treatment. In 1966 there were 276 residential treatment institutions, which cared for only a fraction of the children in need. The staffing patterns include various combinations of child care workers, teachers, social workers, psychiatrists, pediatricians, nurses, and psychologists, making the cost of residential treatment very high.

The design of the building should take into account the physical, cognitive, and emotional needs of children between 6 and 15 years of age. Private or shared bedrooms, separate showers and bath facilities for boys and girls, communal living rooms and dining rooms, safe and easy access to recreational facilities and classrooms, and therapists' offices close to the group living area are some of the minimal requirements.

Indications

Children with antisocial behavior, borderline characters, and aggressive impulse disorders who cannot be managed on an outpatient basis but who do not require a closed-ward environment constitute the majority of children treated in residential settings. The symptoms may include stealing, truancy, running away, fire setting, enuresis, severe learning difficulty, and destructive behavior.

Referral and Intake

Most children who are referred for residential treatment have been seen previously by one or more professional persons. Unsuccessful attempts at outpatient treatment and foster home or other custodial placement often precede residential treatment. The age range of the children varies from institution to institution, but most are between 5 and 15 years of age. Boys are referred more frequently than girls.

An initial review of the data enables the intake staff to determine whether a particular child is likely to benefit from their particular treatment program. It is common to find that, for every child accepted for admission, three are rejected. The next step usually involves interviews with the child and his parents. Psychological testing and neurological examinations are performed when indicated if these have not already been done.

The needs of the child, the skills of the staff, the balance of the patient population, and estimates of the prognosis are some of the variables to be weighed when a child is being considered for admission. The parents may or may not be available for treatment. This evaluation and appraisal process forms the basis on which the staff reaches a decision and makes a tentative treatment plan. A preplacement visit by the child and his family is usually arranged to help prepare the child for admission.

Treatment

The total experience of the residential setting constitutes the treatment of the child.

Group Living

By far the largest amount of time in the child's life in a residential treatment setting is spent in group living. The group living staff members offer a structured environment for the child that constitutes a therapeutic milieu. Tasks are defined within the limits of the child's abilities; incentives, such as increased privileges, encourage the child to progress.

A child often selects one or more staff members with whom to form a relationship through which the child expresses, consciously and unconsciously, many of his feelings toward his parents. Sometimes the group living professional knows enough about the child to make an interpretation to the child when this seems appropriate. However, the professional must be aware of countertransference problems.

To maintain consistency and balance, the group living staff must communicate freely and regularly with each other and with the other professional and administrative staff members of the residential setting, particularly the child's teacher and therapist.

Education

Children in residential treatment frequently have severe learning difficulties, and usually they cannot function in a regular community school. Consequently, a special on-grounds school setting is required. Some of the characteristics of this school include a high teacher-to-student ratio, specialized learning equipment, and a curriculum designed to capture the child's interest and motivate him to begin learning again. The teacher can offer the child a structured environment, a model for identification, and clarifying interpretation of his behavior when appropriate. The teacher must be in free and regular communication with the other professional staff members, including the group living staff and the children's therapists.

Therapy

Traditional modes of psychotherapy have a definite place in residential treatment. These modes include intensive, individual psychotherapy with the child, group therapy with selected children, individual or group therapy or both for parents, and, in some cases, family therapy.

The child relates to the total staff of the setting and, therefore, needs to know that what transpires in the therapist's office is shared with the total professional staff, but will not be revealed to other family members or other children in the residential center. Psychotherapeutic encounters often continue outside the setting of the therapist's office.

Behavior modification principles have also been applied, particularly in group work with children.

Medication is helpful when there is an indication for a particular drug. Methylphenidate has been found helpful for young children with evidence of minimal brain dysfunction. Imipramine has been useful in the management of enuresis. Anticonvulsant medication may be helpful when there is an associated electroencephalographic abnormality suggestive of a seizure disorder. Thioridazine is sometimes useful in children with a borderline diagnosis who are in danger of decompensation because of a particular stress.

Work with the parents is important, both for the parents' sake and because children have strong emotional ties to their parents. The parents may need help in enabling the child to live in another setting.

Communication

To maintain communication, the staff members must meet as a group, without an agenda, at least once a week. The purpose of these meetings is to allow feelings to come to light that may otherwise remain hidden and silently fermenting. Role conflicts, countertransference problems, treatment blind spots, residential center policies, treatment approaches, and work with other agencies are some of the subjects discussed. Greater staff cohesion, collaboration, and commitment occur when all staff members are involved in every aspect of the treatment of the child.

Course of Treatment

Children who enter a residential center may experience anxiety and feelings of loss and some relief. The child may temporarily deal with this anxiety or relief by good behavior and a strong apparent wish to please. This honeymoon period, which may last from a few days to a few months, gives way to the re-emergence of the child's characteristic behavior patterns, albeit in modified form. The slow and difficult task of working through unconscious attitudes and fantasies that perpetuate the child's now maladaptive behavior constitutes a major part of the total therapeutic effort, which may last for 2 or more years. As termination and discharge approach, earlier feelings of loss are often re-evoked, and temporary regression may occur, with heightened acting-out behavior, sometimes of an aggressive kind.

There is no single course of treatment, since the variables are many, including the strengths and weaknesses of the particular child, the strengths and weaknesses of the parents, the skills of staff, and the degree to which a suitable discharge plan can be put into effect.

Evaluation

To monitor the course of treatment, the staff must attend regular comprehensive case review conferences. At such conferences, reports from group living, school, and therapy are presented and discussed, along with additional data derived from neurological examinations and psychological tests. Diagnoses and treatment goals often need to be revised as the child becomes better known to the staff.

Discharge Plans and Follow-up Care

Cure, whatever that may mean, is rarely an attainable goal for children in residential treatment. Improved object relations and social adaptation, ability to function in an outside school and later at work, and the working through of certain kinds of trauma are more realistic goals for the child. Similar goals obtain for the parents.

The range of disposition plans varies according to the outcome. Return to the family with or without further outpatient treatment, day care, placement in a group or foster home, boarding school, further residential treatment in another institution, and custodial care are some common options.

REFERENCES

Allerhand, M. E., Weber, R. E., and Haug, M. *Adaptation and Adaptability: The Bellefaire Follow-up Study.* Child Welfare League of America, New York, 1966.
Hirschberg, J. C. Termination of residential treatment of children. Child Welfare, *49:* 443, 1970.
Hylton, L. F. *The Residential Treatment Center: Children, Programs, and Costs.* Child Welfare League of America, New York, 1964.
Joint Commission on Mental Health of Children. *Crisis in Child Mental Health,* p. 272. Harper & Row, New York, 1970.
Polsky, H., and Claster, D. S. *The Dynamics of Residential Treatment: A Social System Analysis.* University of North Carolina Press, Chapel Hill, 1968.
Reid, J. H., and Hagan, H. R. *Residential Treatment of Emotionally Disturbed Children.* Child Welfare League of America, New York, 1952.

39.5.   DAY TREATMENT

Day Care

Day care programs are designed to provide supplementary stimulation for children whose optimum development is endangered by the lack of such stimulation. Programs that focus on active problem-solving and choice-making processes are preferable to those with fixed curriculums to be learned. The child's individual developmental needs require flexible and creative approaches. The aim of these day care programs is to supplement, rather than replace, the family.

Day Treatment

Day treatment for children consists of a more or less comprehensive program selected from a therapeutic group living experience, psychotherapy—individual, group, joint, or family—education, health care, and psychotropic medication. The primary indication for day treatment is the need for a more structured, intensive, and specialized treatment program than can be provided on an outpatient basis. At the same time, the home in which the child is living should be able to provide an environment that is not destructive to the child's development. The parents are usually involved in the day treatment.

Children likely to benefit from day treatment may have a wide range of diagnoses, including infantile autism, personality disorders, and minimal brain dysfunction or mental retardation. The symptoms, although severe, should not include behavior likely to be destructive.

Because the needs of children who may benefit from day treatment are many, a broad spectrum of day treatment programs is required. Some programs specialize in the special educational and structured environmental needs of the mentally retarded child. Others offer the special therapeutic efforts required for the treatment of the autistic or schizophrenic child. Still others provide the total spectrum of treatment usually found in full residential treatment, of which they may be a part. The school program represents a major component of day treatment.

REFERENCES

Caldwell, B. M., Wright, C. M., Honig, A. S., and Tannenbaum, J. Infant day care and attachment. Am. J. Orthopsychiatry, *40:* 397, 1970.
Dingman, P. R. Day programs for children: A note on terminology. Ment. Hygiene, *53:* 646, 1969.
Donohue, D. T. Establishment of day care programs for the mentally retarded. Child Welfare, *50:* 519, 1971.
Heinecke, C. M., Friedman, L., Prescott, E., Puncel, C., and Sale, J. S. The organization of day care: Considerations relating to the mental health of child and family. Am. J. Orthopsychiatry, *43:* 8, 1973.
La Vietes, R., Cohen, R., Reems, R., and Ronall, R. Day treatment center and school: Seven years experience. Am. J. Orthopsychiatry, *35:* 160, 1965.
Sale, J. S. Family day care: One alternative in the delivery of developmental services in early childhood. Am. J. Orthopsychiatry, *43:* 37, 1973.
Zigler, E. The environmental mystique: Training in the intellect versus development of the child. Child. Educ., *46:* 402, 1970.

39.6. PSYCHIATRY AND THE SCHOOL

Introduction

The purpose of education—from a dynamic, psychiatric point of view—is to give each child those tools that enable the autonomous ego functions to enhance competence, self-worth, and creativity. From society's viewpoint, education provides opportunities to learn the technical skills currently required. For most children, education has had as its function the maintenance of societal norms.

Psychiatry in the schools often functions to help a system that has previously been effective with only cognitive approaches in teaching to recognize the role of feelings in the life of the child and developmentally in the learning process. The increasing need for stimulation not available at home and for socializing experiences not possible in small families has led to great demands for preschool programs.

Child care, early stimulation, development of nurturant child-adult relationships, and socialization need to be provided by persons who understand the developmental tasks of childhood, how they are facilitated, and how learning, curiosity, and competence can be promoted. Conflicts from infancy and early childhood that are not resolved may, to some extent, be ameliorated by the involvement of a child in a school setting that enhances his own sense of self-worth and begins the socialization process, which may not have occurred in a small, disorganized, or fragmented family.

When parents have difficulties in their basic capacities for nurturance and are unable to be very clear and firm with their children, they evoke problems for the child with authority figures in the school. Such problems provide opportunities for resolution of some authority and oppositional behavior problems with teachers. They become new models for the child.

Role of Psychiatric Consultation

Mental health consultation is a method for helping professional colleagues in other professions with their clients' behavioral problems. Educators are concerned with students' behavior that interferes with their own and others' learning in the classroom. The method is an indirect, task-oriented one, not a psychotherapeutic approach. It depends on the development of a colleague relationship between the psychiatrist and the educator, a relationship that reduces the fear of the educator that he will be treated as a patient.

The initial effort of developing a colleague relationship is facilitated by the consultant's statements that, to understand any problem and to begin to think about solutions, certain data must be collected. The basic initial hypothesis is that a child's early life experience provides a basis for later behavior and may be predictive of later behavior. The involvement of the consultee in collecting data from cumulative records, from parents, and when necessary, from such sources as pediatricians and preschools takes time and reinforcement from the consultant.

The student's behavior can then be assessed in terms of the past information and certain patterns tentatively outlined, with reduction of the consultee's sense of blame for current problems. A behavioral data base is established to find out what situations appear to be related to behavior problems and the duration of these problems under varying circumstances.

The third phase is one of hypothesis generation. Both consultant and consultee comb through the data to evolve the most meaningful hypothesis about why the student behaves as he does. From these hypotheses, several ways of testing their relevance evolve. Interventions are planned to test a hypothesis that could reasonably account for most of the behavior. One of several possible interventions is chosen to test how the application of the intervention affects the student. Subsequent meetings are used to evaluate the data from the interventions, to test the hypothesis, and to revise the hypothesis and the interventions based on the new data.

Prevention and the Schools

Prevention of an early intervention in behavior and learning disturbances can be an important school function. Teachers, with minimal help, can diagnose problems in the classroom effectively. The more severe problems require differential diagnosis by specially trained personnel. Currently, psychiatrists are learning to identify problem children on the basis of deficits in their development and their ego capacities for learning and socialization.

Chronic Illness

Child psychiatrists are now involved with pediatricians in comprehensive care clinics, where children with chronic diseases and their families are followed. There is also closer liaison with pediatricians about the emotional impact of illness on children. Perhaps most rewarding has been the mutual education of both psychiatrist and pediatrician about how families and children with chronic illnesses can be helped to face these illnesses more openly. Helping the child, the family, and the school to be clear about the child's abilities to learn and what the actual limitations and expectations are often prevents marginal functioning and increased disability for such a child in school.

Special Education Programs

Emotionally disturbed children and children with retardation, orthopedic, neurological, speech, visual, and auditory handicaps, who often have emotional problems as well, require help for teachers and programs to be effective.

The differentiation between retardation and autism requires consultants experienced in differential diagnosis.

The use of behavior modification techniques has made it possible to alter behavior so that more learning occurs. However, the socialization required for most effective functioning of handicapped children depends on a firm knowledge of child development. Consultants can help parents and teachers understand the feelings of guilt and anger common to both because of the unremitting hard work involved in trying to help the child, the wish for magical cures, and, when difficulties mount, the wish to be rid of the child. The reduction of these painful feelings prevents the child from using adults against each other or using the adults' guilt to avoid the laborious and repetitive learning required for mastery and better functioning.

Psychiatric Disorders

The Joint Commission on Mental Health of Children found in its surveys that between 10 and 12 per cent of all school children had emotional and behavior disorders of sufficient severity to require help outside of the classroom.

Learning Disorders

In disorders of learning, boys are at much higher risk than girls, the ratio being estimated at 8 or 10 to 1. Most disorders are revealed by either withdrawal or hyperactive aggressive behavior that clearly interferes with functioning in the classroom.

Causes. Many learning disorders are related to neurophysiological disturbances of maturation. Maturational lags in cerebral development—implicating sensorimotor, perceptual, and integrative systems—are revealed by problems with auditory, visual, and kinesthetic discrimination and by deficits in memory and problems in symbol formation and receptive and expressive use of language. If not remedied early, these problems are inevitably compounded by severe emotional disturbances. Diagnosis and treatment are often complicated by the emotional overlay and the intrafamilial problems with which these learning disorders are interwoven. Minimal cerebral dysfunctions can result from a variety of insults to the infant's brain in the uterus and in the earliest years of life.

Some psychological disturbances of learning may be linked to the earliest mother-child relationships. Developmental studies indicate the need for predictable and responsive nurturance to permit and encourage ego development, the free use of curiosity, and responsiveness to environmental stimuli necessary to learning.

Diagnosis and Treatment. Diagnosis of learning problems with psychological causes is one of the school psychiatrist's primary functions. He must be involved in continuous in-service training of educators and mental health and health personnel.

The treatment plan must focus on the educational or learning component of the difficulty, so that learning can be enhanced and the student's feelings of self-worth increased, and on other relevant interpersonal methods, such as play and activity groups for young children, therapeutic groups for preadolescents and adolescents, and, when necessary, individual psychotherapy. Behavior modification techniques have proved effective with some learning problems. Brief therapy and crisis interventions are important when abrupt changes in behavior and learning patterns have occurred.

School Phobias

School phobia describes a number of different conditions having in common a refusal to attend school. Most school systems report an incidence of school phobia of 17 cases in 1,000. The incidence statistics reveal three peaks: (1) school entry into kindergarten or first grade and the first separation problems, (2) in the third and fourth grades, when increased demands are made of the students to prove that they have learned, and (3) in junior high school for girls and senior high school for boys, when undressing for gym becomes a problem for some students and leads to refusal to attend school.

Causes. The child's anxiety about separation from his mother, a symbiotic relationship between mother and child, with mutual anxiety about separation, the child's need to avoid deflation of his feelings of omnipotence and inflated sense of achievement promoted by his mother, hostile behavior of teachers in reaction to aggressive and sexual behaviors of the child—all may cause school phobia. In addition, very dependent children may find stern, demanding teachers very frightening and inhibiting of learning and refuse to experience such continued anxiety in school. The fact that school phobia is often related to enuresis, night terrors, and hysterical and psychosomatic symptoms indicates that the school refusal is part of a complex of conflicts. Avoiding school may be a way of avoiding growing up and facing the assertion necessary both at home and in school with peers.

Psychosis with massive anxiety about relationships with others can occur at any developmental stage and lead to refusal to go to school. Adolescence, with its sexual identity and independence problems, frequently highlights psychotic processes, and such decompensation may lead to fear of both peers and adults, with refusal to attend school.

Since the causes of school phobia both developmentally and psychopathologically are varied, each case must be understood in terms of the youngster's previous development and his relations to his mother, father, and siblings and their interactions together as revealed in an evaluation of family dynamics.

Treatment. Most clinicians have emphasized a rapid return to school. However, for the psychotic child, intensive work with the child and parents may be required to be able to return the child to school. Dynamic understanding of the child's problems may lead to family or individual therapy geared to reducing conflicts and the symbiosis between mother and child. The school personnel's attitudes toward vulnerable dependent children who require support and warm relationships as an aid to feeling accepted and believing that one's learning is approved of may also require considerable collaborative work. In puberty, increased sensitivity by gym teachers, counselors, and school nurses to a refusal to undress for gym may avoid forcing the situation and engendering school avoidance.

Various desensitization techniques and behavior modification methods have been used effectively to reduce the fear of school, with early return and often reduction of accompanying symptoms.

Prognosis. Prognosis depends on the underlying causes and the length of time that the student remains absent. Severe psychosomatic problems may continue in those children who are not treated early and may result in continued absence from school because of increasingly severe psychophysiologic problems.

Boys with school refusal seem to have a poorer prognosis than girls, although the frequency of occurrence is about the same. In primitive families or when there is a good deal of psychopathology in the parents, the prognosis is poor.

Poverty and Learning Problems

Children in poverty populations, especially in urban inner cities, are usually raised in family and cultural settings in which there is minimal verbal interaction with parents and little parental interest in the child's early learning. The child enters school with fewer skills in cognitive areas and verbal expression than is expected by the school system. School failure and alienation from teachers and school occur early, and more than half of these children drop out or are expelled for behavior problems before the twelfth grade.

The incidence of maternal and infant malnutrition and premature births is overwhelming in this population, leading to retardation and organic deficits that further complicate learning for up to 20 per cent of these children.

The school psychiatrist who is clear about the issues may help school personnel recognize the psychological problems that the school system engenders in these children. New methods of learning to read and involving children in more interesting and sometimes self-generating curriculum materials have been tried with variable success. A key factor in success has been the degree of parental involvement in the school programs.

Therapeutic and Learning Programs

Psychoeducational programs can be helpful to even very disturbed children. Teaching and learning can be opportunities for providing therapeutic experiences for the child through specially trained educators. Some programs depend on the milieu of special group and individual activities to enhance self-worth and a feeling of competence and to encourage the capacity to relate to peers and adults. Such programs use therapeutic groups, occupational therapy geared to help a child overcome sensorimotor problems, and therapeutic dance, drama, and athletic programs—all geared to fuller expression of feelings and increased physical competence.

College Psychiatry

To a great extent, the issues raised in high school—such as psychotic decompensation, depression, and suicide—are the problems seen in college students. Lack of motivation to do the necessary work when attending college is seen in many young adults.

The first year of college away from home presents problems of separation, making new friends, and coping with the demands of a new environment—academic, social, and sexual. The freedom achieved by being away from home is threatening to many students. Sexual freedom and the freedom of choice may be overwhelming to many students. For many first-year students, the first semester examinations are most threatening as tests of their competence. Failure to do well may result in dropout or serious decompensation. College counseling centers report that the most frequent reason for referral is inability to concentrate and to study consistently. Anxiety and depression are the usual underlying factors.

Students at Risk

The high-risk college students are those who come from rural communities to a large urban college with its competitiveness, students who are pressured by their families for high achievement, students who, although isolated in high school, have had support from the home, and minority students who need to achieve to become more socially mobile or to feel themselves worthy of representing and working for their people. Students from foreign countries and United States minority students frequently cannot cope with the aggressive competition and the isolation from others of similar background who understand their customs, ways of relating, and needs.

In community colleges, which many minority students attend, the high-risk students are those who experience conflict between their former life style and their new way of life. It is difficult for them to schedule themselves and keep their schedules, become responsible for assignments, and abandon their previous gratification-now way of life. The pull between these two life styles is a major cause of anxiety, psychophysiologic symptoms, and antisocial acting out.

Treatment

Most campuses limit therapeutic work to brief therapy. It is important for counselors to have experienced psychiatrists as supervisors for their more difficult treatment cases.

In recent years, group therapy has been frequently used. Young adults find themselves not alone in their problems and concerns, and they can learn about both the causes and the methods of handling problems.

The integration of academic counseling with personal counseling has begun to pick up early troubles before they lead to failure.

Prevention

On many large campuses where students live in dormitories, efforts have been made to include each new student in a living-group experience. In these groups, common problems of entering students are explored with the help of more advanced students, who have experienced these problems firsthand. A buddy system has been effective on several large campuses.

Increased in-service training for dormitory personnel to help them be alert to signs of depression, isolation, loneliness, and anxiety has paid off through earlier therapeutic work with new students.

In off-campus activities—especially working with underprivileged youth, in hospitals, and in other important community services—students find an important esprit de corps with their fellows, socialize more, and feel useful and needed during a period of self-doubt.

Sensitivity training and encounter groups held by senior dormitory personnel with students enhance self-acceptance and socialization of entering students.

REFERENCES

Aries, P. *Centuries of Childhood*. Vantage Books, New York, 1969.

Bateson, G. *Steps to an Ecology of Mind*. Chandler, Scranton, 1972.

Berkovitz, I. H., editor. *Adolescents Grow in Groups*. Brunner/Mazel, New York, 1972.

Berlin, I. N. Crisis intervention and short-term therapy. An approach in a child-psychiatric clinic. In *Children and Their Parents in Brief Therapy*, H. H. Barten and S. S. Barten, editors, pp. 49–62. Behavioral Publications. New York, 1973.

Berlin, I. N. In *Mental Health Consultation to the Schools: Directions for the Future*. BASICO No. 645 (NIMH HSM 42-72-110). May 1973.

Birch, H. G. Functional effects of fetal malnutrition. In *Annual Progress in Child Psychiatry and Child Development*, S. Chess and A. Thomas, editors, p. 96. Brunner/Mazel, New York, 1972.

Bower, E., Shellhamer, T., and Daily, J. School characteristics of male adolescents who later became schizophrenics. Am. J. Orthopsychiatry, *30:* 712, 1960.

Buxbaum, E. Transference and group formation in children and adolescents. Study Child, *19:* 421, 1964.

Caplan, G. *The Theory and Practice of Mental Health Consultation*. Basic Books, New York, 1970.

Coolidge, J. C., Hahn, P. B., and Peck, A. L. School phobia: Neurotic crisis or way of life. Am. J. Orthopsychiatry, *272:* 296, 1967.

Fish, B. The "one child, one drug" myth of stimulants in hyperkinesis. In *Annual Progress in Child Psychiatry and Child Development*, S. Chess and A. Thomas, editors, p. 383. Brunner/Mazel, New York, 1972.

Kagan, J. Reflection-impulsivity and reading ability in primary grade children. Child Dev., *36:* 609, 1965.

Kempe, C. H., and Helfer, R. *Helping the Battered Child and His Family*. J. B. Lippincott, Philadelphia, 1972.

Provence, S. A three-pronged project. Children, *16:* 52, 1969.

Rutter, M. Normal psychosexual development. In *Annual Progress in Child Psychiatry and Child Development*. S. Chess and A. Thomas, editors, p. 64. Brunner/Mazel, New York, 1972.

White, R. W. Competence and the psychosexual stages of development. In *Nebraska Symposium on Motivation*, p. 97. University of Nebraska, Lincoln, 1960.

39.7.   PSYCHIATRIC TREATMENT OF THE ADOLESCENT

Introduction

Until recently, the psychiatric disorders of adolescence received little professional attention. This neglect was partially because of a tendency to regard psychiatric symptoms in the adolescent years as relatively normal, external expressions of necessary internal turbulence during this period of development. However, the untreated or incompletely treated psychiatric disability of adolescence did not disappear with growth. Instead, it became the psychiatric disability of adulthood. In most instances, adolescent emotional disorders reflected basic psychopathology, rather than developmentally induced, time-limited excesses of the growth process.

The period of adolescence may be much less emotionally tumultuous than psychiatric myths have suggested. Only a small minority of youngsters demonstrate definite psychiatric symptoms. The majority show evidence of internal unrest and psychological reorganization, generally limited to a moderate increase in anxiety level and a tendency toward moodiness.

Treatment problems are even more challenging than diagnosis. Most adolescents are referred to treatment by their parents or other adults, often against their conscious desires. The therapist must also deal with the adolescent's increased narcissistic vulnerability. The adolescent tends to disparage, dislike, and discredit the therapist whenever the professional is a source of emotional discomfort and to idealize him during periods when the relationship is gratifying. In psychoanalytic terms, the goal of psychiatric treatment with the adolescent is to strengthen the ego, but the adolescent has a strong need to place and keep the therapist in a superego role. This tendency is magnified by the adolescent's ambivalent wish to relate to the therapist more as a real object than as a transference figure.

Diagnostic Evaluation

Flexibility is the keynote in the psychiatric evaluation of the adolescent patient. The essentials of the diagnostic evaluation include interviews with the youngster and with his parents. In some older adolescents, it may be possible to proceed without talking with the parents, but this is rarely the ideal arrangement. Ancillary studies—such as psychological testing, a neurological examination, an electroencephalogram, a physical examination, or other special procedures—may be needed.

Interviews with the Adolescent

It is usually advisable to initiate the evaluation procedure by interviewing the adolescent. Proceeding in this way not only helps to undercut the adolescent's suspicion that the examiner and his parents are conspiring against him but offers the psychiatrist an opportunity to observe the extent to which the adolescent can take independent responsibility for his adjustment difficulties. The adolescent's personal worries may differ markedly from those presented by the parents. In other instances, there is agreement as to the specifics of the situation but variation as to the priorities of concern. Often, the adolescent has the more accurate understanding of the roots of his difficulties.

Most adolescents seem threatened by the dependency implied in the interview situation.

They explore any latent desires to dominate in the psychiatrist by offering him a variety of authority roles and observing his response. Some patients are so angry, unrealistic, confused, or disorganized that they are unable to provide even a subjective account of their difficulties. Nonpunitive straightforwardness is always an asset in interaction with the adolescent.

Once some degree of rapport is established, the examiner's attention is directed primarily to assessing the adequacy with which the adolescent is coping with his past, his present, and his view of the future. In early adolescence, one anticipates a preoccupation with the regressive reawakening of oedipal and pregenital conflicts, with only tentative, predominantly narcissistic attachments outside the family and an unrealistic view of the future strongly colored by current conflict. By mid-adolescence, one anticipates some resolution of regressive issues and increased interest in real object relations outside the family circle, including a growing focus on solidification of sexual role. In late adolescence and early young adulthood, there should be a stronger movement toward moral and vocational encounters with adult society and the consolidation of conflicts and identity fragments into a coherent and stabilized whole.

It is often useful to concentrate attention on the adolescent's interpersonal relationships. This focus provides one of the most sensitive and comprehensive ways of gaining a rapid understanding of the adolescent's developmental level and areas of psychopathology.

The precipitating event leading to referral can rarely be determined by direct questioning of either the adolescent or his parents. It usually requires careful attention to temporal relationships between occurrences and symptom appearances in the history and sensitivity to the themes presented by both the patient and his parents.

Parental Interviews

The two primary goals in diagnostic interviews with the adolescent's parents are to obtain as much information as possible regarding the developmental history and to assess current family dynamics and the adolescent's role in the family.

Parental memory for the exact chronology and details of the developmental history is notoriously inaccurate, but the style of distortion may tell a great deal about the parental relationship with the child. Differences in the account presented by the two parents separately may represent subtle or gross differences in the way they have perceived and related to their offspring. Extraordinary occurrences such as serious illnesses, prolonged separations from the parents, and intense reactions to such developmental milestones as weaning, toilet training, early separations from the parents tend to be reported fairly accurately. Subtle nauances of early temperamental style may be overshadowed by current parental emotional needs, but extraordinary temperamental deviations tend to be more accurately recalled.

Diagnostic interviews with the parents are also of value in assessing the extent to which the parents require the child's illness for current family homeostasis. Early recognition of such parental needs is essential to appropriate treatment planning.

Ancillary Studies

Psychological testing of the adolescent and sometimes of his parents is most useful if the psychiatric examiner can formulate specific questions that require clarification and if the testing psychologist is experienced in the evaluation of adolescent patients. Psychological evaluation of intellectual level and perceptual skills is essential in all instances of adolescent learning disability or academic failure. Psychological testing may also help the examiner confirm the presence of early psychotic deterioration in youngsters whose surface behavior is more suggestive of a personality disorder or severe neurosis.

Frank discussion of the nature and purposes of the tests is essential. Many adolescents tend to be suspicious of any procedure to obtain information they wish to keep secret.

Postdiagnostic Family Conferences

Adolescents should be included in the reporting and planning conference that normally follows completion of the diagnostic process. In this interview, the examiner attempts to describe his findings, discuss his view of the basic difficulties, encourage family discussion of these ideas, and present treatment recommendations. This post-diagnostic conference is clearly not only a summation of the diagnostic thinking but

a preparation for therapy. It requires a clear understanding of individual and family psychopathology in the specific case, a tactful sensitivity to subtle emotional currents during the interview, and often a willingness to be realistically confronting and firm in the face of unified family denial or hostility.

Treatment

Outpatient Treatment

Most adolescent psychiatric treatment is conducted on an outpatient basis.

Individual psychotherapy. Individual psychotherapy is probably the most frequently used treatment approach with adolescents. Indications for individual work include cases in which it is the primary treatment of choice and cases in which it is a necessary prelude to other treatment approaches.

Some emotional illnesses in adolescence are best understood and approached through an intrapsychic model. These illnesses are characterized by evidences of excessive inhibition, internalized conflicts, and personal discomfort that are clearly experienced by the adolescent. These youngsters need the experience of an intense emotional relationship with an adult therapist in which they can re-experience earlier distortions of their relationships with important authority figures and use the therapist as a new object.

Even for youngsters whose problems require a different approach, a period of individual therapy may be necessary in order to form a working alliance with the patient and his family.

The techniques of individual psychotherapy with the adolescent are basically similiar to those used in dynamic psychotherapy with adults. There are two primary areas of difference: The first consists of the difficulties encountered in attempting to establish a therapeutic relationship that bridges the generation gap. The second concerns the use of the therapeutic alliance rather than the problems involved in its formation. A sparing use of interpretation, frequent confrontation of nonverbal behavior, a comfortable acceptance of exclusion from much of the adolescent's interior life, and a willingness to accept a basically narcissistic transference pattern are needed.

Group Psychotherapy. The tendency of the adolescent to move away from relationships with his parents and other adults and toward a greater involvement in peer relationships has long suggested group psychotherapy as a natural and preferred therapeutic approach. This assumption has not always worked out in practice because of difficulties in establishing a therapeutic alliance with the group leader and problems in the development of cohesion within the group.

Adolescents choose their friends carefully, with an eye not only toward their immediate need for real object relationships but even more with the hope of enhancing their sense of personal worth. A psychotherapy group composed of other youngsters who have admitted some degree of failure in mastering the tasks of adolescence may be viewed as a confirmation of their fears about themselves, rather than as an opportunity for constructive peer interaction.

Group psychotherapy seems to be particularly indicated for youngsters whose problems are primarily the result of interpersonal difficulties in the present. These youngsters tend either to shrink from the age-appropriate involvement with peers, showing a pattern of social isolation, or to choose peer relationships that are valued more for their support of psychopathology than for any potential emotional intimacy. In a successful group, the withdrawn youngster finds support and encouragement for greater peer involvement. The antisocial youngster encounters peer pressures to consider the rights and feelings of others and to confront the personal insecurities and unreasonable expectations that lead him to relate to others in primarily manipulative and exploitative ways.

The basic techniques of group psychotherapy with the adolescent do not differ from the generally accepted techniques used in dynamic group psychotherapy of adults.

Family Therapy. The mechanics of family therapy are dictated by the realities of the case, which may require individual therapy of various family members, use of medication, or temporary removal of the adolescent from the home. At some point, however, it is usually necessary to extend some direct treatment to the family unit as a whole.

Family therapy is particularly indicated when the adolescent is enmeshed in a predominantly satisfying neurotic family homeostasis. Clinical syndromes associated with this type of family situation include adolescent school phobia, schizophrenia, and scholastic underachievement of psychological origin.

Combined Treatment Approaches. Adequate treatment of many adolescent problems requires the flexible application of a variety of approaches. Often, these are most successful in combination. Combined programs require the same therapist to function in both roles or close collaboration between therapists. The aim is for each treatment method to catalyze the other so that the insights and growth experiences in each are additive in their impact on the adolescent patient and his family.

Treatment Outside the Home

Many difficulties require the adolescent's temporary or prolonged removal from his family. The indications are usually related to severe disturbances in impulse control related to psychotic disorganization, inability of the family to provide adequate discipline, or temporary family disruptions. In a smaller number of cases, removal from the home is necessary to interrupt the pattern of excessive closeness within the family that is promoting neurotic or infantile behavior. Suicidal adolescents occasionally require hospitalization for their own protection.

Foster Home and Boarding School Placements. Occasionally, psychiatrists recommend placement of the adolescent in a nontherapeutic alternative living situation. This recommendation is usually based on a psychiatric evaluation that suggests that the adolescent's problems represent a transient situational adjustment that would disappear under different living conditions.

Foster home placement should theoretically offer even more advantages for corrective growth experiences than the relatively impersonal boarding school. However, the practical difficulties in obtaining adequate foster parents who are willing to undertake the management of an adolescent, along with the more pronounced overtones of disloyalty toward the family of origin that acceptance of the foster parents might occasion, makes this placement less practical. It seems to be used primarily in the case of neglected and dependent children who are placed in foster homes for practical, rather than therapeutic, reasons.

Hospitalization and Residential Therapy. The hospitalization of an adolescent, especially for prolonged treatment, has many drawbacks. Not only does it tend to confirm the adolescent's fears that he is uncontrollably insane, but it substitutes a restrictive, structured environment for the independence and autonomy that would be a preferable setting for the unfolding of the adolescent development period. Usually, the adolescent is separated from normal peers and placed in the company of agemates whose problems may be even more serious than his own. Hospitalization is, at least to some extent, an enforced regression that tends to accentuate any dependency problems that the adolescent may be struggling with. Easson states that only the adolescent who can neither handle his inner drives nor use meaningful relationships with other people to promote growth is in need of inpatient treatment.

Brief hospitalization is valuable in a variety of crisis situations, such as acute drug reactions, suicidal or homicidal risks, and acute psychotic episodes. Brief hospitalization can clarify hidden family problems and interrupt defensive acting out. In these crisis situations, hospitalization aims to deal with the emergency with drug therapy, containment, and support to reinstate faltering defenses and avert catastrophe. The period of hospitalization may also promote a trusting relationship between the therapist and his adolescent patient.

Prolonged hospital treatment is usually reserved for youngsters with marked deficiencies in early ego development. These patients require a prolonged corrective living experience that usually includes a significant degree of regression, intense transference feelings toward the hospital staff, and gradual relearning of more appropriate adaptive techniques, internal controls, and skills in interpersonal relationships.

Although extended treatment of this kind is provided in hospital settings, it is more commonly offered in a residential treatment centers. These centers are usually designed to provide a homelike atmosphere, schooling, and social activities.

Inpatient treatment programs for adolescents include recognition of the adolescent's need for vigorous activity, some plan to develop group cohesion among the adolescents, and some system of limitations and privileges designed to control the adolescent tendency to live out problems, rather than discuss them. Programs that emphasize extended hospitalization recognize the importance of parental involvement and offer parents' groups, individual therapy for the parents, and family therapy as part of their treatment program.

Psychopharmacology

The function of the drugs is primarily to control target symptoms that interfere in a marked way with family relationships or the therapeutic process. The symptoms that seem to yield best to medication are excessive motor activity, severe anxiety, some depressive manifestations, and a few specific symptoms, especially enuresis and severe tics.

Drug treatment in the adolescent is complicated by the adolescent's anxiety about his physical functioning and his distrust of adult authority. Side effects of medications may be alarming to the adolescent. Parents may use the prescribed medication as a tool to undermine therapy.

The outpatient administration of drugs to the adolescent patient depends on the strength of the therapeutic alliance. The adolescent must be included in decisions to begin medication and in the continuing assessment of the medication's value. Inpatient treatment allows a greater latitude in the use of drugs.

Minor Tranquilizers. The minor tranquilizers include all the agents typically used to combat anxiety in nonpsychotic adults. Most widely used are the diphenylmethane derivatives, the meprobamates, and the benzodiazepine compounds. There is little evidence that any of these drugs are of significant clinical importance in the management of adolescent psychiatric disorders, but they may have occasional value in brief periods of marked anxiety. Suggestion may be the primary factor when minor tranquilizers appear to be successful.

Major Tranquilizers. The phenothiazine derivatives seem to be as effective in the psychotic adolescent as they are in adults. Excessive aggressiveness, overactivity, and even oppositional behavior may also be diminished by phenothiazine therapy.

Adolescents appear to be more variable than adults in their response to phenothiazines. It is wise to begin therapy with very small doses, which may be gradually increased until therapeutic effectiveness is achieved or until side effects appear.

Antidepressants. Effective antidepressants include the monoamine oxidase inhibitors and the iminodidenzyl derivatives. Imipramine appears to have value in alleviating enuresis. The drug is usually given in a single dose of 25 to 75 mg. at bedtime.

REFERENCES

Easson, W. M. *The Severely Disturbed Adolescent.* International Universities Press, New York, 1969.
Gitelson, M. Character synthesis: The psychotherapeutic problem of adolescence. Am. J. Orthopsychiatry, *18:* 422, 1948.
Masterson, J. F., Jr. *The Psychiatric Dilemma of Adolescence.* Little, Brown, Boston, 1967.
Meeks, J. E. *The Fragile Alliance: An Orientation to the Outpatient Psychotherapy of the Adolescent.* Williams & Wilkins, Baltimore, 1971.
Meeks, J. E. Structuring the early phase of group psychotherapy with adolescents. Int. J. Child Psychother., *2:* 26, 1973.
Offer, D. *The Psychological World of the Teenager: A Study of Normal Adolescent Boys.* Basic Books, New York, 1969.
Proskauer, S., and Rolland, R. S. Youth who use drugs: Psychodynamic diagnosis and treatment planning. J. Am. Acad. Child Psychiatry, *12:* 32, 1973.

40

Child Psychiatry:
Special Areas of Interest

40.1. MATERNAL DEPRIVATION

Introduction

Although the importance of mothering experiences in infancy and early childhood has long been recognized, only in the past quarter of a century has research evidence begun to document the effects on the development of young children of a variety of inadequacies and deviations in maternal care. Bowlby concluded that a warm, continuous relationship with a mother figure is essential for healthy personality development.

Deviations in Maternal Care

Institutionalization

Infants subjected to prolonged residence in poor institutional environments develop intellectual and personality deficiencies and disturbances. Early motor functions that are most dependent on maturation seem to be least affected; cognitive functions, especially language, seem to be most vulnerable. Evidences of intellectual and language retardation appear early in infancy and become intensified with continued institutionalization. Infants growing up in poor institutions often fail to develop normal patterns of social responsiveness; they tend to become withdrawn and apathetic, and frequently they do not develop normal patterns of social discrimination. These early deviations in personal-social behavior are considered precursors of later personality disturbances characterized by poor impulse control, lack of appropriate guilt feelings associated with aggressive and destructive behavior, and an inability to establish close and meaningful interpersonal relationships.

A number of significant variables in institutional environments affect the development of the child, including the amount, the quality, and the variety of sensory and perceptual stimulation provided directly or mediated by the caretaker, the extent of opportunities for acquiring and practicing fine motor skills, the timing and appropriateness of the caretaker's responses to the infant's behavior, the degree of continuity of care provided by a single mother figure, and the quality of affectional interchange with substitute mothers. There appears to be a direct relationship between the extent of intellectual and language retardation and the degree of sensory and verbal stimulation in the institutional environment.

Multiple Mothering

Multiplicity of caretakers tends to create an unpredictable environment for the young child; he has limited opportunities to develop consistent expectations toward one person. Moreover, caretakers are unlikely to adapt their handling to the child's unique characteristics, thus limiting the kinds of reciprocal interactions that are basic to the development of meaningful interpersonal relationships and normal patterns of identification.

Having more than one caretaker is not always associated with severe deprivations or traumatic discontinuities in care. Margaret Mead has suggested that children reared in cultures in which the child care functions are shared by a number of mother figures are better equipped to tolerate separation and often develop subtle and complex personality characteristics, presumably as a consequence of having varied identification figures. The effects of multiple mothering depend on the specific patterns of interaction between child and mother and on the larger social context.

Maternal Separation

Maternal separation frequently precedes deprivation of maternal care, but deprivation experiences are not a necessary or inevitable aftermath of separation. Consistent interaction with one person over a long period of time is one prerequisite for the development of attachment, but probably equally important are the quality and the intensity of the interaction. Among the significant variables are contingent responsiveness to the infant's signals and the sensitivity of the caretaker to the baby's individual characteristics.

A break in the continuity of relationship with a mother figure is a disturbing experience for infants and young children, as evidenced by their behavior at the time and immediately after separation. A three-phase sequence of responses to separation is seen in hospitalized and institutionalized children: protest, despair, and denial-detachment. At first, separated infants tend to show overt protest and active seeking of human contact in an apparent attempt to find a substitute mother. This behavior is usually followed by active rejection of people. Finally, the child withdraws from his environment and shows depressed behavior. Progressively severe depressive reactions occur in children who are placed in impersonal environments without adequate substitute maternal care. Infants who are given individualized substitute maternal care may show similar initial disturbances, but the progression in severity of symptoms is not likely to occur.

The meaning of separation depends on the developmental level of the child. For the young infant, separation may be perceived simply as a global environmental change. The period between 6 months and 2 years appears to be an especially vulnerable one.

The implications of separation experiences for later personality development depend on a number of factors: whether the separation is temporary or permanent, the duration of a temporary separation, the number and character of previous separation experiences, the nature of the substitute caretaking, and the age of the child at the time of separation. Perhaps most significant is the degree of trauma or deprivation subsequent to separation. Brief, temporary separation experiences are not likely to have serious permanent effects, but significant personality disturbances may develop in children who have been subjected to repetitive separations associated with other traumatic and depriving experiences during infancy and early childhood.

Pathological Mother-Child Relationships

Rejection, hostility, and ambivalence on the part of the mother are usually rooted in personality or character disorders. Unlike the experiential deprivations attendant on lack of sufficient interaction with a mother figure or discontinuities in the maternal relationship, these deviations are primarily in the quality of the affectional relationship.

Variables in Maternal Deprivation

Sensory Deprivation

In the course of normal maternal activities, the mother serves both as a source of stimulation and as a medium for bringing the infant into contact with appropriate environmental stimuli, sometimes enhancing and sometimes buffering the intensity of stimulation. Severe sensory and perceptual deprivation in early life may adversely affect the development of the sensory processes and the basic underlying structures in the central nervous system.

Stage of Development

Sensitivity to given kinds of stimulation and vulnerability to specific types of deprivation or stress vary at different developmental periods. For the young infant, giving up a mother figure before a strong dependency relationship has been established is a very different experience from separation during the period when a relationship with the mother is developing or after a focused relationship has been established. Similarly, the young child's reaction to the loss of a mother figure at later developmental periods may vary with the degree of autonomy he has achieved and the stage of object and person permanence.

Individual Differences

There may be individual differences in general susceptibility to stress and differences in sensitivity to particular kinds of stimulation. Recent studies have emphasized the extent to which the infant influences the kind of stimulation he receives and particularly how infant characteristics influence maternal behavior.

Reversibility

Data from recent enrichment studies emphasize the possibility of reversing the severe cognitive and interpersonal damage resulting from extreme deprivation, but the degree of reversibility depends on the extent of the damage and the timing of the therapeutic attempts. From the data, it is not yet possible to specify a developmental point after which therapeutic attempts are unlikely to be successful, but it seems clear that it becomes increasingly difficult with increased age to reverse intellectual deficits and personality distortions.

REFERENCES

Bowlby, J. *Attachment and Loss*, 2 volumes. Basic Books, New York, 1969 and 1973.
Caldwell, B. M. Can young children have a quality life in day care? Young Children, *28:* 197, 1973.
Emde, R. N., Gaensbauer. T. G., and Harmon, R. J. Emotional expression in infancy: A bio-behavioral study. Psychol. Issues, 1974.
Gray, S., and Klaus, R. A. *The Early Training Project: A Seventh Year Report.* John F. Kennedy Center for Research on Education and Human Development, Nashville, 1969.
Hunt, J. McV. *Intelligence and Experience.* Ronald, New York, 1961.
Rutter, M. Parent-child separation: Psychological effects on the children. J. Child Psychol. Psychiatry, *12:* 233, 1971.
Stolz, L. M. Effects of maternal employment on children: Evidence from research. Child Dev., *31:* 749, 1960.
Yarrow, L. J. Separation from parents during early childhood, In *Review of Child Development Research*, M. Hoffman and L. Hoffman, editors, vol. 1, p. 89. Russell Sage Foundation, New York, 1964.
Yarrow, L. J., and Goodwin, M. S. The immediate impact of separation. In *The Competent Infant*, L. J. Stone, H. T. Smith and L. B. Murphy, editors, p. 145. Basic Books, New York, 1973.
Yarrow, L. J., Rubenstein, J. L., Pedersen, F. A., and Jankowski, J. J. Dimensions of early stimulation and their differential effects on infant development. Merrill-Palmer Q., *18:* 205, 1972.

40.2.   CHILD MALTREATMENT AND BATTERED-CHILD SYNDROMES

Introduction

Inhuman cruelty to children appears to be rapidly increasing, and the perpetrators of this crime are, for the most part, the parents themselves. This disease of the maltreatment of children is one aspect of social violence and is symptomatic of an illness that is insidiously creeping into society. Child abuse is a medical-social disease that is assuming epidemic proportions and encompasses a child-rearing pattern that is becoming more entrenched in the population. It is a disease that is not a time-limited phenomenon but, rather, the cause and effect of a cyclical pattern of the violence reflected in all statistics on crime.

Incidence

In 1962 a nationwide survey of hospitals and law enforcement agencies indicated that, in a 1-year period, 749 children were reported as being maltreated; of this number, 78 died, and 114 suffered permanent brain damage. In only a third of these cases did proper medical diagnosis initiate court action.

In New York City there was more than a 500 per cent increase in reported cases of abuse and neglect within the period of 1961 to 1970, and in 1973 more than 19,000 cases of suspected child abuse and neglect were reported to the City Central Registry.

Only a fraction of the neglected and abused children are taken to physicians or hospitals for medical attention. Many of the children seen by physicians go unrecognized, undiagnosed, and, hence, unreported. The true incidence rates and distribution patterns of child abuse and neglect are unknown at this time.

Diagnosis

The neglect and abuse of children denote a situation ranging from the deprivation of food, clothing, shelter, and parental love to incidences in which children are physically abused and mistreated by an adult, resulting in obvious physical trauma to the child and often leading to death. A maltreated child often presents no obvious signs of being battered but has multiple minor physical evidences of emotional and, at times, nutritional deprivation, neglect, and abuse.

The maltreated child is often taken to the hospital or private physician with a history of failure to thrive, malnutrition, poor skin hygiene, irritability, repressed personality, and other signs of obvious neglect. The more severely abused children are seen in hospital emergency rooms with external evidences of body trauma, bruises, abrasions, cuts, lacerations, burns, soft tissue swellings, and hematomas. Hypernatremic dehydration, after periodic water deprivation by psychotic mothers, has been reported as a form of child abuse. Inability

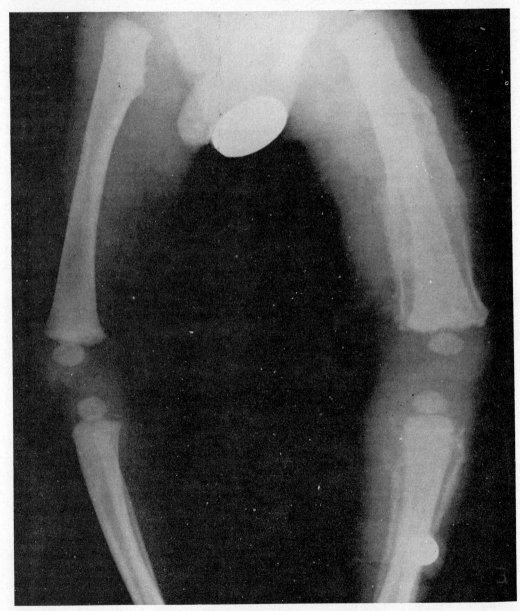

FIGURE 1. Extensive periosteal calcifications of the left femur and left fibula of a 7-month-old boy admitted to the hospital 1 week after inflicted trauma to the left thigh. There is a marked metaphyseal fraying of the distal femur and proximal tibia. (Courtesy of Vincent Fontana, M.D.)

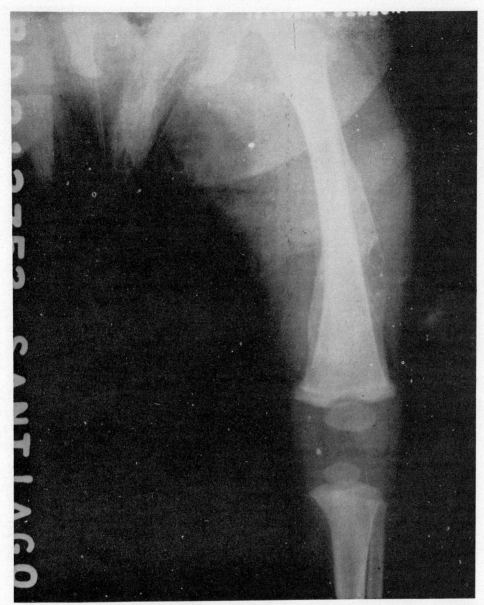

FIGURE 2. X-ray film of a 6-month-old girl taken 4 weeks after an inflicted injury to an extremity, showing extensive reparative changes, new bone formation, external cortical thickening, and "squaring" of the metaphysis. (Courtesy of Vincent Fontana, M.D.)

to move certain extremities because of dislocations and fractures (see Figures 1–3), associated with neurological signs of intracranial damage, can be additional signs of inflicted trauma. Other clinical signs and symptoms attributed to inflicted abuse may include injury to viscera. Abdominal trauma may result in unexplained ruptures of stomach, bowel, liver, or pancreas, with manifestations of an acute abdomen. Those with the most severe maltreatment injuries arrive at the hospital or physician's office in coma or convulsions, and some arrive dead.

Prolonged maternal deprivation of the child can have a serious and lifelong impact on the child's future character structure and can cause a variety of adult disorders, such as hostility,

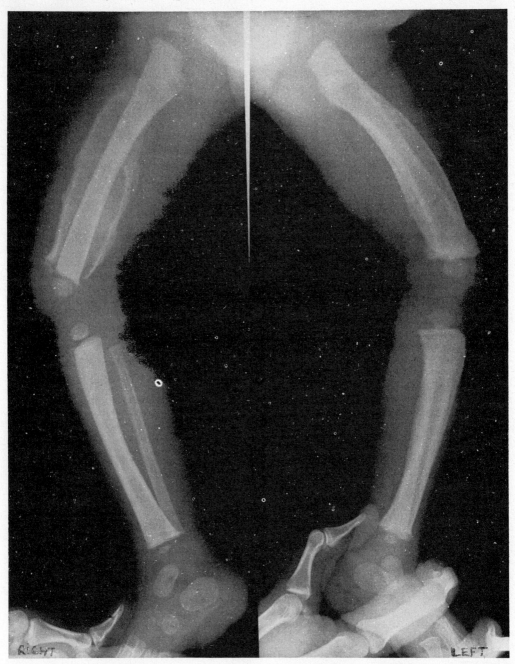

FIGURE 3. Boy, 7 months old, admitted to hospital on several occasions for "accidental" injury to thighs. The left femur shows evidence of periosteal reaction, with calcification and new bone formation 3 to 6 weeks after inflicted trauma. Metaphyseal squaring is also noted. The right femur in the same child shows evidence of more recently incurred injury (1 to 2 weeks), with subperiosteal hemorrhage, some calcification, metaphyseal fragmentation, and chip fractures. (Courtesy of Vincent Fontanta, M.D.)

alcoholism, drug addiction, sexual maladjustment, and inadequate maternal behavior. In addition, inadequate mothering or child neglect stemming from maternal deprivation can result in growth failure, autistic behavior, and retarded mental development in the child.

The only way to establish an unchallengable cause-and-effect relationship between the infant's mothering and his symptoms is to demonstrate significant recovery when the mothering is altered. All infants diagnosed as markedly deprived should have an investigation of the social-environmental condition of the family and the psychological status of the mother to determine the factors responsible for inefficient mothering.

Epidemiology

Children

The children involved in abuse and neglect tend to be very young. Parental neglect and abuse may occur at any age, with an increase of incidence in children under 3 years of age. The children on whom more severe physical injuries are inflicted tend to be younger than those on whom less severe injuries are inflicted.

These maltreated children are perceived as if they had the emotions and motivations of older children and adults. They often are expected to mother the mother, and there is a reversal of roles, with the mother's fears and misperceptions leading to inflicted abuse. Older children are often physically abused because they are found to be unacceptable and offer a threat to the viability of the family unit. The mother justifies her actions on the basis of the child's imperfections, using disciplinary actions that often lead to battering.

Parents

The perpetrator is more often the woman than the man. One parent is usually the active batterer, and the other parent passively accepts the battering. Of the perpetrators, 80 per cent regularly live in the homes of the children they abuse. More than 80 per cent of the children reported in a survey were living with parents married or with parents' substitutes; 50 per cent were living with a single parent. The average age of the mother who inflicted abuse on her

children has been reported to be around 26 years; the average age of the father is 30. The economic circumstances of the 48 families in a recent survey were reported as follows: 56.25 per cent were poor and 39.58 per cent were comfortable.

The battered child is usually the victim of emotionally crippled parents, beginning with unfortunate circumstances surrounding the parents' own childhoods. The battering parent appears to react to the child as a result of past personal experiences of loneliness, lack of protection, and love. Some of these mothers were raised by a variety of foster parents during their own childhoods. These mothers are unable to react normally to the needs of the infant. The abusing parent frequently has a history of having been brutalized himself as a child, and so the pattern of violent behavior perpetuates itself from generation to generation. The parents are usually immature, narcissistic, egocentric, and demanding and show impulsive, aggressive behavior. The parents appear unwilling to accept responsibilities as parents and at times show some signs of rejection of their child.

More than 50 per cent of these abused and neglected children were prematurely born or of low birth weight. These premature children are usually slower in development than the normal newborn. The parents of these infants are often unable to cope with the slow development. Prolonged hospitalization of the infant for treatment of prematurity may have a role in triggering some instances of parental maltreatment.

Divorce, alcoholism, drug addiction, mental retardation, recurring mental illness, unemployment, and financial distress may be important factors in the family structure of the abusing parents. These stress factors may cause the potentially abusive parent to strike out at a special child during a crisis situation.

Physician's Responsibility

Every hospital should have a child abuse committee providing a readily available team of consultants, headed by a capable pediatrician and including a psychiatrist, a social worker, and a hospital administrator. This team must also assume the role of educating their colleagues and the members of allied fields in the community.

TABLE I

Physician's Index of Suspicion

History
  Story told by parents that is at variance with the clinical findings
  Multiple visits to various hospitals
  Familial discord or financial stress
  Reluctance of parents to give information
Physical Examination
  Signs of general neglect, poor skin hygiene, malnutrition, and withdrawn, irritable, repressed personality
  Bruises, abrasions, soft tissue swellings, hematomas, and old healed lesions
  Evidence of dislocations or fractures of the extremities
Radiological manifestations
  Subperiosteal hematomas
  Epiphyseal separations
  Periosteal shearing
  Metaphyseal fragmentation
  Previously healed periosteal reactions
  "Squaring" of the metaphysis

In suspected cases (see Table I) of child abuse and neglect the physician should:

1. Make a suspected diagnosis of maltreatment.

2. Intervene and admit the child to the hospital.

3. Make an assessment—history, physical examination, skeletal survey, and photographs.

4. Report the case to the appropriate department of social service and child protective unit or central registry.

5. Request a social worker report and appropriate surgical and medical consultations.

6. Confer within 72 hours with members of the child abuse committee.

7. Arrange a program of care for the child and parent.

8. Arrange for a social service follow-up.

Treating the parent who neglects, batters, or kills a child is totally inadequate unless it is coupled with a simultaneous concern to ensure future adequate rehabilitation and preventive measures that will help eliminate the psychological and social environmental factors that foster the battering parent syndrome. If these parents are to be given any help, they must be made to recognize their own intrinsic worth and potential as human beings. This can only be accomplished by recognition and cooperative effort by all child-caring professionals and paraprofessionals.

REFERENCES

Fontana, V. J. The "maltreatment syndrome" in children, N. Engl. J. Med., *269:* 1389, 1963.

Fontana, V. J. Which parents abuse their children? Med. Insight, *3:* 16, 1971.
Fontana, V. J. The diagnosis of the maltreatment syndrome in children. Pediatrics, *51* (Suppl.): 780, 1973.
Fontana, V. J. Somewhere a Child is Crying. Macmillan, New York, 1973.
Battered child syndrome and brain dysfunction. J. A. M. A., *223:* 1390, 1973.
Joyner, E. Child abuse: The role of the physician and the hospital. Pediatrics, *51* (Suppl.): 4, 1973.
Kempe, C. H., and Helfer, R. E., editors. *The Battered Child.* University of Chicago Press, Chicago, 1968.
Kempe, C. H., Silverman, F. N., Steele, B. F., Droegemueller, W., and Silver, H. K. The battered child syndrome. J. A. M. A., *181:* 17, 1962.
Paulsen, M. G. Legal protections against child abuse. Children, *13:* 42, 1966.
Savino, A. B., and Sanders, R. W. Working with abusive parents: Group therapy and home visits. Am. J. Nurs., *73:* 482, 1973.
Smith, R. C. New ways to help battering parents. Today's Health, *51:* 57, 1973.
Stern, L. Prematurity as a factor in child abuse. Hosp. Pract., *8:* 117, 1973.

40.3.   DAY CARE PROGRAMS

Introduction

There is no agreed-on definition of the term "day care" other than a service that meets the need of parents to leave their children under the care of others for a period of time during the day. Three centrally important psychiatric aspects must be considered in a discussion of day care: its contribution to the child's mental health or illness, its potential as a social field for mental health assessment and intervention, and its place as part of a total, integrated mental health system. Day care cannot be considered outside the context of child rearing and the social and psychological processes related to it. Day care provides additional social and psychological supports in the child-rearing process beyond those generally offered by parents and family. One needs to know whether day care is causally related to the mental health status of the child and, later, of the adult throughout his life. In the consideration of day care as a potentially important social field for assessment and intervention, the focus of attention is on the opportunity to examine day care programing and the children in such programs for purposes of early diagnosis and possible treatment of a variety of mental health problems.

Day Care in a Mental Health System

The System

It is useful to think of a mental health system as having three interactive levels of care.

The first level is highly integrated in the neighborhood community. It involves a concern with populations of healthy as well as ill persons and consists of programs of prevention and early intervention that are readily placed in naturally occurring social contexts in the community, rather than in clinics and hospitals. Here professional personnel would be employed most effectively in supervisory, training, and back-up consultative roles.

The second level of care consists of more specialized outpatient back-up services. Referral to this second level would be efficiently accomplished after contact at the neighborhood level.

The third level consists of hospitalization and its variations, including partial hospitalization. Both the second and the third levels of care would provide professional consultants to back up the first-level staff working in the neighborhood community. The third level would make use of paraprofessionals, as well as professionals working in ward teams.

Child services need to be built into all three levels, but day care would most reasonably and effectively be part of the first level. Good day care must necessarily reflect the child-rearing attitudes, values, and needs of the community.

Influence on Mental Health

All the psychiatric theories that relate early experience to later mental health or illness emphasize child-rearing. From the psychoanalytic point of view, one can extrapolate the view that day care programs have the potential either to augment the parental resources available to the child and support identity formation and other psychological processes of childhood or be a vehicle for the disruption of these processes and the premature separation of the child from parents and family.

From the viewpoint of social learning theory, day care has similar potential for enhancing as well as inhibiting mental health. The reinforcement of neurotic or socially maladaptive patterns of behavior represents the danger; the

opportunity to reinforce affective interpersonal behaviors represents the potential for good.

From a theoretical causal point of view, then, the assets or limitations of day care can be assessed only in terms of specific characteristics of specific programs. Determining how to develop a good program must take into account the community to be served and must test specific programs in specific populations of children.

Assessment and Intervention

The potential of day care as an arena for assessment and intervention is largely a question of conducting the necessary research. As a basic research model for this population, the community study would appear to offer the best advantage—community studies of preschoolers that are able to define a specific community and to assess the family life and social and cultural context in which the children are to grow and develop. Day care can easily be construed as an educational opportunity and as an economic or vocational opportunity for parents or as a way of augmenting the family's child-rearing resources when a parent becomes disabled.

Child Rearing

The idea that day care programs should take into account the aspirations and concerns of local community residents speaks to the general issue of variations in child rearing. By community is meant a residence area served by local institutions and having some identification as a residence area to the residents and, to a lesser degree, to outsiders.

A local community group of leaders from neighborhood political and social organizations might collaborate with day care center personnel, working out questions of policy, priorities, and recruitment of day care staff. The expertise of childhood specialists would be protected but tempered by the aspirations, values, and concerns of community residents whose children would attend the program. City, state, and federal agencies could play stimulating, standard-setting, and standard-safeguarding roles and could provide some of the necessary funding.

Social and Cultural Context of Day Care

To consider child rearing and day care in a cultural context, one must take into account the many variations in the way in which young children are cared for. Some of the characteristics known to vary from culture to culture are the constellation of adults who are responsible for the child, the amount of mother-child contact, sleeping arrangements, and discipline.

The variations in the adult composition of child-rearing families illustrate the necessity for planning day care programs so that they complement different family structures, as well as various family and community resources. Economic and political influences in the larger society appear to affect modes of child care. And social values concerning child rearing are important in determining how children will be cared for and where the primary responsibility for such care will lie.

Child care also varies from family to family. The personal needs of parents influence child care arrangements, especially in the middle classes of the more affluent, industrialized nations.

Day care design, then, must be closely related to the social context of the particular community that the program will serve. In addition, the design must take into account the fact that values and aspirations are not static; they are changing.

Variations in Day Care Programs

Day care of children in groups is provided in several kinds of settings. Mothers who take a few children not their own into their homes are said to provide family day care. Day care centers are larger operations, usually serving from 20 to 100 children. And residential homes provide 24-hour child care.

Most day care centers serve low-income populations and are likely to be nonprofit institutions; 68 per cent of the families served by nonprofit centers have only one parent. Centers may also be funded by unions, hospitals, or the families they serve. Day care centers tend to provide stability of service and continuity of program philosophy, but they encounter major problems in the maintenance of quality. Heterogeneity of child population is usually considered a value in day care centers, but most centers are ethnically and socio-economically homogeneous.

Family day care may be provided by an individual mother or family operating inde-

pendently, or it may be sponsored by a public or private social agency. Family day care provides 78 per cent of the out-of-home nonrelative care for children under 12 years of age in the U. S. More than 90 per cent of family day care homes lack city or state licenses and are thus free of government regulation. Family day care generally involves fewer children for each available adult and is more easily adapted to young children, sick children, and children with special problems. Such programs provide care for more children under age 3 than do child care centers. The homes involved tend to be located in the child's neighborhood. On the other hand, family day care tends to have a weak educational component or no such component at all, even though the caretakers are generally better educated than are the day care center staff members. Family day care programs serve a population with a slightly higher income level than do day care centers and are usually more expensive than are nonprofit centers, but less expensive than proprietary centers.

Although there are differences between day care centers and family day care, there is also great variation within these two categories in programing, sponsorship, parent participation, and staffing. Programs may be primarily custodial or may include cognitive, social, and mental health components. Existing sponsors include churches, schools, industries, hospitals, labor unions, community groups, participating families, and private entrepreneurial groups. Parent participation ranges from none to active involvement in decision making, teaching, fund raising, and other activities. Large day care centers tend to have more child care professionals on the staff; family day care persons generally lack certification or licenses.

Consequences of Day Care

In one series of studies, children in a foundling home showed strikingly higher death rates than did children in a home for delinquent mothers and children in their own families, outside of institutions. The orphans also showed severe cognitive and emotional deficits. The presence or absence of the mother was considered the major difference. Child care by persons other than the mother was thought to cause serious problems in the child. However, separation from parents for some part of the day is quite different from being cared for entirely in an institution with total deprivation of parental contact. Maternal separation is difficult for the child, but there is no evidence that it must be a serious problem with lasting deleterious results; having close contact with at least one significant person facilitates the separation. Effective intervention is possible if it occurs early enough, and factors other than maternal separation appear to be operating to produce developmental problems with institutionalized children.

One must consider the kind of family that day care is meant to augment in studying the impact of day care. Usually, day care is not planned to replace the mother, but it can be designed to add adult figures who are consistent in the child's environment.

Most of the mothers of children in day care are working or are in training programs. Studies have found no significant differences between children of working mothers and children of nonworking mothers on a variety of cognitive, social, and emotional measures. The mother's attitude is extremely important. A positive attitude toward her work, her child, and life in general is associated with the child's good development; a negative attitude toward working is associated with detrimental effects on the child. Also, the effects of a working mother operate differently on boys and on girls; boys are more likely to suffer negative effects than are girls.

Cognitive Effects

Children cared for outside the home for part of the day do not appear to suffer cognitive deficits. Indeed, the evidence suggests that additional settings, such as day care centers, may promote increased cognitive development and achievement.

Psychological Effects

Day care need not be detrimental to children if it is carefully designed to meet their developmental needs. In fact, some evidence suggests that children may benefit from a day care experience, especially if their home environments are not optimal.

Design and Theory Building

Day care programs should augment the existing child-rearing resources of the family and local community and should be inimately related to the existing child-rearing practices and cultural values of the family, the local community, and the larger society. There are two basic methods of ensuring close integration between day care services and the local community: (1) by providing mechanisms for the local community to be part of the planning, implementation, and evaluation of the program itself, and (2) by gathering information regarding the family and community resources to be augmented and the needs of the children to be served.

Community Participation

Although many day care programs are sponsored by groups outside of local community institutions, the role of the leaders of the local community's social and political organizations must include substantive participation in recruiting day care staff, setting priorities, and designing the program.

The community policy board, set up to govern first-level programing in the local community, has been shown to be a viable mechanism for ensuring participation of local community leaders and consumers in planning and decision-making processes. Sometimes called advisory boards, such groups are valuable if the program requires that planning incorporate local community values and needs. It is particularly important in a program intended for the community's young children that the community see it as its own program. Forming a community board may call for visits by the day care professionals to a variety of local community leaders to achieve the sanction necessary to make a community-based service program work.

Assessment

Adequate knowledge about community resources (institutional and noninstitutional), the kinds of families living in the community and their in-family resources, the local community values, the goals and aspirations the community holds for its children, and the social, cognitive, and mental health status of the children who will be in the program makes it possible to start thinking about program design and to relate day care to other kinds of human services.

One major focus in the assessment of child-rearing resources in the family, local community, and larger society and the assessment of other relevant characteristics of the family and the local community. The other major focus is the child, and this focus presumes that the information system reflects a careful consideration of what desirable outcomes are in the child-rearing process generally and in a day care program specifically.

Mental health may be viewed as having two dimensions. One dimension, the societal dimension, defines desirable outcome on the basis of the tasks society sets for the child in a day care program, in a classroom later on, or in any other social field of importance at a particular stage of life. The specific tasks are defined in each social field by people who are empowered, formally or informally, by society. This societal assessment contrasts with the second dimension of mental health, the person's psychological well-being.

In terms of day care, the assessment of the child may consist of first defining the social tasks expected of the child by the natural raters within that social field and then making the assessment by the natural rater explicit. The assessment of a child's psychological well-being must provide information concerning the symptom status, affective status, and general psychological good feeling of the child.

In day care programs, the technical staff members have a great deal of authority to define what is expected of the children and to assess the adequacy of an individual child's performance. The task-setting process should have input by technical staff, parents, and community leaders. In part, the process reflects the aspirations and values of the community and the particular families served by the program. On the other hand, the task-setting and assessment procedures affect the child's psychological well-being.

REFERENCES

Jay, J., and Birney, R. C. Research findings on the kibbutz adolescent: A response to Bettelheim. Am J. Orthopsychiatry, *43:* 347, 1973.
Kellam, S. G., and Brach, J. D. An approach to community mental health: An analysis of basic problems. Semin. Psychiatry, *3:* 207, 1971.
Kellam, S. G., and Schiff, S. K. An urban community mental health center. In *Mental Health and Urban Social Policy*. L. H. Duhl and R. L. Leopold, editors, p. 113. Jossey-Bass, San Francisco, 1968.
Kellam, S. G., Branch, J. D., Agrawal, K. C., and Ensminger, M. E. *Mental Health and Going to School.* University of Chicago Press, Chicago, 1974.
Keyserling. M. D. *Windows on Day Care.* National Council of Jewish Women, New York, 1972.
Rothman, S. M. Other people's children: The day care experience in America. Public Interest, *30:* 11, 1973.
Sale, J. S. Family day care: One alternative in the delivery of developmental services in early childhood. Am. J. Orthopsychiatry, *43:* 37, 1973.
Schwarz, J. C., Krolick, G., and Strickland, R. G. Effects of early day care experience on adjustment to a new environment. Am. J. Orthopsychiatry, *43:* 340, 1973.
Spiro, M. E. Is the family universal? The Israeli case. In *A Modern Introduction to the Family*, N. W. Bell and E. F. Vogel, editors, rev. ed., p. 68. Free Press of Glencoe (Macmillan), New York, 1968.
Whiting, B., editor. *Six Cultures: Study of Child Rearing.* John Wiley, New York, 1966.

40.4.   TWINS

Introduction

Approximately one in 86 births is a birth of twins; between a third and a fourth of the total twin population is monozygotic. The frequency of twins depends, among other factors, on the socio-economic status and age of the mothers and on the racial background.

Early Development

The somewhat lower performance of twins, as compared with other children, may rest on the fact that very often—in 60 per cent of twin births—twins are born prematurely and may, therefore, have a biological handicap. In addition, there are more often complications during pregnancy and delivery.

Twins also have psychological variables. Personality differences in twins appear during the first years of life and are usually based on which of the pair is active and which is passive at a given time. The active twin may develop more fully the traits of aggressivity and self-reliance, and the other may tend to become altruistic, submissive, and dependent. These features seem at first to be determined by physical differences at birth. But as the weaker child becomes able to bridge this gap or to enjoy certain other advantages, these roles may be reversed.

Twinning

Around the age of 3 or 4, the processes of identification and imitation and the twins' reactions to their mirror images limit the significance of the earlier differences. One twin learns to enjoy the other's activities and to feel the punishment the other receives. This interaction, called "twinning," is an important influence on their further development. At this time, the twins begin to move away from the mother and to establish an independent interplay with each other. This mutual interdependence may result in a lack of individuation and to limitations on their capacity for conceptualization and learning. Twins' intelligence measures are inferior to the levels of matched groups of nontwins. There is also a lag of linguistic development, which seems to be correlated with their difficulty in establishing a mental image of their own bodies (identity).

Mothers' Reactions

Mothers have a natural feeling of pleasure when they are first told that they may expect twins. After the birth, however, they may encounter unanticipated difficulties, which arise from the necessity of having to interact with two children with different characteristics. Some mothers stress these differences. Others treat the two children as one; they thereby feed into the problem of twinning. Later, the tendency of the twins toward closeness to each other may give the mother the feeling of being excluded. If she enjoys the fact that the children demand less of her personal attention, she may foster the twinning reaction; if she resists their exclusion of her, she may find that twins are an exceptional burden. When the differences between the twins are overstressed, thus forcing a polarity of personality characteristics, there is a retardation of individuation and an interference with full development.

Sex

Girls tend to be the dominant partners in opposite-sexed twins during childhood. Twins, especially identical twins, marry less often than do nontwins. However, there may be no greater tendency toward homosexuality among twins.

Recommendations to Assist Development

Twins should always be dealt with in terms of their separate identities. Differences in their tastes, their rhythms, and their perceptions should be recognized and maintained. One should not praise, reward, or punish both twins as a unit. If the twins are placed in separate classes in school, they can receive independent attention and thereby gain in individuation. On the other hand, one should not interfere with their natural closeness by separating them forcefully or too early.

REFERENCES

Alby, J., and Cremieux, R. Les jumeaux (Discussion of R. Zasso: Les jumeaux). Psychiatr. Enfant, 2: 580, 1959.
Benhamin, J. D. Some comments on twin research in psychiatry. In *Research Approaches to Psychiatric Problems: A Symposium*, T. T. Tourlents, editor, p. 92. Grune & Stratton, New York, 1960.
Burlingham, D. *Twins*. International Universities Press, New York, 1952.
Child Study Association. *And Then There Were Two: A Handbook for Mothers*. Child Study Association, New York, 1959.
Leonard, M. R. Problems in identification and ego development in twins. Psychoanal. Study Child, *16:* 300, 1961.

40.5.   CHILDREN'S DREAMS

Content of Dreams

Dreams in a child can have a profound effect on his behavior. During the child's first years, when the differentiation between reality and fantasy has not yet been fully achieved, the dream may be experienced as if it were true or could be true; the child has strong reactions to dreaming, either of pleasure or, as is most often reported, of fears.

The dream content is to be seen in connection with the life experience of the child, his developmental stage, the mechanisms used during dreaming, and the child's sex. To help the child, the therapist must find the relationship between his dreams and the realities of life.

Disturbing dreams reach a peak when the child is 3 years, 6 years, and 10 years old. At the age of 2, the child may dream about being bitten or chased; at the age of 4, there are many animal dreams, and people are introduced who either protect or destroy. At 5 or 6, dreams of getting killed or injured, of flying and being in cars, and of ghosts become more prominent, exposing the role of conscience, of moral values, and of increasing conflicts around these themes. In early childhood, aggressive dreams seem to occur rarely; instead, it is the dreamer who is in danger, which may reflect the child's dependent position.

Dreams and Sleep

At certain periods, a child wakes up from his sleep, disturbed by the content of his dream and extremely frightened; he is unwilling to return to sleep unless he is comforted. Pavor nocturnus is a severe state of fright in which the content of the dream overwhelms reality, so that the child remains frightened by the dream for an extended period of time. During night-terrors, the child remains in this in-between state, from which he cannot be fully aroused and restored to reality. The people around him either are not recognized or else are of minor significance as compared with the impact the dream still has on him. The dream seems to continue, even though the child's eyes are open. The child incorporates some pieces of his actual environment into the dream, or else he projects the dream into his environment.

Between the ages of 3 and 6, it is normal for a child to want to keep his door open or a light burning so that he can maintain contact with his parents or view his room as he knows it to be and not as he fears it to be. At times, he resists going to sleep in order to avoid the dream experience. Disorders associated with falling asleep are, therefore, often connected with the dream experience. Rituals are set up as protective devices designed to make safer the withdrawal from the world of reality into the world of sleep.

When sleep disorders occur as the result of frightening dreams, one must help the child cope with those experiences by directing his inner need into appropriate channels. Symptomatic help, such as sedation, may be useful only to a limited extent. When the child comes into the parental bedroom to seek protection, he should be taken back into his own bed.

Somnambulism is relatively frequent; very often, the content of the dream seems to release motor discharge, and the child tries to go to those persons and places that can offer him protection.

Diagnostic Use of Dreams

Many clinicians consider the dream to be an important source of information for the assessment of internal conflicts, for clues concerning the actual life situation, and for determination of the age appropriateness of the child's development. Of particular significance is the repetitive dream, which affords evidence of a long-standing conflict and aids in the reconstruction of those events that may have contributed to it.

Physiology of Dreaming

The dream-to-sleep ratio is quite stable among adults. In adult life, 20 per cent of sleeping time is given to dreaming. Even in newborns, there is brain activity that is similar to the dreaming sleep. But it is doubtful whether dreaming is possible before speech—that is, before the existence of mental representations of the outside world.

Periods of rapid eye movements (REM) take place about 60 per cent of the time during the first few weeks of life. During the third or fourth year, the REM drops to 20 per cent or less.

REFERENCES

Ames, I. B. *Sleep and Dreams in Childhood.* Macmillan, New York, 1964.
Despert, J. L. Dreams in children of preschool age. Psychoanal. Study Child, *3–4:* 141–180, 1949.
Gesell A., and Ilg, F. L. *The Child From Five to Ten.* Harper & Row, New York, 1946.
Kahn, E., Fisher, C., Edwards, A., and Davis, D. M. A comparison of 24-hour sleep patterns between two- to three-year-old and four- to six-year-old children. Arch. Gen. Psychiatry, *29:* 145, 1973.
Lippman, H. S. The use of dreams in psychiatric work with children. Psychoanal. Study Child, *1:* 233–245, 1945.
MacFarlane, J. W., Allen, L., and Honzik, M. P. *A Developmental Study of the Behavior Problems of Normal Children Between 21 Months and 14 Years.* University of California Press, Berkeley, 1954.

41

Conditions without Manifest Psychiatric Disorder

Introduction

This category is defined by the second edition of the American Psychiatric Association's *Diagnostic and Statistical Manual of Mental Disorders* (DSM-II) as: "conditions of individuals who are psychiatrically normal but who nevertheless have severe enough problems to warrant examination by a psychiatrist. These conditions may either become or precipitate a diagnosable mental disorder."

Marital Maladjustment

The high prevalence of marital maladjustment in American society is indicated by the number of marriage counselors, family counseling agencies, and Dear Abby-type columns, in addition to psychiatrists, dealing specifically with domestic conflicts. One of four marriages in the United States ends in divorce. This fact does not necessarily indicate psychiatric illness in one or both of the partners. Some marriages just cannot last. It is the task of the psychiatrist to help the patient deal with his own conflicts. When a patient presents with specific marital problems, the result of consultation and treatment may be a happier, more fulfilling marriage or a divorce.

One of the evaluations the physician must make is whether the presenting complaint is engendered by the marriage or is part of a greater disturbance. The developmental, family, sexual, personal, and occupational history, as well as the marital history, should be enlightening in this regard.

Marriage involves many stressful situations that tax the adaptive capacities of the partners. If they are of different backgrounds and have been raised within different value systems, conflicts are likely to arise. The areas to be explored include sexual relations; attitudes toward contraception, child bearing, and child rearing; handling of money; relations with in-laws; and attitudes toward social life.

Crises and conflicts in a marriage are often precipitated by the birth of children, especially the first child. On a psychodynamic level, old sibling rivalries may be reactivated; identity problems are precipitated, especially if the couple's own parents were unhealthy models as mates or parents; and competitiveness can arise. On a more superficial level, the birth of a child may herald a change in life style. Often, it means that the wife stops working, leading to a change in environment and status for her and to greater financial strain for the husband.

Economic stresses, moves to new areas, unplanned pregnancies, and abortions may upset a healthy marriage. Differing attitudes toward religion can also present a problem. Complaints of frigidity or impotence by marital partners are usually indicative of deeper disturbances, although sexual dissatisfaction is involved in most cases of marital maladjustment.

The institution of marriage is itself being subjected to stress by cultural changes. Divorce is no longer a stigma. Marriage is no longer an economic necessity or the only acceptable means for achieving consistent sexual satisfaction. Motherhood is less idealized. The extended family is nearly extinct in this country. The nuclear family has come under attack.

Communes, sequential marriages, trial marriages, childless marriages, and marriages without obligations of fidelity are all being suggested as alternative life styles.

Social Maladjustment

This problem, also called culture shock, occurs when a person is suddenly thrust into an alien culture or has divided loyalties to two different cultures. In its most extreme form it means facing new mores and values and unlearning all the automatic daily cues of social behavior. On a less extreme basis, it occurs when young men are drafted into the army, when people change jobs, when families move or experience a significant change in income, when children experience their first day in school, and when black ghetto children are bussed to white middle-class schools. A minimum of culture shock is involved in the time needed to unwind when one first goes on vacation. The shock is lessened if one is not alone in the experience or if there is an overlap in cultures and some habitual forms of behavior can be retained.

Culture shock occurs mildly on a national level in the face of such situations as the energy crisis and government scandals that threaten the nation's confidence in governmental figures.

Immigrants to a country often experience culture shock—both because of the newness of the country they adopt and because of the conflict involved in preferring old, familiar, but different or opposing habits.

The person undergoing culture shock experiences a variety of emotions—isolation, anxiety, and depression, often accompanied by a sense of loss close to mourning. Dependent on the patient's underlying personality structure and ego strengths is the degree of adjustment he can make to his new environment. It is helpful if he can be made aware of what he is feeling and why and then educated about the most puzzling parts of the new culture. Ideally, culture shock should be prepared for in advance.

However, adjustment to a culture is not always identical with mental health. The liberal in Nazi Germany, the escapee from a dictatorship, and the ecologist in an industrial society also deal with culture shock. The goal in therapy is to enable the culture-shocked person to handle the conflict.

Occupational Maladjustment

A healthy adaptation to work provides an outlet for creativity, satisfying relationships with colleagues, pride in accomplishment, and increased self-esteem. Maladaptation can lead to dissatisfaction with self and job, insecurity, decreased self-esteem, anger and resentment.

Occupational boredom *and* dissatisfaction are pervasive among white-collar workers, middle management, and blue-collar workers. The symptoms of job dissatisfaction are a high rate of job changes, absenteeism, mistakes at work, and sabotage.

In reviewing a patient's past work history, a psychiatrist should explore how and why the occupation was chosen. Psychodynamic conflicts can be reflected in the patient's inability to accept the authority of competent superiors or, conversely, on an overdependency on authority figures to fulfill infantile needs. Special problems are the work crises of those facing retirement and the dissatisfaction of the housewife and the minority group member blocked from position or advancement because of sex, race, religion, or ethnic background.

Dyssocial Behavior

Persons classified as exhibiting dyssocial behavior often form the criminal subcultures of society and include racketeers, prostitutes, dope peddlers, and dishonest gamblers.

Unlike antisocial behavior, dyssocial behavior does not preclude a capacity for deep interpersonal relationships and trust, but the early environment of the dyssocial person has usually been such that his loyalty is reserved for his particular subculture—often criminal and predatory in its values and, therefore, antagonistic to the mainstream of society.

The dyssocial personality is not restricted to underprivileged groups; it may develop in the midst of a middle-class or upper-class family. Usually, only one child in the family exhibits this behavior. Frequently, the mother or mothering figure has covertly, often unwittingly, encouraged a kind of acting out for pathological reasons of her own. The dyssocial behavior evolving from this background is usually expressed in only one area, be it stealing, truancy, running away, or promiscuity. Treatment of such cases often means treating the entire family.

In general, the first signs of dyssocial behavior are evident by adolescence. Treatment is effected by removing the patient from his environmental influences and involving him in a warm, accepting, human relationship. Through a good relationship, in either a group or an individual setting, pressure to conform to the standards of society can be exerted. Particularly effective has been the method of giving concrete rewards and emotional support for good behavior, accompanied by the withdrawal of privileges for reversion to dyssocial behavior.

REFERENCES

American Psychiatric Association. *Diagnostic and Statistical Manual of Mental Disorders*, ed. 2. American Psychiatric Association, Washington, 1968.
Fromm, E. *Escape from Freedom*. Rinehart, New York, 1957.
Henderson, D., and Batchelor, I. C. *Textbook of Psychiatry*. Oxford University Press, New York, 1962.
Lidz, T. *The Person*. Basic Books, New York, 1968.
Slater, E., and Roth, M. *Clinical Psychiatry*. Williams & Wilkins, Baltimore, 1969.
United States Department of Health, Education, and Welfare. *Work in America*. Massachusetts Institute of Technology Press, Cambridge, 1973.

42

Community Psychiatry

42.1 COMMUNITY PSYCHIATRY CONCEPTS

Characteristics of Community Psychiatry

Catchment Area

The catchment area, a concept borrowed from the field of public health, is used to implement local service and community orientation. The emphasis on local services requires that there be a means of identifying the community to be served. The catchment area is this community. A catchment area is a designated geographical area having between 75,000 and 200,000 people.

Comprehensive Service

The five required services that are the basis of community mental health are inpatient care, outpatient care, emergency care, partial hospitalization, and community consultation and education programs. The recommended services include specialized diagnostic services, rehabilitation, preadmission and postdischarge services for state hospital patients, research and evaluation programs, and training and education activities.

Continuity of Care

Continuity of care is defined as those program elements most likely to provide linkages between or among the various services of a center. Essentially, the linkages are seen in terms of people and information. Both staff and patients must be able to move easily from one service to another. In like manner, information must move easily from one service to another. Continuity of care also includes liaison between agencies to ensure a minimum of fragmentation and a maximum of optimal care in all areas.

Preventive Psychiatry

There are three types of prevention of mental illness. The first is primary prevention, the elimination of those factors that cause or contribute to the development of disease. Primary prevention is implemented through programs in consultation and education for teachers, clergymen, welfare workers, probation officers, and other groups of community care givers. Members of these groups are most often involved in providing service to people during times of stress and crisis. Consultation by mental health professionals enables these care givers to help their clients handle their crises effectively without the onset of mental disorders.

Secondary prevention is the early detection of disease and the earliest initiation of treatment. The community mental health centers provide secondary prevention by providing readily accessible care for acute illness, often as crisis or emergency care.

Tertiary prevention is the elimination or reduction of residual disability after an illness.

Research

Research on community mental health services consists of investigations of key issues related to the development, organization, and implementation of programs for applying available knowledge to prevent, shorten, or mitigate mental disorders. This research addresses a variety of problems with respect to the availability, communication, and use of this knowledge; the delivery, staffing, and financing of mental health services; and the use of information to improve existing services or to develop new ones.

Evaluation

Evaluation refers to the process of obtaining reliable empirical evidence describing a program's operations and its effect on individuals, institutions, and communities and to the analysis of the data to form valid comparisons of these results with fixed or relative standards for assessing the program's effectiveness. Program evaluation provides feedback to decision makers so that current operating procedures can be modified and future programs can be planned.

Community-Consumer Participation

A primary assumption in the community mental health concept is that the programs should be developed and evaluated according to the needs of the community and that they should remain responsive to the community. This is generally done by electing or appointing a community advisory board, composed of representatives of the catchment population, who work with the mental health professionals in program development. Generally, the board is expected to have control of the center and its programs.

Consultation

Mental health consultation is a helping process, an educational process, and a growth process achieved through interpersonal relationships. Mental health professionals help the care giver agents of a community use mental health principles in their work. The major goals of mental health consultation are to assist care givers in handling certain emotional problems of their clients with greater effectiveness. In addition, the consultant helps care givers recognize the symptoms of mental illness and assists them in making appropriate referrals when required. The mental health consultant does not attempt to teach specialized professional techniques, such as psychodiagnosis and psychotherapy, to the care givers.

Community Psychiatry in Action

Organizational Issues

The organizational models required to provide multiple services to ensure continuity of care often involve the participation of two or more agencies, although some have been formed by the reorganization of a single agency. Typically, several different agencies provide the identifiable center services, and other agencies contribute related or supporting programs. Even when one agency is responsible for the provision of the basic center services, a comprehensive program can be developed only if outside agencies and outside services are also involved.

As community mental health centers have begun to develop in relatively large numbers, a number of common organizational models have emerged. One such model is the consortium or collaboration of private agencies for the purpose of providing services. The community mental health center within a general hospital is another possible organizational model. When a community mental health center is connected with academic psychiatry and other departments of a university concerned with mental health, the emphasis is on an integrated system of service, training, and research.

Sharing of Authority

With the exception of the academic-initiated center, either the multiagency model or the single agency-based or hospital-based model can be initiated by an agency or by the community at large. When a center is agency-initiated, the applying agency or hospital does the planning and generates the grant proposal. Community involvement generally comes a bit later. Even when the community itself has initiated the process, community involvement can be an issue, especially when the community advisory board is composed of members who are not representative of the community at large.

Tension and conflict tend to develop within the center and between the center and outside groups when the vested interests of groups of people differ. In some instances the divisive issue is power; in other instances it is money or the primacy of one group of professionals over others. A community mental health center that proposes shared authority and responsibility, tries to experiment with organizational models that alter traditional relationships between the professions, and attempts to divide service tasks according to ability, rather than professional designation, soon finds itself in an atmosphere of high tension and much conflict. The administrator must address himself to the task of reducing tensions and promoting co-operation if he is not to have total chaos.

Even when the community mental health center is organized as a single agency, there are generally crucial relationships between that agency and other agencies or services. These relationships should be delimited by clearly written and well-defined agreements.

Development of Services

Providing services is the business of the mental health center. Integration of these services generally makes it possible for the patient to be hospitalized for a shorter time and provides support during the patient's re-entry into the community.

An interesting component of the question of development of services is whether or not the medical model is appropriate. A contrasting philosophy takes a behavioral approach. For those who adhere to this philosophy, people exhibiting bizarre or abnormal behavior are not sick but, rather, are under stress and out of phase with those around them. When a nonmedical model is adopted, the emphasis is placed on social engineering and changing behavior, rather than on curing patients. As family members become aware of their involvement in the patient's problem behavior and learn different ways of relating to it, the need for custodial care of the patient is diminished. This kind of handling can facilitate a small inpatient service and reduce the need for back-up services. Sickness requires hospitalization and medical treatment; aberrational behavior may not.

Rather than focus on one or the other of these approaches, most centers have tried to retain the strengths of the medical model while incorporating behavioral modification, new definitions of roles for traditional mental health personnel, and the development of new types of personnel.

Inpatient Services. In the community mental health center many of the traditional principles of inpatient care have been modified to suit a system of integrated services. The aim of the center is to find an alternative to inpatient care if at all possible or, if acute care is required, to return the patient to the community as rapidly as possible and place him in other types of continuing treatment.

Partial Hospitalization. Partial hospitalization programs can be organized in several different ways. One possibility is to combine the day hospital with the inpatient service, so that the two units share the same space and perhaps participate in the same therapeutic programs. Such a program, if properly structured, can stimulate the inpatient service to emphasize more rapid recovery and return to the community. Partial hospitalization is also useful in moving patients out of long-term care facilities because of their adaptability to vocational and resocialization activities.

A number of problems complicate delivery of partial hospitalization services. One of these problems is dependence on transportation, particularly in rural areas. Significant financial stress because of uncertain status with insurance carriers is another problem. Many insurance companies cover mental health for inpatient services, partially cover outpatient services, and leave partial hospital services out entirely.

Outpatient Services. Programs to meet the needs of the community have included group therapy approaches, greater use of paraprofessionals, and the development of systems and organizational structures that extend outpatient services beyond the confines of the traditional clinic setting. Community mental health professionals have come to recognize that the center must often be brought to the patient, rather than the patient coming to the center. The means for bringing the center to the patient include using trained community residents, storefront centers, neighborhood health centers, and mobile units. Other innovations in outpatient services are short-term therapy, walk-in services, and new role definitions for nonmedical staff members.

Emergency Care. Emergency care provides mechanisms for dealing with acute problems at the time they are occurring. The effective reduction in the need for inpatient services depends somewhat on effective crisis intervention, which provides alternatives to hospitalization. In addition, the emergency service can function as the entry point for all patients seeking mental health services. Diagnosis and evaluation can be carried out and the patient referred to the appropriate service. Emergency services can also provide primary treatment for many patients.

Consultation and Education. Consultation and education are indirect services aimed at the prevention of mental disorders in the community. These services are generally involved with other human services in the community, such as schools, the police department, community social services, and care givers. The consultant or consultants, who are mental health specialists, and the consultee or consultees, who play roles in community health, work together to enable the consultee to handle defined problems more effectively. A specific goal is to help key professional workers or key informal care givers become more sensitive to the personal and interpersonal needs of their clients and associates and more comfortable and adept with them within the consultee's accustomed responsibilities and roles.

Members of certain professional groups—such as ministers, physicians, police, welfare caseworkers, school personnel, and public health nurses—and many informal care givers are likely to be called on or to be present at times of stress. These crises provide particularly important opportunities for psychological growth as well as psychological disintegration. The care givers thus have an opportunity to prevent psychological disorders and to promote mental health in a population. Mental health consultation can enhance a person's chances to develop new strengths when he works through a crisis effectively.

Many consultants find that such traditional teaching techniques as lecturing and seminar discussion are useful, especially with groups who expect it, such as policemen and school personnel. The choice of techniques depends on the personality and training of the consultant, the expectations and needs of the consultee, and the phase of consultation. Ideally, consultation is based on the authority of ideas and skills, rather than on institutionalized authority. The consultee should be free to accept or reject the advice of the consultant.

Community Participation

Housing a community mental health center within the imposing edifice of a city hospital reduces its accessibility to the target population, which is composed primarily of inner-city residents who are intimidated by the formality of a hospital.

Establishing community ties depends on knowledge, respect, joint effort, and a host of similar qualities that require new activities, dislocations of routines, conflict, and prolonged divergencies in points of view. A center must interact with the various service systems already established in the community and must identify its role among these established services. And a center must be able to relate to political and socio-economic systems, as well as the populations of the catchment area.

Role of the Community Mental Health Professional

Much has been written in the past few years about the community mental health professional. Above all, the qualities of flexibility and versatility have been stressed. In the interests of reaching out to the community, the constraints of professionalism have been discouraged, and collaboration and teamwork have been encouraged. The basic skills on which the community mental health professional must draw include public health, psychobiological sciences, social sciences, and managerial and political sciences. The community mental health professional often functions as a consultant or teacher. In other instances, he is a therapist or an administrator.

In the traditional clinical setting the psychiatrist or psychologist serves his clients in his quiet office. The community mental health professional, however, deals with his clients not in his territory but in theirs—often busy, public, and uncomfortable surroundings. He must initiate contact with people in their domain. The community mental health professional is less likely to be responding to patients who have requested help than to be involved with populations at risk, consumers, and ordinary citizens.

Clinical training tends to encourage the clinician's acting as a screen that reflects the patient's projections. The clinician is trained to be objective and scientific and not very giving to his patients. In contrast, the mental health professional entering the community must learn to use his skills in a way that is more like ordinary social behavior. Often, he is required to meet agency staff members, community members, and clients openly and with respect. Not only is the community mental health professional confronted by the absence of the patient role, but he is demoted from the leadership position inherent in the medical model. In the community he must interact as a peer with people from various professional backgrounds.

Frequently, community groups respond to the mental health professional with disinterest or open hostility. This reaction can be a major source of anxiety to a clinician used to deference or at least respect from his clients.

Another source of anxiety for the clinically trained community mental health professional can be excessive demands to produce meaningful change. Goals that are quite realistic on a one-to-one clinical basis become unrealistic in a setting in which the client is a group of teachers and the mental health professional is serving as a consultant.

Role of Federal, State, and Local Governments

The 1963 Community Mental Health Center Act was the first mental health legislation that included provisions for Federal support, although that support was only for the construction of centers. Each state had available to it a predetermined portion of the funds appropriated for the program in a given year. Fund allocation to each state was determined on the basis of total population size and socio-economic status. In 1965 Congress adopted legislation authorizing Federal support for the staffing of community mental health centers.

The original goal of the Community Mental Health Center Act of 1963 was to establish 2,000 community mental health centers. In 1973, a total of 398 community centers were in operation, and about 100 more were funded.

The relationships that have developed between state and local mental health agencies are many and varied. This relationship has often been complicated because state and local mental health programs have been under different governmental jurisdictions and have needed to respond to different kinds of sanctions and expectations from their respective governing bodies. Flexibility in the use of staff and physical facilities is essential.

The existence of a host of governments— counties, townships, municipalities, and special authorities of all descriptions—within a single metropolitan community often poses grave problems for the effective performance of governmental functions. The community mental health program may be handicapped in the achievement of its goal of providing comprehensive mental health care co-ordinated with other community activities, such as education, public health, welfare, and housing. In many cases, several authorities compete for the same tax dollar. This competition poses the problem of which unit of government can best assume responsibility for local financial participation.

Until 1963 the responsibility for financing mental health care traditionally fell to the state. The legislation of 1963 and 1965 defined the financial role of the Federal government as that of providing seed money through the grant-in-aid approach. Up to two thirds of the cost of construction is to be raised privately or by public authorities at a local level, and the staffing grants are to decrease from 75 per cent of cost to nothing in a period of 51 months. Although a 1970 amendment increased this time span to 96 months—8 years—an increasing financial responsibility must be assumed by local government.

Local units are reluctant to assume major new responsibilities because they are already seriously underfinanced. At the same time, local governments are hampered in the raising of money by constitutional, statutory, economic, and political impediments. Inequality of local financing means that wealthier areas are able to afford better services; therefore, the insistence on local support is open to serious question.

REFERENCES

Beigel, A., and Levenson, A. I., editors. *The Community Mental Health Center.* Basic Books, New York, 1972.
Bertelsen, K., and Harris, M. R. Citizen participation in the development of a community mental health center. Hosp. Community Psychiatry, *24:* 553, 1973.
Caplan, G. *Principles of Preventive Psychiatry.* Basic Books, New York, 1964.
Connery, R. H. *The Politics of Mental Health.* Columbia University Press, New York, 1968.
Daniels, R. S. Changing human service delivery systems: Their influences on psychiatric training. Am. J. Psychiatry, *30:* 1232, 1973.
Feldman, S., editor. *The Administration of Mental Health Services.* Charles C Thomas, Springfield, Ill., 1973.
Iscoe, I., and Spielberger, C. D., editors. *Community Psychology: Perspectives in Training and Research.* Appleton-Century-Crofts, New York, 1970.
Joint Commission on Mental Illness and Health. *Action for Mental Health.* Basic Books, New York, 1961.

42.2. DEFINITION OF MENTAL HEALTH AND DISEASE

Mental Health

The clinician often defines mental health as resistance to or absence of mental illness. Levinson adopted an ecologically oriented approach; mental health was considered to depend primarily on the way the person felt about himself, other people, and the world, particularly in reference to his own place in it. Special significance was attached to his feelings about earning a living and his responsibilities toward those who depend on him. Karl Menninger's definition of mental health includes the element of happiness. Ginsburg's definition of mental health deals with its relationship to environmental mastery as manifested in three crucial areas of living—love, work, and play.

The polarity of mental health versus mental illness has been used frequently and persistently as the basis for simple definitions of mental health. However, a full description of mental health cannot be provided within this framework. Is one concerned with the sick or the well or both? Can one identify the presick among the well? Is the oft-stated concept that the first responsibility of psychiatrists and physicians is to major mental illness, rather than preventive work, a valid one? Do psychiatrists know enough about prevention to focus on this area?

These questions are not unique to public health psychiatry, nor are they encountered more frequently there. In other areas of specialization, however, they usually take the form of clinical dilemmas that center on an individual patient. In public health psychiatry they emerge as administrative and political issues that are often colored by conflict over control and supervision of finances for program purposes, rather than theoretical and therapeutic considerations.

Problem Areas

Alcoholism and Drug Abuse

Psychiatrists and, increasingly, other physicians have long held alcoholism and drug abuse to be character disorders. Are they one problem or two? Professional thinking about them now emphasizes their similarities.

Clinically, alcoholism is seen as an effect or a cause or both of mental disorder or emotional problems. Administratively, at the state level, alcoholism programs may be independent of or under the aegis of a mental health agency. Programatically, alcoholics may be discouraged from using or actively encouraged to use a variety of mental health services, such as general hospitals, inpatient psychiatric services, and outpatient psychiatric clinics. Legally, alcoholism may be handled under the criminal justice system or may be subject to special medical and rehabilitative procedures.

Drug addiction, on the other hand, was until recently dealt with in less detail and with less structure than alcoholism because it was a problem that fewer—and poorer—people suffered from. Fifteen or 20 years ago, the only significant attention given to drug addiction by social agencies was by police departments in a few large cities and by the Bureau of Narcotics; there, drug addiction was considered a manifestation of criminal behavior, not a mental illness. National voluntary organizations never developed to cope with drug addiction in the same way that they did to deal with alcoholism.

However, research and services connected with alcoholism have not kept pace with those connected with drug addiction during the past decade, perhaps because drug addiction is more closely linked in the public mind with the threatening specter of crime. Federal expenditures on drinking problems have grown to more than $100 million yearly. But by 1973 drug programs had an annual budget of almost $1 billion.

The similarities between alcoholism and drug addiction are becoming more apparent every day. It is logical to assume that their prevention and management in local treatment programs may be joined administratively and legally and dealt with as one problem.

Mental Retardation

At the Federal level, administrative responsibility for various aspects of mental retardation resides in the Office of the Assistant Secretary for Human Development in the Department of Health, Education, and Welfare. The Office of

Mental Retardation is responsible for considering and facilitating all Federal activities dealing with mental retardation, including the President's Committee on Mental Retardation and the National Institute of Child Health and Human Development.

There is considerable variation in the administration of mental retardation programs at the state level. In some instances, departments of mental health bear the major responsibility for mental retardation programs. Other states maintain separate mental health and mental retardation departments. There are variations in local programs that may discriminate for or against services to the mentally retarded. In general, however, a significant proportion of the patient population is not retarded but manifests emotional or psychological problems.

At the clinical and conceptual level, the question of whether mental retardation can ever exist without concomitant emotional problems is a continuing source of controversy. However, mental retardation does represent a significant mental health problem for the family.

Professional and lay groups that have organized independent mental retardation programs object to mental health sponsorship on the grounds that the problems of mental illness are different in certain essential respects from those associated with mental retardation or because of their desire to preserve the critical aspects of visibility, autonomy, and growth potential of their own programs.

Crime and Delinquency

The conviction held by many law enforcement officers and laymen and some psychiatrists that most criminals are not mentally ill and that crime is not a mental health problem clearly precludes a close relationship between this problem area and mental health.

Aging

With the passage of Medicare and the Older Americans Act of 1965, the proper function of mental health in the field of aging has been subjected to intensive examination. Are psychiatrists more appropriately concerned with the aged mentally ill or with the mental health of the aging? The obvious answer is that their concern encompasses both. But whenever the mental health specialist leaves the shelter of the treatment setting and indicates a desire to step out of his traditional role as healer of the mentally ill, he emerges into an arena of conflicting and competing interest groups.

REFERENCES

Ewalt, J. R., and Farnsworth, D. A. *Textbook of Psychiatry.* McGraw-Hill, New York, 1963.
Ginsburg, S. W. The mental health movement and its theoretical assumptions. In *Community Programs for Mental Health,* R. Kotinsky and H. Witmer, editors, p.7. Harvard University Press, Cambridge, 1955.
Jahoda, M. *Current Concepts of Positive Mental Health.* Basic Books, New York, 1958.
Kennedy, J. F. *Message from the President of the United States Relative to Mental Illness and Mental Retardation.* United States Government Printing Office, Washington, 1963.
Levinson, H., Price, R. R., Munden, K. S., Mandl, H. S., and Solley, C. M. *Men, Management, and Mental Health.* Harvard University Press, Cambridge, 1962.
President's Task Force on the Mentally Handicapped. *Action against Mental Disability.* United States Government Printing Office, Washington, 1970.

42.3.   PRIMARY PREVENTION OF MENTAL ILLNESS

Introduction

Prevention of disease is generally a major concern of specialists in public health and preventive medicine. The techniques of public health are relatively new in psychiatry and few psychiatrists have training in public health and are able to use public health techniques.

Public Health Techniques

Public health techniques usually involve providing uniform direct service to all members of a susceptible population to increase resistance to illness, as in vaccination, or to find cases of illness in the early stage, as in tuberculin testing. Public health techniques also provide indirect service that affects every member of the population, as in chlorination of water. These techniques contrast with the traditional individual clinical approach in which individually planned treatment is offered by a physician after a patient develops an illness.

Public health specialists have divided preventive activities into three categories—primary, secondary, and tertiary prevention. Primary prevention involves preventing the occurrence of illness. Secondary prevention involves preventing the development of illness after occurrence. Tertiary prevention involves preventing the sequelae of illness.

The causes of disease are divided into three categories: the host, the agent, and the environment. The host is the person or group of persons, susceptible to the disease. The agent is the major factor, usually external to the host, necessary for the occurrence of the disease. The environment is the collection of all the external factors surrounding the host with the exception of the agent. Public health measures are often directed at strengthening the host against the agent or changing the environment so that it is less hospitable to the agent, rather than directly attacking the agent. In contrast, clinical treatment attempts to counteract the agent directly. Public health psychiatry usually attempts to change the host or the environment.

Primary Prevention and Psychiatry

Primary prevention of mental illness involves the promotion of general mental health and protection against the occurrence of specific diseases.

Promoting Mental Health

Measures undertaken to promote mental health require, first, that there be a definition of mental health so that the health status of a person or of an entire population can be measured. Such definitions do not presently exist; at least, those definitions of mental health that do exist are not generally accepted or amenable to measurement.

Second, interest in promoting mental health as a way of preventing mental illness assumes that mental health and mental illness are opposite ends of a spectrum or that they are mutually exclusive. This dichotomy may be true for many sorts of physical illness, particularly the infectious diseases, but it is questionable for the mental diseases. Regardless of the definition of mental health used, it is possible to find people who meet the definition and yet have symptoms suggesting mental illness. Mental health and mental illness are not mutually exclusive.

A third problem in current efforts to promote mental health is the necessity of accepting the assumption that mental health can be affected by measures undertaken during the lifetime of the person who is the target of the measures. Yet the evidence seems unmistakable that susceptibility to psychosis is influenced, if not determined, genetically, and, it has not been demonstrated that genetic predisposition can be altered. In addition, many psychiatric theories postulate the importance of early childhood events in determining later personality. Clearly, psychotherapy and psychoanalysis undertaken later in life to alter the patterns laid down in childhood can be offered to relatively few people. For most adults, then, according to these theories, fate has been determined and general mental health efforts are useless except to change the veneer that covers basic personality.

At the present state of knowledge of mental health and of public health psychiatry, little prevention of mental illness can be expected from efforts to promote general mental health. Although these efforts may lead to increased happiness or satisfaction in those who are reached by them, mental health promotion programs should not be considered scientifically based, medically related measures but, rather, more in the nature of recreation, entertainment, and moral uplift activities. Efforts of public health psychiatrists and others with similar concerns should be focused on the prevention of specific illnesses, where there seems to be a scientific foundation and much more hope of success.

Preventing Specific Illnesses

Preventive activities for many of the very serious and frightening mental diseases of the past have become so commonplace and effective that one never thinks about them. Other preventive activities, although not yet completely accepted or uniformly carried out by the public, have become so commonplace for professionals that they are no longer of any concern to mental health specialists and now are part of the routine activities of less specialized groups.

In the United States today, it is unusual to find a case of organic brain syndrome resulting from the disease agents that were leading causes of mental hospital admission 50 to 75 years ago—the spirochete of syphilis and vitamin deficiency. Preventive efforts aimed at such diseases have operated so effectively that one tends to take success for granted.

Some chemical agents are still common enough to be worthy of concern as possible causes of organic brain damage. The most notable agents are lead, the hallucinogenic drugs, and intoxicants. The fact that cases resulting from these agents continue to appear indicates a need for preventive efforts; however, the number of cases generated is small.

Crisis Reactions. Crisis or situational reactions are responses to sudden changes in psychological or social environment or status. A person may develop symptoms ranging from mild discomfort not apparent to any observer to the symptoms of the most serious forms of mental illness.

There are two aspects to crisis preparation. The first approach is cognitive and involves presenting factual materials to the person. The second aspect is an emotional or experiential one in which the person is put into stressful situations that he can overcome.

The cognitive aspect consists of a discussion, usually carried out in a group, of the situation that the person will face when he is in the crisis, of techniques others have found effective for making the crisis easier, and of the person's own experiences in mastering previous crises. The person is thus given the opportunity to expand his behavioral repertoire to include techniques that have proved to be effective. He is also told of sources of assistance if he feels overwhelmed during the crisis.

The second aspect involves putting the person through a series of increasingly stressful experiences to the point where he is almost but not quite overwhelmed or disorganized. He is able to overcome each crisis successfully and then go on to the next stage. The person becomes accustomed to dealing with stress, learns about his own reactions under the tutelage of a mental health professional, is able to find and practice techniques that are effective for him in dealing with stress, and is able to build a sense of confidence and self-esteem about his ability to deal with stressful situations. In a real crisis, he knows that he has been through similar experiences many times before and mastered them. He is not likely to lose control or lose hope.

Schizophrenia. All evidence suggests that the rate of schizophrenic breakdown has remained stable for many years and under different circumstances. Experience suggests that the best time for an effective attack on schizophrenia is after it has developed. There seems to be little doubt that there is an inherited tendency toward schizophrenia and that consideration needs to be given to genetic counseling of families in which there is a strong tendency toward schizophrenia. An experiment that needs to be done is a deliberate attempt to involve a group of isolated, friendless adolescents in social interaction, development of friendships, and anticipatory guidance to determine whether illness can be averted.

Senility. Many of the problems of the aged, often considered to result from loss of functioning brain tissue, result from loss of self-esteem, social relationships, responsibilities, and familiar surroundings. The aging person turns inward, becomes depressed, loses his social skills and interests, and falls into a vicious cycle that culminates in a diagnosis of senility.

Effective prevention probably requires a change in life style and attitudes in society so that elderly people have a respected niche and are given a useful, remunerative role. Short of this, young persons can be prepared in advance with the skills, resources, and attitudes necessary to combat the disengagement of old age. These preparations might include encouraging a positive attitude toward aging, fostering skills necessary to become intensively involved in alternative activities once retirement comes, and developing pension programs adequate to support the previous standard of living.

Personality Disturbances. Many personality disturbances result from distorted relationships in childhood. Improved child rearing can reduce the number of people with such disturbances. Orphaned and abandoned children should not be raised in institutions, nor should they be shifted from foster home to foster home. Personality disturbances can be prevented by providing long-term, stable family situations in which children can develop normally.

Child abuse runs in families from generation to generation and is an obvious target for prevention. Treatment of parental impulses toward abuse, while secondary prevention for the parents, acts as primary prevention for their children.

Other Disturbances. Preventive proposals

for other disturbances range from parental psychotherapy and intensive parent education (for the neuroses) through school health education programs (for alcoholism and drug abuse), sterilization (for mental retardation), and involuntary long-term incarceration (for children thought likely to become delinquent). Few of these programs have been evaluated. But a careful weighing of evidence and theory suggests that most of the programs aimed at primary prevention of troublesome, socially disapproved behavior are not effective and not necessarily within the realm of mental health professionals. The target behavior is ill-defined. The proposed prevention programs often have nothing to do with the skills of mental health professionals. And the troublesome behavior is considered troublesome by an almost arbitrary social consensus that can shift suddenly and eliminate the problem.

Conclusion

Primary prevention of mental illness remains for the most part an unproved hope. Major progress has been made against some of the serious mental illnesses of the past, and the potential seems to exist for future progress. Public acceptability remains a major obstacle to other techniques, such as genetic counseling, which may be useful against schizophrenia and other illnesses.

Promotion of general mental health remains at best an uncertain method of preventing mental illness. Mental health may not be related to the occurrence of mental illness, and mental health promotion efforts have such vague objectives that it is difficult to plan and carry out an effective program.

Efforts to expand the number of mental illnesses subject to primary prevention must focus on genuine mental diseases, rather than broad categories of social problems, and must involve specific objectives. The two greatest weaknesses in the area of primary prevention are inadequate definitions of terms and lack of research.

REFERENCES

Caplan, G. *Principles of Preventive Psychiatry*. Basic Books, New York, 1964.
Cumming, E., and Henry, W. E. *Growing Old: The Process of Disengagement*. Basic Books, New York, 1961.
Davis, J. A. *Education for Positive Mental Health: A Review of Existing Research and Recommendations for Future Studies*. Aldine Publishing Company, Chicago, 1965.
Jahoda, M. *Current Concepts of Positive Mental Health*. Basic Books, New York, 1958.
Kempe, C. H., and Helfer, R. E. *The Battered Child*. University of Chicago Press, Chicago, 1968.
Provence, S., and Lipton, R. C. *Infants in Institutions*. International Universities Press, New York, 1967.
Sackler, A. M. One man and medicine, on drugs and good intentions. Hosp. Tribune, Jan. 15, 1973.

42.4.   SECONDARY PREVENTION OF MENTAL ILLNESS

Introduction

Secondary prevention of mental illness involves early diagnosis and treatment to prevent sequelae and limit disability. Most early psychiatric diagnosis and treatment depend on recognition of symptoms in individual cases and then individualized treatment. However, as public health psychiatry develops, more effective mass-screening tools and treatment methods may be found.

Assumptions

Interest in early diagnosis and treatment assumes that the disease in question is treated more easily and the course of disability interrupted more readily if treatment begins in the early stages. It also assumes that treatment of the illness is less stressful and harmful, at least in the long run, than the illness itself.

However, the nature of most mental illnesses when not treated or when treated at different stages is unknown. Without such data, it is impossible to know the effectiveness of early diagnosis and treatment in altering the course of illness or preventing disability. Without administering treatment to a group of healthy people, one cannot know the positive and negative effects of the treatment itself.

Indications and Contraindications

Reactions to severe sudden psychosocial trauma seem to be relieved by early intervention. People in crisis are in great pain, turmoil, and uncertainty. If not helped to regain their equilibrium, they are susceptible to long-term disability.

Phobias and other sorts of disabling fears also seem to be best dealt with as soon as possible after their appearance and before adjustments to them are made. Once the symptomatic person and those around him accept his limitation, it is much harder to generate the psychological momentum necessary to bring about change.

Some cases of schizophrenia do not seem to be affected by treatment at any point, and diagnosis in the early stage simply serves to label the person and confirm his disability in his own eyes and in the eyes of those around him. For a person who cannot be made asymptomatic, the best treatment may be no treatment at all. He simply requires counseling and training in how best to function despite his symptoms.

A disadvantage inherent in early diagnosis is that sometimes the diagnosis must be made on the basis of inadequate information. Some apparently significant symptoms may indicate transient disturbances that will disappear if left alone but that may persist or become distorted if attention is paid to them through treatment.

Secondary Prevention Techniques

Population Screening

Many screening studies have indicated that a surprisingly large proportion of the general population is disabled from psychiatric symptoms. A minimum of 10 per cent of the general American population will report significant psychiatric disability at any one time and, therefore, are possibly in need of treatment. What is not known is what proportion of these persons are amenable to treatment and what proportion will recover without any intervention. Without such information, it may be disastrous to provide mental health services for all persons apparently in need.

Crisis Intervention Services

Crisis intervention includes suicide prevention services using telephone and in-person interviews, teen-age counseling as offered through hot line and drop-in centers, pastoral counseling, brief psychotherapy offered in emergency walk-in clinics, family dispute intervention provided by specially trained policemen, and widow-to-widow programs. All offer service immediately after application; service is brief and focused almost exclusively on the presenting problem. The attempt is not to bring about

major personality change but, instead, to return the person to his previous state of functioning. Usually, no formal diagnosis is made, and there is a deliberate attempt to avoid any sort of patient role or labeling. In many cases the counselors are not mental health professionals but are briefly trained volunteers or members of other occupational groups with little or no professional responsibility for outcome.

Crises and transition states are a normal part of human development. The particular points at which crises occur for any one person depend in large part on his circumstances and his culture. Crises may occur with the sudden illness of the person himself or of a loved one; with the transition from childhood into adolescence, adolescence into adulthood, or adulthood into old age; with induction into the Armed Forces or entrance into college; or with a child's first loss of a tooth or the onset of sexual maturity. The distincitve element of the crisis is that it represents a sudden change in a person's relationship to others, usually because of a change in physical, psychological, or social status and a change in the person's image of himself. This change disrupts old relationships, makes old behavior patterns inappropriate, and leaves him at a temporary loss for direction in his behavior.

Mental illness is more common in certain specific crises. The onset of adolescence, motherhood, and old age are points at which particular forms of psychosis are likely to occur.

Because of the plasticity of the person during the crisis period, the mental health worker seeking to intervene is in a powerful position. Someone in crisis is looking for answers and is likely to accept those offered by the worker. Furthermore, old habits are disrupted and are less likely to interfere with the formation of new ones. On the other hand, if the worker prescribes the wrong treatment, the damage is likely to be far greater and longer lasting.

Mental Health Education

Educating the public to recognize mental illness in the early stages and then to seek help seems logically to be a useful approach for many types of illness. Unfortunately, this assumption has yet to be demonstrated to be true.

Mental health consultation is a special form of mental health education. Here, a mental health professional, usually a clinician with special training in consultation techniques, regularly visits a social service agency to provide information, advice, support, and whatever else may seem appropriate for the workers of that agency as they attempt to deal with the mental health problems of their clients. The clients of all sorts of social service agencies include a large number of people who have serious mental-health-related problems and who could be diagnosed and appropriately offered treatment if they were referred to a mental health service agency. However, if all these people applied for service, the mental health agencies would be overwhelmed and probably paralyzed.

Mental health consultation activities are now carried out with schools, rehabilitation agencies, welfare departments, and police and correctional agencies, and there has been discussion about offering such service to bartenders, pharmacists, and hairdressers. Wherever occupational groups are in contact with large numbers of people under stress or in crisis, there is the opportunity to provide early diagnosis and intervention without the formality and delay of application for service at a mental health agency.

Availability of Services

As service availability increases, utilization rises. This finding suggests that early diagnosis and treatment are facilitated by such availability. Major steps to increase availability have been taken through the funding of community mental health centers by the Federal government and many state governments. The mental health centers themselves have tended to increase availability even further by developing satellites and various outreach measures. The unknown factor is whether the increased utilization is occurring among the groups who need early diagnosis and treatment or whether it is occurring among groups less appropriate for service, such as those who are not really ill.

Conclusion

Secondary prevention of mental illness is generally accepted as an important aspect of mental health services, but whether or not it is in fact important has not yet been clearly demonstrated. There are great gaps in the underlying hypotheses and definitions. Al-

though early diagnosis and treatment seem logical, in some cases they are not effective and are possibly even harmful.

The more serious mental illnesses seem not to be affected by early diagnosis and treatment. The reactive illness—the symptomatic responses to crisis—seem to be far more amenable to early intervention, although formal diagnosis is often neither necessary nor useful. Crucial elements in successful intervention are understanding and making use of the groups with which the person in crisis is affiliated and attempting to relieve or overcome, if only briefly, some of the stresses that have led to his breakdown. Crisis intervention may be best carried out by nonprofessional, briefly trained persons who operate in the environment in which the breakdown occurs.

REFERENCES

Caplan, G. *Principles of Preventive Psychiatry.* Basic Books, New York, 1964.
Glass, A. J. Principles of combat psychiatry. Milit. Med., *117:* 27, 1955.
Levine, M., and Levine, A. *A Social History of Helping Services: Clinic, Court, School, and Community.* Appleton-Century-Crofts, New York, 1970.
Querido, A. The shaping of community mental health care. Br. J. Psychiatry. *114:* 293, 1968.
Zusman, J., and Davidson, D. L. *Practical Aspects of Mental Health Consultation.* Charles C Thomas, Springfield, Ill., 1971.

42.5. TERTIARY PREVENTION OF MENTAL ILLNESS

Introduction

Tertiary prevention of mental illness involves rehabilitation after defect and disability have been fixed. Tertiary prevention of the disability associated with several major mental illnesses has been well demonstrated to be possible.

Many of the symptoms of chronic psychiatric disability result in large part from the treatment offered rather than from the illness itself. When properly treated in the early stages, many psychotic people recover completely. Others recover to the point of being able to live independently except during occasional periods of relapse.

Most serious psychiatric illnesses can result in chronic disability. The factors that lead to deterioration do not differ strikingly from one disease to the next. Principles of rehabilitation similarly are much alike with emphases varying somewhat from disease to disease.

Schizophrenia

The general objective of psychiatric rehabilitation is to produce behavior in the patient that will enable him to resume his function in society. Psychiatric rehabilitation does not involve personality reconstruction or unconscious motivation. Many of the people who are subjects for rehabilitation are ill or have been damaged to the point that they will never be completely free of disability. The objective of rehabilitation is to enable these people to make the best use of what resources they have and to minimize the effects of their disabilities.

It is possible for someone to function in an essentially normal manner—despite the presence of such symptoms as hallucinations and delusions—if he develops secondary mechanisms for reality testing and relating to other people. He must learn to rely on others to give him cues to reality since his own internal mechanisms are not working properly.

Principles of Psychiatric Rehabilitation

Mental illness does not pervade the affected person's behavior. Even the most seriously ill and disabled person makes most of his decisions and relationships on a rational basis. Most seriously ill people are able to care for themselves and adequately meet their own needs in the complex environment of large hospitals. The rehabilitation worker's objective must be to enlarge on this remaining ability to act rationally and to extend the numbers and kinds of decisions that are made in a rational way.

Human behavior can be changed by gradual shaping into completely new responses. This is the opposite of the traditional and unture maxim, "You can't teach an old dog new tricks." However, the complexity of the behavior and the person's ability influence how long it takes to develop the new response. Gradual development must be encouraged.

Human behavior responds to the presence or absence of specific factors in the environment, as well as to the general influence of social pressure. Behavior therapy can rehabilitate patients and produce specific kinds of behavior. The problem is that institutional life is far

simpler than life outside the institution. A method of shaping behavior that is closer to what exists outside the institution is social pressure. The rehabilitation worker makes the patient part of a group and then gets the group to encourage him to act in a particular way.

Social pressure can be inferred from, modified for, and exerted on a patient by observing, modifying, and exerting the group's expectations of that behavior. Staff and patients must demonstrate to disabled people that they expect them to act normally; when such normal behavior does not occur, they must express shock and dismay. Rehabilitation workers should always expect the best and be prepared for the worst.

Since the objective of rehabilitation is to prepare the disabled patient for life outside the institution, the institutional setting must permit and even encourage behavior appropriate for life outside.

Social pressure can be exerted only through involvement in a group and interaction with the members of the group. The greater the person's ties to the group, the greater its influence on him and the more likely his recovery. The first principle of rehabilitation must be to encourage the patient's interaction with other persons. The unwilling patient should be required to spend a certain amount of time in group activities, and the amount of time should be increased as rapidly as possible.

The attitudes and social forces within the group are crucial in determining the behavior of the group members. The rehabilitation worker must see that the groups under his jurisdiction move their members toward recovery, rather than reinforce disability, by mixing normal members into the group. The normal members, simply by acting in socially appropriate ways and using their everyday social skills, encourage rehabilitation of the disabled members. In an institutional setting the most available normal members are the institution staff. To avoid splitting the group, the rehabilitation worker must minimize or eliminate the social barriers between patients and staff.

Practice of Psychiatric Rehabilitation

Psychiatric rehabilitation can be carried out anywhere. The best situation is one in which a small portion of the space and resources of a regular institution of society is devoted to rehabilitation activities. For example, a small fraction of the activities of a Young Men's Christian Association or settlement house might be given over to psychiatric rehabilitation. A part of an industrial plant, a school, a public housing project, or any other major social institution can be used. Such a situation provides a setting conducive to normal behavior, the transition from the rehabilitation service to the normal social institution is eased, the expense of operating the rehabilitation unit is cut, and the problem of integrating patients and normal persons in a single group is reduced.

The patient usually makes a transition from the acute treatment facility, usually the mental hospital ward, to resumption of his normal life through a series of steps. Many patients do not need to go through the full range of transitional services; in fact, many are able to go directly from an acute treatment service back to their previous life. However, others are never able to return to a normal life. These persons should be moved along the system to the point where they are able to get along with the least possible support.

The transitional settings go from more regulation and support to less regulation and support. They go from being completely institutional and populated by a group composed almost exclusively of persons labeled as patients and staff to voluntary settings where there are broad mixtures of people. They also go from being least stressful and most understanding and forgiving of deviant behavior to most stressful and least forgiving.

Alcohol and Drug Abuse

Rehabilitation of alcohol and drug abusers follows similar principles to those discussed above. Again, the problem is social integration and provision of a new social role. Many persons who become disabled as the result of alcohol or drug abuse seem to start out with deficiencies in social skills. The emphasis in rehabilitation, therefore, must be on development of new skills, new associations, and new rewards for behavior.

Unlike psychiatrically disabled people, drug users tend not to be alone; rather they are firmly attached to a drug-using group. Rehabilitation must involve changing their membership to other groups. Groups that have arisen spontaneously to help drug and alcohol users, such as Synanon and Alcoholics Anonymous, develop their own ceremonies, philosophy, ethics, and spiritual life—all offered in contrast to those of the drug or alcohol user's culture.

As with the mentally ill, some alcoholics and drug abusers quite likely will never be rehabilitated to the point of complete integration into normal society. In the facilities available, preparations must be made for each level to be a terminal point for some and transitional for others.

The Aged

The aged mentally disabled differ from other groups in that, for the most part, they have previously had a full range of social skills but have lost these skills through lack of use, depression, and apathy in response to changes in life circumstances and central nervous system tissue damage. Once these skills are lost, it is harder to restore them in the aged because mental resiliency and motivation may not be as great as in younger persons. Reality orientation starts with simple social interaction, such as discussion of the day of the week, the date, and the person's name. It then progresses to more complicated skills, strongly emphasizing repetition.

Conclusion

Modern tertiary prevention of mental illness—rehabilitation of seriously disabled mentally ill persons—is one of the great success stories of psychiatry. The change in appearance of mental hospital patients from 50 years ago to today is so great that it can scarcely be believed. The knowledge to control the worst long-term disabilities is now available. The next pressing problem is to extend rehabilitation services widely into the community.

REFERENCES

Bockoven, J. S. *Moral Treatment in American Psychiatry.* Springer, New York, 1963.

Goffman, E. On the characteristics of total institutions. In *Asylums: Essays on the Social Situation of Mental Patients and Other Inmates,* chap. 1. Anchor Books, New York, 1961.

Gruenberg, E. M. Can the reorganization of psychiatric services prevent some cases of social breakdown? In *Psychiatry in Transition 1966–67,* A. B. Stokes, editor, p. 95. University of Toronto Press, Toronto, 1967.

Gruenberg, E. M., and Zusman, J. Natural history of schizophrenia. Int. Psychiatry Clin., *1:* 699, 1964.

Program Area Committee on Mental Health of the American Public Health Association. *Mental Disorders: A Guide to*

Control Methods. American Public Health Association, New York, 1961.

Taulbee, L. R., and Folsom, J. C. Reality orientation for geriatric patients. Hosp. Community Psychiatry, *17:* 133, 1966.

42.6   MENTAL HEALTH CONSULTATION

Introduction

The Joint Commission on Mental Illness and Health recommended the training of large numbers of mental health counselors who could work under the direction of mental health consultants, giving services to neglected areas. Mental health consultation in the community, together with community education, has been included in the five essential services to be offered by any community mental health center funded by the Federal government.

Mental health consultation is usually defined as the interactions between a consultant and a consultee on behalf of a client. The consultant is a person with specialized knowledge; his consultee requests help in classifying a problem, increasing his skill in handling a disturbance or crisis, or raising the mental health level of a person or group for whom he is responsible. The client can be an individual person, a group, an agency, or an institution.

A consultant acts as a psychological change agent. He deals directly with the consultee but indirectly with the problem. Nevertheless, his focus is on the problem, not on the interpersonal process. It is a content-centered, work-limited process. The relationship is seen as temporary by both parties. The consultant is usually seen as an outsider, not a member of the hierarchy in which the client is centered. The consultee continues to maintain professional responsibility for the client. An important goal, beyond help for the acute problem, is education of the consultee, so that he can handle similar cases better in the future.

Types of Consultation

Client-Centered Case Consultation

This type of consultation usually involves a case with a mental health problem for which a therapist or other responsible party seeks advice. The consultant tries to appreciate exactly what kind of help the consultee wants, then attempts to assist him with diagnosis, case formulation, and treatment plans.

Program-Centered Administrative Consultation

Here, the consultant counsels the consultee not about a single case but about a system or program in the mental health field. The consultant may collect data himself and make observations about the relationships or interactions of staff members and the follow-through of procedures. He may involve himself in a systems analysis of some intensity and duration, especially if the organization is a large clinic, institution, or hospital. Many discussions with the consultee may be necessary, not only to obtain data and viewpoints but to prepare ground work for acceptance of the report. Eventually, the consultant recommends short-term and long-term solutions calculated to improve the mental health potential of the workers and raise the productivity of the institution.

Consultee-Centered Case Consultation

Here, the efforts are centered less on the pathology of the case and more on the difficulties in management of the case resulting from the consultee's inexperience, lack of knowledge, or errors in technique. The most sensitive area for the consultant to deal with is lack of objectivity, since this area often relates to the consultee's own emotional problems or biases that interfere with perception, understanding, or ability to relate to his client. The consultant does not go into the personal roots of the conflict but deals with the effect of these conflicts on work with the client. No attack is made on the consultee's defenses.

Consultee-Centered Administrative Consultation

This form of consultation usually involves a group and requires a series of sessions. There is minimal discussion of private or personal factors. The consultant gives aid in a problem involving leadership or executive performance in relation to a mental health system or organization.

Procedure

Mental health consultation begins with a request from a consultee sanctioned by his agency and his authority figures. The consultant and the consultee meet together over a specific problem with the expectation that the problem can be alleviated or resolved within a short time. Through study, education, or specific actions, the knowledge of both is used to arrive at a reasonable solution.

To be maximally effective, the consultant must maintain objectivity. He must strive for the good will of the organization he serves by maintaining a continuing satisfactory level of sanction from the key figures in the hierarchy. He needs patience to permit the relationship to mature to a point of real effectiveness. He must facilitate, not dominate or make dependent. He cannot be judgmental, delve too deeply into the motivational aspects of the consultee, or practice psychotherapy.

If the consultation proceeds properly, the consultee's anxieties are considerably allayed and his effectiveness thereby increased. Review of the situation with a trained objective person yields considerable clarification in diagnosis and opens up new attitudes, methods of procedures, and avenues of communication.

The treatment model emphasizes medical and psychiatric orientation and training and is client-centered. The preventive model adopts a public health approach, in which program emphasis is on administration, epidemiology, demography, and a knowledge of political structure. The enhancement model focuses on ecology.

Areas of Consultation

Medical, Surgical, and Nursing Services

The psychiatric consultant to the medical and surgical services of a general hospital may function in relation to a puzzling case or program, in relation to a staff person-consultee who works with patients, or in relation to an executive-consultee responsible for the organization of services. Insights gained by social psychiatrists relative to the effect of setting, milieu, and expectation on potential for improvement of mental patients can be translated to life on medical and surgical wards.

Nurses have important emotional problems relating to dirt, body odor, hostility, and perceived immorality and irresponsibility of patients. Nurses cannot be expected to become therapists, but they can, through regular consultations, gain better understanding of mechanisms of denial of aging and death and of resentment in regard to helplessness and dependency. The hostility of relatives can be disturbing. Concepts of grief reaction and the value of expressing feelings, rather than keeping a stiff upper lip, can be helpful, especially when taught by a recognized authority.

Model Cities Programs

Psychiatric consultation to Model Cities programs emerged with the advent of Federal assistance to selected urban centers. Hard survival needs such as housing and jobs receive highest priority; however, as citizens without technical knowledge and expertise begin to think of a better future life, they soon call on mental health professionals for direct service and for consultations.

Schools

Consultations can be with teachers as a group, as individuals seeking general knowledge, or as persons troubled about individual children in their charges. Or the consultations can be with principals and superintendents of schools or with parent groups.

The consultant to the school as a system identifies and strengthens properties conducive to positive mental health and identifies those inimical to mental health. In his discussions, the consultant increases the sensitivity, responsibility, and effectiveness of members of the school community. Roundtable conferences involving several caretakers are encouraged for multiproblem families with an aim toward coordinating therapeutic strategies.

Armed Services

Visits of psychiatrist teams to combat units indicate interest and increase the battalions' hope of solutions. The unit obtains a more objective view of itself. The unit members at all levels are given an opportunity to ventilate frustrations; communication is opened up between high and low levels of command. Distortions are corrected, scapegoating reduced, and positive thinking encouraged.

Other Areas

Reports have been published relating experience in consultation to state rehabilitation agencies, public defender agencies, and theological programs of hospitals and mental health centers—the last carried out by theologians, rather than by psychiatrists. A special field of broad application is crisis intervention.

Research and Educational Potential

The consultant does not have to know all about the field of endeavor in which he is consulting or become an expert in the area in which his consultee is practicing. Instead, he can provide assistance with his general knowledge of psychiatry, psychology, and mental health and with his specific expertness as a consultant trained in objective analysis, development of relationships with consultees, and sensitivity to how anxieties diminish effectiveness. Since every consultation is a learning experience for both parties, the consultant can extend his awareness of problems and activities in the mental health front and open up channels of new information regarding community mental health practices, cultural values and influences, group interrelationships, and social forces leading to disease, crisis, or health. The consultation, therefore, may be useful in many research and educational contexts in addition to its value for service.

Training

Greater emphasis on mental health consultation training may be expected in the future. More and more training programs in psychiatry are making formal attempts to teach consultation. To be prepared for consultation work, the psychiatrist should have considerable experience in psychiatric diagnosis and treatment and intensive grounding in individual and group dynamics. Experience with groups whose values and attitudes are different from the trainee's is worthwhile. An academic background in community and social psychiatry and the social sciences is recommended. Specific training in community psychiatric practice is almost a necessity. Specific consultation activity in several settings under supervision and the opportunity to study and criticize procedures and results and to formulate theoretical views in a seminar-type conference over a considerable period of time are important.

REFERENCES

Bindman, A. J. The clinical psychologist as a mental health consultant. In *Progress in Clinical Psychology*. L. E. Abt and B. F. Reiss, editors. Grune & Stratton, New York, 1966.
Caplan, G. Types of mental health consultation. In *Principles of Preventive Psychiatry*. Basic Books, New York, 1964.
Frankel, F. H. Psychiatric consultation for nursing homes. Hosp. Community Psychiatry, *18:* 331, 1967.
Joint Commission on Mental Illness and Health. *Action for Mental Health Final Report*. Basic Books, New York, 1961.
Mannino, F. V. *Consultation in Mental Health and Related Fields: A Reference Guide*. National Institute of Mental Health, Chevy Chase, 1969.
McClung, F. B., and Stunden, A. A. *Mental Health Consultation to Programs for Children*. National Institute of Mental Health, Chevy Chase, 1970.

43

Military Psychiatry

Introduction

The methods developed for the treatment of combat reactions are fairly simple: The patient must be treated as near as possible to the place where he had his emotional breakdown. The patient must be treated as soon as possible after his breakdown. The patient must expect and be expected to return to his former duty after a short period of self-organization. Rest, food, and reassurance are of great importance. Exhortation, suggestion, and ventilation constitute the principal verbal methods.

Principles

In the military service, the medical evaluation of a person's fitness requires a high regard for functional effectiveness. Anatomical or pathological items may be of some significance, but they have their significance only insofar as they affect one's effectiveness. Compensatory skills developed by strong motivation and persistent application may counterbalance anatomical faults or pathological conditions.

The way in which men are treated and cared for and the manner in which they are led are of crucial importance in determining their emotional fitness and functional effectiveness. Psychiatrists can contribute much to the general development and maintenance of high effectiveness, to the restoration of effectiveness after impairment, and to wise reassignment. The unit is more important than any single person. Mission supersedes safety.

Functions

As chief of mental health services, the psychiatrist is expected to provide for the prevention, diagnosis, and treatment of emotional and personality disorders and mental illness and for the evaluation and disposition of patients. In his staff or advisory functions, the military psychiatrist assists the chief medical officer in advising the commander in matters pertaining to the morale of military personnel and the impact of current policies on the psychological effectiveness of military personnel.

Techniques

Troop clinics assist in classification and assignment and help maladjusted trainees in replacement training centers. They have become true community clinics, serving all elements of their commands. They have a profound effect on hospitalization and treatment patterns.

Military medical regulations for psychiatry foster the outpatient management of emotional disorders, minimize the concept of neurosis as a disabling condition, and emphasize the role of motivation in performance, even where neurosis exists. The mental hygiene consultation service has been charged with interpreting and implementing this policy. Staff clinic members seek and meet adjustment problems at their sources, the units, rather than waiting for patients to come to them, and use a preventive approach to disciplinary problems.

Combat Psychiatry

Prompt evaluation and therapy, good liaison with classification and assignment officers, continuing orientation and support of battalion and regimental medical officers by division psychiatrists, and control of evacuation channels are important in effective combat psychiatry. In most cases, simple measures of rest, sleep, food, and short respite from stress accomplish therapeutic miracles when combined with firm and clearly understood evacuation policies.

The principles of combat psychiatry are:

1. The medical officer functions close to command in preventive medical functions. He moves toward the community's level of need in determining his preventive or societally oriented roles. He emphasizes the public health model that it is not necessary to treat the individual patient, although the model includes the referral of individual patients.

2. Individual treatment is more often suppressive than evocative. The principles applied are those of proximity, immediacy, and expectancy. The model is that of crisis intervention. The psychiatrist must learn about social pathology and must be able to accept the possibility that he is not the key person in a transaction. The treatment team is an interdisciplinary one.

3. Work is field-oriented. Members of the team seek adjustment problems at their sources, the units, and are alert to opportunities for direct communication with military supervisors and the leadership or programming level of the military community for primary preventive work. The individual soldier's symptoms are often a reflection of increased stress within his unit, rather than a manifestation of individual pathology.

4. Special attention is given to the development of congruence in programs. Control of medical evacuation criteria and operations has a high priority. The military community's outside boundaries should be sharply defined in a combat area. Internal relationships, particularly clarity in referral routes for psychiatric consultation, provide practice in experiences that are educational for nonpsychiatric professionals.

As the psychiatrist becomes involved, he begins to have an identification with the group in the same way that he normally acquires an identification with an individual patient. The group becomes his patient, and the efforts of the therapy are directed toward helping the group maintain and improve its performance and adjustment. He identifies himself both with the group and its problems and goals and with the individual patient and his problems and goals.

Unit personnel are the first to deal with the soldier with psychiatric complaints. The most successful programs of forward-area psychiatric treatment place much emphasis on indoctrina-tion of company officers in the proper methods of managing psychiatric complaints at this level. Soldiers with relatively minor psychiatric problems are given suitable help within their own units. Company officers encourage wavering soldiers by exhortation and leadership, by counseling and reassuring, and by making alterations in job assignments in some cases.

The psychiatric casualty first encounters formal medical treatment if he is evacuated to the battalion aid station. Most psychiatric patients admitted to battalion aid stations are soldiers with mild to moderate anxiety states, sometimes complicated by physical exhaustion and the effects of exposure. Although a man may appear to be at the end of his rope one evening, after a good night's rest under sedation in dry clothes, he is often ready and willing to return to his company.

Psychotherapy at the battalion aid station varies with the type of patient and is almost invariably superficial. The attitude of the battalion surgeon is of prime importance in determining the outcome of the case. He must have an air of calm confidence in all his decisions. Ideally, he is firm, yet understanding, so that all his dispositions are regarded as final. His manner and all his remarks indicate that he expects an early return to duty after the soldier has rested. Medical discipline is maintained.

A large group of patients manifest symptoms that consist essentially of no more than the somatic and psychological manifestations of the normal combat fear reaction. These soldiers are treated by proper examination, evaluation, explanation, and reassurance.

Patients with mild to moderate anxiety states with varying degrees of exhaustion and exposure are treated chiefly by sedation and by measures designed to counteract fatigue and exposure. Psychotherapy consists of reassurance, support, and exhortation. After 24 hours, many of these patients feel completely recovered or markedly improved and can be returned directly to duty. Others show little or insufficient improvement and are evacuated for further definitive care by the division psychiatrist.

Certain patients are obviously unsuited for management in the battalion aid station. They exhibit disturbed anxiety states with severe agitation and tension, acute panic states, severe hysterical manifestations, and acute psychoses.

Although evacuation is the only conceivable disposition for such patients, it is important that they be adequately sedated to render their evacuation feasible and nontraumatic.

Toward malingerers, the attitude of the medical officer is one of uncompromising firmness. After careful medical evaluation, he lets the soldier know that he considers the situation trivial and that it does not merit consideration for relief from duty. This is usually sufficient, but, if the soldier persists in his attitude or refuses to accept the situation, reference to the possible consequences of such action usually discourages further attempts.

Habitual stragglers are the apparently willing soldiers who just cannot keep up or who get lost or misunderstand orders or produce any number of other excuses leading to their arrival at the aid station when an attack is just getting under way or is momentarily expected. These men are best managed by providing instructions and, when possible, guides or transportation back to the company in time to make or receive the attack. In this way, they come to realize that the subterfuge does not pay off and entails only additional trouble and risk.

Several principles of therapy have been learned from the trial-and-error experiences of combat psychiatry—decentralization, expectancy, and brief, simplified methods. Decentralization brings treatment to the patient whenever practicable, rather than evacuating psychiatric casualties to a hospital facility. Expectancy refers to the importance of the attitudes displayed by medical personnel when dealing with acute psychiatric disorders; a calm acceptance of the patient's complaints and story of severe battle trauma as being a temporary breakdown from which prompt recovery is expected after a brief respite from battle can produce rapid and dramatic improvement within hours or overnight. Brief, simplified methods of treatment are aimed at a restoration of former competency by a brief removal from battle, along with measures to relieve hunger, fatigue, and other physiological impairments.

Drug Abuse

Studies of servicemen with drug abuse problems identify important differences from civilian addicts. Most of the servicemen are not members of a minority group, are not residents of a ghetto, and have not suffered from discrimi- nation. The family constellation in their homes is not matriarchal. Drug-prone persons often describe the use of heroin as a convenient antidote to the pressures of military life. In a high percentage of cases, the psychodynamics resemble those that account for depressive reactions in other patients. The heroin abuser in military service is so often a polydrug user that methadone substitution is too simplistic a response. Further, the complex issues of extended rehabilitation of the heroin abuser on active duty, through substitution of methadone addiction for heroin addiction, require such restrictions in assignment availability that over-all military mission requirements cannot be satisfied. The service programs are, for the most part, decentralized models that provide on-the-job rehabilitation programs at the military post, seeking to avoid the counterproductive influence of extensive hospitalization and dislocation from work and family.

Clinical Practice Settings

Mental Hygiene Consultation Service

Each major military post and each combat division is assigned a mental hygiene consultation service to provide consultation to and maintain liaison with unit commanders and other military personnel relative to the prevention and treatment of social and emotional problems that interfere with the adequate functioning of military personnel and their dependents. Particularly at posts that provide basic training shortly after induction, this medical facility concerns itself with psychological problems that arise during the transitional period. At such a time, considerable strain is placed on the adaptive resources of the recruit. Unlike adjustment to combat when anxiety is due to external danger, the tensions of the military newcomer originate within the self and are secondary to the blocking of his usual pleasures and desires. The mental hygiene consultation service provides counseling to facilitate the establishment of group identification.

Clinic

Attached to each post and station hospital, the neuropsychiatric outpatient clinic offers direct psychotherapeutic intervention within a framework of established and reciprocal interdisciplinary relationships. Intake procedures ordinarily include participation with the disciplines of psychology and clinical social work. Techniques provided include short-term and long-term supportive psychotherapy, family intervention, couple therapy, and technical liaison with the health nurse to provide clinical supervision of the health nurse's home visit activities for follow-up support of former psychiatric inpatients. Often, the clinic includes neurological diagnostic facilities. This clinic is responsive to dependent and retired persons as an ambulatory care program.

Hospital

Each military post hospital has the capacity for emergency psychiatric admissions for up to 7 days. A number of military hospitals have the specialized mission of providing longer periods of hospitalization and treatment, up to 90 days, and accept patients from smaller hospitals. The large general hospitals have extensive facilities for neuropsychiatric diagnosis and treatment, with authority for up to 180 days of inpatient treatment and rehabilitation. In addition, inpatient consultation service is provided for the nonpsychiatric inpatient population of the hospital.

Military Courts

The military psychiatrist appears infrequently as an expert witness in a court-martial. When he does appear, he is usually called by the prosecution. As a rule, when the defendant, as a result of pretrial psychiatric examination, is found to have a mental disease, defect, or derangement that renders him unable to distinguish right from wrong, adhere to the right, or cooperate in his own defense, he is not brought to trial but is released to the medical authorities for treatment and ultimate disposition. The illness in question is almost invariably of psychotic proportions and not the result of misconduct, such as alcoholic overindulgence.

Special Problems

Fear of Flying

An aviator who examines the risks involved for him and decides to cease his flying duties should not be thought of as having a phobic neurosis. Neither should hysterical neuroses (conversion type) or other neurotic disabilities

be termed phobias, for the psychodynamics and clinical pictures are different. In a phobic neurosis involving flying, the feared situation should be one possessing very little inherent danger. Phobias, then, are rather unusual in military aviators.

It has been proposed that flying phobias are ideal for behavior therapy. Recently, some successes have been reported. Conditioning therapists state that neuroses are persistent, unadaptive habits that have been conditioned. However, flying phobias are often adaptive, rather than maladaptive.

Service in Isolated Areas

Three major dimensions of adaptation to duty in isolated areas have been identified: competence in work performance, social compatability, and emotional composure. The criteria used also include peer nominations, performance ratings by supervisors, and medical symptoms. There is increasing evidence that such evaluations can predict adjustment with high morale and productivity. Even with the best criteria, however, the stress may be psychonoxious for a particular person.

Families of Prisoners of War and the Missing in Action

The families of prisoners experienced a degradation of coping defenses, with a reportedly high incidence of severe, progressive psychological and psychophysiological symptoms. Psychotherapy is often required to respond to stress of functional desertion, ambiguity of role, repressed anger and sexuality, censure, and social isolation. Separation anxiety, role distortion, and sleep disorders are reportedly common in the children of these families. Group therapy is reported to be the treatment of choice.

Reunion after such prolonged husband-father absence has been marked by difficult readjustments for all family members. Added skills acquired during the husband's absence, independent and more decisive life styles, and other changes perceived as constructive may be challenged when the family is reunited. Children have considerable trouble accepting the unknown, unpracticed authority of the returned father. Such families have a high incidence of turmoil and divorce. They require considerable support in the areas of health and adjustment.

Families of the missing in action show increased dependency on alcohol, large fluctuations in body weight, and chronic dysphoric mood problems. The sense of military community membership has been weakened or lost, and the family is embedded in a social limbo in the civilian community, sustained largely by monthly military payments, but without accompanying direction or support. Many such families are paralyzed by the severity of the chronic identity conflicts.

REFERENCES

Artiss, K. L. Human behavior under stress: From combat to social psychiatry. Milit. Med., *128:* 1011, 1963.

Baker, S. L., Cove, L. A., Fagen, S. A., Fischer, E. G., and Janda, E. J. Impact of father absence: Problems of family reintegration following prolonged father absence. Am. J. Orthopsychiatry, *38:* 347, 1968.

Conner, D., and Pearson, M. The development of a MHCS role in race relations. Milit. Med., *138:* 288, 1973.

Crawford, J. V., Morgan, D. W., and Gianturca, D. *Progress in Mental Health Information Systems: Computer Applications.* Ballinger, Cambridge, 1974.

Fiman, B. G., Conner, D. R., and Segal, A. C. A comprehensive alcoholism program in the army. Am. J. Psychiatry, *130:* 532, 1973.

Glass, A. J. Principles of combat psychiatry. Milit. Med., *117:* 27, 1955.

Hall, R. C., and Simmons, W. C. The POW wife: A psychiatric appraisal. Arch. Gen. Psychiatry, *29:* 690, 1973.

Medical Care for Repatriated Prisoners of War: A Manual for Physicians. Center for Prisoner of War Studies, Navy Medical Neuropsychiatric Research Unit, San Diego, 1973.

Medical Department, U. S. Army. *Neuropsychiatry in World War II,* vol. 11. U. S. Government Printing Office, Washington, 1974.

Menninger, W. C. *Psychiatry in a Troubled World.* Macmillan, New York, 1948.

Muston, D. F. *The American Disease.* Yale University Press, New Haven, Conn., 1973.

Perkins, M. E. Preventive psychiatry during World War II. In *Preventive Medicine of World War II,* vol. 3. U. S. Government Printing Office, Washington, 1955.

Zimmerman, F. W., Baker, S. L., and Brown, D. E. *Careers in Military Psychiatry,* vol. 3. D. J. Publications, New York, 1972.

44

Occupational Psychiatry

Introduction

The field of occupational psychiatry is concerned with the adaptation of a person to his work setting. It is concerned with the person who brings his mental disorder to the job and with occupational factors that may contribute to such disability. However, there is equal concern for factors in the work environment that stimulate healthy behavior. Further, concepts of prevention extend to work organization policy, education and training (particularly for management and medical staff), consultation, and early case finding.

Here, the phrase "work organizations" is used to encompass all job situations, be they in the private or public sector, in institutions, in agencies, or on the farm. "Occupational psychiatry" is preferred to "industrial psychiatry" because the latter suggests restriction to jobs in profit-making industries.

Meaning of Work

To the professional, work may well have a meaning different from its meaning to an industrial employee at a fixed station on an assembly line. However, each has a common denominator: change. Much of this change stems from the fact that the work force in Western society is both better educated and more affluent than prior generations. Workers generally realize that society will not let them starve.

The values and ethics of youth in American society have now graduated to the work force, and younger workers are bringing new perspectives. In routine assignments, they have had considerable difficulty in adjusting and have been restless, mobile, changeable, and demand-ing. In the automobile industry, one third of the employees are 30 or younger. Absenteeism has doubled in the past decade. In 1970, there was an absentee rate of 5 per cent midweek and 10 per cent on Mondays and Fridays.

The lack of involvement at work is a major contributing factor to absenteeism and poor work performance. Programs that stimulate employee involvement in the definition and activities of their own work not only enhance job satisfaction and mental health variables, but also stimulate greater productivity. Similarly, work frustrations, job alienation, boredom, and monotony have an adverse impact on employee health, reduce productivity, and have an adverse impact on major satisfaction.

Psychodynamic Concepts

Three major threats to the balance of one's psychological equilibrium are related to occupational stress: the threat of losing control of oneself, a threat to the superego, and the threat of personal physical harm. Fear becomes a problem only when it is prolonged and one cannot escape the threat or when it is irrational. Psychological stress may be defined as the activation of any of these threats, and there is a wide variation in each person's vulnerability. Although some events and circumstances threaten everyone, each person has emotional conflicts, the triggering of which by an environmental event can produce overwhelming anxiety.

There is also a common denominator to most occupational stress from the psychodynamic viewpoint, and that common denominator is change. All change involves loss of some kind—familiar faces, places, pleasures, ways of doing things, or organizational supports. Promotions, demotions, and transfers, however desired, are changes. Change is a threat to the ways people have developed to handle their dependency needs.

Role of the Psychiatrist

The psychiatrist in a work organization spends time with individual employees referred to him by management, by physicians in the medical department, and by members of the personnel department. Many employees that a psychiatrist sees clinically are considered mentally healthy; others are either dissatisfied with their work or angry with their supervisors. Still others may be unhappy at home, disturbed by financial insecurity, or frustrated in the achievement of specific goals. A substantial number have well-established patterns of personality disorder. Some have reacted to trigger situations with emotional and behavioral reactions on the job. Relatively few have major, incapacitating mental disorders.

A substantial number of patients receive definitive therapeutic care. Usually, a patient is seen earlier in the course of his disorder than he might be by a psychiatrist in a different setting. For this reason and because many patients are less seriously disturbed than are those seen in psychiatric settings, therapy is relatively brief.

The psychiatrist is often asked to assist in evaluating prospective employees during preplacement medical examinations. Such a consultation is likely to take place when a job applicant presents a history of serious psychiatric disorder or when the examining physician raises questions about his ability to adapt to the specific assignment in question. Such examination should not be conducted with a view toward excluding an applicant from employment. Rather, the person-environment fit is the question.

The consultant may be called on when the patient is returning to work after having been hospitalized for a mental illness. The questions should relate to how the work environment can be most supportive to assist in rehabilitation.

Occasionally, the psychiatrist helps to arrange for the hospitalization of an employee. When a worker is away from the job because of psychiatric illness, the consultant often maintains contact with his physician, monitoring progress and interpreting medical status to the employer.

Perhaps the most important clinical role is behind-the-scenes work with other physicians and with those in the management hierarchy. The psychiatrist helps them understand and cope with deviant behavior.

The psychiatrist teaches the management of work organizations at all levels. Such education is often aimed at early case finding and may include discussion of the early signs and symptoms of emotional disturbance. Generally in seminar form, the discussions are directed toward increased understanding of the meaning of various patterns of behavior.

Mental health education can easily include informal periodic discussions with small groups of executives. These sessions often help management understand the role that feelings play in decision making. The discussions also further understanding of reactions to stressors at home and at work. The sessions often increase sensitivity to interpersonal and intrapersonal issues involved in the operation of a work organization.

Another aspect of mental health education for administrators includes individual consultation with psychiatrists concerning their own personal reactions to their life situations. Supportive therapy at times of career changes is often of particular value. Promotion, demotion, and job transfer are often threatening and difficult to accept.

The consultant may be called on for comments concerning the human factor in accident prevention, the evolution of personnel policies, and potential changes in benefit plans. Psychiatrists also identify characteristics in the work environment that adversely influence or support healthy behavior.

REFERENCES

Cobb, S. Role responsibility: The differentiation of a concept. Occup. Ment. Health, 3: 1973.

Collins, R. T. *Occupational Psychiatry*. Little, Brown, Boston, 1969.

French, J. R. P. Person role fit. Occup. Ment. Health, 3: 15, 1973.

Group for the Advancement of Psychiatry. *The Application of Psychiatry to Industry*. Group for the Advancement of Psychiatry, New York, 1951.

Kahn, R. L. Conflict, ambiguity, and overload: Three elements in job stress. Occup. Ment. Health, 3: Spring, 1973.

Levi, L. *Society, Stress, and Disease*. Oxford University Press, London, 1972.

1190   Occupational Psychiatry

Levinson, H. A psychoanalytic view of occupational stress. Occup. Ment. Health, *3*: 2, 1973.

McLean, A., editor. *Mental Health and Work Organizations.* Rand McNally, Chicago, 1970.

McLean, A., editor. *Occupational Stress.* Charles C Thomas, Springfield, Ill., 1974.

McLean, A., Dunnington, R. A., and McLean, V. *Selected Bibliography on Occupational Mental Health.* National Institutes of Health, Bethesda, 1965.

Schon, D. A. *Beyond the Stable State.* Random House, New York, 1972.

Schwarz, D. R. Health status assessment: An untapped source of management information. In *Occupational Stress,* A. McLean, editor. Charles C Thomas, Springfield, Ill., 1974.

Taylor, J. C., Landy, J., Levine, M., and Kanath, D. R. *The Quality of Working Life: An Annotated Bibliography 1957 to 1972.* University of California Press, Los Angeles, 1973.

United States Department of Health, Education, and Welfare. *Work in America.* MIT Press, Cambridge, 1973.

45

Clinical Psychology

Introduction

Clinical psychology is directed toward helping persons with behavior disabilities or mental disorders achieve more satisfactory personal adjustment and self-expression. It borders on biology and on sociology. Clinical psychology encompasses large portions of psychopathology, abnormal psychology, and similar areas. It is particularly dependent on personality theory and psychoanalysis for its theoretical underpinnings.

Scope

The activities of clinical psychologists include work in child guidance agencies, psychiatric hospitals, mental hygiene clinics, vocational guidance centers, school systems, student personnel services, prisons, schools for delinquents, general hospitals, neurological and other hospitals for specialized diseases, nursery schools, casework agencies, schools for the handicapped, and a variety of community agencies working with the alcoholic, the aged, the deprived, and other groups.

In a team of psychiatrist, social worker, and psychologist, the clinical psychologist usually contributes the psychological data from psychological tests and situational studies. Problems of intellectual status, developmental stages, special abilities, and defects are usually the concern of the psychologist.

Training

The generally accepted pattern of training of the clinical psychologist is essentially some form of the scientist-professional model proposed in the 1947 report of the Committee on Training in Clinical Psychology of the American Psychological Association. The pattern emphasizes the development of existing university departments as central clinical training centers and encourages the integration of field training centers into the university programs.

The 4-year course of training, which leads to a doctoral degree, is ordinarily followed by 5 years of experience, at least half of which is spent in a recognized field training center. After going through such a program, the candidate is eligible for the examinations of the American Board in Professional Psychology, which issues a diploma of specialization in clinical psychology. After 2 years of postdoctoral experience, he may also be certified in his state.

Diagnostic Procedures

The psychologist depends to some extent on clinical observation, but he places major dependence on testing procedures. To make the tests informative and dependable, three types of controls are set up: pre-examination controls, examination controls, and postexamination controls. These controls are set up to reduce the amount of dependence placed on the observer.

The pre-examination controls involve the standardization of tests with respect to content and method. Controls during the examination are concerned with the determination of where the patient's present performance places him in relation to his own potential present performance and to his underlying capacity. Postexamination controls deal with the problem of norms, relating the performance of the patient to that of other persons in a particular group.

Tests are designed not only to study different functions but also to study various groups of persons. These may include persons in different age ranges; groups of persons with different kinds of handicaps, such as deafness, blindness, psychosis, and neurosis; groups that have special vocational aptitudes or characteristics. Some tests are intended for persons at a high level of functioning, some for persons at a low level. Some tests use language as a means of communication, others deliberately avoid the use of language—using, instead, other symbols of performance. Some tests attempt to get at underlying capacity; others are primarily devoted to a study of nonintellectual or affective aspects. Some are intended for individual administrations, others for groups.

Psychomotor tests generally deal with simple functions, such as steadiness, speed of tapping, and reaction time. Ordinarily, tests of this kind are seldom used in the clinical psychiatric setting except when organic functions appear to be affected or for specific research purposes.

Intelligence tests are the most highly developed tests. There are two major types of intelligence tests: those dealing with composite aspects of intelligence and those dealing primarily with single aspects of intelligence, such as thinking and memory.

Personality tests are mainly of two types: questionnaire and projective. The projective tests are among the most important devices available and have achieved a prominent place among the test batteries used in clinical settings.

Tests of special aptitudes attempt to discover underlying aptitudes for such special fields as art, music, mechanics, medicine, law, and aviation. The test items are based on an analysis of the major functions and skills necessary for the achievement of particular vocational and avocational goals. In the clinical setting, these tests are only moderately important.

Establishing a unified psychological portrait of the patient is best done with a battery of tests. The selection and the administration of a test battery involve sampling (1) in different areas, (2) for content and formal aspects, (3) by overlapping devices, and (4) under conditions of stress as well as under ordinary examination conditions.

Research

The methods of investigation used by the psychologist are not essentially different from those generally used in biology. These methods may be roughly classified as naturalistic observations, seminaturalistic observation, free laboratory, and controlled laboratory.

Naturalistic observation provides for the study of the organism in a relatively free natural habitat in which the widest range of stimuli and responses growing out of the particular setting is observed.

Seminaturalistic observation may be provided for by a natural habitat or by a laboratory situation. In either case the stimuli are varied, and the degrees of freedom of response permitted are considerable. However, some controls and limitations on the situation are set up to direct behavior along certain lines.

In a free laboratory some degree of variation in the stimuli and some degree of freedom of response are maintained but are considerably reduced as compared with the former two methods. Here, the subject is specifically instructed to respond in certain definite ways to the stimuli.

A controlled laboratory carries the degree of control of the situation still further. Here both the stimulus and the response are quite fixed and limited.

The psychologist can also conduct objective studies in the evaluation of the effects of therapies or other observable modifications of behavior. However, the activity of the psychologist should mainly be the exploration of the fundamental aspects of personality, with a view toward developing comprehensive theories of personality.

Therapy

The years have seen a marked change in the formal attitudes taken toward the practice of therapy by psychologists. Many formal reports accept this change in attitude. More important has been the increasing training obtained by psychologists and the competence they have achieved in forms of psychotherapy, ranging from psychoanalysis through nondirective psychotherapy to behavior modification.

Present Picture

Since 1948, the growth of clinical psychology in the United States has been phenomenal. Membership in the division of clinical psychology of the American Psychological Association has increased from 787 in 1948 to more than

3,800 in 1973. The number of schools fully approved by the committee on accreditation of the American Psychological Association has increased from 20 in 1948 to 86 in 1973. An estimated 740 graduate students were enrolled in doctoral training in clinical psychology programs in the academic year 1947–1948, compared with some 5,000 students in 1973. There were 112 fully approved doctoral internship centers in 1973, compared with 27 in 1956. The number of clinical psychologists certified by the American Board of Examiners in Professional Psychology has increased from 234 in 1948 to 1,559 in 1973. At present, 47 states and 6 provinces in Canada have established some form of statutory control—either licensing or certification. Increasing interest is being shown in systematic postdoctoral training.

REFERENCES

American Psychological Association. Report of the Committee on Training in Clinical Psychology, D. Shakow, chairman. Recommended graduate training program in clinical psychology. Am. Psychol., 2: 539, 1947.

Hoch, E. L., Ross, A. O., and Winder, C. L. *Professional Preparation of Clinical Psychologists.* American Psychological Association, Washington, 1966.

Holt, R. R., editor. *New Horizon for Psychotherapy.* International Universities Press, New York, 1971.

Rapaport, D., Gill, M. M., and Shafer, R. *Diagnostic Psychological Testing,* ed. 2, R. R. Holt. ed. International Universities Press, New York, 1968.

Rosenzweig, S. *Psychodiagnosis.* Grune & Stratton, New York, 1949.

Smith, S., and Weiner, I. B. Proceedings of the Menninger Conference on Postdoctoral Education in Clinical Psychology. Monograph No. 17. Menninger Foundation, Topeka, 1973.

Steiner, G. L., and Roth, L. *The Revolution in Professional Training,* ed. 2. National Council on Graduate Education in Psychology, Newark, N. J., 1972–1973.

Weiner, I. B. *Psychodiagnosis in Schizophrenia.* Wiley, New York, 1966.

46

Psychiatric Nursing

Scope and Setting

A 1966 American Nurses Association inventory documented nearly 600,000 actively employed registered nurses. Only 4.5 per cent of these nurses were working in psychiatric-mental health nursing. Of the 26,830 registered nurses in psychiatric-mental health nursing, the majority (88 per cent) were employed by hospitals or other institutions; 5 per cent were employed by schools of nursing, and the remaining 7 per cent were evenly distributed among private-duty nursing, public health agencies, school nursing, industrial settings, and office nursing.

Generalist Nurses

The majority of nurses who work in psychiatric settings are generalists—that is, they have acquired a general undergraduate education in nursing and are licensed to practice as registered nurses. All nursing programs include a course in psychiatric nursing. This introductory course generally includes experience in nursing mentally ill patients in institutional settings, theoretical material on psychiatric diagnostic categories, dynamics of behavior, and principles of therapeutic nursing care. More innovative programs include experience in community mental health settings, work with members of the families of psychiatric patients, and the preventive aspects of mental illness.

In addition most undergraduate programs integrate psychiatric-mental health concepts throughout the student's experiences in school. Seminars on the psychological aspects of disability and disfigurement, care of the dying patient, and psychological responses in medical emergencies are common.

A central role of a generalist nurse in a psychiatric setting is management of the patient's environment. The nurse often has the opportunity to intervene on the spot in behavior that, if ignored or allowed to continue, would perpetuate the patient's pathological condition.

A second major role of the generalist nurse is to carry out brief counseling with patients and families. Such counseling may be formally structured or may take place in informal situations. Usually, the focus of such counseling is on the current life situation of the patient, with an effort being made to help the patient and his family arrive at more viable solutions to their problems. An important feature of the counseling role is to help patients communicate more clearly.

Technical aspects of patient care represent a third major role of the generalist nurse. She manages the distribution of medications, carries out medical treatments, and assists with somatic therapies. Observations regarding the effects of medications and other somatic treatments are reported, and she may recommend changes in treatment plans to the medical team. Another important aspect of her role is the assessment of the patient's physical status.

Assisting patients with many of the activities of daily living is often reminiscent of early mothering experiences. Exploiting this relationship to the fullest can result in considerable therapeutic benefit to the patient.

Health teaching is another important role. The nurse helps patients learn to use the principles of physical and mental hygiene. She instructs patients and their families about drug therapy and answers questions they may have regarding other aspects of psychiatric care.

Clinical Specialists

Education for specialization is at the master's degree level in a program that is usually 1½ to 2 years in length. Most of these programs prepare graduates to work with a variety of psychiatric problems in hospitals, community mental health centers, clinics, schools, and homes. A few programs offer specialization in the psychiatric nursing of children or community mental health nursing.

Preparation by graduate education or comparable supervised experience enables a specialized nurse to engage in psychotherapy of individual patients, groups, and families. The nature of the psychotherapy practiced by nurses varies, depending on the clinical problem, the role of other therapists in the case, the extent of her skill in conducting therapy, and the availability of competent consultation. The development of communication skills and the exploration of interpersonal relationships are emphasized. Techniques have been developed to interrupt and deal with hallucinations, delusions, and suspiciousness. Ways to intervene in high levels of anxiety, aggression, and overdependency have been formulated. The goal of such nursing intervention is usually directed toward behavior change sufficient to permit the patient's return to the community.

Psychiatric nurses now conduct their own groups or serve as co-therapists in mental hospitals, clinics, day care centers, detention homes, prisons, and community centers. Nurses also conduct family therapy in a cotherapist situation or alone.

Nursing's role in crisis intervention and suicide prevention has been expanded with the development of community mental health services. The use of behavior modification is another major development in the role of the clinical specialist in psychiatric nursing.

The shortage of psychiatric nurses requires that an important part of the clinical specialist's role be devoted to supervision, consultation, and education of others who give direct care. The clinical specialist may function as an administrator, a clinical supervisor, or an educator of other nurses and of nonprofessional personnel.

Clinical specialists in psychiatric nursing may conduct clinical studies as the principal investigator or participate as a member of a research team.

REFERENCES

American Nurses Association. *Facts About Nursing: 1970–71 Edition*. American Nurses Association, New York, 1972.

Aquilera, D. C., Messick, J. M., and Farell, M. S. *Crisis Intervention: Theory and Methodology*. C. V. Mosby, St. Louis, 1970.

Bermosk, L. S.. and Morden, M. J. *Interviewing in Nursing*. Macmillan, New York, 1964.

Deloughery, G. W., Gebbie, K. M., and Neuman, B. M. *Community Mental Health Nursing*. Williams & Wilkins, Baltimore, 1971.

Holmes, M. J., and Werner, J. A. *Psychiatric Nursing in a Therapeutic Community*. Macmillan, New York, 1966.

Mereness, D. *Psychiatric Nursing*, 2 vols. Brown, Dubuque, Iowa, 1966.

47

The Middle-Aged

Introduction

The terms "middle age" and "middle life" do not denote precisely specific years. Rather, these terms refer to a process during the middle part of the life span that includes growth and development as well as aging and decline.

Conventionally, ages 40 to 60 or 65 have been considered the middle years. From a strictly chronological point of view, ages 24 to 48 would be the middle years of life. Unlike early child development, this period of life is delineated by no precise physiological phenomena. It has even been argued that the menopause or change of life in women is a disease process rather than a natural middle-aged phenomenon. The definition of middle age must, therefore, be approached from psychosocial and psychodynamic perspectives.

Stage Theories and Psychosocial Crises

Stage theories of development connote a progressive sequence of qualitative changes in either structure or function. Freud's and Abraham's psychosexual, Erikson's psychosocial, and Piaget's cognitive schedules of development are the classic formulations, focusing primarily on child development. Concepts of stage theory are questionable, implying such assumptions as a necessary sequence, universality, and purpose. Middle age is not uniformly characterized by illness, widowhood, empty nests, and becoming a grandparent. Stage theory is most useful in childhood and perhaps has its greatest validity there.

Closely identified with stage theory is the term "crisis," indicating a decisive turning point, the course of which can be toward improvement or deterioration. To students of human development, a crisis provides the possibility for growth as well as for illness.

Six psychological aspects of the life cycle are: (1) the awareness of death, (2) the sense of the life cycle as an unfolding process of change, (3) the sense of human time as distinguished from scientific or objective time, (4) the sense of life experience with broadening perspective, (5) knowledge of age- or time-linked changes, and (6) the idea of sequence or phases or stages. In addition to the subjective sense of the life cycle, there is the actuality of the usual course of the life cycle.

America is middle-age-oriented, in spite of the fact that it is often described as a youth- and child-oriented culture. Much lip service is given to children and young people, but American systems of care, education, and services for them are inadequate and fragmented.

The middle-aged may be looked on as upstarts, incompetents, and usurpers by the old and as objects of rebellion by the young. To the young, the middle-aged are the Establishment, the nay sayers, the rigid protectors of the status quo. The center of political and social power resides in the middle, so it is not surprising that both the young and the old, regarding themselves as out-groups, tend to bear common causes.

Elements of Middle Life

Bodily Changes

Although no precise, identifiable physical changes typify middle age, general trends do occur. The most distinctive feature is the experiencing of various intimations of mortality. Those portents may take the form of increasing development of chronic illnesses, routine medical checkups, an increased reaction time to stimuli, presbycusis, a decreased sense of energy and vigor. People may contribute to a sense of stagnation by their own failure to take good care of their bodies through exercise, relaxation, nutrition, and health care. Men in particular, may first notice bodily declines by way of reduced sexual ability.

Physical changes, even if not directly impairing, may create a variety of psychological and emotional reactions—fear, anxiety, grief, depression, anger. Certain stress illnesses, such as stress polycythemia, commonly occur. Other diseases of diverse origin begin to emerge in the middle years—for instance, pernicious anemia. Twenty-eight million (72 per cent) of those from 45 to 64 are estimated to have one or more chronic conditions.

Women usually experience the menopause between 40 and 50 years of age, averaging 48 to 50. Whether menopause is an ovarian failure due to disease or a natural phenomenon is a matter of some dispute. But the fact of estrogen deficiency and hormonal imbalance is clear. The autonomic nervous system is affected; there is vasomotor instability. Some physicians feel that women should be kept on estrogen more or less continuously all their lives. Men show no decisive evidence of a male equivalent of the climacterium.

Economic Aspects

The middle-aged face extraordinary financial burdens. Middle-aged workers have serious problems with employment. If they are once unemployed, they are unemployed longer than younger people are, get jobs at less pay, and are admitted less frequently to retraining programs.

The middle-aged may be burnt out or bored with their jobs but find themselves trapped. They want to develop new or second careers but have no personal or social sanctions and finances to do so. Moreover, they have collected material possessions that they feel obligated to maintain. They begin to feel that everyone is depending on them for money.

Many middle-aged persons begin to see that they have been living under a dangerous illusion that their Social Security, private pensions, savings, and investments will provide them a decent, secure old age. Neither existent government programs nor personal providence guarantee this. Thus, the middle-aged feel pressure not only by the need to care for their older and younger family members but also by the need to accumulate funds for their own needs in old age.

Social Roles

Social roles tend to become rigidly established. There are fewer options, perhaps none at all, because of responsibilities. There is less freedom in jobs, education, housing location and style, and travel. Roles in the family as parents and as children, in the community, and to one's friends, church, and nation are fairly well demarcated. One's conduct and step-by-step progress in these roles lead to influence and power and to the possibility of entrapment in pursuit of these goals. White men are especially locked into the career ladder, the fulfillment of ambitions. However, it is in the intrapsychic and psychosocial areas that the middle-aged person becomes most profoundly stuck.

Psychological Aspects

A number of critical underlying themes in the middle years appear to be present regardless of marital and family status, gender, or economic level. They are listed in Table I. It is believed that they occur whether or not an external stimulus or crisis is present. However, the means of coping and the kinds of reactions vary.

Middle age has been called the prime of life, the time in most societies when the person attains the height of his power, personal accomplishment, social affiliation, citizenship, and physical maturity. The image of middle life as the prime of life helps offset its negative stereotype of decline. When the achievement of the middle-aged person is essentially in accord with early promise and ambition, it is a period of positive self-confidence, pleasure, and fulfillment. It may also mark an affirmative change in direction.

In old age the autobiographical process appears to manifest itself as a life review, but in middle age it has the quality of stocktaking, giving the opportunity to consider possibilities for alternatives in commitments. The central, profound question is what to do with the rest of one's life. At one extreme, one may close down all possibilities and develop a sense of fatalism; at the other extreme, one may become overex-

TABLE I

Features Salient to Middle Life

Issues	Positive Pole	Negative Pole
Prime of life	Responsible use of power; maturity; productivity	Winner-loser view; competitiveness
Stocktaking	Possibility; alternatives; organization of commitments; redirection	Closure; fatalism
Fidelity	Commitment to self, others, career, society; filial maturity	Hypocrisy; self-deception
Growth-death (to grow is to die); juvenescence and rejuvenation fantasies	Naturality regarding body, time	Obscene or frenetic efforts to be youthful; hostility and envy of youth and progeny; longing
Credulity	Ego beliefs; profound realistic convictions	True believers of the right (past) or left (future); radicalism
Simplification, conservation, and settling-in of persons, time, and places	Centrality, specification, and rootedness of relationships, places, and ideas	Diffusion; confusion; rigidity
Communication complexity (cues)	Abbreviation; matters understood; continuity; picking up where left off	Repetitiveness; boredom; impatience

pansive, as revealed in helter-skelter confusion and disorganization. The erosion of individual omnipotence is necessary to a realistic assessment of the remainder of one's life.

Fidelity is another critical issue. Faithfulness to obligations and observances and loyalty to friends, spouse, and institutions cannot be taken for granted as set for life. Fidelity is an active process, referring to the conscious and unconscious testing of personal, professional, and other commitments. Revisions and entirely new commitments may follow, or old commitments may be more firmly established. The character of the obligation to friend, spouse, or social institution is evaluated, too. The middle-aged person who is not openly concerned with his hypocrisy is in trouble. He is caught in self-deception, and true commitment becomes impossible.

Portents of mortality are ubiquitous. Some people respond naturally and calmly to the reality of the common processes of growing old, auguring disabilities and dying and death. Thoughts of death can be the motivation for constructive change. On the other hand, there may be fantasies of juvenescence and rejuvenation or frenetic and sometimes obscene efforts to be youthful. There may be excessive efforts to

prove one's continuing youth, strength, and virility through activities of possible physical danger to oneself. There may be great hostility toward and envy of youth and one's own progeny. There may be a longing, a nostalgia.

Throughout life one is developing a value system that may be of sufficient depth to warrant the phrase ego beliefs or deep convictions. When this is the case, they are based on profound, realistic evaluation and adoption of an appropriate ethical system that is ego-syntonic and not ego-alien. But one may see extremes—for example, true believers on the right or the left.

Middle age is the period when one frequently feels overwhelmed by stimuli and too many obligations and duties. Often there is an essential joylessness about the middle years. With this comes a kind of weariness, even in success, about doing the same thing over and over again. Feelings of being submerged and engulfed in seemingly insignificant and trivial happenings and structures lead to fatigue and a search for simplicity, for more central roots, and for a conservation of oneself, rather than further diffusion and confusion.

Similarly, there may be a great desire to streamline one's communications. One may cultivate those relationships in which matters are simply understood, in which one can pick up where one left off with old friends, maintaining a kind of continuity. It is possible to do so through the richness of cues. Abbreviations of manner and verbal communication are not as possible with new or younger acquaintances when there is no shared history. On the negative side of the continuum, there are possibilities of repetitiveness, boredom, and impatience.

Men and Women

Only since 1950 have women survived men in the United States. In 1950 there were 99.8 women for every 100 men in the age group 45 to 64. By 1970 there were 109.1 women for every 100 men in that age group. Of 41.8 million persons from 45 to 64 years old, 21.8 million were women, and 20 million were men. This reversal has followed from reduced maternal mortality and reflief from stenuous agricultural labor. Widowhood among women progresses with age at the rate of about 10 per cent a decade. Since women tend to marry older men, in addition to having longer life spans, there are more and more widows beginning in the middle years. For a variety of reasons, from reduced job opportunities to spiraling inflation, destitution joins loneliness in typifying the life of the older woman.

The middle age of men and of women seems to occur at different times. Women experience middle age earlier than men, somewhere at a point when they pass beyond the child-bearing age, whether childless or not, and when the children, if any, leave home. In the case of mothers, they no longer have the responsibilities of parenthood but are now faced with the results of their parental careers. Men, on the other hand, in their work careers tend to experience the issue of success or failure somewhat later.

Middle-class fathers have often abdicated the traditional patriarchal role, which expected responsibility in children and maintained psychological distance from them. The father is simply a regular guy and not a figure of authority. Furthermore, the father is usually interpreted to the child by the mother. When divorce occurs, the father may be still further isolated from his children. The results have been to give children weak models and less self-responsibility.

Until the late 1960's mothers invested themselves in the traditional roles of housewife and mother. These roles are now undergoing re-evaluation and change. Many women are returning to work or are going to work for the first time in middle age. When women achieve equal job opportunities and promotions, they may be subjected to the same stresses as men. There is also the possibility that with equalization between the sexes there will be less pressure on both.

Strong investment in one's physical appearance and functioning are typical of both sexes, spurred on by a culture that admires youth and disparages age. Men fear losing their muscles and hair, women their youthful faces and figures; they associate these losses with sexual unattractiveness and social unacceptability. Both sexes need to develop a variety of satisfactions and skills that are not dependent on an unrealistic attempt to outwit the normal aging process. In women, the menopause has been blamed for a host of ills, both physical and emotional.

Emotional Difficulties and Mental Illness

Episodes of anxiety and depression are omnipresent. Anxiety is customarily connected with threats to one's personal, physical, and social integrity; when threats occur, the resulting anxiety may lead to overreactions, from hypochondria to dogmatism to counterphobia. Depression, on the other hand, follows losses, which can begin to occur with benumbing frequency in the middle years. Losses, like anxiety, may be met with excessive reactions, severe depression, or, less frequently, paranoid projection, replacing the more healthful grieving.

Morbidity and mortality may increase among survivors of a marital union broken by death. Survivors are frequently left guilt-ridden and despairing by the unexpected early deaths of their spouses.

A series of disappointments, worry, and increasing pressure can combine to produce serious mental symptoms. Some persons feel that they have missed out on opportunities or are out of step with what is considered normal.

Grief is a frequent and necessary accompaniment of the middle years. Only after effective grief-work can efforts at restitution begin—to make new beginnings in one's work, to reassay goals, to replace lost loved ones, to experience new facts of personality.

Certain reactions—denial, projection, counterphobia, rigidity—appear to be common in middle life. But these means of avoiding a threat or loss are not satisfactorily protective in helping the person adjust.

With the awareness of bodily changes—whether periodontal disease, rheumatic pains, necessary changes of glasses, decline in hearing, wrinkles, gray hair, or balding—the middle-aged person begins to notice his body more and to monitor its changes. He may practice denial, may take reasonable steps for routine physical checkups, or may become excessively preoccupied with health to the point of hypochondria. Psychosomatic illnesses are common. Oral dependency—obesity, alcoholism, drug misuse and overuse—is frequent.

Some middle-aged women and men seek young lovers, disparage their professions, attack their spouses and the institution of marriage. Some simply drop out. These people are frightened and bored. They feel trapped or imprisoned. They are testing. Middle-life delinquency is one result.

The problems of marriage and divorce are myriad. People often grow, develop, and change at different rates. One spouse may discover that the other is not the same person as when they first married. In truth, both partners have changed and evolved—not necessarily in complementary directions. Certain aspects of marital deterioration and divorce seem related to specific qualities of middle life—the need for change, the weariness with acting responsibly, the fear of facing up to oneself. Some men and women seek a last fling or a last chance to experience something they feel they have missed.

Sexuality in general is a major issue in midlife. Fears and the reality of impotence are a common problem in the middle-age man. The commonest cause of impotence in the middle years is not aging but excessive alcoholic intake, drugs, and stress with fatigue and anxiety; 90 per cent of the cases of chronic impotence are due to psychological rather than organic causes.

Insomnia is often a serious problem in the middle years. Anxiety, guilt, and anger may impair the ability to go to sleep, and depression may cause early awakening. Insomnia and depression may be seen in the hard-striving persons most subject to middle-life depressions.

Psychopathology of all kinds rises with age in both sexes. Depression steadily ascends in incidence. Presenile conditions may emerge in the fifties and leave the patient and his family devastated. Suicide peaks in the 35-to-64 age group in women and the nonwhite population. With white men, suicide rises with age and attains its peak in the 85-plus group. Paranoid states and various forms of depression are common in middle life.

The mental illnesses likely to occur in the middle-aged person are the presenile psychoses, alcoholism, drug addiction, schizophrenic reactions, paranoid states, and depressions, notably including the manic-depressive reaction, especially the depressed type. Involutional depression occurs only in the middle-aged person. This agitated type of depression occurs in a person who has the premorbid personality characteristics of the compulsive or obsessive type—perfectionism, overconscientiousness, and penuriousness.

Therapy

The prospect of therapy in middle age is based on the possibility for change (see Table II). Psychotherapy need be no different for the middle-aged patient than for the patient of any other age. But specific elements in the therapy of the middle-aged derive from the psychosocial and psychodynamic nature of middle life. It is necessary to separate age-specific problems

TABLE II
Elements in the Therapy of the Middle-Aged

Capacity for change
Primary prevention
Maintenance of physical and mental health
Public service and usefulness
Loosening up life
Stocktaking and inventory—pilgrimage, confrontation
Retraining and new careers
Self-help organizations
Traditional individual, group, and family therapies
Marital and sex counseling
Treatment of specific conditions common in the middle-aged, such as the menopause, impotence, insomnia
Broad changes in social policy

from personality problems. In the most general sense, the psychotherapy of the middle-aged is the psychotherapy of re-evaluation (stocktaking and testing of commitments) and possible redirection. The goal of therapy is to bring to consciousness an accurate appraisal of one's self in order to be in a position to elect changes or to stay essentially on course. Typically, there is a desire for selective change.

Classic psychoanalysis should not be ruled out because of middle age. An individual psychotherapeutic program may vary from once weekly up to the frequency of classic psychoanalysis. Support to insight may be in order. Antidepressants and tranquilizers should be used judiciously, if at all, as components in a general treatment plan and as adjuncts to aid healthy persons in periods of stress, not as substitutes for full-scale evaluation or therapy. Family therapy may help in both the evaluation and the process of change and redirection. Group therapy may be particularly useful. Middle-aged people gain a great deal from working in groups composed of different age levels, diverse personality styles, and varied diagnoses.

Mental well-being is closely tied to physical well-being. Any improvement that can be made in the physical condition of the middle-aged patient is helpful. There must be routine periodic checkups, but care must be exercised to avoid iatrogenic hypochondria. Since some of the manifestations of problematic middle age are obesity, drug dependence-addiction, and alcoholism, habit reformation and nutrition must be part of the psychotherapist's program. Working through oral, dependent needs and conflicts is a cornerstone in therapy.

There should be help in the area of sexual difficulties. It is well accepted that sex problems are a critical factor in marital difficulties. There must be work on the development of mutuality and intimacy but also direct work along the behavioral lines of Masters and Johnson. Drug programs must be carefully evaluated with regard to their impact on sexuality.

Relaxation, although difficult for the stressed factory worker and executive alike, should be associated with active participation as well as passive, receptive leisure. The active and passive appreciation of music and the arts are important parts of life and of any therapeutic program.

Insomnia can often be relieved through simple measures, such as relaxation and exercise. A careful, well-established ritual at bedtime can be helpful, including at times a warm tub bath. Sedatives and hypnotics should be left as last resorts, using first a modest amount of wine or warm milk.

Public service helps prepare one for later life and prevents stagnation. Travel is a valuable prescription. Joining certain self-help groups can be important. Women may find it constructive to join women's consciousness-raising sessions because of the special nature of middle age for women. Religious counseling may be useful to the middle-aged.

Therapy in middle age is not only a therapy of inventory and redirection; it is also a therapy dealing with grief and restitution. There is impairment or loss of one's body parts and functions. It is necessary to raise the person's awareness of age changes and to help develop a vigorous acceptance, rather than resignation or a counterphobic reaction. An activist style includes undertaking modifications in attitudes and behavior. Successful psychoanalysis at any age depends on coming to some realistic resolution of the reality of one's own death.

Social Policies

The therapist's efforts to effect many therapeutic suggestions would be helped by pertinent changes in social policy (see Table III). The pressure and the tempo of the culture need to become more relaxed and flexible. Continually available education, opportunities to switch careers, the end of age discrimination in em-

TABLE III
Social Policies for the Middle Years

Take pressure off the middle-aged; change in the cultural tempo
Reorganization of education, work, retirement, and leisure
Enforcement of the Age Discrimination in Employment Act
Diversified income maintenance in old age
Seniority and tenure reform
Day care for children and old people
Life cycle education
Health education in menopause; diet; exercise; illness
Divorce insurance

ployment, and portable retirement pensions would ensure that one is not trapped in a job one can no longer tolerate. There should be reforms in contemporary seniority and tenure systems.

Education, work, and leisure-retirement might be interwoven throughout the course of life. The same amount of support money for education on the one hand and retirement pensions on the other hand could be reallocated to make available continuing education and scattered retirement.

There should be a restyling of income maintenance in old age to mitigate the fears of an insecure old age. Expansion of Social Security to finance divorce has been suggested, as has private divorce insurance. The provision of day care centers for old people, as well as for children, would give greater freedom to the middle-aged. There should be massive public educational programs to reform diet, reduce alcoholism and tobacco usage, and encourage physical fitness.

Education beginning in grammar school could help prepare people to enjoy leisure. The so-called minor subjects of music, physical education, and the arts might well be major subjects. Throughout life there should be life-cycle education.

REFERENCES

Buhler, C. The course of human life as a psychological problem. Human Dev., *2*: 184, 1968.

Butler, R. N., and Lewis, M. I. *Aging and Mental Health: Positive Psychosocial Approaches*. C. V. Mosby, St. Louis, 1973.

Erikson, E. H. Identity and the life cycle, in *Selected Papers*. International Universities Press, New York, 1959.

Levinson, D. J., Darrow, C. M., Klein, E. B., Levinson, M. H., and McKee, B. The psychosocial development of men in early adulthood and the mid-life transition. In *Life History Research in Psychopathology*, vol. 3, D. F. Ricks, A. Thomas, and M. Roff, editors, p. 117. University of Minnesota Press, Minneapolis, 1974.

Lowenthal, M. F., and Chiraboga, D. Transition to the empty nest. Arch. Gen. Psychiatry, *26*: 8, 1972.

Neugarten, B. L., editor, *Middle Age and Aging: A reader in Social Psychology*. University of Chicago Press, Chicago, 1968.

48

Geriatric Psychiatry

Introduction

Old age in itself is not a disease. Geriatric psychiatry deals with the psychopathology attending that period of life that is an end product of an ongoing process. Old age may be considered as yet another of the developmental phases in the life span, developmental in the sense that it is not static, and the defensive responses to the deficits, physical and psychosocial, may be both old and new. Every phase in the human life cycle has specific traumatic elements that are germane and unique to that paticular age group. The same is true of the aged, who have, however, throughout their life accumulated multiple scarring through their exposure to all the sources of human suffering.

Social pressure and inadequate resources create many of the dysfunctional features of old age.

Special Problems

Self-Imagery

The development of a self-image is a dual process, dependent on a mechanism deeply ingrained in one's intrapersonal forces that molds the preception of the self and on one's circumambience—social, psychological, and cultural—that helps shape, polish, constrain, and modify the percept of the self. In most if not all people, the concept of the self as a dynamic force interacting with the environment is more often than not tinged with wish, rather than reality. Thus, the concept of the self is distorted and obscured.

The tragedy of late life is that the legend is running out, and the forces marshaled against the maintenance of an assured image are numerous and often compelling.

Transition

The transition from a well-stabilized psychological maturity of the personality to one of decline starts at various ages, and, although it may have its basis in physical change, it is really a psychological change. When one begins to look back at one's past with fond nostalgia and at the future with apprehension and feelings of insecurity, aging has begun. Human beings between 50 and 60 begin to think about the coming of old age. The gradual change in appearance, the graying of hair, the diminished capacity for physical work, and, above all, the feeling that one's erotic values are diminishing —all are factors in the organism's perception that a peak has been reached and that the descent has begun.

If life has been successful and there is a prospect of continued emotional, economic, and social security, one's value as a personality has not diminished, and one can still enjoy the importance that greater experience and social power bestows on one. When, later on, the impairment of sensory functions, motor performances, and memory functions becomes undeniable and a decline in creative mental capacities becomes obvious to the person himself, a rearrangement in his mental processes must take place. Some revolt by complaining protestations. Others give up completely. And then there are those who attempt to compensate in a world of fantasy.

Physical inadequacy leads to a disquieting insecurity, which is rapidly augmented by the paradox of increasing rigidity in an environment influx that demands constant readaptation. The decrease of ego efficiency in the aged almost invariably calls forth anxiety when readjustment is necessary. To avoid anxiety, the aging organism clings to the plane of adjustment already achieved, no matter how faulty. Change is regarded with suspicion and fear. Rigidity keeps the aged out of step with the ever-changing world and acts to isolate them and add to their insecurity.

Isolation and Aloneness

The term "aloneness" describes the intensely experienced inner affect related to the gradual isolation that takes place in a physical or geographical sense. Aloneness is a result of a number of factors. A real factor is the dispersal and death of friends and members of the family. Each loss necessitates a rearrangement of the equilibrium that one had set up for comfortable functioning. There is no replacement of family, and there are no bidders for the friendship of the aged.

Having no place to go, this freed energy turns inward and is either reinvested in organs or organ systems and appears in the guise of somatic complaints or is experienced as pain and ruminatory recapitulation of a past life experience. The aged then appear to be egocentric, selfish, and preoccupied with the inner rumblings of the self, further alienating others and increasing their isolation and sense of aloneness.

Nor do the losses need to be tangible objects to precipitate grief and depression. An abstraction, if endangered or lost, may be just as catastrophic. Thus, grief over real or abstract losses may be a constant companion of the aging that often takes on the appearance of depression.

Reactions to Losses

Losses may be handled by denial, overcompensatory mechanisms, or projection. Projection is most often expressed by complaints that someone is cheating or lying to them, stealing, or taking things away from them. It is a rebuke and an expression of anger at the facts that internal biological losses are being sustained, that mastery over hitherto controlled functions and impulses is threatened, and that influence over one's family and environment is waning.

Frequently, the aged begin to cling to what seem to be meaningless objects. Hoarding is common. This behavior needs to be understood in the light of ever-increasing losses. The more often the aged person loses close friends, the greater is his need to hold onto inanimate objects with which he has shared common experiences. These objects replace and are substitutes for cherished reunions and memories when very few, if any, friends are left to meet with and reminisce.

Cultural Determinants

Cultural patterns include not only moral standards and mores but also the subtle patterns of motivation and interpersonal relations. Variations in judgment and systems of belief, such as religions and philosophies, are integrated with the other cultural patterns, like child-rearing practices. The values that the child accepts, introjects, and incorporates into himself have much to do with defining his attitude toward aging people and later toward himself as an aging person. If the aged are perceived as unattractive, unproductive, old-fashioned, useless, querulous, and so on, people in their youth absorb these concepts, make them part of themselves, and apply these perceptions to themselves in later life.

Work

Work, no matter how odious an implication it may have for a person, is an enormously prized and meaningful experience to people. A job is part of the identifying data that every human being has. It enables the average person to channel his aggressive impulses into sublimated and acceptable constructive activity. Furthermore, work may supply a person with a reason for existence. Being useful to his family, community, and society and being a productive member of a group may furnish an answer to that ever-recurring question of the meaning of life. Work also enhances a person's erotic value.

Psychodynamic Aspects

Exclusion of Stimuli

The exclusion of stimuli in later life is a psychodynamic defense, an outcome or effect of a psychopathological condition. The perceptual act reflects the psychological point of contact between a person and his internal and external milieu. Its principal function is to convey information from his environment for integration with other psychological functions, such as memory, judgment, and anticipation. Obviously, it also receives and carries information about the nature and consequence of the perceiver's actions. Perception is, thus, a central ingredient in effective adaptation, in the fitting-in process between the person and his environment.

The threat of organ deficits or destruction within, the welling up of heretofore controlled unacceptable impulses, and the all too frequent deterioration of the person's socio-economic status tax the adaptive capacities of the ego to the utmost. To master the threat of the dissolution of its boundaries and to ward off any break with reality, the aging organism, having at its disposal a lowered psychic energy supply and being unable to deal with all stimuli, begins to exclude some stimuli from awareness. Stimuli may be blocked at the point of entry, with a lowered threshold for only those stimuli relevant to one's survival.

Disengagement

The aging process is an inevitable mutual withdrawal, resulting in decreased interaction between the person and society. The aging person begins to disengage from ongoing life processes, often denying their importance or value, so as to prepare himself for the lesser role he is to play in life and for the eventual isolation and aloneness that is death.

Memory Deficits

Memory deficits and the remembrance of things past, although rooted in neuron loss, may also be understood dynamically. Recent memory loss does occur, and it disturbs the elderly, who often view it as the first signs of mental illness, aggravated as the memory loss is by inattention, distractibility, and impatience. Less understood and less troublesome to the observer are the repeated past memories that the elderly seem to relate at the slightest provocation. The memory defect is a defense against the poverty of the present, and the memories retained are those that point up a former mastery of the self and the environment.

Life Review

The tendency of the elderly toward self-reflection and reminiscence is part of a normal life review process brought about by the realization of approaching dissolution and death. The life review is characterized by a progressive return to consciousness of past experiences and a resurgence of unresolved conflicts—in particular, conflicts that can be looked at again and reintegrated. If the integration is successful, it may give new significance and meaning to one's life and prepare one for death by mitigating fear and anxiety.

Dependency

The dependency of the aged can be attributed to somatic changes, intellectual impairment, and socio-economic and personal losses. These changes and losses combine to produce increasing fear, anger, and, above all, helplessness; the need for help from others becomes accentuated. The person's search for another presumed to be stronger and capable of helping and the maneuvers to hold the other in a helpful or potentially helpful relationship are sometimes called dependency or dependency strivings.

Rigidity

Rigidity of the aged has been classified into four types: (1) the diminished capacity for new learning, largely based on irreversible physiological changes, (2) the rut formation that develops through the continued practice of old habits, (3) the protective rigidity against changes, a defense against fear, and (4) the compulsive rigidity of the perfectionistic person. Old people as a group show inflexibility and intellectual impairment. Old persons often place great reliance on already-fixed habitual attitudes and routines for the simple reason that they are incapable of learning, retaining, and using new attitudes and routines without considerable effort.

Depletion and Restitution

Aging may bring with it an accentuation of the role of the enteroceptive apparatus, so that messages or stimuli from within the organism are more quickly perceived, thought about, and responded to than ever before. This process is set in motion by a turning in of the investment of the self in increasing quantities, based on somatic depletion, illness, or pain. This phenomenon explains the increasing narcissistic position assumed as one ages. The middle and later years emerge as an age-specific crisis, a balance between factors of depletion and sources of restitution, both past and present, that each person brings to bear in response to the intensity and new dimension of depletion anxiety. This response depends on social or environmental supports that have been constructed, retained, or abandoned.

Depletion seems to be an intermediate step between depression and other complex conditions subsumed under the term "senility." Because of the convergence of social, environmental, and other forces on the aging organism at a given time, conscious or unconscious messages of depletion are and may be unacceptable to the ego. One may then observe intermittent partial or complete abandonment of external and internal reality. However, energetic depletion can, to some degree, be reversed, aggression neutralized, and restitution made through the emotional refueling of a therapeutic relation.

The decisive roles in the resolution of problems are played by a variety of factors—a life that has a measure of instinctual gratification, the ability to tolerate narcissistic injuries without serious regressive reaction, and a flexible superego structure, tolerant enough to permit some unavoidable modifications of the standards of the preceding year.

Behavior Around Food

The elderly use food as a behavioral symbol and mode of communication. The elderly person's search is for a nourishment that often transcends nutritional vectors. Food may be used as a symbol of the maintenance of the psychological life of a person.

In efforts to provide the aged with a proper diet, people often fail to perceive that it is not what the older person eats but with whom he eats it that is the deciding factor. The failure to adhere to realistic nutritional practices represents a regressive maneuver on the part of the aging organism, a cry for help. The unspoken request is for someone to help him—not so much to provide for him, although that is implicit, but to feed him or eat with him. Conversely, the aged patient may reject food and diets as an indication of his disinterest in all that goes on about him.

Sexual Activity

Advanced chronological age is no barrier to continued sexual activity. When the opportu-

nity and the partners are available, the elderly can and do indulge in and enjoy sexual intercourse well into a ripe old age.

In the absence of opportunity for direct sexual gratification, the need for sexual expression may take on many forms. A national program that had not been visualized as a method of providing physical contact—the foster grandparents program, sponsored by the Administration on Aging—has provided a desirable and sublimated form of intimacy. Mutual trust that is expressed in a meaningful intimacy sublimates and transcends the sexual connotation of the physical contact and closeness.

Attempts to master waning powers over one's environment may take the form of an overt sexual expression, often inappropriate and seemingly bizarre.

Diagnosis

In addition to having symptoms that suggest the presence of more than one psychiatric disorder, elderly patients often suffer from one or more physical illnesses or disabilities. Careful history taking is essential. It is instructive to obtain full knowledge of the patient's background—such as heredity, childhood, work record, sexual and marital experiences—over and above the usual history of physical and emotional health. A supplementary history obtained from members of the family or friends or from those accompanying the patient either before or after the interview is almost an imperative when dealing with the seriously ill aged.

Medical Assessment

A thorough physical examination is mandatory. Toxins of bacterial or metabolic origin are common in old age. Bacterial toxins usually originate in occult or inconspicuous foci of infection, such as unsuspected pneumonic conditions and urinary infections. The commonest metabolic intoxication causing mental symptoms in the aged is uremia; mild diabetes, hepatic failure, and gout may easily be missed as causative agents. Alcohol and drug misuse cause many mental disturbances in late life, but these abuses are more easily determined by history taking.

Cerebral anoxia resulting from cardiac insufficiency or emphysema or both often precipitates mental symptoms in old people. Anoxic confusion may follow surgery, a cardiac infarct, gastrointestinal bleeding, or occlusion or stenosis of the carotid arteries. Nutritional deficiencies may be symptomatic of emotional illness and also cause mental symptoms.

Mental Assessment

Overt behavior may manifest itself in the patient's motor activity, his walk, his expressive movements, and the form of his talk. It can be observed by the examining physician, and the history can be obtained from meaningful others.

Mood disorder may be inferred from the patient's movements. But one must be aware of the presence of euphoria, sadness, despair, anxiety, tension, loss of feelings, a paucity of ideation. The patient often complains of somatic sensations that may be substitutes for an expression of emotional state.

Evaluation of the mental content should be extensive and detailed. One should obtain the patient's own description of his feelings and account of the onset. Melancholy, hypochondriacal, paranoid, grandiose, preoccupied, or suicidal thought may be present. Obsessive and phobic symptoms are common. When an affective disorder appears predominant, pathological ideas may surface through a sense of hopelessness, guilt, self-reproach, depersonalization, or some somatic symptoms. There may be passivity or projective experiences and thoughts.

Abnormalities of cognitive functioning may be the result of many depressive or schizophrenic disturbances, but they are most commonly due to some cerebral dysfunctioning or deterioration. A searching evaluation is necessary. It is important to have a knowledge of the patient's past mental abilities—his school and work history and general level of past achievements and work. Cognitive functions other than memory should be investigated thoroughly, especially when the history suggests the presence of some specific disorder or disability.

Some phenomena—such as perseveration, confabulation, and patchiness of performance —are suggestive of cerebral disorders. But the significance of the affects can be determined only in relation to all other findings. Impairment may be due to temporary cerebral dysfunctioning or to permanent anatomical brain damage. It may also be due to the effects of an emotional disturbance. Mental grasp and comprehension, counting and calculation, concentration, memory retention, immediate recall,

and judgment—all must be appraised within the context of the differentiation of age-relevant behavior from life-long behavior.

Psychological Tests

Psychological tests need not be done in every case. They may be done when there is a question as to differentiation between organic brain disease and depression, although depression may occur as a result of brain damage. The Bender Visual Motor Gestalt is most useful in the assessment of organic change. The Wechsler Adult Intelligence Scale is standardized for intelligence, and there are standardized figures available for older people. In many instances, test analyses do not warrant the time expended in administering the tedious battery of intelligence, personality, and other tests. The psychologist may have difficulty in finding an instrument that works, is appropriate, and can be comfortably administered to the older patient. Some patients may not be interested in being examined; others may offer answers the examiner has previously neither seen nor heard.

Electroencephalography

The basic age-related changes occur along the frequency dimension. The dominant α-rhythm (8 to 12 cycles per second) becomes slower, and there is an accompanying increase in still slower α- (4 to 7 cycles per second) and α- (1 to 3 cycles per second) activity. Although fast β-waves (13 to 25 cycles per second) are prevalent during early senescence, they undergo a decline with advancing age. These changes are usually quite minimal in healthy old people. Elderly patients with various diseases of the nervous and cardiovascular system show more profound alterations. In such cases, the EEG may be dominated by slow, focal and δ-activity, which is significantly associated with impaired cerebral circulation and intellectual deficit. Not all areas of the brain manifest equal degrees of frequency change. Focal slowing is particularly prevalent over the temporal lobe, even in relatively healthy old people. However, diffuse slow activity bears a close relation to intellectual impairment.

Psychiatric Conditions

Mental disorders in old age are quite common. The causes are multiple, complex, and complicated by the frequent presence of organic brain involvement.

Organic Brain Disorders

The organic brain disorders are mental states associated with impairment in function or death of brain tissue. They manifest distinct features: disorientation for time, place, and persons; impairment of intellectual functioning; disturbances and impairment of memory; impairment of judgment; defects in comprehension or grasp; evidence of impaired immediate recall; and emotional lability.

Acute Brain Syndrome. Acute brain syndrome is characterized by its reversibility. It is usually related to an acute febrile, debilitating, or exhausting illness, often accompanied by dehydration or malnutrition.

The precipitating causes are many: infections, fracture, congestive heart failure, coronary thrombosis, drug intoxication, malignancy, electrolyte imbalance, renal disease. The aged may not present the usual defensive reactions against infections, such as fever, tachycardia, or leukocytosis. However, such laboratory studies as blood chemistry and urinalysis may reveal a reversible disorder by indicating the presence of anemias, nutritional deficiencies and so on.

Reversible brain syndrome usually manifests itself at a fluctuating level of awareness, which may vary from a mild confusional state to stupor or active delirium. Occasionally, hallucinatory phenomena are present. At times, the illness is quiet; at other times, it is characterized by restlessness, helpless and bewildered confusion, and a tendency to wander, both physically and verbally. In almost all cases, the presence of acute brain syndrome may be taken as evidence of the simultaneous presence of developing chronic brain syndrome.

There are no consistent or characteristic neuropathological findings in acute brain syndrome. Although mortality rates are substantial—an estimated 40 per cent—those who survive the crisis have a good chance of recovery and return to their home. The reversible brain syndrome can lead to death as a manifestation of the serious physical illness that caused the syndrome or complicated it.

Chronic Brain Syndrome. Chronic brain syndrome can be considered to have emerged when the functional neuronal mass has been decreased to a critical point. Under these circumstances, diffuse brain damage appears to be necessary for the emergence of signs of chronic brain syndrome. Senile brain changes are presumed to be causative factors in the production of the syndrome when there are no other focal neurological signs and no history of a stroke. It most commonly appears after the age of 70. In the eighties it is almost universal, with an insidious and often imperceptible onset.

The old person may pass slowly from normal old age to senile psychosis with no abrupt changes. Early features are errors in judgment, decline in personal care and habits, an impairment in capacity for abstract thought, a lack of interest, and apathy. Many emotional reactions are possible—depression, anxiety, and irritability being the most frequent. A loosening of inhibitions can be an early sign. As deterioration progresses, medical symptoms proliferate, and the traditional signs of organic dysfunction become more evident. Hallucinations may be present, especially at night. Rambling, incoherent speech and fabrication are frequent signs. Sleeplessness and restlessness are common. The patient may wander away from home. Paranoid tendencies may be exacerbated or appear for the first time. Occasionally, one may see manic and hypermanic states.

Functional Disorders

Schizophrenic Syndromes. Schizophrenias in the elderly are marked by disturbances in thinking, mood, and behavior. Hallucinations, delusions, and poor reality testing are characteristic. Paranoid symptoms seem to be a defense against the gradual loss of mastery that the patients experience.

The aged schizophrenics respond quite well to the phenothiazines; however, as in all medication for the elderly, it should be judiciously administered. One should begin with small doses and gradually work up to the tolerance of the individual patient, remembering all the time that the metabolism and the detoxifying aspects of the organism are not as adequately functional in the elderly as in the younger schizophrenic.

Affective Disorders. Affective illnesses—unlike the schizophrenias, which develop slowly—have, as a rule, a sudden onset or develop over a number of months. In a high proportion of cases, the affective illnesses are precipitated by loss or physical illness.

Late-onset depressives, in comparison with early-onset patients, had better adjusted personalities emotionally, socially, and psychosexually. The majority of first depressive attacks, especially severe attacks, appear in the second half of life. The highest first incidence occurs between 55 and 65 in men and between 50 and 60 in women. The onset follows closely the occurrence of some traumatic event—bereavement, the moving away of children, loss of status, retirement from a job, threatened loss through physical illness, the illness of the spouse.

Antidepressant drugs, particularly the tricyclics, have been enormously useful in the therapy of depressive reactions. Medications for the elderly must always be guardedly prescribed and must take into consideration their weight and the presence of any other disease that may mitigate against the proper metabolism and use of the prescribed medication. One should begin with small doses and work up gradually. The tricyclic of choice depends or the tolerance and the response of the patient to that particular medication.

Manic and hypomanic disorders are far less frequent than are depressions. The patient and his family may fail to recognize the hypomanic phase of a bipolar disorder. It may be ascribed to the aggressiveness, overactivity, and poor judgment of a senile brain. It usually follows a depressive reaction, which may have been so brief as to have escaped attention. Hostile or paranoid behavior is usually present. The response to treatment is usually good. Lithium salts have shown a great deal of promise.

Neuroses. The neuroses occupy a conspicuous place in the disorders of later life. The incidence of neuroses is far greater than that of the psychoses, yet little attention is being paid to them because, in the neuroses, there is no total break with reality.

Hypochondriasis. Hypochondriasis is the inordinate preoccupation with one's bodily functions, and it is an especially common disorder in the aged. The symptoms are directed mostly to the organs of ingestion, digestion, and evacuation and to the heart and circulatory system.

With fewer worthwhile things to hold the attention and to divert one from self-concern, it becomes easier to notice and to talk about minor ailments and accidents. In general, the older a person grows, the more experience he has had with illness, operations, and accidents, whether his own or those of other people, and the easier it is for him to feel himself to be ill or in danger. Then, too, bodily concern helps to save face when one is beset by failures.

Despite the fact that heart conditions are more numerous and more often fatal than gastrointestinal disease, the elderly person is usually much more concerned with the latter. This concern is tied in with an unconscious expression of the person's dependency needs. By his unconscious use of physical symptoms, the older person often attempts to regain attention, affection, and domination.

Anxiety States. Since insecurity and realistic anxiety-producing situations are common in later life, anxiety states can easily arise. An anxiety neurosis is characterized by increased muscular tension, with difficulty in relaxation and sleeping, disturbances in the regular rhythm of the heart, gastrointestinal tract and urinary system disturbances, tremors, headaches, excessive perspiration, increased irritability, and a vague sense of impending doom. At times, acute anxiety may arise in the old person because of guilt feelings resulting from hostility toward his family when they fail to understand and meet his needs.

Chronic Fatigue States. These states are difficult to diagnose in the aged patient because it is normal for elderly people to tire more quickly and easily and to recover more slowly and incompletely than do younger ones. Also, as a rule, sleep in old people is shorter and less sound, and they awaken feeling less refreshed and sometimes irritable. Fatigue can, however, be a result of emotional frustration. Whenever the prospect of gratification is small, a person is apt to tire quickly and to remain so until something interesting turns up. Since prospects for gratifying experience wane with the years, easy fatigability is common in this age group. A balanced diet of rest, recreation, and occupation gives a starting point for a successful therapeutic effort.

Compulsive Disorders. The compulsive person can be recognized by his overconscientiousness, perfectionism, orderliness, overattention to details, and doubts about himself and his adequacy. Such symptoms may take the form of excessive cleanliness and orderliness and endless and inflexible rituals to guard against mistakes, danger, or evil thoughts. Repeated acts of a penitential or conciliatory character may appear in elderly people as a result of or as a protection against erratic hostile or vindictive fantasies that arouse guilt in them.

Any attempt to stop these compulsive acts may arouse acute and intolerable anxiety. The attack should be directed at the environment and not at the symptoms themselves.

Hysterical Neuroses. Such neuroses are not common in later years. What one does see is an exaggeration of minor physical symptoms.

Sleep Disturbances. Elderly persons need as much if not more sleep than they did in their earlier mature years. However, complaints about sleeplessness are common. To some extent, these complaints can be traced to sleep disturbances, rather than to sleeplessness. The sleep disturbances may be due to the need for more frequent visits to the bathroom, with resulting problems in again falling asleep. Furthermore, many of the elderly succumb to the practice of taking cat naps during their waking hours, a habit that may interfere with what they describe as a good night's sleep.

When insomnia does occur and is unaccompanied by delirium or a psychotic reaction, it usually responds to chloral hydrate, administered either by capsule or in liquid form. Barbiturates, too, may be used. When insomnia is accompanied by a psychotic or depressive reaction, phenothiazine or tricyclic medication often induces sleep.

Therapy

Remedial measures for most of these difficulties can be gratifying. One must make due allowances for the reduced vigor, agility, and learning capacity of the elderly patient. Beyond that, therapy can be conducted along the lines of therapy at any age level. The therapist has to be more active and more direct than with patients in other age groups, for the exigencies of time demand shorter methods.

First of all, one should assess the physical state of the patient in order to determine how much the aging organism will be able to take.

Second, one must evaluate the patient's suitability for therapy from the viewpoint of his earlier adaptation and maladjustments, his capacity for establishing a workable relation with the therapist, and the degree to which these characteristics are modifiable. And one must determine whether the presenting symptoms are something new in the life of the patient or a continuation of a long-existing neurotic personality structure.

Allow the patient to express himself, to talk about himself and his difficulties. The patient will interpret impatience as a rejection, which cannot be tolerated. The therapist's attitude should be one of respectful attention and thoughtful consideration, despite the fact that the same problem may arise and be discussed over and over again. Empathy—the ability to place oneself in the patient's place without ever identifying with him—and not sympathy is essential. The older person craves respect that will help him bolster his self-esteem.

Allay the anxiety and insecurity of the aging patient, insofar as possible. The helping person must have a genuine fondness for the elderly and a willingness to help them. One must, however, be tactful, for the elderly are proud and do not wish to betray their weakness. Therefore, they should be allowed to gratify their dependency needs in a manner that will not make them feel that they are leaning on another person. A condescending, patronizing attitude on the part of the supporting figure will only tend to accentuate the patient's feelings of inadequacy and insecurity.

Patients should be helped into activities that will tend to enhance their attractiveness—physical and mental. When a person is young, he may be physically attractive. When that youthful attractiveness fails him, achievement in some field of endeavor or continued productivity on a job can enhance his attractiveness. At the same time, the elderly must be helped in accepting gracefully a curtailment of activities when such curtailment will mean redirection into something meaningful and gratifying, rather than merely being out of a job and thus out of life. The therapist should plan their daily activity with them and not for them when life would otherwise become empty. In addition to knowing the patient's own personal and family situation, the therapist should become thoroughly acquainted with the facilities that the community, the church, and social agencies have established for the elderly.

One must bring an optimistic attitude to the psychiatric techniques used in working with old people. One should leave the patient at the end of any interview with the feeling that the contact was a gratifying experience and that something was accomplished during that hour.

The over-all treatment goals with the geriatric patient are to maximize his mental, physical, and social capacities. Remotivation techniques challenge the patient's desire to withdraw from life or to die. He is encouraged to establish new and to re-establish old social relations and to develop and redevelop former interests in church, recreation, games, and household activities in close proximity with other people. He is encouraged to engage in mutual helping relations and to take an active interest in the lives of others.

REFERENCES

Berezin, M. A. Some intrapsychic aspects of aging. In *Normal Psychology of the Aging Process*, N. E. Zinberg and I. Kaufman, editors, p. 93. International Universities Press, New York, 1963.

Butler, R. N., and Lewis, M. I. *Aging and Mental Health*. C. V. Mosby, St. Louis, 1973.

Post, F. *The Clinical Psychiatry of Late Life*. Pergamon Press, London, 1965.

Weinberg, J. Sexual expressions of late life. Am. J. Psychiatry, *126:* 713, 1969.

Weinberg, J. Environment: Its language and the aging. J. Geriatric Soc., *18:* 681, 1970.

Weinberg, J. Some psychodynamic aspects of agedness. In *Aging and the Brain*, vol. 3: *Advances in Behavior Biology*, C. M. Gaitz, editor, p. 209. Plenum Press, New York, 1972.

49

Forensic and Correctional Psychiatry

49.1.   FORENSIC PSYCHIATRY

Introduction

In this society, only the judiciary has the vested right to curtail a person's liberty and rights. One of these rights is the right to privacy. Many criminal and civil law questions necessitate extensive probing into the privacy of a client's psyche. Psychiatrists and psychologists offer valuable understanding and insight but always with the substantial risk of inappropriately and harmfully disturbing privacy. The decision to give up the shroud of privacy lies entirely in the hands of the person concerned, or, if it is to be wrested from him, it may be done only according to due process of law.

At various stages in their historical development, psychiatry and law have converged. Both disciplines are concerned with the social deviant, the person who has violated the "rules" of society and whose behavior presents a problem, not only because it diminishes his ability to function effectively, but because it affects the functioning of the community adversely. Traditionally, the psychiatrist's efforts are directed toward elucidation of the causes, and through prevention and treatment, reducing the self-destructive elements of harmful behavior. The lawyer, as the agent of society, is concerned with the fact that the social deviant represents a potential threat to the safety and security of other people in his environment. Both psychiatry and law seek to implement their respective goals through the application of pragmatic techniques, based on empirical observations.

The Psychiatrist and the Law

Psychiatric Practice: Legal Requirements

The license to practice medicine and surgery which is required in every state of the Union carries with it legal authorization to engage in the practice of psychiatry without prior specialized training. Although a few states make training and certification mandatory for clinical psychologists, for the most part the psychiatrist engaged in the practice of psychotherapy is carrying out a treatment for which no formal training or licensing is required by law. It is illegal to call oneself a psychiatrist without being a physician but anyone can call himself a psychotherapist or a psychoanalyst.

Criminal Law and Psychiatry

According to criminal law, a socially harmful act does not represent the sole criterion of a crime. The objectional act must have been perpetrated deliberately. The criminal must have had a *mens rea*, an evil intent. There cannot be a *mens rea* if the offender's mental status is so deficient, so abnormal, so diseased, as to have deprived him of the capacity for rational intent. The law can be invoked only when an illegal intent is implemented. Neither behavior, however harmful, nor the intent to do harm are, in themselves, grounds for criminal action.

In most American jurisdictions until quite recently, a person could be found not guilty by reason of insanity if he suffered from a mental illness, did not know the difference between right and wrong, and did not know the nature and consequences of his acts.

M'Naughten Rule. The precedent for determining legal responsibility was established in the British courts during 1843. The so-called M'Naughten rule, which has, until recently, determined responsibility in most of the states of the Union, holds that a man is guilty by reason of insanity if he labored under a mental disease such that he was unaware of the nature, quality, and consequences of his act, or if he was incapable of realizing that his act was wrong. Moreover, to absolve a man from punishment, a delusion has to be one which, *if true*, would be an adequate defense. If the *deluded idea* does not justify the crime then presumably the man is to be held responsible, guilty, and punishable. The M'Naughten rule is known commonly as the right-wrong test.

The M'Naughten rule derives from the famous M'Naughten case dating back to 1843. At that time Edward Drummond, the private secretary of Sir Robert Peel, was murdered by Daniel M'Naughten (Figure 1). M'Naughten had been suffering from delusions of persecution for several years. He had complained to many people about his delusional persecutors and finally he decided to correct the situation by murdering Sir Robert Peel. When Drummond came out of Peel's home, M'Naughten shot Drummond, mistaking him for Peel. He was later adjudged insane and committed to a hospital. The case aroused great interest causing the House of Lords to debate the problems of criminality and insanity. In response to questions about what guidelines could be used to determine whether a person should plead insanity as a defense against criminal responsibility, the English judiciary wrote:

1. "To establish a defense on the ground of insanity it must be clearly proved that, at the time of committing the act, the party accused was laboring under such a defect of reason, from disease of the mind, as not to know the nature and quality of the act he was doing, or if he did know it, he did not know he was doing what was wrong."

2. "Where a person labors under partial delusions only and is not in other respects insane" and as a result commits an offense "he must be considered in the same situation as to responsibility as if the facts with respect to which the delusion exists were real."

Irresistible Impulse. In 1922, a committee of jurists in England reexamined the M'Naughten rule and suggested broadening the concept of insanity in criminal cases to further include the concept of the "irresistible impulse." This meant that "a person charged criminally with an offense is irresponsible for his act when the act is committed under an impulse which the prisoner was by mental disease in substance deprived of any power to resist." The courts have chosen to interpret this law in such a way that it has been called the "policeman-at-the-elbow" law. In other words, the court will grant the

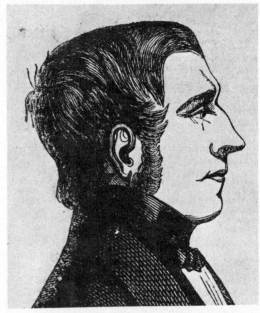

FIGURE 1. Daniel M'Naughten. His 1843-murder trial led to the establishment of rules still generally observed in legal insanity pleas. (Courtesy of Culver Pictures.)

impulse to be irresistible only if it is determined that the accused would have gone ahead with the act even if he had a policeman at his elbow. To most psychiatrists this is an unsatisfactory law because it covers only a small and a very special group of those who are mentally ill.

Durham Rule. In 1954, the case of Durham versus United States, a decision was handed down by Judge David Bazelon in the District of Columbia Court of Appeals that resulted in the product rule of criminal responsibility: "An accused is not criminally responsible if his unlawful act was the product of mental disease or defect."

Lawyers complained of the vagueness in the language of the Durham rule and felt that a lay jury would have great difficulty applying such a rule. This view led to an alternative formulation of the insanity rule, which has come to be known as the ALI (American Law Institute) rule. According to this rule: "(1) A person is not responsible for criminal conduct if at the time of such conduct as a result of mental disease or defect he lacks substantial capacity either to appreciate the criminality of his conduct or to conform his conduct to the requirements of law. (2) As used in this article, the terms 'mental disease or defect' do not include an abnormality manifested only by repeated criminal or otherwise anti-social conduct.'' This standard has been adopted by several courts and has been written into the criminal codes of several states.

Competence to Stand Trial

In all state and Federal jurisdictions, a defendant is deemed incompetent to stand trial if, because of mental illness, he is unable to understand the nature of the legal charges against him and to participate with counsel in his own defense. Initially, all defendants are presumed to be competent, but the prosecutor, the defense counsel, or the court may challenge this presumption. In such an event, the court orders a psychiatric examination to ascertain whether or not the defendant is competent according to the above criteria.

When a person is found incompetent to stand trial, he is usually committed to a state hospital until such a time as his competence has been restored. This procedure has resulted in a large number of persons losing their freedom permanently, even when the issue of whether they committed a crime has remained undetermined.

Juvenile Delinquency and Juvenile Courts

A delinquent act, by legal definition, is any act that would be defined as a crime if it were committed by an adult. In general, juvenile codes apply to any person below the age of majority, although that age varies from state to state.

A juvenile court may take legal jurisdiction of a child on several grounds. The first is that of delinquency. On this basis, the child must be charged with an act that would result in a criminal conviction if he were an adult. The second ground for the juvenile court to take jurisdiction of a child is the neglect jurisdiction. The juvenile court must find that a parent or guardian has neglected a child, physically or emotionally. It may then make a decision to take custody of the child temporarily or permanently, so that it may provide the child with the best possible opportunity to mature into adulthood. The third basis for juvenile court jurisdiction is to find that a child is in need of supervision or has been incorrigible. These cases usually involve runaways or children who

have been brought into court by parents who cannot adequately control them.

Delinquency

In the 1967 case of *in re Gault*, the Supreme Court stated that, under the Consitiution, children have a right to at least the same procedural safeguards as do adults when charged with a crime. The court noted explicitly that juveniles must have appropriate notice to prepare a defense against the charges, the right to representation by counsel, the right to confront witnesses and to cross-examine them, and a right to the privilege against compelled self-incrimination. Psychiatrists, social workers, and psychologists must present their views in the form of expert testimony, adequately tested by the challenge of cross-examination. Mental health staffs must learn how to describe the observational data that lead them to their conclusions, must learn to understand the complexities of such legal evidentiary concepts as hearsay, and, most particularly, must learn how to work with lawyers in ways that will maximize their appropriate and effective communication in the court. The role of both the psychiatrist and the lawyer must be to help the child get appropriate and effective treatment to avoid further psychological and social decompensation.

Neglect

The children who come under the juvenile court's neglect jurisdiction are the children whose parents abandon them, abuse them physically or emotionally, or get into such difficulties that they wind up in prison or a hospital. To take jurisdiction, the court must find that parental care is inadequate and is causing harm to the children. More often than not, these children are from socially disadvantaged groups. When an evaluation is made by persons from disparate social backgrounds, they may or may not understand the qualities of the homes from which these children come. Mothering patterns, disciplinary measures, and appropriate medical care may all be viewed from the vantage point of different value systems.

One issue of central importance is the question of the accuracy of psychiatric predictions. Since psychiatrists do not have a highly reliable predictive capacity, the courts have tended to be conservative and to make the least possible intervention necessary. If psychiatrists become more capable of saying what kinds of behavior signal future serious disability, the courts may then be more willing to interfere in family decision making and to order treatment, despite its attendant risks. Currently when a juvenile court decides to intervene in parents' management of their children, it makes its decision on the basis of the child's best interest.

Battered-child cases are also handled by the juvenile court under its neglect jurisdiction. The battering parents were usually themselves battered as children. As they face the difficulties and frustrations of child rearing, their own traumatic past appears to cause an incapacity to handle the parenting role without occasional outbursts of violence against the child.

The child-abuse statutes were all developed to deal with the legal problem involving doctor-patient confidentiality. In the past, when parents brought their battered children for treatment, the examining physician was prevented in most states from doing anything about the child's plight because of the confidential relationship he had with the parents and because his communications with them were legally privileged. The abuse statutes remove confidentiality and privilege from these cases and often make it a misdemeanor for a physician to fail to report cases that show evidence of unexplained violence on a child. Unfortunately, many of these statutes are written in such a way that, instead of promoting treatment for the child and his family, they provide techniques to obtain evidence that is then used to convict the parents of various crimes against their children.

Persons in Need of Supervision

Children in need of supervision may be brought by their families to the juvenile court, or they may be put into psychiatric treatment. Since their behavior more often than not is precipitated by intrafamilial tension, an alteration of that condition is essential.

When children run away from home, it is usually an unconscious effort on their part to try to bring about some kind of change in the family situation. They may run away to escape parental violence or to disengage themselves from a parent-child incestual involvement. They may be reflecting an adolescent identity struggle

that stimulates an overresponse from their parents. In one of these family crisis moments, the authority of the law may inadvertently interpose changes in the power relationships that virtually foreclose the possibility of appropriate alteration through treatment. When psychiatrists are drawn into this kind of case, they should thoroughly understand the several power alternatives available in order to avoid pressing resolutions that are either therapeutically or legally nonviable. For example, if parents seek to commit a child to a hospital because they cannot manage him and then refuse to be involved in family treatment because they cannot face the fact that they have a hand in the child's problem, the child may run away again. This recurrent behavior may cause the parents to ask the juvenile court to take jurisdiction on grounds of the child's incorrigibility, and the court may commit the child to the very same hospital setting—still without involving the parents.

Because of the nature of the conflicts that lead to incorrigibility, it seems wise for juvenile courts to move swiftly to an evaluation of the parents, long-range capability for carrying out their parenting roles. If the parents do not have such a capacity and if this lack can be demonstrated, the least detrimental alternative would be to work out some alternative parenting procedure for the child as swiftly as possible.

Laws Governing Hospitalization

It is preferable to have a patient enter a mental hospital or the psychiatric inpatient service of a general hospital voluntarily, for the same reasons that his prognosis is better if he enters psychotherapy as an outpatient through his own decision, because he wants to help himself.

All of the states provide for some form of involuntary hospitalization. Such action is usually taken when the psychiatric patient presents a danger to himself and to others in his environment, to the degree that his urgent need for treatment in a closed institution is evident.

The statutes governing hospitalization of the mentally ill have generally been designated as "commitment laws." However, psychiatrists have long considered the term an undesirable one because commitment legally means a warrant for imprisonment. The American Bar Association and the American Psychiatric Association recommended that the term be replaced by the less offensive and more accurate term hospitalization, and this has been done by most states. Although change in terminology will not correct attitudes of the past, emphasis on hospitalization and treatment is more in keeping with the views of psychiatrists toward this process.

There are four procedures of admission to psychiatric facilities that have been endorsed by the American Bar Association as safeguarding civil liberties and ensuring that no individual can be "railroaded" into a mental hospital. While each of the 50 states has the power to enact its own laws regarding psychiatric hospitalization, the procedures outlined are gaining much acceptance.

1. Informal Admission. This form of admission operates on the general hospital model in which the patient is admitted to a psychiatric unit of a general hospital precisely on the same basis as a medical or surgical patient might be admitted. Under such circumstances, the ordinary doctor-patient relationship applies with freedom on the part of the patient to enter and freedom to leave, even against medical advice.

At present there are over 2,000 psychiatric units in general hospitals in the United States in which this procedure may be used. It is estimated that over 90 per cent of all patients could be admitted in this manner.

2. Voluntary Admission (Operates in Psychiatric Hospitals). Under this procedure, the patient applies for admission to any psychiatric hospital in writing. He may come to the hospital on the advice of his personal physician or he may seek help on the basis of his own decision. In either case, the patient is examined by a psychiatrist on the staff of the hospital and is admitted if that examination reveals the need for hospital treatment.

3. Temporary Admission (Emergency Admission or Certificate of One Physician). This category is used for patients who are so senile or confused that they require hospitalization and are not able to make decisions of their own, or for patients who are so acutely disturbed that they must be immediately admitted to a psychiatric hospital on an emergency basis.

Under this procedure a person is admitted to the hospital on the written recommendation of one physician. Once having been brought to the psychiatric hospital, the need for hospitalization must be confirmed by a psychiatrist on the hospital staff.

This procedure is temporary, in that the patient cannot be hospitalized against his will for a period exceeding 15 days.

4. Involuntary Admission (Certificate of Two Physicians). Involuntary admission involves the question of whether or not the patient is a danger to himself, such as in the suicidal patient, or a danger to others, such as in the homicidal patient. Because these individuals do not recognize their need for hospital care, application for admission to a hospital may be made by a relative, or friend.

Once the application is made, the patient must be examined by two physicians and, if they confirm the need for hospitalization, the patient can then be admitted.

There is an established procedure for written notification to the next of kin whenever involuntary hospitalization is involved. Furthermore, the patient has access at any time to legal counsel, who can bring the case before a judge. If hospitalization is not felt to be indicated by the judge, he can order the patient's release from the hospital.

Involuntary admission allows the patient to be hospitalized for 60 days. After that time, the case must be reviewed periodically by a board consisting of psychiatrists, nonpsychiatric physicians, lawyers, and other citizens not connected with the institution, if the patient is to remain hospitalized.

In spite of the clear-cut procedures and safeguards for hospitalization available to the patient, to his family, as well as to the medical and legal profession, involuntary admissions are being reviewed by some as an infringement of civil rights.

A person who has been involuntarily hospitalized and who believes that he should be released has the right to file a petition for a writ of habeas corpus. This legal procedure must be heard by a court at once, regardless of the manner or form in which it is filed. Hospitals are obligated to submit these petitions to the court immediately.

Right to Treatment

Clearly, if the state imposes hospitalization and deprives a person of freedom in order to treat him, there is an implicit right to treatment. In the 1971 Alabama case of Wyatt versus Stickney, a class action against several hospitals in the state mental hospital system on behalf of a group of patients, the court ruled that a plan to provide appropriate treatment must be filed within 90 days, at which time it would set forth a treatment standard. In Appendix A to the opinion in the subsequent 1972 hearing, the court elaborated a highly detailed set of minimum constitutional standards for adequate treatment of the mentally ill. In addition to describing the physical plant, staffing qualifications and ratios, and many other conditions, the court required that there be an individualized treatment plan developed and filed in each patient's chart.

In the 1976 case of O'Connor versus Donaldson, the Supreme Court ruled that harmless mental patients cannot be confined against their will without treatment if they can survive outside. A finding of mental illness alone cannot justify a state's confining a person in a hospital against his will according to the Court. Instead, patients must be considered dangerous to themselves or others. Kopolow had raised the question of the psychiatrists' ability to accurately predict dangerousness and the risk to the psychiatrist who might be sued for monetary damages if a person is deprived of civil rights as a result of this difficulty in accurately assessing dangerousness in some cases.

Civil Competency

In most recent statutes, the issue of hospitalization is sharply separated from that of loss of competency. Hospitalization on a voluntary or involuntary basis does not result in incompetency. A separate hearing on this issue is necessary. If it is felt that the patient lacks the capacity to manage his own affairs, the court so rules after taking evidence on that issue, and it then appoints a guardian to take care of the patients interests. This person has full legal authority to make decisions on behalf of the incompetent person, and it is his duty to concern himself fully with his ward's interests. This concern involves not only managing his property but also making decisions about such things as the granting of treatment consent.

Change of a Child's Parenting Persons

Adoption

When a child is placed for adoption, a parent or both parents have decided that they are unable or unwilling to take up or continue with the parenting function because of illegitimacy, illness, or disinterest. After the parents have given a legally valid consent to have the child placed for adoption, which entails a willingness to end their parental rights, the court responds to a petition for adoption made by those who wish to take over the parental role for such a child. After evaluating all the viable options for the child, the court selects the one most likely to foster the child's interest. The court occasionally asks a psychiatrist to evaluate the potential adoptive parents and perhaps the child to provide information that can help the court make its decision wisely. A crucial psychiatric consideration is that the adoption be carried out while the child is as young as possible and that the adoption be as free from any disruption or tentativeness as it is possible to arrange.

Child-Custody Disputes in Divorce

Whenever a divorce is granted to a couple who have children, the court automatically takes supervisory jurisdiction of the children's interests until they reach majority. A part of every divorce decree for such a couple is a custodial disposition of the children. When the custody of the children is being settled, the lawyers for each parent have always had the ethical duty to seek a resolution in the best interest of the child. But they are also supposed to advance the adversarial position of their respective clients as vigorously as possible, which clearly places counsel in a potential psychological conflict of interest. The end result costs the child several years of existence in a kind of limbo, which is extremely harmful to his healthy growth and development.

Legal Problems and Psychiatric Testimony

Wills

The psychiatrist may be called upon to evaluate a patient's *testamentary capacity*, i.e., his competency to make a will. Three psychological abilities are necessary to demonstrate this competency; the patient must know: (1) the nature and extent of his bounty (property); (2) that he is making a will; and (3) who his natural beneficiaries are—that is, his wife, children, and relatives.

Quite often, when a will is being probated, one of the heirs or some other person challenges the validity of the will. A judgment in such cases must be based on a reconstruction of what the testator's mental state was at the time the will was written. The evidence used to make this reconstruction comes from persons who knew the testator at the time he wrote the will and from expert psychiatric testimony. The expert needs to examine all the data from documents and from the witnesses and then make a reconstruction.

Credibility

Occasionally, a psychiatrist is asked to assist in evaluating the credibility of a witness—in other words, to judge whether the witness is telling the truth. Although it is likely that an expert psychiatrist can observe a witness's behavior and draw some useful inferences that relate to truth telling, he is unlikely to be able to persuade a fact finder. On the other hand, if he uses his impressions to help counsel to cross-examine a witness skillfully in the areas where lying may be taking place, his insights are far more useful.

The Clinical Interview and the Accused

The psychiatrist has no formal role in criminal investigation. He is under no legal or ethical obligation to use his skills to elicit confessions from criminal suspects. If he were to reveal information obtained in a clinical setting, the psychiatrist would rob the psychiatric interview of its essential ingredient: confidentiality.

At times, and with the consent of all concerned, a variety of procedures such as amobarbital (truth serum) interviews or the use of the polygraph (lie detector) may be employed. In general, the results of such interviews are used only to prove innocence rather than guilt.

Competence to Testify

Opposing counsel sometimes maintain that an intended witness is not competent to testify by virtue of his mental state. If the court believes that there is sufficient merit to the challenge, it appoints an expert psychiatrist to examine the potential witness and to offer evidence about whether or not that witness can testify accurately about the relevant issues. This question is relativistic, since a person can have the capacity to talk about some subjects with perfect ease but may become thoroughly disoriented and deranged in relation to others. The expert can often greatly facilitate the court's decision making on the question of admissibility of evidence.

Informed Consent

All medical procedures carried out on a patient have to be done with his informed consent. Occasionally, a question arises as to whether such consent was validly given. There is an analogy to this question in criminal law trials in regard to confession. Confessions may not be coerced; neither may consent be coerced. Occasionally, a psychiatrist is asked to evaluate whether or not any form of coercion was used. The expert may examine the person as thoroughly as he wishes in relation to the process that led to the person's decision to consent or to confess. In the trial, the psychiatrist's testimony describes the process of the consent or the confession, the nature of the person's volition, and the effects of the implied or real pressure placed on him by the circumstances.

Claims for Emotional Damages

There have been an increasing number of negligence suits in which damages are claimed for emotional injuries or so-called traumatic neurosis. With the advent of more dynamic theoretical explanations of injury, it has seemed logical to permit such evidence to go to the jury, where it stands or falls on the merits of its own persuasiveness. Psychiatric expert testimony is often sought.

Legal Obligations of the Psychiatrist

Maintaining the confidentiality of communications between doctor and patient is, first and foremost, an ethical duty. Nowhere is this duty more important than in the psychotherapeutic relationship. The doctor's ethical responsibility is reinforced in law as the legal right to privacy, and an inappropriate revelation may lead to a claim for damages in a tort action for breach of privacy. A psychiatrist may not reveal information about his patient except when he has the legal duty to do so, such as in his obligation to report a battered child.

Privileged communication is purely a legal concept. It exists when there is a statutory bar to testifying about a medically confidential communication in a court of law. When medical privilege exists, the person who is the subject of the confidential information is the only one who can invoke it by objecting to testimony by the doctor. Simply stated, privilege belongs to the patient whereas confidentiality belongs to the doctor.

The usual definition of medical privileged communication is information obtained by a physician during the course of diagnosis or treatment of a patient that is related to diagnostic or treatment needs. If an orthopedic surgeon was treating a patient for a fractured leg and was told that a neighbor had fired the shot that caused the fracture, the surgeon could be forced to testify about who fired the gun because the identity of that person is not required by the surgeon to carry out his medical task. On the other hand, a psychiatrist, who needs total information about his patients in order to carry out his treatment process, is blocked by the medical privilege rule from testifying about anything he heard.

A patient may waive his privilege when he decides that he wishes his physician to testify about information derived from the therapeutic relation. Once the waiver has been given, it is virtually total and covers everything the doctor knows about the patient.

In several situations, there is an automatic waiver. For example, if a person files a suit claiming emotional damages, he must waive privilege in regard to any past psychiatric treatment. A flat refusal by a psychiatrist to testify at all about his patient may cause that patient legal harm and a loss of rights.

Malpractice

Whenever the issue of malpractice arises, the patient has to prove his contention about the physician's negligent medical care by a preponderance of the evidence, and he uses expert testimony to do so. The defendant-psychiatrist then counters by describing his own behavior and probably by bringing expert testimony on his own behalf. Although there is no obligation to maintain patient records, they are legally useful on occasions such as this, when the defendant needs to be able to demonstrate what he did or did not do on some prior occasion. Physicians administering treatment to mentally ill persons must always remember to deal with the informed consent question adequately, especially when they are engaged in any procedure that is risky to the patient.

It is presumed that psychiatrists have special competence to diagnose suicidal risk and to take appropriate preventive measures when such a risk exists. A failure to do so may result in a malpractice action against the psychiatrist. As mentioned above the psychiatrist's ability to predict dangerous behavior—either toward oneself or others—is not as reliable as one might hope.

Problems of Communication

The interpretation of legal language and psychiatric language may differ radically, even when the same words are used. For example, in both psychiatry and law, commitment refers to one of several legally implemented, psychiatrically inspired procedures designed to permit involuntary hospitalization of certain patients. In fact, however, for the lawyer, a commitment is a mittimus, a warrant for imprisonment, whereas for the psychiatrist, the term denotes a "helpful" procedure, in that it facilitates the hospitalization, and appropriate treatment, of a patient who is mentally ill. Other difficulties in terminology that exist are the following: *Insanity* and *lunacy* are legal terms that should be replaced by the term mental illness. The terms *feebleminded* and *weak-minded* should be categorized as mental retardation when applicable. The terms *eloped* and *escaped* to refer to the patient who has left the hospital against medical advice should be abandoned.

Psychiatric Expert Testimony

In legal situations, the psychiatrist functions most of the time in the role of expert witness. Expert witnesses, because of their technical expertise in the field about which they testify, are permitted to express opinions. It is desirable that the psychiatrist deemed by the court to be an expert be certified in psychiatry by the American Board of Psychiatry and Neurology as an absolute minimum.

When a psychiatric expert testifies, he should present his information in three clearly distinguishable portions. First, he should present and discuss his psychological theories as they relate to the legal question at hand. Second, he should describe his data base totally, including such things as exact quotations of things the patient has said, the information about him that has been revealed in documents, and data obtained from his family and significant persons who know him. Third, the diagnostic and legal inferences drawn in relation to the issue at trial should stand clearly apart, so that their logic may be tested thoroughly and without confusion by the fact finders.

During the pretrial conferences with counsel, the psychiatrist should help him prepare to deal with the opposition expert. In addition, the confusion of seemingly disparate expert views can be diminished by taking steps to have them join in their examination and report-writing process.

REFERENCES

Allen, R. C., Ferster, E. Z., and Rubin, J. G. *Readings in Law and Psychiatry*. Johns Hopkins Press, Baltimore, 1968.

Burris, D. S., editor. *The Right to Treatment*. Springer, New York, 1969.

Dawidoff, D. J. *The Malpractice of Psychiatrists*. Charles C Thomas, Springfield, Ill., 1973.

Goldstein, J., Freud, A., and Solnit, A. J. *Beyond the Best Interests of the Child*. Free Press of Glencoe (Macmillan), New York, 1973.

Kopolow, L. E. A review of major implications of the *O'Connor v. Donaldson* decision. Am J. Psychiatry, *133:* 4, 1976.

McGarry, A. L. *Competency to Stand Trial and Mental Illness*. National Institute of Mental Health, Bethesda, Md., 1973.

Rosenheim, M., editor. *Justice for the Child*. Free Press of Glencoe (Macmillan), New York, 1962.

Shartel, B., and Plant, M. L. *The Law of Medical Practice*. Charles C Thomas, Springfield, Ill., 1959.

Watson, A. S. The quest for professional competence: Psychological aspects of legal education. Cincinnati Law Rev., *37:* 91, 1968.

Watson, A. S. *Contested Divorces and Children: A Challenge for the Forensic Psychiatrist*. Appleton-Century-Crofts, New York, 1973.

49.2. CORRECTIONAL PSYCHIATRY

Introduction

Many prisons offer inmates an emotional climate that is destructive to most goals of rehabilitation. Yet all prisons potentially can provide the structure and stability that could lead to the learning of important new skills and ways of relating to people. Since the life histories of most of the inmates reveal significant examples of actual or relative neglect and abandonment and the lack of consistent, caring, responsive environment, the prison setting can offer a new kind of experience.

Inmate Population

There is little agreement about the amount of mental illness within the inmate population. Estimates vary from 10 to 20 per cent to well over 50 to 75 per cent. Most inmates have various difficulties with impulse control.

Many inmates also have long-standing difficulties in establishing permanent relationships. They tend to distrust people, often with good reason, since they have usually come from environments that offered little reward for depending on others and for delaying impulses. Those who become part of the prison population are characterized by a lack of dependability and consistency. Wishes for immediate results make sense in a setting where dependable relationships are rare and where there is little likelihood that long-term delay will lead to experiences of ultimate gratification.

There have often been crucial disturbances within their nuclear families. Abandonment and neglect is a common story, with early losses related to parental separations or death. Alcoholism is frequent in one or both parents; often, the father is absent through separation or alcoholism. Violence can be the usual experience for these children, both at home and in the streets. Many of these children develop a veneer of supercompetence, which can easily disintegrate under stress.

When examined in a court or correctional setting, many of these men and women exhibit a profound distrust, especially of people in authority. They often view themselves as the victims of society and tend to externalize their difficulties. Dyadic relationships arouse severe anxiety in them; they usually flee from these relationships, since they are terrified of their dependency and fantasies of mutual destructiveness. Anxiety and tension are often handled by action or flight.

Chronic offenders usually demonstrate difficulties in the early latency years. Many are hyperactive and unable to learn in school. They soon become truant. The inmates in prison are those who have failed to adapt to or master early, repeated, traumatic experiences and have turned to the correctional system for assistance in controlling impulses.

Treatment Model

Any experience within the prison that is therapeutic to the inmates must relate to the issues of their profound distrust, their difficulties with impulse control, and their lack of ego skills, which include their educational failure and work history deficiencies. Since they have had minimal experiences with caring, consistent people, every contact with the prison staff can provide an opportunity to offer a new kind of relationship. In encounters with the staff, inmates are obviously wary and often distant and provocative. Their early experiences with the prison staff are a testing period to determine whether a specific staff person is consistent and truthful, keeps his promises, and does not retaliate.

The safety and controls of the prison structure help the inmate attend activities and become involved with people, from which he would flee outside of a prison. The staff contacts that become part of the inmate's prison program form the basis for an experience that stresses increasing responsibility.

Inmates' anger and provocativeness and their frequent use of projective mechanisms often set up situations that can lead to destructive confrontation. The ability of the prison staff to understand the significance of such encounters and to weather them without retaliation can set the stage for the inmate's growing capacity to find that his anger does not destroy or lead to his destruction.

The apparent lack of anxiety and depression of the inmate population when not in prison can change when they are confined. In part, their depression can be attributed to the cruel treatment that can occur in prison, their isolation from family members, and their loss of freedom. However, psychotherapeutic work with inmates reveals that this depression also emerges in treatment at the point that they trust their therapist sufficiently to uncover their sense of hopelessness and worthlessness. In addition, the controls in a prison setting may permit the emergence of the depression from which these inmates flee, often through antisocial activity. The quality of the human relationships within the prison then becomes crucial in helping the inmate to bear and work through this depression.

Work with families of inmates can be useful in understanding inmates' present difficulties and resolving future problems. The precipitating stress that led to the crimes of many inmates often occurred in the setting of conflicts within families.

Role of the Psychiatrist

Most psychiatrists working in prisons usually function as consultants or are part of treatment units, often separated from the rest of the prison.

Classification

If prisons wish to offer individualized programs for the inmates, an evaluative procedure is required. A psychiatrist or other mental health professional is in an excellent position to participate with the prison staff in collecting the necessary data for a complete evaluation. Such data include a thorough history that stresses the psychological issues of the inmate's life and his family, educational, and work histories.

Psychotherapeutic Treatment

In addition to the traditional forms of individual and group psychotherapy, behavioral therapy, reality therapy, conjoint family therapy, and self-help groups have been used in the prison setting. The psychiatrist can also be involved in the evaluation and management of patients receiving drugs as part of their treatment in the prison. In addition, the psychiatrist can help evolve a treatment philosophy for working with inmates who misuse drugs or demand drugs to relieve their discomfort.

Training

The psychiatrist and mental health workers provide a professional group with expertise who can serve as a training nucleus for the prison staff. The psychiatrist must be an active, real person with the prison staff, being aware of the fear and distrust that they bring into their contacts with him. Successful experience with the staff often provides the model that they can use in their work with the inmates—caring, respect, and no retaliation. Especially significant is the appreciation of their years of experience and acknowledgment of the unique difficulties of their task.

The mental health professionals within the prison can also help train psychiatric residents, social work students, and psychologists. The structured prison environment allows these students to learn to work with character problems that would often be untreatable outside the prison. Within the prison, issues of trust, confidentiality, and limit setting are seen with an unequaled clarity.

Consultations

The psychiatrist's role as consultant to the superintendent and other administrative personnel can ultimately lead to an identification with the psychiatrist's nonpunitive attitudes and empathic skills. The psychiatrist can offer specific help with the management of suicidal, assaultive, and provocative inmates, and he can use his consultations as another way of educating the staff.

Parole Evaluation

The psychiatrist who understands that many inmates implicitly requested imprisonment through repeated antisocial acts that were manifestations of their serious difficulties in society is also in a position to evaluate changes in the inmate. Although such an evaluation may be relatively crude, it includes a review of the inmate's entire prison program and functioning as well as input from the inmate himself, who can provide important data about his capacities and concerns. It is not unusual for an inmate's behavior to deteriorate before a parole hearing, a possible indication of his inability to tolerate release.

Inmates in group and individual psychotherapy programs within the prison have at times been able to work collaboratively with their therapist in writing a letter to the parole board that expresses their joint opinion about an inmate's readiness for parole, the circumstances in which he is vulnerable, and specific treatment recommendations if parole is granted. Sometimes parole boards make outpatient treatment a mandatory condition of parole based on such letters. When these recommendations convey an understanding of the character problems and ego defects of the inmate, they can lead to a treatment program outside the prison that would otherwise fail.

Innovation

The psychiatrist can assist the staff, inmates, and administration in thinking through the details of innovative programs. In the past decade, increasingly flexible programs have been available to the inmate within the prison structure—halfway houses, work and educational release programs, furloughs, prolonged family visits, and use of former prisoners as personnel in the treatment programs. Each new venture arouses anxieties. The psychiatrist's understanding and his trusting relationships with inmates, staff, and administration can help with the resolution of conflicts and can lead to the implementation of promising programs.

Countertransference

A prison setting that is dominated by a punitive philosophy is especially difficult for a psychiatrist whose training has emphasized humanistic aspects of caring and respect for people. When he sees inmates degraded by personnel, whose sadism may be aroused in part by provocative and sadistic behavior of the inmate, the psychiatrist may feel furious and wish to turn these incidents into confrontations with the administration. However, such responses usually lead to a very short career as a prison psychiatrist.

In his anger at cruelty that he may observe and occasionally experience, the psychiatrist may overidentify with the inmate. By doing so, not only is he potentially harming his relationship with the staff and administration, but he is putting himself in a position that may not be helpful to the inmates. The way in which the psychiatrist manages his own frustration provides a crucial model for the inmate in handling anger and tension.

Another pitfall for the prison psychiatrist is the ease with which it is possible to identify with punitive tendencies of some personnel and inmates. The regressive group phenomenon that can occur in work with provocative inmates or staff can elicit a sadistic side in the psychiatrist. An overidentification with either group places the psychiatrist in a position that heightens its concerns about his neutrality and integrity.

The hopelessness and helplessness of the prisoners, the rigidity of most prison systems, and the apparent lack of change or slow pace of change within the inmates and within the prison personnel can lead to depression in the prison psychiatrist. He may become rigid and nonproductive, similar to many of the people about whom he has felt critical, or he may leave his job and return to a setting where he feels respected and appreciated and where he can see more tangible fruits of his work. Few psychiatrists remain in full-time prison work unless the therapeutic and administrative responsibility they are given or strive for results in a program that verifies their sense of competence, worth, and self-respect.

REFERENCES

Adler, G., and Shapiro, L. N. Psychotherapy with prisoners. In *Current Psychiatric Therapies*. J. Masserman, editor, vol. 9, p. 99. Grune & Stratton, New York, 1969.

Bernabeau, E. P. Underlying ego mechanisms in delinquency. Psychoanal. Q., *27:* 383, 1958.

Halleck, S. L. *Psychiatry and the Dilemmas of Crime*. Harper & Row, New York, 1967.

Kopolow, L. E. A review of major implications of the *O'Connor v. Donaldson* decision. Am. J. Psychiatry, *133:* 4, 1976.

Parker, T. *The Frying-Pan: A Prison and Its Prisoners*. Basic Books, New York, 1970.

Stabenau, J. R., and Pollin, W. Comparative life history differences of families of schizophrenics, delinquents, and "normals." Am. J. Psychiatry, *124:* 1526, 1968.

Stürup, G. K. *Treating the "Untreatable": Chronic Criminals at Herstedvester*. Johns Hopkins Press, Baltimore, 1968.

Vaillant, G. E. Sociopathy as a human process. Mass. J. Ment. Health, *3:* 4, 1973.

50

Administrative Psychiatry

Introduction

Four major conceptual frameworks have been used in thinking about the administration of human organizations: administration as a technological system, administration as a system for policy formulation and decision making, administration as a social process, and administration as a system of responsibility and accountability. All these approaches are intertwined. There may be emphasis placed on one or another, depending on the system involved and on the style and personality of the administrator.

Cost effectiveness in any organization can never be forgotten, and it is becoming more and more prominent in the evaluation and appraisal of institutions for psychiatric care. If many minds are at work in policy development and decision making, this process is usually regarded as a democratic approach worthy of commendation, since in therapeutic organizations the freedom of persons and groups to participate is regarded as a factor in the health and morale of both the persons and the organization. Administration as a social process, which emphasizes the human point of view and the individuality of the people working in the organization, is likely to appeal to psychiatric administrators particularly. In a system of responsibility and accountability, the emphasis is on external relations of the organization.

Or all systems may be regarded as unstable, with disturbances arising from internal or external stresses.

Psychiatrists may find some comfort in viewing the system as an organism subject to health and disease. Like a psychiatrist, a social system clinician may study the system, make a diagnosis as to its needs and problems, identify areas of tension within people and between sections in the organization, bring these groups together, and help them to express problems, to face the sensitive areas in their work, and to become freer with themselves and each other.

The physician trained as a psychiatrist has certain assets when he undertakes the administrative role; on the other hand, his specialty training and professionalism may hamper him. On the positive side is the fact that psychiatric training makes the psychiatrist more sensitive to interpersonal dynamics and more competent to handle interpersonal stresses. On the negative side, the role of an administrator involves qualities for which the psychiatrist is not necessarily trained, or he may be unfit by nature for some critical functions. He is more likely to comprehend individual or small groups than a large system.

Areas of Concern

Law and Psychiatry

No conscientious psychiatric administrator can function nowadays without a thorough mastery of the laws of his locale as to admission and discharge procedures and the rights of patients. He must also know Civil Service laws, rules and regulations protecting employees, and the statutes regulating collective bargaining procedures. In addition, he benefits by studying the mechanisms in his area for the introduction and passage of new legislation, for he may desire to alter or amend existing statutes or to introduce new ones.

Business Administration and Budget

In any organization, efficient business administration is vital to the smooth delivery of services. A business manager of high quality, adequate experience, impeccable integrity, and great flexibility must be appointed to look after supplies, budget and cost control, personnel, physical plant, and other such items supporting direct clinical care. The business executive must take his direction from the over-all administrative head of the institution or organization, usually a clinician. Under no circumstances should final decisions regarding patient care and treatment be left purely to business personnel. Business personnel should be brought early into planning and strategy sessions, so that they may learn how the supervising administrator thinks and what variables and values enter into his decisions.

Budget preparation usually has two components: above-downward guidelines and below-upward preparation. Guidelines emanating from above outline broad policy goals and make fundamental decisions about the over-all distribution of resources. However, detailed budget preparation requires input from persons involved in direct services. Priorities in the final budget should be established by the facility director.

To achieve flexibility, the good administrator attempts to diversify his sources of income. It behooves him, therefore, to become acquainted with all possible sources of aid and to generate projects that will compete successfully for this aid.

Personnel Practices and Labor Relations

Personnel now contributing to the mental health scene are of two types: professionals and nonprofessionals. Professionals seek to develop and enlarge a body of knowledge and theory that pertains to the skills needed to practice in their field, promulgate standards for education and training, promote speciality examinations, confer degrees or certificates, and promulgate rules of conduct. Their loyalties, therefore, are always twofold—to the organization that employs them and to the professional organization with which they are identified or affiliated. The practical administrator recognizes this split loyalty as a fact of life and tries to be aware of the philosophy of each professional organization, its goals and aspirations, and the expectations it may have of its members.

The nonprofessionals in a treatment organization are frequently neglected. Morale is inclined to be low, pay less than adequate, and possibilities for advancement meager or nonexistent. All echelons of workers in a therapeutic organization ought to be in some type of in-service training to maximize their output and to elevate morale. The conscientious executive recognizes the need for education and training involving the broadest possible base of workers.

The executive must enter into regular agreements or contracts that bind him to look after the rights of labor. He can accede to many requests of workers, but he cannot bargain away his basic management rights to administer his organization in the highest professional tradition of service to patients. The conscientious administrator should bring labor into his plans and gain their endorsement, he should bargain in good faith, and he should remain firm where management rights are concerned.

Citizen Involvement

Citizens have served in mental health on three levels: as volunteers, board members, and community groups.

Experience has proved the worth of volunteers as aides to social workers, nurses, laboratory workers, and secretaries; in the organization and leadership of halfway houses and community homes; and in home treatment services.

Board members may be appointed by governors, commissioners, or superintendents, or they may gain office through municipal or county election. They usually receive no compensation, although expenses may be defrayed and a token honorarium is often provided. They serve as advisors, consultants in policy development, visitors to facilities, critics, fund raisers, community ambassadors, guardians of public funds, watchdogs for patient and employee rights, and contributors of their own money and material for good patient care and treatment. They may have participated in the selection of the administrator and he may have to account to them for his conduct in office. On the other hand, they may be purely advisory, with only moral suasion as their main vehicle.

Independent community groups whose concern for the mentally ill is their essential or chief motif and whose role is active advocate on their behalf may be either supporter of administrative plans or friendly adversaries. These organizations include thousands of mental health associations, mental retardation associations, friends and auxiliaries of hospitals, friends of halfway houses and community houses and day centers, associations for mentally ill children, and friends of patient groups of every description. These groups may question the relevance of services given to the needs of the community; the proportion of minority groups, especially blacks and Spanish-speaking people, who receive services or who are hired as personnel to give services; the nature of the collaboration between the professional and the citizen group, especially as it pertains to power in policy development and final decision; and the tactics of change. The administrator must try to work with the most representative, the most rational, and the strongest of the various community elements and to point out the necessity of getting all the community groups together to speak to him with one voice.

Public Relations

Public relations may be divided into internal and external. Internal relations refers to morale and the job satisfaction of people in the employ of the facility. Loyalty, identification, and satisfaction must be cultivated. Discussions by the administrator with employees, a news sheet or house organ to carry messages and communications, public recognition of employees who distinguish themselves on the job, letters of acknowledgment to employees who have won acclaim in the community, and letters of sympathy to those who have suffered misfortune —these yield a substantial return in morale and commitment of workers.

In external public relations and education, the task is to educate the average man to a better understanding of mental disorder, its causes and treatment, and to provide a receptive climate for changing attitudes and reducing the stigma of mental disease. Factual information regarding the facilities that serve the mentally ill must be disseminated and a positive climate established. The application of psychiatric knowledge to such social problems as alcoholism, prejudice, divorce, and deliquency is a continuing interest of the public education effort.

The administrator and the staff of a mental health facility ought to become acquainted with the important members of the press, radio, and television who are responsible for news in their area. All communications ought to be clear, factual, and balanced. When confronted with criticism, the spokesman for the clinic must acknowledge to what extent the criticisms are justified and then present plans for corrective action.

Administrative Styles, Procedures, and Techniques

The basic principles of organizational dynamics include the following: the equating of authority with responsibility, the establishment of clean lines of communication and accountability, the recognition of the practical limits to the span of control, and the centralization of ultimate authority. However, organizations take many forms, and administrators are susceptible to many styles and techniques. As the size of the organization increases, messages must be transmitted through longer and longer lines of communication. The opportunity to meet personally and intimately with the workers diminishes as the organization grows. Large systems become ponderous, respond slowly, are less able to absorb innovation or creative ideas, and rely more heavily on formal structure, delegation of authority, reporting, and accountability.

Tight administrative style is characterized as involving clear-cut delegations of authority and responsibility; an orderly and hierarchical chain of command through which communication flows upward and downward without skipping levels; reliance on formal communication, such as regular meetings, reports, and printed forms; formal expressions of power, such as hearings and written notifications of promotions and dismissals; and reliance on written, explicit rules or on tradition.

By contrast, loose administrative style is characterized by the absence in many areas of clearly designated authority and responsibility; considerable tolerance of role ambiguity and role diffusion; frequent bypassing of the chain of command, both in communications and in authority; informal communication; informal exercise of power; and relatively little reliance on rules and tradition.

Stresses, Strains, and Rewards

Administration is a new world of theory and practice for which one is ill-prepared by the type of formal training granted to professionals in the mental health field. Furthermore, the higher one goes up the management ladder, the more one moves away from the center of professional interest—namely, direct patient care, teaching, and research. The physical and mental demands related to an active, changing organization may be great. The executive must have a lot of regenerative energy, if not boundless and robust health, and a capacity for rapid recovery from frustrations and disappointments so that he can help his staff accept hard realities and move on with vigor. Most professionals shun the limelight to discourage public criticism, especially if given by nonprofessionals ill-equipped to judge them. The administrator is subject to scrutiny by legislative bodies or boards of control, the press, families, mental health associations, and other agencies.

The leader risks the progressive erosion of his reputation. He may be caught in political cross fires between adversary political parties. And he faces a brief tenure and a somewhat uncertain future.

The rewards are the intellectual challenge and joy of mastering new material, the broadening of one's horizons over a larger sector of one's field, the perspective on large areas of health in relation to its sociopolitical determinants, centrality in the arena of action and decision, the power to do a great deal of good for patients and families and colleagues, the control of vast resources, the honing of one's judgment, the greater call on one's personal capacities for performance and achievement.

REFERENCES

Barton, W. E. *Administration in Psychiatry.* Charles C Thomas, Springfield, Ill., 1962.

Barton, W. E. The hospital administrator. Ment. Hosp., *13:* 259, 1962.

Greenblatt, M., Sharaf, M. R., and Stone, E. M. *Dynamics of Institutional Change.* University of Pittsburg Press, Pittsburg, 1971.

Hirschowitz, R. G. Dilemmas of leadership in community mental health. Psychiatr. Q. *45:* 22, 1971.

McGarry, A. L. Overview: Current trends in mental health. Am. J. Psychiatry, *130:* 621, 1973.

Sayre, W. S. Principles of administration. Hospitals, *30:* 34, 1956.

51

Contemporary Issues in Psychiatry

51.1. PSYCHOHISTORY

Freudian Models

Freud's most fundamental historical model is really a prehistorical paradigm: the primeval encounter between father and sons, in which the sons rebel against the father's authority and kill him, with the entire encounter psychologically centered on the Oedipus complex. This model was first put forward in *Totem and Taboo* as an explanation for the origins of society itself and then again in modified form toward the end of Freud's life in *Moses and Monotheism* to account for the origins of Jewish religion and Jewish identity. Freud saw Moses as a kind of foster father, an Egyptian who chose the Jews as his people and gave to them the gift of monotheism, only to be rejected and murdered by his chosen people, his symbolic sons.

Within Freud's prehistorical paradigm there is an iron mold of psychological repetition or repetition-compulsion, enveloping indiscriminately the individual person and the undifferentiated collectivity. When this principle of repetition is seen as the essence of historical experience, there can be nothing new in history.

The second Freudian paradigm is perhaps the more obvious one, the one most likely to come to mind when people think of a psychoanalytic approach to history; that of individual psychopathology. The best known example here is the Bullitt-Freud biography of Woodrow Wilson, a work that Bullitt almost certainly wrote but that exemplifies the Freudian approach. The idea of interpreting the outcomes of major historical events as expressions of the individual psychopathology of a particular national leader, in this case Wilson's struggles with mascu-

linity and his need to fail, was prefigured in Freud's own work—not only in his treatment of men like Leonardo and Dostoevski but also in his general focus on individual psychopathology as existing more or less apart from history. When this second paradigm dominates, the psychopathological idiom for individual development becomes extended to the point where it serves as the idiom for history or psychohistory. When this happens, there is, once more, no history.

These two Freudian paradigms, the prehistorical confrontation and the leader's individual psychopathology, come together in their assumption that, in one way or another, history represents the intrapsychic struggles of the individual person writ large. For instance, the scenario of *Totem and Taboo* includes not only the murderous rebellion against the father and the consuming of the father in the totem feast but the subsequent remorse and residual guilt of the sons and of their sons and daughters ad infinitum, a guilt that reasserts itself periodically in the phenomenon of the return of the repressed. The entire argument derives from an individual psychological model, and the return of the repressed becomes the basis for Freud's view of history as psychological recurrence. And in the individual psychopathological model, it is the aberration of a specific person that is writ large as historical explanation.

No wonder, then, that Freudian models are frustrating to the historian. They interpret but avoid history.

Erikson and the Great Man in History

Erik Erikson has retained a focus on the individual—the great man—and on the kinds of inner conflicts illuminated by the Freudian tradition. But he has placed the great man and psychobiography itself within a specific historical context—the prominent individual in history. With Erikson's elaboration of this paradigm, something approaching a new psychohistory began to take shape.

Erikson's *Young Man Luther* has a direct historical relation to Freud's *Moses and Monotheism*. Freud and Erikson both depicted the great man as a spiritual hero, as a man who achieves an intrapsychic breakthrough.

But Erikson also took several crucial steps away from Freud. Instead of an instinctual idiom—Freud's view of the great man as appealing to instinctual wishes, particularly aggressive ones, and possessing the ability to bring about in the masses a form of instinctual renunciation—Erikson has sought out more specifically historical ground, the intersection of individual and collective histories. Of concern is the great man's monumental struggles with his simultaneous efforts to remake himself and his world. For Luther to emerge from his own identity crisis, he had to bring about a shift in the historical identity of his epoch.

Erikson is forced to recreate certain psychological themes of Luther's early life on the basis of very limited evidence. Problems have also been raised about events in Luther's adult life. And there is the larger question of the extent to which any person, great or otherwise, can exemplify an entire historical epoch or even its major collective psychological struggles.

Shared Themes Model

A recent approach is that of shared psychohistorical themes, as observed in men and women exposed to particular kinds of individual and collective experience. Examples here are Keniston's studies of alienated and then activist American students and Robert Coles's work with children and adults in the midst of racial antagonism and social change.

The shared-themes approach is based on a psychoanalytically derived stress on what goes on inside of people. It moves outward from the individual person in the direction of collective historical experience. It explicitly rejects the 19th century scientific model of man as a mechanism propelled by quantities of energy— energy internally generated by means of instinctual drives, partially held in check by certain defense mechanisms, notably repression, but eventually erupting in the form of various actions of the person directed at his outer environment.

The method is partly empirical, in its stress on specific data from interviews; partly phenomenological or formative, in its stress on forms and images that are simultaneously individual and collective; and partly speculative, in its use of interview data, together with many other observations, to posit relations between man and his history and to suggest concepts that eliminate the artificial separation of the two.

All shared behavior is seen as simultaneously involved in a trinity of universality (that which is related to the psychobiological quests of all men in all historical epochs), specific cultural emphasis and style (as evolved by a particular people over centuries), and recent and contemporary historical influences (the part of the trinity most likely to be neglected in psychological work).

REFERENCES

Bromberg, N. Hitler's childhood. Int. Rev. Psychoanal., 1974
Coles R. *Children of Crisis*, 3 vols. Atlantic-Little, Brown, Boston, 1967–1971.
Erikson, E. H. *Young Man Luther: A Study in Psychoanalysis and History*. W. W. Norton, New York, 1958.
Freud, S. *Moses and Monotheism*. In *Standard Edition of the Complete Psychological Works of Sigmund Freud*, vol. 23. Hogarth Press, London, 1939.
Keniston, K. *The Uncommitted*. Harcourt, Brace & World, New York, 1965.
Kren, G. M., and Rappoport, L. Clio and Psyche. His. Childhood Q., *1:* 151, 1973.
Lifton, R. J. *Death in Life: Survivors of Hiroshima*. Random House, New York, 1968.
Lifton, R. J. *Home From the War: Vietnam Veterans: Neither Victims nor Executioners*. Simon & Schuster, New York, 1973.
Lifton, R. J., and Olson, E., editors. *Explorations in Psychohistory: The Wellfleet Papers*. Simon & Schuster, New York, 1974.
Rieff, P. The meaning of history and religion in Freud's thought. In *Psychoanalysis and History*. B. Mazlish, editor. Grosett & Dunlap, New York, 1971.
Waite, R. G. L. *The Psychopathic God: A Biography of Adolf Hitler*. Basic Books, New York, 1974.

51.2. THE CREATIVE PROCESS

Introduction

The creator of a work of art is usually unaware in his conscious thinking of the mental processes striving for expression before or during the creative effort. Nevertheless, a number of propositions can be offered, as far as present-day knowledge regarding the creative process is concerned.

The role of the unconscious in creativity is of considerable, and in most cases decisive, import.

Human creativity is an innate endowment and, as such, is part of the patrimony of the human race. Its early development—tool making and language, for example—belongs to the realm of evolution and includes the larger problem of how man came to be man.

Creativity, in the sense of original and exceptional achievement, is a relatively rare characteristic of certain persons that, in all probability, is an innate gift. The development and full unfolding of this potential require the presence of internal and external conditions, especially in early life, the confluence of which appear to culminate in the creative process or act.

Individual experiences and influences of various kinds, among them certain types of physical and psychiatric illness, appear to stimulate artistic potentialities in a gifted person. The creative mind is able to absorb, organize or reorganize, and communicate these experiences in a way different from that of the person not thus endowed. Artistic production can be understood as an adaptive phenomenon of a special kind that, albeit rooted in and influenced by the primary process, is oriented toward reality (secondary process).

Body Feelings and Perceptions

Artist-patients who as children sustained injuries or in adulthood were exposed to experiences involving the reactivation of early traumata have shown marked alterations in body tonus and body feelings before and during periods of creative work. These alterations in body tonus have been traced to corresponding changes in self-representation. After the creative job was done, the old feelings of being physically defective and incomplete returned.

Many psychic traumata of early life find a more or less spontaneous solution through mastery in childhood. The presence of an early body defect prevents a spontaneous solution. Rather, the defect tends to remain an area of unresolved conflict through its concreteness, permanence,

narcissistic significance, and resultant cathectic maldistribution. It strongly influences self-representation and the imaginative and symbolic processes, giving rise to a florid and secretive fantasy life. The permanent injury attaches itself to the inner world of self-representations and object-representations, and it tends to intensify personal tensions and the familiar conflictual anxieties—castration fear, aggression, vengefulness, and lifelong rancor—from early life on to the point of massive influence on character formation and ego-superego development. In gifted persons, the urge toward bodily reparation frequently takes the path of creative restitution.

Object Loss and Grief

One of the most profound influences on the creative process is the experience of loss, grief, and death. Within limits, the experience of object loss resembles that of body loss. Indeed, the earliest body and self-image appear to contain close representatives of the outer world (parents and siblings) deep inside. Thus, object loss is bound to affect body imagery and self-representation profoundly.

Object loss is the most frequent factor in the causation of depression. The disappearance of a significant figure, through prolonged absence or death, produces a feeling of body loss. The need for restitution leads to a search for the vanished object, a search that in gifted persons takes the road of creative restitution. This inner search for the lost object or objects is the unconscious force behind creative conceptualizations and the initial step in the direction of creative activity. The special danger for the artist lies in the blurring of the boundary between the self and the object representations, with a resultant break in reality testing.

The Ego

Creative productivity in any field depends on the functioning of the ego and its abilities, the convergence of which in the creative process gives a definite direction and aim to the effort. The ego controls access not only to mobility, use of language, and exercise of personal skills but also to perception, integrative thinking, cognition, volition, reality testing, problem solving, and a variety of other mental faculties. Some of these are autonomous ego functions; others stay close to the primary process, such as fantasies, imagery, and symbol formation. Parts of the ego may lag in their development or may remain fixated on early modes of functioning.

Certain ego functions appear to be better suited for creative activity, facilitating the activation of the creative potential. Restitutive-reparative tendencies can act as autoreconstructive forces. The artist's heightened perceptual and sensorial reactivity to stimuli likewise enhances the task of self-expression. Also, the capacity for symbolization, imaginative think-

ing, and feeling appears to be greater and richer in the artist than in the person not thus endowed. The ego of the artist has the capacity to communicate personal experiences and feelings by the artistic percept. The activation of the creative process is linked to the ego's ability to regress in the service of its creative (or re-creative) strivings to the deeper strata of mental functioning, reaching and tapping their repressed contents without disintegrating under the burden of this voyage into the inner world.

The act of creation may also become a vehicle

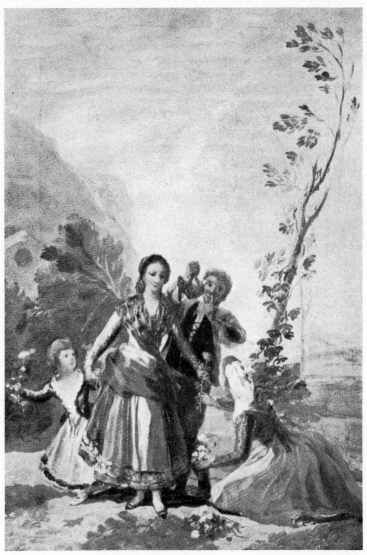

FIGURE 1. "Spring," painted by Goya (1776). (Courtesy of F. Bruckmann, Munich, Germany.)

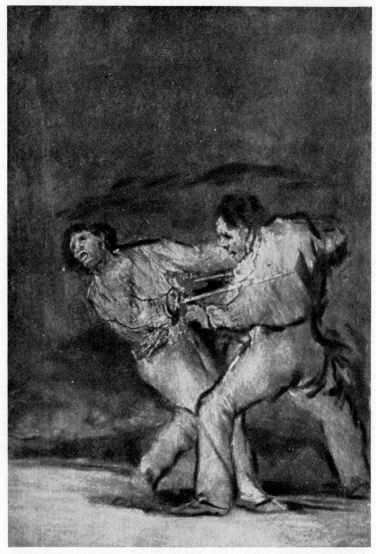

FIGURE 2. "The Duel," by Goya (1810). (Courtesy of F. A. Ackermanns Kunstverlag, Munich, Germany.)

for the discharge of aggression. The artist, by virtue of his creating something new and breaking with established patterns, is often a rebel, both feared and opposed, yet at the same time admired and envied. His regressive involvement may intensify pre-existing psychopathology but may, at the same time, provide an outlet for his conflicts. The synthetic function of the ego aids in uniting such contrasts, reconciling conflicting ideas, and promoting creative activity.

Related to this is the ego's capacity for single-mindedness, isolation, and lonely menta-tion, accompanied by a withdrawal from emotional involvements with the outer world and their replacement, in the psyche, by ideas, projects, and efforts at problem solving.

The affirmation of the artist's own and often fragile self is an important part of the outcome of the creative process. The artistic production gives assurance that the artist is able to produce something new, offers proof to the world and to himself that he is a godlike creator, and confirms his capacity to recreate himself in a perfect form.

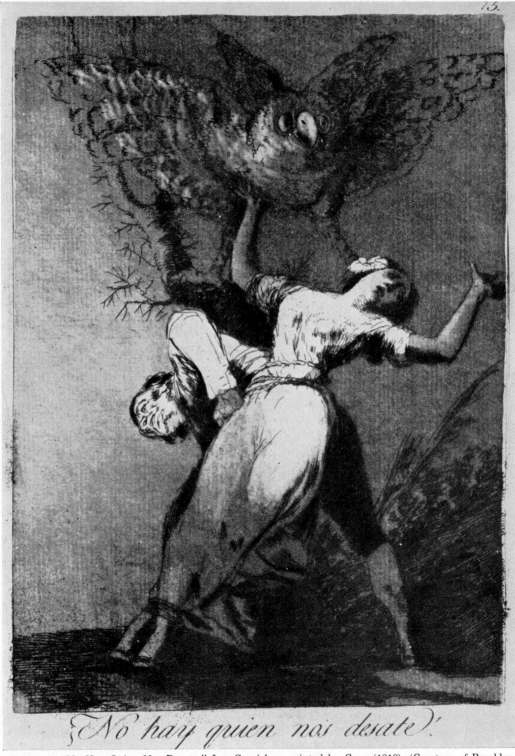

FIGURE 3. "No Hay Quien Nos Desate." Los Caprichos, painted by Goya (1810). (Courtesy of Brooklyn Museum.)

Mental Illness and Creativity

Francisco Goya, the great 18th century painter, had repeated attacks of mental and physical illness that affected his later life and work. During his later years, he suffered recurrent bouts of psychotic depression and hallucinosis. During his early life, Goya had been an outgoing, sensitive, and highly productive (nonschizoid and nondepressive) person. Art critic John Canaday notes that, as he grew older, "a new Goya emerged, Goya the humane and bitter observer, the scourging and despairing delineator of vice and cruelty whose pictures of nightmares explored the most desperate realities." This is seen in the changed nature of his work: the quiet, almost pastoral mood of "Spring" (Figure 1), painted during his younger years in 1776, compared with his later brutal works like "The Duel" and "Los Caprichos" (Figures 2 and 3), painted in 1810. The violent change and insight are dramatic and suggestive of psychosis. Most important, his mental state had been deteriorating and his productivity had been diminishing—which occurs with many artists suffering from mental illness of increasing severity—so that, for periods of several years at a time, he did not paint at all. In the past, schizophrenia and paresis have been suggested as the diseases with which Goya may have been afflicted. However, psychiatrist William Niederland, in a recent study, has concluded that lead poisoning from the white flake paint Goya used, which contained toxic lead carbonate $(2\ PbCO_3Pb(OH)_2)$, probably produced plumbism (lead poisoning) and an organic lead encephalopathy and psychosis. Goya ground his own paints and thereby inhaled, ingested, and absorbed lead. Such a chronic toxic psychosis probably was the cause of the violent change in Goya's work, his decreased productivity, and even his death. With today's modern medical and psychiatric knowledge, it probably could have been prevented or effectively treated.

Vincent Van Gogh is often given as the

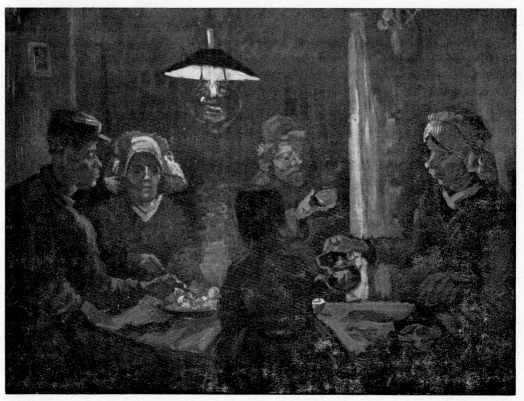

FIGURE 4. "The Potato-Eaters," by Van Gogh (1885). (Courtesy of Rijksmuseum, Kröller-Müller, Otterlo, Holland.)

classic example of schizophrenia and depression affecting an artist's creativity and productivity adversely, causing mental hospitalization, and eventual suicide. Internist Frederick Maire has recently suggested that Van Gogh suffered from glaucoma, which, as he got older, seriously impaired his vision. The knowledge that he was going blind may well have contributed to his severe depression and suicide. That Van Gogh's vision was originally normal is seen in his 1885 painting "The Potato Eaters" (Figure 4), in which one can note the clarity of the lamp light. Signs of glaucoma, suggested by the halo effects around the sun and lamps, increasingly appear in his 1890 works "The Evening" and "The Road with Cypresses." These were painted 1 year before his suicide. At this time, Van Gogh was definitely losing his vision, probably as a result of chronic glaucoma. Recurrent bouts of depressive psychosis seriously diminished his productivity and later caused his death through suicide. Proper treatment of his glaucoma would have probably helped his psychiatric status.

Maire notes that as Van Gogh approached the time when he committed suicide, his last paintings were characteristically dark, suggesting depression, loss of vision, or both.

Neither of the aforementioned studies of Goya and Van Gogh rules out the existence of a concomitant schizophrenic process but certainly blindness due to chronic glaucoma and a lead psychosis would have aggravated that process. Serious psychological disabilities may be produced or aggravated by physical, organic, or mental disturbances, which then affect creativity adversely. With proper medical and psychological treatment, these artists' diseases might well have been ameliorated and their creativity enhanced. Today, in spite of our increased psychiatric and medical knowledge, the destruction and self-destruction of some of the most creative people goes on, unabated—Ernest Hemingway, Sylvia Plath, Cesare Pavese, etc. Many of these tragic deaths might well have been avoided.

Psychiatry's contribution to the creative proc-

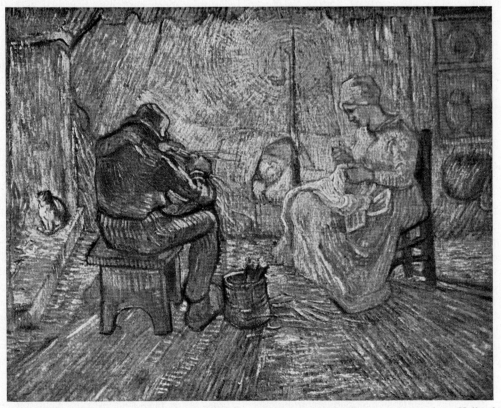

FIGURE 5. "The Evening," by Van Gogh (1889). (Courtesy of Stedelijk Museum, Amsterdam, Holland.)

ess must not only be in the area of further understanding, but also in its perpetuation. Creative people—artists, actors, actresses, writers—should be encouraged to receive adequate psychiatric and medical treatment when emotionally or physically ill, and they should be reassured that treatment will usually nurture and enhance their talent. Because there appears to be an unusually high number of emotionally disturbed individuals in the arts, such reassurance is particularly relevant. This may then allow psychiatry to make a further contribution in aiding some of the most valued members of our society.

REFERENCES

Eissler, K. R. *Leonardo da Vinci.* International Universities Press, New York, 1961.
Freud, S. The ego and the id. In *Standard Edition of the Complete Psychological Works of Sigmund Freud.* Hogarth Press, London, 1927.
Freud, S. Dostoievsky and parricide. In *Standard Edition of the Complete Psychological Works of Sigmund Freud*, vol. 5, pp. 222-242. Hogarth Press, London, 1953.
Greenacre, P. Discussion and comments on the psychology of creativity. J. Child Psychol. Psychiatry. *1:* 129, 1962.
Kubie, L. Unsolved problems concerning the relation of art to psychotherapy. Am. J. Art Ther., *2:* 95, 1973.
Niederland, W. G. Clinical aspects of creativity. Am. Imago, *24:* 6,1967.
Rickman, J. On the nature of ugliness and the creative impulse. In *Selected Contributions to Psychoanalysis*, No. 52, E. Jones, editor, p. 68. Hogarth Press, London, 1957.

51.3.   CONTEMPORARY COMMENT RELEVANT TO MENTAL HEALTH

Alvin Toffler

In *Future Shock*, Alvin Toffler (see Figure 1) —journalist, social commentator, and educator —discusses the social and psychological effects of the technological revolution that characterizes the world today. The enormously rapid changes are producing a disturbing effect on rational thinking, a phenomenon Toffler calls "future shock." Overstimulation and the future shock it produces are evidence in the confusional breakdown in society, the increasingly widespread use of drugs, the rise of mysticism, violence, vandalism, the politics of nihilism, and a pathological apathy and withdrawal in millions of people. This decisional stress and sensory and cognitive overload are producing individual, group, and societal maladaptation.

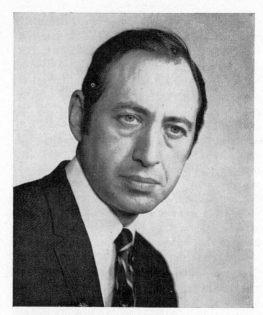

FIGURE 1. Alvin Toffler.

Toffler recommends that people halt the runaway acceleration of society that is producing future shock and that they deal with the problems of ecology, racism, and the revolt of the young. He suggests the possibility of a future-oriented therapy, in which the patient's images of the future are systematically examined for insight into his value system, his fears, and his conflicts.

Kenneth Keniston

In *The Uncommitted*, psychologist Kenneth Keniston (see Figure 2) reports on his study of a group of affluent white undergraduate students at Harvard University who were judged to be severely alienated when evaluated by psychological tests. These students were similar to those alienated youths studied in other sections of society, such as the poor blacks in anthropologist Elliot Liebow's *Talley's Corner*. By alienation, Keniston means that these youths have no connection with their past and no commitment or optimism about the future. They live only in the present, for the present experience. The fathers of these alienated youths were viewed as weak by their children, and their mothers were viewed as dominant women who fragmented their children's self-images into negative self-definitions. The youths turned to fantasy as a means of escape. Keniston sees the cause of this alienation in society's blind acceptance of and drive for change and accomplishment.

Erving Goffman

In his exploration of man as a social being, sociologist Erving Goffman is concerned primarily with personal interaction, nonverbal communication, and the dynamics of people in small group situations. Goffman regards patients as people who have broken both the obvious and the hidden rules of society in such a flagrant manner that they have had to be removed from that society. At the core of mental disorder, says Goffman, is failure to abide by the rules of social interaction. Goffman describes how institutions—and here he means convents, jails, and orphanages, as well as mental hospitals—manipulate the individual person and help transform the self into something public and objective.

Departing from the study of mental illness and stigmatized people, Goffman turns to everyday life, distinguishing important components of human interaction that he calls "gatherings." These are such informal and often fleeting encounters as those in elevator rides, cocktail parties, and passings on the street, in which Goffman says there is a strict formal

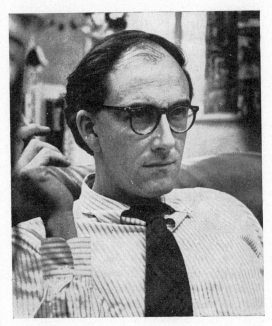

FIGURE 2. Kenneth Keniston. (Courtesy of Charles Moore, Black Star.)

structure. This social theory rests on the notion that all human beings subscribe to fundamental assumptions about unspoken rules underlying even the most insignificant event.

Claude Lévi-Strauss

Anthropologist Claude Lévi-Strauss is the father of structuralism, a method of scientific investigation, a search of "unsuspected harmonies . . . the discovery of a system of relations in a series of objects." Just as the linguist seeks to discover fundamental patterns in all languages and the biologist uses information from the genetic code to explain natural phenomena, Lévi-Strauss tries to find universal laws of human nature.

Likening the human brain to a computer, Lévi-Strauss postulates that the so-called mysteries of human nature are really as yet undiscovered response-and-stimulus patterns. In fact, he says, even the newborn infant has the information codes necessary for discovering all possible kin and myth systems. Thus, man's behavior is not freely initiated; rather, it is a function of the biological structures of his mind.

REFERENCES

Goffman, E. *The Presentation of Self in Everyday Life.* Doubleday, New York, 1959.

Keniston, K. *The Uncommitted: Alienated Youth in American Society.* Harcourt, Brace and World, New York, 1966.

Lévi-Strauss, C. *The Savage Mind.* University of Chicago Press, Chicago, 1962.

Lévi-Strauss, C. *The Elementary Structures of Kinship.* Beacon Press, Boston, 1967.

Liebow, E. *Talley's Corner: A Study of Streetcorner Men.* Little, Brown, Boston, 1967.

Reich, C. *The Greening of America.* Random House, New York, 1971.

Toffler, A. *Future Shock.* Random House, New York, 1971.

51.4. POLITICS

Introduction

The effect of psychiatry on the formulation of public policy and the impact of the political process on psychiatry occur on many levels and in many ways. Psychiatrists and political leaders interact with each other in all the world's power structures, from the World Health Organization to the county board of supervisors. Psychiatrists are called on to advise groups of nations on regional problems of drug abuse, and psychiatrists seek changed program goals or expanded financing from national governments.

International Level

At the pinnacle of international health politics is, at least in theory, the United Nations World Health Organization (WHO). Although its first Director General, Brock Chisholm of Canada, was a psychiatrist, WHO until very recently devoted most of its resources to what it considered the world's most pressing health problems, the struggle against infectious disease and the training of health manpower. In recent years, however, it has recognized the growing importance of mental health as a problem area; in consequence, psychiatrists have come to play a more prominent role in formulating its policies.

Mutinational Level

Because the world is big and diverse, regional groupings of nations have increasingly banded together to focus on problems specific to their regions, including problems of health. Two multinational psychopolitical initiatives may be mentioned, one in the Atlantic area and the other in the Pacific.

In November 1969, the North Atlantic Treaty Organization (NATO) formed a Committee on Challenges for Modern Society (CCMS). Among the several projects adopted by CCMS for study is the rehabilitation of the drug addict. In February 1972, representatives of the United States National Institute of Mental Health (NIMH) presented eight proposals dealing with addict rehabilitation at a CCMS-sponsored meeting. Two of the proposed subprojects, exchange of information and technology for screening urine for drugs of abuse and exchange of information on medical treatment of adverse reactions and toxic drug states, have been initiated.

On the other side of the world, the Pacific Rim Educational Programs for Mental Health (PREP) was organized in June 1973 as a voluntary, nongovernmental, noninstitutional association of mental health educators from Pacific nations. PREP, which is now developing exchanges of information and ideas, seeks to increase communication among mental health educators throughout the Pacific area and to strengthen cooperation among mental health

professionals in medicine, nursing, psychology, social work, and related disciplines.

Bilateral Level

The most publicized of NIMH's bilateral agreements for cooperation in psychiatric research and mental health-related activities is with the Soviet Union. As a result of a 1972 United States-Soviet Union agreement, an NIMH delegation held meetings in September 1972 with senior Soviet scientists in Moscow to discuss the possibilities of joint research in schizophrenia. The delegates agreed to try to standardize the diagnostic descriptions of schizophrenia in its main forms. Advances have already been made in this area through the participation of nine countries, including the Soviet Union and the United States, in a major schizophrenia research program sponsored by WHO and NIMH.

National Level

In 1966 and 1969, the Senate Foreign Relations Committee held hearings on the psychological aspects of international relations and foreign policy. Both hearings were concerned with general psychological principles that may contribute to the conduct of foreign policy and with methods for reducing antagonism among diverse cultural groups.

That political leaders are as susceptible to emotional disturbances as are ordinary citizens and that such disturbances may adversely affect the commonweal has long been recognized, but psychiatrists have written very little about this problem. One of the most recent studies of mental disability in the leader and perhaps the most comprehensive was the Group for the Advancement of Psychiatry's January 1973 report, "The VIP with Psychiatric Impairment."

The question of a candidate's psychiatric fitness for national office has come to the fore in two recent Presidential elections. In 1964, the Republican contender's emotional stability was questioned by word of mouth and in a magazine, against which Senator Barry Goldwater later brought and won a libel action. When a 1972 Democratic Vice Presidential candidate, Senator Thomas F. Eagleton, acknowledged that he had previously been hospitalized for depression and had received shock treatments, psychiatrists almost unanimously confined themselves to general and impersonal comments on depression and its treatment in answering press queries.

An important method of public policy formulation that may involve the psychiatrist is the government commission. Presidential and Congressional commissions are usually formed in response to growing public concern about an issue, which is often catalyzed by the personal interest of a powerful public figure. Once a commission report has been completed, its acceptance depends on whether the commission had the necessary representation to study a problem from all viewpoints and on whether the commission members are considered moderate.

Territorial Issues

Alcoholism and drug abuse have been linked to mental health because they are considered character disorders, yet there are conflicts over definition, therapeutic approaches, programing, and funding among those who say their primary allegiance is to alcoholism, drug abuse, or mental health. The same differing perspectives cut across mental health problems common to all ages, such as schizophrenia, in that some would focus on the mental health of the aging, others on that of adults, and still others on that of children.

Social Issues

Black militants and some physicians think in terms of black mental health; a few women's liberationists set up exclusive categories for women. These special perceptions no doubt have considerable validity, but one may question whether blacks or women in general have mental health problems more peculiar to their groups than the problems that subgroups among blacks and women share with comparable subgroups in the general population.

Behavioral Issues

Every few years several leading social issues of the time seem to become focused in one issue, which may be quite specific and have seemingly little relevance to the broader issues. Such symbolic issues have been called "lightning rods," since they often serve as rallying points for broader problems. In the late 1960's one lightning rod was marijuana. A smaller lightning rod has been violence on television, a reflection in some minds of the violence prevalent in American life. One lightning rod of the early 1970's is psychosurgery, which is a symbol for the pervasive thought control and invasion of privacy that many Americans now fear.

Ethical Issues

The professions have historically drawn up their own ethical codes and disciplined their own members, but their growing impact on society and the failure of some professional bodies to ensure the ethical behavior of their members and to keep their ethical principles abreast of changing political, economic, and social conditions indicate that nonprofessionals may increasingly intervene in professional ethical questions. Senator Edward M. Kennedy, chairman of the Senate Subcommittee on Health, proposed an amendment to the Public Health Service Act that would establish a commission for the protection of human subjects of biomedical research in the Department of Health, Education, and Welfare.

The American Psychiatric Association promulgated the first set of ethical principles specifically for psychiatrists. The principles were in the form of annotations to the American Medical Association's Code of Medical Ethics. Most of the annotations dealt with physician-patient relationships, but several touched on the psychiatrist's behavior in the wider arena of public life.

Extensive attention was given in the code to the question of confidentiality. The code directed that, when a patient authorized the release of confidential information, the psychiatrist should "disclose only information that is immediately relevant to a given situation." The code endorsed a psychiatrist's efforts to resist disclosure of unnecessary data when a court ordered the surrender of information.

The touchy area of public statements by psychiatrists about nonpsychiatric subjects was also dealt with: Psychiatrists should avoid cloaking their public statements with the authority of their profession.

REFERENCES

American Psychiatric Association. *Annotations in the American Medical Association's Code of Medical Ethics.* American Psychiatric Association, Washington, 1973.

Brown B. S., Sirotkin, P. L., and Stockdill, J. W. Psychopolitical perspectives on Federal-state relationships. Am. J. Psychother. 23 645, 1969.

Brown, B. S., Wienchowski, L. A., and Bivens, L. W. *Psycosurgery: Perspective on A Current Issue.* United States Government Printing Office, Washington, 1973.

Group for the Advancement of Psychiatry. *The VIP with Psychiatric Impairment.* Group for the Advancement of Psychiatry, New York, 1973.

National Advisory Commission on Civil Disorders. *Report.* Bantam Books, New York, 1968.

National Commission on the Causes and Prevention of Violence. *To Establish Justice, To Insure Domestic Tranquility.* United States Government Printing Office Washington, 1969.

51.5.   SOCIAL VIOLENCE AND AGGRESSION

Conflict Theory

Research analysts have frequently attempted to break conflict processes down into classifications of properties or typologies or into alternative methods of resolution. Types of information frequently used as organizing variables in analyzing conflicts are: type of conflict, cultural context, data concerning parties involved, history of the conflict and relationship between the parties, costs and benefits of each party, reality or lack of reality of the substance, and mode of intervention.

Some propose that intrapsychic, interpersonal, intergroup, and international conflicts involve the same processes and can benefit from the same analysis. Others insist that the types be separated for analysis on the grounds that little is known as yet about the possibly significant impact of intrapersonal factors on the various types of social conflict. Are groups in conflict affected by pathology in the individual members, indicating psychological analysis, or are they tossed by the winds of social change, indicating economic and political analysis?

Perhaps the most visible consensus underlying theory at this time concerns the validity of transactional approaches in considering conflict. Such an approach assumes that there are multiple causes and sources of behavior outcomes and also assumes that responsive behavior is interlinked in an action-reaction-action cycle, rather than in a two-step action-response behavior. Further, it involves different realms of interacting stimuli—personal, group, and cultural systems meshing with each other and with the external problems (see Figures 1 and 2).

Conflict Regulation by Intervention

Methods for controlling or regulating conflict have been identified as arbitration, mediation, conciliation, negotiation, inquiry, legislation, judicial settlement, informal consensus, the market, violence or force, authoritative command, and varieties of voting procedures. There is general agreement that the particular mode of regulation must be adapted to the nature of the conflict.

The attempt to regulate a conflict by the intervention of a third party flows naturally from an understanding that, left to his own devices, each party to a dispute is motivated only to win his objective.

Conflict regulation is possible only when conflicting sides are organized, united, and responsive to leadership. Weak structure or no structure invites challenges to any agreement made and opens the way for hardliners to object to any compromise. Also, the best chance for the success of intervention occurs when the parties are strongly sensitive to public opinion and are motivated to respond to public attitudes. If the society is already polarized and the disputants appeal to different polarized segments, the problem of resolution becomes very difficult.

Functions of Intervenors

The functions of a conciliating intervenor include easing tensions so that negotiations can begin and the suggestion of measures that may reduce provocative stimuli. In appropriate cases, the conciliator may suggest that amnesty be granted to those involved in illegalities as an inducement to begin negotiations on substantive matters.

The mediator is considered particularly well-endowed if he is seen by all parties to represent the public interest. The moral authority of the public's stake in the conflict can make it possible for parties to the conflict to moderate their stands without losing face or appearing weak.

The mediator should attempt to persuade both sides in the bargaining of desirable reciprocity—a balancing of gains and losses for both sides. The mediator must be able to define the realistic situation to each side, so that neither is tempted to act irrationally or nonrationally. The mediator must be prepared to deal

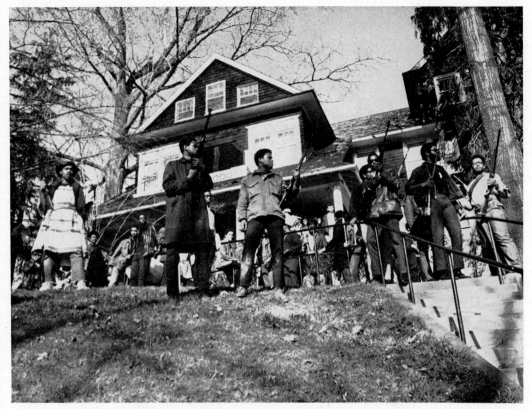

FIGURE 1. Heavily armed black college students guard a building taken overy by students. (Courtesy of Wide World Photos.)

with biased perceptions, distorted communication, and competitive group formations.

The mediator can be a viaduct of information. He can establish physical contacts between adversaries and act as moderator during the initial phase of strong language and immovable position. The mediator can make up an agenda and rules of procedure for negotiations and can suggest terms of agreement that neither side can suggest openly for fear of appearing weak or giving in.

The mediator tries to limit the boundaries of the dispute, even to fractionate it. The mediator may attempt to assess costs for each party and inform the parties so that they can act in their own best interest. His function is not only to help the parties to arrive at a settlement but to terminate the crisis so as to avoid or reduce the threat of violence.

Extended Use and Practice

Institutionalization of the intervention process provides recognition that certain forms of protest are legitimate, provides continued interaction between the parties, and provides regularized procedures for handling changes in goals, power, and conditions in society.

On the international level, relatively few resource people are both talented and trained for the job of intervention. The International Peace Academy has carried out several pilot projects of training and educating representatives sent from many nations to learn peace-related arts and techniques. Its mission is to provide professional training in the arts and sciences of peace.

On the interpersonal level, facilities are localized and are often not able to meet the demand for service. Family and social service agencies are available for help in resolving family conflicts in most metropolitan areas, but auxiliary social services are generally undermanned and overloaded. The National Center for Dispute Settlement, established in 1968 as a division of the American Arbitration Association, provides arbitration services for the settlement of any

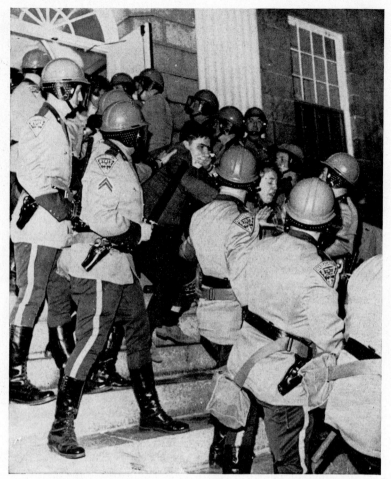

FIGURE 2. State police armed with clubs evict two students from a university building which they held illegally overnight. (Courtesy of Wide World Photos.)

serious dispute—between landlord and tenant, between neighbors, between seller and buyer—-and, under special agreements with the municipal courts, can arbitrate minor criminal cases (misdemeanors) out of court if the parties agree to it.

On a community or intergroup level more has been done to train intervenors than on other levels. The Community Crisis Intervention Center, in St. Louis, and the Community Relations Service, operating mostly within the United States Department of Justice, have played important roles in providing both research support and intervention service in racial and minority group conflicts within many communities. At least 10 nonprofit organizations have been founded since 1960 to provide services or training of mediators for intervention at the community level.

Brainwashing

Definition

Brainwashing is any technique designed to control or manipulate a person's thoughts, feelings, or behavior against the desire, will, or knowledge of the individual involved. Unlike propaganda or advertising, which uses suggestion, brainwashing relies upon both mental and physical coercion to compel or force a person into new ways of thinking, feeling, or behaving.

History

Brainwashing recently came to the attention of the American public in the case of Patricia Hearst, who was accused of various crimes, and was defended by the lawyer F. Lee Bailey, who claimed that she had been the subject of a type of brainwashing—coercive persuasion—which had influenced her behavior. Varieties of brainwashing or coercive persuasion have been recorded throughout history such as the inquisitorial techniques of the auto-da-fé of the Spanish inquisition of the 15th century; the successful attempts by the Nazis during World War II to obtain startling confessions from prisoners; and more recently, the brainwashing used on United States prisoners of war by the Chinese communists in the Korean and Vietnamese wars. Indeed, most credit for perfecting the techniques used in brainwashing is given to the Chinese communists who not only coined the term, but also used the technique extensively on their own people after Mao Tse-tung conquered the mainland in 1949. In so-called "revolutionary universities" thousands of Chinese were introduced into forced indoctrination programs called "thought reform and ideological remolding." Nor is brainwashing unknown to the Russians, who devised their own techniques, which involved the use of drugs, among other things, to forcibly indoctrinate dissidents and nonbelievers of the communist doctrines (see Figure 3).

Vulnerability

According to Lifton, there is no known system that would enable a prospective subject to withstand the rigors of systematic brainwashing, especially as practiced by the Chinese. Generally however, the premorbid personality of those at high risk consists of tendencies toward emotional immaturity with a history of impaired interpersonal relationships going back to childhood. Persons who tend toward passivity with difficulties in assertion are likewise more vulnerable. But, as Sargant has pointed out, a normal person cannot withstand more than 30 continuous days and nights of stress and tension without breaking down during the brainwashing process.

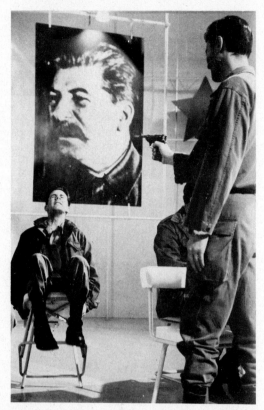

FIGURE 3. In the motion picture, *The Manchurian Candidate*, from which this still photograph is taken, U.S. prisoners of war were brainwashed by their communist captors. The actor holding the gun is being programmed to shoot a fellow prisoner and, after his planned release from captivity, to assassinate an American presidential candidate. (Courtesy of Culver Pictures, Inc.)

Techniques

Various methods used singly, sequentially, or in combination are able to produce the effect desired by the coercers. Among these are isolation, deprivation, repetitive interrogation, threats, self-criticism and group criticism. In controlled experiments, volunteer subjects under conditions of sensory isolation—consisting of visual, auditory, and tactile deprivation for periods of up to 7 days—react with increased suggestibility and show symptoms characteristic of the sensory deprivation state: anxiety, tension, inability to concentrate, vivid sensory imagery sometimes reaching the proportion of hallucinations with delusionary quality, and intense subjective emotions. When deliberately induced, the subject is overwhelmed by feelings of anxiety and fear, and to diminish this terror will usually succumb to suggestions made by the captor. This phase heralds ideological conversion. According to Lifton, the Chinese attacked a prisoner's sense of self by forcing him to criticize both himself, his friends, and his previously held values. This was particularly effective when done in groups. Not only was the person subject to public humiliation, but if the group were composed of others who held beliefs consistent with the sought after ideological conversion, pressure from the other members added to the prisoner's attempt to conform. Additionally, the group might provide approval and positive reinforcement when the subject acknowledged that his beliefs were changing or had changed. The use of a variety of drugs that increased suggestibility, such as sedatives and hypnotics, served in some instances to enhance the process.

Phases

Several workers have described specific phases in brainwashing. Schein has described three: (1) unfreezing, in which the individual is forcibly convinced of the need to change his ideas; (2) changing, during which the indoctrinators introduce the new concepts with which they want to brainwash the individual; and (3) refreezing, where the individual is given a motive and reward to accept and believe the new ideology. Chodoff has outlined four phases of brainwashing: (1) emotional assault, which consists of sensory deprivation, hunger, and sleep deprivation; (2) favors, such as providing food and showing leniency; (3) confession, where the prisoner renounces his past; and (4) re-education, during which the new set of ideas is integrated into the personality.

Treatment

According to Hinkle, as reported in the symposium on methods of forceful indoctrination, published by the Group for the Advancement of Psychiatry, brainwashing methods produce variable changes in attitude and behavior, rather than detectable changes in brain function. Furthermore, these changes are only transient. In a period of months following his release, the individual subjected to such procedures tends to revert to his former personality.

Lifton, who interviewed Westerners who had undergone such treatment and then were released has described a "survivors syndrome" in which the individual attempted to relinquish the effects of brainwashing; but did so with difficulty. Lingering fears, recollection of threats made during the process, combined with susceptibility of the person, and the success of the program, often caused the released prisoner to want to indicate some remaining tie to the behavior and thought patterns set up by their treatment.

As a general rule, the individual's reaction will depend on many factors relating to personality, character, and the immediate situation. Deprograming, the process whereby the person relearns previously held values and re-examines the processes to which he had been subjected, should be carried out in a psychotherapeutic setting characterized by trust, emotional support, and the use of tranquilizers when anxiety is excessive. During restitutive psychotherapy, an exploration of feelings of guilt for having succumbed to the brainwashing technique is necessary. A major mental mechanism used by the victim is that of identification with the agressor which should be brought to conscious awareness during psychotherapy. Environmental modification is often an important and helpful measure and includes working with the patient's immediate family and other people close to him.

REFERENCES

Coser, L. *The Functions of Social Conflict*. Free Press, Glencoe, Ill., 1956.
Coser, L. *Continuities in the Study of Social Conflict*. Free Press of Glencoe (Macmillan), New York, 1967.
Group for the Advancement of Psychiatry. Methods of Forceful Indoctrination Observation and Interviews. Symposium No. 4., GAP, New York, 1956.
Lifton, R. J. *Home From the War*. Simon & Schuster, New York, 1973.
Lifton, R. J. *Thought Reform and the Psychology of Totalism, A Study of "Brainwashing" in China*. W. W. Norton, New York, 1961.
McNeil, E. B., editor. *The Nature of Human Conflict*. Prentice-Hall, Englewood Cliffs, N. J., 1965.
Oberschall, A. *Social Conflict and Social Movements*. Prentice-Hall, Englewood Cliffs, N. J., 1973.
Sargant, W. *Battle for the Mind*. Greenwood. Westport, 1975.
Sargant, W., Slater, E., and Kelley, D. *An Introduction to Physical Methods of Treatment in Psychiatry*, Churchill, Livingstone, Edinburgh, 1972.
Schein, E. *Coercive Persuasion, Sociopsychological Analysis of Brainwashing of American Civilian Prisoners by the Chinese Communists*, W. W. Norton, New York, 1971.
Spiegel, J. P. *Transactions: The Interplay Between Individual, Family, and Society*. Science House, New York, 1971.
Young, O. R. Intermediaries: Additional thoughts on third parties. J. Confl. Res., *16*: 51, 1972.

51.6   INTERRACIAL RELATIONS

White Racism

Some students of the problem believe that white racism is based on whites' delusions about black inferiority, which result from whites' projections of their own unacceptable feelings and drives onto someone with black skin. Because such prejudices are derived from social experiences in a racist society, some investigators view racism as a cultural variant and not as a manifestation of individual psychological disorder. But many black psychiatrists feel that only if white persons see their racism as a mental disturbance will they be motivated to change (see Figure 1).

Other writers have suggested that sexual fears are at the root of white racism and interracial conflict, particularly in America. Blacks have been viewed as animals with insatiable sexual appetites. Whites often used sexual fears to obscure the primary aims of racist practices, which were to keep blacks poor, segregated, uneducated, and powerless.

Some social scientists, believing that racism does not have a strong psychological base, choose to emphasize social and class factors. They believe that white Americans fear the black ghetto life styles, which foster crime, drug abuse, and violence. However, the government and the white community are willing to do little to alleviate the horrendous social conditions that breed crime.

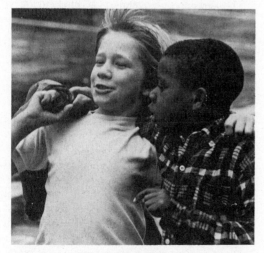

FIGURE 1. Friendship between children. (Courtesy of Bob Adelman for Magnum Photos, Inc.)

Psychiatry and the Black Patient

Many blacks see psychiatrists as agents of the establishment. This view stems in part from the fact that few psychiatrists have paid attention to cultural and social forces that produce mental disorder. Some believe that mental health workers have been more interested in helping blacks to adjust to a racist society than in changing that society.

White psychiatrists are as much a product of society as are other whites, and they have been conditioned by the white supremacist attitudes that dominate cultural experiences. Unfortunately, psychiatric or psychoanalytic training does not purge practitioners of racist beliefs. As a consequence, blacks have suffered discrimination and have been misused and abused by mental health workers.

Professional Prejudices

By catering to a well-to-do clientele, psychiatry has unwittingly expressed a greater commitment to meeting the mental health needs of the white middle class than to satisfying those of minority groups and the poor. As a result, blacks and others have been confined to overcrowded state mental institutions and public clinics. Often the service provided for minorities has been minimal or merely custodial. Because of racial and socio-economic factors, emotionally disturbed blacks have seldom had access to mental health personnel during the early stages of their distress. Frequently, their illnesses have progressed to the stage of incapacitation before services have been provided. Many psychiatric procedures experienced by blacks at the hands of the white establishment have had an aura of criminal proceedings.

Too often, psychiatrists prefer patients who, like themselves, are verbally skillful, educated, and psychologically oriented. Racial and economic discrimination and de facto segregation have allowed countless numbers of social workers, psychologists, and psychiatrists to go through years of training without having black colleagues or seeing any black patients. As a result, most have not had an opportunity to confront their own prejudices or deficits in a cross-cultural contact. Many psychotherapists have unconscious needs to be in helping and controlling roles. They want their patients to accommodate to them or to imitate their style or approach. This kind of relationship between a white therapist and a black patient contains the basic ingredients for a master-slave pattern.

Some professional prejudices are camouflaged in psychiatric jargon that stereotypes minority patients as "hostile," "paranoid," "not motivated for treatment," "possessing a primitive character structure," "not psychologically oriented," "impulse-ridden," and so forth. These categorizations are often code words indicating that someone is not suitable for psychotherapeutic treatment and should be rejected.

Black patients frequently find the white styles and attitudes in public clinics so prohibitive that they avoid seeking help or leave treatment after a short experience.

Cultural Values

The uneven training of many psychiatric workers has made it difficult for them to distinguish deviant, unhealthy behavior from what is merely culturally different behavior. Black youth struggling to cope with a stressful ghetto environment are usually said to be suffering from behavioral disorders. Frequently the effect and not the cause is diagnosed.

Stereotyping

Psychiatrists often view blacks from negative, psychopathological perspectives. Ghettoes have been diagnosed as a tangle of pathology. Black women have been labeled matriarchs, and black men have been termed marginal men. The black family has been diagnosed as disorganized, unstable, and incapable of properly rearing children. Sweeping stereotypes about the black family have been reported by white investigators as a result of cultural biases and inadequate research.

Black Psychiatrists

In 1973, blacks numbered about 450 of about 25,000 practicing psychiatrists in America. Black psychiatrists who had long been restrained and accommodating have grown more assertive and have challenged the traditional assumptions of American psychiatry. Many have seen that a primary aspect of their task as psychiatrists is to change society and bring about full equality for Afro-Americans. They have realized that black mental health is inex-

orably intertwined with racial discrimination and poverty. They are concerned with black victimization by social conditions that lead to greater mental morbidity within the black community. Black mental health workers are currently concerned with the rapidly rising black suicide and homicide rate. These rates are closely related to problems of poverty, unemployment, and the unavailability of good schools and housing among blacks.

REFERENCES

Butts, H. F. White racism: Its origins, institutions, and the implications for professional practice in mental health. Int. J. Psychiatry, 8: 914, 1969.
Comer, J. P. *Beyond Black and White*. Quadrangle Books, New York, 1972.
Genzier, I. L. *Frantz Fanon: A Critical Study*. Pantheon Books, New York, 1973.
Grier, W. H., and Cobbs, P. M. *Black Rage*. Basic Books, New York, 1968.
Pinderhughes, C. A. Racism and psychotherapy. In *Racism and Mental Health*, C. V. Willie, B. M. Kramer, and B. S. Brown, editors, p. 61. University of Pittsburgh Press, Pittsburgh, 1973.
Poussaint, A. F. *Why Blacks Kill Blacks*. Emerson Hall, New York, 1972.
Thomas, A., and Sillen, S. *Racism and Psychiatry*. Brunner-Mazel, New York, 1972.
Thomas, C. S., and Comer, J. P. Racism and mental health services. In *Racism and Mental Health*, C. V. Willie, B. M. Kramer, and B. S. Brown, editors, p. 165. University of Pittsburgh Press, Pittsburgh, 1973.

51.7.   THE WOMEN'S MOVEMENT

Diversity of the Movement

The women's movement is challenging a formidable number of assumptions basic to American society and is challenging them not only at the public, institutional level but at the private, psychological level. Some of these challenges will, in the course of time, prove to be more valid and of greater significance than others.

Issues involving women's occupational roles are those on which most overt action has been centered. These issues are the ones most open to agreement and action. Demands for equal wages for women receive the widest adherence. These are closely followed by demands for equal opportunity, which involves opening professional schools and job-training programs at all levels to women, on a par with men.

Questions involving other segments of woman's role are felt as equally pressing, but they are a great deal less amenable to direct public action or even to agreement on proper action. Much of woman's role has to do with her activities, obligations, and behavior in what is thought of as the private sphere—within the family, as wife and mother.

In terms of her function as wife, some of the questions now being debated are: Is the woman to think of herself mainly as support to her husband? (See Figure 1.) Is his vocation to come first in every case? Is the relation of the family to the community to be maintained by the husband, while the wife's activities are confined to the home or to approved volunteer or leisure-time associations? If not, how are duties and obligations to be divided?

Other obligations considered within marriage deal with sexual relationships. How valid are the traditional mores? Will sexual experience outside marriage enrich or disrupt the union, and can extramarital sex be undertaken by the woman as freely as by the man? How useful and

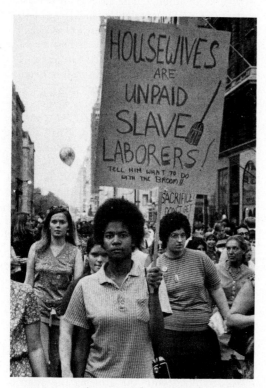

FIGURE 1. Demonstration representing some of the conflicts regarding the status of the housewife. (Courtesy of Burt Glinn for Magnum Photos, Inc.)

advisable are less formal relationships for living together? How is female sexuality conditioned by women's physiology, and does a woman's physiology have a bearing on activities and behavior other than sexual?

Debate over a woman's proper role as wife slips easily into the question of the mother role. Should children be raised primarily by the mother, or should the father also be engaged? Are child care facilities outside the home helpful, baneful, or neutral? What about single-parent families? If women or couples decide to have no children, will their lives be as fulfilled as those of parents, or can psychological difficulties be expected?

The position of women members of minority groups is another factor making for diversity in the women's movement. Black women, in particular, are concerned to define their priorities. Should they support the efforts of black men to step forward to full equality before they insist on their own rights? Have oppression and deprivation produced a family structure differing significantly from the white home, and, if so, what effect does this difference have on the larger social structure? The range of behavior among black women is even wider than that among whites. At one end, women are more numerous among black professionals than among white professionals; at the other end, veiled black women can be seen in America, and some black women argue for polygyny as a deliberate re-creation of the African background.

Another factor making for confusion over priorities is age differences. Older women formed their life styles at a time when traditional roles were less questioned, and it was assumed that marriage and motherhood would set the pattern for their years of maturity. Many are now employed, but they usually see their work as secondary and peripheral to their husbands' careers and, often, to their roles as housewife and homemaker. But young women appear more and more to be looking to a future that will include work and are, therefore, planning their lives differently. Their educational programs are changing, since the prospect of continuing employment makes the early acquisition of professional skills attractive. This change means that women's education increasingly parallels that of men. In addition, the expectation of carrying on a vocation progressively invalidates the old concept that the choice of marriage partner is women's most significant life decision. No longer is a woman's status automatically dependent on that of her husband, for the work that she will very likely undertake serves as another determinant of her position.

The Movement as Response and Reaction

The movement is fundamentally a reaction to drastic social, economic, and cultural changes that have taken place and are still taking place. The validity of the movement derives from its responsiveness to these fundamental shifts in contemporary lives, both social and individual.

Role conflicts can be traced to social shifts. Thus, the changes in women's occupational roles can be understood only in the context of long-term economic trends. Women have worked throughout history, but they have usually done so within a family group, which functioned as an economic unit. The removal of the locus of work from the home has produced increasing strain and faces many women with a dilemma. Their earnings are needed to support the family, but, in order to win these earnings, they must leave the children whose support is sustained by the earnings.

Currently, 50 per cent of women with children between the ages of 6 and 18 hold jobs. Most of them do so because of objective economic need. Six million women are listed in the 1970 census as heads of families. Sixteen million women are cited in Labor Department statistics as contributing the wages that keep their families above the poverty line. One third of married women, aged 20 to 24 with preschool children, in marriages with husbands present, were at work.

Efforts of the women's movement to redefine the mother's and housewife's obligations within the home and to support her by advocating an increase in child care centers outside the home offer an example of response to a pressing existent situation.

Questions Raised

The first question posed by the women's movement for practitioners of psychiatry is one of definition: What is normal?

The second question raised by the movement is, How are norms to be established? Are they to be drawn from innate biological factors, or is normality the product of social training and experiential learning? Most philosophers would doubtless declare that both elements play a part. The thrust of the women's movement here is to lay increased emphasis on the role of social training or acculturation.

Anterior to these questions is the basic postulate of the women's movement, for it explains the need to raise them at all. In the past, women have been held to have special capabilities and disabilities, special characteristics and special limitations. The movement believes in a fundamental equality of talent, mental capacity, and character strength within men and women alike. This equality does not imply sameness. Rather, in its opposition to sex stereotyping, the movement posits individual diversity as great for women as for men. It declares that women's lives, emotions, and aims are as important and significant as those of men.

Both consciously and unconsciously, orthodox psychiatric theory and therapy have approached women as members of the second sex. The male role is seen as primary and that of women as an adjunct. The norm is arrived at by a study of male experience, and treatment is prescribed according to a definition of normality not primary to women but derived by men and male experience. Outdated norms are believed by the movement to diminish or even to undermine the value of therapy.

Another sort of conflict affects women who are strongly motivated to work full-time in fields in which they are competent. They almost always regard themselves as the marriage partner chiefly responsible for the maintenance of the home and the welfare of the family. What comes first, family or career? Either solution sets up its own strains. Psychologically, the personal problem is compounded by the lack of community support in the way of adequate child care centers. Consequently, an increasing number of professional women plan either not to marry or to marry but not bear children. Another reaction is that of women, able to support a child by their own earnings, who have children without marrying.

The option to choose when or whether to bear children has been signally increased by new contraceptive methods. The decline in the birth rate, combined with the growing life span of women, has now reduced the proportionate amount of time spent in actual mothering to an historical low. What effect the drastic shift in occupation from work to home to work again has on the ego identity of women is a question that deserves exploration. This shift clearly invalidates the old proposition that the chief and central role of any woman is motherhood. The right of women to have control of their bodies with the freedom to have abortions is a central issue today (see Figure 2).

Many writers believe that too-rigid sex roles are inhibiting for men as well as women and that greater flexibility would promote the happiness of both sexes. The desire to reach equality but not supremacy is everywhere present in the literature, and fear that the women's movement is working toward a reversal of roles, replacing male by female dominance, cannot be supported.

Effects of Shifts in Sexual Norms

By achieving the ability to support themselves, women have gained immeasurably in independence and, therefore, in their freedom to choose a marriage partner, to abstain from

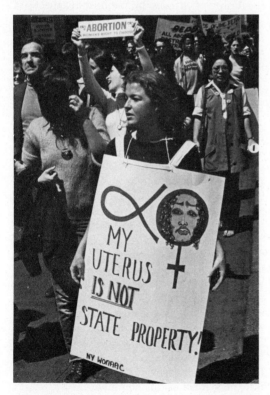

FIGURE 2. A protest about the right to have an abortion. (Courtesy of Charles Gatewood for Magnum Photos, Inc.)

marriage, or to end a marriage that has become painful. Other forces for change in sex behavior are the products of medical technology, like the improved and more widely available methods of contraception, backed up most recently by access to abortion on demand. The effects of the cultural phenomenon denoted by "permissiveness" can be seen in the more frequent involvement in sexual activities at an earlier age by both men and women. These activities are also less confined to a traditional pattern. Various practices once considered perversions are now quite widely accepted. A century ago the pleasures of sex were almost exclusively a male prerogative. Women are now understood to be fully orgasmic. Indeed, women are capable of longer, more sustained, and more quickly repeated orgasm than are men.

But the idea that liberation for women walks hand in hand with the sexual revolution is a mistaken oversimplification. Although a man retains full choice in a sexual encounter, since he can approach the woman or not as he chooses, the woman has not gained full choice, and her decision to say "No" involves her in an apparent personal disparagement of the man. The man's invitation now seems to contain an element of compulsion. Men assume that sexual freedom is as complete for women as it is for themselves, but women do not find this to be the case. Until sexual freedom allows women the right to initiate sexual encounters and to refuse them if they so choose, with equal rights of refusal allowed to men, it cannot be equated with liberation.

The women's movement includes lesbians, fully approves their right to take part in the sexual activity they prefer and to advocate it for others, and supports their insistence on the social acceptability of such a preference. This stand is part of the diversity of the movement, which refuses either to advocate or to condemn any particular form of sexual activity undertaken by consenting adults (see Figure 3).

Effects of Social Change on the Mother Role

The need for mothers to leave the home in order to work if their earnings are necessary for family support is a difficulty in itself. It also points to a wider problem—the current isolation of the family from the wider world of activity. The elimination of the breadwinning father from an effective role in child raising is

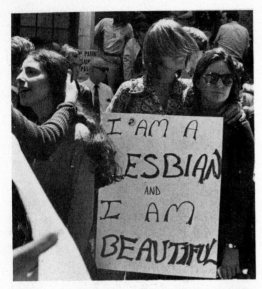

FIGURE 3. Lesbians at a Gay Liberation demonstration in New York City. (Courtesy of Leonard Freed for Magnum Photos, Inc.)

often overlooked, but his absence is as great a historical anomaly as the partially absent mother.

Both young children and youth are growing up without the benefit of a variety of adult role models. Children are becoming increasingly ignorant about the world of paid work. Parents are increasingly replaced by three other socializing agents: the schools, the peer group, and the mass media.

The economic and social factors responsible for the contemporary isolation of families are fundamental reasons for the desire felt by many responsible mothers to engage fathers more deeply in interaction with children, thus preventing dependence on the mother alone, dependence easily productive of intense and binding intimacy. Efforts to overcome family isolation and to provide easy connections with other adults also play a part in the support for adequate child care centers. The endeavor to engage adults other than the mother in active and continuing child care should be seen not as an attempt to replace the mother but, rather, as an effort to support her socializing function.

Psychological difficulties can be induced in the family relationship by isolation from the community and overintimacy within the family group. A consensus points to the danger of confining women to vicarious living through others by binding them to a narrow and isolated home situation. The inability of a woman to gain public reward and acknowledgment of success for individual activity and the injunction to find her reward in the success of husband and children tend to produce a manipulative and devious personality that seeks covert power, since independent open endeavor is denied her. The influence of such a woman on children in her care has sometimes been found to be alienating or even schizophrenegenic. Far from downgrading or belittling the mother role, the women's movement emphasizes the importance of child raising and socialization to the community at large by seeking the participation of others in the process. Such participation provides the positive result of variety in role models and avoids the negative effect of binding the child too tightly within the maternal relationship.

Theoretical Considerations

The work of Freud and his disciples has borne the brunt of attacks by feminists. Aspects of Freud's theory are challenged, first, by the primary postulate of the women's movement—the equal significance of women's lives and experience with men's—and, second, by the evidence of experiential divergence from theory arising from the changes in social circumstances since Freud wrote.

Freud grounded the inferiority of women in their physiological difference from men and saw their recognition of this inferiority as a necessary part of their progress toward maturity (the female castration complex and penis envy), but the women's movement sees female inferiority as attributed to women by dominant men in the social circumstances of a particular time and place. Freudian theory declares the primacy of the man as innate, based on biology. Possession of a penis is the cause of this primacy. The women's movement holds that male primacy is a social construct, fabricated, whether consciously or not, as a means of upholding male dominance in power relationships. Penis envy is not denied, but it is understood as envy of the male position of dominance in society and in the family, and possession of a penis is not the cause but the symbol of this dominance.

Some of Freud's followers, notably Marie Bonaparte and Helene Deutsch, took up a brief suggestion of Freud to the effect that femininity may have "some secret relationship with masochism." The idea that women are by nature masochistic clearly grounds their inferiority even more securely in physiology. This explanation appeared to account both for the high incidence of frigidity noted among women two generations ago and for the concurrent assumption of a self-sacrificial or martyr role of many mothers. In addition, the idea that it is natural for women to wish to suffer justified the existing inferiority of the sex. And the insistence on a passive role for women in sexual activity, tied up with the theory of vaginal orgasm as the only norm, follows from the premise of female masochism.

Challenges to these ideas have arisen over the years. Alfred Adler did not deny to women the common drive toward superiority that he perceived as basic to humanity, although he assumed that the social situation of his time would usually prevent this masculine protest from achieving any real success. Karen Horney declared that, when considering the cause of feminine masochism, "one has to look not for biological reasons but for cultural ones." Horney analyzes the effect of social pressures on women, especially "the cultural situation which has led women to regard love as the only value that counts in life." Horney notes that neurotic fear of aging, which decreases a woman's attractiveness, follows from this, as does a general sense of insecurity and self-devaluation, and, indeed, that "the all-embracing expectations that are joined to love account to some extent for that discontentment with the female role that Freud ascribes to penis-envy," since these expectations are, in the nature of things, rarely achieved in full.

These theoretical difficulties have been reinforced by the actual experience of many women, whose lives no longer conform to the traditional pattern, and by scientific advances. Research into sexual practice and sexual response by Masters and Johnson, has overthrown the assumption of female passivity, of less frequent and lower female response, and of a necessary evolution during maturation in women from clitoral to vaginal orgasm.

REFERENCES

Freeman, J. The origins of the women's liberation movement. In *Changing Women in a Changing Society*, J. Huber, editor, p. 30. University of Chicago Press, Chicago, 1973.

Horney, K. *New Ways in Psychoanalysis*. W. W. Norton, New York, 1939.
Huber, J., editor. *Changing Women in a Changing Society*. University of Chicago Press, Chicago, 1973.
Janeway, E. *Man's World, Woman's Place*. Morrow, New York, 1971.
Johnston, J. *Lesbian Nation: The Feminist Solution*. Simon & Schuster, New York, 1973.
Masters, W. H., and Johnson, V. E. *Human Sexual Response*. Little Brown, Boston, 1966.
Millet, K. *Sexual Politics*. Doubleday, New York, 1970.
Orden, S. R., and Bradburn, N. M. Working Wives and Marriage Happiness. Am. J. Sociol., January, 1969.

51.8. THE URBAN SETTING

Introduction

Urbanization has been called the dominant social, cultural, and ecological process in 20th century America. City life has altered the factors that cause illness and has thus affected the incidence and prevalence of many physical diseases. With respect to mental illness, the consequences of urbanization have been more difficult to discern.

Definitions

The words "urban" and "city" are most frequently used interchangeably for the purpose of differentiating certain populous communities from villages, the countryside, and rural areas. The National Center for Health Statistics conducted a survey in which urban was assigned four possible meanings, based on community size. Cities and suburbs with a collective population of more than 3,000,000 were designated as "giant metropolitan statistical areas." Areas with a population of 500,000 to 3,000,000 were designated "other very large metropolitan statistical areas." The "standard metropolitan statistical areas" contained from 50,000 to 500,000 people, and "other urban areas" were classified as regions with populations of 2,500 to 50,000. Areas of fewer than 2,500 persons were defined as rural.

The urban resident has been characterized as having a group orientation, moving frequently, intensively striving for social prestige and financial success, being strongly influenced by personal contacts, and possessing a highly specialized skill. In terms of mental disorders, the urbanite is more likely to suffer from alcoholic psychoses, general paresis, drug psychoses, paranoia, and neuroses than is the rural resident. Urban residents are admitted to mental institutions in greater proportions than are rural citizens.

Urban Psychosocial Research

Because neuroses have been reported to be more prevalent in urban areas, it has been commonly accepted that neurotic behavior is characteristic of urban living. However, neurotic behavior has been found in members of all societies that have been rigorously studied. Many investigators feel that the inter-relationship of urban life and mental illness is far too complex, the data collection methods too variable, and the data subject to such ambiguous and contradictory interpretation that there has been a reluctance to undertake new studies of socio-cultural and environmental causality of psychiatric disorders in the urban setting.

New Haven Study

Hollingshead and Redlich (1958) conducted a survey of New Haven, Connecticut, and its surrounding region during parts of 1950 and 1951.

Objectives and Methods. The project was primarily concerned with determining the relation of social class to the prevalence of treated illness. Only patients under psychiatric treatment were studied. Thus, the incidence and the prevalence of mental disorders in the general population were not explored. Mental illness treatment methods as they related to social class were of special interest to the researchers.

The data accumulated by the study were intended to prove or disprove the validity of several basic hypotheses:

Position in the class structure is related to the prevalence of treated mental illness.

Position in the class structure is related to the types of diagnosed psychiatric disorders.

Position in the class structure is related to social and psychodynamic factors in the development of psychiatric disorders.

Mobility in the class structure is related to the development of psychiatric difficulties.

Five substudies were developed to gather the data. These studies included a census of psychiatric patients, a survey of the population at large, a study of psychiatrists, a study of the community, and a controlled case study. Hollingshead and Redlich also divided the study population into distinct categories, based on life-styles and cultural characteristics. These categories ranged from class I, representing persons from the upper sociocultural stratum, to class V, representing the least skilled and least educated persons in the population.

Findings. Analysis of the data revealed definitive relationships between social class and various aspects of the psychiatric process, beginning with the nature of the initial referral for treatment. Among those persons classified as neurotics entering treatment for the first time, for example, the referrals by private physicians were much greater in classes I and II (52.5 per cent) than in class V (13.9 per cent). The police and the courts referred no one from classes I and II, but they referred 13.9 per cent of class V.

With respect to the five initial hypotheses, it was found that an inverse relationship existed between social class and mental illness; that neuroses were more prevalent in classes I and II and fell as the class level fell, but psychoses were most markedly increased among the lower classes; that social class was related to the site, duration, and nature of psychiatric therapy; and that observed relations between socio-cultural variables and the prevalence of treated disorders do not establish that socio-cultural variables are essential and necessary conditions in the causation of mental disorders.

Midtown Manhattan Study

A team under the direction of a psychiatrist, Thomas A. C. Rennie, designed and conducted a survey involving a sample of 1,660 adults drawn from a specific section of New York City.

Objectives and Methods. The general objectives of the study were to estimate the mental health of a geographically defined population, the majority of whom had never been psychiatric patients, and to determine the possible influence of demographic factors and social and personal experiences on mental health and mental illness. In contrast to the New Haven study, the sample population in the Midtown project were not necessarily persons under past or present psychiatric care. Moreover, the Midtown project made a major effort to estimate reliably and objectively the mental health of each respondent. The vehicle for obtaining a mental health rating was a questionnaire-guided interview conducted by nonpsychiatrists. However, determinations made by psychiatrists during examinations of clinical patients were incorporated into the data. In this fashion a comprehensive mass of information was obtained, so that the presence or absence of psychiatrically significant symptoms could be determined. Four final mental health rating levels were developed:

Well: no evidence of symptom formation.

Mild: mild symptom formation but functioning adequately.

Moderate: moderate symptom formation with no apparent interference with life adjustment.

Impaired: Marked—moderate symptom formation with some interference in life adjustment. Severe—serious symptom formation, yet functioning with some difficulty. Incapacitated—serious symptom formation, functioning with great difficulty or unable to function.

These mental health ratings became the principal psychiatric referrant for correlation with socio-cultural factors in the published study (Srole et al., 1962). The ratings were analyzed for their relationship to age, sex, marital status, own socio-economic status, generation in America, religious origin, and ethnic origin.

Findings. It was observed that there is a rise in mental disorder or poor mental health as age increases. Respondents in their fifth decade of life were, collectively, 15 per cent well and 31 per cent impaired. The youngest persons studied, from age 20 to 29, were judged 24 per cent well and 15 per cent impaired. Perhaps the most dramatic conclusions of the project was that, over-all, only 19 per cent of the study population was considered well and that only 18 per cent displayed no symptoms of mental disorder. On the continuum, the largest number (36 per cent) suffered from mild symptom formation, with 34 per cent categorized as being a probable neurotic type.

Another specific finding was related to socioeconomic status, which was calculated from occupation, education, income, and rent. The highest stratum showed about six times as many members in the well group and less than a quarter as many in the impaired group as did the lowest stratum. Socio-economic status appeared to be the most important single variable. In the study, the presence of symptoms was not taken as an indication of a disorder. It was observed, however, that those with the largest number of symptoms would most likely be diagnosed as having a mental disorder if they were seen by a psychiatrist.

Stirling County Study

Alexander H. Leighton headed a psychiatric epidemiological study of Stirling County, a Canadian county of 20,000 persons. Unlike the New Haven and Midtown Manhattan surveys, the Stirling County population was primarily rural, being mostly scattered in small villages of a few hundred, with one town of 3,000 and a good many isolated farms. A sample of 1,010 adults was drawn.

Objectives and Methods. Psychiatric assessment was made through the use of questionnaire interviews. These interviews, conducted by nonpsychiatrists, were supplemented by additional data-gathering techniques. Classifications were developed to express various aspects of mental illness. One classification, for example, expressed the degree of certainty felt by the evaluators that the person did or did not show psychiatric disorder. "A" meant almost certain psychiatric disorder, "B" meant probable psychiatric disorder, "C" meant doubtful disorder, and "D" meant the person showed no evidence of disorder. A second scale showed major symptom categories. Included were psychophysiological, psychoneurotic, sociopathic, mental deficiency, personality disorder, brain syndrome, and psychosis.

Of particular interest to the researchers was Leighton's theory of social integration and disintegration as factors in mental illness. This hypothesis stated that a social environment that adequately fulfills its incumbents' needs (integrated) is associated with less psychiatric disorder than is an environment that does not (disintegrated). It stated, as well, that prolonged and severe noxious social conditions within a community will cause disintegration.

Findings. As reported by Murphy (1971), the study found that communities in Stirling County showed a significant correlation between disintegration and prevalence of psychiatric symptoms. The conditions of poverty, secularization, and cultural confusion were three criteria used to identify community disintegration.

Like the Midtown Manhattan study, the Stirling County study found that only about 20 per cent of the population could be said with certainty to be free of symptoms of mental disorder. Women showed considerably more psychiatric disorder than did men. Forty per cent of women were in class A, and 25 per cent in class B; only 15 per cent were believed to be in class D. Twenty-one per cent of the men were in class A, and 26 per cent in class B; 20 per cent of the men were considered symptom free. In terms of symptom categories, the survey found that 66 per cent of the men and 71 per cent of the women suffered from psychophysiological symptoms. Psychoneurosis was found in 44 per cent of the men and 64 per cent of the women. Age was found to be a factor, with psychiatric disorders increasing with age. The study also disclosed a linear relation between mental health and economic position.

Other Studies

The pioneer study of Faris and Dunham has been particularly influential. This survey reported that first hospital admissions for schizophrenia were highest among persons from the central sections of Chicago, the lowest socioeconomic sections of the city. It was also reported that rates of admission decreased as one moved away from the central areas and into the more affluent and prestigious communities. These findings gave rise to what is termed the drift hypothesis. According to this theory, the environment in the central city does not produce the disease but, rather, acts as a magnet, drawing schizophrenics who are in the process of decompensating. By the time the illness is most severe and hospitalization is required, they have drifted into the core city. Some studies, such as those by Clauson and Kohn (1959) in Hagerstown, Maryland, failed to show a relation between schizophrenia and the central city.

In part, the difficulties in properly interpreting the meaning of research data are a consequence of the problems in psychiatric diagnostic classification and of the differences in methods and terminology that make findings difficult to compare.

Issues in Urban Psychiatry

Antiurban Bias

Antiurban bias manifests itself in numerous disparaging commentaries on the character of cities and city dwellers. When this prejudice is injected into psychiatric and social science research, national attitudes and social policy regarding mental illness are influenced.

A national survey of 6,672 adults conducted by the National Center for Health Statistics found that the largest urban areas had lower incidence rates of age-adjusted symptoms than did smaller urban-rural areas. Rural women were found to be the most symptomatic of all groups surveyed. The mobile, organized society may, indeed, be psychologically eugenic in comparison with the restrictive, immobile, rural society.

Poverty

Most current concepts about the interplay among poverty, mental health, and mental illness are founded on theoretical psychological models, experimental observations of monkeys, empirical observations by those who work with the poor, and psychosocial research. The psychosocial studies most consistently, although not conclusively, suggest a relationship between poverty and psychopathology.

Poverty is conventionally defined in terms of a family's financial resources. However, most workers agree that this arbitrary form of definition is inadequate and unrealistic. The related variables of low income, family size, age, low occupational level, high unemployment rate, local cost of living, and geographic location have come to be used in measuring poverty.

Being poor is a universal phenomenon; it is found in all societies, in the countryside as well as the city. Nevertheless, since World War II poverty has become associated with the urbanite, the black, and the aged.

Social isolation is commonly invoked as the single most pathogenic consequence of poverty. The poor, it is contended, are restricted in experiences that are necessary for normal maturation. Deprived of parental intimacy, adequate peer interaction, and intellectual stimulation, the person growing up in poverty is isolated from those factors that shape an adequate personality and may, in fact, experience intractable emotional trauma.

In regard to the variables at each stage of development that predispose a person to develop along the unhealthy pathways, the preponderant psychological and sociological observations suggest that these conditions are more pervasive among the poor than among the affluent.

Mental health workers have attempted to describe those personality traits and mental disorders that are most frequent among the poor. The poor are said to be (1) physical and visual, rather than aural, (2) content-centered, rather than form-centered, (3) externally oriented, rather than introspective, (4) problem-centered, rather than abstract-centered, (5) inductive, rather than deductive, (6) spatial, rather than temporal, (7) slow, careful, patient, perservering (in areas of importance), rather than quick, facile, clever, (8) games-and-action-oriented, rather than test-oriented, (9) expressive-oriented, rather than instrumental-oriented, (10) geared to one-tract thinking and unorthodox learning, rather than other-directed flexibility, and (11) prone to use words in relation to action, rather than being word-bound.

The poor are also characterized as being impulsive; oriented in terms of time to the present and, to a lesser extent, the immediate past, a fact that manifests itself in failure to plan for the future and to delay gratification; and resigned and fatalistic, a fact that results in a tolerance of somatic and psychological pathology far in excess of that accepted by the more affluent.

The Affluent Urbanite

Data indicate high rates of participation by well-salaried, highly skilled, and well-educated persons in psychiatric processes. In urban centers, where these professionals are concentrated, the question has arisen as to whether psychiatry is a major force in promoting social change or social stability. Most knowledgeable observers believe that the social influence of psychiatry is too small to be noticeable.

More than half of the nation's psychiatrists practice in the five states that contain the nation's largest cities—New York, Pennsylvania, Massachusetts, Illinois, and California. In New York, psychiatrists represent 10.5 per cent of all physicians. One can only wonder as to the potential or real impact of so substantial a segment of the medical community on society.

Teaching Hospitals

The most commonly heard criticism of the psychiatric services in the teaching hospital involves the concept of institutional isolation within the community. There is inadequate articulation and responsiveness on the part of the university medical facility to the geographic community. This situation is ascribed to the general tendency of the teaching faculty to identify their functions and roles with institutional goals and objectives, which may be at variance with the requirements of the community.

REFERENCES

Abrams, C. *The Language of Cities.* Viking Press, New York, 1971.
Dohrenwend, B. P., Chin-Song, E. T., Egri, G., Mendelsohn, F. S., and Stokes, J. Measures of psychiatric disorder in contrasting class and ethnic groups. In *Psychiatric Epidemiology,* E. H. Hare and J. K. Wing, editors, p. 159. Oxford University Press, London, 1970.
Fishbein, M. The hazards of consulting a psychiatrist. Med. World News, *14:* 52, 1973.
Fromm, E. *The Anatomy of Human Destructiveness.* Holt, Rinehart & Winston, New York, 1973.
Hollingshead, A. B., and Redlich, F. C. *Social Class and Mental Illness: A Community Study.* John Wiley, New York, 1958.
Huffine, C. L., and Craig, T. J. Social factors in the utilization of an urban psychiatric emergency service. Arch. Gen. Psychiatry, *30:* 249, 1974.
Kaplan, S. R., and Roman, M. *The Organization and Delivery of Mental Health Services in the Ghetto.* Praeger, New York, 1973.
Knowles, J. The unseen ostrich in our teaching hospitals. Prism, *1:* 13, 1973.
Kolb, L. C. *Modern Clinical Psychiatry.* W. B. Saunders, Philadelphia, 1973.
Kristol, I. The suburbanized world. Psychol. Today, *7:* 72, 1974.
Lemkau, P. V. The epidemiological study of mental illness and mental health. Am. J. Psychiatry, *3:* 801, 1955.
Reed, S., Myers, F. S., and Schenidemandel, P. L. *Health Insurance and Psychiatric Care: Utilization and Cost.* American Psychiatric Association, Washington, 1972.
Srole, L. Urbanization and mental health: Some reformations. Am. Sci., *60:* 576, 1972.

51.9. DELIVERY SERVICE SYSTEMS

Market Sector

If a good or service is acquired in the private sector, costs and benefits can be construed narrowly. Only the parties directly involved in a transaction—the buyer and the seller—are concerned with the outcome. Under conditions of competition, with large numbers of buyers and sellers in the market, costs and benefits to the traders are embodied, respectively, in the supply and demand functions.

Where the supply and demand curves intersect is the equilibrium, the optimum, most efficient solution when the assumptions of competition apply. The essential assumptions include large numbers of knowledgeable buyers and sellers in a market, goods or services of standard quality, and the absence of appreciable effects on third parties. Even when these assumptions are satisfied, the most efficient economic solution is not synonymous with the most desirable solution, for the existing distribution of income and purchasing power may be held to be unfair. The solution that is deemed most desirable is the one associated with the preferred income distribution, which is a value judgment, external to economics.

The opposite pole of a group of competitive sellers is a single seller, a monopoly. The price is higher under monopoly than under competition, quantity is lower, profits persist longer, and power is exercised.

Intermediate between competition and monopoly lie other market structures, such as monopolistic competition and oligopoly (few sellers). For these market structures, the price and quantity solutions are uncertain, with a good deal depending on the particular institutional arrangements and circumstances.

In the health field, economists have been especially intrigued by the sliding scale of fees, under which patients are charged for services in accordance with their estimated ability to pay. Some economists view this practice as evidence of monopoly, since only monopolists can exercise price discrimination between customers. Others see it as a private philanthropic activity, in which the physician takes it upon himself to mitigate the effects of income differentials among his patients. The sliding scale has lost ground in the health field because of its incompatibility with health insurance.

Public Sector

In the health field, there was relatively little purchase of services by government funds before the creation of Medicare and Medicaid in 1965. The criteria for production by government became superior efficiency of operation, after allowing for the possible cost of regulating private producers; the unavailability of facilities in the private sector; and sheer propriety, as in the administration of the machinery of justice.

In this country the health services market is displaced by the nonprofit institution more often than by the government. The nonprofit hospital has played a modest role in the provision of mental health services, even in recent years. Major reliance for service was put on the state mental hospital system. City government provided emergency services and triage services for the state hospitals in the psychiatric units of large municipal hospitals for the sick poor. The Federal government provided long-term psychiatric care for some veterans.

In the mid-1950's came the policies and practices that reduced the total patient load in state mental hospitals, cut the size of each hospital, increased the numbers of discharged patients in the community, and activated a search for alternative modalities and facilities to care for mentally ill patients in the community. The shifts in site of treatment were associated and compatible with the uncoupling of the sources of financing and production of services.

As long as government financing and production were tied together, there was little occasion to undertake certain functions that government often assumes in the health services—regulation and planning. Government agencies do not impose regulatory sanctions on themselves.

In the 1950's, as the state hospital system shrank in size and other facilities and programs gained in importance, it became necessary to assume some regulatory supervision over the new facilities and programs, especially since they were recipients of state funds. Planning came to mean taking the actions of others into account and coordinating with them. Planning must go beyond the most efficient solution in terms of dollar cost and take account of such external effects on a geographic area as are brought about by the concentration in it of large numbers of discharged hospital patients or drug addicts under treatment.

Cost-Benefit Analysis

Cost-benefit analysis, which is an analytical model for the public sector akin to supply-demand analysis in the private sector, is a systematic approach to calculating all the prospective benefits and costs of a proposed public program. Costs include both private costs and government costs. More important, costs and benefits of persons not directly involved in the particular transaction are included. And taking cognizance of costs and benefits into the future makes obvious sense. It precludes establishing new programs on a small scale as an entering wedge for large ones not yet acknowledged just as much as it prevents discrimination against programs that take time to mature.

Link Between Inputs and Outputs

For a study to serve the purpose of a cost-benefit analysis, there must be an effective link between program costs and benefits, between inputs and outputs. The crucial question to be decided is: What is the expected yield of the proposed program relative to its costs? A given program may be worthwhile at its existing level, but expansion would be a dubious venture because marginal cost exceeds marginal benefit.

Quantitative knowledge of the effects of health services on health status seldom exists. When two facilities, such as state mental hospitals and psychiatric units in general hospitals, are compared with respect to cost and duration of absence from employment, it is necessary to determine that they treat patients with the same types of condition and prognosis. Without that premise, the comparison is faulty, perhaps invalid, and it affords an unsound base on which to erect a policy.

The unique characteristics of the mental health services pose extra difficulties for the economist. Figures on incidence are less precise than for other segments of the health services industry. Prognosis of the natural history of disease is more uncertain. There is less agreement among experts on what constitutes effective treatment. Outcome measures are more ambiguous.

Cost-Effectiveness Analysis

The principal source of difficulty in performing cost-benefit analysis in the health field lies in valuing intangible benefits. Even when the effects of a program on mortality, morbidity, and disability are ascertained, what value is to be put on the reduction in discomfort, pain, or grief? What cost-benefit analysis requires is the preparation of such estimates for all alternative programs under consideration so that the program that yields the largest net benefit (benefits minus costs) may be chosen.

Accordingly, it becomes more practical to use cost-effectiveness analysis, accepting the limitation that priorities cannot be derived from the analysis. In cost-effectiveness analysis, all benefits are counted and measured in physical units, and all costs are included, but benefits are not valued.

REFERENCES

Cochrane, A. L. *Effectiveness and Efficiency.* Nuffield Provincial Hospitals Trust, London, 1971.

Klarman, H. E. *The Economics of Health.* Columbia University Press, New York, 1965.

Klarman, H. E. Application of cost-benefit analysis to health systems technology. In *Technology and Health Care Systems in the 1980's*, M. F. Collen, editor, p. 225. United States Government Printing Office, Washington, 1973.

Rice, D. P. *Estimating the Cost of Illness.* United States Government Printing Office, Washington, 1966.

Samuelson, P. A. *Economics*, ed. 9. McGraw-Hill, New York, 1973.

Sloan, F. A. *Planning Public Expenditures on Mental Health Service Delivery.* New York City Rand Institute, New York, 1971.

51.10. HEALTH INSURANCE

Present Coverage of Mental Disorders

As of 1969, more than 63 per cent of the civilian population of all ages had some coverage under private insurance plans for hospital care of mental illness—at minimum, a few days in a psychiatric unit of a general hospital—and 37 per cent had some coverage for out-of-hospital care. The comparable figures for nonpsychiatric illness were 78 per cent and 43 per cent. The benefits for mental illness are in most cases less generous than those offered for other illnesses. The difference is least in regard to hospital care and greatest for ambulatory care. In regard to in-hospital care, there are often fewer days of coverage, special limits on the type of institution in which the care may be provided, or special restrictions governing the number of days between admissions. In regard to ambulatory care, there is sometimes a limit on the number of visits to a psychiatrist during a given time period or a ceiling on the amount of fees covered.

Blue Cross and Blue Shield plans cover 35 to 40 per cent of all persons having some hospital coverage for mental illness and about 20 per cent of those having out-of-hospital coverage. Commercial insurance company plans cover 55 to 60 per cent of all those with some hospital coverage and more than two thirds of those with coverage for out-of-hospital care. Independents cover the rest of the insured population. These independents include community group practice plans, employer-employee-union plans, and medical group clinics.

As of July 1, 1971, all 74 Blue Cross plans in the United States provided some coverage of mental conditions for at least some of their subscribers. The benefits for mental illness were usually less extensive than the benefits for other illnesses; the discrimination was especially severe when the patient was confined to a private mental hospital and even more severe when he was in a public mental hospital.

Of the 72 Blue Shield plans, 63 covered physicians' services for mental illness in the hospital under their most widely held contract in 1968. Nearly half of the 63 plans that gave some coverage provided benefits for the same number of days as for other illnesses. Of the 33 providing lesser benefits, the days of care ranged from 10 during the lifetime of the subscriber to 70 days per admission; the most common benefit was 30 days during a 1-year period.

At the end of 1970, Blue Cross reported that 14.3 million persons were covered under supplementary certificates, mainly those offered jointly with Blue Shield, for outpatient psychiatric benefits.

Basic hospital policies written by insurance companies almost always provide the same benefits for mental illness as for other illnesses, and almost universally benefits are provided in all types of hospitals, although not in institutions caring primarily for alcoholics or drug addicts. Days of care range from 31 to 365, with most policies covering 7 to 120 days. Under basic medical expense policies, physicians' in-hospital visits for persons with a psychiatric diagnosis are covered on the same basis as for any other illness. However, since the benefits are usually fixed amounts per day, they may meet less of a psychiatrist's charges than, for example, the charges of an internist.

Under the major medical policies, the coverage of hospital care and physicians' services in the hospital is almost universally the same for mental illness as for other illnesses. However, coverage of out-of-hospital physicians' services is usually on a lower scale than for other illnesses; most policies provide only 50 per cent reimbursement, and many policies place special limits on the number of visits, charge per visit, and maximum benefits payable.

Group practice plans have been slower than the Blue Cross and Blue Shield plans and the commercial insurance companies to offer substantial mental illness benefits, especially for outpatient treatment. Most of the group practice plans provide fewer hospital benefits for mental illness than for other conditions; some provide benefits only in general hospitals; others provide benefits in mental hospitals but limit care to 30 or 45 days. Virtually all the plans provide some outpatient psychiatric benefits. Some provide these benefits to all subscribers; others provide benefits only to those who have purchased riders or special contracts. Some provide coverage for an unlimited number of visits without a direct charge to the patient; others provide coverage for a limited number of visits at no direct charge but perhaps only $5 a visit for additional visits. Some provide coverage for only a limited number of visits. Almost all, in one way or another, exclude psychoanalysis or the treatment of conditions not thought to be susceptible to improvement through short-term terapy.

The Civilian Health and Medical Program of the Uniformed Services (CHAMPUS), administered by the Department of Defense, provides medical care to dependents of members of the uniformed services and to retired military personnel and dependents of retired and deceased personnel. Care is provided for nervous, mental, and emotional disorders on the same basis as for all other conditions, except that beneficiaries who require continuous hospitalization for more than 45 days must have CHAMPUS approve a plan for the management of the condition. Since January 1, 1967, a special program has been in effect for the care, including institutional residential care, of moderately or severely mentally retarded dependents of active-duty personnel.

Utilization

The cost of providing broad benefits for mental disorders under health insurance has not been astronomical, as some once feared it would be. In most cases the cost is less than 10 per cent of the cost of care for all conditions. In community group practice plans that provide all necessary outpatient care of mental conditions other than psychoanalysis or other long-term therapy, the cost of maintaining the psychiatric department is usually less than 5 per cent of the cost of providing services for all conditions.

The conclusion that the cost of care for mental disorders under health insurance falls within a range that makes such coverage feasible finds additional confirmation from the fact that, in 1968, total estimated expenditures, public and private, for all care for recognized mental conditions in the United States was about $4 billion or about $20 per person. This figure was about 7 per cent of total national health expenditures, public and private, which were $57 billion or $285 per person.

National Health Insurance

Almost all the many bills for national health insurance introduced in the early 1970's had limits on the number of in-hospital days and on the number of physician visits for the treatment of mental illness that did not apply to other illnesses.

The American Medical Association's Medicredit proposal is for a voluntary plan with tax credits provided against individual income taxes to offset the cost of private health insurance purchased by the taxpayer and with the government paying the full premium for those people with incomes below a certain level. No special limits on psychiatric benefits are included.

The Kennedy-Griffith Health Security Bill would provide for a compulsory plan financed by a payroll tax and general Federal revenues. Covering the entire range of personal health service, it would be administered by the Federal government and would have no deductibles or co-insurance. The mental health benefits, more restrictive than those for other illnesses, would include a 45-day in-hospital benefit and a limit of 20 out-patient visits if the service was furnished by a private practitioner but no limit if the service was obtained in certain types of organized settings.

The National Health Insurance Partnership Act, introduced in 1971, included physicians'

services "except when provided by a psychiatrist." This exclusion applied to both inpatient and outpatient services.

The Department of Health, Education, and Welfare has been working on a new proposal, but only its general outlines had been revealed by December 1973, and it had not been introduced as a bill. Under this proposal, employers would be required to offer their employees a minimum health insurance plan and to pay a fixed percentage of the premiums. There would be no limit on hospital services or physician services with the exception of certain specified preventive services and services in cases of mental illness. In-hospital care of mental illness would be limited to 30 days, and outpatient care would be limited to the cost of 15 visits if the care were provided by a private practitioner or of 30 visits if the outpatient service was provided in an organized community setting. Covered services would be subject to deductibles and co-insurance. There would be another program, with similar benefits, for those not in employee groups.

REFERENCES

American Hospital Association. *Hospital Utilization, 1972.* American Hospital Association, Chicago, 1973.

Arnhoff, F. N., and Kumbar, A. H. *The Nation's Psychiatrists—1970 Survey.* American Psychiatric Association, Washington, 1973.

Auster, S. L. Insurance coverage for "mental and nervous conditions": Developments and problems. Am. J. Psychiatry, *126:* 698, 1969.

Avnet, H. H. *Psychiatric Insurance.* Group Health Insurance, New York, 1962. Follmann, J. F. *Insurance Coverage for Mental Illness.* American Management Association, New York, 1970.

Hunter, H. R., Plaska, M., Pinzow, B., and Nesbitt, M. *Development of Alternatives for an Evaluation of the Cost and Effectiveness of Inclusion of Mental, Dental, and Pharmaceutical Benefits in Health Maintenance Organizations—Final Report for Mental Health Component.* American Public Health Association, Washington, 1973.

Mueller, M. S. Private health insurance in 1971: Health care services, enrollment, and finances. Social Security Bull., *36:* 3, 1973.

National Center for Health Statistics. *Utilization of Short-Stay Hospitals by Diagnosis, U.S. 1971.* United States Department of Health, Education, and Welfare, Washington, 1973.

Reed, L. S. *Utilization of Care for Mental Disorders under the Blue Cross and Blue Shield Plan for Federal Employees, 1972.* American Psychiatric Association, Washington, 1973.

Reed, L. S., Myers, E. S., and Scheidemandel, P. L. *Health Insurance and Psychiatric Care: Utilization and Cost.* American Psychiatric Association, Washington, 1972.

Schedemandel, P. L., Kanno, C. K., and Glasscote, R. M., *Health Insurance for Mental Illness.* Joint Information Service of the American Psychiatric Association and the National Association for Mental Health, Washington, 1968.

51.11. SOCIO-ECONOMIC CONSIDERATIONS

Social Parameters

World War II was the watershed for American psychiatry. The rejection of 1 million young men for military service because of emotional instability and the premature separation of an equal number for similar reasons forced the nation to re-evaluate its earlier beliefs about mental illness. A new generation of psychiatrists and young physicians who had become interested in psychiatry became convinced that mental illness could be treated and that treatment, often relatively short, could be efficacious. And the attitudes of the American public that had led to the isolation of the emotionally ill, reinforced by a pessimistic view of their recovery, gave way to a belief that psychiatry could cure many of the severely disturbed and could reduce the incidence and prevalence of mental disorders and disabilities.

The federal government established the National Institute of Mental Health after the war and provided increasingly large sums for research, development, and training. And state legislators were prodded to appropriate more resources for the care and treatment of the mentally ill.

One goal of the mental health reformers was to transform the state mental hospitals from holding facilities to active treatment centers. Second, the reformers argued for the expansion of psychiatric units in general hospitals. A third goal was the expansion of clinic facilities. Fourth, the reformers pressed for a shift in favor of preventive services. Closely associated was a new emphasis on rehabilitation.

The reformers were successful in shifting the locus of inpatient treatment from the state-county hospital to the general hospital. They were even more successful in shifting the emphasis from inpatient to outpatient services.

Finances and Personnel

In 1956, the daily maintenance expenditure per patient in public hospitals was just above $3. In 1970 the figure was about $15. Between 1956 and 1970 the public mental hospital full-time equivalent personnel per 100 resident patients increased from 27 to 67, about 250 per cent. These increased state expenditures were possible because of substantial gains in taxpayers' real income and corresponding gains in state revenues, which permitted the typical legislature to increase funding for its state mental hospitals from $3.95 to $9.30 per capita total population, about 240 per cent, at the same time that the proportion of such expenditures declined from about 3.3 per cent of general state expenditures to 2.2 per cent.

In 1970, about one third of the almost 16,000 full-time or equivalent psychiatrists employed in all mental health facilities were employed in public mental hospitals, where they treated both inpatients and outpatients. In addition, the state mental hospitals employed about 2,000 physicians other than psychiatrists. About 75 hours of physician time were allotted each week to 100 patients in state hospitals, 45 minutes per patient per week.

The data for 1968 show that 8,000 of the total of 32,000 full-time or equivalent psychologists in mental health facilities worked in the state hospital system, as did 4,500 of the total 15,000 social workers and half of the total 36,000 registered nurses. Slightly more than 50 per cent of all full-time personnel are practical nurses, aides, attendants, and other mental health workers. Slightly more than a third are administrative, clerical, and maintenance personnel. The total professional group accounts for only slightly more than 13 per cent of the total. On the average, state and county mental hospitals operated with about two-thirds of a full-time employee for every resident patient.

Treatment in the Community

Inpatient Services

Psychotropic drugs, active programs aimed at early discharge, increased resources, community services for discharged patients, and tighter controls over admissions of the aged into the system transformed state hospitals. The number of patients treated in the psychiatric units of general hospitals doubled between 1955 and 1969 as a result of many of the same forces. In addition, the willingness of Blue Cross, commercial insurance, Medicare, and Medicaid to cover a substantial part of short-term psychiatric patient costs in a general hospital accelerated the willingness of community hospitals to develop or expand treatment facilities.

In 1970-1971, the 600,000 patients who were

discharged from general hospital psychiatric units had an average stay of 11 days, which was only about 3 days above the average for all general hospital patients. About 40 per cent of the psychiatric patients were discharged within the first week and 75 per cent within 3 weeks, a clear indication that the general hospital had not become a holding place for chronic patients.

Outpatient services

Between the mid-1950's and the end of the 1960's, there was approximately a fivefold increase in the number of patients treated on an outpatient basis—fourfold if allowance is made for the increase in the population base. In 1972 about 2.3 million people received some type of treatment or service in an outpatient facility; this figure represents 55 per cent of all persons who sought psychiatric help during the course of the year.

Clinics are by far the largest provider of outpatient services. In 1970, of about 1,100 clinics, 927 admitted about 450,000 new patients, who, together with those already on the rolls, made a total of 5,530,000 visits. The average clinic had one psychiatrist, two psychologists, and three social workers. These three major disiplines accounted for about 85 per cent of all professional personnel.

Community mental health centers have expanded rapidly since the passage of the enabling legislation in the early 1960's. In July 1972 there were about 500 centers across the country; 325 were in full operation. In 1971 about one patient in four receiving outpatient treatment was cared for by a community mental health center, and one in six of all patients treated during the course of the year was treated in whole or in part by a community center.

The Federal government contributed about 30 per cent of the $255 million spent by community centers, state governments contributed about 33 per cent, and local governments contributed about 11 per cent. Patient fees accounted for almost all the remainder, with direct payments amounting to 8 per cent and most of the rest coming from insurance, Medicare, and Medicaid payments.

A 1970 survey of the nation's almost 26,000 psychiatrists reported that the private office was the primary locus of psychiatric practice, followed in order by general hospitals, state mental hospitals, and medical schools.

Socio-Economic Characteristics of Patients

There was relatively little difference between the sexes in total admissions to psychiatric facilities in 1970. The ratio of male to female admissions was 96 to 100. However, in the state system, the male admission rate was 50 to 100 per cent higher than the female rate in every age group except that of persons over 65. In sharp contrast, the male rate was much below the female rate (70 to 100) of admissions to general hospital inpatient units and to private hospitals. Men were also less frequent users of outpatient services; the ratio was about 85 to 100. The principal explanations for the sex differences lie in the much higher admissions of men to state hospitals for alcohol and drug abuse; the much higher rate among women of depressive disorders, which can often be effectively treated in general hospitals; the lower labor force participation rates of women, which are likely to explain in part their greater use of outpatient services.

There are striking differences in the median ages of persons who seek outpatient and inpatient treatment. The clinic population is in its twenties; those requiring hospitalization average about 40.

About one third of all the men who sought psychiatric assistance in 1970 had never married, and only two of five were then living with their wives. Less than half of those women who sought treatment were then married. State mental institutions are characterized by a differentially high proportion of single persons.

About two of five men and one of three women in state hospitals have not gone beyond grammar school. In contrast, psychiatric patients who make use of outpatient facilities are only a shade below the educational norm for the community.

Among discharges from general hospitals, the nonwhite-to-white ratio is 1.3 to 1.0. However, the male rate of 1.7 to 1.0 is responsible for this racial disparity; nonwhite women have a ratio of 0.9 to 1.0 to their white counterparts. Outpatient services were used more heavily by nonwhite women.

Role of the Federal Government

When the National Institute of Mental Health was established in 1946, its primary missions were research and training; relatively small sums were available for developmental projects. The primary commitment of the Federal government for direct care of the mentally ill continued to be the Veterans Administration. In fiscal year 1972, the total obligations for psychiatric services of the V.A. totaled $465 million.

Medicare-Medicaid represented a departure. The Federal government assumed new but limited commitments for the psychiatric care of the aged, but it specifically excluded the use of Medicaid funds for the care of patients below the age of 65 in state mental hospitals. The 1972 budget discloses Federal obligations under the Medical Services Administration of the Department of Health, Education, and Welfare of $563 million. Another $300 million of HEW funds were obligated for rehabilitation and for the assistance of community mental health centers. The Health Services and Mental Health Administration (National Institute of Mental Health and various special programs) had a budgetary obligation of $392 million, bringing HEW's total to $1.255 billion.

A rough estimate of the obligating authority for mental health expenditures for 1972 totaled $2.9 billion, but, if the drug abuse and alcoholism programs and the research and training funds of the National Institute of Mental Health are included, the expanded total is $3.450 billion.

REFERENCES

Kanno, C. K. *Eleven Indices: An Aid in Reviewing State and Local Mental Health and Hospital Programs.* Joint Information Service of the American Psychiatric Association and the National Association for Mental Health, Washington, 1971.
Mechanic, D. *Mental Health and Social Policy.* Prentice-Hall, Englewood Cliffs, N. J., 1969.
National Institute of Mental Health, *Statistical Notes, 30–86: 1970–1973.*
Public Health Service National Center for Health Statistics. *Facts of Life and Death.* United States Government Printing Office, Washington, 1970.
Reed, L. S., Myers, E. S., and Scheidemandel, P. L. *Health Insurance and Psychiatric Care: Utilization and Cost.* American Psychiatric Association, Washington, 1972.
Sloan, F. A. *Planning Public Expeditures on Mental Health Service Delivery.* Rand Institute, New York, 1971.

51.12. RELIGION

Introduction

From the psychological point of view, perhaps the most striking feature of religion is its universality. There are few societies in which religion plays no significant role, and there are relatively few persons who, at one time or another, have not experienced some religious stirring. From this universality one must infer that religion performs some adaptive function, that it is invoked to satisfy one or more universal human needs.

Psychodynamics of Religious Practice

Obsessive-Compulsive Neurosis

Freud observed the similarity of obsessive actions and religious practices—the fixed, stereotyped, and rigid character of the behavior in each, the fact that the behavior of each seems to be meaningless, and the anxiety that follows each when the specific action in question is not performed or is performed imprecisely. Starting from clinical inferences that obsessions and compulsions represent efforts to reinforce the control of instinctual impulses that are threatening to escape from control, he proposed that religious rituals serve the same purpose. The chief difference between the two is that, in the case of neurotic compulsions, it is a sexual impulse that threatens to escape, but in the case of religious ritual, it is an antisocial act. In the case of mental illness, control is exerted intrapsychically on oneself; in the case of religion, control is imposed by society on the person, although it is subsequently accepted into the person's system of self-controls.

Phobia

The phobic patient avoids situations that symbolize to him sexual temptation or opportunity. Religious discipline also imposes stringent prohibitions. Religious persons develop aversions that are almost phobic in intensity toward situations that offer the temptation to violate these prohibitions. However, the phobic person avoids sexual experience because the prospect of it fills him with anxiety; the pious person avoids those situations in which he would be tempted to violate religious discipline and thereby incur the anxiety that such a violation would incur.

Hysteria

The classical hysterical attack represents a flight from genital sexuality by a dramatic disability but with symbolic sexual gratification demonstrated by the hysterical movement or paralysis. In formal, institutionalized Western religions, behavior resembling hysterical attacks is not commonly described, although it is often elicited in certain fundamentalists, revivalist sects. However, mystical trance states have been described frequently. They often resemble an attack of hysteria and sometimes may even betray symbolic sexual content. In some non-Western religions and in some revivalist services even today, trance states are deliberately induced.

Depression

Of all forms of mental illness, depression probably elicits most of the behavior that suggests religion in both form and content. However, this behavior appears much less commonly in the definitive depressive state than in one of the clinical states that precede it and that constitute part of the struggle against it. Many persons, when they feel the first stirrings of discomfort due to threatening depression, respond with exuberant, pleasure-seeking behavior. Excessive self-indulgence is seldom recommended in Western religion, but, in unfamiliar religions or anomalous deviations, sexual excess and perversion are recommended as intermediary steps toward achieving mystical union with God.

The prospect of depression frequently motivates a person to attach himself in a dependent way to a parental protector. The clinging may take the form of devout adherence to God, but it is usually associated with meticulous adherence to the rules of a religious community.

The new religious faith in many instances is other than the one in which the person was reared. Therefore, the conversion is usually an affront to one's parents. This shift is not an easy one because it involves the complete repudiation of one's way of life and an admission of guilt. Generally, these conversions are temporary. Occasionally, however, when this experience occurs in a person of leadership potential and in times of social turmoil, that person may create and lead a new religious movement.

When neither self-indulgence nor clinging succeeds in containing the advance of the depression, the person must suddenly detach himself from those to whom he had been clinging and, in fact, turn against them. When the religious community is repudiated, a negative conversion is seen.

Religion provides mechanisms for both intensifying guilt and alleviating it. It creates guilt by setting high standards of behavior and pointing up transgressions. It provides a number of methods of alleviating guilt: confession, prayer, acts of good work, and charity. Guilt appears with pathological intensity in states of definitive depression.

Schizophrenia

The aspect of religion that corresponds psychodynamically to schizophrenia is otherworldliness or transcendentalism. Transcendentalism finds its most explicit expression in mysticism.

The mystical trance resembles a kind of hysterical transport or brief psychotic dissociation. The trance is ordinarily induced by observing a regimen, usually of abstinence and asceticism or, in other cultures, of excessive sexual indulgence. It may be invited by long periods of mediation. The person experiences the state passively. Descriptions of the trance state consistently refer to striking sensory experiences. The trance state, at its beginning, is sometimes associated with anxiety. As it approaches its climax, the person usually describes a feeling of great pleasure, often called bliss or ecstasy.

The schizophrenic is apt to announce that the world has come to an end, that it is destroyed in a conflagration or in a war. He then becomes aware that the world and life are being renewed, often by virtue of some act of his. A similar mechanism can be recognized in instances of drug-induced hallucinatory experiences. The drug is taken in an attempt to alleviate anguish or depression. The hallucinations induced resemble those described in the mystical trance.

Paranoia

Less dramatic than the trance state but more influential in determining the person's fate is the mystical way of life. The person who adopts the mystical way of life may display a general behavior pattern that is little, if at all, different from that of others. The difference lies in how he experiences his life. Doing the same mundane things that everyone else does, he feels himself to be in direct contact with divinity. For the mystic, the world of consensual reality is flavored by the transcendent world. It is the quality of transcendence that lends his life meaning, pleasure, and reality, even though this whole dimension is invisible to others.

The psychopathological analogue to this state of mind is paranoia. The paranoiac, too, walks with one foot in consensual reality and the other in his own private universe, which he considers the ultimate reality. He can arrange his responses to the outside world so that they seem appropriate. Yet he knows that these things that others regard as ordinary and unremarkable have meanings. One may regard both these states as states of partial dissociation. The two states differ in that the mystical way of life affords gratification and pleasure, but the paranoiac sees the world as hostile.

Religion and Society

Some of the functions of religion arise from its role in community organization. Religion provides rites and ceremonies to facilitate the induction of the young into the adult community. It validates marriage and divorce. Its rituals encourage identification of the individual members with one another and subservience to traditional leadership and its current representatives. It discourages intragroup dissension by interdicting incest and murder, and it surrounds these two principal offenses with an elaborate code of morality and ethics. The observance of this code deters the pursuit of individual advantage at the expense of other members of the group.

Pastoral Counseling

The pastoral function of the clergyman in the United States extends to the function of assisting the individual member of the religious congregation to deal with serious problems that he cannot resolve alone and that may cause anguish and damage. The pastoral function includes visiting the ill, comforting the mourner, encouraging the widow, and helping the orphan. The term "counseling" involves consultation for the purpose of helping the troubled person solve a specific presenting problem. It may be a marital problem, a parent-child problem, a problem of conflict among siblings, or a complaint of feelings of guilt or anxiety.

Those who are seriously mentally ill seldom go for counseling. Sometimes, a person fighting depression goes to a clergyman. An occasional paranoiac asks the clergyman to alter the religion or attacks the religious authority in conformity with his delusion. Of those who are not grossly ill, many show some sort of personality disorder, character disorder, mild depression, or sexual inhibition. Most of these persons will not see a psychiatrist.

In their counseling, some clergymen offer spiritual guidance, others offer advice on how to get along with family and neighbors, and still others offer psychoanalytically oriented discussions and advice. They may suggest psychiatric consultation or discuss the case with a psychiatrist they trust.

REFERENCES

Freud, S. Totem and taboo. In *Standard Edition of the Complete Psychological Works of Sigmund Freud*, vol 13, p. 61. Hogarth Press, London, 1955.
Freud, S. Obsessive actions and religious practices. In *Standard Edition of the Complete Psychological Works of Sigmund Freud*, vol. 9, p. 117. Hogarth Press, London, 1959.
Freud, S. Civilization and its discontents. In *Standard Edition of the Complete Psychological Works of Sigmund Freud*, vol. 21, p. 64. Hogarth Press, London, 1961c.
Freud, S. Moses and monotheism. In *Standard Edition of the Complete Psychological Works of Sigmund Freud*, vol. 23, p. 7. Hogarth Press, 1964.
Freud, S., and Pfister, O. *Psychoanalysis and Faith: The Letters of Sigmund Freud and Oskar Pfister*. H. Meng and E. L. Freud, editors, Basic Books, New York, 1963.
Group for the Advancement of Psychiatry. *The Psychic Function of Religion in Mental Illness and Health*, Report No. 67. Group for the Advancement of Psychiatry, New York, 1968.

51.13. PARAPROFESSIONALS

Introduction

Here a paraprofessional is defined as a person who has not obtained a degree in one of the usual mental health professions, although he may have a degree in the arts or from some professional school other than those serving the mental health group.

Who They Are

About 42 per cent of community mental health center staffs in 1969 were composed of paraprofessionals. The paraprofessionals come from every walk of life. They usually have a high school education but not necessarily so; many programs aid workers in obtaining a high school equivalency diploma before going on to further education. Paraprofessionals may have several years of college and occasionally a baccalaureate degree. There is a likelihood that, in the urban scene, they are indigenous to the area.

Where They Work

Most programs that employ large numbers of paraprofessionals are located in inner-city areas. The facilities often serve areas undergoing deterioration or disorganization.

Paraprofessionals are also employed in the more conventional mental health establishments, such as ambulatory care divisions, inpatient partial hospitals, and the various categorical programs—addiction, alcoholism, mental retardation, and geriatric programs.

What They Do

Early in the nonprofessional movement, the bridging-expediter function was an unmet role and, hence, was a natural role for this new type of worker. Later, the caretaker and helping person roles, all of which could easily be taught, were appropriate to the new group. The unique aspect of the workers was that the majority came from the same socio-economic class and from the same community as the patients, and they were aware of the patients' problems in living. In the Western Psychiatric Institute's Community Mental Health-Mental Retardation Center, the roles listed in Table I were delineated as being performed or participated in by paraprofessionals.

Training and Education

Of the many criticisms of the paraprofessional movement, the most often voiced include lack of adequate supervision and inadequate training or education for the roles the nonprofessionals have been assigned or have assumed.

In the beginning of the movement, the emphasis was on the indigenous nonprofessional. At the Lincoln Hospital Mental Health Clinic, there was a prejob period of 3 weeks to orient workers to the operational tasks and to learn about roles vis-à-vis the agencies in the community and the client. This phase was followed by a 3-week intensive training program of a mixed on-the-job and didactic nature. After this 6-week period, ongoing training continued, and an attempt was made to refine interviewing skills and to teach new skills as they seemed appropriate to the aide's level of development. This ongoing training occupied about a fifth of the aide's time—1 day a week. This pattern has been the one followed by many programs in the early phases.

TABLE I

Roles of Paraprofessionals in Western Psychiatric Institute's Community Mental Health-Mental Retardation Center

Reception center	Initial screening, supervised testing
	Crisis intervention where social factors seem most significant
Inpatient	Milieu therapy
	Social relationship therapy
	Caretaking
Day hospital	Milieu therapy
	Social relationship therapy
	Companionship
	Caretaking
Mental retardation	Social relationship
	Caretaking
	Activities therapy (activity group therapy)
	Mental retardation expediting in neighborhoods
	Tutoring
	Training
	House parents
Addiction services	Counseling—individual and group
	Rehabilitation
	Job training and retaining
Neighborhood teams	Liaison with other units
	Generalist activities with all ages—individual counseling, group counseling, socializing, activity groups (particularly with children), tutoring, and home visiting
	Consultation with school and community groups
	Community activities

One of the glaring deficiencies of in-service or on-the-job training is that it does not provide a true career ladder and has a tendency to lock one into a particular establishment or forces the worker to resign and seek out one of the established professional career lines for advancement.

Attempts at more formal education, such as the 2-year training of housewives who were college graduates, were made in the early 1960's. These programs have graduated limited numbers and, although not the answer, have stimulated the paraprofessional movement.

Other training programs have used the college graduate manpower pool to recruit students. In a program in the Georgia Mental Health Center, college graduates majoring in the social sciences who have a desire to work with people are given a year-long intensive educational experience consisting of both practical and didactic work.

Another trend is the associate-of-arts degree. The first program of this nature was developed by Purdue University. The program attempted to educate and train a middle-level or preprofessional mental health worker for a vocation and not a job. Since an associate degree was involved, general educational requirements had to be met, and a broad social-psychological base in the understanding of human behavior had to be developed. In addition to the didactic program, a practicum in a variety of mental health facilities was made available.

The current trend appears to be toward the community college with an associate-of-arts degree. In 1972, the 2-year college programs had grown to 140, nearly all in community colleges, although schools of the allied health professions and a few universities have been involved. In general, curriculum time is divided into one-third general studies, one-third mental health courses; and one-third practicum or field experiences.

Collaborative planning with various participating agencies results in future employment potential. Graduates of these programs are found in nearly every type of care-giving program. The success of this movement depends on the ability of the mental health establishments to set up jobs for these workers.

Problems

Numbering nearly 100,000, the paraprofessionals make up half of the care givers in the mental health field. These persons are at many levels of education and training.

In the beginning of the nonprofessional movement, when the persons being hired came from the poor themselves, great emphasis was placed on the uniqueness of this type of mental health worker. He appeared to perform some functions that persons in the usual professional categories could not. It was felt that some of these functions were not teachable but were a part of the nonprofessional's personality, his relationship with the client and his problems, and his ability to provide an acceptable model for the patient or client. Many persons glorified the role of the indigenous nonprofessional worker, assigning abilities that either did not exist or were greatly exaggerated. These high expectations could not be met, and the professionals who were already somewhat threatened became more negative in their opinions. This disillusionment is not as true of the programs for the middle-level worker, with their more clearly defined goals and roles and more structured and unified educational programs.

The question of supervision is an important one for which there is no easy answer. What type? By whom? How much? Obviously, it varies from worker to worker, depending on his level of sophistication and training and the tasks he performs. There must be sufficient supervision to enable the worker to feel comfortable with what he is doing. Most paraprofessionals accept supervision from professionals if the professional has a relatively egalitarian approach to the wide range of professionals and nonprofessionals in the field. The availability of the professional is important.

The professionals who promote programs where paraprofessionals are involved must believe in the paraprofessionals' ability and efficacy in the mental health care delivery system. If a professional's persuasion is that the only effective therapy is carried out by professionals and that the use of the paraprofessional is largely expedient, the use and role of the paraprofessional will be vastly different from what it would be if the professional were devoted to helping develop the unique aspects of the paraprofessional through the full range of programing for primary, secondary, and tertiary prevention of mental disorders.

Career ladders must be built to enable those who wish to remain paraprofessionals to advance in status and income. A way must be found to provide quality education that enables the paraprofessional to be prepared for entrance into professional schools if he desires.

A national schema for licensing or certification would perhaps be ideal. This schema would ensure that a status existed that would enable the paraprofessional to change locations and not be penalized because his training and education took place outside the state to which he moved. Unless paraprofessionals are used to the highest level that their education has prepared them for, their training will be a waste of time and money.

REFERENCES

American Psychiatric Association. Position paper on community mental health centers. Am. J. Psychiatry, *130:* 239, 1973.

Baltimore, C. F., and Wolford, J. A. The nondegree community mental health worker and the community. In *The Community Mental Health Center: Strategies and Programs*, A Beigel and A. I. Levenson, editors, p. 397. Basic Books, New York, 1972.

Grosser, C., Henry, W. E., and Kelly, J. G. *Nonprofessionals in the Human Services* Jossey-Bass, San Francisco, 1969.

McPheeters, H. L., King, J. B., and Teare, R. J. The middle-level mental health worker. Hosp. Community Psychiatry, *23:* 329, 1972.

Pattison, M. E., and Elpers, J. R. A developmental view of mental health manpower trends. Hosp. Community Psychiatry, *23:* 325, 1972.

Pearl, A., and Riessman, F. *New Careers for the Poor: The Nonprofessional in Human Services*. Free Press, New York, 1965.

Position paper on community mental health centers. Am. J. Psychiatry, *130:* 239, 1973.

Rogeness, G. H., and Bednar, R. A. Teenager helper: A role in community mental health. Am. J. Psychiatry, *130:* 933, 1973.

Sobey, F. *The Nonprofessional Revolution in Mental Health.* Columbia University Press, New York, 1970.

51.14. ETHICS

Introduction

Ethics is defined in the dictionary as "the discipline dealing with what is good and bad and with moral duty and obligation." In normal usage ethics is more applied to professional behavior, and morals has more of a religious connotation and pertains particularly to sexual conduct.

A new set of rules of evidence, adopted by the United States Supreme Court, includes a clarification of the limits of doctor-patient confidentiality in Federal court proceedings. Rule 504, concerning the psychotherapist-patient privilege, stipulates that "a patient has a privilege to refuse to disclose and to prevent any other person from disclosing confidential communications, made for the purposes of diagnosis or treatment of his mental or emotional condition, including drug addiction, among himself, his psychotherapist, or persons who are participating in the diagnosis or treatment under the direction of the psychotherapist, including members of the patient's family."

Psychiatric Ethics

The psychiatric profession annotated the principles of medical ethics of the American Medical Association as they are applicable to the practice of psychiatry and published them in September 1973. These annotations include comments regarding such topics as the doctor-patient relationship, continuing education, professional competence, contract practice, income, psychiatric records, anonymity, and income sources. The comment on sex is the one direct, unequivocal, short-sentence principle. Section 1, paragraph 2 reads: "Sexual activities with a patient are unethical." Procedures for handling complaints on ethical conduct accompany the annotations.

Psychiatry realizes more than any other profession that ethical behavior changes with the time and the place according to conditions and consequences and that particular duties or changes or conditioned complexes give rise to a particular consequence or group of consequences. The application of ethics cannot be seen as static; it will always be secondary to and lagging behind the scientific development. It will respond more to the wisdom of the many than to the knowledge of the few. When dealing with ethics, one borrows from many imperative sources—for example, from the religious beliefs of the group to which he belongs and under whose auspices he was brought up.

No longer can one abide by the exclusive protection of the right of the individual patient. To the rights of the individual, one must add the rights of the group, and sometimes collective right becomes imperative. In assessing the need for hospitalization, the psychiatrist has to take into consideration the possibilities of emotional contagion and the possibilities of familial and group psychological trauma that psychological symptoms in one member of the family or the group may provoke.

In 1948 the Geneva Convention adopted a Neo-Hippocratic Oath for the medical profession, and in 1949 the World Medical Association voted in London a code of international medical ethics. The fundamentals can be summarized in a phrase secondary to *primum non nocere;* "Protect and prolong the life of human beings." General guidelines for use in the physician's own personal code of ethics can be simply stated in the dictum, "Do for your patient as you would like others to do for you." The care of the individual patient poses ethical problems in such areas as examination, information, confidentiality, choice of treatment, hospitalization, suicidal or homicidal possibilities, destructive behavior, and drugs.

Personal Code of Ethics

The development of ethics as part of the human psyche is ascribed to the superego. Superego development is late, incomplete, and increasingly complicated. The investigator, the policeman, the accusatory voice, the judge, and the hangman are not internalized in the same way in everyone. The psychiatrist's original bent for medicine and his later involvement in psychiatry may pertain to specific characterological aspects of a special personality profile with superego specifics.

Ethics is ultimately a study of human behavior, and human behavior can be evaluated only in the framework of its motivations.

Professional Code of Ethics

In psychiatry, the ethics of the relationship with a patient borrows heavily from the long-established rules of the medical profession. But it is not clear whether the acceptance of the patient dates from the time the appointment is made or from the time of the appointment itself, with its therapeutic contract and the development of some kind of therapeutic alliance. It is the responsibility of the psychiatrist to train, assist, and supervise answering services and secretaries for the strict maintenance of confidentiality. The one-to-one relationship established with the psychiatrist makes adherence to confidentiality extremely important. The necessary intensity of the therapeutic relationship may tend to activate sexual and other fantasies on the part of both, but the one-to-one situation has served as a model from which most ethical solutions derive.

The collection and banking of data, the present capacity for easy and total reproduction of documents, total-memory machines, eavesdropping apparatus, and tape recordings bring new problems. Recent developments outside the profession, including the increased use of subpoenas to produce patient records in court, have made a revision in the principle of confidentiality obligatory. Not taking notes or not keeping records is not a plausible solution. The fight for private records must go on, in spite of adverse court decisions. Records, once taken, must be kept in a safe place.

Interviews are frequently taped or videotaped. This practice is permissible in teaching and research situations, but it should not become an everyday occurrence. Taping telephone conversations with patients without their knowledge and permission is prohibited by law.

Patients must be apprised of the full connotations of waiving the privilege of privacy. On examinations done to determine suitability for various jobs or to determine legal competence, the psychiatrist must describe the nature, purpose, and lack of confidentiality of the examination to the patient at the beginning of the examination.

Rules on charging for a missed appointment, specifying fees, and extending professional courtesy are easy to promulgate and observe, but the nuances involved will never be covered by a code. The personal ethics of the physician must guide his conduct. The legal responsibilities involved in stopping treatment for nonpayment have to be taken into consideration.

Hospitalized patients, outpatient clinics, follow-up clinics, the drug scene, college and university services, and payment by third parties complicate the ethical aspect of the doctor-patient relationship. Most of the time the contract for services exists before the relationship starts, and policies are in effect regarding such matters as records, procedure, and discharge. Sometimes these policies are obsolete or do not conform with the psychiatrist's personal ethical commitment; at other times a professional preaches one set of rules and practices according to another set of rules.

If the ethical problems of relations with one's own profession are difficult, the ethical problems of relations with other professions and some paraprofessions are even more difficult. In some instances, the law declares that any services given by other professionals must be under the constant supervision of a psychiatrist, who carries the legal responsibility for their actions. In some places new laws permit the direct practice of certain therapies by psychologists. Apart from the legal implications, the decision to delegate certain functions and the evaluation and supervision of others need constant study to decide what to delegate, how much, and to whom.

Redefining mental health to encompass the gamut of the human condition and redefining alcoholics and drug users as sick have added new burdens on the limited supply of competent health manpower. It has become inexpedient for the psychiatrist to assume direct services to his clients. The delegation of responsibility for cases and the supervision of others have become psychiatric ethical problems.

Hospitalization

The decision whether or not to hospitalize, the evaluation of suicidal and homicidal possibilities, and the evaluation of the result of hospitalization on social and professional grounds are always ethical problems. The law attempts to provide guidelines for the hospitalization of the legally insane, and these guidelines have to be constantly revised. Accusatory voices are raised against too much and too long hospitalization, even to the use of habeas corpus, peer review boards, and defenders from other professions on the civil rights scene. Weekend passes, coed activities, mixing patient populations, protests—these are other areas for ethical concern.

Setting rules for divergent age groups has to be stressed; an adolescent patient population is not the same as an older group. The differences between the community's rules and laws and those observed inside the walls of the hospital are not easily understood. When the patient's welfare and the psychiatric administrator's legal responsibility are in conflict, the ethical issue is formidable.

Drug addicts, especially the hard-core and long-term users, form a patient population that has to be dealt with on terms that are different from those used with the usual patient population. The physical facilities have to be different, and keeping control of the drug traffic in the hospital is always a serious problem. Hospital drug populations are usually young populations, with problems inherent to that age group. Their viewpoints and practices on the outside prove to be constant stresses in the hospital situation.

Economics

The ethical problem of direct fees is nonexistent if psychiatrists abide by a per-hour basis for charging. Unfortunately, drug dispensing, rapid encounter groups, infrequent contacts, and undue use of ancillary personnel to perform functions that are charged for at a psychiatrist-fee level are getting the upper hand in psychiatric practices.

It is the responsibility of the psychiatrist to prevent misuse and overuse of psychiatric service. The dependent patient must not be allowed to prolong treatment interminably.

Ethics and the Law

Professional ethical considerations are sometimes directly opposed to legal mandates and have to be resolved individually. For decades psychiatrists fell back on the M'Naughten rule of jurisprudence. Different happenings in various quarters brought a reappraisal of the whole situation. To mention only some of the most important: the Durham decision on the substantive test of insanity, the nature and extent of psychiatric testimony in cases raising the insanity defense, a person's legal right to adequate treatment if he is involuntarily confined, criteria for the hospitalization of senile patients, and the evaluation and definition of dangerousness. Thomas Szasz argues that psychiatrists have no place in the courts of law and that all forced confinement of people because of mental illness is unjust. Arguments accumulate on both sides of the questions about confinement, suicide prevention, and abortion.

Institutions

The hospitalization of voluntary and involuntary patients under the same roof complicates the setting of rules, regulations, and ethical standards. Should any sexual behavior between consenting adults be permitted, avoided, or prosecuted? If such behavior is permitted between patients, is it permitted between patients and staff? The protection of the personal property of the patient has not always been a well-documented concern. In the name of precaution, patients are often subjected to harsh rules and deprived of the simplest forms of human dignity. Informing patients of their rights is rarely done properly and consistently. A patient's right to refuse treatment and other measures imposed on him is never clearly stated. Patients are rarely informed of the disposition of their belongings or of the possibility of having contacts with the outside, and there is too much reliance on verbal information being given not by the psychiatrist but by others among the hospital personnel. Permitting the use of certain therapies, with a knowledge that other, preferred forms of therapy are not available in that situation, poses a problem of large ethical dimensions.

Records and Confidentiality

What records does one keep? For how long? How should they be disposed of? When? By whom?

It facilitates matters and indirectly takes the ethical question into account if unused or unserviceable records and papers are eliminated permanently every 5 to 10 years. Every psychiatrist should have, preferably in writing, a set of orders regarding the disposition of his records and an appointed person to carry out such orders after his death. A law firm, a personal lawyer, a colleague, or a group of colleagues could be used for such purposes.

Clinic and hospital records are public property and are treated as such, but some confidential papers of ongoing cases may pose ethical questions. It is easy for controversial material to get into a school record. This record usually accompanies the student not only through his school years but well into his adult years, ready to deprive him of important college or job opportunities that are far removed from the event recorded. It falls to the psychiatrist to set rules and regulations in ethical matters. Some school systems are applying different standards of availability to different sets of student records (a set that would be kept confidential and a set of more public information, such as grades) and with different lifetime schedules (to be destroyed or to be kept after the student has left the school).

Increasingly, forms standardized for insurance and for entrance to colleges, professions, jobs, and clubs include questions about past mental illness, hospitalization, outpatient treatment, use of ataraxics, psychotherapy, psychoanalysis, and psychiatric consultations. Information about treatment is completely different ethically from information about diagnosis and hospitalization. How to answer the questions of concerned parties about a psychotic patient may be easy; but how to answer questions about the consultation of a well-adapted, healthy adolescent may prove distressing. To answer evasively may not be realistic. To answer outright may be unlawful.

The practitioner must make up his own mind how to deal with this problem.

Relations with Others

When referring a case, the psychiatrist must know the other physician's professional capacity and his availability.

Psychiatrists, because of the broad spectrum of their expertise, are subject to innumerable pressures by the news media to make statements in distantly related fields. Ad hoc statements are usually lacking in precision, even when produced by the most knowledgeable persons in the field; but the real danger exits when a professional naively attempts to give opinions on broad subjects and in fields other than his own.

The division of responsibility between trainee and supervisor required for training purposes has to safeguard the welfare of the patient. Confidentiality in the training situation is complicated because videotape and closed-circuit television are useful in training but call for new ethical considerations. Patients are not always informed that they are being used for training purposes.

The problem of informed consent by psychotic patients and the criminally insane should constantly be under careful surveillance. Experimenting with human beings solely for scientific interest must always be weighed against the aspects of discomfort or even cruelty visited on the patient.

New Techniques

As some techniques of group therapy evolved and the movement acquired momentum, the spectrum became complicated with encounter groups, sensitivity groups, and marathon groups. Most of the time, the training of practitioners of these modalities is meager or nonexistent, therapeutic indications and contraindications are not established, and no evaluation is made. Walk-in clinics, store-front clinics, and other services must be evaluated carefully.

Group treatment of couples for specific sexual difficulties and some variations of the Masters and Johnson techniques can easily run into problems with the community. To provide, directly or indirectly, sexual partners of various ages and both sexes also presents pointed ethical questions. The production of sexual educational material (films and photographs) of individuals and groups, although under the aegis of science, raises questions about the ethical aspects of information, consent, usage, and basic respect for individual privacy.

Behavior-modification techniques have been questioned vigorously. Controversy has been aroused by the use of electrical stimulation of the central nervous system in operant conditioning to modify behavior. Behavior-modification techniques, when used to modify group behavior, can become powerful tools. In unscrupulous hands these techniques might lead to sinister uses.

REFERENCES

American Psychiatric Association. *Constitution and By-laws.* American Psychiatric Association, Washington, 1973.
Hardin Branch, C. H. Princples of medical ethics with annotations especially applicable to psychiatry. Am. J. Psychiatry, *130:* 9, 1973.
Chavez, I. Ética, deontología, y responsibilidad del médico contemporáneo. J. Puerto Rico Med. Assoc. *62:* 5, 1970.
Menninger, K. A. Psychological factors in the choice of medicine as a profession. Bull. Menninger Clin. *21:* 51, 1957.
Sore, M. F., and Golan, S., editors. *Current Ethical Issues in Mental Health.* National Institute of Mental Health, Rockville, Md., 1970.
Silving, H. Psychoanalysis and the criminal law. Crim. Law, Criminol. Polit. Sci., *51:* 19, 1960.
Szasz, T. S. *The Myth of Mental Illness.* Harper & Row, New York, 1961.

51.15. PARAPSYCHOLOGY

Parapsychology

Parapsychology or psychic research borders on physics and biology as well as on the behavioral sciences. Its subject matter is the study of interactions between organisms and their external environment, including other organisms, that are not mediated by recognized sensorimotor functions of the organism.

Such interactions are divided into input-output types. The input form, generally called extrasensory perception (ESP), involves the acquisition of information concerning external states, objects, or events under conditions that prohibit the involvement of receptor organs. Psychokinesis (PD) is the output form, consisting of influences exerted by a person on some aspect of his external environment without the use of known motor (output) functions.

Experimental evidence exists for several modalities of ESP, based on characteristics of the target information. Telepathy is ESP of subjective states or cognitive contents in another person. ESP of objective conditions or events is called clairvoyance. In addition to contemporaneous ESP of subjective and objective events, evidence has been produced for noninferential prediction of future states or events, which is termed precognition.

It has become customary to refer to these extrasensory and motor functions generally as psi phenomena. Psi is here used as a less committal equivalent to the popular usage of "psychic." Embedded in this usage is the hypothesis of an underlying common basis for the various psi modalities. Supporting evidence for this hypothesis consists of laboratory comparisons in which, for example, telepathic and clairvoyant responses were found to co-vary with experimental conditions, such as stimulant and depressant drug treatments.

Surveys of American psychologists indicate increasing acceptance of ESP research, especially among younger members of the profession. The Parapsychological Association, an international society of professional research workers engaged in parapsychological research was admitted.

Psychokinetic Effect

The experimental investigation of psychokinesis began at Duke in the mid-1930's with dice-throwing tests in which subjects attempted to mentally influence the fall of specific die faces or combinations. The evidence for PK in these studies consisted of two effects: statistically highly significant deviations from chance expectancy and significant and highly consistent declines in scoring. Independent replications of these wishing-with-dice experiments have confirmed the decline effect tendency for subjects to deteriorate in their dice-willing success over a period of effort. PK effects have more recently been produced with completely automated electronic test equipment.

Attitudinal and Personality Factors

The subject's attitudes toward ESP, the ESP task he is required to perform, and the experimenter with whom he interacts during the task have been found to interact significantly with success in psi tasks. The ESP test scores of believers are significantly higher than those of disbelievers. Similar attitudinal factors have been found in classroom studies of teacher-pupil relations. Pupils who liked and were liked by their teachers (who administered the tests) obtained significantly higher ESP scores than pupils who disliked and were disliked by their teachers.

The search for personality correlates of psi has generated a sizable literature. The most consistent finding is a positive relationship between ESP scores and various measures of extroversion. Questionnaire measures of anxiety and neuroticism correlate negatively with ESP guessing success, whereas creativity and frequency of dream recall are positively related with ESP. General intelligence has not been found to be correlated strongly or reliably with ESP success.

Altered States of Consciousness

The most frequently reported mediator of spontaneous ESP effects is dreaming. A series of experimental studies employing electrophysiological sleep-monitoring techniques to detect dream episodes has been reported in which a sensorially isolated agent attempted to transmit salient aspects of randomly chosen target pictures to a sleeping subject during periods of dreaming. In these studies, target pictures were rated against verbatim dream reports on a blind basis for correspondences. Significant ESP target incorporation has been reported in 9 of 12 published studies.

Experimental studies comparing ESP success in hypnotic and nonhypnotic conditions indicate that hypnosis affects ESP performance, but the specific facilitative factors have not yet been identified. Cortical inhibition, induced through sensory deprivation and feedback regulation of electroencephalographic α density, appears positively related to ESP success, although the work in this area must still be regarded as inconclusive.

Psi Effects in Infrahuman Subjects

Experimental studies of psi functioning in lower animals have involved a wide variety of methods and species. In the most convincing studies small rodents (mice or gerbils) were placed in a special cage and presented with an extrasensory shock-avoidance task. A random number generator passed an electric current through one of two floor grids in the cage. The animal could avoid being shocked by precognitively anticipating which side would receive the current. Photocell sensors tracked trial-to-trial movements, permitting automatic recording of binary hits and misses. Trials were selected in which the animal's behavior was not rigidly stimulus-bound or stereotyped, since it was hypothesized that such random behavior trials would be more amenable to psi influence. The results for selected random behavior trials have been consistently significant in eight American replications of the original French work.

Parapsychology and Psychiatry

Psychoanalysis

Ehrenwald suggested that some of the symptoms of schizophrenia could be understood as a failure on the part of the patient to ward off heteropsychic or telepathically perceived information arising from the unconscious or preconscious of others. The misinterpretation of such content as autopsychically derived (arising from one's own unconscious or preconscious) reinforces paranoid and grandiose ideation. Ehrenwald developed the view that any handicap or defect prepared the way for telepathic functioning. He also called attention to the resemblance between the fragmentation and displacement effects that characterize the efforts of precipients trying to reproduce target material and the kind of disorganization noted in the drawings of brain-damaged patients.

Servadio emphasized the relationship between transference and thought transference, stressing the unconscious, emotionally colored bridging function of each. Telepathy takes place when, in the course of an impelling transference, the element of frustration occurs, blocking communication and forcing the patient into a more regressive state, one that favors the reinstatement of an archaic mode of communication. Servadio also stressed countertransferential factors and noted that telepathy occurs when there is a dovetailing of the analyst's emotional patterns with those of the patient.

Eisenbud emphasized the frequency and range of psi events in the psychoanalytic setting. He traced out the dynamic interconnections between the patient's telepathic comment or dream and the relevent events in his own life.

He was sensitive not only to telepathic exchanges between his patients and himself but also among his patients as they unconsciously acted out elements of earlier family conflicts. Eisenbud regarded psi effects as a ubiquitous, ever-active component of daily life.

Precognition in dreams is far more frequent in anecdotal reports than is the telepathic dream. A number of accounts have appeared describing the occurrence of precognitive dreams in the course of therapy, accounts that the authors regarded as genuinely precognitive rather than explainable in terms of latent dynamics or telepathy.

Presumptively Telepathic Dreams

The criteria useful in identifying a dream as presumptively telepathic are as follows:

1. When correspondences between dream elements and objective events occur, these correspondences should be both unusual and of a noninferential character. The dream element should be one not ordinarily occurring in dreams or in the dreams of the particular patient. The objective event to which it refers should be one that could not have been inferred by the patient from his knowledge of the therapist or known on the basis of nonverbal cueing.

2. A close temporal relationship should exist between the occurrence of the patient's dream and the events in the life of the therapist that are mirrored in the dream.

3. The linkage or correspondence to be established must exist not only at the manifest level but also at the level of psychological meaning.

Character Traits of Telepathic Dreamers. Patients who report the most striking and frequent telepathic incidents tend to be withdrawn and schizoid in makeup, so that telepathy, when it does occur, appears to break through a compulsively maintained isolation. Under experimental conditions, healthier and more outgoing people do better than more constricted and narcissistic people.

Dynamics. Telepathic rapport seems to occur in response to what the patient experiences as a temporary loss of contact with the therapist. The patient appears to be sensitive to the loss, and his response in the form of a comment or dream incorporating telepathic content pertaining to the therapist dramatically refocuses attention on the patient. It serves the dual purpose of establishing the patient's

awareness of the therapist's dereliction and challenging the therapist to acknowledge the part his own difficulties are playing in the analysis.

Those therapists who are interested and oriented to the occurrence of the telepathic dream seem to encounter such dreams more often than do more skeptical colleagues. The problem may be not one of the frequency of the occurrence of the psi event but, rather, the failure to recognize it as such.

The spontaneous occurrence of telepathy in crisis situations suggests that in some way the mobilization of vital needs is implicated. Motivational systems close to the core of the person come into operation in the dream. Dreaming as a state of heightened activation suggests that a vigilance function is operative, oriented more to the detection of threats to the symbolic system linking the person to his social milieu than to the detection of threats involving his state of bodily intactness. In the dreaming state, one has the possible advantages of an altered state of consciousness combined with a state of high arousal and one in which basic motivational systems are activated. While a person is dreaming, his conscious experience is organized along lines of emotional contiguity, rather than spatial and temporal contiguity. To accommodate the reality of telepathic phenomena, one would have to postulate that the affective scanning that takes place as dreaming occurs can, when the occasion calls for it, bridge a spatial gap and incorporate information arriving independently of any known communication channel or energy system. At these moments, the dreamer seems able to incorporate transpersonal as well as personal content into his dream.

Implications. The clarification of the dynamics underlying the patient's instrumental use of the telepathy maneuver may expose more sharply than under any other circumstances the way in which a particular transference-countertransference difficulty may be blocking therapeutic progress.

At a theoretical level, the study of psi events may have a bearing on the understanding of altered states of consciousness, particularly those states in which, as in dreaming, attention is withdrawn from the outside world. Transpersonal information gathering is apt to occur when significant relations are threatened, impaired, or destroyed. The existence of a relationship between dreams and psi events presents an opportunity to learn more about both.

REFERENCES

Braud, W. G., and Braud, L. W. Preliminary explorations of psi-conductive states: Progressive muscular relaxation. J. Am. Soc. Psychol Res., *67:* 26, 1973.
Ehrenwald, J. *New Dimensions of Deep Analysis*. Allen and Unwin, London, 1954.
Eisenbud, J. *Psi and Psychoanalysis*. Grune & Stratton, New York, 1970.
Freud, S. Psychoanalysis and telepathy. In *Psychoanalysis and the Occult*, G. Devereux, editor, p. 56. International Universities Press, New York, 1953.
Honorton, C., Drucker, S., and Hermon, H. Shifts in subjective state and ESP under conditions of partial sensory deprivation. J. Am. Soc. Psychical Res., *67:* 191, 1973.
Kanthamani, B., and Rao, K. Personality characteristics of ESP subjects. IV. Neuroticism and ESP. J. Parapsychol., *37:* 37, 1973.
Levy, W., Davis, J., and Mayo, A. An improved method in a precognition test with birds. J. Parapsychol., *37:* 83, 1973.
Pratt, J., Rhine, J. B., Smith, B., Stuart, C., and Greenwood, J. *Extra-sensory Perception after Sixty Years*. Holt, Rinehart and Winston, New York, 1940.
Rao, K. *Experimental Parapsychology*. Charles C Thomas, Springfield, Ill., 1966.
Ullman, M., and Krippner, S. *Dream Studies and Telepathy*. Parapsychology Foundation, New York, 1970.
Ullman, M., Krippner, S., and Vaughan, A. *Dream Telepathy*. Macmillan, New York, 1973.

51.16.   TRANSCENDENTAL MEDITATION AND OTHER NONPROFESSIONAL PSYCHOTHERAPIES

Introduction

Nonprofessional modes of psychotherapy have increased steadily in the United States during recent years. Some nonprofessional approaches to psychological self-improvement are apparently benign. Some may actually be beneficial. Others can pose definite risks for those who are lured by their promises. All represent a potential hazard if pursued as a substitute for professional care because of the danger that serious psychiatric symptoms will be misunderstood, ignored, or even temporarily relieved but to the neglect of progressive underlying pathology, organic or functional. Furthermore, the patient often attributes to his putative healer qualities of professional responsibility, such as confidentiality, that are legally not required and, in fact, not obtained. In addition, there is a tendency among nonprofessional mental healers to assume that their method has near-universal applicability.

Today it is a widely accepted that powerful psychophysiologic forces, many of them latent under ordinary conditions, can be mobilized and used under the force of powerful suggestion, keen expectation, and the human body's still uncalculated potentialities for the maintenance of health and life. Some of the most successful nonprofessional healing and self-improvement programs offer a judicious combination of old-fashioned religious and modern scientific or science-fiction formulations.

Scientology

The Church of Scientology began nearly 25 years ago as a pseudoscientific healing cult, primarily directed toward psychiatric and psychosomatic disorders. Its founder, a former engineer and science-fiction writer named L. Ron Hubbard, called his system dianetics, a precedure that seemed to include popular elements of psychoanalysis (tracing all troubles back to infancy, even to the womb), hypnosis (including a dianetic reverie to get on the time track to the past), cybernetics (obtaining information from a mental file clerk out of memory banks), and catharsis (undamming mental energy by clearing away inhibitory engrams, with resultant relief and even—if totally cleared—permanent cure and subsequent full utilization of all personal potentialities).

Today branches are found in most American cities. Los Angeles alone is said to have 75,000 members, and 5.5 million members worldwide were claimed in 1972. Dianetics was occasionally in trouble with the law because of statutes concerning the practice of medicine. However, scientology is now immune from legal interference because Hubbard and his attorneys succeeded in getting it classified as a religion. The official hostility of scientology toward the medical establishment in general, as exemplified by the American Medical Association, is exceeded only by its open warfare with psychiatry. The Church of Scientology is now a multimillion-dollar enterprise, growing steadily in power and respectability and openly using its special brand of nonprofessional psychotherapy or mental healing without interference, beyond the reach of malpractice lawsuits.

Other Organizations

Some organizations offer procedures that are directed at highly defined problems or symptoms, such as smoking, overeating, alcohol abuse, drug addiction, and sexual inadequacies. Weight-Watchers, Alcoholics Anonymous, and Synanon are three highly successful examples. Others strive generally for the restoration or maintenance of health, regardless of the nature of the disease or complaint in the particular case. Still others seek a general state of self-improvement.

Transcendental Meditation

Transcendental Meditation (TM) incorporates many of the historically typical components of a successful nonprofessional healing enterprise; a charismatic founder and leader (Maharishi Mahesh Yogi); an appealing but global body of theory that partakes of both science and mystique (the science of creative intelligence); a parental enterprise representing the founder's original organizational effort (the Spiritual Regeneration Movement); derivative organizations (such as the Student's International Meditation Society); and the establishment of a major institution for the promulgation of the belief, the promotion of the movement, and the diversification of its enterprises (Maharishi International University).

Technique

Maharishi Mahesh Yogi defines the technique as "turning the attention inwards toward the subtle levels of a thought until the mind transcends the experience of the subtlest states of the thought and arrives at the source of thought." Maharishi, an honorary title meaning "great sage" or "world teacher," describes the meditation as an effortless, automatic mental technique in which the mind settles down to finer states of thought.

The meditator usually sits comfortably in a chair, with eyes closed, and allows the sound of a selected Sanskrit word—his Mantra, given to him during his initiation—to echo in his mind at will. He avoids pursuing any special line of thought, maintains an alert but relaxed state of mind, and permits all intruding thoughts to fragment or refine themselves until there are no longer any specific ideas at all, only an experience of transcendent awareness or pure consciousness. From time to time, specific thoughts return, only to dissolve again peacefully.

This meditative state is usually practiced for about 20 minutes, twice a day. During meditation, there is likely to be a considerable degree of bodily relaxation, with a slowing of pulse and respiratory rates, an elevation of galvanic skin resistance, a diminution of blood lactate, and other signs of decreased metabolic activity. At the end of each session, there is typically described a sense of refreshment, alertness, and well-being. Those who practice the procedure twice daily over a period of months commonly report an over-all rise in spirits, energy, and morale. Routine tasks are accomplished with more relish and effectiveness. Various bad habits and unhealthy practices, such as the use of tobacco and alcohol and drug abuse, seem to fade away without special effort. Creativity is said to increase, chronic tension and neurotic symptoms to diminish, and a sense of peace and benevolence toward others to emerge gradually.

The expansion of consciousness that occurs during meditation carries over into ordinary activity. Meanwhile, the deep relaxation provided twice daily by TM relieves any stress that accumulates during the day.

Western Uses

Recent efforts have been made to incorporate TM into hospital psychiatry in three ways; first, as a self-improvement technique for members of the staff, second, as an adjunct to more traditional therapies, and third, as an alternative to other means of treatment. Preliminary results suggest that TM may be useful in all these connections. Patients who can become significantly involved in TM are more likely to be discharged from the hospital and are less likely to require readmission. There is also some evidence that TM decreases the amount of psychotropic medication required. The adjunctive usefulness of TM seems to hold, regardless of diagnostic categories.

Effects

During TM, the respiration becomes shallow. Both oxygen consumption and carbon dioxide production decrease markedly. There is no change in the respiratory quotient. Arterial pH and base excess decrease slightly. Blood lactate falls.

Researchers have shown qualitative and quantitative changes in the EEG during TM. Of special interest is the apparent nonpathological increase in interhemispherical synchronization or coherence, which occurs at different, regular frequency bands during various stages of meditation.

TM appears to be acceptable to many persons who were once much involved in drug abuse or the counterculture. Preliminary results in several studies suggest that TM may have value as a treatment modality for alcoholics, addicts, and others with volitional disorders, such as heavy smokers and the obese.

Several recent articles relate the practice of TM to reduced nervousness or anxiety and increased self-actualization. Experimental clinical studies also suggest the potential usefulness of TM in bronchial asthma and other disorders having significant psychosomatic components.

REFERENCES

Adler, H. M., and Hammett, V. B. Crisis, conversion, and cult formation: An examination of a common psychosocial sequence. Am. J. Psychiatry, *130:* 861, 1973.

Banquet, J. P. Spectral analysis of the EEG in meditation. Electronceph. Clin. Neurophysiol., *35:* 143, 1973.

Calestro, K. M. Psychotherapy, faith healing, and suggestion. Int. J. Psychiatry, *1:* 83, 1972.

Forem, J. *Transcendental Meditation: Maharishi Mahesh Yogi and the Science of Creative Intelligence.* E. P. Dutton, New York, 1973.

Gelhorn, E., and Kiely, W. F. Mystical states of consciousness: Neurophysiological and clinical aspects. J. Nerv. Ment. Dis., *154:* 339, 1972.

Hall, J. H. Scientologists making impact on West side. Los Angeles Times, May 6, 1973.

Maharishi Mahesh Yogi. *The Science of Being and Art of Living.* International SRM Publication, London, 1966.

Mitchell, E. D. The Institute of Noetic Sciences. Psychic. July/August 1973.

Rose, L. *Faith Healing.* Penguin Books, England, 1971.

St. Clair, D. *The Psychic World of California.* Bantam, New York, 1973.

Sykes, D. E. Transcendental meditation as applied to criminal justice reform, drug rehabilitation, and society in general. U. Md. Law Forum, *3:* 37, 1973.

Tart, C. T., editor. *Altered States of Consciousness.* Wiley, New York, 1969.

Wallace, R. K., and Benson, H. The physiology of meditation. Sci. Am., *226:* 84, 1972.

Wolf, R. Mind over matter for better health. Prevention, *25:* 128, 1973.

Zullo, A. Relax with transcendental meditation. Marriage, *55:* 10, 1973.

51.17. PSYCHIATRY IN THE FUTURE

Validity

Controversy exists and will continue to exist about whether there actually are mental ailments or whether psychiatrists deal with socially defined forms of undesirable deviance for purposes of labeling to achieve social control. Is there just one mental illness, or are there several? The effectiveness of treatment modalities in regard to outcome remains in the foreground of discussions.

Certainly, new models of normal and abnormal behavior and of intervention will be developed. These models will be characterized by a synthesis of seemingly disparate or artificially separate ideas. Thus, there is the fruitless struggle of counterposing individual and family approaches versus societal approaches. Both must be synthesized in a joint structure, such as community mental health centers.

New complex models will have to incorporate impressive advances in genetics in addition to those of neurophysiology, development, and neurochemistry. Further, important developments will investigate how learning, memory, and affect can be influenced by various psychological, pharmacological, and other means.

At the same time, existing forms of treatment will be expanded and contracted, depending on outcome evaluation and influences from such outside sources as government policy, national health insurance, and public popularity. Many expect, under the pressure of national health insurance, greater emphasis on brief psychotherapy, brief hospitalization, and group psychotherapy. Family therapy and marital therapy will have particular importance because of the changing societal values about religion, family structure, marriage, and other social systems.

Group therapy has advanced within the past decade and will continue to do so. Training in group process theory and technique will parallel training in the individual therapy methods. The variety of group approaches that exists at the present time indicates that no one approach is superior to the other, but the success of the group method of treatment indicates that— with appropriate leadership, selection, and organization—groups of people can be of immense help to one another. A future form of group therapy will consist of persons who have mastered and adjusted to a particular problem in living or life-style—vocational, social, sexual, interpersonal—gathering together in small groups under appropriate conditions to help others similar to themselves.

One of the fields that has grown tremendously in the past few years has been that of sex therapy, as pioneered by Masters and Johnson.

The technique has been of value for a great many sexually dysfunctional people. Much has yet to be determined about the long-term results of this therapy and still more about its indications and contraindications. It is probable that, as with all new therapies, the number for whom it is useful will diminish considerably, as will the enthusiasm with which it is presently offered. But its place in the choice of effective therapeutic techniques will certainly remain secure. Of particular concern will be the training and qualifications of the practitioners. At the present time, this training is deficient, and qualifications have not been set.

There has been a decrease in interest in formal psychoanalytic training by residents in psychiatry and a decrease in the number of patients receiving long-term formal psychoanalysis or psychoanalytic psychotherapy. Many training centers have integrated psychoanalytic training into the structure of residency training programs, and most educators are satisfied that a personal analysis and close supervision of the resident's cases in treatment are sufficient as a replacement for the traditional psychoanalytic institute training.

Just as many psychiatric residents resist the long and expensive training programs for psychoanalysis, many patients resist the long and expensive course of psychoanalysis. Session length has been significantly diminished by an increasing number of therapists, and the frequency of treatment in a week has been cut even more. The future seems to inciate that psychoanalytic theory will be largely integrated into psychiatry and that psychoanalytic therapy will be absorbed into a new type of psychotherapy, one that uses an eclectic approach.

Applications of new discoveries in basic behavioral sciences should emerge as innovations in therapy. Biofeedback is one illustration. New pharmacological agents with different chemical configurations will be discovered, and the use of such naturally occurring substances as hormones, vitamins, and prostaglandins will be explored. A renewed attempt to discover the mechanism of the excellent results of electroconvulsive therapy in depression may be undertaken to replicate the results without using the total procedure.

Factors in the social management of patients in and out of the hospital will augment the discoveries of the postwar period in regard to open hospitalization, therapeutic communities, social breakdown syndrome, and community care

Equity

The denial of excellent mental health care has been redefined by the public from a misfortune to an injustice. Equality in the delivery of mental health services is demanded by those who are poor and by members of minority groups. There are also geographic inequities; many areas of the country are poorly served.

If hospitalization is necessary the deprived are the ones who end up in state hospitals. And the deprived are most evident among those turned out into the streets or into rundown motels and hotels.

National health insurance and health maintenance organizations (HMO) will be expected to solve many of these problems. The development of a national health insurance program, including mental health coverage, seems to be a certainty, but its exact form and implementation will emerge slowly. The hospitalization coverage will be enacted without too much argument, but much controversy will continue for some time in regard to office and outpatient coverage.

Solo private practice will continue, but group arrangements, public and private of many sorts, will expand. The end of the 1970's may well see demands for the placement of all physicians on salary in order to control costs.

Extension and improvement of coverage will be actively sought by health consumer groups. They will also pressure for a role in monitoring and evaluation, which has been the exclusive domain of the professions in peer review and professional standards review organizations (PSRO). Furthermore, the issue of ensuring high-quality psychiatric care by further expansion of board certification—as of 1974, only 38 per cent of all American psychiatrists are board certified, the lowest percentage of any medical specialty—and the need for more and better continuing education programs in psychiatry, leading to periodic recertification, are all related and pressing problems.

Equity will depend largely on an adequate supply of professionals. The limitation of Federal funding for psychiatric training programs will prove to be a major hindrance and may prove to be disatrous. The 1970's will witness two countervailing manpower trends; increasing the supply of psychiatrists and other professionals by increasing the number of medical school graduates and by expanding programs on the one hand and, on the other hand, serious attempts to limit the number of graduates of foreign medical schools, who increasingly dominate the staffs of state hospitals and other installations.

Legitimacy

Voluntary and involuntary hospitalization, commitment procedures, the right to treatment, the extent of confidentiality and privilege, and conflicts of interest inherent in the role of those providing services have been criticized.

Historically, deviants have been labeled as criminal or sick or both. Often, the labeling has, as its purpose, social control. Social change and broader psychiatric knowledge have resulted in such actions as the removal of homosexuality from the diagnositic manual of psychiatric disorders by the board of trustees of the American Psychiatric Association and the subsequent referedum on the issue by the membership. Such controversies will continue. Many are mindful of allegations concerning the involuntary psychiatric hospitalization of political dissidents in the Soviet Union.

The development of national health insurance, HMOs, PSROs and vast computer data banks containing information on millions of Americans makes the issue of confidentiality an escalating source of apprehension.

The conflict between researchers who desire an unfettered opportunity to pursue their investigations and those who fear abuse of the civil liberties of patients, as well as actual harm, is an ongoing one. Increased sensitivity and education on both sides will be necessary as negotiations in regard to legislation take place.

Roles

The last issue is the need to arrive at some agreement in regard to the appropriate roles of those engaged in the mental health care system. In 1970 about 75 per cent of those who needed care from mental health professionals apparently received no attention. Providing care for more people will require not only the maximum effort of all available mental health professionals but the training and employment of many times the number presently available.

REFERENCES

Eisenberg, L. The future of psychiatry. Lancet, *1:* 1371, 1973.
Engel, G. The best and the brightest: The missing dimension in medical education. Pharos, *36:* 129, 1973.
Freedman, A. M. Critical psychiatry. Hosp. Community Psychiatry, *24:* 819, 1973.
Freud, A. *Difficulties in the Path of Psychoanalyses: A Confrontation of Past with Present Viewpoints.* International Universities Press, New York, 1969.
Hofling, C. K., and Meyers, R. W. Recent discoveries in psychoanalysis. Arch. Gen. Psychiatry, *5:* 518, 1972.
Kaplan, H. I., and Sadock, B. J. *Comprehensive Group Psychotherapy.* Williams & Wilkins, Baltimore, 1971.
Kuhn, T. S. *The Structure of Scientific Revolutions.* ed. 2. Chicago University Press, Chicago, 1970.
Schaar, J. H. The case for patriotism. In *American Review*, T. Solotaroff, editor, ed. 17, p. 59. Bantam Books, New York, 1973.

Glossary of Psychiatric Terminology

Aberration, mental. Pathological deviation from normal thinking. Mental aberration is not related to a person's intelligence. *See also* Mental illness.

Ablutomania. Excessive interest in bathing and cleaning oneself. It is common in obsessive-compulsive neurosis.

Abnormal. Deviating from the average or normal.

Abreaction. A process by which repressed material, particularly a painful experience or a conflict is brought back to consciousness. In the process of abreacting, the person not only recalls but relives the repressed material, which is accompanied by the appropriate affective response. *See also* Catharsis.

Abscess, brain. An inflammation resulting in pus in a part of the brain. Both psychotic and nonpsychotic conditions can be caused by a brain abscess.

Abstinence. Refraining from the use of certain substances, such as food or drugs. In psychoanalysis, abstinence refers to refraining from sexual intercourse.

Abstraction. The ability to generalize thinking and to form ideas that are apart from particular instances or material objects; not concrete. In schizophrenia, abstraction is impaired.

Abulia. Inability to make decisions; lack of will.

Abuse, drug. *See* Drug abuse.

Acalculia. A learning or speech disorder in which the patient cannot perform arithmetic operations.

Acarophobia. Fear of small objects, like insects, worms, and such nonliving items as pins and needles.

Acatalepsia. Inability to reason or comprehend.

Acataphasia. A speech disorder in which the patient expresses himself with words that sound like the ones he means to use but that are not appropriate to his thoughts. He may also use totally inappropriate expressions.

Acathexis. Lack of feeling associated with an ordinarily emotion-charged subject. In psychoanalysis, acathexis denotes the patient's detaching or transferring of affect from thoughts and ideas. *See also* Cathexis.

Accelerated interaction. An alternate term for marathon group session. *See also* Group marathon.

Accident prone. The tendency to have accidents as a result of psychological causes.

Acenesthesia. Loss of sensation of physical existence.

Achluophobia. Fear of the dark.

Acid. Slang for lysergic acid diethylamide (LSD).

Acromegaly. Hyperpituitarism that results in certain body structures being oversized. It is often associated with somnolence and moodiness.

Acrophobia. Fear of high places.

Acting out. An action rather than a verbal response to an unconscious instinctual drive or impulse that brings about temporary partial relief of inner tension. Relief is attained by reacting to a present situation as if if were the situation that originally gave rise to the drive or impulse.

Active therapist. Type of therapist who makes no effort to remain anonymous but is forceful and expresses his personality definitively in the therapy setting. *See also* Passive therapist.

Activity group therapy. A type of group therapy introduced and developed by S. R. Slavson and designed for children and young adolescents, with emphasis on emotional and active interaction in a permissive, nonthreatening atmosphere. The therapist stresses reality testing, ego strengthening, and active interpretation.

Actualization. Process of mobilizing one's potentialities or making them concrete. *See also* Individuation.

Aculalia. Nonsense speech characterized by little or no comprehension.

Acute brain disorder. An impairment of tissue function that can be reversed and from which the patient may recover.

Acute confusional state. A stress reaction common in adolescence and often associated with new surroundings or new demands. Frustration and rage yield to despair and loneliness, which usually pass as the person adjusts to his situation.

Acute situational or stress reaction. A severe emotional reaction resulting from extreme environmental stress, such as death, disaster, or similar life situations.

Adaptation. An attempt to conform to the environment through alloplasty and autoplasty. The goal of adaptation is adjustment. *See also* Alloplasty, Autoplasty.

Adaptational approach. An approach used in analytic therapy. Consonant with Sandor Rado's formulations on adaptational psychodynamics, therapy focuses on the maladaptive patterns used by patients in the treatment sessions, on how these patterns developed, and on what the patients must do to overcome them and stabilize their functioning at self-reliant, adult levels.

Addiction. Habituation to the use of a drug, the deprivation of which gives rise to symptoms of distress and an irresistible impulse to take the drug again.

Adjustment. A person's relation to his society and to his inner self.

Adler, Alfred (1870–1937). Viennese psychiatrist and one of Freud's original followers. Adler broke off from Freud and introduced and developed the concepts of individual psychology, inferiority complex, and overcompensation.

Adolescence. Period of growth from puberty to maturity. The beginning of adolescence is marked by the appearance of secondary sexual characteristics, usually at about age 12, and the termination is marked by the achievement of sexual maturity at about age 20. *See also* Psychosexual development.

Adrenergic. Relating to the sympathetic nerve fibers.

Adynamia. Weakness and fatigability. *See also* Asthenic personality.

Aerophagia. Excessive swallowing of air.

Affect. Emotional feeling tone attached to an object, idea, or thought. The term includes inner feelings and their external manifestations. *See also* Inappropriate affect, Mood.

Affect, blunted. A disturbance of affect manifested by dullness of externalized feeling tone. Observed in schizophrenia, it is one of that disorder's fundamental symptoms, according to Eugen Bleuler.

Affect-fantasy. According to Jung, an emotion-laden fantasy.

Affective interaction. Interpersonal experience and exchange that are emotionally charged.

Affective psychosis. A psychosis in which disturbance of mood is the primary characteristic; disturbances in thinking and behavior are the secondary characteristics.

Aftercare. After hospitalization, the continuing program of rehabilitation designed to reinforce the effects of therapy and to help the patient adjust to his environment.

Ageusia. Lack of the sense of taste. It is common in certain psychiatric conditions, particularly depression.

Aggression. Forceful, goal-directed behavior that may be verbal or physical. It is the motor counterpart of the affects of rage, anger, and hostility.

Aggression, identifying with. *See* Identification with the aggressor.

Aggressive drive. Destructive impulse directed at oneself or another. It is also known as the death instinct. According to contemporary psychoanalytic psychology, it is one of the two basic drives; sexual drive is the other one. Sexual drive operates on the pleasure-pain principle, whereas aggressive drive operates on the repetition-compulsion principle. *See also* Aggression, Libido theory.

Agitation. State of anxiety associated with severe motor restlessness.

Agnosia. Disturbance of perception characterized by inability to recognize a stimulus and interpret the significance of its memory impressions. It is observed in patients with organic brain disease and in certain schizophrenics, hysterics, and depressed patients.

Agoraphobia. Fear of open places.

Agranulocytosis. A rare, serious side effect occuring with some of the psychotropic drugs. The condition is characterized by sore throat, fever, a sudden sharp decrease in white blood cell count, and a marked reduction in the number of granulocytes.

Agraphia. State of being unable to write.

Agromania. Excessive interest in living along or in rural seclusion; it is sometimes associated with schizophrenia.

Aichmophobia. Fear of pointed objects, usually expressed as a fear that the person will use the object against someone else.

Ailurophobia. Fear of cats.

Akathisia. Condition characterized by an inability to remain in a sitting posture, motor restlessness, and a feeling of muscular quivering, which may be a side effect of phenothiazine medication.

Akinesia. Lack of physical movement. In psychiatry, akinesia is often seen in conjunction with a lack of mental activity, as in the extreme immobility of catatonic schizophrenia.

Alcoholic psychoses. Mental disorders that result from alcoholism and involve organic brain damage. *See also* Delirium tremens, Korsakoff's psychosis, Hallucinosis.

Alcoholics Anonymous (AA). An organization of alcoholics formed in 1935. It uses certain group methods, such as inspirational-supportive techniques, to help rehabilitate chronic alcoholics.

Alcoholism. Excessive dependence on or addiction to alcohol, usually to the point that the person's physical and mental health is threatened or harmed.

Alexia (dyslexia). Loss of the power to grasp the meaning of written or printed words and sentences.

Algophobia. Fear of pain.

Alienation. A psychiatric term used variously to describe a person's feelings of detachment from his self or society, to denote one's avoidance of emotional experiences, or to describe a person's efforts to estrange himself from his own feelings.

Alienist. A psychiatrist who offers expert opinion about a person's mental health or sanity. The term is now obsolete.

Allergic jaundice. *See* Jaundice, allergic.

Alliance. *See* Therapeutic alliance, Working alliance.

Alloplasty. Adaptation that involves altering the external environment. *See also* Autoplasty.

Allport's group relations theory. Gordon W. Allport's theory that a person's behavior is influenced by his personality and his need to conform to social forces. It illustrates the interrelationship between group therapy and social psychology. For example, dealing with bigotry in a therapy group enhances the opportunity for therapeutic experiences because it challenges the individual patient's need to conform to earlier social determinants or to hold on to familiar but restrictive aspects of his personality.

Alpha feedback. A technique in which a patient is made conscious of his restful state, characterized by alpha waves, in an attempt to condition the brain to remain in the alpha state. By means of electronic methods or transcendental meditation, the patient learns to become aware of his departure from the alpha state and makes a conscious effort to return to it. *See also* Alpha state, Biofeedback, Mantra.

Alpha state. A state in which the brain is in an awake yet relaxed and peaceful condition, characterized by alpha waves. *See also* Alpha feedback, Biofeedback, Mantra.

Alternating role. Pattern characterized by periodic switching from one type of behavior to another.

Altruism. Regard for and dedication of the welfare of others. The term was originated by Auguste Comte (1798–1857), a French philosopher. In psychiatry the term is closely linked with ethics and morals. Freud recognized altruism as the only basis for the development of community interest; Bleuler equated it with morality.

Alzheimer's disease. A disease characterized by progressive mental deterioration; usually considered a presenile dementia.

Ambivalence. Presence of strong and often overwhelming simultaneous contrasting attitudes, ideas, feelings, and drives toward an object, person, or goal. The term was coined by Eugen Bleuler, who differentiated three types; affective ambivalence; intellectual ambivalence, and ambivalence of the will.

Amentia. Lack of intellectual development as a result of inadequate brain tissue. *See also* Dementia.

American Psychiatric Association. The most important and largest professional organization of American physicians who specialize in the practice of psychiatry. The organization was founded in 1844 as the Association of Medical Superintendents of American Institutions for the Insane. In 1891 the name was changed to the American Medico-Psychological Association and in 1921 to its present name.

Amimia. Lack of ability to make gestures or to comprehend those made by others.

Amines. Organic compounds derived from ammonia by replacing hydrogen atoms with hydrocarbon radicals.

Amnesia. Disturbance in memory manifested by partial or total inability to recall past experiences.

Amnesia, retrograde. *See* Retrograde amnesia.

Amok. A condition usually associated with Malayan men, consisting of a sudden, unprovoked outburst of wide rage, usually resulting in homicide.

Amphetamine. A central nervous system stimulant. Its chemical structure and action are closely related to ephedrine and other sympathomimetic amines. *See also* Sympathomimetic drug.

Anaclitic. Depending on others, especially the infant on the mother. Anaclitic depression in children results from the absence of mothering.

Anaclitic therapy. A form of psychotherapy characterized by allowing the patient to regress and used mainly in the treatment of psychophysiological disorders.

Anal erotism. *See* Anal phase.

Anal phase. The second stage in psychosexual development. It occurs when the child is between the ages of 1 and 3. During this period the infant's activities, interests, and concerns are centered on his anal zone, and the pleasurable experience felt in this area is called anal erotism. *See also* Infantile sexuality, Genital, Latency, Oral, and Phallic phases.

Analgesia. State in which one feels little or no pain.

Analysand. In psychiatry, the one who is being analyzed.

Analysis. *See* Psychoanalysis.

Analysis in depth. *See* Psychoanalysis.

Analysis of transference. *See* Psychoanalysis.

Analysis of variance. A statistical technique by which sets of measurements are investigated to find out to what extent they are determined by experimental influences or chance influences.

Analytic psychology. Carl Jung's system of psychology, characterized by a belief in the collective unconscious or objective psyche, the archetype, and the complex. *See also* Jung, Carl Gustav.

Anamnesis. A patient's medical history, particularly used in connection with the patient's own recollections.

Anancasm. Repetitious or stereotyped behavior or thought, usually used as a tension-relieving device.

Anancastic personality. *See* Obsessive-compulsive personality.

Androgyny. A combination of female and male characteristics in one person. *See also* Bisexuality.

Anesthesia. Absence of sensation.

Anhedonia. State of being unable to experience pleasure. *See also* Hedonism.

Anima. According to Jungian psychology, the person's inner self, as opposed to the persona or self that he presents to the outside world. *See also* Jung, Carl Gustav.

Anorexia nervosa. A serious and sometimes life-endangering condition characterized by self-imposed severe dietary limitation, usually resulting in serious malnutrition and malaise.

Antabuse (disulfiram). A drug used in the treatment of alcoholics. By altering the metabolism of alcohol, it produces unpleasant physical sensations that discourage the patient from further use of alcohol.

Anthropology. The scientific study of primitive societies.

Antianxiety drug. Drug used to reduce pathological anxiety and its related symptoms without influencing cognitive or perceptual disturbance. It is also known as a minor tranquilizer and an anxiolytic drug. Meprobamate derivatives and diazepoxides are typical antianxiety drugs.

Anticholinergic effect. Effect due to a blockade of the cholinergic (parasympathetic and somatic) nerves. It is often seen as a side effect of phenothiazine therapy. Anticholinergic effects include dry mouth and blurred vision. *See also* Paralytic ileus.

Antidepressant drug. Drug used in the treatment of pathological depression. It is also known as a thymoleptic drug and a psychic energizer. The two main classes of antidepressant drugs are the tricyclic drugs and the monoamine oxidase inhibitors. *See also* Hypertensive crisis, Monoamine oxidase inhibitor, Tinnitus, Tricyclid drug.

Antimanic drug. Drug, such as lithium, used to alleviate the symptoms of mania. Lithium is particularly effective in preventing relapses in manic-depressive illness. Other drugs with antimanic effects are haloperidol and chlorpromazine.

Antiparkinsonism drug. Drug used to relieve the symptoms of parkinsonism and the extrapyramidal side effects often induced by antipsychotic drugs. The antiparkinsonism drug acts by diminishing muscle tone and involuntary movements. Antiparkinsonism agents include benztropine, procyclidine, biperiden, and trihexyphenidyl. *See also* Cycloplegia, Mydriasis.

Antipsychotic drug. Drug used to treat psychosis, particularly schizophrenia. It is also known as a major tranquilizer and a neuroleptic drug. Phenothiazine derivatives, thioxanthene derivatives, and butyrophenone derivatives are typical antipsychotic drugs. *See also* Autonomic side effect, Dyskinesia, Extrapyramidal effect, Major tranquilizer, Parkinsonism-like effect, Reserpine, Tardive oral dyskinesia.

Antisocial personality. A disorder characterized by inability to get alone with other members of society and by repeated conflict with individual persons and groups.

Antlophobia. Fear of floods.

Anxiety. Unpleasurable affect consisting of psychophysiological changes in response to an intrapsychic conflict. In contrast to fear, the danger or threat in anxiety is unreal. Physiological changes consist of increased heart rate, disturbed breathing, trembling, sweating, and vasomotor changes. Psychological changes consist of an uncomfortable feeling of impending danger, accompanied by overwhelming awareness of being powerless, inability to perceive the unreality of the threat, prolonged feeling of tension, and exhaustive readiness for the expected danger. *See also* Basic anxiety, Fear.

Anxiety neurosis. A neurosis characterized by panic and anxious overconcern.

Anxiolytic drug. *See* Antianxiety drug.

Apathetic withdrawal. *See* Withdrawal.

Apathy. Want of feeling or affect; lack of interest and emotional involvement in one's surroundings. It is observed in certain types of schizophrenia and depression.

Apgar scores. Measurements taken 1 and 5 minutes after birth to determine physical normality in the neonate. The scores are based on color, respiratory rate, heart beat, reflex action, and muscle tone. Used routinely, they are particularly useful in detecting the effects on the infant of drugs taken by the pregnant mother.

Aphasia. Disturbance in speech due to organic brain disorder. It is characterized by an inability to express thoughts verbally. There are several types of aphasia: (1) motor aphasia: inability to speak, although understanding remains; (2) sensory aphasia: inability to comprehend the meaning of words or the use of objects; (3) nominal aphasia: difficulty in finding the right name for an object; (4) syntactical aphasia: inability to arrange words in proper sequence.

Aphasia, central. *See* Central aphasis.

Aphasia, syntactical. *See* Central aphasia.

Aphonia. Loss of voice.

Apoplexy. A sudden loss of consciousness due to cerebral hemorrhage or embolus or thrombus of an artery of the brain.

Apperception. Awareness of the meaning and significance of a particular sensory stimulus as modified by one's own experiences, knowledge, thoughts, and emotions. *See also* Perception.

Apraxia. Loss of the ability to make voluntary goal-directed movements.

Aptitude tests. Tests used to evaluate a person's interests, talents, and skills; they are particularly valuable in vocational counseling.

Art therapy. Treatment procedure that uses the spontaneous creative work of the patient. For example, group members make and analyze drawings, which are often expressions of their underlying emotional problems.

Arteriosclerotic cardiovascular disease. A metabolic disturbance characterized by degenerative changes involving the blood vessels of the heart and other arteries, mainly the arterioles. Fatty plaques deposited within the blood vessels gradually obstruct the flow of blood. Organic brain syndrome may develop when cerebral arteries are involved in the degenerative process.

Assertive training. A behavior therapy technique in which the patient is trained to respond to people and situations with a direct and honest expression of his or her feelings, whether positive or negative. In this way, appropriate interpersonal responses are learned.

Association. Relation between ideas and feelings.

Asthenic personality. A disorder characterized

by lack of enthusiasm, fatigability, lack of capacity for enjoyment, and low tolerance for stress.

Asyndesis. A disorder of language, commonly seen in schizophrenia, in which the patient combines unconnected ideas and images.

Ataractic drug. *See* Major tranqulizer.

Ataxia. Lack of coordination, either physical or mental. In neurology, it refers to loss of muscular coordination. In psychiatry, the term intrapsychic ataxia refers to lack of coordination between feelings and thoughts; the disturbance is found in schizophrenia.

Attention. Concentration; the aspect of consciousness that relates to the amount of effort exerted in focusing on certain aspects of an experience.

Attitude. Preparatory mental posture with which one receives stimuli and reacts to them.

Atypical child. A term describing a child with distorted personality development; often used in connection with brain-damaged or autistic children.

Auditory hallucination. False auditory sensory perception.

Aura. The warning sensations that an epileptic usually feels just before a seizure.

Authenticity. Quality of being authentic, real, and valid. In psychological functioning and personality, it applies to the conscious feelings, perceptions, and thoughts that a person expresses and communicates. It does not apply to the deeper, unconscious layers of the personality.

Authority figure. A real or projected person in a position of power; transferentially, a projected parent.

Authority principle. The idea that each member of an organizational hierarchy tries to comply with the presumed or fantasied wishes of those above him while those below him try to comply with his wishes.

Autism. *See* Autistic thinking.

Autistic thinking. A form of thinking in which the thoughts are largely narcissistic and egocentric, with emphasis on subjectivity rather than objectivity and without regard for reality. The term is used interchangeably with autism and dereism. *See also* Narcissism.

Autochthonous idea. An idea brought about purely by the psyche, without any basis in terms of reality. In the paranoid personality the idea often takes the form of a revelation.

Autoerotism. Sexual arousal of self without the participation of another person. The term, introduced by Havelock Ellis, is at present used interchangeably with masturbation. In psychoanalysis, autoerotism is considered a primitive phase in object-relationship development preceding the narcissistic stage. In narcissism there is a love object, but there is no love object in autoerotism.

Automatism. Undirected behavior that is not controlled by conscious thought.

Automysophobia. Fear of smelling bad or of being unclean.

Autonomic nervous system. The part of the nervous system that functions outside of consciousness and that directs such functions as breathing, heart rate, and digestion.

Autonomic side effect. Disturbance of the autonomic nervous system, both central and peripheral. It may be a result of the use of antipsychotic drugs, particulary the phenothiazine derivatives. The autonomic side effects include hypotension, hypertension, blurred vision, nasal congestion, and dryness of the mouth. *See also* Mydriasis.

Autoplasty. Adaptation that involves altering one's self. *See also* Al;oplasty.

Auxiliary ego. In psychodrama, a person, usually a member of the staff, trained to act out different roles during a psychodramatic session to intensify the therapeutic situation. The trained auxiliary ego may represent an important figure in the patient's life. He may express the patient's unconscious wishes and attitudes or portray his unacceptable self. He may represent a delusion, hallucination, symbol, ideal, animal, or object that makes the patient's psychodramatic world real, concrete, and tangible.

Auxiliary therapist. Co-therapist. *See also* Co-therapy.

Average. A central value in a frequency distribution around which other values are distrib-

uted. Three kinds of averages are the mode, the median, and the mean.

Aversion stimulus. *See* Conditioned reinforcer.

Aversive therapy. A form of conditioning whereby a patient is made to associate an unpleasant or painful experience with undesirable behavior in an effort to eliminate the undesirable behavior patterns.

Aypnia. Insomnia; inability to sleep.

Barbiturate. Highly addictive central nervous system depressant derived from barbituric acid. Phenobarbital and pentothal are among the best known barbiturates.

Basic anxiety. As conceptualized by Karen Horney, the mainspring from which neurotic trends get their intensity and pervasiveness. Basic anxiety is characterized by vague feelings of loneliness, helplessness, and fear of a potentially hostile world. *See also* Anxiety, Fear.

Battered child syndrome. Physical damage to a child sustained as a result of repeated beating, usually by a parent.

Beard, George M. (1839–1883). American psychiatrist who in 1869 introduced the term "neurasthenia."

Beers, Clifford W. (1876–1943). Author of *A Mind That Found Itself* (1909), the book that is generally considered to have founded the mental hygiene movement.

Behavioral psychotherapy. A type of therapy that focuses on overt and objectively observable behavior, rather than on thoughts and feelings. It aims at symptomatic improvement and the elimination of suffering and maladaptive habits. Various conditioning and anxiety-eliminating techniques derived from learning theory are combined with didactic discussions and techniques adapted from other systems of treatment. A major worker in this field is Joseph Wolpe.

Behavioral sciences. Those scientific disciplines that deal with man's relationships, experiences, and values; they include sociology, psychology, and anthropology.

Behaviorism. The psychological theory of John B. Watson that is concerned with measurable and observable data, rather than with ideas and emotions.

Bender, Lauretta (1897–   ). American psychiatrist who has done extensive work in the fields of child psychiatry, neurology, and psychology.

Bender-Gestalt test. A psychological test that measures the subject's ability to reproduce from memory a set of geometric designs. It is useful for measuring visuomotor co-ordination and thus for detecting brain damage.

Berne, Eric (1910–1970). American psychiatrist. He was the founder of transactional analysis, which is used in both individual and group therapy.

Bestiality. Sexual deviation in which a person engages in sexual relations with an animal.

Biodynamics. System of psychoanalytic psychiatry introduced by J. H. Masserman.

Biofeedback. A technique in which a patient is made aware of unconscious or involuntary physiologic processes in an effort to control them. Fluctuations in these processes are seen as responses and may be appropriately reinforced. A patient may learn to control inner organ functions, even though he may not consciously understand how this control is being effected. *See also* Alpha feedback.

Bipolar depression. A depressive illness that is marked by depression and a history of manic episodes. *See also* Hypomania, Unipolar depression.

Birth trauma. Otto Rank's term to describe what he considered the basic source of anxiety in human beings, the birth process.

Bisexuality. Existence of the qualities of both sexes in the same person. Freud postulated that both biologically and psychologically the sexes differentiated from a common core, that differentiation between the two sexes was relative, rather than absolute, and that regression to the common core occurs to varying degrees in both normal and abnormal conditions. An adult person who engages in bisexual behavior is one who is sexually attracted to and has contact with members of both sexes. He is also known in lay terms as an AC-DC person. *See also* Androgyny, Heterosexuality, Homosexuality, Latent homosexuality, Overt homosexuality.

Black-patch syndrome. A psychosis induced by sensory isolation as result of eye-patches used after cataract surgery.

Blank screen. Neutral backdrop in which the patient projects a gamut of transferential irrationalities. The passivity of the analyst allows him to act as a blank screen.

Bleuler, Eugen (1857–1939). Swiss psychiatrist known for his important studies in schizophrenia, which term he preferred over the earlier term "dementia praecox."

Blind spot. In psychiatry, an area of someone's personality that he is totally unaware of. These unperceived areas are often hidden by repression so that he can avoid painful emotions. In both group and individual therapy, such blind spots often appear obliquely as projected ideas, intentions, and emotions.

Blocking. Involuntary cessation of thought processes or speech because of unconscious emotional factors. It is also known as thought deprivation.

Blunted affect. *See* Affect, blunted.

Body contact-exploration maneuver. Any physical touching of another person for the purpose of becoming more aware of the sensations and emotions aroused by the experience. The technique is used mainly in encounter groups.

Body image. One's image, conscious and unconscious, of one's own body at any particular time.

Body language. The system by which a person expresses his thoughts and feelings by means of his bodily activity.

Borderline state (borderline psychosis). A state in which the symptoms are so unclear or transient that it is difficult to classify the patient as psychotic or nonpsychotic.

Bradylalia. Abnormally slow speech, common in depression.

Bradylexia. Inability to read at normal speed. It may be associated with organic or psychological causes or with a combination of both.

Brain waves. *See* EEG.

Brainwashing. Any technique designed to manipulate human thought or action against the desire, will, or knowledge of the person involved. It usually refers to systematic efforts to indoctrinate nonbelievers.

Breuer, Josef (1842–1925). Viennese physician with wide scientific and cultural interests. His collaboration with Freud in studies of cathartic therapy was reported in *Studies on Hysteria* (1895). He withdrew as Freud proceeded to introduce psychoanalysis, but he left important imprints on that discipline, such as the concepts of primary and secondary processes.

Brief psychotherapy. A form of psychotherapy in which the sessions are limited to 10 to 15 in number and during which time attempts to modify behavior occur. This approach is used in both individual and group settings.

Brigham, Amariah (1798–1849). One of the founders of the American Psychiatric Association and the first editor of its journal.

Brill, A. A. (1874–1948). First American analyst (1908). Freud gave him permission to translate several of his most important works. He was active in the formation of the New York Psychoanalytic Society (1911) and remained in the forefront of propagators of psychoanalysis as a lecturer and writer throughout his life.

Brooding compulsion. *See* Intellectualization.

Bulimia. Hunger characterized by a voracious appetite. A bulemic episode may be followed by intentional vomiting by some persons.

Burned-out anergic schizophrenic. A chronic schizophrenic who is apathetic and withdrawn, with minimal florid psychotic symptoms but with persistent and often severe schizophrenic thought processes.

Burrow, Trigant L. (1875–1951). American student of Freud and Jung who coined the term "group analysis" and later developed a method called phyloanalysis. Much of Burrow's work was based on his social views and his opinion that individual psychotherapy places the therapist in too authoritarian a role to be therapeutic. He formed groups of patients, students, and colleagues who, living together in a camp, analyzed their inteactions.

C.A. Abbreviation for chronological age. *See also* I.Q.

Cacodemonomania. A condition in which the patient thinks he is possessed by a devil or other evil spirit.

Carbon dioxide therapy. A rarely used form of treatment in which carbon dioxide gas is used to induce unconsciousness.

Care and protection proceedings. Judicial intervention designed to protect the health, education, and welfare of a child when his parents or guardians are remiss in their care of the child.

Carebaria. Sensation of discomfort or pressure in the head.

Castration anxiety. Fears concerning the loss or injury of the genitalia.

Castration complex. A group of ideas during a phase of the oedipal cycle in which a child experiences anxiety concerning punishment by castration because of his passionate and sexual attachment to his mother and his desire to eliminate and replace his father. The complex is ideally resolved when the child relinquishes his love for his mother to protect himself from castration and identifies with his father, internalizing his father's prohibitions and restraints.

Catalepsy. *See* Cerea flexibilitas.

Cataphasia. *See* Verbigeration.

Cataplexy. Temporary loss of muscle tone, causing weakness and immobilization. It can be precipitated by a variety of emotional states.

Catastrophic anxiety. The anxiety associated with organic brain syndromes when the patient is aware of his defects in mentation. The anxiety can be overwhelming.

Catathymia. A situation in which elements in the unconscious are sufficiently affect-laden to produce changes in conscious functioning.

Catatonic state (catatonia). A state characterized by muscular rigidity and immobility. It is usually associated with schizophrenia.

Catchment area. The area bounded by lines on a map that represents the number of people to be served by a particular community mental health center.

Catecholamine. Monoamine containing a catechol group that has a sympathomimetic property. Norepinephrine, epinephrine, and dopamine are common catecholamines.

Categorical thought. A term introduced by Piaget to refer to abstract thinking. *See* Secondary process.

Catharsis. Release of ideas, thoughts, and repressed materials from the unconscious, accompanied by an affective emotional response and release of tension. Commonly observed in the course of treatment, both individual and group, it can also occur outside therapy. *See also* Abreaction, Conversational catharsis.

Cathexis. In psychoanalysis, a conscious or unconscious investment of the psychic energy of a drive in an idea, a concept, or an object.

Causalgia. Burning pain that may be either organic or psychic in origin.

Central aphasia. Syntactical aphasia. A condition in which difficulty in understanding spoken speech is due to a lesion in the temporoparietal region of the brain. The aphasis is associated with a gross disorder of thought and expression; comprehension is impaired, although speech is fluent. Generally, reading and writing are less affected when done silently. The patient may have difficulty evoking words for actions, qualities, and objects. Speech is characterized by grammatical and verbal confusions. In severe cases the patient may lapse into unintelligible jargon.

Central nervous system (CNS). The spinal cord and brain.

Central tendency. *See* Average.

Centripetal. In psychiatry, connoting treatment or approaches that focus on minute analysis of the psyche.

Cephalalgia. Violent headache occurring in infectious diseases or in tension states.

Cerea flexibilitas. Condition in which a person maintains the body position into which he is placed. It is a pathological symptom observed in severe cases of catatonic schizophrenia. It is also known as "waxy flexibility" and "catalepsy."

Cerebral arteriosclerosis. Hardening of the arteries of the brain, it may lead to an organic psychosis.

Cerebral dominance. *See* Dominance.

Character. An attribute, trait, or definite and distinct feature of the personality.

Character defense. A trait of personality that serves an unconscious defensive purpose.

Character disorder. A pattern of personality characterized by maladaptive, inflexible behavior.

Charcot, Jean M. (1825–1893). French neurologist noted for describing hysteria and treating it by means of hypnosis. Freud based much of his early work on Charcot's pioneer studies in hysteria.

Chemotherapy. *See* Drug therapy.

Chi square. A statistical technique whereby variables are categorized in order to determine whether a distribution of scores is due to chance or to experimental factors.

Child abuse syndrome. *See* Battered child syndrome.

Child analysis. Application of psychoanalytic principles to the treatment of the child.

Chlorpromazine. A phenothiazine derivative used primarily as an antipsychotic agent and in the treatment of nausea and vomiting. The drug was synthesized in 1950 and was used in psychiatry for the first time in 1952. At present, chlorpromazine is one of the most widely used drugs in medical practice.

Cholinergic. Relating to parasympathetic nerve fibers.

Chromosome. The microscopic portion of each body cell that contains the genes.

Chronophobia. Fear of time; sometimes called prison neurosis, since almost all prisoners are affected by it in some fashion. It is characterized by panic, anxiety, and claustrophobia.

Circadian rhythm. Cyclical variations in emotional and physiologic functions that occur in 24-hour cycles. These cycles are regulated by an inner clock that has become embedded in human physiology through evolution. Circadian rhythms are believed to be intrinsic in every cell and to persist under all conditions. *See also* Infradian rhythm, Ultradian rhythm.

Circumstantiality. Disturbance in the associative thought processes in which the patient digresses into unnecessary details and inappropriate thoughts before communicating the central idea. It is observed in schizophrenia, obsessional disturbances, and certain cases of epileptic dementia. *See also* Tangentiality, Thought process disorder.

Classical conditioning response conditioning. A procedure through which a response of the autonomic nervous system occurs in the presence of a stimulus that does not normally elicit this response. In the procedure, a neutral stimulus is habitually presented immediately before a stimulus that does elicit the desired response. Gradually, the autonomic response occurs in the presence of the neutral stimulus even when the other stimulus is not present. *See also* Conditioned reinforcer, Conditioned stimulus, Conditioning therapy, Discrimination, Discriminative stimulus, Eliciting stimulus, or Extinction, Operant conditioning, Unconditioned stimulus.

Claustrophobia. Fear of closed places.

Client-centered psychotherapy. A form of psychotherapy, formulated by Carl Rogers, in which the patient or client is believed to possess the ability to improve. The therapist merely helps him clarify his own thinking and feeling. The client-centered approach in both group and individual therapy is democratic, unlike the psychotherapist-centered treatment methods.

Climacteric. The menopause in women. Sometimes used to refer to the same age period in men.

Clouding of consciousness. Disturbance of consciousness characterized by unclear sensory perceptions.

Coefficient of correlation. A statistical term referring to the relation between two sets of paired measurements. Correlation coefficients—which may be positive, negative, or curvilinear, depending on whether the variations are in the same direction, the opposite direction, or both directions—can be computed in a variety of ways. The most common is the product-moment method referred to as *r*. Another method is rank correction (*p*). Correlation coefficients are intended to show degree of relation, but they do not mean that one variable causes the other.

Coexistent culture. Alternative system of values, perceptions, and patterns for behavior. The group experience leads to an awareness of other systems as legitimate alternatives to one's own system.

Cognition. Mental process of knowing and becoming aware. One of the ego functions, it is closely associated with judgment. Groups that study their own processes and dynamics use more cognition than do encounter groups, which emphasize emotions. Also known as thinking.

Cognitive. Related to the processes of reasoning, comprehension, judgment, and memory, as opposed to the emotional and conative processes.

Cognitive development. The achievement of such mental abilities as conscious thought, problem-solving skills, and intellectual activities. At maturity, these cognitive abilities permit one to test strategies, construct logical principles, handle abstract relationships, conjecture, and think hypothetically.

Cohesion. *See* Group cohesion.

Coitus interruptus. Sexual intercourse that is interrupted before the man ejaculates.

Cold turkey. Abrupt withdrawal from opiates without the benefit of methadone or other drugs. The term was originated by drug addicts to describe their chills and consequent gooseflesh. This type of detoxification is generally used by abstinence-oriented therapeutic communities.

Collaboration. A term used by Harry Stack Sullivan to connote sensitivity to the needs of another person.

Collective experience. The common emotional experiences of a group of people. Identification, mutual support, reduction of ego defenses, sibling transferences, and empathy help integrate the individual member into the group and accelerate the therapeutic process. S. R. Slavson, who coined the phrase, warned against letting the collective experience submerge the individuality of the members or give them an opportunity to escape from their own autonomy and responsibility.

Collective unconscious. Psychic contents outside the realm of awareness that are common to mankind in general, not to one person in particular. Jung, who introduced the term, believed that the collective unconscious is inherited and derived from the collective experience of the species. It transcends cultural differences and explains the analogy between ancient mythological ideas and the primitive archaic projections observed in some patients who have never been exposed to these ideas.

Coma. A profound degree of unconsciousness with minimal or no detectable responsiveness to stimuli. It is seen in conditions involving the brain, such as head injury, cerebral hemorrhage, thrombosis and embolism, and cerebral infection; in such systemic conditions as diabetes; and in drug and alcohol intoxication. In psychiatry, comas may be seen in severe catatonic states.

Coma vigil. A profound degree of unconsciousness in which the patient's eyes remain open but there is minimal or no detectable evidence of responsiveness to stimuli. It is seen in acute brain syndromes secondary to cerebral infection.

Combat fatigue. A strong physical and mental reaction to the stresses of military battle.

Combined therapy. A type of psychotherapy in which the patient is in both individual and group treatment with the same or two different therapists. In marriage therapy, it is the combination of married couples' group therapy with either individual sessions with one spouse or conjoint sessions with the marital pair. *See also* Conjoint therapy, Co-therapy, Family therapy, Marriage therapy, Quadrangular therapy.

Command automatism. Condition closely associated with catalepsy in which suggestions are followed automatically.

Command negativism. *See* Negativism.

Commitment. The legal process by which a person is confined to a mental hospital, usually against his will.

Communion. The union of one living thing with another or the participation of a person in an organization. It is a necessary ingredient in individual and group psychotherapy and in sensitivity training. Both the leader-therapist and the patient-trainee must experience communion for a successful learning experience to occur.

Community. *See* Therapeutic community.

Community psychiatry. Psychiatry focusing on the detection, prevention, and early treatment of emotional disorders and social deviance as they develop in the community, rather than as they are perceived and encountered at large, centralized psychiatric facilities. Particular emphasis is placed on the environmental factors that contribute to mental illness.

Compensation. Conscious or, usually, uncon-

scious defense mechanism by which a person tries to make up for an imagined or real deficiency, physical or psychological, or both.

Competency to stand trial. A legal term denoting that the state of mind of a defendant at the time of his trial is such that he is aware of the nature of the charge against him and the consequences of a possible conviction and that he possesses the faculties to aid his defense counsel. *See also* Criminal responsibility, Durham decision, Insanity defense, Irresistible impulse test, Mens rea, M'Naghten rule.

Competition. Struggle for the possession or use of limited goods, concrete or abstract. Gratification for one person largely precludes gratification for another.

Complementarity of interaction. A concept of bipersonal and multipersonal psychology in which behavior is viewed as a response to stimulation, and interaction replaces the concept of reaction. Each person in an interactive situation plays both a provocation role and a responsive role.

Complex. A group of interrelated ideas, mainly unconscious, that have a common affective tone. A complex strongly influences the person's attitudes and behavior.

Compliance. In psychiatry, neurotic oversubmissiveness, often associated with obsessive-compulsive neurosis.

Compression. The process by which such conditions as fractures, blood clots, and tumors exert pressure on the brain, spinal cord, or nerve fibers.

Compulsion. Uncontrollable impulse to perform an act repetitively. It is used as a way to avoid unacceptable ideas and desires. Failure to perform the act leads to anxiety. *See also* Obsession.

Compulsion, repetition. *See* Repetition compulsion.

Compulsive personality. A type of personality characterized by rigidity, overconscientiousness, extreme inhibition, and inability to relax.

Conation. That part of a person's mental life concerned with his strivings, instincts, drives, and wishes as expressed through his behavior.

Concordance. A term used in studies of twins

to describe traits that are similar in each. The highest level of concordance is found in monozygotic (one-egg) twins.

Concussion. A brain injury, usually involving unconsciousness, caused by a blow on the head.

Condensation. A mental process in which one symbol stands for a number of others.

Conditioned reinforcer. A stimulus used to strengthen a response. If the stimulus strengthens the immediately preceding response by adding to the environment, it is termed a positive reinforcer. If the stimulus strengthens the response immediately preceding it by subtracting from the environment, it is termed a negative reinforcer or aversion stimulus. When a stimulus has gained reinforcing power it did not have before, it is called a conditioned reinforcer. *See also* Classical conditioning, Conditioned stimulus, Conditioning therapy, Differential reinforcement, Extinction, Operant conditioning, Reinforcement, Schedule of reinforcement, Unconditioned stimulus.

Conditioned stimulus. An environmental event that was formerly neutral but, as a result of behavioral therapy, now elicits an autonomic response because of its association with an unconditioned stimulus. *See also* Classical conditioning, Conditioned response, Conditioning therapy, Discrimination, Discriminative stimulus, Eliciting stimulus, Operant conditioning, Unconditioned stimulus.

Conditioning. Procedure designed to alter behavioral potential. There are two main types of conditioning: classical and operant. Classical or Pavlovian conditioning pairs two stimuli, one adequate, such as offering food to a dog to produce salivation, and the other inadequate, such as ringing a bell, which by itself does not have an effect on salivation. After the two stimuli have been paired several times, the dog responds to the inadequate stimulus (ringing of bell) by itself. In operant conditioning a desired activity is reinforced by giving the subject a reward every time he performs the act. As a result, the activity becomes automatic without the need for further reinforcement.

Conditioning, classical. *See* Classical conditioning.

Conditioning, instrumental. *See* Instrumental conditioning.

Conditioning, operant. *See* Operant conditioning.

Conditioning, Pavlovian. *See* Classical conditioning.

Conditioning, response. *See* Classical conditioning.

Conditioning therapy. A form of learning in which actions either lead to a reward or prevent an unpleasant stimulus, thereby changing behavior by reinforcement or extinction. The simplest application is the removal of behavior that poses a problem by, for example, avoidance of a painful electric shock or the extinguishing of delusional statements by ignoring them and by responding to normal statements only. *See also* Classical conditioning, Conditioned reinforcer, Conditioned stimulus, Discrimination, Discriminative stimulus, Extinction, Operant conditioning.

Confabulation. Unconscious filling of gaps in memory by imagining experiences that have no basis in fact. It is common in organic brain syndromes. *See also* Fabulation, Paramnesia.

Confidentiality. Aspect of medical ethics in which the physician is bound to hold secret all information given him by the patient. Legally, certain states do not recognize confidentiality and can require the physician to divulge such information if needed in a legal proceeding.

Conflict. Clash of two opposing emotional forces. *See also* Extrapsychic conflict, Intrapsychic conflict.

Conflict-free area. Part of one's personality or ego that is well integrated and does not cause any conflicts, symptoms, or displeasure.

Confrontation. Act of letting a person know where one stands in relation to him, what one is experiencing, and how one perceives him. Used in a spirit of deep involvement, this technique is a powerful tool for changing relationships; used as an attempt to destroy another person, it can be harmful. In group and individual therapy, the value of confrontation is likely to be determined by the therapist. *See also* Encounter group, Existential psychotherapy.

Confusion. Disturbance of consciousness manifested by a disordered orientation in relation to time, place, or person.

Congenital. Referring to conditions present at birth, including hereditary conditions and those resulting from prenatal development or the process of birth itself.

Cojoint therapy. A type of marriage therapy in which a therapist sees the partners together in joint sessions. This situation is also called triadic or triangular, since two patients and one therapist work together. *See also* Combined therapy, Family therapy, Marriage therapy, Quadrangular therapy.

Conscience. The part of the self that judges one's own values and performance. It is often used synonymously with superego.

Conscious. One division of Freud's topographical theory of the mind. The content of the conscious is within the realm of awareness at all times. The term is also used to describe a function of organic consciousness. *See also* Preconscious, Unconscious.

Consciousness. *See* Sensorium.

Consensual validation. The continuous comparison of the thoughts and feelings of group members toward one another that tend to modify and correct interpersonal distortions. The term was introduced by Harry Stack Sullivan to refer to the dyadic therapeutic process between doctor and patient. Previously, Trigant Burrow referred to consensual observation to describe this process, which results in effective reality testing.

Constitution. The inherent physical and psychological makeup of a person.

Constitutional types. Categories of types based on physical and psychological characteristics. Such scholars as Galen, Kretschmer, and Sheldon formulated sets of major types.

Contagion. Force that operates in large groups or masses. When the level of psychological functioning has been lowered, some sudden upsurge of anxiety can spread through the group, speeded by a high degree of suggestibility. The anxiety gradually mounts to panic, and the whole group may be simultaneously affected by a primitive emotional upheaval.

Contemporaneity. Here-and-now.

Contract. Explicit, bilateral commitment to a well defined course of action. In group or individual therapy, the therapist-patient contract is to attain the treatment goal.

Control group. In an experimental design, the group in which a condition or factor being tested is deliberately omitted. For example, in a study measuring the effects of a new drug, the control group may be given a placebo, instead of the drug. *See also* Experimental group.

Conversational catharsis. Release of repressed or suppressed thoughts and feelings in group and individual psychotherapy as a result of verbal interchange.

Conversion. An unconscious defense mechanism by which the anxiety that stems from an intrapsychic conflict is converted and expressed in a symbolic somatic symptom. See in a variety of mental disorders, it is particularly common in hysterical neurosis.

Conversion, somatic. *See* Somatic conversion.

Convulsive disorders. The centrencephalic seizures, grand mal and petit mal, and the focal seizures of Jacksonian and psychomotor epilepsy.

Coping mechanisms. Unconscious and conscious ways of dealing with stress without changing one's goals.

Coprolalia. The use of vulgar, obscene, or dirty words. It is observed in some cases of schizophrenia. The word is derived from the Greek words *kopros* (excrement) and *lalia* (talking). *See also* Gilles de la Tourette's disease.

Coprophagia. Eating filth or feces.

Coprophilia. Excessive interest in filth or feces.

Corrective emotional experience. Re-exposure under favorable circumstances to an emotional situation that the patient could not handle in the past. As advocated by Franz Alexander, the therapist temporarily assumes a particular role to generate the experience and facilitate reality testing.

Co-therapy. A form of psychotherapy in which more than one therapist treat the individual patient or the group. It is also known as combined therapy, cooperative therapy, dual leadership, multiple therapy, and three-cornered therapy.

Counterphobia; counterphobic. Denoting a state of actual preference on the part of a phobic person for the very situation he fears.

Countertransference. Conscious or unconscious emotional response of the therapist to the patient. It is determined by the therapist's inner needs, rather than by the patient's needs, and it may reinforce the patient's earlier traumatic history if not checked by the therapist.

Creativity. Ability to produce something new. Silvano Arieti describes creativity as the tertiary process, a balanced combination of primary and secondary processes, whereby material from the id are used in the service of the ego.

Cretinism. Mental and physical retardation resulting from severe thyroid deficiency in infancy and childhood.

Criminal responsibility. A legal term denoting the culpability of an accused person at the time of the alleged crime. If it can be proved that, at the time of the crime, the defendant lacked the ability to form a criminal intent (mens rea), the plea of criminal insanity may be entered. *See also* Competency to stand trial, Durham decision, Insanity defense, Irresistible impulse test, Mens rea, M'Naghten rule.

Crisis intervention. A brief therapeutic approach used in the emergency rooms of general or psychiatric hospitals that is ameliorative, rather than curative, of acute psychiatric emergencies. Often, treatment factors focus on environmental modification, although interpersonal and intrapsychic factors are also considered. Individual, group, family, or drug therapy is used within a time-limited structure of several days to several weeks.

Crisis-intervention group psychotherapy. Group therapy aimed at decreasing or eliminating an emotional or situational crisis.

Crisis, therapeutic. *See* Therapeutic crisis.

Critical ratio. In a statistical study involving 30 or more subjects, the ratio that is used to determine whether differences found between two items are larger than could be expected from chance. *See also* T ratio.

Cross-cultural psychiatry. The comparative study of mental illness and health among various societies around the world.

Cultural deprivation. Restricted participation in the culture of the larger society.

Cultural psychiatry. A form of social psychiatry involving the diagnosis and treatment of the mentall ill in relation to their cultural environments. The cultural environment may vary so greatly from one culture to another that a form of behavior pathological in one society is acceptable in another.

Cunnilingus. Use of the mouth or tongue to stimulate the female genitalia.

Current material. Data from present interpersonal experiences. *See also* Genetic material.

Cushing's syndrome. Hyperadrenocorticism, named for American neurologist Harvey W. Cushing (1869–1939). The disorder is characterized by muscle wasting, obesity, osteoporosis, atrophy of the skin, and hypertension.

Cybernetics. The scientific study of regulatory mechanisms such as thermostats.

Cyclazocine. A narcotic antagonist that blocks the effects of heroin but does not relieve heroin craving. It has been used experimentally with a limited number of drug addicts in research programs.

Cycloplegia. Paralysis of the muscles of accommodation in the eye. It is observed at times as an autonomic side effect of phenothiazine and antiparkinsonism drugs.

Cyclothymic personality. A personality disorder in which the patient experiences regularly alternating periods of elation and depression, usually not related to external circumstances.

Da Costa's syndrome. Neurocirculatory asthenia; also called "soldier's heart."

Dance therapy. Nonverbal communication through rhythmic body movements; used to rehabilitate people with emotional or physical disorders. Pioneered by Marian Chase in 1940, this method is used in both individual and group therapy.

Day hospital. A hospital setup whereby a patient spends the day in the hospital and returns home at night.

Death instinct. *See* Aggressive drive.

Decompensation. In medical science, the failure of normal functioning of an organ, as in cardiac decompensation; in psychiatry, the breakdown of the psychological defense mechanisms that maintain the person's optimal psychic functioning. *See also* Depersonalization.

Decomposition. In psychiatry, the breaking up of a person into several identities. Paranoid schizophrenics are known to attribute their persecutions to separate entities derived from the same person.

Defense mechanism. Unconscious intrapsychic process. Protective in nature, it is used to relieve the anxiety and conflict arising from one's impulses and drives. *See also* Compensation, Conversion, Denial, Displacement, Dissociation, Idealization, Identification, Incorporation, Intellectualization, Introjection, Projection, Rationalization, Reaction formation, Regression, Repression, Sublimation, Substitution, Symbolization, Undoing.

Defensive emotion. Strong feeling that serves as a screen for a less acceptable feeling, one that would cause a person to experience anxiety if it appeared. For example, expressing the emotion of anger is often more acceptable to a patient than expressing the fear that his anger covers up. In this instance, anger is defensive.

Déjà entendu. Illusion of auditory recognition. *See also* Paramnesia.

Déjà pensé. A condition in which a thought never entertained before is incorrectly regarded as a repetition of a previous thought.

Déjà vu. Illusion of visual recognition in which a new situation is incorrectly regarded as a repetition of a previous experience. *See also* Paramnesia.

Delirium. A disturbance in the state of consciousness that stems from an acute organic reaction characterized by restlessness, confusion, disorientation, bewilderment, agitation, and affective lability. It is associated with fear, hallucinations, and illusions.

Delirium tremens. An acute psychotic state, usually occurring after a prolonged, copious, and severe period of drinking alcohol.

Delirium verborum. Psychiatric state in which the patient is excessively talkative.

Delusion. A false fixed belief not in accord with one's intelligence and cultural background. Types of delusion include the following. *Delusion of control:* false belief that one is being manipulated by others; *delusion of grandeur:* exaggerated concept of one's importance; *delusion of infidelity:* false belief that one's lover is unfaithful—it is derived from pathological jealousy; *delusion of persecution:* false belief that

one is being harrassed; *delusion of reference:* false belief that the behavior of others refers to oneself—a derivation from ideas of reference in which the patient falsely feels that he is being talked about by others; *delusion of self-accusation:* false feeling of remorse; *paranoid delusion:* oversuspiciousness leading to false persecutory ideas or beliefs.

Dementia. Organic loss of mental functioning.

Dementia praecox. An early term to describe what is now known as schizophrenia.

Denial. An unconscious defense mechanism in which an aspect of external reality is rejected. At times it is replaced by a more satisfying fantasy or piece of behavior. The term can also refer to the blocking of awareness of internal reality. It is one of the primitive or infantile defenses.

Dependence on therapy. Patient's pathological need for therapy, created out of the belief that he cannot survive without it.

Dependency. A state of reliance on another for psychological support. It reflects needs for security, love, protection, and mothering.

Depersonalization. Sensation of unreality concerning onself, parts of oneself, or one's environment. It is seen in schizophrenics, particularly during the early stages of decompensation. *See also* Decompensation.

Depression. In psychiatry, a morbid state characterized by mood alterations, such as sadness and loneliness; by low self-esteem associated with self-reproach; by psychomotor retardation and at times agitation; by withdrawal from interpersonal contact and at times a desire to die; and by such vegetative symptoms as insomnia and anorexia. *See also* Grief.

Deprivation, emotional. *See* Emotional deprivation.

Depth psychology. Psychology that has to do with unconscious rather than conscious processes.

Descriptive psychiatry. A form of psychiatry that focuses on readily observable external factors. It is instrumental in referring Kraepelin's systematized descriptions of mental illnesses.

Desensitization. A method of behavior therapy that is often used in dealing with phobias, insomnia, and frigidity. It involves deep-muscle relaxation, the establishment of anxiety hierarchies, and the use of relaxation to combat anxiety-evoking stimuli. *See also* Operant conditioning.

Deterioration. The increasing severity of a clinical condition. It is usually indicated by a progressive impairment of function.

Determinism. The concept that states that psychic events are not random happenings but have a discoverable cause or causes. Freud demonstrated that even human dreams, slips of the tongue, and other parapraxes are determined by discoverable causes.

Detoxification. Removal of the toxic effects of a drug. It is also known as detoxication. *See also* Cold turkey, Methadone.

Developmental disability. A disability that originates before the patient reaches the age of 18 and that is projected to continue for an indefinite period of time. To be considered a disability, it must constitute a substantial handicap, as mental retardation does.

Deviation. A statistical measure representing the difference between an individual value in a set of values and the mean value in that set.

Diagnostic and Statistical Manual of Mental Disorders. A handbook for the classification of mental illnesses. Formulated by the American Psychiatric Association, it was first issued in 1952 (DSM-I). The second edition (DSM-II), issued in 1968, correlates closely with the World Health Organization's *International Classification of Diseases.*

Dialogue. Verbal communication between two or more persons.

Differential reinforcement. A technique in conditioning therapy in which desirable behavior is followed by a positive reinforcer; an undesirable response is followed by a negative reinforcer. *See also* Conditioned reinforcer, Conditioning therapy, Extinction, Operant conditioning, Reinforcement, Schedule of reinforcement.

Differentiation. *See* Individuation.

Dipsomania. Morbid, irrepressible compulsion to drink alcoholic beverages.

Disability, learning. *See* Learning disability.

Discrimination. The process by which a person responds differently to stimuli. In the conditioning setting the desired response usually occurs. However, in an environment free from the conditioned stimulus or the unconditioned stimulus, the desired response is unlikely to occur. A patient conditioned for response at the professional center responds with maximum results in those reinforced surroundings; the same patient is unlikely to respond at all in his or her home environment. *See also* Classical conditioning, Conditioned reinforcer, Conditioned stimulus, Conditioning therapy, Desensitization, Differential reinforcement, Discriminative stimulus, Operant conditioning.

Discriminative stimulus. An environmental event that becomes correlated to a reinforcer in conditioning therapy. If one person always rewards an animal when the task is performed correctly, that person becomes correlated with the reward and can evoke the desired behavior with or without the reward. The person is the discriminative stimulus. *See also* Classical conditioning, Conditioned reinforcer, Conditioned stimulus, Conditioning therapy, Differential reinforcement, Discrimination, Eliciting stimulus, Operant conditioning, Unconditioned stimulus.

Disinhibition. Withdrawal of inhibition. Chemical substances, such as alcohol, can remove inhibitions by interfering with unctions of the cerebral cortex. In psychiatry, disinhibition leads to the freedom to act on one's own needs, rather than to submit to the demands of others.

Disintegration. Psychic disorganization.

Disorientation. Inability to judge time, space, and personal relations. It is characteristic of most acute and chronic brain disorders.

Displacement. An unconscious defense mechanism by which the affective component of an unacceptable idea or object is transferred to an acceptable one.

Disposition. Sum total of a person's inclinations as determined by his mood.

Dissociation. An unconscious defense mechanism by which an idea is separated from its accompanying affect, as seen in hysterical dissociative states; an unconscious process by which a group of mental processes is split off from the rest of a person's thinking, resulting in an independent functioning of this group of processes and thus a loss of the usual interrelationships.

Distortion. Misrepresentation of reality. It is based on unconsciously determined motives.

Distractibility. Inability to focus one's attention.

Dix, Dorothea Lynde (1802–1887). A former schoolteacher who devoted her life to improving institutional care for the mentally ill.

Dizygotic twins. Twins who are fraternal in that they develop from two separate ova. Monozygotic twins are identical in that they develop from one ovum.

DNA (deoxyribonucleic acid). Chemical found in the nucleus of cells; the essential substance in the genes which is responsible for inheritance.

Doctor-patient relationship. Human interchange that exists between the person who is sick and the person who is selected because of training and experience to heal.

Dominance. In neurology, the natural tendency for one half of the brain to be more active and important than the other half in some functions. In genetics, the tendency for one gene to express itself in a person, regardless of its pairing with a gene that would have expressed itself differently.

Double bind. Two conflicting communications from another person. One message is usually nonverbal and the other verbal. For example, parents may tell a child that arguments are to be settled peacefully and yet battle with each other constantly. The concept was formulated by Gregory Bateson.

Double blind study. A study in which one or more drugs and a placebo are compared in such a way that neither the patient nor the persons directly or indirectly involved in the study know which is being given to the patient. The drugs being investigated and the placebo are coded for identification.

Double personality. *See* Multiple personality.

Down's syndrome (mongolism). A congenital syndrome involving mental retardation, thick tongue, epicanthal folds, stubby fingers, simian creases on the hands and the feet, and short stature.

Drawing test. Any of a variety of psychological tests in which the subject is asked to draw certain familiar objects, such as people, trees, and houses. Attitudes and feelings are often revealed in the way the subject depicts these objects.

Dread. Anxiety related to a specific danger, as opposed to anxiety, which is usually regarded as objectless.

Dream. Mental activity during sleep that is experienced as though it were real. A dream has both a psychological and a biological purpose. It provides an outlet for the release of instinctual impulses and wish fulfillment of archaic needs and fantasies unacceptable in the real world. It permits the partial resolution of conflicts and the healing of traumata too overwhelming to be dealt with in the waking state. And it is the guardian of sleep, which is indispensable for the proper functioning of mind and body during the waking state. *See also* Hypnagogic hallucination, Hypnopompic hallucination, Paramnesia.

Dreamy state. Altered state of consciousness likened to a dream situation. It is accompanied by visual, auditory, and olfactory hallucinations and is believed to be associated with temporal lobe lesions. *See also* Marijuana.

Drive. A mental constituent, believed to be genetically determined, that produces a state of tension when it is in operation. This tension or state of psychic excitation motivates the person into action to alleviate the tension. Contemporary psychoanalysts prefer to use the term "drive," rather than Freud's term "instinct." *See also* Aggressive drive, Instinct, Sexual drive.

Drug abuse. The use of drugs for other than legitimate medical purposes. Also known as substance abuse.

Drug dependence. Habitual need for drugs, with or without physiological addiction.

Drug therapy. The use of chemical substances in the treatment of illness. It is also known as chemotherapy. *See also* Maintenance drug therapy.

DSM. *See* Diagnostic and Statistical Manual of Mental Disorders.

Dual-sex therapy. A specific form of psychotherapy developed by William Masters and Virginia Johnson in which treatment is focused on a particular sexual disorder. The crux of the program is the "round-table session" in which a male and female therapy team suggest special exercises prescribed for the couple and to diminish fears of sexual performance felt by both sexes, and to facilitate communication in sexual and nonsexual areas.

Durham decision. A legal decision handed down in 1954 by the U.S. Court of Appeals for the District of Columbia. The decision held that "an accused is not criminally responsible if his unlawful act was the product of mental disease or mental defect." The American Law Institute has replaced this rule with Section 4.01 of the Penal Code, which states that "a person is not responsible for criminal conduct if at the time of such conduct as a result of mental disease or defect he lacks substantial capacity either to appreciate the criminality of his conduct or to conform his conduct to the requirements of the law." *See also* Competency to stand trial, Criminal responsibility, Insanity defense, Irresistible impulse test, Mens rea, M'Naghten rule.

Dyad. A pair of persons in an interactional situation, such as husband and wife, mother and father, co-therapists, or patient and therapist.

Dyadic session. Psychotherapeutic session involving only two persons, the therapist and the patient.

Dynamic psychiatry. A form of psychiatry that involves the study of the emotional processes, their origins, and their mental mechanisms. It is based on the principles of dynamics, which implies progression or regression in the changing factors of human behavior and motivation.

Dynamic reasoning. Formation of all the clinical evidence gained from free-associative anamnesis into a psychological reconstruction of the patient's development. Term used by Franz Alexander.

Dysarthria. Speech impairment usually due to organic disorder of the speech organs or nervous system.

Dyskinesia. Involuntary stereotyped, rhythmic muscular activity, such as a tic or a spasm. It is sometimes observed as an extrapyramidal side effect of antipsychotic drugs, particularly the phenothiazine derivatives. *See also* Tardive oral dyskinesia.

Dyslalia. Speech impairment caused by a defect in the speech organs.

Dyslexia. Reading disability in which the patient is unable to understand the written word. It is not related to intelligence.

Dyspareunia. Physical pain in sexual intercourse experienced by women; usually emotionally caused.

Dysphagia. Difficulty in swallowing.

Dyssocial behavior. Formerly known as sociopathic behavior; the behavior pattern of such marginal criminal types as racketeers, prostitutes, and illegal gamblers. *See* Antisocial personality.

Dystonia. Extrapyramidal motor disturbance consisting of uncoordinated and spasmodic movements of the body and limbs, such as arching of the back and twisting of the body and neck. It is observed as a side effect of phenothiazine drugs and other major tranquilizers. *See also* Tardive oral dyskinesia.

Echolalia. Repetition of another person's words or phrases. It is a psychopathological symptom observed in certain cases of schizophrenia, particularly the catatonic types. Some authors consider this behavior to be an attempt by the patient to maintain a continuity of thought processes. *See also* Gilles de la Tourette's disease.

Echopraxia. Imitation of another person's movements. It is a psychopathological symptom observed in some cases of catatonic schizophrenia.

Ecology. The study of the symbiotic relationships between organisms and their environments. As related to human beings, ecology deals with the effect of environment and human institutions on humans.

Ecstasy. Affect of intense rapture.

ECT (electroconvulsive therapy). A treatment, usually for depression, that uses electric current to induce unconsciousness and convulsive seizures.

Educable. Capable of some degree of learning. Usually, one is considered educable if his or her I.Q. exceeds 50 and if he or she is expected to achieve the equivalent of a fourth or fifh-grade education, which may include the learning of enough skills for self-support.

EEG (electroencephalogram). A recording of the electrical impulses emanating from the brain.

Ego. One of the three components of the psychic apparatus in the Freudian structural framework. The other two components are the id and the superego. Although the ego has some conscious components, many of its operations are automatic. It occupies a position between the primal instincts and the demands of the outer world; therefore, it serves to mediate between the person and external reality. In so doing, it performs the important functions of perceiving the needs of the self, both physical and psychological, and the qualities and attitudes of the environment. It evaluates, coordinates, and integrates these perceptions so that internal demands can be adjusted to external requirements. It is also responsible for certain defensive functions to protect the person against the demands of the id and the superego. It has a host of functions, but adaptation to reality is perhaps the most important one. *See also* Reality testing.

Ego analysis. The psychoanalytic study of the manner in which the ego operates.

Ego-coping skill. Adaptive method or capacity developed by a person to deal with or overcome a psychological or social problem.

Ego defense. *See* Defense mechanism.

Ego-dystonic. Repugnant to or at variance with the ego.

Ego function. *See* Executive ego function.

Ego ideal. Part of the ego during its development that eventually fuses with the superego. It is a social as well as a psychological concept, reflecting the mutual esteem and the disillusionment in child-parent and subsequent relationships.

Ego model. A person on whom another person patterns his ego.

Ego state. In Eric Berne's structural analysis, a state of mind and its related set of coherent behavior patterns. It includes a system of feelings directly related to a given subject. There are three ego states: parent, adult, and child.

Ego-syntonic. Acceptable to the aims of the ego.

Egocentric. Refers to a person who is self-centered, preoccupied with his own needs, selfish, and lacking interest in others.

Egomania. Pathological self-preoccupation or self-centeredness. *See also* Narcissism.

Eidetic image. Visualization of objects previously seen or imagined.

Eitingon, Max (1881–1943). Austrian psychoanalyst. An emissary of the Zurich school, he gained fame as the first person to be analyzed by Freud in a few sessions in 1907. Later, he became the first chief of the Berlin Psychoanalytic Clinic, a founder of the Berlin Psychoanalytic Institute, and a founder of the Palestine Psychoanalytic Society.

Elaboration. The unconscious process of embellishing the symbolic content of a dream.

Elation. Affect characterized by euphoria, confidence, and enjoyment. It is associated with increased motor activity.

Electrocardiographic effect. Change seen in recordings of the electrical activity of the heart. It is observed as a side effect of phenothiazine derivatives, particularly thioridazine.

Electroconvulsive treatment (ECT). *See* Shock treatment.

Electroencephalograph (EEG). Apparatus that records the electrical activity of the brain.

Electromyograph (EMG). Apparatus that records the electrical activity of the muscles.

Eliciting stimulus. An environmental event that produces an autonomic response. Eliciting stimuli include both unconditioned and conditioned stimuli. *See also* Classical conditioning, Conditioned stimulus, Discriminative stimulus, Operant conditioning, Unconditioned stimulus.

Elopment. The unauthorized departure of a patient from a mental health care facility. The term should be replace by the phrase "left hospital against medical advice."

Emotion. *See* Affect.

Emotional deprivation. Lack of adequate and appropriate interpersonal or environmental experiences, or both, especially in the early developmental years. Emotional deprivation is caused by poor mothering or by early separation from the mother.

Emotional insight. *See* Insight.

Emotional support. Encouragement, hope, and inspiration given to one person by another.

Empathy. Ability to put oneself in another person's place, get into his frame of reference, and understand his feelings and behavior objectively. It is one of the major qualities in a successful therapist, facilitator, or helpful group member. *See also* Sympathy.

Encephalitis. An acute or chronic inflammation of the brain.

Encephalopathy. Degenerative disease of the brain.

Encopresis. Involuntary passage of feces, usually occuring at night or during sleep.

Encounter group. A form of sensitivity training that emphasizes the experiencing of individual relationships within the group and that minimizes intellectual and didactic input. It is a group that focuses on the present, rather than concerning itself with the past or outside problems of its members. J. L. Moreno introduced and developed the idea of the encounter group in 1914.

Endocrine disorders. Malfunction of any of the endocrine glands. In psychiatry, of particular interest is the relation between an endocrine disturbance and an emotional and behavioral disturbance.

Engram. According to the mnemic hypothesis, the physical trace left on the protoplasm of an organism by the repetition of stimuli; acquired habits may thus be transmitted to descendants.

Entropy. A turning inward of energy; a diminished capacity for change, particularly with regard to the aging process.

Enuresis. Bed wetting.

Epidemiology. In psychiatry, the study of the prevalence and distribution of mental disorder within a particular population.

Epigenesis. A term introduced by Erikson to refer to the stages of ego and social development.

Epilepsy. A disorder characterized by the periodic appearance of a recurring pattern of short-lived disturbances of consciousness. The disease may have no apparent organic cause, or it may be due to organic lesions.

Epileptic dementia. A form of epilepsy that is accompanied by progressive mental and intellectual impairment. Some believe that the circulatory disturbances during epileptic attacks cause nerve cell degeneration and lead to dementia.

Epinephrine. A sympathomimetic agent. It is the chief hormone secreted by the adrenal medulla. In a state of fear or anxiety, the physiological changes stem from the release of epinephrine. Also known as adrenaline, it is related to norepinephrine, a substance presently linked with mood disturbances in depression.

Eremophobia. Fear of being by oneself.

Ergasia. Adolf Meyer's term for a person's total activity, as opposed to the functioning of parts of the whole.

Erikson, Erik (1902–   ). Psychoanalyst who has developed a theory to explain ego development and psychosexual development in terms of social adaptation as they relate to Freud's formulations.

Erogenous zone. *See* Erotogenic zone.

Eros. *See* Sexual drive.

Erotic. Related to the pleasurable sensations or the instinctual qualities of sexual love or desire. When describing the physical, erotic most frequently refers to body zones, such as the oral, anal, and genital zones. It may also be used to define psychic structures or objects related to sexual pleasure.

Erotogenic zone (erogenous zone). An area of the body susceptible to erotic arousal, particularly the oral, anal, and genital areas.

Erotomania. Pathological preoccupation with sexual activities or fantasies.

Erythrophobia. Fear of blushing.

Ethnocentrism. Conviction that one's own group is superior to other groups. It impairs one's ability to evaluate members of another group realistically or to communicate with them on an open, equal, and person-to-person basis.

Ethology. The study of animals in their natural habitat and the kind of behavior that is specific to a species.

Etiology. The study of the causes of a disease.

Euergasia. Word used by Adolf Meyer to mean normal mental functioning.

Eunuch. A man whose gonads have been removed before puberty, thus causing him to develop the secondary sex characteristics of a woman.

Euphoria. An altered state of consciousness characterized by an exaggerated feeling of well-being that is inappropriate to apparent events. It is often associated with opiate, amphetamine, and alcohol abuse.

Evasion. Act of not facing up to or of strategically eluding something. It consists of suppressing an idea that is next in a thought series and replacing it with another idea closely related to it. Evasion is also known as paralogia and perverted logic.

Exaltation. Affect consisting of intense elation and feelings of grandeur.

Executive ego function. A psychoanalytic term used to describe the ego's management of mental mechanisms to meet the organism's needs.

Exhibitionism. A form of sexual deviation characterized by a compulsive need to expose one's body, particularly the genitals.

Existential psychotherapy. A type of therapy that puts the emphasis on confrontation, primarily in the here-and-now interaction, and on feeling experiences, rather than on rational thinking. Little attention is given to patient resistances. The therapist is involved on the same level and to the same degree as the patient. It is based on existential philosophy which holds that man has the responsibility for his own existence.

Exogenous psychosis. *See* Organic brain syndrome.

Exorcism. A magical practice in which mystical incantations are invoked to remove demons that are alleged to have entered the mind.

Experiencing. Feeling emotions and sensations as opposed to thinking; being involved in what is happening, rather than standing back at a distance and theorizing.

Experimental group. In an experimental design, the group to which the treatment under study is administered. *See also* Control group.

Explosive personality. A personality disorder in which the person strikes out in an extremely angry and hostile fashion, usually in contrast to his normal behavior.

Extended family therapy. A type of family therapy that involves family members, beyond the nuclear family, who are closely associated with it and affect it. *See also* Network, Social network therapy.

Extinction. In conditioning, the return to a preconditioned state. When a response is not followed by a reinforcer, it eventually returns to its level of strength before it was altered. Behavior that has been subjected to extinction is termed extinguished behavior. *See also* Classical conditioning, Conditioned reinforcer, Conditioning therapy, Differential reinforcement, Operant conditioning, Reinforcement.

Extinguished behavior. *See* Extinction.

Extrapsychic. The ralationship between the mind (psyche) and the environment.

Extrapsychic conflict. Conflict that arises between the person and his environment. *See also* Intrapsychic conflict.

Extrapyramidal effect. Bizarre, involuntary motor movement. It is a central nervous system side effect, sometimes produced by antipsychotic drugs. *See also* Dyskinesia.

Extrasensory perception. Experiencing of an external event by means other than the five senses. Telepathy—perception of another person's thoughts—and clairvoyance—perception of outside events—are two kinds of extrasensory perception; abbreviated as ESP.

Extroversion. The state of one's energies being directed outside oneself. *See also* Introversion.

Fabulation. A term used by Adolf Meyer to mean fabrication. *See also* Confabulation.

Family neurosis. Emotional maladaptation in

which a person's psychopathology is unconsciously interrelated with that of the other members of his family.

Family therapy. Treatment of a family in conflict. The whole family meets as a group with the therapist and explores its relationships and process. The focus is on the resolution of current reactions to one another, rather than on individual members.

Fantasy. Daydream; fabricated mental picture or chain of events. A form of thinking dominated by unconscious material and primary processes, it seeks wish fulfillment and immediate solutions to conflicts. Fantasy may serve as the matrix for creativity or for neurotic distortions of reality.

Father surrogate. Father substitute. In psychoanalysis, the patient projects his father image onto another person and responds to that person unconsciously in an inappropriate and unrealistic manner, with the feelings and attitudes that he had toward his real father.

Fausse reconnaissance. False recognition. *See also* Paramnesia.

Faute de mieux. Literally, "for want of anything better," connoting in psychiatry a person's choosing a homosexual relationship when no partner of the opposite sex is available.

Fear. Unpleasurable affect consisting of psychophysiological changes in response to a realistic threat or danger to one's existence. *See also* Anxiety.

Federn, Paul (1871–1950). Austrian psychoanalyst, one of Freud's earliest followers, and the last survivor of the original Wednesday Evening Society. He made important original contributions to psychoanalysis, such as the concepts of flying dreams and ego feelings, and he was instrumental in saving the minutes of the Vienna Psychoanalytic Society for subsequent publication.

Feeblemindedness. An obsolete term for mental retardation.

Feedback. Expressed response by one person or a group to another person's behavior.

Fellatio. Use of the mouth or tongue to stimulate the male genitalia.

Ferenczi, Sandor (1873–1933). Hungarian psychoanalyst, one of Freud's early followers, and a brilliant contributor to all aspects of psychoanalysis. His temperament was more romantic than Freud's, and he came to favor more active and personal techniques, to the point that his adherence to psychoanalysis during his last years was questioned.

Fetishism. The process of achieving sexual excitement and gratification by substituting an inanimate object—such as a shoe, piece of underwear, or other article of clothing—for a human love object.

Field theory. Concept postulated by Kurt Lewin that a person is a complex energy field in which all behavior can be conceived of as a change in some state of the field during a given unit of time. Lewin also postulated the presence within the field of psychological tensions—that is, states of readiness or preparation for action. The field theory is concerned essentially with the present field, the here-and-now. The theory has been applied by various individual and group psychotherapists.

Fixation. The arrest of psychosexual development at any stage before complete maturation; a close and paralyzing attachment to another person, such as mother or father. *See also* Oral, Anal, and Phallic phases.

Flagellantism. The process by which sexual partners are aroused and gratified by whipping or being whipped.

Flexibilitas, cerea. *See* Cerea flexibilitas.

Fliess, Wilhelm (1858–1928). Berlin nose and throat specialist. He shared an early interest with Freud in the physiology of sex and entered into a prolonged correspondence that figures importantly in the records of Freud's self-analysis. Freud was influenced by Fliess's concept of bisexuality and his theory of the periodicity of the sex functions.

Flight of ideas. Rapid succession of thoughts without logical connections.

Floccillation. Aimless plucking or picking, usually at bedclothes or clothing. It is common in senile psychosis and delirium.

Flooding. A technique in behavior therapy that is used in the treatment of phobic and maladaptive anxieties. Either real or imaginary oppressive stimuli are presented in intense forms; if the technique is successful, the undesirable emotional responses cease after several trials.

Focal conflict theory. Theory elaborated by Thomas French in 1952 that explains the current behavior of a person as an expression of his method of solving currently experienced personality conflicts that originated very early in his life; he constantly resonates to these early life conflicts.

Folie à deux. Emotional illness shared by two persons. If it involves three persons, it is referred to as folie à trois, etc.

Forensic psychiatry. The branch of psychiatry that is concerned with legal aspects of mental illness.

Forepleasure. The sexual play that precedes sexual intercourse.

Formal operations. Jean Piaget's label for the complete development of a person's logical thinking capacities.

Formication. A form of paresthesia in which there is a sensation of ants running over the skin. It is most commonly found in delirium tremens and cocainism.

Foulkes, S. H. (1923–   ). English psychiatrist and one of the organizers of the group therapy movement in Great Britain. His work combines Moreno's ideas—the here-and-now, the sociogenesis, the social atom, the psychological network—with psychoanalytic views. He stresses the importance of group-as-a-whole phenomena. *See also* Group analytic psychotherapy, Network.

Free association. Investigative psychoanalytic technique devised by Freud in which the patient seeks to verbalize without reservation or censorship the passing contents of his mind. The conflicts that emerge while fulfilling this task constitute resistances that are the basis of the analyst's interpretations. *See also* Conflict.

Free-floating anxiety. Pervasive, unrealistic fear that is not attached to any idea or alleviated by symptom substitution. It is observed particularly in anxiety neurosis, although it may be seen in some cases of latent schizophrenia.

Frequency distribution. A statistical description of raw data in terms of the number of cases that fall into each interval within a set of data. Frequency distribution is often presented graphically in the form of a frequency histogram or frequency polygram.

Freud, Sigmund (1856–1939). Austrian psychiatrist and the founder of psychoanalysis. With Josef Breuer, he explored the potentialities of cathartic therapy, then went on to develop the analytic technique and such fundamental concepts of mental phenomena as the unconscious, infantile sexuality, repression, sublimation, superego, ego, and id formation and their applications throughout all spheres of human behavior.

Frigidity. In the female, lack of sexual response or feeling, ranging from complete anesthesia to incomplete climax.

Frotteur. A person who becomes sexually aroused by rubbing up against someone, usually without specific genital contact, as in a crowd.

Frustration. The thwarting of an impulse or drive. The ability to tolerate frustration and delay gratification is considered a sign of maturity and good ego strength.

Fugue. A long period in which a person has almost complete amnesia for his past. Habits and skills are usually unaffected. He leaves home and starts a new life with different conduct. Afterward, earlier events are remembered, but those of the fugue period are forgotten.

Fulfillment. Satisfaction of needs that may be either real or illusory.

Functional. Referring to bodily changes not attributable to known organic alterations.

Fusion. A term used in psychoanalysis to mean the joining together of instincts.

Galactorrhea. Excessive or spontaneous flow of milk from the breast. It may be a result of the endocrine influence of phenothiazine drugs.

Galvanic skin response. *See* GSR

Gamophobia. Fear of marriage.

Ganser's syndrome. A rare disease, most often observed in prisoners, in which the patient replies to questions with utterly incorrect and often ridiculous replies, even though he has understood the sense of the question.

Gargoylism. A rare metabolic disorder characteristic of Hurler's disease, that becomes evident in infancy. The affected person resembles a dwarf with hideously deformed facial features, a bovine expression, a protruding tongue, and general maldevelopment of the facial bones. Victims of this disease are mentally retarded to some degree.

Gender identity. An inner sense of maleness or femaleness that is formed at a very early age and is reinforced by social expectations and later by bodily changes. It is a concept of masculinity or femininity, rather than male or female, which is related to biological implications, not social implications. *See also* Gender role.

Gender role. The sex-related public image that a person presents to others and to himself or herself. It publicly declares the person to be a man or a woman. *See also* Gender identity.

General adaptational syndrome (GAS). Hans Selye's term for the response of the body to major stress passing through the alarm reaction, resistance, and finally, exhaustion.

General paralysis (general paresis). Organic brain syndrome caused by a chronic syphilitic infection.

General systems theory. A theory that sees all events as part of a network of interlocking systems in which the behavior of each system is determined by its characteristics and components and is defined by the larger systems of which it is a component. In psychiatry, this theory gives rise to a view of the personality as a whole composed of many integrated systems that affect human behavior and must be treated as such.

Generalization. The process of arriving at a group of conclusions or judgments on the basis of a limited sampling. A schizophrenic patient often indulges in overgeneralization and tends to see the concrete as an abstract.

Genes. The basic units of heredity contained within the chromosomes of cells.

Genetic counseling. The presenting and discussing of the scientific factors involved in inherited pathological conditions. The counselor investigates a couple's genetic background, indicates to the prospective parents how likely or unlikely they are to transmit certain characteristics, and in many cases helps them make appropriate plans based on all available scientific evidence.

Genetic material. Data out of the personal history of the patient that are useful in developing an understanding of the psychodynamics of his present adaptation. *See also* Current material.

Genital phase. The final stage of psychosexual development. It occurs during puberty. In this stage the person's psychosexual development is so organized that he can achieve sexual gratification from genital-to-genital contact and has the capacity for a mature, affectionate relationship with someone of the opposite sex. *See also* Infantile sexuality, Anal, Oral, Phallic, and Latency phases.

Genotype. Term that refers to the genetic inheritance of a person, the set of genes that he receives from both parents at the time of conception.

Geriatrics. Branch of medicine that deals with the aged and the problems of aging; also called gerontology and geropsychiatry.

Gerontology. The study of aging and the aged.

Gestalt therapy. Type of psychotherapy that emphasizes the treatment of the person as a whole—his biological component parts and their organic functioning, his perceptual configuration, and his interrelationships with the outside world. Gestalt therapy, developed by Frederic S. Perls, can be used in either an individual or a group therapy setting. It focuses on the sensory awareness of the person's here-and-now experiences, rather than on past recollections or future expectations. Gestalt therapy uses role-playing and other techniques to promote the patient's growth process and to develop his full potential.

Gilles de la Tourette's disease. A rare illness that has its onset in childhood. First described by a Paris physician, Gilles de la Tourette, the illness is characterized by involuntary muscular movements and motor incoordination, accompanied by echolalia and coprolalia. It is considered by some to be a schizophrenic condition.

Globus hystericus. A hysterical symptom in

which the person feels as if he had a lump in his throat.

Glossolalia. Unintelligible jargon.

Go-around. Technique used in group therapy in which the therapist requires each member of the group to respond to another member, a theme, or an association. This procedure encourages the participation of all members in the group.

God complex. A belief sometimes seen in therapists that one can accomplish more than is humanly possible or that one's word should not be doubted. The God complex of the aging psychoanalyst was first discussed by Ernest Jones, Freud's biographer. *See also* Mother Superior complex.

Grand mal. The major form of epilepsy, in which gross seizures are accompanied by loss of consciousness.

Grandiose. Characterized by an exaggerated perception of one's importance, abilities, or identity. Grandiose may be accompanied or manifested by delusions of power, fame, or wealth.

Gray-out syndrome. A psychosis that occurs in pilots flying in the stratosphere, out of sight of the horizon.

Grief. Alteration in mood and affect consisting of sadness appropriate to a real loss. *See also* Depression.

Group. *See* Therapeutic group.

Group analytic psychotherapy. A type of group therapy in which the group is used as the principal therapeutic agent and all communications and relationships are viewed as part of a total field of interaction. Interventions deal primarily with group forces, rather than with individual forces. S. H. Foulkes applied the term to his treatment procedure in 1948. It is also known as therapeutic group analysis. *See also* Phyloanalysis, Psychoanalytic group psychotherapy.

Group cohesion. Effect of the mutual bonds between members of a group as a result of their concerted effort for a common interest and purpose. Until cohesiveness is achieved, the group cannot concentrate its full energy on a common task.

Group dynamics. Phenomena that occur in groups; the movement of a group from its inception to its termination. Interactions and interrelations among members and between the members and the therapist create tension, which maintains a constantly changing group equilibrium. The interactions and the tension that they create are highly influenced by individual members' psychological make-up, unconscious instinctual drives, motives, wishes, and fantasies. The understanding and effective use of group dynamics are essential in group treatment. It is also known as group process. *See also* Psychodynamics.

Group pressure. Demand by group members that individual members submit and conform to group standards, values, and behavior.

Group psychotherapy. A type of psychiatric treatment that involves two or more patients participating together in the presence of one or more psychotherapists, who facilitate both emotional and rational cognitive interactions to effect changes in the maladaptive behavior of the members.

GSR (galvanic skin response). Measurement of a person's response to certain emotional stimuli by means of his skin resistance to electric current.

Guilt. Affect associated with self-reproach and need for punishment. In psychoanalysis, guilt refers to a neurotic feeling of culpability that stems from a conflict between the ego and the superego. It begins developmentally with parental disapproval and becomes internalized as conscience in the course of superego formation. Guilt has normal psychological and social functions, but special intensity or absence of guilt characterizes many mental disorders, such as depression and antisocial personality, respectively. Some psychiatrists distinguish shame as a less internalized form of guilt.

Gustatory hallucinations. False sense of taste.

Gynephobia. Fear of women.

Gyrectomy. A form of psychosurgery in which portions of the frontal cortex are removed in such a way that the normally functioning gyri are left intact.

Habit. A repetitive learned response. Common habits are nail biting and thumb sucking.

Halfway house. A facility for mental patients who no longer need the full facilities of a hospital but are not yet ready to return to their communities.

Hallucination. A false sensory perception without a concrete external stimulus. It can be induced by emotional and by organic factors, such as drugs and alcohol. Common hallucinations involve sights or sounds, although any of the senses may be involved. *See also* Auditory, Gustatory, Hypnagogic, Hypnopompic, Kinesthetic, Lilliputian, Tactile, and Visual hallucinations.

Hallucinogenic drug. *See* Psychotomimetic drug.

Hallucinosis. A state in which a person experiences hallucinations while he is fully conscious.

Haloperidol. An antipsychotic agent of the butyrophenone class of drugs.

Haphephobia. Fear of being touched.

Haplology. Rapid speech in which syllables are left out. It is common in certain manias and in schizophrenic conditions.

Health Maintenance Organization (HMO). A type of group practice composed of physicians and other health-related professionals that is aimed at maintaining the health of those it serves, as well as treating their illnesses.

Healthy identification. Modeling of oneself, consciously or unconsciously, on another person who has a sound psychic makeup. The identification has constructive purposes. *See also* Imitation.

Hebephrenia. A complex of symptoms considered a form of schizophrenia. *See also* Schizophrenia.

Hedonism. Seeking after pleasure.

Herd instinct. Desire to belong to a group and to participate in social activities. Wilfred Trotter used the term to indicate the presence of a hypothetical social instinct in man. In psychoanalysis, herd instinct is viewed as a social phenomenon, rather than as an instinct. *See also* Aggressive drive, Sexual drive.

Here-and-now. Contemporaneity. *See also* There-and-then.

Here-and-now approach. A technique that focuses on understanding the interpersonal and intrapersonal responses and reactions as they occur in the ongoing treatment session. Little or no emphasis is put on past history and experiences.

Hermaphrodite. A person who has both female and male sexual organs, usually with one sex dominating.

Heroin. A potentially addicting opiate. It is the substance most commonly used by narcotics addicts, who crave larger and larger amounts to achieve the same narcotic and analgesic effects.

Heterosexuality. Sexual attraction or contact between opposite-sex persons. The capacity for heterosexual arousal is probably innate, biologically programed, and triggered in very early life, perhaps by olfactory modalities, as seen in lower animals. *See also* Bisexuality, Homosexuality.

Heterozygous. A term used in genetics when both a dominant gene and a recessive gene are necessary to produce a trait.

Heuristic. A quality that encourages a person to discover something for himself or herself.

Histrionic personality disorder (hysterical personality). A condition in which the patient, usually an immature and dependent person, exhibits unstable, overreactive, and excitable behavior that is aimed at gaining attention, although the person may not be aware of this aim.

Holism. In psychiatry, the study of a person as a distinctive entity, rather than as a collection of various characteristics.

Holophrastic. The use of a single word to express a combination of ideas. Schizophrenics are known for this type of language expression.

Homeostasis. The tendency to maintain a constant balance among bodily processes to ensure optimal functioning.

Homosexual panic. Sudden, acute onset of severe anxiety, precipitated by the unconscious fear or conflict that one may be a homosexual or act out homosexual impulses. *See also* Homosexuality.

Homosexuality. Sexual attraction or contact between same-sex persons. Some authors distinguish two types; overt and latent. *See also* Bisexuality, Heterosexuality, Inversion, Lesbianism.

Honesty. Forthrightness of conduct and uprightness of character; truthfulness. In therapy, honesty is a value manifested by the ability to communicate one's immediate experience, including inconsistent, conflicting, or ambivalent feelings and perceptions. *See also* Authenticity.

Horney, Karen (1885–1952). Psychiatrist and psychoanalyst, whose theory of neurosis and therapy included a philosophy of human nature and morality and that focused on a drive toward self-realization. Her emphasis was on the environmental and cultural determinants of neurosis.

Hospital addiction. *See* Munchausen syndrome.

Humiliation. Sense of disgrace and shame frequently experienced by depressed patients.

Huntington's chorea. A hereditary and progressive central nervous system disease characterized by jerking motions and progressive mental deterioration.

Hydrocephalus. Increased amount of cerebrospinal fluid in the skull.

Hydrotherapy. External or internal use of water in the treatment of disease. In psychiatry, the use of wet packs to calm an agitated psychotic patient was formerly a popular treatment modality.

Hyperactivity. Increased muscular activity. The term is commonly used to describe a disturbance found in children that is manifested by constant restlessness and movements executed at a rapid rate. The disturbance is believed to be due to brain damage, mental retardation, or emotional or physiological disturbance. It is also known as hyperkinesis.

Hyperalgesia. Unusual sensitivity to pain.

Hyperkinesis. *See* Hyperactivity.

Hypermnesia. Exaggerated degree of retention and recall. It is observed in schizophrenia, the manic phase of manic-depressive illness, organic brain syndrome, drug intoxication induced by amphetamines and hallucinogens,

hypnosis, and febrile conditions. *See also* Memory.

Hyperorexia. Extreme hunger. *See also* Bulimia.

Hyperpragia. Excessive thinking and mental activity, generally associated with the manic phase of manic-depressive illness.

Hypersomnia. Excessive sleep lasting from many hours to several days. It is characterized by extreme difficulty in awakening from nocturnal sleep and by confusion after awakening. Hypersomniac patients should be evaluated to determine whether a significant neurological or psychological disorder exists.

Hypertensive crisis. Severe rise in blood pressure that can lead to intracranial hemorrhage. It is occasionally seen as a side effect of certain antidepressant drugs.

Hyperventilation. Overbreathing, often caused by anxiety, in which a lack of carbon dioxide in the blood produces such symptoms as lightheadedness, numbness in the extremities, and faintness.

Hypesthesia. Diminished sensitivity to tactile stimulation.

Hypnagogic hallucination. False sensory perception that occurs just before falling asleep. *See also* Hypnopompic hallucination.

Hypnoanalysis. The use of hypnosis in psychoanalysis to gain access to unconscious processes that the patient cannot reveal by means of ordinary therapeutic maneuvers.

Hypnodrama. Psychodrama under hypnotic trance. The patient is first put into a hypnotic trance. During the trance he is encouraged to act out the various experiences that torment him.

Hypnoid state. A term introduced by Freud describing an alteration of consciousness that occurs characteristically in hysteria during periods of emotional stress. It is characterized by heightened suggestibility and provides a basis for hysterical somatic symptom formation.

Hypnopompic hallucination. False sensory perception that occurs just before full wakefulness. *See also* Hypnagogic hallucination.

Hypnosis. Artificially induced alterations of consciousness of one person by another. The subject responds with a high degree of suggestibility, both mental and physical, during the trance-like state.

Hypnotic. A drug that is used for the express purpose of producing sleep.

Hypochondriasis (hypochondriacal neurosis). Exaggerated concern with one's physical health. The concern is not based on real organic pathology.

Hypomania. An abnormal emotional state or mood that is intermediate between normal euphoria and mania. It is associated with bipolar depression.

Hypotension, orthostatic. *See* Orthostatic hypotension.

Hypothesis, null. *See* Null hypothesis.

Hysterical anesthesia. Disturbance in sensory perception characterized by absence of sense of feeling in certain areas of the body. It is observed in certain cases of hysterical neurosis, particularly the conversion type, and it is believed to be a defense mechanism.

Hysterical neurosis. A neurosis that occurs in response to emotional stress and involves a sudden loss or impairment of function. It may be of the conversion type, in which the senses of the voluntary nervous system are involved, or of the dissociative type, in which the person's state of consciousness is affected.

Hysterical personality. *See* Histrionic personality disorder.

I-It. Philosopher Martin Buber's description of damaging interpersonal relationships. If a person treats himself or another person exclusively as an object, he prevents mutuality, trust, and growth. When pervasive in a group, I-It relationships prevent human warmth, destroy cohesiveness, and retard group process. *See also* I-Thou.

I-Thou. Philosopher Martin Buber's conception that man's identity develops from the true sharing by persons. Basic trust can occur in a living partnership in which each member identifies the particular real personality of the other in his wholeness, unity, and uniqueness. In groups, I-Thou relationships promote warmth, cohesiveness, and constructive group process. *See also* I-It.

Iatrogenic illness. A disease accidentally caused or aggravated by a physician.

ICT (insulin coma therapy). A form of shock treatment in which large amounts of insulin are given to a psychotic, usually a schizophrenic, patient in order to induce a coma. The therapy was introduced by Manfred Sakel.

Id. Part of Freud's concept of the psychic apparatus. According to his structural theory of mental functioning, the id harbors the energy that stems from the instinctual drives and desires of a person. The id is completely in the unconscious realm, unorganized and under the influence of the primary processes. *See also* Conscious, Ego, Preconscious, Primary process, Superego, Unconscious.

Idea of reference. Misinterpretation of incidents and events in the outside world as having a direct personal reference to oneself. Occasionally observed in normal persons, ideas of reference are frequently seen in paranoid patients. *See also* Projection.

Idealization. A defense mechanism in which a person consciously or, usually, unconsciously overestimates an attribute or an aspect of another person.

Ideational shield. An intellectual, rational defense against the anxiety that a person would feel if he became vulnerable to the criticisms and rejection of others. As a result of his fear of being rejected, he may feel threatened if he criticizes another person, an act that is unacceptable to him. In both group and individual therapy, conditions are set up that allow the participants to lower this ideational shield.

Idée fixe. A fixed idea that is recurrent and most often associated with obsessional states.

Identification. An unconscious defense mechanism in which a person incorporates into himself the mental picture of an object and then patterns himself after this object; seeing oneself as like the person used as a pattern. It is distinguished from imitation, a conscious process. *See also* Healthy identification, Imitation, Role.

Identification with the aggressor. An unconscious process by which a person incorporates within himself the mental image of a person who represents a source of frustration from the outside world. A primitive defense, it operates in the interest and service of the developing ego. The classic example of this defense occurs toward the end of the oedipal stage, when the male child, whose main source of love and gratification is the mother, identifies with his father. The father represents the source of frustration, being the powerful rival of the mother; the child cannot master or run away from his father, so he is obliged to identify with him. *See also* Psychosexual development.

Identity, gender. *See* Gender identity.

Identity crisis. A chaotic sense of self, a disorientation regarding one's true self and one's role in society.

Idiopathic. Without known cause.

Idiot. *See* Mental retardation.

Idiot-savant. A mentally retarded person who is able to perform unusual mental feats, usually involving complicated puzzle solving or calculations based on numbers or calendar dates.

Idiotropic. Egocentric; introspective.

Ileus, paralytic. *See* Paralytic ileus.

Illuminism. A state of hallucination in which the patient carries on conversations with imaginary supernatural creatures.

Illusion. False perception and misinterpretation of an actual sensory stimulus.

Imago. A Jungian term referring to an idealized, unconscious mental image of a key person in someone's early life.

Imbecile. *See* Mental retardation.

Imitation. In psychiatry, a conscious act of mimicking another person's behavior pattern. *See also* Healthy identification, Identification.

Impasse. *See* Therapeutic impasse.

Impetus. In psychoanalytic psychiatry, the force or energy behind a particular drive.

Impotence. Inability to achieve an erection of the penis.

Imprinting. The phenomenon of learning based on an animal's early environmental experiences. A biologically predetermined response to a specific stimulus is induced thereby; a term used in ethology.

Improvisation. In psychodrama, the acting out of problems without prior preparation.

Impulse. Unexpected, instinctive urge motivated by conscious and unconscious feelings over which the person has little or no control. *See also* Drive, Instinct.

Impulsion. The blind following of internal drives without regard for social acceptance or pressure from the superego. Impulsion is normally seen in young children. In adults it is common in those with weak defensive organizations; in such cases it tends to be a symbolic phenomenon.

Inadequate personality. A personality disorder characterized by emotional and physical instability. The person is unable to deal with the normal vicissitudes of life.

Inappropriate affect. Emotional tone that is out of harmony with the idea, object, or thought accompanying it.

Incest. Sexual activity between members of a family. Common patterns are father-daughter, mother-son, and between siblings. Incest may also be homosexually oriented.

Incoherence. Communication that is disconnected, illogical, and incomprehensible.

Incompetence. A legal term suggesting thought processes that are inadequate for sound judgment and that lead to abnormal behavior.

Incorporation. An unconscious defense mechanism in which an object representation is assimilated into oneself through symbolic oral ingestion. One of the primitive defenses, incorporation is a special form of introjection and is the primary mechanism in identification.

Individual psychology. Holistic theory of personality developed by Alfred Adler. Personality development is explained in terms of adaptation to the social milieu (life style), strivings toward perfection motivated by feelings of inferiority, and the interpersonal nature of the person's problems. Individual psychology is applied in group psychotherapy and counseling by Adlerian practitioners.

Individual therapy. A type of psychotherapy in which a professionally trained psychotherapist treats one patient who either wants relief from disturbing symptoms or improvement in his ability to cope with his problems. This one therapist-one patient relationship, the traditional dyadic therapeutic technique, is opposed to other techniques that deal with more than one patient. *See also* Group psychotherapy, Psychotherapy.

Individuation. A Jungian term: differentiation, the process of molding and developing the individual personality so that it is different from the rest of the group. *See also* Actualization.

Indoklon therapy. A kind of shock treatment in which a convulsive seizure is induced by the drug Indoklon, which is inhaled.

Indoles. A group of biogenic amines, some of which affect the workings of the central nervous system.

Ineffability. An ecstatic state in which the person insists that his experience is inexpressible and indescribable, that it is impossible to convey what it is like to one who never experienced it.

Infancy. The childhood period of helplessness and marked dependency; generally the first year of life.

Infantile autism (Kanner's disease). A syndrome that develops before the age of 3 years. It is characterized by withdrawal, an obsessive need for sameness, and mutism.

Infantile dynamics. Psychodynamic integrations, such as the Oedipus complex, that are organized during childhood and continue to exert unconsciously experienced influences on adult personality.

Infantile sexuality. Freudian concept regarding the erotic life of infants and children. Freud observed that, from birth, infants are capable of erotic activities. Infantile sexuality encompasses the overlapping phases of psychosexual development during the first 5 years of life and includes the oral phase (birth to 18 months), when erotic activity centers on the mouth; the

anal phase (ages 1 to 3), when erotic activity centers on the rectum; and the phallic phase (ages 2 to 6), when erotic activity centers on the genital region. *See also* Psychosexual development.

Inferiority complex. Concept originated by Alfred Adler that everyone is born with inferiority or a feeling of inferiority secondary to real or fantasied organic or psychological inadequacies. How this inferiority or feeling of inferiority is handled determines a person's behavior in life. *See also* Masculine protest.

Infradian rhythm. Cyclical variations in emotional and physiologic functions that occur in cycles of less than 24 hours. *See also* Circadion rhythm, Ultradian rhythm.

Inhibition. The depression or arrest of a function; suppression or diminution of outgoing impulses from a reflex center. The sexual impulse, for example, may be inhibited because of psychological repression.

Inner-directed person. A person who is self-motivated and autonomous and is not easily guided or influenced by the opinions and values of other people. *See also* Other-directed person.

Insanity. A legal term, now generally obsolete, denoting certain kinds of mental illness or disturbance.

Insanity defense. A legal plea that a person may not be convicted of a crime because of his insanity, which is defined by various legal standards based on court definitions and rulings. The major premise is that the accused person lacks the intent to harm because of his mental state and, therefore, cannot be held criminally responsible. *See also* Competency to stand trial, Criminal responsibility, Durham decision, Irresistible impulse test, Mens rea, M'Naghten rule.

Insecurity. Feelings of helplessness and inadequacy in the face of anxieties about one's place, one's future, and one's goals.

Insight. Conscious awareness and understanding of one's own psychodynamics and symptoms of maladaptive behavior. It is highly important in effecting changes in the personality and behavior of a person. Most therapists distinguish two types: (1) intellectual insight: knowledge and awareness without any change of maladaptive behavior; (2) emotional or visceral insight: awareness, knowledge, and understanding of one's own maladaptive behavior, leading to positive changes in personality and behavior.

Insomnia. A pathological inability to sleep.

Instinct. A basic, inborn drive.

Instrumental conditioning (Operant conditioning). A process in which reinforcers follow the behavior of an animal or person to determine if the behavior is more or less likely to occur in the future. *See also* Conditioned reinforcer, Differential reinforcement, Operant conditioning, Reinforcement.

Insulin coma therapy. A form of psychiatric treatment originated by Manfred Sakel in which insulin is administered to the patient to produce coma. It is used in certain types of schizophrenia. *See also* Shock treatment.

Intake. The initial interview between a patient and a member of a psychiatric team. The term is usually used in connection with admission to a mental health facility.

Integration. The absorbing into the personality and the use of data and experience during the various phases of human development.

Intellectual insight. *See* Insight.

Intellectualization. An unconscious defense mechanism in which reasoning or logic is used in an attempt to avoid confrontation with an objectionable impulse or affect. It is also known as brooding and thinking compulsion.

Intelligence. Capacity for understanding, recalling, mobilizing, and integrating constructively what one has learned and for using it to meet new situations.

Intermission. In psychiatry, the interval between attacks of a particular syndrome. When it is not certain that the symptoms will return, the interval is called a remission. *See also* Remission.

Interpersonal conflict. *See* Extrapsychic conflict.

Interpersonal psychiatry. Dynamic-cultural system of psychoanalytic therapy based on Harry Stack Sullivan's interpersonal theory. Sullivan's formulations were couched in terms of a person's interactions with other people. In group psychotherapy conducted by practitioners of this school, the focus is on the patients' transactions with one another.

Interpersonal skill. Ability of a person in relationship with others to express his feelings appropriately, to be socially responsible, to change and influence, and to work and create. *See also* Socialization.

Interpretation. A psychotherapeutic technique used in psychoanalysis, both individual and group. The therapist conveys to the patient the significance and meaning of his behavior, constructing into a more meaningful form the patient's resistances, defenses, transferences, and symbols (dreams). *See also* Clarification.

Interpretation of Dreams, The. Title of a book by Freud. Published in 1899, this work was a major presentation not only of Freud's discoveries about the meaning of dreams—a subject hitherto regarded as outside scientific interest—but also of his concept of a mental apparatus that is topographically divided into unconscious, preconscious, and conscious areas.

Intrapsychic ataxia. *See* Ataxia.

Intrapsychic conflict. Conflict that arises from the clash of two opposing forces within oneself. It is also known as intrapersonal conflict. *See also* Extrapsychic conflict.

Introjection. An unconscious defense mechanism in which a psychic representation of a loved or hated object is taken into one's ego system. In depression, for example, the emotional feelings related to the loss of a loved one are directed toward the introjected mental representation of the loved one. *See also* Identification, Incorporation.

Intropunitive. Turning anger inward on oneself, commonly observed in depressed patients.

Introversion. A turning in to one's self, accompanied by lack of interest in the outside world. *See also* Extroversion.

Inversion. Synonym for homosexuality. Inversion was the term used by Freud and his predecessors. There are three types: absolute, amphigenous, and occasional. *See also* Homosexuality, Latent homosexuality, Overt homosexuality.

Involutional melancholia (involutional psychotic reaction). Depression occurring most commonly in late middle age or the menopausal period, characterized by isomnia, anxiety, and sometimes by paranoid ideas. There is usually no history of previous mental disorder.

I.Q. (intelligence quotient). A measure of intelligence, based on psychological tests, that is calculated as follows: I.Q. = mental age (MA)/chronological age (CA) × 100.

Irresistible impulse test. A legal test used to determine whether a person may be held responsible for a crime. If he acted under an impulse that he was unable to control because of his mental disease, he is not criminally responsible. This test is no longer valid in most states. *See also* Competency to stand trial, Criminal responsibility, Durham decision, Insanity defense, Mens rea, M'Naghten rule.

Isolation. To set apart an idea from the attached feeling tone.

Isophilic. Term used by Sullivan to mean liking or feeling affectionate toward people of the same sex, without the genital aspects of homosexuality.

Jamais vu. False feeling of unfamiliarity with a real situation that one has experienced. *See also* Paramnesia.

Janet, Pierre (1859–1947). The last great representative of the French school of psychiatry; known for his concept of psychological automatism and for his interest in cases of multiple personalities.

Jaundice, allergic. Yellowish staining of the skin and deeper tissues, accompanied by bile in the urine secondary to a hypersensitivity reaction. An obstructive type of jaundice, it is occasionally detected during the second to fourth week of phenothiazine therapy.

Jones, Ernest (1879–1958). Welsh psychoanalyst and one of Freud's early followers. He was an organizer of the American Psychoanalytic Association in 1911 and of the British Psychoanalytical Society in 1919 and a founder and long-time editor of the journal of the International Psychoanalytical Association. He was the author of many valuable works, the most important of which is his three-volume biography of Freud.

Judgment. Mental act of comparing or evaluating choices within the framework of a given set of values for the purpose of electing a course of action. Judgment is said to be intact if the course of action chosen is consistent with reality; judgment is said to be impaired if the chosen course of action is not consistent with reality.

Jung, Carl Gustav (1875–1961). Swiss psychiatrist and psychoanalyst. He founded the school of analytic psychology. *See also* Collective unconscious.

Kinesthetic hallucination. False perception of muscular movement. An amputee may feel movement in his missing limb; this phenomenon is also known as phantom limb.

Kinesthetic sense. Sensation in the muscles, as differentiated from the senses that receive stimulation from outside the body.

Kirkbride, Thomas S. (1809–1883). One of the 13 original founders of the American Psychiatric Association; noted for his 1854 manual advocating reform in the design of institutions for the mentally ill.

Klein, Melanie (1882–1960) British psychoanalyst and child analyst whose theories of early development were often at variance with those of the more orthodox Freudian school.

Kleptomania. Pathological compulsion to steal. In psychoanalytic theory, it originates in the infantile stage of psychosexual development.

Koro. An acute anxiety reaction characterized by the patient's fear that his penis is shrinking and may disappear into his abdomen, in which case he will die. This psychogenic disorder is found only among the people of the Malay archipelago and among the South Chinese.

Korsakoff's psychosis. A syndrome usually associated with alcoholism and characterized by confusion, disorientation, and amnesia with confabulation.

Kraepelin, Emil (1865–1926). The last representative of the predynamic school of psychiatry; noted for his classification systems and for his differentiation between dementia praecox (schizophrenia) and manic-depressive psychoses.

Kretschmer, Ernest (1888–1964). German psychiatrist noted for his theories of the relation of physique to character and personality.

La belle indifférence. Attitude of calm that contrasts sharply with the extent of the patient's disability.

Labile. Unstable; characterized by rapidly changing emotions.

Labyrinthine. A type of schizophrenic speech characterized by aimless wandering from subject to subject, with no apparent associative connections.

Lalophobia. Fear of speaking.

Lapsus calmi. A slip of the pen. *See also* Lapsus linguae.

Lapsus linguae. A slip of the tongue.

Latah. A disorder found principally among the Malaysian people and characterized by either a sudden onset of unusual and inappropriate motor and verbal manifestations or by an echo reaction, in which the victim is compelled to imitate any words or actions to which he is exposed. In both forms the affected person cannot control or inhibit his behavior.

Latency phase. Stage of psychosexual development extending from age 5 to the beginning of adolescence at age 12. Freud's work on ego psychology showed that the apparent cessation of sexual preoccupation during this period stems from a strong, aggressive blockade of libidinal and sexual impulses in an effort to avoid the dangers of the oedipal relationship. During the latency period, boys and girls are inclined to choose friends and join groups of their own sex. *See also* Identification with the aggressor, Psychosexual development.

Latent content. The hidden or unconscious meaning of symbolic representations, especially in fantasies and dreams.

Latent homosexuality. Unexpressed conscious or unconscious homoerotic wishes that are held in check. Freud's theory of bisexuality postulated the existence of a constitutionally determined, although experientially influenced, instinctual masculine-feminine duality. Normally, the opposite-sex component is dormant, but a breakdown in the defenses of repression and sublimation may activate latent instincts and result in overt homoeroticism. Many writers have questioned the validity of the theory of a universal latent homoeroticism. *See also* Bisexuality, Homosexuality, Overt homosexuality.

Leadership role. Stance adopted by the therapist in conducting a group. There are three main leadership roles: authoritarian, democratic, and laissez-faire. Any group—social, therapeutic, training, or task-oriented—is primarily influenced by the role practiced by the leader.

Learning disability. An impairment of the capacity for scholastic development up to the level appropriate to the child's intellectual endowment as a result of inefficiencies in information processing. The disability is caused by some disorder in cerebral function, rather than by emotional, social, or intellectually factors. Dyslexia, dysgraphia, and dyscalculia are learning disabilities.

Lesbianism. Female homosexuality. About 600 B. C. on the island of Lesbos in the Aegean Sea, the poetess Sappho encouraged young women to engage in mutual sex practices. Lesbianism is also known as Sapphism. *See also* Bisexuality, Homosexuality, Latent and Overt homosexuality.

Lewin, Kurt (1890–1946). German psychologist who emigrated to the United States in 1933. His work on the field theory has been useful in the experimental study of human behavior in a social situation.

Libido theory. Freudian theory of sexual instinct, its complex process of development, and its accompanying physical and mental manifestations. Before Freud's introduction and completion of the dual instinct theory (sexual and aggressive) in 1920, all instinctual manifestations were related to the sexual instinct, making for some confusion at that time. Current psychoanalytic practice assumes the existence of two instincts: sexual (libido) and aggressive (death). *See also* Aggressive drive, Sexual drive.

Life instinct. *See* Sexual drive.

Life lie. A contrary-to-fact conviction around which a person structures his life philosophy and attitudes.

Lifwynn Foundation. Organization established by Trigant Burrow in 1927 as a social community in which the participants examined their interactions in the daily activities in which they were engaged. Lifwynn is currently under the direction of Hans Syz, M.D., in Westport, Conn.

Lilliputian hallucination. False perception

that persons are reduced in size. *See also* Micropsia.

Lithium therapy. The treatment of manic or hypomanic states with lithium salts.

Lobotomy. Neurosurgical procedure in which one or more nerve tracts in a lobe of the cerebrum are severed. Prefrontal lobotomy is the ablation of one or more nerve tracts in the prefrontal area of the brain. It is used in the treatment of certain severe mental disorders that do not respond to other treatments. The procedure, introduced by Egas Moniz, is also called leukotomy.

Locus. Anatomical place of origin.

Logorrhea. Copious, pressured, coherent speech. It is observed in manic-depressive illness, manic type. Logorrhea is also known as tachylogia, verbomania, and volubility.

Logotherapy. Existential analysis based on spiritual values, rather than psychobiological laws.

LSD (lysergic acid diethylamide). A potent psychotogenic drug discovered in 1942. LSD produces psychotic-like symptoms and behavior changes, including hallucinations, delusion, and time-space distortions.

Lust dynamism. A term used by Sullivan to describe clearly stated sexual desires and abilities.

Lysergic acid diethylamide. *See* LSD.

Macropsia. False perception that objects are larger than they really are. *See also* Micropsia.

Magical thinking. A notion that thinking something is the same as doing it. It is common in dreams, in certain mental disorders, and in children.

Maintenance drug therapy. A stage in the course of chemotherapy. After the drug has reached its maximal efficacy, the dosage is reduced and sustained at the minimal therapeutic level that will prevent a relapse or exacerbation.

Major tranquilizer. Drug that has antipsychotic properites. The phenothiazines, thioxanthenes, butyrophenones, and reserpine derivatives are typical major tranquilizers, which are also known as ataractics, neuroleptics, and antipsychotics. *See also* Dystonia, Minor tranquilizer.

Maladaptive way. Poorly adjusted or pathological behavior patern.

Malingering. Feigning disease.

Mania. A state of excessive excitability, agitation, and hyperactivity, commonly seen in the manic phase of manic-depressive illness.

Manic-depressive illness. A major disorder in which there are severe changes of mood and usually a tendency to remission and recurrence. In the manic state, the patient is overrelated and hyperactive; in the depressed type, the patient suffers from a depressed mood, anxiety, and possible physical slowing down that can lead to stupor. In the circular form of the disorder, the affected person has at least one of each kind of episode.

Manifest content. That part of a dream or fantasy that a person remembers and reports. *See also* Latent content.

Mannerism. Stereotyped involuntary activity that is peculiar to a person.

Mantra. A syllable or word, usually meaningless, that is used by a person in transcendental meditation. Its function is to relax the person's mind by repetition until the person enters the alpha state. If disruptive thoughts invade the alpha state, the person begins repeating the mantra again. *See also* Alpha feedback, Alpha state.

MAO inhibitor. *See* Monoamine oxidase inhibitor.

Marathon. Group meeting that usually lasts from 8 to 72 hours, although some sessions last for a week. The session is interrupted only for eating and sleeping. The leader works for the development of intimacy and the open expression of feelings. The time-extended group experience culminates in intense feelings of excitement and elation. Group marathon was developed by George Bach and Frederick Stoller.

Marijuana. Dried leaves and flowers of *Cannabis sativa* (Indian hemp). It induces somatic and psychic changes in man when smoked or ingested in sufficient quantity. The somatic changes include increased heart rate, rise in blood pressure, dryness of the mouth, increased appetite, and occasional nausea, vomiting, and diarrhea. The psychic changes include dreamy state level of consciousness, disruptive chain of ideas, perceptual disturbances of time and space, and alterations of mood. In strong doses, marijuana can produce hallucinations and, at times, paranoid ideas and suspiciousness. It is also known as pot, grass, weed, tea, and Mary Jane.

Marital counseling. Process whereby a trained counselor helps married couples resolve problems that arise and trouble them in their relationship. The theory and techniques of this approach were first developed in social agencies as part of family casework. Husband and wife are seen by the same worker in separate and joint counseling sessions that focus on immediate family problems.

Marital therapy. *See* Marriage therapy.

Marriage therapy. A type of family therapy that involves the husband and the wife and focuses on the marital relationship, which affects the individual psychopathology of the partners. The rationale for this method is the assumption that psychopathological processes within the family structure and in the social matrix of the marriage perpetuate individual pathological personality structures, which find expression in the disturbed marriage and are aggravated by the feedback between partners.

Masculine identity. Well developed sense of gender affiliation with males.

Masculine protest. Adlerian doctrine that depicts a universal human tendency to move from a passive and feminine role to a masculine and active role. This doctrine is an extension of his ideas about organic inferiority. It became the prime motivational force in normal and neurotic behavior in the Adlerian system. *See also* Adler, Alfred; Inferiority complex.

Masculinity-femininity scale. Any scale on a psychological test that assesses the relative masculinity or femininity of the testee. Scales vary and may focus, for example, on basic identification with either sex or preference for a particular sex role.

Masochism. A sexual deviation in which sexual gratification is derived from being maltreated by the partner or oneself. It was first described by an Austrain novelist, Leopold von Sacher-Masoch (1836–1895). *See also* Sadism, Sadomasochistic relationship.

Masturbation. *See* Autoerotism.

Maximum security unit. That part of an institution for the mentally ill reserved for those who have committed crimes or who are considered dangerous to others.

McNaughton rule. *See* M'Naghten rule.

Mean. A statistical measurement derived from adding a set of scores and then dividing by the number of scores. *See also* Average.

Mean deviation. A statistical measure of variation determined by dividing the sum of deviations in a set of variables by the number of cases involved. *See also* Deviation.

Median. In a set of measurements, the middle value. For example, in the series 1, 3, 5, 7, 9, the number 5 is the median value. *See also* Average.

Medicare. A government program of supplementary medical and hospital insurance incorporated into the Social Security system by Congressional amendments in 1965. The beneficiaries are the aged, who, through Medicare, receive ordinary benefits in general hospitals but are limited to a lifetime benefit of 190 days in psychiatric hospitals.

Megalomania. Morbid preoccupation with expansive delusions of power and wealth.

Melancholia. Old term for depression that is rarely used at the present time. As used in the term "involutional melancholia," it refers to a morbid state of depression and not to a symptom.

Melancholia agitata. Agitated depression, usually used in connection with senile psychosis.

Memory. Ability to revive past sensory impressions, experiences, and learned ideas. Memory includes three basic mental processes: registration: the ability to perceive, recognize, and establish information in the central nervous system; retention: the ability to retain registered information; and recall: the ability to retrieve stored information at will. *See also* Amnesia, Hyperamnesia, Paramnesia.

Menarche. The onset of menstruation.

Mendacity. Pathological lying.

Mens rea. A legal term referring to the intent to

harm. In court, the term is used to pursue the question of the defendant's criminal responsibility. *See also* Competency to stand trial, Criminal responsibility, Durham decision, Insanity defense, Irresistible impulse test, M'Naghten rule.

Mental aberration. *See* aberration, mental.

Mental age. A measure of mental ability as determined by standard psychological tests. *See also* I.Q.

Mental health. A state of emotional well-being in which a person is able to function comfortably within his society and in which his personal achievements and characteristics are satisfactory to him.

Mental illness. Psychiatric disease included in the list of mental disorders in the *Diagnostic and Statistical Manual of Mental Disorders*, published by the American Psychiatric Association, and in the *Standard Nomenclature of Diseases*.

Mental ratardation. Subnormal general intellectual functioning that may be evident at birth or may develop during childhood. Learning, social adjustment, and maturation are impaired, and emotional disturbance is often present. The degree of retardation is commonly measured in terms of I.Q.: borderline (68–85), mild (52–67), moderate (36–51), severe (20–35), and profound (under 20). Obsolete terms that are still used occasionally are idiot (mental age of less than 3 years), imbecile (mental age of 3 to 7 years), and moron (mental age of 8 years).

Mental status. The results of a psychiatric examination in which a patient's general health, speech patterns, physical appearance, general mood, and other such characteristics are considered.

Mescaline. A hallucinogenic drug obtained from the peyote cactus.

Mesmerism. Hypnotism.

Metapsychology. A branch of psychology that constitutes the interface between suprasensory, esoteric, and suprarational manifestations of consciousness and psychology. These manifestations include parapsychology, transcendental meditation, biofeedback, mysticism, and psychic phenomena that may be relevant to the theory and practice of psychiatry.

Methadone. Methadone hydrochloride, a long acting synthetic narcotic developed in Germany as a substitute for morphine. It is used as an analgesic and in detoxification and maintenance treatment of opiate addicts.

Methadone maintenance treatment. Long term use of methadone on a daily basis to relieve narcotic craving and avert the effects of narcotic drugs.

Metonymy. A speech disturbance common in schizophrenia in which the affected person uses a word or term that is related to the proper one but is not quite right or appropriate.

Metrazol shock treatment. A rarely used form of treatment in which a convulsive seizure is induced by injection of the drug Metrazol.

Meyer, Adolf (1866–1950). American psychiatrist known for the concept of psychobiology. Instead of emphasizing symptoms, Meyer focused on the types of reaction manifested by the whole person in terms of his total life experience.

Microcephaly. A condition in which the head is unusually small as a result of defective brain development and premature ossification of the skull.

Micropsia. False perception that objects are smaller than they really are. *See also* Lilliputian hallucination, Macropsia.

Migraine. A severe one-sided headache, often accompanied by nausea and disturbed vision; it may be associated with emotional conflicts.

Milieu therapy. Treatment that emphasizes appropriate socioenvironmental manipulation for the benefit of the patient. The setting for milieu therapy is usually the psychiatric hospital.

Minimal brain dysfunction. A behavior pattern of childhood characterized by learning problems, hyperactivity, irritability, and short attention span. It is believed to be due to diencephalic dysfunction.

Minnesota Multiphasic Personality Inventory (MMPI). Questionnaire type of psychological test for ages 16 and over, with 550 true-false statements that are coded in 14 scales, ranging from a social to a schizophrenia scale. Group and individual forms are available.

Minor tranquilizer. Drug that diminishes tension, restlessness, and pathological anxiety without any antipsychotic effect. Meprobamate and diazepoxides are typical minor tranquilizers.

Minutes of the Vienna Psychoanalytic Society. Diary of Freud's Wednesday Evening Society (after 1910 the Vienna Psychoanalytic Society) as recorded by Otto Rank, the paid secretary between 1906 and 1915.

Mitchell, S. Weir (1830–1914). American neurologist known for his concept of rest treatment to cure "anemia of the brain."

Mixoscopia. A sexual perversion in which a person attains orgasm by watching his or her love object make love with another person.

MMPI. *See* Minnesota Multiphasic Personality Inventory.

M'Naghten rule. A legal rule, which still pertains in most states, that is based on rulings of the English House of Lords in 1843. The original rulings stated that any person accused of a crime would not be held responsible if he "was labouring under such defect of reason, from disease of the mind, as not to know the nature and quality of the act; he was doing, or if he did know it, that he did not know he was doing what was wrong." *See also* Competency to stand trial, Criminal responsibility, Durham decision, Insanity defense, Irresistible impulse test, Mens rea.

Mode. In a set of measurements, that value that appears most frequently. *See also* Average.

Mongolism. *See* Down's syndrome.

Monoamine oxidase inhibitor. Agent that inhibits the enzyme monoamine oxidase (MAO), which oxidizes such monoamines as norepinephrine and serotonin. Some MAO inhibitors are highly effective as antidepressants. *See also* Tricyclic drug.

Monomania. Morbid mental state characterized by preoccupation with one subject. It is also known as partial insanity.

Monozygotic twins. *See* Dizygotic twins.

Mood. Feeling tone that is experienced by a person internally. Mood does not include the external expression of the internal feeling tone. *See also* Affect.

Moral treatment. Humane treatment of the mentally ill. To counteract the remarkably inhumane treatment of the mentally ill in the eighteenth century, psychiatrists such as Philippe Pinel in France and Benjamin Rush in the United States advocated kindness, removal of restraints, attention to religion, and the performance of useful task in the treatment setting.

Moses and Monotheism. Title of a book by Freud published in 1939. In this book Freud undertook a historical but frankly speculative reconstruction of the personality of Moses and examined the concept of monotheism and the abiding effect of the patriarch on the character of the Jews. One of Freud's last works, it bears the imprint of his latter-day outlook and problems.

Mother Superior complex. Tendency of a therapist to play the role of the mother in his relations with his patients. The complex often leads to interference with the therapeutic process. *See also* God complex.

Mother surrogate. Mother substitute. In psychoanalysis, the patient projects his mother image onto another person and responds to that person unconsciously in an inappropriate and unrealistic manner, with the feelings and attitudes that he had toward his real mother.

Motivation. Force that pushes a person to act to satisfy a need. It implies an incentive or desire that influences the will and causes the person to act.

Mourning. *See* Grief.

Multiple ego states. Many psychological stages, relating to different periods of one's life or to different depths of experience. These states may be of varying degrees of organization and complexity, and they may or may not be capable of being called to awareness consecutively or simultaneously.

Multiple personality. The existence of two or more distinct and separate subpersonalities in one person. The original personality is referred to as the primary personality; the split-off personality is called the secondary personality; the third personality is called the tertiary personality; and so on.

Multiple therapy. *See* Co-therapy.

Munchausen syndrome. A term denoting

chronic abuse of hospitals. The syndrome, also known as hospital addiction and polysurgery, is characterized by repeated hospital admissions and treatment of illnesses that the patient knows do not exist.

Mutism. *See* Stupor.

Mydriasis. Dilation of the pupil. The condition sometimes occurs as an autonomic side effect of phenothiazine and antiparkinsonism drugs.

Mysophobia. Fear of germs and dirt.

Nalline test. The use of Nalline, a narcotic antagonist, to determine abstinence from opiates. An injection of Nalline precipitates withdrawal symptoms if opiates have been used recently. The most important use of Nalline, however, is as an antidote in the treatment of opiate overdose.

Narcissism. Self-love. It is linked to autoerotism but is devoid of genitality. The word is derived from Narcissus, a Greek mythology figure who fell in love with his own reflected image. In psychoanalytic theory, it is divided into primary and secondary types. Primary narcissism refers to the early infantile phase of object relationship development, when the child has not differentiated himself from the outside world. All sources of pleasure are unrealistically recognized as coming from within himself, giving him a false sense of omnipotence. Secondary narcissism results when the libido once attached to external love objects is redirected back to the self. *See also* Autistic thinking, Autoerotism.

Narcolepsy. Sudden irresistible desire to sleep while sedentary.

Narcosis. Drug-induced stupor.

Narcosynthesis. Psychoanalysis with the patient sedated.

Narcotic blockade. The use of certain drugs to inhibit the effects of narcotics, such as heroin, and thus to aid in the treatment of opiate addicts.

Narcotic hunger. A physiological craving for a drug. It appears in abstinent narcotic addicts.

National Training Laboratories. Organization started in 1947 at Bethel, Maine, to train professionals who work with groups. Interest in personal development eventually led to sensitivity training and encounter groups.

Natural group. Group that tends to evolve spontaneously in human civilization, such as a kinship, tribal, or religious group. In contrast are various contrived groups or aggregates of people who meet for a relatively brief time to achieve some goal.

Necromania. Pathological preoccupation with dead bodies. Also called necrophilia.

Negative reinforcer. *See* Conditioned reinforcer.

Negativism. Verbal or nonverbal opposition to outside suggestions and advice. It is also known as command negativism.

Neologism. New word or condensation of several words formed by the patient in an effort to express a highly complex idea. It is often seen in schizophrenia.

Neoplasm. A new growth; a tumor.

Network. The persons in the patient's environment with whom he is most intimately connected. It frequently includes the nuclear family, the extended family, the orbit of relatives and friends, and work and recreational contacts. S. H. Foulkes believes that this dynamically interacting network has a fundamental significance in the production of illness in the patient. *See also* Extended family therapy, Social network therapy.

Neurasthenia. A neurotic condition characterized by complaints of chronic weakness, easy fatigability, and sometimes exhaustion.

Neuroleptic. *See* Antipsychotic drug, Major tranquilizer.

Neurologist. A physician who specializes in diseases of the nervous system.

Neurology. The medical specialty that deals with organic diseases of the nervous system.

Neuropsychiatry. The medical specialty that combines psychiatry and neurology.

Neurosis. Mental disorder characterized by anxiety. The anxiety may be experienced and expressed directly, or, through an unconscious psychic process, it may be converted, displaced, or somatized. Although neuroses do not manifest depersonalization or overt distortion of reality, they can be severe enough to impair a person's functioning. The neuroses, also known as psychoneuroses, include the following types: anxiety, hysterical, phobic, obsessive-compulsive, depressive, neurasthenic, depersonalization, and hypochondriacal.

Niemann-Pick disease. A progressive metabolic disease resulting in death within 2 years of onset and characterized by mental deterioration, blindness, and skin discoloration.

Night hospital. A part time hospital facility in which patients function in the outside world during the day but return to the hospital at night.

Nihilism. The notion that the self or part of the self does not exist.

Nondirective approach. Technique in which the therapist follows the lead of the patient in the interview, rather than introducing his own theories and directing the course of the interview. This method is applied in both individual and group therapy.

Norepinephrine (noradrenaline). A catecholamine that functions as a neurohumoral mediator liberated by postganglionic adrenergic nerves. It is also present in the adrenal medulla and in many areas in the brain, with the highest concentration in the hypothalamus. A disturbance in the metabolism of norepinephrine is considered to be an important factor in the causation depression. *See also* Serotonin.

Nosology. The science of the classification of diseases.

Nuclear family. Immediate members of a family, including the parents and the children. *See also* Extended family therapy, Network, Social network therapy.

Null hypothesis. The assumption that any observable difference between two random samplings of a statistical population is the result of chance.

Nurse, psychiatric. Part of the mental health team, usually in an institutional setting. She works with patients in the hospital milieu; today the psychiatric nurse often carries out individual, family, and group psychotherapy.

Nymphomania. Morbid, insatiable need in women for sexual intercourse. *See also* Satyriasis.

Object relation. An emotional attachment between one person and another, as opposed to the feelings that one has for oneself.

Obsession. Persistent idea, thought, or impulse that cannot be eliminated from consciousness by logical effort. *See also* Compulsion.

Obsessive-compulsive personality. A personality disorder in which the person is excessively perfectionistic, overconscientious, and usually overinhibited.

Occupational therapy. A form of therapy in which the patient is encouraged to perform useful tasks, usually in a social setting with other patients and hospital personnel.

Oedipus complex. A distinct group of associated ideas, aims, instinctual drives, and fears that are generally observed in children when they are from 3 to 6 years of age. During this period, which coincides with the peak of the phallic phase of psychosexual development, the child's sexual interest is attached chiefly to the parent of the opposite sex and is accompanied by aggressive feelings and wishes about the parent of the same sex. One of Freud's most important concepts, the Oedipus complex, was discovered in 1897 as a result of his self-analysis. *See also* Totem and Taboo.

Ogre. In structural analysis, the child ego state in the father that supersedes the nurturing parent and becomes a pseudoparent.

Oligophrenia. Mental retardation.

Onanism. Coitus interruptus or masturbation.

Ontogenic. Having to do with a person's biological development.

Operant conditioning. B. F. Skinner's term for the procedure through which the activities of an animal or a person are shaped in desired ways by reinforcement. When the animal or the person spontaneously performs the desired action, the experimenter rewards him, thus encouraging him to repeat the action. *See also* Classical conditioning, Conditioned reinforcer, Conditioned stimulus, Conditioning therapy, Densensitization, Differential reinforcement, Discriminative stimulus, Eliciting stimulus,

Extinction, Reinforcement, Schedule of reinforcement, Unconditioned stimulus.

Oral dyskinesia, tardive. *See* Tardive oral dyskinesia.

Oral phase. The earliest stage in psychosexual development. It lasts through the first 18 months of life. During this period the oral zone is the center of the infant's needs, expression, and pleasurable erotic experiences. It has a strong influence on the organization and development of the child's psyche. *See also* Infantile sexuality, Anal, Genital, Latency, and Phallic phases.

Organic brain syndrome (OBS). A psychotic or nonpsychotic disorder caused by impaired brain tissue function.

Organic disease. An illness that is caused by actual structural or biochemical change in an organ or tissue.

Orgasm. Sexual climax.

Orientation. State of awareness of one's relationships and surroundings in terms of time, place, and person.

Orthomolecular psychiatry. A form of psychiatry that uses the megavitamin approach. This form of treatment assumes that emotional and, perhaps, other illnesses are due to biochemical abnormalities that cause an increased need in the patient for certain vitamins. The treatment's efficacy is thus far unproved.

Orthopsychiatry. A combined mental hygiene approach using psychiatry, psychology, and other sciences to promote healthy emotional development and growth.

Orthostatic hypotension. Reduction in blood pressure brought about by a shift from a recumbent to an upright position. It is observed as a side effect of several psychotropic drugs.

Other-directed person. A person who is readily influenced and guided by the attitudes and values of other people. *See also* Inner-directed person.

Overcompensation. The process by which a person exaggerates his power and dominance in an effort to make up for real or imagined inadequacies or feelings of inferiority.

Overdetermination. The ascribing of many meanings to the elements of a dream or neurotic symptom.

Overt homosexuality. Behaviorally expressed homoeroticism, as distinct from unconsciously held homosexual wishes or conscious wishes that are held in check. *See also* Homosexuality, Latent homosexuality.

Pain-pleasure principle. A psychoanalytic concept stating that, in man's psychic functioning, he tends to seek pleasure and avoid pain.

Panic. An acute, intense attack of anxiety, associated with personality disorganization. Some writers use the term exclusively for psychotic episodes of overwhelming anxiety. *See also* homosexual panic.

Panphobia. Fear of everything.

Pantomime. Gesticulation; psychodrama without the use of words.

Paralogia. *See* Evasion.

Paralysis agitans. *See* Parkinsonism.

Paralytic ileus. Intestinal obstruction of the nonmechanical type, secondary to paralysis of the bowel wall, that may lead to fecal retention. It is a rare anticholinergic side effect of phenothiazine therapy.

Paramnesia. Disturbance of memory in which reality and fantasy are confused. It is observed in dreams and in certain types of schizophrenia and organic brain syndromes. *See also* Confabulation, Déjà entendu, Déjà vu, Fausse reconnaissance, Jamais vu, Retrospective falsification.

Paranoia. A psychosis characterized by a complicated, highly elaborate delusional system, which is often developed logically from the distortion of a real event. Although the psychosis is usually long-term, it may not interfere with other aspects of the patient's psychic functioning.

Paranoid. A psychiatric syndrome marked by the presence of systematized delusions, with few other signs of disorganization.

Paranoid delusion. *See* Delusion.

Paraphrenia. A chronic schizophrenic condition that is characterized by the presence of well systematized delusions, which often remain unchanged in content for years.

Parapraxis. Slips of the tongue motivated by unconscious thoughts.

Parapsychology. A branch of psychology that concerns itself with extranormal events, including clairvoyance, precognition, and telepathy. *See also* Extrasensory perception.

Parasympathetic nervous system. The part of the autonomic nervous system that controls the life-sustaining organs of the body.

Parataxic distortion. Term used by Harry Stack Sullivan to describe certain perceptual distortions, particularly regarding interpersonal relationships, with which a person seeks to defend himself against anxiety.

Parental rejection. Denial of affection and attention to a child by one or both parents. The child develops great affect hunger and hostility, which are directed either outwardly in the form of tantrums, or inwardly toward himself in the form of allergies or other disorders.

Paresthesia. Strange feelings on the skin, including burning, tickling, and tingling.

Parkinsonism. Syndrome characterized by rhythmical muscular tremors known as pill rolling, accompanied by spasticity and rigidity of movement, propulsive gait, droopy posture, and mask-like facies. It is usually seen in later life as a result of arteriosclerotic changes in the basal ganglia.

Parkinsonism-like effect. Symptom that is a frequent side effect of antipsychotic drugs. Typical symptoms are motor retardation, muscular rigidity, alterations of posture, tremor, and autonomic nervous system disturbances. *See also* Phenothiazine derivative.

Partial hospitalization. A system of treating mental illness in which the patient is attached to a hospital on a part time basis. *See also* Day, Night, and Weekend hospital.

Partial insanity. *See* Monomania.

Passive-aggressive personality. A personality disorder in which the patient shows his aggressive feelings in passive ways, such as obstructionism, pouting, and stubbornness.

Passive therapist. Type of therapist who remains inactive but whose presence serves as a stimulus for the patient in the group or individual treatment setting. *See also* Active therapist, Nondirective approach.

Pavlov, Ivan Petrovich (1849–1936). Russian neurophysiologist famous for his work in conditioning. *See also* Conditioning.

Pavor nocturnus. Nightmare.

Pecking order. Hierarchy or sequence of authority in an organization or social group.

Pederasty. Anal intercourse between a man and a boy.

Pedophilia. A sexual deviation in which a child is used for sexual purposes.

Penis envy. A concept developed by Freud that maintains that the woman envies the man for his possession of a penis. It is sometimes used to refer to a woman's generalized envy of the man.

Perception. Mental process by which data—intellectual, sensory, and emotional—are organized meaningfully. Through perception a person makes sense out of the many stimuli that bombard him. It is one of the many ego functions. Therapy groups and T-groups aim to expand and alter perception in ways conducive to the development of the potential of each participant. *See also* Agnosia, Apperception, Clouding of consciousness, Ego, Hallucination, Hysterical anesthesia, Memory.

Perceptual expansion. Development of one's ability to recognize and interpret the meaning of sensory stimuli through associations with past experiences with similar stimuli. Perceptual expansion through the relaxation of defenses is one of the goals in both individual and group therapy.

Perseveration. Pathological repetition of the same response to different questions.

Persona. In Jungian psychology, the term for the outside personality that a person presents to the world, as opposed to his inner self or anima. *See also* Anima.

Personal growth laboratory. A sensitivity training laboratory in which the primary emphasis is on each participant's potentialities for creativity, empathy, and leadership. In such a laboratory, the facilitator encourages most modalities of experience and expression, such as art, sensory stimulation, and intellectual, emotional, written, oral, verbal, and nonverbal expression. *See also* National Training Laboratories.

Personality. Habitual configuration of behavior of a person, reflecting his physical and mental activities, attitudes, and interests and corresponding to the sum total of his adjustment to life.

Personality disorder. Mental disorder characterized by maladaptive patterns of adjustment to life. There is no subjective anxiety, as seen in neurosis, and no disturbance in the capacity to recognize reality, as seen in psychosis. The types of personality disorders include passive-aggressive, antisocial, schizoid, hysterical, paranoid, cyclothymic, explosive, obsessive-compulsive, asthenic, and inadequate.

Perversion. Deviation from the expected norm. In psychiatry, it commonly signifies sexual perversion. *See also* Sexual deviation.

Perverted logic. *See* Evasion.

Phallic overbearance. Domination of another person by aggressive means. It's generally associated with masculinity in its negative aspects.

Phallic phase. The third stage in psychosexual development. It occurs when the child is from 2 to 6 years of age. During this period, the child's interest, curiosity, and pleasurable experiences are centered on the penis in boys and the clitoris in girls. *See also* Infantile sexuality, Anal, Genital, Latency, and Oral phases.

Phantasy. *See* Fantasy.

Phantom limb. *See* Kinesthetic hallucination.

Phenomenology. The study of man's consciously reported experiences. It is associated with existential psychiatry.

Phenothiazine derivative. Compound derived from phenothiazine. It is particularly known for its antipsychotic property. As a class, the phenothiazine derivatives are among the most widely used drugs in medical practice, particularly in psychiatry. Chlorpromazine, triflupromazine, fluphenazine, perphenazine, and thioridazine are some examples of phenothiazine derivatives. *See also* Anticholinergic effect, Autonomic side effect, Electrocardiographic effect, Mydriasis, Paralytic ileus, Parkinsonism-like effect.

Phenotype. A person's outer attributes. *See also* Genotype.

Pheromones. Chemicals secreted by an individual and received by a second individual, usually of the same species, which releases in the latter a specific pattern of behavior or developmental process, also known as ectohormones.

Phobia. Pathological fear associated with some specific type of stimulus or situation. *See also* Acrophobia, Agoraphobia, Ailurophobia, Algophobia, Claustrophobia, Erytophobia, Mysophobia, Panphobia, Xenophobia, Zoophobia.

Phyloanalysis. A means of investigating disorders of human behavior, both individual and collective, resulting from impaired tensional processes that affect the organism's internal reaction as a whole. Trigant Burrow adopted the word to replace his earlier term, "group analysis," which he first used in 1927 to describe the social participation of many persons in their common analysis. Because group analysis was confused with group psychotherapy of the analytic type, Burrow changed his nomenclature to phyloanalysis.

Piaget, Jean (1896–   ). Swiss psychologist who has described the cognitive development in children, based on direct observation.

Pica. A hunger for substances generally not fit to eat, such as paint containing lead and clay.

Pick's disease. A presenile degenerative brain disease. *See also* Alzheimer's disease.

Pinel, Phillipe (1746–1826). French reformer in the field of mental illness; known for his work in abolishing restraints on hospitalized mental patients.

PKU (phenylketonuria). A congenital metabolic disease that, if untreated in infancy, leads to mental retardation.

Placebo. Inert substance prepared to resemble the active drug being tested in experimental research. It is sometimes used in clinical practice for a psychotherapeutic effect. The response to the placebo may represent the response due to the psychological effect of taking a pill and not to any pharmacological property.

Play therapy. Type of therapy used with children, usually of preschool and early latency ages. The patient reveals his problems on a fantasy level with dolls, clay, and other toys. The therapist intervenes opportunely with helpful explanations about the patient's responses and behavior in language geared to the child's comprehension. *See also* Activity group therapy.

Pleasure principle. In psychoanalytic theory, the notion that a person tries to gain pleasure and gratification and to avoid pain and discomfort.

Pleonexia. A psychiatric disorder in which the patient has excessive needs to acquire wealth or objects.

Pluralism. In psychiatry, the notion that multicausal factors affect behavior.

Polyphagia. Pathological overeating.

Polysurgery. *See* Munchausen syndrome.

Porphyria. A metabolic disease that is accompanied by abdominal pain and certain mental symptoms.

Positive reinforcer. *See* Conditioned reinforcer.

Postpartum psychosis. A psychotic reaction to the experience of childbirth.

Potency. A male's ability to perform the sexual act.

Pratt, Joseph H. Boston physician born in 1842 and generally considered to be the first pioneer in group psychotherapy in America. He is known for his work with tuberculous patients (1900–1906). He formed discussion groups to deal with the physical aspects of tuberculosis. Later, these groups began discussing the emotional problems that stemmed from the illness.

Preconscious. In psychoanalysis, one of the three divisions of the psyche, according to Freud's topographical psychology. The preconscious includes all ideas, thoughts, past experiences, and other memory impressions that can be consciously recalled with effort. *See also* Conscious, Unconscious.

Prefrontal lobotomy. *See* Lobotomy.

Pregenital. In psychoanalytic theory, the oral

and anal periods, before the genitals become a dominating force in sexual development.

Prejudice. Adverse judgment or opinion formed without factual knowledge. Elements of irrational suspicion or hatred are often involved, as in racial prejudice.

Preoccupation of thought. *See* Trend of thought.

Primal father. Hypothetical head of the tribe. He is depicted by Freud in *Totem and Taboo* as slain by his sons, who subsequently devour him in a cannibalistic rite. Later, he is promoted to a god. The son who murders him is the prototype of the tragic hero, and the memory of the crime is perpetuated in the conscience of the person and of the culture.

Primal scene. In psychoanalysis, the real or fantasied observation by a child of sexual intercourse, particularly between his parents.

Primal therapy. A system of psychotherapy developed by Arthur Janov, in which the patient undergoes a short period (2 to 3 weeks) of intensive individual therapy, preceded by a 24-hour period of isolation and followed by a few months of group therapy with other postprimal patients. During the therapy the patient is encouraged to experience a series of what Janov calls primals, in which the patient relives the prototypical traumatic events that originally crystallized his suffering and thereby created his neurosis.

Primary gain. The reduction of tension or conflict through neurotic illness.

Primary process. In psychoanalysis, the mental process directly related to the functions of the id and characteristic of unconscious mental activity. The primary process is marked by unorganized, illogical thinking and by the tendency to seek immediate discharge and gratification of instinctual demands. *See also* Secondary process.

Prince, Morton (1854–1929). American psychiatrist known for his study of multiple personalities.

Prison psychosis. Psychotic reaction to incarceration or to the prospect of incarceration.

Projection. Unconscious defense mechanism in which a person attributes to another the ideas, thoughts, feelings, and impulses that are part of his inner perceptions but that are unacceptable to him. Projection protects the person from anxiety arising from an inner conflict. By externalizing whatever is unacceptable, the person deals with it as a situation apart from himself. *See also* Blind spot.

Projective test. Loosely structured psychological test that requires the subject to reveal his own feelings, personality, or psychopathology. Examples include the Rorschach and Thematic Apperception Test.

Prototaxic. A term introduced by Harry Stack Sullivan to refer to primitive illogical thought processes. *See* Primary process.

Pseudoaggression. A neurotic defense in which the patient denies his basic masochistic feelings and displays them, instead, as false aggression.

Pseudoauthenticity. False or copied expression of thoughts and feelings.

Pseudocollusion. Sense of closeness, relationship, or cooperation that is not real but is based on transference.

Psyche. Greek work for the mind.

Psychiatrist. A medical doctor whose speciality is the study and treatment of mental disorders. After receiving the M.D. degree the psychiatrist spends 1 year as an intern and 3 years as a resident in a hospital setting. When he passes the written and oral examinations of the *American Board of Psychiatry and Neurology* He becomes a *Diplomate in Psychiatry* and is said to be "board-certified."

Psychiatry, cultural. *See* Cultural psychiatry.

Psychiatry, descriptive. *See* Descriptive psychiatry.

Psychiatry, dynamic. *See* Dynamic psychiatry.

Psychiatry, orthomolecular. *See* Orthomolecular psychiatry.

Psychic determinism. Freudian adaptation of the concept of causality. It states that all phenomena and events have antecedent causes that operate on an unconscious level, beyond the control of the person involved.

Psychoactive drug. Drug that alters thoughts, feelings, or perceptions. Such a drug may help a person in either individual or group therapy overcome depression, anxiety, or rigidity of thought and behavior while he learns new methods of perceiving and responding.

Psychoanalysis. Freud's method of psychic investigation and form of psychotherapy. As a technique for exploring the mental processes, psychoanalysis includes the use of free association and the analysis and interpretation of dreams, resistances, and transferences. As a form of psychotherapy, it uses the investigative technique, guided by Freud's libido and instinct theories and by ego psychology, to gain insight into a person's unconscious motivations, conflicts, and symbols and thus to effect a change in his maladaptive behavior. Several schools of thought are loosely referred to as psychoanalytic at present. Psychoanalysis is also known as analysis in depth and its practioners are known as psychoanalysts.

Psychoanalytic group psychotherapy. A major method of group psychotherapy, pioneered by Alexander Wolf and based on the operational principles of individual psychoanalytic therapy. Analysis and interpretation of a patient's transferences, resistances, and defenses are modified to take place in a group setting. Although strictly designating treatment structured to produce significant character change, the term encompasses the same approach on groups conducted at more superficial levels for lesser goals.

Psychobiology. Term introduced by Adolf Meyer and referring to the study of the human being as an integrated unit, incorporating both psychological and biological functions.

Psychodrama. Psychotherapy method originated by J. L. Moreno in which personality makeup, interpersonal relationships, conflicts, and emotional problems are explored by means of dramatic methods. The therapeutic dramatization of emotional problems includes: (1) protagonist or patient, the person who presents and acts out his emotional problems with the help of (2) auxiliary egos, persons trained to act and dramatize the different aspects of the patient that are called for in a particular scene in order to help him express his feelings, and (3) director, leader, or therapist, the person who guides those involved in the drama for a fruitful and therapeutic session.

Psychodynamics. Science of the mind, its mental processes, and affective components that influence human behavior and motivations. *See also* Group dynamics, Infantile dynamics.

Psycholinguistics. The study of factors that affect communication and general understanding of verbal information.

Psychological defense system. *See* Defense mechanism.

Psychological procedure. Any technique intended to alter a person's attitude toward any perception of himself and others. *See also* Group psychotherapy, Psychoanalysis, Psychotherapy.

Psychologist. A person, usually with an advanced degree (M.A., Ph.D.), who specializes in the study of mental processes and the treatment of mental disorders.

Psychometry. The science of measuring mental and psychological functioning and capacity.

Psychomotor. The combined effect of physical and emotional activity, which may be retarded —that is, slowed down—or excited—that is, accelerated.

Psychomotor stimulant. Drug that arouses the patient through its central excitatory and analeptic properties. Amphetamine and methylphenidate are drugs in this class.

Psychopathic personality. *See* Antisocial personality.

Psychopathology. Branch of science that deals with morbidity of the mind.

Psychopharmacology. The study of how certain drugs affect mental and behavioral processes.

Psychophysiological disorder. Mental disorder characterized by physical symptoms of psychic origin. It usually involves a single organ system innervated by the autonomic nervous system. The physiological and organic changes stem from a sustained emotional disturbance. It was previously known as psychosomatic disorder.

Psychosexual development. Maturation and development of the psychic phase of sexuality from birth to adult life. Its phases are oral, anal, phallic, latency, and genital. *See also* Identification with the aggressor, Infantile sexuality.

Psychosis. Mental disorder in which a person's mental capacity, affective response, and capacity to recognize reality, to communicate, and to relate to others are impaired enough to interfere with his capacity to deal with the ordinary demands of life. The psychoses are subdivided into two major classifications according to their origin: psychoses associated with organic brain syndromes and functional psychoses.

Psychosomatic illness. *See* Psychophysiological disorder.

Psychosurgery. Treatment of emotional disorders by surgical procedures on the brain. *See also* Lobotomy, Topectomy.

Psychotherapy. Form of treatment for mental illness and behavioral disturbances in which a trained person establishes a professional contract with the patient and through definite therapeutic communication, both verbal and nonverbal, attempts to alleviate the emotional disturbance, reverse or change maladaptive patterns of behavior, and encourage personality growth and development. Psychotherapy is distinguished from such other forms of psychiatric treatment as the use of drugs, surgery, electric shock treatment, and insulin coma treatment.

Psychotic depressive reaction. A depressed state after a particular experience.

Psychotomimetic drug. Drug that produces psychic and behavioral changes that resemble psychosis. Unlike other drugs that can produce organic psychosis as a reaction, a psychotomimetic drug does not produce overt memory impairment. It is also known as a hallucinogenic drug. Lysergic acid diethylamide (LSD), tetrahydrocannabinol, and mescaline are examples of psychotomimetic drugs.

Psychotropic drug. Drug that affects psychic function and behavior. Also known as a phrenotropic drug, it may be classified as an antipsychotic drug, antidepressant drug, antimanic drug, antianxiety drug, or hallucinogenic drug. *See also* Agranulocytosis, Orthostatic hypotension.

Pyromania. A compulsion to set fires.

Quadrangular therapy. A type of marital therapy that involves four people: the Married pair and each spouse's therapist.

Random. A statistical term that means occurring by chance or without attention to selection or planning.

Range. In a statistical study, a measure of variation determined by the end point values. For example, in a group of people aged 32, 34, 41, 53, 62, the range would be 30 (62 – 32).

Rank, Otto (1884–1939). Austrian psychoanalyst. He was one of Freud's earliest followers and the longtime secretary and recorder of the minutes of the Vienna Psychoanalytic Society. He wrote such fundamental works as *The Myth of the Birth of the Hero.* He split with Freud on the significance of the birth trauma, which he used as a basis of brief psychotherapy.

Rapport. Conscious, harmonious accord that usually reflects a good relationship between two persons. In a group, rapport is the presence of mutual responsiveness, as evidenced by spontaneous and sympathetic reaction to each other's needs, sentiments, and attitudes. *See also* Countertransference, Transference.

Rapture-of-the-deep syndrome. A psychosis induced by sensory deprivation that occurs in scuba and deep-sea divers. It is often associated with excessive blood levels of nitrogen, known as nitrogen narcosis.

Rationalization. An unconscious defense mechanism in which an irrational behavior, motive, or feeling is made to appear reasonable. Ernest Jones introduced the term.

Ray, Issac (1807–1881). One of the original 13 founders of the American Psychiatric Association; famous for his *Treatise on Medical Jurisprudence of Insanity* (1837).

Reaction formation. An unconscious defense mechanism in which a person develops a socialized attitude or interest that is the direct antithesis of some infantile wish or impulse in the unconscious. One of the earliest and most unstable defense mechanisms, it is closely related to repression; both are defenses against impulses or urges that are unacceptable to the ego.

Reality. The totality of objective things and factual events. Reality includes everything that is perceived by a person's special senses and is validated by other people.

Reality principle. In psychoanalytic theory, the principle that represents the demands of the outside world and that modifies the demands of the pleasure principle. *See also* Pleasure principle.

Reality testing. Fundamental ego function that consists of the objective evaluation and judgment of the world outside the self. By interacting with his animate and inanimate environment, a person tests its real nature, as well as his own relation to it. How the person evaluates reality and his attitudes toward it are determined by early experiences with the significant persons in his life. *See also* Ego.

Recall. Process of remembering thoughts, words, and actions of a past event in an attempt to recapture what actually happened. It is part of the complex mental function known as memory. *See also* Amnesia, Hypermnesia.

Reciprocal inhibition and desensitization. A kind of behavior therapy in which a person is conditioned to associated comfortable, supportive surroundings with anxiety-producing stimuli and thus to modify the adverse affects of these stimuli.

Recognition. *See* Memory.

Reconstructive Psychotherapy. A form of therapy that seeks not only to alleviate symptoms but to produce alterations in maladaptive character structures and to expedite new adaptive potentials. This aim is achieved by bringing into consciousness an awareness of the insight into conflicts, fears, inhibitions, and their derivatives. *See also* Psychoanalysis.

Re-enactment. In psychodrama, the acting out of a past experience as if it were happening in the present, so that a person can feel, perceive, and act as he did the first time.

Registration. *See* Memory.

Regression Unconscious defense mechanism in which a person undergoes a partial or total return to earlier patterns of adaptation. Regression is observed in many psychaitric conditions, particularly schizophrenia.

Regressive-reconstructive approach. A psychotherapeutic procedure in which regression is made an integral element of the treatment process. The original traumatic situation is reproduced to gain new insight and to effect significant personality change and emotional maturation. *See also* Psychoanalysis, Reconstructive psychotherapy.

Reik, Theodore (1888–1969). Psychoanalyst and early follower of Freud, who considered him one of his most brilliant pupils. Freud's book *The Question of Lay Analysis* was written to defend Reik's ability to practice psychoanalysis without medical training. Reik made many valuable contributions to psychoanalysis on the subjects of religion, masochism, and technique. *See also* Third ear.

Reinforcement. In behavior therapy, a method of strengthening a response by using an unconditioned stimulus along with a conditioned stimulus. *See also* Conditioned reinforcer, Conditioning therapy, Differential reinforcement, Extinction, Operant conditioning, Schedule of reinforcement.

Reinforcer, conditioned. *See* Conditioned reinforcer.

Relatedness. Sense of sympathy and empathy with regard to others, sense of oneness with others. It is the opposite of isolation and alienation.

Reliability. The degree to which a test produces the same results on repeated administrations.

REM sleep. The so-called deep sleep period during which the sleeper exhibits rapid eye movements (REMs); believed to account for one fifth to one fourth of total sleep time.

Remission. Partial or complete disappearance of the symptoms of a disorder. *See also* Intermission.

Remotivation. A group treatment technique used with withdrawn patients in mental hospitals.

Repetition compulsion. The irresistible urge to re-enact or redramatize an early emotional experience, regardless of the ability of this act to bring about pleasure. The effect is often a painful one.

Repetitive pattern. Continual attitude or mode of behavior characteristic of a person and performed mechanically or unconsciously.

Repression. An unconscious defense mechanism in which a person removes from consciousness those ideas, impulses, and affects that are unacceptable to him. A term introduced by Freud, it is important in both normal psychological development and in neurotic and psychotic symptom formation. Freud recognized two kinds of repression: (1) repression proper —the repressed material was once in the conscious domain; (2) primal repression—the repressed material was never in the conscious realm. *See also* Suppression.

Repressive-inspirational group psychotherapy. A type of group therapy in which discussion is intended to bolster patients' morale and help them avoid undesired feelings. It is used primarily with large groups of seriously regressed patients in institutional settings.

Reserpine. An alkaloid extracted from the root of the *Rauwolfia serpentina* plant. It is used primarily as an antihypertensive agent. It was formerly used as an antipsychotic agent because of its sedative effect.

Residential treatment facility. A center where the patient lives and receives treatment appropriate for his particular needs. A children's residential treatment facility ideally furnishes both educational and therapeutic experiences for the emotionally disturbed child.

Resistance. A conscious or unconscious opposition to the uncovering of the unconscious. Resistance is linked to underlying psychological defense mechanisms against impulses from the id that are threatening to the ego.

Response conditioning. *See* Classical conditioning.

Responsibility, criminal. *See* Criminal responsibility.

Retardation. Slowness of development or progress. In psychiatry, there are two types, mental retardation and psychomotor retardation. Mental retardation refers to slowness or arrest of intellectual maturation. Psychomotor retardation refers to slowness or slackened psychic activity or motor activity or both; it is observed in pathological depression.

Retention. *See* Memory.

Retroflexion. A psychoanalytic term used notably by Rado to describe the turning of rage onto oneself.

Retrograde amnesia. Loss of memory extending back to events and facts that predate the onset of the memory loss.

Retrospective falsification. Recollection of false memory. *See also* Paramnesia.

Reversal. In psychoanalysis, an instinct's change from passive to active or from active to passive, as when a destructive instinct changes from masochism to sadism or vice versa.

Rhythm, circadian. *See* Circadian rhythm.

Rhythm, infradian. *See* Infradian rhythm.

Rhythm, ultradian. *See* Ultradian rhythm.

Right to treatment. The concept that a person who is involuntarily committed to a mental institution has the right to treatment that may realistically be expected to provide a cure or an improvement in his or her mental condition.

Rigidity. A term used in psychiatry to mean a person's resistance to change.

Ritual. Automatic activity of psychogenic or cultural origin.

RNA. Ribonucleic acid, which is manufactured by DNA and is important in memory function. *See also* DNA.

Role. Pattern of behavior that a person takes. It has its roots in childhood and is influenced by significant people with whom the person had primary relationships. When the behavior pattern conforms with the expectations and demands of other people, it is said to be a complementary role. If it does not conform with the demands and expectation of others, it is known as a noncomplementary role. *See also* Identification, Injunction, Therapeutic role.

Role, gender. *See* Gender role.

Role playing. Psychodrama technique in which a person is trained to function more effectively in his reality roles, such as employer, employee, student, and instructor. In the therapeutic setting of psychodrama, the protagonist is free to try and to fail in his role, for he is given the opportunity to try again until he finally learns new approaches to the situation he fears, approaches that he can then apply outside.

Rorschach test. A projective test in which the subject reveals his attitude and emotions by responding to a set of inkblot picutres.

Rush, Benjamin (1745–1813). The father of American psychiatry whose text, *Medical Inquiries and Observations Upon the Diseases of the Mind* (1812), was the only American textbook on psychiatry until the end of the 19th century.

Sadism. A sexual deviation in which sexual gratification is achieved by inflicting pain and humiliation on the partner. Donatien Alphonse François de Sade (1740–1814), a French writer, was the first person to describe this condition. *See also* Masochism, Sadomasochistic relationship.

Sadomasochistic relationship. Relationship in which the enjoyment of suffering by one person and the enjoyment of inflicting pain by the other person are important and complementary attractions in their ongoing relationship. *See also* Masochism, Sadism.

Sanatorium. An institution where patients are treated for chronic physical or mental diseases or where they are attended to during a period of recuperation.

Satyriasis. Morbid, insatiable sexual needs or desires in men. It may be caused by organic or psychiatric factors. *See also* Nymphomania.

Schedule of reinforcement. The pattern by which a reinforcer follows a particular operant response. The reinforcer does not have to follow the particular response each time. Usually the reinforcement is done intermittently by and has no adverse affect on the maintenance of the response. *See also* Conditioned reinforcer, Differential reinforcement, Operant conditioning, Reinforcement.

Schilder, Paul (1886–1940). American neuropsychiatrist. He started the use of group psychotherapy at New York's Bellevue Hospital, combining social and psychoanalytic principles.

Schizocaria. An acute form of schizophrenia, sometimes called "catastrophic schizophrenia," in which the patient's personality deteriorates rapidly.

Schizoid personality. A personality disorder in which the person is shy, oversensitive, and sometimes eccentric. People with schizoid personalities are usually detached and seemingly unemotional in the face of upsetting events and experiences.

Schizophrenia. Mental disorder of a psychotic

level, characterized by disturbances in thinking, mood, and behavior. The thinking disturbance is manifested by a distortion of reality, especially by delusions and hallucinations, accompanied by a fragmentation of associations that results in incoherent speech. The mood disturbance is manifested by inappropriate affective responses. The behavior disturbance is manifested by ambivalence, apathetic withdrawal, and bizarre activity. Formerly known as dementia praecox, schizophrenia as a term was introduced by Eugen Bleuler. The causes of schizophrenia remain unknown. The types of schizophrenia include simple, hebephrenic catatonic, paranoid, schizoaffective, childhood, residual, latent, and chronic undifferentiated types and acute schizophrenic episode.

School phobia. A term that describes a young child's sudden fear of and refusal to attend school; usually considered a manifestation of separation anxiety.

Schreber case. One of Freud's cases. It involves the analysis in 1911 of Daniel Paul Schreber's autobiographical account, *Memoirs of a Neurotic*, Published in 1903. Analysis of these memoirs permitted Freud to decipher the fundamental meaning of paranoid processes and ideas, especially the relationship between repressed homosexuality and projective defenses.

Scotoma. In psychiatry, a person's blind spot in his psychological awareness.

Screen memory. A memory that serves as a cover-up for an associated painful memory.

Screening. Initial patient evaluation that includes medical and psychiatric history, mental status evaluation, and diagnostic formulation to determine the patient's suitability for a particular treatment modality.

Secondary gain. The obvious advantage that a person gains from his illness, such as gifts, attention, and release from responsibility. *See also* Primary process.

Secondary process. In psychoanalysis, the mental process directly related to the functions of the ego and characteristic of conscious and preconscious mental activities. The secondary process is marked by logical thinking and by the tendency to delay gratification by regulation of discharge of instinctual demands. *See also* Primary process.

Sedative. Drug that produces a calming or relaxing effect through central nervous system depression. Some drugs with sedative properties are barbiturates, chloral hydrate, paraldehyde, and bromide.

Selective inattention. An aspect of attentiveness in which a person blocks out those areas that generate anxiety.

Self-analysis. Investigation of one's own psychic components. It plays a part in all analysis, although to a limited extent, since few people are capable of sustaining independent and detached attitudes to the degree necessary for this approach to be therapeutic.

Self-awareness. Sense of knowing what one is experiencing; for example, realizing that one has just responded with anger to another group member as a substitute for the anxiety left when he attacked a vital part of one's self-concept. Self-awareness is a major goal of all therapy, individual and group.

Self-discovery. In psychoanalysis, the freeing of the repressed ego in a person who has been brought up to submit to the wishes of the significant others around him.

Self-realization. Psychodrama technique in which the protagonist enacts, with the aid of a few auxiliary egos, the plan of his life, no matter how remote it may be from his present situation. For instance, an accountant who has been taking singing lessons, hoping to try out for a musical comedy part in summer stock and planning to make the theater his life's work, can explore the effects of success in this venture and of possible failure and return to his old livelihood.

Senile dementia. An organic brain syndrome associated with aging and marked by some degree of mental deterioration, accompanied by childish behavior, self-centerdness, and difficulty in dealing with new experiences.

Sensation. Feeling of impression when the sensory nerve endings of any of the six senses —taste, touch, smell, sight, kinesthesia, and wound—are stimulated.

Sensitivity training group. Group in which members seek to develop self-awareness and an understanding of group processes, rather than to gain relief from an emotional disturbance.

See also Encounter group, Personal growth laboratory, T-group.

Sensorium. Theoretical sensory center located in the brain that is involved with a person's awareness about his surroundings. In psychiatry, it is often referred to as consciousness.

Sensory deprivation. Lack of external stimuli and opportunity for the usual perceptions. Loss of such senses as hearing and vision, may occur either experimentally or accidentally and may lead to panic, delusions, and other such reactions.

Separation anxiety. An infant or child's fear and apprehension upon being removed from the parent or parent figure.

Serotonin. A monoamine that is believed to be a neurohumoral transmitter. It is found in the serum and, in high concentrations, in the hypothalamus of the brain. Recent pharmacological investigations link depression to disorders in the metabolism of serotonin and other biogenic amines, such as norepinephrine.

Sexual deviation. Mental disorder characterized by sexual interests and behavior other than what is culturally accepted. Sexual deviation includes sexual interest in objects other than a person such as bestiality; bizarre sexual practices, such as necrophilia; and other sexual activities that are not accompanied by copulation. *See also* Bestiality, Exhibitionism, Homosexuality, Masochism, Sadism.

Sexual drive. On of the two primal instincts (the other is the aggressive drive), according to Freud's dual instinct theory of 1920. It is also known as eros and life instinct. Its main goal is to preserve and maintain life. It operates under the influence of the pleasure-unpleasure principle. *See also* Aggressive drive, Libido theory.

Shock treatment. A form of psychiatric treatment with a chemical substance (ingested, inhaled, or injected) or sufficient electric current to produce a convulsive seizure and unconsciousness. It is used in certain types of schizophrenia and mood disorders. Shock treatment's mechanism of action is still unknown. It was introduced by Cerletti and Bini.

Sibling rivalry. Competition among children for the attention, affection, and esteem of their parents. The children's jealousy is accompanied by hatred and death wishes toward each other.

The rivalry need not be limited to actual siblings; it is a factor in both normal and abnormal competitiveness throughout life.

Skinner, B. F. (1904–). American behavioral psychologist and author, noted for his theories of operant conditioning. *See also* Operant conditioning.

Slavson, S. R. (1890–). American theoretician who pioneered in group psychotherapy based on psychoanalytic principles. In his work with children, from which he derived most of his concept, he introduced and developed activity group therapy. *See also* Collective experience.

Sleep. A temporary physiologic state of unconsciousness, characterized by a reversible cessation of the person's waking sensorimotor activity. A biological need, sleep recurs periodically to rest the whole body and to regenerate neuromuscular tissue. *See also* Dream.

Social adaptation. Adjustment to the whole complex of interpersonal relationships; the ability to live and express oneself in accordance with society's restrictions and cultural demands. *See also* Adaptational approach.

Social control. Influence exerted by a society or its subgroups to induce to conform to the established expectations and requirements of that society.

Social instinct. *See* Herd instinct.

Social network therapy. A type of therapy in which the therapist assembles all the persons—relatives, friends, social relations, work relations—who have emotional or functional significance in the patient's life. Some or all of the social network may be assembled at any given time. *See also* Extended family therapy.

Social psychiatry. Branch of psychiatry interested in ecological, sociological, and cultural variables that engender, intensify, or complicate maladaptive patterns of behavior and their treatment.

Social therapy. A rehabilitation form of therapy with psychiatric patients. The aim is to improve social functioning. Occupational therapy, therapeutic community, recreational therapy, milieu therapy, and attitude therapy are forms of social therapy.

Social worker, psychiatric. A skilled professional, trained in social work, who works with psychiatrists, usually in an institutional setting. The social worker evaluates family, environmental, and social factors in the patient's illness; may work in intake and reception with new patients; and may follow up and counsel after discharge. All these activities are incorporated in the technique of case work. Psychiatric social workers also carry out individual, family, and group psychotherapy and participate in community organization.

Socialization. Process of learning interpersonal and interactional skills according to and in conformity with one's society. In a group therapy setting, it includes a member's way of participating both mentally and physically in the group. *See also* Interpersonal skill.

Sociogram. Diagrammatic portrayal of choices, rejections. and indifferences of a number of persons involved in a life situation.

Sociology. The scientific study of group life and social organization.

Sociometric distance. The measurable degree of perception that one person has for another. It can be hypothesized that the greater the sociometric distance between persons, the more inaccurate is their social evaluation of their relationship.

Sociometrist. Social investigator engaged in measuring the interpersonal relations and social structures in a community.

Sodomy. Anal intercourse.

Somatic conversion. The manifestation of a deep-seated neurotic disorder by a bodily dysfunction or disorder.

Somnambulism. Sleepwalking; motor activity during sleep. It is commonly seen in children. In adults it is observed in persons with schizoid personality disorders and certain types of schizophrenia.

Speech disturbance. A term that encompasses any of a variety of verbal or nonverbal communication disorders not due to impaired function of speech muscles or organs of articulation. *See also* Aphasia, Alexia, Agraphia, Amimia, Apraxia.

Standard deviation. A statistical measure of variation derived by squaring each deviation in a set of scores, taking the average of these squares, and taking the square root of the result. The standard deviation, represented by σ, the Greek letter sigma, is one of the most useful measures of variation, since it is helpful in other statistical computations.

Standard error. In statistics, a measure of how much variation in test results is due to chance and error and how much is due to experimental influences. The standard error of the mean is arrived at by dividing the standard deviation by the square root of the numbers of measures or, when the number of measures is less than 30, by the square root minus 1.

Stanford-Binet intelligence scale. A primarily verbal test administered individually to children and adults. *See also* I.Q., Mental age.

Startle reaction. A reflex response to a sudden intense stimulus, consisting of a diffuse motor response involving flexion movements of the trunk and extremities (hence, in German, *Zusammenschreken* reflex) and associated with a sudden increase in the level of consciousness. It occurs in normal persons and in acute anxiety neuroses.

Statistical significance. A measure of the reliability of a statistical measure.

Statistics, psychiatric. *See* Analysis of variance, Average, Central tendency, Chi square, Coefficient of correlation, Control group, Critical ratio, Deviation, Experimental group, Frequency distribution, Mean, Mean deviation, Median, Mode, Range, Standard deviation, Standard error, Statistical significance, T ratio, Variance, Variation.

Status value. Worth of a person in terms of such criteria as income, social prestige, intelligence, and education. It is considered an important parameter of one's position in the society.

Stekel, Wilhelm (1868–1940). Viennese psychoanalyst. He suggested the formation of the first Freudian group, the Wednesday Evening Society, which later became the Vienna Psychoanalytic Society. A man given to intuition, rather than to systematic research, his insight into dreams proved stimulating and added to the knowledge of symbols. Nevertheless, his superficial wild analysis proved incompatible with the Freudian school. He introduced the word "thanatos" to signify death wish.

Stereotypy. Continuous repetition of speech or physical activities. It is observed in cases of catatonic schizophrenia.

Stimulant. Drug that affects one or more organ systems to produce an exciting or arousing effect, increase physical activity and vivacity, and promote a sense of well-being. There are, for example, central nervous system stimulants, cardiac stimulants, respiratory stimulants, and psychomotor stimulants.

Stimulus, conditioned. *See* Conditioned stimulus.

Stimulus, discriminative. *See* Discriminative stimulus.

Stimulus, eliciting. *See* Eliciting stimulus.

Stimulus, unconditioned. *See* Unconditioned stimulus.

Stress immunity. Failure to react to emotional stress.

Stroke. General term for a cerebrovascular accident, apoplexy, or any hemorrhage or softening of the brain as a result of certain kinds of damage to the cerebral arteries. Paralysis, aphasia, and coma are among the neurological symptoms that may result.

Structured interactional group psychotherapy. A type of group therapy developed by Harold Kaplan and Benajmin Sadock in which the therapist provides a structural matrix of the group's interactions, the most important of which is that a different member of the group is the focus of the interaction in each session.

Studies on Hysteria. Title of a book by Josef Breuer and Sigmund Freud. Published in 1895, it described the cathartic method of treatment and the beginnings of psychoanalysis. It demonstrated the psychological origins of hysterical symptoms and the possibility of effecting a cure through psychotherapy.

Stupor. Disturbance of consciousness in which the patient is nonreactive to and unaware of his surroundings. Organically, it is synonymous with unconsciousness. In psychiatry, it is referred to as mutism and is commonly found in catatonia and psychotic depression.

Subcoma insulin treatment. A form of shock treatment in which instead of being used to induce coma, insulin is given to produce sleepiness and to produce in the patient a sense of well-being.

Subconscious. Once used to mean the preconscious and the unconscious but now obsolete in psychiatry.

Subjectivity. Qualitative appraisal and interpretation of an object or experience as influenced by one's own feelings and thinking.

Sublimation. An unconscious defense mechanism in which unacceptable instinctual drives are diverted into personally and socially acceptable channels. Unlike other defense mechanisms, sublimation offers some minimal gratification of the instinctual drive or impulse.

Substitution. An unconscious defense mechanism in which a person replaces an unacceptable wish, drive, emotion, or goal with one that is more acceptable.

Succinylcholine. A powerful muscle relaxant used in anesthesia and in electroconvulsive treatment.

Suggestibility. State of compliant responsiveness ot an idea or influence. It is commonly observed among persons with hysterical traits.

Sullivan, Harry Stack (1894–1949). American psychiatrist. He is best known for his interpersonal theory of psychiatry. *See also* Consensual validation.

Superego. One of the three component parts of the psychic apparatus. The other two are the ego and the id. Freud created the theoretical condept of the superego to describe the psychic functions that are expressed in moral attitudes, conscience, and a sense of guilt. The superego results from the internalizatin of the ethicatl standards of the society in which the person lives, and it develops by identification with the attitudes of his parents. It is mainly unconscious and is believed to develop as a reaction to the Oedipus complex. It has a protective and rewarding function, referred to as the ego ideal, and a critical and punishing function, which evokes the sense of guilt.

Supportive psychotherapy. A form of psychotherapy that seeks to reinforce the patient's defenses and to provide him with reassurance, rather than to probe deeply into his conflicts.

Suppression. Conscious act of controlling and inhibiting an unacceptable impulse, emotion, or idea. Suppression is differentiated from repression in that the latter is an unconscious process.

Surrogate parent. An authority figure who functions as a parent as far as the child's feelings and responses are concerned.

Symbiosis. A dependent relationship between two mentally ill persons who reinforce each other's pathology.

Symbolization. An unconscious defense mechanism whereby one idea or object comes to stand for another because of some common aspect or quality in both. Symoblization is based on similarity and association. The symbols formed protect the person from the anxiety that may be attached to the original idea or object. *See also* Defense mechanism.

Sympathetic nervous system. The part of the autonomic nervous system that helps a person deal with threatening situations by preparing his body for fight or flight.

Sympathomimetic drug. Drug that mimics the actions of the sympathetic nervous system. Examples are amphetamine and epinephrine.

Sympathy. Sharing of another person's feelings, ideas, and experiences. As opposed to empathy, sympathy is not objective. *See also* Identification, Imitation.

Symptom. Any morbid phenomenon or departure from the normal in function, appearance, or sensation experienced by the patient and indicative of disease.

Symptom formation. *See* Symptom substitution.

Symptom substitution. Unconscious psychic process in which a repressed impulse is indirectly released and manifested through a symptom. Such symptoms as obsession, compulsion, phobia, dissociation, anxiety, depression, hallucination, and delusion are examples of symptom substitution. It is also known as symptom formation.

Syncretic-thought. A term introduced by Jean Piaget to describe concrete, particular thinking. *See also* Primary process.

Syndrome, Munchausen. *See* Munchausen syndrome.

Syntactical aphasia. *See* Central Aphasia.

Syntaxic thought. A term introduced by Harry Stack Sullivan to describe logically, goal-directed, reality-oriented thinking. *See also* Secondary process.

Syntropy. A term used by Adolf Meyer to characterize healthy or wholesome relationships.

Syphilis. A venereal disease that can lead to an organic psychosis if it is left untreated.

Systematic desensitization. *See* Desensitization.

T-group (training group). A type of group that emphasizes training in self-awareness and group dynamics.

T ratio. In a statistical study involving fewer than 30 subjects, the ratio that is used to determine whether differences found between two items are larger than could be expected from chance. *See also* Critical ratio.

Tachylogia. *See* Logorrhea.

Tactile hallucination. False sense of touch.

Talion. Retribution, as represented in the Biblical quotation, "An eye for an eye, a tooth for a tooth."

Tangentiality. Disturbance in the associative thought processes in which the patient is unable to express his idea. In contrast to circumstantiality, the digression in tangentiality is such that the central idea is not communicated. It is observed in schizophrenia and certain types of organic brain disorders. Tangentiality is also known as derailment. *See also* Circumstantiality.

Tardive oral dyskinesia. A syndrome characterized by involuntary movements of the lips and jaw and by other bizarre involuntary dystonic movements. It is an extrapyramidal effect occurring late in the course of antipsychotic drug therapy.

Target patient. Group member who is preceptively analyzed by another member. It is a term used in the process of going around in psychoanalytically oriented groups.

Task-oriented group. Group whose main energy is devoted to reaching a goal, finding a solution to a problem, or building a product. Distinguished from this type of group is the experiential group, which is mainly concerned with sharing whatever happens.

TAT (Thematic Apperception Test). A projective psychological test in which the subject supplies interpretations of a series of life situation drawings, based on his own feelings and attitudes.

Temperament. Inborn, constitutional predisposition to react in a specific way to stimuli. Termperament varies from person to person.

Tension. An unpleasurable alteration of affect characterized by a strenuous increase in mental and physical activity.

Thanatos. Death wish. *See also* Stekel, Wilhelm.

Theater of Spontaneity (Stegreiftheater). Theater in Vienna that improvised group processes and that was developed by J. L. Moreno.

Therapeutic agent. Anything—a person or a drug—that promotes healing in a maladaptive person. In group therapy, it refers mainly to people who help others.

Therapeutic alliance. Conscious relationship between therapist and patient in which each implicitly agrees that they need to work together by means of insight and control to help the patient with his conflicts. It involves a therapeutic splitting of the patient's ego into observing and experiencing parts. A good therapeutic alliance is especially necessary during phases of strong negative transerence to keep the treatment going.

Therapeutic atmosphere. All therapeutic, maturational, and growth-supporting agents—cultural, social, and medical.

Therapeutic community. Ward or hospital treatment setting that provides an effective environment for behavioral changes in patients through resocialization and rehabilitation.

Therapeutic crisis. Turning point in the treatment process. An example is acting out, which, depending on how it is dealt with, may or may not lead to a therapeutic change in the patient's behavior. *See also* Therapeutic impasse.

Therapeutic group. Group of patients joined together under the leadership of a therapist for the purpose of working together for psycho-

therapeutic ends—specifically, for the treatment of each patient's emotional disorders.

Therapeutic impasse. Deadlock in the treatment process. Therapy is in a state of imminent failure when there is no further insight or awareness and when sessions are reduced to routine meetings of patient and therapist. Unresolved resistances and transference and countertransference conflicts are among the common causes of this pehnomenon. *See also* Therapeutic crisis.

Therapeutic role. Position in which one aims to treat, bring about an improvement, or provide alleviation of a distressing condition or state.

There-and-then. Past experience, rather than immediate experience. *See also* Here-and-now.

Thinking. *See* Cognition.

Thinking compulsion. *See* Intellectualization.

Thinking through. The mental process that occurs in an attempt to understand one's own behavior and gain insight from it.

Third ear. Ability to make use of intuition, sensitivity, and awareness of subliminal cues to interpret clinical observations of individual and group patients. First introduced by the German philosopher Friedrich Nietzsche, the term was later used in analytic psychotherapy by Theodor Reik.

Third nervous system. Burrow's conception of a nervous system based on function, rather than anatomy.

Thought deprivation. *See* Blocking.

Thought process disorder. A symptom of schizophrenia that involves the intellectual functions. It is manifested by irrelevance and incoherence of the patient's verbal productions. It ranges from simple blocking and mild circumstantiality to total loosening of associations, as in word salad.

Three Essays on the Theory of Sexuality. Title of a book by Freud published in 1905. It applied the libido theory to the successive phases of sex instinct maturation in the infant, child, and adolescent. It made possible the integration of a vast diversity of clinical observations and promoted the direct observation of child development.

Tic. Involuntary, spasmodic, repetitive motor movement of a small segment of the body. Mainly psychogenic, it may be seen in certain cases of chronic encephalitis.

Timidity. Inability to assert oneself for fear of some fancied reprisal, even though there is no objective evidence of potential harm.

Tinnitus. Noises in one or both ears, such as ringing and whistling. It is an occasional side effect of some of the antidepressant drugs.

Toilet training. The program of teaching a child to control the bladder and bowel functions. The attitudes of both parent and child regarding this period may have important psychological implications for the child's later development.

Topectomy. A psychosurgical procedure performed in some cases on chronic psychotic patients.

Totem and Taboo. Title of a book by Freud published in 1913. It applied his concepts to the data of anthropology. He was able to afford much insight into the meaning of tribal organizations and customs, especially by invoking the Oedipus complex and the characteristics of magical thought as he had discovered them from studies of the unconscious. *See also* Oedipus complex, Primal father.

Toxic psychosis. A psychosis caused by toxic substances produced by the body or introduced into it in the form of chemicals or drugs.

Trainer. Professional leader or facilitator of a sensitivity training or T-group; teacher or supervisor of a person learning the science and practice of group therapy.

Training group. *See* T-group.

Trance. A sleep-like state of reduced consciousness.

Tranquilizer. Psychotropic drug that induces tranquility by calming, soothing, quieting, or pacifying, without clouding the consciousness. The major tranquilizers are antipsychotic drugs, and the minor tranquilizers are antianxiety drugs.

Transaction. Interaction that arises when two or more persons have an encounter. In transactional analysis, it is considered the unit of social interaction. It involves a stimulus and a response.

Transactional analysis. A system introduced by Eric Berne that centers on the study of interactions going on in the treatment sessions. The system includes four components: (1) structural analysis of intrapsychic phenomena; (2) transactional analysis proper, the determination of the currently dominant ego state (parent, child, or adult) of each participant; (3) game analysis, identification of the games played in their interactions and of the gratifications provided; and (4) sceipt analysis, uncovering of the causes of the patient's emotional problems. Transactional analysis is used in both individual and group psychotherapy.

Transference. Unconscious phenomenon in which the feelings, attitudes, and wishes originally linked with important figures in one's early life are projected onto others who have come to represent them in current life. *See also* Countertransference, Rapport, Transference neurosis.

Transference neurosis. A phenomenon occurring in psychoanalysis in which the patient develops a strong emotional attachemnt to the therapist as a symoblized nuclear familial figure. The repetition and depth of this misperception or symbolization characterize it as a transference neurosis. In transference analysis, a major therapeutic technique in both individual therapy and group therapy, the therapist uses transference to help the patient understand and gain insight into his behavior.

Transsexualism. The desire to change one's sex. Some transsexuals, many of whom have adopted the role of the opposite sex since childhood, have been treated successfully with sex-changing surgical procedures, accompanied by intensive hormonal therapy and psychotherapy.

Transvestitism (transvestism). Dressing in clothing of the opposite sex, usually associated with homosexuality and the desire to be accepted as a member of the opposite sex.

Trauma. In psychiatry, a significant, upsetting experience or event that precipitates or aggravates a mental disorder.

Trend of thought. Thinking that centers on a particular idea associated with an affective tone.

Triad. Father, mother, and child relationship projectively experienced in group therapy. *See also* Nuclear family.

Trichotillomania. Morbid compulsion to pull out one's hair.

Tricyclic drug. Antidepressant drug believed by some to be more effective than monamine oxidase inhibitors. The tricyclic drugs (imipramine and amitriptyline) are presently the most popular drugs in the treatment of pathological depression.

Trisomy. A chromosomal aberration in which there are three chromosomes instead of the two in the usual set of chromosomes.

Tuke, William (1732–1819). A pioneer in the treatment of mental patients without the use of physical restraints.

Tyramine. A sympathomimetic amine that is believed to influence the release of stored norepinephrine. Its degradation is aided by monoamine oxidase. The use of monoamine oxidase inhibitors in the treatment of depression prevents the degradation of tyramine. The simultaneous ingestion of food containing tyramine may cause a sympathomimetic effect, such as an increase in blood pressure, that could be fatal.

Ultradian rhythm. Cyclical variations in emotional and plupiologic physiologic functions that occur in cycles of more than 24 hours. *See also* Circadian rhythm, Infradian rhythm.

Ululation. The incoherent crying of a psychotic or hysterical patient.

Unconditioned reflex. An automatic response to a stimulus, such as salivation upon seeing food.

Unconditioned stimulus. An environmental event that normally evokes an autonomic response. For example, the presentation of food (an unconditioned stimulus) usually elicits salivation (an autonomic response) in a hungery animal. *See also* Classical conditioning, Conditioned stimulus, Discriminative stimulus, Eliciting stimulus, Operant conditioning.

Unconscious. 1. (Noun) Structural division of the mind in which the psychic material—primitive drives, repressed desires, and memories—is not directly accessible to awareness. 2. (Adjective) In a state of insensibility, the absence of orientation and perception. *See also* Conscious, Preconscious.

Underachievement. Failure to reach a biopsychological, age-adequate level.

Underachiever. Person who manifestly does not function up to his capacity. The term usually refers to a bright child whose school test grades fall below expected levels.

Undoing. An unconscious defense mechanism by which a person symbolically acts out in reverse something unacceptable that has already been done. A primitive defense mechanism, undoing is a form of magical expiatory action. Repetitive in nature, it is commonly observed in obsessive-compulsive neurosis.

Unipolar depression. A depressive illness that is marked by recurrent depression with a history of manic episodes. *See also* Bipolar depression.

Vaginismus. Vaginal spasm that causes pain during sexual intercourse. It may be due to psychological causes.

Validity. The degree to which a given measure does indicate a particular quality or attribute that it attempts to measure.

Variable. A characteristic that can assume different values in different experimental situations. An independent variable is a characteristic set up by the experimenter to determine the outcome of the experiment. A dependent variable is linked to another condition in the experiment.

Variance. A statistical measure arrived at by squaring all the deviations in a set of measures, summing them, and then dividing them by the number of measures. Variance is a useful concept because other statistical computations are based on it and because it is helpful in analyzing how much variation is due to experimental influence and how much to chance or error influence.

Variation. A statistical term referring to different results obtained in measuring the same phenomenon. Variation may be association with known variables within the data or with chance variables that result from error or chance.

Vasectomy. A means of male sterilization in which the seminal ducts are tied off, eliminating the production of sperm. Potency and sexuality are unaffected.

Verbal technique. Any method of group or individual therapy in which words are used. The major part of most psychotherapy is verbal.

Verbigeration. Meaningless repetition of words or phrases. Also known as cataphasia, it is a morbid symptom seen in catatonic schizophrenia.

Verbomania. *See* Logorrhea.

Vienna Psychoanalytic Society. An outgrowth of the Wednesday Evening Society, an informal group of Freud's earliest followers. The new name was acquired and a reorganization took place in 1910, when the society became a component of the newly formed International Psychoanalytical Society. Alfred Adler was president from 1910 to 1911, and Freud was president from 1911 until it was disbanded by the Nazis in 1938.

Visual hallucination. False visual perception.

Volubility. *See* Logorrhea.

Voyeurism. A morbid desire to look at sexual organs or sexual acts.

WAIS (Wechsler Adult Intelligence Scale). An intelligence test specifically for adults.

Waxy flexibility. *See* Cerea flexibilitas.

Wednesday Evening Society. A small group of Freud's followers who in 1902 started meeting with him informally on Wednesday evenings to receive instructions in psychoanalysis. As the society grew in numbers and importance, it evolved in 1910 into the Vienna Psychoanalytic Society.

Weekend hospital. A form of partial hospitalization in which the patient spends only weekends in the hospital and functions in the outside world during the week.

Weyer, Johann (1515–1588). Dutch physician considered by some to be the first psychiatrist. His interest in human behavior led to his writing *De Praestigiis Daemonum* (1563), a landmark in the history of psychiatry.

White, William Alanson (1870–1937). An early exponent of psychoanalysis in this country.

White-out syndrome. A psychosis that occurs in Arctic explores and mountaineers who are exposed to the lack of diverse stimuli in the snow-clad environment.

Withdrawal. Act of retreating or going away. Observed in schizophrenia and depression, it is characterized by a pathological retreat from interpersonal contact and social involvement, leading to self-preoccupation.

Withdrawal symptoms. Vomiting, trembling, profuse sweating, and other physical and emotional symptoms brought on by withdrawal from addictive or habituating drugs.

Wittels, Fritz. (1880–1950). Austrian psychoanalyst. One of Freud's early followers, he wrote a biography of him in 1924 during a period of estrangement, when he was under the influence of Wilhelm Stekel. Later, a reconciliation took place, and Freud conceded that some of Wittels' interpretations were probably correct.

Word salad. An incoherent mixture of words and phrases. This type of speech results from a disturbance in thinking. It is commonly observed in far-advanced states of schizophrenia.

Working alliance. Collaboration between the group as a whole and each patient who is willing to strive for health, growth, and maturation with the help of the therapist. *See also* Therapeutic alliance.

Working out. Stage in the treatment process in which the personal history and psychodynamics of a patient are discovered.

Working through. Process of obtaining more and more insight and personality changes through repeated and varied examination of a conflict or problem. The interactions between free association, resistance, interpretation, and working through constitute the fundamental facets of the analytic process.

Xenophobia. Fear of strangers.

Zoophobia. Fear of animals.

Index